Self Assessment & Review

MEDICINE

By

Mudit Khanna

M.S (Orth), MRCS(ed), M.Ch (Orth,U.K)

Consultant

Adult Reconstructive / Joint Replacement Surgery

WOCKHARDT Hospital, Goa

India

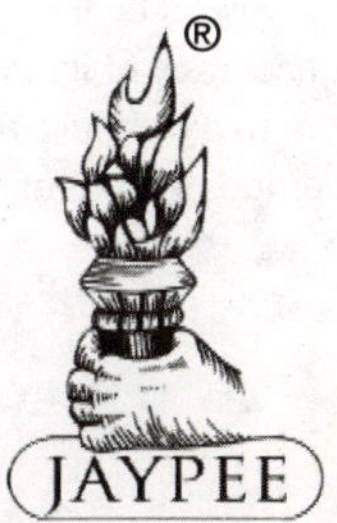

JAYPEE BROTHERS MEDICAL PUBLISHERS (P) LTD

New Delhi • London • Philadelphia • Panama

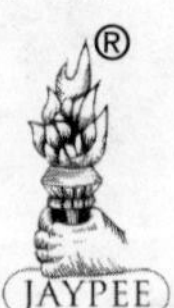

Jaypee Brothers Medical Publishers (P) Ltd

Headquarters
Jaypee Brothers Medical Publishers (P) Ltd
4838/24, Ansari Road, Daryaganj
New Delhi-110 002, India
Phone: +91-11-43574357
Fax: +91-11-43574314
Email: jaypee@jaypeebrothers.com

Overseas Offices

J.P. Medical Ltd
83 Victoria Street, London
SW1H 0HW (UK)
Phone: +44-2031708910
Fax: +02-03-0086180
Email: info@jpmedpub.com

Jaypee-Highlights Medical Publishers Inc.
City of Knowledge, Bld. 237, Clayton
Panama City, Panama
Phone: + 507-301-0496
Fax: + 507-301-0499
Email: cservice@jphmedical.com

Jaypee Medical Inc.
The Bourse
111 South Independence Mall East
Suite 835, Philadelphia, PA 19106, USA
Phone: + 267-519-9789
Email: joe.rusko@jaypeebrothers.com

Jaypee Brothers Medical Publishers (P) Ltd
17/1-B Babar Road, Block-B, Shaymali
Mohammadpur, Dhaka-1207
Bangladesh
Mobile: +08801912003485
Email: jaypeedhaka@gmail.com

Jaypee Brothers Medical Publishers (P) Ltd
Shorakhute, Kathmandu
Nepal
Phone: +00977-9841528578
Email: jaypee.nepal@gmail.com

Website: www.jaypeebrothers.com

Website: www.jaypeedigital.com

Inquiries for bulk sales may be solicited at: jaypee@jaypeebrothers.com

Self Assessment and Review Medicine

Sixth Edition: **2012**

Seventh Edition: **2013**

ISBN : 978-93-5090-728-3

Printed at Sanat Printers, Kundli

Dedicated to My Parents

"My thoughts bear an indelible imprint of their vision"

Preface

The structure of Postgraduate Entrance Examinations has undergone a dramatic change over past year with the pattern of examinations moving from a *'Paper Based' 'All India Postgraduate Examination'* to a *'Computer based' NEET* test.

While All India Institute of Medical Sciences (AIIMS) conducted the earlier test, National Board of Examinations (NBE) conducts the present examination 'NEET'.

Postgraduate Entrance Examination whether *AIPGME* OR *NEET* remains our battleground and the dates of the battle has already been decided!

Five long years has been time long enough for each one of us to realize our potential strengths and weaknesses. Nevertheless, this year is qualitatively unlike the past, for it carries with it, an invisible force of strength, unprecedented energy and firmness of purpose like never before. As if our latent capacities were lying in a state of inactivity, only to reemerge and domineer over our weakness and distractions.

Our vigor, durability, toughness is all put to test but the vehemence to succeed or the fear of failure drives us on. As if we reinvented the essence of the golden words

"When the going gets tough the tough gets going"

FRIENDS !

It would certainly be an understatement, if I say that it is strategy that sees you through in this most bewildering examination rather than the genius in you or the amount of core knowledge that you possess.

The most brilliant of students you have always feared and envied are often left dismayed, surprised, and shocked at their performance results, while the most average ones have been seen to become the ideals of those setting their first foot forward into this blind race.

Most of us and you too must have wondered

What is it after-all… that turned this average guy into a marvelous performer?

FIRST: is the 'will to succeed' **flanked by** courage, faith **and** confidence **in your own vision.**

> *'If you have the will to win, you have achieved half your success;*
> *If you don't, you have achieved half your failures.'*
>
> — *David Ambrose*

Never dismiss the possibility of success as a distant dream or a matter of chance. Eliminate all tendencies to take a gloomy or cynical view of affairs. Always choose to take a look at the better side of things. Keep your mind 'solution focused' rather than 'problem focused'.

> *'What the caterpillar calls the end of the world the master calls the butterfly'*

SECOND: is effort, persistence and determination; NO QUITTING

There is certainly no route to success in a PG entrance examination without the cornerstone of exhausting relentless effort that leaves you thoroughly worn out.

'Destiny is not a matter of chance, it is a matter of choice;
It is not a thing to be waited for, it is a thing to be achieved' —*Williams Jennings Bryan*

The route to success is difficult and long and often just before every big achievement, every great accomplishment, comes anxiety with a fear of failure and discouragement.

Persistence—that is the key, and you must hold on, with the faith that your resolution and firmness would generate sufficient amount of energy to help you sail past this one year.

'Stick to the fight when you are hardest hit, it's when things go wrong that you must not quit.'

THIRD: and foremost is Strategy!

Strategy is the distinction between knowledge and wisdom.

Analysis and maximum revelation out of the same raw stock in our grey matter is what sets those who perform apart from those who fail to perform with an equal effort. While effort friends, provides the foundation without which the tomb of your success would never build, it is strategy, that sets your structure apart from those of others.

What then should be your strategy?

In the simplest words the answer to the above question lies in the following line:

Try and know all what has been asked previously, the most recent questions being the most important.

All the best!

MUDIT KHANNA

From the Publisher's Desk
We request all the readers to provide us their valuable suggestions/errors (if any) *at:*
jaypeemcqproduction@gmail.com

A Few Words to Share

Dear Friends,

The structure of Postgraduate Entrance Examinations has undergone a dramatic change over past year with the pattern of examinations moving from a *'Paper Based' 'All India Postgraduate Examination (AIPGME)* to a *'Computer based' NEET* test. While All India Institute of Medical Sciences (AIIMS) conducted the earlier test, National Board of Examinations (NBE) conducts the present examination 'NEET'. This has not only brought about a change in the preparatory content but also a change to the best approach to the same content.

To help you prepare for the test in a more efficient manner we have made certain key changes in the format of the book.

1. We have edited the content in the book to provide *'Essential Revision Notes'* before each chapter. This will allow the student to revise all relevant and important 'key' themes much quicker and in a more structured and coordinated manner.
2. We have included the latest years of DNB Questions to broaden the relevant question bank besides the latest questions from All India Post Graduate Examinations (AIPGME) and the All India Institute of Medical Examinations (AIIMS).

The Present Book

- Approaches 'medicine' systematically by dividing its contents into clinical chapters and further into sequential topics and themes.
- Gives an elaborate overview of the most significant themes within each chapter.
- Explains each theme and complements it with high-yield facts.
- Provides the most essential facts in flow diagrams and tabulation with an 'easy-to-remember' format.
- Provides an effective Revision tool in the form of 'Essential Revision Notes' before each chapter covering all major themes.
- Includes a vast bank of previously asked questions from various Entrance examinations.

In the present edition we have not deleted content from the explanatory answers primarily to allow the reader, to choose an 'Antegrade' approach (*First read the Essential Revision Notes-Theory and then attempt answering the questions*) or a 'Retrograde' approach (*First attempt answering the questions with detailed explanatory answers, and then revise the theory from the Essential Revision Notes-Theory section in the book*). We do understand that this approach has led to repetition of content within the same book, but the objective for the same has been to make it relatively easy for the reader to understand and integrate the content in a more efficient manner. We are open to suggestions and would welcome and appreciate any suggestions to improve the book further, by deleting or adding further content as desired.

Wishing you all the very best

Dr Mudit Khanna

Acknowledgments

"To Dear God, whose eternal blessings and divine presence helps us to fulfill all our goals".

When emotions are profound, words sometimes are not sufficient to express our thanks and gratitude. I express my sincere thanks to all people who have helped and provided consistent enthusiasm and encouragement in bringing out this work.

I would like to take this opportunity to offer my special thanks to Mr Habil Khorakiwala, Ms Zahabiya Khorakiwala, MrArvind Baganiya and the entire family of Wockhardt Group of Hospitals for their constant inspiration and support right from the time, I joined the department of Orthopedics at Wockhardt Hospital, Goa.

I will always remain grateful and obliged to my consultants in the UK with particular reference to Prof. David Rowley, Dr BN Muddu, Dr R Sofat, Dr R Sharma who have been a great source of inspiration throughout my postgraduate training in the UK.

Expressions and emotions fail to find words to express thanks to my parents. I thank them for being a constant source of inspiration and motivation. Their confidence in me has always propelled me to work harder.

My wife Diksha and daughter Vanya - words are hard to find, when it comes to highlighting their role, in the making of this book. I thank them for always standing by my side.

I express my special thanks to all my friends, especially Dr Anurag Shukla, Dr Yogesh Chaudhuri, Dr Sachin Jadhav, Dr Minal Jadhav, Dr Saurabh Agarwal, Dr Gunjan, Dr Chitwan, Dr Ashish Gupta and Dr Amit Tripathi for their presence and support at all times.

Special thanks to Shri Jitendar P Vij, Group Chairman and Mr Bhupesh Arora, General Manager Publishing M/s Jaypee Brothers Medical Publishers (P) Ltd, New Delhi, India for their inspiring guidance and suggestions that helped me a lot in accomplishing this huge task.

Sincere thanks are also extended to Mr Sayeed and Mr Saleem and M/s Compsphere for their technical help and layout design. Their committed effort in presenting this work on paper is deeply appreciated.

I am highly grateful to the readers of the previous editions for their creative criticism, overwhelming response, immediate acceptance of the overall contents of the book and for their queries and suggestions.

The last but not the least, I gratefully acknowledge and thank in anticipation, all readers who, I am confident, will act and continue to act as a guiding torch in improving and upgrading the content of this book.

Friends your feedback and suggestions are always welcome at **muditkhanna@yahoo.com**

MUDIT KHANNA

M.S (Orth), MRCS(ed), M.Ch (Orth,U.K)

Consultant

Adult Reconstructive / Joint Replacement Surgery

WOCKHARDT Hospital

Goa

Contents

***

Hematology

ESSENTIAL REVISION NOTES

Classification of Anemia

Morphological Classification of Anemia

MCV (Mean Corpuscular Volume)	MCHC (Mean Corpuscular Hb concentration)
• Mean Corpuscular Volume refers to the average size of the RBC (volume). • MCV is usually expressed in femtoilitres (fl) • Normal MCV varies from 79.0 to 93.3 fl *(H 18th/3587)* Raised MCV: *Macrocytic* Normal MCV: *Normocytic* Reduced MCV: *Microcytic*	• Mean Corpuscular Haemoglobin Concentration (MCHC) refers to the average concentration of Hb in the RBC (MCHC describes the colour of the RBC) • MCHC is usually expressed in pg/dl • Normal MCHC varies from 32.3 to 35.9 pg/dl *(H 18th/3587)* Raised MCHC: *Hyperchromic* Normal MCHC: *Normochromic* Reduced MCHC: *Hypochromic*

Morphological Classification of Anemia based on MCV and MCHC

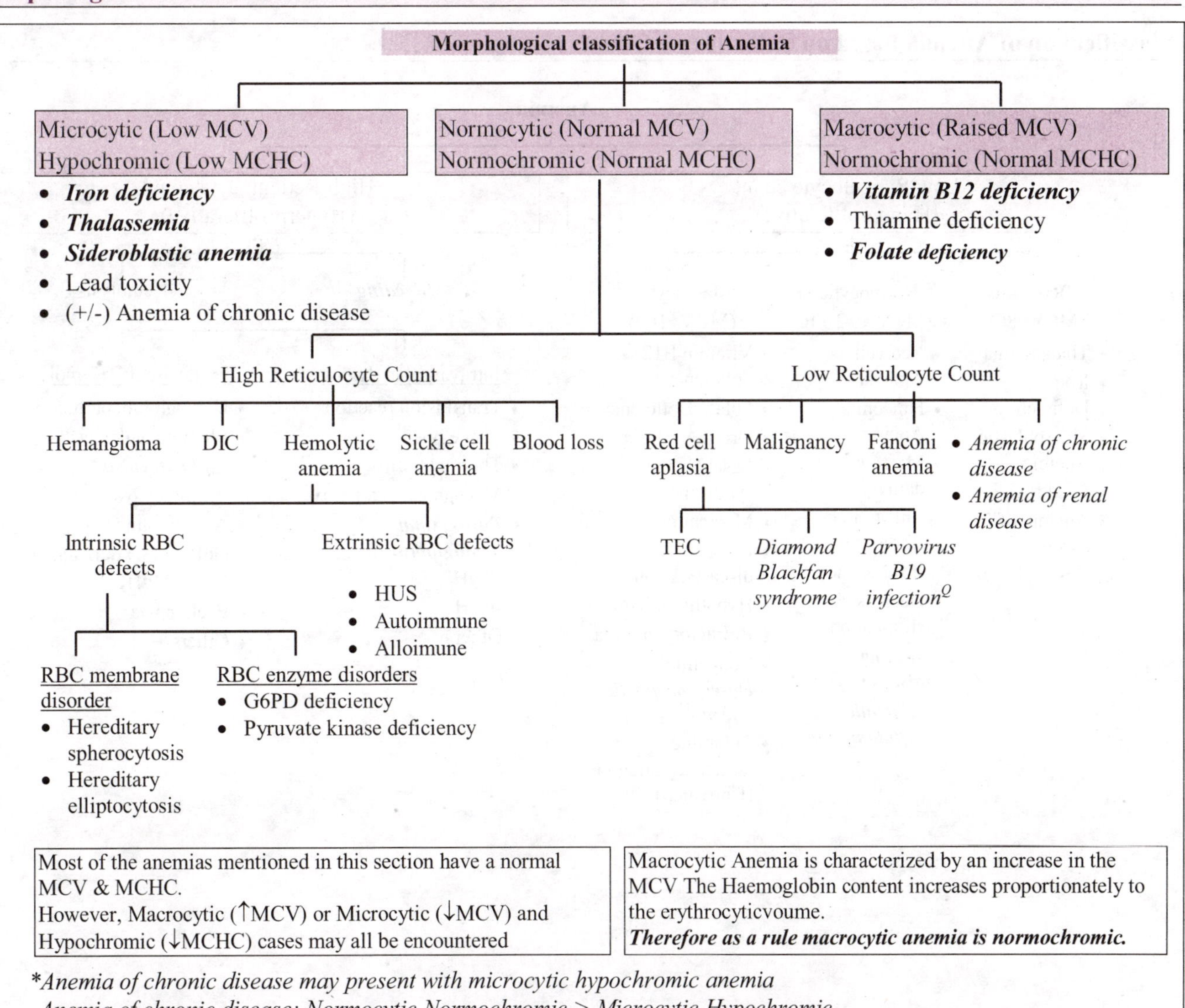

**Anemia of chronic disease may present with microcytic hypochromic anemia*
Anemia of chronic disease: Normocytic Normochromic > Microcytic Hypochromic

Classification of Anemia based on MCV and Red Cell Distribution Width (RDW)

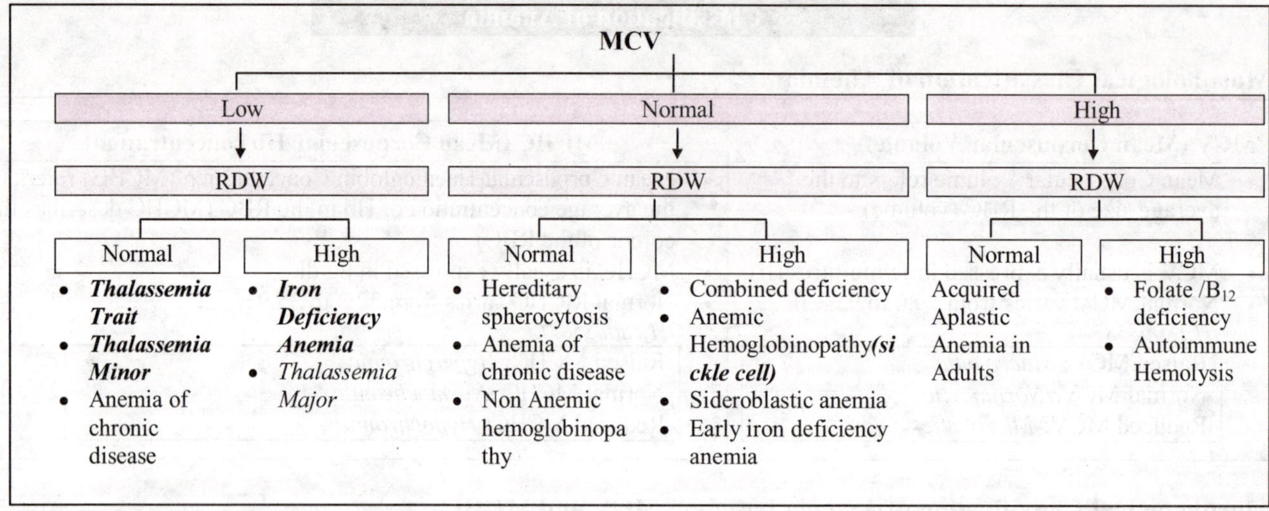

Classification of Anemia based on Reticulocyte Count

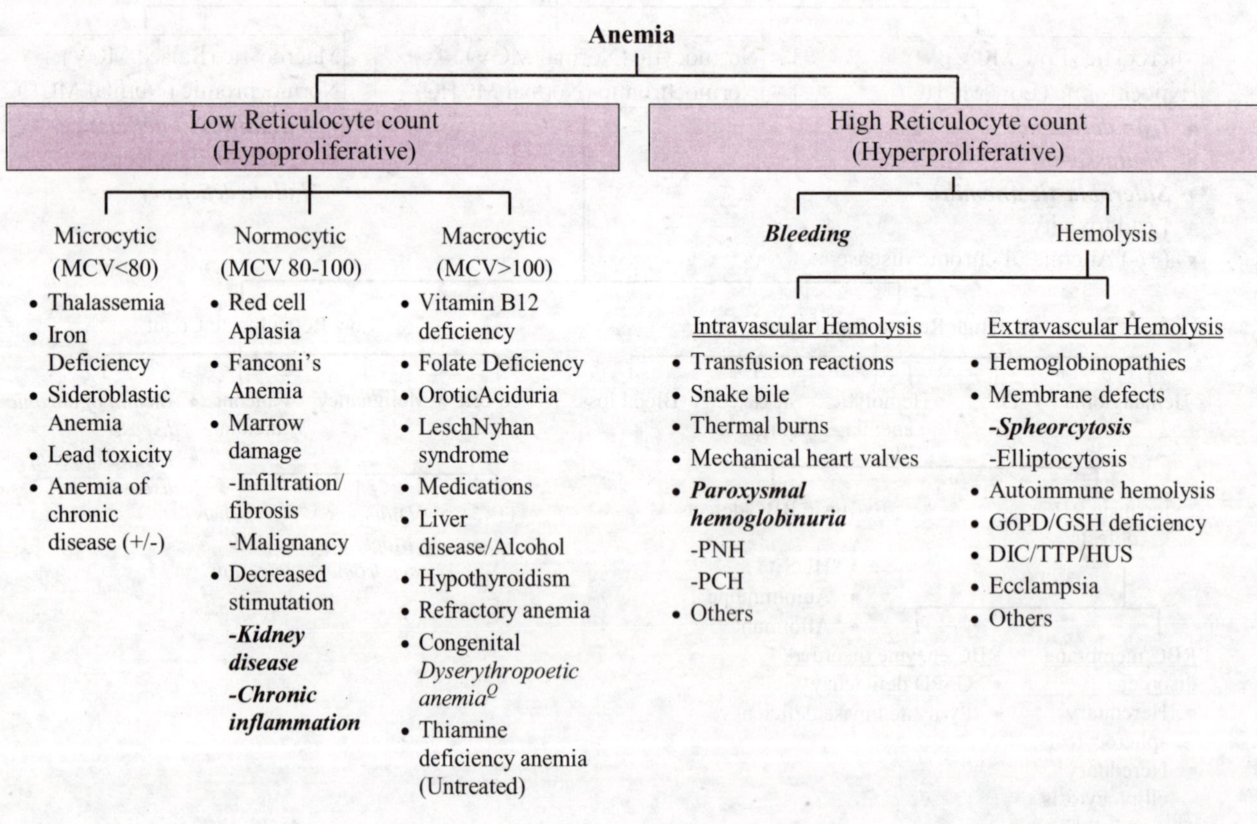

Hypochromic Microcytic Anemias

Causes of Microcytic hypochromic Anemia

Causes of microcytic hypochromic anaemia
• *Iron deficiency anaemia*
• *Thalassemia*
• *Sideroblasticanaemia*
• *Lead poisoning*
• *Anemia of chronic disease (+/-)*

Differential Diagnosis of Microcytic Hypochromic Anemia

Condition / Test (normal values)	Iron deficiency	Thalassemia	Sideroblastic anemia	Anemia of chronic disease
Smear	Microcytic hypochromic	Microcytic hypochromic	Microcytic hypochromic	Normocytic normochromic > Micro/hypochromic (but Micro/Hypo may be present)
Serum iron (50-150μg/dl)	Low (<30)	Normal	Normal	↓ (<50)
TIBC (300-600 μg/dl)	High (>360)	Normal	Normal (Chandrasoma Taylor)	↓ (<300)
% Saturation (30-50%)	< 10 (↓ed)	N or ↑ed (30-80)	N or ↑ (30-80)	↓ (10-20)
Ferritin (μg/l) (50-200 μg/L)	< 15 (↓ed)	↑ (50-300)	↑ (50-300)	Normal or ↑ (30-200)
Hemoglobin pattern	Normal	Abnormal	Normal	Normal
Free Erythrocyte Protporphrin	↑ed	Normal	↑ed	↑ed
RDW	↑ed	Normal	Normal	Normal

Microcytic Hypochromic Anemias are typically associated with a Normal or High Red Cell Distribution Width and normal or High Free Erythrocyte Protoporphyrin

Microcytic Hypochromic anemias are not associated with Low Red Cell Distribution Width and Low Free Erythrocyte Protoporphyrin

Hypochromic microcytic anemia with ↓serum iron and ↑TIBC: iron Deficiency Anemia

Hypochromic microcytic anemia with ↓ serum iron and ↓TIBC : Anemia of Chronic disease

Causes of Macrocytic Anemias

Causes of Macrocytic anemia
1. *Vit. B_{12} deficiency*
2. *Folic acid deficiency*
3. *Oroticaciduria*
4. *Nitrous oxide inhalation*
5. *Liver disease*
6. *Hypothyroidism*
7. *Thiamine deficiency*

Hemolysis and Hemolytic Anemias

Intravascular Hemolysis vs Extravascular Hemolysis

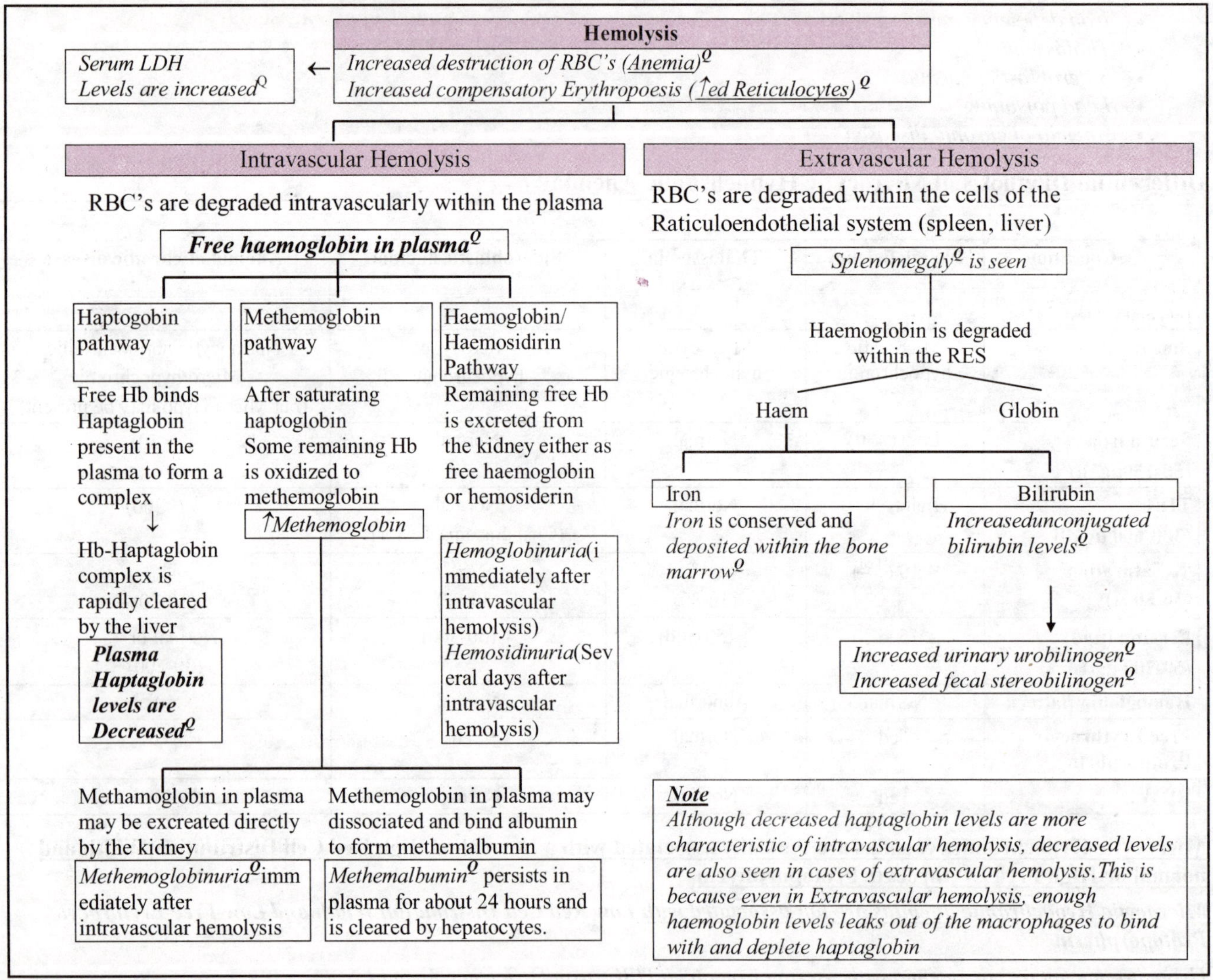

Laboratory Evaluation of Haemolysis

	Extravascular	Intravascular
Hematologic		
Routine blood film	Polychromatophilia	Polychromatophilia
Reticulocyte count	↑	↑
Bone marrow examination	Erythroid hyperplasia	Erythroid hyperplasia
Plasma or serum		
Bilirubin	↑ Unconjugated	↑ Unconjugated
Haptoglobin	↓	Absent
Plasma hemoglobin	N - ↑	↑↑
Lactate dehydrogenase	↑ (Variable)	↑↑ (Variable)
Urine		
Bilirubin	0	0
Hemosiderin	0	+
Hemoglobin	0	+ in severe cases

Intravascular Hemolysis vs Extravascular Hemolysis

Intravascular Hemolysis vs Extravascular Hemolysis

Causes of intravascular hemolysis	Causes of extravascular hemolysis
• Blood transfusion - ***ABO mismatched transfusion*** - Infected blood • *Thermal burns* • *Snake bites* • *Sepsis* - Bacterial / parasitic infections - Clostridial sepsis - Malaria - Bartonellosis - *Mycoplasma pneumoniae* • *Mechanical heart valves* • ***Paroxysmal hemoglobinuria*** - PNH - PCH	• Blood and viral infections - Malaria - *Mycoplasma pneumoiae* - Infectious mononucleosis • Drug-induced hemolysis - G6PD/GSH deficiency - Autoimmune drug reactions - Strong oxidant drugs/chemicals • Autoimmune hemolysis - Warm-reacting (IgG) AIHA - Cold-reacting (IgM) AIHA • Hemoglobinopathies - ***Thalassemia*** • Membrane structural defect - Hereditary sperocytosis - Hereditary spherocytosis - Acanthocytosis • Environmental disorders - Malignancy/DIC - TTP/HUS - Eclampsia or Preeclampsia

Characteristic features of Hemolytic Anemia:

Increased red cell breakdown	Compensatory increase red cell production
• *↓Hemoglobin (Anemia)* • Serum bilirubin is ↑ed *(Unconjugated bilirubin ↑ed)Q* • *Urine urobilinogen is ↑edQ* • *Fecal stercobilinogen is ↑edQ* • *Hemoglobinemia / HemoglobinuriaQ* • *MethemoglobinemiaQ* • ***↓ Haptoglobin*** ***Hemoglobin binding proteins Q such as Haptoglobin and Hemopexin are reduced or absent. Q*** • ***HemosiderinuriaQ*** • *Plasma Lactic dehydrogenase Q (LDH) is ↑ed* • *↑ AST*	• *Reticulocyte **count is** ↑ed Q* • *Routine blood film shows a variety of abnormal morphological types of red cells Q* - *Schistocytes* - ***SpherocytesQ** etc.* • *Bone narrow*↑ MCV / ↑ MCH (The increased number of reticulocytes is associated with an increased MCV) • Macrocytes, Polychromasia& sometimes nucleated red cells in smear • *Shows erythroid hyperplasia with raised iron stores. Q* • *X Rays of bones show:* - ***Evidence** of expansion of marrow space, especially in tubular bones & in skull Q* - ***Bossing** of skull Q*

Both intravascular and extravascular hemolysis are characterized by elevated reticulocyte counts

High Reticulocyte count Reticulcyte production index >2.5

Hereditary Spherocytosis

HS is characterised by defect in one of the proteins in the cytoskeleton of Red cell membrane, leading to loss of membrane, and hence ***decreased ratio of surface area to volume*** *and consequently spherocytosis.*

- ***Hereditary spherocytosis is inherited as an Autosomal Dominant Trait***[Q]
- ***Most common membrane defect is that of Ankyrin***

Proteins that may be defective in Hereditarysphenocytosis

Protein Defects causing Hereditary Spherocytosis: Ankyrin> Protein 3 ≥Spectrin>Palladin

Proteins that may be defective in Hereditarysphenocytosis

• ***Ankyrin***: *(Most common defect)*[Q]	:	(Defective in about 50% of cases)
• ***Protein 3:(Anion transport channel)***	:	(Defective in about 25% of cases)
• ***Spectrin***: (Spectrin or αspectrin)	:	(Defective in most of remaining 25% of cases)
• ***Palladin***:*(Protein 4.2)*[Q]	:	(Rare defect, but may cause H. S)

- ***One characteristic clinical presentation is Striking splenomegaly***[Q]***(Anemia, Splenomegaly and Jaundice)***
- ***One characteristic Laboratory abnormality in HS is 'Increased Osmotic Fragility'***

Characteristic Laboratory abnormalities

- ***The mean corpuscular volume (MCV) : is decreased***[Q]
- ***The mean corpuscular Hb. concentration (MCHC) : is increased***[Q]
- ***Osmotic fragility is : increased***[Q]

Osmotic Fragility

Osmotic fragility of red cells is defined as the ease with which red cells are ruptured (hemolysed) when they are exposed to hypotonic solution.

Osmotic fragility test assesses the integrity of the membrane of red cells.

Increased Osmotic Fragility	Decreased Osmotic Fragility
Cells which have a lower surface to volume ratio such as spherocytes from any cause have increased osmotic fragility Conditions • ***Hereditary spherocytosis (HS)*** • Autoimmune Hemolytic Anemias (AIHA) • Hemolytic Disease of new born • Malaria • Severe pyruvate kinase deficiency • Other conditions in which spherocytes are found in the blood	Cells which have a high surface to volume ratio such as thin/hypochromic/target cells have decreased osmotic fragility. • ***Thalassemia*** *(otherhemoglobinopathieseg. HbC, HbS)* • *Iron deficiency anemia* • ***Sickle cell anemia*** • *Post splenectomy* • *Reticulocytosis* • *Other conditions in which thin/target cells are found in the blood.*

- ***Treatment of Choice for Hereditary Spherocytosis is 'Splenectomy'***[Q]

Sickle Cell Disease/Anemia

Sickle Cell Anemia is characterized by increased number of 'Sickled' red blood cells in the circulation. These sickled cells are more fragile (increased mechanical fragility: hemolysis) than normal red blood cells and tend to incresase the viscosity of blood (ischemia and infarction)

Mutation causing Sickle Cell Disease:

The sickle cell anemia is caused by a mutation in the beta globin gene that changes the sixth amino acid from glutamic acid to valine in the beta chain of HbA ($\alpha_2\beta_2$).

Designation	Mutation
HbS (Sickle) ($\beta^{6Glu} \rightarrow$ Val)	Replacement of Glutamate by Valine at position 6 beta chain of HbA
HbC ($\beta^{6Glu} \rightarrow$ Lys)	Replacement of Glutamate by Lysine at position 6 on beta chain of HbA
HbE ($\beta^{26Glu} \rightarrow$Lys)	Replacement of Glutamate by Lysine at position 26 on beta chain of HbA

Clinical Manifestations of Sickle Cell Disease:

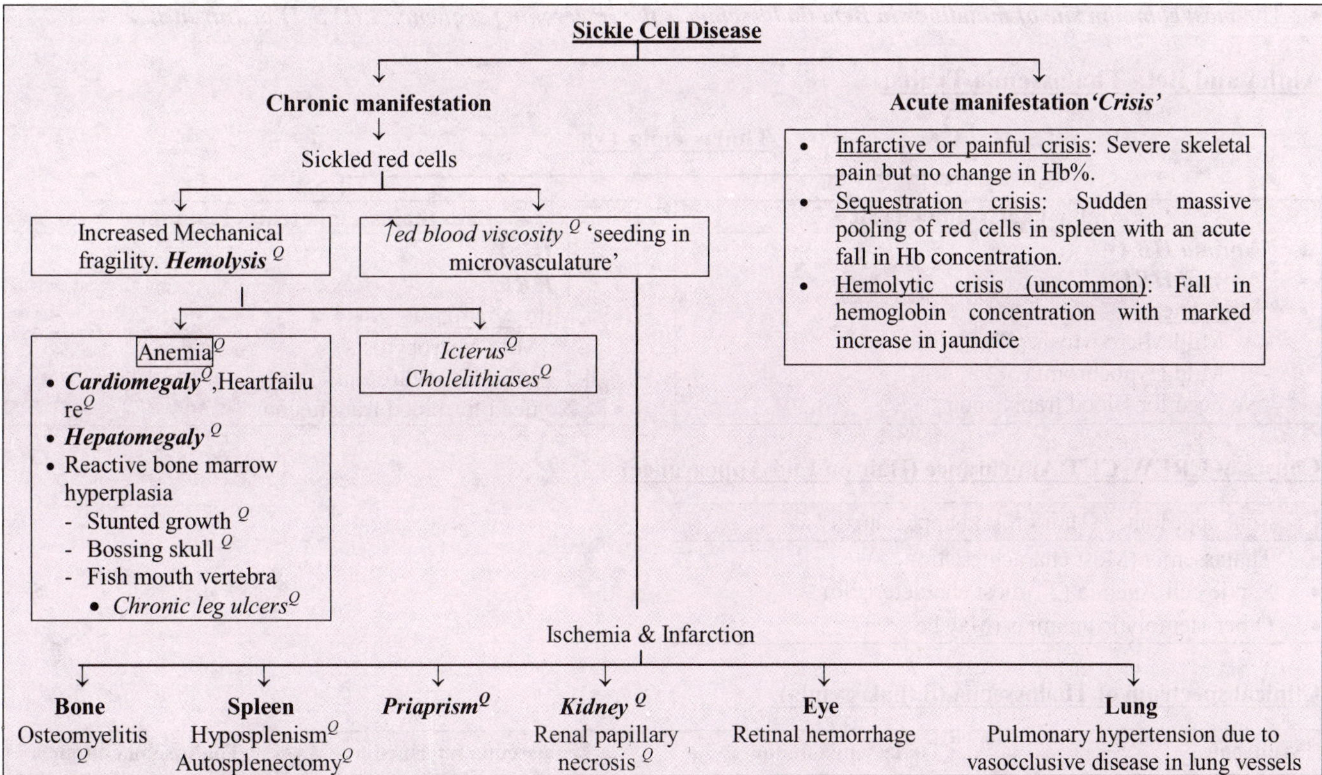

Factors favouring Sickling Crisis:

Factors favouring polymerization: Q

1. **<u>Hypoxia</u>**Q : (2,3 diphosphoglycerate increases polymerization Q)
2. **<u>Acidosis</u>**Q : decreased pH enhances polymerization Q
3. **<u>Haemoglobin</u>** concentration Q: Higher concentration leads to increased polymerization Q
4. **<u>Combination of HbS with other haemoglobins</u>**: This depends on the extent of homology with other haemoglobins. Descending order of ability to copolymerization are HbS, C, D, O, Arab, A, J & F ***(Least with HbF)***

Thalassemias

- Thalassemias are characterized by *decreased rate of synthesis of Hb chains* [Q]that are *structurally normal* [Q]

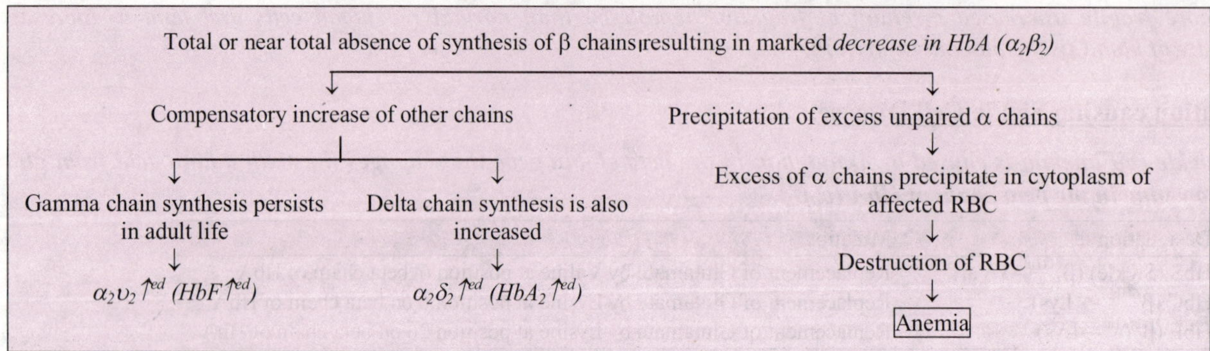

- *β-thalassemia or Cooley's anemia is the commonest thalassemia*
- Most types of Beta thalassemia are caused by point mutations affecting one or few bases.
- The ***most common site of mutations in Beta thalassemia is the intervening sequence 1 (IVS-1) or Intron 1***

Alpha and Beta Thalassemia Traits:

Thalassemia Trait

Alpha Thalassemia Trait	Beta thalassemia trait (T. minor)
• ***Normal HBA_2*** • ***Normal HBF*** • Mild Anemia - Mild Microcytosis - Mild Hypochromia • No need for Blood transfusion	• ↑ ***HBA_2*** • ↑ ***HBF*** • Mild Anemia - Mild Microcytosis - Mild Hypochromia • No need for blood transfusion

Causes of CREW-CUT Appearance (Hair on End Appearance):

Crew cut appearance (Hair on End appearance)
• Thalassemia (Most charachteristic) • Sickle cell Anemia (2nd most characteristic) • Other Hemolytic anamias (May be seen)

Clinical spectrum of Thalassemia (β thalassemia):

Syndrome	Thalassemia major (Serious homozygos form)	Thalassemia intermedia (They are also homozygos)	Thalassemia minor (heterozygos form)
General characteristic	• Presentation in early infancy with: - Progressive pallor - Hepatosplenomegaly - Bony changes • Invariably fatal during first few years of life if left untreated (Require repeated blood transfusions)	• Patient present somewhere between the two extremes with variable clinical manifestations of - Progressive pallor - Hepatosplenomegaly - Bony changes • These patients maintain hemoglobin levels between 6-10 g/dl and lead their life fairly comfortably. These patients may need occasional transfusions but are not dependent on blood transfusions for their survival.	• Presents late and patient can lead a practically normal life except for mild persistent anemia • These patients are not dependent on blood transfusions

Clinical Features			
• Severity of disease	++++	++	±
• Growth and development	Impaired	-	-
• Splenomegaly	++++	++	-
• Jaundice	++	+/-	-
• Skeletal changes	+++	+	-
• Thalassemia facies	+++	+	-
Haematological findings			
• Anaemia Hb gm/dl	< 7 (severe)	7-10 (moderate)	>10
• Microcytosis	+++	++	+
• Hypochromia	+++	++	+
• Basophilic stippling	++	+	+
• Anisopoikilocytosis	+++	++	±
• Target cells	+++	++	+
• Nucleated red cells	+++	+/- occasional	-
• Reticulocytes	2-15	2-10	< 5
• HbF	30-90%	20-100%	0-5%
• HbA_2	<3.5%	<3.5%	3.5-8%
• B.M. Iron	++++	++	±
• Iron overload	+	-	-
• Life expectancy	20-28 YEARS	Normal	Normal

Autoimmune Hemolytic Anemias

Classification of Autoimmune Hemolytic Anemias

Depending upon reactivity of autoantibodies these are divided into two types

Warm antibody hemolytic anemia	*Cold antibody hemolytic anemia*
Antibodies here react at room temperature and are mainly of IgG type [Q]	Antibodies here react better at temperatures lower than 37^0C, and are mainly IgM [Q][An exception is cold reactive antibodies of IgG [Q] type in Paroxysmal cold hemoglobulinuria] [Q]
Causes :	*Causes :*
1. Idiopathic 2. Lymphomas : CLL [Q], Non-Hodgkins, etc. 3. SLE [Q]and other Collagen Vascular Diseases [Q] 4. Drugs : e.g. α Methyldopa [Q]	1. Acute : Mycoplasma Infection [Q]Infectious mononucleosis [Q] 2. Chronic : Idiopathic [Q] 3. Paroxysmal cold hemoglobinuria[Q]
Mechanism of Hemolysis :	*Mechanism of Hemolysis :*
Human red cells cooled with IgG are trapped by splenic macrophages - Red cell destruction	Antibodies of IgM type bind on Red cell surface and cause agglutination. Hemolytic effect is mediated through fixation of C3 to RBC surface. [Q]
Diagnosis :	*Diagnosis :*
Positive direct Coomb's test, at 37^0C for presence of warm antibodies on surface of Red cell. [Q] Positive Indirect Coomb's test at 37^0C for presence of large quantities of warm antibodies in serum. [Q]	Positive direct Coomb's test for detection of C3 on the red cell surface, but IgM responsible for coating on red cells is not found. [Q]

Microangiopathic Hemolytic Anemias

Classification and/or causes of Microangiopathic Hemolytic Anemias:

Classification of Microangiopathic Hemolytic Anemia
Primary
• **Thrombotic thrombocytopenic purpura**
• **Hemolytic uremic syndrome**
Secondary
• **Associated with disseminated intravascular coagulation**
Infections (sepsis)
Shiga-type toxins
HIV
Snake venoms
Abruptio placentae
• **Associated with hypertension**
Malignant hypertension
Preclampsia, eclampsia,
HELLP syndrome
• **Associated with malignancy**
Adenocarcinomas; gastrointestinal, breast, lung
• **Associated with drugs and/or radiation**
Antineoplastic agents
Radiation nephritis and chemotherapy in organ transplantation
Ticlopidine
• **Associated with immunologic disorders/Vasculitis**
Acute glomerulonephritis
SLE
Polyarteritisnodosa
Scleroderma
Other vasculitis
• **Associated with congenital malformations**
Cavernous hemangioma (Kasabach-Meritt syndrome)
Hemangioendothelioma of the liver
• **Associated with antiphospholipid syndrome** (*NMS Medicine*)
• **Associated with Prosthetic valves** (*Harrison/CMDT*) (Pathologically Macroangiopathic – *Rubin's Pathology*)

Important causes of Microangiopathic Hemolytic Anemias
• ***TTP***
• ***HUS***
• ***DIC***
• *Vasculitis (Collagen Vascular Disorders)*
• *Malignant Hypertension/Eclampsia/**HELLP***
• *Disseminated carcinomatosis (Metastasis)*
• *Drugs / Radiation*
• *Antiphospholipidsyndrome(NMS Medicine)*
• *Prosthetic Heart Valve*
(PathologicallyMacroangiopathic – *Rubin's*)

Patients with microangiopathic hemolytic anemias are usually thrombocytopenic

(due to consumption of Platelets).

Evan's syndrome (combination of ITP and Autoimmune Hemolytic Anemia (AIHA))

- *Evan's Syndrome refers to a combination of Idiopathic Thrombocytopenic Purpura (ITP) and Autoimmune Hemolytic Anemia (AIHA) in the absence of an underlying cause / disease.*
- The occurence of thrombocytopenia may coincide with episodes of hemolysis or may arise as separate episodes.
- Evan's syndrome is more common in children
- Evan's syndrome tends to be resistanct to management of Warm AIHA or ITP
- ***Evans syndrome presents with 'Thrombocytopenia' and 'Immune Hemolysis'.***

Evan's syndrome does not present with microangiopathic features or fragmented RBCs.

PNH: Paroxysmal Nuctunalhaemoglobinuria

PNH is an Acquired[Q] Intracarpuscular[Q] disorder, acquired at stem cell level[Q] by loss characterised by undue sensitivity of red blood cell's membrane to complement[Q]

Common manifestations: PNH : Three common manifestation

Hemolytic Anemia

↓

Because of increased activation of complement and complement mediated destruction

↓

Hemoglobinemia[Q]
Hemoglobinuria[Q]
Hemosiderinuria[Q]
Elevated LDH[Q]

Venous Thrombosis

Activation of complement indirectly stimulates platelet aggregation and hypercoagulability (thus thrombosis despite thrombocytopenia)

Deficient Hematopoesis

Probably due to defect at stem cell level

↓

Pancytopenia/Aplastic anemia-H16th/ 618
- ↓ Granulocytes
- Thrombocytes (thrombocytopenia)

Why is it called Paroxysmal Nocturnal haemoglobinuria?
Basis :*Acidification enhances activity of complement*

During night when one sleeps **(noctunal)** → Relative Hypoxia → Acidosis → Enhanced complement activity

↓

Paroxysm of **Haemoglobinuria**identified by passage of brown urine in morning. ← Complement mediated destruction of red blood cells

Red Cell Membrane is **deficient in two factors** which result in increased activation of complement

1. **DAF**[Q] : Decay accelerating factor that activates decay of complements
2. MIRL CD 59 : inhibits membrane attack complex

Conditions associated with decreased and increased Leukocyte Alkaline Phosphatase Scores (LAP Score)

Conditions with decreased LAP scores	Conditions with increased LAP scores
1. P.N.H. [Q]	1. Polycythemia [Q]
2. C.M.L. [Q]	2. Leukemoid reaction [Q]
	3. Infection [Q]

1

Hematology

Aplastic Anemia and Myelodysplastic Syndrome

Differential diagnosis of Pancytopenia

Pancytopenia with Hypocellular Bone Marrow
Acquired aplastic anemia
Constitutional aplastic anemia
(Fanconi's anemia, dyskeratosiscongenita)
Some myelodysplastic syndromes
Rare aleukemic leukemia (AML)
Some acute lymphoid leukemia
Some lymphomas of bone marrow

Hypocellular bone marrow ±Cytopenia
Q fever
Legionnaires' disease
Anorexia nervosa, starvation
Mycobacteria

Pancytopenia with Cellular Bone Marrow

Primary bone marrow diseases	*Secondary to systemic diseases*
Myelodysplasia syndromes	Systemic lupus erythematosus
Paroxysmal nocturnal hemoglobinuria	Hypersplenism
Myelofibrosis	***B_{12}, folate deficiency (Megaloblastic Anemia)***
Some aleukemic leukemia	Overwhelming infection
Myelophthisis	Alcohol
Bone marrow lymphoma	Brucellosis
Hairy cell leukemia	Sarcoidosis
	Tuberculosis
	Leishmaniasis

Fanconi's Anemia:

Fanconi's Anemia (F A)

- *Autosomal Recessive*[Q]
- *Positive Family History*[Q]

- Inherited *chromosomal instability syndrome*[Q]
- The diagnosis of FA is based on the demonstration of increased chromosomal breakage in the presence of DNA cross- linking agents such as mitomycin C (MMC) or Diepoxybutane (DEB)

Progressive Bone Marrow Failure

- ***Pancytopenia with hypocellular marrow***
- *Aplastic Anemia* ***(Normochromic-Normocytic)*** *(May be Normochromic Macrocytic)*

Congenital Anomalies

- Skeletal
  Short stature
  Radial ray anomalies (thumbs, hands, radii)
  Hip and spine anomalies
- Skin
  Hyperpigmentation (café au lait spots)
  Hypopigmentation
- Genitourinary
  Renal structural anomalies
  Hypogonadism
- Craniofacial
  Microcephaly
  Ophthalmic anomalies (microphthalmia, epicanthal folds)
  Otic anomalies (external and middle ear anomalies, deafness)
- Gastrointestinal malformations
  Esophageal atresia or tracheoesophageal fistula
  Imperforate anus
- Cardiac malformations

Increased Risk of Malignancy

- *Fanconi's anemia is a premalignant state.*
- Patents with FA are at increased risk of developing Myelodysplasia (MDS) or *Acute Myeloid Leukemia (AML)*[Q]
- Patients with FA are at increased risk of developing *solid tumours*[Q] particularly squammous cell carcinoma of the head and neck, skin, GIT & genital tract

Sideroblastic Anemia

What are Sideroblasts

Sideroblasts are Erythroblasts (Red blood cell precursors) that contain iron (ferritin) granules in their cytoplasm. The iron in these cells is normally located in the cytoplasm away from the nucleus (and stains positive for prussian blue).

In normal bone marrow sideroblasts constitute 20- 40% (approx 1/3rd) of red blood cell precursors

What are Ringed Sideroblasts

Ringed sideroblasts are abnormal sideroblasts seen in conditions with disturbed haem synthesis. In these cells iron accumulates within the mitochondria, surrounds the nucleus and does not progress into haemoglobin

Ringed sideroblasts are defined as Nucleated Red blood cells (Erythroblasts) containing five or more granules and encircling at least two – thirds of the nucleus.

Ring sidroblasts are pathological and their presence suggests a diagnosis of sideroblastic anemia whether congenital or acquired

What are the conditions associated with Ringed Sideroblasts

Ringed Sideroblasts may be seen in all causes of sideroblatic anemia whether Congenital or Acquired but are most often associated with Myelodysplastic syndromes

Causes of Sideroblastic Anemia (Ringed Sideroblasts in Bone Marrow)

1. Hereditary Sideroblastic Anemia
2. Acquired Sideroblastic Anemia
   - Primary (Acquired) SideroblasticAnemia***(Myelodysplastic Syndromes)***
   - Secondary (Acquired) SidroblasticAnemia : Secondary to
   - Alcohol (Alcohol induced sidroblasticanemia)[Q]
   - Lead (Lead induced sideroblasticanemia)[Q]
   - Zinc (Zinc induced sidroblasticanemia)[Q]
   - Drugs such as INH, pyrizinamide, cycloserine, chloramphenical etc.
   - Other Myeloprolifirative disorders and Myelofibrosis
3. Others (Rare)
   - Thiamine responsive megaloblastic anemia
   - Pearson's syndrome
   - Hypothermia
   - Certain Haemoglobinopathies

Myeloproliferative disorders

Differential Diagnosis of Myeloproliferative disorders

Myeloproliferative disorders classically include:

- Polycythemia vera[Q]
- Idiopathic myelofibrosis[Q]
- Essential thrombocytosis[Q]
- Chronic myeloid leukemia[Q]

Condition	WBCount	Hematocrit/Red cell mass	Platelet count	Red cell morphology
CML	↑↑	N	N or ↑	N
Myelofibrosis	N or ↓or ↑	N or ↓	↓or N or ↑	Abnormal
Polycythemia	N or ↑	↑	N or ↑	N
Essential Thrombocytosis	N or ↑	N	↑↑	N

Polycythemia Vera
Neoplasm arising in multipotent elements

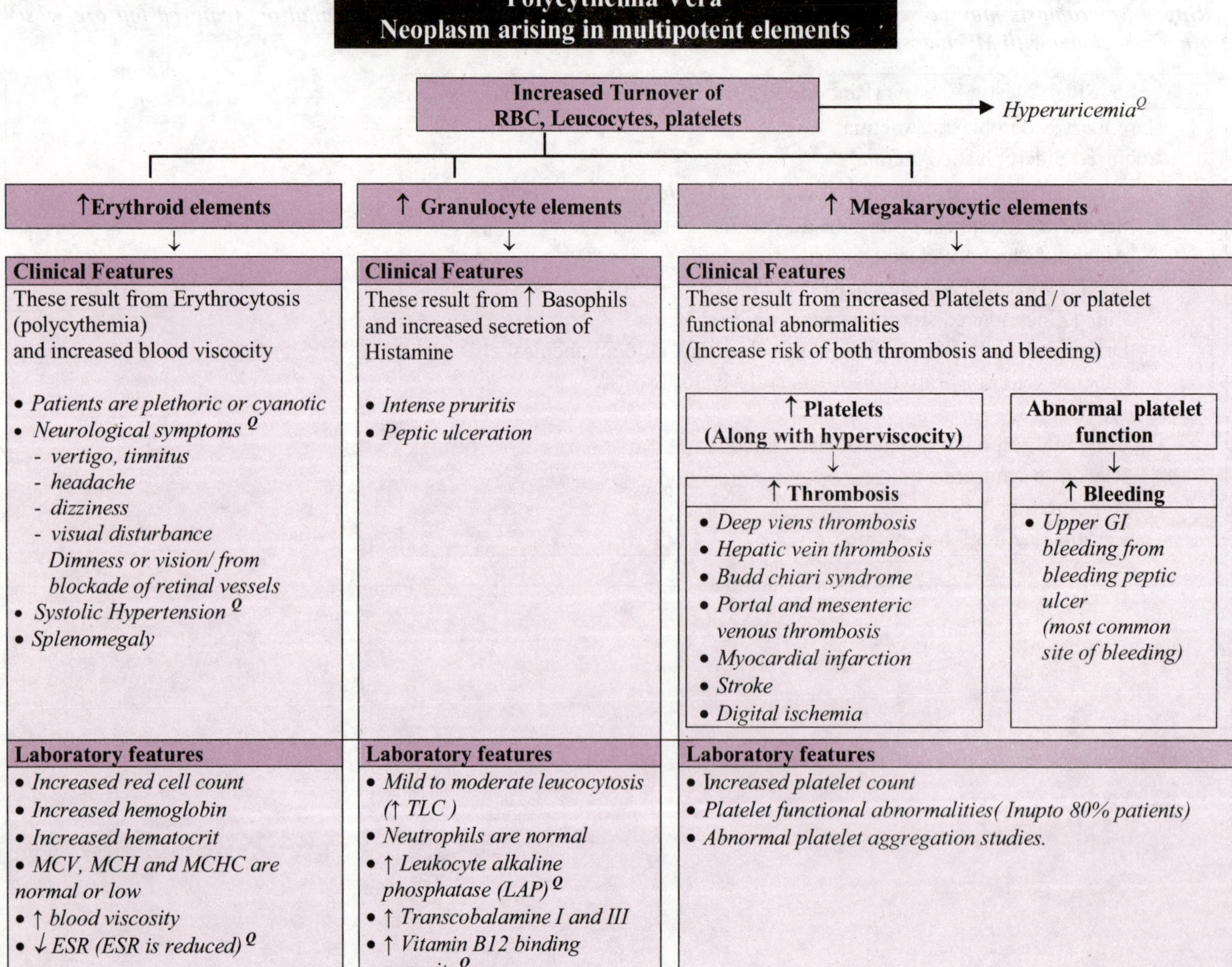

Various major and minor criteria used for the diagnosis of polycythemia vera in various classification systems
(WHO criteria (revised and old)/ Polycythemia vera study group criteria)

Major	Minor
• ***JAK2 V617F mutation*** • *Hemoglobin >18.5 g/dL in men, 16.5 g/dL in women* • *Increased red blood cell mass* • *Splenomegaly* • *Clonal genetic abnormality other than Philadelphia chromosome or BCR/ABL in marrow* • *Endogenous erythroid colony formation in vitro* • *Normal arterial O2 saturation (>92%)*	• ***Thrombocytosis*** *(> 400 × 10^9/L)* • ***Leucocytosis*** *(WBC > 12 × 10^9/L)* • ***Increased leukocyte alkaline phosphatase*** *(LAP > 100U)* • *Increased serum B12/binders (B12 > 900 pg/ml; unbound B12 binding capacity > 2200 pg/ml)* • *Low serum erythroprotein levels.* • *Panmyelosis with prominent erythoid and megakaryocytic hyperplasia on bone marrow biopsy.*

Revised WHO criteria (Proposed) for the diagnosis of Polycythemia vera

Revised WHO criteria (Proposed) for the diagnosis of Polycythemia vera

Major Criteria

- Hemoglobin > 18.5 g/dl in men, > 16.5 g/dl in women or evidenced on increased red cell volume
- ***Presence of JAK2 mutation***

Minor Criteria

- Hypercellular bone marrow biopsy with panmyelosis with prominent erythroid, granulocytic, and megakaryocytic hyperplasia
- Low serum erythropoietin level
- Endogenous erythroid colony formation in vitro.

WHO Criteria for the diagnosis of Plycythemia Vera (Prior to the proposed new criterion)

WHO Criteria*(Previous)* **for the diagnosis of Plycythemiavera**

Major Criteria

- Red blood cell mas > 25% above mean normal predicted value, or Hb > 18.5 g/dl in men, 16.5 g/dl in women.
- Splenomegaly on palpation
- Clonal genetic abnormality other than Philadelphia chromosome or BCR/ABL in marrow.
- Endogenous erythroid colony formation in vitro

Minor Criteria

- Thrombocytosis > 400 × 10^9/L
- WBC > 12 × 10^9/L
- Panmyelosis with prominent erythroid and megakaryocytic hyperplasia on bone marrow biopsy.
- Low serum erythropoietin levels.

Tumors associated with Polycythemia Vera

Tumors associated with polycythemia veraare:

- Hypernephroma
- Hepatoma
- Adrenal adenoma
- Pheochromocytoma
- ***Cerebellar Haemangioblastoma***
- Uterine fibromyoma
- Meningioma

Myelofibrosis

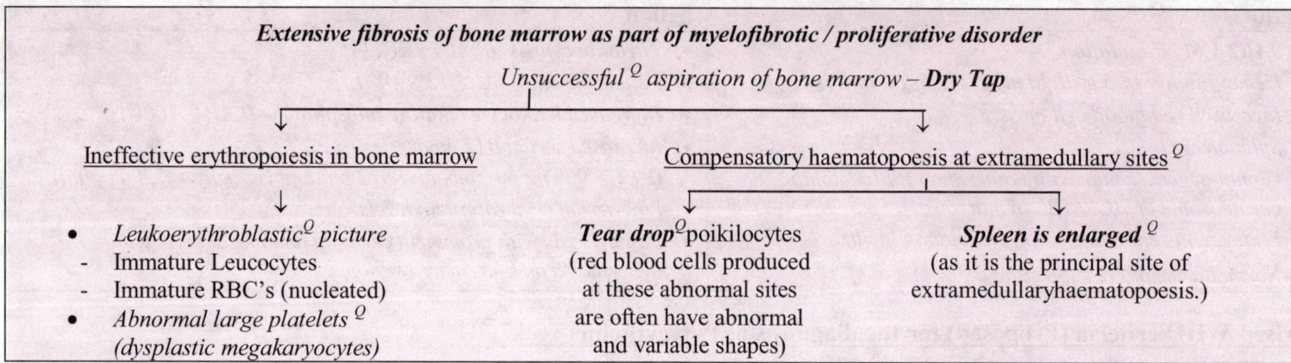

Most characteristic are the Laboratory findings and the *triad of*[Q]

a. Tear drop poikilocytes[Q]
b. Leukoerythroblastic blood i.e. immature leukocytes and nucleated (immature) RBC's [Q]
c. Giant abnormal platelets [Q]

Biopsy of bone marrow to detect reticular or collagen fibrosis is essential for diagnosis. [Q]

Essential thrombocytosis

(essentialthrombocythaemia; idiopathic thrombocytosis; hemorrhagic thrombocythaemia)

Essential thrombocytosis is a myeloproliferative disorder characterized by overproduction of platelets without a definable cause.

Clinical features

Symptoms

- Haemorrhagictendencies : Easy bruising [Q]
- Thrombotic tendencies :Microvascular occlusions
  - Erythromelalgia
  - Migraine (headache)
  - Transient ischemic attacks

Signs

- Splenomegaly : usually mild/moderate *massive splenomegaly is more characteristic of other myeloproliferative disorders.*

Laboratory Diagnostic features

- Elevated platelet count is hallmark (often $>1000\times10^3/\mu L$)
- Haematocrit and RBC morphology normal
- WBC count is mildly elevated/normal (mildneutrophillicleucocytosis)
- LAP is normal or elevated
- Philadelphia chromosome is absent

Management in a symptomatic patient

Elevated platelet count in asymptomatic patient

- No therapy is recommended because agents used in treatment place the patient at risk of developing acute leukemia

↓

Therapy with risk of acute leukemia

- Radioactive phosphorus
- Hydroxyuria
- Alkylating agents

Management in symptomatic patient

Elevated platelet count in symptomatic patients

- Symptoms must be clearly identified to be a consequence of elevated platelet count

↓

Platelet reduction

- IFN a
- Anagrelide
- Hydroxyurea: *should be considered only if the above agents are not effective or tolerable*

.- Harrison

Lymphomas and Chronic Leukemias

Hodgkin's Disease/ Lymphoma

Hodgkin's Disease

Classical Hodgkin's Disease	Histogenetically distinct subtype of HodgkinsDisease
Variants/Subtypes	Variant/Subtype
Mixed cellularity *Nodular sclerosis* *Lymphocyte Rich* *Lymphocyte Depletion*	*Lymphocyte predominant* *(Nodular Lymphocyte Predominant)*
Characterized by:	Characterized by
• *Frequent Reed sternberg cells* • *Characteristic immunophenotype* *CD 15 positive; CD 30 positive* *CD 45 Negative*	• *Rare Reed Sternberg cells* (Frequent Lymphocytic and Histocytic variants (Popcorn cells)) • Characteristically different immunophenotype *CD 15 Negative : CD 30 Negative* *CD 45 Positive*

Characteristic R.S cells are less frequent in nodular sclerosis variant of Hodgkins but these cells are characteristically positive for CD 15 and CD 30 and negative for CD 45

The Hodgkin's lymphomas may be classified into four subtypes according to the Rye's classification.

Hodgkins lymphoma subtypes in order of frequency

1. *Nodular sclerosis (30-60%)*
2. *Mixed cellularity (20-40%)*
3. *Lymphocyte predominance (< 10%)*
4. *Lymphocyte depleted (< 10%)*

Note: WHO classification recognizes another subtype of Hodgkins called 'Lymphocyte Rich' subtype

The most common subtype of Hodgkin's Lymphoma is 'Nodular Sclerosis'

Incidence: NS > MC > LP > LD

Prognosis of Hodgkin's Lymphoma Variants:

Variant	5 years survival
Lymphocyte predominance	*90%*
Nodular sclerosis	*70%*
Mixed cellularity	*50%*
Lymphocyte depletion	*40%*

Lymphocyte predominant type of Hodgkins lymphoma is associated with the best prognosis.

Prognosis: LP > NS > MC > LD

Variants of Reed Sternberg cells:

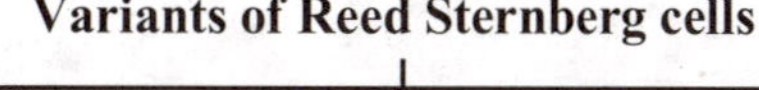

Variants of Reed Sternberg cells

Lacunar variant	Mononuclear variant	Lymphohistiocytic variant (Popcorn cell; L and H cells)
R.S cells variant with a folded or multilobate nuclei and abundant pale cytoplasm which gives the appearance of a nucleus silting in an empty hole (lacunae) on histological sections	R.S cell variant with a single round or oblong nucleus	R.S cell variant with multiple folded or convoluted nuclear contour resembling a popcorn kernel (popcorn cell variant)
↓	↓	↓
Characteristically seen in	Characteristically seen in	Characteristically seen in
Nodular Sclerosis subtype	*Mixed cellularity subtype* *Lymphocyte Rich Subtype*	*Lymphocyte predominance variant*

Remember one Reed Sternberg Variant and one characteristic of each variety

Hodgkins lymphoma subtypes	Red Sternberg cells variant	Charachterisitic feature
Nodular sclerosis	Lacunar cells [Q]	*M.C. type (all over the world)* [Q]
Mixed cellularity	Mononuclear variant[Q]	*M.C. type in India* [Q]
Lymphocyte predominance	Popcorn cell [Q] (Lymphocytic variant)	*Best prognosis* [Q]
Lymphocyte depleted	Reticular variant (more cellular)	*Worst prognosis* [Q]

Hodgkins Lymphoma	Immunopheno type	Association with EBV	Read Sternberg Cell variant[Q]
Nodular Sclerosis	**CD15 + , CD30 +**	EBV – Ve[Q]	Lacunar cells[Q] (Occasional R-S-cells)
Mixed cellularity	**CD15 + , CD30 +**	EBV + Ve[Q] (70%)	Classic Reed Sternberg cells[Q]
Lymphocyte depletion	**CD15 + , CD30 +**	EBV +Ve[Q]	Reticular variant[Q] (Frequent R-S cells)
Lymphocyte Predominance	CD15 –ve, CD30-ve CD20 +ve, CD45+ve (H17th)	EBV – Ve[Q]	Popcorn cell variant[Q]

Prognostic Factors In Hodgkin's Lymphoma:

Prognostic factors in Hodgkins lymphoma

Poor prognostic factors for advanced disease

- Male Gender
- Age>45 years
- Stage IV Disease
- Serum Haemoglobin < 10g
- Serum Albumin < 4 g
- WBC count > 15,000/mm^3
- Absolute lymphocyte count <600mm^3

These factor predict relapse of advanced disease

Poor prognostic factors in Localized disease

- Male Gender
- Age >50 years
  Histological subtype (mixed cellularity and lymphocyte Depletion)
- Elevated ESR
- Mediastinal mass >1/3 of thoracic diameter (Mediastinal/thorax ratio > 35%)
- Number of involved sites with the same side of diaphragm > 4
- Presence of systemic symptoms ('B' symptoms)

These factors predict prognosis in patients with clinical stages I and II in Hodgkin's disease.

Treatment of Hodgkin's Lymphoma:

Treatment of Hodgkin's Lymphoma

Classical Hodgkin's Lymphoma		Nodular Lymhocyte predominant Hodgkin's Lymphoma	
Limited Stage Disease	Advanced Disease	Limited Stage Disease	Advanced Disease
(Favourable/unfavourable) (Stage I, II)	Stage III, IV	Stage I, II	Stage III, IV
Combined Modality treatment with Radiotherapy and chemotherapy is the treatment of choice Limited Stage Disease (I, II) is primarily managed by a combination of chemotherapy (CT) and Radiotherapy (RT) (CT→RT)	Chemotherapy is the treatment of choice Advanced stage disease is primarily managed by chemotherapy Radiotherapy may be used in advanced disease for bulky disease or residual disease after chemotherapy (PTO)	Radiotherapy alone is the treatment of choice (Involved Field RT or Regional RT may be used) *Some clinicians favour no treatment and merely close follow up*	Chemotherapy is the treatment of choice Advanced stage disease is primarily managed chemotherapy *RT may be used in advanced disease for palliation only and in selected cases after chemotherapy.*
CT + RT	CT (± RT)	RT	CT (± RT)

Non-Hodgkin's Lymphoma

Classification of Non-Hodgkin's Lymphoma:

Classification of Non Hodgkin Lymphoma	
B cell Neoplasms	**T cell Neoplasms**
Neoplasms of immature B cells	Neoplasms of immature T cells
Precursor B cell Acute Lymphoblastic leukaemia / lymphoma	Precursor T-cell Acute Lymphoblastic leukaemia / Lymphoma
Neoplasms of mature B cells	Neoplasms of mature T cells / NK cells

• ***Burkitt'slymphoma***[Q]
• ***Hairy cell leukemia***[Q]
• ***Mantle cell lymphoma***[Q]
• Solitary plasmacytoma / Multiple Myeloma[Q]
• Small lymphocytic lymphoma / Chronic lymphocytic leukaemia (CLL)
• Follicular lymphoma
• Diffuse large B cell lymphoma
• Extranodal marginal zone lymphoma (MALT Type)
	• Mycosis fungoides : Cutaneous T cell lymphoma
	• Adult T cell lymphoma / Leukemia
	• Anaplastic Large T cell / Null cell Lymphoma
	• Peripheral T cell Lymphoma
	  o Angioimmunoblastic Lymphoma
	  o ***Angiocentric Lymphoma***(Extra-nodal T/NK cell Lymphoma
	  o Enteropathy type intestinal lymphoma
	  o Hepatosplenic lymphoma
	  o Subcutaneous Panniculitis - like lymphoma
	• T cell granular lymphocytic lymphoma

Burkitt's Lymphoma

Translocations in Burkitt's Lymphoma

Burkitt's lymphoma / leukemias are associated with reciprocal translocations involving the ***c-myc gene on chromosome 8***

Most common Translocation (70% cases)	Less common translocations
t (8; 14): c- myc gene on chromosome 8 and IgHheavy chain on chromosome 14	**t (8; 22)** c- myc gene on chromosome 8 and λ-light chain on chromosome 22 **t (2; 8) :** c- myc gene on chromosome 8 and κ-light chain on chromosome -2

Hairy cell leukemia:

Hairy cell leukemia is a rare but distinctive form of chronic B cell leukemia that derives its name from the appearance of fine 'hair like projections'[Q] on the leukaemic cells (large B cells)

• **Characteristic cytochemical feature:**	Presence of tartrate resistant acid phosphatase 'TRAP' [Q] in neoplastic B cells
• **Cellular features/ Markers**[Q]	• Hairy cells express the pan B cell markers CD 19 and CD 20 and monocyte associated antigen CD 11 • Plasma cell associated antigen (PCA-1) is also present – Robbins • Expression of **CD 25**, IL2 and specific adhesion molecules – Harrison 14th/695
• **Clinical features** result largely from infiltration of bone marrow liver and spleen	• Present predominantly in the older age group > 40 years[Q] • Massive splenomegaly[Q] (hepatomegaly is less common) • Lymphadenopathy • Pancytopenia[Q] • Recurrent infections
• **Treatment**[Q]	• Current treatment of choice is with purine analogues – Cladribine[Q] • Other drugs used - Pentostotin[Q] - Interferon α[Q] • Splenectomy used to be the standard treatment earlier

Mantle cell lymphoma

Presents in the middle aged and the elderly (Mean Age = 63 yrs– *Harrison 16th/ 648*).

Clinical profile
- Painless lymphadenopathy - Splenomegaly - Occasional GI involvement

Immunocytochemical profile of Mantle Cell Lymphoma

CD markers	SURFACE immunoglobulins	Translocation
• Cells are positive for PAN B markers D 19, CD 2, CD 22, CD 24 • Cells are positive for CD 5 • Cells are negative for CD 23 • Cells are negative for CD 10	• Moderately high levels of surface immunoglobulins heavy chains IgM &IgD • B cells present bright K positivity (either K or λ light chain may be present)	t (11; 14) translocation 14 t (11; 14) translocation leads to increased expression of cyclin D1

Coexpression of CD19 and CD5 suggests a diagnosis of Mantle Cell Lymphoma or CLL:

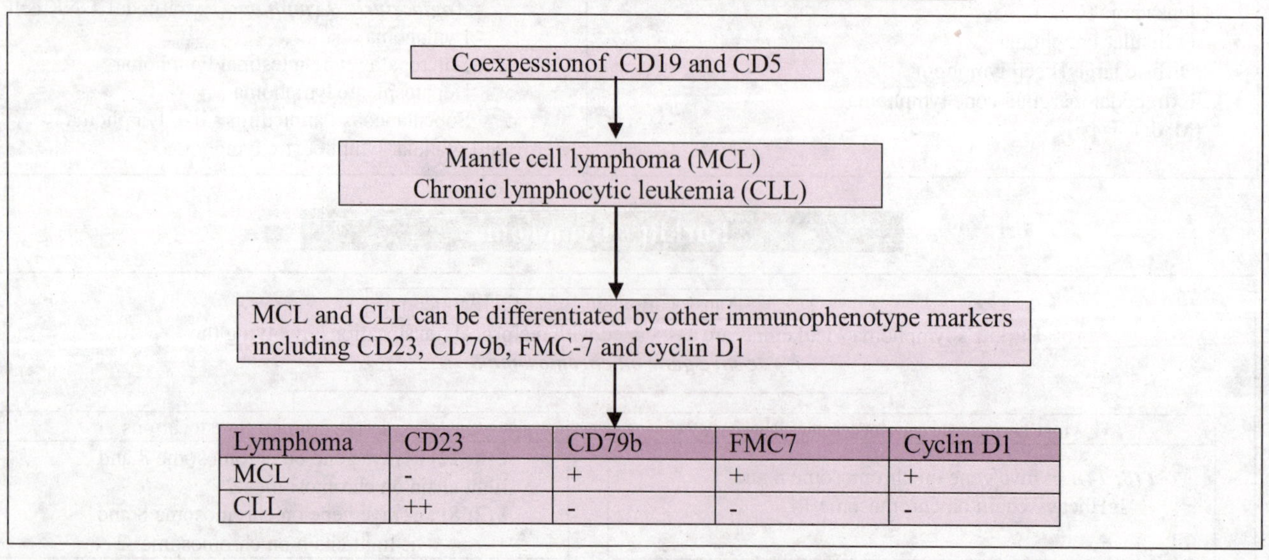

Lymphoma	CD23	CD79b	FMC7	Cyclin D1
MCL	-	+	+	+
CLL	++	-	-	-

Chronic Lymphocytic Leukemia

Chronic Lymphocytic Leukemia (CLL)

Chronic lymphocytic leukemia/small lymphocytic lymphoma (CLL/SLL) is tumor composed of monomorphic small B lymphocytes in the peripheral blood, bone marrow and lymphoid organs (spleen and lymph nodes).

WHO considers both CLL and SLL as a single entity with different presentations. Small lymphocytic lymphoma (SLL) is considered as a tissue equivalent of chronic lymphocytic leukemia (CLL). The CLL/SLL tumor cells coexpress CD5 and CD23.

Pripheral blood picture

- **Peripheral smear**
  - **RBCs:** Show normocytic normochromic anemia or rarely hemolytic blood picture.
  - **WBCs:** Total leukocyte count is increased and varies from 20-50 x 109/L.

    Differential Leukocyte Count:

    Lymphocytosis is the characteristic feature and absolute lymphocyte count should be more than 5 x 109/L. *Usually absolute lymphocyte count above 10 x 109/L is common at the time of diagnosis.*

    Lymphocytes constitute more than 50% of the white cells and may reach up to 90-98% with resultant neutropenia (lymphocytes 70-98% and polymorphs 2-30%).

    Smudge cells: Smudge cells or basket cells are disintegrated lymphocytes and represent the spread out nuclear material observed in the peripheral blood film. They are due to rupture of the neoplastic lymphoid cells while making the peripheral smear due to its fragile nature.
  - **Platelets:** Initially the platelet count is normal. The bone marrow infiltration as well as autoimmune destruction of platelets associated with hypersplenism may result in decreased platelet count and a count below 100 x 109/L is associated with a worse prognosis.

Hemoglobin: Usually below 13 gm/dL and as the disease progresses, it may decrease below 10 gm/dL. This is due to marrow failure and associated autoimmune hemolysis may also be contributory, when present.

Bone marrow

- **Cellularity:**hypercellular marrow.
- **Erythropoiesis:** Erythropoiesis is normal. Patients are prone to develop autoimmune diseases, most commonly directed against red cells or platelets. Such cases which result in hemotytic anemia show normoblasticerythroid hyperplasia.
- **Myelopoiesis:**Myelopoies is is normal in the initial stages of the disease.
- **Megakaryopoiesis:**Mega karyopoiesis is within normal limits.

As the neoplastic lymphocytes increase in number, they replace the normal cells of erythroid, myeloid and megakaryocytic series in the bone marrow. This results in anemia, neutropenia and thrombocytopenia and indicates that the disease is advancing.

Special Tests

Antiglobulin (Coombs) Test

About 15 to 20% of patients manifest autoimmune hemolytic anemia and have positive direct Coombs test.

Immunophenotype

The tumor cells in CLL/SLL express the pan-B cell markers CD19 and CD20.

B cell CLL is characterized by aberrant expression of

T cell antigen CD5 (found only in a small subset of normal B cells). There is also weak expression of monoclonal surface immunoglobulin with k or l light chains.

Cytogenetic Abnormalities

Chromosomal translocations are rarely observed in both CLL and SLL. The common mutations associated are deletions of l3q14.3, 11q22-23, and 17p13.

About 20% of CLL show trisomy I2.

Clinical Presentation of CLL:

Clinical Presentation

- ***Age:*** Most of the patients at the time of diagnosis are between 50-60 years of age.
- ***Sex:*** More common in males than in females with a ratio of 2:1.

Asymptomatic	Non specific symptoms	Symptoms from splenomegaly
About 25% of patients are often asymptomatic and are detected either because of nonspecific symptoms or routine blood examination for some other disease	• Fatigue • Malaise • Weight loss • Anorexia	• ***Generalized lymphadenopathy:*** Initially the cervical lymph nodes are enlarged and in later stages there may be generalized lymphadenopathy. Involved nodes are rubbery, discrete, non-tender, small and mobile. • ***Splenomegaly and hepatomegaly:*** This is observed in very few cases. Infiltration by CLL cells is seen in the splenic white and red pulp and in hepatic portal tracts resulting in enlargement of both organs. • ***Immunological defects:*** CLL/SLL disrupts normal immune function, the mechanisms of which are not known. The pathogenic lgGs are produced by non-neoplastic, self-reactive B cells rather than tumor cells resulting in the following: **Immune deficiency:**Hypogammaglobulinemia is common and is responsible for increased risk of opportunistic infections. **Autoimmunity:**Patients may develop systemic autoimmune diseases, especially hemolytic anemia or thrombocytopenia due to autoantibodies.

Course and Prognosis of CLL:

Course is variable and depends on Clinical stage of disease.

Prognostic Factors of CLL

- *Plasma β2 microglobulin level:* High levels are associated with a poor prognosis.
- *Presence of deletions of 11q and l7p*: Worse prognosis.
- *Bone marrow trephine biopsy*: Pattern of marrow infiltration.
- *Nodular and interstitial pattern of infiltration* has better prognosis than mixed and diffuse types.
- *Lack of somatic hypermutation:* Worse prognosis

Progression and Transformation of CLL:

CLL/SLL may transform to more aggressive tumors. These transformations are probably due to additional mutations resulting in rapid growth and are indicative of poor prognosis.

B cell Prolymphocytic Transformation

Transformation to B cell prolymphocytic leukemia is extremely rare. It is characterized by:

- Appearance of "prolyrnphocytes" in the peripheral blood (>10%).
  These prolymphocytes are large cells with a single prominent centrally placed nucleolus
- Worsening of cytopenias
- Increasing splenomegaly.

Transformation to Diffuse Large B cell Lymphoma (Richter syndrome) (Found in 5 to l0% of patients)
Characterized by the development of a rapidly enlarging mass within a lymph node or the spleen.

Chronic Myeloid Leukemia (CML)

What is Chronic Myeloid Leukemia:

CML

Chronic myeloproliferative disorder from neoplastic transformation of a bone marrow stem cell that still retains capacity to differentiate along erythrocytic, megakaryocytic and granulocytic or monocytic lines.

Pripheral blood picture

- StrikingLeucocytosis (Elevated WBC count)
  Both immature and mature farms in different Stages of maturation may be seen But ***Blood picture is dominated by Mature forms and precursor in the intermediate stages of differentiation***
  (Neutrophils, Metamyelocytes and Myelocytes)

  Immature forms are less numerous
  Blasts <5%
  Promyelocytes<10%

  (Cells are usually present in direct degree to the stage of maturation)

  BasophillsEosinophils may be increased
  - Elevated Basophils (often present)
  - Elevated Eosinophils (less common)
- **Thrombocytosis**
  Elevated platelet count if often present.Platelet count may be normal or sometimes elevated to strikingly high levels
- **Erythrocytes**
  Red blood cell morphology is normal.
  Patient is usually not anemic or only mildly anemic

Bone marrow

- Bone marrow is hypercellular with left shifted myelopoesis
- Myeloid: Erythroid ratio is increased
- Myeloblasts comprises less than 5% of marrow cells

Special Tests

- Cytogenetic Analysis for PhiladelphiaChromosome
  A small chromosome 22 caused by t (9; 22) translocation that results in bcr/abl fusion gene
- Reduced Leukocyte alkaline phosphatase levels(↓LAP)
  This indicates that although the total number of granulocytes is increased they are functionally impaired
- Serum levels of vitamin B_{12}proteins is ↑ed binding.

Clinical Presentation in CML:

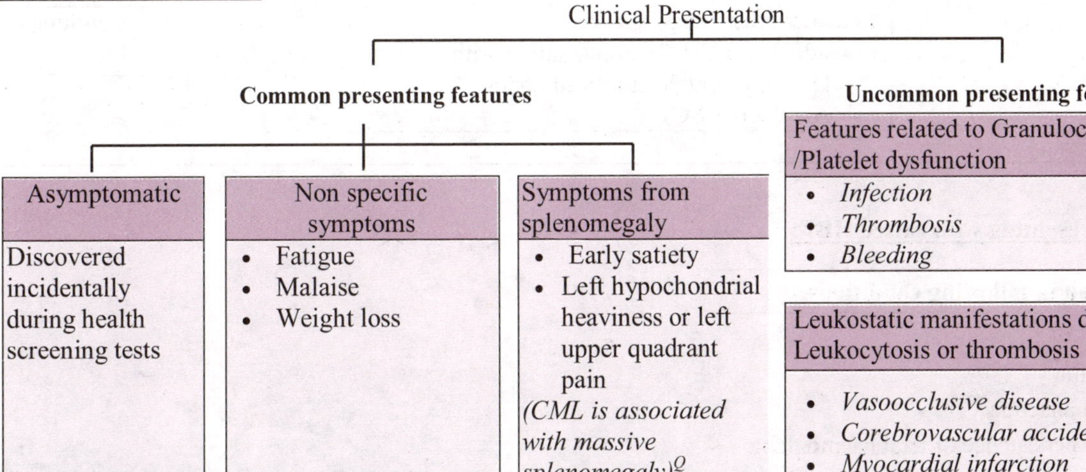

Physical examination : Physical signs

- Splenomegaly (mild, moderate, massive), and sternal tenderness are characteristic
- Mild hepatomegaly may be present &lymphademopathy is unusual

Treatment of CML

- The only curative treatment for CML is Allogenic Stem Cell Transplantation (SCT) (Allogenic bone marrow transplantation) [Q]
- The treatment of choice for CML is also Allogenic Stem Cell Transplantation (SCT) (Allogenic bone marrow transplantation) [Q]
- ***The drug treatment of choice for CML is Imatinib*** [Q]
- ***The initial treatment of choice for CML is drug treatment with Imatinib***
- *Interferon alpha (IFN α) used to be the drug treatment of choice for CML when Imatinab was not available*

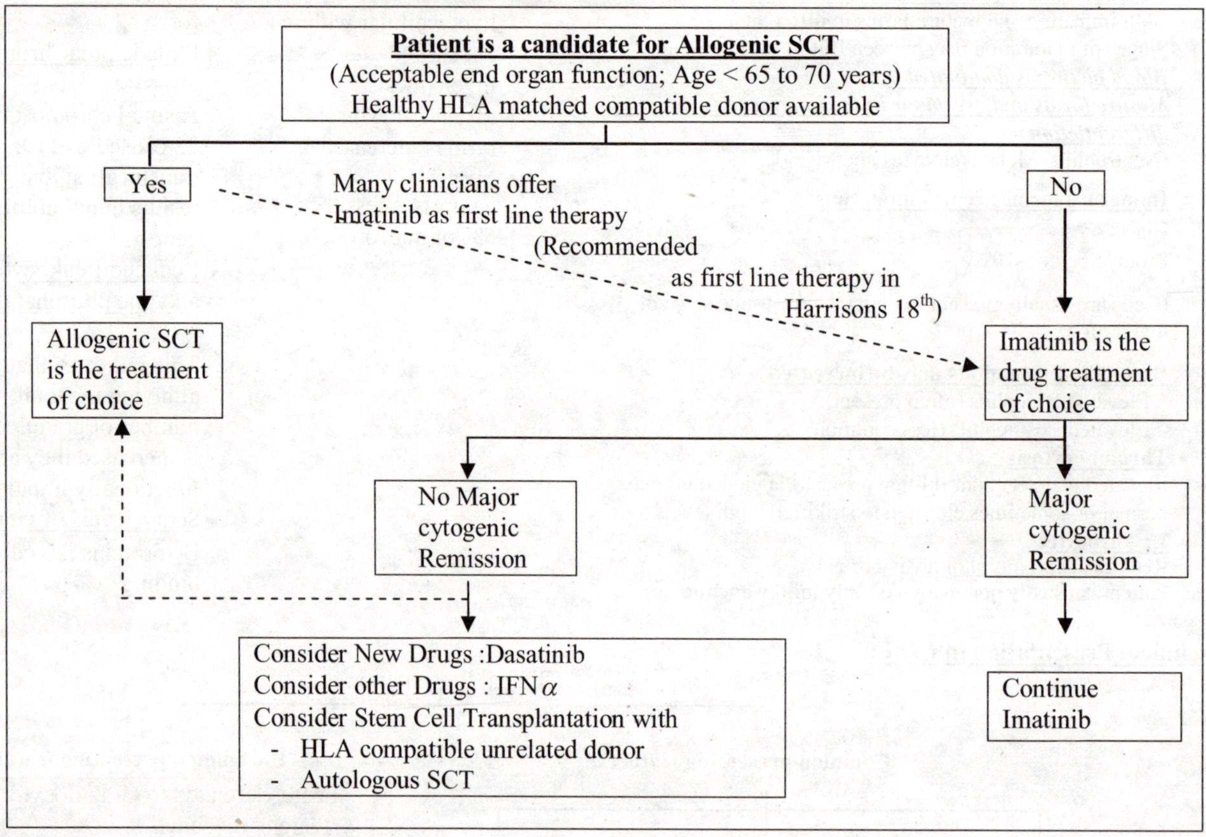

Conditions presenting with raised HBF:

HbF is raised in following conditions
• *Juvenile CML* [Q]
• βthalossemia [Q]
• Sickle cell anaemia [Q]
• Heriditary persistence of fetal haemoglobin (HPFF)

Mycosis Fungoides

Mycosis fungoides is synonymous with Cutaneous T cell lymphoma.

Clinical presentation and course:

- Mycosis fungoides***has an indolent course.***
  Most affected individuals have disease that remains localized to the skin for many years.
  It begins on the skin and may involve only the skin for years or decades
- Presentation is with localized or generalized erythematous / eczematous skin lesions.
  Skin lesion progress from 'patch' stage to 'plaque stage' to cutaneous 'tumors' stage.
- Metastasis occurs in advanced stages :

To lymph nodes	Peripheral circulation
	Sezary syndrome (Erythroderma and Circulating tumor cells) Seeding of the blood by melanoma cells is accompanied by diffuse erythema and scaling of the entire body surface (erythroderma).

Histology

Sezary - Lutzner cells	***PautrierMicroabscesses***
• Histological hall mark of Mycosis fungoides • These are T helper cell (CD4 positive)	Sezary - Lutzner cells characterstically form band like aggregates within the superficial dermis and invade the epidermis as single cells or small clusters called Pautrier'sMicroabscesses.

Treatment (Mycosis fungoides is not easily amenable to treatment)

- ***The treatment of Mycosis fungoides is complex. Even early and aggressive treatment has not been proved to cure or prevent progression of the disease***. *-CMDT*
- *Cure has been possible with radiotherapy only in rare patients with early stage mycosis fungoides.*
- *Most of thetreatment for mycosis fungoides are 'palliative'.*

Acute Leukemias

Acute Lymphoid Leukemia (ALL)

Classification of Acute Lymphoid Leukeia (ALL):

Immunologic Subtype	% of Cases	FAB Subtype	Cytogenetic Abnormalities
Pre-B ALL	75	L1, L2	t(9;22), t(4, 11), t(1; 19)
T Cell ALL	20	L1, L2	14q 11 or 7q34
BCell ALL	5	L3	t(8; 14), t(8; 22), t(2;8)

Immunophenotypic classification for ALL

FAB classification	Immunologic classification	Phenotype	Incidence (% cases)		Cytogenetic Abnormalities
Pre-B Cell	Early Pre-B	CD19, CD20-/+, CD10, CD34, TdT	55	75	t(9;22), t(4, 11), t(1; 19)
	Pre-B	CD19, CD20+/-, CD10, CD34-, cIgM, Tdt+/-	20		
B cell	B cell	CD19, CD20, CD22, CD10+/-, CD34-, Tdt-, sIg	5		14q 11 or 7q34
T cell	T cell	CD1, CD2, CD3, CD5, CD7, CD10+/-, CD34-/+, Tdt, dual CD4/CD8	20		t(8; 14), t(8; 22), t(2;8)

Prognostic factor for ALL:

Determinants	**Favourable**	**Unfavrourable**
White blood cell count	Low WBC count*	High WBC count*
Age	***3-7 yrs***	***<1, > 10 yr***
Gender	Female	Male
Ethnicity	White	Black
Node, Liver, spleen enlargement	Absent	Massive
Testicular enlargement	***Absent***	***Present***
Central nervous system leukemia	Absent	Overt (blasts + pleocytosis)
FAB morphological features	L1	L2
Ploidy	Hyperdiploidy	Hypodiploidy< 45
DNA index	> 0.16	< 0.16
Cytogenenetic markers	Trisomies 4, 10 and/or 17 t(12;21) (telaml 1)	t(9; 22) [bcrabl] t(4; 11) [mll af4] t(1; 19)
Time to remission	< 14 d	> 28 d
Minimal residual disease	$< 10^{-4}$	$> 10^{-3}$
Immunophenotype	Early Pre-B cell	T cell

High WBC count is associated with a poor prognosis

Initial leukocyte count at diagnosis has proved to be an important prognostic factor in virtually every ALL study. Different studies (textbooks) quote different values for the initial WBC count that is associated with a poor prognosis but uniformly a high WBC count carries a poor prognosis.

Different text books	Favourable WBC count	Unfavourable WBC count
Wintrobe's Hematology	*< 10,000*	*> 20,000*
Hoffman Hematology	*< 50,000*	*> 50,000*
Manual of Clinical oncology	*<30,000*	*>30,000*
Inference	***Low WBC count***	***High WBC count***

Acute Myeloid Leukemia (AML)

Prognostic Feature in Acute Myeloid Leukemia:

Factor	Favourable	Unfavourable
Clinical		
Age	*<45 yr*	*<2yr, >60yr*
ECOG performance status	*0-1*	*>1*
Leukemia	*De novo*	*Antecedent hematologic disorder, myelodysplasia, myeloproliferative disorder*
Infection	*Absent*	*Present*
Prior chemotherapy	*No*	*Yes*
Leukocytosis	*<25,000/mm3*	*>100,000/mm2*
Serum LDH	*Normal*	*Elevated*
Extramedullary disease	*Absent*	*Present*
CNS disease	*Absent*	*Present*
Cytoreduction	*Rapid*	*Delayed*
Morphology		
Auer rods	*Present*	*Absent*
Eosinophils	*Present*	*Absent*
Megaloblasticerythroids	*Absent*	*Present*
Dysplastic megakaryocytes	*Absent*	*Present*
FAB type	*M2, M3, M4*	*M0, M6, M7*
Surface/enzyme markers		
Myeloid	*CD34-, CD14-, CD13-*	*CD34+*
HLA-DR	*Negative*	*Positive*
TdT	*Absent*	*Present*
Lymphoid	*Cd2+*	*CD7+, CD56+ Biphenotypic (2 or more lymphoid markers)*
MDR-1	*Absent*	*Present*
Cytogenetics		
Cytogenetics	*t(15;17), t(8;21), inv(16)*	*-7, del(7q), -5, del(5q), 3q21 and 3q26 abnormalities, complex karyotypes*
Molecular markers		
Fms-related tyrosine kinase-3 mutation	*Absent*	*Present*
Ecotropic viral integration site 1 expression	*Absent*	*Present*
Mixed-lineage leukemia partial tandem duplication	*Absent*	*Present*
Nucleophosphin mutation	*Present*	*Absent*
CCAAT/enhancer-binding protein-α mutation	*Present*	*Absent*
Brain and acute leukemia cytoplasmic gene expression	*Absent*	*Present*
Vascular endothelial growth factor expression	*Absent*	*Present*

Auer Rods and Acute Myeloid Leukemia (AML)

Auer Rods are crystalline, refractile, azurophilic rod shaped structures made from alignment of granules that are typically seen in AML (may be seen in refractory anemia with excess blasts in transformation)

- *Auer Rods are most frequently seen in AML-M3 (95-100%) and AML-M2 (70%)*[Q]
- *Auer Rods are absent by definition in AML-M0*[Q]
- *Auer Rods are usually not seen in AML-M5a and AML-7*[Q]

Auer Rods in AML

Most Frequently seen in (Typical Findings)	Absent in (By Definition)	May be seen in other subtypes(30-50%)
• AML M3 (95-100%) • AML M2 (70%)	AML – M0 Usually not seen in AML 5a and AML 7	*AML M1* *AML M4* *AML M6*

Plasma cell dyscrasias

Expansion of single clone of immunoglobulins secreting cells and a resultant increase in serum levels of a single homgenous immunoglobulin or its fragments.

Myeloma

- **Multiple Myeloma**: Multiple tumerous masses of plasma cells, scattered throughout the skeletal system
- **Solitary plasmacytoma**: Solitary Neoplastic mass of plasma cells found in the bone or soft tissue

Waldenstrommacroglobulinemia

- Diffuse infiltrate of Neoplastic B cells throughout bone marrow and lymph nodes, liver and spleen
- Neoplastic B cells produce only IgM. i.e. monoclonal component = IgM

Heavy chain disease

- Characterized by elevated levels in blood and urine of a specific heavy chain of immuno-globulins

Monoclonal gammopathy of undetermined significance (MGUS). This is the most common monoclonal gammopathy.

Multiple Myeloma

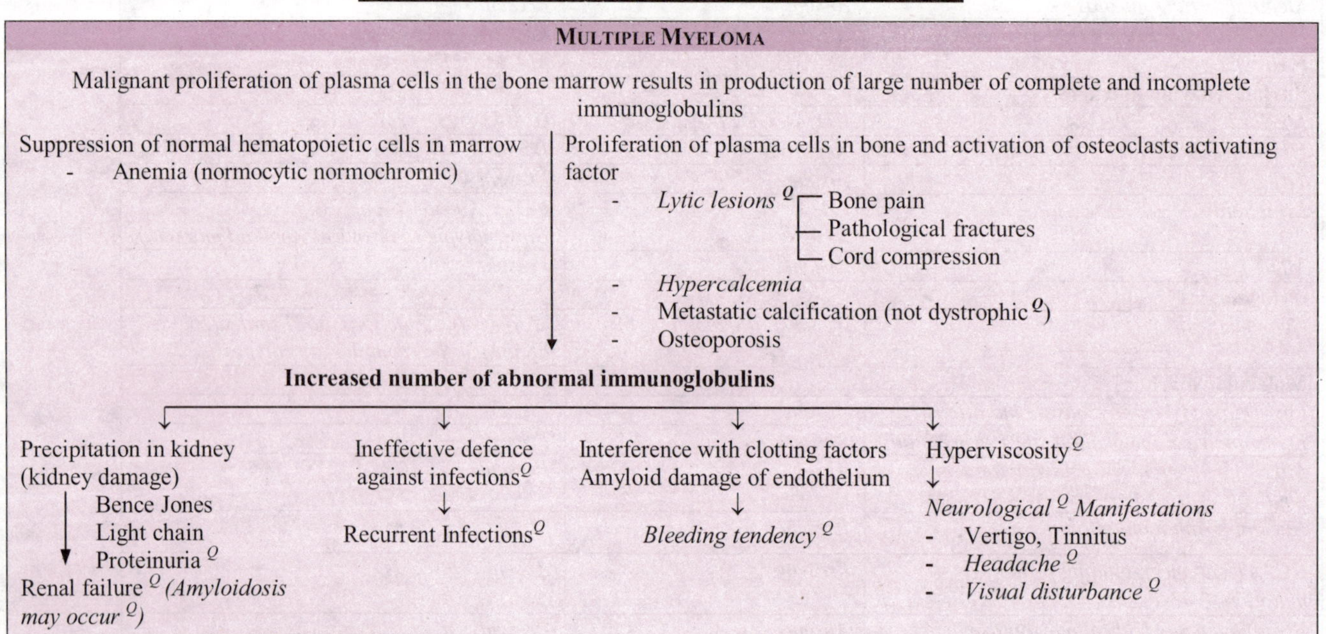

The Classic Triad of Multiple Myeloma

The classic triad of myeloma is:
a) *Marrow plasmacytosis> 10%*
b) *Lytic bone lesions*
c) *Serum or urine 'M' component*

Diagnosis and Staging of Multiple Myeloma (The Durie and Salmon myeloma diagnostic criteria)

- The Durie and Salmon myeloma diagnostic criteria are used widely in the United States and have been validated by large multicenter trials.
- The diagnostic criteria are divided into major and minor.
  The diagnosis of Multiple Myeloma requires a minimum of one major and one minor criterion or three minor criteria as defined in the table below
- Once the diagnostic criteria for multiple myeloma are met, Durie-Salmon clinical staging can be used to determine the stage of disease.

Criteria for Diagnosis of Multiple Myeloma

Major criteria

1. *Plasmacytomas on tissue biopsy*
2. *Bone marrow plasmacytosis (> 30% plasma cells)*
3. *Monoclonal immunoglobulin spike (M spike) on serum electrophoresis:*
   IgG > 3.5 g/dl or
   IgA > 2.0 g/dl
   κ or λ light-chain excretion > 1.0 g/d on 24-h urine protein electrophoresis.

Minor criteria

a. *Bone marrow plasmacytosis (10-30% plasma cells)*
b. *Monoclonal immunoglobulin spike present but of lesser magnitude than in 3*
c. *Lytic bone lesions*
d. *Normal IgM <50mg/dl or*
   Normal IgA <100 mg/dl or
   Normal IgG <600 mg/dl.

Any of the following sets of criteria will confirm the diagnosis.

Any two major criteria
Major criterion 1 plus minor criterion b, c or d
Major criterion 3 plus minor criterion a or c
Minor criteria a, b and c or a, b and d

Comparisonof MGUS, Indolent myeloma and Smoldering myeloma:

	MGUS	SMM	IMM	Multiple Myeloma
Plasma cell (BM)	<10%	10-30%	>30%	>30%
M-component	IgG<3.5, IgA<2	IgG>3.5, IgA>2	IgG 3.5-7, IgA 2-5	IgG >3.5/dl; IgA >2g/dl
Lytic bone lesion	None	None	≤3	Present
Symptoms/Infection - *Anemia* - *Renal insufficiency* - *Hypercalcemia*	None	None	None	Present

Disorders of Bleeding and Coagulation

Coagulation Cascade

Factors involved in exclusively Intrinsic Pathway

- *Factor XII*
- *Factor XI*
- *Factor IX*
- *Factor VIII*

Prekallekrein
HMW kininogen

Factors involved in exclusively in Extrinsic Pathway

- ***Factor VII***
- TissueThromboplastin (Formerly called Factor III)

APTT

Measure the time required to generate Thrombin and Fibrin polymers via the intrinsic and common pathway

Intrinsic pathway + Common Pathway

APTT assays thus reflect the activity of
XII, XI, IX, VIII + X, V, II, I

Factors Involved in Common Pathway

Factor X
Factor V
Factor II
Factor I
Factor XIII

PTT

Measures the true required to generate thrombin and fibrin polymers via the extrinsic and common pathway

Extrinsic pathway + Common Pathway

PTT assays thus reflect the activity of
VII + X, V, II, I

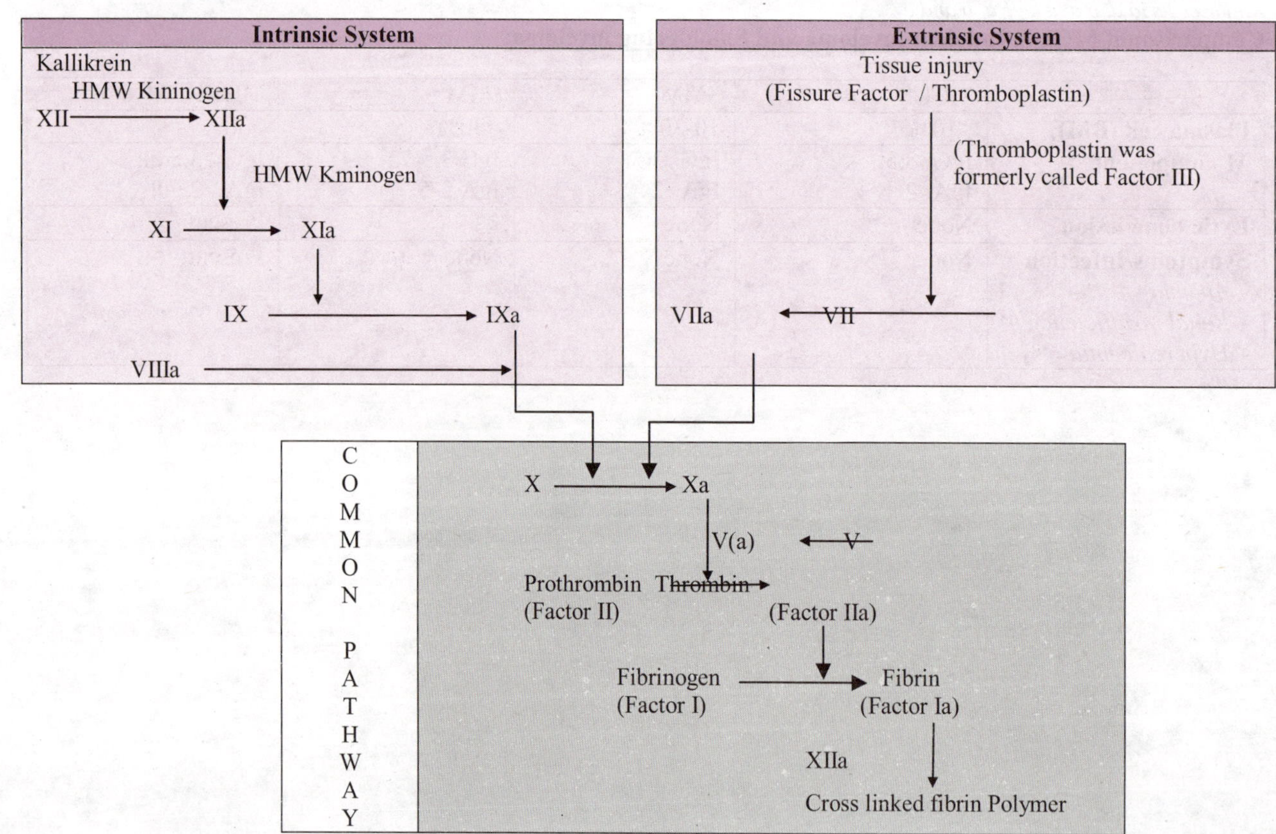

Approach to a patient with isolated prolongation of activated Partial Thromboplastin time (aPTT)

- The Partial Thromboplastin Time (aPTT) is a performance indicator measuring the efficacy of both the '*intrinsic system*' *and the 'common' coagulation pathway.*
- ***Isolated prolongation of aPTT (normal PT)*** may indicate:
  - *Coagulation Factor Deficiency (Factor VIII, IX, XI, XII, Prekallikrein, HMWK)*
  - *Presence of Antiphospholipid Antibodies especially Lupus Anticoagulant*
  - *Use of heparin (or contamination of sample with Heparin)*
  - *Specific coagulation factor Inhibitors (factor VIII inhibitor or Factor IX or XI (rare) inhibitor)*
- The ***presence or absence of bleeding manifestation*** even after major surgery may narrow down the differential diagnosis.

Isolated Prolongation of aPTT with no bleeding manifestation	Isolated prolongation of aPTT with bleeding manifestation
• Specific Coagulation Factor Deficiencies - *Factor XII Deficiency* - *Prekallekrien* - *HMW Kininingogen Defect* • ***Presence of Lupus Anticoagulant***	• Specific Coagulation Factor Deficiencies - *Factor VIII defect* - *Factor IX defect* - *Factor XI defect* • Specific Coagulation Factor Inhibitors - *Factor VIII inhibitor* - *Factor IX inhibitor or Factor XI inhibitor*

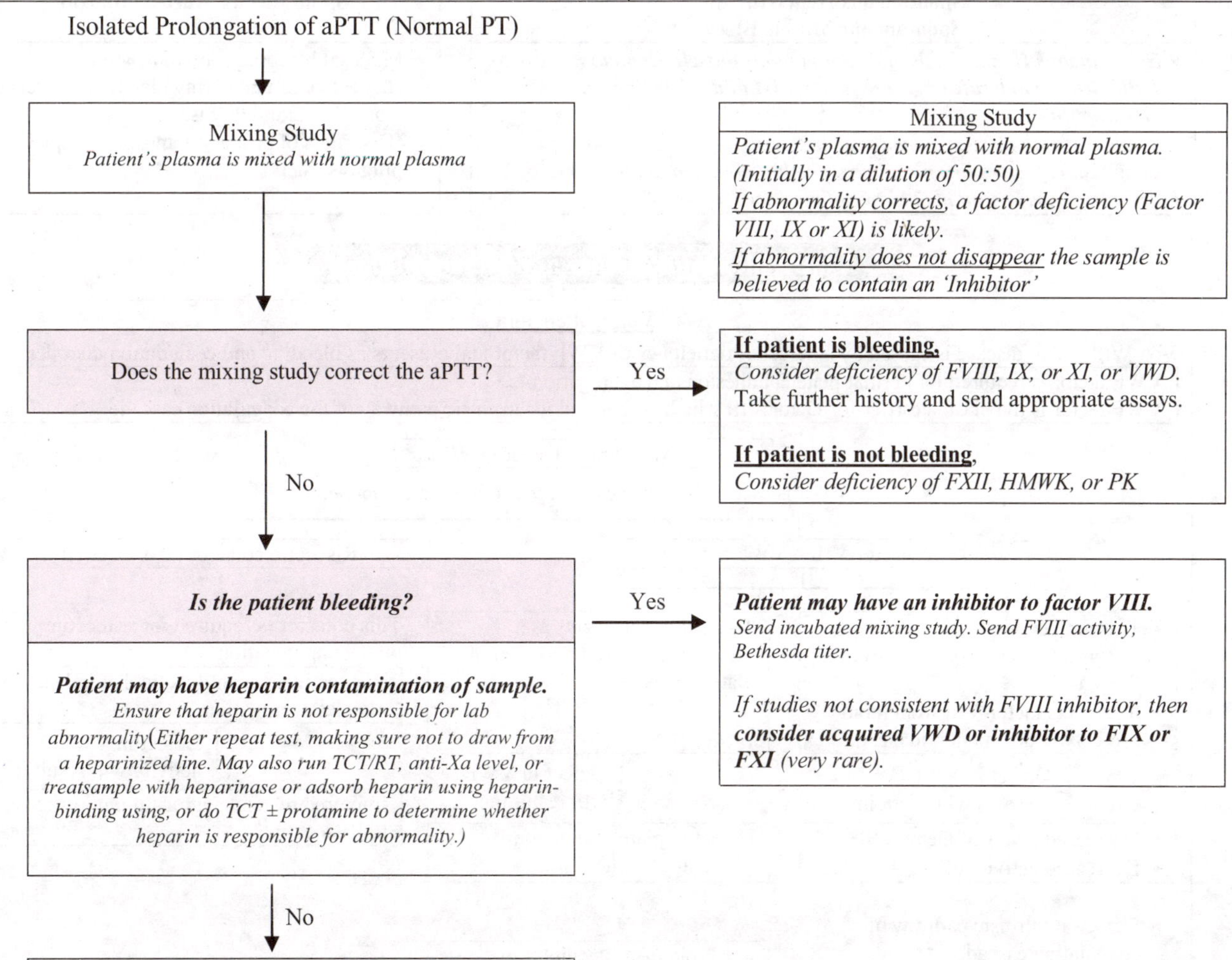

Causes of isolated Prolongation of PT

Cause of Isolated prolongation of PT (CMDT)
Vitamin K deficiency
Warfarin therapy
Liver disease
Factor VII deficiency

Causes of Prolonged PT and APTT

Causes of Prolonged PT and APTT

- Coagulation Factor Deficiency (Factor II, V, X or fibrinogen)
- Use of oral anticoagulants (Warfarin)
- Disseminated Intravascular coagulation
- Severe vitamin K deficiency
- Liver Disease (Severe Hepatic Insufficiency)
- Heparin in sample (at high concentrations only)

(Heparin is typically associated with prolonged APTT & normal PT)

Bleeding and Coagulation Disorders

Spontaneous Hemarthrosis Spontaneous Muscle Bleed	Spontaneous Mucosal Bleeding
• ***Spontaneous Hemarthosis and spontaneous muscle Hematomas are a hallmark of moderate or severe factor VIII and IX deficiency (Hemophilia)*** • *These can also be seen in moderate or severe deficiencies of other coagulation factors like fibrinogen, prothrombin and factor V, VII, & X* • *These are rarely seen in other bleeding disorders.*	• Mucosal bleeding symptoms are more suggestive of underlying platelet disorders or Von Willebrand disease (Disorders of primary hemostosis or platelet plug disorders)

Von Willebrand disease and Hemophillia

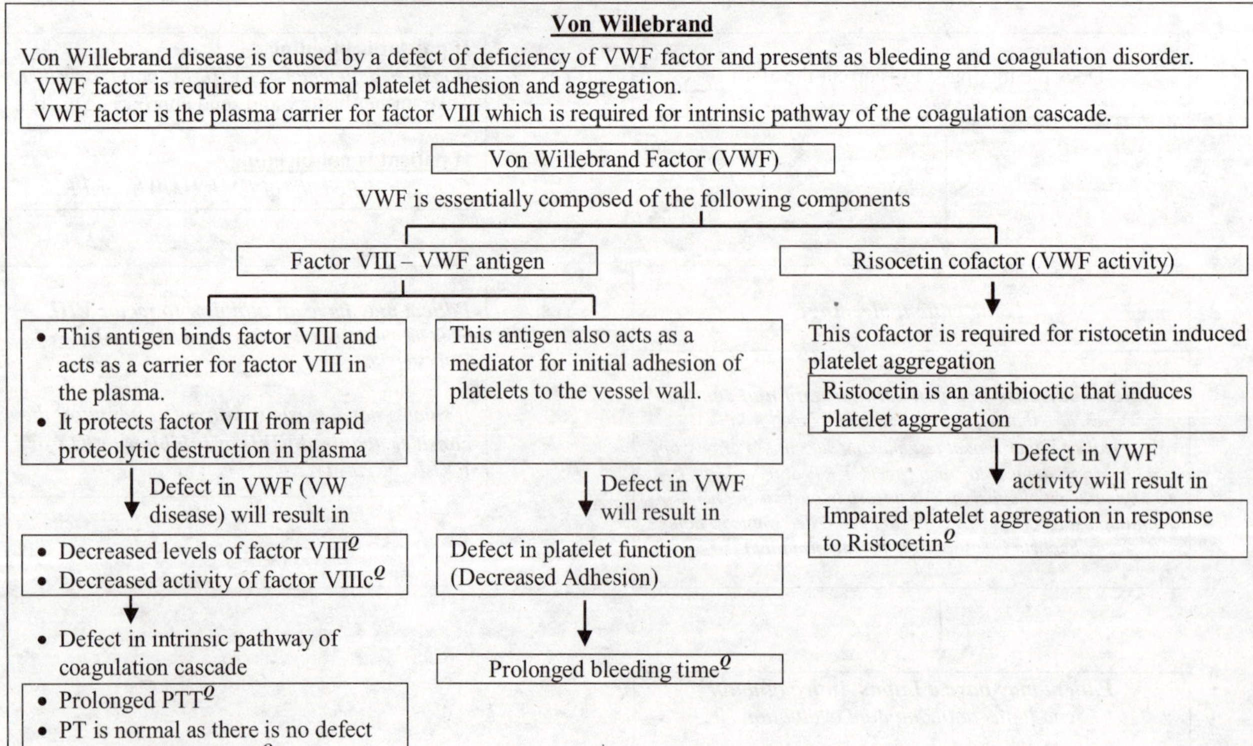

Features of VWF and differences with Haemophilia A

Feature	Hemophilia A	Von Willebrand Disease
Inheritance	***Sex linked*** Clinical disease limited to Men /boys ***(Extremely rare in females)***	***Autosomal (Most commonly A-dominant)*** Clinical disease may be seen in both boys & girls
Factor VIIIc	Decreased	Decreased
VWF	Normal	Decreased
Ristocetin cofactor	Normal	Decreased
Common Presentation	Features of clotting disorder Skin/Mucosal bleeding – ***Hemarthrosis ++***	Features of bleeding disorder ± clotting disorder Skin/Mucosal bleeding + ***Hemarthrosis+***
Bleeding Time	Normal	Prolonged
APTT	***Prolonged***	***Prolonged (may be normal)***
PT	***Normal***	***Normal***
Thrombin Time	Normal	Normal
Fibrinogen	Normal	Normal
Platelet aggregation in Response to Ristocetin	Normal	Decreased

Differences betweenHaemophilia A and Hemophilia B

	Haemophilia A (Classical hemophilia)	Haemophilia B (Christmas disease)
Defect	Deficiency of coagulant subunit of factor i.e (VIII c) Factor VIII = VIII c + VWF	Deficiency/absence of factor IX.
Pathway of coagulation affected	Intrinsic Pathway	Intrinsic pathway
Whole blood clotting time	↑	↑
PTT	↑	↑
PT	N	N
BT	N	N
Platelet count	N	N
Tourniquet test	N	N

1

Hematology

Disorders of Platelet Number and Function

Thrombocytopenia

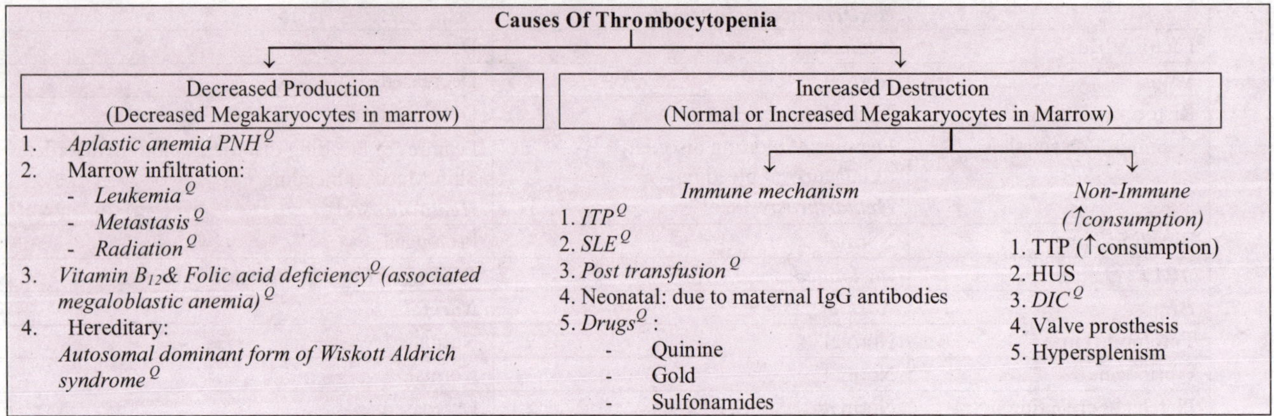

Disorders of Platelet Function

Classification of congenital disorder of platelet function:

1. Defects in platelet-vessel wall interaction (disorders of adhesion)
   - ***(a) VonWillebrand disease (deficiency or defect in plasma vWF)***
   - ***(b) Bernard-Soulier syndrome (deficiency or defect in GPIb)***
2. Defects in platelet-platelet interaction (disorders of aggregation)
   - *(a) Congenital afibrinogenemia (deficiency of plasma fibrinogen)*
   - ***(b) Glanzmannthrombosthenia (deficiency or defect in GPIIb-IIIa)***
3. Disorders of platelet secretion and signal transduction
   - *(a) Storage pool deficiency*
   - *(b) Quebec platelet disorder*
   - *(c) Chediak Higashi syndrome*
   - *(d) Gray Platelet syndrome*
   - ***(e) Wiskott-Aldrich syndrome***
4. Disorders of platelet coagulation – protein interaction
   - *(a) Defect in facorVa-Xa interaction on platelets (Scott syndrome)*

Wiskot Aldrich syndrome:

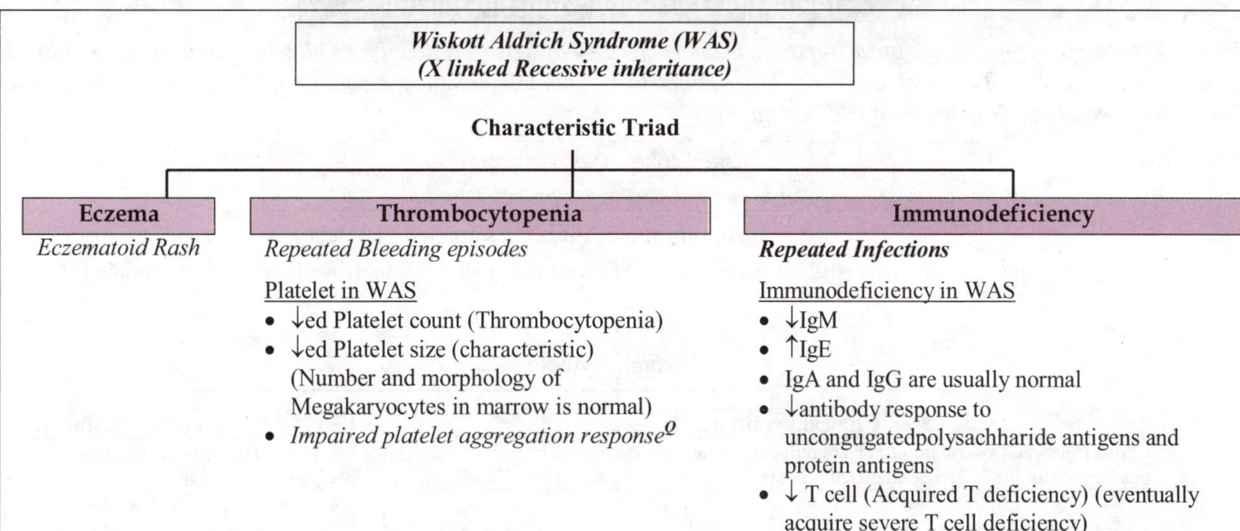

Bernard SoulierSyndrome andGlanzmann'sthrombasthenia

(Intrinsic platelet defects to adhesion and aggregation.)
Platelet adhesion and aggregation are modulated by glycoprotein receptors located on platelet surface.

GpIb / Ix	GpIIb / IIIa complex
• Mediates ***platelet adhesion*** • *VWF facilitates* platelet adhesion by binding to this receptor	• Mediates ***platelet aggregation*** • *Fibrinogen facilitates* platelet aggregation via sites on this receptor

Loss or defect in above glycoprotein receptors leads to rare platelet disorders causing bleeding

Bernard Soulier Syndrome	Glanzmann'sthrombasthenia
• Autosomal recessive disorder • Deficiency / dysfunction of GpIb / Ix Receptor • ***Platelets cannot adhere*** to subendothelium because of lack of above receptors for VWF which mediates platelet adhesion • ***Platelet aggregation to largely normal platelet aggregation is normal in response to standard agonists (collagen ADP, thrombin / but platelet fail to aggregate in response to ristocetin as it acts by a different mechanism*** Other laboratory parameters • ***Thrombocytopenia may be present*** • ***Platelets on smears are abnormally large*** • Bleeding time is abnormally prolonged • VWF factor levels in plasma are normal Clinical presentation • Recurrent episodes of severe mucosal haemorrhage	• Autosomal recessive disorder • Deficiency / dysfunction of GpIIb / III a complex • ***Platelets cannot aggregate*** because of lack of above receptors for fibrinogen which form the bridges between platelets during aggregation. • ***Platelet aggregation is largely abnormal. Platelet fail to aggregate in response to standard agonists, (ADP, collagen, thrombin) as these require fibrinogen binding, but aggregate normally to ristocetin as it cause platelet clumping by a different mechanism.*** Other laboratory parameters • Platelet number is usually normal • Platelet morphology is usually normal • Bleeding time is abnormally prolonged • VWF factor level in plasma are normal Clinical presentation • Recurrent episodes of severe mucosal hemorrhage

Note :VonWillebrand's disease : ***Platelet aggregation studies with standard agonists ADP, collagen, thrombin are normal but platelet aggregation in response to ristocetin may be subnormal (CMDT 2006 / 524).***

1

Hematology

Idiopathic Thrombocytopenic Purpura

Idiopathic thrombocytopenic purpura *is a disease characterized by severe reduction of platelet numbers, caused by immune destruction of platelets. The mechanism of ITP appears to be immune complexes containing antibodies, which react with platelets and lead to their immunological destruction.*

Immune Thrombocytic Purpura (ITP)
(Idiopathic Thrombocytopenic Purpura)

Autoimmune Antibodies against Platelets

From response to ***previous viral infection***[Q] (Acute ITP) or From underlying immune dysregulation (chronic ITP)

↓

Platelet destruction

Thrombocytopenia

Clinical manifestations

Clinical signs and symptoms of ITP are reflective of thrombocytopenia (Bleeding manifestations due to decreased platelet count)

Characteristic Clinical Features

Bleeding and haemorrhages from small venules or capillaries
- *Spontancouspetechiae*
- *Spontaneous echymoses*
- *Spontancous mucosal bleeding*
- *Easy Bruisibility*
- *Spleen is normal in size*

Clinical features that are characteristically unusual and suggest the possibility of other diagnosis

- *Frequent Bleeding and haemorrhages from larger veins and arteries and bleeding into joints (Suggest coagulation disorders)*
- *Splenomegaly and Lymphadenopathy are unusual/rare and their presence should lead one to consider other diagnosis.*

Laboratory Features

- Isolated thrombocytopenia
- Platelet Antibodies
- Normal or increased number of megakaryocytes on bone marrow examination

Features of bleeding disorder
- Bleeding time is prolonged
- Tests of coagulation are essentially normal
  - Normal PT
  - Normal APTT
  - Normal Fibrinogen
  - Normal Fibrinogen Degradation products
  - Normal levels of coagulation factors

'Hepatomegaly, splenomegaly and lymphadenopathy are notably absent in ITP, and their presence should initiate an investigation for other possible underlying illnesses associated with thrombocytopenia'- Oski's 2nd/463

Features of Acute and Chronic Idiopathic Thrombocytopenic Purpura (ITP):

ITP occurs in two forms, namely acute ITP and chronic ITP. Acute ITP and chronic ITP differ in incidence, prognosis and therapy

Features	Acute ITP	Chronic ITP
Peak age of incidence	Children, 2-6 yr	Adults 20-40 yr
Sex predilection	None	3:1 female to male
Antecedent infection	Common 1-3 wk before	Unusual
Onset of bleeding	Abrupt	Insidious
Hemorrhagic bullae in mouth	Present in severe cases	Usually absent
Platelet count	<20,000 /µl	30,000-80,000/µl
Eosinophilia and lympocytosis	Common	Rare
Duration	2-6 wk; rarely longer	Months or years
Spontaneous remission	Occur in 80% of cases	Uncommon

Treatment Modalities for ITP:

Common Treatment Modalities for ITP *(Platelet count <20,000/µl or significant mucosal bleeding)*
- *Corticosteroids*
- *IV Immunoglobulins / gamma globulins*
- *Additional Immunosupressive agents (Rituximab / Anti CD 20 Antibody)*
- *Splenectomy*

Thrombotic Thrombocytopenic Purpura

Thrombotic Thrombocytopenic purpura is a disorder of 'vessel wall'^Q characterised by lesions in arteriolar walls ^Q in various organs that initiate formation of **localised platelet thrombi and fibrin deposits at various sites.**

Clinical Pentad of TTP

Microangiopathic Hemolytic Anemia^Q (Coomb's negative)	Thrombocytopenia^Q (due to consumption of platelets)	Decreased Renal Function^Q (due deposits in the Renal Vasculature.)	Disturbed Neurological function^Q	Fever
- Haemolysis^Q - Fragmentation ^Q of RBC's - Increased LDH (elevated due to intra- vascular hemolysis)^Q			Characteristically diffuse and non focal eg. - Confusion - Aphasia - Alteration in consciousness	

Tests of coagulation are essentially normal ^Q
- Normal PT ^Q
- Normal APTT ^Q
- Normal Fibrinogen concentration ^Q
- Normal Fibrin degradation Products ^Q

Thus: PENTAD as mentioned above + normal coagulation tests: PATHOGNOMIC OF TTP

DIC or Disseminated Intravascular Coagulation

DIC or Disseminated Intravascular Coagulation, is a complex thrombohaemorrhagic disorder characterized by the following sequence of events in general:

Events
1. Intravascular activation of coagulation by *both intrinsic and extrinsic mechanism.* ^Q 2. A thrombotic phase 3. Consumption phase, wherein most coagulation factors and platelets are consumed. 4. Stage of secondary fibrinolysis, at site of intravascular coagulation.
Laboratory findings are in accordance with the above pathogenic mechanisms :
1. *Platelets count, coagulation factors and fibrinogen level: are decreased* ^Q or 'consumed'. As a result of above: The *bleeding time as well as the coagulation time both are prolonged* ^Q therefore - *PTT: increased Q* - *PT: increased* ^Q - *Thrombin time : increased* ^Q 2. Increased secondary fibrinolysis accounts for - *raised plasmin levels* ^Q - *raised levels of fibrin degradation product (FDP).* ^Q 3. The thrombolic phase accounts for *features of microangiopathichaemolytic anemia.* ^Q - *presence of schistiocytes, spherocytes, burr cells, halmet cells in the peripheral film.* ^Q
Some question asked:
• Most important treatment is : finding a reversible cause and *treatment of the cause* ^Q • *Finding in DIC, that correlates best and most closely with bleeding is : fibrinogen level* ^Q • Most common site for thrombin formation in DIC is : Brain ^Q(Brain > heart > lung > kidney > adrenal > liver) • DIC is related to 2 very important endocrine manifestations : a. *Adrenals - FredrichHausen Syndrome.* ^Q b. *Pituitary - Sheehan's Syndrome.* ^Q

Antiphospholipid syndrome (APS)

Antiphospholipid syndrome (APS)

- Defined by a clinical association of antiphospholipid antibodies and Hypercoagulability
- Considered a systemic autoimmune disease which is charachterized by recurrent thrombosis or pregnancy complications, along with the presence of Antiphospholipid antibodies.

Primary APS : No cause is identified

Secondary APS : Defined cause like SLE is identified

Important Clinical Features

Vascular Thrombosis

- *Recurrent arterial or venous thrombosis* in any tissue or organ is the *most common presentation*

Pregnancy morbidity

- *Recurrent spontaneous Abortions*[Q]
- *Pregnancy induced Hypertension*[Q] *(Preeclampsia and ecelampsia)*
- *Placental Insufficiency/Abruption*[Q]
- *Intrauterine Growth Retardation*[Q]

Important Laboratory Features

- *Elevated Anticardiolipin antibodies* [Q] *(IgG or IgM)* [Q]
- *Elevated Anti β -2 glycoprotein-1 Antibody* [Q]
- *Presence of Lupus Anticogulant (LA) in plasma* [Q]
- *Thrombocytopenia* [Q]
- *Haemolytic anemia* [Q]

Venous thrombosis
(More common)

- *DVT is the most*[Q] *common manifestation*
- *Pulmonary Embolism*[Q]
- Pulmonary hypertension from thromboembolic disease

Arterial thrombosis
(less common)

CNS	Heart	Lungs	Kidney	Bones	Others
Stroke[Q] (Cerebral vessel occlusion)	*Myocardial infarction*[Q] (coronary occlusion)	*Pulmonary Hypertension*[Q] (Pulmonary artery occlusion)	Glomerular Thrombosis *Renal Artery thrombosis*[Q]	*Avascular*[Q] *Necrosis*	

Diagnostic Criteria for Antiphospholipid Syndrome

Definitive Antiphospholipid Syndrome is said to be present if atleast one of the clinical criteria and one of the laboratory criteria are met

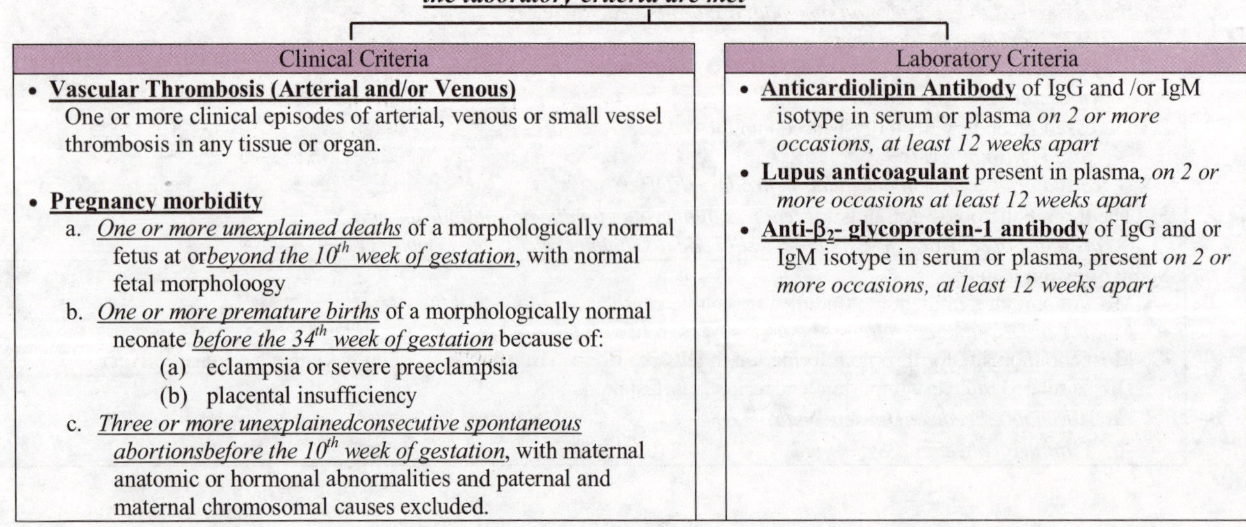

Clinical Criteria	Laboratory Criteria
• **Vascular Thrombosis (Arterial and/or Venous)** One or more clinical episodes of arterial, venous or small vessel thrombosis in any tissue or organ. • **Pregnancy morbidity** a. *One or more unexplained deaths* of a morphologically normal fetus at or*beyond the 10th week of gestation*, with normal fetal morphology b. *One or more premature births* of a morphologically normal neonate *before the 34th week of gestation* because of: (a) eclampsia or severe preeclampsia (b) placental insufficiency c. *Three or more unexplainedconsecutive spontaneous abortionsbefore the 10th week of gestation*, with maternal anatomic or hormonal abnormalities and paternal and maternal chromosomal causes excluded.	• **Anticardiolipin Antibody** of IgG and /or IgM isotype in serum or plasma *on 2 or more occasions, at least 12 weeks apart* • **Lupus anticoagulant** present in plasma, *on 2 or more occasions at least 12 weeks apart* • **Anti-β_2- glycoprotein-1 antibody** of IgG and or IgM isotype in serum or plasma, present *on 2 or more occasions, at least 12 weeks apart*

'The mainstay of treatment of Antiphospholipid Syndrome is Warfarin' – Harrison

Bleeding manifestations due to vitamin deficiency

Vitamin K dependent Coagulation Factors / Proteins :

Vitamin K dependent Coagulation Factors / Proteins

- Six proteins involved in clotting require conversion of a number of glutamic acid residues to γ - carboxyglutamic acid residues before being released into circulation
- This process of γ (gamma) carboxylation occurs in the liver and requires vitamin k and hence these proteins are called vitamin – K dependent
- These include coagulation factors II, VII, IX and X as well as protein C and protein S.

Vitamin K dependent proteins involved in clotting
• ***Coagulation Factor II*** [Q] ***(Prothrombin)***
• ***Coagulation Factor VII*** [Q] ***(Proconvertin)***
• ***Coagulation Factor IX*** [Q] ***(Christmas factor)***
• ***Coagulation factor X (Stuart Prover Factor)***
• *Protein C* [Q]
• *Protein S* [Q]

Bleeding manifestations due to vitamin deficiency

VITAMIN C	VITAMIN K
• Vitamin C is required for synthesis of collagen which forms part of capillary walls. • Vitamin C deficiency leads to increased capillary wall fragility and hence increased manifestations of haemorrhagic areas such as– - *over lower extremities* [Q] - *around hair follicles* [Q] - *nailbeds* [Q]	• Vitamin K dependent factors include Factor II, VII, IX, X • In vitamin K deficiency bleeding occurs due to lack of coagulation factors
• Patient presents with - increased bleeding time [Q] - normal PTT, PT, TT [Q] - normal clotting time [Q]	• Patient presents with - increased clotting time [Q] - increased PTT, PT, TT [Q] - normal bleeding time [Q]

Conditions predisposing to Thrombosis

Abnormality	Arterial	Venous
Factor V Leiden mutation	—	+
Prothrombin	—	+
Antithrombin III	—	+
Protein C	—	+
Protein S	—	+
Homocysteinemia	+	+
Antiphospholipid syndrome	+	+

Most common genetic cause for thrombophilia	:	*Factor V Leiden*
Most common congenital cause of venous thrombosis	:	*Factor V Leiden*
Most common hereditary blood coagulation disorder	:	*Factor V leiden*

1

Hematology

Methaemoglobinemia

Methaemoglobinemia

- Methaemoglobinemia is an uncommon but distinct cause of central cyanosis in the absence of hypoxemia or cardio vascular compromise
- Methaemoglobinemia occurs when a significant concentration of hemoglobin (Hb) is oxidized to methaemoglobin (Met Hb)

> *When the haemmoety (iron atoms) of Hb molecule encounter a strong oxidizing agent iron loses an electron and switches from the Ferrous (2^+) to Ferric (3^+) state turning Hb to 'Met Hb'*

- Methaemoglobin has such high oxygen affinity that virtually no oxygen is delivered

Presentation

- Methaemoglobinemia most commonly presents as *cyanosis unresponsive to supplemental oxygen*

> The most notable physical examination finding is generalized cyanosis which can manifest as muddy brown dark mucus membranes before proceding to global skin discolaration

- 'The charachteristic***muddy appearance(chocolate brown)*** of freshly drawn blood can be a critical clue'

- Harrison's 18th/858

*Blood appears dark brown, brownish, muddy or chocolate in colour immediately after withdrawal. In contrast to normal venous blood, the color does not change with addition of oxygen or agitation in the air'- *Diffirential diagnosis in Internal Medicine (Thieme) 2007/709*

> Methaemoglobinemia>15% cause symptoms of cerebral ischaemiaMethaemoglobinemia> 60% is usually lethal

Diagnosis

- *The best diagnostic test for Methaemoglobinuria is 'Methaemoglobin Assay'*

Treatment

- The most effective emergency management for methaemaglobinemia is *administration of Methylene blue*[Q] which serves as an antidote (introvenous)

> *Methylene blue is not effective in patients with methaemoglobinemia due to Hemoglobinopathy M*[Q] *(Haemoglobin M)*
> Methylene blue is *contraindicated in patients with G6 PD deficiency*[Q] since it can cause severe hemolysis due to its potential for oxidation

QUESTIONS

Hypochromic Microcytic Anemias

Differential Diagnosis/Approach

1. Which of the following conditions is associated with microcytic hypochromic anemia: *(AIIMS Dec 94)*
   A. Sickle cell Anemia
   B. Thallassemia
   C. Fanconi's anemia
   D. Hereditary spherocytosis
2. All of the following cause microcytic hypochromic anaemia, *except*: *(AIIMS Dec 97)*
   A. Lead poisoning
   B. Thalassemia
   C. Iron deficiency
   D. Fanconi's anemia
3. All of the following cause Microcytic Hypochromic anemia *except:* *(AI 1995/AIIMS 1997)*
   A. Lead poisoning
   B. Thalassemia
   C. Iron deficiency anemia
   D. Fanconi's anemia
4. Which of the following are not associated with microcytic hypochromic RRCs on Peripheral smear?
   A. Iron Deficiency Anemia *(PGI 2009)*
   B. Lead
   C. Sideroblastic anemia
   D. Sickle Cell Anemia
   E. Hereditary spherocytosis
5. Which of the following is not expected in a case of Microcytic Hypochromic Anemia: *(DNB 2009)*
   A. Reduced serum Iron
   B. Reduced Total RBC distribution Width
   C. Normal Ferritin levels
   D. Increased TIBC
6. Which of the following is not expected in a case of Microcytic Hypochromic Anemia *(DNB 2008)*
   A. Reduced serum iron
   B. Increased serum ferritin level
   C. Decreased TIBC
   D. Decreased Free Erythrocyte protoporphyrin
7. A patient presents with Microcytic Hypochromic anemia. Serum iron levels and TIBC are decreased. Likely diagnosis is:
   A. Iron deficiency anemia
   B. Anemia of chronic disease
   C. Thalassemia
   D. Sideroblastic anemia
8. Anemia of Chronic disease can be differentiated from Iron deficiency anemia by: *(PGI 2009)*
   A. ↑ TIBC
   B. ↓ TIBC
   C. ↑ S.ferritn
   D. ↓ Fe store in marrow
   E. ↓ Ferritin
9. A 29 year old woman was found to have a hemoglobin of 7.8 g/dl. with a reticulocyte count of 0.8%. The peripherial blood smear showed microcytic hypochromic anemia, Hemoglobin A2 and hemoglobin F levels were 2.4% and 1.3% respectively. The serum iron and the total iron binding capacity were 15 micro g/dl, and 420 micro g/dl, respectively. The most likely cause of anemia is:
   A. Iron deficiency anemia. *(AIIMS Nov 02)*
   B. Beta-thalassemia minor.
   C. Sideroblastic anemia.
   D. Anemia due to chronic infection.
10. A child presents with hypochromic microcytic anemia, with normal levels of free Erythrocyte Protoporphyrin The most likely diagnosis is: *(AI 92)*
    A. Iron deficiency anemia
    B. Lead toxicity
    C. Thalassemia
    D. Anemia of chronic disease
11. A 16 year old young girl presents with a history of fatiguability weakness and lethargy. Complete Blood picture (CBC) reveals Haemoglobin of 7.0, MCV of 70, MCH of 20 pg/cell and Red cell Distribution Width (RDW) of 20. The most likely diagnosis is:
    A. Iron Deficiency Anemia *(AI 2010)*
    B. Thalassemia Minor
    C. Thalassemia Major
    D. Sickle cell trait
12. A child has Hb-6.5 gm%, MCV-65, MCH-15 and protoporphyria with red cell distribution width much less is most likely to be suffering from :
    A. Thalassemia *(AIIMS June 2000)*
    B. Iron deficiency anaemia
    C. Porphyria
    D. Megaloblastic anaemia
13. A nine month old boy of Sindhi parents presented to you with complaints of progressive lethargy, irritability & pallor since 6 months of age. Examination revealed severe pallor. Investigation showed Hb-3.8 mg%; MCV-58 fl; MCH-19.4 pg/cell. Blood film shows osmotic fragility is normal (target cells and normoblasts). X-ray skull shows expansion

of erythroid marrow. Which of the following is the most likely diagnosis? *(AI 2004)*

A. Iron deficiency anemia
B. Acute lymphoblastic anemia
C. Hemoglobin D disease
D. Hereditary spherocytosis

14. A 30 year old female being evaluated for anemia reveals the following indices: RBC count = 4.5 x 1012/L; MCV 55fl; TLC 8000. There is no history of blood transfusion. Which of the following is the most likely diagnosis: *(AIIMS Nov 2011)*

A. Iron Deficiency Anemia
B. Thalassemia major
C. Thalassemia minor
D. Megaloblastic anemia

15. Elevated serum ferritin, serum iron and percent transferrin saturation are most consistent with the diagnosis of : *(AI 2004)*

A. Iron deficiency anemia
B. Anemia of chronic disease
C. Hemochromatosis
D. Lead poisoning

Iron Deficiency Anemia

16. All of the following are causes of iron deficiency anemia, Except: *(PGI June 01)*

A. Chronic renal failure
B. Celiac Sprue
C. Hookworms
D. Carcinoma colon

17. A patient with anemia has the following indices. MCV = 60; Hb = 5gm%; MCHC = 20. The most likely cause of his anemia is: *(PGI Dec 2000)*

A. Phenytoin
B. Blind loop syndrome
C. Hookworm infectino
D. CRF

18. Iron absorption is increased in all except: *(PGI Dec 01, June 03)*

A. Iron deficiency
B. Pregnancy
C. Hypoxia
D. Alkaline pH of stomach
E. Ferrous iron salts

19. Which of the following findings is diagnostic of iron deficiency anemia : *(AI 2007)*

A. Increased TIBC, decreased serum ferritin
B. Decreased TIBC, decreased serum ferritin
C. Increased TIBC, increased serum ferritin
D. Decreased TIBC, increased serm ferritin

20. The earliest sign of iron deficiency anaemia:

A. Increase in iron binding capacity
B. Decrease in serum ferritin level
C. Decrease in serum iron level
D. All the above *(AIIMS Feb 1997)*

21. Which of the following statements about iron deficiency anemia is true:

A. Decreased TIBC
B. Increased Ferritin levels
C. Bone marrow iron is decreased after serum iron is decreased
D. Bone marrow iron is decreased earlier than serum iron

22. Most sensitive and specific test for diagnosis of iron deficiency is: *(AI 2003, AI 2001)*

A. Serum iron levels
B. Serum ferritin levels
C. Serum transferrin receptor population
D. Transferrin saturation

23. Best marker for iron deficiency is: *(DNB 2012)*

A. Serum iron
B. Serum ferritin
C. Total Iron Binding capacity
D. Transferrin saturation

24. The most suitable test to assess iron stores is:

A. Serum iron *(DNB 2010)*
B. Serum Ferritin
C. TIBC
D. Transferrin saturation

25. Which is not seen in Iron deficiency anaemia:

A. Hyper-segmented neutrophils *(AI 2000)*
B. Microcytosis preceeds hypochromia
C. MCHC < 50%
D. Commonest cause of anaemia in India

26. Which of the following is true about oral therapy for iron deficiency anemia: *(PGI Dec 05)*

A. In 300 mg elemental iron given 100 mg get absorbed
B. Reticulocytosis appears in one to 2 weeks and then peaks in 3-4 weeks
C. Hemoglobin levels are usually corrected in six months of initiating therapy
D. Decrease in absorption with improvement of symptoms
E. Stop the Rx after normalizing the Hb

27. Iron overload occurs in all, *except* :

A. Thalassemia *(AIIMS Sept 96)*
B. Myelodysplastic syndrome
C. Polycythemia vera
D. Sideroblastic anaemia

Anemia of Chronic Disease

28. Which of the following is true about Anemia of Chronic Disease: *(DNB 2012)*

A. Increased TIBC
B. Normal serum iron levels
C. Normal or increased serum ferritin
D. Increased Transferrin saturation

29. A 25-year-old lady on treatment for Rheumatoid Arthritis has the following laboratory findings. Hemoglobin of 9 gm/dL; MCV-50 fl; Ferritin 200µg/L; TIBC 274 µg/dL; Serum iron 30µg/dL. What is the likely diagnosis: *(AIIMS Nov 2011)*
   A. Iron Deficiency Anemia
   B. Anemia of Chronic Disease
   C. Thalassemia Minor
   D. Autoimmune Hemolytic Anemia

30. All are true regarding Anaemia of Chronic Diseases, *except* : *(AIIMS 1999)*
   A. Decreased serum Fe
   B. Decreased Ferritin
   C. Decreased Total Fe Binding Capacity
   D. Increased Bone Marrow Fe

31. Seen in chronic inflammatory anemia is: *(PGI Dec 99)*
   A. Serum iron ↓, S. ferritin ↑ and transferrin ↓
   B. Serum iron ↑, S. ferritin ↑ and transferrin ↑
   C. Serum iron ↓, S. ferritin ↓ and transferrin ↑
   D. Serum iron ↑, S. ferritin ↓ and transferrin ↓

32. True regarding anaemia of chronic disease are all *except* : *(AI 2000)*
   A. Decreased TIBC
   B. Increased macrophage iron in marrow
   C. Decreased serum ferritin level
   D. Decreased serum iron level

33. Anemia of chronic disease is characterized by all, except *(AIIMS May 94)*
   A. Decreased serum iron
   B. Increased total iron binding capacity (TIBC)
   C. Increased serum ferritin
   D. Increased macrophage iron in bone marrow

Anemia of Chronic Renal Failure

34. All of the following are true about Anemia of chronic failure Except: *(PGI Dec 05)*
   A. Normocytic normochromic anaemia
   B. Erythropoietin improves the symptom
   C. Dialysis worsens anemia of renal failure
   D. Anemia is proportional to the kidney disease

35. Anemia in chronic renal failure (CRF) is due to: *(PGI June 01)*
   A. Decreased erythropoietin production
   B. Iron deficiency
   C. Hypoplastic bone marrow
   D. Decreased Vit B12
   E. Decreased folate levels

Sideroblastic Anemia

36. Not present in Sideroblastic anaemia is : *(AIIMS Feb 97)*
   A. Microcytic anaemia
   B. Decreased transferrin saturation
   C. Sideroblast cells in blood smear film
   D. Ineffective erythropoiesis

37. A patient presents with increased serum iron, decreased TIBC, increased percent saturation and increased serum ferritin. Most probable diagnosis is :
   A. Anemia of chronic disease : *(AIIMS Nov. 2006)*
   B. Sideroblastic anemia
   C. Iron deficiency anemia
   D. Thalassemia minor

Megaloblastic Anemia

38. Which of the following types of anemia is associated with a Raised MCV and Normal MCHC: *(AI 2012)*
   A. Sideroblastic anemia
   B. Vitamin B12 and Folic acid deficiency
   C. Beta thalassemia
   D. Iron deficiency anemia

39. Macrocytic anemia may be seen with all of the following conditions *except* :
   A. Liver disease *(AI 1998, AIIMS 1996)*
   B. Copper deficiency
   C. Thiamine deficiency
   D. Orotic aciduria

40. Megaloblastic anemia may be caused by all of the following *except* : *(AI 1997)*
   A. Phenytoin
   B. Methotrexate
   C. Pyrimethamine
   D. Amoxycilline

41. Megaloblastic anemia due to folic acid deficiency is commonly due to: *(AI 2006)*
   A. Inadequate dietary intake
   B. Defective intestinal absorption
   C. Absence of folic acid binding protein in serum
   D. Absence of glutamic acid in the intestine

42. Megaloblastic anemia in blind loop syndrome is due to: *(AI 99)*
   A. Vitamen B_{12} malabsorption
   B. Bacterial overgrowth
   C. Frequent diarrhoea
   D. Decrease iron intake

43. Thiamine deficiency is known to occur in all of the following *except*: *(AI 2003)*
   A. Food Faddist
   B. Homocystinemia
   C. Chronic alcoholic
   D. Chronic heart failure patient on diuretics

44. Deficiency of the 'intrinsic factor of Castle' causes:
   A. Microcytic anemia *(AI 95)*
   B. Pernicious anemia
   C. Cooley's anemia
   D. Aplastic anemia

45. Shilling's test is used to determine deficiency of
   A. Vitamin B12 *(DNB 2012)*
   B. Vitamin B6
   C. Folic Acid Deficiency
   D. Vitamin D Deficiency

46. A patient has Hb 6gm%, folic acid 8 ng/ml, vitamin B12 60pg/ml, serum iron 160µg/dl, and MCV-104. The diagnosis is: *(AIIMS Nov 99)*
A. Iron deficiency anemia
B. Vitamin B12 deficinecy
C. Folic acid deficiency
D. Pyridoxine deficiency

47. A Patient presents with macroglossia and loss of tongue papilla. His Hb is 11.5 and MCV is 100. What should be the next step in investigating this patient?
A. B_{12} estimation *(AI 2008)*
B. Brush biopsy of the lesion
C. Fluconazole treatment
D. Incision biopsy

48. Megaloblastic anemia should be treated with both folic acid vitamin B_{12} because : *(AI 2008)*
A. Folic acid alone causes improvement of hematologic symptoms but worsening of neurological symptoms
B. It is a Co factor
C. It is enzyme
D. None of the above

Hemolytic Anemias

General Features

49. All of the following cause intravascular hemolysis, Except:
A. Mismatched Blood transfusion
B. Snake bite
C. Thalassemia
D. Paroxysmal Nocturnal Hemoglobinuria (PNH)

50. Hemoglobinuria may be seen in all of the following conditions Except:
A. Mismatched Blood transfusion
B. Paroxysmal cold hemoglobinuria
C. Thermal burns
D. Hereditary spherocytosis

51. Haemoglobinuria does not occur in :
A. $CuSO_4$ poisoning *(AIIMS Feb 97)*
B. Snake bite
C. Mismatched blood transfusion
D. Thalassemia

52. Haptaglobin levels are decreased in: *(AI 1996)*
A. A mismatched transfusion reactions
B. Thalassemia
C. G 6PD deficiency
D. All of the above

53. Chronic Hemolysis from which of the following conditions may be associated with iron deficiency:
A. Paroxysmal cold Haemoglobinuria *(AI 97)*
B. Thalassemia
C. Hereditary spherocytosis
D. G 6 PD deficiency

54. All of the following are features of hemolytic anemia Except: *(PGI June 04)*
A. Decreased RBC life span
B. Decreased Haptoglobin
C. Unconjugated hyperbilirubinemia
D. Bilirubin in urine
E. Altered Erythroid and Myeloid ratio

55. All are seen in Hemolytic anemia *except:*
A. Hemosiderinuria *(AI 1996)*
B. Reticulocytosis
C. Spherocytosis
D. Increased haptoglobin

56. Hemolytic anemia may be characterized by all of the following except- *(AIIMS May 05)*
A. Hyperbilirubinemia
B. Reticulocytosis
C. Hemoglobinuria
D. Increased plasma haptoglobin level

57. All are features of hemolytic anaemia except:
A. Thrombocytopenia *(AIIMS Dec 95)*
B. Hemosiderinuria
C. Decreased haptoglobin
D. Raised indirect bilirubin

58. Features seen in hemolytic anemia are all except:
A. Tear drop and Burr cells *(AIIMS May 07)*
B. ↓ Haptoglobin
C. Reticulocytosis
D. Hemoglobinuria

59. Reticulocytosis is NOT a feature of: *(AIIMS Dec 94)*
A. Paroxysmal nocturnal hemoglobinuria
B. Following acute bleeding
C. Hereditary spherocytosis
D. Anemia in CRF

60. Reticulocytosis is seen in all except: *(AIIMS May 07)*
A. P.N.H
B. Hemolysis
C. Nutritional anemia
D. Dyserythropoietic syndrome

61. Reticulocytosis is NOT a feature of *(AIIMS Dec 94)*
A. Paroxysmal nocturnal hemoglobinuria
B. Following acute bleeding
C. Hereditary spherocytosis
D. Anemia in CRF

Hereditary Spherocytosis

62. The following protein defects can cause hereditiary spherocytosis except : *(AI 07)*
A. Anykyrin
B. Palladin
C. Glycophorin C
D. Anion transport protein

63. Features of hereditary spherocytosis include all of the following *except* : *(AI 1998)*
A. ↑Osmotic fragility
B. ↑MCHC
C. ↑MCV
D. Decrease surface area per unit volume

64. Osmotic fragility is increased in: *(PGI June 98)*
A. Sickle cell anemia
B. Thalassemia
C. Hereditary spherocytosis
D. Chronic lead poisoning

65. Decreased osmotic fragility is seen in (select two options): *(PGI Dec 2000)*
A. Herediatry spherocytosis
B. Sickle cell ds
C. Autoimmune hemolytic anemia
D. Thallasemia

66. Aplastic anemia in hereditary spherocytosis precipitated by- *(PGI Dec 05)*
A. Parvo virus
B. HIV
C. Adenovirus
D. Influenza virus
E. Measles virus

67. Splenectomy is most useful in : *(AI 1998)*
A. Thrombocytopenia
B. Hereditary spherocytosis
C. H.S. purpura
D. Sickle cell anemia

G6 PD Deficiency

68. Hemolysis in G6PD may be caused by all Expect: *(AI 2008)*
A. Primaquine
B. Chloroquine
C. Pyrimethamine
D. Quinine

69. Which doesn't cause hemolysis in G6 PD deficiency: *(PGI Dec 99)*
A. Oestrogen
B. Salicylates
C. Primaquine
D. Nitrofurantoin

70. Primaquine may cause hemolysis in : *(AI 1998)*
A. G-6-PD deficiency
B. NADP-deficiency
C. Methemoglobin reductase deficiency
D. Crabb's disease

Hemoglobinopathies: Sickle Cell Anemia

71. The primary defect which leads to sickle cell anemia is-
A. An abnormality in porphyrin part of hemoglobin
B. Replacement of glutamate by valine in B-chain of HbA
C. A nonsense mutation in the B-chain of HbA
D. Substitution of valine by glutamate in the A chain of HbA

72. Which of the following is not seen in a chronic case of Sickle cell anemia : *(AI 1996)*
A. Hepatomegaly
B. Pulmonary hypertension
C. Cardiomegaly
D. Splenomegaly

73. All are true for sickle cell anemia, *except*
A. Pulmonary arterial hypertension
B. Fish vertebra *(AIIMS May 94)*
C. Leukopenia
D. Increased size of heart

74. All of the following statements are true about sickle cell disease *except* *(AI 2004)*
A. Patient may require frequent blood transfusions
B. Acute infection is the most common cause of mortality before 3 years of age.
C. There is positive correlation between conc. HBS and polymerization of HBS.
D. Patient presents early in life before 6 months of age.

75. All of the following are true about sickle cell disease, except: *(PGI June 2008)*
A. Mutation in α chain
B. Symptoms ameliorated by HbF
C. Venoocclusive cries is cause of morbidity
D. Bone pain is presenting feature

76. Commonest acute presentation of sickle cell anaemia is: *(AIIMS Dec 98)*
A. Priapism
B. Bone pain
C. Fever
D. Splenomegaly.

77. Heterozygous sickle cell anemia gives protection against: *(AI 2010)*
A. G6PD
B. Malaria
C. Thalassemia
D. Dengue fever

78. Which of the following is not seen on hemoglobin electrophoresis in sickle cell anemia: *(AI 2001)*
A. HbA
B. HbA2
C. HbF
D. HbS

79. Sickle cell trait patient do not have manifestations as that of Sickle cell disease, because : *(AIIMS 2001)*
A. 50% HbS is required for occurrence of sickling
B. HbA prevents sickling
C. HbS is less than 50% & HbA has low affinity for HbS

D. HbA prevents polymerization of Hbs

80. The mother has sickle cell disease; Father is normal; Chances of children having sickle cell disease and sickle cell trait respectively are : *(AI 2001)*
A. 0 and 100%
B. 25 and 25%
C. 50 and 50%
D. 10 and 50%

81. Crew haircut appearance in X-rays skull and Gandy gamma bodies are seen in- *(AIIMS Nov 93)*
A. G6-PD deficiency
B. Hodgkin's lymphoma
C. Hereditary spherocytosis
D. Sickle cell anaemia

82. Sickle cell Anemia leads to resistance towards
A. P. Falciparum *(DNB Dec 2009)*
B. P. Ovale
C. P. Malariae
D. P. Vivax

Hemoglobinopathies: Thalassemias

83. In Beta thalassemia, there is : *(AIIMS May 01)*
A. Increase in beta chain, decrease in alpha chain
B. Decrease in beta chain, increase in alpha chain
C. Decrease in beta chain, decrease in alpha chain
D. Increase in beta chain, increase in alpha chain

84. The most common mulations in Beta thalassemia involves
A. Intron-1
B. Intron-22
C. 619 bp deletion
D. 3.7 bp deletion

85. A 25-year female presented with mild pallor and moderate hepatosplenomegaly. Her hemoglobin was 92 dl/L and fetal hemoglobin level was 65%. She has not received any blood transfusion till date. She is most likely to be suffering from: *(AIIMS Nov 02)*
A. Thalassemia major
B. Thalassemia intermedia.
C. Hereditary persistent fetal hemoglobin, homozygous state.
D. Hemoglobin D, homozygous state.

86. A 21 year old male presents to the emergency department with sever anemia and haemoglobin levels of 5 gm/dl. He gives a history of similar presentation in the past which wave adequately managed by a single blood transfusion. He has not required any further blood transfusions till date. Most probable diagnosis is:
A. Thalassemia major
B. Thalassemia Minor
C. Thalassemia intermedia
D. Autoimmune hemolytic anemia

87. A 23 years old asymptomatic female pilot has MCV-70, ferritin – 100g/L, Hb-10gm%, what is the cause:
A. Thalassemia trait *(AI 2009)*
B. B_{12} def
C. Folate def
D. Iron def

88. All of the following arc true about β thalassemia trait, Except: *(PGI June 2008)*
A. Microcytic hypochromic picture
B. ↑ed HbA2
C. ↑ed HbF
D. Patient requires blood transfusion

89. All are true about β - thalassemia trait Except:
A. ↑ HbF *(PGI June 04)*
B. ↑HbA_2
C. Microcytosis
D. Severe anaemia

90. True about α-thalassemia trait : *(PGI June 06)*
A. Increased HbF
B. Increased HbA2
C. Microcytosis
D. Severe anemia

91. A 32-year-old female, asymptomatic, not requiring blood transfusion, presents with Hb 13.0 gm/dl. Her HbF levels are 95%, Hb A_2 1.5%. Which of the following is the most likely diagnosis *(AIIMS May 04)*
A. Hereditary persistence of fetal hemoglobin
B. Beta homozygous thalassemia
C. Thalassemia intermedia
D. Beta heterozygous thalassemia

92. A child aged 2 year presents with nonspecific symptoms suggestive of anemia. On peripheral blood smear target cells are seen. He has hypochromic mic-zrocytic picture and Hb of 6 gm. He also has 'a positive family history' Next investigation of choice is *(AI 01)*
A. Hb electrophoresis
B. Coombs test
C. Liver function tests
D. Osmotic fragility test

93. The peripheral blood smear of a patient shows features of thalassemia, also presented with anaemia. Family history is also +ve. The investigation done to establish the diagnosis is: *(AIIMS 1999)*
A. ESR estimation
B. Blood spherocyte estimation
C. Bone marrow aspiration
D. Hb-electrophoresis

94. Diagnosis of beta Thalassemia is established by:
A. NESTROFT Test.
B. Hb A_1 C estimation.
C. Hb electrophoresis.
D. Target cells in peripheral smear.

95. A 5 year old girl came with history of progressively increasing pallor since birth and hepatosplenomegaly.

Which of the following is the most relevant test for achieving diagnosis : *(AI 2004)*
A. Hb electrophoresis
B. Peripheral smear examination
C. Osmotic fragility test
D. Bone marrow examination

96. Hair on end appearance is seen in X-rays skull in: *(AIIMS June 97)*
A. Thalassemia
B. Hydrocephalus
C. Chronic malaria
D. Sickle cell analuria

97. Haemoglobin F is raised in: *(AIIMS Dec 97)*
A. Juvenile chronic myeloid leukemia
B. Hereditary spherocytosis
C. Congenital red cell aplasia
D. Mysthania gravis

98. HbA2 levels are increased in all Except: *(PGI June 02)*
A. Alpha Thalassemia
B. Beta Thalassemia
C. Sickle cell anemia
D. Megaloblastic Anemia
E. Hyperthyroidism

Autoimmune Hemolytic Anemia

99. Warm autoimmune hemolytic anaemia may be seen in all of the following conditions *except* : *(AI 1997)*
A. Systemic lupus erythematous
B. α-Methyl dopa therapy
C. Non hodgkin's lymphoma
D. Mycoplasma pneumonia

100. Cold haemagglutinin is associated with- *(AI 97)*
A. Anti IgM
B. Anti IgG
C. Anti IgA
D. Donath landsteiner antibody

101. Autoimmune hemolytic anemia is seen in *(AIIMS May 94)*
A. Sickle cell anemia
B. Chronic lymphocytic leukemia (CLL)
C. Acute myelocytic leukemia (AML)
D. Multiple myeloma

102. Autoimmune hemolytic anemia is associated with malignancy of which lineage : *(AI 2007)*
A. T cell
B. B cell
C. Pre B cell
D. Pre T cell

103. Autoimmune haemolytic anemia is seen in: *(AI 2001)*
A. ALL
B. AML
C. CLL
D. CML

104. Coomb's +ve Hemolytic Anaemia is seen in *except* : *(AI 2000)*
A. Alcoholic cirrhosis
B. Chronic active hepatitis
C. Primary biliary cirrhosis
D. Primary sclerosing cholangitis

105. Coombs positive hemolytic anemia associated with: *(AI 2009)*
A. TTP
B. PAN
C. SLE
D. HUS

106. All of the following conditions are associated with coombs positive hemolytic anemia Except *(AI 2009)*
A. Thrombatic Thrombocytopenic purpura (TTP)
B. Scleroderma
C. SLE
D. PAN

107. Which of the following conditions is associated with Coomb's positive hemolytic anaemia:
A. Thrombotic thrombocytopenic purpura.
B. Progressive systemic sclerosis. *(AIIMS May 03)*
C. Systemic lupus erythematosus.
D. Polyarteritis nodosa

108. A 20 years old female presenting with anemia, mild jaundice for 2 years, peripheral smear showing spherocytes, the best investigation to be done is: *(AIPGMEE 08)*
A. Reticulocyte count
B. Osmotic fragility test
C. Coombs test
D. Bone marrow aspiration

109. A 23 Year old female presents with anemia and jaundice for 2 years. Peripheral smear shows spherocytes. The best investigation to be done is : *(AIIMS Nov. 2006)*
A. Reticulocyte Count
B. Osmotic Fragility Testing
C. Coombs Test
D. Bone Marrow Aspiration

Microangiopathic Hemolytic Anemia

110. All of the following are causes of fragmented RBC in peripheral blood Except: *(PGI June 05, 02)*
A. Microangiopathic hemolytic anemia
B. D.I.C
C. Hemophilia-A
D. Malignant hypertension
E. HELLP syndrome

111. A 25-year-old pregnant lady presents with thrombocytopenia (Platelet count < 50,000) and fragmented RBC's in peripheral smear. Which of the following is the least likely differential diagnosis? *(AI 2012)*
A. Thrombotic Thrombocytopenic Purpura (TTP)
B. Disseminated Intravascular Coagulation (DIC)
C. HELLP syndrome
D. Evan's syndrome

112. The differential diagnosis of micro-angiopathic anemia includes all Except: (PGI Dec. 05)
A. Sepsis
B. Hemolytic uremic syndrome
C. MI
D. Eclampsia
E. Scleroderma

113. Microangiopathic Hemolytic anemia is seen in all Except: (AIIMS Nov 2009)
A. TTP
B. Metallic heart valve
C. Microscopic polyangitis
D. Anti-phospholipid syndrome

114. Microangiopathic hemolytic anemia is seen in all Except:
A. HUS (PGI June 01, 00)
B. ITP
C. Malignant hypertension
D. Prosthetic valves
E. TTP

Proxysmal Nocturnal Hemoglobinuria (PNH)

115. PNH is associated with all of the following conditions, *except*: (AI 2002)
A. Aplastic anemia
B. ↑ed LAP scores
C. Venous thrombosis
D. Iron deficiency anemia

116. All of the following can be associated with PNH Except: (AI 2009)
A. Cerebral thrombosis
B. Budd chiari syndrome
C. Pancytopenia
D. Massive splenomegaly

117. All are true regarding paroxysmal nocturnal haemoglobinuria, *except*: (AIIMS Dec 91)
A. Haemosiderinuria
B. Pancytopenia
C. Increased alkaline phosphatase
D. Cellular marrow

118. A stem cell disorder affecting all the three cell lines platelets, RBCs and leucocytes is : (AIIMS May 01)
A. Hemolytic anaemia
B. Paroxysmal cold haemoglobinuria
C. Paroxysmal nocturnal haemoglobinuna
D. Blackfan Diamond syndrome

119. All of the following are true about PNH, Except:
A. Hypocellular marrow (PGI Dec 2000)
B. Budd-chirai syndrome
C. Thrombosis
D. LAP score low

120. Which of the following is NOT seen in Paroxysmal Nocturnal Hemoglobinuria : (AIIMS Nov. 2000)
A. Thrombosis
B. Hemosiderinuria
C. Decreased LDH
D. Thrombocytopenia

121. PNH is associated with a deficiency of : (AI 2010)
A. DAF
B. MIRL
C. GPI Anchored protein
D. All of the above

122. PNH is associated with deficiency of: (AI 2010)
A. DAF (Decay accelerating factor)
B. MIRL (Membrane inhibitor of reactive lysis)
C. GPI Anchored Proteins (Glycosyl phosphatidyl Inositol anchored proteins)
D. LFA (Lymphocyte function associated antigen)

123. HAM test is based upon : (AIIMS Nov06)
A. GPI Anchor Proteins
B. Complement
C. Spectrin protein
D. Mannose binding proteins

Aplastic Anemia and Myelodysplastic Syndrome

Aplastic Anemia and Pancytopenia

124. All the following are examples of diseases causing Aplastic anemia *except*: (AI 1995)
A. PNH
B. Hepatitis
C. Pregnancy
D. Cold hemoglobinuria

125. Aplastic anemia is seen in all of the following except:
A. PNH (PGI Dec 03)
B. Chloramphenicol
C. Hepatitis A
D. HIV-1
E. Parvovirus

126. Pancytopenia with cellular marrow is seen in:
A. PNH (AI 2007)
B. G6PD deficiency
C. Acquired aplastic anemia
D. Thalassemia

127. Pancytopenia with hypercellular marrow may be seen due to all of the following except: (DNB 2011)
A. Myelodysplasia
B. Paroxysmal Nocturnal Hemoglobinuria
C. Dyskeratosis congenita
D. Sarcoidosis

128. Which of the following causes of Anemia is associated with a Hypoplastic marrow: (AI 2012)
A. Fanconi's Anemia
B. Paroxysmal Nocturnal Hemoglobinuria (PNH)
C. Hypersplenism

D. Myelofibrosis

129. Pancytopenia with hypercellular bone marrow is seen in: *(AI 2007)*
A. PNH
B. Megaloblastic anemia
C. Acquired aplastic anemia
D. Thalessemia

130. Pancytopenia with Cellular marrow is seen in all except : *(AIIMS Nov. 2006)*
A. Megaloblastic Anemia
B. Myelodysplasia
C. PNH
D. G6PD Deficiency

131. Pancytopenia with a cellular marrow is seen in all except: *(AIIMS Nov 07)*
A. PNH
B. Megaloblastic anemia
C. Myelodysplastic syndrome
D. Dyskeratosis congenita

132. All of the following are causes of pancytopenia with cellular bone marrow except:
A. Paroxysomal noctural hemoglobinuria
B. Dyskeratosis congenita
C. Megaloblastic anemia
D. Hairy cell leukemia

133. Pancytopenia with cellular marrow is seen in all Except: *(AI 2008)*
A. Megaloblastic anemia
B. Myelodysplasia
C. Paroxysmal nocturnal hemoglobinuria
D. G6 PD deficiency

134. Vasanti, a 25-year-old-girl, presents with complaints of fever and weakness. On examination there is splenomegaly of 3 cm below the costal margin. Hb is 8 gm/dL, TLC is 3,000/mm^3, platelet count is 80,000/mm^3. Which of the following is the least likely diagnosis : *(AIIMS Nov. 2000)*
A. Acute lymphocytic leukemia
B. Anemia of chronic disease
C. Aplastic anemia
D. Megaloblastic anemia

135. All of the following statements about Fanconi's anemia are true, Except. *(AI 2010)*
A. Autosomal dominant inheritance
B. Hypocellular Bone Marrow
C. Congenital Anomalies
D. Usually normocytic / macrocytic cell morphology

136. True about aplastic anemia is all Except:
A. Splenomegaly *(PGI June 05)*
B. Reticulocytopenia
C. Thrombocytopenia
D. Neutropenia

137. A pt with an Hb of 6, WBC count of 2000, has a normal Different count except for having 6% blasts; platelets are reduced to 80,000; moderate splenomegaly is present; possible diagnosis is:
A. Leukemia *(AI 2001)*
B. Aplastic anemia
C. Hemolysis
D. ITP

138. A patient aged 63 years, is diagnosed to have severe aplastic anemia. HLA compatible sibling is available. The best option of treatment is : *(AIIMS May. 06)*
A. Anti-thymocyte globulin followed by cyclosporine
B. A conventional bone marrow transplantation from the HLA identical sibling
C. A non-myeloablative bone marrow transplantation from the HLA identical sibling
D. Cyclosporine

139. A 20 yrs adult presents with severe hypoplastic anemia. What is most effective treatment :
A. α-interferon *(AI 2002)*
B. IL-2
C. ATG therapy
D. Bone marrow transplantation

Myelodysplastic Syndrome

140. Ring sideroblasts are characteristically seen in:
A. Myelodysplastic syndrome (MDS) *(AI 2008)*
B. Acute Lymphoid Leukemia (ALL)
C. Acute Myeloid Leukemia (AML)
D. Anemia of chronic disease

141. In which of the following age group myelodysplastic syndrmome (MDS) are most common: *(AI 06)*
A. 2-10
B. 15-20
C. 5q
D. >50

142. Which is the most common cytogenetic abnormality in adult myelodysplastic syndrome (MDS) - *(AI 04)*
A. Trisomy 8
B. 20q-
C. 5q-
D. Monosmy 7

Myeloproliferative Disorders

General/Classification

143. Which of the following is NOT a myeloproliferative disease: *(AIIMS Nov. 2000)*
A. Polycythemia rubra vera
B. Acute myeloid leukemia
C. Chronic myeloid leukemia
D. Essential thrombocytosis

144. A patient with Myeloproliferative syndrome presents with decreased while cell count and decreased platelets The most likely diagnosis is: *(AI 1993)*
A. Chronic myeloid leukemia
B. Myelofibrosis
C. Polycythemias vera
D. Essential thrombocytosis

145. Massive Splenomegaly is least likely to be associated with which of the following Myeloproliferative disorders: *(AI 2012)*
A. Chronic Myeloid Leukemia (CML)
B. Polycythemia Vera (PV)
C. Essential Thrombocytosis (ET)
D. Primary Myeloproliferative (PMF)

146. Laboratory evaluation for the differential diagnosis of chronic myeloproliferative disorders includes all the following except- *(AIIMS Nov 04)*
A. Chromosomal evaluation
B. Bone marrow aspiration
C. Flow-cytometric analysis
D. Determination of red blood cell mass

147. Laboratory evaluation for the differential diagnosis of chronic myeloproliferative disorders includes all the following *except* : *(AIIMS Nov.2004)*
A. Chromosomal evaluation
B. Bone marrow aspiration
C. Flow-cytometric analysis
D. Determination of red blood cell mass

Polycythemia

148. All of the following are the causes of relative polycythemia *except*: *(AI 2005)*
A. Dehydration.
B. Dengue haemorrhagic fever.
C. Gaisbock syndrome.
D. High altitude.

149. A 59-year-old male came with Hb 18.0 gm/dl on three occasions. The resident doctor wants to exclude Polycythemia Vera. Which of the following is the most relevant investigation : *(AIIMS May 04)*
A. Hematocrit
B. Total leukocyte count
C. Red cell mass
D. Reticulocyte count

150. Secondary Polycythemia may be seen in:
A. Cor pulmonale *(DNB 2012)*
B. Congestive cardiac failure
C. Acyanotic congenital heart disease
D. All of the above

151. Which of the following factors can differentiate primary polycythemia from secondary polycythemia.
A. Increased Red cell mass
B. Arterial oxygen tension <90% on room air
C. Pruiritis
D. Hypertension

152. Erythropoietin is increased in all except :
A. Hepatocellular carcinoma
B. Renal cell carcinoma
C. Cerebellar Hemangioblastoma
D. Pancreatic carcinoma

153. Which of the following is not commonly seen in Polycythemia Vera ? *(AI 2002)*
A. Thrombosis
B. Hyperuricemia
C. Prone for acute leukemia
D. Spontaneous severe infection

154. True about polycythemia rubra vera is all Except:
A. Bleeding *(PGI Dec 97)*
B. Thrombosis
C. ↓ed ESR
D. Infection

155. In Polycythemia vera, all the following are seen *except* : *(AIIMS May 01)*
A. Thrombocytopenia
B. Increased GI bleed
C. Thrombosis
D. Transient visual loss

156. All of the following are seen in polycythemia rubra vera *except* : *(AIIMS Nov. 2000)*
A. Increased Vit B_{12} binding capacity (>9000 micromols/dL)
B. Decreased LAP Score
C. Leucocytosis
D. Increased platelets

157. Which of the following is a major criteria for diagnosis of poycythemia vera: *(AI 2010)*
A. Presence of JAK-2 mutation
B. Low Erythropoetin levels
C. High Leucocyte Alkaline Phosphatase (↑LAP score)
D. Thrombocytosis

158. Which is not seen in polycythemia vera :
A. Increased Vit B_{12} binding capacity
B. Increase erythropoietin level
C. Increase RBC count *(AIIMS Feb 97)*
D. Ocular congestion

159. Tumor associated with polycythemia is :
A. Sarcoma *(AI 2001, AI 1995)*
B. Pituitary adenoma
C. Cerebellar haemangioblastoma
D. None of the above.

Myelofibrosis

160. A patient has the following findings-splenomegaly, low RBC count, normal WBC, and platelet count and peripheral blood smear shows tear drop cells.

Repeated BM aspiration is unsuccessful. The probable diagnosis is: *(AIIMS 1999)*
A. Thalassemia
B. Chronic myeloid leukemia
C. Iron deficiency anaemia
D. Myelofibrosis

161. A pt. being investigated for anemia has a dry marrow tap; peripheral smear reveals tear drop cells; likely diagnosis is: *(AI 2001)*
A. Leukemia
B. Lymphoma
C. Myelofibrosis
D. Polycythemia rubra vera

162. Leukoerythroblastic picture may be seen in all of the following, *except*: *(AI 2003)*
A. Myelofibrosis
B. Metastatic carcinoma
C. Gaucher's disease
D. Thalassemia

Essential Thrombocytosis

163. A 45 year old female patient presents with symptoms of easy bruisability and frequent headaches. Physical examination show a moderate splenomegaly. Blood counts shows a normal leucocyte count and a platelet count of 1000×10^3/cu mm. The leucocyte alkaline phosphatase score is normal. Which one of the following is the drug of choice for the treatment of this patient? *(AIIMS Nov 03)*
A. Hydroxyurea
B. Radioactive phosphorus
C. Anagrelide
D. Interferon alpha

164. A patient presents with a platelet count of 700 x 109/L with abnormalities in size, shape and granularity of platelets. WBC count is 12 x 109/L, hemoglobin is 11g/dl and Philadelphia chromosome is absent. The most likely diagnosis would be:
A. Polycythemia vera *(AIIMS May. 2006)*
B. Essential thrombocythemia
C. Chronic myeloid leukemia
D. Leukemoid reaction

Lymphomas & Chronic Leukemias

Hodgkin's Lymphoma

165. The subtype of Hodking's disease, which is histogentically distinct from all the other subtypes, is-
A. Lymphocyte predominant *(AI 05)*
B. Nodular sclerosis
C. Mixed cellularity
D. Lymphocyte depleted

166. Cells characteristic of Hodgkin's disease are:
A. Lacunar cells
B. Red-Stemberg cells
C. Giant cells
D. Eosinophils

167. The lymphocytic and histiocytic variant of Reed-Sternberg cell is seen in: *(AIIMS Nov 05)*
A. Follicular center lymphoma
B. Lymphocyte depleted Hodkin's disease
C. Nodular sclerosis Hodkin's disease
D. Lymphocyte predominant Hodkin's disease

168. Hodgkin's lymphoma of the nodular subtype is associated with: *(AIIMS June 1992)*
A. Lacunar cells
B. Popcorn cells
C. Reticular variant
D. None of the above

169. Most common type of Hodgkin's lymphoma is :
A. Nodular sclerosis *(AI 1996)*
B. Lymphocyte predominance
C. Mixed cellularity
D. Lymphocyte depletion

170. Most common type of hodgkin's lymphoma in India is : *(AI 1998)*
A. Nodular sclerosis
B. Lymphocyte predominance
C. Mixed nodulatory
D. Lymphocyte depletion

171. Which of the following types of Hodgkins lymphomas is associated with a good prognosis
A. Lymphocyte Predominance *(DNB Dec 2010)*
B. Lymphocyte Depletion
C. Nodular sclerosis
D. Mixed cellularity

172. Best prognostic type of Hodgkin's lymphoma is :
A. Lymphocytic predominant *(AIIMS June 1998)*
B. Lymphocytic depletion
C. Mixed cellularity
D. Nodular sclerosis

173. Classical markers for Hodgkin's disease is-
A. CD 15 and CD 30 *(AIPGMEE 08)*
B. CD 15 and CD 22
C. CD 15 and CD 20
D. CD 20 and CD 30

174. Diagnosis of Hodgkins disease is based on all of the following, except: *(PGI Dec 1999)*
A. Reed- Sternberg cells
B. Reactive cellular background
C. Atypical cells in backgriound
D. D. CD 30 positivity

175. All are true regarding Hodgkin's lymphoma, *except* :
A. CNS is the commonest site of involvement
B. Characteristic cell is a Reed Sternberg cell
C. Mediastinal involvement is common in nodular--sclerosis type. *(AI 2000)*
D. Eosinophils, plasma cells and neutrophils increase.

176. The paraneoplastic syndrome associated with Hodgkin's disease is : *(AIIMS Nov. 05)*
A. Nephrotic syndrome
B. Retinopathy
C. Cerebellar degenerative disease
D. Acanthosis nigricans

177. All of the following are the good prognostic features Hodgkin's disease except: *(AI 04)*
A. Haemoglobin>10 gm/dl
B. WBC count<15000/mm3
C. Absolute lymphocyte count<600/ul
D. Age < 45 yrs

178. All of the following are poor prognostic factors for Hodgkin's disease, Except: *(PGI Dec 01)*
A. Younger age
B. Systemic manifestations
C. Lymphocyte depletion
D. Mediastinal disease
E. Stomach involvement

179. A patient presents to the hospital for percistant fever and significant weight loss for the post two months. On examination he is observed to have cervical and axillary lymphadenopathy. Other examination and investigations are unremarkable. Biopsy from the cervical nodes is performed and returns positive for Hodgkin's Lymphoma. The patient can be staged as haring: *(AI 1997)*
A. Stage II A
B. Stage II B
C. Stage II A
D. Stage II B

180. A patient with Hodgkin's lymphoma is having a single cervical lymphnode. Biopsy showed lymphocyte predominant variant. Which of the following is the treatment of choice:
A. Chemotherapy with Radiotherapy
B. Chemotherapy only *(AIIMS Nov 2000)*
C. Radiotherapy only
D. No treatment needed

181. A patient with Hodgkin's lymphoma presents with isolated cervical lymphadenopathy. Biopsy from the lesion shows characteristic lacunar cells. The treatment of choice for this patient is:
A. Chemotherapy with Radiotherapy
B. Chemotherapy alone
C. Radiotherapy alone
D. No treatment needed

182. True for Hodgkin's stage IA is: *(PGI Dec 05)*
A. Chemotherapy is best
B. Radiotherapy is best
C. Total radiation therapy is best treatment
D. Fever and wt loss is always present

183. Treatment of choice in Hodgkin's Lymphoma is:
A. CHOP *(PGI Dec 06)*
B. MOPP
C. ABVD
D. MOPP and ABVD hybrid

184. All of the following statements about Treatment of Hodgkin's lymphoma are true, Except: *(PGI June 07)*
A. ABVD is the most commonly used Regimen
B. Sterility is more frequent after ABVD than MOPP
C. Combination chemotherapy is the mainstay of treatment in Advanced Hodgkin's disease
D. WBC count > $15000/mm^3$ is a poor prognostic factor

Non Hodgkins Lymphoma and Leukemia

185. The classification proposed by the International Lymphoma Study Group for non-Hodgkin's lymphoma is known as: *(AI 2005)*
A. Kiel classification.
B. REAL classification.
C. WHO classification.
D. Rappaport classification.

186. Which of the following is not a B-cell neoplasm?
A. Hairy cell leukemia *(AIIMS May 06)*
B. Angiocentric lymphoma
C. Mantle cell lymphoma
D. Burkitt's lymphoma

187. Plasmacytoid Lymphomas may be associated with:
A. IgG *(AI 2010)*
B. IgM
C. IgA
D. IgE

188. "International prognostic index" for lymphoma includes the following prognostic factors except:
A. Stage of disease *(AI 2009)*
B. Number of extralymphatic sites involved
C. LDH
D. Hemoglobin and Albumin

189. 'Intermediate form' of Non hodgkin's lymphoma is :
A. Small non cleaved cell *(AI 1999)*
B. Diffuse, small cleaved cell
C. Lymphoblastic
D. Large cell immunoblastic

190. Intermediate grade of NHL are all *except* : *(AI 2000)*
A. Diffuse small cell cleaved
B. Diffuse large cell l
C. Mycosis fungoides
D. Diffuse mixed

191. Most malignant form of NHL is : *(AI 1998)*
A. Diffuse large cell
B. Small cell lymphocytic lymphoma
C. Follicular cleavage
D. Large cell follicular

Burkitt's Lymphoma

192. In Burkitts lymphoma, translocation seen is chromosome *(AIIMS May 01)*
A. 12 - 14 translocation
B. 8 - 14 translocation

C. 4 - 8 translocation
D. 12 - 18 translocation

193. Translocation t(2:8)(p12:q24) is associated with:
A. Chronic Myeloid Leukemia (CML) *(AI 2010)*
B. Acute Myeloid Leukemia (AML)
C. T cell – ALL
D. Burkitt's Lymphoma

194. Burkitt's Lymphoma is associated with which of the following viruses *(DNB 2012)*
A. EBV
B. HTLV-1
C. HHV- 8
D. Adenovirus

195. Burkitt's Lymphoma is associated with: *(AI 2010)*
A. t (8:14)
B. t (11:14)
C. t (15:17)
D. t (14:18)

196. All of the following statements about Burkitt's lymphoma are true, Except: *(PGI June 02)*
A. B cell lymphoma
B. 8, 14 translocation
C. Can present as an abdominal mass
D. Radiotherapy is the treatment of choice

Hairy Cell Leukemia

197. All of the following statements about Hairy cell leukaemia are true except: *(AI 2004)*
A. Splenomegaly is conspicuous
B. Results from an expansion of neoplastic T lymphocytes
C. Cells are positive for Tartrate Resistant Acid phosphatase
D. The cells express CD25 consistently

198. 'Hairy cell leukemia' is a Neoplastic proliferation of : *(AI 1999)*
A. T. cells
B. B. cells
C. Myeloid cells
D. Macrophages

199. CD 19 positive, CD22 positive, CD103 positive monoclonal B-cells with bright kappa positivity were found to comprise 60% of the peripheral blood lymphoid cells on flow cytometric analysis in a 55 year old man with massive splenomegaly and a total leucocyte count of 3.3 x 10^9/L. Which one of the following is the most likely diagnosis?
A. Splenic lymphoma with villous lymphocytes
B. Mantle cell lymphoma *(AIIMS Nov. 2004)*
C. B-cell prolymphocytic leukemia
D. Hairy cell leukemia

200. 'Which of the following is NOT used in treatment of hairy cell leukemia: *(AIIMS Feb 97)*
A. Steroid
B. Pentostatin
C. Splenectomy
D. Alpha-interferon

201. Treatment of choice in hairy cell leukemia is:
A. Steroid *(AI 1995)*
B. Cladribine
C. Splenectomy
D. Pentostatin

Mantle Cell Lymphoma

202. A 63 year old man presents with splenomgaly and lymphadenopathy. Immunophenotype was positive for CD19, CD79b and FMC7. The most likely diagnosis is: *(AIIMS May 01)*
A. Hairy cell leukemia
B. Mantle cell Lymphoma (MCL)
C. Chronic Lymphocytic Leukemia (CLL)
D. Follicular Lymphoma

203. A 63-year old man presented with massive splenomegaly, lymphadenopathy and a total leucocyte count of 17000 per mm^3. The flow cytometery showed CD 19 positive, CD 5 positive, CD 23 negative, monoclonal B-cells with bright kappa positively comprising 80% of the peripheral blood lymphoid cells. The most likely diagnosis is:
A. Mantle cell lymphoma *(AI 2003)*
B. Splenic lymphoma with villous lymphocytes
C. Follicular lymphoma
D. Hairy cell leukemia

Chronic Lymphocytic Leukemia (CLL)

204. Chronic Lymphocytic Leukemia (CLL) is associated with:
A. Individuals > 50 years of age
B. Mature small lymphocytes in peripheral smear
C. Hepatosplenomegaly and lymphadenopathy
D. All of the above

205. 80 year old, asymptomatic man present with a Total Leucocyte Count of 1 lakh, with 80% lymphocytes and 20% PMC's. What is the most probable diagnosis? *(AI 2005)*
A. HIV
B. CML
C. CLL
D. TB

206. All of the following are true about Chronic Lymphocytic Leukemia, Except: *(PGI 2008)*
A. Diagnosed on routine blood tests
B. Leukocytosis is prominent
C. Can present as acute leukemia
D. T lymphocyte CLL is more common

207. 80 year old, asymptomatic man present with a Total Leucocyte Count of 1 lakh, with 80% lymphocytes and 20% PMC's. What is the most probable diagnosis? *(AI 2007)*
A. HIV
B. CML
C. CLL
D. TB

208. A 48 years of woman was admitted with a history of weakness for two months. On examination cervical lymph nodes were found enlarged and spleen was palpable 2 cm below the costal margin. Her hemoglobin was 10.5g/dl. Platelet count 237×10^9/L, and total leukocyte count 40×10^9/L, which include 80% mature lymphoid cell with coarse clumped chromatin. Bone marrow revealed a nodular lymphoid infiltrate. The peripheral blood lymphoid cells were positive for CD19, CD5, CD20 and were negative for CD79B and FMC(-7). Which one of the following statements is not true about this disease?
   A. Trisomy 12 correlates an aggressive clinical course
   B. Abnormalities of 13q 14 are associated with long term survival *(AIIMS Nov 2004)*
   C. Case with 11q22-23 deletions have excessive lymphadenopathy
   D. t(11;14) translocation is present in most of the cases

209. A 48 year old women was admitted with a history of weakness for two months. On examination, cervical lymph nodes were found enlarged and spleen was palpable 2 cm below the costal margin. Her hemoglobin was 10.5 g/dl, platelet count 2.7×109/L and total leukocyte count 40×10^9/L, which included 80% mature lymphoid cells with coarse clumped chromatin. Bone marrow revealed nodular lymphoid infiltrate. The peripheral blood lymphoid cells were positive for CD 19, CD 5, CD20 and CD23 and were negative for CD79B and FMC-7.
   The histopathological examination of the lymph node in this patient will most likely exhibit effacement of lymph node architecture by *(A.I.2005)*
   A. A pseudofollicular pattern with proliferation centers
   B. A monomorphic lymphoid proliferation with a nodular pattern.
   C. A predominantly follicular pattern
   D. A diffuse proliferation of medium to large lymphoid cells with high mitotic rate.

210. A 48 year old woman was admitted with a history of weakness for two months. On examination, cervical lymph nodes were found enlarged and spleen was palpable 2 cm ptatelet count 237 X 109L and total leukocyte count 40 x coarse clumped chromatin. Bone marrow revelaed a nodular lymphoid infiltrate. The peripheral blood lymphoid were negative for CD 19, CD5, CD 20 and CD 23 and were negative for CD 79 B and FMC - 7. *(AIIMS Nov. 05)*
   What is the most likely diagnosis?
   A. T- cell rich B - cell lymphoma with leukemic spill over in blood.
   B. Chronic lymphocytic leukemia
   C. Mantle cell lymphoma
   D. A definite diagnosis can not be made in this patient without lymph node biopsy

Chronic Myeloid Leukemia (CML) and CMML

211. Peripheral smear with increased neutrophils, basophils, eosinophils, and platelets is highly suggestive of- *(AIIMS May 06)*
   A. Acute myeloid leukemia
   B. Acute lymphoblastic leukemia
   C. Chronic myelogenous leukemia
   D. Myelodysplastic syndrome

212. A 60 year old man presented with fatigue, weight loss and heaviness in left hypochondrium for 6 months. The hemogram showed Hb. 10gm/dL, TLC 5 lakhs/mm^3, platelet count 4 lakhs/mm^3, DLC; neutrophil 55%, lymphocutes 4%, monocytes 2%, basophils 6%, metamyelocytes 10%, myelocytes 18%, promyelocytes 2% and blast 3%. The most likely cytogenetic abnormality in this case is:
   A. t (1; 21) *(AIIMS May 03)*
   B. t (9; 22)
   C. t (15; 17)
   D. Trisomy 21

213. In a patient suffering from chronic myeloid leukemia, Hb falls from 11g% to 4g% in a short span of time, and splenomegaly occurs. The cause could be (select two options)- *(PGI June 02)*
   A. Accelerated phase
   B. CML in blast crisis
   C. Ineffective erythropoesis
   D. Myelofibrosis

214. Which one of the following is not a criterion for making a diagnosis of chronic myeloid leukemia in accelerated phase : *(AIIMS Nov 2004)*
   A. Blasts 10-19% of WBC's in peripheral blood
   B. Basophils 10-19% of WBC'S in peripheral blood
   C. Increasing spleen size unresponsive to therapy
   D. Persistent thrombocytosis (>1000 x 10^9/L) unresponsive to therapy

215. Leukocyte alkaline phosphate is increased in all, *except* *(AIIMS May 94)*
   A. Polycythemia vera
   B. CML
   C. Myelofibrosis
   D. Myeloid metaplasia

216. Which of these is true regarding CML : *(AIIMS 1999)*
   A. Size of splenomegaly indicates prognosis
   B. Phagocytic activity of WBC is reduced
   C. Sudan black stain is specific for myeloblast
   D. Myeloblast, granuloblast and lymphoblast become PH chromosome +ve. –ve following remission

217. All of the following are features of juvenile CML *except:* *(AI 94)*
   A. Thrombocytopenia
   B. Fetal Hb is increased

C. Philadelphia chromosome is positive
D. Lymphadenopathy

218. Haemoglobin F is raised in: *(AIIMS Dec 97)*
A. Juvenile chronic myeloid leukemia
B. Hereditary spherocytosis
C. Congenital red cell aplasia
D. Myasthenia gravis

219. Initial treatment recommended for newly diagnosed patient with CML is:
A. Allogenic Bone Marrow Transplantation
B. Imatinib Mesylate Therapy
C. TNF-α
D. IFN-α

220. Drug of choice for chronic myeloid Leukemia (CML) is: *(AI 2008)*
A. Hydroxyurea
B. Imatinib
C. Inflliximab
D. IFN

221. Drug of choice for treatment of CML is: *(DNB)*
A. Imatinib
B. Hydroxyurea
C. IFN-Alfa
D. Infliximab

222. Best Rx for CML is: *(PGI Dec 98)*
A. Autologous BMT
B. Allogenic BMT
C. Alpha Interferon
D. Hydroxyurea

223. Which of the following is not compatible with a diagnosis of chronic myelomonocytic leukemia? *(AIIMS Nov 03)*
A. Peripheral blood monocytosis more than 1×109L
B. Absence of Philadelphia chromosome
C. More than 20% blasts in blood or bone marrow
D. Absent or minimal dysplasia in myeloid lieages.

Mycosis Fungoides

224. Mycosis fungoides which is not true
A. It is the most common form of cutaneous lymphoma *(AI 2007)*
B. Pautriers microabscess
C. Indolent course and easily amenable to treatment
D. Erythroderma seen and spreads to peripheral circulation

Acute Leukemia

General Characteristics

225. The marker for B lymphocyte is-
A. CD 19
B. CD 68
C. CD 34
D. CD 4

226. Which of the following is a pan-T lymphocyte marker: *(AI 2003)*
A. CD2
B. CD3
C. CD19
D. CD25

227. Marker specific for myeloid lineage- *(AIIMS Nov 95)*
A. CD33
B. CD14
C. CD13
D. MPO

228. Memory T cells can be identified by using the following marker *(AI 2003)*
A. CD45RA
B. CD45RB
C. SD45RC
D. CD45RO

229. Which of the followings combinations of cytogenetic abnormality and associated leukemia/lymphoma is incorrect? *(AIIMS Nov 2004)*
A. t (8:14): Burkitts lymphoma
B. t (15:17) : AML-M3
C. t (9:22) : CML
D. t (9:20) : ALL

Acute Lymphoid Leukemia (ALL)

230. The most common type of ALL is:
A. Pre B cell ALL
B. T cell ALL
C. B cell ALL
D. Biphenotypic ALL

231. Which of the following presents as mediastinal enlargement:
A. Promyelocytic Leukemia
B. CML
C. ALL
D. Diffuse histiocytic lymphoma

232. A17-year-old boy presented with TLC of 138×10^9/ L with 80% blasts on the peripheral smear. Chest X-ray demonsnstrated a large mediastinal mass. Immunophenotyping of this patent's blasts would most likely demonstrate: *(AIIMS May 2006)*
A. No surface antigens (null phenotype)
B. An immature T cell phenotype (Tdt/CD34/CD7 positive)
C. Myeloid markers, such as CD13,CD33 and Cd15
D. B cell markers, such as CD19,CD20 and CD22

233. All of the following are good prognostic factors for childhood. ALL except: *(AIIMS May 02, AI 07)*
A. Hyperdiploidy
B. Female sex
C. Pre B cell ALL
D. t (12 : 21) translocation

234. Good prognostic Factors for ALL include all of the following, Except: *(DNB 2011)*
A. Hyperdiploidy
B. Female sex

C. Pre B cell ALL
D. t (12 : 21) translocation

235. Which of the following is a poor prognostic factor for childhood ALL. *(AIIMS Nov 09)*
A. Total Leukocyte count 4000-100,000
B. Age < 2 years
C. Testicular involvement
D. Blasts in peripheral smear

236. Which of the following is a good prognostic factor in ALL: *(PGI 2008)*
A. High WBC count
B. Male sex
C. Age < 2 years
D. Hyperdiploidy

237. Lasparaginase is particularly used in which type of leukemia- *(AI 1996)*
A. AML
B. CML
C. ALL
D. CLL

238. Treatment of choice in intracranial ALL is:
A. A. Intrathecal methotrexate *(PGI June 99)*
B. Vincristine and prednisolone
C. Intrathecal vincristine
D. Prednisolone

239. In which of the following types of leukemia is methotrexate administered for CNS prophylasxis:
A. ALL
B. AML
C. CLL
D. CML

240. All of the following drugs are used in management of ALL Except: *(PGI June 02)*
A. Methotrexate
B. All – trans retinoic acid
C. Prednisolone
D. L-Asparginase
E. Vincristine

241. A four year old boy was admitted with a history of abdominal pain and fever for two months maculo papular rash for ten days, and dry cough, dyspnea and wheezing for three days. One examination liver and spleen were enlarged 4 cm and 3 cm respectively below the costal margins. His hemoglobin was 10.0 g/dl, platelet count 37×109/L and total leukocyte count 70 × 109L, which included 80% eosinophils Bone marrow examination revealed a cellular marrow comprising of 45% blasts and 34% Eosinophils and eosinophilic precursors. The blasts stained negative for myeloperoxidase and non-specific esterase and were positive for CD19, CD10, CD22 and CD20. Which of the following is the most likely diagnosis?
A. Biphenotypic acute leukemia (lymphoid and eosinophil lineage *(AIIMS Nov 2004)*
B. Acute eosinophilic leukemia
C. Acute lymphoblastic leukemia with hypereosinophilic syndrome
D. Acute myeloid leukemia with eosinophilia

242. A four year old boy was admitted with a history of abdominal pain and fever for two months, maculopapular rash for ten days, and dry cough, dyspnea and wheezing for three days. On examination, liver and spleen were enlarged 4 cm and 3 cm respectively below the costal margins. His hemoglobin was 10.0 g/dl, platelet count 37×10^9/L and total leukocyte count 70×10^9/L, which included 80% eosinophils. Bone marrow examination revealed a cellular marrow comprising 45% blasts and 34% eosinophils and eosinophilic precursors. The blasts stained negative for myeloperoxidase and non-specific esterase and were positive for CD19, CD10, CD22 and CD20. Which one of the following statements in not true about this disease? *(AI 2005)*
A. Eosinophils are not part of the Neoplastic clone.
B. t(5:14) rearrangement may be detected in blasts.
C. Peripheral blood eosinophilia may normalize with chemotherapy.
D. Inv (16) is often detected in the blasts and the eosinophils.

Acute Myeloblastic Leukemia (AML)

243. Which of the following is a poor prognostic factor in Acute Myeloid Leukemia (AML)
A. Monosomy *(AIIMS Nov 2010)*
B. Deletion of X or Y chromosome
C. t (8; 21) translocation
D. Nucleophosphin mutation

244. Auer Rods are most frequently seen in which subtype of AML *(DNB 2012)*
A. M0
B. M 3
C. M 5
D. M 7

245. Auer Rods are typically not seen in: *(DNB 2012)*
A. AML – M0
B. AML – M2
C. AML – M3
D. AML – M1

246. All of the following are poor prognostic factors for acute myeloid leukemias, *except*: *(AI 2003)*
A. Age more than 60 years
B. Leucocytes count more than 1,00,000/μl
C. Secondary leukemias
D. Presence of t(8:21)

247. A child with Acute myeloid Leukemia presents with Hyperleukocytosis. Treatment includes all of the following, Except:
A. IV fluids
B. Allopurinol
C. Alkalinization
D. Immediately start induction chemotherapy

248. Poor prognosis in AML is indicated by: *(AI 2008)*
A. Inversion 16
B. Translocation 15/17 (t15; 17)
C. Normal cytogenecity
D. Monosomy 7

249. AML with worst prognosis is :
A. 8/21 translocation *(AIIMS Nov 2006)*
B. Inversion 16
C. Normal Cytogenetics
D. Monosomy 7

250. In PML, all of the following are seen except :
A. Retinoic acid is used in treatment
B. 15/17 translocation *(AI 2007)*
C. CD 15/34 both seen in same cell
D. Associated with DIVC

251. A 15-years-old boy presented with one day history of bleeding gum,subconjunctival bleed and purpuric rash. Investigations revealed followed results:Hb- 6.4 gm/dl; TLC-26, 500/mm3 platelet 35,000 mm3; prothrombin time-20 sec with a control of 13 sec; partial thromboplastin time-50sec; and Fibrinogen 10mg/dL.Peripheral smear was suggestive of acute myeloblastic leukemia. Which of the following is the most likely? *(AIIMS May 2006)*
A. Myeloblastic leukemia without maturation
B. Myeloblastic leukemia with maturation
C. Promyelocytic leukemia
D. Myelomonocytic leukemia

252. Arsenic is used in treatment of: *(AIIMS May 07)*
A. Acute promyelocytic leukemia
B. A.L.L
C. CML
D. Transient myeloproliferative disorder

Biphenotypic Leukemia

253. In a patient with acute leukemia, immunophenotype pattern is CD 19+ve, CD 10+ve, CD33+ve, CD13+ve. He may probably have- *(AIIMS May 04)*
A. Biphenotypic leukemia
B. ALL
C. AML-M2
D. AML-Mo

Plasma Cell Disorders / Multiple Myeloma

254. All the following are seen in Multiple myeloma *except:* *(AI 1995)*
A. Visual Disturbance
B. Bleeding tendency
C. Proteinuria
D. Dystrophic calcification

255. All of the following are seen in multiple myeloma except:
A. Visual Disturbance
B. Proteinuria
C. Bleeding tendency
D. Dystrophic calcification

256. Which of the following is the least common feature of Multiple Myeloma: *(AI 2012)*
A. Bone pain
B. Normocytic Normochromic Anemia
C. Susceptibility to bacterial infection
D. Hyperviscosity syndrome

257. Which of the following is not a major criteria for diagnosis of multiple myeloma? *(AI 2006)*
A. Lytic bone lesions
B. Plasmacytoma on tissue biopsy
C. Bone marrow plasmacytosis > 30%
D. 'M' spike > 3g% for Ig G, > 2g% for IgA

258. Which is not a minor criteria of Multiple Myeloma?
A. Multiple lytic lesions *(AIIMS Nov 2008)*
B. Plasmacytosis > 20%
C. Plasmacytoma in tissue
D. S. IgG > 3gm, IgA > 1.5

259. **All of the following are minor criteria for multiple Myeloma, Except** *(AIIMS Nov 2010)*
A. Plasmacytosis 20%
B. Multiple lytic lesions
C. Plasmacytoma on tissue biopsy
D. Monoclonal Ig spike < 2g/dl for IgA and < 3.5 for IgG

260. All seen in multiple myeloma, *except* :
A. Lytic bone lesion *(AIIMS May 95*
B. Hypercalcemia
C. Plasmacytosis of bone marrow > 2%
D. Decreased serum alkaline phosphatase activity

261. All the following are true about multiple myeloma *except:* *(AI 1994)*
A. Osteolytic bone disease
B. t(8-14) translocation
C. Light chain proliferation
D. Bence-Jones proteins in urine

262. True about Myeloma is all, *except* *(AIIMS Nov 01)*
A. Plasma cell clonal proliferation
B. Common after 50 yrs of age
C. Amyloidosis can occur
D. Protein casts in urine are made up of complete Ig chains

263. Commonest site of lytic lesion, in multiple myeloma is
A. Vertebral column *(AIIMS Dec 97)*
B. Femur
C. Clavicle
D. Pelvis

264. Which of the following may be seen in Multiple Myeloma: *(PGI June 05)*
A. Decreased Calcium
B. Sclerotic bone lesion
C. Bone deposition
D. Renal failure

265. The following is the least useful investigation in multiple myeloma : *(AI 2007)*
A. ESR
B. X-Ray
C. Bone scan
D. Bone marrow biopsy

266. An elderly male presents with headache, recurrent infections and multiple punched out lytic lesions of x-ray skull. The investigation that will best help in establishing a diagnosis is: *(AI 2009)*
A. Protein Electrophoresis
B. Serum calcium
C. Alkaline phosphatase levels
D. Acid phosphatase levels

267. Which is not seen in multiple myeloma :
A. Anemia *(AIIMS Feb 97)*
B. Increased alkaline phosphatase
C. Hypercalcemia
D. ↑ed ESR

268. True regarding multiple myeloma is all. *except* :
A. Bone pain *(AI 1998)*
B. Lytic lesions
C. Increased alkaline phosphatase
D. Tarterate resistance acid phosphatase positive

269. Raised serum alkaline phosphatase is seen in all, *except* *(AIIMS Dec 94)*
A. Paget's disease
B. Multiple myeloma
C. Osteomalacia
D. Hyperthyroidism

270. Which one of the following is not a feature of multiple mycloma?
A. Hypercalcemia
B. Anemia
C. Hyperviscosity
D. Elevated alkaline phosphatase

271. Maximum ESR is seen in : *(AI 1998)*
A. CHF
B. Polycythemia vera
C. Multiple myeloma
D. Sickle cell anemia

272. In multiple myeloma following are seen except:
A. Anion gap raised *(PGI Dec 97)*
B. Lytic bone lesion
C. Polyarticular pain
D. M spike present with polyarticulopathy

273. Multiple myeloma is characterized by all except:
A. Presence of light chains *(PGI 2000)*
B. Monoclonal gammopathy
C. Polyclonal gammopathy
D. Hypergammaglobulinemia

274. True about Multiple myeloma are all Except:
A. Bence Jones protein in urine *(PGI 2000)*
B. Hypogammaglobulinemia
C. Amyloidosis
D. Plasmacytosis < 10%
E. Renal failure

275. Russell bodies are found in- *(AI 96)*
A. Multiple Myeloma
B. Gonadal tumor
C. Parkinsonism
D. Intracranial neoplasms

276. Russell body is found in- *(AIIMS June 97, AI 95)*
A. WBC
B. RBC
C. Mast cells
D. Plasma cells

277. All of the following are poor prognostic factors in Multiple Myeloma, Except: *(PGI June 99)*
A. Azotemia
B. Hypocalcemia
C. ↑ LDH
D. Chromosoma 13 deletion
E. High M component production

278. A patient of multiple myeloma presents with bony lesions. What is the best marker for prognosis of the disease: *(AIIMS June 99; AIIMS 2000)*
A. Bone marrow plasma cell
B. Serum calcium level
C. Beta 2 microglobulin
D. Beta 1 microglobulin

279. A 58 years old woman, who had backache and recurrent chest infections for 6 months, develops sudden weakness of the legs and urinary retention. Her investigations show hemoglobin of 7.3 gm/dl, serum calcium 12.6 mg/dl, phosphate 2.5 mg/dl, alkaline phosphatse 100 u/l, serum albumin 3 gm/dl, globulin 7.1 gm/dl, and urea 178 mg/dl. What is the most likely diagnosis ? *(AI 06)*
A. Lung cancer
B. Disseminated tuberculosis
C. Multiple myeloma
D. Osteoporosis

280. Ramla, 65 yrs old male, presents with low back pain especially at L3, anaemia and fatigability. His investigation profile reveals – Hb = 7 gm%, TLC-9000/cmm, DLC -N- 55%, L-30%, M-10%, E-1%, B-2%, Serum proteins-8 gm %, ratio-2.9/5.9, ESR-90 and serum creatinine-3.2 mg%. Likely diagnosis is :
A. Waldenstroms macroglobulinemia
B. Multiple myeloma *(AIIMS Nov 01)*
C. TB spine
D. Secondaries in spine

281. Which of the following drugs is not used for the management of multiple myeloma *(DNB)*
A. Bortezomib
B. Hydroxyurea
C. Melphelan
D. Cyclophosphamide

282. All of the following drugs are used in the treatment of Multiple myeloma, Except: *(PGI 09)*
A. Bortezomib
B. Melphelan
C. Hydroxyurea
D. Cyclophosphamide

Multiple Myeloma Variance and Other Plasma Cell Disorders

283. True about smoldering myeloma is: *(PGI June 2008)*
   A. Monoclonal gammopathy
   B. Lytic bone lesion
   C. Hypercalcemia
   D. Bone Marrow Plasma cell < 10%
284. An 80 year old asymptomatic woman was detected to have a monoclonal spike on serum electrophoresis (IgG levels 1.5 g/dl). Bone marrow revealed plasma cells of 8%. The most likely diagnosis is: *(AI 2004)*
   A. Multiple myeloma
   B. Indolent myeloma
   C. Monoclonal gammopathy of unknown significance
   D. Waldenstorm's macroglobulinemia
285. Ramesh 60 years, presents with generalized bone pain. On examination there is elevated ESR of 100 mm, serum globulin 7, lytic lesions in the skull, serum creatinine of 3.5 mg/dL and serum calcium of 11 mg/dL. What is the most likely diagnosis :
   A. Waldenstrom's macroglobulinemia
   B. Multiple myeloma *(AIIMS Nov. 2000)*
   C. Hyperparathyroidism
   D. Osteomalacia
286. Which of the following statement is not true?
   A. Patients with IgD myeloma may present with no evident M-spike on serum electrophoresis.
   B. A diagnosis of plasma cell leukemia can be made if circulating peripheral blood plasmablasts comprise 14% of peripheral blood white cells in a patient with white blood cell count of 1×10^9/L and platelet count of 88×10^9/L. *(AI 2005)*
   C. In smoldering myeloma plasma cells constitute 10-30% of total bone marrow cellularity.
   D. In a patient with multiple myeloma, a monoclonal light chain may be detected in both serum and urine
287. Franklin's disease is associated with :*(AIIMS May 95)*
   A. Gamma heavy chain disease
   B. Multiple myeloma
   C. Alpha heavy chain disease
   D. Waldenstorm's macroglobulinemia

Bleeding / Coagulation Disorder

General

288. Vitamin K dependent coagulation factors include:
   A. II and III *(AI 2010)*
   B. IX and X
   C. III and V
   D. VIII and XII
289. Vitamin K-dependent factor is-
   A. II
   B. III
   C. IV
   D. VI
290. Which is most likely to be increased in Vit K deficiency: *(AI 2000)*
   A. P.T.T.
   B. P.T.
   C. Platelet count
   D. Fibrinogen time
291. Feature of hemorrhagic disease of new born is-
   A. Prolonged prothrombin time *(AIIMS June 97)*
   B. Defective platelet count
   C. Prolonged bleeding time
   D. Prolonged thrombin time
292. A 78 year old man who lives alone and prepares his own food is found to have ecchymotic patches over posterior aspect of his lower extremities. He has haemorrhagic areas around hair follicles, hair are fragmented and splinter haemorrhages are present in nail beds and several hematomas are present in the muscles of arms and legs. PT and CT are normal. This clinical syndrome is most likely due to :
   A. Vitamin K deficiency *(AIIMS Nov 99)*
   B. Vitamin C deficiency
   C. Pyridoxine deficiency
   D. Vitamin A deficiency
293. A patient is on aspirin, what will be the finding?
   A. Prolonged BT *(AI 2007)*
   B. Prolonged PT
   C. Prolonged APTT
   D. Prolonged CT
294. Platelet function may be assessed by (select two options): *(PGI Dec 02)*
   A. Platelet adhesion Assays
   B. BT
   C. CT
   D. PTT
   E. APTT
295. Which of the following is not involved in intrinsic pathway? *(AI 2009)*
   A. Factor XII
   B. Factor XI
   C. Factor IX
   D. Factor VII
296. Which of the following helps in bridging the fibrin in a clot and stabilizes the clot? *(AI 2009)*
   A. Factor XIII
   B. Factor V
   C. Factor VIII
   D. Factor III
297. Converging point of both pathway in coagulation is at: *(PGI June 99)*
   A. Factor VIII
   B. Stuart factor X
   C. Factor IX
   D. Factor VII

298. Which of the following may present with isolated prolongation of prothrombin time (PT):
A. Factor VIII deficiency
B. Factor VII deficiency
C. Factor XII deficiency
D. Factor IX deficiency

299. A patient has normal PT and Platelet Count. The aPTT is increased and factor VIII levels are observed to be 60 Iu/dL (60%). There is no associated history of bleeding even after a surgical procedure. The most likely diagnosis is: *(AIIMS Nov 2011)*
A. Factor IX deficiency
B. Factor VIII inhibitors
C. Lupus anticoagulant
D. Thalassemia

300. Both PT and APTT are prolonged in
A. Factor II Deficiency
B. Thrombocytopenia
C. Factor VII Deficiency
D. Heparin Therapy

301. A child underwent a tonsillectomy at 6 years of age with no complications. He underwent a preoperative screening for bleeding at the age of 12 years before an elective laparotomy, and was found to have a prolonged partial thromboplastin time but normal Prothrombin time. There was no family history of bleeding. The patient is likely to have-
A. Acquired vitamin K deficiency
B. Acquired liver disease *(AIIMS Nov 2004)*
C. Factor XII deficiency
D. Mild hemophilia A

302. A 35 year old lady presents with an isolated prolongation of aPTT. Prothrombin time (PT) and platelet count are normal and there is no obvious bleeding tendency. Two years back, she was operated for cholecystectomy and had no adverse bleeding episode. Which of the following should be the next step in evaluating this patient
A. Factor VIII Assay *(AIIMS Nov 2010)*
B. Platelet aggregation test
C. Russell viper venom assay
D. Ristocetin cofactor assay

303. Which of the following statements about coagulation factor VII is not true *(AI 2009)*
A. Deficiency is inherited as an Autosomal Recessive trait
B. Deficiency is associated with prolonged APTT
C. Deficiency can be managed by Fresh Frozen plasma
D. Has a shorter half life in comparison to Hageman factor (XII)

304. Spontaneous muscle bleeding is typically seen in:
A. Hemophilia *(DNB 2009)*
B. Afibrinogenemia
C. Von Willebrand's disease
D. Scott's syndrome

Hemophilia

305. True about Haemophilia A are all *except* :
A. PTT increased *(AI 2001)*
B. PT increased
C. Clotting time is increased.
D. Serum levels of factor VIII are decreased.

306. Hemophilic A has following diagnostic features except- *(AI 97)*
a) ↓ VIII factor
b) ↑ PTT
c) ↑ PT
d) Normal BT

307. All are true about hemophilia, *except*
A. Increased Bleeding time (BT)
B. Decreased factor VIII *(AIIMS May 94)*
C. Decreased factor IX
D. Increased partial thromboplastin time (PTT)

308. Which of the following feature may be used to differentiate hemophilia A from von Willebrand disease.
A. Bleeding time
B. Prothrombin time
C. Partial thromboplastin time
D. Factor VIII levels

309. In a patient of Hemophilia to be taken for dental extraction true is all, *except* *(AIIMS Nov 01)*
A. All patients should be screened for HIV
B. Extraction should be done under general anaesthesia and skilled anaesthetic care
C. Factor VIII or cryoprecipitate can be needed
D. Dose of Lignocaine required for anaesthesia is same as that for normal individuals

Von Willebrands Factor (VWF) Disease

310. The coagulation profile in a 13-year old girl with Menorrhagia having Von Willebrands disease is:
A. Isolated prolonged PTT with a normal PT
B. Isolated prolonged PT with a normal PTT
C. Prolongation of both PT and PTT
D. Prolongation of thrombin time

311. True about Von Willebrand's disease is all *except* :
A. Increased bleeding time *(AIIMS 2000)*
B. Factor VIII c levels are decreased in circulation.
C. Increased platelet aggregation in response to Ristocetin
D. APTT is increased

312. True about Von Willebrand's disease is all *except* :
A. Increased bleeding time *(AIIMS 2000)*
B. Factor VIII c levels are decreased in circulation.
C. Defect in VWF is detected by ristocetin
D. APTT is increased

313. A seven year old girl presents with repeated episodes of bleeding into joints. APTT is prolonged and PT is normal. The most likely diagnosis is. *(AI 2009)*
A. Factor VIII deficiency (Hemophilia A)
B. Factor VII deficiency
C. Von Willebrand Disease
D. Factor XII deficiency

314. Best assay for deficiency of von Willebarnd factor is: *(PGI Dec 01)*
A. Bleeding time
B. BT + APTT
C. BT + APTT + vWF-ristocetin factor assay
D. PT

315. The commonest mode of inheritance of Von Willebrand's disease : *(AIIMS Dec 97)*
A. Codominant
B. Autosomal recessive
C. Autosomal dominant
D. X-linked recessive

Platelet Function Disorders

316. All of the following are inherited platelet function disorders Except:
A. Bernard Soulier syndrome
B. Glanzman Thrombasthenia
C. Wiskott Aldrich Syndrome
D. Von-Willebrand disease
E. Weber-Christian disease

317. Wiskott Aldrich syndrome is characterized by all Except: *(AIIMS Nov 2009)*
A. Thrombocytopenia
B. Autosomal recessive
C. Failure of aggregation of platelets in response to agonists
D. Eczema

318. A patient presents with Thrombocytopenia, eczema and recurrent infection. The most probable diagnosis is: *(DNB Dec 2009)*
A. Wiskott Aldrich syndrome
B. Chediak-Higashi syndrome
C. Job's syndrome
D. Bruton's Agammaglobulinemia

319. All of the following statements about Wiskott-Aldrich syndrome are true, Except *(AIIMS NOV 2008)*
A. Autosomal Recessive disorder
B. Eczematous Rash
C. Impaired platelet aggregation in response to agonist
D. Thrombocytopenia

320. The presence of small sized platelets on the peripheral smear is characteristic of: *(AIIMS Nov. 03)*
A. Idiopathic thrombocytopenic purpura
B. Bernard soulier syndrome
C. Disseminated intravascular coagulation
D. Wiskott Aldrich syndrome

321. Which is not true regarding Bernard soulier syndrome?
A. Ristocetin aggregation is normal *(AI 2007)*
B. Aggregation with collagen and ADP is normal
C. Large platelets
D. Thrombocytopenia

Thrombocytopenia and Purpura

322. Thrombocytopenia is not seen in: *(AI 1996)*
A. H.S. purpura
B. DIC
C. Leukemia
D. Metastasis

323. All of the following can cause megakaryocytic thrombocytopenia, except- *(AIIMS Nov 04)*
A. Idiopathic thrombocytopenic purpura
B. Systemic lupus erythematosus
C. Aplastic anemia
D. Disseminated intravascular coagulation (DIC)

324. Thrombocytopenia occurs in all *except*: *(AI 2001)*
A. Henoch schonlein purpura
B. TTP
C. DIC
D. Wiskott Aldrich syndrome

325. Platelet count is decreased in all of the following condition *except*: *(AIIMS Dec 98)*
A. H. S. Purpura
B. Idiopathic thrombocytopenic purpura
C. Thrombotic thrombocytopenic purpura
D. Systemic lupus erythematosus

326. Auto immune destruction of platelets is seen in
A. SLE
B. Chronic Lymphocytic leukemia
C. HIV
D. All the above

327. Autoimmune destruction of platelet is seen in :
A. SLE *(AIIMS May 95)*
B. Rheumatoid arthritis
C. Reiter disease
D. Polyarteritis nodosa

328. Palpable purpura could occur in the following conditions, *except*: *(AI 2005)*
A. Thrombocytopenia.
B. Small-vessel vasculitis.
C. Disseminated gonococcal infection.
D. Acute meningococcemia.

329. Palpable purpura is seen in *(AIIMS May 94)*
A. Idiopathic thrombocytopenic purpura (ITP)
B. Scurvy
C. Henoch Sconlein Purpura
D. Monoclonal cryoglobulinemia

Idiopathic Thrombocytopenic Purpura (ITP)

330. Cause of ITP is : *(AIIMS Feb 97)*
   A. Vasculitis
   B. Antibody to vascular epithelium
   C. Antibody to platelets
   D. Antibody to clotting factors

331. Idiopathic thrombocytopenic purpura is associated with all of the following Except:
   A. Splenomegaly
   B. Mucosal bleeding
   C. Thrombocytopenia
   D. Increased megakaryocytes

332. Which of the following statements about Acute Immune Thrombocytopenic Purpura is not true:
   A. Autoimmune Mediated *(PGI 09)*
   B. Massive Splenomegaly
   C. Increased Megakaryocytes in marrow
   D. IV immunoglobulins may be required
   E. Usually self limiting condition

333. A six year old boy presents with echymoses and petichiae all over the body 2 weeks after an upper respiratory tract infection Abdominal examination is unremarkable with no hepatosplenomegaly All of the following statements about the affecting condition are true Except: *(AIIMS Nov 99)*
   A. Bleeding into the joints is a common manifestation
   B. Bone marrow will show increased megakaryocytes
   C. Platelet count is decreased
   D. Condition resolves spontaneously in 80% of patients in 2 to 6 weeks

334. All of the following features about Idiopathic Thrombocytopenia are true, Except:
   A. Acute ITP is often proceded by Viral infections
   B. Chronic ITP is common in females
   C. Spontaneous remission is common in Chronic ITP
   D. Acute ITP is more common in children

335. The following laboratory determinants is abnormally prolonged in ITP : *(AI 2002)*
   A. APTT
   B. Prothrombin time
   C. Bleeding time
   D. Clotting time

336. Platelet transfusion is not indicated in: *(AI 1996)*
   A. Dilutional Thrombocytopenia
   B. Immunogenic Thrombocytopenia
   C. Aplastic Anemia
   D. DIC

Thrombotic Thrombocytopenic Purpura (TTP)

337. All of the following feature may be seen in thrombotic thrombocytopenic purpura, *except* :
   A. Fever *(AI 2002)*
   B. Haemolysis
   C. Hypertension
   D. Low platelets count

338. All of the following statements about Thrombotic thrombocytopenic purpura (TTP) are true, Except :
   A. Microangiopathic Hemolytic Anemia
   B. Thrombocytopenia
   C. Normal complement levels
   D. Grossly abnormal coagulation tests

339. All of the following are features of Thrombotic Thrombocytopenic purpura, Except *(AIIMS June 90)*
   A. Fever
   B. Hemolysis
   C. Hypertension
   D. Low platelet count

340. A person presents with fever and altered consciousness. Investigations reveal anemia with fragmented red blood cells, platelet count of 20,000/mm^3, serum creatinine of 3.0 mg % and normal PT and aPTT.
   Which of the following is the most appropriate treatment for the patient: *(PGI 09)*
   A. Plasma Exchange Therapy
   B. Corticosteroids and Intravenous Immunoglobulins
   D. Anticoagulation with Heparin
   E. Platelet transfusion

341. All of the following are used in the treatment of Thrombotic Thrombocytopenic Purpura, Except.
   A. Plasmapharesis *(PGI -09)*
   B. Corticosteroids
   C. Immunotherapy
   D. Heparin
   E. Platelet transfusion

Disseminated Intravascular Coagulation (DIC)

342. Causes of DIC include: *(PGI Dec 04)*
   A. Leukemia
   B. Masive transfusion
   C. Abruptio placentae
   D. All of the above

343. Causes of DIC include: *(PGI Dec 05)*
   A. Lymphoma
   B. Leukemia
   C. Adenocarcinoma Prostate
   D. Snake venom
   E. All of the above

344. False statement regarding DIC is: *(AI 2001)*
   A. Thrombocytopenia
   B. Decreased fibrinogen
   C. Decreased PTT
   D. Increased PT

345. The following is the finding seen in DIVC :
A. Increased fibrinogen , increased antithrombin III, increased thrombin-antithrombin III complexes
B. Increased FDP, decreased PT, increased antithrombin III *(AI 2007)*
C. Increased FDP, prolonged PT, increased thrombin-antithrombin complexes
D. Increased FDP, prolonged PT, reduced Platlets

346. The most sensitive test for DIC is: *(AI 2001)*
A. Serum fibrinogen levels
B. Serum levels of fibrin degradation products (FDP)
C. Prolonged PT and PTT
D. Thrombocytopenia

347. Bleeding in DIC is most closely related to:
A. Raised fibrin degradation products level in blodd
B. Prolong prothrombin time *(AIIMS June 98)*
C. Low serum fibrinogen level
D. Raised thrombin time

348. DIC is commonly seen in-
A. MI AML
B. M2 AML
C. M3 AML
D. M4 AML

349. Disseminated intravascular coagulation (DIC) differs from thrombotic thrombocytopenic purpura. In this reference the DIC is most likely characterized by:
A. Significant numbers of schistocytes
B. A brisk reticulocytosis *(AI 2004)*
C. Decreased coagulation factor levels
D. Significant thrombocytopenia

Hypercoagulable States / Thrombosis

General

350. All are hypercoagulable states, except :
A. Protein C resistance *(AIIMS June 98)*
B. Factor V Leiden deficiency
C. Antiphospholipid antibody
D. Polycythemia

351. All of the following conditions are associated with venous and arterial thrombotic events, except: *(AIIMS May 2011)*
A. Paroxysmal Nocturnal Haemoglobinuria (PNH)
B. Disseminated Intravascular Coagulation
C. Idiopathic Thrombocytopenic Purpura (ITP)
D. Heparin Induced Thrombocytopenia (HIT)

352. All of the following conditions predispose to thrombosis *except*: *(AIIMS Dec 98)*
A. Paroxysmal nocturnal hemoglobinuria
B. Homocystinurea
C. Hypomagnesemia
D. Behcets syndrome

353. Coagulation defects associated with ↑ed coagulation are seen in:
A. ↑ Protein C *(PGI Dec 06)*
B. ↑ Protein B
C. ↑ Anti thrombin III
D. Dysfibrinogenemia

354. Hypercoagulability due to defective factor V gene is called : *(AIIMS Nov. 03)*
A. Lisbon mutation
B. Leiden mutation
C. Antiphospholipid syndrome
D. Inducible thrombocytopenia syndrome

355. Most common inherited thrombotic disorder is :
A. Protein C deficiency *(PGI Dec. 05)*
B. Protein S deficiency
C. Factor V leiden mutation
D. Prothrombin gene mutation
E. tPA deficiency

356. Predisposing factor for arterial thrombosis:
A. AT III deficiency *(PGI Dec. 04)*
B. Protein S deficiency
C. Protein C deficiency
D. Homocystenemia

357. All of the following are aquired causes of Hypercoagulability, Except *(AI 2009)*
A. Infection
B. Inflammatory Bowel disease
C. Myeloproliferative disorders
D. Prolonged surgery > 1 hour

358. Causes of Deep venous thrombosis include all of the following, Except. *(AI 2009)*
A. Diabetes Mellitus
B. Oral contraceptives
C. Paroxysmal Nocturnal Hemoglobinuria (PNH)
D. Prolonged surgery

359. A patient is admitted with 3rd episode of deep venous thrombosis. There is no history of any associated medical illness. All of the following investigations are required for establishing the diagnosis *except* :
A. Protein C deficiency *(AIIMS Nov 2004)*
B. Antithrombin III deficiency
C. Antibodies to factor VIII
D. Antibodies to cardiolipin

Antiphospholipid Syndrome

360. Anti Phospholipid Syndrome (APS) is associated with all of the following Except: *(AI 2008)*
A. Pancytopenia
B. Recurrent abortions
C. Venous thrombosis
D. Pulmonary hypertension

361. Antiphospholipid Antibody (APLA) syndrome is associated with all of the following except: *(AI 2010)*
A. Bleeding disorders
B. Thrombotic disorders
C. Coagulation disorders
D. Recurrent fetal loss

362. All of the following statements about Antiphospholipid Antibody Syndrome (APLAb) are true, Except : *(AI 2010)*
A. Single titre of Anticardiolipin is diagnostic
B. Commonly presents with recurrent fetal loss
C. May cause pulmonary hypertension
D. Warfarin is given as treatment

363. The following condition is not associated with an Anti-phopholipid syndrome: *(AI 2002)*
A. Venous thrombosis
B. Recurrent foetal loss
C. Thrombocytosis
D. Neurological manifestations

364. All are true regarding lupus anticoagulant except- *(AIIMS Sep 96)*
A. Thrombocytosis
B. Increased abortions
C. Rashes
D. Arterial thrombosis

365. All are true regarding Lupus anticoagulant, EXCEPT- *(AIIMS Nov 93)*
A. Increased abortions
B. Arterial thrombosis
C. Rashes
D. Increased PT

366. All of the following statements about Lupus Anticoagulant are true, Except. *(AI 2009)*
A. May present with an isolated prolongation of APTT
B. May present with Recurrent Abortions
C. May occur with minimal clinical manifestations
D. Thrombotic spells can be followed by severe life threatening haemmorrhage

367. Lupus anticoagulants may cause all of the following except:
A. Recurrent abortion
B. False+ve VDRL results
C. Increase prothrombin time
D. Arterial thrombosis

368. Which of the following is recommended in a woman with Antiphospholipid Antibodies and history of prior abortions / still birth: *(AI 2010)*
A. Aspirin only
B. Aspirin + Low molecular weight Heparin
C. Aspirin + Low molecular weight Heparin + Prednisolone.
D. No Treatment

Hemolytic Uremic Syndrome

369. All of the following statements are true about Hemolytic uramic syndrome except- *(AI 97)*
A. Uraemia
B. Hypofibhrinogenemia
C. Thrombocytopenia
D. Positive coomb's test

370. Shigella associated hemolytic uramic syndrome is associated with all of the following except-
A. Hyperkalemia
B. Thrombocytopenia
C. Neurological symptom
D. Renal micro thrombi

Budd Chiari Syndrome

371. Commonest cause of Budd Chiari syndrome is- *(AI 97)*
A. Valve in the IVC
B. Hepatocellular carcinoma
C. Paroxysmal nocturnal hemoglobinuria
D. Renal cell carcinoma

372. Most common cause of Budd Chiari syndrome is: *(AIIMS May 94)*
A. Idiopathic
B. Valves in hepatic veins
C. Hepatocellular carcinoma
D. Thrombosis of hepatic veins

373. In Budd Chiari syndrome, the site of venous thrombosis is-
A. Infrahepatic inferior vena cava
B. Infrarenal inferior vena cava
C. Hepatic veins
D. Portal veins

374. What is the most common cause for Budd chiary syndrome- *(AIIMS Nov 2000)*
A. Right ventricular failure
B. PNH
C. Valve in hepatic veins
D. Polycythemia vera

Blood Transfusion

375. Which of the following statements about Acute Hemolytic blood transfusion reactions is true:
A. Complement mediated Hemolysis is seen
B. Type III Hypersensitivity is responsible for most cases *(PGI June 04)*
C. rarely life threatening
D. Renal blood flow is always mainatained
E. No need for stopping transfusion

376. True about Blood transfusions (select two options) : *(PGI June 98)*
A. Antigen 'D' determines Rh positivity
B. Febrile reaction is due to HLA antigens
C. Anti-D is naturally occurring antibody
D. Cryoprecipitates contains all coagulation factors

377. MC blood transfusion reaction is- *(AI 2008)*
A. Febrile nonhemolytic transfusion reaction
B. Hemolysis
C. Transmission of infections
D. Electrolyte imabalnce

378. All of the following infections may be transmitted via blood transfusion, except: *(AI 2002)*
A. Parvo B-19
B. Dengue virus
C. Cytomegalo virus
D. Hepatitis G virus

379. All of the following viruses may be transmitted by blood transfusion Except: *(AIIMS May 09)*
A. Parvovirus B-19
B. Hepatitis G
C. Epstein Bar virus
D. Cytomegalovirus

380. Which of the following is the least likely complication after massive blood transfusion: *(AIIMS May 09)*
A. Hyperkalemia
B. Citrate toxicity
C. Hypothermia
D. Metabolic Acidosis

381. All of the following are major complications of massive transfusion, except: *(AI 2006)*
A. Hypokalemia
B. Hypothermia
C. Hypomagnesemia
D. Hypocalcemia

382. Which of the following investigations should be done immediately to best confirm a non matched blood transfusion reaction: *(AI 2010)*
A. Indirect Coomb's test
B. Direct Coomb's test
C. Antibody in patient's serum
D. Antibody in donor serum

383. Blood components products are: *(PGI Dec 05)*
A. Whole blood
B. Platelets
C. Fresh frozen plasma
D. Leukocyte reduced RBC

384. Cryoprecipitate contains all except- *(AIIMS Nov 07)*
A. Factor VIII
B. Factor IX
C. Fibrinogen
D. VWF

385. Arterial blood Gas analysis in a bottle contaiing heparin causes a decrease in value of :
A. pCO_2
B. HCO_3^-
C. pH
D. All of the above

Miscellaneous

386. A patient with blood pressure of 90/60 mm Hg presents with pronounced cyanosis. Blood drawn from peripheral veins is observed to be chocolate brown in colour. The most likely diagnosis is:
A. Methaemoglobinemia
B. Hypovolemic shock
C. Cardiogenic shock
D. Hemorrhagic shock

387. Low Erythropoetin levels are seen in: *(DNB 2012)*
A. Aplstic Anemia
B. Renal failure
C. Obesity
D. Hepatoma

388. While handling a febrile neutropenic patient all are essential *except* : *(AI 1998)*
A. Repeated hand washing of hospital person
B. White cell infusion
C. Prophylactic antibiotic
D. Colony stimulating factor for macrophages

389. All of the following are Preleukemic conditions, Except: *(AIIMS 2011)*
A. Paroxysmal Nocturnal Haemoglobinuria (PNH)
B. Paroxysmal Cold Haemoglobinuria (PCH)
C. Myelodysplasia
D. Aplastic anemia

390. Splenomegaly is least likely to be associated with:
A. Chronic Myeloid Leukemia (CML)
B. Polycythemia Rubra Vera *(AIIMS Nov 2010)*
C. Myelofibrosis
D. Primary Thrombocytosis

391. Which of the following drugs is recommended for the treatment of Heparin Induced thrombocytopenia *(AI 2010)*
A. Abciximab
B. Lepirudin
C. Warfarin
D. Alteplase

ANSWERS, REFERENCES, EXPLANATIONS AND RELEVANT HIGH YIELD FACTS

Hypochromic Microcytic Anemias

Differential Diagnosis/Approach

1. **Answer is B (Thallassemia):** Harrison 18th/p 887, 889 *Harrisons 17th/663,665; Harrisons 16th/617,619; Board Review Series (BRS) Pediatrics (2004)/394*

Thalassemia is associated with Hypochromic Microcytic Anemia.

Hereditary spherocytosis, sickle cell anemia and fanconi's anemia are associated with normocytic normochromic anemia

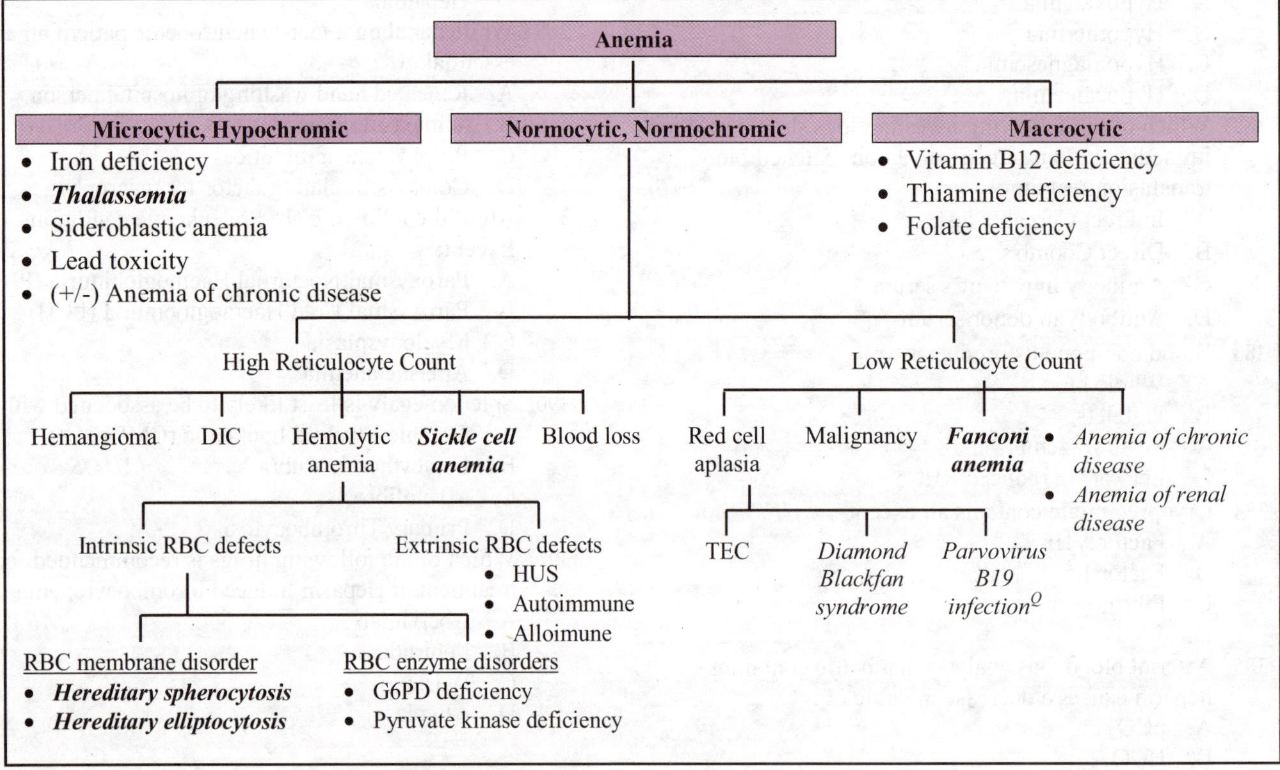

Note:

*Anemia of chronic disease may present with microcytic hypochromic anemia

Anemia of chronic disease: Normocytic Normochromic > Microcytic Hypochromic

2. **Answer is D (Fanconi's anemia):** Harrison 18th/p 847, 848 *Refer previous question; Harrison 15th/ 663, Harrison 17th/ 631, 632; API edn 8th/ 796*

Fanconi's anemia is a congenital disorder responsible for a form of aplastic anemia. It is a cause of normocytic normochromic anemia, and not microcytic hypochromic anemia.

Causes of microcytic hypochromic anaemia
• *Iron deficiency anaemia*
• *Thalassemia*
• *Sideroblastic anaemia*
• *Lead poisoning*
• *Anemia of chronic disease (+/-)*

3. **Answer is D (Fanconi's Anemia):** Harrison 18th/p 847, 848 *Harrison 15th/ 663, Harrison 17th/ 631, 632; API edn 8th/ 796;*

Refer previous question

Fanconi's anemia is congenital disorder responsible for a form of aplastic anemia. It does not produce a microcytic hypochromic picture. It causes a normocytic normochromic anemia.

Causes of Microcytic Hypochromic Anemia
• *Iron deficiency anemia* • *Thalassemia* • *Sideroblastic anemia* • *Lead poisoning* • *Anemia of chronic disease (+/-)*

Lead poisoning

- Lead causes inhibition of several enzymes involved in haem synthesis including ALA synthetase and leads to sideroblastic anemia with a microcytic hypochronic anemia.
- The characteristic haematological features of lead poisoning include: *Kumar Clark 15th/ 416*

- Sideroblastic anemia Q
- Haemolysis Q
- Punctate basophilia Q

4. **Answer is D and E (Sickle cell Anemia; Herediatry Spherocytosis):** Harrison 18th/p 848 *Harrison 17th/632*

Sickle cell anemia and Hereditary Spherocytosis do not cause microcytic hypochromic anemia

Causes of Microcytic Hypochromic Anemia
• *Iron deficiency anemia* • *Thalassemia* • *Sideroblastic anemia* • *Lead poisoning* • *Anemia of chronic disease (+/-)*

5. **Answer is B (Reduced Total RBC distribution width)**

Microcytic Hypochromic Anemias are typically associated with a Normal or High Red Cell Distribution Width

Condition / Test (normal values)	Iron deficiency	Thalassemia	Sideroblastic anemia	Anemia of chronic disease
Smear Microcytic (MCV<80)	Microcytic hypochromic	Microcytic hypochromic	Microcytic hypochromic	Normocytic normochromic > Micro/hypochromic (but Micro/Hypo may be present)
Serum iron (50-150µg/dl)	Low (<30)	Normal	Normal	↓ (<50)
TIBC (300-360 µg/dl)	High (>360)	Normal	Normal (Chandrasoma Taylor)	↓ (<300)
% Saturation (30-50%)	< 10 (↓ed)	N or ↑ed (30-80)	N or ↑ (30-80)	↓ (10-20)
Ferritin (µg/l) (50-200 µg/L)	< 15 (↓ed)	↑ (50-300)	↑ (50-300)	Normal or ↑ (30-200)
Hemoglobin pattern	Normal	Abnormal	Normal	Normal
Free Erythrocyte Protporphrin	↑ed	Normal	↑ed	↑ed
RDW	↑ed	Normal	Normal	Normal

6. **Answer is D (Decreased Free Erythrocyte protoporphyrin):**

Free Erythrocyte protoporphyrin is typically normal in Thalassemia while it is increased in other forms of Microcytic Hypochronic anemias like iron deficiency anemia, sideroblastic anemia and anemia of chronic disease.

Hematology

1

Microcytic Hypochromic Anemias are typically associated with a Normal or High Red Cell Distribution Width

Condition / Test (normal values)	Iron deficiency	Thalassemia	Sideroblastic anemia	Anemia of chronic disease
Free Erythrocyte Protporphrin	↑ed	Normal	↑ed	↑ed

7. Answer is B (Anemia of chronic disease): Harrison 18th/p 848 *Harrison 17th/ 631*

Hypochromic microcytic anemia with decreased serum iron and decreased TIBC is characteristic of anemia of chronic disease.

Hypochromic microcytic anemia with ↓serum iron and ↑TIBC: iron Deficeincy Anemia
Hypochromic microcytic anemia with ↓ serum iron and ↓ TIBC : Anemia of Chronic disease

Condition / Test (normal values)	Iron deficiency	Thalassemia	Sideroblastic anemia	Anemia of chronic disease
Serum iron (50-150μg/dl)	Low (<30)	Normal	Normal	↓ (<50)
TIBC (300-600 μg/dl)	High (>360)	Normal	Normal (Chandrasoma Taylor)	↓ (<300)

8. Answer is B & C(↓ TIBC;↑Ferritin): Harrison 18th/p 848 *Harrison 17th/632*

Anemia of chronic disease is associated with decreased TIBC and increased serum Ferritin while Iron deficiency anemia is associated with Increased TIBC and reduced serum Ferritin

<u>Differential diagnosis of Microcytic Hypochromic Anemia</u>

Parameters	Iron deficiency	Chronic Inflammatory
Smear	Microcytic hypochromic + target cell	Normocytic Normochromic > Microcytic Hypochromic
Se Fe	< 30 (↓)	↓ (< 50)
TIBC	***> 360 (↑)***	***↓ (< 300)***
Saturation	< 10 (↓)	↓ (10-20)
Ferritin	< 15 (↓)	↑ (30-200)
Free Erythrocyte Protporphrin	***↑ed***	***↑ed***

9. Answer is A (Iron deficiency anemia): Harrison 18th/p 847 *Harrison 16th edn /591; Harrison 17th edn /631*

Hypochromic microcytic anemia with decreased serum iron and an increased total iron binding capacity (TIBC) suggests a diagnosis of 'iron deficiency anemia'

Parameter	Normal index	Patient in question	Inference
Hb	Male 14-18 g/dl Female 12-16 g/dl	7.8 g/dl	↓
Serum Iron	50-150 μg/dl	15 μg/dl	↓
% Saturation	30-50%	-	-
Serum Ferritin	50-200 μg/L	-	-
Total iron binding capacity	300-600 μg/dl	420 μg/dl	↑
HbA_2	1.5 to 3.5% of total Hb.	2.4%	N
HbF	<2% of total Hb.	1-3%	N

<u>Remember:</u>

- ***Hypochromic microcytic anemia with decreased serum iron and increased TIBC is iron deficiency anemia***[Q]
- ***Hypochromic microcytic anemia with decreased serum iron and decreased TIBC is anemia of chronic disease***[Q]

Differential diagnosis of Microcytic Hypochromic Anemia

Parameters	Iron deficiency	Thalassemia	Sideroblastic	Chronic Inflammatory
Smear	Microcytic hypochromic + target cell	Microcytic hypochromic	Variable	Normocytic
Se Fe	< 30 (↓)	N	N	↓ (< 50)
TIBC	> 360 (↑)	N	N	↓ (< 300)
Saturation	< 10 (↓)	↑ (30-80)	↑ (30-80)	↓ (10-20)
Ferritin	< 15 (↓)	↑ (50-300)	↑ (50-300)	↑ (30-200)

10. Answer is C (Thalassemia): *Harrisons 16th/589; Pediatric complaints and diagnostic dilemmas by Ludwig and Shah (2003)/275; Interpretation of Diagnostic tests by Wallach/400*

Erythrocyte protoporphyrin levels are characteristically normal in Thalassemia

Free Erythrocyte Protoporphyrin is a useful screening test for microcytic hypochromic anemias. Free Erythrocyte protoporphyrin levels are increased in iron deficiency anemias, lead poisoning many cases of sideroblastic anemia and anemias of chronic disease. Erythrocyte protoporphyrin levels are normal in Thalassemias.

Parameter	Iron Deficiency	Lead Poisoning	Thalassemia trait	Chronic disease
Free Erythrocyte Protoporphyrin (FEP)	↑ed	↑ed	Normal	↑ed

11. Answer is A (Iron Deficiency Anemia): *Wintrobe's Hematology 12th/795,4; Harrison's Manual of Oncology (2007)/ 138*

Microcytic Hypochronic Anemia (↓MCV, ↓MCH) with an elevated Red cell distribution width *(Nomal RDW < 14.5%)* ***suggests a diagnosis of Iron deficiency anemia***

'Among microcytic anemias, the red cell distribution width (RDW) distinguishes between iron deficiency anemia (↑RDW) and thalassemia (Normal RDW)' - Harrison's Manual of Oncology (2007)/138

'RDW is particularly useful in characterizing microcytic anemia, allowing to distinguish between uncomplicated iron deficiency anemia (High RDW, Normal to Low MCV) and uncomplicated heterozygous thalassemia (Normal RDW, Low MCV)' - Wintrobe's Hematology 12th/ - 4

Red Cell Distribution Width (RDW) and Evaluation of Anemia

- *Red cell distribution width is a measure of anisocytosis and quantitates cellular volume heterogeneity*
- *An increased RDW suggests a state of increased anisocytosis as seen early in iron deficiency anemia,* and is especially useful in charachterizing microcytic anemias.
- MCV and RDW, together can be used to classify various types of anemias
- *The normal RDW is less than 14.5%*
- *Anisocytosis is an early and prominent finding in iron deficiency,* often detectable before significant microcytosis, hypochromia or anemia is apparent and hence *RDW tends to be elevated early in iron deficiency anemia. In contrast, anisocytosis tends to be mild or absent in Thalassemia.*
- *An increased RDW tends to be 90% to 100% sensitive for iron deficiency anemia (Although it is only 50% to 70% specific).*

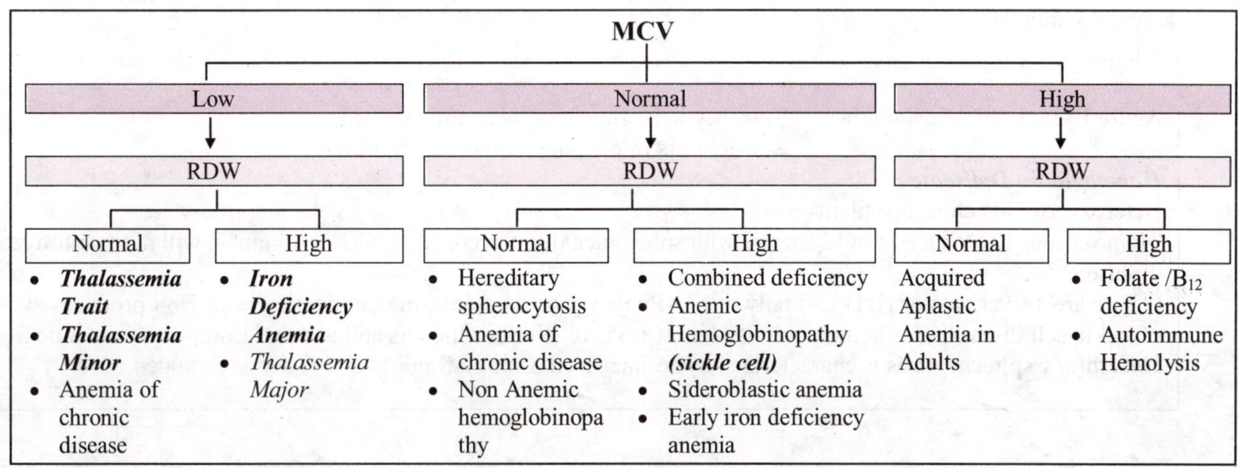

Note: ***Although a high RDW may be seen in Thalasemia major, the clinical presentation of this patient with haemoglobin of 7.0 at the age of 16 years is not consistent with a diagnosis of Thalassemia major.***

1

Hematology

12. Answer is B (Iron deficiency): Harrison 18th/p 847, 848 *Harrison 16th edn /589, 590; Harrison 17th edn /631, 632*

Microcytic hypochromic anemia with increased levels of red cell protoporphyrin suggests a diagnosis of iron deficiency anemia.

Parameter	Normal	Patient	Inference
Hb	13-18 g/dl	6.5	↓ed (Anemia)
MCV	86-98 μm^3	65	↓ed (microcytosis)
MCH	28-33 g/dl	15	↓ed (hypochromia)

Protoporphyrin is an intermediate in the pathway of heme synthesis. Under conditions in which synthesis of heme is impaired, protoporphyrin accumulates within the red cell. Protoporphyrin levels thus determine a state of iron deficiency i.e. when there is inadequate iron to combine with protoporphyrin to form haem, the levels of protoporphyrin increases.

Normal	Iron deficiency (↑ed)
30 µg/dl of red cells	100 µg/dl of red cells

- Microcytic hypochromic anemia with increased levels of red cell protoporphyrin is characteristic of iron deficiency anemia, but may also be seen in lead poisoning, anemia of chronic diseases and many cases of sideroblastic anemia.
- Red cell protoporphyrin will not be increased in Thalassemia as serum iron is normal or increased in them.

13. Answer is A (Iron deficiency anemia) : *Read text below*

Parameter	Normal	Patient in question	Inference
Hb	13 – 16 gm %	3.8 gm %	Anemia
MCV	79-93.3 fl	58 fl	Microcytic
MCH	26.7-31.9 pg/cell	19.4 pg/cell	Hypochromia
Inference	**Hypochromic Microcytic Anemia**		

The peripheral blood smear in patient with iron deficiency anemia:

- Microcytosis
- Hypochromia
- Poikilocytosis & Anisocytosis (with increasing iron deficiency the RBC's become deformed and misshappen) -*Nelson*
- Normoblasts : 'The bone marrow reveals a mild to moderate increase in erythropoetic activity manifested by increased number of normoblasts. - *Robbins*

Controversy 'Target cells' :

According to Harrison's text, target cells are not seen with iron deficiency anemia, but CMDT states :
'Severe iron deficiency will produce bizzare peripheral blood smear with severely hypochromic cells, target cells, hypochromic pencil shaped cells and occassionally small number of nucleated red blood cells." – CMDT 2004/464

I would thus conclude that target cells are unusual with iron deficiency and when present should suggest either a globin chain production defect one of thallassemia or liver disease. Neverthless occasional target cells may be seen with iron deficiency anemia.

Excluding other three options :

Acute Lymphoblastic anemia : - Normocytic Normochromic anemia is seen
- Normoblasts in peripheral blood are unlikely

Haemoglobin D disease :
Heterozygos D is clinically silent
'Homozygous D produces a mild anemia with splenomegally. Severe anemia (Hb 3.8 gm%) will not result from HbD disease.
[There are 16 variants of HbD and only one D-Punjab (Los Angeles), in combination with HbS produces symptoms of sickle cell disease. This hemoglobin is seen in 1-3% of Western Indians and in some Europeans with a tie to India]
Hereditary spherocytosis is characterized by an increased osmotic fragility and is hence excluded.

14. Answer is C (Thallassemia minor): *Refer text below*

The patient in question has a microcytic anemia (excludes Megaloblastic anemia) and has never required blood transfusion (excludes Thalassemia major). This patient may therefore have either an Iron deficiency anemia or Thalassemia minor.
Microcytic anemia (MCV 55 fl) with a normal RBC count (4.5 x 10^{12}/L) favours a diagnosis of Thalassemia minor over Iron Deficiency Anemia.

Thalassemia minor is typically characterized by a normal or elevated RBC count while in Iron deficiency anemia the RBC count is significantly reduced.

Approach

Parameter	Normal values	Patient values	Interpretation	Mentzer's Index	
RBC count	(M) 4.3 – 5.6 x 10^{12}/L (F) 4.0 – 5.2 x 10^{12}/L	4.5 x 10^{12}/L (F)	*Normal range*	*MCV/RBC Count*	***A value of Mentzer index below 13 is highly predictive of Thalassemia***
MCV	79 – 93.3 fl	55 fl	*Reduced MCV (Microcytic Anemia)*	*55/4.5 =12.22 (<13)*	

<u>The patient in question has a microcytic anemia with a normal Red cell count and has never required a blood transfusion</u>

The patient in question may have either an Iron Deficiency Anemia or Thalassemia Minor

Megaloblastic Anemia *can be excluded since the MCV is reduced* **Thalassemia Major** *can be excluded since the patient has never required blood transfusion to the age of 30*

<u>Special parameters to distinguish Thalassemia Minor from Iron Deficiency Anemia</u>

Special Parameters	**Thalassemia Minor**	**Iron Deficiency Anemia**
Red Cell Distribution width (RDW)	*Normal*	*High*
Free Erythrocyte Protoporphyrin (FEP)	*Normal*	*High*
Red Blood Cell Count	*Normal or Increased*	*Reduced*

<u>Several Red Cell indices</u> may help to distinguish Iron deficiency Anemia from Thalassemia minor and various formulas have been evolved to make this distinction.
*The most commonly used index is the **<u>Mentzer Index</u>**, which utilizes MCV and Red cell Count.*

Mentzer Index = MCV / Red Cell Count

<u>Mentzer Index</u> utilizes the finding that the Red Cell counts are higher in Thalassemia minor in comparison to Iron deficiency anemia to distinguish these two causes of microcytic hypochromic anemia.

Since RBC count is higher in Thalassemia minor the Mentzer Index will be low. *Since RBC count is lower in Iron deficiency anemia the Mentzer Index will be high*	*Mentzer Index = MCV / RBC Count*

Index	Thalassemia Minor	Iron Deficiency Anemia
Mentzer Index (MCV/RBC count)	*< 13*	*> 13*

A value of Mentzer index below 13 is highly predictive of Thalassemia.

15. Answer is C (Haemochromatosis): *Harrison 16th edn /2259, 663, 2302, 590; Harrisons 17th edn /2432, 2433, 631*

None of the conditions other than haemochromatosis present with an increased serum iron along with an increased serum ferritin and percent saturation of transferrin.

<u>Haemochromatosis</u> is a disorder of iron storage in which an in appropriate increase in intestinal iron absorption results in deposition of excessive amounts of iron in parenchymal cells with eventual tissue damage and impaired function of organs.
Diagnosis is established after assessment of parenchymal iron stores.

Parameter	Haemochromatosis	Iron deficiency anemia	Anemia of chronic disease
Serum iron	Increased	Low	Decreased
% saturation of transferrin	↑ed : > 50% saturation	↓ed : < 10 % saturation	Decreased
Serum ferritin	↑ed	Decreased	Normal or Increased

Lead poisoning may present with :

- A normocytic normochromic anemia [Q] with basophilic stippling [Q].
- Microcytic hypochromic picture may be seen
- Elevated free erythrocyte protophyrin may be seen

Iron Deficiency Anemia

1

16. Answer is A (Chronic renal failure): *Refer text below*

Chronic Renal failure causes a normocytic normochromic anemia due to deficiency of Erythropoetin.
Iron deficiency anemia may develop in patients with chronic renal failure who are on dialysis because of the blood lost in the dialysis equipment.

However, chronic renal failure remains the single best answer of exclusion.

Hematology

Causes of iron deficiency anemia

Blood Loss		Diet
• Gastrointestinal bleeding - Hemorrhoid - Angiodysplasia of the colon - Hereditary, hemorrhagic, teleangiectasia syndrome (Osler-Weber-Rendu syndrome) - Peptic ulcer - Nonsteroidal, anti-inflammatory drugs - Oral anticoagulation - Hiatal hernia - Meckel diverticulum - Diverticulosis of the colon - Intestinal polyps - ***Carcinoma*** - Inflammatory bowel disease - Hookworm: Nector Americanus, Ancylostoma duodenale - Shistosoma: S. Mansoni, S. hematobium - Trichuris	• Menstruation • Frequent blood donations • Erythrocyturia: bladder neoplasm • Hemoglobinuria - Paroxysmal, nocturnal hemoglobinuria - Erythrocyte fragmentation in prosthetic heart valves • Factitious anemia • Intravenous and intra-arterial drug abuse • ***Hemodialysis*** • Nosocomial blood loss due to frequent venisection	**Malabsorption** • Achlorhydria • Chronic, atrophic gastritis -Gastric resection and bypass -Vagotomy -Intestinal bypass operations • ***Celiac disease (=nontropical sprue)*** • Tropical sprue **Increased iron requirements** • Pregnancy and lactation • Growth

17. Answer is C (Hookworm infection): *Refer text below*

The indices of the patient in question suggests a diagnosis of Microcytic Hypochromic anemia. The single best cause for his anemia is a Hookworm infection which causes an iron deficiency anemia due to persistant gastrointestinal blood loss.

Phenytoin and Blind loop syndrome are causes for Macrocytic anemias

CRF causes a normocytic normochromic anemia.

18. Answer is D (Alkaline pH): Harrison 18th/p 845 *Harsh Mohan 4th/316, Harrison 17th/629, 630*

Iron absorption is increased by acidic pH of stomach and not by an alkaline pH.

Factors that enhance / reduce iron absorption

	Enhanced absorption	Reduced absorption
Dietary factors	• Increased heme iron • Increased animal food • ***Ferrous iron salts***	• Decreased heme iron • Decreased animal foods • Ferric iron salts
Luminal factors	• ***Acid pH*** • Low molecular weight soluble chelates	• ***Alkaline pH (e.g. pancreatic secretion)*** • Insoluble iron complexes
Systemic factors	• ***Iron deficiency*** • Increased erythropoesis • ***Pregnancy*** • ***Hypoxia***	• ***Iron overloaded*** • Decreased erythropoiesis • Inflammatory disorders

19. Answer is A (Increased TIBC decreased serum Ferritin) ; Harrison 18th/p 847 *Harrison 16th edn /592; Harrison 17th edn /631*

Iron deficiency anemia is associated with increased TIBC, decreased serum Ferritin.

Serum iron	**TIBC**	**Transferrin saturation**	**Ferritin**
Serum iron reflects the amount of circulating iron bound to transferrin	TIBC is an indirect measure of the circulating transferrin	This is a measure of transferrin saturated with iron and is given by : Serum iron/TIBC x 100	Within cells iron is stored complexed to protein as ferritin
Normal range of serum iron is 50 to 150 μg/dL	Normal range for TIBC is 300 to 360 μg/dl	Normal transferrin saturation ranges between 25 – 50%.	Normal values for serum ferritin depend on age and gender Adult males 100mg/L Adult females 30 μg/L.
Iron deficiency anemia is associated with ***decreased serum iron levels of < 30 μg/dL***	Iron deficiency anemia is associated ***with increased TIBC > 360 μg/dl***	Iron deficiency anemia is associated with ***decreased transferrin saturation below 18%*** *(< 10%; H16th / table)*	Iron deficiency states are associated with ***decreased serum ferritin to <15 μg/dl.***

20. Answer is B (Decrease in serum ferritin): *Harrison 16th edn /630; Chandrasoma Taylor 3rd/687*

The first stage of iron deficiency is depletion of iron stores which is associated with a decrease in levels of serum ferritin levels only. *As long as some stores are still available, other indices viz. SI, TIBC, Red cell Protoporphyrin levels continue to be within normal limits.*

21. Answer is D (Bone marrow iron is decreased earlier than serum iron): Harrison 18th/p 846 *Harrison 17th/630*

Serum levels of iron decrease after bone marrow iron is decreased.

As long as iron stores are present (serum ferritin, bone marrow iron), and can be mobilised, the serum iron, Total Iron Binding Capacity (TIBC) and red cell protoporphyrin levels remain within normal limits.

Iron deficiency anemia is associated with decreased ferritin levels and an increased TIBC.

22. Answer is B (Serum ferritin levels): Harrison 18th/p 846 *Harrisons 16th/ 589; Harrison 17th edn / 630*

Iron deficiency is best detected by measurement of serum ferritin.

'The test of choice for screening and diagnosis of iron deficiency is the serum ferritin. Ferritin is the storage protein of iron which correlates best with marrow iron stores. The test is highly sensitive and specific for the diagnosis of iron deficiency' -'Primary care medicine' 6th/632

1

Hematology

'Serum Ferritin indicates the iron store status and decreased serum ferritin is the first most sensitive and specific test for iron deficiency. The levels <15µg/L indicate depletion of iron stores and is diagnostis of iron deficiency (normal 15-300 µg/L)' - Essentials in Hematology & Clinical Pathology (JP) 2012/22

This is so because:

- The first stage of iron deficiency is depletion of iron stores which is associated with a decrease in levels of serum ferritin levels only.
- As long as some stores are still available, other indices viz. SI, TIBC, Red cell Protoporphyrin levels continue to be within normal limits.
- As the patients are not anemic yet, RBC morphology is essentially normal.

Remember

- Iron is stored as Ferritin
- Ferritin found in circulation is in equilibrium with tissue ferritin
- Serum Ferritin levels fall as iron stores are depleted

23. Answer is B (Serum ferritin): *Harrison's 18th/847*

Serum ferritin levels are the best marker for assessment of iron deficiency.

24. Ans. Answer is B (Serum Ferritin): *Harrison's 18th/847*

The most suitable test to assess iron status in serum Ferritin.

'Under steadystate conditions the serum ferritin is the most convenient laboratory test to estimate iron stores as the serum ferritin levels correlate with total iron body stores' - Harrison

25. Answer is A (Hypersegmented neutrophils): *Harrison 18th/846, 847; Harrison 17th/630, 631; API 8th/794, 795, 796*

***Hypersegmented neutrophils are a feature of megaloblastic anemia, and not iron deficiency anemia. This is such a characteristic finding, that a single cell with a nucleus of six or more lobes Q should raise immediate suspicion of a megaloblastic anemia** – Harrisons 16th/ 605*

- Iron deficiency anemia is the commonest cause of anemia in India.
- It is a hypochromic, microcytic anemia and MCHC may well be less than 50% (Hypochromia).
- Initially cells tend to be microcytic and not hypochromic thus microcytosis precedes hypochromia. At lower haemoglobin levels both microcytosis and hypochromia become pronounced – *Harrison 16th/ 589*

26. Answer is D (Decrease in absorption with improvement of symptoms): Harrison 18th/p 848, 849 *Harrison 17th/632; Kelley's Essential of Internal Medicine 2nd/508*

***'Percentage absorption of iron falls progressively as iron deficiency is corrected'**-Kelly's Essentials of Internal Medicine 2nd/508*

***'As the hemoglobin levels rise, erythropoietin stimulation decreases and the amount of iron reabsorbed is reduced'** .*
– Harrison 17th/632

Oral therapy for iron deficiency anemia

- A dose of 300mg of elemental iron is given per day in divided doses
- ***300mg of elemental iron gives about 50mg of absorbed iron per day** (and not 100 mg of absorbed iron)*
- ***Typically the reticulocyte count should begin to increase in 4-7 days after initiation of therapy and peak at 1½ weeks** (not at 3-4 weeks)*
- ***Typically the Hb levels should be fully corrected within 1 month of initiating therapy in the absence of continuing blood loss** (and not after six months).*
- ***Treatment should not be stopped after normalizing of Hb, but continued for an additional 4 to 6 months to replenish body iron stores.***

27. Answer is C (Polycythemia vera): Harrison 18th/p 846, 900, 3162 *Harrison 17th edn /630, 673 2430;(table 351-1)*

Increased erythropoetin leads to increased haematopoasis and an increased demand for iron producing a state of iron deficiency. Polycythemia vera being a state of increased erythropoetin is a cause of iron deficiency rather than iron overload.

Iron overload states *(Harrison 16th/336-1t)*

Iron loading anaemias	Chronic liver disease	Hereditary hemochromatosis	Dietary iron overload
• *Thalassemia major* • *Sideroblastic anaemia* • *Chronic hemolytic anaemias* • *Transfusional and parenteral iron overload*	• *Hepatitis C* • *Alcoholic cirrhosis (advanced)* • *Non alcoholic steatohepatitis* • *Porphyria cutanea tarda* • *Post portocaval shunting*		

Anemia of Chronic Disease

28. Answer is C (Normal or increased serum ferritin): *Harrison 17th /631*

Anemia of chronic disease is associated with normal or increased serum Ferritin.

Anemia of chronic disease is associated with decreased serum iron, decreased TIBC, decreased % saturation and normal or increased serum Ferritin levels.

Test (normal values) \ Condition	Iron deficiency	Thalassemia	Sideroblastic anemia	Anemia of chronic disease
Smear	Microcytic hypochromic	Microcytic hypochromic	Microcytic hypochromic	Normocytic normochromic > Micro/hypochromic (but Micro/Hypo may be present)
Serum iron (50-150μg/dl)	Low (<30)	Normal	Normal	↓ (<50)
TIBC (300-360 μg/dl)	High (>360)	Normal	Normal (Chandrasoma Taylor)	↓ (<300)
% Saturation (30-50%)	< 10 (↓ed)	N or ↑ed (30-80)	N or ↑ (30-80)	↓ (10-20)
Ferritin (μg/l) (50-200 μg/L)	< 15 (↓ed)	↑ (50-300)	↑ (50-300)	Normal or ↑ (30-200)
Hemoglobin pattern	Normal	Abnormal	Normal	Normal
Free Erythrocyte Protporphrin	↑ed	Normal	↑ed	↑ed
RDW	↑ed	Normal	Normal	Normal

29. Answer is B (Anemia of Chronic Disease): *Repeat*

Microcytic anemia (MCV < 80) with decreased Serum Iron and decreased TIBC suggest a diagnosis of Anemia of Chronic Disease.

Hypochromic microcytic anemia with ↓***Serum Iron and ↑TIBC***	*Iron Deficeincy Anemia*
Hypochromic microcytic anemia with ↓ ***Serum Iron and ↓ TIBC***	*Anemia of Chronic disease*

30. Answer is B (Decreased Ferritin): *Harrison 18th/849; 15th/ 665; 16th/ 590, 591; 17th edn / 633*

Anemia of chronic disease is characterised by a block in delivery of iron from the reticulo-endothelial system to the erythroid progenitors. Consequently ***patients have normal to increased iron stores in the marrow and a normal or increased, ferritin level.*** *Because of the block in delivery, serum iron levels fall and so does the TIBC and transferrin saturation.*

Laboratory parameters in Anemia of chronic disease

Smear	SI (µg/dl)	TIBC (µg/dl)	Percent saturation (%)	Ferritin (µg/dl)	Hb pattern
Normocytic normochromic or Microcytic hypochronic	< 50 (↓)	300 (↓)	10-20 (↓)	30-200 (↑)	Normal

Remember again:

- *Low serum iron with an increased TIBC is : iron deficiency anemia* Q
- *Low serum iron with a decreased TIBC is : anemia of chronic disease.* Q

31. Answer is A (Serum iron ↓, S. ferritin ↑, transferritin ↓): Harrison 18th/p 849 *Harrison 17th/633*

Anemia of chronic inflammations is associated with decreased serum iron, decreased transferrin levels (↓TIBC) and normal or increased ferritin levels.

32. Answer is C (Decreased serum ferritin level): Harrison 18th/p 849 *Harrison 16th/ 590, 591; Harrison 17th edn / 633; Chandrasoma Taylor 3rd/ 388; See previous questions also.*

Serum ferritin level is increased in patients with anaemia of chronic disease.

33. Answer is B (Increased total iron binding capacity): Harrison 18th/p 849 *Harrison 15th edn /665, 666; Harrison 16th edn/590, 591, 592; Harrison 17th edn /633; Chandrasoma Taylor 3rd/ 388*

Total iron binding capacity is decreased in patients with anaemia of chronic disease.

Anemia of Chronic Renal Failure

34. Answer is C (Dialysis worsens anemia of renal failure): Harrison 18th/p 850 *Harrison 17th/634; Williams Hematology /452*

Dialysis has little effect with regard to correcting the anemia of chronic renal failure.

Dialysis may improve the anemia of renal disease but it does not usually worsen it.

Anemia of chronic renal failure

- *It is normocytic normochromic, hypoproliferative anemia*
- ***The level of anemia correlates with the severity of renal failure***
- *The anemia is primarily due to a failure to produce adequate amounts of Erythropoetin and a reduction in red cell survival.*
- *Patients usually present with normal serum iron, TIBC & ferritin levels*
- ***Erythropetin therapy is the mainstay of treatment (improves symptoms)***
- ***Dialysis per se tyopically has little effect with regard to correcting the anemia.***
  Peritoneal dialysis (ambulatory) usually improves anemia while hemodialysis may cause an associated iron deficiency anemia.

35. Answer is A (Decreased Erythropetin Production): Harrison 18th/p 850 *Harrison 17th/633*

The Anemia of chronic renal failure is primarily due to failure to produce adequate amounts of Erythropetin (EPO) and a reduction in red cell survival.

Anemia in chronic renal failure is usually not caused by iron deficiency
Patients with anemia of chronic renal failure usually have normal levels of serum iron, serum TIBC and serum ferritin. *Iron deficiency anemia may however be seen in some patients with CRF who are maintained on chronic hemodialysis due to loss through the dialysis procedure.*
Anemia of chronic renal failure is not caused by deficiency of vitamin B12 or folate deficiency
Anemia of chronic renal failure is not caused by a Hypoplastic bone marrow.

Sideroblastic Anemia

36. Answer is B (Decreased transferrin saturation): Harrison 18th/p 848 *Harrison 16th/ 589, 590; Harrison 17th edn /632; Chandrasoma Taylor 3rd/ 388*

High or normal transferrin saturation is found in sideroblastic anaemia.

Sideroblastic anemia: is an uncommon form of anemia characterized by the presence of a large no of sideroblasts in the bone marrow.

Sideroblasts: are erythroid precursors with demonstrable Cytoplasmic iron Q.
*Ring sideroblasts*Q are normoblasts in which the amount of iron is so greatly increased that it appears as Cytoplasmic granules arranged in a complete ring around the nucleus.

Defect: *There is a defect in incorporating iron into the haemoglobin molecule within the erythrocyte.*

Laboratory parameters in Sideroblastic Anemia:

Smear	SI (μg/dl)	TIBC (μg/dl)	Saturation	Ferritin (μg/dl)	Marrow
Hypochromic microcytic or ****Dimorphic*** Q *picture*	Normal or ↑ed	Normal	Normal or ↑ed	Increased	Sideroblasts

****Dimorphic*** Q*: mixture of hypochromic microcytic and macrocytic erythrocytes*

37. Answer is B (Sideroblastic anemia) : Harrison 18th/p 848 *Harrison 17th edn /632; Repeat*

The association of Increased serum iron, Increased percent saturation and Increased serum ferritin is consistent with the presentation of Sideroblastic anemia..

The TIBC in Sideroblastic anemia is usually normal (Harrison), but it may also be decreased or low.
Sideroblastic anemia is the single best answer of choice.

Megaloblastic Anemia

38. Answer is B (Vitamin B12 and Folic acid deficiency): *Repeat*

Raised MCV (Macrocytic) and normal MCHC (Normochromic) suggests a diagnosis of Macrocytic Normochromic anemia seen most characteristically with vitamin B12 and Folic acid deficiency.

Iron deficiency anemia, Beta-thalassemia and Sideroblastic anemia are all Microcytic (Low MCV) Hypochromic (Low MCHC) anemias.

MCV (Mean Corpuscular Volume)	MCHC (Mean Corpuscular Hb concentration)
• Mean Corpuscular Volume refers to the average size of the RBC (volume). • MCV is usually expressed in femtoilitres (fl) • Normal MCV varies from 79.0 to 93.3 fl *(H 18th/3587)* Raised MCV: Macrocytic Normal MCV: Normocytic Reduced MCV: Microcytic	• Mean Corpuscular Haemoglobin Concentration (MCHC) refers to the average concentration of Hb in the RBC (MCHC describes the colour of the RBC) • MCHC is usually expressed in pg/dl • Normal MCHC varies from 32.3 to 35.9 pg/dl *(H 18th/3587)* Raised MCHC: Hyperchromic Normal MCHC: Normochromic Reduced MCHC: Hypochromic

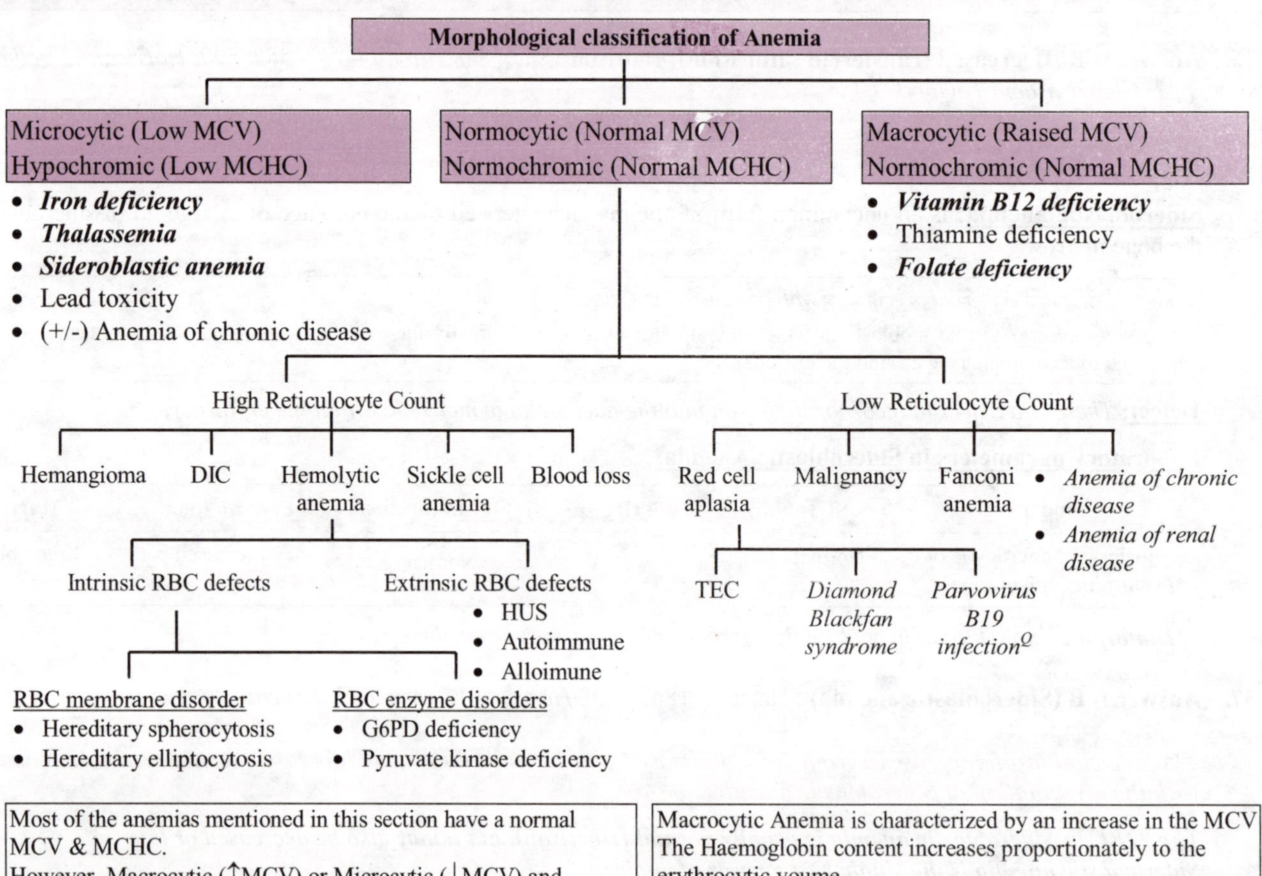

39. Answer is B (Copper deficiency): Harrison 18th/p 862 *Nelson 15th/ 408; Harrison 14th/ 657, Harrison 15th/ 679, 675, 468, Harrison 17th/643;(table 100-1); Chandrasoma Taylor 3rd/ 379, 382*

Cu deficiency has not been mentioned to cause megaloblastic picture. It causes a normocytic hypochromic picture.

- **Orotic acid** is an intermediate metabolite in the synthesis of pyrimidines. Orototic aciduria is a rare disorder in children, resulting from block of further metabolism of orotic acid.

  Affected children have megaloblastic anemia that is unresponsive to Vit C, Vit B12 and folic acid.
- **Thiamine deficiency** may be associated with 'thiamine responsive anemia'. In the untreated state this ***gives rise to a megaloblastic anemia***. - *Nelson 15th/173*
- **Liver disease** may give rise to ***megaloblastic anemia***, by interferring with storage and metabolism of fat soluble vitamin B_{12}.

Causes of Macrocytic anemia
1. Vit. B_{12} deficiency
2. Folic acid deficiency
3. Orotic aciduria
4. Nitrous oxide inhalation
5. Liver disease
6. Hypothyroidism
7. Thiamine deficiency

40. Answer is D (Amoxycilline): Harrison 18th/p 862 *Harrison 14th/ 426, 633, Harrison 15th/ 675; Harrison 16th/ 601; Harrison 17th/643*

All options other than Amoxycylline are mentioned as causes for megaloblastic anemia.

Megaloblastic Anemia is caused by :	
1. Phenytoin Q 2. Primidone Q 3. Phenobarbitone Q 4. Nitrous oxide	5. Folate antagonists : (inhibiters of dehydrofolate reductase) - *Harrison 14th / 653* - Methotrexate Q - Pyrimethamine Q - Pentamidine Q - Triamterine Q - Triamethoprim Q - Cotrimaxazole Q
Also, Drugs that inhibit DNA synthesis may cause Megaloblastic Anemia - *Harrison 14th/ 653*	
- **Purine Antagonist** : 6-Mercaptopurine, Azathioprine Q - **Pyrimidine antagonist** : 5FU, cystosine arabinose Q - **Others** : Procarbazine, hydroxyurea, acyclovir, zidovudine. Q	

41. Answer is A (Inadequate dietary intake): *Harrison 16th/603*

Folic acid deficiency most commonly results from either decreased dietary intake or increased metabolic demand. Amongst the options provided decreased dietary intake is the single best answer.

Megaloblastic anemia

Cobalamine deficiency	Folate deficiency
Most common cause is Malabsorption *'The dietary intake of cobalamine is more than adequate for body's requirement except in complete vegetarians and their breast fed infants.* ***Thus deficiency of cobalamine is almost always due to malabsorption'*** – *Harrison 16th/603*	Most common cause is either decreased dietary intake or increased metabolic demand. *The dietary intake of folic acid is marginal in many parts of the world. Furthermore because the body's stores of folate are low,* ***folic acid deficiency can arise rather suddenly during periods of decreased dietary intake or increased metabolic demand'*** – *Harrison 16th/603*

42. Answer is B (Bacterial overgrowth): *Harrison 16th/1773-74; Love&Bailey 23rd/1031*

Vitamin B_{12} deficiency in blind loop syndrome is not due to defect in the absorption process of vit B_{12} but due to competitive uptake of vit B_{12} by colonizing bacteria and hence decreased availability of vit B_{12} for absorption.
In Blind loop syndrome, malabsorbtion occurs secondary to bacterial overgrowth.

The possible mechanism causing malabsorption are :

1. *Bacterial deconjugation of bile salts :* In contrast to conjugated bile salts, unconjugated bile salts may be absorbed in the proximal small bowel resulting in decreased intraluminal concentration of bile salts in Jejunum.
   This leads to impaired micelle formation and hence fat malabsorption.
2. Utilization of vit B_{12} by bacteria: The impaired absorbtion of vit B_{12} is not related to above disturbed bile salt metabolism, but appears to be due to uptake of vit B_{12} by microorganisms i.e. competition for vit B_{12} by bacteria.
3. Injury to the mucosal absorptive surface.

Remember:

- Blind loop in the *upper intestine* : defect is chiefly of Fat malabsorption / Steatorrhea[Q]
- Blind loop in the *lower intestine* : There is Vitamin B_{12} deficiency / Megaloblastic anemia[Q]

43. Answer is B (Homocystinemia): *Harrison 18th/p 594, 595, 3218; 16th/ 1422, 1423, 403; 17th/ 441, 442, 2470, 2473*

All options other than homocyctinemia have been clearly mentioned as causes of thiamine deficiency.

Causes of thiamine deficiency – *Harrison*

1. **Malnutrition** [Q]
2. **Dietry habits** particularly in the far-east where *polished rice* [Q] deficient in thiamine is the major dietry component.
3. **Alcoholics and food faddists** [Q]**:** *In western nations the wide spread use of thiamine enriched flour limits the presence of deficiency primarily to alcoholic and food faddists – Harrison 15th/ 14th*
4. **Chronic heart failure** [Q]**:**
   - The measurement of thiamine pyrophosphate effect can biochemically quantitate thiamine stores.
   - An elevated TPPE indicative of thiamine deficiency has been found in 20 to 90% of patients with chronic heart failure.
   - The deficiency appears to result from both, reduced dietry intake and a diuretic induced increase in urinary excretion of thiamine - *Harrison*

44. Answer is B (Pernicious Anemia): *Robbin's 7th/639*

Deficiency of Intrinsic factor leads to a specific form of vitamin B12 deficiency megaloblastic anemia called 'Pernicious Anemia'.

Pernicious Anemia also known as Addison's Anemia is a megaloblastic anemia due to deficiency of intrinsic factor (secreted by parietal cells of gastric mucosa) that is essential for vitamic B12 absorption.

Note:

'Intrinsic factor' was first described by castle & coworkers and hence intrinsic factor is also called Intrinsic factor of Castle.

45. Answer is A (Vitamin B_{12}): *Harrison 17th /1878*

Shilling's test is done to determine the cause of cyanocobalamine deficiency (Vitamin B_{12}).

Schilling test is abnormal in conditions that affect cobalamine absorption including Pernicious anemia, Chronic Pancreatitis, Bacterial overgrowth syndrome and Ileal dysfunction.

Conditions with Abnormal Schilling's Test (Abnormal Cobalamine Absorption)
Pernicious anemia
Chronic Pancreatitis
Achlorhydria
Bacterial overgrowth syndrome
Ileal dysfunction

Schilling Test:

- Schilling test is performed to determine the cause of cobalamine malabsorption (Vit B12 malabsorption).
- Since cobalamine absorption requires multiple steps including gastric, pancreatic and ileal processes, the Schilling test can also be used to assess the integrity of these other organs.
- The Schilling test is performed by administering Co58-labeled cobalamin orally and collecting urine for 24h

  1 mg of cobabmine is administed intramuscularly one hour after ingestion of the Radiolabelled cobalamine. This is done to ensure saturation of cobalamine binding sites in the liver as urinary excretion of cobalamine will reflect cobalamine absorption only provided that intrahepatic binding sites of cobalamine are fully occupied. Once intrahepatic binding sites of cobalamine are saturated all absorbed radiolabelled cobalamine will be excreted in urine

- The ***Schilling test may be abnormal (defined as less than 10 percent excretion in 24h) in conditions that affect cobalamine absorption including Pernicious anemia, Chronic Pancreatitis, Bacterial overgrowth syndrome and Ileal dysfunction.***

- The etiology for an abnormal Schilling test may be deduced by administering Co58-labeled cobalamin with intrinsic factor, pancreatic enzymes or after 5 day course of antibiotics. Differential Results of Schilling Test in various diseases associated with cobalamin malabsorption may thus help establish the diagnosis.

Diagnosis	**^{58}Co-Cbl**	**With Intrinsic Factor**	**With Pancreatic Enzymes**	**After 5 Days of Antibiotics**
Pernicious anemia	*Reduced*	*Normal*	*Reduced*	*Reduced*
Chronic pancreatitis	*Reduced*	*Reduced*	*Normal*	*Reduced*
Bacterialovergrowth	*Reduced*	*Reduced*	*Reduced*	*Normal*
Ileal disease	*Reduced*	*Reduced*	*Reduced*	*Reduced*

1

Hematology

46. Answer is B (vitamin B_{12} is Deficiency): Harrison 18th/p 870 *Harrisons 16th/605,606; 17th/650; Harrison Appendix A for Reference values*

Presence of anemia (Hb= 6gm%) Macrocytosis (MCV=104) and decreased vitamin B12 levels (B12=60 pg/ml) suggests a diagnosis of megaloblastic anemia due to vitamin B12 deficiency.

Reference values from Harrison's Appendix A

Parameter	Normal Values	Patient value	Inference
Hb	13-18 g/dl	6 gm/dl	Anemia
HCV	79-93.3/L	104 fL	Macrocytosis
Vitamin B12	>250 pg/ml	60 pg/ml	Vitamin B12 deficiency
Folic Acid	5.4-18.0 ng/ml	8 ng/ml	Normal folate levels
Iron	30-160 µg/dl	160 µg/dl	Normal

The patient in question, thus has a macrocytic anemia due to vitamin B12 deficiency.

47. Answer is A (B_{12} Estimation) : *Harrisons 16th/602, 603; Other references with text*

***Increased MCV** (normal MCV = 79- 93.3), **Anemia** (Normal Hb = 12 –16.2) and **characteristic oral manifestation (macroglossia and Atrophy of Papillae) suggest the diagnosis of vitamin B_{12} deficiency. The next best step is to confirm the diagnosis by estimating vitamin B_{12} levels**.*

Oral Manifestations of vitamin B_{12} deficiency : *Color Atlas of Oral Diseases by Scully & Welbury (1994)/109*

- Tongue may be large (*'**Macroglossia**'*^{Q})-*Greenberg's Text-Atlas of Medicine/744*
- Tongue may be smooth due to **loss of papillae** *(Atrophic Glossitis)*^{Q}
- Tongue may show red patches on red lines on the ventrum *(Moeller's glossitis)*
- Tongue may be red and inflamed *(Sore tongue)*^{Q}
- *Angular cheilitis* may be associated
- *Oral ulcers* may be seen

Tongue in vitamin B_{12} deficiency
Macroglossia^{Q}
Atrophic glossitis^{Q}
Moeller's glossitis
Sore tongue^{Q}
Beefy tounge^{Q}

48. Answer is A (Folic acid alone causes improvement in hematologic in symptoms but worsening of neurological symptoms): *Harrison 18th/871; Robbins 7th/642, 643; Harrisons 17th/ 651*

*Megaloblastic anemia may be caused by a deficiency of vitamin B12 (cobalamine) or deficiency of folate. Unless it is clearly established, which of the two deficienceis / folate or cobalamine) is the cause anemia treatment should include administration of both folic acid and vitamin B_{12}. **If only folic acid is administered in a patient with megaloblastic anemia due to vitamin B12 deficiency, worsening of neurological symptoms (cobalamine neuropathy) is seen despite an improvement in the hematological symptoms (anemia)***

*'Although prompt hematologic response heralded by reticulocytosis follows the administration of folic acid, it should be cautioned that **the hematologic symptoms of a vitamin B_{12} deficiency anemia also respond to folate therapy. However folate does not prevent and may even exacerbate the progression of neurological deficits typical of vitamin B_{12} deficiency states'** – Robbins 6th/643*

*Before large doses of folic acid are given, cobalamine deficiency must be excluded and if present corrected, otherwise **cobalamine neuropathy may develop despite a response of the anemia of cobalamine deficiency to folate therapy** – Harrisons 17th/651*

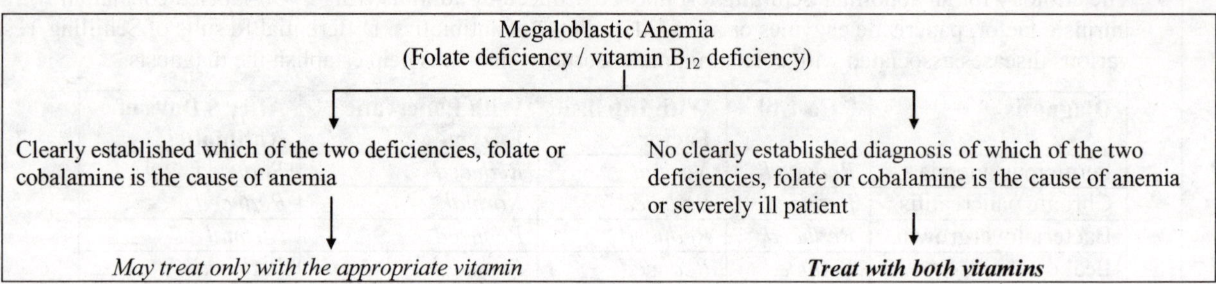

Hemolytic Anemias

General Features

49. Answer is C (Thalassemia): *Hematology in Clinical Practice 4th/142, 143*

Hemoglobinopathies including thalassemia cause extravascular hemolysis and not intravascular hemolysis.

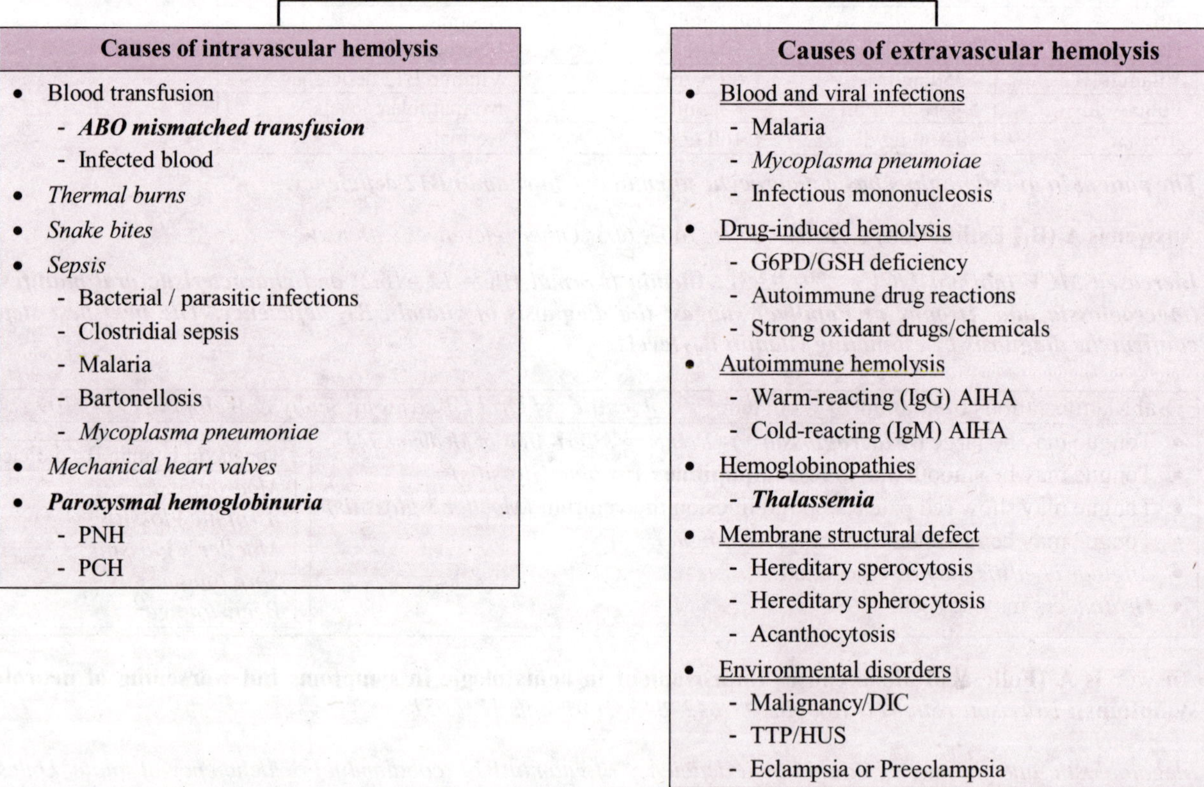

50. Answer is D (Hereditary Spherocytosis): *Hematology in clinical practice 4th/142,143; Refer previous questions*

Hemoglobinuria is a feature of intravascular hemolysis. Amongst the options provided hereditary spherocytosis is a cause for extravascular hemolysis and is therefore not associated with hemoglobinuria.

Urine	Extravascular hemolysis	Intravascular hemolysis
Hemosiderin	0	+
Hemoglobin	0	+ in severe cases

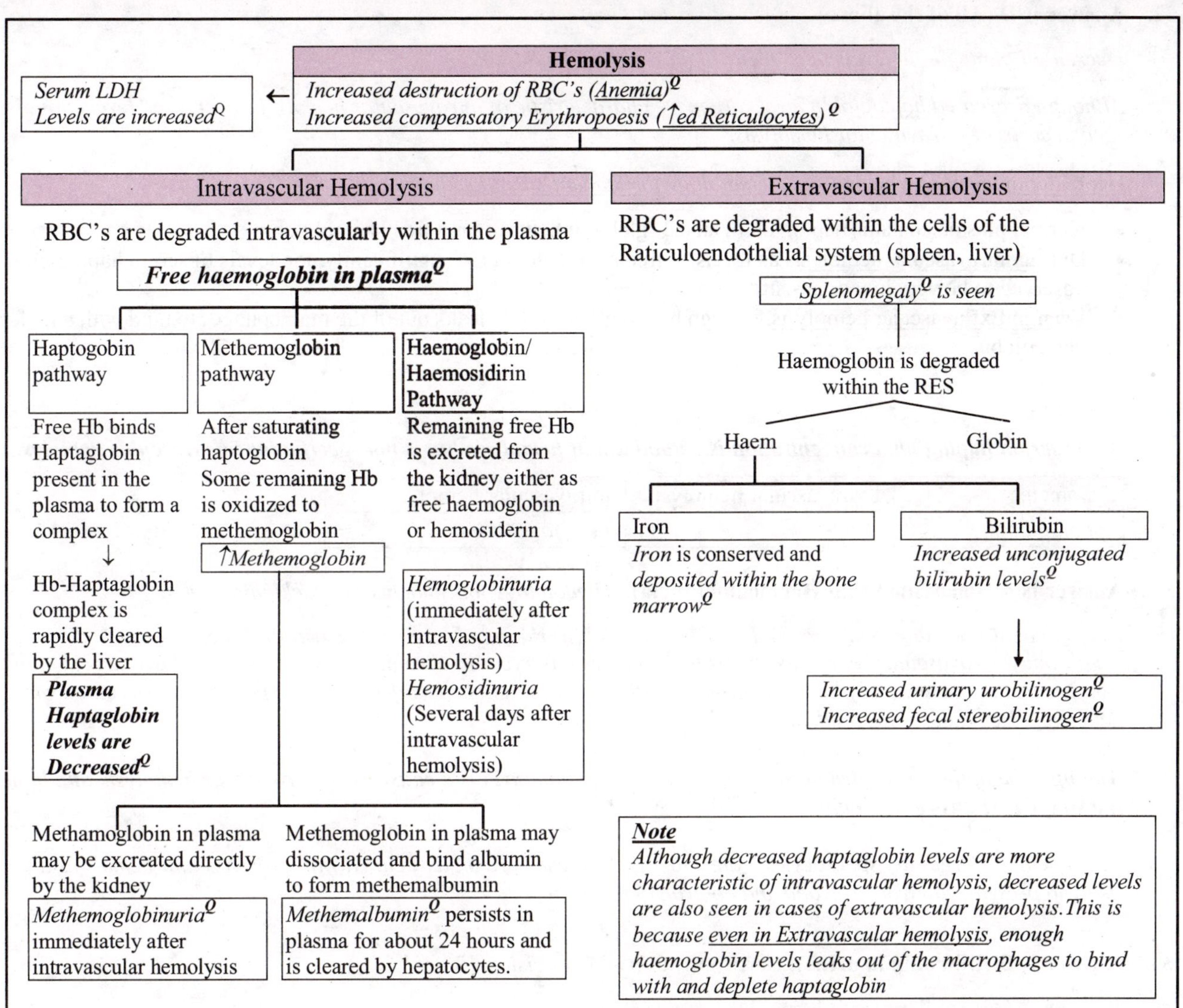

51. Answer is D (Thalassemia): *Harrison 16th/ 607; 17th/ 652; API 8th/ 809; Chandrasoma Taylor 3rd/ 391*

Haemoglobinuria is a feature of intravascular hemolysis. Amongst the options provided thalassemia is the only cause for extravascular hemolysis all others being causes for intravascular hemolysis.

Laboratory Evaluation of Haemolysis

	Extravascular	Intravascular
Hematologic		
Routine blood film	Polychromatophilia	Polychromatophilia
Reticulocyte count	↑	↑
Bone marrow examination	Erythroid hyperplasia	Erythroid hyperplasia
Plasma or serum		
Bilirubin	↑ Unconjugated	↑ Unconjugated
Haptoglobin	↓	Absent
Plasma hemoglobin	N - ↑	↑ ↑
Lactate dehydrogenase	↑ (Variable)	↑ ↑ (Variable)
Urine		
Bilirubin	0	0
Hemosiderin	0	+
Hemoglobin	0	+ in severe cases

52. **Answer is D (All of the above)**

Decreased haptaglobin levels may occur in all cases of hemolysis.

Although decreased haptaglobin levels are more characteristic of intravascular hemolysis, decreased levels are also seen in cases of extravascular hemolysis.

Heptaglobin levels and hemolysis *(Hematology for Student's by Mackinney (2003)/78,79*

- Normal plasma contains haptoglobin, an α2- globulin that can bind free haemolglobin
- During intravascular hemolysis as levels of free haemoglobin rise significantly, the levels of serum haptoglobin are observed to be very low or absent
- Even in Extravascular hemolysis, enough haemoglobin levels leaks out of the macrophages to bind with and deplete haptaglobin

Therefore

A low serum haptaglobin concentration is a good test of hemolysis but is not specific for intravascular hemolysis.

Parameter	Extravascular hemolysis	Intravascular hemolysis
Haptaglobin	*Low*	*Very low/Absent*

53. **Answer is A (Paroxsmal cold Haemoglobinuria):** *Hematology for Students by Mackinney (2003)/79*

Chronic hemolysis due to paroxysmal cold Haemoglobinuria may be associated with iron deficiency
'In chronic extravascular hemolysis iron is tenaciously conserved. In chronic intravascular hemolysis large amounts of iron are lost in the urine as free haemoglobin, muthemoglobin and hemosiderin and the patient may become iron deficient'- Hematology for Students.

Amongst the options provided paroxysmal cold haemoglobinuria is a cause for intravascular hemolysis and hence the single best answer of choice

Thalassemia, Hereditary spherocytosis and G6-PD deficiency are all associated with extravascular hemolysis and are likely to present with iron overload and not iron deficiency

54. **Answer is D (Bilirubin in urine):** Harrison 18th/p 873 *Harrision 17th/652*

Presence of bilirubin in urine is not a feature of Hemolytic Anemias.
Presence of bilirubin in urine indicates the presence of conjugated bilirubin in the plasma. Hemolytic anemias are associated with unconjugated hyperbilirubinemia not conjugated hyperbilirubinemia.

Features of Hemolytic Anemia

Features due to Increased Hemolysis (*↓ed RBC life span*)	Features due to Erythropoetic response of the bone marrow
• *Hemoglobin : reduced* • ↑ ***unconjugated bilirubin*** • ↑ *LDH* • ↑ *AST* • ↓ ***Haptoglobin*** • ↑ *Urobilinogen in urine (& stool)* • ↑ *Stercobilinogen in stool* • *Hemoglobinuria (intravascular hemolysis)*	• ↑ Reticulocytes (Reticulocytosis) • ↑ MCV / ↑ MCH (The increased number of reticulocytes is associated with an increased MCV) • Macrocytes, Polychromasia & sometimes nucleated red cells in smear • ***Erythroid Hyperplasia in marrow (Myeloid Erythroid Ratio is decreased)***

55. **Answer is D (Increased Haptoglobin):** Harrison 18th/p 873 *Harrison 17th/ 652; Harsh Mohan 4th/ 356*

Hemoglobin binding proteins such as Haptoglobin are reduced or absent. *- Harsh Mohan 4th / 356*

Characteristic features of Hemolytic Anemia:

Increased red cell breakdown	Compensatory increase red cell production
• Serum bilirubin is ↑ed *(unconjugated bilirubin ↑ed)*Q • *Urine urobilinogen is ↑ed Q* • *Fecal stercobilinogen is ↑ed Q* • *Hemoglobinemia / Hemoglobinuria Q* • *Methemoglobinemia Q* • ***Hemosiderinuria** Q* • ***Hemoglobin binding proteins** Q **such as Haptoglobin and Hemopexin are reduced or absent.** Q* • *Plasma Lactic dehydrogenase Q (LDH) is ↑ed*	• *Reticulocyte **count is** ↑ed Q* • *Routine blood film shows a variety of abnormal morphological types of red cells Q* - *Schistocytes* - ***Spherocytes** Q etc.* • *Bone narrow shows erythroid hyperplasia with raised iron stores. Q* • *X Rays of bones show :* - ***Evidence** of expansion of marrow space, especially in tubular bones & in skull Q* - ***Bossing** of skull Q*

56. Answer is D (Increased plasma Haptaglobin levels): *Repeat*

Hemolytic anemia are associated with decreased or absent levels of plasma haptaglobin.
Hyperbilirubinemia, Reticulocytosis and Hemoglobinuria are charachteristic features of hemolytic anemias.

57. Answer is A (Thrombocytopenia) : *Repeat*

Thrombocytopenia is not a feature of hemolytic anemia.
Decreased levels of serum haptaglobins, hemosidinuria and raised levels of indirect bilirubin are recognized feature of hemolytic anemias.

58. Answer is A (Tear drop cells are Burr cells) : *Refer text below*

Tear drop cells and Burr cells are not characteristic of hemolytic anemias.
Decreased levels of haptagobin, Reticulocytosis and haemoglobinuria are characteristic features of hemolytic anemia.

Burr cells and Tear Drop cells- *'Pathology of Bone marrow and Blood cells (2004)'*

Burr Cells may be seen in cases of microangiopathic hemolytic anemia but the presence of burr cells alone is not characteristic of a hemolytic anemias.

Burr cells (Echnocyte)

Burr cells are an acquired RBC membrane abnormality with short evenly spaced spicules.

They may be seen in

- *Renal failure (Uremia) – Characteristic feature*
- Liver disease
- Burns
- Pyruvate kinase deficiency
- Gastric ulcers
- Cancer
- *Microangiopathic Hemolytic Anemias*

Tear drop cells are drop shaped cells characteristic of marrow fibrosis.
They are not a characteristic feature of hemolytic anemias.

Tear Drop cells (Dacrocytes)

Tear Drop cells are drop/ tear shaped RBC's characteristically seen in conditions associated with marrow fibrosis or extramedullary hemotopaesis

They may be seen in

- Myelofibrosis
- Myelodysplastic syndrome
- Sideroblastic anemia
- Metastatic marrow infiltration
- These may also be seen in thalassemia, pernicious anemia and iron deficiency anemia

Note

Fragmented Erythrocytes seen in microangiopathic hemolytic anemia

- Helmet cells[Q]
- Burr cells[Q]
- Schistocytes[Q]

Taken from Heptinstall's pathology of the kidney 6th/703.

59. Answer is D (Anemia of chronic Renal Failure): *Refer previous questions*

Anemias of chronic renal failure and chronic disease are associated with low or normal reticulocyte counts. Elevated reticulocyle count is a feature of hyperproliferative anemias including PNH, hereditary spherocytosis and anemia after blood loss.

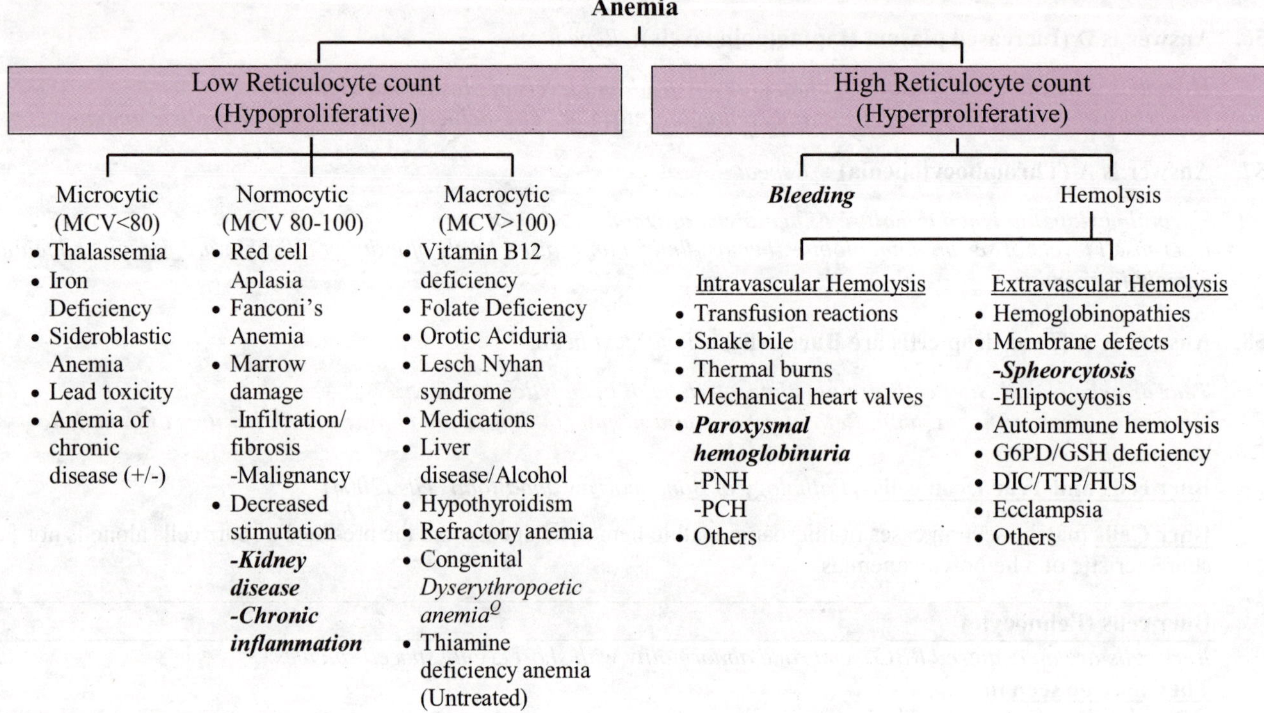

60. Answer is both C and D (Nutritional Anemia and Congenital dyserythropoeitic anemia): *Harrisons 16th/334; Refer previous question*

Nutritional anemia is associated with normal/Low Reticulocyte count. Increased reticulocyte count (Reticulocytosis) is not a feature of nutritional anemias.

Nutritional Anemia

Anemia resulting from deficiency of important nutrients in diet is called Nutritional anemia. Nutritional anemia is most commonly seen secondary to deficiency of Iron (Iron deficiency anemia) and vitamin B12 and Folic acid (Megaloblastic anemia). Both iron deficiency anemia and megaloblastic anemia are associated with low reticulocyte count.

Congenital Dyserythropoetic Anemia (CDA's) (Essential Hematology by Moss 4th/97)

Congenital dyserythropoetic anemias are a group of hereditary refractory anemias characterized by ineffective erythropoesis.

The reticulocyte count in these disorders in characteristically low (to normal for the degree of anemia).

Paroxysmal Nocturnal haemoglobinuria (PNH)

Paroxysmal Nocturnal Haemoglobinuria is associated with Intravascular hemolysis and is a known cause for elevated Reticulocyte count.

Hemolysis

Both intravascular and extravascular hemolysis are characterized by elevated reticulocyte counts

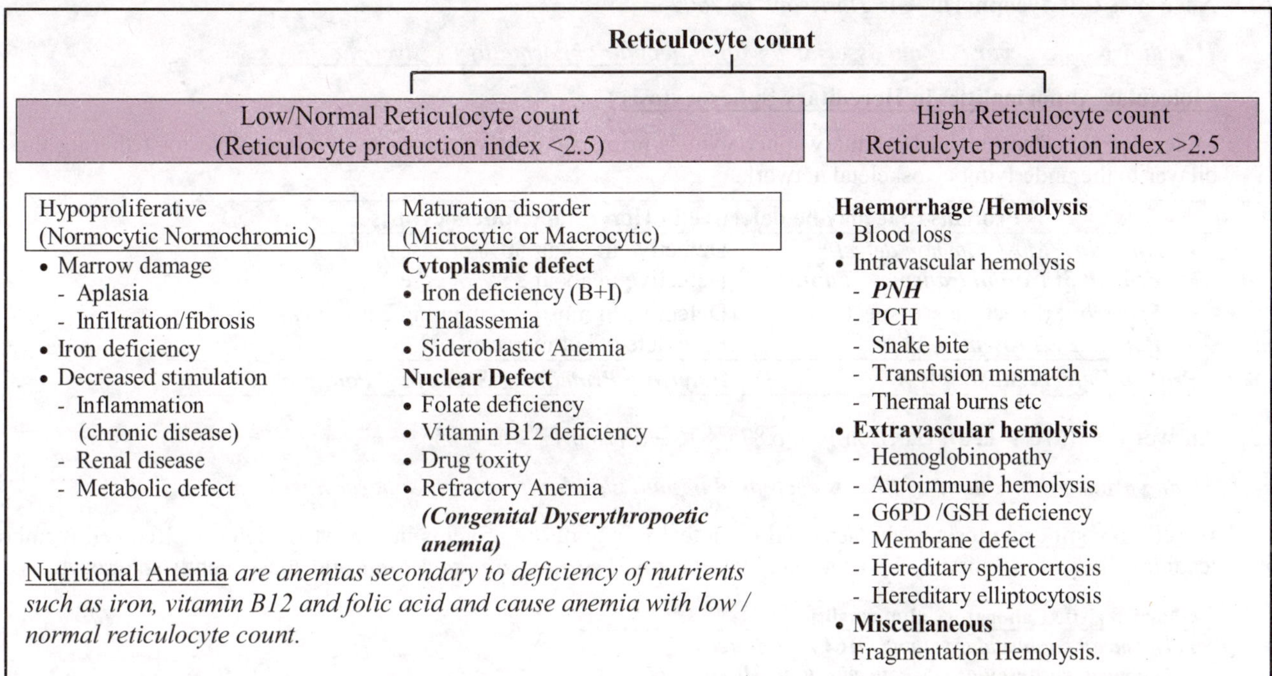

61. Answer is D (Anemia in C.R.F.): Harrison 18th/p 850, 885, 886 *API 6th/ 856, API 7th/ 923; Harrison 17th/ 633, 634, 662; CMDT 2008/430*

Anemia of chronic disease is associated with a normal / low Reticulocyte count.

Reticulocytes are young red cells with presence of nuclear remnants in the cytoplasm. Their number gives an estimate of the adequacy of marrow response to anaemia.

Reticulocyte count (Normal is 0.5 to 1.5% of all red cells):

High Reticulocyte Count	Low Reticulocyte Count
1. Haemolysis from any cause eg. Haemolytic anemias including hereditary Spherocytosis & PNH.	1. Aplastic anemia
2. Bleeding (Blood loss)	2. Nutritional deficiency anemia.

Note: Reticulocytosis occurs in nutritional anemias as soon as treatment is started.

Diagnostic approach based on assessment of reticulocyte count in patients with normal or low MCV

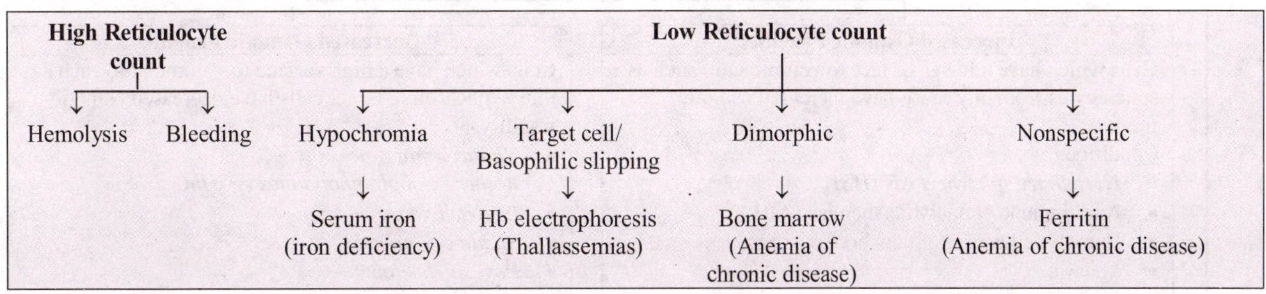

Hereditary Spherocytosis

62. Answer is C (Glycophorin–C): *Harrisons 16th/609*

Hereditary spherocytosis is not associated with molecular abnormality in Glycophorin – C.

Molecular Abnormalities in Hereditary Spherocytosis

Molecular abnormalities in Hereditary spherocytosis primarily involve the proteins responsible for tethering the lipid bilayer to the underlying cytoskeletal network.

Proteins that may be defective in Hereditary sphenocytosis		
• ***Ankyrin***: *(Most common defect)*Q	:	(Defective in about 50% of cases)
• ***Protein 3***: ***(Anion transport channel)***	:	(Defective in about 25% of cases)
• ***Spectrin*** : (Spectrin or α spectrin)	:	(Defective in most of remaining 25% of cases)
• ***Palladin*** : *(Protein 4.2)*Q	:	(Rare defect, but may cause H. S)
Protein Defects causing H.S	:	***Ankyrin > Protein 3 ≥ Spectrin > Palladin***

63. Answer is C (MCV ↑ed): Harrison 18th/p 875, 876 *Harrison 17th/ 654, 655;*

Mean corpuscular volume of RBC is decreased in patients with hereditary spherocytosis.

Hereditary spherocytosis is characterised by defect in one of the proteins in the cytoskeleton of Red cell membrane, leading to loss of membrane, and hence ***decreased ratio of surface area to volume*** and consequently spherocytosis.

Characteristic Laboratory abnormalities
- ***The mean corpuscular volume (MCV) : is decreased*** Q
- ***The mean corpuscular Hb. concentration (MCHC) : is increased*** Q
- ***Osmotic fragility is : increased*** Q

Remember the following also :

• *Hereditary spherocytosis is inherited as*	:	*Autosomal dominant* Q
• *Most common membrane defect is that of*	:	*Ankyrin* Q
• *One characteristic clinical presentation is*	:	*Striking splenomegaly* Q *(anemia, splenomegaly, jaundice)*
• *Treatment of choice is*	:	*Splenectomy* Q

64. Answer is C (Hereditary spherocytosis): Harrison 18th/p 875 *'A manual of Laboratory and Diagnostic Tests' 8th/116, 117; Harrison 17th/654*

Hereditary spherocytosis is characteristically associated with an increased osmotic fragility.

Osmotic Fragility

Osmotic fragility of red cells is defined as the ease with which red cells are ruptured (hemolysed) when they are exposed to hypotonic solution.
Osmotic fragility test assesses the integrity of the membrane of red cells.

Increased Osmotic Fragility	Decreased Osmotic Fragility
Cells which have a lower surface to volume ratio such as spherocytes from any cause have increased osmotic fragility Conditions • ***Hereditary spherocytosis (HS)*** • Autoimmune Hemolytic Anemias (AIHA) • Hemolytic Disease of new born • Malaria • Severe pyruvate kinase deficiency • Other conditions in which spherocytes are found in the blood	Cells which have a high surface to volume ratio such as thin/hypochromic/target cells have decreased osmotic fragility. • ***Thalassemia*** *(other hemoglobinopathies eg. HbC, HbS)* • *Iron deficiency anemia* • ***Sickle cell anemia*** • *Post splenectomy* • *Reticulocytosis* • *Other conditions in which thin/target cells are found in the blood.*

65. Answer is B and D (Sickle cell ds and Thalassemia): *'Practical Physiology by Pal and Pravati 2nd/104; Manual of Laboratory and Diagnostic Tests 8th/116, 117; Refer previous question*

Hemoglobinopathies with increased target cells such as sickle cell disease, Thalassemias, HbC disease etc are associated with decreased osmotic fragility.

Hereditary spherocytosis and Autoimmune Hemolytic Anemias are characteristically associated with an increased osmotic fragility.

66. Answer is A (Parvovirus): *Robbins 7th/627*

Aplastic crisis is usually triggered by an acute parvovirus infection.

67. Answer is B (Hereditary spherocytosis): *Harrison 18th/876; Harrison 15th/ 682, 16th/ 608; 17th/ 654*

Splenectomy is curative in hereditary spherocytosis.

Splenectomy is carried out in all symptomatic patients Q because of the potential for gall stones and stones and episodes of bone marrow hyperplasia or hemolytic crisis Q

- It reliably corrects the anemia and RBC survival often becomes normal or nearly so.
- The operative risk is low.

Remember

Splenectomy is not carried out in young children Q (preferably postponed until age 4) in order to minimize the risk of severe infections Q with gram positive encapsulated organisms.

G6 PD Deficiency

68. Answer is C (Pyrimethamine): Harrison 18th/p 879 *Harrisons 17th /657*

***Primaquine** is associated with definite risk, **Chloroquine** is associated with possible risk and **Quinine** is associated with doubtfull risk of inducing clinical hemolysis in persons with G6PD deficiency.*

***Pyrimethamine** is not mentioned in the list of drugs that carry risk of hemolysis and is the single best answer of exclusion*

Drugs that carry risk of clinical hemolysis in persons with G6PD deficiency: *(Harrison)*

Agent	Definite risk	Possible risk	Doubtful risk
Antimalarials	**Primaquine** Dapsone/Chlorproguanil	**Chloroquine**	**Quinine**
Sulphonamides/Sulphones	Sulphametoxazole Others Dapsone	Sulfasalazine Sulfadimidine	Sulfisoxazole Sulfadiazine
Antibacterial/Antibiotics	Cotrimoxazole Nalidixic acid Nitrofurantoin Niridazole	Ciprofloxacin Norfloxacin	Chloramphenicol p-Aminosalicylic acid
Antipyretic/analgesics	Acetanilide Phenazopyridine (Pyridium)	Acetylsalicylic acid high dose (>3 g/d)	Acetylsalicylic acid <3 g/d Acetaminophen Phenacetin
Others	Napthalene Methylene blue	Vitamin K analogues Ascorbic acid >1 g Rasburicase	Doxorubicin Probenecid

69. Answer is A (Oestrogen): Harrison 18th/p 879 *Harrison 17th/657*

Oestrogen is not included in the list of drugs that carry rick of hemolysis in patients with G-6 PD deficiency.

***Primaquine** and **Nitrofurantoin** are associated with definite risk while **salicylates** are associated with a possible risk of hemolysis in G6 PD deficient patients.*

Hematology 1

70. Answer is A (G-6 PD deficiency): Harrison 18th/p 878, 879 *Harrison 15th/ 685, Harrison 16th/ 611; Harrison 17th/ 657 (Add table 101.5)*

Erythrocytes are vulnerable to oxidative injuries by a variety of endogenous and exogenous oxidants. Glucose 6-PD, prevents such oxidative damage by maintaining the supply of reduced glutathione which inactivates such oxidants. In the absence of G 6 PD therefore patient may experience an acute hemolytic crisis within hours of exposure to oxidants stress.

Drugs causing hemolysis in subjects deficient in G6PD are :	
1. *Antimalarials : Primaquine*	5. *Antiarrhythmics : Procanamide, Quinidine* Q
2. Sulfonamides : Cotrimoxazole	6. *Dapsone* Q
3. *Nitrofurantoin, Nalidixic acid* Q	7. *Vit C, Vit K, Probenecid, Furazolidone* Q
4. *Analgesics : Aspirin, Phenocetin* Q	

Hemoglobinopathies: Sickle Cell Anemia

71. Answer is B (Replacement of glutamate by valine in beta chain of Hb): *Harrison 18th/p 854; 17th/637 639 Robbins 7th/628*

The sickle cell anemia is caused by a mutation in the beta globin gene that changes the sixth amino acid from glutamic acid to valine in the beta chain of HbA ($\alpha_2\beta_2$).

Designation	Mutation
HbS (Sickle) ($\beta^{6Glu} \rightarrow$ Val)	Replacement of Glutamate by Valine at position 6 beta chain of HbA
HbC ($\beta^{6Glu} \rightarrow$ Lys)	Replacement of Glutamate by Lysine at position 6 on beta chain of HbA
HbE ($\beta^{26Glu} \rightarrow$Lys)	Replacement of Glutamate by Lysine at position 26 on beta chain of HbA

72. Answer is D (Splenomegaly): Harrison 18th/p 855 *Harrison 17th/ 638; Read text*

"Sickle cell anemia is characterized by Hyposplenism /Autosplenectomy (not Splenomegaly)".

Repeated episodes of splenic infarction cause the spleen to be reduced to small calcified remnant – a phenomenon that has been termed as 'Autosplenectomy'."

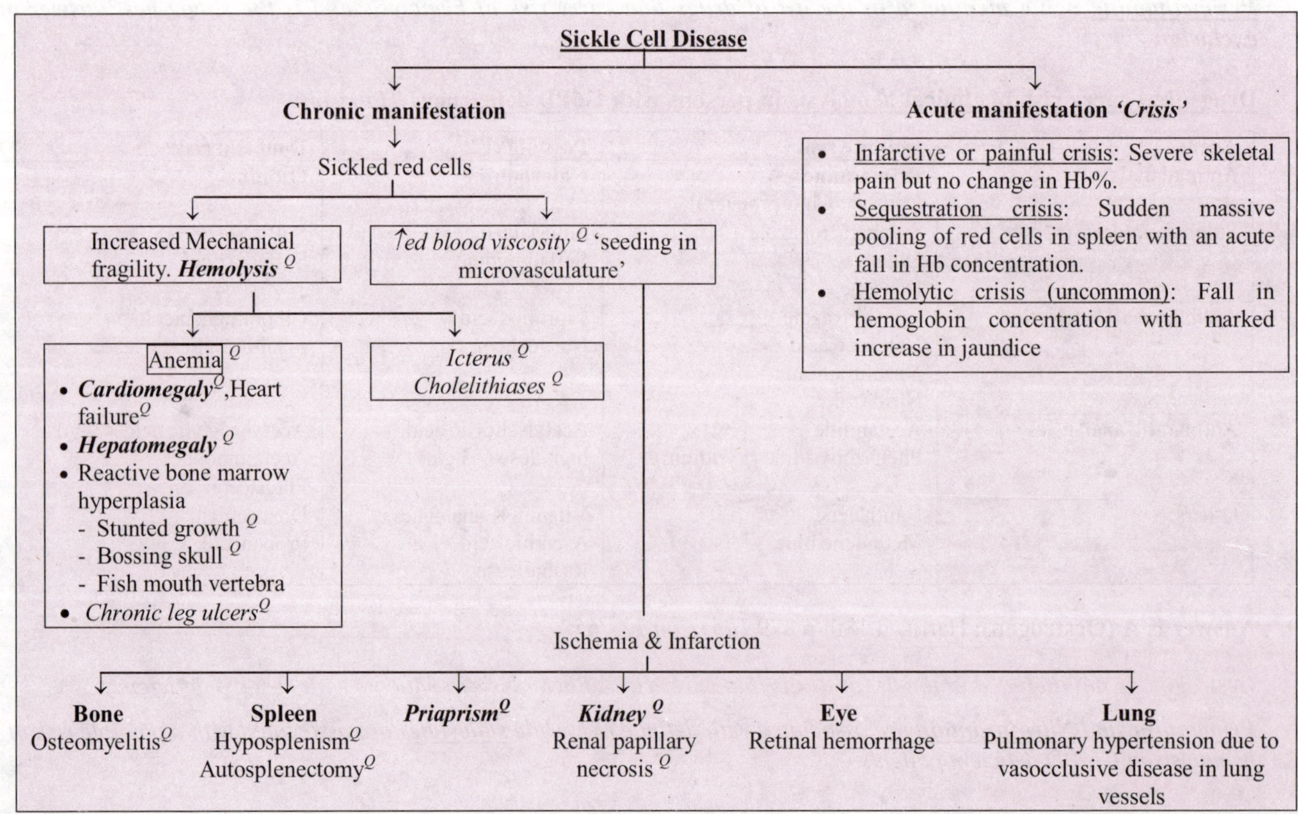

73. Answer is C (Leukopenia): Harrison 18th/p 855 *Harrison 17th/ 637, 638;CMDT to be added; Read reference below*

Sickle cell anemia is associated with granulocytosis (leukocytosis) and not leukopenia.

- The ***white blood cell count is characteristically elevated*** to 12,000-15,000/μL. – *CMDT 2003 / 481.*
- Chronic acute or subacute pulmonary crisis (pulmonary vasocclusive disease) lead to pulmonary hypertension and cor pulmonale – *Harrisons 16th/ 596*
- The heart is enlarged with a hyperdynamic precordium and systolic murmurs – *CMDT 2003 / 481*
- Reactive hyperplasia of bone marrow with associated widening of medullary cavities produces a characteristic 'biconcave vertebra' i.e. fish mouth vertebra.

74. Answer is D (Patient presents early in life before 6 months of age): Harrison 18th/p 855, 856 *Harrison 17th edn /637,638; Nelson 17th edn 1624*

- ***Affected newborn seldom exhibit clinical features of sickle cell disease. Anemia develops over the first 2-4 months paralelling the replacement of much of the fetal haemoglobin by HbS. Clinical manifestations are uncommon before 5-6 months of age'*** – *Nelson 17th / 1624*
- The most important factor which affects the rate and degree of sickling (polymerization) ***is amount of HbS*** and its interaction with other Haemoglobin chains – *Robbins*

Factors favouring polymerization: Q
1. **Hypoxia** Q : (2,3 diphosphoglycerate increases polymerization Q)
2. **Acidosis** Q : decreased pH enhances polymerization Q
3. **Haemoglobin** concentration Q: Higher concentration leads to increased polymerization Q
4. **Combination of HbS with other haemoglobins**: This depends on the extent of homology with other haemoglobins. Descending order of ability to copolymerization are HbS, C, D, O, Arab, A, J & F ***(Least with HbF)***

- Acute splenic sequestration has a peak incidence between 6 months and 3 years and can be rapid in onset and lead to death. ***The most common cause of mortality is sepsis*** and acute chest syndrome'-*Nelson 17th/ 1626*
- ***Chronic transfusion therapy*** (repeated blood transfusions) has been used to decrease the frequency of crisis and may be useful in some severely affected patients - *Harrison*

75. Answer is A (Mutation in α chain): Harrison 18th/p 855, 854 *Harrison 17th/637, 638; Robbin's 7th/629*

Sickle cell disease is caused by a mutation in the β globin gene that codes for β chain and not by a mutation in the 'α-chain'.

Sickle cell disease is caused by a mutation in the β gene (H17th/637)

- The sickle cell syndrome is caused by a mutation in the β chain from glutamic acid to valine ($\alpha 2\beta 2^{6Glu\text{-}val}$)

Severity of sickle cell disease may be decreased by HbF (Robbins/Internal Medicine)

- Fetal Hemoglobin (HbF) inhibits the polymerization of HbS (Robbins)
- By inhibiting polymerization of HbS, HbF diminishes the severity of sickle cell disease – Internal Medicne 5th/659 Patients with higher HbF levels have fewer pain episodes and longer survival – Internal Medicine 5th/659
- 'Through uncertain mechanisms, Hydroxyurea causes an increase in the levels of HbF in red cells. This may in part, be responsible for the mechanism of action of Hydroxyurea in sickle cell disease.
- Efforts are currently being directed towards gene therapy that would increase the production of HbF.

Venoocclusive crisis is a cause of morbidity (H 17th/638; Robbins 7th/632)

Venoocclusive disease in sickle cell syndrome is a major cause of morbidity as it leads to repeated episodes of painful ischemia – painful crisis

'Some patients are crippled by repeated vaso-occlusive crisis' – Robbin's.

Bone pain may by the presenting feature *(H17th/638; Robbin's 7th/631)*

Painful bone crisis may be the presenting feature.

This is extremely common in children and difficult to distinguish from acute osteomyelitis.

1

Hematology

76. Answer is B (Bone pain): Harrison 18th/p 855 *Harrisons 17th/638*

'Recurrent episodes of painful crisis are the most common clinical manifestations' *– Harrisons 16th/ 596*
Pain can develop almost anywhere in the body and may persist for a variable period. Among the options provided 'bone pain' is one such manifestation of 'painful crisis' and is thus the option of choice.
These painful crises are produced as a result of intermittent episodes of vasoocclusion in connective tissue and musculoskeletal structures producing painful ischaemia.

77. Answer is B (Malaria): *Robbins 8th/387, 645; Robbins 7th / 402, 628*

Heterozygous Sickle Cell Anemia confers protection against Malaria.

Sickle cell trait (HbS trait) confers resistance against Malaria in Heterozygotes (*Robbins 7th / 402, 628*)
The possession of the sickle cell allele protects these individuals against malaria because the parasite dies when potassium leaks out of RBCs as they become sickle shaped.
*'**HbS trait causes parasites to grow poorly or die at low oxygen concentrations** perhaps because of low potassium levels caused by potassium efflux from red cells on haemoglobin sickling' - Robbins*

*'In certain populations in Africa the prevalence of Heterozygosity is as high as 30%. This high frequency probably stems from **protection afforded by HbS against falciparum malaria'**. – Robbins 8th/645*

78. Answer is A (HbA): Harrison 18th/p 852, 854 *Harrison 17th edn /635, 637; Read text below*

There are no β chains in sickle cell anemia (homozygos) and therefore no HbA ($\alpha_2\beta_2$)

Sickle cell anemia is the prototype of *Structural Haemoglobinopathies* ᵠ characterised by production of structurally abnormal Hb chain.

It is caused by substitution of valine for glutamic acid at position 6 of **β chains.** ᵠ

HbA is $\alpha_2\ \beta_2$. It thus needs to have both α and β chains.

β chains however are defective in sickle cell disease such that :
- In hetrozygotes or sickle cell trait : 40% chains are defective
- In homozygotes or sickle cell disease : 100% chains are defective.

In other words ***there are no β chains in sickle cell anemia (homozygos) and therefore no HbA.***

HbA_2 is $\alpha_2\delta_2$ and HbF is $\alpha_2\ \gamma_2$

There is *no underlying defect in δ chains or γ chains in sickle cell disease and hence HbF and HbA2 may well be seen.*

79. Answer is C (HbS is less than 50% and HbA has low affinity for HbS): *Robbins 7th/629*

*The most important factor affecting the rate and degree of sickling is the amount of HBs and its interaction with other hemoglobin chains in the cell. Patients with sickle cell trait (heterozygotes) have 40% of haemoglobin in the form of HbS, the rest being HbA, which interacts only with HbS when deoxygenated. **Both the low concentration of HbS and the presence of interfering HbA act to prevent effective HBs aggregation and polymerization and thus red cells in sickle cell trait (heterozygotes) do not sickle.** – Robbins*

80. Answer is A (0 and 100): Harrison 18th/p 855 *Harrison 17th edn /638; Too obvious for reference*

If the mother has sickle cell disease 'SS' and father is normal 'AA' all the offsprings will be 'SA'. Thus % of sickle cell disease (SS) will be zero and that of sickle cell trait (SA) will be 100%.

Well the answer is fairly obvious but for those who still want an explanation, I will give it a try :
- Sickle cell disease is the homozygous state of HbS (SS) where S stands for gene coding HbS.
- Sickle cell trait is the heterozygous state of HbS (SA) where A stands for Absent gene.
- Normal individual has no gene for HbS (AA).

If the mother has sickle cell disease 'SS' and father is normal 'AA' all the offsprings will be 'SA'. Thus % of sickle cell disease (SS) will be zero and that of sickle cell trait (SA) will be 100%.

81. Answer is D (Sickle cell Anemia): *Robbins 7th/630; Outlines in pathology (2005)/80,82,199*

Sickle cell Anemia is the single best answer of choice.

Crew cut appearance of skull and Gamma Gandy bodies in the spleen may be observed in several causes of hemolytic anemias but are most characteristic of sickle cell anemia amongst the options provided.

***Crew cut appearance** is most characteristic of Thalassemia and Sickle cell anemia.*

Crew cut appearance (Hair on End appearance)

- Thalassemia (Most charachteristic)
- Sickle cell Anemia (2nd most characteristic)
- Other Hemolytic anamias (May be seen)

Hair on End appearance / crew cut appearance of skull results from expansion of marrow with bone resorption and secondary new bone formation because of compensatory hyperplasia of erythroid progenitors and may hence be seen in several causes of hemolytic anemias.

Gamma Gandy bodies are most characteristic of congestive splenomegaly but may be seen in hemolytic anemias especially sickle cell anemia

Gamma Gandy bodies (calcium and hemosidrn deposits in spleen)

- Congestive spleenomegaly / portal hypertension. (most characteristics)
- *Hemolytic Anemias (Most characteristic of sickle cell anemia)*
- Hematochromatosis

82. Answer is A (P. Falciparum): *'Lecture Notes on Tropical Medicine' (John Wiley & Sons)2009/62*

Sickle cell Anemia confers resistance against P. Falciparum.

Innate Traits that offer resistance against malaria

- ***The Sicke Cell Haemoglobin trait confers resistance against P. Falciparum*ᵠ.**
  Individuals with sickle cell trait are resistant to the lethal effects of P. Falciparum. These individual may still develop infection with P. Falciparum but the trait prevents development of high parasitemia and prevents development of deadly complication of Falciparum malaria.

There is now evidence that G-6PD difficiency and β thalassemia trait also offer resistance against P. falciparum but such evidence is less striking than with sickle cell trait.

- ***The Duffy gene null allele confers resistance against P. vivax*ᵠ.**
  Duffy antigens act as outside receptors for P. vivax. Without the Duffy antigens P. vivax canot intrude humans. This is believed to account for natural resistance of people of subsaharan African origin who lack the Duffy antigen

Hemoglobinopathies: Thalassemias

83. Answer is B (Decrease in β chain, increase in alpha chain): Harrison 18th/p 858, 859 *Harrison 17th edn /640,641; Robbins 7th/632*

'The abnormality in Beta thalassemia is diminished synthesis of structurally normal Beta globin chains with unimpaired synthesis of alpha chains' *– Robbins 7th/ 632*

Thalassemias

Characterized by *decreased rate of synthesis of Hb chains* ᵠ that are *structurally normal* ᵠ.
β thalassemia or Cooley's anemia is the commonest thalassemia.

Characterized by:

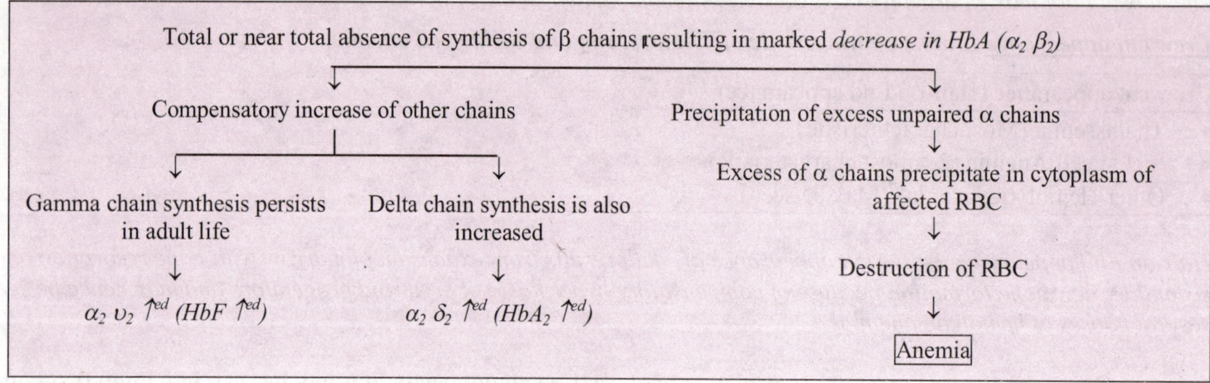

84. Answer is A (Intron-1): *Hematology by Hoffman 4th/559,560*

The most common mutation in beta thalassemia involves the intervening sequence 1 (IVS-1) or the intron-1

Mutations in Beta Thalassemia

- Most types of Beta thalassemia are caused by point mutations affecting one or few bases.
- A given mutation usually occurs within only one racial group and within a given racial group, five or six specific mutations usually accounts for more than 90% of cases of Beta-thalassemia.
- ***The most common site of mutations in Beta thalassemia is the intervening sequence 1 (IVS-1) or Intron 1***

85. Answer is B (Thalassemia intermedia): Harrison 18th/p 859 *Harrison 17th/641; Nelson Pediatrics 16th/1479-1484; Nelson 17th/ 1630.*

Presence of pallor and hepatosplenomegaly in a patient presenting late and capable of survival without blood transfusions is most suggestive of a diagnosis of thalassemia intermedia.
Due to abnormal synthesis of HbA, HbF is increased. (60-80%)

Clinical spectrum of Thalassemia (β thalassemia):

Syndrome	Thalassemia major (Serious homozygos form)	Thalassemia intermedia (They are also homozygos)	Thalassemia minor (heterozygos form)
General characteristic	• Presentation in early infancy with: - Progressive pallor - Hepatosplenomegaly - Bony changes • Invariably fatal during first few years of life if left untreated (Require repeated blood transfusions)	• Patient present somewhere between the two extremes with variable clinical manifestations of - Progressive pallor - Hepatosplenomegaly - Bony changes • These patients maintain hemoglobin levels between 6-10 g/dl and lead their life fairly comfortably. These patients may need occasional transfusions but are not dependent on blood transfusions for their survival.	• Presents late and patient can lead a practically normal life except for mild persistent anemia • These patients are not dependent on blood transfusions
Clinical Features			
• Severity of disease	++++	++	±
• Growth and development	Impaired	-	-
• Splenomegaly	++++	++	-
• Jaundice	++	+/-	-
• Skeletal changes	+++	+	-
• Thalassemia facies	+++	+	-

Haematological findings			
• Anaemia Hb gm/dl	< 7 (severe)	7-10 (moderate)	>10
• Microcytosis • Hypochromia	+++ +++	++ ++	+ +
• Basophilic stippling • Anisopoikilocytosis • Target cells • Nucleated red cells • Reticulocytes	++ +++ +++ +++ 2-15	+ ++ ++ +/- occasional 2-10	+ ± + - < 5
• HbF • HbA_2	30-90% <3.5%	20-100% <3.5%	0-5% 3.5-8%
• B.M. Iron • Iron overload • Life expectancy	++++ + 20-28 YEARS	++ - Normal	± - Normal

86. Answer is C>D (Thalassemia Intermedia > Auto immune Hemolytic anemia): *Harrisons 16th/612; Robbins 7th/634 Textbook of Emergency pediatric medicine 5th/934; Nelson 18th/2043*

Both Thalassemia Intermedia and Autoimmune hemolytic anemias, may present with a haemoglobin of 5gm/dl in an adult patient. Adequate response with a single blood transfusion in the past favours a diagnosis of Thalassemia intermedia over AIHA, and is hence the single best answer of choice.

Thalassemia Intermedia *patients usually have a moderate hemolytic anemia with Haemoglobin levels between 6 to 10 gm/dl.Patients with thalassemia intermedia are not transfusion dependent and present later in life as they are capable of maintaining a haemoglobin level of greater than 6 gm without transfusion. However because of their constant dependence on a compensatory increase in red cell production, these patients are subject to exacerbations in their anemia (Hb<6gm/dl) during febrile or other illness, perioperatively or during pregnancy. Occasional blood transfusions in such patients may be required when there is a fall in the haemoglobin levels.*

The patient in question is 21 years old and has a history of single blood transfusion in the past. He has now presented with a possible acute exacerbation of his anemia with a haemoglobin level of 5g/dl. His presentation is thus consistent with a diagnosis of thalassemia intermedia which is the single best answer of choice

Autoimmune Hemolytic Anemias

Autoimmune Hemolytic Anemias may occur at all ages but are more common in adults. In many cases anemia is profound with haemoglobin levels < 6gm/dl

However patients with Auto immune hemolytic anemia are usually managed by glucocorticoids and not by blood transfusion. Such patients may be managed by blood transfusion if anemia is severe, but the patient is unlikely to stay asymptomatic after a single blood transfusion without receiving definitive therapy in the form of glucocorticoids splenectomy or immunosupressive medications

The patient in question is 21 years old and has presented to the emergency department with haemoglobin level of 5g/dl. This is consistent with a presentation of Autoimmune Hemolytic Anemia.

However the patient in question turned asymptomatic after receiving a single blood transfusion in the past which is unlikely with an autoimmune process. Thalassemia intermedia is therefore the better answer of exclusive.

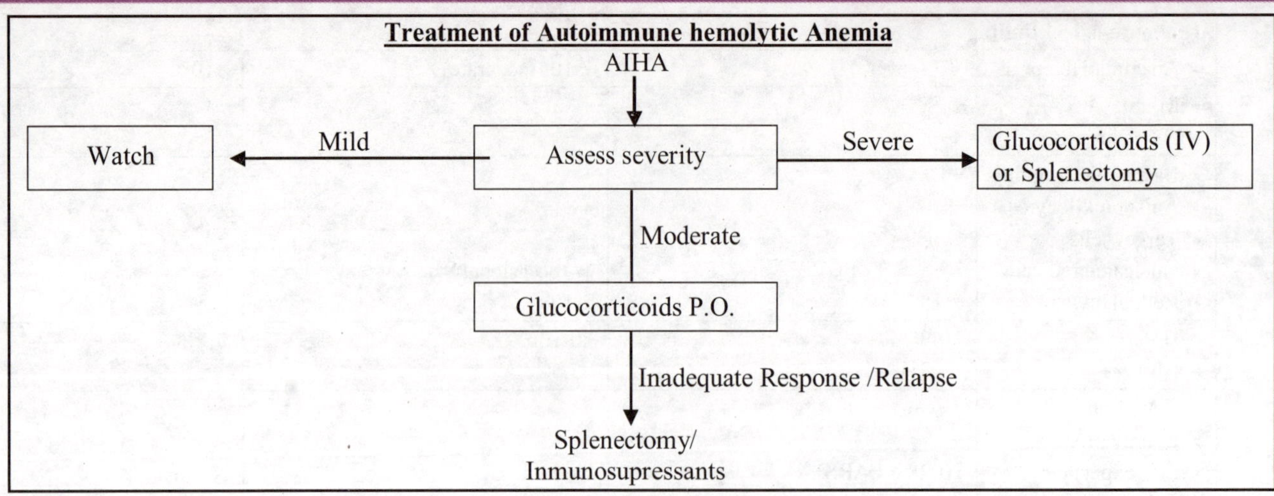

Note

Patients with severe anemic may require blood transfusions that are usually only for transient benefits – Nelson

Thalassemia Minor *does not present with severe anemia with haemoglobin levels of 5g/dl. Thalassemia minor can therefore be excluded in this patient.*

Thalassemia major *patients are transfusion dependent and require regular and multiple blood transfusion's by the time they reach 21 years of age thalassemia major can therefore be excluded in the patient*

Syndrome	Genotype	Anemia	Treatment
Thalassemia Minor	Heterozygous	Mild Anemia or normal Hb (Hb > 10 gm /dl) Asymptomatic	No treatment
Thalassemia Intermedia	Homozygous	Moderate Anemia (Hb= 6-10 gm/dl) Present later in life (adolescent/adult) without need of regular transfusion	Intermittent transfusions during exacerbations of anemia.
Thalassemia Major	Homozygous	Severe anemia (Hb< 7gm/dl) Present in infancy	Regular blood transfusions

87. Answer is A (Thalassemia Trait): *Harrison 18th/ 847; 17th/631, 640, 641; Hoffman 4th/575*

Mild degree of Microcytic Anemia (MCV=70) with normal ferritin levels (100μg/L) suggests a diagnosis of thalassemia trait.

Parameter	Normal Index	Patient in question	Inference
Hb	Male: 14-18g/dl Female: 12-16g/dl	Female with 10g/dl	*Mild Anemia*
Ferritin	50-200 μg/dl	100 μg/dl	*Normal*
MCV	86-98 fl	70 fl	*Microcytosis*
The patient in question has a microcytic anemia with normal ferritin levels			

Thalassemia trait and Iron deficiency anemia may present with microcytic anemia, but Iron deficiency Anemia is associated with decreased Ferritin levels. The patient in question has normal / increased Ferritin levels and hence she is unlikely to have an iron deficiency anemia.

The patient in question is thus most likely a patient of Thalassemia Trait

Parameter	Iron deficiency	Thalassemia Trait (Minor)
Smear	Microcytic Hypochromic	Microcytic hypochromic (Mild)
MCV (86-98 fi)	↓ed	↓ed
Serum iron	↓ed (<30)	Normal
TIBC	↑ed (>360)	Normal
Saturation	↓ed (<10)	↑ (30-80)
Ferritin	↓ed (<15)	↑ or (Normal Range in Minor/Trait)

Vitamin B12 deficiency and Folate deficiency cause Megaloblastic or Macrocytic anemia with increase MCV.

These anemias can be excluded as patient has a decreased MCV

88. Answer is D (Patient requires blood transfusion): Harrison 18th/p 859 *Harrison 17th/641; Hoffman 4th/575*

Most patients with β thalassemia trait are asymptomatic and have minimal or mild anemia. These patients do not require blood transfusions.

β Thalassemia Trait (Thalassemia - Minor):

- Thalassemia Trait results from inheritance of single β thalassemia allele.
- Most patients are asymptomatic and do no require treatment.
- The Hemoglobin levels average 1-2g/d lower than that seen in normal persons.
- It results in mild hypochromic microcytic anemia

Red cells are characteristically Hypochromic MCH < 26 pg
Red cells are characteristically Microcytic MCV < 75 fl

- Smear shows varying number of target cells, prokaryocytes, ovalocytes and basophilic stippling
- Red cells protoporphyrin levels are normal (elevated in Iron deficiency anemia)
- Diagnosis is established in most cases by Hb electrophoresis
  HbA2 levels are elevated (usually upto twice the normal (normal = 1.5 – 3.5%))
  HbF levels are elevated (may be normal <2% or moderately elevated 2.1 –5%)
- Reticulocytes count is usually normal
- Osmotic fragility is decreased
- Most patients are asymptomatic and do not require any treatment.

89. Answer is D (Severe anemia): *Refer previous question*

β Thalassemia trait is associated with mild anemia and not severe anemia.

Thalassemia Trait

Alpha Thalassemia Trait	Beta thalassemia trait (T. minor)
• ***Normal HBA_2***	• ↑ ***HBA_2***
• ***Normal HBF***	• ↑ ***HBF***
• Mild Anemia	• Mild Anemia
- Mild Microcytosis	- Mild Microcytosis
- Mild Hypochromia	- Mild Hypochromia
• No need for Blood transfusion	• No need for blood transfusion

90. Answer is C (Microcytosis): *Harrison 18th/859; Harrison 17th/641*

Alpha thalassemia trait exhibit mild microcytosis
HbF and HbA2 levels are normal and there is generally no anemia (mild anemia may be present)
'Persons with alpha thalassemia trait may exhibit mild hypochromia and microcytosis usually without anemia, HbA2 and HbF levels are normal' – Harrison 17th/641

91. Answer is A (Hereditary persistence of fetal hemoglobin): *Harrison 18th/ 859; 17th/642; Nelson 17th/1630; CMDT 2005/467*

Persistance of 95% of haemoglobin in the fetal form (HbF) in an adult who is asymptomatic and requires no blood transfusion suggests a diagnosis of hereditary persistence of fetal haemoglobin.

A combination of 95% HbF and 1.5% HbA2 may also be seen in Thalassemia intermedia. Although thalassemia intermedia does not require blood transfusion, ***it is not asymptomatic****.*

Hereditary persistence of Fetal haemoglobin syndromes *are a form of thalassemia with decreased production of either or both β & δ globin chains.*

The characteristic features are :
• Continued synthesis of high levels of HbF in adult life.
• (A mutation lead to decreased synthesis of β and δ globins).
• Haemoglobin electrophoresis reveals only HbF
• Clinically the patient is asymptomatic
• Mild anemia and slight microsytosis may be preserved

Hemoglobin levels in various thalassemias - *CMDT*

	Beta globin genes	HbA	HbA_2	HbF
Normal	*Homozygous β*	**97-99 %**	**1-3%**	**< 1%**
Thalassemia major	*Homozygous β°*	**0%**	**4-10 %**	**90-96 %**
Thalassemia major	*Heterozygous $β^+$*	**0-10 %**	**4-10%**	**90-96 %**
Thalassemia Intermedia	*Homozygous $β^+$ (mild)*	**0-30 %**	**0-10%**	**60-100%**
Thalassemia minor	*Heterozygous β°*	**80-95 %**	**4-8%**	**1-5%**
	Heterozygous $β^+$	**80-95 %**	**4-8%**	**1-5%**

A combination of 95% HbF and 1.5% HbA2 may only be seen in Thalassemia intermedia

1

92. Answer is A (Haemoglobin electrophoresis) : *Chandrasoma Taylor 2nd/386*

Presence of hypochromic microcytic anemia. Target cells on peripheral smear and positive family history suggest a diagnosis of Thalassemia.

Hemoglobin electrophoresis should always be the first investigation to include/exclude thalassemias.

Hematology

Thallassemia

- Thallassemias are characterised by *decreased rate of synthesis*[Q] of Hb chains that are *structurally normal*[Q]
- Thallassemia symdromes are common in persons with Mediterranean, African, Asian ancestary and *show marked familial tendencies*[Q]
- **β thallassemia or *Cooley's anemia***[Q] is the *commonest type*[Q]
- β thallassemia major is characterised by
  - Total or near total absence of synthesis of β chains, resulting in marked ***decrease in HbA ($α_2β_2$) levels***[Q]
  - Gamma chain synthesis then persists into adult life resulting in ***elevated HbF ($α_2γ_2$) levels*** [Q]
  - Delta chain synthesis is also increased to compensate for β chains resulting in ***elevated HbA_2 ($α_2δ_2$) levels***[Q]
- Excess free α chains precipiate in cytoplasm of affected RBC and result in their destruction which contributes to ***anemia (decreased Hb).*** [Q]
- The peripheral blood picture shows : - ***Microcytic hypochromic anemia*** [Q]
  - Anisocytosis (marked) [Q]
  - ***Target cells (numerous)*** [Q]
  - Reticulocytosis and nucleated red cells. [Q]
- Diagnosis is ***established by Haemoglobin electrophoresis*** which shows : [Q]
  - Elevated HbF and HbA_2 with greatly decreased or absent HbA.

***Target cells** are formed due to increased ratio of RBC surface area to volume. Seen in Haemoglobin disorders such as: Thallassemia, HbS, HbC etc, Liver disease.*

93. Answer is D (Hb-electrophoresis): Harrison 18th/p 854, 859 *Harrison 17th edn /637, 641; Read text below*

Hemoglobin electrophoresis documenting elevated HbF & HbA_2 with greatly decreased or absent HbA point towards a diagnosis of β thalassemia.

- ***Thalassemia is a quantitative defect in Hb characterized*** by lack of certain types of globin chains and compensatory increase in other globin chains.
  Electrophoretic techniques used for routine hemoglobin analysis help in quantification and identification of various hemoglobins.
- Thalassemia, the commonest thalassemia for example can be detected by electrophoretic demonstration of the following characteristics:
  Total absence of synthesis of β chain : Marked decrease in HbA ($α_2β_2$)
  Compensatory increase of α & delta chains : ↑HbF ($α_2υ_2$); ↑HbA_2 ($α_2δ_2$)

94. Answer is C (Hb electrophoresis) : Harrison 18th/p 854, 859 *Harrison 16th/599, 608; Harrison 17th edn /637, 641; CMDT 2005/466; CMDT 09/432*

'The diagnosis of thalassemia syndromes is best established by Hb electrophoresis.'

Thalassemia is a quantitative defect in Hb characterized by lack of certain types of globin chains and compensatory increase in other globin chains. These changes form the basis of electrophoretic investigations and are diagnostic of respective thalassemia syndromes.

NESTROFT test : *Naked **E**ye **S**ingle **T**ube **R**ed Cell **O**smotic **F**ragility **T**est is used for screening of thalassemia but is not diagnostic.*

HBAIC : Estimation of glycated haemoglobin is used for estimating long term Glucose control in diabetics. It has no role in thalassemia.

Target cells **:** May be seen in thalassemia but do not establish diagnosis of thalassemia.

Target Cells
Thalassemia
Haemoglobin C, s etc.
Liver diseases

95. Answer is A (Hb electrophoresis): Harrison 18th/p 854, 859 *Harrison 17th/637, 641; Nelson Pediatrics 16th/1479-1484; Nelson 17th/1630*

Progressive increasing pallor along with hepatosplenomegaly in a five year old girl is consistent with a diagnosis of thalassemia. (Thalassemia intermedia)

'Haemoglobin electrophoresis' is the test of choice for diagnosing this condition and hence is the option of choice here.

Medullary and extramedullary erythropoiesis leads to expansion of bone marrow space causing a characteristic hemolytic facies with frontoparental, occipital bossing, malar prominence and malocclusion of teeth and complications that include distortion of ribs and vertebra, pathological fractures of the long bones, splenomegaly and its complications – hypersplenism, hepatomegaly gallstone and leg ulcers.

96. Answer is A (Thalassemia): *Rotations 7th/634,635; Essential Radiology (2006)/536; Rudolph Pediatrics 21st/1537; Musculoskeletal Imaging by Bohndorf (2001)/214*

Hair on end appearances may be seen in both sickle cell anemia and thalassemia, but it is more characteristic of thalassemia major which is the single best answer of choice

Hair on End appearances (Crew cut appearance) of the cranial vault

- Hair an end appearance refers to the presence of multiple vertical striations through expanded marrow (widened diploic space) as a result of subperiosteal bone growth in a series of vertical striations
- This is produced as a result of marrow hyperplasia and may be observed in conditions.
- Associated with marrow hyperplasias secondary to hemolytic anemia.
- ***Its presence is considered characteristic of thalassemia but it may also be seen in sickle cell anemia and other causes of hemolytic anemia including hereditary spherocytosis and G-6po deficiency.***

Hair on end appearance is also called crew cut appearance

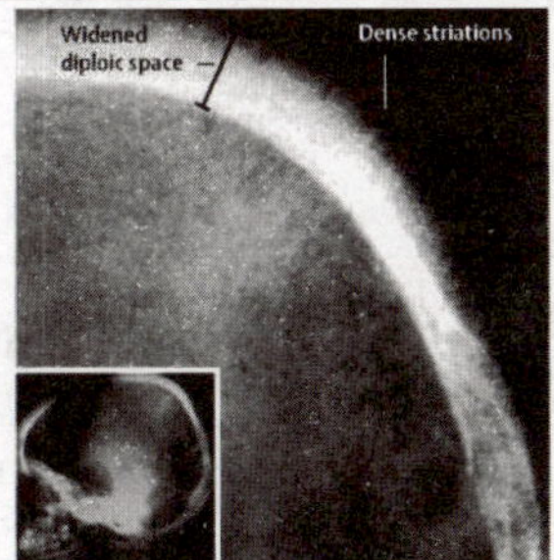

Thalassemia. Typical 'hair-on-end' skull

1

Hematology

97. Answer is A (Juvenile CML): *Ghai 6th/569; Interpretation of diagnostic tests 8th/411, 412*

Fetal Haemoglobin levels (HbF) are increased in most cases of Juvenile CML – Ghai 6th/569

Causes of Raised HbF levels (Interpretation of Diagnostic Test 8th/411, 412)

- Haemoglobinopathies
  - β thalassemia major
  - β thalassemia minor
  - Sickle cell disease
- Hereditary Persistance of HbF
- Anemia:
  - Non Hereditary refractory normoblastic anemia
  - Pernicious anemia
  - Aplastic anemia
- ***Leukemia specially Juvenile Myeloid Leukemia***
- Multiple myeloma
- Molar pregnancy
- Patients with Trisomy 13 or Trisomy 21 (Down's syndrome)
- Some chronic viral infections (eg CMV, EBV)

98. Answer is A (Alpha Thalassemia): *Disorders of Hemoglobin 1st (2001)/212, 213*

Alpha Thalassemia are associated with reduced levels of HbA2

Causes of Increased HbA2 levels	Causes of Decreased HbA2 levels
• *Beta thalassemia*	• *Iron deficiency Anemia*
• *Sickle cell anemia*	• ***Alpha thalassemia***
• *Megaloblastic anemia*	• *Delta thalassemia*
• *Hyperthyroidism*	• *Sideroblastic anemia*
• *Unstable Hemoglobinopathies*	• *Myelodysplastic syndromes*
• *Malaria (doubtfull cases)*	• *Acute myelocytic leukemia (minor reduction)*
	• *Hb Lepore*

Autoimmune Hemolytic Anemia

99. Answer is D (Mycoplasma Pneumonia): *Harrison 18th/ 882; 16th/612, 613, 614; 17th/ 660; API 8th edn/ 810, 811*

Mycoplasma pneumoniae infections are associated with a cold antibody haemolytic anemia

Autoimmune hemolytic anemias are characterized by formation of autoantibodies against patient's own red cells.

Depending upon reactivity of autoantibodies these are further divided into two types.

Warm antibody hemolytic anemia	***Cold antibody hemolytic anemia***
Antibodies here react at room temperature and are mainly of IgG type Q	Antibodies here react better at temperatures lower than 37°C, and are mainly IgM Q [An exception is cold reactive antibodies of IgG Q type in Paroxysmal cold hemoglo bulinuria] Q
Causes :	*Causes :*
1. Idiopathic 2. Lymphomas : CLL Q , Non-Hodgkins, etc. 3. SLE Q and other Collagen Vascular Diseases Q 4. Drugs : e.g. α Methyldopa Q	1. Acute : Mycoplasma Infection Q Infectious mononucleosis Q 2. Chronic : Idiopathic Q 3. Paroxysmal cold hemoglobinuria Q
Mechanism of Hemolysis :	*Mechanism of Hemolysis :*
Human red cells cooled with IgG are trapped by splenic macrophages - Red cell destruction	Antibodies of IgM type bind on Red cell surface and cause agglutination. Hemolytic effect is mediated through fixation of C3 to RBC surface. Q
Diagnosis :	*Diagnosis :*
Positive direct Coomb's test, at 37°C for presence of warm antibodies on surface of Red cell. Q Positive Indirect Coomb's test at 37°C for presence of large quantities of warm antibodies in serum. Q	Positive direct Coomb's test for detection of C3 on the red cell surface, but IgM responsible for coating on red cells is not found. Q

100. Answer is A (IgM antibodies) : Harrison 18th/p 882 *Harrison 17th/660 , Harrison 16th/613, 612*

Antibodies that bind with antigens better at temperature lower than 37°C are called Cold reactive antibodies. These antibodies are usually IgM antibodies.

IgM cold- reacting antibodies readily agglutinate RBC's and are called cold agglutinins.

Warm Antibody Hemolytic Anemia	*Cold Antibody Hemolytic Anemia*
• Antibodies here bind with antigens (on RBC) at body temperature (37°C) • These antibodies are called warm antibodies and are **nearly IgG** (Rarely IgM or IgA)	• Antibodies here bind with antiens (on RBC) better at temperatures lower than 37°C • These antibodies are called cold reactive antibodies and are **usually IgM** ***(Rarely IgG antibodies eg. The Donath Landsteiner Antibody of 'Paroxysmal cold Haemoglobinuria***[Q])
Causes	*Causes*
1. Idiopathic 2. Lymphomas: CLL [Q], Non-Hodgkins, etc 3. SLE [Q] and other Collagen Vascular Diseases 4. Drugs: eg. α Methyldopa[Q]	1. Acute: Mycoplasma infection [Q] Infectious mononucleosis [Q] 2. Chronic : Idiopathic [Q] 3. Paroxysmal cold hemoglobinuria [Q]
Mechanism of Hemolysis	*Mechanism of Hemolysis*
Human red cells cooled with IgG are trapped by splenic macrophages – red cell destruction	Antibodies of IgM type bind on Red cell surface and cause agglutination. Hemolytic effect is mediated through fixation of C3 to RBC surface.[Q]
Diagnosis	*Diagnosis*
Positive direct Coomb's test, at 37°C for presence of warm antibodies on surface of Red cell.[Q] Positive Indirect Coomb's test at 37°C for presence of large quantities of warm antibodies in serum. [Q]	Positive direct Coomb's test for detection of C3 on the red cell surface but IgM responsible for coating on red cells is not found. [Q]

Note

Donath Landsteiner antibody of Paraxysmal Cold Haemoglobinuria is a rare IgG type of cold reactive antibody. But the term 'cold agglutinins' is generally used for only the IgM cold reacting antibodies that readily agglutinate Red Blood cells

'IgM Cold reacting antibodies readily agglutinate RBC and are called cold Aglutinins' - Harrisons 16th/613

IgM antibody is therefore the single best answer of choice.

101. Answer is B (Chronic lymphatic leukemia): *Harrison 18th/p 882; 16th/ 612; Harrison 17th/ 660; API 8th edn/ 810, 811*

Leukemias specially of the CLL type are associated with Autoimmune hemolytic anemia *– Harrison*

Hemolysis due to Antibodies:

Warm-Antibody immunohemolytic anemia	Cold-Antibody immunohemolytic Anemia
1. Idiopathic 2. Lymphomas: Chronic lymphocytic leukemia, non-Hodgkin's lymphomas, Hodgkin'd disease (infrequent) 3. SLE and other collagen-vascular diseases 4. Drugs (a) α-Methyldopa type (autoantibody to Rh antigens) (b) Penicillin type (stable hapten) (c) Quinidine type (unstable hapten) 5. Postviral infections 6. Other tumors (rare)	1. Cold agglutinin disease (a) Acute: Mycoplasma infection, infectious mononucleosis (b) Chronic: Idiopathic, lymphoma 2. Paroxysmal cold hemoglobinuria

102. Answer is B (B cell type) : Harrison 18th/p 926, 927 *Harrison 16th 648, 612; 17th/ 693; CMDT 2006/495, 506; CMDT 2008/449; 09/455*

The diagnosis of typical B cell CLL should be considered in a patient presenting with an autoimmune hemolytic anemia or autoimmune thrombocytopenia. *– Harrison 16th / 648*

Autoimmune hemolytic anemia (AIHA) and Lymphoid malignancies

Autoimune hemolytic anemias may be seen in association with Leukemias specially of the B cell CLL type and with Lymphomas especially of the Non Hodgkins type.

Leukemias and AIHA	Lymphomas & AIHA
Characteristically seen in association with Chronic Lymphocytic Leukemia (***Typical B cell CLL)***[Q]	More commonly seen in association with Non Hodgkin's Lymphoma, but may also be seen with Hodgkins type.
(CLL is a clonal malignancy of B cell)[Q]	***Non Hodgkins(NHL) > Hodgkins (infrequent)***
Autoantibodies are mainly ***IgG type***[Q] and hemolytic anemias are accordingly classified as ***warm antibody type***	Autoantibodies are *usually IgG* (warm antibodies) but cold Antibody type (IgM) hemolytic anemias may also be seen .
	Warm antibody type > Cold Antibody (infrequent) type

103. Answer is C (CLL): *Harrison 14th/ 666; Harrison 16th/ 612; Refer previous question*

Leukemias specially of the CLL type are associated with Autoimmune hemolytic anemia - Harrison

Autoimmune hemolytic anemia of the warm antibody type are caused by leukemias specially of the chronic lymphocytic type & Non Hodgkin lymphoma

104. Answer is A (Alcoholic cirrhosis): *Harrison 16 th edn/ 612; API 8th edn/ 810, 811; Read text below*

Coomb's positive hemolytic anemia may be seen in autoimmune conditions. All options other than alcoholic cirrhosis may have autoimmune etiologies and hence, may very well have coomb's positive haemolytic anemia as a feature.

Anemias which occur due to autoimmune destruction of RBCs are called autoimmune hemolytic anemia. The autoimmune destruction of RBC's is caused by the presence of autoantibodies against R.B.C.

Coomb's test is used to detect the presence of these autoantibodies. ***So autoimmune hemolytic anemias are also known as coomb's positive hemolytic anemias.***

105. Answer is C (SLE): *Harrison 16th/612; API 8th/810; Hoffman's 4th/693, 695*

Coombs positive hemolytic anemia is a feature of autoimmune hemolytic anemia and is characteristically seen in SLE.

Polyarteritis Nodosa (PAN) may also be associated with a Coombs positive hemolytic anemia. However this association is rare, and more commonly patients with PAN present either with an anemia of chronic disease or a microangiopathic hemolytic anemia.

TTP and HUS are characteristically associated with Coombs negative microangiopathic hemolytic anemias.

106. Answer is A (Thrombotic Thrombocytopenic Purpura): *Harrisons 16th/612; API 8th/810*

Thrombotic Thrombocytopenic purpura is associated with Coombs negative hemolytic anemia

Coomb's positive hemolytic anemia is a feature of Autoimmune Hemolytic anemias*, SLE and other collagen vascular diseases including PAN, and scleroderma may be associated with warm antibody autoimmune hemolytic anemias and hence may present with Coomb's positive hemolytic anemia.*

Thrombotic Thrombocytopenic purpura is not associated with immune mediate hemolysis and hence it is associated with Coomb's negative hemolytic anemia

Collagen vascular diseases associated with Autoimmune Hemolytic Anemias (AIHA) (Warm Antibody Type)

Common	Less Common/Rare
SLE	• Rheumatoid Arthritis • PAN • Scleroderma • Sjogren's syndrome

107. Answer is C (systemic lupus erythematosis) : *Harrisons 16th/612; Hoffman's 4th/693,695*

Coomb's positive hemolytic anemia is a feature of autoimmune vascular disease and may also be seen in SLE and other Collagen Vascular diseases including PAN and Systemic sclerosis.

However amongst the options provided coombs positive hemolytic anemia is most commonly associated with SLE which is the single best answer of exclusion.

Autoimmune hemoletic anemias are associated with 'collagen vascular diseases especially systemic lupus Erythematosis'– Harrisons

Autoimmune hemolytic anemia are associated with 'autoimmune diseases particularly Systemic Lupus Erythematosis' -Hoffman.

108. Answer is C (Coomb's test) : *Harrison 18th/p 875, 881; 17th/ 634, 635, 659, Harrisons 16th/ 608, 609; CMDT 09/436*

Presence of anemia and jaundice together with spherocytes in peripheral smear is consistent with a diagnosis of both hereditary spherocytosis and auto immune hemolytic anemias.

The onset of symptoms at 40 years of age favours an acquired etiology and suggests a presumptive diagnosis of Acquired Autoimmune Hemolytic anemias. Nevertheless, mild cases of Hereditary spherocytosis may also first present in young adults and even later in life (Harrison) ***Coomb's test is the single best investigation for such patients as it can clinch the diagnosis of Autoimmune Hemolytic anemias and establish the distinction between the two probable diagnosis.***

According to Harrison text:

'Hereditary spherocytosis must be distinguished primarily from the spherocytic hemolytic anemias associated with RBC antibodies'

Coomb's test is positive in immune spherocytic hemolytic anemias and it is negative in hereditary spherocytosis

- "The diagnosis of immune spherocytosis is readily established by a positive coomb's test" – Harrison
- "Coomb's test is negative in hereditary spherocytosis" CMDT 06

Osmotic fragility *test will be positive in both hereditary spherocytosis and immune spherocytic hemolytic anemias. "Increased osmotic fragility merely reflects the presence of spherocytes and does not distinguish hereditary spherocytosis from other spherocytic hemolytic disorders such as autoimmune hemolytic anemia" – CMDT 06/491*

Coomb's test *is the single best next investigation here as it will* ***establish the distinction****.*

Note: Presence of spherocytes in the peripheral blood smear does not necessarily imply hereditary spherocytosis

Causes of spherocytosis in peripheral smear / Spherocytic hemolytic anemia
• Hereditary spherocytosis
• Immunohemolytic anemias (Autoimmune hemolytic anemias)
• In association with hemolysis induced by splenomegaly in patients with cirrhosis
• Clostridial infections
• Certain snake envenomations
• G6PD deficiency (few spherocytes)

109. Answer is C (Coombs test) : Harrison 18th/p 851, 852, 879 *Harrison 17th/ 654, 655, 659;API 8th/809, 810, CMDT 2008 / 430, 431; CMDT 09/436*

Presence of anemia and jaundice together with spherocytes in peripheral smear is consistent with the diagnosis of both 'hereditary spherocytosis' and 'immunohemolytic anemias'. ***Coomb's test*** *is the single best next investigation here as it will* ***establish the above distinction.***

According to Harrisons text:

'Hereditary spherocytosis must be distinguished primarily from the spherocytic hemolytic anemias associated with RBC antibodies.'

Coomb's test is positive in immune spherocytic hemolytic anemias and it is negative in hereditroy spherocytosis.

o *"The diagnosis of immune spherocytosis is readily established by a positive coomb's test." - Harrison*

o *"Coomb's test is negative in hereditary spherocytosis." CMDT 06*

Osmotic fragility test will be positive in both hereditary spherocytosis and immune spherocytic hemolytic anemias.

"Increased osmotic fragility merely reflects the presence of spherocytes and does not distinguish hereditary spherocytosis from other spherocytic hemolytic disorders such as autoimmune hemolytic anemia." - CMDT 06 / 491

Coomb's test *is the single best next investigation here as it will* ***establish the above distinction.***

Causes of spherocytes in peripheral smear / Spherocytic hemolytic anemia

- Hereditary spherocytosis.
- Immunohemolytic anemias (Autoimmune hemolytic anemias).
- In association with hemolysis induced by splenomegaly in patients with cirrhosis.
- Clostridial infections.
- Certain snake envenomations.
- G6PD deficiency (few spherocytes).

1

Hematology

Microangiopathic Hemolytic Anemia

110. Answer is C (Hemophilia - A): *Harrison 18th/ 883; 17th/658; CMDT 2007/533; 2009/442, 436; William's Manual of Hematology 6th/118*

Hemophilia A is not a cause for microangiopathic hemolytic anemia or fragmented RBC's in peripheral blood.

Classification of Microangiopathic Hemolytic Anemia

Primary

- **Thrombotic thrombocytopenic purpura**
- **Hemolytic uremic syndrome**

Secondary

- **Associated with disseminated intravascular coagulation**
  - Infections (sepsis)
  - Shiga-type toxins
  - HIV
  - Snake venoms
  - Abruptio placentae
- **Associated with hypertension**
  - Malignant hypertension
  - Preclampsia, eclampsia,
  - HELLP syndrome
- **Associated with malignancy**
  - Adenocarcinomas; gastrointestinal, breast, lung
- **Associated with drugs and/or radiation**
  - Antineoplastic agents
  - Radiation nephritis and chemotherapy in organ transplantation
  - Ticlopidine
- **Associated with immunologic disorders/Vasculitis**
  - Acute glomerulonephritis
  - SLE
  - Polyarteritis nodosa
  - Scleroderma
  - Other vasculitis
- **Associated with congenital malformations**
  - Cavernous hemangioma (Kasabach-Meritt syndrome)
  - Hemangioendothelioma of the liver
- **Associated with antiphospholipid syndrome** (*NMS Medicine*)
- **Associated with Prosthetic valves** (*Harrison/CMDT*) (Pathologically Macroangiopathic – *Rubin's Pathology*)

111. Answer is D (Evan's syndrome): *Wintrobe's Hematology 12th/968; Harrison 17th/658; Harrison 18th/881; William's Obstetrics 21st/577*

Evan's syndrome is not a microangiopathic hemolytic condition and does not present with fragmented RBCs in the peripheral smear.

Presence of fragmented RBC's in the peripheral smear suggests the diagnosis of a micro-angiopathic process (Microangiopathic Hemolytic Anemia). The fragmentation of RBC's is caused by fibrin deposits in small blood vessels, which cause mechanical hemolysis. Patients with microangiopathic hemolytic anemias are usually thrombocytopenic (due to consumption of Platelets).

Microangiopathic Hemolytic anemia (fragmented RBC) and Thrombocytopenia are typically seen in TTP, HUS, DIC and HELLP syndrome besides several other conditions.

Evan's syndrome (combination of ITP and Autoimmune Hemolytic Anemia (AIHA))

- *Evan's Syndrome refers to a combination of Idiopathic Thrombocytopenic Purpura (ITP) and Autoimmune Hemolytic Anemia (AIHA) in the absence of an underlying cause / disease.*
- The occurence of thrombocytopenia may coincide with episodes of hemolysis or may arise as separate episodes.
- Evan's syndrome is more common in children
- Evan's syndrome tends to be resistanct to management of Warm AIHA or ITP
- ***Evans syndrome presents with 'Thrombocytopenia' and 'Immune Hemolysis'.***

Evan's syndrome does not present with microangiopathic features or fragmented RBCs.

TTP, DIC and HELLP syndrome all may present with microangiopathic features (fragmented RBC's) and thrombocytopenia

Microangiopathic Hemolytic Anemias
• ***TTP***
• ***HUS***
• ***DIC***
• *Vasculitis (Collagen Vascular Disorders)*
• *Malignant Hypertension/Eclampsia/**HELLP***
• *Disseminated carcinomatosis (Metastasis)*
• *Drugs / Radiation*
• *Antiphospholipid syndrome(NMS Medicine)*
• *Prosthetic Heart Valves* (Pathologically Macroangiopathic – *Rubin's Pathology*)

Patients with microangiopathic hemolytic anemias are usually thrombocytopenic *(due to consumption of Platelets).*

112. Answer is C (Myocardial Infarction): Harrison 18th/p 883 *CMDT 2007/533; 2009/442, 436; Harrison 17th/658; William's Hematology 6th/118*

Myocardial Infarction is not a cause for microangiopathic hemolytic anemia.

113. Answer is None or B (None or Metallic Heart Valve): *Rubin's Pathology 5th/878; William Manual of Hematology Nathan and Osk's Hematology 7th/643; NMS Medicine 5th/348*

'Metallic heart valves' is the single best answer of exclusion.

Pathologically Prosthetic Heart valves are associated with macroangiopathic hemolytic anemias and not microangiopathic hemolytic anemias.

TTP, Antiphospholipid syndrome, vasculitis syndromes (including MPA) and mechanical heart valves may all give rise to hemolytic anemia due to red cell fragmentation. Most textbooks do not make a distinction between macroangiopathic and microangiopathic hemolytic syndromes and club all causes into the category of microangiopathic hemolytic anemias (including prosthetic valve hemolytic anemias)

However in strict terminology microangippathic hemolytic anemias result from cell fragmentation that occurs in the microcirculation.

Red cell fragmentation hemolytic anemias from prosthetic heart valves is strictly/pathologically a macroangiopathic hemolytic anemia and hence the single best answer of exclusion.

Mechanical Red Cell Fragmentation Syndromes

Macroangiopathic (large vessel)	**Microangiopathic (small vessel)**
Direct Red Cell trauma from an abnormal vascular surface. • ***Prosthetic Heart Valves***^{Q} • ***Synthetic vascular grafts***^{Q} Large vessel disorders that may cause shearing of Erythrocytes • *Cavernous Hemangioma* (Kasabach-Merritt syndrome)	Abnormalities in microcirculation that cause turbulent blood flow • *DIC* • *TTP* • *HUS* • *Vasculitis (Collagen Vascular Disorders)* • *Malignant Hypertension/Eclampsia* • *Disseminated carcinomatosis (Metastasis)* • *Drugs / Radiation* • *Antiphospholipid syndrome*

Antiphospholipid syndrome and microangiopathic hemolytic anemia

Microangiopathic hemolytic anemias has been found in association with the antiphospholipid antibody syndrome.
– NMS Medicine 5th/348

Note:

Both Harrison and CMDT classify Hemolysis in association with prosthetic heart valves as microangiopathic hemolytic anemia and hence 'none' would probably be the correct answer.

114. Answer is B (ITP): Harrison 18th/883; *17th/658; CMDT 2007/533; 2009/442, 436; William's Hematology 6th/118*

Idiopathic thrombocytopenic purpura is not a cause for microangiopathic hemolytic anemia.

Note:

Pathologically Prosthetic Heart valves are associated with macroangiopathic hemolytic anemias and not microangiopathic hemolytic anemias.However, most textbooks do not make a distinction between macroangiopathic and microangiopathic hemolytic syndromes and club all causes into the category of microangiopathic hemolytic anemias (including prosthetic valve hemolytic anemias)

Both Harrison and CMDT classify Hemolysis in association with prosthetic heart valves as microangiopathic hemolytic anemia and hence prosthetic valves is not excluded in this answer.

Proxysmal Nocturnal Hemoglobinuria (PNH)

115. Answer is B (Increased LAP scores): *Harrison 18th/883, 884; 16th/ 616; 17th/ 660, 661; CMDT 2008/432; 2009/437*

PNH is associated with a decreased Leukocyte Alkaline phosphase (LAP) score

PNH: Paroxysmal Nuctunal haemoglobinuria: *Review*

PNH is an Acquired ^{Q} Intracarpuscular ^{Q} disorder, acquired at stem cell level ^{Q} by loss characterised by undue sensitivity of red blood cell's membrane to complement ^{Q}

Common manifestations: PNH : Three common manifestation

Hemolytic Anemia	**Venous Thrombosis**	**Deficient Hematopoesis**
↓ Because of increased activation of complement and complement mediated destruction ↓ *Hemoglobinemia* ^{Q} *Hemoglobinuria* ^{Q} *Hemosiderinuria* ^{Q} ***Elevated LDH*** ^{Q}	Activation of complement indirectly stimulates platelet aggregation and hypercoagulability (thus thrombosis despite thrombocytopenia)	Probably due to defect at stem cell level ↓ Pancytopenia/Aplastic anemia-H16th/ 618 - ↓ Granulocytes - Thrombocytes (thrombocytopenia)

Why is it called Paroxysmal Nocturnal haemoglobinuria? **Basis** : *Acidification enhances activity of complement*
During night when one sleeps **(noctunal)** → Relative Hypoxia → Acidosis → Enhanced complement activity ↓ **Paroxysm** of **Haemoglobinuria** identified by passage of brown urine in morning. ← Complement mediated destruction of red blood cells
Red Cell Membrane is **deficient in two factors** which result in increased activation of complement 1. **DAF** [Q] : Decay accelerating factor that activates decay of complements 2. MIRL CD 59 : inhibits membrane attack complex

116. Answer is D (Massive splenomegaly): *Harrison 18th/883, 884, 887; 17th/660, 661; Williams 7th/470; 'Blood' by Handin 2nd/326*

PNH is usually not associated with a massive splenomegaly

'Splenomegaly is present in some patients with PNH, but the enlargement of spleen is usually quiet modest'.

– Williams Hematology 7th/470

Venous Thrombosis is a common manifestation/complication of PNH

Venous Thrombosis

Abdominal veins are the most common site of venous thrombosis in PNH	Cranial vein are the second most common site of venous thrombosis after abdominal veins- *'Blood' 2nd/326*
• ***Classic site of thrombosis is the Hepatic vein causing Budd Chiari syndrome.*** • Splenic veins, portal vein, mesenteric vessels, renal vein and inferior venacava may also be involved.	***Frank Cerebral thrombosis is a grave complication of PNH.*** *– William's Hematology 7th/471*

PNH is associated with Pancytopenia (Harrison 17th/663)
PNH is a cause for Pancytopenia with a cellular marrow.

117. Answer is C (Increased alkaline phosphatase): *See previous question*

PNH is associated with a decreased leukocyte alkaline phosphate scape.
Remember the following fact to answer several questions in our kind of examinations by the principle of exclusion:

Conditions with decreased LAP scores	Conditions with increased LAP scores
1. P.N.H. [Q]	1. Polycythemia [Q]
2. C.M.L. [Q]	2. Leukemoid reaction [Q]
	3. Infection [Q]

118. Answer is C (Paroxysmal Nocturnal haemoglobinuria): Harrison 18th/p 883, 884 *Harrison16th/616; Harrison17th/660, 661; Robbins illustrated 5th/619, Robbins 7th/636*

Paroxysmal nocturnal haemoglobinuria (PNH) results from an acquired somatic mutation on the pleuripotent stem cells. Hence all its clonal progeny i.e. red cells, white cells and platelets are affected *- Robbins 7th/ 636*

Paroxysmal nocturnal haemoglobinuria: is an acquired *clonal disease* that is associated with abnormality of complement regulation. *This defect affects the Pluripotent stem cells & the clonal progeny of these stem cells. Red cells, white cells & platelets thus all are affected.*

Paroxysmal cold haemoglobinuria, Blackfan Diamond syndrome (pure red cell aplasia) and hemolytic anemias *characteristically involve the red cell lineage only.*

119. Answer is A (Hypercellular marrow): *Refer text below*

PNH is associated with a normocellular or hypercellular marrow and not with a hypocellular marrow.

PNH is associated with an increased incidence of venous thrombosis and may lead to Budd-Chirai syndrome.
PNH is associated with decreased LAP scores.

120. Answer is C (Decreased LDH): Harrison 18th/p 883, 884 *Harrison 16th/616; 17th/ 660, 661; Robbins illustrated 6th/681, Robbins 7th/ 630*

Because of increased activation of complement and complement mediated destruction of RBC there occurs intravascular hemolysis and an elevated LDH is seen.

Paroxysmal nocturnal haemoglobinuria may have thrombosis and thrombocytopenia both, as is depicted in the previous explanations.

121. Answer is D (All of the above): *Harrison 18th/p 883, 884; 17th/ed 660, 661 Wintrobe's Hematology 12th/1002;*

PNH is associated with a deficiency of GPI anchored proteins including DAF and MIRL

PNH is associated with a deficiency of GPI Anchored proteins

DAF (CD55) and MIRL (CD59) are the most important GPI Anchored proteins that may be deficient in PNH.

Since option 'D' allows us to select all the above options and we are not forced to select one single best protein 'Option D' becomes the answer of choice.

Glycosyl phosphatidylinositol (GPI) anchored proteins and PNH

- PNH is primarily associated with a deficiency of GPI anchored proteins on hemotopoetic cells
  All proteins that are deficient in PNH are GPI Anchored and all GPI anchored proteins that are expressed by hematopoietic cells are deficient in PNH' – *Wintrobe's*
- The most important GPI anchored proteins that are causally related to PNH are the complement regulatory proteins that result in abnormal susceptibility of erythrocytes to complement mediated lysis.

GPI Anchored complement regulatory proteins
Decay accelerating factor (DAF – CD 55)
Membrane Inhibitor of Reactive Lysis (MIRL – CD59)

- However several other GPI anchored proteins may be deficient in PNH and currently the list of proteins deficient in PNH numbers more than 20

GPI Anchored Proteins Deficient in PNH	
• Leukocyte alkaline phosphatase	• CD66b (formerly CD67)
• Acetylcholinesterase	• CD66c
• Decay accelerating factor (DAF, CD55)	• p50-80
• Membrane inhibitor of reactivity lysis (MIRL, CD59)	• CD24
• FcγRIIIb (CD16b)	• CD48
• Lymphocyte function-associated antigen 3 (LFA-3, CD58)	• Thy-1 (CD90)
• Endotoxin-binding protein (CD14)	• CD109
• Campath 1 (CD52)	• CD157
• 5'-ectonucleotidase (CD73)	• GP500
• Urokinase plasminogen activator receptor (CD87)	• GP175
• JMH-bearing protein (CD108)	• Folate receptor
	• Cellular prion protein

122. Answer is C (GPI Anchored Proteins): Harrison 18th/p 883, 884 *Wintrobe's 12th/ 1002; Harrison's 17th/ed 660, 661*

All of the proteins mentioned as options (DAF, MIRL and LFA) may be deficient in PNH and all of these proteins are GPI anchored proteins. ***Since we have to chose a single best answer amongst the options provided, GPI Anchored proteins becomes the answer of choice.***

'All proteins that are deficient in PNH are GPI Anchored and all GPI – Anchored proteins that are expressed by hematopoetic cells are deficient in PNH' - Wintrobe's Hematology

All proteins deficient in PNH are GPI anchored proteins and hence GPI anchored proteins is the single best answer of choice

123. Answer is B (Complements): Harrison 18th/p 884 *Harrison 16th / 616; Harrison 17th/ 661*

HAM test is based upon susceptibility of RBC's to complement mediated lysis in patients with PNH.

HAM test is used for the diagnosis of PNH (Paroxysmal Nocturnal Haemoglobinuria). HAM test (Acidified serum lysis test) demonstrates lysis of RBC after activation of complement by acid. ***In acidified serum complement is activated by the alternate pathway.*** *In patients with PNH, RBC are unusually susceptible to complement, and undergo lysis when incubated with acidified fresh serum.*

Diagnosis of PNH

Flow cytometry	Demonstration of Lysis of RBC after complement activation
▪ ***Test of Choice*** ▪ Analyses GPI - Linked proteins - CD 59 - DAF (CD55) ▪ These proteins block activation of complement on cell surface. Their absence accounts for sensitivity of RBC to complement lysis	▪ Ham Test (complement activation by acid) ▪ Sucrose lysis test (complement activation by reduction in ionic strength)

Aplastic Anemia and Myelodysplastic Syndrome

Aplastic Anemia and Pancytopenia

124. Answer is D (Cold haemoglobinuria): Harrison 18th/p 888; table 107.2 *Harrison 16th/ 618; 17th/ 663; table 1022; Chandrasoma Taylor 3rd/ 381*

Paroxysmal Cold Hemoglobinuria is a form of immune mediated hemolytic anemia and is not a form of aplastic anemia.

Pregnancy, PNH and hepatitis have all been mentioned as causes of Aplastic anemia.

Classification Of Aplastic Anemia And Cytopenias :

Acquired **Aplastic Anemia**	***Inherited*** **Aplastic Anemia**
Radiation	Fanconi's anemia
Drugs and chemicals	Dyskeratosis congenita
Regular effects	Shwachman-Diamond syndrome
Idiosyncratic reactions	Reticular dysgenesis
Viruses	Amegakaryocytic thrombocytopenia
Epstein-Barr virus (infectious mononucleosis)	Familial aplastic anemias
Hepatitis (non-A, non-B, non-C hepatitis)	Preleukemia (monosomy 7, etc.)
Parvovirus B19 (transient aplastic crisis. PRCA)	Nonhematologic syndrome
HIV-1 (AIDS)	(Down's Dubowitz, Seckel)
Immune diseases	
Eosinophilic fasciitis	
Hypoi-immunophilic globulinemia	
Thymoma/thymic carcinoma	
Graft-versus-host disease in Immunodeficiency	
Paroxysmal nocturnal hemoglobinuria	
Pregnancy	
Idiopathic	

125. Answer is C (Hepatitis A): Harrison 18th/p 887, 888 *Harrison 17th/663, 664*

Aplastic anemia is associated with Non-A, Non-B, Non-C, Hepatitis and not with Hepatitis A

Parvovirus B19, HIV-1, Chloramphenicol and PNH are all associated with Aplastic anemia.

126. Answer is A (PNH) : Harrison 18th/p 883, table 107.1 *Harrison 16th / 617; 17th / 663; table 102-1*

Amongst the options provided PNH is the single best answer of choice.

Differential diagnosis of Pancytopenia

Pancytopenia with Hypocellular Bone Marrow
Acquired aplastic anemia
Constitutional aplastic anemia
(Fanconi's anemia, dyskeratosis congenita)
Some myelodysplastic syndromes
Rare aleukemic leukemia (AML)
Some acute lymphoid leukemia
Some lymphomas of bone marrow

Hypocellular bone marrow ± Cytopenia
Q fever
Legionnaires' disease
Anorexia nervosa, starvation
Mycobacteria

Pancytopenia with Cellular Bone Marrow	
Primary bone marrow diseases	*Secondary to systemic diseases*
Myelodysplasia syndromes	Systemic lupus erythematosus
Paroxysmal nocturnal hemoglobinuria	Hypersplenism
Myelofibrosis	***B_{12}, folate deficiency (Megaloblastic Anemia)***
Some aleukemic leukemia	Overwhelming infection
Myelophthisis	Alcohol
Bone marrow lymphoma	Brucellosis
Hairy cell leukemia	Sarcoidosis
	Tuberculosis
	Leishmaniasis

127. Answer is C (Dyskeratosis Congenita): *Harrison's 18th/887*

Dyskeratosis congenita (constitutional aplastic anemia) is associated with Pancytopenia and a Hypocellular bone marrow

Myelodysplasia, PNH and Sarcoidosis may all be associated with Pancytopenia and a cellular bone marrow

Differential diagnosis of Pancytopenia

Pancytopenia with Hypocellular Bone Marrow
Acquired aplastic anemia
Constitutional aplastic anemia
(Fanconi's anemia, dyskeratosis congenita)
Some myelodysplastic syndromes
Rare aleukemic leukemia (AML)
Some acute lymphoid leukemia
Some lymphomas of bone marrow

Hypocellular bone marrow ± Cytopenia
Q fever
Legionnaires' disease
Anorexia nervosa, starvation
Mycobacteria

Pancytopenia with Cellular Bone Marrow	
Primary bone marrow diseases	*Secondary to systemic diseases*
Myelodysplasia syndromes	Systemic lupus erythematosus
Paroxysmal nocturnal hemoglobinuria	Hypersplenism
Myelofibrosis	***B_{12}, folate deficiency (Megaloblastic Anemia)***
Some aleukemic leukemia	Overwhelming infection
Myelophthisis	Alcohol
Bone marrow lymphoma	Brucellosis
Hairy cell leukemia	Sarcoidosis
	Tuberculosis
	Leishmaniasis

128. Answer is A *(Fanconi's Anemia): Harrison 18th/887*

Constitutional Aplastic Anemias like Fanconi's Anemia are associated with a Hypoplastic Marrow

Myelofibrosis, Paroxysmal Nocturnal Hemoglobinuria (PNH) and Hypersplenism are all associated with a cellular marrow.

Differential diagnosis of Pancytopenia

Pancytopenia with Hypocellular Bone Marrow
Acquired aplastic anemia
Constitutional aplastic anemia
***(Fanconi's anemia**, Dyskeratosis congenita)*
Some myelodysplastic syndromes
Rare aleukemic leukemia (AML)
Some acute lymphoid leukemia
Some lymphomas of bone marrow

Hypocellular bone marrow ± Cytopenia
Q fever
Legionnaires' disease
Anorexia nervosa, starvation
Mycobacteria

Pancytopenia with Cellular Bone Marrow

Primary bone marrow diseases	*Secondary to systemic diseases*
Myelodysplasia syndromes	Systemic lupus erythematosus
Paroxysmal nocturnal hemoglobinuria	***Hypersplenism***
Myelofibrosis	B_{12}, folate deficiency (Megaloblastic Anemia)
Some aleukemic leukemia	Overwhelming infection
Myelophthisis	Alcohol
Bone marrow lymphoma	Brucellosis
Hairy cell leukemia	Sarcoidosis
	Tuberculosis
	Leishmaniasis

129. Answer is Both B and A (B > A): Harrison 18th/p 884, 887 *Harrison 16th / 616; Harrison17th/661, 663; Robbins 7th / 638; CMDT 2006 / 491; CMDT 2009/437; Read previous question*

According to the reference table from Harrison, both Megaloblastic anemia and PHN may present with pancytopenia and cellular bone marrow. Bone marrow in megalobastic anemia is almost always hypercellular while in cases of PHN this may be normocelllar, hypercellular or hypocellular. Thus megalobastic anemia is the single best answer of choice here.

Note that a 'Cellular bone marrow' is not synonymous with a 'Hypercellular' marrow. Even a 'Normocellular' marrow is classified as a 'Cellular' marrow. The question is specific for hypercellular marrow.

PNH	Megaloblastic anemia
*'Bone marrow may appear **normocellular**'* (H16th/ 616) *(ie. cellular but not necessarily hypercellular)* *'Bone marrow morphology is variable and may show either generalized **hypoplasia** or erythroid **hyperplasia**' – CMDT 2006 / 49)* ***It may thus be hypocellular, normocellular or hypercellular***	***'Bone marrow is hypercellular** with a decrease myeloid / erythroid ratio and abundant stainable iron' – Harrison 16th / 606* ***'Marrow is usually markedly hypercellular** due to incrase number of all types of myeloid precursors which may completely replace the fatty marrow' – Robbin's 7th / 638*

130. Answer is D (G6PD deficiency) : Harrison 18th/p 887, 888 *Harrison 16th / 617, Harrison17th/663; (table 94-1) : Refer previous question*

PNH, megaloblastic anemia, and Myelodysplasia may all present with pancytopenia and cellular marrow. G6PD deficiency is not associated with Pancytopenia and cellular marrow.

131. Answer is D (Dyskeratosis congenita): Harrison 18th/p 887 *Harrisons 17th/663; Harrisons 16th/617*

Dyskeratosis congenita is associated with Pancytopenia and a hypocellular marrow.

132. Answer is B (Dyskeratosis congenita): Harrison 18th/ 887 *Harrisons 17th/663; Harrisons 16th/617*

Dyskeratosis congenita is associated with Pancytopenia and a hypocellular marrow.

133. Answer is D (G-6PD Deficiency) : Harrison 18th/ 887 *Harrisons 17th/663, Harrisons 16th/617*

Glucose – 6 – PD Deficiency is not associated with Pancytopenia and a cellular marrow
Myelodysplasias, PNH and Megaloblastic anemia (Vit B_{12}, Folate deficiency) may present with Pancytopenia and a cellular marrow.

Differential Diagnosis of Pancytopenia

Pancytopenia with Hypocellular Bone Marrow
Acquired aplastic anemia
Constitutional aplastic anemia
(Fanconi's anemia, dyskeratosis congenita)
Some myelodysplasia syndromes
Rare aleukemic leukemia (AML)
Some acute lymphoid leukemia
Some lymphomas of bone marrow

Hypocellular bone marrow ± Cytopenia
Q fever
Legionnaires' disease
Anorexia nervosa, starvation
Mycobacteria

Pancytopenia with Cellular Bone Marrow	
Primary bone marrow diseases	***Secondary to systemic diseases***
Myelodysplasia syndromes	*Systemic lupus erythematosus*
Paroxysmal nocturnal hemoglobinuria	*Hypersplenism*
Myelofibrosis	***B_{12}, folate deficiency (Megaloblastic Anemia)***
Some aleukemic leukemia	*Overwhelming infection*
Myelophthisis	*Alcohol*
Bone marrow lymphoma	*Brucellosis*
Hairy cell leukemia	*Sarcoidosis*
	Tuberculosis
	Leishmaniasis

134. Answer is C (Aplastic anemia): *Harrison 16th/ 617, Harrison17th/606; Robbins: Read text below.*

Patient in question has anemia with pancytopenia and an enlarged spleen. Presence of an enlarged spleen makes aplastic anemia the least likely diagnosis. *All other conditions mentioned as options may present with both pancytopenia and splenomegaly.*

Parameters	Normal	Patient in question	**Inference**
Hb	12-18 g/dl	8 gm/dl	*Anemia*
TLC	4000-11000 / mm^3	3000/ mm^3	*Granulocytopenia*
Platelet Count	130,000-400000/mm^3	80,000/mm^3	*Thrombocytopenia*
Spleen size	Not enlarged	Enlarged	*Splenomegaly*

- **Aplastic anemia** may present with anemia and pancytopenia but not with an associated enlarged spleen. *'If splenomegaly is present the diagnosis of aplastic anemia is seriously questioned.' - Robbins*
- **Megaloblastic anemia:** Besides ineffective synthesis and increased hemolytic destruction of red blood cells, there also occurs premature destruction of granulocytes and platelet resulting in Leucopenia and thrombocytopenia – Pancytopenia (Robbins) An enlarged spleen may be associated.
- **Leukemia** : Aleukemic form of Acute Lymphocytic leukemia also explains both – pancytopenia and hepatosplenomegaly
- **A chronic disease** associated with splenomegaly also explains pancytopenia as a sequels to increased destruction as a manifestation of 'HYPERSPLENISM' (increased sequestration and destruction of cells in sinusoids of an enlarged spleen).

135. Answer is A (Autosomal dominant inheritance): *Harrison's 17th/-665; API Textbook of Medicine 8th/828, 829; Wintrobe's Hematology 12th/1173, 1174*

Fanconi's anemia is primarily inherited as an autosomal recessive disorder and not as an autosomal dominant disorder

Fanconi's Anemia is inherited as an Autosomal Recessive / X- Linked disorder
There are currently 13 known subtypes of fanconi's Anemia. With the exception of one subtype (Subtype B) which is X-linked recessive, all other subtypes of Fanconi's anemia follow an ***autosomal recessive pattern of inheritance.***

- Wintrobe's Hematology

<u>Fanconi's Anemia is associated with Pancytopenia and Hypocellular Bone Marrow</u>

'Once pancytopenia develops, the bone marrow is hypocellular' – *API Textbook of medicine*

Fanconi's anemia is associated with *progressive bone marrow failure*[Q]

Pancytopenia[Q] develops insidiously and presents in most cases between the ages of 5 and 10 years

Bone marrow may show *normal cellularity initially*, however with progressive bone marrow failure pancytopenia develops and the bone marrow *becomes hypocellular*.

<u>Fanconi's anemia is usually normochronic, normocytic or macrocytic</u>

Fanconi's anemia is a form of inherited hypoproliferative aplastic anemia.

'The hypoproliferative anemias are normochromic, normocytic or macrocytic and are charachterized by a low reticulocyte count' – Harrison's 17th/663

Fanconi's Anemia	*Normochromic- Normocytic > Normochromic – Macrocytic*

<u>Fanconi's Anemia is associated with several congenital disorders</u>

Fanconi's Anemia manifests as congenital developmental anomalies, progressive pancytopenia and an increased risk of malignancy- Harrison's 17th/665

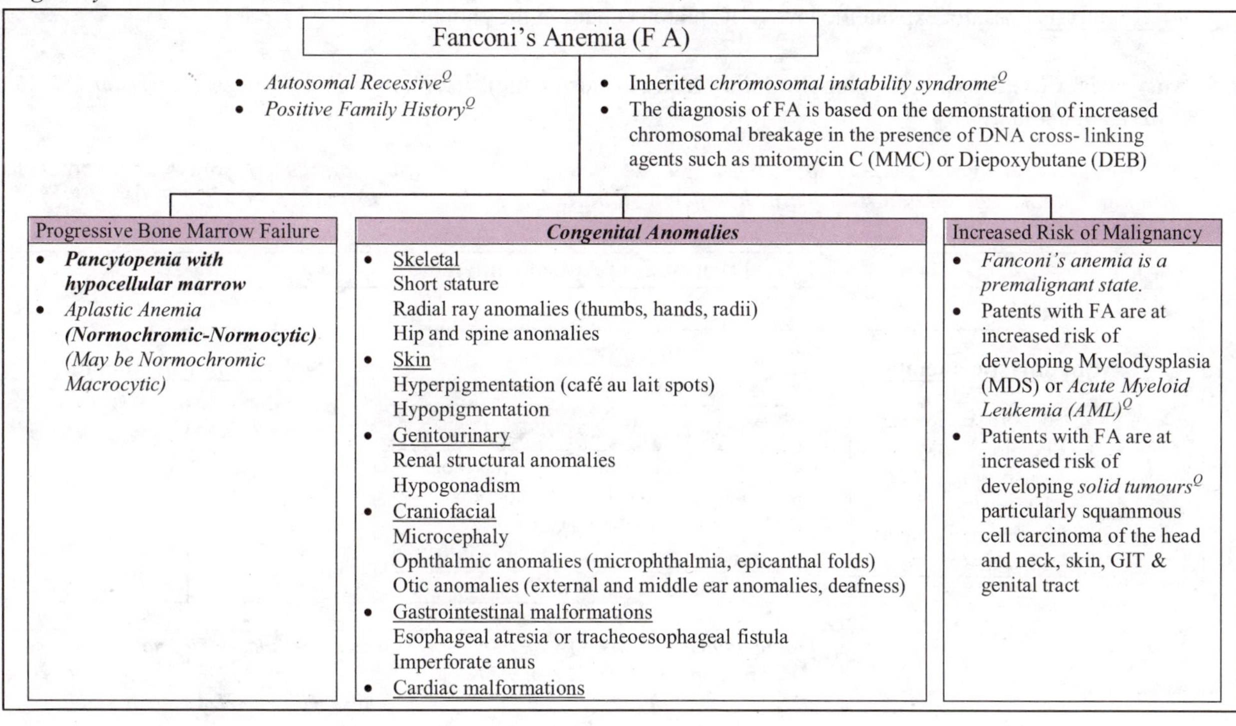

136. Answer is A (Splenomegaly): *Robbins 7th/648*

Splenomegaly is characteristically absent in Aplastic Anemia

'Splenomegaly is characteristically absent. If present, the diagnosis of aplastic anemia should be seriously questioned'
- *Robbins*

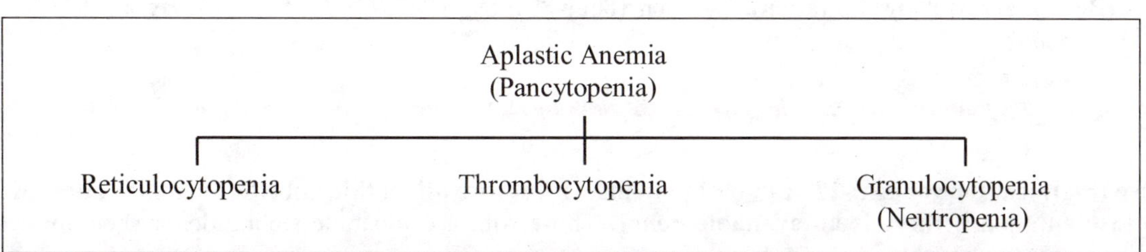

137. Answer is A (Leukemia): *Reference alongside; Robbins 7th/648, 652*

The presence of Pancytopenia and 6% blasts in peripheral blood is enough to support the diagnosis of aleukemic leukemia. *Presence of splenomegaly eliminates aplastic anemia & ITP as the possibilities and hemolysis does not explain the low WBC and platelet count in the patient.*

- **Leukemia:** Although leukemia usually presents with an elevated WBC count the presence of Pancytopenia and 6% blasts in peripheral blood is enough to support the diagnosis of aleukemic leukemia. Some patients with aleukemic leukemia present with pancytopenia without circulating blasts. The diagnosis of leukemia in such patients should however be ideally made only once, a marrow blast count is done and it comes out to be > 30%.
- **Presence of splenomegaly eliminates aplastic anemia & ITP as the possibilities.**
  - Splenomegaly & Lymphadenopathy are extremely uncommon in **ITP** & their presence should lead one to consider other possible diagnosis – *Robbins 7th/652*
  - Splenomegaly is characteristically absent in **aplastic anemia** and if present the diagnosis of aplastic anemia should be seriously questioned - *Robbins 7th/648*
- **Hemolysis** does not explain the low WBC platelet count in the patient.

138. Answer is A (Antithymocyte globulin followed by cyclosporine): *Harrison 18th/p 891, 892; Harrison 17th/666, 667; CMDT 2008/438;2009/443*

'For adults over age 50 years or those without HLA matched siblings, the treatment of choice for severe Aplastic anemia is immunosupression with antithymocyte globulin (ATG) plus Cyclosporine' *-CMDT 2006 / 498*

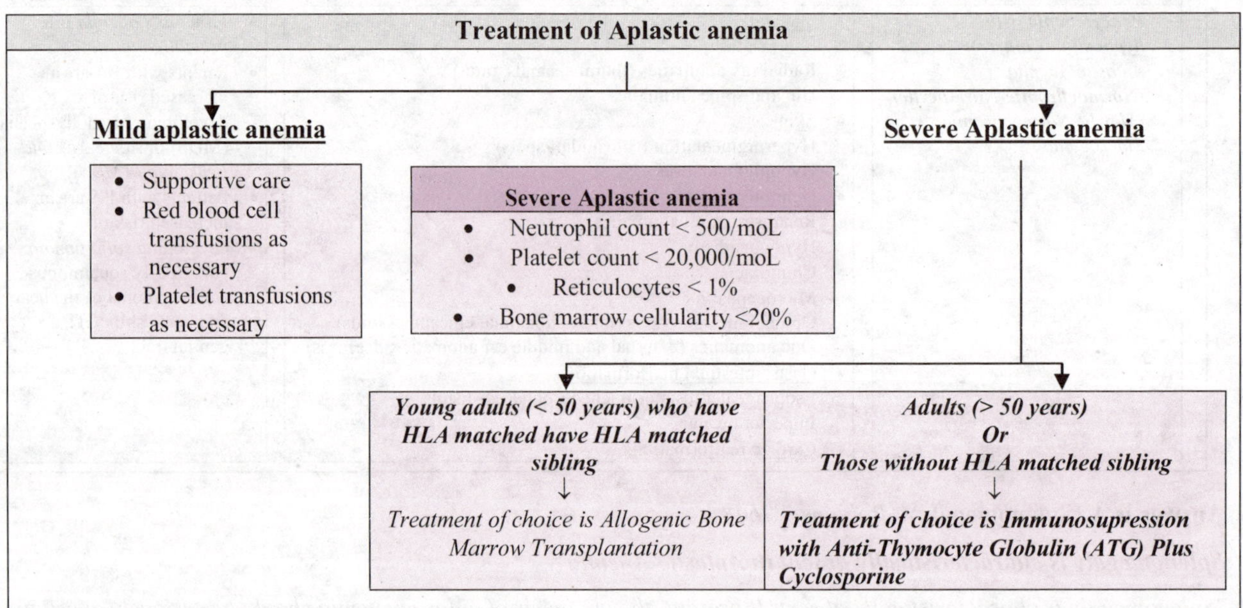

139. Answer is D (Bone marrow transplantation): Harrison 18th/p 891, 892 *Davidson 18th/ 769; Harrison 16th/ 621, Harrison 17th/ 666, 667*

'Bone marrow transplantation is the best therapy for the young patient with a fully histocompatible sibling donor.'
– Harrisons 16th/ 621

The curative treatment for young (<20 year-old) patients with severe idiopathic aplastic anemia is allogenic bone marrow transplantation if there is an available donor. Those with a compatible sibling donor should proceed to transplantation as soon as possible. – *Davidson.*

Myelodysplastic Syndrome

140. Answer is A (Myelodysplastic Syndrome (MDS): Harrison 18th/p 455 *Harrisons 17th /361, Williams Hematology 7th/374, 823*

'Based on the distinctive finding of ringed sideroblasts on the marrow iron stain, patients are diagnosed as having sideroblastic anemia – almost always reflecting myelodysplasia' – *Harrisons*

Ringed Sideroblasts are a charachteristic bone marrow finding in Myelodysplasia

What are Sideroblasts
Sideroblasts are Erythroblasts (Red blood cell precursors) that contain iron (ferritin) granules in their cytoplasm. The iron in these cells is normally located in the cytoplasm away from the nucleus (and stains positive for prussian blue). In normal bone marrow sideroblasts constitute 20- 40% (approx 1/3rd) of red blood cell precursors
What are Ringed Sideroblasts
Ringed sideroblasts are abnormal sideroblasts seen in conditions with disturbed haem synthesis. In these cells iron accumulates within the mitochondria, surrounds the nucleus and does not progress into haemoglobin Ringed sideroblasts are defined as Nucleated Red blood cells (Erythroblasts) containing five or more granules and encircling at least two – thirds of the nucleus. Ring sidroblasts are pathological and their presence suggests a diagnosis of sideroblastic anemia whether congenital or acquired
What are the conditions associated with Ringed Sideroblasts
Ringed Sideroblasts may be seen in all causes of sideroblatic anemia whether Congenital or Acquired but are most often associated with Myelodysplastic syndromes

Causes of Sideroblastic Anemia (Ringed Sideroblasts in Bone Marrow)
1. Hereditary Sideroblastic Anemia 2. Acquired Sideroblastic Anemia • Primary (Acquired) Sideroblastic Anemia ***(Myelodysplastic Syndromes)*** • Secondary (Acquired) Sidroblastic Anemia : Secondary to - Alcohol (Alcohol induced sidroblastic anemia)Q - Lead (Lead induced sideroblastic anemia)Q - Zinc (Zinc induced sidroblastic anemia)Q - Drugs such as INH, pyrizinamide, cycloserine, chloramphenical etc. - Other Myeloprolifirative disorders and Myelofibrosis 3. Others (Rare) - Thiamine responsive megaloblastic anemia - Pearson's syndrome - Hypothermia - Certain Haemoglobinopathies

141. Answer is D (> 50 years): *Harrison 16th/624; API 7th/958*

Idiopathic MDS is a disease of the elderly. The mean age of onset is 68 years.

Myelodysplastic Syndromes

(Disease of the elderly with mean onset > 68 years)
Heterogenous group of haematological disorder

Characterized by	Classified as
- Peripheral blood cytopenias - Trilineage dysplastic changes - Hypercellular bone marrow - Propensity to undergo transformation into Acute Myeloid LeukaemiaQ.	**The French American British Group has classified this disorder into 5 pathological entities** - Refractory Anemia - Refractory Anemia with ring sideroblasts - Refractory Anemia with Excess blasts - Refractory Anemia with Excess blasts in transformation - Chronic Myelomonocytic Leukaemia

142. Answer is C (5q-): *'Myelodysplastic Syndromes' by John Bennett (2002)300; Childhood Leukemias' 2nd/549*

'Monosomy 7 is by far the most common cytogenetic abnormality in children (pediatric MDS) whereas 5q- is observed most frequently in adults' *– Myelodysplastic Syndromes by John Bennett (2002)/300*

Cytogenetic Abnormalities in MDS: Facts to Remember
Monosomy 7 is the most frequent cytogenetic abnormality in children.[Q]
Deletion 5q (5q-) is the most frequent cytogenetic abnormality in adults[Q].
Trisomy 8 is the most frequent trisomy[Q].

Differences between Myelodysplastic Syndromes in children and Adults
('Myelodysplastic Syndromes' 2002/300; 'Childhood Leukemias' 2nd/549)

Feature	Children	Adults
• Frequency	Less common	More common
• Presence of sideroblasts	Uncommon (<2%)	More common (≈25%)
• Cytogenetic Abervations		
-7/7q-	Most common (≈30%)	Less common (≈10%)
-5/5q-	Uncommon (≈1-2%)	Most common (≈20%)

Myeloproliferative Disorders

General/Classification

143. Answer is B (Acute myeloid leukemia): *Harrison 18th/ 898;Harrison 15th/701, Harrison 16th/626; Harrison 17th/ 672*

The myeloproliferative disorders are characterized pathophysiologically by clonal expression of a multipotent hematopoitic progenitor cell with the overproduction of one or more of the formed elements of Blood. ***These disorders may transform into acute leukemia naturally or as a consequence of mutagenic treatment.***

Myeloproliferative disorders classically include:
- Polycythemia vera[Q]
- Idiopathic myelofibrosis[Q]
- Essential thrombocytosis[Q]
- Chronic myeloid leukemia[Q]

144. Answer is B (Myelofibrosis): *CMDT 2008/440*

Myelofibrosis may be associated with decreased white cell count and decreased platlet counts. Myelofibrosis is an established cause for panyctopenia with cellular marrow

Condition	WBCount	Hematocrit/Red cell mass	Platelet count	Red cell morphology
CML	↑↑	N	N or ↑	N
Myelofibrosis	N or ↓ or ↑	N or ↓	↓ or N or ↑	Abnormal
Polycythemia	N or ↑	↑	N or ↑	N
Essential Thrombocytosis	N or ↑	N	↑↑	N

145. Answer is C (Essential Thrombocytosis (ET)): *Harrison 18th/903*

Essential Thrombocytosis is not associated with massive splenomegaly.

'Physical Examination in Essential Thrombocytosis is generally unremarkable except ***occassionally for mild splenomegaly****. Massive splenomegaly is indicative of another Myeloproliferative disorder in particular PV, PMF or CML'. – Harrison 18th/903*

'Splenomegaly in Essential Thrombocytosis is seen in less than 30% of patients, and when palpable the spleen is usually not enlarged more than 4 cm below the left costal margin'. – 'Blood: Principles and Practice of Hematology' 2nd/414

Condition	WBCount	Hematocrit/Red cell mass	Platelet count	Red cell morphology	Splenomegaly
CML	↑↑	N	N or ↑	N	***Massive***
Myelofibrosis	N or ↓or ↑	N or ↓	↓or N or ↑	Abnormal	***Massive***
Polycythemia	N or ↑	↑	N or ↑	N	***Moderate (Massive in late stages)***
Essential Thrombocytosis	N or ↑	N	↑↑	N	***Mild***

146. Answer is C (Flow-cytometric analysis): *Hematology in Clinical Practice 4th/222, 223; Williams 7th/28; Wintrobe's Atlas of Clinical Hematology 2006/217*

Amongst the options provided flow cytometry analysis is the least commonly employed laboratory test for the evaluation of myeloproliferative syndromes and has only limited application and selective indications for its use.

Flow cytometry analysis is the single best answer of choice.
Complete blood picture including Red cell mass / Hematocrit estimation, Bone marrow aspirate studies and chromosomal Studies are key investigations for the differential diagnosis of chronic myeloproliferative disorders.

Laboratory studies in the diagnosis of Myeloproliferative Syndromes

Key laboratory Tests

- **Blood counts and general blood picture evaluation including hematocrit / Red cell mass measurements and Red cell morphology**

Condition	WBCount	Hematocrit/Red cell mass	Platelet count	Red cell morphology
CML	↑↑	N	N or ↑	N
Myelofibrosis	N or ↓ or ↑	N or ↓	↓ or N or ↑	Abnormal
Polycythemia	N or ↑	↑	N or ↑	N
Essential Thrombocytosis	N or ↑	N	↑↑	N

Abnormal Red cell morphology includes tear drop cells, schistocytes etc
An elevated red cell mass is important to distinguish polycythemia vera from other myeloproliferation disorders.

- **Marrow Aspirate and Biopsy**
These are considered *essential investigations* for the diagnosis of Myeloproliferative disorders.
Bone marrow aspirate (dry tap) is particularly important to distinguish myelofibrosis from other mycloproliferative disorders.

- **Chromosomal studies (karyotyping) for cytogenetic abnormalities**
Chromosomal *studies are important*, particularly to distinguish CML from other causes of myeloproliferative disorders

CML philadelphia chromosome (9:22)

Optimal/Other laboratory Tests

Flow cytometry

Flow cytometry may be used in the assessment and diagnosis of myelodysplastic and myeloproliferative disorders, but this approach is controversial' – *William's hematology 7th/28*

'Flow cytometry may be used in cases of Myeloproliferative syndromes in cases in which cytogenetic studies fail to detect a clonal karyotype abnormality - *Wintrobe's atlas of hematology (2006)/217*

147. Answer is C (Flow cytometry) : Harrison 18th/p 898 *Read text below : Harrison 16th/626-631; Harrison 17th/ 672-676*

All investigations other than flow cytometry mentioned in the options are indicated useful tests for diagnosis of respective myeloproliferative disorder.

Myeloproliferative disorder	Useful tests
Polycythemia vera	Elevated Red cell mass / with normal erythropoetin levels
Chronic myeloid leukemia	Chromosomal demonstration of Philadelphia chromosome or bcr /abl translocation
Chronic idiopathic Myelofibrosis	Dry tap on bone marrow aspiration alongwith characteristic peripheral blood picture
Essential thrombocytosis	Elevated Platelet count with cytogenetic evaluation to rule out CML or other myelodysplastic disorder

Polycythemia

148. Answer is D (High altitude) : Harrison 18th/p 456, 898 *Harrison 16th/336, 627; Harrison 17th/ 362, 363, 672*

High altitude is associated with physiological increase in erythropoetin levels and leads to absolute polycythemia and not relative polycythemia.

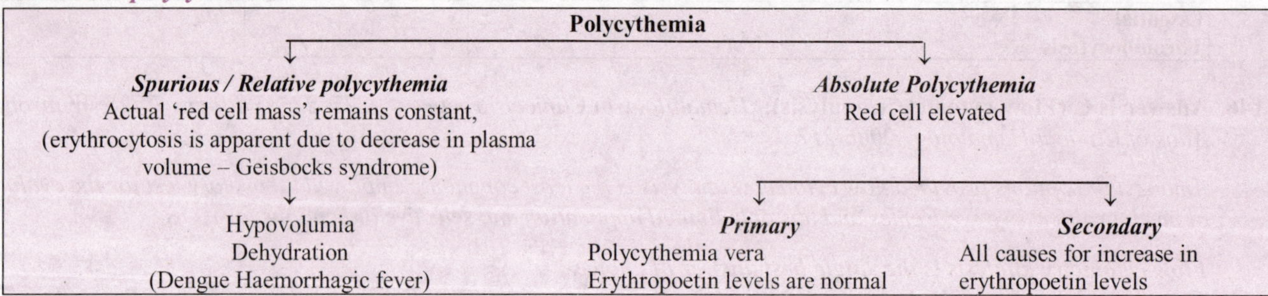

***Relative erythrocytosis due to reduction in plasma volume alone is also known as stress or spurious erythrocytosis or 'Geisbock's syndrome'** – Harrison 16th/627*

149. Answer is C (Red cell mass) : Harrison 18th/p 899 *Harrison 15th/ 702, 703, Harrison 16th/ 627, 628; Harrison 17th/ 672, 673*

When confronted with an elevated Haemoglobin or Haematocrit the first step should be to determine whether this increase is due to absolute erythrocytosis or relative erythrocytosis.

Absolute erythrocytosis	Relative/ spurious erythrocytosis
True increase in red cell mass	Apparent increase in red cell mass due to reduction in plasma volume

***'Red cell mass' is the investigation of choice to determine such distinction.** Once 'red cell mass' determination confirms absolute erythrocytosis, a diagnosis of polycythemia vera can be established by demonstrating absence of elevation in serum erythropoetin levels.*

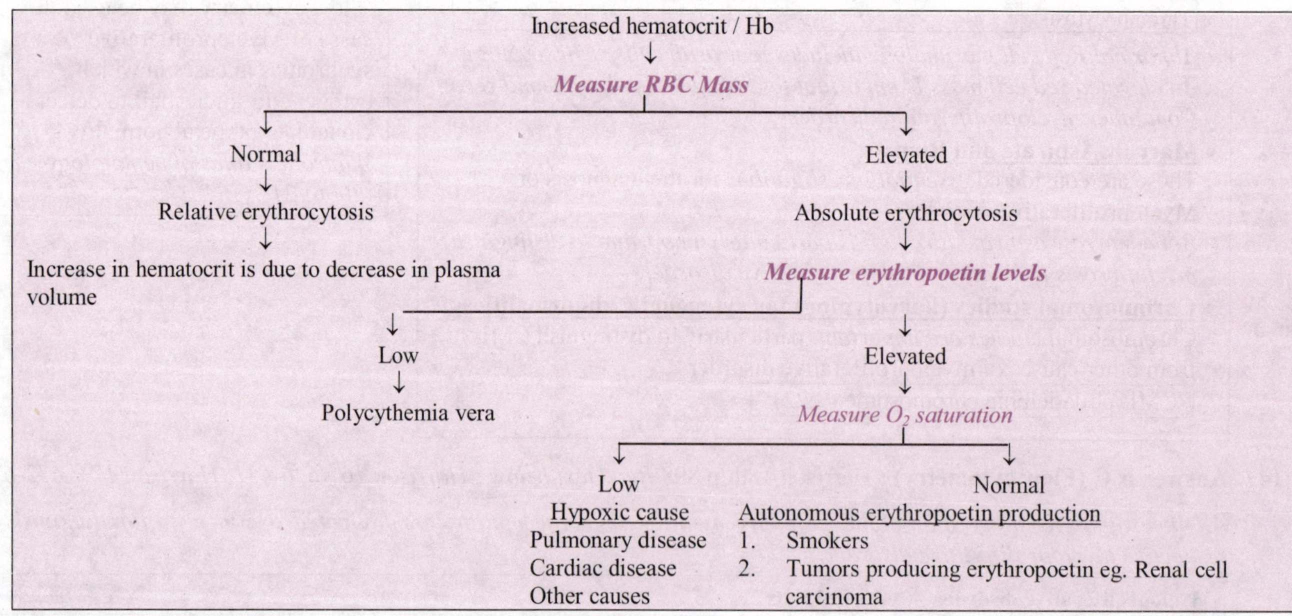

150. Answer is A (Cor pulmonale): *Wintrobe's 12th/1263*

Secondary polycythemia due to decreased tissue oxygenation may be seen in chronic corpulmonale.

Polycythemia may also be seen in association with cyanotic congenital heart diseases.

Secondary Polycythemia (Absolute Erythrocytosis)

Physiologically Appropriate Polycythemia (Secondary to decreased tissue oxygenation or hypoxic erythrocytosis)	Physiologically inappropriate polycythemia (Secondary to appropriate erythropoietin production or response)
• High-altitude erythrocytosis (Monge disease) • Pulmonary disease - Chronic cor pulmonale - Ayerza syndrome • Cyanotic congenital heart disease • Hypoventilation syndromes - Primary alveolar hypoventilation - Pickwickian syndrome, Ondine curse - Positional desaturation - Sleep apnea • Abnormal hemoglobins - Inherited - Acquired: Drugs and chemicals, carboxyhemoglobin • Familial polycythemia	• Tumors, cysts, hemangiomas, and so forth • Androgen abuse • Erythropoietin abuse • Familial polycythemia

151. Answer is B (Arterial oxygen tension < 90% on room air): Harrison 18th/p 899 *Harrison 17th/672, 363*

Arterial oxygen tension < 90% on room air indicate a secondary cause of polycythemia from either heart or lung disease

Primary polycythemia (Polycythemia vera) is characteristically associated with a normal arterial oxygen saturation >92% on room air.

Both primary and secondary polycythemia will have an elevated red cell mass.

Pruritis and Hypertension are consequences of increased red cell mass and the resultant hyperviscocity, and may hence be seen in both forms of polycythemia.

A summary of significant differences between Polycythemia Vera and Other Types of Polycythemia

Findings	Polycythemia vera	Secondary polycythemia
Red cell mass	*Increased*	*Increased*
Erythropoietin	Decreased or absent	Normal or increased
Arterial oxygen saturation	***Normal***	***Decreased or normal***
Erythrocyte sedimentation rate	Decreased	Normal
Leukocyte alkaline phosphate stain	Increased	Normal
Vitamin B12 binding capacity	Increased	Normal
Total leukocytes	Increased (Leukocytosis)	Normal
Total Platelets	Increased (Thrombocytosis)	Normal
Basophil count	Increased	Normal
Blood histamine	Increased	Normal
Serum iron	Decreased	Normal or increased
Splenomegaly	Present	Absent
Marrow	Panhyperplasia	Erythroid hyperplasia

152. Answer is D (Pancreatic carcinoma) : Harrison 16th / 569, 627; *Harrison 17th/ 621, 673*

Ectopic production of erythropoietin by cancer cells cause most paraneoplastic erythrocytosis. Cancers typically associated with this syndrome include Renal cancer, Hepatocarcinoma and cerebellar hemangioblastomas.

Syndrome	Protein	Cancers typically associated with syndrome
Erythrocytosis *Paraneoplastic syndrome*	***Erythropoetin***	• ***Renal cancers*** • ***Hepatocarcinoma*** • ***Cerebellar hemangioblastoma***

Tumours associated with Erythrocytosis : *Harrison 16th / 627*	
• ***Hypernephroma***	• Adrenal adenoma
• ***Hepatoma***	• Pheochromocytoma
• ***Cerebellar Hemangiblastoma***	• Meningioma
	• Uterine fibromyoma

153. Answer is D (Spontaneous severe infection): Harrison 18th/p 898, 899 *Harrison 15th/ 701, Harrison 16th/ 627; Harrison 17th/ 672, 673*

All options other than spontaneous severe infections have been mentioned as common associations with Polycythemia vera.

Polycythemia vera:

Polycythemia is a disorder of multipotent haematopoetic progeniter cells, characterised by :

- overproduction of phenotypically normal red cells, granulocytes and platelets.
- In absence of recognizable physiological stimulus.

Polycythemia Vera

↓ ↓ ↓

Increase In Blood Viscosity
- Neurological symptoms [Q]
  - vertigo, tinnitus
  - headache
  - visual disturbance
- Systolic Hypertension [Q]
- Venous or arterial thrombosis [Q]
- Digital ischaemia
- Easy bruising, epistaxis or gastrointestinal haemorrhage.

Increased Turnover of RBC, Leucocytes, platelets

↓

increased uric acid [Q]

increased histamine release

↓

- Peptic ulcer disease [Q]
- Pruritis [Q]

Myeloproliferative Syndrome [Q]

May transform into acute Leukemia naturally or as a consequence of mutagenic treatment.

Note:

Polycythemia is associated with an increased risk of both thrombosis and bleeding.

154. Answer is D (Increased Infection): Harrison 18th/p 899, 900 *Harrison 17th/672, 673; Harrison 16th/627, 628; Harrison 15th/702*

Polycythemia vera is not associated with an increased predisposition to infections.

ESR levels are characteristically normal or reduced

'ESR' is characteristically low or normal. If this is abnormal another diagnosis or a complication shiuld be considered'

- Diagnostic Hematology

Polycythemia vera is associated with an increased incidence of both thrombosis and bleeding

Both arterial and venous thrombosis may be seen in Polycythemia vera.

Paradoxically patients may show a tendency of bleeding and bruising, mainly due to platelet of dysfunction.

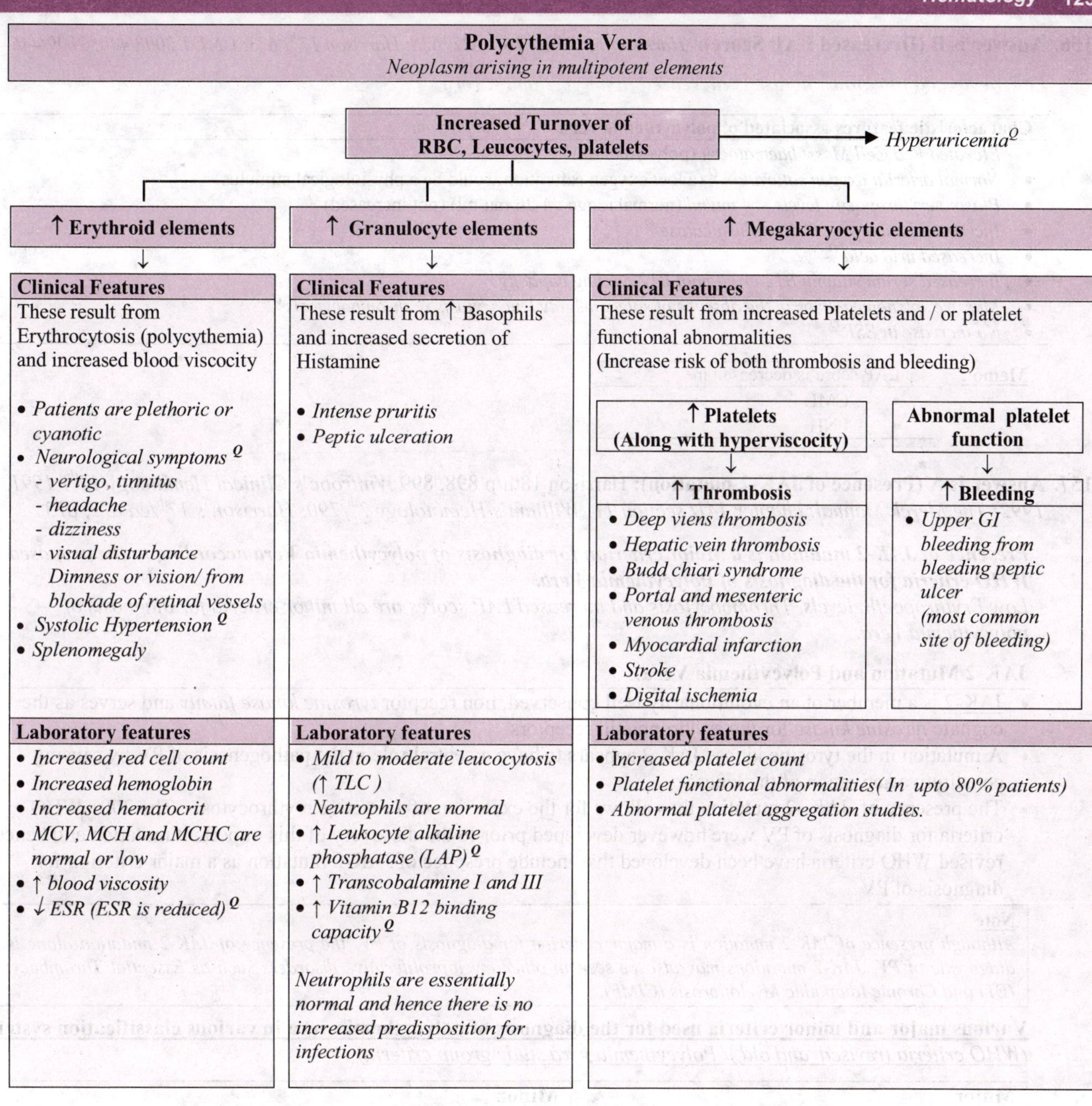

155. Answer is A (Thrombocytopenia): Harrison 18th/p 899, 900 *Harrison 15th/ 702; Harrison 16th/627; Harrison 17th/ 672, 673*

Polycythemia vera is associated with thrombocytosis and not thrombocytopenia

Polycythemia vera is associated with thrombocytosis and not thrombocytopenia

Polycythemia Vera is an acquired myeloproliferative disorder that is characterised by *overproduction* of *three hematopoitic cell lines*[Q] with *predominant elevation in RBC's*[Q].

Thus there is overproduction of granulocytes, red cells and platelets. Overproduction of platelets results in thrombocytosis. Thrombocytopenia is not seen.

Polycythemia vera is associated with an increased incidence of both thrombosis and bleeding

Both arterial and venous thrombosis may be seen in Polycythemia vera.

Paradoxically patients may show a tendency of bleeding and bruising, mainly due to platelet of dysfunction.

Transient visual loss may be seen in polycythemia vera as a manifestation of associated hyperviscosity syndrome.

156. Answer is B (Decreased LAP Score): *Harrison 15th/ 702, 16th/ 627, 628; Harrison 17th/ 673; CMDT 2008/440; 2009/446*

Leucocyte alkaline phosphatase is increased in polycythemia vera

Characteristic features associated of polycythemia vera *** *V. important*
• *Elevated Red Cell Mass/ haematocrit* (polycythemia) Q • *Normal arterial oxygen saturation* Q (a low oxygen saturation would be a physiological stimulus) • *Plasma erythropoetin levels < 4 mu/ml* (normal range : 4-26 mu/ml) (not increased) Q • *Increased Leucocyte alkaline phosphatase* Q • *Increased uric acid* Q- • *Increased serum vitamin B12 or vitamin B12 binding capacity* Q • *Massive splenomegaly or in the absence of splenomegaly leucocytosis & thrombocytosis* Q • *No increase in ESR* Q

1

Memo :

LAP score is decreased in
• CML
• PNH

157. Answer is A (Presence of JAK-2 mutation): Harrison 18th/p 898, 899 *Wintrobe's Clinical Hematoogy 12th/ 1991, 1992; The Merck Manual: chapter 141/ section 11; William's Hematology 7th/790; Harrison's 17th/ed 672, 673*

Presence of JAK-2 mutation is a Major criterion for diagnosis of polycythemia Vera according to the proposed new WHO criteria for the diagnosis of Polycythemia Vera.

Low Erythropoetin levels, Thrombocytosis and increased LAP scores are all minor criteria for diagnosis of polycythemia Vera.

JAK-2 Mutation and Polycythemia Vera

- JAK-2 is a member of an evolutionarily well conserved, non receptor *tyrosine kinase family* and serves as the cognate *tyrosine kinase* for the erythropoietin receptors
- A mutation in the tyrosine kinase JAK-2 appears to have a central role in the pathogenesis of PV by causing constitutive activation of the kinase
- The presence of JAK -2 mutation thus allows for the exclusion of a reactive erythrocytosis. The 2001 WHO criteria for diagnosis of PV were however developed prior to the discovery of this important mutation and hence revised WHO criteria have been developed that include presence of JAK-2 mutation as a major criterion for diagnosis of PV

Note
Although presence of JAK-2 mutation is a major criterion for diagnosis of PV, the presence of JAK-2 mutation alone is not diagnostic of PV. JAK-2 mutations may also be seen in other myeloproliferative disorders such as Essential Thrombocytosis (ET) and Chronic Idiopathic Myelofibrosis (CIMF).

Various major and minor criteria used for the diagnosis of polycythemia vera in various classification systems
(WHO criteria (revised and old)/ Polycythemia vera study group criteria)

Major	Minor
• ***JAK2 V617F mutation*** • *Hemoglobin >18.5 g/dL in men, 16.5 g/dL in women* • *Increased red blood cell mass* • *Splenomegaly* • *Clonal genetic abnormality other than Philadelphia chromosome or BCR/ABL in marrow* • *Endogenous erythroid colony formation in vitro* • *Normal arterial O2 saturation (>92%)*	• ***Thrombocytosis*** *(> 400 × 10^9/L)* • ***Leucocytosis*** *(WBC > 12 × 10^9/L)* • ***Increased leukocyte alkaline phosphatase*** *(LAP > 100U)* • *Increased serum B12/binders (B12 > 900 pg/ml; unbound B12 binding capacity > 2200 pg/ml)* • *Low serum erythroprotein levels.* • *Panmyelosis with prominent erythoid and megakaryocytic hyperplasia on bone marrow biopsy.*

Revised WHO criteria (Proposed) for the diagnosis of Polycythemia vera

Revised WHO criteria (Proposed) for the diagnosis of Polycythemia vera
Major Criteria • Hemoglobin > 18.5 g/dl in men, > 16.5 g/dl in women or evidenced on increased red cell volume • ***Presence of JAK2 mutation***

Minor Criteria
• Hypercellular bone marrow biopsy with panmyelosis with prominent erythroid, granulocytic, and megakaryocytic hyperplasia
• Low serum erythropoietin level
• Endogenous erythroid colony formation in vitro.

WHO Criteria for the diagnosis of Plycythemia Vera (Prior to the proposed new criterion)

WHO Criteria *(Previous)* for the diagnosis of Plycythemia vera
Major Criteria
• Red blood cell mas > 25% above mean normal predicted value, or Hb > 18.5 g/dl in men, 16.5 g/dl in women.
• Splenomegaly on palpation
• Clonal genetic abnormality other than Philadelphia chromosome or BCR/ABL in marrow.
• Endogenous erythroid colony formation in vitro
Minor Criteria
• Thrombocytosis > 400 × 10^9/L
• WBC > 12 × 10^9/L
• Panmyelosis with prominent erythroid and megakaryocytic hyperplasia on bone marrow biopsy.
• Low serum erythropoietin levels.

158. Answer is B (Increased erythropoieten level): Harrison 18th/p 899 *Harrison 16th/ 627; Harrison 17th/ 672, 673*

Polycythemia vera is characterized by an increase in red cell mass without any increase in level of erythropoietin. *In fact* ***erythropoietin level is decreased*** *due to feedback by increased erythrocytes.*
The plasma erythropoetin level is a useful diagnostic test in patients with isolated erythrocytosis, because an elevated level excludes polycythemia vera as the cause for erythrocytosis.

159. Answer is C (Cerebellar haemangioblastoma): *Harrison 18th/899; 14th/ 680; 15th/ 702, 16th/ 627; Harrison 17th/ 673*

Tumors associated with polycythemia vera are :	
• Hypernephroma	• ***Cerebellar Haemangioblastoma***
• Hepatoma	• Uterine fibromyoma
• Adrenal adenoma	• Meningioma
• Pheochromocytoma	

Myelofibrosis

160. Answer is D (Myelofibrosis): Harrison 18th/p 901 *Harrison 16th/628,629; 17th/674,675; CMDT 08,442,443; 2009/448; Chandrasoma Taylor 3rd/ 421*

Presence of dry tap (unsuccessful aspiration), tear drop cells and splenomegaly all suggest a diagnosis of myelofibrosis.

Myelofibrosis: *Review*

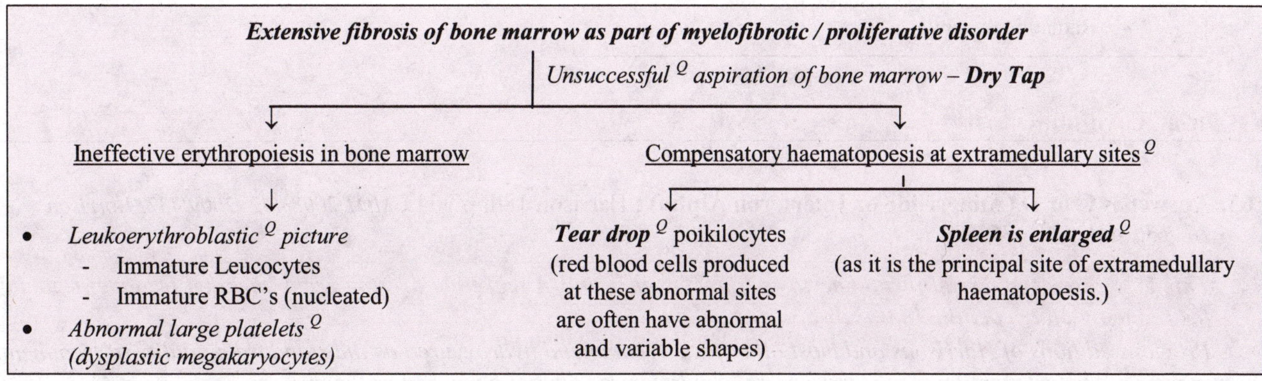

161. Answer is C (Myelofibrosis): Harrison 18th/p 901 *Harrison 16th/ 628, 629; Harrison 17th/ 674, 675 Chandrasoma Taylor 3rd/ 421*

Presence of a dry tap from the marrow and tear drop cells in the peripheral smear suggests the diagnosis of myelofibrosis.

- Because of the fibrotic nature of this disorder, bone marrow aspiration is generally unsuccessful and yields a '***dry tap***'.
- ***Tear drop cells*** are suggestive of extra medullary haematopoesis as in spleen.

Most characteristic are the Laboratory findings and the *triad of* Q
a. Tear drop poikilocytes Q
b. Leukoerythroblastic blood i.e. immature leukocytes and nucleated (immature) RBC's Q
c. Giant abnormal platelets Q

Biopsy of bone marrow to detect reticular or collagen fibrosis is essential for diagnosis. Q

162. Answer is D (Thalassemia): Harrison 18th/p 896, 901, 902 *Harrison 15th/ 700, 701, 703; Harrison 16th/ 626, 629; Harrison 17th/ 669, 670, 674, 675*

Leukoerythroblastosis is usually accompanied by fibrosis of the bone marrow and may be seen in all conditions associated with primary or secondary myelofibrosis / myelophthesis. Amongst the options provided all conditions other than thalassemia may produce fibrosis in the marrow and may produce a leukoerythroblastic picture.

Leucoerythroblastosis:

- Refers to the presence of a variable number of immature erythroid and myeloid cells in circulation.
- This picture is indicative of ineffective erythropoesis in the normal marrow and extension of haematopoesis into extramedullary sites such as spleen, liver and Lymphnodes.
- It is usually accompanied by fibrosis of the bone marrow.

Causes include:

Primary Myelofibrosis
Secondary myelofibrosis or Myelophthesis

- Infections:
  - T.B. fungal, HIV etc.
- Tumors:
  - Metastastic carcinomas
  - Lymphomas e.g. Hodgkins
  - Leukaemias e.g. CML, AML, Hairy cell.
  - Plasma cell disorders :
  - Multiple Myeloma
  - Polycythemia vera
- Lipid deposition:
  - Gaucher's disease
- Radiation therapy

Essential Thrombocytosis

163. Answer is C or D (Anagrelide or Interferon Alpha) : Harrison 18th/p 904 *CMDT 2008/442; 2009/437; Harrison 16th/630, 631; 17th/ 676, 677*

This is a case of essential thrombocytosis. Interferon α and Anagrelide are the recommended treatment modalities for reducing platelet count in this disorder.

Previous editions of Harrisons and most other texts recommend hydroxyurea as the standard modality of treatment, but in view of the text mentioned in Harrisons 16th, hydroxyurea cannot be picked as the answer.

Essential thrombocytosis

(essential thrombocythaemia; idiopathic thrombocytosis; hemorrhagic thrombocythaemia)

Essential thrombocytosis is a myeloproliferative disorder characterized by overproduction of platelets without a definable cause.

Clinical features	Laboratory Diagnostic features
Symptoms • Haemorrhagic tendencies : Easy bruising Q • Thrombotic tendencies : Microvascular occlusions - Erythromelalgia - Migraine (headache) - Transient ischemic attacks Signs • Splenomegaly : usually mild/moderate *massive splenomegaly is more characteristic of other myeloproliferative disorders*.	• Elevated platelet count is hallmark (often $>1000\times10^3/\mu L$) • Haematocrit and RBC morphology normal • WBC count is mildly elevated/normal (mild neutrophillic leucocytosis) • LAP is normal or elevated • Philadelphia chromosome is absent
Management in a symptomatic patient	**Management in symptomatic patient**
Elevated platelet count in asymptomatic patient • No therapy is recommended because agents used in treatment place the patient at risk of developing acute leukemia ↓ Therapy with risk of acute leukemia • Radioactive phosphorus • Hydroxyuria • Alkylating agents	Elevated platelet count in symptomatic patients • Symptoms must be clearly identified to be a consequence of elevated platelet count ↓ Platelet reduction • IFN a • Anagrelide • Hydroxyurea: *should be considered only if the above agents are not effective or tolerable* *.- Harrison*

164. Answer is B (Essential thrombocythemia) : *CMDT 2008 / 441, 442; 2009/447; Robbins 7th / 700*

Since all Myeloproliferative disorders can be associated with Thrombocytosis, Essential Thrombocytosis is a diagnosis of exclusion. The absence of an elevated Haemoglobin makes Polycythemia unlikely (Polycythemia is associated with increased Hb) and the absence of Philadelphia chromosome makes a diagnosis of CML unlikely. . ***The patient in question has an elevated platelet count (> 600 x 10^9/L) and only mild elevation of WBC count (12 x 10^9/L both of which are consistent with a diagnosis of Essental thrombocythemia / thrombocytosis.***
Essential Thrombocytosis is the single best option of exclusion.

Essential Thrombocytosis - CMDT / Robbins	Myeloprotiferative Disorders
• Diagnosis of exclusion • ***Elevated Platelet count is the hall mark (usually >600 x 10^9/L)*** • ***White cell count is only mildly elevated*** • Haematocrit is normal • Philadelphia chromosome absent	Chronic Myeloid leukaemia Polycythemia vera Essential thrombocytosis Myelofibrosis

	White cell count	Haematocrit	Platelet count	Red cell morphology	pH chromosome
CML	↑↑	N	N or ↑	N	+ve
Myelafibrosis	N or ↓ or ↑	N or ↓	↓ or N or ↑	Abnormal	-nt
Polycythemia vera	N or ↑	↑ (↑Hb)	N or ↑	N	-nt
Essential Thrombocytosis	N or ↑	N	↑↑	N	-nt

Robbins 7th / 619 : Polycythemia : ***The Haemoglobin concentration ranges from 14 to 28 gm/dL with Haematocrit values of 60% or more.***

Presence of Markedly elevated Platelet count and mild elevation of white cell count in the absence of raised Haemoglobin levels suggests a diagnosis of essential thrombocytosis by exclusion.

Lymphomas & Chronic Leukemias

Hodgkin's Lymphoma

165. Answer is A (Lymphocyte predominant): Harrison 18th/p 935 *Harrisons 17th/699; Robbins 7th/689*

Lymphocyte predominant Hodgkin's disease is now recognized as an entity distinct from classical hodgkin's disease. Nodular Lymphocyte predominant hodgkins disease has a number of characteristic that suggest its relationship to Non-Hodgkins lymphoma

Hodgkin's Disease

Classical Hodgkin's Disease	**Histogenetically distinct subtype of Hodgkins Disease**
Variants/Subtypes	Variant/Subtype
Mixed cellularity *Nodular sclerosis* *Lymphocyte Rich* *Lymphocyte Depletion*	*Lymphocyte predominant* *(Nodular Lymphocyte Predominant)*
Characterized by:	Characterized by
• *Frequent Reed sternberg cells* • *Characteristic immunophenotype* *CD 15 positive; CD 30 positive* *CD 45 Negative*	• *Rare Reed Sternberg cells* (Frequent Lymphocytic and Histocytic variants (Popcorn cells)) • Characteristically different immunophenotype *CD 15 Negative : CD 30 Negative* *CD 45 Positive*

Characteristic R.S cells are less frequent in nodular sclerosis variant of Hodgkins but these cells are characteristically positive for CD 15 and CD 30 and negative for CD 45

166. Answer is B (Read Sterberg cells): *Robbins 7th/686*

Hodgkin's Lymphoma is characterized morphologically by the presence of distinctive neoplastic giant cells called Read – Sternberg cells *-Robbins 7th/686*

167. Answer is D (Lymphocyte Predominant Hodgkin's disease): *Robbins 7th/687,688,689)*

Lympho-Histiocytic variants (L and H cells) have a delicate multilobed nucleus resembling a popcorn kernel and are also called popcorn cells.

Lymphohistiocytic variants are specific to lymphocyte predominance subtype of Hodgkin's Lymphoma.

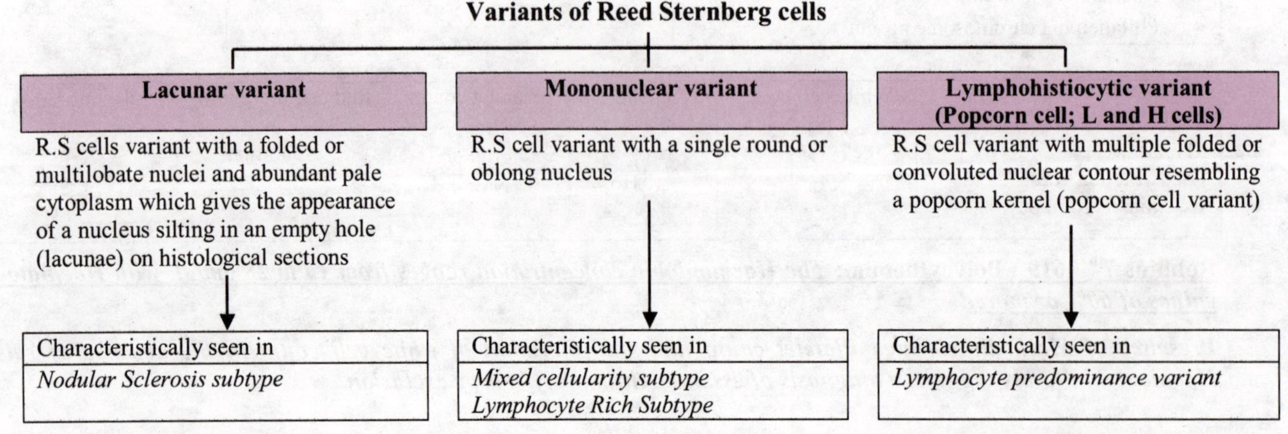

168. Answer is A (Lacunar cells): *Read text below*

Lacunar cells are characteristic of nodular subtype of Hodgkins lymphoma.

Hodgkins lymphoma subtypes	Red Sternberg cells variant
Nodular sclerosis	Lacunar cells [Q]
Mixed cellularity	Mononuclear variant[Q]
Lymphocyte predominance	Popcorn cell [Q] (Lymphocytic variant)
Lymphocyte depleted	Reticular variant (more cellular)

169. Answer is A (Nodular sclerosis): Harrison 18th/p 934 *Harrison 17th / 699; API 8th / 903; Chandrasoma Taylor 3rd/ 457, 458*

Nodular sclerosis is the most common subtype worldwide.

The Hodgkin's lymphomas may be classified into four subtypes according to the Rye's classification.

Hodgkins lymphoma subtypes in order of frequency
1. Nodular sclerosis (30-60%)
2. Mixed cellularity (20-40%)
3. Lymphocyte predominance (< 10%)
4. Lymphocyte depleted (< 10%)

Incidence: NS > MC > LP > LD

Note: WHO classification recognizes another subtype of Hodgkins called 'Lymphocyte Rich' subtype

170. Answer is C (Mixed cellularity): *Chandrasoma Taylor 3rd/ 459; API 6th/ 928; API 8th/903*

'While nodular sclerosis is the most common subtype in the developed countries, the mixed cellularity type is most common in developing countries.' *- API 6th/928*

As the questions specifically asks about the most common variant in India mixed cellularity is undoubtedly the single best answer.

171. Answer is A (Lymphocyte Predominance): *Chandrasoma Taylor 3rd/ 459*

Lymphocyte predominant type of Hodgkins lymphoma is associated with the best prognosis.

Variant	5 years survival
Lymphocyte predominance	*90%*
Nodular sclerosis	*70%*
Mixed cellularity	*50%*
Lymphocyte depletion	*40%*

Prognosis: LP > NS > MC > LD

Remember one characteristic each, of each variety

• Lymphocytic predominant	*Best prognosis* [Q]
• Mixed cellularity	*M.C. type in India* [Q]
• Lymphocytic depleted	*Worst prognosis* [Q]
• Nodular sclerosis	*M.C. type (all over the world)* [Q]

Note: *WHO classification recognizes another subtype of Hodgkins Lymphoma called 'Lymphocyte Rich' subtype.*

172. Answer is A (Lymphocyte predominance): *Chandrasoma Taylor 3rd/ 459*

Lymphocyte predominant type of Hodgkins lymphoma is associated with the best prognosis.

Variant	5 years survival
Lymphocyte predominance	90%
Nodular sclerosis	70%
Mixed cellularity	50%
Lymphocyte depletion	40%

Prognosis: LP > NS > MC > LD

Remember one characteristic each, of each variety

• Lymphocytic predominant	*Best prognosis* [Q]
• Mixed cellularity	*M.C. type in India* [Q]
• Lymphocytic depleted	*Worst prognosis* [Q]
• Nodular sclerosis	*M.C. type (all over the world)* [Q]

Note: *WHO classification recognizes another subtype of Hodgkins Lymphoma called 'Lymphocyte Rich' subtype.*

173. Answer is A (CD15 and CD30): *Robbins 7th/688, Harrisons / 16th /655*

The tumor cells in Hodgkins Lymphoma are characteristically positive for CD15 and CD30 and negative for CD45.
– Robbins 7th/688

Lymphocyte predominance Hodgkins Lymphoma is the only histological subtype that does not express CD15 and CD30. This subtype expresses CD45 and is often considered as an entirely distinct category from classical Hodgkin's disease (Harrisons)

Hodgkins Lymphoma	Immunopheno type	Association with EBV	Read Sternberg Cell variant[Q]
Nodular Sclerosis	**CD15 + , CD30 +**	EBV – Ve[Q]	Lacunar cells[Q] (Occasional R-S-cells)
Mixed cellularity	**CD15 + , CD30 +**	EBV + Ve[Q] (70%)	Classic Reed Sternberg cells[Q]
Lymphocyte depletion	**CD15 + , CD30 +**	EBV +Ve[Q]	Reticular variant[Q] (Frequent R-S cells)
Lymphocyte Predominance	CD15 –ve, CD30-ve CD20 +ve, CD45+ve ($H17^{th}$)	EBV – Ve[Q]	Popcorn cell variant[Q]

174. Answer is C (Atypical cells): *Robbin's 7th/686, 687*

Atypical cells may be seen in some variants of Hodgkin's disease but they are not required for the diagnosis of Hodgkin's disease

Diagnosis of Hodgkin's disease

Histopathological (In all cases)

Identification of R-S cells and their variants in the appropriate reactive cellular background remains the diagnostic sine qua non – 'Blood' 2nd/841

Reed Sternberg cells/Variants
Reactive cellular background

Although RS cells are requisite for the diagnosis they must present in an appropriate background of non-neoplastic inflammatory cells (lymphocytes, plasma cells, eosinophils)

Immunohistochemical markers (In difficult cases)

Immunohistochemical markers on tissue sections of biopsy material for CD 15 & CD30 provides vital clues in establishing diagnosis in difficult cases.

The tumor cells have a characteristic immunophenotypes: Positive for CD15 and CD30 and negative for CD45

Except lymphocyte predominant variant which is CD15 & CD30 negative CD45 positive

175. Answer is A (CNS is the commonest site of involvement) : Harrison 18th/p 934 *Harrison 14th/ 708, Harrison 15th/ 725, Harrisons 16th/ 654; Harrisons 17th/ 699; API 8th/ 903; Chandrasoma Taylor 3rd/ 456, 457, 459*

CNS involvement is an uncommon feature of Hodgkins disease

CNS involvement is an uncommon feature with Hodgkins disease: This may occur as :

- Sudden spinal cord compression in advanced progressive disease.
- Headache and visual disturbance in very rare patients with intra-cranial Hodgkins disease.

Reed stern berg cell is the characteristic cell in Hodgkins, and the diagnosis of Hodgkins Lymphoma is still based entirely upon histological examination & the finding of classic Reed-Sternberg cell or one of its variants is considered essential for diagnosis.

Plasms cells, Eosinophils and Neutrophils are seen in the reactive background

Histology in Hodgkins shows distinctive Reed Sternberg cells (few) that are admixed with variable number of Lymphocytes, plasma cells, histocytes, eosinophills neutrophils and fibroblasts.

Mediastinal involvement is particularly common with nodular sclerosis variant.

Certain Distincitive Features Seen In Nodular Sclerosis Variant

- it is the most common variant. Q
- it is the only variant more common in females. Q
- mediastinal involvement is particularly common. Q
- large Reed Sternberg cell variants - 'Lacunar cells' Q - are present on histology.
- it has a good prognosis Q {2nd best, following Lymphocyte predominance (best)}

176. Answer is C (Cerebellar degenerative disease): Harrison 18th/p 934 *Harrison 16th/572-573; Harrison 17th / 699*

Hodgkin's Lymphoma is associated with prominent or pure paraneoplastic cerebellar degeneration.

Cancer	Syndrome	Antibody
Hodgkins Lymphoma	Paraneoplastic cerebellar degeneration (PCD)	Anti Tr.

Paraneoplastic Cerebellar degeneration

Pure crebellar degeneration
- Breast and Gynaecological cancers (Anti Yo Antibodies)
- Hodgkins Lymphoma (Anti Tr Antibodies)

Subacute Cerebellar degeneration
- Small cell carcinoma lung
- Thymoma
- Neuroblastoma

177. Answer is C (Absolute lymphocyte count < 600/mm3): *'Blood' by Handen, Lux and Stossel (2002)/852,854; Hoffman 4th/1351,1352; William's 7th/1473*

An absolute Lymphocyte count of <600 is a poor prognostic factor in Hodgkin's lymphoma.

Prognostic factors in Hodgkins lymphoma

Poor prognostic factors for advanced disease
- Male Gender
- Age>45 years
- Stage IV Disease
- Serum Haemoglobin < 10g
- Serum Albumin < 4 g
- WBC count > 15,000/mm^3
- Absolute lymphocyte count < 600mm^3

These factor predict relapse of advanced disease

Poor prognostic factors in Localized disease
- Male Gender
- Age >50 years
- Histological subtype (mixed cellularity and lymphocyte Depletion)
- Elevated ESR
- Mediastinal mass >1/3 of thoracic diameter (Mediastinal/thorax ratio > 35%)
- Number of involved sites with the same side of diaphragm > 4
- Presence of systemic symptoms ('B' symptoms)

These factors predict prognosis in patients with clinical stages I and II in Hodgkin's disease.

178. Answer is A (Younger age): *Refer previous questions*

Young age < 45 years is a good prognostic feature. Old age (> 50 years) is a poor prognostic factor

Lymphocyte depletion subtype, presence of mediastinal disease and systemic manifestation *are all established poor prognostic factors*

Stomach involvement *reflects advanced stage of disease and is likely to be associated with a poor prognosis.*

179. Answer is B (stage IIB): Harrison 18th/p 924 *Harrisons 17th/691*

The patient is presenting with involvement of two lymph node regions on the same side of diaphragm (stageII) along with presence of systemic symptoms (Group B). This patient can thus be staged as having stage II B disease.

THE ANN ARBOR STAGING SYSTEM FOR HODGKIN'S DISEASE

Stage	Definition
I	Involvement of a single lymph node region or lymphoid structure (e.g., spleen, thymus, Waldeyer's ring)
II	Involvement of two or more lymph node regions on the same side of the diaphragm (the mediastinum is a single site; hilar lymph nodes should be considered "lateralized" and, when involved on both sides, constitute stage II disease)
III	Involvement of lymph node regions or lymphoid structures on both sides of the diaphragm
III-1	Subdiaphragmatic involvement limited to spleen, splenic hilar nodes, celiac nodes, or portal nodes
III-2	Subdiaphragmatic involvement includes paraaortic, iliac, or mesenteric nodes plus structures in III-1
IV	Involvement of extranodal site(s) beyond that designated as"E" more than one extranodal deposit at any location Any involvement of liver or bone marrow.
A	No symptoms
B	Unexplained weight loss of >10% of the body weight during the 6 months before staging investigation Unexplained persistent, or recurrent fever with temperatures >38°C during the previous month Recurrent drenching night sweats during the previous month
E	Localized, solitary involvement of extralymphatic tissue, excluding liver and bone marrow.

180. Answer is C (Radiotherapy only): Harrison 18th/p 935 *Harrisons 17th/700; William's Hematology 7th/1470*

Regional Radiotherapy is the treatment of choice for localized/limited stage disease nodular lymphocyte predominant hodgkin's Lymphoma

'Nodular lymphocyte predominant Hodgkins lymphoma NLPHL presents as asymptomatic limited stage disease in most patients. Most patients present with peripheral lymph nodes in neck, axilla or groin and are classified as limited stage IA disease. Because of the low likelihood of occult disease and tendency of disease to remain localized for years, regional RT is considered treatment of choice'.-Williams 7th/1471

The patient in question presents with a single cervical lymph node and hence can be classified as having stage 1A disease with nodular lymphocyte predominant Hodgkin's lymphoma. Regional RT is the treatment of choice for such patients

Treatment of Hodgkin's Lymphoma

Classical Hodgkin's Lymphoma		Nodular Lymhocyte predominant Hodgkin's Lymphoma	
Limited Stage Disease	Advanced Disease	Limited Stage Disease	Advanced Disease
(Favourable/unfavourable) (Stage I, II)	Stage III, IV	Stage I, II	Stage III, IV
Combined Modality treatment with Radiotherapy and chemotherapy is the treatment of choice Limited Stage Disease (I, II) is primarily managed by a combination of chemotherapy (CT) and Radiotherapy (RT) (CT→RT)	Chemotherapy is the treatment of choice Advanced stage disease is primarily managed by chemotherapy Radiotherapy may be used in advanced disease for bulky disease or residual disease after chemotherapy (PTO)	Radiotherapy alone is the treatment of choice (Involved Field RT or Regional RT may be used) *Some clinicians favour no treatment and merely close follow up*	Chemotherapy is the treatment of choice Advanced stage disease is primarily managed chemotherapy *RT may be used in advanced disease for palliation only and in selected cases after chemotherapy.*
CT + RT	CT (± RT)	RT	CT (± RT)

181. Answer is A (Chemotherapy with Radiotherapy): Harrison 18th/p 934 *Harrisons 17th/699: Williams 7th/1469-1471*

Combined modality treatment with Chemotherapy and Radiotherapy is the treatment of choice in limited stage (stage I,II) Hodgkin's lymphoma with a classical Histological subtype.

Patient has limited Stage I Hodgkin's Lymphoma

Patient in question presents with involvement of single lymph node region and hence can be staged as having stage I (Limited) disease.

Stage I	Disease Involvement of single lymph node region.

Patient has a classical Hodgkin's Lymphoma of nodular sclerosis subtype
The presence of frequent Lacuner cells suggests a diagnosis of nodular sclerosis

Hodgkins lymphoma

Classical Hodgkin's	Non classical Hodgkins
Nodular sclerosis (Lacunar cells) Mixed cellularity (Mononuclear cells) Lymphocyte rich (Mononuclear cells) Lymphocyte depletion	Nodular lymphocyte predominance Hodgkins NLPHL (popcorn cell/lymphohistiocytic cell)

The treatment of choice for limited Stage I Classical Hodgkins Lymphoma is combined modality therapy with Chemotherapy and Radiotherapy

182. Answer is B (Radiatiotherapy is best): Harrison 18th/p 934 *Harrison 17th/; CMDT 2008/453; 2009/459*

Patients with localized stage IA disease are best treated with Radiation therapy to involved fileds.

Initial treatment with a brief course chemotherapy before radiuotherapy may improve the outcome, however, amongst the options provided the treatment of choice remains radiotherapy.

Treatment of Hodgkins Disease

Stage I (A) and Stage II (A)	Stage III and Stage IV and patient with group B symptoms
Corner stone of treatment is Radiotherapy to involved field *Initial treatment with a brief course of chemotherapy improves outcome* *Treatment of choice is a brief course of chemotherapy followed by Radiotherapy to sites of node involvement*	***Cornerstone of treatment is combination chemotherapy*** *Radiotherapy may be administered after chemotherapy in those who obtain only a poor partial response, but it has not shown to improve outcome in patients who achieve complete remission after combination chemotherapy.*

183. Answer is C (ABVD): Harrison 18th/p 934 *Harrison 17th/Manual of Oncology 6th/443*

ABVD is the chemotherapy regimen of choice in Hodgkins lymphoma

'Chemotherapy with ABVD is considered the standard first line treatment for most patients and is superior to MOPP in efficacy and toxicity profile'- Manual of Clinical Oncology 6th/443

Regimen	Agents	Comments
ABVD	Doxorubicin Bleomycin Vinblastine Dacarbazine	• *First line treatment of choice* • *Most popular regimen in United States* • *More effective than MOPP* • *Lesser incidence of Sterility and secondary malignancies than MOPP* • *More satisfactory than MOPP and ABVD in alternating cycles or MOPP/ABV Hybrid*
MOPP	Mechlorethamine Vincristine Procarbozine Prednisolone	• *Less effective and more toxic than ABVD* • *Higher incidence of sterility and secondary malignancies than ABVD*

Stanford V	• Doxorubicin • Bleomycin • Vinblastine • Mechlorethamine • Vincristine • Prednisolone • Etoposide + Radiotherapy	• *Excellent results but still under investigations/ Trial*
BEACOPP		• *Popular in Europe* • *Not fully evaluated*

184. Answer is B (Sterility is more frequent complication of ABVD than MOPP): Harrison 18th/p 935 *Harrison 17th/699; Harrison 's Manual of Oncology (2007)/218*

Sterility is more frequent complication of MOPP than ABVD.

Infertility and Treatment of Hodgkins Lymphoma

- Infertility is a concern for all patients undergoing treatment
- Risk of infertility is age related – Risk is increased in old age (younger patients are more likely to recover fertility)
- ***Risk of infertility is more with MOPP than ABVD***
  (*Treatment with ABVD rather than MOPP increases the chances to retain fertility* - Harrison)

Non Hodgkins Lymphoma and Leukemia

185. Answer is B (REAL Classification) : *Robbins 7th/668; AJC Cancer staging Handbook API 8th/905*

In 1994, a group of hematopathologists, oncologists and molecular biologists came together (International Lymphoma Study Group) and introduced a new classification, called the 'Revised European-American Classification of Lymphoid Neoplasms (REAL).

WHO has now reviewed and updated the real classification resulting in inclusion of additional rare entities.

WHO Classification / Modified 'REAL' Classification	
I. Precursor B-cell Neoplasm Precursor-B lymphoblastic leukemia/lymphoma **II. Peripheral B-Cell Neoplasms** Chronic lymphocytic leukemia/small lymphocytic lymphoma B-cell prolymphocytic leukemia Lymphoplasmacytic lymphoma Splenic and nodal marginal zone lymphomas Extranodal marginal zone lymphomas Mantle cell lymphoma Follicular lymphoma Marginal zone lymphoma Hairy cell leukemia Plasmacytoma/plasma cell myeloma Diffuse large B-cell lymphoma Burkitt lymphoma **III. Precursor T-Cell Neoplasms** Precursor-T lymphoblastic leukemia/lymphoma	**IV. Peripheral T-Cell and NK-Cell Neoplasms** T-cell prolymphocytic leukemia Large granular lymphocytic leukemia Mycosis fungoides/Sezary syndrome Peripheral large cell lymphoma, unspecified Anaplastic large cell lymphoma Enteropathy-associated T-cell lymphoma Hepatosplenic γδ T-cell lymphoma Adult T-cell leukemia/lymphoma NK/T-cell lymphoma, nasal type NK cell leukemia **V. Hodgkins Lymphoma** Classical subtypes - Nodular sclerosis - Mixed cellularity - Lymphocyte-rich - Lymphocyte depletion Lymphocyte predominance

186. Answer is B (Angiocentric Lymphoma) : Harrison 18th/p 920 *Robbins 7th / 671; Harrison 16th / 654; Harrison 17th / 688*

Angiocentric Lymphoma is a type of T cell lymphoma that has been linked to the Epstein Barr Virus.

Angiocentric Lymphoma has been classified as a Peripheral T cell Lymphoma : - *Harrison 16th*
'Extranodal T/NK cell lymphoma of nasal type has also been called angiocentric lymphoma' - Harrison
(Also called Lethal Midline granuloma)

Classification of Non Hodgkin Lymphoma	
B cell Neoplasms	**T cell Neoplasms**
Neoplasms of immature B cells	Neoplasms of immature T cells
Precursor B cell Acute Lymphoblastic leukaemia / lymphoma	Precursor T-cell Acute Lymphoblastic leukaemia / Lymphoma
Neoplasms of mature B cells	Neoplasms of mature T cells / NK cells
• ***Burkitt's lymphoma***[Q] • ***Hairy cell leukemia***[Q] • ***Mantle cell lymphoma***[Q] • Solitary plasmacytoma / Multiple Myeloma[Q] • Small lymphocytic lymphoma / Chronic lymphocytic leukaemia (CLL) • Follicular lymphoma • Diffuse large B cell lymphoma • Extranodal marginal zone lymphoma (MALT Type)	• Mycosis fungoides : Cutaneous T cell lymphoma • Adult T cell lymphoma / Leukemia • Anaplastic Large T cell / Null cell Lymphoma • Peripheral T cell Lymphoma o Angioimmunoblastic Lymphoma o *Angiocentric Lymphoma* (Extra-nodal T/NK cell Lymphoma) o Enteropathy type intestinal lymphoma o Hepatosplenic lymphoma o Subcutaneous Panniculitis - like lymphoma • T cell granular lymphocytic lymphoma

187. Answer is B (IgM): Harrison 18th/p 942, 943 *Harrison's 17th/-706 ' Surgicla pathology of Head & Neck' by Barnes 2nd/ 1270, 1271*

Plasmacytoid Lymphomas may be associated with a monoclonal IgM paraprotein (Waldenstrom's Macroglobulinemia).

Plasmacytoid Lymphocyte Type Malignant Lymphoma / Plasmacytoid Lymphoma

- This is a ***B cell neoplasm***[Q] that is associated with plasmacytoid differentiation of lymphocytes
- Plasmacytoid lymphocytes are transitional forms between lymphocytes and plasma cells
- ***These may be associated with a monoclonal IgM paraprotein and are thus considered the histological counterparts of Waldenstrom's Macroglobulinemia***
- Synonyms include immunocytoma

  Kiel Classification : Malignant Lymphoma, Lymphoplasmacytoid immunocytoma
  REAL Classification: Lymphoplasmacytoid Lymphoma / Immunocytoma
- These are ***low grade lymphoid neoplams***[Q] that occur in middle aged or older individuals.

188. Answer is D (Hemoglobin and Albumin) Harrison 18th/p 925 *'Harrison 17th Ed / 692*

'International prognostic index' does not include Hemoglobin and Albumin as prognostic factors.

Prognostic Factors according to International Prognostic Index for NHL

1. *Age*[Q] : *(Age ≤ 60 years carries adverse prognosis)*
2. *Stage*[Q] : *(Ann Arbor stage III or IV carries adverse prognosis)*
3. *LDH levels*[Q] : *(Elevated LDH levels above normal carry adverse prognosis)*
4. *Performance status*[Q] : *(P.S ≥ 2 (ECOG) or ≤ 70 (Karnofsky) carries adverse prognosis)*
5. *Number of Extranodal sites involved*[Q] : *(>1 extranodal site* involvement carries adverse prognosis)

International Prognostic Index for NHL

Five clinical risk factors:

- *Age ≥ 60 years*
- *Serum lactate dehydrogenase levels elevated*
- *Performance status ≥ 2 (ECOG) or ≤ 70 (Karnofsky)*
- *Ann Arbor stage III or IV*
- *> 1 site of extranodal involvement*

189. Answer is B (Diffuse, small cleaved cell): *Robbins 5th/638, Robbins 7th/does not mention the working formulation*

Working formulation of NHL for clinical usage is as follows:

Low grade
1. Small lymphocytic Q
2. Follicular, predominantly small cleaved cell Q
3. Follicular, mixed, small cleaved and large cell. Q
Intermediate grade
1. Follicular predominantly large cell Q
2. Diffuse small cleaved cell
3. Diffuse mixed small and large cell.
4. Diffuse large cell.
High grade
1. Large cell immunoblastic Q
2. Lymphoblastic Q
3. Small non cleaved cell. Q

Note that all varieties of diffuse fall in the intermediate grade category only.

190. Answer is C (Mycosis fungoides): *Repeat Harrison 15th/ 724; Robbins 5th/ 638; (Harrison 16th/ Robbins 7th/ does not mention the working formulation)*

Mycosis fungoides is included in the Miscellaneous group. Q ***It does not fall in the intermediate grade.***
All' diffuse' fall into intermediate grade. Intermediate grade includes only one more variant, which is follicular, large cell.

Intermediate grade includes:

1. Diffuse small cleaved Q
2. Diffuse mixed small and large cell Q
3. Diffuse large cell, and Q
4. Follicular large cell Q

191. Answer is A (Diffuse large cell): *Repea Harrison 15th/ 724; Robbins 5th/ 638t*

Diffuse large cell lymphoma is the most malignant, amongst the options provided.
Although Follicular large cell and Diffuse varieties are both classified in the intermediate grade of the 'working formulation of NHL', in general, ***'lymphomas with a follicular histological pattern are of a lower grade (longer survival times) than those with a diffuse pattern'*** *– (Chandrasoma Taylor 2nd/ 439)*

Burkitt's Lymphoma

192. Answer is B (8 – 14 translocation): Harrison 18th/p 931 *Harrison 17th / 696; Chandrasoma Taylor 3rd/ 296*

Presence of t (8; 14) or one of its variants t (2; 8) or t (8; 22) can be confirmatory *– Harrison 16th/ 652.*

Important translocation to be remembered

Translocation	Associated Malignancy
t 8 – 14	Burkitt's lymphoma Q ALL (FAB type L3) Immunoblastic B cell lymphoma Q
t 15-17	Promyelocytic Leukemia Q (M_3- AML)
t 4 – 11	ALL Q
t 11 – 14	CLL Q, *Mantle cell lymphoma*
t 14 – 18	B cell lymphomas Q

193. Answer is D (Burkitt's Lymphoma): Harrison 18th/p 931, 923 *Harrison's 17th/696, 690; Wintrobe's Hematology 12th/2082, 1604; Atlas of Hematologic Neoplasms by Tsieh Sun/26; Cancer Cytogenetics by Heim, Mitelman 3rd/326; Clinical Malignant Hematology by Sekeres, Kalaycio, Bolwell 1st (2007)/114*

Translocation t(2:8)(p12:q24) is associated with Burkitt's lymphoma / leukemia.

'The hallmark of Burkitt lymphoma is the t(8;14)(q24;q32) and its variants, t(2;8)(p12; q24) and t(8;22)(q24;q11)'.
-Cancer Cytogenetics by Heim, Mitelman 3rd/326; Clinical Malignant Hematology by Sekeres, Kalaycio, Bolwell 1st (2007)/114

'Demonstration of very high proliferative fraction and the presence of the t(8;14) or one of its ***variants t(2;8)*** *or t(8:22) can be confirmatory of Burkitt's lymphoma / leukemia'* - *Harrison's 17th/696*

Neoplasm	Translocation	Genes involved
Burkitt	*t(8;14)(q24:q32) most common*^{Q}	*c-MYC: IgH (heavy chain)*
	t(2;8)(p12;q24)	*Igκ: c-MYC (light chain)*
	t(8;22)(q24:q11)	*c-MYC : Igλ (light chain)*

194. Answer is A (t(8:14)): Harrison 18th/p 931, 923 *Harrison's 17th/696, 690*

t (8; 14) is the most common translocation seen in association with Burkitt's Lymphoma

'Demonstration of very high proliferative fraction and the presence of the ***t (8; 14)*** *or one of its variants t (2; 8) or t(8:22) can be confirmatory of Burkitt's lymphoma / leukemia'* - *Harrison's 17th/696*

Translocations in Burkitt's Lymphoma

Burkitt's lymphoma / leukemias are associated with reciprocal translocations involving the ***c-myc gene on chromosome 8***

Most common Translocation (70% cases)	Less common translocations
t (8; 14): c- myc gene on chromosome 8 and IgH heavy chain on chromosome 14	**t (8; 22)** c- myc gene on chromosome 8 and λ-light chain on chromosome 22 **t (2; 8) :** c- myc gene on chromosome 8 and κ-light chain on chromosome -2

195. Answer is A (EBV): *Harrison 17th /689; Harrison's 18th/921*

Burkitt's Lymphoma is typically associated with Epstein Barr virus (EBV).

EBV is associated with upto 95% of cases of Endemic Burkitt's Lymphoma.
EBV is associated with approximately 30% of cases of Sporadic Burkitt's Lymphoma and Immune Deficiency associated Burkitt's Lymphoma.

Infectious Agents Associated with the Development of Lymphoid Malignancies

Infectious Agent	Lymphoid Malignancy
Epstein-Barr virus	• *Burkitt's lymphoma* • *Post–organ transplant lymphoma* • *Primary CNS diffuse large B cell lymphoma* • *Hodgkin's disease* • *Extranodal NK/T cell lymphoma, nasal type*
HTLV-I	• *Adult T cell leukemia/lymphoma*
HIV	• *Diffuse large B cell lymphoma* • *Burkitt's lymphoma*
Hepatitis C virus	• *Lymphoplasmacytic lymphoma*
Helicobacter pylori	• *Gastric MALT lymphoma*
Human herpesvirus 8	• *Primary effusion lymphoma* • *Multicentric Castleman's disease*

CNS, central nervous system; HIV, human immunodeficiency virus; HTLV, human T cell lymphotropic virus; MALT, mucosa-associated lymphoid tissue; NK, natural killer.

196. Answer is D (Radiotherapy is the treatment of choice): Harrison 18th/p 931 *Harrison 17th/; Robbins 7th/678*

The treatment of choice for Burkitt's Lymphoma is chemotherapy and not Radiotherapy.

'Burkitt's lymphoma responds well to short term high dose chemotherapy. Treatment of Burkitt's lymphoma in both children and adults should begin within 48 hours of diagnosis and involves the use of intensive combination chemotherapy regimens' – Harrisons

Burkitt's Lymphoma is a B cell lymphoma
Burkitt's Lymphoma are tumors of mature B cells – Robbins 7th/677

t (8;14) translocation is the most common translocation in Burkitt's Lymphoma
Burkitt's lymphomas are associated with translocation of the c-MYC gene on chromosome 8.
Translocation
t (8; 14)
t (8; 22)
t (2; 8)

Burkitt's Lymphoma may present with an abdominal mass

- Most Burkitt's Lymphoma presents at extranodal sites but may present with lymphadenopathy
  Extranodal sites of involvement include the mandible and abdominal viscera
  'Burkitt's Lymphomas may present with peripheral lymphadenopathy or an intraabdominal mass' – Harrison
- CNS involvement is frequent
  The disease is rapidly progressive and has a propensity to metastasize to CNS, prophylactic therapy to CNS is therefore mandatory.
- *Burkitt's Lymphoma is the most rapidly progressive human tumor* – Harrison

Hairy Cell Leukemia

197. Answer is B (Results from an expansion of Neoplastic T lymphocytes): *Repeat: Harrison's 15th/725;Robbins 6th/668*

Hairy cell leukemia isa 'B' cell neoplasm and is characterized by expansion of neoplasticB cells (not T lymphocytes)

Hairy cell leukemia:
Hairy cell leukemia is a rare but distinctive form of chronic B cell leukemia that derives its name from the appearance of fine 'hair like projections'Q on the leukaemic cells (large B cells)

• **Characteristic cytochemical feature:**	Presence of tartrate resistant acid phosphatase 'TRAP' Q in neoplastic B cells
• **Cellular features/ Markers**Q	• Hairy cells express the pan B cell markers CD 19 and CD 20 and monocyte associated antigen CD 11 • Plasma cell associated antigen (PCA-1) is also present – Robbins • Expression of **CD 25**, IL2 and specific adhesion molecules – Harrison 14th/695
• **Clinical features** result largely from infiltration of bone marrow liver and spleen	• Present predominantly in the older age group > 40 yearsQ • Massive splenomegalyQ (hepatomegaly is less common) • Lymphadenopathy • PancytopeniaQ • Recurrent infections
• **Treatment** Q	• Current treatment of choice is with purine analogues – CladribineQ • Other drugs used - PentostotinQ - Interferon αQ • Splenectomy used to be the standard treatment earlier

198. Answer is B (B Cells): Harrison 18th/p 920 *Harrison 16th/ 652; Harrison 17th/ 688; Robbins 6th/ 668, Robbins 7th/ 683*

Hairy Cell Leukemia is a rare but distinctive B-cell neoplasm.

Hairy cell leukemia review :

Presentation **is with a triad of :**
1. Splenomegaly Q : often massive. However hepatomegaly is less common while lymphadenopathy is rare. 2. Pancytopenia Q and thereby, resulting infections. 3. Vasculitis like syndrome Q : Erythema nodosum and cutaneous nodules due to perivasculitis and PAN.
Course : Hairy cell leukemia follows an indolent course. Q

199. Answer is D (Hairy cell leukemia) : Harrison 18th/p 920 *Harrison 17th/ 697;CMDT 2008/450; 2009/456; Robbins 7th/683*

Presence of massive splenomegaly, and granulocytopenia, alongwith characteristic immunophenotypic features (specially CD103) suggests the diagnosis of Hairy cell leukemia. CD103 is exclusively positive in Hairy cell leukemia and thus leaves no doubt as regards the correct diagnosis.

Immunophenotypic features of Hairy cell leukemia.

CD markers	Surface immunoglobulins
Pan B cell markers : CD 19, CD 20	Heavy chain : IgG
Monocytic associated antigen : CD11c, CD25, CD103	Light chain : γ or λ

	SIg	CD5	CD10	CD11c	CD19	CD20	CD22	CD23	CD25	CD103
Hairy cell leukemia	-/+	-/+	-	++	+	+	++	-/+	+	++
Mantle cell lymphoma	+	++	-	-	+	+	+	-/+	-	-
CLL	+/-	++	-	-/+	+	+/-	-/+	++	-/+	-
Prolymphocytic leukemia	++	+	-	-/+	+	+/-	+	+/-	-	-
Splenic marginal lymphoma	+	-/+	-/+	+	+	+	+/-	-/+	-	-
Lympho- plasmacytoma	+/-	-/+	-	-	+	-/-	+/-	-/+	+/-	-

200. Answer is A (Steroid): Harrison 18th/p 931, 932 *Harrison 16th/ 652; Harrison 17th/ 697; Robbins 7th/ 683*

Steroid has no role in treatment of hairy cell leukemia.
Cladribine is the drug of choice. Clinical complete remissions with cladribine occur in majority of patients and long-term disease free survival is frequent.

Treatment of hairy cell leukemia is chemotherapy with
• Cladribine : Drug of choice. • *Alpha-interferon* Q • *Pentostatin* Q

Splenectomy *used to be the standard treatment* of cytopenias resulting from Hairy cell leukemia

201. Answer is B (Cladribine): Harrison 18th/p 931, *Harrison 15th/ 724, Harrison 16th/ 652; Harrison 17th/ 697; CMDT 2005/ 494; 2009/456*

"The treatment of choice is Cladribine Q (2 chlorodoxy adenosine) 0.14 mg /kg daily for 7 days" *– CMDT*
This is a relatively non-toxic drug that produces benefit in 95% of cases, and complete remission in more than 80%

Mantle Cell Lymphoma

202. Answer is B (Mantle cell Lymphoma): *Handbook of Human Immunology 2nd/245; Williams 7th/1347; Hoffman's 4th/1381*

Coexpression of the B lymphocyte lineage marker CD 19 and T lymphocyte marker CD5 is unique to CLL and mantle cell Lymphoma. CLL can be differentiated from MCL be expression of CD79b and FMC-7 both of which are absent in CLL and positive in MCL- *Handbook of clinical immunology 2nd/245*

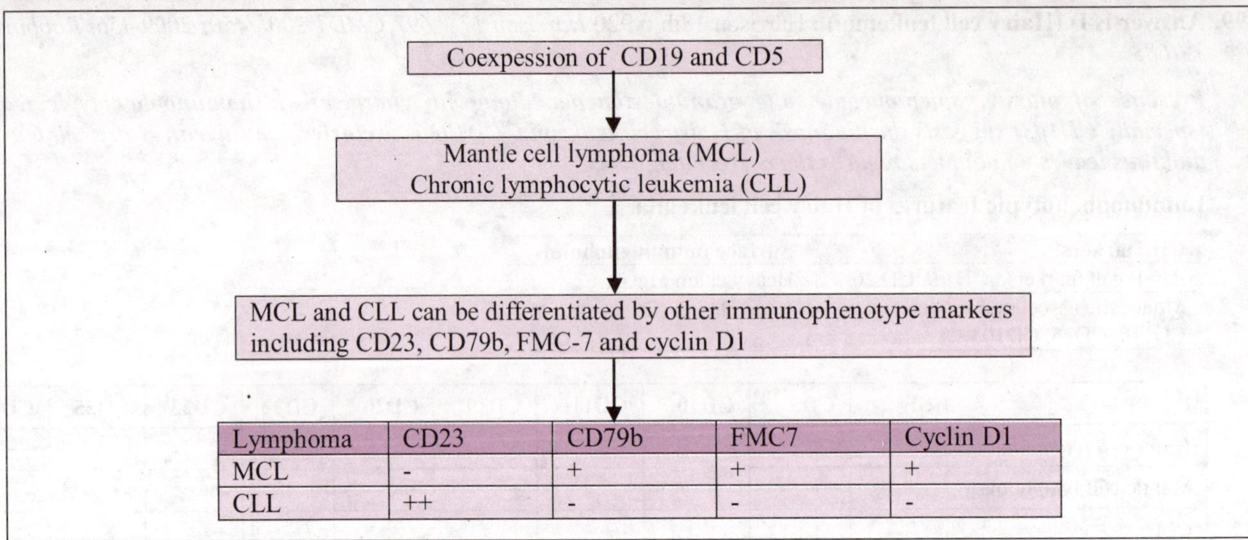

Lymphoma	CD23	CD79b	FMC7	Cyclin D1
MCL	-	+	+	+
CLL	++	-	-	-

'CLL can be differentiated from MCL by expression of CD79b and FMC-7 both of which are absent in CLL/SLL and bright in MCL' -Handbook of human Immunology 2nd/245

'In contrast to CLL B cells mantle cell Lymphoma cells do not express CD23' – Williams 7th/1351

203. Answer is A (Mantle cell lymphoma): Harrison 18th/p 928, 929 *Ackerman surgical pathology 8th/ 1721; Neoplastic histopathology 2nd/ 789; Robbins 7th/ 683; Harrisons 16th/ 648, 650; Harrison 17th/ 693, 694, 695*

The given clinical profile is suggestive of mantle cell lymphoma as explained below.

Mantle cell lymphoma

Presents in the middle aged and the elderly (Mean Age = 63 yrs – *Harrison 16th/ 648*).

Clinical profile
- Painless lymphadenopathy - Splenomegaly - Occasional GI involvement

Immunocytochemical profile of Mantle Cell Lymphoma

CD markers	SURFACE immunoglobulins	Translocation
• Cells are positive for PAN B markers D 19, CD 2, CD 22, CD 24 • Cells are positive for CD 5 • Cells are negative for CD 23 • Cells are negative for CD 10	• Moderately high levels of surface immunoglobulins heavy chains IgM & IgD • B cells present bright K positivity (either K or λ light chain may be present)	t (11; 14) translocation 14 t (11; 14) translocation leads to increased expression of cyclin D1

Chronic Lymphocytic Leukemia (CLL)

204. Ans. Answer is D (All of the above): *Harrison 18th /926; Wintrobe's Atlas of Clinical Hematology (2007)/138; Essentials in Hematology and clinical pathology' by Naik, Ras, Gupta (JP) 2012/202, 205, 204*

CLL is commonly seen in individuals > 50 years (median age is about 65 year) and are typically chrachterized by the presence of increased number of mature small lymphocytes in the peripheral smear. Hepatosplenomegaly and lymphadenopathy may be seen.

'The physical examination may be unremarkable but common findings are hepatosplenomegaly and enlarged non tender, firm mobile lymph nodes in the cervical axillary and inguinal areas' - Wintrobe's Atlas of clinical Hematology

Diagnostic criteria of CLL are (Wintrobe's Atlas of Clinical Hematology)
1. An absolute Lymphocytosis > 5x 10^9/L
2. > 30% Lymphocytosis in a normocellular or hypercellular bone marrow
3. Monoclonal B cells with low levels of surface immunoglobulins and CD5 positivity

205. Answer is C (CLL) : *Harrison 16th / 648; CMDT 2006 / 510; 2009/454-455*

Incidental finding of Lymphocytosis (80,000/mcL) in an elderly and asymptomatic patient suggests the diagnosis of CLL.

Why is CLL the single best answer of choice here ?

- *'CLL is a disease of older patients wth 90% of cases occurring after the age of 50 years and median age of presentation is 65 years'. – CMDT*

  The patient in question is aged 80 years and hence falls in the bracket of CLL.
- *'Typical B cell CLL is often found incidentally when a complete blood count is done for another reason'. – Harrison 16th / 648*

  The patient in question is asymptomatic and the findings represent incidental observation on a full blood count done for an obscure reason.
- *'The hallmark of CLL is absolute lymphocytosis. White cell count is usually greater than 20,000/mcL may be markedly elevated to several 100,000/mcL. Usually 75-80% of circulating cells are lymphocytes'. – CMDT*

  The patient in question is presenting with a white cell count of 100,000/mcL and 80% of circulating cells are lymphocytes. This finding is consistent

206. Answer is D (T lymphocyte CLL is more common): Harrison 18th/p 926, 927 *Harrison 17th/693; Clinical Malignant Hematology 1st (2007)/254*

The most common form of CLL is a B-cell CLL.

The most common form of Chronic Lymphocytic leukemia is a B-cell CLL
B cell CLL is more common than T cell CLL.

CLL is diagnosed on routine blood tests/Leukocytosis
Typical (B cell) CLL is often found incidentally when a complete blood count is done for another reasons.
The diagnosis is usually made when an increased number of circulating lymphocytes (↑ WBC count) is found on routine complete blood counts.

CLL does not normally present as an acute Leukemia
Transformation of CLL into acute Leukemias has been reported in a few studies but such transformation is extremely rare, and there is no convincing evidence that CLL ever transforms into an Acute Leukemia.

'There is no convincing evidence that CLL ever transforms into ALL' – Clinical Malignant Hematology 1st (2007)/254

207. Answer is C (CLL) : Harrison 18th/p 919, 921 *Harrison 16th / 648; Harrison 17th / 687, 691; API 8th/901; CMDT 2006 / 510; 2009/454-455*

Incidental finding of Lymphocytosis (80,000/mcL) in an elderly and asymptomatic patient suggests the diagnosis of CLL.

Why is CLL the single best answer of choice here ?

- *'CLL is a disease of older patients wth 90% of cases occurring after the age of 50 years and median age of presentation is 65 years'. – CMDT*

  The patient in question is aged 80 years and hence falls in the bracket of CLL.
- *'Typical B cell CLL is often found incidentally when a complete blood count is done for another reason'. – Harrison 16th / 648*

  The patient in question is asymptomatic and the findings represent incidental observation on a full blood count done for an obscure reason.

1

Hematology

- *'The hallmark of CLL is absolute lymphocytosis. White cell count is usually greater than 20,000/mcL may be markedly elevated to several 100,000/mcL. Usually 75-80% of circulating cells are lymphocytes'. – CMDT* ***The patient in question is presenting with a white cell count of 100,000/mcL and 80% of circulating cells are lymphocytes. This finding is consistent with the blood picture of CLL.***

208. Answer is D (t(11,14) translocation is present in most of the cases): Harrison 18th/p 923 *CMDT 2008/449; Washington manual of oncology 2nd/325; Postgraduate Hematology 4th/627; Robbins 7th/674; Harrison 17th/690; Wintrobe's 11th/2434*

The profile of this patient is consistent with a diagnosis of CLL (Refer previous question)

t (11;14) translocation is characteristic of Mantle cell lymphoma and not CLL. The most common genetic abnormality in CLL are deletions on the long arm of chromosome 13 (13q14)

Genetic Abnormalities in CLL and Associated Prognosis

Genetic Abnormalities with good Prognosis	
13q14 deletion	Good Prognosis ***Long term survival***

Genetic Abnormalities with poor prognosis	
Chromosome 11 deletion (11q22-23 deletion)	• Poor prognosis • Younger age • ***Bulky lymphadenopathy*** • Reduced survival
Chromosome 17 detection (17 p 21 detection)	• Poor Prognosis • Poor Response to therapy • Transformation
Chormone 12 Trisomy (Trisomy 12)	• Poor prognosis • Atypical morphology • ***Aggressive course/Progressive*** • High proliferation rate

209. Answer is A (A pseudofollicular pattern with proliferation centres): *William's 7th/1347; Hoffman's 4th/1381; Robbins 7th/673,674; Handbook of Human Immunology 2nd/245*

Coexpression of CD19 and CD 5 together with negative CD 79 and FMC7 markers suggest a diagnosis of chronic lymphocytic leukemia (CLL)

The histapathological examination of lymph nodes in CLL shows characteristic effacement of normal nodal architecture by diffuse proliferation and infiltration of small round lymphocytes (and not medium to large lyumphocytes). Pseudofollicular growth centres or proliferation centres are present in most cases and when present proliferation centres are considered pathognomic of CLL/SLL

Approach to the question

What is the diagnosis of the patient in question?
The patient in question is case of CLL

CLL is characterized by coexpression of CD5 and CD19[Q]
CLL is characteristically positive for CD23 and usually negative for CD7/9b and FMC7[Q]

Lymphoma	CD5	CD19	CD20	CD23	CD79b	FMC7
CLL	+	+	+/-	+	-	-

What are the histopathological characteristics of CLL?
Histopathological Features of CLL *(Robbins/Williams/Haffman)*

- *Lymph nodes in patients with CLL characteristically are diffusely infiltrated with monomorphic small round lymphocytes that efface the normal node architecture*

Diffuse effacement by a predominant population of small lymphocytes

- *The predominant cell is a small lymphocyte with clumped nuclear chromatin.*

These cells may be mixed with variable number of larger cells called prolymphocytes, but the predominant cells remain small lymphocytes.

- *Pseudofollicular growth centres or proliferation centres are present in most cases.*
Proliferation centres are clusters of prolymphocyte appearing cells that form aggregates or pseudofollicles, and so called because they contain a large number of mitotically active cells.

When present proliferation centres are considered pathognomic of CLL/SLL*-Robbins 7th/673*

1

210. Answer is B (Chronic Lymphocytic Leukemia): *CMDT' 2006/510;2008/449; 2009/455; Refer previous question*

Coexpression of the B Lymphocyte lineage marker CD 19 and the T lymphocyte marker CD 5 is unique to CLL and Mantle cell Lymphoma.
CD 23 is expressed by CLL and not by Mantle cell Lymphomas.
CLL cells are also negative for CD 79B and FM 7 and hence CLL is the answer of choice.

	CD5	CD9	CD23
Mantle cell Lymphoma	++	++	+-/+
CLL	++	++	++

Mantle cell Lymphoma also tend to express higher levels of CD79a and CD79b than CLL.

Chronic Myeloid Leukemia (CML) and CMML

211. Answer is C (Chronic myelogenous leukemia): Harrison 18th/ p915 *CMDT 2008/444; CMDT 2009/449; Harrisons 17th/684*

Peripheral blood picture with excessive number of granulocytes, basophills and eosinophils is characteristic of chronic myeloid leukemia (CML). CML is also often associated with an elevated platelet count (thrombocytosis) sometimes to strikingly very high levels. Chronic myelocytic leukemia is the single best answer of choice.

CML

Chronic myeloproliferative disorder from neoplastic transformation of a bone marrow stem cell that still retains capacity to differentiate along erythrocytic, megakaryocytic and granulocytic or monocytic lines.

Pripheral blood picture

- Striking Leucocytosis (Elevated WBC count)
Both immature and mature farms in different Stages of maturation may be seen But
Blood picture is dominated by Mature forms and precursor in the intermediate stages of differentiation
(Neutrophils, Metamyelocytes and Myelocytes)

Immature forms are less numerous
Blasts <5%
Promyelocytes <10%

(Cells are usually present in direct degree to the stage of maturation)

Basophills Eosinophils may be increased
- Elevated Basophils (often present)
- Elevated Eosinophils (less common)

- **Thrombocytosis**
Elevated platelet count if often present. Platelet count may be normal or sometimes elevated to strikingly high levels
- **Erythrocytes**
Red blood cell morphology is normal.
Patient is usually not anemic or only mildly anemic

Bone marrow

- Bone marrow is hypercellular with left shifted myelopoesis
- Myeloid: Erythroid ratio is increased
- Myeloblasts comprises less than 5% of marrow cells

Special Tests

- Cytogenetic Analysis for Philadelphia Chromosome
A small chromosome 22 caused by t (9; 22) translocation that results in bcr/abl fusion gene
- Reduced Leukocyte alkaline phosphatase levels (↓LAP)
This indicates that although the total number of granulocytes is increased they are functionally impaired
- Serum levels of vitamin B_{12} proteins is ↑ed binding.

212. Answer is B (t (9; 22): Harrison 18th/p 915 *CMDT 2008/444; CMDT 2009/449; Harrisons 17th/684; Refer previous question*

The patient in question is a case of chronic myeloid leukemia (CML)
And the characteristic cytogenetic abnormality in CML is the t (9; 22) translocation resulting in the Philadelphia chromosome
The diagnosis of CML is suggested by the characteristic laboratory feature (strikingly elevated WBC count with mature forms dominating the picture, associated basophilia and less that 5% blasts and promyelocytes) and supported by the clinical features (non specific symptoms of fatigue and weight loss along with heaviness in left hypochondrium suggesting massive splenomegaly which is characteristic of CML)

Cytogenetic Abnormality in CML

- CML is characterized by a reciprocal translocation between chromosome 9 and 22 t (9:22)
- This translocation results in the fusion of BCR gene on chromosome 22 with ABL gene (protoncogene) located on chromosome 9 forming the BCR-ABL fusion gene

The abl gene on chromosome 9 is translocated to bcr site on chromosome 22

- The bcr-abl gene is the hallmark of CML and may be detected in peripheral blood

Refer previous question for characteristic laboratory findings in CML

Clinical Presentation in CML

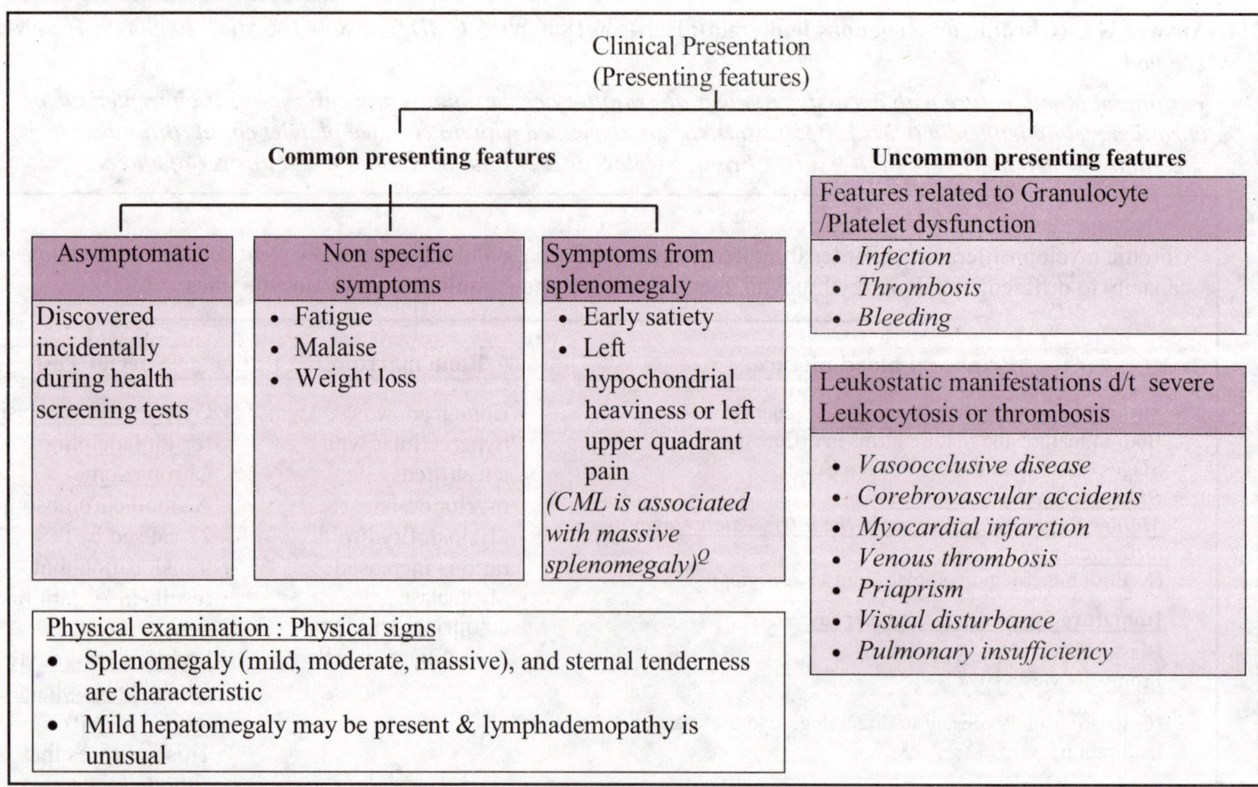

213. Answer is A and B (Accelerated phase and Blast crisis): Harrison 18th/p 915 *Refer text below; Harrison 17th/684; manual of Clinical Oncology 5th/504*

The natural history of CML is a triplastic process. Most patients present in a chronic phase and may progress to an accelerated phase or blast phase.

*'Evolution of accelerated or blast phase from the chronic phase is suggested by the **development of anemia,** thrombocytopenia, leukocytosis with immature myeloid cells or basophilia, **increasing splenomegaly** or recurrent contitutional symptoms while on therapy'. – Manual of Clinical Oncology 6th/504*

214. Answer is D (Persistant thrombocytosis > 1000 x 10^9/L positive to therapy): *Harrison 17th/ 684; API 7th/957*

Accelerated phase is associated with thrombocytopenia (<100 x 10^9/L) and not thrombocytosis.

Although multivariate analysis derived criteria also place blood or marrow basophils > 20% in disease criteria, other criteria do consider marrow and peripheral basophills > 10% as a criteria and hence option (D) is the single best answer here.

***Accelerated phase of CML*:** It is defined by the development of increasing degrees of anemia unaccounted for by bleeding or chemotherapy and is defined by several criteria.

Multivariate analysis derived criteria	Other commonly used criteria
Cytogenetic clonal evolution *Blood or marrow blasts between 10 and 20%* ***Blood or marrow basophills > 20%*** *Platelet count < 100 x 10^9/L unrelated to therapy*	*Splenemegaly unresponsive to therapy* Increasing drug dosage requirement Marrow reticulum or collagen fibrosis Marrow or peripheral blasts > 10% *Marrow or peripheral basophills ± eosinophills ≥ 10%* Triad of WBC > 50 x 10^9/L, hematocrit < 25% and *platelets < 100 x 10^9/L not controlled with therapy* Unexplained fever or bone pain

215. Answer is B (CML): Repeat

Leucocyte alkaline phosphatase is characteristically low in chronic myeloid leukemia.

Leucocyte Alkaline phosphatase is decreased in
• **CML** (chronic myeloid leukemia)
• **PNH** (Paroxysmal nocturnal hemoglobinuria)

216. Answer is A (Size of splenomegaly indicates prognosis): Harrison 18th/p 915 *Harrison16th/638;17th/683,684; Chandrasoma Taylor 3rd/ 420*

- ***Splenomegaly or size of enlarged spleen is used as a prognostic indicator in CML as part of the 'Sokal index'.***

Sokal index: Prognosis in CML – *Harrison 15th/ 712*
1. % of Circulating blasts
2. Spleen size
3. Platelet count
4. Age
5. Cytogenetic clonal evaluation

- In CML, the dominant cell lines in the peripheral blood and bone marrow are – myelocytes, metomyelocytes and granulocytes.

  The Philadelphia chromosome is present in all these cell lineages and *remains detectable even after remission of the CML – Chandrasoma Taylor 3rd/ 420.*
- Phagocytic functions are usually normal at time of diagnosis and remain normal during the chronic phase-*Harrison 15th/ 711*

Remember
• Q Leucocyte alkaline phosphatase is characteristically Low Q in CML.
• Q Serum levels of vit B_{12} and vit B_{12} binding proteins are ↑ed Q

- Myeloblastic cells are Sudan black positive.

217. Answer is C (Philadelphia chromosome is positive) : *Ghai 5th / 465*

Juvenile CML is mostly seen in children below 2 years of age. Philadelphia chromosome is negative and leukocyte count is less than 100'000/mm3. *– Ghai*

Features	Adult CML	Juvenile CML
• Age	- 10-12 years	- < 2 years
• Bleeding manifestation	- Absent	- Frequent
• ***Thrombocytopenia***	- Uncommon	- Frequent
• Rash	- Absent	- Frequent
• ***Lymphadenopathy***	- Rare	- Frequent
• Splenomegaly	- Marked	- Variable
• WBC count at diagnosis	- > 100'000	- < 100'000
• WBC type	- Granulocyte	- Monocyte
• Normoblastic	- Unusual	- Common
• ***HbF***	- Normal	- Increased
• Immunoglobulins	- Normal	- Increased
• Muramidase levels	- Normal	- Increased
• Response to Busulphan	- Good	- Poor
• Survival	- 2.5-3 years	- 9 months

218. Answer is A (Juvenile CML): *Ghai 6th/569; Other texts*

Fetal haemoglobin (HbF) values are elevated in most cases of juvenile CML – Ghai 6th/569

HbF is raised in following conditions

- *Juvenile CML*Q
- β thalossemiaQ
- Sickle cell anaemiaQ
- Heriditary persistence of fetal haemoglobin (HPFF)

219. Answer is B (Imatinib Mesylate Therapy): *Harrison's 18th/915*

Harrison's 18th edition recommends starting treatment of newly diagnosed CML with TK inhibitors (Imatinib) and reserving alloginic transplantation for those who develop Imatinib resistance.

'The therapy of CML is changing rapidly because we have a proven curative treatment (allogenic transplantation) that has significant toxicity and a new targeted treatment (imatinib) with outstanding outcome based on 8 year follow up data. We recommend starting with TK inhibitors (Imatinib) and reserving allogenic transplantation for those who develop imatinib resistance' -Harrison's 18th

Note:

- *The only curative treatment for CML is Allogenic stem cell Transplntation*
- *The treatment of choice in CML is Allogenic BMT*Q
- *The drug treatment of choice in CML is Imatinib*Q
- *Initial treatment recommended for newly diagnosed patient with CML is Imatinib.*

Treatment of CML

- The only curative treatment for CML is Allogenic Stem Cell Transplantation (SCT) (Allogenic bone marrow transplantation)Q
- The treatment of choice for CML is also Allogenic Stem Cell Transplantation (SCT) (Allogenic bone marrow transplantation)Q
- ***The drug treatment of choice for CML is Imatinib*** Q
- *Interferon alpha (IFN α) used to be the drug treatment of choice for CML when Imatinab was not available*

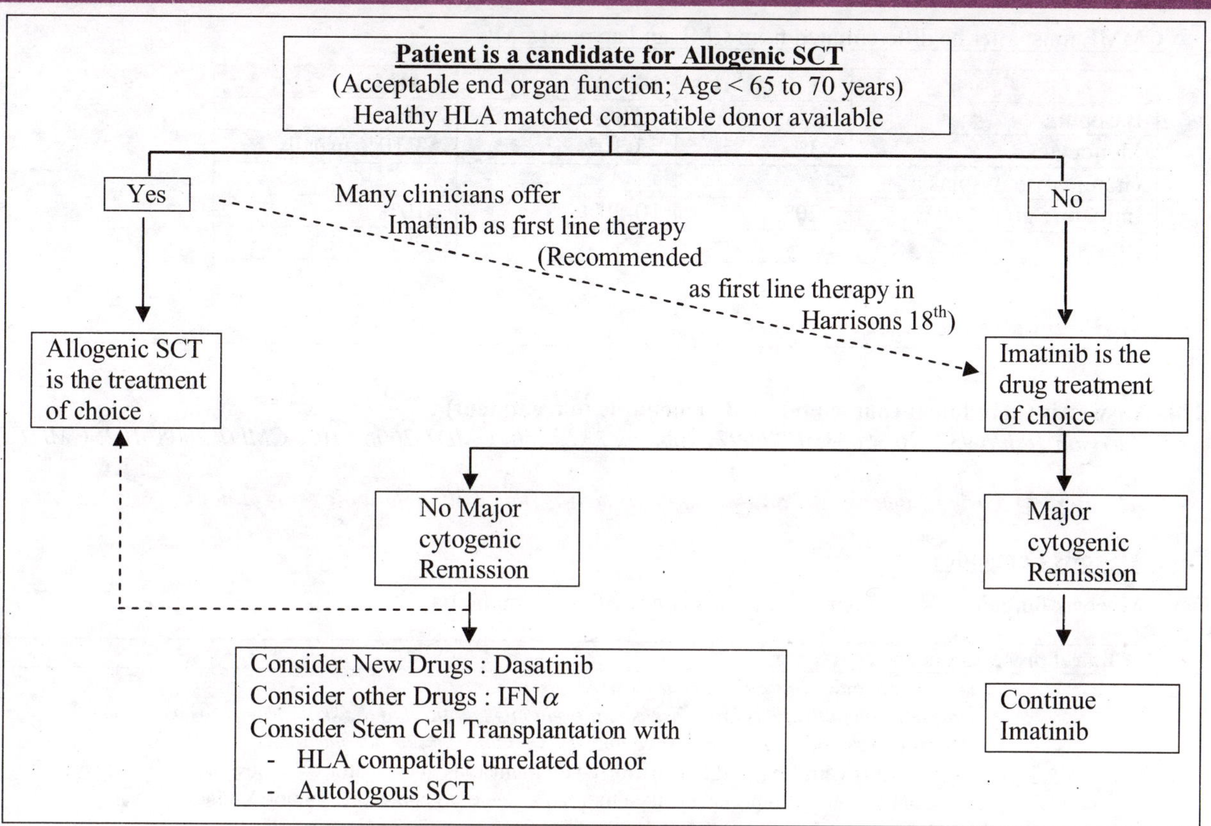

220. Answer is B (Imatinib): *Harrisons 17th; CMDT 2008/444; CMDT 2009/450*

Imatinib mesylate is the drug of choice for management of Chronic Myeloid Leukemia.

221. Ans. Answer is A (Imatinib): *Harrison 17th /685; Harrison's 18th/915*

The drug of choice for drug treatment of CML is Imatinib mesylate.

222. Answer is B (Allogenic BMT): Harrison 18th/p 915 *Harrisons 17th/685; CMDT 2008/444; CMDT 2009/450*

The only curative treatment for CML is Allogenic stem cell Transplntation

Note:

- *The treatment of choice in CML is Allogenic BMT*
- *The drug treatment of choice in CML is Imatinib*

223. Answer is C (More than 20% blasts in blood or bone marrow):
Wintrobe's atlas of clinical hematology 1st (2006) /133,134

Chronic myelomonocytic leukemia (CMML) is characterized by less than 20% blasts in peripheral blood or bone marrow.

Diagnostic Criteria for Chronic Myelomonocytic Leukemia according to WHO

- It is a chronic disorder (a variant of C.M.L)
- Middle aged and elderly males are usually affected
- ***Persistent peripheral blood monocytosis is >1×10⁹/L.***
- Absence of Philadelphia chromosome or BCR/ABL rearrangement
- ***Blasts are less than 20% in peripheral blood or bone marrow.***
- Dysplasia in one or more myeloid lineages, or ***in the absence of dysplsia, CMML can be diagnosed***, if all other criteria are met together with either of the following
  - Presence of clonal cytogenetic abnormality
  - Monocytosis has been persistent for at least 3 months and all other causes of monocytosis have been excluded.

CMML must after be differentiated from CML and atypical CML

	CGL (CML)	aCML	CMML
Basophils	>2%	<2%	<2%
Monocytes	<3%	>3-10%	>3-10% usually
Granulocyte dysplasia	-	++	+
Immature granulocytes	>20%	10-20%	<10%
Blasts	<2%	>2%	<2%

Mycosis Fungoides

224. Answer is C (Indolent course and easily amenable to treatment) :
Harrison 18th/p 932; 16th / 653; 17th/ 697; Robbins 7th / 1250; CMDT 2006 / 106; CMDT 2008/ 102; CMDT 2009/108

Although Mycosis fungoides has an indolent course it is not easily amenable to treatment.

Mycosis Fungoides

Mycosis fungoides is synonymous with Cutaneous T cell lymphoma.

Clinical presentation and course :

- Mycosis fungoides ***has an indolent course.***
  Most affected individuals have disease that remains localized to the skin for many years.
  It begins on the skin and may involve only the skin for years or decades
- Presentation is with localized or generalized erythematous / eczematous skin lesions.
  Skin lesion progress from 'patch' stage to 'plaque stage' to cutaneous 'tumors' stage.
- Metastasis occurs in advanced stages :

To lymph nodes	Peripheral circulation
	Sezary syndrome (Erythroderma and Circulating tumor cells) Seeding of the blood by melanoma cells is accompanied by diffuse erythema and scaling of the entire body surface (erythroderma).

Histology

Sezary - Lutzner cells	***Pautrier Microabscesses***
• Histological hall mark of Mycosis fungoides • These are T helper cell (CD4 positive)	Sezary - Lutzner cells characterstically form band like aggregates within the superficial dermis and invade the epidermis as single cells or small clusters called Pautrier's Microabscesses.

Treatment (Mycosis fungoides is not easily amenable to treatment)

- ***The treatment of Mycosis fungoides is complex. Even early and aggressive treatment has not been proved to cure or prevent progression of the disease.*** *-CMDT*
- *Cure has been possible with radiotherapy only in rare patients with early stage mycosis fungoides.*
- *Most of the treatment for mycosis fungoides are 'palliative'.*

Acute Leukemia

General Characteristics

225. Answer is A (CD 19) : *Robbins 7th/670; Blood by Handin Lux and Stossel 2nd/46*

CD 19 is a marker for B lymphocytes.

Markers for various lineage

Lymphoid lineage		Myeloid lineage
B Lineage	T Lineage	Myeloid Lineage
CD79a	*CD3 (m/cyt)*	*Anti-MPO (monoclonal)*
cyt IgM	*Anti-TCR α/β*	*MPO cytochemistry*
cyt CD22	*Anti-TCR γ/δ*	
CD19	*CD2*	*CD117*
CD10	*CD5*	*CD13*
CD20	*CD8*	*CD33*
	CD10	*CD65s*
		Anti-MPO (polyclonal)
	TdT	*CD14*
TdT	*CD7*	*CD15*
CD24	*CD1a*	*CD64*

226. Answer is A and B (CD2 and CD3): *Robbins 7th/670: Refer previous question; Medical Immunology 5th/179*

CD2 and CD3 are pan T cell markers.

Important Tcell markers

Pan Tcell markers	Subset Markers
Markers that are common to all cells of a given type	*Markers that are present only on a subset of population of cells in a given lineage*
Pan T cell markers include	Subset T cell markers include
CD2	*CD4*
CD3	*CD8*
CD5	
CD7	

Note that their specificity is not absolute because CD2 is also expressed by NK cells and CD3 by a special subpopulation of NK cells.

227. Answer is D (MPO): *Refer previous question*

MPO (myeloperoxidase) is a marker for myeloid lineage

Important Marker for Myeloid lineage
AntiMPO (monoclonal)
MPO cytochemistry
CD117
CD13
CD33
CD65s
Anti-MPO (polyclonal)
CD14
CD15
CD64

228. Answer is D (CD 45RO): *Harrison 15th/1808*

CD Marker	T cell
CD 45 RA	subset T, medullary thymocytes "naïve" T cells
CD 45 RB	All leukocytes
CD 45 RC	subset T, medullary thymocytes, "naïve" T cells
CD 45 RO	subset T, cortical thymocytes, **"memory"** T cells

229. Answer is D (t(9; 20): ALL): *Harrison 17th / 690; Chandrasoma Taylor 3rd /296; Robbins 7th /314*

Acute Lymphoblastic leukemia (ALL) may be associated with t(4;11), t(9;22) or t(8; 14) but association with t(9; 20) is not seen.

Type of Leukemia	Translocation	Deletion (-) / Trisomy (+)
Chronic myelocytic leukemia (CML)	t(9; 22)[1]Philadelphia chromosome	-
Acute Myoblastic Leukemia (AML)	t(8; 21), t(9;22)	+8, 7-, 5-, 7q, 5q-
Acute Monocytic Leukemia	t(9; 11), t(11; 23)	-
Acute Promyelocytic leukemia (M3)	t(15; 17)	
Acute lymphoblastic leukemia (ALL)	t(4; 11), t(9; 22), t(8; 14)	20q-
Chronic lymphocytic leukemia (CLL)	-	+12
Erythroleukemia	-	7q-, 5q-
Polycythemia Rubravera	-	20q-

Acute Lymphoid Leukemia (ALL)

Hematology

230. Answer is A (Pre-B cell ALL): Harrison 18th/p 919 *Harrisons 17th/687*

Pre B-cell ALL are the commonest types of Acute Lymphoplastic leukemias and account for upto 75% of all ALL

Classification of Acute Lymphoid Leukeia (ALL)

Immunologic Subtype	% of Cases	FAB Subtype	Cytogenetic Abnormalities
Pre-B ALL	75	L1, L2	t(9;22), t(4, 11), t(1; 19)
T Cell ALL	20	L1, L2	14q 11 or 7q34
BCell ALL	5	L3	t(8; 14), t(8; 22), t(2;8)

231. Answer is C (ALL): Harrison 18th/p 932 *Harrisons 17th/697; CMDT 2008/447; Robbins 7th/670; NMS Rediatrics 4th/533,534*

The presence of a mediastinal mass is a characteristic feature of 'T' cell ALL.

'Precursor T cell ALL is most often found in young men presenting with a large mediastinal mass' – Harrison

A young adolescent male presenting with a mediastinal mass is most often a precursor T cell ALL.

Characteristic Features of T cell ALL (20% of ALL)

- *Occurence in older children (adolescents) and adults*
- *Predilection for males*
- *Presence of anterior mediastinal mass in upto half of the cases at presentation (thymic mass)*
- *Early central nervous system involvement*
  (Early dissemination to meninges and testes)
- *High WBC count often greater than 100,000/mm^3*

232. Answer is B (An immature T cell phenotype-Tdt/CD34/CD7 positive): Harrison 18th/p 932 *CMDT 2009/452, 453 Harrisons 17th/697; Blood by Hadden & Stossel 1st/44*

The presence of a mediastinal mass in a young adolescent male suggests the diagnosis of precursor T cell ALL. Precursor T cell ALL is phenotypically characterized by an immature T cell phenotype and is positive for TDT and CD7 and may be positive for CD34.

The patient in question has a Tcell ALL (Precursor T cell ALL)

Patient is presenting with characteristic clinical features of T cell ALL

- *Occurance in an adolescent age group (17 year old)*
- *Occurance in a male (predilection for males)*
- *Presence of a mediastinal mass*
- *High WBC count > 100,000/mm3*

Presursor T cell ALL will show an immature T cell Phenotype and will be positive for CD7 and Td t

Immunophenotypic classification for ALL

FAB classification	Immunologic classification	Phenotype	Incidence (% cases)		Cytogenetic Abnormalities
Pre-B Cell	Early Pre-B	CD19, CD20-/+, CD10, CD34, TdT	55	75	t(9;22), t(4, 11), t(1; 19)
	Pre-B	CD19, CD20+/-, CD10, CD34-, cIgM, Tdt+/-	20		
B cell	B cell	CD19, CD20, CD22, CD10+/-, CD34-, Tdt-, sIg	5		14q 11 or 7q34
T cell	T cell	CD1, CD2, CD3, CD5, CD7, CD10+/-, CD34-/+, Tdt, dual CD4/CD8	20		t(8; 14), t(8; 22), t(2;8)

233. Answer is C (Pre B cell ALL): *Devita 6th/2240, 2237; Nelson 17th/1695; Ghai 6th/563; Harrison 16th ; Wintrobe's 11th/2145, 2142; Hoffman 4th/1159*

Hyperdiploidy, Female sex and translocation t (12, 21) are associated with good prognosis.
Pre B cell ALL may be associated with a poor prognosis and is the single answer of exclusion.

Hyperdiploidy Female sex and translocation t (12, 21) are associated with good prognosis.

Prognostic factor for ALL:

Determinants	**Favourable**	**Unfavrourable**
White blood cell count	Low WBC count*	High WBC count*
Age	***3-7 yrs***	***<1, > 10 yr***
Gender	Female	Male
Ethnicity	White	Black
Node, Liver, spleen enlargement	Absent	Massive
Testicular enlargement	***Absent***	***Present***
Central nervous system leukemia	Absent	Overt (blasts + pleocytosis)
FAB morphological features	L1	L2
Ploidy	Hyperdiploidy	Hypodiploidy < 45
DNA index	> 0.16	< 0.16
Cytogenenetic markers	Trisomies 4, 10 and/or 17 t(12;21) (tel aml 1)	t(9; 22) [bcr abl] t(4; 11) [mll af4] t(1; 19)
Time to remission	< 14 d	> 28 d
Minimal residual disease	$< 10^{-4}$	$> 10^{-3}$
Immunophenotype	Early Pre-B cell	T cell

Pre B cell ALL is often associated with an unfavourable prognosis (although it may be associated with a favourable outcome)

Pre B cell ALL has been associated with a poorer outcome compared to Early Pre B cell ALL. – *Wintrobe's*

Hematology

1

Hematology

Immunophenotype and Prognosis

Early Pre B cell ALL	Pre B cell ALL	Mature B cell ALL	T cell ALL
Early Pre B cell All comprises about 2/3 cases of childhood ALL and is associated with a favourable prognosis.	Pre B cell ALL account for 20% of childhood ALL and have ***been associated with a poorer outcome compared to Early Pre B cell ALL.***	Mature B cell ALL in uncommon in children and accounts for 1-2% of childhood ALL. It is characterized by L3 FAB morphology ***and has a poor prognosis.***	T cell ALL accounts for 15% of ALL in children T cell ALL was (previously) ***associated with a poor prognosis*** but *recent use of more intensive therapeutic regimen has resulted in survival approaching that of Non T cell ALL.*
Most Early Pre B cell ALL are CALLA positive. CALLA expression does not appear to have independent prognosis significance.			

234. Answer is C (Pre B cell ALL): *Devita 6th/2240, 2237; Nelson 17th/1695; Ghai 6th/563; Harrison 16th ; Wintrobe's 11th/2145, 2142; Hoffman 4th/1159*

Hyperdiploidy, Female sex and translocation t (12, 21) are associated with good prognosis.

Pre B cell ALL may be associated with a poor prognosis and is the single answer of exclusion.

Hyperdiploidy Female sex and translocation t (12, 21) are associated with good prognosis.

Prognostic factor for ALL:

Determinants	**Favourable**	**Unfavrourable**
White blood cell count	Low WBC count*	High WBC count*
Age	***3-7 yrs***	***<1, > 10 yr***
Gender	Female	Male
Ethnicity	White	Black
Node, Liver, spleen enlargement	Absent	Massive
Testicular enlargement	***Absent***	***Present***
Central nervous system leukemia	Absent	Overt (blasts + pleocytosis)
FAB morphological features	L1	L2
Ploidy	Hyperdiploidy	Hypodiploidy < 45
DNA index	> 0.16	< 0.16
Cytogenenetic markers	Trisomies 4, 10 and/or 17 t(12;21) (tel aml 1)	t(9; 22) [bcr abl] t(4; 11) [mll af4] t(1; 19)
Time to remission	< 14 d	> 28 d
Minimal residual disease	$< 10^{-4}$	$> 10^{-3}$
Immunophenotype	Early Pre-B cell	T cell

Pre B cell ALL is often associated with an unfavourable prognosis (although it may be associated with a favourable outcome)

Pre B cell ALL has been associated with a poorer outcome compared to Early Pre B cell ALL. – *Wintrobe's*

Immunophenotype and Prognosis

Early Pre B cell ALL	Pre B cell ALL	Mature B cell ALL	T cell ALL
Early Pre B cell All comprises about 2/3 cases of childhood ALL and is associated with a favourable prognosis. *Most Early Pre B cell ALL are CALLA positive. CALLA expression does not appear to have independent prognosis significance.*	Pre B cell ALL account for 20% of childhood ALL and have ***been associated with a poorer outcome compared to Early Pre B cell ALL.***	Mature B cell ALL in uncommon in children and accounts for 1-2% of childhood ALL. It is characterized by L3 FAB morphology ***and has a poor prognosis.***	T cell ALL accounts for 15% of ALL in children T cell ALL was (previously) ***associated with a poor prognosis*** but *recent use of more intensive therapeutic regimen has resulted in survival approaching that of Non T cell ALL.*

235. Answer is C (Testicular involvement): *Refer text below*

Testicular involvement / enlargement is a typical poor prognostic factor for childhood ALL

Age < 2 years versus Testicular Involvement

Typically Age < 1 year is considered a poor prognostic factor

Although Age < 2 year has been mentioned as a poor prognostic factor in certain textbooks including Hoffman's Hematology (4th/1158) most textbooks use the criteria of Age < 1 year to define a poor prognostic factor
Since testicular involvement provided amongst the option is an established poor prognostic factor, this is selected as the single best answer of choice.

236. Answer is D (Hyperdiploidy): *Hoffman 4th/1159; Wintrobe's 11th/2145, 2142*

Hyperdiploidy is associated with a good prognosis

Hyperdiploidy is associated with a good prognosis

Patients with hyperdiploidy (>50 chromosomes) or DNA index > 0.16 have a favourable prognosis – Hoffman's 4th/1158
Age < 2 years has a poor prognosis
Patients who are very young (< 2 years) and older patients (> 10 years) tend to have a worse prognosis-Hoffman's 4th/1158

Although most textbooks use the criteria of Age < 1 year to define a poor prognostic factor, Age < 2 year has been mentioned as a poor prognostic factor in certain textbooks including Hoffman's Hematology (4th/1158) ***Since Hyperdiploidy provided amongst the option is an established good prognostic factor, this is selected as the single best answer of choice.***

High WBC count is associated with a poor prognosis

Initial leukocyte count at diagnosis has proved to be an important prognostic factor in virtually every ALL study. Different studies (textbooks) quote different values for the initial WBC count that is associated with a poor prognosis but uniformly a high WBC count carries a poor prognosis.

Different text books	Favourable WBC count	Unfavourable WBC count
Wintrobe's Hematology	*< 10,000*	*> 20,000*
Hoffman Hematology	*< 50,000*	*> 50,000*
Manual of Clinical oncology	*<30,000*	*>30,000*
Inference	***Low WBC count***	***High WBC count***

Male sex is associated with a poor prognosis
'Female patients have a rare favourable prognosis' – Hoffman 4th/1158

237. Answer is C (ALL): *Ghai 6th/565*

L- Asparginase is particularly used in treatment of ALL

238. Answer is A (Intrathecal methotrexate): *Cancer Chemotherapy : Medicine outlinr series 2nd/167; Ghai 6th/564; Harrison 17th/1734*

Intrathecal Methotrexate is the chemotherapy of choice for intracranial manifestation of Acute Leukemia

Treatment of choice for intracranial ALL

Combination of intrathecal methotrexate and cranial irradiation.

Agents used for Intrathecal chemotherapy
Methotrexate
Cytarabine
Thiotepa

Note: Intrathecal Cytarabine may be as effective as intrathecal methotrexate

239. Answer is A (ALL): *Ghai 6th/564; Clinical Hematology and Oncology 1st (2003)/554, 560*

Preventive treatment or CNS prophylaxis against the possibility of later central nervous system involvement is routinely administered in both children and adults with Acute Lymphoblastic Leukemia (ALL).
The concept of CNS prophylaxis in ALL is based on the fact that most children with ALL have subclinical CNS involvement at the time of diagnosis. The meninges harbour occult leukemic cells and act as a sanctuary site where leukemia cells are protected from systemic chemotherapy because of blood brain barrier.

Note:
CNS Relapse is very uncommon in AML.

240. Answer is B (All – trans-retinoic acid): *Ghai 6th/565, 567*

All – trans- retinoic acid is used in the treatment of M3 subset (Acute Promyelocytic leukemia) of Acute Myeloid Leukemia (AML) and not in ALL

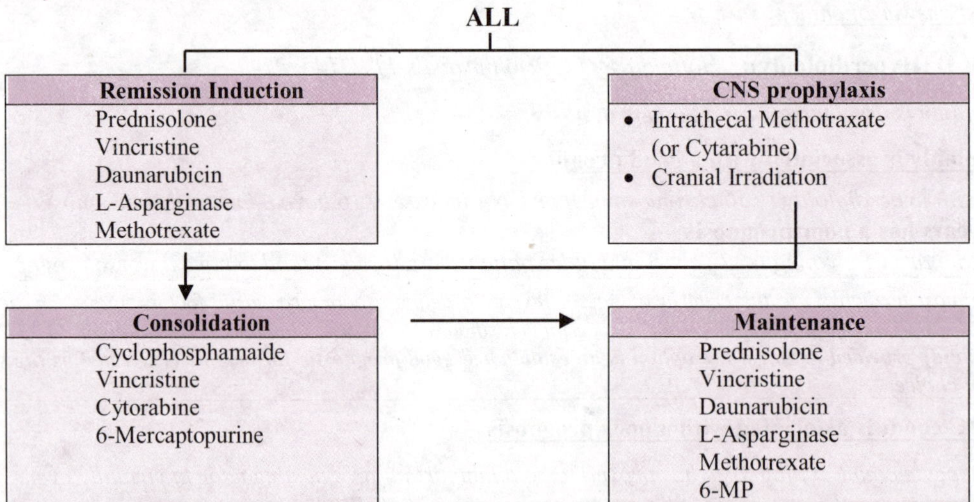

241. Answer is C (Acute lymphoblastic leukemia with hypereosinophilic syndrome): *Refer text below*

The immunophenotypic markers in the question are specific for lymphoid lineage alone and not for myeloid series.

Presence of immunophenotypic marker for myeloid lineage is essential before considering a diagnosis of biphenotypic leukemias, or Acute Eosinophilic leukemia (Eosinophils belong to the myeloid series) or Acute myeloid leukemia

The patient in question has positive markers for lymphoid series in isolation (CD19,CD10,CD20 and CD22) and hence the single answer by exclusion is Acute Lymphoblastic leukemia (lymphoid series) with hypereosinophilic syndrome.

Biphenotypic Acute Leukemia **Acute Eosinophilic leukemia** **Acute myeloid leukemia**	→	*Diagnosis requires immunophenotypic markers of Myeloid lineage The patent in question stained negative for MPO and NSE and shows no positive markers for Myeloid lineage and hence a diagnosis of these malignancies can be excluded.*

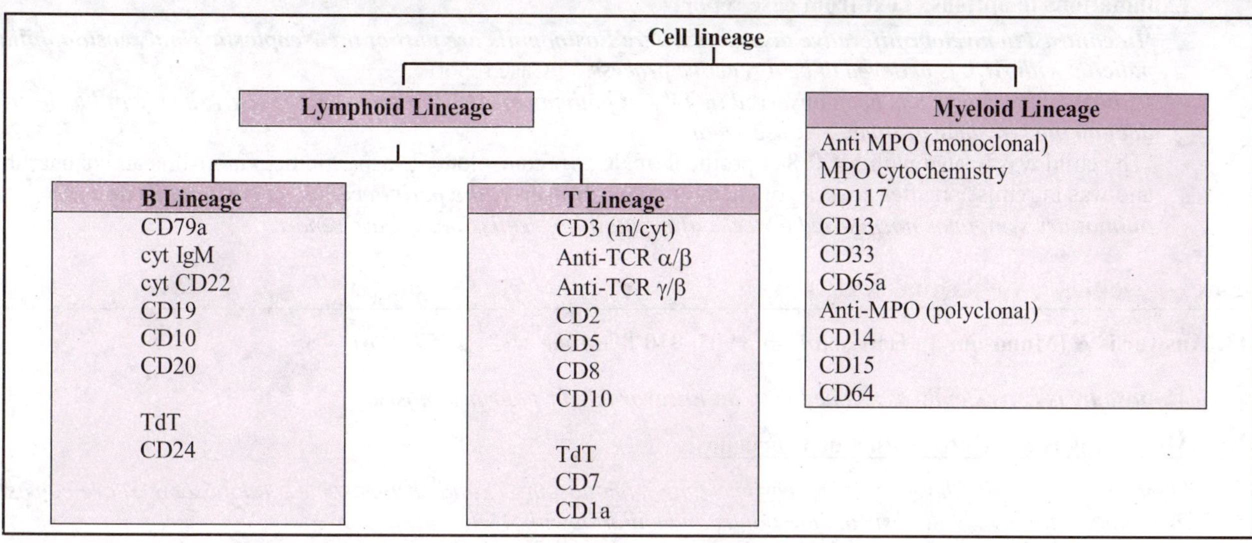

242. Answer is D (Inv (16) is often detected in the blasts and the eosinophils):

This is a case of ALL with hypereosinophillic syndrome. Inv (16) is associated with AML and not ALL, *and therefore represents the incorrect statement amongst the option.*

Wonder why such questions are set at all: This questions has been taken from a case report published in 'Annals jouranal of Haematology', authored by the faculty at AIIMS, who believed that 'the case represents the first report of the coexistance of granular ALL and hypereosinophillic syndrome'. It is difficult to understand what the faculty of the examination section at AIIMS expects out of undergraduates. Personally I believe that such questions are a mockery at the tremendous efforts each candidates puts up in preparation leading to the examinations.

Abstract Title: Granular acute lymphoblastic leukemia with hypereosinophilic syndrome.

Journal Source: Ann Hematol. 2000 May;79(5):272-4.

Authors: Jain P, Kumar R, Gujral S, Kumar A, Singh A, Jain Y, Dubey S, Anand M, Arya LS.

A four-year-old boy presented with marked peripheral blood eosinophilia (absolute eosinophil count of 54 x 10(9)/1), features of hypereosinophilic syndrome, and acute lymphoblastic leukemia (ALL-L2), the latter characterized by the presence of granular blasts. Blasts were negative for myeloperoxidase, non-specific esterase, acid phosphatase, periodic-acid Schiff stain, and toluidine blue. They exhibited an early pre-B immunophenotype (TdT, CD19, CD10, CD20 and CD22 positive) and stained negative for T (CD7, CD2, CD5 and CD3) and myeloid markers (MPO, CD33 and CD13). Chromosomal analysis revealed a normal karyotype. To the best of our knowledge, this case represents the first report of the coexistence of granular ALL and hypereosinophilic syndrome.

I do not have the permission to elaborate the entire case report, therefore, I shall be citing the relevant text, only, however, I do recommend each one of you to read the entire article as this question has also been asked in AIIMS/2004 with different options and may as well be twisted and repeated in future.

Why ALL

- Blasts were negative for myeloperoxidase and non specific esterase

Type	Myeloperoxidase	Sudan black
AML	–	–
ALL	+	+

- Presence of positive immunological markers CD 19, CD 20, CD 22 indicate a cell Lineage ALL

Immunological markers for Bcell Lineage ALL:	CD19, CD 20, CD 22, CD 79a, cCD 22, cCD 79a

Why Hypereosinophillic Syndrome: Option A Explanation

- Idiopathic hypereosinophillic syndrome is a rare condition characterized by extremely high levels of peripheral blood eosinophil counts. (80% of (70×10^9) Leucocytes were eosinophils in this patient)
- Clinical picture of dry cough, dyspnea, wheezing etc is further suggestive of HES.
- *This is differentiated from eosinophillic leukaemia by the* ***absence of eosinophilic blast cells.*** *(Text from case report: for option A)*

1

Hematology

Explanations to options: Text from case report

- ***'In contrast to myeloproliferative disorders where Eosinophils are part of the Neoplastic clone, eosinophilia in patients with ALL is believed to be a reactive process.'*** – Case report
- ***'A normal karyotype has been observed in 45% of patients of ALL/Eo and t (5:14) rearrangement has been documented in same of them.'*** – *Case report*
- 'The child was treated with MCP-841 protocol of NC2 (prednisolone, L-asparginine, vincristine and daunarubicin) and was in remission after 4 weeks of chemotherapy. ***However, the peripheral blood eosinophils and the pulmonary symptoms normalized 6 weeks after attaining remission.*** – *Case report.*

Acute Myeloblastic Leukemia (AML)

243. Answer is A (Monosomy) : Harrison 18th/p 905, 910 *Wintrobe's 12th/1859, 1861*

Monosomy is consistently associated with an unfavorable or poor prognosis.

Monosomy is associated with a poor prognosis

Monosomy especially those involving chromosome 7 (monosomy 7) and chromosome 5 (monosomy 5) are consistently associated with poor prognosis in both adults and children with AML

Deletion of X or Y chromosome is associated with a favorable / intermediate prognosis

'Monosomy of the X chromosome in a female patient (loss of the Y chromosome) is the most common whole chromosome loss identified in pediatric patients with AML. This numeric abnormality is usually associated with t(8; 21) translocation and AML M2 which carry a good prognosis' - 'Childhood Leukemias' by Puri 2nd/253

'Loss of Y and X chromosomes are most frequently observed in patients with t(8; 21) which carries a favourable prognosis' - 'Blood: Principles and Practice of Hematology' 2nd/108

Nucleophosphin mutation is associated with a favorable prognosis

Factor	*Favourable*	*Unfavourable*
Nucleophosphin mutation	Present	Absent

t (8; 21) translocation is associated with a favorable prognosis

Factor	*Favourable*	*Unfavourable*
Cytogenetics	t(15;17), ***t(8;21),*** inv(16)	-7, del(7q), -5, del(5q), 3q21 and 3q26 abnormalities, complex karyotypes

Prognostic Feature in Acute Myeloid Leukemia:

Factor	**Favourable**	**Unfavourable**
Clinical		
Age	*<45 yr*	*<2yr, >60yr*
ECOG performance status	*0-1*	*>1*
Leukemia	*De novo*	*Antecedent hematologic disorder, myelodysplasia, myeloproliferative disorder*
Infection	*Absent*	*Present*
Prior chemotherapy	*No*	*Yes*
Leukocytosis	*<25,000/mm3*	*>100,000/mm2*
Serum LDH	*Normal*	*Elevated*
Extramedullary disease	*Absent*	*Present*
CNS disease	*Absent*	*Present*
Cytoreduction	*Rapid*	*Delayed*
Morphology		
Auer rods	*Present*	*Absent*
Eosinophils	*Present*	*Absent*
Megaloblastic erythroids	*Absent*	*Present*
Dysplastic megakaryocytes	*Absent*	*Present*
FAB type	*M2, M3, M4*	*M0, M6, M7*

Surface/enzyme markers		
Myeloid	*CD34-, CD14-, CD13-*	*CD34+*
HLA-DR	*Negative*	*Positive*
TdT	*Absent*	*Present*
Lymphoid	*Cd2+*	*CD7+, CD56+* *Biphenotypic (2 or more lymphoid markers)*
MDR-1	*Absent*	*Present*
Cytogenetics		
Cytogenetics	*t(15;17), t(8;21), inv(16)*	*-7, del(7q), -5, del(5q), 3q21 and 3q26 abnormalities, complex karyotypes*
Molecular markers		
Fms-related tyrosine kinase-3 mutation	*Absent*	*Present*
Ecotropic viral integration site 1 expression	*Absent*	*Present*
Mixed-lineage leukemia partial tandem duplication	*Absent*	*Present*
Nucleophosphin mutation	*Present*	*Absent*
CCAAT/enhancer-binding protein-α mutation	*Present*	*Absent*
Brain and acute leukemia cytoplasmic gene expression	*Absent*	*Present*
Vascular endothelial growth factor expression	*Absent*	*Present*

244. Answer is B (M3): *Surgical Pathology of Head & Neck (volume 2) by Barnes (CRC Press) 2001/1343*

Auer Rods are most frequently seen in AML – M3 (FAB).

Auer Rods and Acute Myeloid Leukemia (AML)

Auer Rods are crystalline, refractile, azurophilic rod shaped structures made from alignment of granules that are typically seen in AML (may be seen in refractory anemia with excess blasts in transformation)

- *Auer Rods are most frequently seen in AML-M3 (95-100%) and AML-M2 (70%)*[Q]
- *Auer Rods are absent by definition in AML-M0*[Q]
- *Auer Rods are usually not seen in AML-M5a and AML-7*[Q]
- *Auer Rods may be seen in other subtypes of AML in < 30-50% of cases*

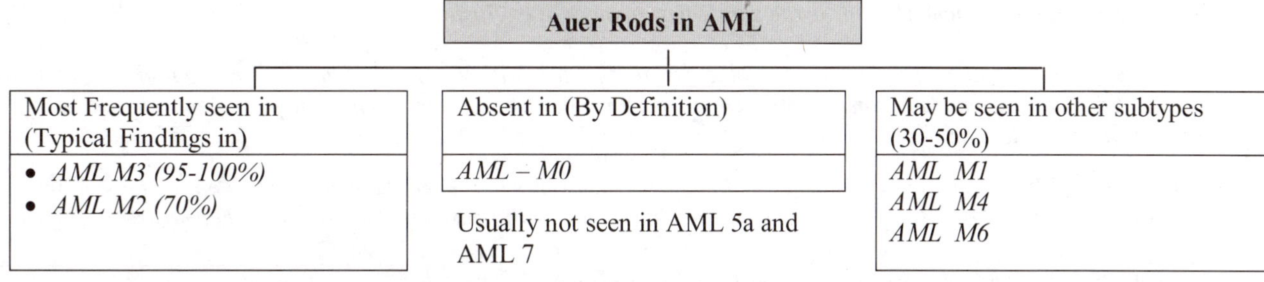

245. Answer is A (AML – M0): *Surgical pathology of Head & Neck (2001)/1343*

Auer Rods by definition are absent in AML-M0.

'Auer Rods by definition are absent in AML-M0 and usually not seen in AML-M5a and AML-M7. Auer rods are most often present in AML-M3 (95-100%) and AML-M2 (70%) and are seen in 30-50% of the other subtypes'

- Surgical Pathology of Head & Neck

246. Answer is D (Presence of t 8 : 21): *Harrisons 16th/634; Harrison 17th/677,678,680; CMDT 2008/448; CMDT 2009/453*

Patients with t (8, 21), t (15 : 17) or inv (16) have extremely good prognosis

The single most important prognosis factor is attainment of complete remission. [Q]

The Likelihood of entering complete remission and hence the prognosis is determined by the following factors :

Age of Diagnosis :

- ***> 60 years has a poor prognosis***
- Chronic intercurrent ***disease***, acute medical problems with increasing age are associated with poor prognosis.

Chromosome findings :

Prognosis	Chromosome Findings
Good	t (8 : 21), t (15 : 17), inv (16)
Moderate	No cytogenetic abnormality
Poor	Monosomy 5 and 7, Complex karyotype, Inv(3)

Presenting Leucocyte count :

- A high presenting Leucocyte count is an independent prognostic factor
- Duration of CR is inversely related to presenting Leucocyte count

  Among patients with ***hyperleucocytosis (>100,000/μg)*** early central nervous system bleeding and pulmonary leukostasis and Late relapse contribute to poor outcome.

Prolonged symptomatic interval with cytopenias - Antecedent hematological disorder

- Poor prognosis is seen in patients with anemia, Leukopenia, thrombocytopenia for duration of more than 1 month before diagnosis.
- Poor prognosis is seen in patients with **secondary Leukemias** developing after treatment with cytotoxic agents / irradiation.

Other Prognostic features :

- FAB classification
- Characteristics of Leukaemic cells : e.g. *Auer Rods* [Q] *- poor prognosis*
- Expression of *MDRI Gene* [Q] *- poor prognosis*

247. Answer is D (Immediately start induction chemotherapy): *Harrison's Manual of Oncology 1st/207; 'Treatment of Acute Leukemia' br Pei 1st/259; 'Hematology-Oncology Therapy' 1st/220*

Immediate treatment of Hyperleukocytosis is leukocytoreduction which is generally achieved by Leukopharesis or administration of Hydroxyurea.
Induction chemotherapy is initiated early in treatment after attempts at leukocytoreduction but not immediately.

Immediate induction chemotherapy is the single best answer of exclusion.

Immediate Administration of induction chemotherapy to a patient with hyperleukocytosis carries a high risk of Acute tumor lysis syndrome and hence induction chemotherapy is often not initiated immediately but generally follows attempts at cytoreduction.

IV hydration, Allopurinol and alkalinization of urine are measures to reduce the metabolic complications of tumor lysis syndrome and are indicated as preventive measures in patients with Leukostasis and hyperleukocytosis.

Hyperleukocytosis and Leukostasis (Independent poor prognostic factor in acute leukemia)

- Hyperleucocytosis is a condition in which patients with acute leukemia present with an extraordinary high leukocyte count usually greater than 100,000.

  The high number of circulating blasts increase the blood viscocity and predispose to the development of Leukostasis.
- Leukostasis refers to sludging of leukemia blasts in the microcirculation leading to obstruction of small vessels especially in the cerebral and pulmonary circulations.
- Once identified leukostasis requires immediate and effective treatment to lower the blast count rapidly.

Treatment of Hyperleukocytosis

Immediate Cytoreduction /Leukoreduction	Initiation of Induction Chemotherapy	Supportive / Preventive of Complications
Leukostasis requires immediate and effective treatment to lower the blast count. This may be achieved by Leukopharesis Hydroxyurea	• Initiation of chemotherapy is also critical for the treatment of Leukostasis since blasts removed from circulation by cytoreduction are rapidly replaced by blasts from bone marrow. However *Induction chemotherapy is not initiated 'immediately' but generally follows attempts at cytoreduction.* *Early chemotherapy is advised but not necessarily 'immediate' chemotherapy.*	• IV hydration • Allopurinol • Alkalinization of urine } To prevent complication of tumor lysis syndrome *Initiation of induction chemotherapy carries the risk of Acute Tumor lysis syndrome and hence these supportive measures are instituted.*

248. Answer is D (Monosomy 7): *Harrisons 16th /634; CMDT 2006/509; CMDT 2009/453; Hematology by Hoffman 4th/1128*

Monosomy 7 is associated with a very poor prognosis. Patients with t (8, 21), t (15; 17) and inv (16) have a good prognosis.

Cytogenic studies are most powerful prognostic factors (CMDT)

Good Prognosis	Moderately favourable prognosis	Poor prognosis
• t(8:21) • Inv (16) (p13, q22) • t(15; 17)	• No cytogenic abnormality	• Complex karyotype • Monosomy 7 (-7) • Monosomy 5 • Del 5q • 3q rearrangement • Inv. (3) • FLT3 internal tandem duplication

249. Answer is D (Monosomy 7) : Harrison 18th/p 910 *Harrison 16th /634; Harrison 17th/680; CMDT 2008/448; CMDT 2009/453; Repeat*

***Patient with a complex karyotype, inv (3), or -7 (monosomy) have a poor prognosis.* - Harrison**

250. Answer is C (CD15 / 34 both seen in same cell) : Harrison 18th/p 905, 906, 912 *Harrison 16th /632-634; Harrison 17th/ 678, 682; Robbins 7th /693; CMDT 2006/508-509; Ghai 6th / 567; CMDT 2008/446*

CD15 and CD34 are not associated with Acute Promyelocytic leukemia.

Acute promyelocytic Leukaemia (PML : FAB M3)
• This is a type of Acute Myeloid Leukaemia (AML) and has been classified as the M3 category according to the FAB morphological classification.[Q] • It constitutes 5 – 10% of all AML (Robbin's / Ghai)
Pathological characteristic of PML
• It is ***characterized by the chromosomal translocation t(15;17)***[Q] *– CMDT* • ***t(15;17) translocation*** produces a fusion gene (PML-RAR)involving the Retinoic Acid Receptor gene and Promyelocytic Leukemia (PML) gene. This PML – RaR fusion protein tends to suppress gene transcription and blocks differentiation of cells. ***This block can be overcome with pharmacological doses of retinoic acid*** (Harrison). • *Most cells are hypergranular*[Q] promyelocytes often with many Auer rods per cell.

Presentation characteristic / Specific features of PML
• Patients of PML are younger (median age 35 – 40 years) – Robbin's • ***Incidence of Disseminated Intravascular Coagulation (DIVC) is*** high in patient with PML. *–Robbin's DIC may occur with any subgroup of AML but is especially common in acute PML (M3)*–Ghai
Treatment specific to PML subject
All-Trans Retinoic Acid (ATRA/Tretinoin) • ***The treatment of patient with PML has been dramatically improved by the use of All – Trans – Retinoic acid.*** *This agent is an analog of vitamin A that leads to terminal differentiation of occult promyelocytic leukemia cells. - CMDT* • *Remission in PML is induced by All – Trans-Retinoic acid as a single agent –Ghai* Arsenic Trioxide Arsenic Trioxide produces meaningful response in upto 85% of patients refractory to tretinoin

1

251. Answer is C (Promyelocytic Leukemia): Harrison 18th/p 907 *Hematology by Hoffman 4th/1087; Harrisons 17th/679: Appendix A2*

Acute promyelocytic Leukemia (APL) characteristically presents with Thrombocytopenia, prolonged PT, Prolonged PTT, hypofibrinogenemia and increased levels of fibrin degradation product as it is associated with a high incidence of DIC.

The patient in question is presenting with an elevated PT, elevated PTT, Thrombocytopenia (platelets 35,000) and decreased fibrinogen levels (Normal fibrinogen levels = 233-496 mg/dl) All these features are characteristic of DIC which is a common mode of presentation in APL. APL is the single best answer of choice.

Characteristic presentation of APL

- Patients are typically younger than other subtypes of AML
- Patients typically present with bleeding tendencies and/or DIC (as DIC is common in APL)

Features of DIC
Thrombocytopenia *Prolonged prothrombin time (PT)* *Prolonged Partial Thromboplastin Time (PTT)* *Increased Fibrin Degradation products (N=0-1 ug/ml)* *Decreased Fibrinogen levels (N=233-496 mg/dl)*

Hematology

252. Answer is A (Acute promyelocytic leukemia): Harrison 18th/p912, 913 *Harrisons 16th/636; 17th/682; CMDT 2008/448; CMDT 2009/453*

Arsenic trioxide has been approved for the treatment of relapsed disease in Acute promyelocytic leukemia (PML).
– CMDT

Treatment of Acute Promyelocytic Leukemia (M3-FAB-AML)

Acute promyelocytic leukemia is treated differently from all other subtypes of AML and has become the most curable type of AML of adults.

Treatment Agents

Chemotherapy	All-Trans Retinoic Acid (ATRA) (Vitamin A/Tretinoin)	Arsenic Trioxide
Standard chemotherapy especially Anthracycline antibiotics	• ATRA has revolutionized the treatment of PML • ATRA is capable of inducing Complete Remission as a Single agent in PML • ATRA is part of induction therapy in PML (along with an anthracycline antibiotic for chemotherapy)	• ***Arsenic trioxide has been approved for the treatment of relapsed disease in APL*** • *Arsenic trioxide can provide meaningful response in upto 85% of patients refractory to tretinoin*

Biphenotypic Leukemia

253. Answer is A (Biphenotypic leukemia): *Principles and Practice of Pediatric Oncology 5th/172 Wintrobe's 11th/2108 Blood by Hadden Lux and Stossel 1st/492*

Biphenotypic leukemias are leukemias that express features of more than one lineage. The patient in question has a rare leukemia that expresses both, myeloid antigens (CD 33 and CD 13) and Lymphoid antigens of B cell lineage (CD 10 and CD 19) and hence can be described as a Biphenotypic leukemia.

Biphenotypic Leukemias

- Biphenotypic Leukemias are rare acute leukemias that express both myeloid and lymphoid associated antigens to a degree that no single lineage can be assigned.
- Scoring systems have been proposed to more precisely defines biphenotypic leukemias and to distinguish these cases from 'ALL with myeloid antigen expression' or 'AML with lymphoid antigen expression'

Scoring System for Biphenotypic Acute Leukemia

Points	B Lineage	T Lineage	Myeloid Lineage
2	CD79a Cyt IgM Cyt CD22	CD3 (m/cyt) Anti-TCR α/β Anti-TCR γ/δ	Anti-MPO (monoclonal) MPO cytochemistry
1	CD19 CD10 CD20	CD2 CD5 CD8 CD10	CD117 CD13 CD33 CD65s Anti-MPO (polyclonal)
0.5	TdT CD24	TdT CD7 CD1a	CD14 CD15 CD64

M, membrane; cyt, cytoplasm; MPO, myeloperoxidase
A diagnosis of biphenotypic acute leukemia requires a score of more than 2 points for the myeloid and one of the lymphoid lineages.

The patient in question scores two points for myeloid lineage and two points for lymphoid B cell lineage and hence can be classified as a Biphenotypic Leukemia

Plasma Cell Disorders / Multiple Myeloma

254. Answer is D (Dystrophic classification): Harrison 18th/p 938, 939; *16th/ 657, 658, 659; Harrison 17th/ 702, 703*

Multiple myeloma is associated with hypercalcemia and as a result metastatic calcification may occur. Dystrophic calcification is not a feature.

Pathogenetic evolution of other symptoms can be understood from the following chart:

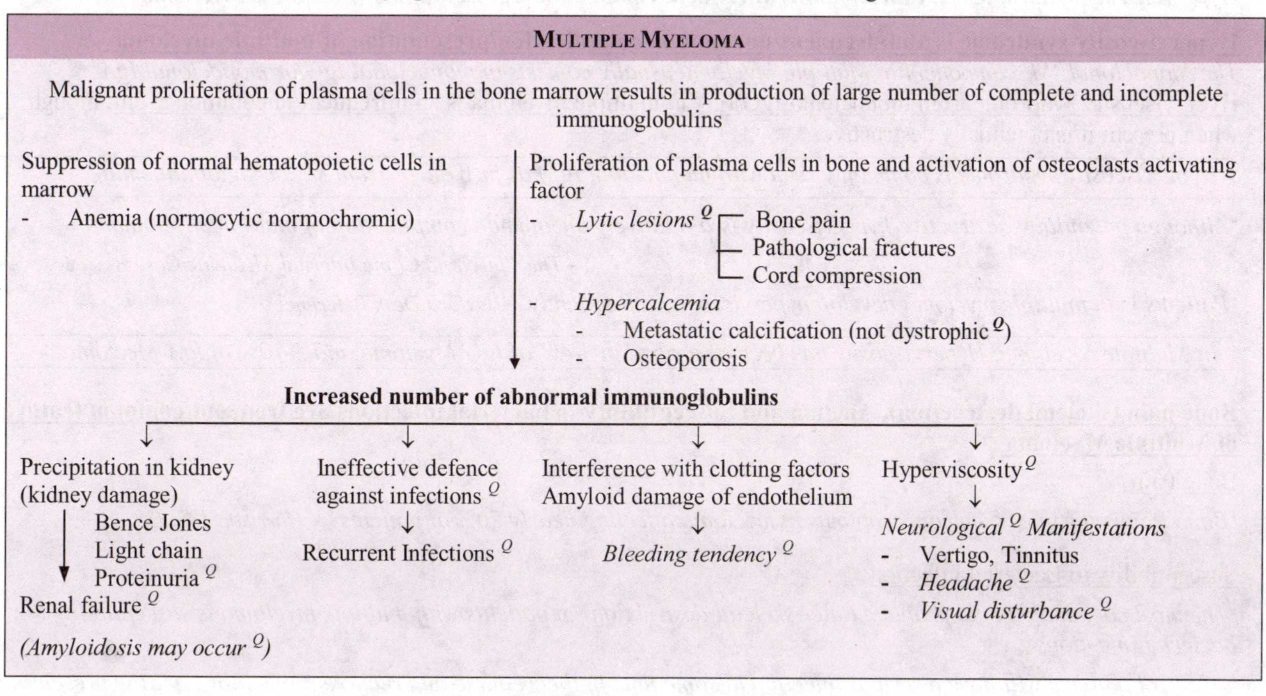

255. Answer is D (Dystrophic calcification): *Text below*

Multiple myeloma may be associated with metastatic calcification (not dystrophic calcification).

Multiple myeloma is associated with hypercalcemia and as a result metastatic calcification may occur. Dystrophic calcification is not a feature.

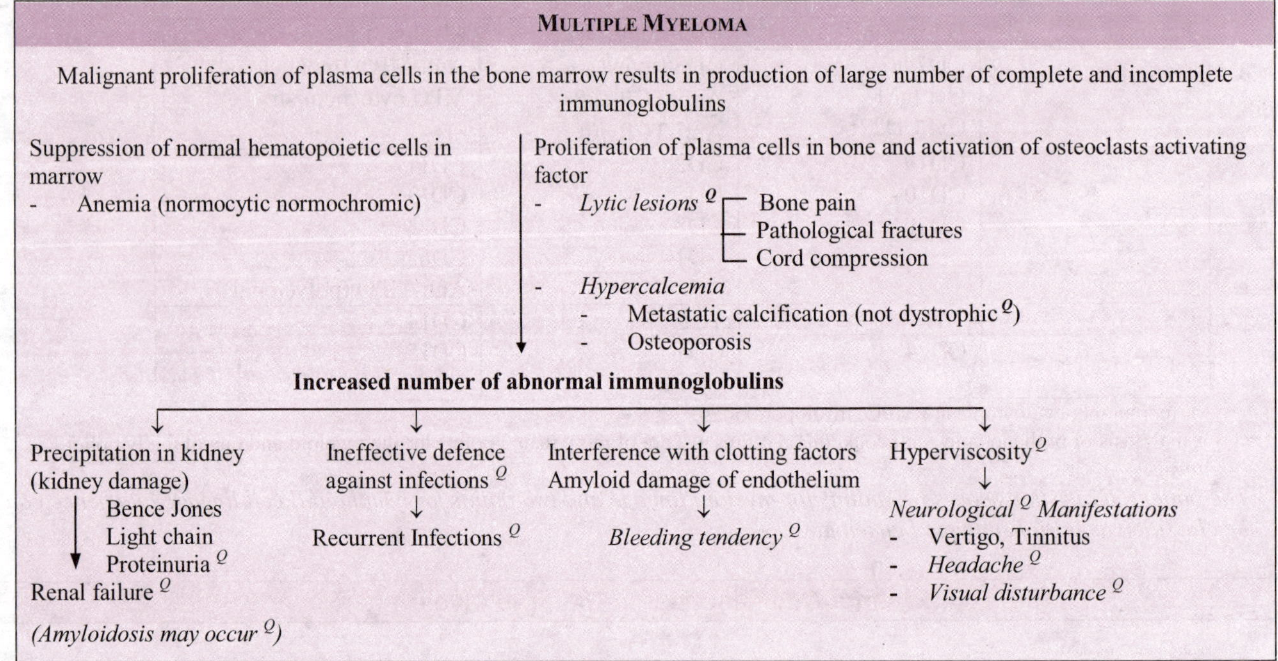

256. Answer is D (Hyperviscosity syndrome): *Harrison 18th/938, 939; 'The Cleveland Clinical Internal Medicine Case Reviews' (Lippincott Williams) 2003/page 141 (MCQ); Oxford Desk Reference: Oncology (2011)/509*

Hyperviscosity syndrome is an uncommon /infrequent complication/presentation of Multiple myeloma.

Hyperviscosity syndrome is an infrequent/uncommon complication/presentation of multiple myeloma

The Monoclonal 'M' component in Multiple Myeloma usually consists of monoclonal IgG or monoclonal IgA. Hyperviscosity syndrome from monoclonal IgG/IgA in multiple myeloma is an infrequent/uncommon event, though when present it is potentially destructive.

Hyperviscosity syndrome is commonly seen with monoclonal IgM as in Waldenstrom's Macroglobulinemia

'Although potentially destructive hyperviscosity is a relatively uncommon complication of multiple myeloma'

– The Cleveland Clinic Internal Medicine Case Review

'Patients with multiple myeloma develop hyperviscosity infrequently' – Oxford Desk Reference

In Multiple Myeloma, Hyperviscosity has been described in 3-4% of IgG Myeloma and 5-10% of IgA Myeloma.

Bone pain (skeletal destruction), Anemia and Susceptibility to bacterial infections are frequent/common features of Multiple Myeloma

Bone Pain

'Bone Painis the most common symptoms in myeloma affecting nearly 70% of patients' – Harrison 18th/938

Susceptibility to Bacterial Infection

'The most common clinical problem (after skeletal destruction) in patients with multiple myeloma is susceptibility to bacterial infections'

'>75% of patients will have a serious infection at some time in their course and recurrent infections are the presenting feature in approximately 25% of patients.' – Harrison 18th/938

Anemia

'Normocytic Normochromic anemia is present in approximately 80% of myeloma patients' – Harrison 18th/939

Clinical Feature of M. Myeloma	Approximate frequency
Bone pain/skeletal Destruction	~ 70% (***Most common presenting feature***)
Recurrent bacterial Infection	~> 25% (*Presenting feature in > 25%*)
Renal failure	~> 25% (*Renal Failure occurs in ~ 25% of MM patients*)
Hypercalcemia	~ 25% (*About 25% of patients develop Hypercalcemia at some stage of disease. It is the most common cause of Renal failure in MM patient*)
Anemia (Normocytic Normochromic)	~ 80% (*Normocytic Normochromic anemia occurs in approx. 80% of patients.* It is usually not a presenting feature.)

257. Answer is A (Lytic bone lesions): *'Blood' by Handin 2nd/890; Hematology in Clinical Practice 4th/306*

Multiple Myeloma is now widely defined in accordance with the Durie and Salmon diagnostic criteria .The diagnostic criteria are divided into major and minor criteria. ***Lytic bone lesions constitute minor criteria in accordance with the classification system. All other options are part of the major criteria that define multiple myeloma.***

Diagnosis and Staging of Multiple Myeloma (The Durie and Salmon myeloma diagnostic criteria)

- The Durie and Salmon myeloma diagnostic criteria are used widely in the United States and have been validated by large multicenter trials.
- The diagnostic criteria are divided into major and minor.
  The diagnosis of Multiple Myeloma requires a minimum of one major and one minor criterion or three minor criteria as defined in the table below
- Once the diagnostic criteria for multiple myeloma are met, Durie-Salmon clinical staging can be used to determine the stage of disease.

Criteria for Diagnosis of Multiple Myeloma

Major criteria

1. *Plasmacytomas on tissue biopsy*
2. *Bone marrow plasmacytosis (> 30% plasma cells)*
3. *Monoclonal immunoglobulin spike (M spike) on serum electrophoresis:*
   IgG > 3.5 g/dl or
   IgA > 2.0 g/dl
   κ or λ light-chain excretion > 1.0 g/d on 24-h urine protein electrophoresis.

Minor criteria

a. *Bone marrow plasmacytosis (10-30% plasma cells)*
b. *Monoclonal immunoglobulin spike present but of lesser magnitude than in 3*
c. *Lytic bone lesions*
d. *Normal IgM <50mg/dl or*
   Normal IgA <100 mg/dl or
   Normal IgG <600 mg/dl.

Any of the following sets of criteria will confirm the diagnosis.

Any two major criteria
Major criterion 1 plus minor criterion b, c or d
Major criterion 3 plus minor criterion a or c
Minor criteria a, b and c or a, b and d

258. Answer is C (Plasmacytoma on Tissue Biopsy): *'Blood' by Handin 2nd/890; Hematology in Clinical Practice 4th/306*

Plasmacytoma on tissue biopsy is a major criterion for diagnosis of Multiple Myeloma and not a minor criterion.

Criteria for Diagnosis of Multiple Myeloma

Major criteria

1. *Plasmacytomas on tissue biopsy*
2. *Bone marrow plasmacytosis (> 30% plasma cells)*
3. *Monoclonal immunoglobulin spike (M spike) on serum electrophoresis:*
   IgG > 3.5 g/dl or
   IgA > 2.0 g/dl
   κ or λ light-chain excretion > 1.0 g/d on 24-h urine protein electrophoresis.

Minor criteria
a. *Bone marrow plasmacytosis (10-30% plasma cells)*
b. *Monoclonal immunoglobulin spike present but of lesser magnitude than in 3*
c. *Lytic bone lesions*
d. *Normal IgM <50mg/dl or*
Normal IgA <100 mg/dl or
Normal IgG <600 mg/dl.
Any of the following sets of criteria will confirm the diagnosis.
Any two major criteria
Major criterion 1 plus minor criterion b, c or d
Major criterion 3 plus minor criterion a or c
Minor criteria a, b and c or a, b and d

259. Answer is C (Plasmacytoma on tissue biopsy): *Refer Previous Question; William's Hematology 7th/1507*

Plasmacytoma or tissue biopsy is a major criterion for diagnosis of multiple myeloma (and not a minor criterion)

260. Answer is C (Plasmocytosis > 2%): *Harrison 18th / 940; 15th/ 730; Harrison 16th/ 659; Harrison 17th/ 703, 704*

Diagnosis of Multiple Myeloma requires plasmacytosis of > 10%.

The classic triad of myeloma is:
a) *Marrow plasmacytosis > 10%*
b) *Lytic bone lesions*
c) *Serum or urine 'M' component*

261. Answer is B (t (8-14) translocation): Harrison 18th/p 938 *Harrison 15th/ 729, 16th/ 657; Harrison 17th/ 702, 703*

- A variety of chromosomal alterations have been found in patients with Multiple myeloma. The most common translocation is t (11; 14) (q 13; q32). 13q14 deletions and 17p13 deletions and 11q abnormalities predominate. ***Translocation t(8-14) has not been mentioned.***
- Complete Immunoglobulin chain comprises of both heavy chains and light chains. But ***in Multiple myeloma there is excess production of light chains*** Q over heavy chains.
  These light chains are eliminated in urine as Bence Jones protein. Q
  Protein cast in urine are thus made up of light chains only Q (not complete immunoglobulin chains).
- ***'Bone lesions in multiple myeloma are lytic in nature*** and are rarely associated with osteoblastic new bone formation.' – *Harrison.*
  Bone lesions in MM are caused by the proliferation of tumor cells and activation of osteoclasts that destroy the bone.
  'Bone pain is the most common symptom in MM affecting 70% of patients Q*' - Harrison*

262. Answer is D (Protein casts in urine are made up of complete Ig chains): *Harrison 16th/657, 658, 659; 17th/ 703, 704*

Protein casts in urine are made up of light chains only and not complete I g chains.

- Complete lg chain comprises of both heavy chain & light chain.
  In Multiple myeloma there is ***excess production of light chains*** *over heavy chains. These light chains are eliminated in urine as* ***Bence Jones Protein.***
- Multiple myeloma represents a clonal proliferation of plasma cells derived from a single clone.
  - Thus there is an elevation of only one chain of immunoglobulins which forms the 'M' component with a reciprocal depression of other classes of immuno globulins.
  - The M component is most commonly formed by IgG.
  - Serum protein electrophoresis thus shows a monoclonal spike corresponding the this M component.
- It is rare under age of 40 and the median age at diagnosis in 68 years.
- Amyloid glomerulopathy may occur – Harrisons.

263. Answer is A (Vertebral column): *Robbins 6th/ 664; 7th/679*

The commonest site of involvement in multiple myeloma is vertebral column.

<u>Although any bone may be involved, the following order of involvement is most often seen.</u>

Vertebral column (66%) > Ribs (44%) > Skull(41%) > pelvis (28%) > femur (24%) > clavicle(10%) > scapula(10%)

264. Answer is D (Renal failure): Harrison 18th/p 938, 939 *Harrison 17th/703, 702, 704*

Renal failure occurs in nearly 25% of Myeloma patients and some renal pathology is noted in over half. *–Harrison 17th/703*

<u>Multiple Myeloma is associated with Lytic bone lesion and Bone Resorption</u>
The bone lesions of Myeloma are caused by activation of osteoclasts that destroy bone and suppression of osteoblasts that form bone.
Bone lesions are thus lytic in nature and not sclerotic.
There is a net resorption of bone and not bone deposition.

<u>Multiple Myeloma is associated with Hypercalcemia and not Hypocalcemia</u>
Hypercalcemia is caused by substantial mobilization of calcium from bone due to associated bony lysis.

265. Answer is C (Bone scan) : Harrison 18th/p 940, 941 *Harrison 16th / 658, 659; Harrison 17th/ 703, 704, 705; Other references*

Bone scans are least useful for diagnosis of Multiple Myeloma. Cytokines secreted by myeloma cells suppress osteoblastic activity therefore typically no increased uptake is observed.

In multiple myeloma the osteoblastic response to bone destruction is negligible. The bone scan therefore is often normal or may show areas of decreased uptake (photopenia).It has been found to be less useful in diagnosis than plain radiography.

Diagnosis of Multiple Myeloma (*Harrison 16th & Others)*

Serum Markers	**Urine examination**	**Skeletal survey**	**Bone marrow aspire biopsy**
▪ **Full blood count / Differential count** -Anemia [Q] ▪ **Biochemical profile :** –↑ serum calcium –↑ urea / creatinine –↑ uric acid ▪ **Albumin / Globulin Ratio** : Reversed ▪ ***ESR : Elevated*** ▪ **Quantitative Ig levels (IgG, IgA, IgM)** -Elevated Myeloma protein -Supressed non myelomatous Ig ▪ **Serum Protein electrophoresis** -Characteristic M spike ▪ **Serum Alkaline Phosphatase***: Normal* ▪ **β2 microglobulin** *:* *Most important predictor of outcome.* ▪ **C – Reactive protein & IL6 levels** : *-CRP is useful as a prognostic marker* -CRP is surrogate marker of IL6 activity (IL6 is often referred to as plasma cell growth factor)	<u>**24 hour urine**</u> <u>**specimen**</u> to <u>quantitate</u> <u>protein excretion</u> (> 1g protein /24 hour is a major ciriteria for diagnosis <u>**Urine protein**</u> <u>**electrophoresis**</u> to identity Bence Jones protein	<u>**X rays**</u> Perform complete skeletal series including skull chest, pelvis, spine & long bones -Lytic bones -Diffuse osteopenia <u>**MRI scan**</u> MRI is useful in symptomatic patients with normal radiographs Sensitive means to document cord or root compression	• Calculate % of plasma cells in marrow <u>**aspirate**</u> (Normal < 3%) • Look for a sheets or clusters of plasma cells in biopsy specimens. • Cytogenetic analysis of bone marrow may give prognostic information (Abnormalities of chromosome 13 eg. C13q deletion indicates poor prognosis.)

<u>Note :</u>

- *Serum M component is most commonly IgG [Q] (IgG (53%), IgA (25%), IgD (1%)*
- *Bence Jones proteins are light chain protein only [Q].*

266. Answer is A (Protein Electrophoresis): Harrison 18th/p 938, 940, 941 *Harrison's 17th/703, 704, 705*

Presence of symptoms of hyperviscocity syndrome (Headache), recurrent infections (ineffective defense against infections) and multiple punched out lytic lesions in the skull suggest a diagnosis of Multiple myeloma

Protein electrophoresis will help demonstrate a characteristic 'M spike' and help in establishing the diagnosis of multiple myeloma.

Serum Calcium is likely to be elevated while serum alkaline phosphatase levels are likely to be normal. Although both serum calcium and serum alkaline phosphatase levels may be done to support a diagnosis of Multiple Myeloma, demonstration of the charachteristic 'M spike' on protein electrophoresis is the single preferred investigation.

Classic Triad of Multiple Myeloma	Relevant investigations
• Marrow plasmacytosis > 10%	(*Bone Marrow examination*: Not provided in options)
• Lytic bone lesions	(*X-Ray skull*: Already performed in patient)
• Serum/urine M component	(***Protein Electrophoresis***: *Suggested next investigation*)

267. Answer is B (Increased in alkaline phosphatase): Harrison 18th/p 939, 940 *Harrison 16th/ 659; Harrison 17th/ 704*

Serum alkaline phosphatase is usually normal even with extensive bone involvement because of the absence of osteoblastic activity *– Harrison 16th/ 659*

Laboratory parameters in multiple myeloma :

- Anaemia: Normocytic normochromic
- ESR[Q] : markedly increased
- Hypogammaglobulinemia[Q]
- Monoclonal spike on Serum protein electrophoresis - Monoclonal Gammopathy (M Band)
- Bone marrow replacement of normal marrow elements by plasma cells.
- Bence Jones Proteinuria: Light chain proteinuria (inclomplete IgG)
- Uric Acid level : Elevated due to increased cell turnover
- Serum calcium : Elevated
- Alkaline phosphatase : Normal
- Neutropenia & Thrombocytopenia rare

268. Answer is C (Increased alkaline phosphatase): Harrison 18th/p 938, 939, 940 *Harrison 15th/ 730, Harrison 16th/ 659; Harrison 17th/ 703, 704*

Serum Alkaline phosphatase is usually normal even with extensive bone involvement because of absence of osteoblastic activity *– Harrisons 16th/ 659*

- Bone pain is the most common symptom in myeloma [Q]
- Bone lesions are lytic in nature and are rarely associated with osteoblastic new bone formation. Therefore

- Radioisotope bone scanning is less useful in diagnosis than plain radiography [Q]
- No hot spot is seen on bone scan [Q]
- Alkaline phosphatase (marker of osteoblastic activity) is not raised.

269. Answer is B (Multiple myeloma): Harrison 18th/p 940, 2529 *Harrison 15th/ 730, Harrisons 16th/ 659, 181; Harrison 17th/704, 1925*

Serum alkaline phosphatase *is usually normal in multiple myeloma.*

Alkaline phosphatase consists of many distinct isoenzymes and can be elevated in a number of conditions affecting Liver, Bone, placenta & small intestine.

Causes of elevated alkaline phosphatase

Physiological:	Liver derived Alkaline phosphatase:
• Patients over age > 60 y • Individuals with blood group O & B after a fatty meal • Adolescents and children undergoing rapid bone growth. • Late in normal pregnancy.	• Elevation of less than three times normal can be seen in any liver disease • Elevation of rather than four times normal suggests - Cholestatic liver disease - Infiltrative liver disease eg. cancer.
Bone derived Alkaline phosphatase:	**Miscellaneous conditions:** (Isolated elevation of serum alkaline phosphatase)
• Elevation suggests increased bone turn over / increased osteoblastic activity such as - Paget's disease - Rickets & osteomalacia	1. Hodgkin's disease 2. Diabetes 3. Hyperthyroidism 4. Congestive heart failure 5. Inflammatory bowel disease.

270. Answer is D (Elevated alkaline phosphatase): *Refer previous question .*

Serum alkaline phosphatase is characteristically normal even with extensive bone involvement because of absence of osteoblastic activity *– Harrison*
Anemia, Hypercalcemia and Hyperviscocity are recognized features of multiple myeloma.

271. Answer is C (Multiple myeloma): Harrison 18th/p 940 *Harrison 15th/ 728; Harrisons 16th/ 659 ; 17th/ 704;*

Hematology manual KGMC

ESR is elevated in multiple myeloma *– Harrisons 16th/ 659*

Conditions with decreased ESR that need to be remembered	
1. *Polycythemia* Q	3. *Sickle cell anemia* Q
2. *CHF* Q	4. *Afibrinogenimea*
Conditions with increased ESR that need to be remembered :	
1. *Pregnancy* Q	5. *Leucocytosis* Q
2. *Menstruation* Q	6. *New born* Q
3. *Multiple myeloma* Q	7. *DLE* Q
4. *Anemia other than sickle cell* Q	

272. Answer is A (Anion Gap Raised): *Refer text below; High Yield 'Acid Base Balance' 2nd/10*

Multiple Myeloma is associaitd with decreased Anion Gap.

Causes of Decreased Anion Gap
• Hypoalbuminemia • Multiple Myeloma and other paraproteinemic states like Waldenstorm's macroglobulinemia • Lithium intoxication / Bromide intoxication

Decreased Anion Gap is rare / uncommon and occurs due to accumulation of positively charged unmeasured cations which lower the anion gap
This is important as it may mask a significant anion gap acidosis.

273. Answer is C (Polyclomal gammapathy): Harrison 18th/p 937, 940 *Harrison 17th/701*

Mulitple Myeloma is characterized by monoclonal gammapathy and not polyclonal gammapathy.

Multiple myeloma represents a malignant proliferation of plasma cells derived from a single clone (monoclonal) – Harrison 17th/701

Bone marrow cells are monoclonal – Harrison 17th/703

274. Answer is D (Plasmacytosis < 10%): *Harrison 17th/703; Internal Medicine 5th/565; Clinical Hematology and Oncology 1st (2003)/202; Clinical Laboratory Medicine 6th/347*

Multiple myeloma is characteristically associated with Plasmacytosis >10%.

Multiple myeloma may be associated with both Hypogammaglobulinemia and Hypergammaglobulinemia.

Electrophoresis Pattern in Multiple Myeloma

Monoclonal Hypergammaglobulinemia (M spike)	Hypogammaglobulinemia
This is the characteristic electrophoresis pattern in Myeloma	• About 10-20% of multiple myeloma patients present with Hypogammaglobulinemia on electrophoresis. • This configuration is suggestive of light chain variant of multiple myeloma in which Bence Jones proteins are excreted into urine without a serum myeloma protein being evident with routine electrophoresis techniques.

'Multiple Myeloma results in hypergammaglobulinemia of a specific class of immunoglobulins. Hypogammaglobulinemia also justifies a search for myeloma especially for the possibility of light chain disease.'

– *Guide to Diagnostic Testing 1st (2002)/259*

Multiple Myeloma may be with Bence Jones Proteins, Amyloidosis & Renal failure

275. Answer is A (multiple mycloma): *Robbins 7th/680*

Russell bodies are intracytoplasmic inclusion bodies seen in within plasma cells in multiple mycloma

Characteristic Pathological features of multiple myeloma
(Not specific for multiple myeloma and may also be seen in benign disorders)

Cell types/shapes	Inclusion Bodies
• Plasma blasts • Bizzare multinucleated cells • Flame cells (cells with cherry red cytoplasm) • Mott cells (cells with multiple blue grape like cytoplasmic droplets)	• Russell bodies (intracyloplasmic) • Dutcher bodies (nuclear) • Inclusions of fibrils, crystalline rods and globules

276. Answer is D (Plasma cells): *Robbins 7th/680*

Russel bodies are intracytoplasmic inclusion bodies seen within plasma cells in patients with multiple myeloma.

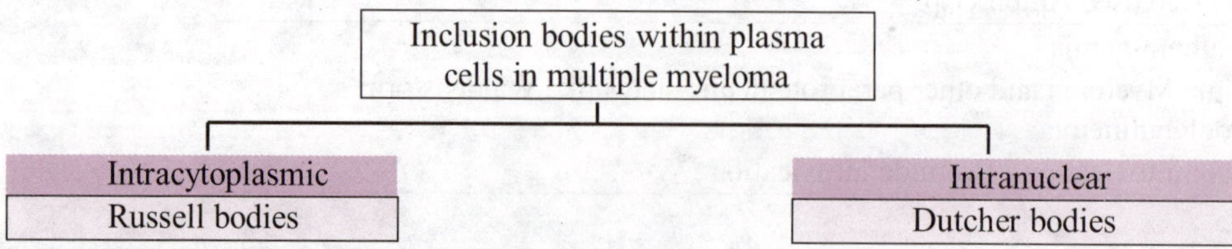

277. Answer is B (Hypocalcemia): Harrison 18th/p 940 *Harrison 17th/704; Clinical Malignant Hematology 1st (2007)/916; 'manual of Clinical Oncology' 6th/482, 483*

Hypercalcemia is associated with a poor prognosis in Multiple Myeloma and not hypocalcemia.
Azotemia (↑ creatinine), ↑ LDH, Chromosome 13q deletion and High M component production are all established poor prognostic factors.

Poor prognostic factors in Multiple Myeloma

Stage Related Factors	Independent factors
Stage III disease : High Tumor Burder • Hb < 8.5 g/dl • Hypercalcemia (Ca > 12 mg/dl) • Advanced Lytic bine lesions • High M component production IgG > 7g/dl IgA > 5g/dl Urine light chains > 12g/24 hrs Subclassification based on serum creatinine levels • Serum creatinine > 2 mg/dl	• β2 microglobulin (single most important factor) • ↓ Serum albumin • ↑ LDH • ↑ labeling index (%age of cells undergoing mitosis) • ↑ CRP or IL6 • ↑Hepatocyte growth factor, TGF (β) or syndecan – 1 • Plasmoblastic morphology • Genetic Abnormalities - Hyperploidy - Chromosome 13 deletion (and chromosome 17 p deletion) - t(4; 14), t(14; 16), t(11; 4) translocation - RAS & P53 mutations.

278. Answer is C (β_2 microglobulin): *Harrison 18th/p 941 Harrison 15th/ 731; Harrison 16th/ 659; Harrison 17th/ 704*

***Serum β_2 microglobulin is the single most powerful predictor of survival and can substitute for staging**-H-16th*

β_2 microglobulin level	Median survival
< 0.04 g/L	Median survival of 43 months
>0.04 g/L	Median survival of only 12 months.

279. Answer is C (Multiple myeloma): Harrison 18th/p 938, 940 *Harrison 16th/658; Harrison 17th/ 703, 704*

Backache and Recurrent infections in the backdrop of normal alkaline phosphatase levels and a reversed albumin globulin ratio (A : G ratio) is highly suggestive of the diagnosis of multiple myeloma.

Interpretation of information provided in the question

Clinical information

Infomation	Interpretation
• Backache	• Bony pains
• Weakness of legs & urinary retention	• Cord compression
• Chest infection (recurrent)	• Ineffective defence against infection

Laboratory parameters

Parameter	Normal	Patients	Interpretation
• Haemoglobin	12 - 16gm	7.3	***Anemia***
• Serum Ca^{++}	9.0 - 10.5mg/dl	12.6	***Hypercalcemia***
• Alkaline phosphatase	30-120 U/l	100	***Normal***
• Albumin	3.5 - 5.5 gm/dl	3.0	Normal
• Globulin	2.0 - 3.5 gm/dl	7.1	***Elevated***
• Urea	20 - 40 mg/dl	178	Elevated

Both clinical findings and laboratory data suggest the diagnosis of Multiple Myeloma

- Serum Alkaline Phosphatase is usually normal even with extensive bone involvement.– *Harrison*
- Serum Albumin is normal or low, Total protein is normal or raised.– *Kumar 5th/501*

280. Answer is B (Multiple myeloma): *Harrison 18th/940, 941 Harrison 15th/ 728, Harrison 16th/ 659; Harrison 17th/ 704*

This is a 65 year old patient presenting with low back pain along with-a reversed A: G ratio. This indicates an excess of globulin fraction or a possible gammopathy. These findings along with an elevated ESR and Renal involvement (indicated by increased creatinine levels) suggest a diagnosis of Multiple Myeloma.

281. Answer is B (Hydroxyurea): *NCCH Clinical Practice Guidelines in oncology; Harrison's 18th/941, 942*

Hydroxyurea is not recommended for the management of multiple myeloma

Chemotherapeutic Agents Recommended in the management of multiple myeloma

- *Bortezomib*
- *Cyclophosphamide*
- *Doxorubicin*
- *Vincristine*
- *Lenalidomide*
- *Thalidomide*
- *Melphelan*
- *Dexamethasone / Prednisolone*
- *Interferon (Maintenance)*

1

Hematology

The most commonly used chemotherapy agents in non-transplant and transplant candidates and in relapsed or refractory myeloma, based on the *2007 National Comprehensive Cancer Network (NCCN) guidelines*

Primary Induction therapy for transplant candidates	Primary Induction Therapy for non-transplant Candidates
• *Bortezomib/dexamethasone (category 1)* • *Bortezomib/cyclophosphamide/dexamethasone* • *Bonezomib/doxorubicin/dexamethasone (category 1)* • *Bortezomib/enalidomide*[e]*/dexamethasone (category 2B)* • *Bortezomib/thalidomide/dexamethasone (category 1)* • *Dexamethasone (category 2B)* • *Lenalidomide*[e]*/dexamelhasone (category 1)* • *Liposomal doxorubicin/vincristine/dexamethasone (DVD) (category 2B)* • *Thalidomide/dexamethasone (category 2B)*	• *Bortezomib/dexamethasone* • *Dexamethasone (category 2B)* • *Lenalidomide/low-dose dexamethasone (category 1)* • *Liposomal doxorubicin/vincristine/dexamethasone (DVD) (category 2B)* • *Melphalan/prednisone (MP)* • *Melphalan/prednisone/bortezomib (MPB) (category 1)* • *Melphalan/prednisone/thalidomide (MPT) (category 1)* • *Melphalan/prednisone/lenalidomide (MPL)* • *Thalidomide/dexamethasone (category 2B)* • *Vincristine/doxorubicin/dexamethasone (VAD) (cateoorv 2B)*
Maintenance Therapy	**Salvage**
• *Interferon (category 2B)* • *Lenalidomide*[f] • *Steroids (category 2B)* • *Thalidomide (category 1) ± prednisone (category 2B)*	• *Repeat primary induction therapy (if relapse at > 6 mo)* • *Bendamustine (category 2B)* • *Bortezomib*[g] *(category 1)* • *Bortezomib/dexamethasone* • *Borlezomib/lenalidomide/dexamethasone (category 2B)* • *Bortezomib/liposomal doxorubicin*[g] *(category 1)* • *Cyclophosphamide-VAD* • *Cyclophosphamide/bortezomib/dexamethasone*[h] • *Cyclophosphamide/lenalidomide/dexamethasone*[h] • *Dexamethasone* • *Dexamethasone/cyclophosphamide/etoposide/cisplatin (DCEP)* • *Dexamethasone/thalidomide/cisplatin/doxorubicin/ cyclophosphamide/etoposide (DT-PACE)* • *High-dose cyclophosphamide* • *Lenalidomide/dexamethasone (category 1)* • *Lenalidomide* • *Thalidomide* • *Thalidomide/dexamethasone*

[a]*Selected, but not inclusive of all regimens →Thalidomide/dexamethasone*
[b]*Treatments are listed alphabetically and do not imply preference.*
[c]*Recommend herpes zoster prophylaxis for patients treated with bortezomib*
[d]*Prophylactic anticoagulation recommended for patients receiving thalidomide-based therapy or lenalidomide with dexmethasone.*
[f]*Lenalidomide as maintenance has been evaluated in three independent randomized clinical trials. Results from each of these trials show improvements in TTP. The panel felt that this warranted inclusion: however, this recommendation remains Category 2A since these results have not undergone full peer review and safety/efficacy data are still preliminary.*
[g]*Bortezomib/liposomal doxorubicin is prefered to bortezumib single agent*
[h]*These are representative regimens combining standard agents with novel agents.*

Note: All recommendations are category 2A unless otherwise indicated.
Clinical Trials: NCCN believes that the best management of any cancer patient is in a clinical trial. Participation in clinical tirals is especially encouraged.

282. Answer is C (Hydroxyurea): *Harrison's 17th/705.*

Hydroxyurea is not used in the management of Multiple Myeloma.

Multiple Myeloma Variance and Other Plasma Cell Disorders

283. Answer is A (Monoclonal gammopathy): Harrison 18th/p 940 *Hariosn 17th/704*

Smoldering myeloma is a variant of multiple myeloma and is associated with a monoclonal gammopathy

Smoldering Myeloma

- Smoldering Myeloma is an asymptomatic variant of multiple myeloma (Monoclonal gammopathy)
- These patients have a higher levels of M-component and marrow plasmacytosis than patients with **MGUS** (Monoclonal Gammopathy of Unknown Significance), and fulfill the minimal criteria for diagnosis of plasma cell myeloma, but are asymptomatic and have no lytic bone lesions or other clinical features of Myeloma.

Diagnostic Criteria for Smoldering Myeloma (Asymptomatic Myeloma)

M protein is serum > 30g/L (>3g/dl)

Bone marrow clonal plasma cell (Plasmacytosis) ≥ 10%

No myeloma related organ or tissue impairment

- *No lytic bone lesions*
- *No myeloma related symptoms*
  - *- No renal insufficiency*
  - *- No Anemia*
  - *- No Hypercalcemia*

Comparisonof MGUS, Indolent myeloma and Smoldering myeloma:

	MGUS	SMM	IMM	Multiple Myeloma
Plasma cell (BM)	<10%	10-30%	>30%	>30%
M-component	IgG<3.5, IgA<2	IgG>3.5, IgA>2	IgG 3.5-7, IgA 2-5	IgG >3.5/dl; IgA >2g/dl
Lytic bone lesion	None	None	≤3	Present
Symptoms/Infection - *Anemia* - *Renal insufficiency* - *Hypercalcemia*	None	None	None	Present

284. Answer is C (Monoclonal gammopathy of unknown significance): Harrison 18th/p 940 *Harrison 16th/ 65; Harrison 17th/ 704, 706*

'Patients with monoclonal gammopathy of uncertain significance have < 10% bone marrow plasma cells, and < 3g / dl of M component', *- Harrison 15th / 730*

Presence of 8% bone marrow plasma cells and 1.5 gm/dl of M component in the form of IgG in this patient thus lead us to the above diagnosis.

Plasma cell dyscrasia : Monoclonal gammopathies : Paraproteinemias : dysproteinemias

These are monoclonal neoplasms characterized by expansion of a single clone of immunoglobulin secreting cells (plasma cells) and result in increase in serum levels of a single homogenous 'immunoglobulin' or – its fragments (light chains or heavy chains).

The most important differential diagnosis in patients with multiple myeloma involves their distinction from individuals with MGUS or Benign monoclonal gammopathy:

Parameters	Multiple myeloma	Monoclonal gammopathy of undetermined significance
1. Age Q	> 50 years	> 50 years
2. Incidence Q	Less common	More common
3. Plasma cells Q (%age)	> 10%	< 10%
4. M component Q (concentration : g/dl)	> 3g/dl	< 3g/dl
5. Benze Jones Q proteins	Present	No urinary Bence Jones proteins

6. Clinical features Q	Lytic bones lesions Hypercalcemia Renal failure Anemia	No Lytic bony lesions Q No hypercalcemia Q No renal failure Q No anemia Q
7. Labelling index Q (Thymidine)	> 1%	< 1%
8. Plasma cell - acid phosphatase - glucoronidase	 High High	 Low Low
9. Treatment	Required	No therapy required

Woldenstorm's macroglobulinemia: is also a monoclonal gammopathy and is characterized by neoplasm of lymphoplasma cytoid cells that secrete IgM

M component is only IgM and not IgG.

This is characterized clinically by
- Lymphadenopathy - Hepatosplenomegaly - Hyperviscosity syndrome

Indolent multiple myeloma (IMM):

Lies in the spectrum between MM and MGUS

Unlike MGUS, patients with IMM have -	Unlike MM patients with IMM
> 10% plasma cells > 3g / dl of M protein	- are Asymptomatic - Patients have mild non progressive anemia but no bone lesions, hypercalcemia or renal failure - Progress to overt MM in < 1 years

285. Answer is B (Multiple myeloma): Harrison 18th/p 938, 940, 941 *Harrison 15th/ 729, Harrison 16th/ 658, 659, 661; Harrison 17th/ 703, 704; 705*

This is a 60 year patient presenting with generalized bone pain and lytic lesion in skull with blood parameters indicating a markedly raised ESR, Hypercalcemia, Hyperglobulinemia and raised serum creatinine. All these suggest a diagnosis of multiple myeloma.

	Patient	Normal	Interpretation & inference
Age	60 years	-	60 years
ESR	100	< 15 (male)	Markedly increased
Serum globulin	7	2.5 to 3.5	Increased
Serum creatinine	3.5	< 1.5 mg/dl	Increased: Renal failure
Serum calcium	11.0	9 mg/dl	Increased hypercalcemia

Distinguishing features between W. Macroglobulinemia from multiple myeloma

- **Does not cause lytic bone lesions**
- **Does not cause hypercalcemia* serum calcium is usually not elevated***
- **Serum 'M' component is IgM**
  - IgM being large in size undergoes Less renal excretion
  - Renal disease is not common Q
  - Serum creatinine is usually not elevated.
- Hepatomegaly, splenomegaly and lymphadenopathy are common unlike in multiple myeloma where they are uncommon.
- Symptoms due to hyperviscocity are more prominent as compared to those in multiple myeloma
  - Epistaxis visual disturbance and neurological symptoms are more common.
  - Rouleaux formation and positive Coombs test are more common.

286. Answer is B (A diagnosis of plasma cell leukemia ......): *Wintrobe's haematology 11th/ 2620, 2593*

'Plasma cell leukaemia' by definition is characterized by more than 20% plasma cells in the peripheral blood. The patient in question has 14% plasma blasts in peripheral blood and thus does not classify as a plasma cell leukaemia.

Distinguishing features in various types of plasma cell disorders:

Plasma cell leukaemia (Rare form of plasma cell disorder) *Wintrobe's 11th/ 2620*

- ***More than 20% plasma cells*** in the peripheral blood
- Absolute plasma cell count of more than 2×10^9/L

IgD Myeloma *(Wintrobe's 11th/ 2592)*

- Accounts for approximately 2% of all cases of myeloma
- Presence of Monoclonal IgD in the serum usually indicates IgD myeloma
- ***Present with a small bond or no evident M-spike on serum protein electrophoresis.***
- Higher incidence of renal insufficiency, Amyloidosis and proteinuria than IgG / IgA myeloma.
- Higher incidence of Extramedullary involvement and inferior survival rates.

Monoclonal gammopathy of undetermined significance

- Serum monoclonal protein < 3 g/dl
- No anemia, renal failure, or hypercalcemia
- Bone lesions absent on radiographic bone survey
- Bone marrow < 10% plasma cells.

Smoldering multiple myeloma

- Serum monoclonal protein (≥ 3 g/dl) or ***≥ 10% marrow plasma cells*** or aggregates on biopsy, or both
- No anemia, renal failure, or hypercalcemia attributable to myeloma

Multiple myeloma

- ***Monoclonal protein presents in serum or urine***
- ≥ 10% marrow plasma cells on biopsy of histologic evidence of plasmacytoma
- Plus one or more more of the following
  - Anemia
  - Lytic lesions or osteoporosis and ≥30% plasma cells in marrow
  - Bone marrow plasma cell labeling index >1%
  - Renal insufficiency
  - Hypercalcemia

Criteria for diagnosis of Monoclonal Gammopathy of Undetermined Significance, Smoldering Multiple Myeloma and Multiple Myeloma, According to Kyle and Greipp-Wintrobes.

287. Answer is A (Gamma heavy chain disease): Harrison 18th/p 943, 944 *Harrison 17th/ 707; Read text below*

Franklin's disease is a gamma heavy chain disease.

Heavy chain diseases: Characterized by elevated levels of a specific heavy chain of immuno-globulins in blood or urine.

Gamma chain	Seen in elderly resemble lymphoma. Franklin's disease
Alpha chain	*Saligmann's disease* is the most common example
mμ chain	Rarest form seen in patients with CLL

Plasma cell dyscrasias :

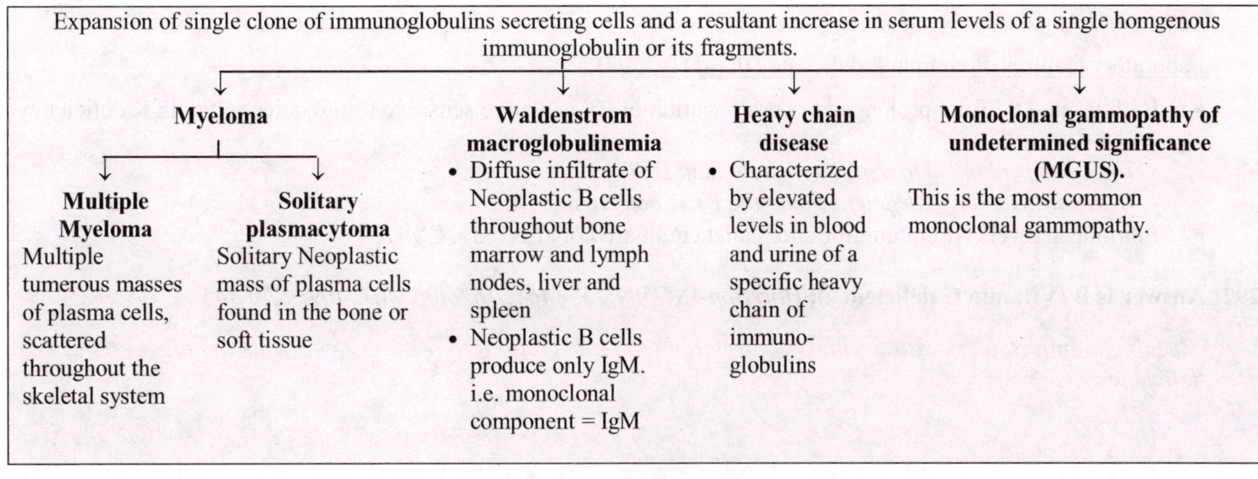

Bleeding / Coagulation Disorder

General

288. Answer is B (IX and X): *Ganong 23rd/535, Chaudhry physiology 6th/73*

Vitamin K dependent coagulation factors include coagulation factor II, VII, IX and X.

Vitamin K dependent Coagulation Factors / Proteins

- Six proteins involved in clotting require conversion of a number of glutamic acid residues to γ - carboxyglutamic acid residues before being released into circulation
- This process of γ (gamma) carboxylation occurs in the liver and requires vitamin k and hence these proteins are called vitamin – K dependent
- These include coagulation factors II, VII, IX and X as well as protein C and protein S.

Vitamin K dependent proteins involved in clotting
• ***Coagulation Factor II*** [Q] ***(Prothrombin)*** • ***Coagulation Factor VII*** [Q] ***(Proconvertin)*** • ***Coagulation Factor IX*** [Q] ***(Christmas factor)*** • ***Coagulation factor X (Stuart Prover Factor)*** • *Protein C* [Q] • *Protein S* [Q]

289. Answer is A(II): *Refer text below; CMDT 2008/466; CMDT 2009/481*

Vitamin K dependent factors include factors II, VII IX and X

Vitamin K dependent factors: Factor II, VII, IX, X

290. Answer is B (P.T.): *CMDT 2008/466; CMDT 2009/481; Read text below*

Although PT and PTT both will be affected PT is the single best answer as explained below.

Vit K dependent factors : Factor II, VII, IX & X [Q]

Therefore both intrinsic & extrinsic mechanisms of the coagulation cascade are affected. (Refer previous questions) PT & PTT both will be prolonged.

However, *factor VII has short t½ & so PT is the first to be prolonged (even in mild vit. K deficiency)*

Later, factors II, IX & X will also fall, causing PTT to be prolonged. PT is thus the better choice out of PT and PTT.

291. Answer is A (Prolonged prothrombin time): *Ghai 6th/31; CMDT 2008/466,467; CMDT 2009/481*

Hemorrhagic disease of new born results from a deficiency of vitamin K.

Prothrombin time is the single best laboratory test to detect vitamin K deficiency as vitamin k deficiency may present with isolated prolongation of PT

Laboratory features of vitamin k deficiency (CMDT-2008)

- Both PT and PTT are prolonged but prolongation of PT is a more sensitive test to detect vitamin K deficiency than PTT
  - *The PT is prolonged to a greater extent than PTT*
  - *With mild vitamin K deficiency only the PT is defective*
- Fibrinogen level, Thrombin time and platlet count are not affected – CMDT

292. Answer is B (Vitamin C deficiency): *Harrison 18th/599;15th/ 464; 16th/406, 407, 409; 17th/ 445*

Bleeding manifestations with normal prothrombin time and clotting time almost confirms the diagnosis of vitamin C deficiency.

Bleeding manifestations due to vitamin deficiency

VITAMIN C	VITAMIN K
• Vitamin C is required for synthesis of collagen which forms part of capillary walls. • Vitamin C deficiency leads to increased capillary wall fragility and hence increased manifestations of haemorrhagic areas such as– - *over lower extremities*[Q] - *around hair follicles*[Q] - *nail beds*[Q]	• Vitamin K dependent factors include Factor II, VII, IX, X • In vitamin K deficiency bleeding occurs due to lack of coagulation factors
• Patient presents with - increased bleeding time [Q] - normal PTT, PT, TT [Q] - normal clotting time[Q]	• Patient presents with - increased clotting time[Q] - increased PTT, PT, TT[Q] - normal bleeding time[Q]

293. Answer is A (Prolonged bleeding time (BT) : *Robbins 7th / 653; KDT 5th / 172;*

Bleeding time is indicative of function of platelets. Aspirin ingestion results in defective platelet function and hence the deranged parameter will be Bleeding time. PT, APTT and Clotting time (CT) are parameters of coagulation defects, and will be normal in isolated disorders of platelet function.

'Ingestion of Aspirin and other Nonsteroidal Antiinflammatory drugs, significantly prolongs the bleeding time'.
– Robbin 7th / 653

'Aspirin even in small doses irreversibly inhibits TxA2 synthesis by platelets. ***Thus it interferes with platelet aggregation and bleeding time is prolonged to nearly twice the normal value'****-KDT 5th / 172*

Note:

- *Aspirin* ***irreversibly***[Q] ***inhibits COX –1 and COX*** *– 2. (Harrison)*
  COX inhibition leads to prevention of TXA2 synthesis and impairment of platelet secretion and aggregation
- *The effect of aspirin on platelet function* ***occur within 1 hour and lasts for the duration of the affected platelet's life span ie. 1 week.***[Q] *– Harrison*

294. Answer is A and B (Platelet adhesion Assays and BT): *Refer text below*

Platelet function may be assessed by 'Bleeding time' and Platelet Adhesion Assays.

295. Answer is D (Factor VII) : *Refer text below; Ganong 22nd/ 542; Robbins 7th / 128; Clinical Hematology 4th / 355*

Factor VII is involved in the extrinsic pathway of coagulation and plays no role in the intrinsic pathway.

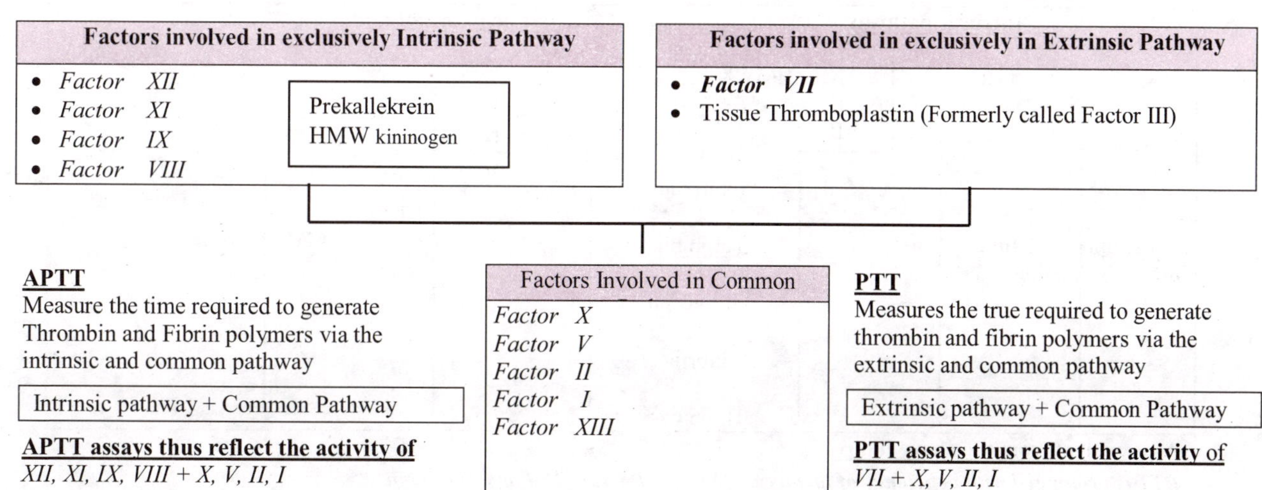

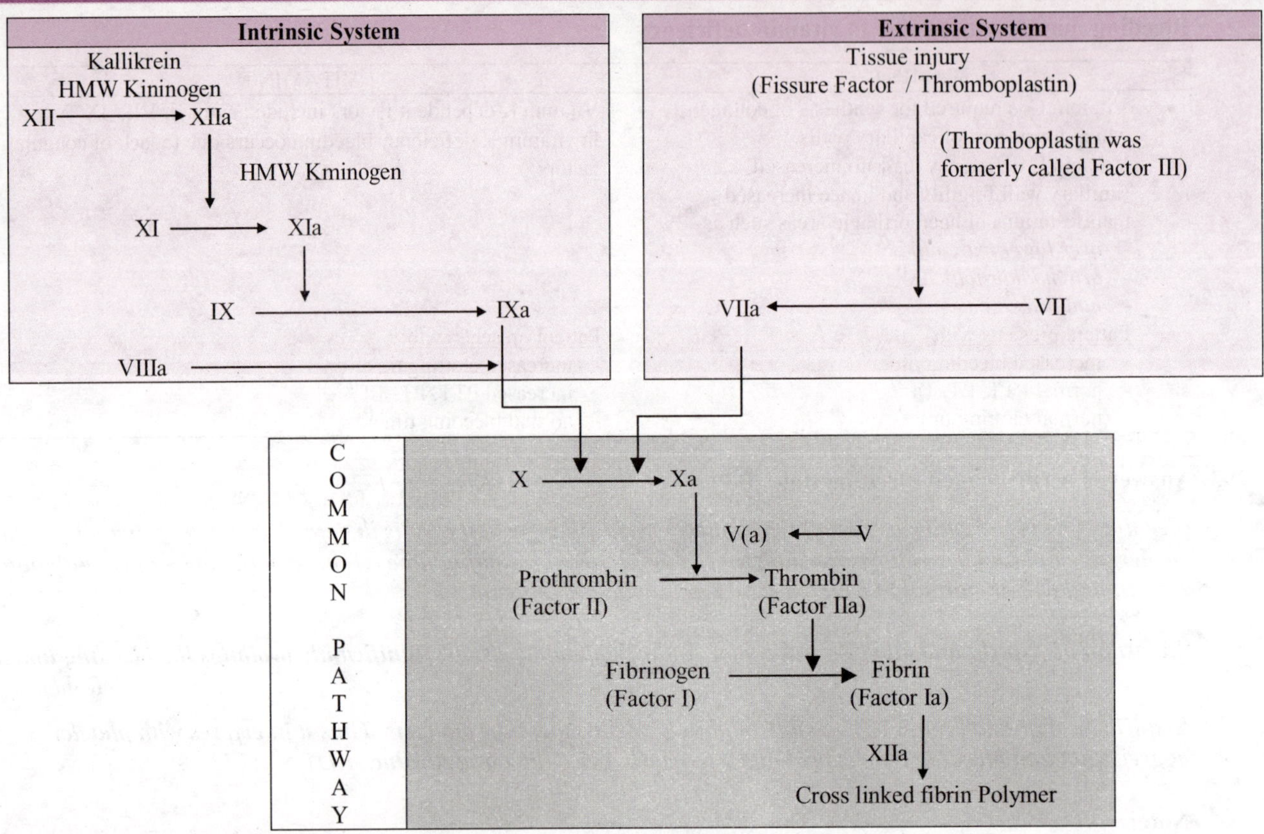

296. Answer is A (Factor XIII) : *Ganong 22nd/ 543; Harrisons 17th /364;Refer previous question*

Factor XIII is also known as fibrin stabilizing factor. Activated factor XIII (XIIIa) covalently cross links and stabilizes the fibrin clot *– Harrison*

*The fibrin is initially a loose mesh of interlacing strands. It is converted into a dense, tight aggregate (Stabilization) by the formation of covalent cross linkages. This reaction is **catalyzed by activated factor XIII** and requires calcium.*

-Harrison

297. Answer is B (Stuart factor X): *Refer text below: Refer previous question*

The extrinsic and Intrinsic pathways in coagulation converge at the stuart factor X.

Understanding the coagulation cascade:

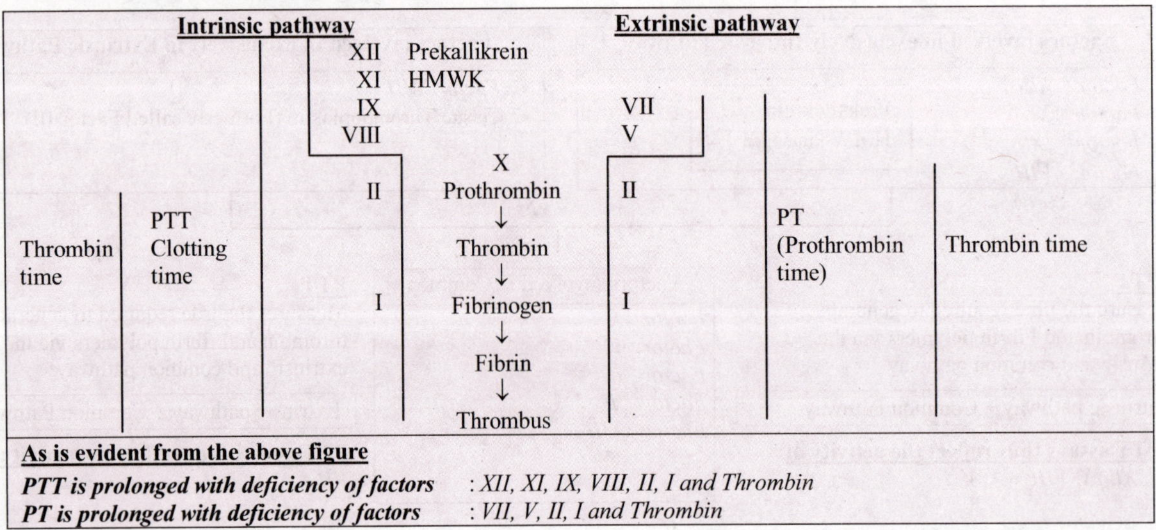

298. Answer is B (Factor VII deficiency): *CMDT 2008/467; Refer previous question*

Factor VII deficiency may present with isolated prolongation of prothrombin time.

Deficiency of factor VIII, IX and XII may present with isolated prolongation of Partial Thromboplastin Time (APTT) and not isolated prolongation of prothrombin time (PT)

Cause of Isolated prolongation of PT (CMDT)
Vitamin K deficiency
Warfarin therapy
Liver disease
Factor VII deficiency

299. Answer is C (Lupus Anticoagulant): *Practical Hemostasis and Thrombosis; Harrison's 17th/369; Wintrobe's 12th/1447-1453; 'Clinical Anesthesia' 6th (Lippincott William's)/187, 'Complications in Surgery' by Doherty (2006)/187*

Isolated prolongation of aPTT with no clinical history of bleeding suggests the presence of Lupus anticoagulant or deficiency of contact factors (Factor XII, Prekallikrein or HMWK)

'If there is no bleeding history, but the APTT alone is prolonged, the most likely cause of prolonged aPTT is a lupus anticoagulant' - *'Complications in Surgery' by Doherty (2006)/187*

Approach to a patient with isolated prolongation of activated Partial Thromboplastin time (aPTT)

- The Partial Thromboplastin Time (aPTT) is a performance indicator measuring the efficacy of both the '*intrinsic system' and the 'common' coagulation pathway.*
- ***Isolated prolongation of aPTT (normal PT)*** may indicate:
  - *Coagulation Factor Deficiency (Factor VIII, IX, XI, XII, Prekallikrein, HMWK)*
  - *Presence of Antiphospholipid Antibodies especially Lupus Anticoagulant*
  - *Use of heparin (or contamination of sample with Heparin)*
  - *Specific coagulation factor Inhibitors (factor VIII inhibitor or Factor IX or XI (rare) inhibitor)*
- The ***presence or absence of bleeding manifestation*** even after major surgery may narrow down the differential diagnosis.

Isolated Prolongation of aPTT with no bleeding manifestation	Isolated prolongation of aPTT with bleeding manifestation
• Specific Coagulation Factor Deficiencies - *Factor XII Deficiency* - *Prekallekrien* - *HMW Kininինogen Defect* • ***Presence of Lupus Anticoagulant***	• Specific Coagulation Factor Deficiencies - *Factor VIII defect* - *Factor IX defect* - *Factor XI defect* • Specific Coagulation Factor Inhibitors - *Factor VIII inhibitor* - *Factor IX inhibitor or Factor XI inhibitor*

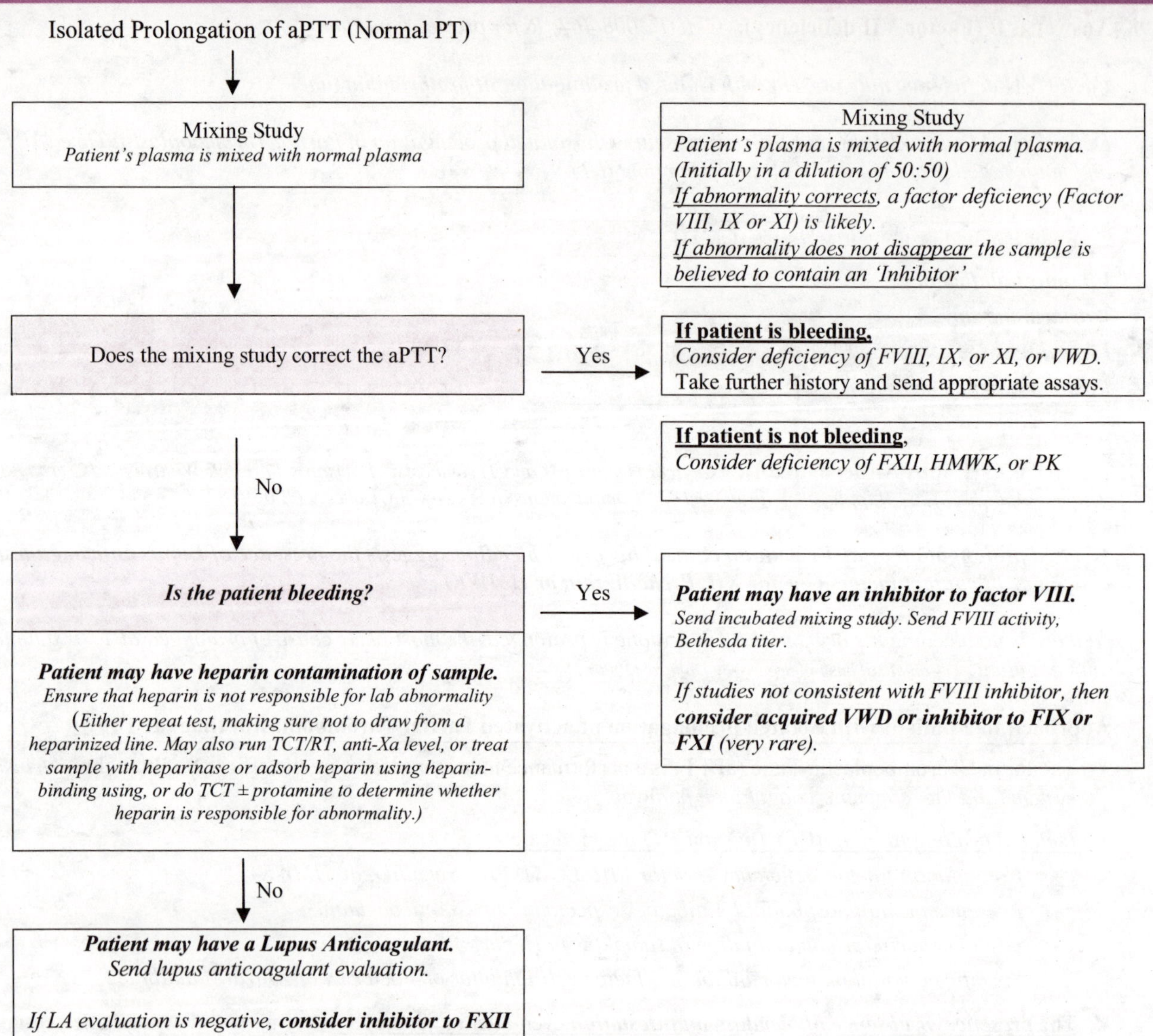

300. Answer is A (Factor II Deficiency): *Refer text below*

Prolongation of both PT and APPT is typically seen in deficiency of factors involved in the common pathway, namely factor II, factor V and factor X (and fibrinogen).

Heparin in clinical concentrations is typically associated with isolated prolongation of APTT while PT is normal because heparin acts on the intrinsic pathway. (However Heparin at very high concentrations within the sample may cause prolongation of both PT & APTT).

Causes of Prolonged PT and APTT
• *Coagulation Factor Deficiency (Factor II, V, X or fibrinogen)*
• *Use of oral anticoagulants (Warfarin)*
• *Disseminated Intravascular coagulation*
• *Severe vitamin K deficiency*
• *Liver Disease (Severe Hepatic Insufficiency)*
• *Heparin in sample (at high concentrations only)*
(Heparin is typically associated with prolonged APTT & normal PT)

301. Answer is C (Factor XII deficiency) : *Nelson 17th/1660; See previous questions*

Isolated prolongation of PTT suggest a defect in the intrinsic pathway of coagulation cascade only, and leaves us with the possibility of either factor XIII deficiency or Haemophilia A (Factor VIII deificiency).

Absence of clinical bleeding even after major surgery like tonsillectomy suggests a classical deficiency of contact factor XII.

Isolated elongation of aPTT with bleeding manifestations	Isolated prolongation of aPTT without bleeding manifestations
Factor VIII defect Factor IX defect Factor XI defect	Factor XII defect Prekallikrein defect HMW kininogen defect

Non bleeding disorder / Deficiency of the contact factors

- Contact factors function at the step of initiation of intrinsic pathway of the clotting cascade and include the following :

Contact factors
Factor XII Prekallikrein High Molecular Weight Kininogen (HMWK)

- Deficiency of these factors is characterized by –
  - Isolated prolonged of PTT
  - Absence of clinical bleeding
- These patients do not need treatment if major surgery is indicated.

A paradoxical situation in which these is an extremely prolonged PTT but no evidence of clinical bleeding suggests a deficiency of contact factors.

302. Answer is C (Russell viper venom assay): *Harrison 18th/464; 17th/369; Wintrobe's 12th/1447-1453; 'Clinical Anesthesia' 6th (Lippincott William's)/187, 'Complications in Surgery' by Doherty (2006)/187*

'If there is no bleeding history, but the APTT alone is prolonged, the most likely cause of prolonged aPTT is a lupus anticoagulant' - 'Complications in Surgery' by Doherty (2006)/187

Russell Viper Venom assay is done to establish the presence of lupus anticoagulant and is the single best answer amongst the options provided.

Isolated prolongation of aPTT with no clinical history of bleeding suggests the presence of Lupus anticoagulant or deficiency of contact factors (Factor XII, Prekallikrein or HMWK)

No options are provided to detect deficiency of contact factors in this question and hence Russell Viper Venom assay is the answer of choice here

Factor VIII deficiency, Defect in platelet aggregation and vWF disease all lead to variable amount of clinical bleeding

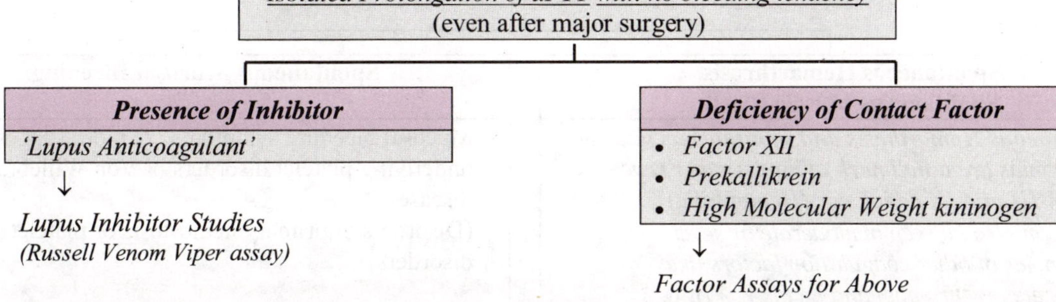

'If there is no bleeding history, but the APTT alone is prolonged, the most likely cause of prolonged aPTT is a lupus anticoagulant' - 'Complications in Surgery' by Doherty (2006)/187

Tests for Lupus Anticoagulant (Lupus Inhibitor studies)
• *Lupus Anticoagulant test* • ***Dilute Russell Viper Venom Time (d RVVT)*** • *Kaolin Clotting time* • *Tissue Thromboplastin Time* • *Platelet Neutralization test*

303. Answer is B (Deficiency is associated with prolonged APTT): Harrison 18th/p 973 *Harrison's 17th/725*

Factor VII deficiency is associated with isolated prolongation of PT, APTT is normal in Factor VII deficiency

Genetic and laboratory characteristic of inherited coagulation disorders

Clotting factor deficiency	Inheritance	Prevalence in General Population	Laboratory Abnormality[a] aPTT	PT	TT	Minimum Hemostatic levels	Treatment	Plasma Half-Life
Fibrinogen	AR	1 in 1,000,000	+	+	+	100 mg/dL	Cryoprecipitate	2-4 d
Prothrombin	AR	1 in 2,000,000	+	+	-	20-30%	FFP/PCCs	3-4 d
Factor V	AR	1 in 1,000,000	+/-	+/-	-	15-20%	FFP	36 h
Factor VII	***AR***	***1 in 500,000***	**-**	**+**	**-**	***15-20%***	***FFP/PCCs***	***4-6 h***
Factor VIII	X-linked	1 in 5,000	+	-	-	30%	FVIII concentrates	8-12 h
Factor IX	X-linked	1 in 30,000	+	-	-	30%	FIX concentrates	18-24 h
Factor X	AR	1 in 1,000,000	+/-	+/-	-	15-20%	FFP/PCCs	40-60h
Factor XI	AR	1 in 1,000,000	+	-	-	15-20%	FFP	40-70h
Factor XII	***AR***	***ND***	**+**	**-**	**-**	***b***	***b***	***60 h***
HK	AR	ND	+	-	-	*b*	*b*	150 h
Prekallikrein	AR	ND	+	-	-	*b*	*b*	35 h
Factor XIII	AR	1 in 2,000,000	-	-	+/-	2-5%	Cryptoprecipitate	11-14d

a Values within normal range (-) or prolonged (+)
b No risk for bleeding, treatment is not indicated

HK, high-molecular weight kininogen; AR, autosomal recessive; aPTT, activated partial thromboplastin time; PT, prothrombin time; TT, thrombin time; ND, not determined; FFP, fresh frozen plasma; PCCs, prothrombin complex concentrates.

304. Answer is A (Hemophilia) : *Harrison's 18th/460; Hemotasis and Thrombosis : Back Principles & clinical Practice' by Colman (Lippincott Williams) 5th/1148*

Spontaneous Hemarthrosis and spontaneous muscle hematomas are charachteristic of moderate or severe congenital factor VIII or IX deficiency (Hemophilia).

Spontaneous bleeding may also be seen in Afibrinogenemia, Von willebrand disease and Scott's syndrome (defect in platelet's activated surface that promotes thrombin formation), but it is most charachteristic (Hallmark) of Hemophillia or factor VIII & IX Deficiency.

Bleeding Disorders

Spontaneous Hemarthrosis Spontaneous Muscle Bleed	Spontaneous Mucosal Bleeding
• ***Spontaneous Hemarthosis and spontaneous muscle Hematomas are a hallmark of moderate or severe factor VIII and IX deficiency (Hemophilia)*** • *These can also be seen in moderate or severe deficiencies of other coagulation factors like fibrinogen, prothrombin and factor V, VII, & X* • *These are rarely seen in other bleeding disorders.*	• Mucosal bleeding symptoms are more suggestive of underlying platelet disorders or Von Willebrand disease (Disorders of primary hemostosis or platelet plug disorders)

Primary Hemostatic (Platelet Plug) Disorders

Defects of Platelet Adhesion
• *Von Willebrand disease* • *Bernard-Soulier syndrome (absence of dysfunction of GpIb-IX-V)*
Defects of Platelet Aggregation
• *Glanzmann's thrombasthenia (absence or dysfunction of GpIIbIIIa)* • *Afibrinogenemia*
Defects of Platelet Secretion
• *Decreased cyclooxygenase activity* • *Granule storage pool defects* • *Non-specific inherited secretory defects* • *Non-specific drug effects* • *Uremia* • *Platelet coating (e.g., paraprotein, penicillin)*
Defect of Platelet Coagulant Activity
• *Scott's syndrome*

Hemophilia

305. Answer is B (PT is increased): *Harrison 18th/974, 975; Harrison 17th / 726; Chandrasoma Taylor 3rd/ 428, 429*

It is PTT which is affected (increased) and not PT (unaffected).

Haemophilia A occurs *due to deficiency or reduced activity of factor VIII* (antihaemophilic factor). *Factor VIII is involved in the intrinsic pathway which is measured by PTT and not in extrinsic pathway which is measured as PT.*

Understanding the coagulation cascade:

Intrinsic pathway | **Extrinsic pathway**

XII Prekallikrein
XI HMWK
IX | VII
VIII | V
X
II Prothrombin II
↓
Thrombin
↓
I Fibrinogen I
↓
Fibrin
↓
Thrombus

Thrombin time | PTT Clotting time | PT (Prothrombin time) | Thrombin time

As is evident from the above figure

PTT is prolonged with deficiency of factors : *XII, XI, IX, VIII, II, I and Thrombin*
PT is prolonged with deficiency of factors : *VII, V, II, I and Thrombin*

306. Answer is C (↑ PT) : *Repeat AI-2001*

Hemophilia A is associated with a defect in intrinsic pathway of clotting cascade and hence PT is essentially normal.

307. Answer is A (Increased bleeding time): Harrison 18th/p 974 *Harrison 15th/ 751; Harrison 16th/680, 681; Harrison 17th / 726 Chandrasoma Taylor 3rd/ 428, 429, 430; CMDT 2003 / 512; CMDT 2008/ 463, 464; CMDT 2009/478*

Haemophilia is a disorder of coagulation (bleeding time unaffected) affecting the intrinsic pathway (prothrombin time unaffected).

	Haemophilia A (Classical hemophilia)	Haemophilia B (Christmas disease)
Defect	Deficiency of coagulant subunit of factor i.e (VIII c) Factor VIII = VIII c + VWF	Deficiency/absence of factor IX.
Pathway of coagulation affected	Intrinsic Pathway	Intrinsic pathway
Whole blood clotting time	↑	↑
PTT	↑	↑
PT	N	N
BT	N	N
Platelet count	N	N
Tourniquet test	N	N

308. Answer is A (Bleeding time) : *Refer text below*

Bleeding time is prolonged in von Willebrand disease, but normal in Hemophilia A

Both conditions present with decreased levels of factor VIII normal PT and elevated PTT and hence these features cannot be used to differentiate between hemophilia A and von Willebrand disease.

Features of VWF and differences with Haemophilia A

Feature	Hemophilia A	Von Willebrand Disease
Inheritance	Sex linked	Autosomal (Most common is A.dominant)
Factor VIIIc	Decreased	Decreased
VWF	Normal	Decreased
Ristocetin cofactor	Normal	Decreased
Common Presentation	Features of clotting disorder Skin/Mucosal bleeding – Hemarthrosis ++	Features of bleeding disorder ± clotting disorder Skin/Mucosal bleeding + Hemorthrosis+
Bleeding Time	Normal	Prolonged
APTT	Prolonged	Prolonged (may be normal)
PT	Normal	Normal
Thrombin Time	Normal	Normal
Fibrinogen	Normal	Normal
Platelet aggregation in Response to Ristocetin	Normal	Decreased

309. Answer is B (Extraction should be done under General Anaesthesia): *Harrison 17th /727; Lee's Synopsis of Anaesthesia 12th/422&420, 752*

'In dentistry Surgery, General Anaesthesia is contraindicated in patients with Hemophilia' - Lee's

Von Willebrands Factor (VWF) Disease

310. Answer is A (Isolated prolonged PTT with a normal PT): *Refer previous questions*

Von Willebrand disease is characterized by prolonged bleeding time and a prolonged PTT. The prothrombin time is normal.

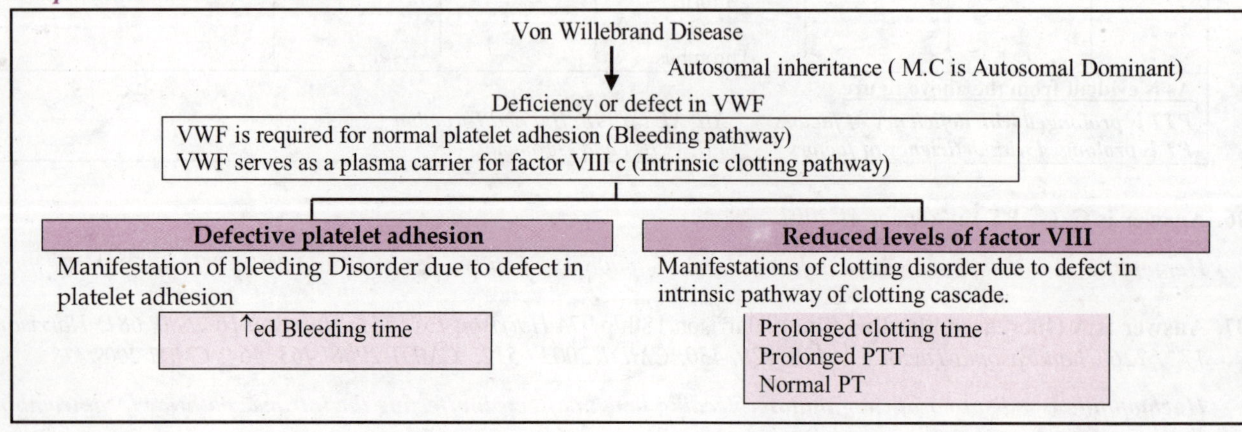

311. Answer is C (Increased platelet aggregation in response to Ristocetin): *Read text below.*

Von Willebrand disease is characterized by decreased (impaired) platelet aggregation in response to Ristocetin.

Deficiency of Factor VIII is characteristic of hemophilia and not VWF disease. ***VWF however serves as a carrier for factor VIII c and its deficiency therefore leads to decreased availability of factor VIII c at the site of injury.*** *Decaresed level of factor VIII c in the circulation may therefore be explained by a deficiency of vW factor.*

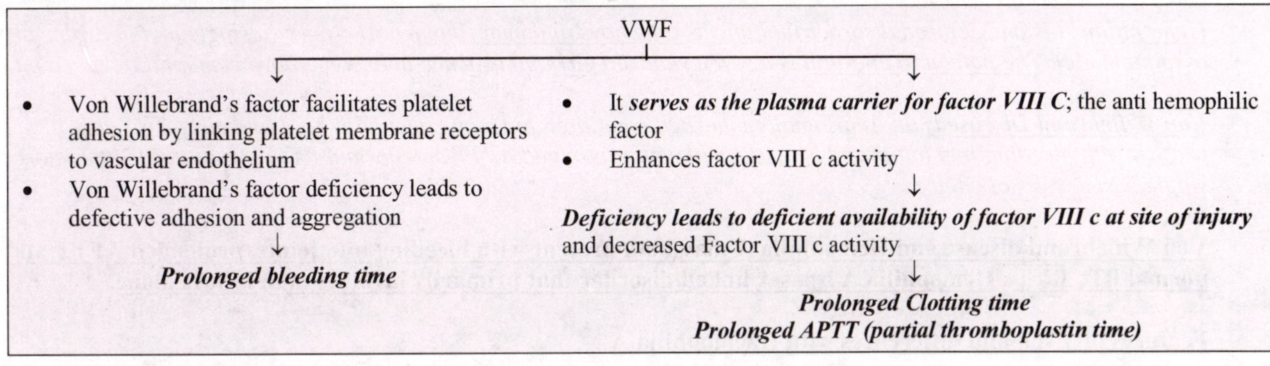

In vitro platelet aggregation is tested by addition of ristocetin an antibiotic. Ristocetin test is used for diagnosis of VWF disease by demonstrating decreased aggregation.

312. Answer is None (All statements are true): *Read text below*

Von Willebrand disease is associated with decreased levels of VWF and factor VIII in circulation. Bleeding time and APTT are prolonged. Platelet aggregation in response to ristocetin is abnormal which indicates a deficit in VWF or Ristocetin cofactor.

Von Willebrand

Von Willebrand disease is caused by a defect of deficiency of VWF factor and presents as bleeding and coagulation disorder.

VWF factor is required fir normal platelet adhesion and aggregation.
VWF factor is the plasma carrier for factor VIII which is required for intrinsic pathway of the coagulation cascade.

Von Willebrand Factor (VWF)

VWF is essentially composed of the following components

Factor VIII – VWF antigen

- This antigen binds factor VIII and acts as a carrier for factor VIII in the plasma.
- It protects factor VIII from rapid proteolytic destruction in plasma

↓ Defect in VWF (VW disease) will result in

- Decreased levels of factor VIII^Q
- Decreased activity of factor VIIIc^Q

↓

- Defect in intrinsic pathway of coagulation cascade
- Prolonged PTT^Q
- PT is normal as there is no defect in extremely pathway^Q

This antigen also acts as a mediator for initial adhesion of platelets to the vessel wall.

↓ Defect in VWF will result in

Defect in platelet function (Decreased Adhesion)

↓

Prolonged bleeding time^Q

Risocetin cofactor (VWF activity)

↓

This cofactor is required for ristocetin induced platelet aggregation

Ristocetin is an antibioctic that induces platelet aggregation

↓ Defect in VWF activity will result in

Impaired platelet aggregation in response to Ristocetin^Q

1

Hematology

313. Answer is C (Von Willebrand disease): *Harrison's 17th/725,726; Clinical Hematology 4th/381; Nelson's 17th/1660*

Bleeding into joints along with normal PT and prolonged APTT in a girl/female suggest a diagnosis of Von Willebrand disease

Bleeding into joints along with prolonged APTT and normal PT may be seen in Factor VIII deficiency (Hemophilia A) and Von Willebrand disese.

***Hemophilia** A is an X Linked disorder that affects only boys and men (Women who carry a single mutated gene are asymptomatic). The patient in question is a seven year old **girl** and is hence unlikely to have hemophilia A.*

***Von Willebrand Disease** is an Autosomally inherited condition and may affect both boys and girls. This condition may present with bleeding into joints and is associated with prolonged APTT and normal PT. VWF disease is therefore the single best answer of choice*

Von Willebrand disease and Hemophilia A may both present with bleeding into joints, prolonged APTT and normal PT BUT Hemophilia A is a sex linked disorder that primarily involves males /boys alone.

Features of VWF and differences with Haemophilia A

Feature	Hemophilia A	Von Willebrand Disease
Inheritance	***Sex linked*** Clinical disease limited to Men /boys ***(Extremely rare in females)***	***Autosomal (Most commonly A-dominant)*** Clinical disease may be seen in both boys & girls
Factor VIIIc	Decreased	Decreased
VWF	Normal	Decreased
Ristocetin cofactor	Normal	Decreased
Common Presentation	Features of clotting disorder Skin/Mucosal bleeding – ***Hemarthrosis ++***	Features of bleeding disorder ± clotting disorder Skin/Mucosal bleeding + ***Hemarthrosis+***
Bleeding Time	Normal	Prolonged
APTT	***Prolonged***	***Prolonged (may be normal)***
PT	***Normal***	***Normal***
Thrombin Time	Normal	Normal
Fibrinogen	Normal	Normal
Platelet aggregation in Response to Ristocetin	Normal	Decreased

Factor VII deficiency is associated with an isolated prolongation of PT (APTT is normal)

Causes of isolated prolongation of PT (CMDT):
Factor VII deficiency
Vitamin K deficiency
Warfarin therapy
Liver disease

Factor XII deficiency may present with an isolated prolongation of APTT (normal PT) but this condition is not associated with clinical Bleeding tendencies (Nelson/Clinical Hematoloy)

'Factor XII deficiency is a rare hereditary defect of coagulation factors in which no clinical bleeding tendancies are apparent' - Clinical Hematology

Isolated elongation of APTT with bleeding manifestations	Isolated prolongation of APTT without bleeding manifestations
Factor VIII defect	*Factor VII defect*
Factor IX defect	*Prekallekrein defect*
Factor XI defect	*HMW Kininogen defect*

314. Answer is C (BT + APTT + vWF-ristocetin factor assay): Harrison 18th/p 973, 974 *Refer previous question*

Estimation of BT, APTT and VWF-Ristocetin factor assay would provide the maximal information to aid a diagnosis of VWF disease (amongst the options provided)

315. Answer is C (Autosomal dominant): Harrison 18th/p 971 *Harrison 15th/ 747; Harrison 16th/676; Harrison 17th / 723; CMDT 2008/461*

There are 3 major forms of Von WilleBrand's disease and with one exception i.e. type III all forms are inherited as autosomal dominant trait- *Harrison 16th/676*

Von WilleBrand's disease is the most common hereditary coagulation disorder characterized by a quantitative or qualitative defect in Von Willebrand's factor

Factor VIII circulates in blood as a complex with vWF

Property	VWF	Factor VIII
Gene	Located on Q chromosome XII	Located on Q X chromosome
Inheritance	Autosomal dominant Q	Sex linked Q
Synthesis	Endothelial cells, megakaryocytes platelets (not in liver cells) Q	In liver cells Q
Function	Facilitate the adhesion of platelets to subendothelial collagen	Activation of factor X in coagulation cascade.
Disease	V. W. disease	Hemophillia

Platelet Function Disorders

316. Answer is E (Weber-Christian disease): *Harrison 18th/971; Harrison 17th/719, 723; 'Platelet' 2nd/826*

Weber Christian Disease is not an inherited disorder of platelet function.

Weber Christian Disease is a relapsing febrile nodular non suppurative panniculitis characterized by multiple recurrent subcutaneous nodules, with accompanying fever. The laboratory abnormalities include elevated ESR, Anemia, Leucopenia or leucocytosis, depression of complements and evidence of circulating immune complexes.

Classification of congenital disorder of platelet function:

1. Defects in platelet-vessel wall interaction (disorders of adhesion)
   - ***(a) von Willebrand disease (deficiency or defect in plasma vWF)***
   - ***(b) Bernard-Soulier syndrome (deficiency or defect in GPIb)***
2. Defects in platelet-platelet interaction (disorders of aggregation)
   - *(a) Congenital afibrinogenemia (deficiency of plasma fibrinogen)*
   - ***(b) Glanzmann thrombosthenia (deficiency or defect in GPIIb-IIIa)***
3. Disorders of platelet secretion and signal transduction
   - *(a) Storage pool deficiency*
   - *(b) Quebec platelet disorder*
   - *(c) Chediak Higashi syndrome*
   - *(d) Gray Platelet syndrome*
   - ***(e) Wiskott-Aldrich syndrome***
4. Disorders of platelet coagulation – protein interaction
   - *(a) Defect in facor Va-Xa interaction on platelets (Scott syndrome)*

317. Answer is B (Autosomal Recessive): *Harrison 17th/2060; Hoffman 4th/847*

Wiskot Aldrich syndrome is an X linked Recessive syndrome and not an autosomal recessive syndrome.

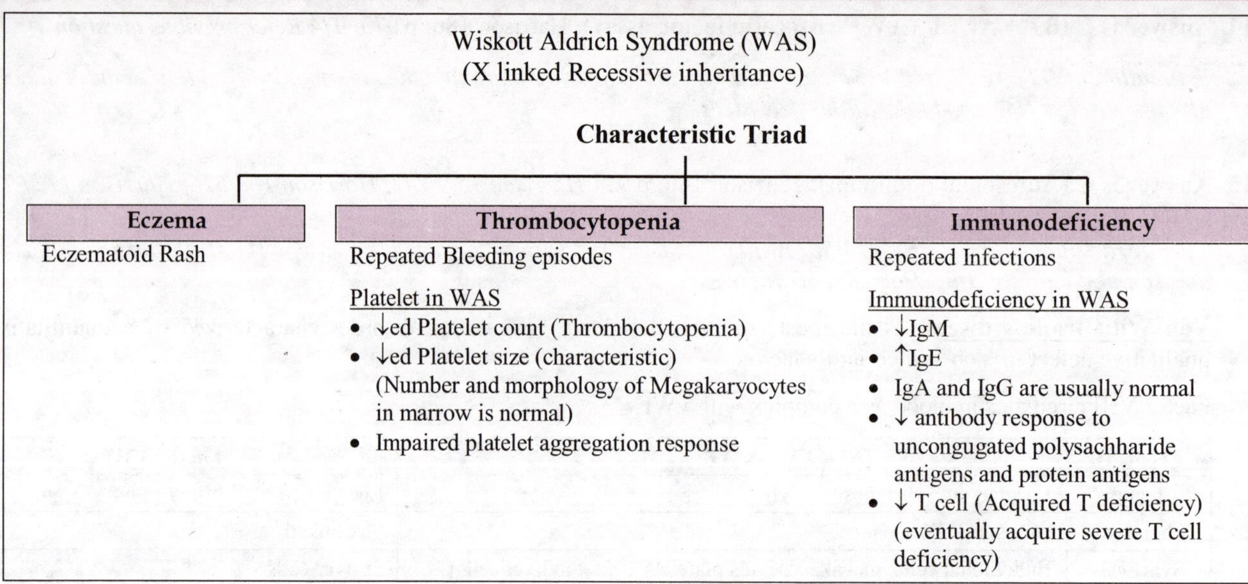

<u>Wiskott Aldrish Syndrome is associated with an impaired platelet aggregation response.</u>

'Several platelet abnormalities have been reported in Wiskott Aldrich syndrome including impaired aggregation responses'- 'Hemostasis & Thrombosis' 5th/967

318. Answer is A (Wiskott Aldrich syndrome): *Harrison 17th/2060; Hoffman 4th/847*

Thrumbocytopenia, Eczema and Recurrent Infections (Immunodeficiency) represents the charachteristic triad of Wiskott – Aldrich syndrome.

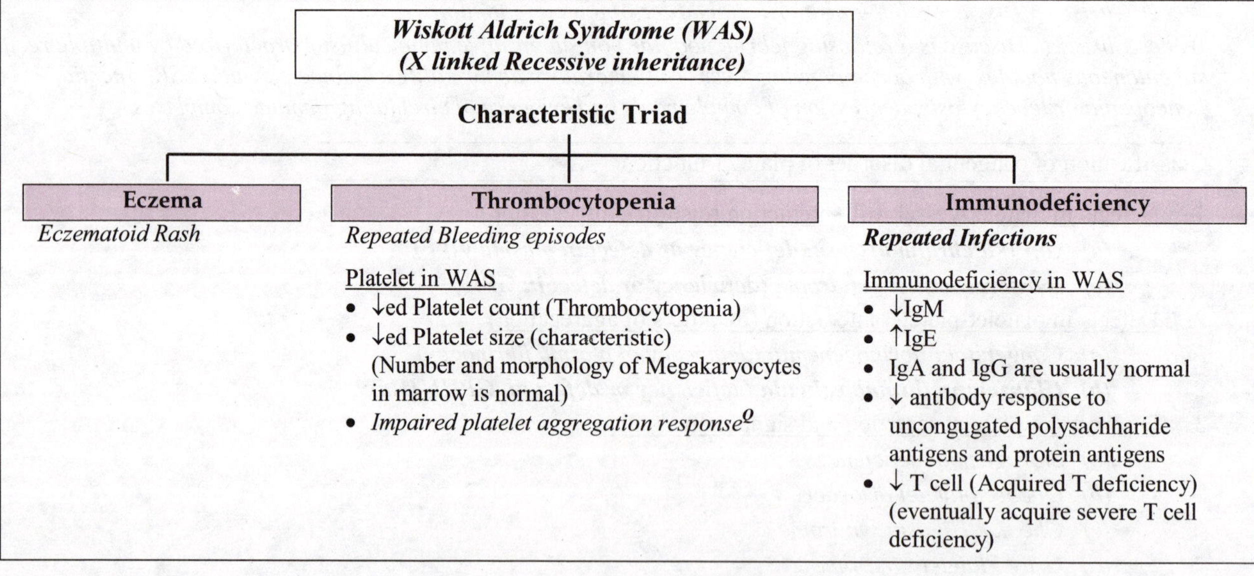

319. Answer is A i.e. (Autosomal Recessive disorder): *Harrison's 17th/ 2060; Hoffman's 4th/847*

Wiskott-Aldrich syndrome is an X-Linked Recessive Syndrome and not an Autosomal Recessive disorder

Eczema, Thrombocytopenia and Impaired Platelet Aggregation response are typical presenting features of Wiskott-Aldrich syndrome (Refer table in previous question)

320. Answer is D (Wiskott Aldrish Syndrome): Harrison 18th/p 2702, 2703 *Hoffman 4th/848; Harrison 17th/2060*

Small sized platelet is a characteristic feature of Wiskott Aldrich Syndrome.

'Platelet size is characteristically small, a feature that is highly specific for Wiskott Aldrich Syndrome'.
-Hoffman 4th/848

'Platelets in Wiskott Aldrich Syndrome are small and have a reduced half life' – Harrison

Platelets in Wiskott Aldrich Syndrome
• ↓ed Platelet count (Thrombocytopenia) • ↓ed Platelet size (characteristic) (Number and morphology of Megakaryocytes in marrow is normal) • Impaired platelet aggregation response

321. Answer is A (Ristocetin Aggregation is normal): *Harrison 16th /678; CMDT 2006/525; 2008/463; 2009/476*

'Bernard – Soulier platelets react normally to all stimuli except Ristocetin' *– Harrison 16th / 678*
'Platelet aggregation is normal in response to standard agonists (Collagen,ADP,Thrombin), but platelets fail to aggregate in response to ristocetin' *– CMDT 2006 / 525*

Intrinsic platelet defects to adhesion and aggregation.

Platelet adhesion and aggregation are modulated by glycoprotein receptors located on platelet surface.

GpIb / Ix	GpIIb / IIIa complex
• Mediates ***platelet adhesion*** • *VWF facilitates* platelet adhesion by binding to this receptor	• Mediates ***platelet aggregation*** • *Fibrinogen facilitates* platelet aggregation via sites on this receptor

Loss or defect in above glycoprotein receptors leads to rare platelet disorders causing bleeding

Bernard Soulier Syndrome	Glanzmann's thrombasthenia
• Autosomal recessive disorder • Deficiency / dysfunction of Gp Ib / Ix Receptor • ***Platelets cannot adhere*** to subendothelium because of lack of above receptors for VWF which mediates platelet adhesion • ***Platelet aggregation to largely normal platelet aggregation is normal in response to standard agonists (collagen ADP, thrombin / but platelet fail to aggregate in response to ristocetin as it acts by a different mechanism*** Other laboratory parameters • ***Thrombocytopenia may be present*** • ***Platelets on smears are abnormally large*** • Bleeding time is abnormally prolonged • VWF factor levels in plasma are normal Clinical presentation • Recurrent episodes of severe mucosal haemorrhage	• Autosomal recessive disorder • Deficiency / dysfunction of Gp IIb / III a complex • ***Platelets cannot aggregate*** because of lack of above receptors for fibrinogen which form the bridges between platelets during aggregation. • ***Platelet aggregation is largely abnormal. Platelet fail to aggregate in response to standard agonists, (ADP, collagen, thrombin) as these require fibrinogen binding, but aggregate normally to ristocetin as it cause platelet clumping by a different mechanism.*** Other laboratory parameters • Platelet number is usually normal • Platelet morphology is usually normal • Bleeding time is abnormally prolonged • VWF factor level in plasma are normal Clinical presentation • Recurrent episodes of severe mucosal hemorrhage

Note :Von Willebrand's disease : ***Platelet aggregation studies with standard agonists ADP, collagen, thrombin are normal but platelet aggregation in response to ristocetin may be subnormal (CMDT 2006 / 524).***

Thrombocytopenia and Purpura

322. Answer is A (H. S. Purpura): Harrison 18th/p 2797 *Harrisons 16th/ 341 t; Harrisons 17th/ 2128; API 8th /839 Chandrasoma Taylor 3rd/ 427*

H. S. Purpura is characterized by bleeding tendency due to vasculitis. Thrombocytes remain unaffected.

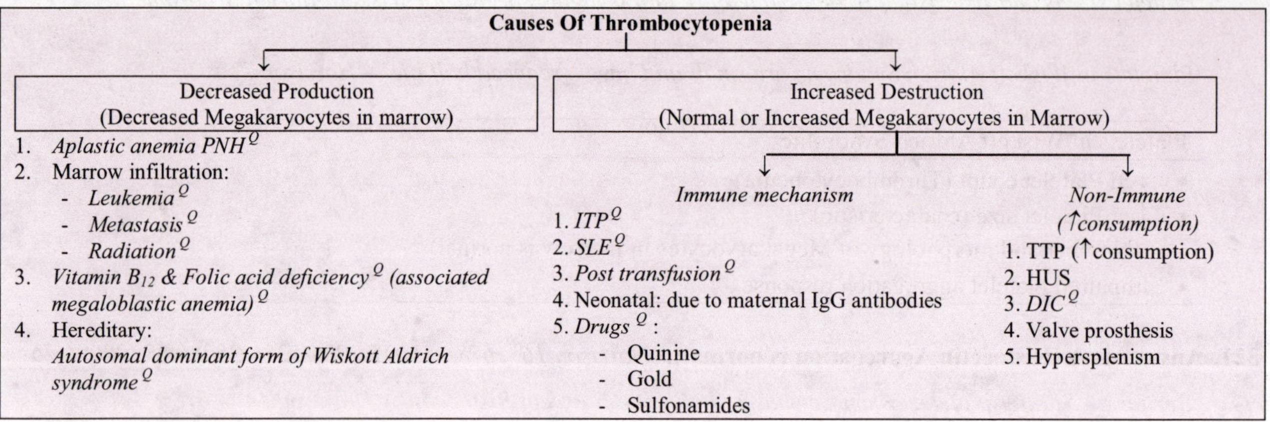

323. Answer is C (Aplastic Anemia): *Harrisons 16th/674,341; Refer previous question*

Amegakaryocytic Aplastic anemia is characterized by decreased or absent megakaryocytes (platelet precusors) and indicates a defect in production of platelets.

Amongst the options provided only aplastic anemia is associated with decreased production of platelets and causes amegakaryocytic thrombocytopenia.

The most common causes of thrombocytopenia with decreased number of megakaryocytes in marrow are aplastic anemia, marrow fibrosis and infiltration of marrow with malignant cells (Harrison)

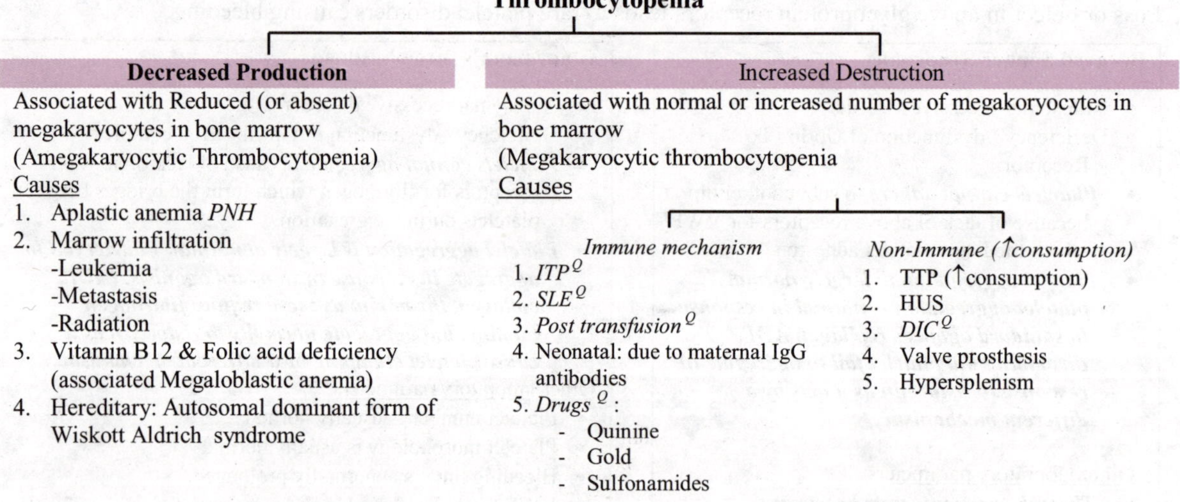

324. Answer is A (Henoch Schonlein Purpura): Harrison 18th/p 2797 *Harrison 16th/ 341, 17th / 2128; API 8th /839, Chandrasoma Taylor 3rd/427*

The mechanism of ecchymosis or purpura in Henoch Schonlein is vasculitis. There is no thrombocytopenia. All other options are known causes of thrombocytopenia.

For details on Henoch Shonlein purpura refer the chapter on 'Connective tissue and metabolism'.

325. Answer is A (H. S. Purpura): Harrison 18th/p 2797 *Harrison 17th / 2128; API 8th /839, Chandrasoma Taylor 3rd/427; Refer previous table*

The mechanism of ecchymosis or purpura in Henoch Schonlein is vasculitis. There is no thrombocytopenia. All other options are known causes of thrombocytopenia.

326. Answer is D (All of the above): *Lecture notes in Hematology 7th/168; Wintrobe's 11th/*

SLE CLL and HIV may all cause autoimmune destruction of platelets or immune thrombocytopenia

Cause of Autoimmune Thrombocytopenia

Idiopathic	Secondary
Immune Thrombocytopenic purpura (ITP)	• Connective tissue disorders (Specially SLE) • Lymphoproliferative disorders (Lymphoma, CLL) • Infections (example HIV infection) • Drugs • Solid tumors

327. Answer is A (SLE): *Harrison 16th / 341; (Refer Previous table)*

SLE is characterized by antiplatelet antibody mediated autoimmune destruction of platelets.

328. Answer is A (Thrombocytopenia) : *Harrison 18th/421; Harrisons 16th/ 309; Harrison 17th/ 334*

'Thrombocytopenia is associated with non palpable purpura'. *– Harrison 16th/309*

Causes of palpable purpura :

Emboli (bacterial fungal or parasitic)	Vasculitis
Acute meningococcemia Disseminated gonococcal infection[Q] Rocky mountain spotted fever Ecthyema gangrenosum	Leucocytoclastic vasculitis (predominantly cutaneous vasculitis) Henoch – Schonlein pupura Polyarteritis nodosa

Causes of Non palpable pupura:

Primary cutaneous disorders	Systemic diseases				
	Clotting disturbance	*Vascular fragility*	*Thrombosis*	*Emboli*	*Possible immune complex*
Trauma Solar purpura Steroid purpura Capillaritis Livedoid vasculitis	Thrombocytopenia (including ITP) Abnormal platelet function Clotting factor defects	Amyloidosis Ehlers-Danlos syndome Scurvy	Disseminated intravascular coagulation Monoclonal cryoglobulinemia Thrombotic thrombocytopenic purpura Warfarin reaction	Cholesterol Fat	Gardner-Diamond syndrome Waldenstrom's hypergammaglobulinemic purpura

329. Answer is C (H. S. Purpura): Harrison 18th/p 422, 2797 *Harrison 16th/ 309; Harrison 17th/ 335, 2128*

Henoch Sconlein Purpura is associated with palpable purpura *without thrombocytopenia*[Q]

Idiopathic Thrombocytopenic Purpura (ITP)

330. Answer is C (Antibody to platelets): *Harrison 17th / 721; Chandrasoma Taylor 3rd/ 425, Robbins 6th/ 635-636, 7th/ 651*

'There are two clinical subtypes of primary ITP, acute and chronic, both are autoimmune disorders in which platelet destruction results from the formation of antiplatelet antibodies' *– Robbins 7th/ 651*

Idiopathic thrombocytopenic purpura *is a disease characterized by severe reduction of platelet numbers, caused by immune destruction of platelets. The mechanism of ITP appears to be immune complexes containing antibodies which react with platelets and lead to their immunological destruction.*

331. Answer is A (Splenomegaly): *Robbins 7th/651,652; Ghai 6th/324*

Splenomegaly and lymphadenopathy are rare in primary Idiopathic Thrombocytopenic purpura and their presence should lead one to consider other possible diagnosis *– Robbins*

ITP

Clinical manifestations	
Clinical signs and symptoms of ITP are reflective of thrombocytopenia (Bleeding manifestations due to decreased platelet count)	
Characteristic Clinical Features	***Clinical features that are characteristically unusual and suggest the possibility of other diagnosis***
Bleeding and haemorrhages from small venules or capillaries • *Spontancous petechiae* • *Spontaneous echymoses* • *Spontancous mucosal bleeding* • *Easy Bruisibility* • *Spleen is normal in size*	• *Frequent Bleeding and haemorrhages from larger veins and arteries and bleeding into joints (Suggest coagulation disorders)* • *Splenomegaly and Lymphadenopathy are unusual/rare and their presence should lead one to consider other diagnosis.*

Laboratory Features
• Isolated thrombocytopenia • Platelet Antibodies • Normal or increased number of megakaryocytes on bone marrow examination Features of bleeding disorder • Bleeding time is prolonged • Tests of coagulation are essentially normal - Normal PT - Normal APTT - Normal Fibrinogen - Normal Fibrinogen Degradation products - Normal levels of coagulation factors

332. Answer is B (Massive splenomegaly) : *Refer Previous Question*

Immune Thrombocytopenic Purpura is not associated with massive splenomegaly

'*Hepatomegaly, splenomegaly and lymphadenopathy are notably absent in ITP, and their presence should initiate an investigation for other possible underlying illnesses associated with thrombocytopenia'- Oski's Essential Pediatrics 2nd/463*

Acute ITP is considered a self limiting condition

'Immune Thrombocytopenic purpura is a self limiting condition and most children will have normal platelet count within 8-12 weeks even without treatment' – 'Pediatrics: A concise Text' by Kabro & Srivastava 1st/164

'*Acute ITP in children frequently has a benign course with an excellent prognosis. More than 50% of untreated children with ITP recover within 4 weeks without treatment and more than 80% recover 6 months' – Oski's 2nd/463*

Intravenous immunoglobulins may be required for treatment of ITP

'Intravenous Immunoglobulin is a useful modality for treatment of ITP' -Oski's 2nd/464

Common Treatment Modalities for ITP *(Platelet count <20,000/μl or significant mucosal bleeding)*
• *Corticosteroids* • *IV Immunoglobulins / gamma globulins* • *Additional Immunosupressive agents (Rituximab / Anti CD 20 Antibody)* • *Splenectomy*

Immune Thrombocytic Purpura (ITP)
(Idiopathic Thrombocytopenic Purpura)

Autoimmune Antibodies against Platelets

From response to ***previous viral infection***[Q] (Acute ITP) or From underlying immune dysregulation (chronic ITP)

↓ *Platelet destruction*

Thrombocytopenia

Clinical Features	Laboratory Features
• Bleeding from skin (purpura) and mucosal sites (most prominent symptom) -Ecchymoses / Petichiae -Bruising -Gum bleeding -Epistaxis • Bleeding into the CNS (most feared complication) Rare (<1%) *Bleeding into Joints (Hemarthrosis) is unusual* *Hepatomegaly, splenomegaly & Lymphadenopathy are notably absent*	• *↓ Platelet count* • *Platelet antibodies +nt* • *Normal / ↑ed megakaryocytes in marrow* • *↑Bleeding time* • *Normal coagulation tests* - *PT normal* - *PTT normal* - *CT normal* - *Fibrinogen / FDP Normal* - *Coagulation factors normal*

333. Answer is A (Bleeding into joints is a common manifestation): *Robbins 7th/651,652; Ghai 6th/329*

The patient in question is presenting with Acute Idiopathic Thrombocytopenic Purpura (ITP) Bleeding into joints is an uncommon manifestation of ITP.

Bleeding into joints is commonly seen in coagulation disorders and not in bleeding disorders (platelet disorders) like ITP

Thrombocytopenia, increased number of megakaryocytes and spontaneous remission in 80% of cases are characteristic features of Acute ITP.

Features of Acute ITP

Characteristics	Feature
Peak Age incidence	2-6 years
Sex predilection	None
Presenting features	• *Preceding/Antecedent viral infection seen in about 50% of cases* • *Bleeding from mucosal surfaces with frequent petichea and echymoses* ***Bleeding into joints is unusual*** • Spleen is normal is size ***No Hepatosplenomegaly or Lymphadenopathy***
Laboratory features	• ***Thrombocytopenia*** • Platelet Antibodies (Antibodies against platelets) • ***Normal or Increased megakaryocytes in marrow*** • Prolonged Bleeding time • Normal tests for Coagulation - PT Normal - PTT Normal - Fibrinogen Normal - FDP Normal - Coagulation factors Normal
Course and Prognosis	Self Limiting Course ***Spontaneous remission is seen in 80% of cases in 4-6 weeks***

334. Answer is C (Spontaneous remission is common in chronic ITP): *Ghai 6th/324; Wintrobe's 11th/1534*

Spontaneous remission is common in Acute Form of ITP but it is an uncommon feature of chronic ITP

Idiopathic/immune Thrombocytopenic purpura
ITP occurs in two forms, namely acute ITP and chronic ITP
Acute ITP and chronic ITP differ in incidence, prognosis and therapy

Features of Acute and Chronic Idiopathic Thrombocytopenic Purpura (ITP)

Features	Acute ITP	Chronic ITP
Peak age of incidence	Children, 2-6 yr	Adults 20-40 yr
Sex predilection	None	3:1 female to male
Antecedent infection	Common 1-3 wk before	Unusual
Onset of bleeding	Abrupt	Insidious
Hemorrhagic bullae in mouth	Present in severe cases	Usually absent
Platelet count	<20,000 / μl	30,000-80,000/μl
Eosinophilia and lympocytosis	Common	Rare
Duration	2-6 wk; rarely longer	Months or years
Spontaneous remission	Occur in 80% of cases	Uncommon

335. Answer is C (Bleeding time): Harrison 18th/p 460 *Harrison 17th / 366; See text below*

Bleeding time is indicative of function of platelets. ***In any form of thrombocytopenia it is platelets that are affected and hence the deranged parameter would be bleeding time.***

PT, APTT and Clotting time are parameters of coagulation disorders and not bleeding disorders. These parameters will be normal in disorders of platelet function.

336. Answer is B (Immunogenic Thrombocytopenia): Harrison 18th/p 968 *Harrison 15th/ 747; Harrisons 16th/675; Harrison 17th / 722*

Immunogenic thrombocytopenias are caused by immune mediated destruction of platelets and therefore platelet supplementation is unlikely to benefit.

Hemorrhage in a case of immunogenic thrombocytopenia such as Idiopathic Thrombocytopenic Purpura (ITP) is **controlled by** -

- Glucocorticoids
- Intravenous Immunoglobulins
- Splenectomy

Thrombotic Thrombocytopenic Purpura (TTP)

337. Answer is C (Hypertension): *Harrison 18th/969, 970; 16th/678, 679; 17th / 722, 723; CMDT 2008/459; CMDT 2009/472*

Blood pressure is normal in Thrombotic Thrombocytopenic purpura.

Thrombotic Thrombocytopenic purpura is a disorder of 'vessel wall' Q characterised by lesions in arteriolar walls Q in various organs that initiate formation of **localised platelet thrombi and fibrin deposits at various sites.**

Clinical Pentad of TTP

Microangiopathic Hemolytic Anemia Q (Coomb's negative)	**Thrombocytopenia** Q (due to consumption of platelets)	**Decreased Renal Function** Q (due deposits in the Renal Vasculature.)	**Disturbed Neurological function** Q	**Fever**
- Haemolysis Q - Fragmentation Q of RBC's - Increased LDH (elevated due to intra- vascular hemolysis) Q			Characteristically diffuse and non focal eg. - Confusion - Aphasia Alteration in consciousness	

Tests of coagulation are essentially normal Q
- Normal PT Q - Normal APTT Q - Normal Fibrinogen concentration Q - Normal Fibrin degradation Products Q

Thus: PENTAD as mentioned above + normal coagulation tests: PATHOGNOMIC OF TTP

338. Answer is D i.e. (Grossly abnormal coagulation tests): Harrison 18th/p 969 *Harrison's 17th /722, 723; Refer previous question*

Tests of coagulation are essentially normal in Thrombotic Thrombocytopenic Purpura (TTP).

Clinical Pentad + Normal Tests for coagulation : TTP

Clinical Pentad of TTP
• *Microangiopathic Hemolytic Anemia* • *Thrombocytopenia* • *Decreased Renal function* • *Disturbed Neurological function* • *Fever*

339. Answer is C (Hypertension): *Refer Previous question*

Hypertension is not a typical feature of TTP

Fever, Hemolysis (microangiopathic intravascular hemolysis) and Low platelet count (Thrombocytopenia) are part of the 'pentad' of TTP

340. Answer is A (Plasma Exchange Therapy): *Harrison 18th/p 970 Harrison's 17th/ 723*

Plasma Exchange Therapy is the treatment of choice for TTP

Pentad of Fever, Microangiopathic Hemolytic Anemia, Thrombocytopenia (platelets count = 20,000), Renal Failure (↑serum creatinine) and Neurological dysfunction (altered consciousness) together with normal tests of coagulation (normal PT and aPTT) confirms a diagnosis of Thrombotic Thrombocytopenic Purpura. Plasma Exchange forms the mainstay of treatment of TTP.

'Plasma Exchange remains the mainstay of treatment of TTP' – Harrison's 17th/723

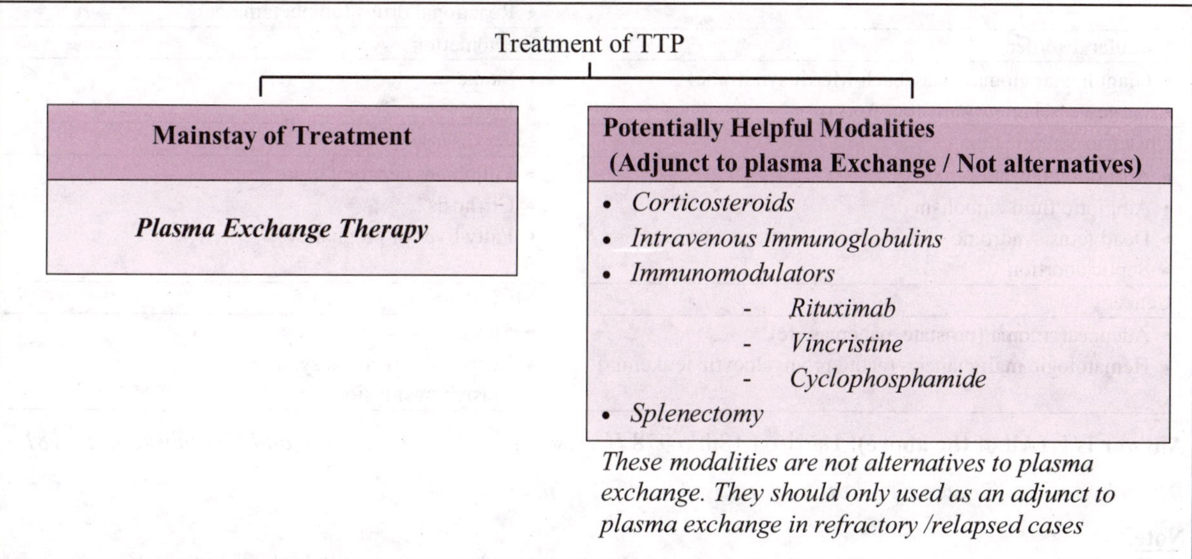

341. Answer is D & E (Heparin & Platelet transfusion): *'The Cleveland Clinic Internal Medicine Case Review' (2003)/153*

Heparin and platelet transfusions are not used in the treatment of Thrombotic Thrombocytopenic Purpura

Heparin and platelet transfusions are not used in treatment of TTP

'Heparin is not indicated in the treatment of TTP-HUS. Platelet transfusion is also not indicated and may worsen neurological symptoms and renal dysfunction. Platelet transfusion can lead to the geeration of new or expanding thrombi, as the infused platelets are transfused' - *Cleveland Clinic Internal Medicine Case Reviews (2003)/153*

Plasmapharesis, Corticosteroids and Immunotherapy may be used in treatment of TTP

Plasmapharesis forms the mainstay of treatment for TTP. Corticosteroids and Immunotherapy may be used as adjuncts to plasma exchange in refractory /relapsed cases.

Disseminated Intravascular Coagulation (DIC)

342. Answer is D (All of the above): Harrison 18th/p 978 *Harrison 17th/34*

DIC may be associated with all of the options provided in the question.

Common Clinical causes of Disseminated Intravascular Coagulation:

Sepsis	Immunologic disorders
• Bacterial • Staphylococci, streptococci, pneomococci, meningococci, gram-negative bacilli • Viral • Mycotic • Parasitic • Rickettsial	• Acute hemolytic transfusion reaction • Organ or tissue transplant rejection • Graft-versus-host disease
Trauma and tissue injury	**Drugs**
• Brain injury (gunshot) • Extensive burns • Fat embolism • Rhabdomyolysis	• Fibrinolytic agents • Aprotinin • Warfarin (especially in neonates with protein C deficiency) • Prothrombin complex concentrates • Reactional drugs (amphetamines)
Vascular disorders	**Evenomation**
• Giant hemangiomas (Kasabach-Merrit syndrome) • Large vessel aneurysms (eg. Aorta)	• Snake • Insects
Obstetric complications	**Liver disease**
• Abruptio placentas • Amniotic fluid embolism • Dead fetus syndrome • Septic abortion	• Fulminant hepatic failure • Cirrhosis • Fatty liver of pregnancy
Cancer	**Miscellaneous**
• Adenocarcinoma (prostate, pancreas etc) • Hematologic malignancies (acute promyelocytic leukemia)	• Shock • Respiratory distress syndrome • Masive trasnfusion

343. Answer is E (All of the above): Harrison 18th/p 978 *Harrison 17th/729; Thrombosis and Hemmorhage 3rd/781*

DIC may be associated with all of the options provided in the questions.

Note:
Although Lymphoma is not mentioned as a cause in Harrison's text, it is an established cause for DIC.

Common Neoplastic causes of DIC - *Thrombosis & Hemorrhage 3rd/781*

Solid Tumors	Leukemia
• Adenocarcinoma (prostate, pancreas etc) • Lymphoma	• Acute Promyclocytic Leukemia (characteristic) • Acute Myelogenous • Chronic Myelogenous • Acute Lymphoblastic • Others

344. Answer is C (Decreased PTT): Harrison 18th/p 979 *Harrison 17th / 729; CMDT 2003 / 516-18; 2005/511-513; 2008/467, 468; CMDT 2009/474*

PTT is increased in DIC

DIC or Disseminated Intravascular Coagulation, is a complex thrombohaemorrhagic disorder characterized by the following sequence of events in general :

Events
1. Intravascular activation of coagulation by *both intrinsic and extrinsic mechanism.* Q
2. A thrombotic phase
3. Consumption phase, wherein most coagulation factors and platelets are consumed.
4. Stage of secondary fibrinolysis, at site of intravascular coagulation.

Laboratory findings are in accordance with the above pathogenic mechanisms :
1. *Platelets count, coagulation factors and fibrinogen level: are decreased* Q or 'consumed'. As a result of above: The *bleeding time as well as the coagulation time both are prolonged* Q therefore - *PTT: increased Q* - *PT: increased* Q - *Thrombin time : increased* Q 2. Increased secondary fibrinolysis accounts for - *raised plasmin levels* Q - *raised levels of fibrin degradation product (FDP).* Q 3. The thrombolic phase accounts for *features of microangiopathic haemolytic anemia.* Q - *presence of schistiocytes, spherocytes, burr cells, halmet cells in the peripheral film.* Q
Some question asked: • Most important treatment is : finding a reversible cause and *treatment of the cause* Q • *Finding in DIC, that correlates best and most closely with bleeding is : fibrinogen level* Q • Most common site for thrombin formation in DIC is : Brain Q (Brain > heart > lung > kidney > adrenal > liver) • DIC is related to 2 very important endocrine manifestations : a. *Adrenals - Fredrich Hausen Syndrome.* Q b. *Pituitary - Sheehan's Syndrome.* Q

345. Answer is D (Increased FDP, prolonged PT, Reduced platelets): *Harrison 18th/p 979; 16th / 683; Harrison 17th / 729*

The laboratory manifestation of DIC include ***thrombocytopenia (Reduced platelets), prolonged PT****, PTT and thrombin time (TT). Reduced fibrinogen levels from depletion of coagulation protein and* ***elevated FDP*** *from intense secondary fibromolysis - Harrison*

346. Answer is B (Serum FDP): *Harrisons 17th/729*

The most sensitive test for DIC is the FDP level *– Harrisons*

FDP levels and DIC – Harrison

- The most sensitive test for DIC is the FDP level
- DIC is an unlikely diagnosis in the absence of normal FDP
- The D-Dimer test is a specific test for detection of FDP and indicates that the cross linked fibrin has been digested by plasmin

Note

Because fibrinogen has a prolonged half life, plasma levels diminish acultely in only severe cases of DIC.
Low fibrinogen levels predict the tendency of bleeding in DIC

Q Most sensitive test for DIC is – Elevated FDP levels Q Most sensitive test for DIC that predicts tendency of bleeding in - Serum Fibrinogen levels

347. Answer is C (Low serum fibrinogen level): Harrison 18th/p 979 *Harrisons 16th/684*

Finding in DIC that corvelates relates to bleeding tendency is serum fibrinogen levels

'Low fibrinogen levels predicts more bleeding'- *Harrison*

348. Answer is C (M3-AML): *Ghai 6th/567; Repeat; Robbins*

DIC or DIVC may occur in any subgroup of AML but is especially common in Acute Promyelocytic Leukemia or M3-AML of FAB classification.

349. Answer is C (Decreased coagulation factor levels): Harrison 18th/p 969, 970, 979 *Harrison 17th / 722, 723, 729; Refer previous two questions*

While coagulation factors are characteristically consumed (decreased) in case of DIC their levels are essentially normal in case of TTP

Hypercoagulable States / Thrombosis

General

350. Answer is B (factor V Leiden deficiency): *Harrison 16th/342*

Factor V Leiden mutation (or ↑ Factor V Leiden levels) are associated with a hypercoaguable state and not a Factor V Leiden deficiency.

Inherited	Acquired
• Defective inhibition of coagulation factors - Factor V Leiden (resistant to inhibition by activated protein C) - Antithrombin III deficiency (or resistance) - Protein C deficiency (or resistance) - Protein S deficiency (or resistance) - Prothrombin gene mutation (G20210A) • Impaired clot lysis - Dysfibrinogenemia - Plasminogen deficiency - tPA deficiency - PAI-I excess • Uncertain mechanism - Homocystinuria	• Diseases or syndromes - Lupus anticoagulant/anticardiolipin antibody syndrome - Malignancy - Myeloproliferative disorder - Thrombotic thrombocytopenic purpura - Estrogen treatment - Hyperlipidemia - Diabetes mellitus - Hyperviscosity - Nephrotic syndrome - Congestive heart failure - Paroxysmal nocturnal hemoglobinuria • Physiologic states - Pregnancy (especially postpartum) - Obesity - Postoperative state - Immobilization - Old stage

351. Answer is C (Idiopathic Thrombocytopenic Purpura (ITP)): *Harrisons 17th/367, 741*

Idiopathic Thrombocytopenic Purpura (ITP) is an immune complex mediated thrombocytopenia characterized by varying degrees of bleeding manifestations due to destruction of platelets. ITP is not associated with an increased incidence of venous and/or arterial thrombosis.

Paroxysmal Nocturnal Haemoglobinuria (PNH), Diseminated Intravascular Coagulation (DIC) and Heparin Induced Thrombocytopenia (HIT) are all associated with increased risk of venous and/or arterial thrombotic events.

Risk factors for Thrombosis:

Venous	Venous and Arterial
Inherited	**Inherited**
Factor V Leiden	*Homocystinuria*
Prothrombin G20210A	*Dysfibrinogenemia*
Antithrombin deficiency	
Protein S deficiency	
Elevated F VIII	
Acquired	**Acquired**
Age	*Malignancy*
Previous thrombosis	*Antiphospholipid antibody syndrome (APLA)*
Immobilization	*Hormonal therapy*
Major surgery	*Polycythemia vera*
Pregnancy &puerperium	*Essential thrombocythemia*
Hospitalization	***Paroxysmal nocturnal hemoglobinuria (PNH)***
Obesity	Thrombotic thrombocytopenic Purpura *(TTP)*
Infection	***Heparin-induced thrombocytopenia (HIT)***
APC resistance, nogenetic	***Disseminated intravascular cogulation (DIC)***
Unknown[a]	**Mixed (Inherited and acquired)**
Elevated factor II, IX, XI	*Hyperhomocysteinemia*
Elevated TAFI levels	
Low levels of TFPI	

[a]Unknown whether risk is inherited or acquired.

Note APC, activated protein C; TAFI, thrombin-activatable fibrinolysis inhibitor; TFPI, tissue factor pathway inhibitor.

Note : Heparin induced Thrombocytopenia is more commonly associated with Thrombosis than Bleeding

Heparin induced Thrombocytopenia is more commonly associated with Thrombosis than Bleeding

- Heparin induced thrombocytopenia should be included in the differential diagnosis of conditions that produce thrombosis despite thrombocytopenia.
- ***Despite thrombocytopenia bleeding is rare in HIT.***
  On the contrary HIT is more related to thrombosis, which often leads to initial recognition of this condition (HIT).

  'Thrombosis often leads to initial recognition of HIT. Bleeding is rare despite thrombocytopenia'

  - Essentials of Emergency Medicine (2006)/286

Thrombocytopenia with Thrombosis
DIC
TTP
HUS
HIT

- *Thrombosis* in Heparin Induced Thrombocytopenia is *caused by the generation of prothrombotic platelet microparticles that promote thrombin generation.*

HIT is an antibody – mediated process that is triggered by antibodies directed against neoantigens on PF4 that are exposed when heparin binds to this protein. These antibodies (usually IgG type) bind simultaneously to heparin PF4 complex and to platelet Fc receptors. Such binding activates the platelets and generates platelet microparticles. Circulating microparticles are prothrombotic because they express anionic phospholipids on their surface and can bind clotting factors and promote thrombin generation.

- **Features of Heparin-Induced Thrombocytopenia**

Features	**Details**
Thrombocytopenia	*Platelet count of ≤100,000/□L or a decrease in platelet count ≥ 50%*
Timing	*Platelet count falls 5-10 days after starting heparin*
Type of heparin	*More common with unfractionated heparin than with low-molecular-weight heparin*
Type of patient	*More common in surgical patients than medical patients; more common in women than in men.*
Thrombosis	*Venous thrombosis more common than arterial thrombosis*

352. Answer is C (Hypomagnesemia): *Harrison 15th/ 359, Harrison 16th/ 342; Harrison 17th/ 367*

All conditions other than hypmagnesemia are known predisposing causes of thrombosis.

353. Answer is D (Dysfibrinogenemia): *Harrison 16th/342*

Dysfibrinogenemia is associated with a hypercoagulable state.
Deficiency of Protein C, Protein S and Antithrombin III are associated with hypocoagulable states and not their elevated levels (↑)

354. Answer is B (Leiden mutation): *Harrison 16th/342; Refer text below*

Hypercoagulability due to defective Factor V gene is called 'Leiden mutation' and is named after the city in which it was described.

Factor V Leiden
- Factor V Leiden is a variant (mutated) of normal clotting factor V and differs from normal clotting factor V by a single nucleotide.
- While Factor V Leiden is completely normal in terms of its ability to prevent bleeding, the one amino acid difference makes Factor V Leiden resistant to being degraded by activated protein C and protein S.
- Consequently factor V Leiden persists in the circulation longer and contributes to formation of blood clots.
- Factor V Leiden mutation is the most common underlying genetic cause of thrombophilia (venous thrombosis)
- Factor V Leiden mutation poses a life long risk of deep venous thrombosis.

355. Answer is C (Factor V Leiden Mutation): *William's 7th/1984; The Five Minute Clinical Consult (2009)/470; Clinical Hematology 4th/386*

Factor V Leiden mutation is the most common inherited thrombotic disorder

Most common genetic cause for thrombophilia	:	*Factor V Leiden*
Most common congenital cause of venous thrombosis	:	*Factor V Leiden*
Most common hereditary blood coagulation disorder	:	*Factor V leiden*

356. Answer is D (Homocystenemia): *Harrison 16th/686*

Homocystenemia is associated with increased risk of arterial thrombosis.

Deficiency of AT III, Protein C and Protein S predisposes to venous thrombosis and not arterial thrombosis.

Abnormality	Arterial	Venous
Factor V Leiden mutation	—	+
Prothrombin	—	+
Antithrombin III	—	+
Protein C	—	+
Protein S	—	+
Homocysteinemia	+	+
Antiphospholipid syndrome	+	+

357. Answer is None or A (Infection) : *CMDT 2003 / 468 ' Principles of pharmacology' by Golan, Armstrong 2nd/397, The Washington Manual of Hematology and Oncology' (2003) / 27*

Infection has not been mentioned as a direct cause of hypercoagulability in any standard textbook and is the single best answer of exclusion.

Acquired Condition	Mechanism of Hyper Coagulability
• Antiphospholipid syndrome	• Autoantibodies to negatively charged phospholipids →↑platelet adhesion
• Heparin-induced thrombocytopenia	• Antibodies to platelet factor 4 → platelet activation
• Malignancy	• Tumor cell induction of tissue factor expression
• ***Myeloproliferative syndromes***	• Elevated blood viscosity, altered platelets
• Nephrotic syndrome	• Loss of antithrombin III in urine↑. Fibrinogen,↑ platelet activation
• Oral contraceptive use, estrogen replacement therapy	• ↑Hepatic synthesis of coagulation factos and/or effects of estrogen on endothelium (effect may be more prominent in patients with underlying primary hypercoagulability)
• Paroxysmal nocturnal hemoglobinuria	• Unknown, possibly "leaky" platelets
• Postpartum period /Pregnancy	• Venous stasis, increased coagulation factors, tissue trauma
• ***Surgery /trauma (postoperative period)***	• Venous stasis, immobilization, tissue injury
• ***Inflammatory Bowel Disease***	• Increased inflammatory mediators down regulate thrombomodulin leading to impaired generation of APC. • Elevated levels of factor VIII, Fibrinogen; ↓ Protein S activity.

Prolonged surgery *has been directly mentioned in association with hypercoagulable states in some standard text books including 'Washington Manual of Hematology and Sub specialty consult'*

Also 'postoperative state' is an established cause of hypercoagulability (CMDT) and hence prolonged surgery has been included as a correct option.

358. Answer is A (Diabetes Mellitus) : Harrison 18th/p 883, 987 *Harrisons 17th / 632, 732, 660; CMDT 2008 / 468)*

Diabetes Mellitus has not been mentioned as a risk factor for deep venous thrombosis.

Prolonged surgery and OCP usage are established risk factors.
PNH is associated with hypercoagulability (CMDT 2008) and an increased risk of deep venous thrombosis.

Acquired	Inherited	Mixed/Unknown
Orthopedic surgery	*Antithrombin deficiency*	*High levels of factor VIII*
Neurosurgery	*Protein C deficiency*	*High levels of factor IX*
Major abdominal surgery	*Protein S deficiency*	*High levels of fibrinogen*
Major trauma	*Factor V Leiden (FVL)*	*High levels of TAFI*
Central venous catheters	*Prothrombin 20210A*	*Low levels of TFPI*

Malignancy	*Non-O blood group*	*APC resistance in the absence of FVL*
Antiphospholipid syndrome	*Dysfibrinogenemia*	*Hyperhomocysteinemia*
Puerperium	*Factor XIII 34val*	*High levels of PCI (PAI-3)*
Prolonged bed rest		
Pregnancy		
Obesity		
Plastercast		
Oral contraceptives		
Hormonal replacement therapy		
Myeloproliferative disorders		
Polycythemia vera		
Long-haul travel		
Age		
***PNH** (Harrison's 17th/632)*		

TAFI, thrombin activable fibrinolysis inhibitors; TFPI, tissue factor pathway inhibitor; PCI, protein C inhibitor; PAI-3, plasminogen activator inhibitor-3; APC, activated protein C

359. Answer is C (Antibodies to factor VIII) : Harrison 18th/p 986, 987 *Harrison 16th/e 686; 17th/ 367,732,733,734; CMDT 2008/465; CMDT 2009/480*

Antibodies to factor VIII should be suspected in a disorder presenting with 'bleeding' and not in presenting with recurrent thrombosis.

- *'Antibodies against factor VIII should be suspected in any acquired severe bleeding disorder associated with a prolonged PTT' – CMDT*
- *Factor VIII antibodies are distinguished from lupus anticoagulant by presence of clinical bleeding.' – CMDT*

Approach to Patient presenting with deep venous thrombosis

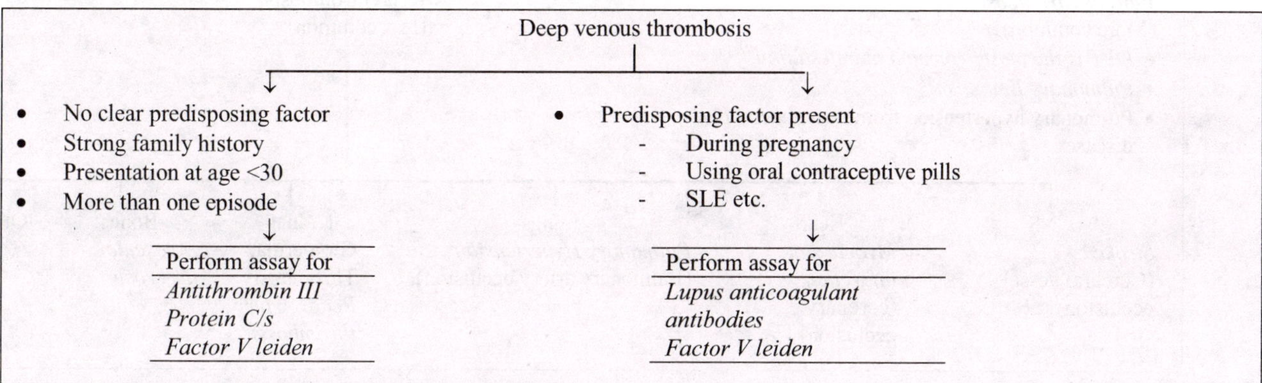

Major coagulation defects associated with venous thrombosis
Factor V leiden (commonest association with DVT)
Antithrombin III deficiency
Protein C deficiency
Protein S deficiency
Prothrombin gene mutation
Homocyteinemia
Antiphospholipid antibody

Homocyteinemia and Antiphospholipid antibodies are also associated with arterial thrombi (others being associated with venous thrombosis only).

Antiphospholipid Syndrome

360. Answer is A (Pancytopenia): *Harrison 18th/987; 17th/732, 1579, 2082; API textbook Medicine 8th/306, 307*

Venous thrombosis, recurrent abortions and pulmonary hypertension are recognized clinical manifestations of Antiphospholipid Syndrome (APS).

***Anti phospholipid syndrome has also not been listed as a cause for Pancytopenia.** Antiphospholipid syndrome may lead to thromboytopenia in (40- 50% cases) and hemolytic anemias in 14-25% of cases but leucopenia has not been mentioned in association with Anti phospholipid syndrome.*

Pancytopenia is the single best answer of exclusion.

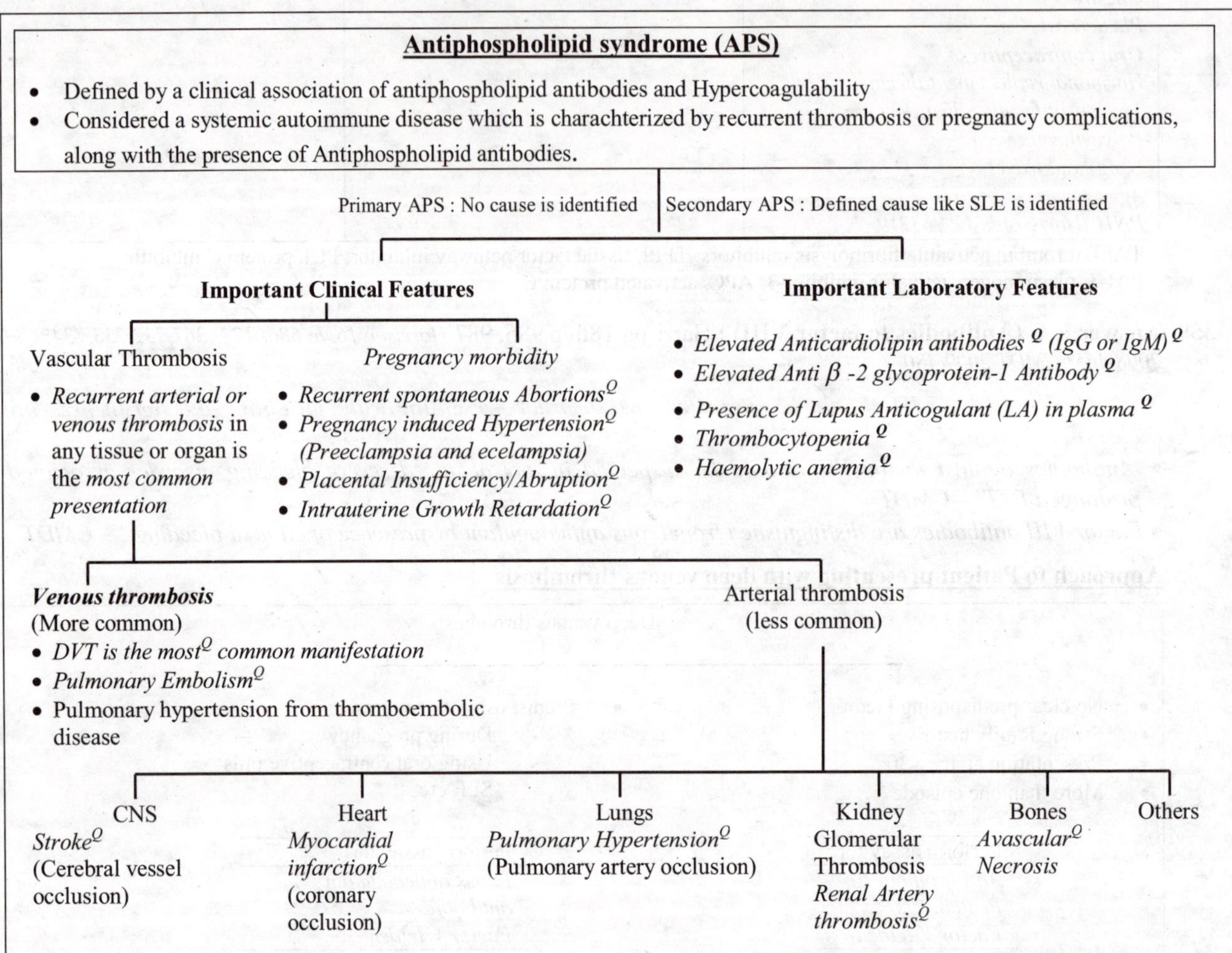

361. Answer is A (Bleeding disorders): Harrison 18th/p 987, 2734 *API Textbook of Medicine 8th/ed 306, 307; Harrison's 17th/ 732, 1579, 2082; 'Current Diagnosis and Treatment in Rheumatology' 2nd/219*

Antiphospholipid Antibody Syndrome is associated with thrombotic disorders and not bleeding disorders

Antiphospholipid Antibody syndrome (APLA) is primarily a disorder of coagulation resulting in a hypercoagulation state. ***Manifestations of Antiphospholipid Antibody syndrome including recurrent thrombosis and fetal loss result from the hypercoagulable state. Bleeding disorders are not seen.***

362. Answer is A (Single titre of Anticardiolipin is diagnostic): Harrison 18th/p 987, 2734 *API Textbook of Medicine 8th/ed 306, 307; Harrison's 17th/ 732, 1579, 2082; 'Current Diagnosis and Treatment 'Rheumatology' 2nd/219*

Single titre of anticardiolipin antibodies does not establish a diagnosis of APLAb syndrome
Laboratory criteria require anticardiolipin antibodies to be present on 2 or more occasions at least 12 weeks apart.
A Definite diagnosis of Antiphospholipid Syndrome requires at least one clinical criteria and one laboratory criteria to be met.

Diagnostic Criteria for Antiphospholipid Syndrome

Definitive Antiphospholipid Syndrome is said to be present if atleast one of the clinical criteria and one of the laboratory criteria are met

Clinical Criteria	Laboratory Criteria
• **Vascular Thrombosis (Arterial and/or Venous)** One or more clinical episodes of arterial, venous or small vessel thrombosis in any tissue or organ. • **Pregnancy morbidity** a. *One or more unexplained deaths* of a morphologically normal fetus at or *beyond the 10th week of gestation*, with normal fetal morpholoogy b. *One or more premature births* of a morphologically normal neonate *before the 34th week of gestation* because of: (a) eclampsia or severe preeclampsia (b) placental insufficiency c. *Three or more unexplained consecutive spontaneous abortions before the 10th week of gestation*, with maternal anatomic or hormonal abnormalities and paternal and maternal chromosomal causes excluded.	• **Anticardiolipin Antibody** of IgG and /or IgM isotype in serum or plasma *on 2 or more occasions, at least 12 weeks apart* • **Lupus anticoagulant** present in plasma, *on 2 or more occasions at least 12 weeks apart* • **Anti-β_2- glycoprotein-1 antibody** of IgG and or IgM isotype in serum or plasma, present *on 2 or more occasions, at least 12 weeks apart*

Recurrent fetal loss is a common manifestation of Antiphospholipid Syndrome

Recurrent fetal loss is an established Pregnancy associated morbidity of Antiphospholipid syndrome and is included in the diagnostic criteria (Refer previous question)

Antiphospholipid Syndrome may cause Pulmonary Hypertension

Pulmonary hypertension may be seen as a consequence of recurrent subclinical pulmonary emboli (Refer previous question)

Warfarin is used in the treatment of Antiphospholipid Syndrome

'The mainstay of treatment of Antiphospholipid Syndrome is Warfarin' - Harrison

363. Ans is C (Thrombocytosis): *Dutta 5th 1364: 4th/364*

Antiphospholipid syndrome is associated with thrombocytopenia and not thrombocytosis.

Common obstetric complications associated with antiphospholipid syndrome are:
1. Recurrent fetal loss[Q]   2. IUGR[Q]   3. Pregnancy associated hypertension[Q]   4. Placental abruption[Q]   5. Recurrent thrombotic events[Q]   6. Thrombocytopenia[Q] (and not thrombocytosis).

364. Answer is A (Thrombocytosis): *Refer previous question*

Antiphospholipid syndrome secondary to lupus anticoagulant is associated with thrombocytopenia and not thrombocytosis

365. Answer is D or none(Increased PT or none): *CMDT 2008/469; Thrombosis and Hemorrhage' 3rd/326; CMDT 2009/735*

The Lupus Anticoagulant typically causes an isolated prolongation of APTT. Prothrombin time is usually normal although slight prolongation in PT may also be observed

Lupus anticoagulant should be suspected in cases of markedly prolonged PTT without clinical bleeding and normal or slightly elevated PT- CMDT

<u>Lupus Anticoagulant</u>

- Lupus anticoagulant is an 'antiphospholipid' seen in about 5 to 10% of cases of SLE
- The term 'anticoagulant' is a misnomer as LA acts as a procoagulant casuing increased tendency of thrombosis and does not act as an anticoagulant.

> *'It is mistermed as an 'anticoagulant' because it causes prolongation of PTT in the vitro PTT assay'*
> *(This prolongation is produced because lupus anticoagulant being an antiphospholipid binds to the phospholipid used in vitro PTT assays)*
> *PT is usually not affected by the lupus anticoagulant.*

- Lupus anticoagulant is a cause for antiphospholipid syndrome and may present with recurrent thrombosis and pregnancy related morbidity including Recurrent abortions.
- Being an antiphospholipid, presence of lupus anticoagulant cause a false positive VDRL test for syphilis

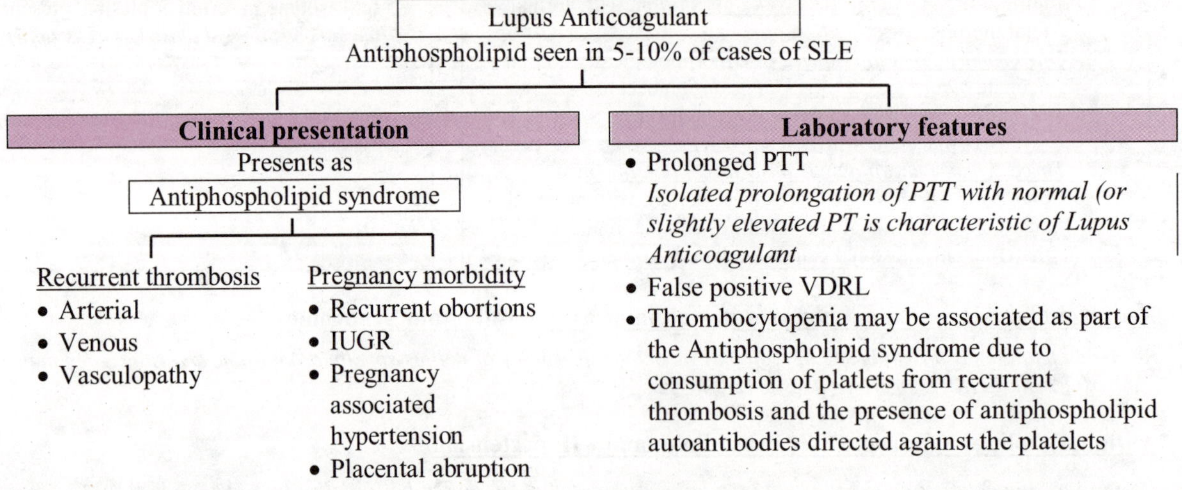

366. Answer is D (Thrombotic spells can be followed by severe life threatening haemmorrhage): *William's Hematology 7th/1763; Current Rheumatology 2nd/218; Samter's Immunologic Disease 6th/573*

Bleeding episodes after Thrombotic spells may occur as a result of consumptive Thrombocytopenia. However such bleeding episodes are rare even with severe thrombocytopenia and do not lead to life threatening haemorrhage. Catastrophic Life threatening Antiphospholipid Syndrome results from rapid onset thrombosis and ischemia in multiple organ systems and not from severe bleeding.

<u>Bleeding is rarely associated with Lupus Anticoagulant</u>

Lupus Anticoagulant may cause thrombocytopenia, but bleeding complications secondary to thrombocytopenia are rare & severe life threatening bleeding due to Lupus anticoagulant has not been reported in any standard text book.

'Although Thrombocytopenia is a common finding in patients with APS, bleeding complications are rare, even with severe thrombocytopenia Bleeding in an APS patient should trigger evaluation for the presence of antiprothrombin antibodies and other disorders that may affect hemostasis, such as DIC & Uremia' - William's Hematology

'Bleeding is unsual in APS despite the prolongation of in vitro clotting time. When bleeding is present it suggests the presence of antiprothrombin antibody with hypoprothrombinemia but it may rarely be caused by thrombocytopenia'.

- Samter's Immunologic diseases

367. Answer is C or None (Increased PT or None): *Harrison 18th/p 1385; Harrison 15th/685; 16th/982, 685; Harrison 17th/1043*

Prothrombin time is usually not affected by Lupus Anticoagulant.

- ***The Lupus Anticoagulant typically causes an isolated prolongation of APTT. Prothrombin time is usually normal although slight prolongation in PT may also be observed***

'Lupus anticoagulant should be suspected in cases of markedly prolonged PTT without clinical bleeding and normal or slightly elevated PT'- CMDT

- The presence of LA activity may predispose patients to **venous and arterial thromboembolism** and may cause mid trimester **abortions** – Harrisons 16th/685
- VDRL tests for syphillis are non specific tests, detecting anticardiolipin antibodies.
  Lupus anticoagulants are family of antiphospholipid antibodies of the same class and ***may give a false positive VDRL.***

Causes of false positive VDRL reactions:

Acute false positive (< 6 months)	Chronic false positive (≥ 6 months)
• Recent viral infection / immunization	• Aging
• Genital herpes	• Autoimmune disorders
• Human immunodeficiency virus	• SLE
• Malaria	• RA
• Parentral drug use	• Parentral drug use.

368. Answer is B (Aspirin + Low molecular weight Heparin): *Harrison's 17th/ 2082; Speroff's Clinical Gynaecological endocrinology & Infertility 7th/1083, 1084*

The recommended treatment for women with recurrent pregnancy loss associated with antiphospholipid syndrome includes combined Aspirin and Heparin therapy.

'In pregnant SLE patients with Antiphospholipid antibodies and prior fetal loss, treatment with heparin (standard or low –molecular- weight) plus low dose aspirin has been shown in prospective controlled trials to increase significantly the proportion of live births'. – Harrison's 17th/2082

'Combined aspirin and heparin therapy has proven effectiveness and is the preferred treatment for women with recurrent pregnancy loss associated with antiphospholipid syndrome' - Speroff 7th/1084

Antiphospholipid syndrome in pregnancy

- The risk of pregnancy loss in women with APS and prior pregnancy loss may exceed 60%
- History of recurrent fetal loss in a pregnant woman with Antiphospholipid antibodies is an indication of treatment during pregnancy as these are identifiable and treatable immunologic disorders
- **Treatment options** include Antiplatelet agents such as Aspirin, Anticoagulants such as Heparin / LMWH, and corticosteroids
  Aspirin along with Heparin / LMWH *is the recommended treatment of choice.*
  Corticosteroids should be avoided if possible. If required to control maternal SLE, these should be used at the lowest effective doses for the shortest time required.

Hemolytic Uremic Syndrome

369. Answer is D (Positive Coomb's test) : *CMDT 2001 / 544; CMDT 2003/508; Harrison 16th/679; 15th/750, 690*

Coomb's test is characteristically negative in patients with HUS.

Hemolytic Uremic Syndrome is characterised by a microangiopathic hemolytic anemia, and thrombocytopenia. The LDH is usually elevated out of proportion to degree of hemolysis, and the coomb's test is negative.

Coagulation test are normal with the exception of elevated fibrin degradation products Q ***(explains hypofibrinogenemia)*** *- normal coagulation results exclude DIC.* Q

Remember the following essentials of diagnosis :

1. *Microangiopathic hemolytic anemia* Q *(coomb's negative).* Q
2. ***Thrombocytopenia*** Q
3. ***Renal failure*** Q
4. *Elevated LDH* Q
5. ***Normal coagulation tests (exclude DIC)*** Q ***(an exception is elevated FDP)*** Q

370. Answer is A or None (Hyperkalemia or None) : *Harrison 14th/959; Harrison 15th/745, 977*

Hyperkalemia is the single best answer of exclusion.

HUS may occur with Shigella Dysentriae type I.

Clinical features in HUS due to shigella as mentioned in *(Harrison 14th/959)* include :

- Oliguria progressing to anuria and *renal failure*[Q]
- Drop in hematocrit progressing to severe *anemia and CHF*[Q]
- ***CNS abnormalities include - encephalopathic symptoms***
  - seizures
  - altered consciousness
  - bizzare posturing
- Laboratory : - Profound *hyponatremia*[Q] and severe *hypoglycemia*[Q] may be seen
  - Leukamoid reactions with *increased leucocyte counts*[Q] may be seen
  - *Thrombocytopenia*[Q] is common

Although one might argue that hyperkalemia may as well be a feature of HUS on account of renal failure, I have excluded it because all other options have been mentioned directly in the standard Harrison text.

Budd Chiari Syndrome

371. Answer is C (Paroxymal nocturnal hemoglobinuria): *Harrison 16th/1862; Robbins 547*

PNH is the most common cause of Budd Chirai syndrome amongst the options provided.

- ***Most common cause of Budd chiari syndrome is - thrombosis of hepatic vein***[Q]

This is seen in the setting of : - *polycythemia rubra vera*[Q]
- *myeloproliferative syndrome*[Q]
- ***Paroxysmal nocturnal hemoglobinuria***[Q]
- Oral contraceptive use
- Hyercoagulable states

- ***It may also result from obstruction of venacava.***[Q]

This may be seen in the setting of :
- invasion of IVC by tumor such as hepatocellular carcinoma.
- Idiopathetic membranous obstruction of IVC is the most common cause of this syndrome in Japan.

372. Answer is D (Thrombosis of hepatic veins): *Harrisons 17th/1950; Harrisons 16th/1862*

The most common cause of Budd Chiari syndrome is thrombosis of hepatic veins *– Harrisons*

373. Answer is C (Hepatic vein): Harrison 18th/p 2561 *Harrison's 16th/1863; 15th/1759: See previous question*

Budd chiari syndrome is characterized by post sinusoidal obstruction outside the liver at the level of hepatic veins.
– Harrison's 15th/1759

374. Answer is D (Polycythemia vera): *Harrisons 17th/267.268; Harrisons 16th/1862; Robbins Pathology Illustrated 6th/883*

Polycythemia vera is the most common cause for Budd chirai syndrome amongst the options provided.

Blood Transfusion

375. Answer is A (Complement mediated Hemolysis is seen): *Refer text below*

Acute Hemolytic Transfusion reactions following Blood transfusion are Type II hypersensitivity reactions caused most often by complement mediated hemolysis. These reactions are often life threatening and complications include Oliguria and acute renal failure (decreased renal blood flow).
Treatment involves immediate termination of transfusion.

376. Answer is A and B (Antigen 'D' determines Rh positivity and Febrile reaction is due to HLA antibodies): *Harrison 18th/p 953, 955 Ananthanarayan 7th/186, 187; Harrison 17th/711, 710*

Rh positive or nregative depends on the presence or absence of antigen D (Rh D) on red cells. *- Ananthanarayanan*
Febrile (non hemolytic) transfusion reactions are caused by antibodies directed against donor leukocytes and HLA antigen may mediate these reactions *– Harrison 17th/711*

Anti-D is not a naturally occurring Antibody
'There are no natural anti – Rh (anti - D) antibodies in the serum' – Ananthanarayanan

Cryoprecipitate does not contain all coagulation factors
Cryoprecipitate is a source for fibrinogen, factor VIII and Von-Willebrand factor (VWF) – Harrison 17th/710

377. Answer is A (Febrile Non Hemolytic Reaction) : Harrison 18th/p 953 *Harrisons 17th/711, Harrisons 16th/665*
The most frequent reactions associated with the transfusion of cellular blood components is a Febrile Non Hemolytic Transfusion Reaction (F N H T R).

Febrile Non Hemolytic Transfusion Reactions (F N H T R)

Etiology	Clinical presentation	Prevention and Treatment
• *These reactions are most commonly caused by* antibodies directed against donor leukocytes and HLA antigens[Q] • *These may also be caused by cytokines released from cells within stored blood* • *Patients at risk include*[Q] Multiply transfused patients[Q] Multiparous women[Q]	• *These reaction are characterized by chills and rigors and ≥ 1°C rise in temperature* • *Diagnosis is usually made by excluding other causes of fever in a transfused patient*	• *Most reactions are mild and do not require any further investigations or treatment* • *Their incidence and severity may be reduced by:* - *Use of leucocyte reduced blood products* - *Premedication with acetaminophen or other antipyretic agents*

378. Answer is B (Dengue Virus): *Harrison's 16th/666*

Dengue virus has not been mentioned as an infectous viral complication of blood transfusion.

Viruses associated with blood transfusion:

Hepatitis C virus
Hepatitis G virus
Hepatitis B Virus
HIV Type I
HTLV Type I
Cytomegalovirus [Q]
Parvovirus B-19[Q]
West Nile Virus
Human Herpes Virus (HHV)[Q]

Hepatitis C virus : *Most common cause of transfusion associated viral hepatitis* [Q]
Hepatitis G virus : *Is a blood borne agent whose modes of transmission have not been defined adequately but tend to parallel those of HCV infection.* [Q]

379. Answer is None or C (None >> EBV): Harrison 18th/p 954, 956, 957 *Ananthnarayanan 8th/475; 'Microbiology in Blood Transfusion' by Barbara 1st/211, Harrison's 17th/710, 711, 712*

Parvovirus B-19, Hepatitis G, Cytomegalovirus and Epstein Bar virus may all be transmitted by blood transfusion.
Transfusion transmitted EBV is however a rare event and may hence be selected as the single best answer by exclusion.

EBV and Blood Transfusion (Morbidity following EBV Transfusion is Rare)

'*EBV infection may also follow blood transfusion or marrow transfusion but these are rare* events' – *Ananthanarayan 8th/131*

'*Although transfusion associated EBV is rare, it is nevertheless well documented*' - *Microbiology in Blood Transfusion 1st/211*

380. Answer is D (Metabolic Acidosis) : '*Handbook of Transfusion Medicine' by Hillyer (2001)/194*

Massive blood transfusion is usually associated with metabolic alkalosis rather than metabolic acidosis
Hyperkalemia, Citrate toxicity and Hypothermia are established complications of massive blood transfusion

Metabolic acidosis / Alkalosis after Massive Blood Transfusion

Banked / stored blood is acidic because of accumulated red cell metabolites. However the actual acid load to the patient is minimal. The acid load on massive blood transfusion is quickly countered by the effect of citrate infusion as citrate is normally metabolized to sodium bicarbonate. It is therefore more common for massively transfused patients to exhibit metabolic alkalosis rather than metabolic acidosis.

Patients with massive transfusion may present with initial metabolic acidosis, however metabolic alkalosis is more frequent once citrate is metabolized in liver to bicarbonate.

381. Answer is A (Hypokalemia): *Harrison's 16th/666; Transfusion Practices by American College of Anaesthetics 3rd/20, 21*

Massive transfusions are associated with risk of hyperkalemia and not hypokalemia.

Massive transfusions: Defined as acute replacement of more than one blood volume within several hours.

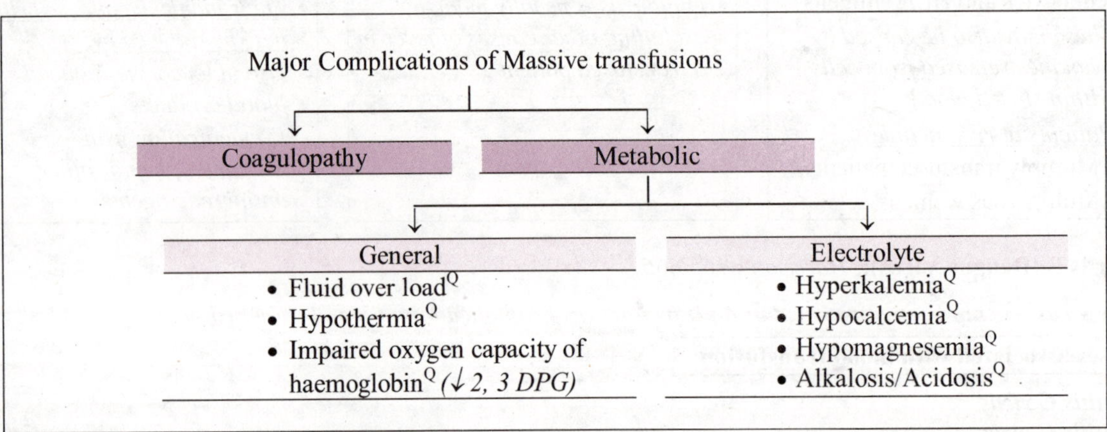

Hypothermia: 'Refrigerated (4°C) or frozen (-18°C) blood components can result in hypothermia when rapidly infused' – *Harrison*

Hyperkalemia, Hypocalcemia & Hypomagnesemia: *Transfusion Practices by American College of Anaesthetics 3rd/20, 21*

The potential metabolic problems resulting from blood transfusion are hyperkalemia, hypocalcemia and hypomagnesemia' – *Transfusion Practice – American society of Anesthesiologists 3rd/20, 21*

- **Hyperkalemia:**
  Potassium increases in the plasma of stored blood as potassium leaves viable erythrocytes.
  However, hyperkalemia is rarely a problem in adults for two reasons:
  - there is very little plasma in Red Blood Cells and
  - the potassium that is present leaves the intravascular space of the recipient and rapidly moves intracellularly.

  Neonates and patients in renal failure are at increased risk of hypokalemia.
- **Hypocalcemia:**
  Citrate present in anticoagulant preservative solutions chelates calcium and causes hypocalcemia

- **Hypomagnesemia:**
  Citrate also has an affinity for the magnesium ion and the occurrence of hypomagnesemia in the setting of massive transfusion has been reported.

- **Alkalosis/Acidosis**
  Stored blood is acidic (pH of 6.6 to 6.9) due to citric acid in the antocoagulant and the accumulation of carbondioxide and lactic acid from erythrocyte metabolism.

Metabolic acidosis / Alkalosis after Massive Blood Transfusion
Banked / stored blood is acidic because of accumulated red cell metabolites. However the actual acid load to the patient is minimal. The acid load on massive blood transfusion is quickly countered by the effect of citrate infusion as citrate is normally metabolized to sodium bicarbonate. ***It is therefore more common for massively transfused patients to exhibit metabolic alkalosis rather than metabolic acidosis.***
Patients with massive transfusion may present with initial metabolic acidosis, however metabolic alkalosis is more frequent once citrate is metabolized in liver to bicarbonate.

- **Citrate Toxicity:**
  Citrate toxicity occurs when ionized calcium is significantly reduced by citrate present in anticoagulant preservative solutions and thereby inhibits the coagulant cascade.

382. Answer is B (Direct Coomb's test): *Harrison 18th/p 954 ; 17th/710; 'Clinical Hematology & Oncology' (Churchill Livingstone) 2003/433*

A direct Coomb's test or direct antiglobulin test (DAT) on post-transfusion blood sample from patient should be done to detect antibodies directed against the transfused red blood cells

A positive direct antiglobulin test (positive direct Coomb's test) that develops during a red blood cell transfusion or immediately following a transfusion strongly suggests that the patient has an antibody directed against the transfused red cells. This is consistent with a hemolytic transfusion reaction.

Blood bank related action for every suspected case of mismatched blood transfusion

- Every suspected case of mismatched blood transfusion *should be reported* to the blood bank.
- A correctly labeled post transfusion blood sample and any untransfused blood should be sent back to the blood bank for analysis.
- ***At the blood bank the post transfusion specimen should be tested for evidence of hemolysis*** *(serum haptaglobin, LDH, hemoglobin and bilirubin)* **and *a direct antiglobulin test (direct Coomb's test) should be performed*.**
  A positive direct Coomb's test confirms the presence of antibodies / complement directed against the transfused RBCs and confirms a hemolytic transfusion reaction.

383. Answer is E (All of the above): Harrison 18th/p 952, 953 *Refet text below; Harrison 17th/709, 710*

Commonly used blood components

Product	Description	Common Indications
Whole Blood *1 unit = 450 ml ± 45ml*	No elements removed Contains RBC, WBC, plasma and platelets (WBC & platelets may be nonfunctional) Deficienct in factors V & VII	• Not for routine use • Acute, massive bleeding • Open heart surgery • Neonatal total exchange
Packed Red Cells (PRBC) *1 unit = 250 – 300 ml*	Most plasma, WBC, platelets removed; 1 unit should raise HCT 3%	• Replacement in chronic and acute blood loss, GI bleeding, trauma
Leukocyte -Poor Red cells (Leukocute reduced) Red cells *1 unit = 200-250 ml*	Most WBC removed by filtration to make it less antigenic $< 5 \times 10^6$ WBC, few platelets, minimal plasma	• Potential renal transplant patients • Previous febrile transfusion reactions • Patients requiring multiple transfusions (leukemia etc)
Washed RBCs *1 unit = 300 ml*	Like leukocyte-poor red cells, but WBC almost completely removed $< 5 \times 10^6$ WBC, no plasma	• As for leucocyte poor red cells, but very expensive and much more purified.
Granulocytes, Phoresis *1 unit = 220 ml*	Some RBC, $> 1 \times 10^{10}$ PMN/unit, Lymphocytes, platelets	

Platelets (smple unit) *1 pack = about 50 ml*	1 "pack" should raise count by 5000-8000 "6 pack" means a pool of platelets from 6 units of blood. > 5 x 10^{10} platelets unit, contains RBC, WBC	• Decreased production or destruction (aplastic anemia, acute leukemia, post-chemo etc) • Counts <5000-10,000 (risk of spontaneous hemorrhage) • Counts 10,000-30,000 if risk of bleeding (headache, GI losses, contagious petechiae) or active bleeding • Counts <50,000 for major surgery • Usually not indicated in ITP or TTP unless life-threatening bleeding or preoperative status.
Platelets (Phoresis unit) *1 unit = 300 ml*	> 3 x 10^{10} platelets/unit	May be HLA matched
Leukocyte- Reduced Platelets	As above, but < 5 x 10^6 WBC/unit	• May decrease febrile reaction and CMV transmission, alloimmunization to HLA antigens
Cryoprecipitate ("Cryo") *1 unit = 10 ml*	Contains factors VIII, XIII, von Willebrand factor and fibrinogen	• Hemophilia A (factor VIII deficiency), when safer factor VIII concentrate not available; • von Willebrand disease, fibrinogen deficiency
Fresh frozen Plasma (FFP) *1 unit* =150-250 ml (400-600 ml if single-donor pheresis)	Contains factors II, VII, IX, X, XI, XII, XIII and heat labile V and VII About 1 h to thaw	• Emergency reversal of warfarin • Massive transfusion (>5 L in adults) • Hypoglobulinemia (IV immune globulin preferred) • Suspected or documented coagulopathy (congenital or acquired) with active bleeding or before surgery • Clotting factor replacement when concentrates unavailable • Not recommended for volume replacement

384. Answer is B (Factor IX): *Harrisons 16th/664*

Cryoprecipitate is not a source for factor IX

Cryoprecipitate is a source for
Fibrinogen[Q]
Factor VIII[Q]
VWF[Q]

Cryoprecipitate also contains factor XIII (I), and fibroructin

- Cryoprecipitate is ideal for supplying fibrinogen to the volume deficient patient
- Cryoprecipitate is indicated for factor VIII deficiency (Hemophilia A) when fresh Frozen plasma is not available
- Cryoprecipitate may also supply VWF to patients will dysfunctional (type II) or absent (type III) von Willebrand disease

385. Answer is D (All of the above): *Clinical Laboratory Medicine 6th/396; Pulomary Respiratory Therapy Secrets 2nd (2001)/27*

Dilution of a sample with heparin can cause erroneously low value for pH, pCO_2 and HCO_3^-.

Heparin and Blood Gas Measurements

- Heparin is the preferred anticoagulant for blood gas specimens
- Heparin is used in blood gas syringes to avoid coagulation of the blood sample, as clots interfere with the function of the blood gas analyzer. Heparinization of blood sample also limits the deposition of proteins on the electrodes.
- ***However excess heparin can affect blood gas analysis by lowering the PaCO2 and calulcated HCO3- by dilutional effect and the pH as heparin is acidic.***

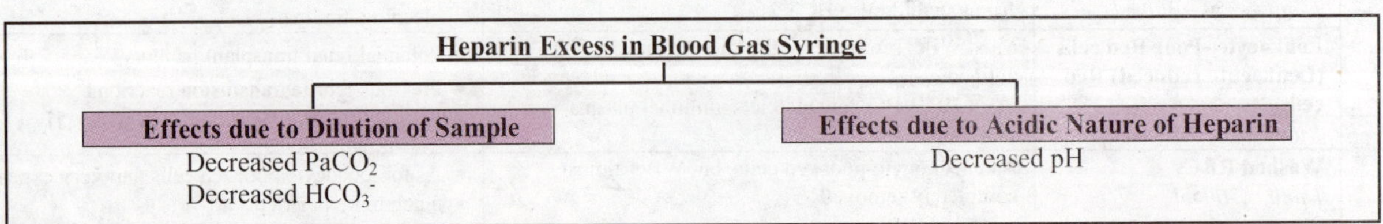

Miscellaneous

386. Answer is A (Methaemoglobinemia): *Harrison 18th /857,858*

Pronounced cyanosis together with chocolate brown colour of freshly drawn blood suggests a diagnosis of methaemoglobinemia

Methaemoglobinemia

- Methaemoglobinemia is an uncommon but distinct cause of central cyanosis in the absence of hypoxemia or cardio vascular compromise
- Methaemoglobinemia occurs when a significant concentration of hemoglobin (Hb) is oxidized to methaemoglobin (Met Hb)

> *When the haem moety (iron atoms) of Hb molecule encounter a strong oxidizing agent iron loses an electron and switches from the Ferrous (2^+) to Ferric (3^+) state turning Hb to 'Met Hb'*

- Methaemoglobin has such high oxygen affinity that virtually no oxygen is delivered

Presentation

- Methaemoglobinemia most commonly presents as *cyanosis unresponsive to supplemental oxygen*

> The most notable physical examination finding is generalized cyanosis which can manifest as muddy brown dark mucus membranes before proceding to global skin discolaration

- 'The charachteristic ***muddy appearance (chocolate brown)*** of freshly drawn blood can be a critical clue' *- Harrison's 18th/858*

*Blood appears dark brown, brownish, muddy or chocolate in colour immediately after withdrawal. In contrast to normal venous blood, the color does not change with addition of oxygen or agitation in the air'- *Diffirential diagnosis in Internal Medicine (Thieme) 2007/709*

> *Methaemoglobinemia >15% cause symptoms of cerebral ischaemia*
> *Methaemoglobinemia > 60% is usually lethal*

Diagnosis

- *The best diagnostic test for Methaemoglobinomia is 'Methaemoglobin Assay'*

Treatment

- The most effective emergency management for methaemaglobinemia is *administration of Methylene blue*[Q] which serves as an antidote (intravenous)

> *Methylene blue is not effective in patients with methaemoglobinemia due to Hemoglobinopathy M*[Q] *(Haemoglobin M)*
> Methylene blue is *contraindicated in patients with G6 PD deficiency*[Q] since it can cause severe hemolysis due to its potential for oxidation

Outline of The Four Main Pathways to MetHb Production

1. Congenitally abnormal hemoglobin: Hemoglobin M
   - Hemoglobin M is passed as an autosomal dominant trait affecting either the alpha or beta chain of hemoglobin; homozygous Hb M affecting both alpha and beta chains is incompatible with life.
   - Amino acid substitution (often a tyrosine for histidine) near the heme iron facilitates iron oxidation.
2. Inherited enzyme deficiencies: NADH-dependent cytochrome b_5 -reductase and cytochrome b_5 deficiency.
   - Deficiency of either cytochrome b_5 or its reducing enzyme, cytochrome b_5-reductase, decreases reduction of MetHb back to Hb
3. Nitrite (NO_2), other oxidants and oxygen-reducing compounds
   - Nitrites are a common oxidizing source of MetHb production.
   - Reducing agents paradoxically produce methemoglobinemia by reducing oxygen to a free radical or water to H_2O_2, which then oxidizes hemoglobin.
4. "Sensitive" hemoglobin: Blue baby syndrome
   - Bacteria in the immature gastrointestinal tracts of infants convert nitrate (NO_3) to the powerful oxidant nitrite (NO_2).
   - Infants have a relative NADH-dependent reductase deficiency (only 50% of adult levels) and are more susceptible to oxidative injury.

387. Answer is B (Renal failure)

Renal Failure is associated with reduced erythropoietin levels due to decreased production of erythropoietin by the diseased kidney.

The kidney is the primary site of erythropoietin production producing more than 85 percent of total erythropoietin. Chronic Renal failure is associated with severe anemia. The most important contributor to the anemia of chronic renal failure is insufficient production of Erythropoetin.

Patients with inflammatory disorders (Anemia of chronic disease) also have inappropriately low levels of Erythropoetin. Examples include Rheumatoid arthritis, some forms of Cancer and AIDS. This is believed to result from suppression of EPO gene expression by inflammatory cytokines in these disorders.

Causes of Anemia in Chronic Renal Failure and other Chronic Diseases

- *Decreased production of Erythropoetin*[Q]
- *Reduced survival of RBCs*[Q]
- *Impaired flow of iron from bone marrow macrophages to erythroblasts.*

388. Answer is B (White cell infusion): Harrison 18th/p 476 *Read text below : Harrison 14th/ 359, 541; Harrison 17th/ 379*

While all might be used, the best to be eliminated here is a 'white cell transfusion' as its exact role is yet to be established. White cell infusion (transfusion) as a measure is still controversial- *Harrison*

- Neutropenic patients are highly susceptible to infections, and therefore, ***surgical cleanliness*** is the first step to ensuring a decreased infection potential - ***Repeated hand washing***
- ***Prophylactic antibiotics*** are certainly required. Patients with luekopenias and leukocyte dysfunction often have delayed inflammatory responses to infection. Therefore clinical manifestations may be minimal despite overwhelming infection. *This necessitates early and prompt institution of prophylactic antibiotics at the earliest suspected sign of infection. Prolonged antibiotics are often required.*
- ***Recombinant G-CSF and M-CSF*** is indicated in the management of certain forms of *neutropenia due to depressed production.* These enhance granulocyte recovery specially that after chemotherapy and consequently shorten the period of maximal vulnerability to fatal infections.
- *Other agents* used include *INF* which non specifically enhance phagocytic cell function and *short courses of Glucocorticoids.*
- ***White cell infusion (transfusion) as a measure is still controversial- Harrison***

Thus while all might be used, the best to be eliminated here is a 'white cell transfusion' as its exact role is yet to be established, and its role is still controversial.

389. Answer is B (Paroxysmal Cold Haemoglobinuria (PCH)): *Harrisons 18th/882, 883, 895*

Paroxysmal Cold Hemoglobinuria (PCH) is a benign self-limiting autoimmune hemolytic anemia. PCH does not undergo leukemic transformation and is hence not considered a Preleukemic condition. Recovery is the rule in Paroxysmal Cold Hemoglobinuria.

Paroxysmal Nocturnal Haemoglobinuria may be considered a Preleukemic condition

'PNH may evolve into Aplastic anemia and PNH may manifest itself in patients who previously have Aplastic Anemia. ***Rarely (estimated 1-2% of all cases) PNH may terminate in Acute Myeloid Leukemia'.*** *– Harrison 18th/883*

Myelodysplasia (Myelodysplastic Syndrome) is a Preleukemic condition

'Myelodysplastia is a clonal hematopoietic stem cell disorder leading to impaired cell proliferation and differentiation Cytogenetic abnormalities are found in approximately one half of patients and some of the same specific lesions are also seen in frank leukemia. ***The type and number of cytogenetic abnormalities strongly correlate with the probability of leukemic transformation*** *and survival' – Harrison 18th/895*

Aplastic Anemia may be considered a Preleukemic condition

'Recent studies have shown that long term survivors of acquired aplastic anemia may be at high risk of subsequent malignant diseases or late clonal hematological diseases often years after successful immunosuppressive therapy. ***One Hypothesis has postulated that aplastic anemia is a Preleukemic condition****'.*

– 'Clinical Hematology' (Lippincott- Williams) 4th/123

390. Answer is D (Primary Thrombocytosis): Harrison 18th/p 470, 903 *Harrison's 17th/374, 676*

Splenomegaly is least likely to be associated with Primary Thrombocytosis amongst the options provided

CML, Polycythemia Vera and Myelofibrosis are characteristically associated with massive splenomegaly.

Primary Thrombocytosis is only occasionally associated with mild splenomegaly and hence is the single best answer of choice

Primary Thromobcytosis is only occasionally associated with mild splenomegaly

'Physical examination is generally unremarkable, except occasionally for mild splenomegaly'-Harrison's 17th/676

CML, Polycythemia Vera and Myelofibrosis are associated with massive splenomegaly - *Harrison's 17th/374*

Diseases associated with massive splenomegaly *(Harrison's 17th/374)*
• ***Chronic myelogenous leukemia***
• *Lymphomas*
• *Hairy cell leukemia*
• ***Myelofibrosis*** *with myeloid metaplasia*
• ***Polycythemia Vera***
• *Gaucher's disease*
• *Chronic lymphocytic leukemia*
• *Sarcoidosis*
• *Autoimmune hemolytic leukemia*
• *Diffuse splenic hemangiomatosis*

391. Answer is B (Lepirudin): *Goodman & Gillman's Manual of Pharmacology (2007) 955; 'Clinical Hematology & Oncology' by Furie (2003) /488.*

Lepirudin (direct thrombin inhibitor) is a recommended agent for Heparin induced thrombocytopenia and thrombosis.

Currently Recommended Agents for Heparin Induced Thrombocytopenia

- ***Lepirudin*** *(Direct Thrombin Inhibitor)*
- *Argatroban (Direct Thrombin Inhibitor)*
- *Danaparoid (Mixture of Non Heparin Glycosaminoglycans)*

Bivalirudin (Direct thrombin inhibitor) is under evaluation for HIT

Heparin Induced Thrombocytopenia (HIT)

- Heparin Induced Thrombocytopenia is an important complication / adverse effect of Heparin administration that necessitates use of alternative agents to treat or prevent thrombus formation
- HIT is usually seen as a complication of the use of unfractionated heparin but may also be seen with the use of LMWH
  HIT may be non immune mediated (Type I, Mild) or immune mediated due to development of antibodies (Type 2/ Significant)

Type I	Type II
Non immune mediated	*Immune mediated*
Benign	*Severe*
Mild Thrombocytopenia	*Significant thrombocytopenia*
Heparin Therapy may be continued	*Heparin must be discontinued immediately*

- Heparin Induced thrombocytopenia Type II is a serious form of HIT that can result in serious complications
- The diagnosis of Immune mediated HIT depends on clinical criteria with confirmation by specific laboratory tests

Clinical Criteria for Immune Mediated (Type II) HIT
• Thrombocytopenia < 150, 000/µl or a 50% decrease from pretreatment values
• Thrombocytopenia follows heparin exposure by at least 5 days (Time taken to form antibodies)
• Reasonable exclusion of other clinical causes of thrombocytopenia
• *Onset of new thrombotic event or extension of previous thrombosis*

- **Management of HIT (Immune mediated)**
- Direct Thrombin Inhibitors
  Lepirudin and Argobatran along with Danaparoid are the recommended alternative anticoagulants for patients with Heparin Induced thrombocytopenia.
  Direct thrombin inhibitors (Lepirudin and Argobatram) are usually preferred but all three drugs are effective anticoagulants and the choice of drug depends on personal experience and patient characteristics like hepatic or renal insufficiency and desired route of administration
- Heparin administration *should be stopped immediately.*
- Low Molecular Weight Heparin (LMWH) *should not be substituted* because it may cross react with antI-heparin antibodies
- Warfarin *should not be used* until the thrombocytopenia is resolved and the patient is adequately anticoagulated with another agent. Warfarin may precipitate venous limb gangrene or multicentric skin necrosis in patients with HIT

Comparison of Danaproid, Lepirudin, and Argatroban for the treatment of Heparin induced Thrombocytopenia			
	Danaproid	**Lepirudin**	**Aragtroban**
Mechanism of action	Primarily inhibits Xa in a complex with Antithrombin III	Directly inhibits thrombin	Directly inhibits thrombin
Administration	IV or SC	IV	IV
Half-life	24 hours	13 hours	30 minutes
Reversible	No	No	No
Monitoring	Anti-Xa activity using a danaproid standard	aPTT	aPTT
Use in pregnancy	Several reported cases	No reported experience	No reported experience
Dose adjustment for renal failure	Yes, monitor Xa activity dosely in patients with renal insufficiency	Yes, monitor Xa activity closely in patients with renal insufficiency	No
Special considerations	Cross- reacts with heparin-induced antibodies in some cases	Antibodies may develop to lepirudin and prolong the half –life	

All three drugs are anticoagulant in patients with heparin-induced thrombocytopenia. The choice of drug depends on personal experience and patient characteristics such as renal or hepatic insufficiency, desired route of administration.

Cardiovascular System

ESSENTIAL REVISION NOTES

Arterial and Venous Pulses

Types of Pulses

Pulses alternans [Q]	Bisferiens pulse [Q]	Pulsus paradoxus [Q]	Dicrotic pulse [Q]
• Regular alteration of pressure in pulse with regular rhythm (single peak) • Seen in - LVF [Q] - May be seen in all conditions leading to LVF	• Two systolic peaks • Seen in - Aortic regurgitation[Q] ± AS - Hypertrophic cardiomyopathy [Q]	• Normal decrease in systolic pressure during inspiration is accentuated [Q] • Seen in - Pericardial tamponade [Q] - S.V.C. obstruction [Q] - COPD/Acute Severe Asthma - Constrictive pericarditis - Pulmonary embolism - Hypovolemic shock	• Has two palpable waves are in systole and one in diastole. • Seen in - Dilated cardiomyopathy

Jugular Venous Pulse (JVP)

Jugular venous pulse:

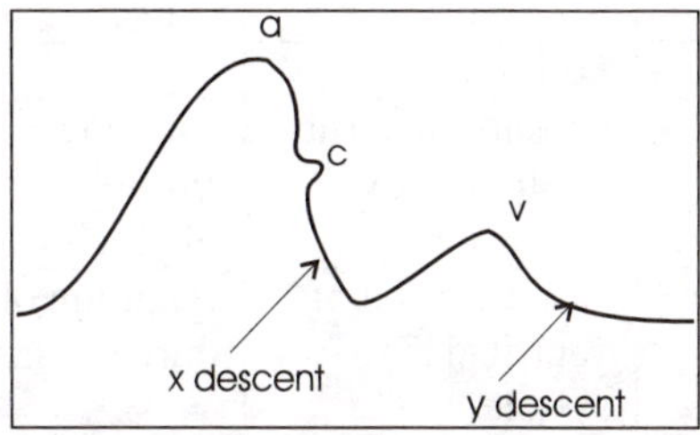

Various Waveforms in Jugular Venous Pulse

<table>
<tr><td>a waves :</td><td colspan="2">Due to distention produced by right atrial contraction.</td></tr>
<tr><td>c waves :</td><td colspan="2">Are positive waves produced by bulging of tricuspid valve into right atrium during right ventricular isovolumetric contraction.</td></tr>
<tr><td>v waves:</td><td colspan="2">Due to increasing volume of blood in the right atrium during ventricular systole when the tricuspid valve is closed.</td></tr>
<tr><td rowspan="5">a – x descent:</td><td colspan="2">Due both to atrial relaxation and to the downward displacement of the tricuspid valve during ventricular systole.</td></tr>
<tr><td>Accentuated in</td><td>Reduced with</td></tr>
<tr><td rowspan="3">• Constrictive pericarditis
• Cardiac temponade
• Restrictive cardiomyopathy</td><td>• Right ventricular dilatation</td></tr>
<tr><td>Reversed with</td></tr>
<tr><td>• Tricuspid Regurgitation</td></tr>
<tr><td rowspan="3">v – y descent:</td><td colspan="2">By the opening of the tricuspid valve and the subsequent rapid inflow of blood into the right ventricle.</td></tr>
<tr><td>Accentuated in</td><td>Reduced with</td></tr>
<tr><td>• Tricuspid regurgitation
• Constrictive pericarditis</td><td>• Tricuspid stenosis
• Right / Atrial Myxoma
(Suggests obstruction to right ventricular filling)</td></tr>
<tr><td>y – a descent:</td><td colspan="2">Due to continuous diastolic inflow of blood into great veins, right atrium and ventricle, which are all in free communication during diastole.</td></tr>
</table>

'a' waves in Jugular Venous Pulse

Large 'a' waves :	Cannon 'a' waves :	Absent 'a' waves :
• ***Tricuspid stenosis*** [Q] • Pulmonary stenosis [Q] • ***Pulmonary hypertension*** [Q]	• Regularly - During ***junctional rhythm*** [Q] • Irregularly - Atrioventricular dissociation with ventricular tachycardia - *Complete heart block* [Q]	*Atrial fibrillation* [Q]

Prominent x descent and y descent

Feature	Tamponade	Constrictive pericarditis	Restrictive cordiomyopathy	RVMI
Prominent y descent	***Absent***	Usually present	Rare	*Rare*
Prominent x descent	Present	Usually present	Present	*Rare*

Cardiac Auscultation: Heart Sounds and Murmurs

Heart Sounds

Feature	1st heart sound	2nd heart sound	3rd heat sound	4th heart sound
Character	High pitched (lower than S_2) Slightly prolonged "lub"	High pitched (higher than S_1) Shorter "dup"	Soft low pitched weak rumbling	Low pitched heart sound
Duration	0.14 second	0.11 sec	0.1 sec	-
Frequency	25-45 Hz	50 Hz	-	***< 20 Hz*** [Q]
Cause	Sudden closure of mitral & tricuspid valves	Closure of aortic & pulmonary valves	***Rapid ventricular filling*** [Q] d/t inthrushing of blood from atria	***Ventricular filling*** [Q] d/t atrial contraction causing inthrushing of blood
Timing	Start of ventricular systole	Just after end of ventricular systole	Begining of middle third of diastole	Immediately before 1st heart sound (presystolic)
Heard	Better heard with Diaphram	Better heard with Diaphram	***Better heard with the Bell***	***Better heard with the Bell***

S_3 & S_4 can often not be heard with a stethoscope (ear) [Q] and require phonocardiogram
S_3 often and S_4 sometimes can be recorded in phonocardiorgam

The first and second heart sounds and opening snaps are heard better with the diaphragm, and low-pitched sounds such as the third or fourth heart sound are beter heard with the bell of stethoscope – Hutchisons 20th / 174

First Heart Sound (S1)

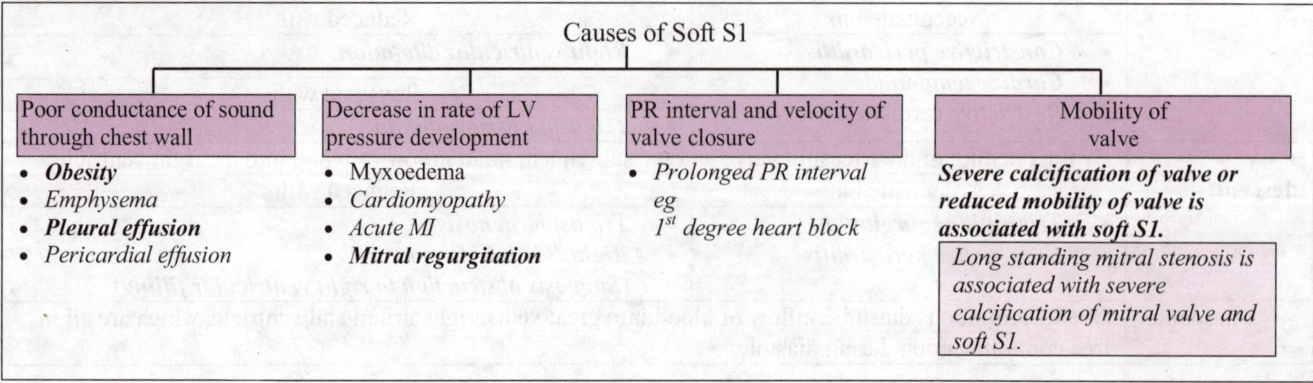

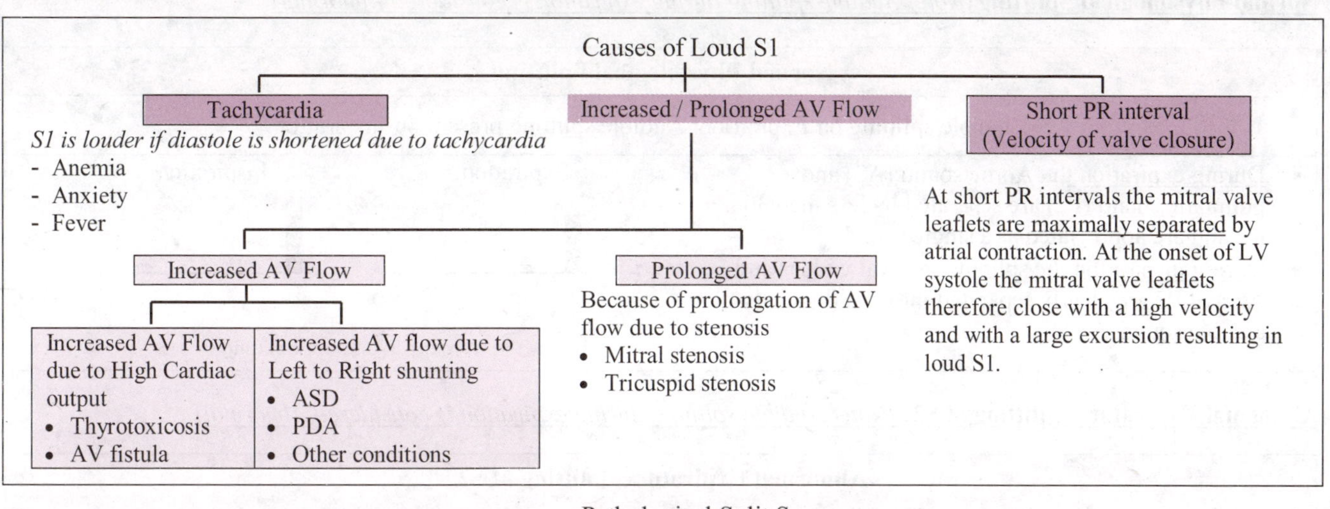

Pathological Split S_1

Normal splitting (T1 follows M1 after a longer gap : M1 T1)	Reverse splitting (T1 precedes M1 : T1 M1)
• Right Bundle Branch Block	• ***Left Bundle Branch Block***
• LV pacing	• RV pacing
• Ectopic beats and Idioventricular rhythms originating in Left Ventricle	• Ectopic beats and Idioventricular rhythms originating in Right ventricle
• Ebstein's anomaly	• ***Severe Mitral Stenosis and Atrial Myxoma***

Second Heart Sound (S2)

Causes of Single S2 (No Splitting)

Causes of single S_2

Conditions causing Delayed Aortic Closure

All conditions associated with delayed A_2 can produce a single S_2 when the splitting interval becomes less than 30ms

Causes of Delayed A2

- Delayed electrical activation of the right ventricle
  - Complete RBBB (proximal type)
  - Left ventricular paced beats
  - Left ventricular ectopic beats
- Prolonged right ventricular mechanical systole
  - Acute massive pulmonary embolus
  - Pulmonary hypertension with right heart failure
  - ***Pulmonic stenosis*** with intact septum (moderate to severe)
- Decreased impedence of the pulmonary vascular bed (increased hangout)
  - Normotensive atrial septal defect
  - Idiopathic dilation of the pulmonary artery
  - ***Pulmonic stenosis*** (mild)
  - Atrial septal defect
  - Unexplained AES in normal subjects

Conditions in which one component of S_2 is either absent or inaudible

Conditions in which one component of S_2 is either absent or in audible will produce a single S_2

- ***Severe TOF***
- Severe semilunor valve stenosis
  - severe AS
  - ***severe PS***
- ***Pulmonic valve atresia***
- Tricuspid valve atresia
- Eisseminger syndrome

Semilunar valves include Aortic valve, Pulmonary valve and trancal valves

Condition resulting in inability to hear the fainter of the two components of the sound (usually P_2)

These conditions also produce a single S_2

- Emphysema
- Obesity
- Respiratory noise

Normal Physiological Splitting *(Note: Audible splitting during expiration is considered Abnormal)*

Normal Physiological Splitting
No audible splitting on Expiration; Audible splitting present on Inspiration.

- During expiration the Aortic sound (A2) and pulmonic sound (P2) are separated by less than 30 ms and are appreciated as a single sound
- During inspiration the splitting interval widens and A2 and P2 are clearly separated into two distinctly audible sounds.

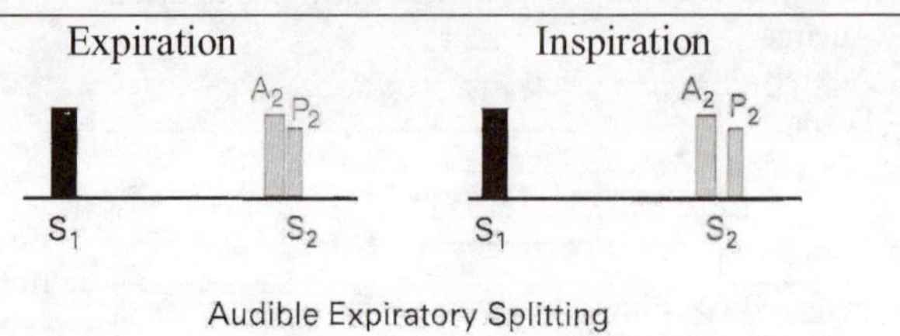

Abnormal Expiratory Splitting of S2: *(Note: Audible splitting during expiration is considered Abnormal)*

Abnormal Expiratory Splitting of S2 *(Audible splitting during expiration is considered Abnormal)*
Audible splitting during both expiration and inspiration

- Wide physiological splitting
- This is caused by delayed P2/early A2

Expiration Inspiration

A_2 P_2 A_2 P_2

S_1 S_2 S_1 S_2

- Reversed Splitting
- This is caused by delayed A2/early P2

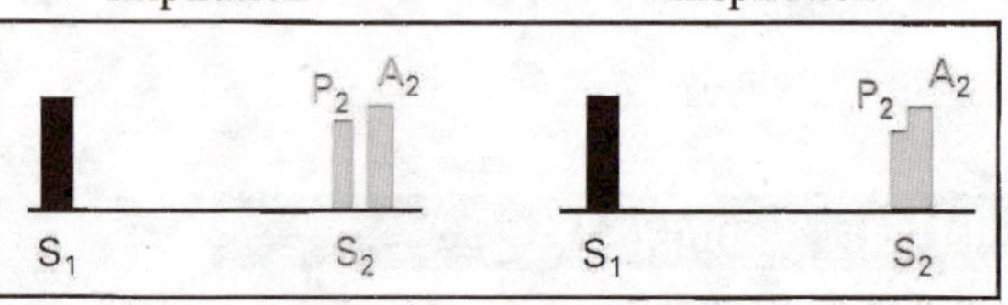

This is associated with Paradoxical movements i.e. P2 moves towards A2 with inspiration and hence splitting interval narrows with inspiration.

Wide Physiologic Splitting of the second Heart Sound
Delayed pulmonic closure
• Delayed electrical activation of the right ventricle
- Complete RBBB (proximal type) - Left ventricular paced beats - Left ventricular ectopic beats
• Prolonged right ventricular mechanical systole
- Acute massive pulmonary embolus - Pulmonary hypertension with right heart failure - Pulmonic stenosis with intact septum (moderate to severe)
• Decreased impedence of the pulmonary vascular bed (increased hangout)
- Normotensive atrial septal defect - Idiopathic dilation of the pulmonary artery - Pulmonic stenosis (mild) - ***Atrial septal defect*** - Unexplained AES in normal subjects
Early aortic closure
• Shortened LVET - ***Mitral regurgitation*** - ***Ventricular septal defect***

Reversed Splitting of the second Heart Sound
Delayed aortic closure
• Delayed electrical activation of the left ventricle
- Complete LBBB (proximal type) - Right ventricular paced beat - Right ventricular ectopic beats
• Prolonged left ventricular mechanical systole

- Complete LBBB (peripheral type)
- Left ventricular outflow tract obstruction
- Hypertensive cardiovascular disease
- Arteriosclerotic heart disease
  - Chronic ischemic heart disease
  - Angina pectoris

• Decreased impedance of the systemic vascular bed (increased hangout)
- Poststenotic dilation of the aorta secondary to aortic stenosis or regurgitation - Patent ductus arteriosus
Early pulmonic closure
• Early electrical activation of the right ventricle - Wolff-Parkinson-White syndrome, type B

Fixed Wide-Spitting of S2

Causes of Fixed (wide) split
• ***ASD (Most characteristic cause for wide fixed splitting)*** • Pulmonic Stenosis • *Acute Right Heart Failure (Pulmonary Embolism)*

Third Heart Sound (S3)

- *It is a low frequency sound*[Q]
- *It is a diastolic heart sound that occurs shortly after S2*[Q]
- *It occurs during rapid filling of the ventricles (termination of rapid filling)* [Q]
- *It is best heard at the apex in the left lateral position*[Q]
- *It is better heard with the bell of the stethoscope*[Q]

Causes of Physiological and Pathological Third Heart Sounds (S3)

Third Heart Sound (S_3): Ventricular Diastolic Gallop, Protodiastolic Gallop, and Pericardial Knock

Physiologic S_3	Pathologic S_3

• Children
• High cardiac output
- ***Atheletes*** [Q]
- *Fever* [Q]
- *Pregnancy* [Q]
- *Thyrotoxicosis* [Q]
- *AV fistulas* [Q]
	• ***Ventricular dysfunction (LVF/RVF)*** – poor systolic function, increased end-diastolic and end-systolic volume, decreased ejection fraction, and high filling pressure.
	- Idiopathic dilated cardiomyopathy
	- *Ischemic heart disease*
	- Valvular heart disease
	- Congenital heart disease
	- Systemic and pulmonary hypertension
	• Excessively rapid early diastolic ventricular filling
	- Hyperkinetic states
	  - Anemia
	  - Thyrotoxicosis
	  - Arteriovenous fistula
	- Atrioventricular valve incompetence
	- ***Left to right shunts (VSD, PDA and ASD)***
	• Restrictive myocardial or pericardial disease
	• ***Constrictive pericarditis (pericardial knock)***
	• Restrictive cardiomyopathy
	• Hypertrophic cardiomyopathy.

Pathological Third Heart Sound (S3) may be associated with Constrictive Pericarditis

Constrictive pericarditis is characterixstically associated with pericardial knock which is a distinct form of third heart sound (S_3)

'Pericardial knock is S_3 that occurs earlier *(0.1 to 0.12 after A2) and is higher pitched than normal. Its presence depends upon the restrictive effects of the adherent pericardium which halts diastolic filling abruptly'* – Harrison

Congenital Heart Diseases associated with Loud S3

Congenital Heart Diseases associated with Loud S3
• *Ventricular septal Defect (VSD)*[Q] • *Patent Ductus Arteriosus (PDA)*[Q] • *Atrial Septal Defect (ASD)* [Q]

Fourth Heart Sound (S4)

- Fourth Heart sound occurs in association with an *effective atrial contraction*[Q]
  (It is presumably caused by inrush of blood into the ventricles when the atria contracts and hence it is also called the 'Atrial Heart Sound')
- ***It is heard during the ventricular filling phase of the cardiac cycle (Presystolic[Q] heart sound)***
- ***It is low pitched (frequency usually 20 cycle/sec or less-(Guyton)***
- ***It is not audible to the unaided ear***
  Normally the fourth heart sound can almost never be heard even with a stethascope because of its weakness and low frequency *(Guyton)*
- S4 becomes audible when diminished ventricular compliance increases the resistance to normal filling
  When audible the S4 is *best heard with the bell of the stethescope*[Q]
- Loudest (Best heard) at the Left ventricular Apex when the patient is in left Lateral position
- It is accentuated by mild isotonic or isometric exercises in the supine position

Causes of Pathological Fourth Heart sound

Fourth Hearth Sound (S4), Atrial Diastolic gallop, and Presystolic Gallop:

Decreased ventricular compliance

- Ventricular hypertrophy
  - Left or right ventricular outflow obstruction
  - Systemic or pulmonary hypertension
  - Hypertrophic cardiomyopathy
- Ischemic heart disease
  - Angina pectoris
  - Acute myocardial infarction
  - Old myocardial infarction
  - Ventricular aneurysm
- Idiopathic dilated cardiomyopathy

Excessively rapid late diastolic filling secondary to:

- Vigorous atrial systole
- Hyperkinetic states
  - Anemia
  - Thyrotoxicosis
- Arteriovenous fistula
- Acute atrioventricular valve incompetence

Arrhythmias

- Heart block

Note:

Physiologic S4 may be recordable in patients with increasing age ***but is rarely audible***

Added Heart Sounds

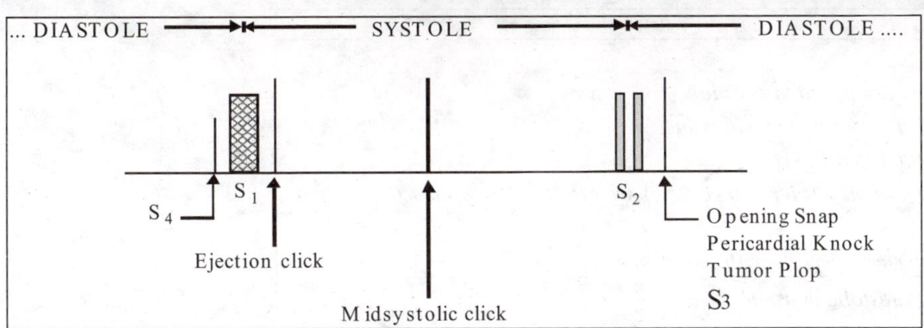

Diastolic vs Systolic added Heart Sounds

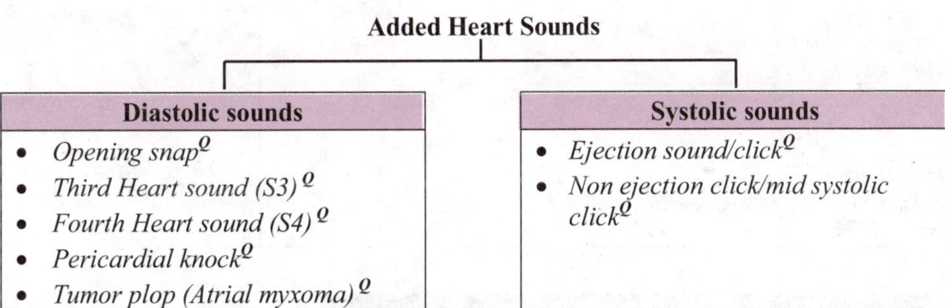

Location of Added Heart Sounds in systole/diastole

Shortly after S1 [Q]	Shortly before S1 [Q]	Between S1 & S2 [Q]	Shortly after S2 [Q]
Ejection click	*Fourth heart sound*	*Midsystolic click*	*Opening snap* *Pericardial knock* *Tumor plop* *S3*

Features of Added Sounds

Ejection Click	Opening Snap	Pericardial knock	Tumor Plop
• *Sharp, High pitched sound* [Q]	• Brief, *High pitched sound* [Q]	• A third heart sound that is *higher pitched than normal* (S3 is low pitched).	• Tumor plop is a characteristic *low pitched sound* [Q]
• Audible during *early systole* [Q] *(Immediately after S1)*	• Audible during *early diastole* [Q] *(Between 0.04 to 0.12 sec after A2)*	• Audible during *early diastole* [Q] *(Within 0.01 to 0.12 sec after A2)*	• Audible during *early or mid diastole* [Q]
• *Seen in Aortic stenosis* [Q], *Pulmonary stenosis* [Q], *Hypertension* [Q] *and is produced due to sudden opening of semilunar valves in conditions where this opening is delayed.*	• *Seen in stenosis of AV valves (Mitral stenosis* [Q] > Tricuspid stenosis)	• Seen in *constrictive pericarditis* [Q] and produced due to sudden deceleration of venticular filling because of restrictive effect of adherent pericardium.	• Seen in conditions like *atrial myxoma* [Q] and produced due to the tumor abruptly stopping as it strikes the ventricular wall

Opening Snap

Opening snap

- ***Brief high pitched sound***
- *Heard in early **diastole** (Ejection sound are heard in systole)*
- *It is usually due to **stenosis of an (A.V.)** most often mitral value.*
- *It **follows second heart sound,** A_2 by 0.05 to 0.12 sec.*
- *It is generally best heard at **lower left sternal border** and radiates well to the base of heart*
- *It is best heard during expiration*
- *The time interval between A_2 and O_s varies inversely with the severity of M.S.*
- *It is followed by low pitched rumbling diastolic murmur*

Opening snap indicates that :

- *M.S. is organic (and significant)* Q
- *Valve cusps are pliable* Q
- *High atroventricular pressure gradient is present* Q
- *Severe, AR, MR, AF, SABE are absent.* Q

Note:

- *O.S. may also be audible in tricuspid stenosis*
- *O.S. of tricuspid stenosis occurs later in diastole than the mitral O.S*

Cardiac Murmurs

Classification and Types of Systolic murmurs

Holosystolic /pan systolic murmurs	Midsystolic murmurs ejection systolic murmurs		Early systolic murmurs
Begin with S_1 and end after S_2	***Starts shortly after S_1 and ends before S_2***		***Begin with first heart sound and end in midsystole***
• VSD • Mitral Regurgitation • Tricuspid Regurgitation • Aortopulmonary shunts	**Aortic** Aortic stenosis Coarctation Aneurysm PDA High output states	**Pulmonary** P. stenosis P. hypertension P. artery dilatation ASD High output states	• VSD - Large VSD with pulmonary hypertension - *V. small muscular VSD* • ***Tricuspid regurgitation*** in absence of Pul. Hypertension • Mitral regurgitation in a non compliant left atrium as in ***papillary muscle dysfunction***

Differentiation of systolic murmurs base don changes in their intensity from physiologic maneuvers

Maneuver	HOCM	AS	MR/VSD	MVP	TR	Flow
Valsalva's maneuver	↑	↓	↓	↑	↓	↓
Stand	↑	-	-	↑	-	↓
Squat	↓	-	-	↓	-	↑
Handgrip/TAO	↓	-	↑	↑	-	↓
Inspiration	-	-	-	-	↑	- or ↑
Post-PVC	↑	↑	-	-	-	↑

AS= aortic stenosis; Flow = benign flow murmur; HOCM = hypertrophic obstructive cardiomyopathy; MR = mitral regurgitation; MVP = mitral valve prolapse; PVC = pressure ventricular contraction; TAO = transient arterial occlusion; TR = tricuspid regurgitation; VSD = ventriocular septal defect; ↑ = increased in murmur intensity; ↓ = decreased in murmur intensity; - = no predictable change

Murmur in Aortic Regurgitation :

Typical **diastolic murmur** of Chronic AR	**Midsystolic** ejection murmur	Austin flint murmur (**diastolic**)
• High pitched, blowing, decrescendo diastolic murmur • Heard best in the third I.C.S. along the left sternal border Note: With marked post stenotic dilatation of aorta the murmur may be loudest in the 2nd or 3rd right interspace – *API 7th/ 420*	• Resembles murmur of AS but is higher pitched, shorter and less rasping • Heard best at the base of heart and is transmitted along the carotids	• Soft, low pitched rumbling middiastolic • Heard best at the apex • Produced by diastolic displacement of anterior leaflet of mitral valve by AR stream

Murmur of Mitral Stenosis

Low pitched^Q, rumbling^Q diastolic murmur^Q with 'Pre-systolic accentuation' heard best at the apex in left lateral recumbent position^Q.

Carey Coomb's Murmur and Austin Flint Murmur

Carey Coomb's Murmur	**Austin Flint Murmur**
• Low pitched (soft) • Delayed diastolic (Middiastolis) • Mitral • Associated with Acute Rheumatic carditis **Attributed to :** • Inflammation of mitral valve cusps • Excessive left atrial blood flow as consequence of mitral regurgitation	• Low pitched (soft) • Delayed diastolic (Middiastolic / Late diastolic) • Mitral • Associated with Aortic Regurgitation **Attributed to :** • Anterior mitral valve leaflet when blood enters the left ventricle simultaneously from both the aortic route and the left atrium

"Carey Coomb's murmur is a delayed diastolic mitral murmur." - *Ghai 6th / 376*

Remember:

Low pitched, delayed diastolic mitral murmur in association with Rheumatic fever: Carey Coomb's murmur.
Low pitched, delayed diastolic mitral murmur is association with severe chronic AR: Austin Flint murmur.

Common condition producing acute MR include
- Rupture of chordae tendnae
- ***Papillary muscle dysfunction*** or rupture following MI
- Infective endocarditis

Causes of Continuous Murmurs

Causes of Continuous Murmur (Hurst)

Continuous Murmur caused by Blood flow	**Continuous murmurs caused by high-to low-pressure shunts**	**Continuous murmurs secondary to localized arterial obstruction**
• Venous hum • Mammary soufflé • Hemangioma • Hyperthyroidism • Acute alcoholic hepatitis • Hyperemia of neoplasm - hepatoma - renal cell carcinoma - paget disease	Systemic artery to pulmonary artery - Patient ductus arteriosus - Aortopulmonary window - Truncus arteriosus - Pulmonary atresia - Anamolous left coronary - Bronchiectasis - Sequestration of the lung Systemic artery to right heart - Ruptured sinus of Valsalva - Coronary artery fistula Left-to-right atrial shunting - Lutembacher syndrome - Mitral atresia plus atrial septal defect Venovenous shunts - Anomalous pulmonary veins - Portosystemic shunts Arteriovenous fistula (systemic or pulmonic)	• Coarctation of the aorta • Branch pulmonary stenosis • Carotid occlusion • Celiac mesenteric occlusion • Renal occlusion • Femoral occlusion • Coronary occlusion

ELECTROCARDIOGRAM (ECG)

The Cardiac Axis

The Cardiac Axis

- The cardiac axis refers to the mean direction of the wave of ventricular depolarization in the vertical plane measured from a zero reference point
- The zero refrence point looks at the heart from the same view point as lead I
- An axis lying above this line is given a negative number while an axis lying below this line is given a positive number
- *Theoretically the cardiac axis may lie anywhere between +180 to -180*

Normal AXIS

Normal cardiac axis flows down and towards the left lower aspect of the heart between – 30 and +90

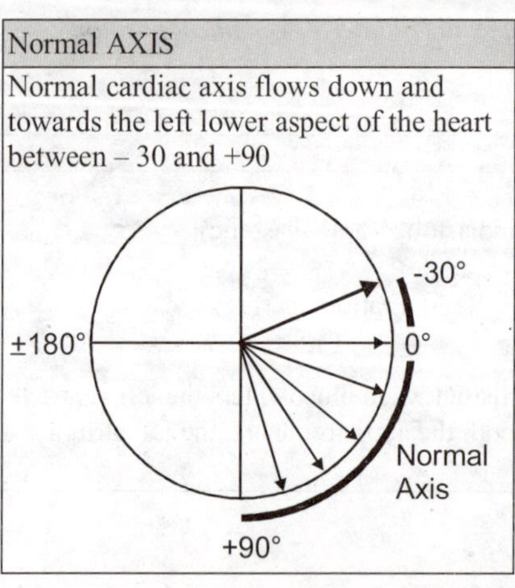

Left Axis Deviation

Cardiac axis flow is upward and towards the left upper half of the heart between -30 and -90

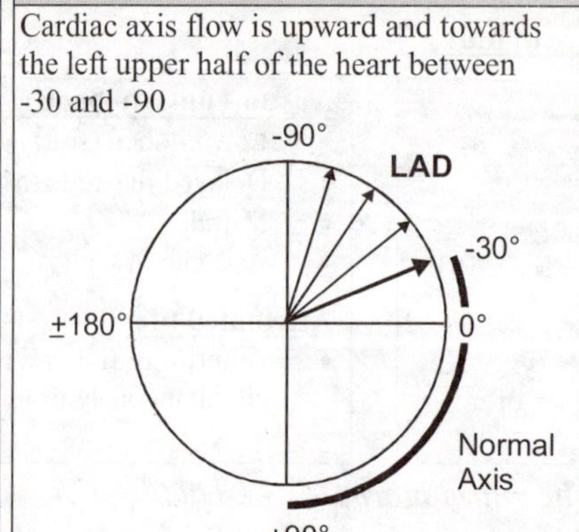

Right Axis Deviation

Cardiac axis flow is downwards and towards the right part of the heart between +90 and +/- 180

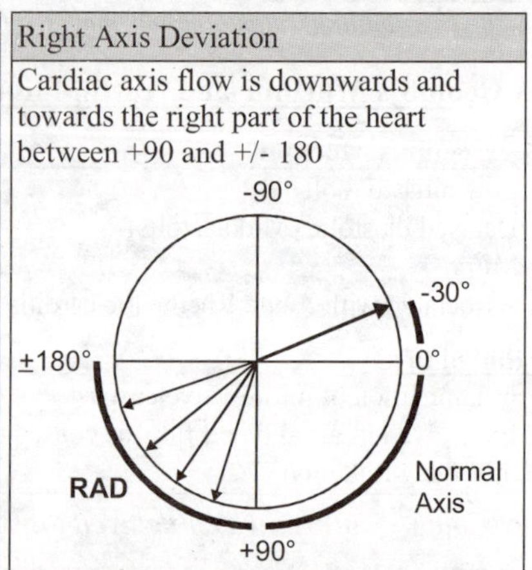

Extreme Right Axis Deviation

When flow of cardiac axis is upward and to the right between +/-180 and -90

- The standard cardiac axis is determined using Lead I and Lead II

Normal Axis	Left Axis Deviation	Right Axis Deviation
-30 to +90 Positive in Lead I Positive in Lead II	-30 to -90 Positive Lead I Negative in Lead II	+90 to ±180 Negative in Lead I Positive or Negative in Lead II

- The Cardiac Axis in Different Leads

	Normal Axis	Right axis deviation	Left axis deviation
Lead I	Positive	Negative	Positive
Lead II	Positive	Positive or negative	Negative
Lead III	Positive or negative	Positive	Negative

Note:
Lead I : POSITIVE BETWEEN -90 TO +90 (CLOCKWISE) Lead II : POSITIVE BETWEEN -30 TO +150 (CLOCKWISE) Lead III : POSITIVE BETWEEN +30 TO -150 (CLOCKWISE)

QRS Complex

QRS Complex Voltage

Low QRS voltage on ECG

Low QRS voltage or ECG
QRS amplitude <5 mm on all limb leads
QRS amplitude < 10 mm on all precordial leads

- Diagnostic criteria for Low QRS voltage include QRS complex amplitude < 5mm in all limb leads (*when this is the case the amplitude in each of the precordial leads (V) is usually less than 10 mm, but this is not necessary for the diagnosis)*
- Low QRS voltage should be considered a description and not a diagnosis (it may be a normal variant)

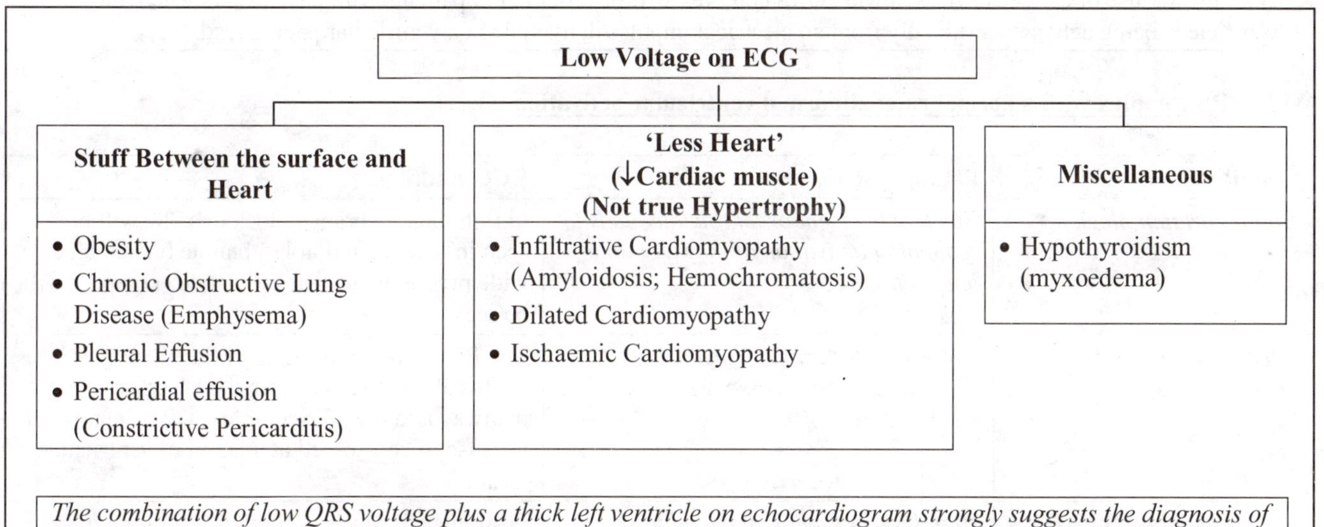

The combination of low QRS voltage plus a thick left ventricle on echocardiogram strongly suggests the diagnosis of infiltrative cardiomyopathy like cardiac amyloidosis. The increased thickness is the amyloid. It is not muscle (not true hypertrophy), does not depolarize and therefore adds nothing to QRS voltage.

QRS Complex Duration

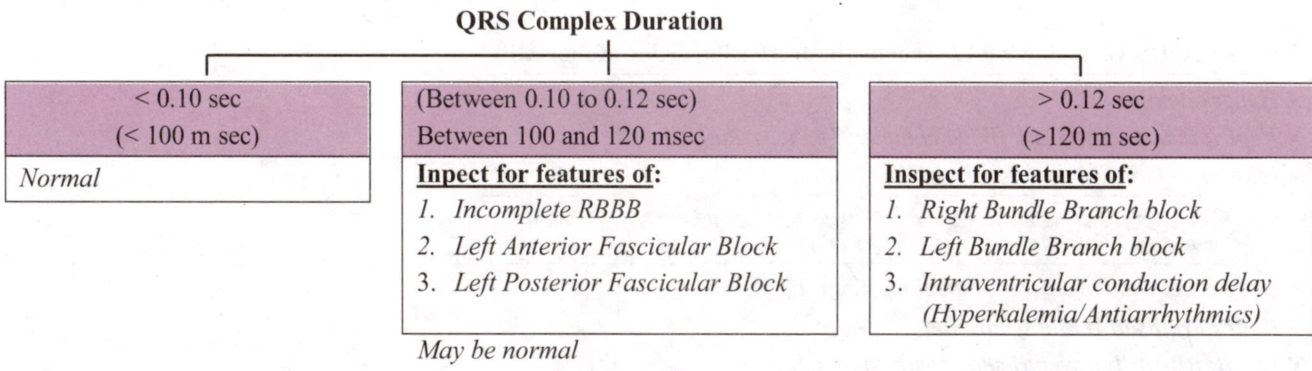

Any QRS complex Duration > 0.12 seconds is abnormal. There are no exceptions to this rule (A QRS complex Duration < 0.12 seconds may be normal)

QRS complex: Wide or Narrow

- QRS complex represents ventricular depolarization and QRS interval represents the duration of ventricular depolarization.

> The normal QRS interval (QRS duration) is less than 0.10 to 0.11 seconds.

- If the QRS complex is less than 0.12 second, ventricular depolarization is more or less occurring normally over the His-Purkinje system.
- There are several causes for a wide QRS complex, which result from abnormal activation of the ventricles.
- ***Most commonly, a wide QRS complex is due to abnormal conduction over the right or left bundle due to block or delay of ventricular activation***.
- Rarely, a wide QRS complex is observed because the ventricles are being activated via both the His-Purkinje system and an accessory pathway.
- With greater use of cardiac devices, a wide QRS complex will be observed in patients with pacemakers where the ventricle is being activated artificially from an electrical impulse delivered via a ventricular pacing lead.

Wide QRS complex with a normal rate: abnormal ventricular activation

Condition	Pathophysiology	ECG findings
Bundle branch block	*Block in the right or left bundle leads to sequential activation of the right and left ventricles*	In right bundle branch block an rSR' will be seen in lead V_1 and in left bundle branch block a wide predominantly negative QRS complex will be seen
Accessory pathway	*The ventricles are activated by both the AV node and an accessory pathway*	The PR interval will be short due to early ventricular activation from the accessory pathway and the QRScomplex will be abnormal because of cell-to-cell activation of ventricular tissue
Hyperkalemia	*High levels of potassium lead to slow ventricular depolarization*	Prominent T waves will often be observed
Ventricular rhythm	*A site within the ventricles drives ventricular depolarization*	P waves will not precede the QRS complexes
Ventricular paced rhythm	*Similar to the ventricular rhythm*	A pacing artifact will be observed

Causes of QRS Widening ≥ 0.12 seconds (in decreasing order of mortality)

- ***Hyperkalemia***
- ***Ventricular Tachycardia (Wide complex Tachycardia)***
- *Idioventricular Rhythm including heart blocks*

> *Wide QRS complex may be seen in Mobitz Type II second degree block and incomplete Third Degree Blocks but lacks certainity*

- *Drug effects and overdoses (especially Tricyclics)*
- ***Wolf Parkinson White syndrome***
- *LBBB; RBBB; Intraventricular conduction delay*
- *Ventricular premature contraction*
- *Aberrantly conducted complexes*

QT Interval

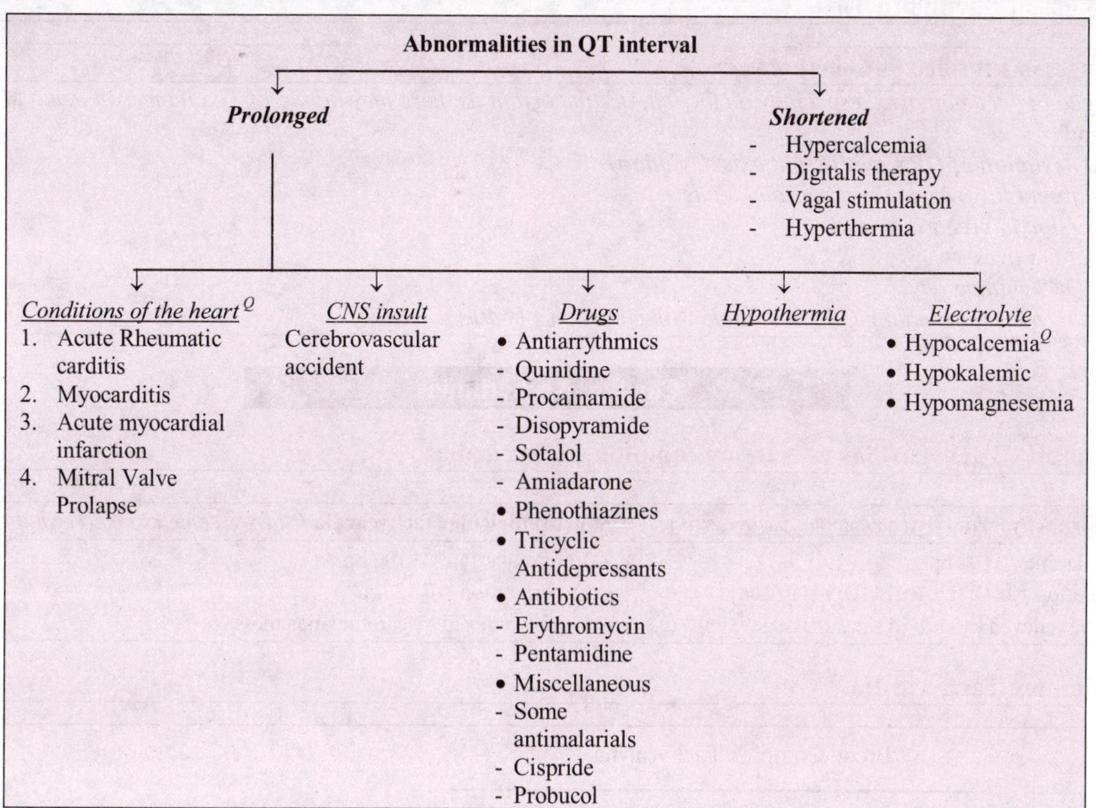

ST Segment

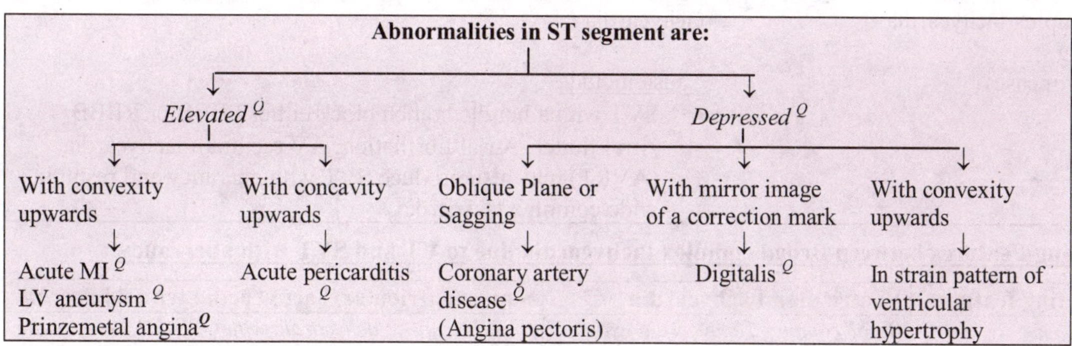

ECG Changes in Hypokalemia and Hyperkalemia

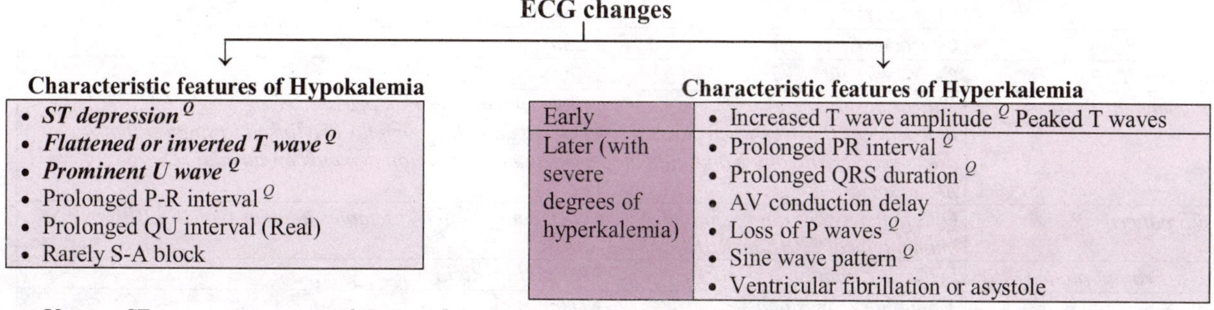

Prominent U wave, ST segment sagging and T-wave flattening or inversion are characteristic features of Hypokalemia. *Hypokalemia may also present with a apparently prolonged QT interval on ECG. However this apparently prolonged QT interval is in* reality the QU interval that mimics a prolonged QT interval due to fusion of T-U waves.

ECG changes in Pneumothorax

ECG Changes in left sided Pneumothorax

ECG changed in pneumothorax, especially on the left, are important as there may mimic ECG, changes of acute MI

These include

Right ward deviation of QRS axis (Right axis deviation)

Decreased/absent R waves in the precordial leads

T wave inversion in precordial leads

Pathological Q waves

Decreased QRS voltage

Electrical alternans (alternating QRS amplitude with each heart beat)

Cardiac Arrhythmias

Broad Complex Tachycardias vs Narrow complex Tachycardias

Ventricular tachycardia (Broad complex tachycardia)	**Supraventricular tachycardia** *(Narrow complex tachycardia)*
• Ventricular rate > 100 bpm • QRS duration > 0.12 sec. (>.14 sec.- Harrison)[Q] • Cannot be relieved by carotid sinus massage. [Q]	• Ventricular rates > 100 bpm [Q] • QRS duration < 0.12 sec. • Can be relieved by carotid sinus message [Q]

Broad Complex Tachycardia

Broad Complex Tachycardia

Ventricular Tachycardia

VT is the most common cause of Broad complex tachycardia accounting for >80% of cases

Supraventricular Tachycardia with abberancy

SVT with abberancy accounts for 15-20% cases of broad complex tachycardia

Cause include

- SVT with a bundle branch block either LBBB or RBBB
- Atral flutter, Atrial fibrillation, AV reentrant tachycardia (AVRT) may also produce SVT with aberancy and result in wide complex tacycardia.

Distinguishing Features between Broad complex tachycardia due to VT and SVT with aberrancy

Differentiating features	Ventricular Tachycardia	Supraventricular Tachycardia with Abaerrancy
• *QRS duration*	*Broad complex Tachycardia with QRS duration usually greater that 0.14 seconds* *QRS ≥ 0.14 sec*	*Broad complex tachycardia with QRS duration usually between 0.12 sec to 0.14 seconds* *QRS ≤ 0.14 sec.*
• *Fusion Beats*	*Characteristic of VT*	*Absent*
• *Capture Beats*	*Characteristic of VT*	*Unusual*
• *AV dissociation*	*Characteristic of VT*	*Absent*
• *Independent P waves*	*May be seen* *Independent P waves when present are characteristic of VT and indicate AV dissociation*	*Independent P work's are not seen* *P wave and QRS complex are linked to suggest that ventricular activation depends on atrial discharge*
• *QRS pattern*	*QRS pattern does not resemble /mimic typical LBBB or RBBB*	*QRS pattern often resembles /mimics typical LBBB or RBBB*
• *Axis (Frontal plane QRS)*	*Left axis deviation (< - 30°)*	*Normal or Right ward*
• *QRS morphology in V1*	*Monophasic or Biphasic*	*Triphasic*
• *R/S Ratio in V6*	*<1*	*>1*
• *Vagal manuvres*	*No effect*	*Slowing or termination of tachycardia by vagal manuvres*

ECG Features of Torsades de Pointes

Characteristics of *Torsades de pointes*

- Polymorphic QRS complexes that change in amplitude
- Cycle length giving the appearance of oscillations around the baseline.
- Marked QT prolongation [Q]

WPW Syndrome

WPW syndrome : Accessory AV Pathways

- WPW syndrome or 'Prexcitation syndrome' is charachterized by the presence of *tachyarrythmias*[Q] due to an *accessory conducting pathway*[Q] between atrium and ventricle
- WPW abnormality occurs when an impulse reaches the atria or ventricles earlier than would be expected if the impulse traveled by way of normal specialized conducting tissue *(Pre excitation)* [Q]

- When atrial impulse activates the entire or some part of ventricle
- When ventricular impulse activates the entire or some part of the atrium

Epidemiology

- ***Incidence varies from 0.1 to 3.0/1000 in apparently healthy subjects (Average = 1.5/1000)***
- It may be found in all ages (Neonates to Elderly)
- Prevalence decreases with age apparently because of loss of preexcitation
- ***It is more common in Males***
- Most adults with WPW syndrome have normal heart
  (However various acquired and congenital defects may be associated specially Ebstein's anomaly, MVP and cardiomyopathics)

Electrocardiographic features

Three basic features typify the ECG abnormalities with usual form of WPW syndrome

- Short PR interval (PR interval <120 ms during sinus rhythm)[Q]
- Wide QRS complex (>120 ms) with a slurred slowly rising upstroke (delta wave) [Q]
  The terminal portion of QRS complex is usually normal as conduction through bundle of His usually catches up with preexcitation
- Secondary ST-T changes[Q] that are generally directed to an opposite direction to the major Delta/ QRS vectors

Note

- **Fusion beats**: [Q] If the accessory pathway is capable of anteprade conduction, the typical QRS complex represents a 'Fusion beat' as a result of depolarization of the ventricle in part by the wave travelling from the accessory pathway and in part by wave travelling from normal AV nodal pathway
- **Normal p wave**[Q] – Since the atrial activation is normal, the P wave is usually normal

Cardiac Conduction Blocks

First Degree AV Block

First Degree AV Block

First degree AV block is charachterized by a delay in conduction across the conducting tissue (prolonged PR interval)

Features

- *PR interval is prolonged (>0.20 seconds)*[Q]
- *PR interval is constant (at the prolonged duration)* [Q]
- *Rhythm is regular* [Q]
- *Each P wave is followed by a QRS complex* [Q]
- *QRS complex morphology / duration is usually normal* [Q]

Second Degree AV block

Second Degree AV Block

Second degree AV block is characterized by intermittent failure of conduction from atria to ventricles

Type I (Mobitz) / Wenchebeck Type

This is charachterized by progressive prolongation of PR interval prior to a non conducted P wave

Features

- *Atrial Rhythm regular* [Q]
- *Ventricular Rhythm irregular* [Q]
- *Atrial rate exceeds ventricular rate* [Q]
- *PR internal varies* [Q]
- *PR progressively gets longer until a QRS is dropped* [Q]
- *QRS morphology is often normal* [Q]

Type II (Mobitz)

This is charachterized by constant PR interval prior to a non conducted P wave

Features

- *Atrial Rhythm regular* [Q]
- *Ventricular Rhythm Regular (unless conduction rations vary)* [Q]
- *Atrial Rate exceeds ventricular rate* [Q]
- *PR interval is constant* [Q]
  PR interval does not get progressively longer and a QRS is dropped suddenly
- *QRS morphology is usually abnormal* [Q] *(rarely normal)*

Third Degree AV Block

Third Degree AV Block: Complete AV Block

Third degree AV block or complete AV block is charachterized by complete failure of conduction from atria to ventricles. (Atria and ventricles are under the control of separate pacemakers).

Features

- *Atrial Rhythm regular* [Q]
- *Ventricular Rhythm regular* [Q]
- *Atrial rate exceeds ventricular rate* [Q] *(The inherent rate of ventricular pacemaker is slower)*
- *PR interval varies* [Q] *(variable)*
- *P waves have no constant relationship to QRS complexes* [Q] *(AV dissocation)*
- *QRS complex morphology may be abnormal* [Q]

AV Blocks classified based on PR Interval

PR Interval

Constant	Variable
• First degree block • Second Degree – Mobitz II	• Second degree – Mobitz I • Third degree block

PR constant (First-degree) (First-degree)	PR varies (Second-degree, Mobitz 1)
PR constant	*PR varies*
PR prolonged	*PR progressively gets longer until a QRS is dropped*
Regular atrial rhythm; *Regular ventricular rhythm*	*Regular atrial rhythm;* *Irregular ventricular rhythm*
(Second –degree, Mobitz II)	**(Third- degree)**
PR constant	*PR varies*
PR normal or prolonged *Two or three P waves (possibly more) to each QRS*	*P waves have no constant relationship to QRS (found hidden in QRS complexes and T waves)*
Regular atrial rhythm; Regular ventricular rhythm (unless conduction ratios vary)	*Regular atrial rhythm;* *Rgular ventricular rhythm*

AV CONDUCTION BLOCKS: Review

Name	Rhythm	Rate (beats/minute)	P waves (lead II)	PR Interval	QRS complex
First-degree atrio-ventricular (AV) block	Regular	That of underlying sinus rhythm; both atrial and ventricular rates will be the same	***Sinus origin; one P wave to each QRS complex***	Prolonged (more than 0.20 second); remains constant	Normal (0.10 second or less)
Second-degree AV block, Mobitz I	Atrial: regular Ventricular: irregular	Atrial: that of underlying sinus rhythm Ventricular: depends on number of impulses conducted through AV node: ***will be less than atrial rate***	Sinus origin	Varies; progressively lengthens until a P wave isn't conducted (P wave occurs without the QRS cmplex); a pause follows the dropped QRS complex	Normal (0.10 second or less)
Second-degree AV block, Mobitz II	Atrial: regular ventricular: usually regular, but may be irregular if conductions ratios vary	Atrial: that of underlying sinus rhythm Ventricular: depends on number of Impulses conducted through AV node; will be ***less than atrial rate***	Sinus origin: two or three P waves (sometimes more) before each QRS complex	Normal or prolonged; remains constant	Normal if block at level of bundle of His; ***Wide if block in bundle branches***
Third-degree AV block	Atrial: regular Ventricular: regular	Atrial: that of underlying sinus rhythm Ventricular:40 to 60 if paced by AV junction; 30 to 40 (sometimes less) if paced by ventricles; will be less than atrial rate	Sinus P waves with ***no constant relationship to the QRS complex***; P waves found hidden in QRS complexes and T waves	Varies greatly	Normal if block at level of AV node or bundle of His; wide if block in bundle branches

No constant Relationship between P wave and QRS complex is a feature of Third degree or complete heart block.
One P wave to each QRS complex is a feature of First degree block

Heart Failure

Features of Left Heart Failure and Right Heart Failure

Left heart failure

- Left heart failure is defined as a clinical syndrome where the dominant feature is fluid congestion in the lungs (pulmonary) rather than in the systemic circulation
- The pulmonary capillary wedge pressure is typically elevated (↑PCWP)
- Predominant symptoms are related to passive congestion of lungs and pulmonary edema
- Dyspnea
- Orthopnea
- Paroxysmal Nocturnal Dyspnea (PND)
- Cough with Pink Frothy Sputum
- Rales / Crackles

Right heart failure

- Right heart failure is defined as a clinical syndrome where the dominant feature is fluid congestion in the systemic circulation.
- The pulmonary capillary wedge pressure is normal (Normal PCWP) unless Right heart failure is caused secondary to left sided heart failure (↑ed PCWP)
  (PCWP is not elevated in isolated Right heart failure)
- Predominant symptoms are related to passive systemic congestion
- Peripheral Edema
- Ascitis
- Congestive hepatomegaly (may be pulsatile)
- Congestive splenomegaly
- Weight gain
- Nocturia
- Raised JVP
- Positive Hepatojugular reflex

Valvular Heart Diseases

Mitral stenosis

Auscultatory findings and Xray Features of Mitral Stenosis

Mitral stenosis

Auscultatory findings	X Ray findings
• S_1 : *accentuated.* • S_2 : *Normally split S_2 with accentuated P_2*[Q] • **Murmur :** *Low pitched*[Q], *rumbling*[Q] *diastolic murmur*[Q] *with 'Pre-systolic accentuation' heard best at the apex in left lateral recumbent position*[Q]. • **Opening snap:** *brief, high pitched*[Q], *early diastolic*[Q] *sound, best heard at the lower left sternal border*[Q].	• *Straightening of the left border of cardiac silhouette*[Q] • *Prominence of main pulmonary artery*[Q] • *Dilation of upper lobe pulmonary veins*[Q] • *Kerley B lines*[Q] • *Backward displacement of the esophagus*[Q]

Features Suggesting severity of Mitral Stenosis

Features suggesting severe MS are :
1. *Proximity of S2 - O.S. gap* [Q], *and*
2. *Longer duration of mid-diastolic murmur* [Q]

Mitral Regurgitation

Features Suggesting severity of Mitral Stenosis

Severity of Mitral Regurgitation : Features indicating increased severity:
• ***Presence of Left ventricular S_3 or an inflow rumble at the apex***
• *Harsh Decrescendo murmur with lot of low and medium frequencies*
• *Wide split S_2 due to early A_2 (not caused by P_2 delay) in presence of MR*

Severity of Mitral Regurgitation:

1. If the murmur is harsher and has a lot of low and medium frequencies. It usually indicates a lot of flow and therefore will imply significant regurgitation.

   A harsh decrescendo mitral regurgitation murmur is usually indicative of severe regurgitation because the decrscendo effect is caused by early buildup of a very high v wave pressure in the left atrium resulting from a severe degree of regurgitation. Thus decreasing the gradient in late systole

   (If the murmur, on the other hand, is all pure high frequency and confined only to late systole. Then it must indicate a high pressure difference between the left ventricle and the left atrium and therefore only mild regurgitation).
2. When the mitral regurgitation is severe, the volume overload on the left ventricle will be high, resulting in an enlarged left ventricle. This may be reflected in a displaced hyperdynamic wide –area left ventricular apical impulse. In addition, the hyperdynamic left ventricle will have rapid ejection. This will make the A2 occur early. Resulting in a wide-split S2. Thus, a wide –split S2 in the presence of mitral regurgitation is a sign of severe regurgitation if the wide split is not caused by P2 delay.
3. In addition, severe regurgitation because of the volume load effect will have a torrential inflow through the mitral valve during diastole. This will set up the necessary conditions for the production of an S3 or a mid –diastolic inflow rumble. The presence of an S3 or an inflow rumble at the apex will, therefore, be a sign of significant mitral regurgitation as well.

Note

Loudness and duration of Mitral regurgitation murmur does not always correlate with the severity of the regurgitation

Mitral Valve Prolapse (MVP)

Mitral Valve Prolapse Review

- Also known as *'Barlow's syndrome'* [Q] or *'Billowing mitral valve'* [Q] or *'Floppy valve syndrome'* [Q].
- It is most common in *females* [Q]
  Most commonly seen in young adults (15 to 50 years)
  (MVP may be seen in older individuals > 50 yrs. When seen in older individuals most patients are males and MR is more common and severe and requires surgical treatment)
- Inheritance in familial cases is *autosomal dominant* [Q].
- Clinical course is usually benign
  - Patients are *usually asymptomatic* [Q]
  - Patients may present with *non specific chest pain, dyspnea, fatigue and palpitations.* [Q]
- Auscultatory findings are characteristic and most important :
  - Characteristic *mid systolic* [Q] or late systolic *non ejection* [Q] *clicks* [Q] which may be *multiple* [Q]
  - Late systolic ejection murmur (Often but not always)
  - Accentuation of findings by *Valsalva and standing.* [Q]
  - Diminished by *squatting and isometric exercises.* [Q]
- Diagnosis :
  - *Investigation of choice is echocardiography.* [Q]
  - *ECG in most cases is normal.* [Q]
- Pathological Findings:
  - ***Myxomatous degeneration of mitral valve (less commonly in tricuspid and aortic valves)***
  - Elongated, Redudant or Ruptured chordae tendinae
    (patients with ruptured chordae tendinae are usually symptomatic with significant regurgitation – MR)
  - Dysfunction and ischaemia of papillary muscles
  - Progressive dilatation and calcification of mitral valve annulus
- Complications :
  - *M.R* [Q].
  - *Arrythmias* [Q]
  - *Sudden death* [Q]
  - *Transient ischemic attack* [Q]
  - *Infective endocarditis* [Q]

Atherosclerosis

Major Risk Factors for Atherosclerosis

Major risk Factors for Atherosclerosis - *Harrisons*

- *Cigarette smoking*
- *Hypertension (BP > 140/90mm/hg) or (on Antihypertensive medication)*
- ***Low HDL cholesterol***
- Diabetes mellitus
- Family history of CHD
- Age (Men > 45 years; Women ≥ 55 years)
- Life style risk factors
  Obeity (BMI > 30 kg/m²)
  Physical inactivity
  Atherogenic diet

Emerging risk factors

- Lipoprotein (a)
- ***Homocystine***
- Prothrombotic factors (Fibrinogen)
- Pro inflammatory factors
- Impaired fasting glucose
- Subclinical atherogenesis

Risk Factor and Relative Risk of Future Cardiovascular adverse events

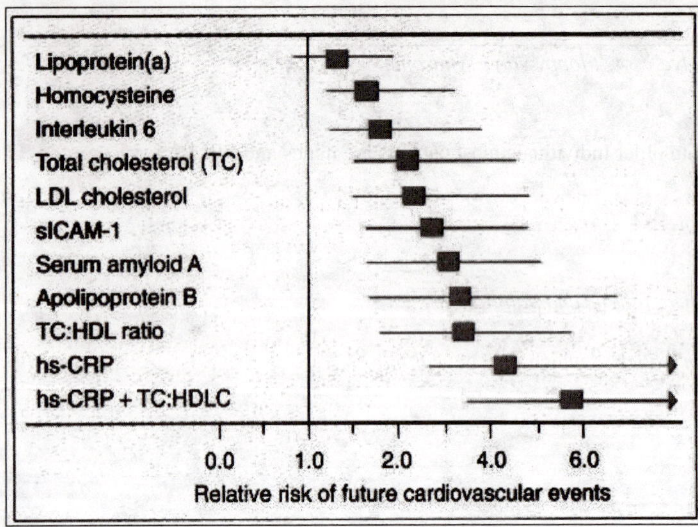

hsCRP, high reactivity C-reactive protein;
siCAM-1, soluble intercellular adhesion molecule-1;
HDLC, high density lipoprotein cholesterol

Lipid Fractions and Relative Risk of Future Cardiovascular adverse events

Relative risk for future cardio vascular events	Lipid Fractions and Lipid Ratios
Decreasing Predictivity of Risk	• *Total chotesterol: HDL Cholestrol Ratio (TC: HDLC)* • *Apopratein B100: HDL Cholesterol Ratio (APo B100: HDLC)* • *LDL Cholesteral : HDL Cholesterol Ratio (LDLC: HDLC)* • *Apoprotein B100: Apoprotein A-1 (APO B100: APO A1)* • *Non HDL Cholesterol fraction* • *Apolipoprotein B-1 Fraction* • *HDL cholesterol Fraction* • *Total cholesterol Fraction* • *Apolipoprotein A1 Fraction* • *LDL cholesterol Fraction*

Type of Hyperlipidemia and Risk of Coronary Artery Disease

Condition	Risk Of Coronary Artery Disease
Type I (Familial Hyper Chylomicronemia)	*Not increased*
Type II A (Familial Hyper Cholesterolemia)	Accelerated
Type II B (Familial Combined Hyperlipidemia)	Accelerated
Type III (Familial Dysbetalipoprotenemia	Accelerated
Type IV (Familial Hyper Triglyceredemia)	Accelerated
Type V (Familial Mixed Hypertriglyceredemia)	***Not increased***

Myocardial Infarction

Universal Defination of Myocardial infarction

Universal Defination of Myocardial infarction

Myocardial infarction related to ischemia due to primary coronary event (plaque rupture) ***or imbalace between oxygen demand and supply*** (coronary spasm, hypotension etc)	***Myocardial Infarction related Sudden Cardiac Death*** (Death occuring before blood samples could be obtained, or at a time before the appearance of cardiac biomarkers in the blood.)	***Myocardial Infarction associated with PCI*** (in patients with normal baseline troponin values)	***Myocardial infarction associated with CABG*** (in patients with normal baseline troponin values,)
Detection of rise and/or fall of cardiac biomarkers (preferably troponin) with at least one value above the 99th percentile of the upper reference limit (URL) together with evidence of myocardial ischaemia with at least one of the following: • Symptoms of ischaemia • ECG changes indicative of new ischaemia [new ST-T changes or new left bundle branch block (LBBB)] • Development of pathological Q waves in the ECG • Imaging evidence of new loss of viable myocardium or new regional wall motion abnormality.	*Sudden, unexpected cardiac death, involving cardiac arrest, often with :* • ***Symptoms suggestive of myocardial ischaemia***, and accompanied by • New ST elevation, or new LBBB, and/or • Evidence of fresh thrombus by coronary angiography and/or at autopsy,	• ***By convention, increases of biomarkers greater than 3 x 99th percentile*** *URL have been designated as defining PCI-related myocardial infarction.*	• ***By convention, increases of biomarkers greater than 5 x 99th percentile*** URL plus either new pathological Q waves or new LBBB, or angiographically documented new graft or native artery occlusion, or imaging evidence of new loss of viable myocardium have been designated as defining CABG-related myocardial infarction.

Criteria For Prior Myocardial Infarction

Criteria for prior myocardial infarction
Any one of the following criteria meets the diagnosis for prior myocardial infarction • Development of new pathological Q waves with or without symptoms • Imaging evidence of a region of loss of viable myocardium that is thinned and fails to contract, in the absence of a non-ischaemic cause. • Pathological findings of a healed or healing myocardial infarction.

Taken from :Expert Consensus Document Circulation 2007 (American Heart Association Journals); 'ECS-ACCF-AHA-WHF Universal Definition of Myocardial Infarction'; http://circ.ahajournals.org/content/116/22/2634.full.pdf

The frequency of critical narrowing of arterial trunks and corresponding sites of myocardial lesions

The frequency of critical narrowing of arterial trunks

Common	Uncommon	Rare (Never Encountered)
• Left anterior descending (LAD) artery (40-50%) • Right coronary artery (30-40%) • Left circumflex coronary artery (15-20%)	• Left main coronary artery • Secondary branches e.g. - Diagonal branches of LAD artery - ***Marginal branches***	• Penetrating intramyocardial branches of coronary arteries

Left anterior discending (LAD) (Br. of LCA) 40 to 50% (Most common)	Right coronary artery (RCA) 30-40 %	Left circumflex (br. of LCA) 15 to 20%
Anterior wall of L.V. near apex *Anterior portion of ventricular septum*	*Inferior/Posterior wall of L.V* *Post. portion of ventricular septum* *Inferior/posterior right ventricular free wall in some cases*	*Lateral wall of left ventricle except the apex*

Cardiac Enzymes and Myocardial Infarction

Enzyme	Seen at	Peaks at	Returns to Normal	Other features
CPKMB	2-4 hrs[Q]	24 hr[Q]	72 hr[Q]	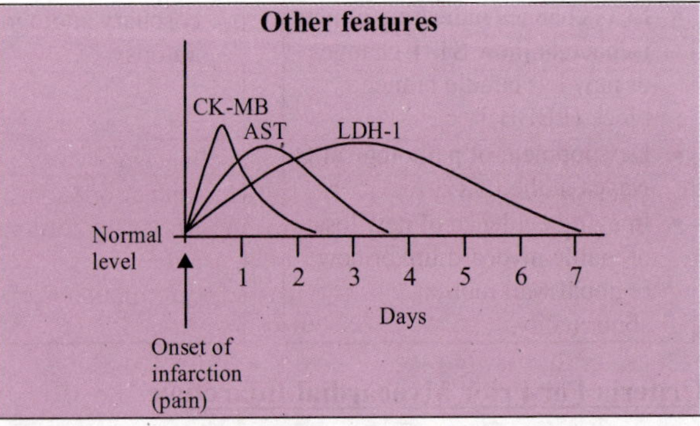
LDH	24 hr	4-5 days	After 10 days[Q]	
AST or SGOT	Within 12 hr	48 hrs	4-5 days[Q]	

LDH and AST are non specific and there use now is limited

Management of Myocardial Infarction

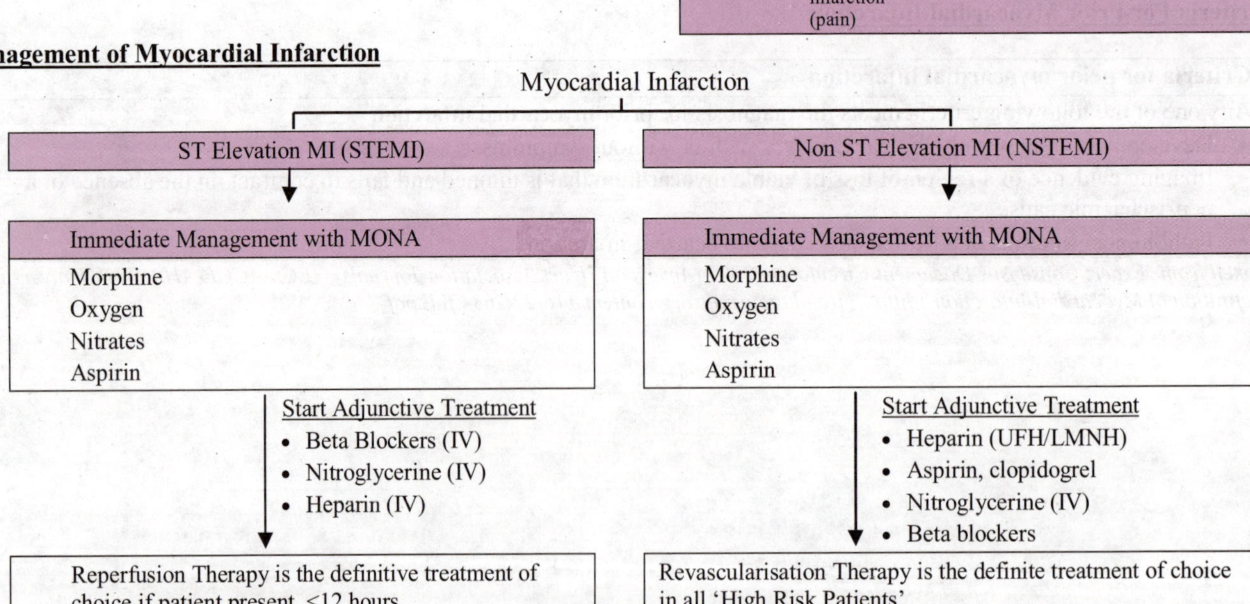

Cardiomyopathy

Symptomatic Cardiomyopathy

Dilated cardiomyopathy	Restrictive Cardiomyopathy	Hypertrophic cardiomyopathy
Dominant Feature is systolic dysfunction (contractile dysfunction)	*Dominant Feature is diastolic dysfunction*	*Dominant Feature is diastolic dysfunction*
Ejection Fraction <30%	**Ejection Fraction > 30-50%**	**Ejection Fraction >60%**
'Decreased systolic function charachterizes dilated cardiomyopathy' - H18th	*'Restrictive cardiomyopathy is dominated by abnormal diastolic function'- H18th*	*'Hypertrophic cardiomyopathy is characterized hemodynamically with diastolic dysfunction'- H18th*

Presentation with Symptomatic Cardiomyopathy:

Features	Dilated	Restrictive	Hypertrophic
Ejection fraction (Normal 55%)	Usually <30%	Usually >30 – 50%	Usually >60%
Left ventricular diastolic dimension (Normal <55mm)	>= 60 mm	<60 mm (May be decreased)	Often decreased
Left ventricular wall thickness	Decreased	Normal or increased	Markedly increased
Atrial size	Increased	Increased; may be massive	Increased
Valvular regurgitation	Related to annular dilation; Mitral appears earlier, during decompensation; Tricuspid regurgitation in late stages	Related to endocardial involvement; Frequent mitral and tricuspid regurgitation, rarely severe	Related to valve-septum interaction; Mitral regurgitation
Common first symptoms	Exertional intolerance	Exertional intolerance, Early fluid retention	Exertional intolerance; May have chest pain
Congestive symptoms*	Left before right, except right prominent in young adults	Right often dominates	Left-sided congestion may develop late
Arrhythmia	Ventricular tachyarrhythmia; Conduction block in Chagas' disease, and some families. Atrial fibrillation.	Ventricular uncommon except in sarcoidosis Conduction block in sarcoidosis and amyloidosis. Atrial fibrillation.	Ventricular tachyarrhythmias; Atrial fibrillation

*Left-sided symptoms of pulmonary congestion: dyspnea on exertion, orthopnea, paroxysmal nocturnal dyspnea.
*Right-sided symptoms of systemic venous congestion: discomfort on bending, hepatic and abdominal distention, peripheral edema.

Hypertrophic Obstructive Cardiomyopathy (HOCM)

Distinctive Pathophysiological features include

Heterogeneous hypertrophy of LV

Septal Hypertrophy

- Pattern of hypertrophy is distinctive
- ***Asymmetrical septal hypertrophy*** is characteristic
- Thickness of ventricular septum is disproportionately increased when compared with the free wall

Dynamic LV outflow obstruction

- Dynamic LV outflow obstruction: it is related to narrowing of the subaortic area as a consequence of opposition of anterior mitral valve leaflet against the hypertrophied septum in midsystole. The concept is termed ***systolic anterior motion (SAM)*** of mitral valve.
- Dystolic dysfunction: The ubiquitous pathophysiological abnormality is not systolic but rather ***diastolic dysfunction*** - *Harrison*

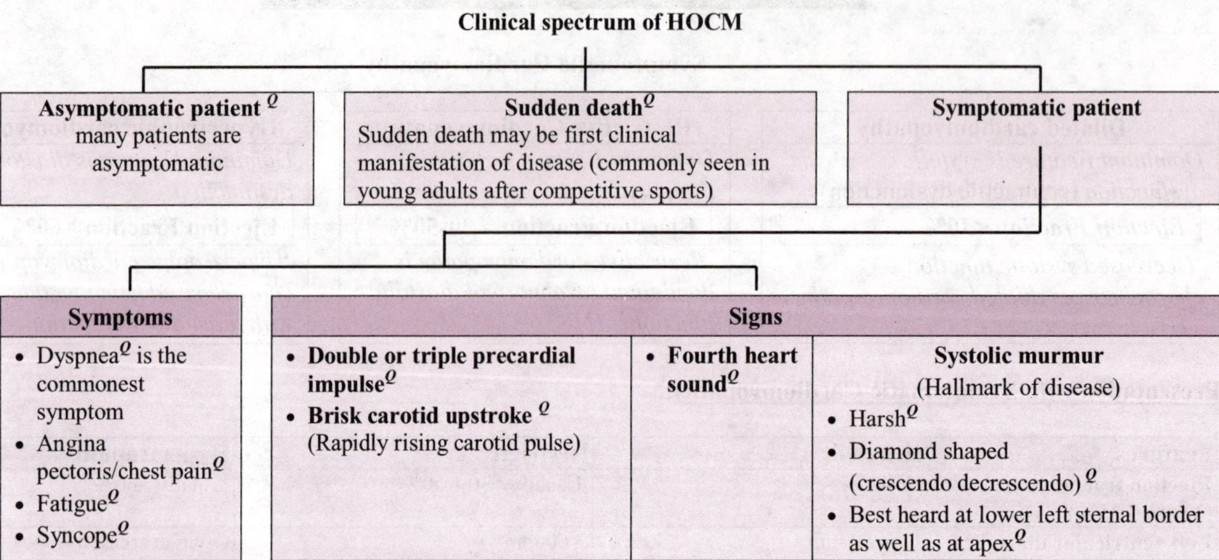

Condition which increase obstruction & intensity of murmur	Conditions which decrease obstruction & intensity of murmur
Factors that increase myocardial contractility • *Exercise*[Q] • *Sympathomimetic Amines*[Q] • *Digitalis Glycosides*[Q] **Factors which decrease Ventricular volume** • *Valsalva maneuver*[Q] • *Sudden standing*[Q] • *Nitroglycerine*[Q] • *Amyl nitrite*[Q] • *Tachycardia*[Q] **Decreased aortic impedance & afterload**	**Factors that decrease myocardial contractility** • Beta blockers • Calcium channel blockers **Factors which increase Ventricular volume** • *Augmentation of venous return by passive leg raising*[Q] • *Expansion of Blood Volume*[Q] • *Supine* ***Position***[Q] **Increased aortic impedance & afterload:** • *Elevation of Arterial pressure by phenylephrine*[Q] • *Sustained hand grip*[Q] • *Squatting*

Management of HOCM

- Avoidance of strenuous physical activity
- **Beta Blockers** should be the initial drug [Q] in symptomatic individuals. They reduce:
  - *Heart rate*
  - *Blood pressure*
  - *Stiffness of left ventricle*
  - *Fatal arrythmias*
- **Calcium channel Blockers**[Q] (verapamil and diltiazem) are alternative drugs.
  - They reduce-stiffness of ventricle
  - Elevated diastolic pressures
- **Amiadarone** may be used to reduce arrythmias.
- **Surgical myomectomy**

Cardiac Tamponade, Constrictive Pericarditis, Restrictive Cardimyopathy and Right Ventricular MI

Characteristic	Tamponade	Constrictive Pericarditis	Restrictive Cardiomyopathy	RVMI
Clinical				
Pulsus paradoxus	**Common**	**Usually absent**	**Rare**	**Rare**
Jugular veins				
Prominent y descent	Absent	Usually present	Rare	Rare
Prominent x descent	Present	Usually present	Present	Rare
Kussmaul's sign	**Absent** (Rare)[Q]	**Present**	**Present**	**Present**
Third heart sound	Absent	Absent	Rare	May be present
Pericardial knock	Absent	Often present	Absent	Absent
Electrocardiogram				
Low ECG voltage	May be present	May be present	May be present	Absent
Electrical alternans	**May be present**	**Absent**	**Absent**	**Absent**
Echocardiography				
Thickened pericardium	Absent	Present	Absent	Absent
Pericardial calcification	Absent	Often present	Absent	Absent
Pericardial effusion	Present	Absent	Absent	Absent
RV size	Usually small	Usually normal	Usually normal	Enlarged
Myocardial thickness	Normal	Normal	Usually increased	Normal
Right atrial collapse and RVDC	**Present**	**Absent**	**Absent**	**Absent**
Increased early filling, ↑ mitral flow velocity	Absent	Present	Present	May be present
Exaggerated respiratory variation in flow velocity	Present	Present	Absent	Absent
CT/MRI				
Thickened/calcific pericardium	Absent	Present	Absent	Absent
Cardiac catheterization				
Equalization of diastolic procedures	Usually present	Usually present	Usually absent	Absent or present
Cardiac biopsy helpful?	No	No	Sometimes	No

*RV, right ventricle; RVMI, right ventricular myocardial infarction; RVDC, right ventricular diastolic collapse; ECG, electrocardiograph.

Note:

*'A positive Kussmaul's sign is rare in cardiac tamponade. Its presence suggests that an organizing process and epicardial constriction are present in addition to effusion' – Harrisons

Hypertensive Emergencies and Urgencies

Hypertensive Crisis

Hypertensive Emergencies

- Marked elevation of Blood pressure with rapidly evolving end organ damage.
- No fixed Blood pressure cut off values are defined but, in general the blood pressure values are as follows.

  Diastolic BP> 120; Systolic BP>220
- Rapid /Immediate reduction of blood pressure is indicated in these patients
- Blood pressure should be controlled within hours (Preferably within 1 hours)
- Intensive monitoring in a critical care setting is mandatory

Hypertensive urgencies

- Marked elevation of blood pressure without rapidly evolving end organ damage
- No fixed blood pressure cut off values are defined but in general the blood pressure values may approach the same range as seen in hypertensive emergencies
- Lowering of blood pressure is essential but immediate very rapid reduction is often not required
- Blood pressure should be controlled over a period of hours or days (Preferably within 24 hours)
- Intensive monitoring in a critical care setting is not always required

  If the patient is asymptomatic or clinically stable the patient can be managed as an outpatient with dose follow up within days without an intensive monitoring setting usually with oval medications – Hurst 12th/1625

Commonly used Drugs in the Management of Hypertensive Crisis

Common Intravenous Agents
(Used for Hypertensive Emergencies)

Diuretics

Furosemide

Vosodilators

Sodium Nitroprusside
Nitroglycerine
Fenoldapam
Nicardipine
Hydralazine
Enolaprilant

Adrenergic Inhibitors

Phentolamine
Esmolol
Metaprolol
Labetolol
Urapidil

Common Oral Agents
(Used for Hypertensive Urgencies)

Nifedipine (Not Recommended now)
Nicardipine
Israpidine
Clonidine
Coptopril
Labetolol
Hydralazine
Nitroglycerine

**** Nifedipine should be used with great caution 'if at all' according to the US F.D.A.'***

Renovascular Hypertension/ Renal Artery Stenosis

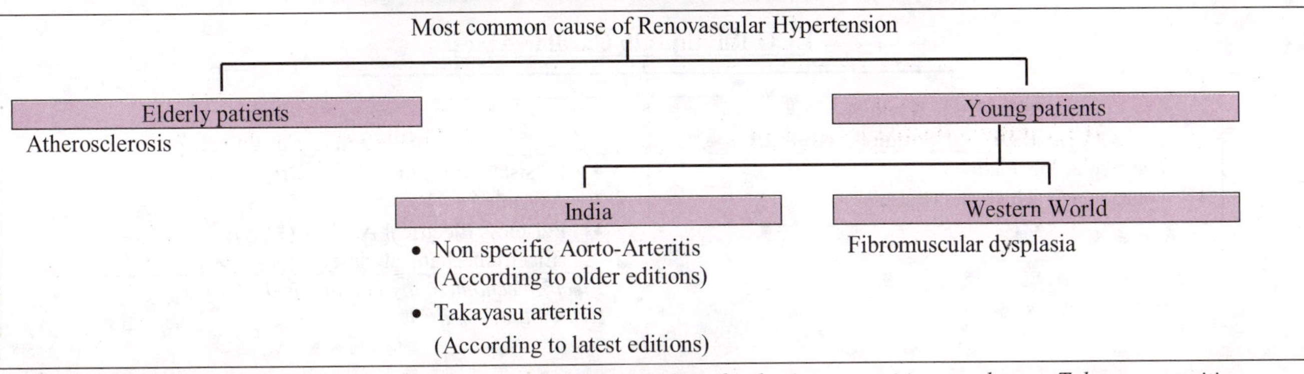

The non specific aorto-arteritis causing renal artery stenosis is now believed to be Aorto-arteritis secondary to Takayasu arteritis

Renal Artery Stenosis: Review

- Renal Artery stenosis is an important cause of Renovascular Hypertension
- ***Bilateral involvement is seen in half of the affected cases (50%)***

Etiology

- Atherosclerotic disease : This is the most common cause in middle aged /elderly patients
- Fibromuscular Dysplasia : ***This is the most important cause in young females***

Presentation

- Hypertension
  - Abrupt onset of hypertension
  - Acceleration of previously well controlled hypertension
  - Refractory Hypertension
- Features of increased sympathetic neural activity (which is associated with Renovascular disease)
  - Flushing
  - Loss of nocturnal BP decrease
  - Putonomic instability
  - Rapid BP swings
- Progressive Renal failure / Azotemia

Diagnosis

Magnetic Resonance Angiography (MRA)	Contrast Enhanced Arteriography
MRA is the most sensitive (>90%) and specific (95%) non invasive test for the diagnosis of RAS	Contrast enhanced angiography is the most definitive (but invasive) diagnostic procedure for diagnosis of RAS

Management

Medical Therapy with ACE Inhibitors or Angiotensin Receptor Blockers

Indications	Contra indications
Unilateral Renal artery Stenosis - With hypertension & normal renal function (more effective than other antihypertensives) - With hypertension & abnormal renal function (beneficial effect on survival without affecting renal function) - With hypertension, diabetes, proteinuria and normal or abnormal renal function (effective antihypertensives)	**Bilateral Renal Artery stenosis** ACE inhibitors or Angiotensin receptor blockers are contraindicated in patients with Bilateral renal artery stenosis or stenosis in a solitary kidney as their use in such patients leads to worsening of renal failure (These patients are especially sensitive to decline in intraglomerular pressure)

Note

Acute Renal Failure / Worsening of Renal Failure with Angiotension Receptor Inhibitors is a diagnostic clue to the diagnosis of renal artery stenosis (indicates bilateral disease)

Surgical Therapy with Angioplasty + Stent placement

Should be considered only after optimal medical therapy has failed to achieve goal BP or resulted in a > 30% increase in serum creatinine

Cardiac Arrest

ECG Rhythms in Cardiac Arrest

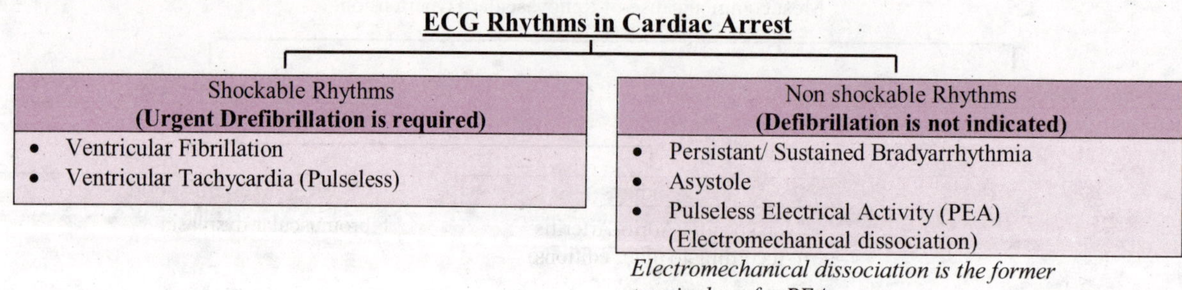

Electromechanical dissociation is the former terminology for PEA

Management of Cardiac Arrest

Cardiac Arrest
↓
Is monitor/Defibrillator Attached
- No → Start basis life support (CPR) and attach Monitor/Defibrillator
- Yes ↓

Assess Rhythm ? Shockable

Shockable Rhythm → Shockable Rhythm (VF,VT)
↓
Immediate defibrillation within 5 min of onset
Brief CPR before defibrillation for delay ≥5 min
↓ **Fail**
Continue CPR, intubate, IV access
↓ **Fail**
Epinephrine, 1 mg IV; or Vasopressin, 40 units IV once
Repeat epinephrine q 3-5 min
↓ **Fail**
Defibrillate, 360 J with 30 to 60 s
↓ **Fail**
Epinephrine , ↑dose | Antiarrhythmics | $NaHCO_3$, 1 meq/kg ($\uparrow K^+$)
↓
Amiodarone: 150mg over 10 min, 1mg/min
Lidocaine: 1.5 mg/kg; repeat in 3-5 min
Magnesium sulfate: 1-2 gm IV (polymorphic VT)
Procainamide: 30 mg/min, to 17 mg/kg (monomorphic VT)
↓ ↑
Defibrillate, 360 J: Drug – Shock – Drug - Shock

Non Shokable Rhythm → Non shockable Rhythm (Asystole, Bradyarrhythmia, PEA)
↓
CPR, Intubate, IV access
Identify and treat causes
↓
Epinephrine 1 mg iv (repeat) - Atropine (1mg iv repeat) - Sodium Bicarbonate (1meq/Kg iv)
Consider pacing – External or Pacing wire

Coarctation of Aorta:

Clinical presentation :

- Most patients are asymptomatic [Q]
- Symptomatic patients usually present with :
  - *Headache, dizziness,* [Q]
  - Epistaxis
  - *Cold extremities, and weakness in the legs* [Q]
  - ***Claudication with exercise*** [Q]
- Hypertension in upper extremities with marked diminution of pulsation in lower extremities. [Q]
- Mid systolic or continuous murmur over anterior part of chest and back [Q]
- Enlarged and pulsatile collateral vessels in intercostal spaces anteriorly in axilla or posteriorly in interscapular area[Q]
- Upper extremity and thorax may be more developed than lower extremities. [Q]

Investigations :

- ECG: shows L.V. Hypertrophy [Q]
- Radiography :
  - *Indentation of aorta at site of coarctation and '3 sign' on paramediastinal shaddon are almost pathogenic.* [Q]
  - *Notching* (erosion) of inferior surfaces of ribs. [Q]

Complications :

- Cerebral aneurysms and haemorrhage [Q]
- Rupture of aorta
- Left ventricular failure [Q]
- Infective endocarditis [Q]

Treatment :

- Is surgical *resection* [Q] of 'coarctation' and end to end anastomosis
  Remember that HT may not be corrected even after surgical correction of the 'coarctation'. [Q]

Few other questions :

Most common site [Q] of coarctation of aorta	:	*distal to origin of left subclavian artery.* [Q]
Most common associated cardiac anomaly [Q]	:	*bicuspid aortic valve.* [Q]
May be associated with [Q]	:	*Turner's syndrome.* [Q]

Associated anomalies with coarctation of Aorta [Q]

- **Bicuspid Aortic valve[Q] (commonest)**
- PDA[Q]
- VSD[Q]
- Tubular hypoplasia of aortic arch[Q]
- Aortic stenosis[Q] (valvular / subvalvular)

Other Associated lesions that have been asked previously

- Mitral valve abnormalities
(Subvalvular mitral ring /parachute mitral valve)
- Turner's syndrome[Q]

Shone complex[Q]

Coarctation of Aorta
+
Left sided obstructive lesions
(Mitral valve abnormalities and subaortic stenosis)

Marfan Syndrome and associated Cardiac Lesions

Marfan's syndrome is a genetic disorder of the connective tissue of the body manifested principally by changes in the skeleton, eye and cardiovascular system

Mutation in the fibrillary gene Q (15 q 21.1) Q
↓
Loss of fibrillary fibre base for deposition of elastin
↓
Alteration in connective tissue in various parts of the body particularly in

Skeletal changes of marfans syndrome:
- *Patients are usually tall* Q
- *Have long limbs* Q
- *The ratio of upper segment to lower segment is usually* ***2 SDs below*** *the mean for age, race &sex*
- *Arachnodactyly (fingers are long and slender, spider like in appearance)* Q
- *Pectus Excavation, Pectum Carinatum.* Q
- *Scoliosis, Kyphosis* Q

Cardiovascular changes Q
- *Dmitral valve prolapse &* Q
- *Mitral valve progresses to* ***Mitral valve Regurgitation***
- *Aortic aneurysm occurs it can leads to* ***Aortic Regurgitation.***

Associated changes
- *Spontaneous pneumothorax* Q
- *Inguinal & incisional hernias*
- *Striae may occur over the shoulders & buttocks.*

Ocular changes Q
- *Dislocation of the lens* Q
- *Elongation of globe (Myopia)* Q
- *Retinal detachment.* Q

Atrial Myxoma

Sporadic myxomas:	Familial myxomas:
• Are solitary Q • Located in Atria, most commonly in the left Q • Unlikely to have post-op recurrence Q • Occur in younger individuals Q	• Are multiple Q • More likely to have post op recurrence Q

Presentation is highly dependent on position of tumour and hence it is intermittent and sudden in onset. *(As a result of changes in tumor position with gravity).*

Cardiac signs and symptoms	Non cardiac signs and symptoms
- Picture of Mitral valve disease - Characterised by low pitched sound– 'tumor plop' Q (audible during early or mid diastole).	- **Peripheral or pulmonary emboli** Q - **Fever** : Prolonged pyrexia of unknown origin Q - **Clubbing** Q - Raynaud's Phenomenon Q - Anemia/polycythemia or thrombocytopenia / thrombocytosis Leucocytosis - Elevated ESR Q - Rash Q - Weight loss, cachexia, malaise, arthralgia

Rheumatic Fever

World Health Criteria for the diagnosis of Rheumatic fever

World Health Criteria for the diagnosis of Rheumatic fever and rheumatic heart disease	
Major manifestations	• *Carditis* • *Polyarthritis* • *Chorea* • *Erythema marginatum* • *Subcutaneous nodules*
Minor manifestations	• Clinical: fever, polyarthralgia • Laboratory: elevated erythrocyte sedimentation rate or leukocyte count • Electrocardiogram: prolonged P-R interval *@1992 Revised Jones criteria do not include elevated leucocyte count as a laboratory minor manifestation (but do include elevated C-reactive protein)*
Supporting evidence of a preceding streptococcal infection within the last 45 days	• Elevated or rising anti-streptolysin O or other streptococcal antibody, or • A positive throat culture, or • Rapid antigen test for group A streptococcus, or • Recent scarlet fever *@1992 Revised Jones criteria do not include recent scarlet fever as supporting evidence of a recent streptococcal infection*

Diagnostic Categories	Criteria
Primary episode of rheumatic fever	*Two major or one major two minor manifestations plus evidence of preceding group A streptococcal infection*
Recurrent attack of rheumatic fever in a patient without established rheumatic heart disease	*Two major or one minor manifestations plus evidence of preceding group A streptococcal infection*
Recurrent attack of rheumatic fever in a patient with established rheumatic heart disease	*Two minor manifestations plus evidence of preceding group A streptococcal infection*

Pathological Manifestations of Acute Rheumatic Fever

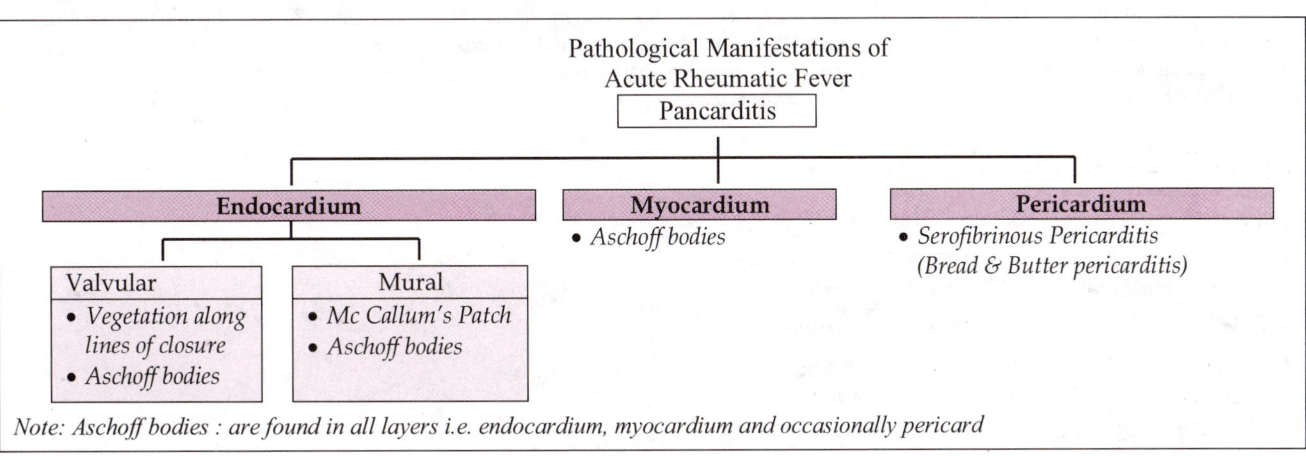

Infective Endocarditis

The Duke Criteria for the Clinical Diagnosis of Infective Endocarditis:

Major Criteria
1. Positive blood culture
• Typical microorganism for infective endocarditis from two separate blood cultures • Viridans streptococci, *Streptococcus gallolyticus*, HACEK group, *Staphylococcus aureus*, *or* • Community-acquired enterococci in the absence of a primary focus, *or* • Persistently positive blood culture, defined as recovery of a microorganism consistent with infective endocarditis from: • Blood cultures drawn >12 h apart; *or* • All of 3 or a majority of 4 separate blood cultures, with first and last drawn at least 1 h apart • Single positive blood culture for *Coxiella burnetii* or phase I IgG antibody titer of >1:800
2. Evidence of endocardial involvement
• ***Positive echocardiogram***[b] • Oscillating intracardiac mass on valve or supporting structures or in the path of regurgitant jets or in implanted material, in the absence of an alternative anatomic explanation, *or* • Abscess, *or* • New partial dehiscence of prosthetic valve, *or* • New valvular regurgitation (increase or change in preexisting murmur not sufficient)
Minor Criteria
1. Predisposition: predisposing heart condition or injection drug use 2. Fever 38.0°C (100.4°F) 3. Vascular phenomena: major arterial emboli, septic pulmonary infarcts, mycotic aneurysm, intracranial hemorrhage, conjunctival hemorrhages, Janeway lesions 4. Immunologic phenomena: glomerulonephritis, Osler's nodes, Roth's spots, ***rheumatoid factor*** 5. Microbiologic evidence: positive blood culture but not meeting major criterion as noted previously[c] or serologic evidence of active infection with organism consistent with infective endocarditis

[a]Definite endocarditis is defined by documentation of two major criteria, of one major criterion and three minor criteria, or of five minor criteria.

[b] Transesophageal echocardiography is recommended for assessing possible prosthetic valve endocarditis or complicated endocarditis.

[c]Excluding single positive cultures for coagulase-negative staphylococci and diphtheroids, which are common culture contaminants, and organisms that do not cause endocarditis frequently, such as gram-negative bacilli.

Note: HACEK, *Haemophilus* spp., *Aggregatibacter actinomycetemcomitans*, *Cardiobacterium hominis*, *Eikenella corrodens*, *Kingella* spp.

Risk of infective endocarditis in various lesions:

High Risk	Moderate Risk	Low Risk
• *Prosthetic heart value* • *Tetralogy of fallot* • *PDA* • *A regurgitation* • *A stenosis* • *Coarctation of Aorta* • *VSD* • *Mitral regurgitation*	• *MVP + M.R.* • *T. stenosis* • *T. Regurgitation* • *P. Stenosis* • *M. Stenosis*	• *ASD* • *MVP without MR*

Differetial Diagnosis of Vegetations in various Cardiac Lesions

Rheumatic Fever	Non bacterial Thrombotic (Marantic Endocarditis)	Libman Sack's Endocarditis (SLE)	Infective Endocarditis
• Small • Warty, verrucous • Usually Firm May be friable (but less than those of NBTE) (embolization rare)	• Small (but larger than those of rheumatic) • Friable (embolization common)	• Medium sized(small) • Flat, Verrucous,Irregular • Usually Firm; occasionally friable (embolization rare)	• Large, Bulky • Irregular • Friable *(most friable)*[Q] (embolization common)
• Along lines of closure	• Along lines of closure	• On surface of cusps Both surfaces may be involved most common being the undersurface, less often on mural endocardium • In pockets of valves	• Irregular vegetations on valve cusps that can extend onto the chordae. • Less often on mural endocardium
• Sterile (no organisms)	• Sterile	• Sterile	• Non-sterile (bacteria)
• Non destructive Valve perforation : no Mural involvement: rare	• Non destructive Valve perforation : no Mural involvement: rare	• Destructive Valve perforation : no Mural involvement: common	• Destructive Ulcerates or perforates underlying valve (or myocardium)
• Seen in Rheumatic fever	• Seen in hyper coagulable states e.g. cancer, promyelocytic leukemia increased estrogenic state	• Seen in SLE	• Seen in Infective endocarditis

Most common site:

- ***Most common site*** *for vegetations in Libman Sack's endocarditis are the A-V values, mitral and tricuspid.*
- ***Most common site*** *for vegetations in NBTE is mitral and less often aortic and Tricuspid.*
- ***Most common site*** *for vegetations of RF is mitral followed by combined mitral and aortic.*

Cardiac Cycle

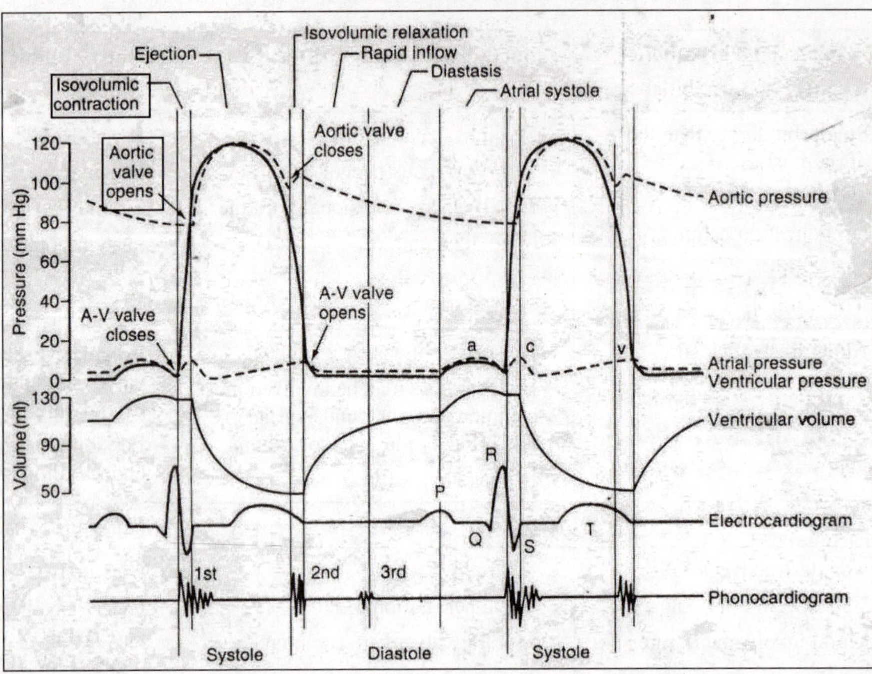

Valvular event (valves)	Cardiac events	ECG	JVP (Jugular venous Pressure curve)
Opening of AV valve[Q]	***End of isovolumic relaxation phase***[Q]	***End of T wave***[Q] ***(phase b/w T wave and new p wave)***	***V-Y descent***[Q]
Closure of AV valve	- End of diastole - Beginning of isovolumic contraction	Later half of R wave	End of 'x' descent
Opening of semilunar valve	*End of isovolumic contraction*[Q]	ST segment	Peak of 'C' wave
Closure of semilunar valve	- Beginning of isovolumic relaxation phase - Beginning of diastole	Later half of T wave	

QUESTIONS

Arterial Pulses

Pulsus Bisferiens

1. Pulsus bisiferiens is seen in all, EXCEPT:
   A. Aortic regurgitation + Aortic stenosis
   B. Aortic regurgitation *(AIIMS May 93)*
   C. Hypertrophic cardiomyopathy
   D. Tetralogy of Fallot
2. Bisfiriens pulse is seen in all Except: *(PGI Dec 05)*
   A. AS + AR
   B. AR
   C. Hypertrophic cardiomyopathy
   D. TOF
3. Pulsus bisferiens is best felt in :
   A. Carotid artery *(AIIMS Nov 98/ June 98)*
   B. Brachial artery
   C. Radial artery
   D. Femoral artery

Pulsus paradoxus

4. Pulsus paradoxus is seen in all *except* :
   A. IPPV *(AIIMS June 98)*
   B. COPD
   C. Cardiac Temponade
   D. Constrictive pericarditis
5. Pulsus paradoxus is present in all Except:
   A. Emphysema *(PGI Dec 05)*
   B. Pulmonary embolism
   C. Hypovolemic shock
   D. Hypertrophic cardiomyopathy
6. True about pulsus paradoxus is – *(PGI June 98)*
   A. Arm-tongue circulation time is increased
   B. ↑ Stroke volume
   C. Seen in constrictive pericarditis
   D. ↑ HR
7. Pulsus paradoxus is seen in (select three correct options)– *(PGI June 06)*
   A. Cardiac tamponade
   B. Constrictive pericarditis
   C. HOCM
   D. AR
   E. Severe asthma

Pulsus alternans

8. Pulsus alternans occurs in – *(PGI-June 98)*
   A. Constrictive pericarditis
   B. Viral myocarditis
   C. Hypokalemia
   D. MI

Miscellaneous Pulses

9. Water hammer pulse is seen in- *(AIIMS May 07)*
   A. Aortic stenosis
   B. Aortic regurgitation
   C. Aortic stenosis and Aortic regurgitation
   D. Mitral regurgitation
10. Double apical impulse is seen in – *(PGI Dec-98)*
    A. MR
    B. AR
    C. AS
    D. MS

Jugular Venous Pulse (JVP)

11. All of the following phases of the jugular venous pulse and their causes are correctly matched, *except*:
    A. ‘c’ wave - onset of atrial systole *(AI 2002)*
    B. ‘a-x’ descent - atrial relaxation
    C. ‘v-y’ - emptying of blood from right atrium into right ventricle
    D. ‘y-a’ ascent - filling of the right atrium from the vena cava
12. Which of the following is the correct statement regarding findings in JVP *(AI 2002)*
    A. Cannon wave : Complete heart block
    B. Slow vy descent : Tricuspid regurgitation
    C. Giant c wave : Tricuspid stenosis
    D. Increased JVP with prominent pulsations : SVC obstruction
13. Giant 'a' waves in JVP occur in *all except:*
    A. Junctional rhythm *(AI 1996)*
    B. Pulmonary hypertension
    C. Tricuspid regurgitation
    D. Complete heart block
14. In the JVP, ‘a’ waves are absent in : *(AI 1994)*
    A. Atrial fibrillation
    B. Mitral stenosis
    C. Tricuspid atresia
    D. Sick sinus syndrome
15. ‘C’ wave in JVP is due to- *(AIIMS Nov 07)*
    A. Atrial contraction
    B. Tricuspid valve bulging into right atrium
    C. Right atrial filling
    D. Rapid ventricular filling
16. C wave in JVP indicates: *(AI 2009)*
    A. Atrial contraction
    B. Bulging of tricuspid valve
    C. Ventricle systole
    D. Rapid ventricular filling

17. Typical JVP finding in cardiac tamponade – *(PGI-June-2000)*
 A. Absent 'Y' descent
 B. Prominent 'a' wave
 C. Absent 'a' wave
 D. Prominent 'Y' wave

Pulse Pressure

18. Pulse pressure is: *(AIIMS May 93)*
 A. 1/3 diastolic + 1/2 systolic B.P.
 B. 1/2 diastolic + 1/3 systolic B.P.
 C. Systolic – diastolic B.P.
 D. Diastolic + 1/2 systolic B.P.
19. Wide pulse pressure may be seen in all Except: *(AI 1991)*
 A. Aortic Regurgitation
 B. PDA
 C. Complete Heart Block
 D. Congestive Heart failure

Cardiac Auscultation: Heart Sounds and Murmurs

First Heart Sound (S1)

20. All of the following are true about S1, except: *(AI 1991)*
 A. Lower frequency than S_2
 B. Caused by closure of mitral valve
 C. Heard at the end of ventricular systole
 D. Better heard with diaphragm of stethoscope
21. First heart sound is soft in all, *except*: *(AIIMS Dec 95)*
 A. Short PR interval
 B. Ventricular septal defect
 C. Mitral regurgitation
 D. Calcified valve
22. Causes of soft S1 include: *(PGI June 97)*
 A. Long standing severe MS
 B. Obesity
 C. Mitral Regurgitation
 D. Pleural effusion
 E. All of the above
23. All of the above Loud S_1 is caused by (select two correct options): *(PGI Dec 04)*
 A. Calcified mitral valve.
 B. MVP
 C. Short Pr interval
 D. Tachycardia
 E. Dilatation or widening of mitral valve after valvotomy
24. Loud S1 in Mitral stenosis is caused by: *(PGI June 99)*
 A. Prolonged flow through mitral valve
 B. 1st degree heart block
 C. Calcification of the valve
 D. Immobilization of valve
25. Reverse splitting of first heart sound in heard in (select two correct options): *(PGI June 04)*
 A. RBBB
 B. LBBB
 C. Tricuspid stenosis
 D. AR
 E. Atrial myxoma

Second Heart Sound (S2)

26. Wide split S2 occurs in: *(AIIMS May 93)*
 A. VSD (ventricular septal defect)
 B. Mitral stenosis
 C. ASD (Atrial septal defect)
 D. Coarctation of aorta
27. Wide-split second heart sound is seen in (select two options) – *(PGI Dec 02)*
 A. ASD
 B. LBBB
 C. PDA
 D. MR
 E. PS
28. Wide-splitting of S_2 is seen in (select three correct options): *(PGI Dec 06)*
 A. ASD
 B. MR
 C. PDA
 D. PS
 E. LBBB
29. Fixed splitting of S2 may be seen in all except: *(PGI June 95)*
 A. Pulmonary embolism
 B. PS
 C. ASD
 D. LBBB
30. Reverse splitting of S2 is seen in all except (select two options): *(PGI Dec 05)*
 A. LBBB
 B. WPW type A
 C. LV pacing
 D. Systemic hypertension
 E. Post-stenotic dilatation in AS
31. Single second heart sound is seen in (select three options): *(PGI Dec 04)*
 A. TOF
 B. Pulmonary arterial hypertension
 C. Pulmonary atresia
 D. Corrected TGA
 E. Severe pulmonary stenosis
32. Loud pulmonary component of second heart sound heard in (select two options) – *(PGI June 04)*
 A. Pulmonary hypertension
 B. TOF
 C. Eissenmenger's syndrome
 D. Pulmonary stenosis
 E. AS

Third Heart Sound (S3)

33. Third heart sound is seen in all *except* : (AIIMS Dec 98)
    A. Athletes
    B. Mitral stenosis
    C. Constrictive pericarditis
    D. LVF
34. All of the following statements about third Heart sound (S3) are true, except: (AI 2010)
    A. Occurs due to rapid filling of the ventricles during atrial systole
    B. Seen in in Constrictive Pericarditis
    C. Seen in Atrial Septal Defect (ASD)
    D. Seen in Ventricular Septal Defect (VSD)
35. True about third heart sound is – (PGI Dec-98)
    A. Absent in Chr. Constrictive pericarditis
    B. Absent in aortic aneurysm
    C. Absent in MS
    D. Normal physiologically in Athletes

Fourth Heart Sound (S4)

36. Which of the following is true about fourth heart sound 'S4' : (AI 07)
    A. Can be heard by the unaided ear
    B. Frequency is greater than 20 Hz
    C. Heard during ventricular filling phase
    D. Heard during ventricular ejection phase
37. S4 is seen in all of the following, Except: (AIIMS May 94)
    A. Thyrotoxicosis
    B. Acute MI
    C. Atrial fibrillation
    D. Hypertrophic cardiomyopathy
38. S_4 is not seen in : (AIIMS May 95)
    A. Ventricular aneurysm
    B. Mitral regurgitation
    C. Hypertrophic cardiomyopathy
    D. Hypertension

Added Sound

39. All of the following heart sounds occur shortly after S_2 *except*: (AI 2003)
    A. Opening snap
    B. Pericardial knock
    C. Ejection click
    D. Tumor plop
40. Following is true regarding opening snap : (AIIMS Nov 02)
    A. It is a high-pitched diastolic sound.
    B. It s due to opening of stenosed aortic valve.
    C. It indicates pulmonary arterial hypertension.
    D. It preceedes the aortic component of second heart sound.
41. All of the following sounds are diastolic sounds, Except: (PGI- Dec-06)
    A. S3
    B. S4
    C. Opening snap
    D. Ejection chick
42. Systolic thrill in left 2nd and 3rd intercostals space may be seen in all of the following, Except (AI 2009)
    A. Subpulmonic VSD
    B. Pulmonic stenosis
    C. Ebstein's anomaly
    D. Pink TOF

Cardiac Murmur

43. An early systolic murmur may be caused by all of the following except: (AI 2003)
    A. Small ventricular septal defect
    B. Papillary muscle dysfunction
    C. Tricuspid regurgitation
    D. Aortic stenosis
44. All of the following murmurs may be heard in patients with aortic regurgitation *except* : (AIIMS Nov 02)
    A. High-pitched decrescendo diastolic murmur.
    B. Soft, low pitched mid distolic rumbling murmur.
    C. Mid-systolic ejection flow murmur
    D. Pansystolic murmur.
45. Mid-diastolic Murmur with presystolic accentuation is typically seen in: (DNB)
    A. Mitral stenosis
    B. Mitral Regurgitation
    C. Aortic stenosis
    D. MVP
46. Which of the following murmurs increase with Valsalva maneuver? (AIIMS Nov 2010)
    A. MR
    B. VSD
    C. AS
    D. HOCM
47. A young patient presents with a systolic murmur at the apex. The murmur increases on both handgrip and valsalva maneuver. Which of the following conditions is most likely? (AI 04)
    A. HOCM
    B. AS
    C. MVP
    D. VSD
48. Which of the following murmurs increase with valsalva maneovre (AIIMS May 09)
    A. Mitral stenosis
    B. HOCM
    C. Mitral Regurgitation
    D. Aortic stenosis

49. What is false in relation to Carey Coombs Murmur?
A. Delayed Diastolic Murmur *(AIIMS Nov 06)*
B. Seen in Rheumatic Fever
C. Associated with AR
D. Low Pitched Murmur

50. Carey coomb murmur is seen in – *(PGI Dec 97)*
A. Severe mitral stenosis
B. Acute rheumatic carditis
C. Pure aortic regurgitation
D. Severe pulmonary HT

51. Continuous murmur is found in all, EXCEPT:
A. Mitral stenosis with mitral regurgitation
B. Patent ductus arteriosus *(AIIMS May 93)*
C. Rupture of sinus of Valsalva
D. Systemic arteriovenous (AV) fistula

52. Continuous murmur is seen in all the following *except:* *(AI 1995)*
A. Aortic sinus of valsalva rupture
B. Coarctation of Aorta
C. AV malformations
D. Peripheral pulmonary stenosis

53. A continuous murmur is heard in all of the following conditions except: *(AIIMS May 05)*
A. Ventricular septal defect with aortic regurgitation
B. Patent ductus arteriosus
C. Coronary arteriovenous fistula
D. Venous hum

54. Continuous murmur is present in (select two options)
A. PDA *(PGI June 06)*
B. AS with AR
C. Shunt between pulmonary & subclavian artery
D. VSD with AR

55. Continuous murmur is found in (select three options)
A. AS combined with AR *(PGI Dec 04)*
B. Systemic A V fistula
C. PDA with reversal f shunt
D. Aortopulmonary window
E. Rupture of sinus valsalva

56. A new systolic murmur after Acute myocardial infarction may be due to all of the following Except:
A. Complete heart block *(AIIMS May 1993)*
B. Rupture of Interventricular septum
C. Papillary muscle dysfunction
D. Ischemic cardiomyopathy

Cardiovascular Clubbing

57. Cardiovascular causes of digital clubbing include all of the following Except:
A. Infective Endocarditis
B. Arteriovenous Fistulos
C. Tricuspid Atresia
D. Aortic Dissection

Electrocardiogram and Arrhythmias

General

58. Normal Axis of the heart is best described as being between:
A. – 30 to +90
B. + 30 to -90
C. – 30 to -90
D. +90 to ±180

59. Left Axis Deviation is seen as
A. A. Positive in Lead I and Positive in Lead II
B. B. Positive in Lead I and Negative in Lead II
C. C. Negative in Lead I and Negative in Lead II
D. D. Negative in Lead I and positive in Lead II

60. P wave is due to: *(AI 99)*
E. Atrial depolarization
F. Atrial repolarization
G. Ventricular depolarization
H. Ventricular repolarization

61. QRS complex indicates- *(AI 98)*
A. Atrial repolarization
B. Atrial depolarization
C. Ventricular repolarization
D. Ventricular depolarization

62. A QRS duration between 100 and 120 milliseconds suggests all of the following, Except: *(DNB)*
A. Normal
B. Left anterior Fascicular Block
C. Left posterior Fascicular Block
D. Left Bundle Branch Block

63. Wide QRS complex ≥ 0.12 seconds may be seen in all of the following EXCEPT: *(DNB)*
A. Hyperkalemia
B. Wolf Parkinson White Syndrome
C. Ventricular Tachycardia
D. Left Anterior Fascicular Block

64. Wide QRS complex is typically seen in
A. Bundle Branch block
B. Sick sinus sydrome
C. Mobitz Type I block
D. Mobitz Type II block

65. The ECG of a 40 year old male was recorded using standard bipolar limb leads. The sum of voltage of the three standard leads was found to be 5 millivolts. This indicates: *(AIIMS May 05)*
A. A normal heart
B. Right ventricular hypertrophy
C. Left ventricular hypertrophy
D. Increased cardiac muscle mass

66. Low QRS voltage on ECG indicates: *(DNB 2009)*
A. Pulmonary embolism
B. Pericardial effusion
C. Cor pulmonale
D. Infective endocarditis

67. Low QRS voltage on ECG with left ventricular hypertrophy on Echocardiography suggests a diagnosis of:
A. Pericardial effusion
B. Cardiac Amyloidosis
C. Corpulmonale
D. Infective endocarditis

ST Segment

68. ST elevation is seen in all of the following conditions *except* : *(AIIMS 2002)*
A. Myocardial infarction
B. Coronary artery spasm
C. Constrictive pericarditis
D. Ventricular aneurysm

69. All of the following may cause ST segment elevation on EKG, except : *(AI 2005)*
A. Early repolarization variant.
B. Constrictive pericarditis.
C. Ventricular aneurysm.
D. Prizmetal angina.

70. What is diagnostic of fresh myocardial infarction in ECG : *(AIIMS May 95)*
A. QT interval prolongation
B. P mitrale
C. ST segment elevation
D. ST segment depression

QT Interval

71. QT prolongation is seen in all, *except* :
A. Hypothermia *(AIIMS June 2000)*
B. Digitalis toxicity
C. Hypocalcemia
D. Romanowand syndrome

72. QT interval is shortened in- *(AI 95)*
A. Hypocalcaemia
B. Hypokalemia
C. Hypercalcemia
D. Hyperkalemia

73. Hypercalcemia in ECG is diagnosed by:
A. Increased QT interval *(PGI Dec-99)*
B. Decreased QT interval
C. Increased PR interval
D. Tall T waves

74. Hypocalcemia is characterized by all of the following features except- *(AI 03)*
A. Numbness and tingling of circumoral region
B. Hyperactivity tendon reflexes
C. Shortening of Q-T interval in ECG
D. Carpopedal spasm

Hypo/Hyperkalemia

75. All are ECG changes in hypokalemia, *except*:
A. U wave *(AIIMS Dec 97)*
B. ST segment sagging
C. T-wave flattening or inversion
D. QT interval prolongation

76. The following ECG findings are seen in Hypokalemia: *(AI 2007)*
A. Increased PR interval with ST depression
B. Increased PR interval with peaked T wave
C. Prolonged QT interval with T wave inversion
D. Decreased QT interval with ST depression

77. All of the following are the electrocardiographic features of Hyperkalemia, except- *(AIIMS May 04)*
A. Prolonged PR interval
B. Prolonged QT interval
C. Sine wave patterns
D. Loss of P waves

78. All of the following may occur due to hyperkalemia, except : *(AI 06)*
A. Prolonged PR interval
B. Prolonged QRS interval
C. Prolonged QT interval
D. Ventricular asystole

Digitalis Toxicity

79. All of the following electrocardiographic findings may represent manifestations of digitalis intoxication, *except*: *(AIIMS Nov 99)*
A. Bigeminy
B. Junctional tachycardia
C. Atrial flutter
D. Atrial tachycardia with variable block

Miscellaneous

80. In left sided massive pneumothorax, ECG shows all, except- *(AIIMS May 94)*
A. Left axis deviation
B. Absent R wave
C. Pathological Q waves
D. Precordial T wave inversion

81. Which of the following ECG changes is least likely in a patient with left pneumothorax : *(AIIMS Nov. 2000)*
A. Inversion of T wave
B. Left axis deviation
C. Small R wave
D. Electrical alternans

Arrhythmias

AF and PSVT

82. Atrial fibrillation may occur in all the following conditions, except- *(AIIMS May 03)*
    A. Mitral stenosis
    B. Hypothyroidism
    C. Dilated cardiomyopathy
    D. Mitral regurgitation
83. A chronic alcoholic develops palpitations suddenly after alcohol binge. Which of the following arrythmia is most commonly associated with alcohol binge in the alcoholics? *(AIIMS Nov 01)*
    A. Ventricular fibrillations
    B. Verticular premature contractions
    C. Atrial flutter
    D. Atrial fibrillation
84. All of the following are true about Atrial Fibrillation, Except
    A. ↑ risk of thromboembolism
    B. digoxin for treatment
    C. anticoagulation not required
    D. aspirin given
85. A person with mitral regurgitation and atrial fibrillation presents with syncope. On examination the person has a heart rate of 55. What is the most probable cause ? *(AI 2007)*
    A. Digitalis toxicity
    B. Incomplete heart block
    C. Stroke
    D. Subarachnoid Haemorrhage
86. In a patient with chronic atrial fibrillation with a regular beat of 60/min, the most probable cause is : *(AIIMS May 01)*
    A. Sleep
    B. Digitalis toxicity
    C. Sino nodal block
    D. Hypothyroidism
87. Drug of choice in PSVT is : *(AI 1998)*
    A. Amiodarone
    B. Lingnocaine
    C. Quinidine
    D. Adenosine
88. Drug of choice for Paroxysmal Supraventricular Tachycardia (PSVT) is: *(DNB June 2010)*
    A. Metaprolol
    B. Amiadarane
    C. Adenosine
    D. Lidocaine
89. What is the drug of choice to control supraventricular tachycardia : *(AIIMS Nov. 05)*
    A. Adenosine
    B. Propranolol
    C. Verapamil
    D. Digoxin

VT, VF and PVCs

90. All of the following features can differentiate between ventricular tachycardia and supraventricular tachycardia *except*: *(AIIMS Nov 98)*
    A. QRs < 0.14 seconds
    B. Ventricular rate > 160/min
    C. Variable first heart sound
    D. Relieved by carotid sinus massage
91. In a patient with wide-complex tachycardia, the presence of all of the following in the ECG indicates ventricular tachycardia except *(AIIMS Nov 03)*
    A. Atrioventricular dissociation
    B. Fusion beats
    C. Typical right bundle branch block
    D. Capture beats
92. Broad complex tachycardia due to ventricular a tachycardia is suggested by (select three correct options): *(PGI –1994)*
    A. Fusion Beats
    B. AV dissociation
    C. Capture Beats
    D. Termination of tachycardia by carotid massage
    E. Triphasic QRS in V1
93. Ventricular Tachycardia is represented by all, Except: *(PGI 1996)*
    A. Wide QRS complex
    B. AV dissociation
    C. Capture Beats
    D. Fusion beats
    E. Typical RBBB QRS complex
94. Which of the following statements about Premature Ventricular Beats is false: *(PGI 1997)*
    A. Sequential depolarization of ventricles
    B. Wide, Bizzare, Notched QRS complexes
    C. Prevalence decreases with age
    D. Palpitations is a common presenting feature
95. All of the following are features of Premature Ventricular Complexes, Except *(AI 1993)*
    A. Wide QRS complex
    B. Absent P wave
    C. Complete compensatory pause
    D. Prolonged PR interval
96. Which of the following is the most characteristic EKG finding of ventricular premature beats (select one single best correct option): *(PGI- June-04)*
    A. Fusion beat
    B. Narrow QRS complex
    C. AV Dissociation
    D. Wide QRS complex
    E. Capture beat
97. All of the following may be seen in ventricular premature beats, Except: *(PGI June 04)*
    A. Fusion beat
    B. Narrow QRS complex

C. AV Dissociation
D. Wide QRS complex
E. Capture beat

98. Accelerated Idioventricular Rhythm (AIVR) is the most common arrhythmia associated with:
A. Dilated cardiomyopathy *(AI 2010)*
B. Myocardial Reperfusion
C. Digitalis Intoxicatiun
D. Myocarditis

Torsades De Pointes

99. Feature of Torsade de pointes is: *(AIIMS Dec 97)*
A. Wide QRS complex
B. Short QRS complex
C. Prolonged QTc interval
D. Short QTc interval

100. Congenital long QT syndrome can lead to-
A. Complete heart block *(AIIMS May 2003)*
B. Polymorphic ventricular tachycardia
C. Acute myocardial infarction
D. Recurrent supraventricular tachycardia

101. Torsade-de-pointes is caused by – *(PGI June 99)*
A. Hypermagnesemia
B. Metabolic acidosis
C. Hypomagnesmia
D. Metabolic alkalosis

WPW Syndrome

102. WPW syndrome is caused by: *(DNB 2012)*
A. Bundle Branch Block
B. Right sided accessory pathway
C. Ectopic pacemaker in atrium
D. Left bundle Branch block

103. The most common accessory pathways leading to WPW syndrome is:
A. Left free wall
B. Posteroseptal
C. Right free wall
D. Anteroseptal

104. The most common reentrant tachycardia associated with WPW syndrome is *(PGI 2012)*
A. Orthodromic AV reentry
B. Antidromic AV reentry
C. Rapidly conducting AF
D. None

105. All are ECG findings in Wolf Parkinson's white syndrome, *except* : *(AIIMS Feb 97)*
A. Narrow QRS complexes
B. Normal QT interval
C. Slurred and tall QRS
D. Short PR interval

106. All of the following statements about WPW syndrome are true, Except: *(PGI Dec 05)*
A. More common in females
B. Rt ventricular aberrant is commonly seen
C. Incidence ↓ with age
D. Heart is structurally normal
E. Incidence is 0.3 to 0.7%.

107. The drug of choice in patients with Wolff-Parkinson-White syndrome with atrial fibrillation is-
A. Digitalis *(AIIMS Nov 03)*
B. Procainamide
C. Verapamil
D. Adenosine

108. Radiofrequency ablation is done for :
A. Ventricular tachycardia *(AIIMS June 98)*
B. PSVT
C. WPW
D. Atrial tachycardia

Heart block and Conduction Disturbance

109. All of the following are features of Mobitz Type I block, except: *(AI-1992)*
A. Constant PR interval
B. Normal QRS morphology
C. Regular Atrial Rhythm
D. Atrial rate > ventricular rate

110. Constant PR interval is seen in: *(PGI-1997)*
A. First degree block
B. Second degree – Mobiz type I block
C. Second degree – Mobitz type II block
D. Third degree block

111. Which of the following may be seen in second degree Heart block (select three options): *(PGI Dec 05)*
A. Change in QRS complex morphology
B. Atrial rate more than ventricular rate
C. Prolonged conduction time
D. One P wave to each QRS complex
E. No constant Relationship between P wave and QRS complex

112. True statement regarding Atrioventricular block with atrial tachycardia is : *(AIIMS Nov 98)*
A. Seen in WPW syndrome
B. Is a complication of pacemaker
C. Can occur in normal person occasionally.
D. Seen in Digitalis toxicity with K^+ depletion.

113. In the treatment of severe bradycardia, all of the following can be the best modality of treatment except:
A. Atropine *(AIIMS Nov. 05)*
B. Pacing
C. Isoproterenol
D. Diltiazem

Miscellaneous

114. Athletic syndrome is characterized by: *(PGI June 99)*
   A. Increased amplitude of QRS
   B. Tachycardia
   C. Decreased QT interval
   D. U-waves

Congestive Heart Failure and PCWP

115. All the following are features of right sided heart failure, Except: *(AI 2009)*
   A. Increased PCWP
   B. Pulsatile liver
   C. Increased JVP
   D. Positive hepatojugular reflex
116. All of the following are true about Right Ventricular Infarcts, Except *(DNB 2012)*
   A. Nocturia
   B. Hepatomepaly
   C. Ascitis
   D. Normal JVP
117. Which of the following is not a major Framingham criteria in CHF: *(AIIMS Nov 2008)*
   A. Cardiomegaly
   B. Paroxysmal nocturnal dyspnea
   C. S3 gallop
   D. Hepatomegaly
118. Left ventricular Hypertropy is caused by all, Except:
   A. M.S (Mitral stenosis) *(AIIMS Nov 09)*
   B. A. S (Aortic Stenosis)
   C. M.R (Mitral Regurgitation)
   D. A. R (Aortic Regurgitation)
119. CCF is associated with increase in all the following except: *(AI 2007)*
   A. Right atrial mean pressure
   B. Serum Sodium
   C. Urea
   D. Nor epinephrine
120. Positive hepatojugular reflux is found in conditions except: *(AI 2009)*
   A. Tricuspid regurgitation
   B. Right heart failure
   C. Decreased after load
   D. PS
121. Positive Hepatojugular Reflux is found in all of the following conditions, except: *(AIIMS May 2011)*
   A. Tricuspid Regurgitation
   B. Precapillary Pulmonary Hypertension
   C. Right Ventricular Infarction
   D. Decreased After-load
122. Enlarged Pulsative liver with ascitis is typically seen in: *(AIIMS May 2011)*
   A. Tricuspid Regurgitation (TR)
   B. Mitral Regurgitation (MR)
   C. Mitral stenosis
   D. Pulmonary stenosis (PS)
123. Left atrial filling pressure closely approximates-
   A. Pulmonary capillary wedge pressure
   B. Central venous pressure *(AIIMS May 93)*
   C. Intrapleural pressure
   D. Intracranial pressure
124. A Patient comes with sudden respiratory distress. On examination, bilateral basal crepts are present over chest suggestive of pulmonary edema. Alveolar wedge pressure is normal. The likely cause is-
   A. Narcotic overdose *(AIIMS June 2000)*
   B. Congestive heart failure
   C. Myocardial infarction
   D. Cardiogenic shock
125. Normal PCWP with pulmonary oedema is seen in-
   A. Left atrial myxoma *(AIIMS June 98)*
   B. High altitude
   C. Pulmonary vein obstruction
   D. Pulmonary artery obstruction.
126. Pulmonary edema associated with normal PCWP is observed. Which of these is not a cause: *(AI 01)*
   A. High altitude
   B. Cocaine overdose
   C. Post cardiopulmonary bypass
   D. Bilateral renal artery stenosis
127. A 45-year-old woman underwent a modified radical mastectomy 4 years ago. She was treated for multiple bone metastases with cyclophosphamide, doxorubicin, and fluorouracil for 6 months. She is complaining of exertion on exercise, swelling of the legs, and swelling around eyes in the morning. On examination, she has bilateral rales in the lungs, S1, S2 audible, S3, S4 gallop present. Her BP is 149/117 mm Hg, PR is 80/min, and RR is 18/min. What is the most likely cause for her cardiac condition?
   A. Systolic dysfunction CHF *(AIIMS May 06)*
   B. Drug induced cardiac toxicity
   C. Metastatic cardiac disease
   D. Pneumonia
128. 4. All of the following are used in the initial management of acute life threatening cardiogenic pulmonary edema, except: *(AI 2012)*
   A. Digoxin
   B. Morphine
   C. Furosemide
   D. Positive Pressure Ventilation
129. All of the following medications may be used in congestive cardiac failure, Except *(AIIMS Nov 09)*
   A. Spironolactone
   B. Nitrates
   C. Nesiritide
   D. Trimetazidine
130. All of the following are true about starting beta-blocker therapy in cases of CHF, Except
   A. They should be initiated at the effective doses

B. They should be gradually increased over weeks
C. Special precautions should be taken in NYHA class III & IV *(AIIMS Nov 2010)*
D. Carvedilol and Metoprolol are the preferred drugs

131. In a patient with chronic congestive cardiac failure, all of the following drugs prolong survival *except :*
A. Metoprolol *(AIIMS May 04)*
B. Carvedilol
C. Enalapril
D. Digoxin

132. All of the following statements about digitalis are true *except* : *(AI 1997)*
A. Excretion is mainly renal
B. Oral absorption is good
C. Actively metabolized in liver
D. Lipid soluble

133. Digoxin toxicity is enhanced by all, *except*:
A. Quinidine *(AIIMS Dec 97)*
B. Hypokalemia
C. Hypomagnesemia
D. Hepatic dysfunction

134. All of the following may precipitate digitalis toxicity *except* : *(AI 1997)*
A. Hypocalcemia
B. Hypokalemia
C. Hypomagnecemia
D. Hypothyroidism

135. Treatment of digoxin over dose includes administration of all of the following *except* :
A. Potassium *(AI 1997)*
B. Lignocaine
C. Phenyton
D. Hemodialysis

136. Following are used in treatment of digitalis toxicity except- *(AI 95)*
A. Potassium
B. Lignocaine
C. Fabparticles
D. Hemodialysis

137. All the following are radiological features of Chronic Cor pulmonale *except :* *(AI 1996)*
A. Kerley B lines
B. Prominent lower lobe vessels
C. Pleural effusion
D. Cardiomegaly

Vulvar Heart Disease

Mitral Stenosis

138. Area of mitral orifice in adults is: *(AIIMS Dec 94)*
A. 6-8 cm^2
B. .5-2 cm^2
C. 4-6 cm^2
D. 1-4 cm^2

139. Mitral stenosis is associated with : *(AI 1997)*
A. Right ventricular hypertrophy
B. Left ventricular hypertrophy
C. Left axis deviation
D. QRS complex

140. Mid diastolic Murmur with presystolic accentuation is typically seen in:
A. Mitral stenosis
B. Mitral Regurgitation
C. Aortic stenosis
D. MVP

141. All of the following may be seen as severity of mitral stenosis increases Except *(DNB Dec 2011)*
A. Pulsatile liver
B. Atrial fibrillation
C. Opening snap delayed from S2
D. Length of murmur is prolonged

142. Severity of mitral stenosis is assessed by:
A. Loud opening snap *(AI 1998)*
B. Length of murmur *(AIIMS May 03)*
C. Loud S_1
D. Splitting S_2

143. Severity of mitral stenosis is assessed by (select two options): *(PGI June 02)*
A. Loud S_1
B. S_2-OS gap
C. Prolonged diastolic murmur
D. S_3
E. S_4

Mitral Regurgitation

144. Severity of Mitral Regurgitation may be judged by
A. Intensity of murmur
B. Duration of murmur
C. Left ventricular S_3
D. Loud S_1

145. The severity of mitral regurgitation is decided by all of the following clinical findings *except*:
A. Presence of mid-diastolic murmur across mitral valve. *(AIIMS May 03)*
B. Wide split second heart sound.
C. Presence of left ventricular S3 gallop.
D. Intensity of systolic murmur across mitral valve

146. A 59 year old man with severe myxomatous mitral regurgitation is asymptomatic, with a left ventricular ejection fraction of 45% and an endsystolic diameter index of 2.9 cm/m2. The most appropriate treatment is: *(AI 2005)*
A. Mitral valve repair or replacement
B. No treatment
C. ACE inhibitor therapy
D. Digoxin and diuretic therapy

2

Cardiovascular System

Mitral Valve Prolapse (MVP)

147. A young asymptomatic female is observed to have a Midsystolic Click on routine examination. Valves are likely to show *(AI 2010)*
A. Myxomatous degeneration
B. Aschoff bodies
C. Calcific degeneration
D. Ruptured chordae tendinae

148. All of the following statements about mitral valve prolapse are true except: *(AIIMS Nov 93)*
A. It is more common in females
B. Most patients are symptomatic
C. It has a benign clinical course
D. Transient cerebral ischemic is a know complication

149. True regarding Mitral valve prolapse syndrome is all, EXCEPT- *(AIIMS Nov 93)*
A. More common in female
B. Mostly symptomatic
C. High incidence of arrhythmia
D. Transient cerebral ischemia can occur

150. All of the following are true for mitral valve prolapse, except- *(AI 06)*
A. Transmission may be as an autosomal dominant trait
B. Majority of the case present with features of mitral regurgitation
C. The valve leaflets characteristically show myxomatous
D. The disease is one of the common cardiovascular manifestations of Marfan's Syndrome

151. A 26 yr old asymptomatic woman is found to have arrthymias and a systolic murmur associated with midsystolic clicks; which investigation would you use: *(AI 2001)*
A. Electrophysiological testing
B. Tc scan
C. Echocardiography
D. Angiography

152. A female patient Chandani develops chest pain which is not associated with exercise and chest auscultation shows multiple non ejection clicks. The investigation which is used to diagnose the disease is : *(AIIMS June 99)*
A. Echocardiography
B. Pyrophosphate scan
C. Thallium 201 scan
D. ECG

Aortic Stenosis

153. Angina pectoris and Syncope are most likely to be associated with: *(AI 1994)*
A. Mitral stenosis
B. Aortic stenosis
C. Mitral regurgitation
D. Tricuspid stenosis

154. A 63 year old man present with a triad of angina, syncope and congestive heart failure. Which of the following valvular heart lesion can be suspected :
A. Mitral stenosis *(AIIMS Nov. 05)*
B. Tricuspid regurgitation
C. Aortic stenosis
D. Aortic regurgitation

155. In severe aortic stenosis true finding is :
A. Late systolic ejection click. *(AIIMS Nov 98)*
B. Heaving with outward apex
C. ST segment changes in ECG
D. Loud S_2

156. Which of the following physical signs is seen in a patient with severe aortic stenosis: *(AIIMS 2002)*
A. Opening snap
B. Diastolic rumble
C. Holosystolic murmur
D. Delayed peak of systolic murmur

157. Exercise testing is absolutely contraindicated in which one of the following: *(AI 2003)*
A. One week following myocardial infarction
B. Unstable angina
C. Aortic stenosis
D. Peripheral vascular disease

158. Calcification of the aortic valve is seen in :
A. Aortic stenosis *(AI 95)*
B. Aortic regurgitation
C. Marfan's syndrome
D. Hurler's syndrome

159. A 50-year-old asymptomatic man with established aortic stenosis undergoes Exercise Stress testing according to Bruce Protocol. The stress test was terminated at 11 minutes due to development of fatigue and dyspnea. Regional pressure gradient was observed to be 60 mm Hg between the two sides of the aortic valve. What is the best management.
A. Angiogram *(AIIMS Nov 2011)*
B. Aortic valve replacement
C. Aortic Balooning
D. Observation

Aortic Regurgitation

160. Acute Aortic regurgitation is seen in all the following *except:* *(AI 1994)*
A. Marfan's syndrome
B. Acute myocardial infarction
C. Bacterial endocarditis
D. Ankylosing spondylitis

161. Aortic regurgitation does NOT occur in :
A. Acute MI *(AIIMS Sept 96)*
B. Marfan's syndrome
C. Rheumatic heart disease
D. Infective endocarditis

162. All of the following murmurs may be heard in patients with aortic regurgitation *except* : *(AIIMS Nov 02)*
A. High-pitched decrescendo diastolic murmur.
B. Soft, low pitched mid distolic rumbling murmur.
C. Mid-systolic ejection flow murmur
D. Pansystolic murmur.

163. A 35 year old athlete has height 184 cm., arm span 194 cm., pulse rate 64/min., BP 148/64 mm Hg. Chest auscultation reveals long diastolic murmur over right 2nd intercostal space on routine examination. The probable diagnosis is : *(AIIMS June 99)*
A. Aortic regurgitation
B. Atrial septal defect
C. Ebstein anomaly
D. Coarctation of aorta

164. A young basketball player with ht 188 cm and arm span 197 cm has a diastolic murmur best heard in second right intercostal space: likely cause of murmur is: *(AI 2001)*
A. AS
B. Coarctation of aorta
C. AR
D. MR

165. LVH is commonly seen with : *(AI 1999)*
A. Pure mitral stenosis
B. ASD with fossa-ovalis
C. Aortic incompetance
D. Carcinoid syndrome

Pulmonic Stenosis

166. Obstruction in pulmonary stenosis may occur at the following sites : *(AI 97)*
A. Supravalvular
B. Valvular
C. Subvalvular
D. All of the above

167. Peripheral pulmonic stenosis is associated with (select two options): *(PGI June 02)*
A. Subaortic stenosis
B. Takayasu's arteritis
C. William syndrome
D. Coarctation of syndrome
E. Rubella

Tricuspid Regurgitation

168. The most common cause of tricuspid regurgitation is secondary to – *(AI-03)*
A. Rheumatoid heart disease
B. Dilatation of right ventricle
C. Coronary artery disease
D. Endocarditis due to intravenous drug abuse

169. Hepatomegaly with liver pulsation indicates: *(AI 2009)*
A. TR
B. MR
C. Pulmonary hypertension
D. MS

Ischemic Heart Disease and Atherosclerosis

Risk Factors / Atherosclerosis:

170. All of the following are risk factors for atherosclerosis except : *(AI 06)*
A. Increased waist - hip ratio
B. Hyperhomocysteinemia
C. Decreased fibrinogen levels
D. Decreased HDL levels

171. Best predictor for future risk of cardiovascular events, amongst the following is: *(AI 2009)*
A. hs CRP
B. Lipoprotein 'a'
C. Homocysteine
D. Interleukin 6

172. Which of the following is the best marker to predict future cardiac events *(DNB June 2012)*
A. hs CRP
B. Homocystine
C. Interleuken-6

173. The amino acid which is associated with atherosclerosis is : *(AIIMS May 2006)*
A. Lysine
B. Homocysteine
C. Cysteine
D. Alanine

174. Risk factors for coronary artery disease (CAD) (select two options)– *(PGI June 01)*
A. High HDL
B. Low LDL
C. Increased homocysteine levels
D. Decreased fibrinogen levels
E. Increased lipoproeins

175. Predisposing factors for coronary artery disease include, all Except: *(PGI Dec 02)*
A. Homocysteinemia
B. ↑ Lipoprotein B
C. ↑ Fibrinogen
D. ↑ plasminogen activator inhibitors 1

176. Raised serum level of lipoprotein-(a) is a predictor of *(AI 03)*
A. Cirrhosis of liver
B. Rheumatic arthritis
C. Atherosclerosis
D. Cervical cancer

177. Which of the following increases the susceptibility to coronary artery disease : *(AI 03)*
A. Type V hyperlipoproteinaemia
B. Von willebrands disease
C. Nephrotic syndrome
D. Systemic lupus erythematosus

178. In an old patient, the best indicator of probability of developing cardiovascular disease can be calculated by- *(AIIMS May 02)*
A. LDL/HDL ratio.
B. Triglycerides
C. Total cholesterol
D. Serum LDL

179. Most important predictor of coronary artery disease is: *(AIIMS May 09)*
A. VLDL
B. LDL
C. Chylomicron
D. LDL/HDL

180. All of the following dietary goals are recommended for patients with high risk of coronary heart disease, Except: *(AI 2011)*
A. LDL cholesterol < 100 mg/dl
B. Saturated fat < 7 % of total calories
C. Salt restriction < 6 gm/day
D. Avoid Alcohol

181. Which of the following dietary interventions has shown to reduces mortality in patients with coronary heart disease.- *(AIIMS May 07)*
A. High Fibre diet
B. Steral Esters
C. Potassium supplements
D. Omega 3 polysaturated fatty acids

182. A patient with hypertriglycerdemia is treated with Omega -3- polyunsaturated fatty acids. Treatment with omega-3- polyunsaturated fatty acids, will have the following effect on lipid profile: *(AIIMS Nov 2006)*
A. Increased LDL and Increased total cholesterol
B. Decreased LDL and Decreased total cholesterol
C. Increased LDL and Decreased total cholesterol
D. Decreased LDL and Increased total cholesterol

183. Which of the following statements about Atherosclerosis is true: *(AIIMS May 2011)*
A. Intake of Unsaturated Fatty Acids is associated with decreased risk
B. Extent of lesions in veins is similar as that in arteries
C. Thoracic Aorta is more commonly involved than abdominal aorta
D. Hypercholesterolemia alone does not increase the risk of atherosclerosis per se

Myocardial Infarction / Angina

184. All of the following statements about Universal Definition of Myocardial Infarction are true, Except: *(AIIMS Nov 2011)*
A. Sudden, unexpected Cardiac death with symptoms of Ischemia.
B. Elevation of cardiac biomarkers with new regional wall motion abnormality
C. Three times increase in Troponin levels after Percutaneous Coronary Intervention (PCI)
D. Three times increase in Troponin levels after Coronary Artery Bypass Grafting (CABG)

185. Most common site of myocardial infraction is: *(AI 98)*
A. Anterior wall of left ventricle
B. Posterior wall of left ventricle
C. Posterior wall of right ventricle
D. Inferior wall of left ventricle

186. The most common site for myocardial infarction is : *(AI 96)*
A. Left atrium
B. Left ventricle
C. Right atrium
D. Right ventricle

187. The most common site of Myocardial infarction is: *(AI 94)*
A. Anterior wall
B. Interventricular septum
C. Posterior wall
D. Inferior wall

188. All of the following arteries are common sites of occlusion by a *except*: *(AIIMS May 2005)*
A. Left anterior descending
B. Right coronary artery
C. Circumflex coronary artery
D. Marginal artery

189. Which of the following ECG findings is associated with acute myocardial Infarction *(DNB 2012)*
A. Elevation of S wave
B. Prolonged QT interval
C. Tall T waves with increased amplitude
D. Prolonged PR interval

190. ECG is poor in detecting ischemia in areas supplied by which of the following vessels: *(AI 2011)*
A. Left Anterior Descending (LAD)
B. Left Circumflex (LCx)
C. Left Coronary Artery (LCA)
D. Right Coronary Artery (RCA)

191. Which of the following ECG leads is most sensitive in detecting intraoperative myocardial ischemia
A. Lead I
B. Lead II
C. Lead V_1
D. Lead V_2
E. Lead V_5

192. A 60 year old man presents with chest pain with last 6 hours and is diagnosed as acute myocardial infarction. Angiography showed involvement of anterior descending branch of left coronary artery. The most probable site of infarct is : *(AIIMS May 01)*
A. Anterolateral wall
B. Posterior wall
C. Inferior wall
D. Septal

193. A 70 year old male patient presented to the emergency department with pain in epigastrium and

difficulty in breathing for 6 hours. On examination, his heart rate was chest examination was normal. The patient has been taking omeprazole for gastresophageal reflux disease for last 6 months. What should be the intial investigation :

A. An ECG *(AIIMS Nov. 05)*
B. An upper GI endoscopy
C. Urgent ultrasound of the abdomen
D. An x-ray chest

194. In stable angina : *(AIIMS Nov 03)*
A. CK-MB is elevated
B. Troponin I is elevated
C. Myoglobin is elevated
D. The levels of cardiac markers remain unchanged.

195. What is diagnostic of fresh myocardial infarction in ECG: *(AIIMS May 95)*
A. QT interval prolongation
B. P mitrale
C. ST segment elevation
D. ST segment depression

196. ST elevation and hyperacute T waves in precordeal leads V1 to V6 and in lead aVL indicates:
A. Anterolateral wall MI *(PGI Dec 2000)*
B. Posterior wall MI
C. Inferior MI
D. Lateral wall MI

197. In MI, which enzyme is raised in 4 to 6 hrs. & decreases in 3 to 4 days : *(AIIMS Nov. 2000)*
A. SGOT *(AIIMS June 98)*
B. LDH
C. CPK
D. SGPT

198. A patient presents 12 hours following a Myocardial infarction. Test of choice : *(AIIMS June 98)*
A. Lactate dehydrogenase
B. Cardiac troponins
C. Creatinine phosphokinase
D. Myoglobin

199. Troponin - T is a marker of : *(AIIMS May 2004)*
A. Renal disease
B. Muscular disease
C. Cirrhosis of liver
D. Myocardial infarction

200. Troponin-T is preferable to CPK-MB in the diagnosis of acute myocardial infarction (MI) in all of the following situations except: *(AI 2003)*
A. Bedside diagnosis of MI
B. Postoperatively (after CABG)
C. Reinfarction after 4 days
D. Small infarcts

201. Which of the following is the preferred marker for detecting Acute STEMI in Atheletes: *(AI 2012)*
A. CK-MB
B. Troponin T/I
C. C-Reactive Protein
D. LDH

202. Reperfusion is believed to restore contractile function of: *(AIIMS May 2011)*
A. Stunned Myocardium
B. Hibernating Myocardium
C. Ischemic non-viable myocardium
D. Non ischemic viable myocardium

203. Agent of first choice in an acute attack of Prinzmetal's angina is: *(AI 1995)*
A. Diltiazem
B. Nitrates
C. Propranolol
D. Verapamil

204. The best possible intervention for acute myocardial infarction is: *(AIIMS May 2005)*
A. Streptokinase
B. Streptokinase and aspirin
C. Early primary coronary intervention
D. Streptokinase and heparin

205. 40 year old male patient presents to the Emergency department with central chest pain for 2 hours. The ECG shows ST segment depression and cardiac troponins are elevated. Patient has a positive history of previous PCI 3 months back. He is administered Aspirin, Clopidogrel, Nitrates and LMWH, in the Emergency Department and shifted to the coronary are unit. The best recommended course of further action should include
A. Immediate Revascularization with Thrombolytics
B. Early Revascularization with PCI
C. Continue conservative management and monitoring of cardiac enzymes and ECG
D. Continue conservation management and plan for delayed Revascularization procedure after patient is discharged

206. A 50 year old man with a history of smoking, hypertension, and chronic exertional angina develops several daily episodes of chest pain at rest compatible with cardiac ischemia. The patient is hospitalized. All the following would be part of an appropriate management plan *except* : *(AIIMS Nov 99)*
A. Intravenous heparin
B. Aspirin
C. Intravenous nitroglycerin
D. Lidocaine by bolus infusion

207. A patient present with acute anterior wall infarction and hyotension. Which will be the immediate treatment modality for this atient : *(AI 2007)*
A. Intra aortic balloon counter pulsation
B. Anticoagulation
C. Thrombolytic therapy
D. Primary antioplasty

208. A patient presents with intense chestpain of 2 hrs duration. ECG shows ST depression in leads I and V1

to V4. There is associated T inversion and CPK-MB is elevated. All of the following should be included in the management of this patient, Except:
A. Nitroglycerine drip (PGI June 2000)
B. Aspirin
C. Coronary angiography
D. Streptokinase
E. I.V. metoprolol

209. A 40 years old male, chronic smoker comes with acute epigastric discomfort, for past one hour. ECG showing ST segment elevation in inferior leads. What is the immediate intervention? *(AIIMS Nov 07)*
A. Aspirin
B. Thrombolytic therapy
C. IV pantoprazole
D. Beta blockers

210. All of the following drugs are used in the management of acute myocardial infarction, *except*:
A. Tissue Plasminogen activator
B. Intravenous beta blockers
C. Acetylsalicylic acid *(AIIMS May 04)*
D. Calcium channel blockers

211. In MI following are used Except: *(PGI Dec 97)*
A. Fibrinolytics
B. Plasminogen activator inhibitor
C. Anti thrombin
D. Platelet inhibitor

212. Allof the following are used in the management of acute myocardial infarction Except: *(PGI Dec 01)*
A. Aspirin
B. Heparin
C. Alteplase
D. Warfarin

213. Streptokinase and Urokinase are contraindicated in:
A. Intracranial malignancy *(AI 2010)*
B. Pulmonary Embolism
C. AV fistula
D. Thrombophlebitis

214. All of the following are complications of streptokinase, Except: *(PGI June 01)*
A. Joint pain
B. Inctracranial bleed
C. Fever
D. Anaphylaxis
E. Hypotension

215. A patient with acute inferior wall myocardial infarction has developed shock. Which of the following is the most likely cause of shock
A. Cardiac rupture *(AIIMS May 04)*
B. Interventricular septal perforation
C. Papillary muscle rupture
D. Right ventricular infarction

216. A previously healthy 58 years old man is admitted to the hospital because of an acute inferior myocardial infarction. Within several hours, he becomes oliguric and hypotensive (blood pressure is 90/60 mmHg). Insertion of a pulmonary artery (Swan-Ganz) catheter reveals the following pressures: pulmonary capillary wedge-4 mm Hg; pulmonary artery- 22/4 mmHg: and mean right atrial- 11 mmHg. This man would best be treated with : *(AIIMS Nov 99)*
A. Fluids
B. Digoxin
C. Dopamine
D. Intraaortic balloon counter pulsation

217. In a pt of acute inferior wall MI; best modalitiy of rx is: *(AI 2001)*
A. IV fluids
B. Digoxin
C. Diuretics
D. Vasodilators

218. In a pt of acute inferior wall MI; best modalitiy of rx is: *(AI 2001)*
A. IV fluids
B. Digoxin
C. Diuretics
D. Vasodilators

219. A patient had an inferior wall myocardial infarction and was in shock. The reason for the patient being in shock is:- *(AIIMS May 02)*
A. Mitral regurgitation
B. Infarction causing septal defect
C. Right ventricular infarction
D. Decreased ejection fraction from left ventricle

220. In a patient with myocardial infarction the valvular lesion commonly seen in:- *(AIIMS May 02)*
A. Aortic stenosis
B. Mitral regurgitation
C. Aortic regurgitation
D. Septal defect

221. Ramkumar a 70 year old hypertensive male was admitted in the intensive care unit with transmural anterolateral myocardial infraction. His condition was stable till fifth day of admission, when he developed a pericardial friction rub and pleuritic chest pain which persisted despite narcotic and steroid therapy. On the seventh morning, he suddenly developed marked hypotension. On examination there was marked distension of the jugular veins, accompanied with electromechanical dissociation. Most likely, the patient had developed : *(AIIMS Nov 02)*
A. Severe acute mitral regurgitation.
B. Ventricular septal rupture.
C. Right ventricular infarction.
D. External cardiac rupture.

222. A new systolic murmur after Acute myocardial infarction may be due to all of the following Except:
A. Complete heart block *(AIIMS May 1993)*
B. Rupture of Interventricular septum
C. Papillary muscle dysfunction
D. Ischemic cardiomyopathy

223. True about Dressler.'s syndrome is all, except :
A. Occurs with in hours after myocardial infarction
B. Recurrence may be seen
C. Chest pain is common *(AIIMS June 98)*
D. Responds well to salicylates

224. Which of the following tests is used to detect reversible myocardial ischemia *(AIIMS May 09)*
A. Angiography
B. Thallium scan
C. MUGA
D. Resting Echocardiography

225. Which test is performed to detect reversible myocardial ischemia? *(AIIMS May 03)*
A. Coronary angiography.
B. MUGA scan.
C. Thallium scan.
D. Resting echocardiography.

226. Which of the following drugs has been linked with increased cardiac mortality: *(AI 2012)*
A. Rofecoxib
B. Metoprolol
C. Losartan
D. Nicorandil

227. Following an attack of myocardial infarction the mortality and morbidity of the patient is indicated by
A. Ventricular extra systole *(AIIMS June 2000)*
B. Left ventricular ejection fraction
C. Duration of syncope
D. Percentage of narrowness of coronary artery

Cardiomyopathy/HOCM

228. Cardiomyopathy may be seen in all of the following except : *(AIIMS May 2006)*
A. Duchene muscular dystrophy
B. Friedrich's ataxia
C. Type II glycogen storage disease
D. Alkaptonuria

229. Contractile Dysfunction is the dominant feature of which of the following types of cardiomyopathies
A. Dilated cardiomyopathy *(DNB 2012)*
B. Restrictive cardiomyopathy
C. Hypertrophic cardiomyopathy
D. Infiltrative cardiomyopathy

230. Which one of the following is the most common cause for 'Restrictive cardiomyopathy' :
A. Alcohol *(AIIMS May 04)*
B. Hemochromatosis
C. Amyloidosis
D. Sarcoidosis

231. A 25 years old basket ball player suddenly collapsed while undergoing an athletic event and died. At autopsy the septum was hypertrophied. The most probable diagnosis is- *(AIPGMEE 08)*
A. HOCM
B. Right ventricular conduction Abnormality
C. Epilepsy
D. Snake bite

232. A 26 year old man died suddenly during sporting activity. At autopsy the heart revealed chamber and septum Hypertrophy. The most likely diagnosis is
A. HOCM *(AIIMS May 09)*
B. DCM
C. Arrhythmogenic cardiac problem
D. Restrictive cardiomyopathy

233. All are true about Hypertrophic Obstructive Cardiomyopathy, *except* : *(AI 2000)*
A. β agonist are useful
B. Asymmetrical hypertrophy of septum
C. Dynamic L.V. outflow obstruction
D. Condition improves on passive leg raising

234. A 16 year old male is referred by high school coach for a physical examination before joining the football team. His elder brother had died suddenly during football practise, no autopsy was done. The patient has a loud systolic murmur on chest auscultation. All of the following would be constant with hypertrophic cardiomyopathy, *except* : *(AIIMS Nov 99)*
A. A crescendo-decrescendo systolic murmur
B. Murmur radiating to neck
C. Brisk carotid upstroke
D. Increase in murmur during valsalva or standing

235. All are true about hypertrophic cardiomyopathy, *except* : *(AIIMS 1996)*
A. Systolic dysfunction
B. Concentric hypertrophy
C. Diastolic dysfunction
D. Double apical impulse

236. The murmur of hypertrophic obstructive cardiomyopathy is decreased in which of the following: *(AIIMS Nov. 2000)*
A. Supine position
B. Standing position
C. Valsalva maneuver
D. Amyl nitrate inhalation

237. A 68-year old man who has had a recent syncopal episode is hospitalized with congestive heart failure. His blood pressure is 160/80 mmHg. His pulse rate is 80 beats per minute, and there is a grade III/IV harsh systolic murmur. An echocardiogram shows a disproportionately thickened ventricular septum and systolic anterior motion of the mitral valve. Which of the following findings would most likely be present in this man : *(AIIMS Nov 99)*
A. Radiation of the murmur to the neck.
B. Decrease of the murmur with hand grip
C. Delayed carotid upstroke
D. Reduced left ventricular ejection fraction

238. Which of the following drugs are contraindicated in HOCM *(DNB 2009)*
A. Verepamil
B. Propanalol

C. Digoxin
D. None of the above

239. The 9 month old child of a diabetic mother presents with tachypnea and hepatomegaly. Echocardiography of the heart showed normal cardiac morphology with asymmetric septal hypertrophy. Which of the following you will give to treat this child : *(AIIMS Nov. 2000)*
A. Digoxin
B. Frusemide
C. Propranolol
D. Isoptin

240. Aggravation of symptoms of angina in a patient when given nitrates is seen in : *(AIIMS June 2000)*
A. Aortic regurgitation
B. Mitral regurgitation
C. Single left coronary artery stenosis
D. Idiopathic hypertrophic subaortic stenosis

241. A 35-year-old farmer consulted a local medical practitioner for recurrent attacks of chest pain. His elder brother had similar complaints and had died suddenly at the age of 40 years. The farmer was advised to take nitroglycerine sublingually at the time of pain. However, the patient finds that the intensity of pain is increased by nitroglycerine. Most probably, he is suffering from : *(AIIMS Nov 02)*
A. Subacute bacterial endocarditis involving the aortic valve.
B. Hypertrophic obstructive cardiomyopathy.
C. Degenerative mitral regurgitation.
D. Chronic Type A dissection of aorta.

242. All are the true regarding hypertrophic obstructive cardiomyopathy, *except*: *(AIIMS Dec 97)*
A. Digitalis is useful
B. Left ventricular outflow obstruction
C. Asymmetrical septal thickness
D. Double apical impulse

Pericardial Disease

Cardiac Tamponade

243. All of the following are seen in cardiac tamponade *except*: *(AI 2004)*
A. Pulsus paradoxus
B. Diastolic collapse of right ventricle on echocardiogram
C. Electrical alternans
D. Kussmaul's sign

244. All of the following may be seen in patients of cardiac tamponade except: *(AI 06)*
A. Kussmaul's sign
B. Pulsus paradoxus
C. Electrical alternans
D. Right ventricular diastolic collapse on echocardiogram

245. All are features, seen in cardiac tamponade, *except*: *(AIIMS Dec 95)*
A. Raised JVP
B. Kussamaul sign
C. Rapid y descent
D. Pulsus paradoxus

246. Pulsus paradoxus is a characteristic feature of: *(AIIMS Dec 92)*
A. Constrictive pericarditis
B. Cardiac Tamponade
C. Hypertrophic obstructive cardiomyopathy
D. Restrictive cardiomyopathy

247. Beck's Triad is seen in: *(AI 2010)*
A. Constrictive Pericarditis
B. Cardiac tamponade
C. Right ventricular Myocardial Infarction (RVMI)
D. Restrictive Cardiomyopathy

248. Beck's triad of cardiac tamponade includes all, Except: *(AI 1991)*
A. Hypotension
B. Increased JVP
C. Muffled Heart sounds
D. Tachycardia

249. Beck's triad of cardic tamponade includes (select three correct options): *(PGI Dec 03)*
A. Hypotension
B. Neck vein distension
C. Paradoxical pulse
D. Silent heart
E. Tachycardia

250. A pt presents with engorged neck veins, BP 80/50 and pulse rate of 100 following blunt trauma to the chest : Diagnosis is: *(AI 2001)*
A. Pneumothorax
B. Right ventricular failure
C. Cardiac tamponade
D. Hemothorax

251. A young motorist suffered injuries in a major road traffic accident. He was diagnosed to have fracture of left femur and left humerus. He was also having fractures of multiple ribs anteriorly on both the sides. On examination the blood pressure was 80/60 mm Hg. and heart rate was 140/minute. The patient was agitated, restless, and tachypenic. Jugular veins were distended. Air entry was adequate in both the lung fields. Heart sounds were barely audible. Femoral pulses were weakly palpable but distally no pulsation could be felt. On priority basis, the immediate intervention would be :
A. Rapid blood transfusion. *(AIIMS Nov 02)*
B. Urgent pericardial tap.
C. Intercostal tube drainage on both the sides.
D. Fixation of left femur & repair of femoral artery

252. A post-operative cardiac surgical patient developed sudden hypotension, raised central venous pressure, pulsus paradoxus at the 4th post operative hour. The most probable diagnosis is:

A. Excessive mediastinal bleeding (AI 2003)
B. Ventricular dysfunction
C. Congestive cardiac failure
D. Cardiac tamponade

253. Kussmaul's sign is NOT seen in (AI 2001)
A. Restrictive cardiomyopathy
B. Constrictive pericarditis
C. Cardiac tamponade
D. RV infarct

254. A 30 year male patient presents to the emergency department with ahistory of acute breathlessness. On examination, JVP is increased and an inspiratory decline in systolic blood pressure of 14mm Hg is observed. Which of the following statements about the condition is true: (PGI June 2008)
A. Kussmaul's sign
B. Low ECG voltage
C. Prominent 'y' descent
D. Thickened Pericardium

255. Electric alternans is seen in: (AI 1995)
A. Cardiac tamponade
B. Restrictive cardiomyopathy
C. Constructive pericarditis
D. Right Ventricular MI (RVMI)

Constrictive Pericarditis

256. Haemorrhagic pericarditis occurs in all of the following conditions *except*.: (AIIMS May 03)
A. Transmural myocardial infarction.
B. Dissecting aneurysm of aorta.
C. Metastatic disease of pericardium.
D. Constrictive pericarditis.

257. Which of the following is least likely to cause constrictive pericarditis? (AIIMS Nov. 03)
A. Tuberculous pericardial effusion
B. Staphylococcal effusion
C. Post cardiac surgery
D. Acute rheumatic fever

258. All of the following statements about chronic constrictive pericarditis are true except
A. Commonest cause in India is 'Idiopathic'
B. Kussmaul's sign is present (PGI Dec 99)
C. Ascitis is not in proportion to edema
D. Right ventricular End Diastolic pressure is raised

259. All of the following are features of constrictive pericarditis Except: (PGI Dec 99)
A. Ascitis
B. Retractile Apex
C. Pericardial knock
D. Acute pulmonary Edema

260. During ventricular pressure pulses square root wave is seen in – (PGI Dec-98)
A. ASD
B. MVPS
C. Dilated cardiomyopathy
D. Constrictive pericarditis

261. Restrictive cardiomyopathy may be differentiated from constrictive pericarditis by the following features (select two options): (PGI June 02)
A. Diastolic pressures are equalized
B. Pericardial effusion
C. Thick pericardium is present
D. RV size

262. Rapid X descent unlikely in (PGI Dec 99)
A. Constrictive pericarditis
B. Cardiac tamponade
C. RVMI
D. Restrictive cardiomyopathy

Hypertension

General

263. Management of uncomplicated essential hypertension is: (DNB 2009)
A. No need to treat
B. Diet modification and exercise
C. Diet modification, exercise & drugs
D. Drugs alone

264. All of the followed drug combinations may be recommended for initial for management of hypertension, Except: (AI 1991)
A. ACE inhibitors and Belablockers
B. ACE inhibitors and calcium channel blockers
C. Diuretics and ACE inhibitors
D. Diuretic and Betablockers

265. First line drug choice for management of hypertension in patients with angina: (DNB)
A. Beta Blockers
B. ACE Inhibitors
C. Calcium Channel Blockers
D. Hydralazine

266. A hypertensive diabetic is having proteinuria, antihypertensive of choice is: (AIIMS May 95)
A. Propanolol
B. Clonidine
C. Enalaprilat
D. Alpha methyldopa

267. An elderly patient presents with hypertension and diabetes, proteinuria without renal failure. Antihypertensive of choice is: (AIIMS Nov 93)
A. Furosemide
B. Methyldopa
C. Enalapril
D. Propranolol

268. A young patient presented with blood pressure of 190/120 mm of Hg without any clinical symptom and fundus examination is normal, treatment of choice: (PGI June 03)
A. Oral Nitroglycerine
B. I.V. Nitroglycerine
C. Oral Enalapril
D. IV Enalarpil
E. Sublingual short acting Nifedipine

269. Monogenic AD cause of HTN? *(PGI 2009)*
A. 17- α Hydroxylase deficiency
B. Gordon's Syndrome
C. Pregnancy Exacerbated HTN
D. Glucocortiocoid responsive HTN
E. Glucocorticoid Remediable Aldosteronism

Hypertensive Crisis

270. Rapid Reduction of blood pressure is indicated in : *(AI 1991)*
A. Acute Aortic Dissection
B. Hypertensive Encephalopathy
C. Intracercbral haemorrhage
D. All of the above

271. Which of the following statements regarding hypertensive crisis is false: *(AIIMS Nov 1992)*
A. Hypertensive urgency is characterized by marked elevation of blood pressure and rapidly evolving end organ damage.
B. Hypertensive emergencies require immediate reduction of blood pressure within minutes
C. Hypertensive urgencies may be managed without extensive monitoring on an outpatient basis.
D. None of the above

272. All the following agents may be used for the management of hypertensive crisis Except: *(AIIMS May 1992)*
A. Furosemide
B. Nitroglyarine
C. Indapamide
D. Esmolal

273. A male patient presents with headache, profuse sweating and palpitations with a blood pressure of 180/120 mm Hg. The drug of choice would be *(DNB 2009)*
A. Nifedipine
B. Labetalol
C. Prazocin
D. Phenoxy benzamine

274. All of the following drugs can be used in the management of hypertensive crises Except- *(AIIMS May 1994)*
A. Hydralazene
B. Trimethophan
C. Nifedipine
D. Indapamide

275. All of the following are used for hypertensive emergencies, Except:
A. Fenoldapam
B. Nitroglycerine
C. Nitroprusside
D. Clonidine

276. All of the following are useful intravenous therapy for hypertensive emergencies except- *(AIIMS May 03)*
A. Fenodopam
B. Uradipil
C. Enalaprilat
D. Nifedipine

277. A patient presents with headache and profuse sweating. On examination his blood pressure is recorded as 200/120 mm Hg. Which of the following agents are not preferred (Select three best options) *(PGI 2009)*
A. Nifedipine
B. Sodium nitroprusside
C. Phenoxybenzomine
D. Methyldopa
E. Labetalol

278. In Accelerated HTN what is metabolic defect: *(PGI June 2000)*
A. Normal non-ionic metabolic acidosis
B. Ionic gap met acidosis
C. Hypomagnesemia
D. Metabolic alkalosis

Renovascular Hypertension

279. Which of the following is the most specific and sensitive screening test for Renovascular Hypertension. *(AIIMS May 01)*
A. HRCT
B. CT Angiography
C. Captopril enhanced radionucleatide scan
D. MRI

280. Which of the following is the most specific screening test for renovascular hypertension: *(PGI 2008)*
A. Magnetic Resonance Angiography (MRA)
B. Spiral Computed Tomographic Angiography (CT Angiography)
C. Captopril induced Radionucleotide Scan (Captopril Renogram)
D. Duplex Doppler Ultrasonography

281. A 20 year old female presents with a blood pressure of 160/110 mm Hg. Clinical examination reveals a bruit in both flanks. Which of the following statements about this patient is not true (select one option) *(PGI 09)*
A. Enalapril may deteriorate renal function
B. Most definitive diagnostic procedure is contrast enhanced angiography
C. Condition is nearly always bilateral
D. Surgical intervention may be used
E. Fibromuscular dysplasia is the likely cause in this patient

282. Most common cause of renal artery stenosis in young adults in India is: *(AIIMS Dec 97)*
A. Atherosclerosis
B. Non specific aorto-arteritis
C. Fibro muscular dysplasia
D. None of the above

283. Renal artery stenosis may occur in all of the following except: *(AI 2006)*
A. Atherosclerosis
B. Fibromuscular dysplasia
C. Takayasu's arteritis
D. Polyarteritis nodosa

Pulmonary Hypertension

284. In primary pulmonary hypertension basic abnormality in gene lies in: *(AIIMS May 07)*
   A. Bone morphogenetic protein receptor II
   B. Endothelin
   C. Homebox gene
   D. PAX – 11

285. Not seen in pre capillary pulmonary hypertension:
   A. ↑ pressure in pulm. circulation *(PGI June 98)*
   B. ↑ capillary pressure
   C. Rt-vent.hypertrophy
   D. ↑ Pulmonary wedge pressure

286. Precapillary Pulmonary hypertension is caused by all Except: *(PGI June 03)*
   A. Mitral stenosis
   B. Pulmonary vasculitis
   C. Primary pulmonary hypertension
   D. Thromboembolism

287. All are causes of pulmonary hypertension except-
   A. Hyperventilation *(AIIMS Nov 07)*
   B. Morbid obesity
   C. High altitude
   D. Fenfluramine

288. Pulmonary hypertension may occur in all of the following conditions except- *(AIIMS Nov 06)*
   A. Toxic oil syndrome
   B. Progressive systemic sclerosis
   C. Sickle cell anemia
   D. Argemone mexicana poisoning

289. Pulmonary hypertension in COPD is due to all, Except: *(PGI Dec 97)*
   A. Hypoxia
   B. Pulmonary vasoconstriction
   C. High lung volume
   D. Bronchoconstriction

Aortic Dissection

290. A 50 year old man, an alcoholic and a smoker presents with a 3 hour history of increasing shortness of breath. He started having this pain while eating, which was constant and radiated to the back and interscapular region. He was a known hypertensive. On examination, he was cold and clammy with a heart rate of 130/min, and a BP of 80/40 mmHg. JVP was normal. All peripheral pulses were present and equal. Breath sounds were decreased at the left lung base and chest x-ray showed left pleural effusion. Which one of the following is the most likely diagnosis? *(AI 2005)*
   A. Acute aortic dissection.
   B. Acute myocardial infarction.
   C. Rupture of the esophagus.
   D. Acute pulmonary embolism.

291. Manifestation of Acute Dissection include all of the following, Except: *(PGI June 01)*
   A. Pericardial effusion
   B. AR
   C. MR
   D. AMI
   E. Limb ischemia

292. All of the following factors predispoase to Aortic dissection, Except: *(PGI June 02)*
   A. Systemic hypertension
   B. Coarctation of aorta
   C. In Ist trimester pregnancy
   D. Takayasu's arteritis
   E. Marfan syndrome

293. All of the following agents may be used in the treatment of Aortic dissection, Except (select two options): *(PGI Dec 05)*
   A. Propanolol
   B. Diazoxide
   C. Na nitroprusside
   D. Hydralazine
   E. Labetolol

Cardiopulmonary Resuscitation

294. A young patient sustains cardiac arrest, in the medical ward. Immediate defibrillation is advised when the ECG shows: *(AI 1992)*
   A. Ventricular Tachycardia
   B. Asystole
   C. Electromechanical dissociation
   D. Persistant Bradyarrhythmia

295. True regarding cardio pulmonary resuscitation is: *(AIIMS Dec 98)*
   A. Most common presentation in ECG is asystole
   B. Compression to ventilation ratio is 5:1
   C. Adrenaline is given if cardioversion fails
   D. Calcium gluconate is given immediately

296. All of the following may be used in the treatment of cardiac arrest following ventricular fibrillation, Except (Select two best options) *(PGI 09)*
   A. Atropine
   B. External cardiac pacing
   C. Epinephrine
   D. Antiarrhythmic agents
   E. Vasopressin

297. True regarding cardio pulmonary resuscitation is– *(AIIMS Dec 97)*
   A. Most common presentation in ECG is asystole
   B. Compression to ventilation ratio is 5:1
   C. Adrenaline is given if cardioversion fails
   D. Calcium gluconate is given immediately

298. Asynchronous cadioversion is given in: *(AIIMS Nov 98)*
A. AF
B. Ventricular fibrillation
C. Atrial flutter
D. Ventricular tachycardia

299. What would be the first line of treatment is a patient who develops ventricular fibrillation after intravenous injection of potassium chloride- *(AIIMS May 2004)*
A. Cardiac massage
B. I.V Adrenaline
C. Defibrillation
D. IPPV

300. The best chances of recovery after successful cardiopulmonary resuscitation are seen in: *(AI 1993)*
A. Ventricular Tachycardia
B. Ventricular Fibrillation
C. Asystole
D. Electromechanical dissociation

301. In cardio pulmonary resuscitation, calcium can be given in all, EXCEPT- *(AIIMS Dec 97)*
A. Hypocalcemia
B. Hypokalemia
C. Hyperkalemia
D. Calcium channel blocker

Cardiac Tumors

302. Most common tumour of heart is: *(AI 99)*
A. Myxoma
B. Rhabdomyosarcoma
C. Fibroma
D. Leiomyosarcoma

303. The commonest tumor of the myocardium is : *(AI 94)*
A. Myxoma
B. Rhabdomyoma
C. Sarcoma
D. Fibroma

304. Which of the following statements about atrial myxomas is true *(DNB 2011)*
A. Most common in Left Atrium
B. More common in Males
C. Distant metastasis are seen
D. Most myxomas are familial

305. All of the following statement about atrial myxomas are true, except: *(DNB 2011)*
A. Most common site is Left Atrium
B. Most common in young individuals
C. Distant metastasis are rare
D. Most myxomas are familial

306. All of the following are clinical features of myxoma, *except* : *(AI 2002)*
A. Fever
B. Clubbing
C. Hypertension
D. Embolic phenomenon

307. True statement about cardiac myxoma is : *(AI 1999)*
A. Commonest site is left atrium
B. Rarely reoccurs after excision
C. Distant metastasis are seen
D. More common in females

308. Gradient in pulmonary artery wedge pressure and left ventricular end diastolic pressure is seen in
A. Aortic regurgitation *(AIIMS June 2000)*
B. Constrictive pericarditis
C. Left atrial myxoma
D. Pulmonary thromboembolism

Rheumatic Fever

309. Which is a minor criteria for diagnosis of RF according to modified Jones criteria?
A. ASO titre *(AI 2007)*
B. Past History of Rheumatic Fever
C. Fever
D. Subcutaneous nodules

310. Which of the following is a minor criteria for diagnosis of Rheumatic Fever (RF) according to modified Jones criteria? *(AI 2007)*
A. ASO titre
B. Past History of Rheumatic Fever
C. Fever
D. Subcutaneous nodules

311. Which of the following is not included in Jone's Major Criteria *(AIIMS Nov 2010)*
A. Pancarditis
B. Chorea
C. Subcutancous nodule
D. High ESR

312. Major criteria of Rheumatic fever include (select three options) –
A. Chorea
B. Erythema nodosum
C. Arthritis
D. Fever
E. Carditis

313. True about acute rheumatic fever (select three options) *(PGI Dec-02)*
A. Chorea
B. Erythema nodosum
C. Arthritis
D. Caused by antecedent α - hemolytic streptococcus infection
E. Carditis

314. Characteristic feature of Rheumatic carditis is : *(AI 99)*
A. Pericarditis
B. Endocarditis
C. Myocarditis
D. Pancarditis

315. A 10 year old boy, Pappu, died of acute rheumatic fever. All the following can be expected at autopsy except : *(AI 02)*
A. Ashoff nodules
B. Rupture of chordae tendinae

C. Mc Callum patch
D. Fibrinous pericarditis

316. Diagnostic feature in rheumatic heart disease is : *(AI 97)*
A. Aschoff's nodule
B. Mc Callman patch
C. Adeno Carcinoma
D. Alveolar cell Carcinoma

317. Aschoff's nodules are seen in : *(AI 05)*
A. Subacute bacterial endocarditis
B. Libman-sacks endocarditis
C. Rheumatic carditis
D. Nonbacterial thrombotic endocarditis

318. McCallum's patch is diagnostic of : *(AI 95)*
A. Infective endocarditis
B. Rheumatic endocarditis
C. Myocardial infarction
D. Tetralogy of fallout (TOF)

319. All are true about rheumatic fever, *except* :
A. Common in poor socioeconomic group
B. Develops after streptococcal pharyngitis
C. Communicable disease *(AIIMS June 99)*
D. Seen in 5-15 year of children

320. True about Rheumatic fever – *(PGI Dec 03)*
A. Chorea is aggravated during pregnancy
B. Chorea & arthritis co-existing
C. Subcutaneous nodules are tender
D. Erythema multiforme seen

321. True statement about Rheumatic fever in children (select two options)– *(PGI Dec- 03)*
A. Polyarthritis
B. Caused by α hemolytic streptococci
C. Erythem marginatum is most common manifestation
D. MC valve involvement is Mitral
E. Erythema marginatum is common in face

322. True about Erythema Marginatum in Acute Rheumatic fever is: *(PGI Dec 01)*
A. Pruiritic
B. Commonly involves face
C. Common manifestation of Acute Rheumatic fever
D. Usually associated with carditis

323. True about subcutaneous nodule in Rheumatic fever (select two options)- *(PGI Dec 03)*
A. Non tender
B. Most common manifestation
C. Present in extensor surfaces
D. Associated with arthritis

324. Earliest valvular lesion in a case of acute rheumatic fever is- *(AIIMS May 94)*
A. Mitral regurgitation (MR)
B. Aortic Regurgitation (AR)
C. Mitral stenosis (MS)
D. Aortic Stenosis (AS)

Congenital Heart Disease

General

325. The commonest mode of inheritance of congenital heart disease is *(AI 2002)*
A. Autosomal dominant
B. Autosomal recessive
C. Sex linked dominant
D. Multifactorial

326. Cardiac abnormality seen with Noonan's syndrome is: *(AIIMS May 95)*
A. VSD
B. ASD
C. Pulmonary stenosis
D. Coarctation of aorta

327. Differential cyanosis is seen in: *(AI 1996)*
A. ASD
B. VSD
C. PDA
D. All of the above

328. Pressure difference of 5mm Hg between the two upper limbs occurs in which congenital heart disease:
A. TOF
B. TGA
C. HOCM
D. Supra –valvular aortic stenosis

329. Congenital heart disease associated with decreased pulmonary blood flow - *(PGI Dec 04)*
A. Truncus arteriosus
B. TAPVC
C. Ebstein's anomaly
D. Complete TGA
E. Single ventricle with pulmonary stenosis

330. All of the following are cyanotic heart diseases, Except : *(PGI June 05)*
A. TOF
B. PDA
C. Tricuspid Atresia
D. Eisenmenger's complex

331. All can cause recurrent pulmonary infection except: *(AIIMS Sep 96)*
A. VSD
B. Recurrent LVF
C. TOF
D. ASD

Tetralogy of Fallot

332. The following features are true for tetralogy of Fallot, *except*: *(AI 2006)*
A. Ventricular septal defect
B. Right ventricular hypertrophy
C. Atrial septal defect
D. Pulmonary stenosis

333. Essential criteria for TOF includes all except – *(AIIMS Nov 07)*
A. Valvular stenosis
B. Infundibular stenosis
C. Over riding of aorta
D. RVH

334. Which of the following is a component of Pentalogy Of Fallot: *(AI 2007)*
A. Atrial Septal Defect (ASD)
B. Patent Ductus Arteriosus (PDA)
C. Coarctation of Aorta (COA)
D. Left Venticular Hypertrophy (LVH)

335. All of the following statements about Tetralogy of fallot are true, Except
A. JVP is normal
B. Second Heart sound is single
C. Ejection systolic murmur is third left intercostal space
D. First Heart sound is soft

336. All of the following are true regarding Tetralogy of fallot except – *(AIIMS May 05)*
A. Ejection systolic murmur in second intercostal space
B. Single second heart sound
C. Predominantly left to right shunt
D. Normal jugular venous pressure

337. In which of the following a 'Coeur en Sabot' shape of the heart is seen: *(AI 2004)*
A. Tricuspid atresia
B. Ventricular septal defect
C. Transposition of great arteries
D. Tetralogy of Fallot

338. Blalock and Taussig shunt is done between: *(AI 2006)*
A. Aorta to pulmonary artery
B. Aorta to pulmonary vein
C. Subclavian artery to pulmonary vein
D. Subclavian vien to artery

339. Potts shunt is : *(AI 2001)*
A. Rt subclavian artery to rt pulmonary artery
B. Descending aorta to left pulmonary artery
C. Left subclavian to left pulmonary artery
D. Ascending aorta to right pulmonary artery

340. Fallots tetralogy manifestation (select two options) – *(PGI June 06)*
A. Left axis deviation
B. Left ventrucular hypertrophy
C. VSD
D. Blalock taussig shunt is between pulmonary artery & subclavian artery
E. Morphine is contraindicated in cyanotic spells

Atrial Septal Defect

341. A young female presents with history of dyspnoea on exertion. On examination, she has wide, fixed split S2 with ejection systolic murmur (III/VI) in left second intercostal space. Her EKG shows left axis deviation. The most probable diagnosis is : *(AIIMS May 03)*
A. Total anomalous pulmonary venous drainage.
B. Tricuspid atresia. *(AIIMS May 04)*
C. Ostium primum atrial septal defect.
D. Ventricular septal defect with pulmonary arterial hypertension.

342. All of the following are true about ASD *except*: *(AI 2001)*
A. Right atrial hypertrophy
B. Left atrial hypertrophy
C. Right ventricular hypertrophy
D. Pulmonary hypertension

343. True about ASD : *(AI 1998)*
A. Foramen ovale is patent
B. Left parasternal heeve is due to increased pulmonary artery flow
C. S_2 is wide and variable
D. Systolic murmur is due to rapid flow of blood across the shunt.

344. Presence of a pansystolic murmur of Mitral Regurgitation with left axis deviation in a patient with ASD suggest: (DNB)
A. TGA
B. Ostium secondum with floppy mitral valve
C. Ostium primum with floppy mitral valve
D. Pulmonary Hypertension

345. In which of the following conditions left atrium is not enlarged: *(AI 2006)*
A. Ventricular septal defect
B. Atrial septal defect
C. Aortopulmonary window
D. Patent ductus arteriosus

Ventricular Septal Defect (VSD)

346. True about V.S.D. is, all *except* : *(AIIMS June 97)*
A. Small hole closes spontaneously
B. Defect is usually in membranous part
C. Endocarditis is commonest complication
D. Pulmonary oligemia in chest X-ray

Patent Ductus Arteriosus (PDA)

347. Differential cyanosis is seen in: *(AI 1996)*
A. ASD
B. VSD
C. PDA
D. All of the above

348. True statement about Ductus Arteriosus is : *(AI 2000)*
A. It undergoes anatomic closure within 24 hrs of birth
B. Forms the ligamentum venosum in later life
C. It is induced to close by high levels of prostaglandins
D. May cause a machinary murmur by its patency.

349. MC cause of death in adult with PDA is – (PGI Dec 99)
A. CCF
B. Infective endocarditis
C. Rupture
D. Embolism

Tricuspid Atresia

350. All of the following are characteristics features of Tricuspid Atresia Except: (AIIMS Dec 98)
A. Left Axis deviation
B. Right ventricular hypoplasia
C. Pulmonary vascularity is diminished
D. Splitting of S_2

351. A five year old child presents with Left ventricular hypertrophy and central cyanosis. What is the most probable diagnosis? (AIIMS Nov 2000)
A. Tricuspid atresia
B. Eisenmenger syndrome
C. Tetrology of Fallot
D. Total anomalous pulmonary venous drainage

352. A child presents with LVH and pulmonary complications. ECG shows left axis deviation. Most likely diagnosis is: (AI 2001)
A. TOF
B. Tricuspid atresia
C. TAPVC
D. VSD

353. Right axis deviation is seen in all except – (AIIMS June- 98)
A. VSD
B. Tricuspid atresia
C. Pulmonary atresia
D. ASD

Coarctation of Aorta

354. A patient complains of intermittent claudication, dizziness and headache; likely cardiac lesion is: (AI 2001) (AIIMS Nov 2000)
A. TOF
B. ASD
C. PDA
D. Coarctation of aorta

355. A 1-month-old boy is referred for failure to thrive. On examination, he shows feature of congestive failure. The femoral pulses are feeble as compared to branchial pulses. The most likely clinical diagnosis is: (AI 2006)
A. Congenital aortic stenosis
B. Coarctation of aorta
C. Patent ductus arteriosus
D. Congenital aortoiliac disease

356. A 27 year old man in noted to have blood pressure of 170/100 mmHg. He has prominent aortic ejection click and murmurs heard over the ribs on the both sides anteriorly and over the back posterioly. In addition.the pulses in the lower extremities are feeble and he complains of mild claudication with exertion. The most likely diagnosis is (AIIMS Nov 04)
A. Artial septal defect
B. Aortic stenosis
C. Coarctation of the aorta
D. Cardiomyopathy

357. A 4 1/2- year-old girl always had to wear warm socks even is summer season. On physical examination, it was noticed that she had high blood pressure and her femoral pulse was weak as compared to radial and carotid pulse. A chest radiograph showed remarkable notching of ribs along with their lower borders. This was due to: (AIIMS Nov 02)
A. Femoral artery thrombosis.
B. Coarctation of aorta.
C. Raynaud's disease.
D. Takayasu's arteritis.

358. A Ten year old boy presents to the pediatric emergency unit with seizures. Blood pressure in the upper extremity measured as 200/140 mm Hg. Femoral pulses were not palpable. The most likely diagnosis amongst the following is: (AI 2010)
A. Takayasu Aortoarteritis
B. Renal parenchymal disease
C. Grandmal seiures
D. Coarctation of Aorta

359. A child presented with headache, dizziness, intermittent claudication with occassional dyspnoea. The most probable diagnosis in : (AI 1999)
A. ASD
B. PDA
C. TOF
D. Coarctatation of aorta

360. A 20 year young man presents with exert ional dyspnoea, headache, and giddiness. On examination, there is hypertension and LVH. X-ray picture shows notching of the anterior ends of the ribs. The most like diagnosis is : (AI 2002)
A. Phaeochromocytoma
B. Carcinoid syndrome
C. Coarctation of the aorta
D. Superior Mediastinal syndrome

361. All the following findings would be expected in a person with coarctation of the aorta *except* :
A. A systolic murmur across the anterior chest and back and a high-pitched diastolic murmur along the left sternal border
B. B. A higher blood pressure in the right arm than in the left arm (AIIMS Nov 99)
C. Inability to augment cardiac output with exercise
D. Persistent hypertension despite complete surgical repair

2

Cardiovascular System

362. True about co-arctation of aorta : *(AI 1999)*
   A. Most common site is distal to the origin of the left subclavian artery
   B. Most common age of presentation is at 15-20years
   C. Superior rib notching is due to erosion by dilated collateral vessels
   D. Right ventricular hypertrophy is prominent

363. Which condition is most commonly associated with coarctation of aorta? *(AI 2008)*
   A. PDA
   B. Bicuspid aortic valve
   C. Aortic stenosis
   D. VSD

364. Coarctation of Aorta is most commonly associated with: *(AI 2011)*
   A. Bicuspid Aortic valve
   B. Patent Dustus Arteriosus (PDA)
   C. Ventricular Septal Defect (VSD)
   D. Atrial Septal Defect (ASD)

365. Coarctation of aorta is associated with all, *except*: *(AIIMS June 98)*
   A. Turner's syndrome
   B. Bicuspid aortic valve
   C. Pulmonary stenosis
   D. Atresia of aortic arch

366. Coarctation of aorta may be associated with all of the following *except* : *(AI 1997) (AIIMS 1995)*
   A. Bicuspid aortic valve
   B. Turner's syndrome
   C. Renal artery stenosis
   D. PDA

367. Coarctation of the aorta is common in which syndrome: *(AI 1995)*
   A. Down's
   B. Turner's
   C. Klinefelter's
   D. Noonan's

368. Inferior Rib notching is seen in all except- *(AIIMS June 2000)*
   A. Coarctation of aorta
   B. Classical blalock tausing operation
   C. SVC obstruction
   D. Neurofibromatosis

369. Ribnotching of 4-9th ribs with double bulging is seen in : *(AI 1998)*
   A. Aortic aneurysm
   B. Aortic dessection
   C. Co-arctation of aorta
   D. Diaphragmatic hernia

370. All of the following causes death in coarctation of Aorta except: *(PGI June 2000)*
   A. Infective endocarditis
   B. CCF
   C. Intra cranial hemorrhage
   D. Anterior MI

Total Anomalous Pulmonary Venous Connection (TAPVC)

371. The most common type of total anomalous pulmonary venous connection is: *(AI 2005)*
   A. Supracardiac.
   B. Infracardiac.
   C. Mixed.
   D. Cardiac.

372. All of the following statements regarding total anomalous pulmonary connection are true except: *(AI 97)*
   A. The total pulmonary venous blood reaches the right atrium
   B. Always associated with a VSD
   C. The oxygen saturation of the blood in the pulmonary artery is higher than that in the aorta
   D. Infracardiac type is always obstructive

Transposition of Great Vessels (TGV)

373. A five day old, full term male infant was severely cyanotic at birth. Prostaglandin E was administered initially and later ballooned atrial septosomy was done which showed improvement in oxygenation. The most likely diagnosis of this infant is : *(AI 2004)*
   A. Tetralogy of Fallot
   B. Transposition of great vessels
   C. Truncus Arteriosus
   D. Tricuspid Atresia

Anamolous Coronary Artery

374. A neonate has recurrent attacks of abdominal pain, restless irritability and diaphoresis on feeding. Cardiac auscultation reveals a nonspecific murmur. He is believed to be at risk for M.I. Likely diagnosis here is: *(AI 2001)*
   A. ASd
   B. VSd
   C. TOF
   D. Anomalous coronary artery

Eissenmerger's Syndrome

375. Eisenmenger syndrome is characterized by all except: *(AI 2005)*
   A. Return of left ventricle & right ventricle to normal size.
   B. Pulmonary veins not distended.
   C. Pruning of peridpheral pulmonary arteries.
   D. Dilatation of central pulmonary arteries.

Miscellaneous

376. The heart lesion *not* found in Congenital Rubella infection is: *(AI 1995)*
   A. ASD

B. VSD
C. PDA
D. PS

377. Sustained severe hypertension in children is most commonly suggestive of: *(AI 1995)*
A. Coarctation of aorta
B. Pheochromocytoma
C. Renal paranchymatous disease
D. Drug induced

378. NADA's criteria are used for: *(AI 1996)*
A. Assessment of child for degree of dehydration
B. Assessment of child for degree of malnutrition
C. Assessment of child for presence of heart disease
D. Assessment of child for degree of mental retardation

Endocarditis

379. Diagnostic criterion for Infective Endocarditis include all, Except: *(DNB June 2011)*
A. Positive Echocardiogram
B. Positive Blood culture
C. Raised ESR
D. Positive Rheumatoid Factor

380. Infective endocarditis is least likely to occur in:
A. Atrial septal defect *(AIIMS June 97)*
B. Small ventricular septal defect
C. Mitral valve prolapse *(AIIMS June 98)*
D. Tetrology of Fallot's *(AIIMS May 01)*

381. Which of the following is least likely to be associated with Infective Endocarditis: *(AI 2012)*
A. Small ASD
B. Small VSD
C. Mild MR
D. Mild MS

382. Bacterial endocarditis is rarely seen in- *(AI 96)*
A. VSD
B. PDA
C. MVP
D. secundum ASD

383. Infective endocarditis is commonly seen in all except-
A. Small VSD *(AIIMS June 98)*
B. Tetralogy of fallot
C. PDA
D. ASD

384. Infective endocarditis is least common in-
A. Mitral stenosis *(AIIMS Nov 93)*
B. Aortic stenosis
C. VSD
D. ASD

385. Least common site for vegetation is-
A. Aortic Stenosis (AS) *(AIIMS May 94)*
B. Mitral Stenosis (MS)
C. Mitral Regurgitation (MR)
D. Atrial Septal Defect (ASD)

386. Least common cause of endocarditis is:
A. A.S.D *(AIIMS June 97)*
B. P.D.A
C. T.O.F.
D. V.S.D.

387. Infective endocarditis is most commonly seen in:
A. ASD *(AIIMS Feb 97)*
B. VSD
C. PDA
D. Pulmonary stenosis.

388. Endocarditis is most commonly seen in :
A. Mitral stenosis *(AIIMS May 95)*
B. Mitral regurgitation
C. Mitral valve prolapse
D. Tricuspid stenosis

389. Mitral valve vegetations do not usually embolise to :
A. Lung *(AI 2001) (AIIMS Nov 2001)*
B. Liver
C. Spleen
D. Brain

390. Most common heart valve involved in IV drug user is: *(AIIMS Feb 97)*
A. Mitral valve
B. Aortic valve
C. Pulmonary valve
D. Tricuspid valve

391. A woman has septic abortion done; vegetation on tricuspid valve is likely to go to: *(AI 2001)*
A. Septic infarcts to lung
B. Liver
C. Spleen infarcts
D. Emboli to brain

392. Osler's nodes are seen at : *(AIIMS June 98)*
A. Heart
B. Knee joint
C. Tip of Palm & Sole
D. Anterior abdominal wall

393. Roth's spots are seen in:
A. Infective Endocarditis
B. Rheumatic Endocarditis
C. Central Retinal Arterial Occlusion (CRAO)
D. Typhoid

394. Not a feature of infective endocarditis is :
A. Myocardial abscess *(AIIMS Feb 97)*
B. Vegetations along cusps
C. Thrombus in left atria
D. Perforation of cusp

395. Which of the following is least likely to cause infective endocarditis : *(AI 06)*
A. Staphylococcus albus
B. Streptococcus faecalis
C. Salmonella typhi
D. Pseudomonas aeruginosa

396. Bacterial endocarditis is most commonly caused by –
A. α -Hemolytic Streptococci *(AI 06)*
B. β -Hemolytic Streptococci

C. Staphylococcus aureus
D. Cardiobaterium
E. Staph epidermidis

397. A patient with a prosthetic heart valve develops endocarditis eight months after valve replacement. Most likely organism responsible is: *(AIIMS Nov 2010)*
A. Staphylococcus Aureus
B. Staphylococcus Epidermidis
C. Streptococcus Viridans
D. HACEK group

398. Acute Infective Endocarditis with abscess formation is most commonly associated with *(DNB 2012)*
A. Listeria
B. Staphylococcus
C. Streptococcus
D. Enterococcus

399. Antiboiotic Prophylaxis for infective endocarditis is indicated in:
A. Isolated secundum ASD
B. Mitral valve prolapse without regurgitation
C. Prior coronary artery bypass graft
D. Coarctation of aorta

400. In a patient of heart disease antibiotic prophylaxis for dental extraction is
A. Amoxycillin
B. Imipenam
C. Gentamycin
D. Erythromycin

401. Which of the following have most friable vegetation: *(AI 2010)*
A. Infective endocarditis
B. Libman Sack's endocarditis
C. Rheumatic heart disease
D. SLE

402. Vegetations on undersurface of A.V. valves are found in: *(AI 2001)*
A. Acute Rheumatic corditis
B. Limban Sack's endocarditis
C. Non thrombotic bacterial endocarditis
D. Chronic rheumatic carditis

403. Libman Sack's Endocarditis is seen in: *(DNB June 2012)*
A. SLE
B. Rheumatic Fever
C. Carcinoid
D. Infective Endocarditis

404. Flat vegetations in pockets of valves are due to : *(AI 2000)*
E. Rheumatic heart disease
F. Libman sacks Endocarditis
G. NBTE
H. Infective endocarditis

405. Site of lesion in endocarditis of RHD is – *(PGI Dec-97)*
A. Along line of closure of valves
B. Both sides of valves
C. Valve cusps
D. Free margin of valves

406. Firm warty vegetations along the line of closure of valves is due to : *(AI 2000)*
A. Rheumatic heart disease
B. Libman Sacks Endocarditis
C. NBTE
D. Infective Endocarditis

Cardiac Involvement in Carcinoid Syndrome

407. Carcinoid syndrome produces valvular disease primarily involving- *(AIIMs May 05)*
A. Pulmonary valves
B. Tricuspid valves
C. Mitral valves
D. Aortic valves

408. Charachteristic pathological finding in carcinoid heart disease is: *(AI 2010)*
A. Fibrous endocardial thickening of Right ventricle, Tricuspid valve & Pulmonary valve
B. Endocardial thickening of Tricuspid valve with severe Tricuspid Stenosis
C. Collagen rich, elastic deposits in endocardium of right ventricle and Pulmonary valve
D. Calcification of Tricuspid and Pulmonary valve

409. Carcinoid syndrome produces valvular disease primarily involving: *(AIIMS May 04)*
A. Venous valves
B. Tricuspid valve
C. Mitral valve
D. Aortic valve

410. In carcinoid syndrome, the aprt of heart mostly affected is: *(PGI Dec 97)*
A. Outflow tract of RV
B. Inflow tract of RV
C. Inflow tract of LV
D. Outflow tract LV

Sudden Cardiac Death

411. Sudden cardiac death may occur in all of the following except : *(AI 06)*
A. Dilated cardiomyopathy
B. Hypertrophic cardiomyopathy
C. Eisenmenger's syndrome
D. Ventricular septal defect

Miscellaneous

412. S.A. node acts as a pacemaker of the heart because of the fact that it: *(AI 05)*
A. Is capable of generating impulses spontaneously
B. Has rich sympathetic innervations
C. Has poor cholinergic innervations
D. Generates impulses at the highest rate

413. Highest rate of impulse generation is given in:
A. SA node
B. AV node
C. Bundle of HIS
D. Purkinje system

414. Highest conduction rate in m/s is observed in: *(AI 1995)*
A. SA node
B. AV node

C. Bundle of His
D. Purkinje system

415. Speed of conduction is fastest in: *(PGI Dec 05)*
A. AV node
B. SA node
C. Bundle of His
D. Purkinje system
E. Ventricular muscle

416. Least conduction velocity is seen in: *(PGI Dec 98)*
A. AV node
B. Purkinje fibres
C. Bundle of his
D. Ventricular myocardial fibres

417. Which of the following is the order of activation after stimulation of Purkinji fibrs is : *(AIIMS Dec 95)*
A. Septum –> Endocardium –> Epicardium
B. Endocrdium –> Septum –> Epicardium
C. Epicardium –> Septum –> Endocardium
D. Septum –> Epicardium –> Endocardium

418. The right coronary artery supplies all of the following parts of the conducting system in the heart except:
A. SA Node *(AI 2003)*
B. AV Node
C. AV Bundle
D. Right Bundle branch

419. If circumflex artery gives the posterior intervenetricular branch, this circulation is described as:
A. Right dominance *(AIIMS Nov 07)*
B. Left dominance
C. Codominance
D. Undetermined

420. During the cardiac cycle the opening of the aortic valve takes place at the : *(AI 04)*
A. Beginning of systole
B. End of isovolumetric contraction
C. End of diastole
D. End of diastasis

421. At the end of isometric relaxation phase :
A. Atrioventricular valves open *(AI 2000)*
B. Atrioventricular valves close
C. Corresponds to peak of "C" wave in JVP
D. Corresponds to T wave in ECG

422. Of the following which one correlates with isovolumic contraction phase: *(AIIMS June 98)*
A. AV opening and aortic and pulmonary valve closure
B. AV closure and aortic & pulmonary valve opening
C. Both valves are closed
D. Both valves are open

423. Isovolumic relaxation phase of the cardiac cycle ends with : *(AI 1998)*
A. Peak of 'C' waves
B. Opening of A.V. valve
C. Closure of semilunar valve
D. Beginning of 'T' wave

424. Cardiac index in a normal person is
A. 2.1 *(TN 96, Kerala 95, KA 99, UP 02)*
B. 3.2
C. 4.6
D. 5.9

425. Cardiac output in L/min divided by heart rate equals:
A. Cardiac efficiency *(AI 1995)*
B. Mean stroke volume
C. Cardiac index
D. Mean arterial pressure

426. Mean arterial pressure is : *(AI 1996)*
A. Systolic + (Diastolic BP)/2
B. Systolic + 1/3rd Pulse pressure
C. Diastolic + (Systolic BP)/2
D. Diastolic + 1/3rd Pulse pressure

427. Mean arterial pressure is calculated as:
A. (SBP + 2DBP)/3 *(AIIMS Nov 06)*
B. (DBP + 2SBP)/3
C. (SBP + 3DBP)/2
D. (DBP + 3SBP)/2

428. Blood pressure is defined as the product of:
A. Systolic pressure × pulse *(PGI Dec 98)*
B. Diastolic pressure × pulse rate
C. Pulse pressure × pulse rate
D. Cardiac output × peripheral resistance

429. SI unit for measuring Blood Pressure is: *(AI 02)*
A. Torr
B. mmHg
C. kP_a
D. Barr

430. The blood pressure measured by a sphygmomanometer
A. Is lower than the intraarterial pressure *(AI 08)*
B. Is higher than the intraarterial pressure
C. Is same as the intraarterial pressure
D. Is the same with different cuff sizes

431. True about blood pressure measurement is all/except:
A. Cuff width should be 40% of arm circumference
B. Diastolic blood pressure is indicated by fourth Korotkoff sound *(AIIMS May 07)*
C. Small cuff measures spuriously elevated Diastolic blood pressure
D. Monkenberg sclerosis causes pseudohypertension

432. Spuriously high BP is seen in A/E:
A. Auscultatory gap *(AIIMS May 01)*
B. Small cuff
C. Thick calcified vessels
D. Obesity

433. Which is true about measurement of BP with syphgnomonmeter versus intraarterial pressure measurements: *(AI 2001)*
A. Less than intravascular pressure
B. More than intravascular pressure
C. Equal to intravascular pressure
D. Depends upon blood flow

434. All of the following statements regarding subendocardial infarction are true, except: *(AI 06)*
A. These are multifocal in nature
B. These often result from hypotension or shock
C. Epicardities is not seen
D. These may result in aneurysm

435. A 45 year old male had severe chest pain and was admitted to the hospital with a diagnosis of acute Myocardial Infarction. Four days later he died and autopsy showed Transmural coagulative necrosis. Which of the following microscopic features will be seen on further examination *(AI 2009)*
A. Fibroblasts and collagen
B. Granulation tissue
C. Neutrophilic infiltration surrounding coagulative necrosis
D. Granulomatous inflammation.

436. A 60 year old male presented with acute chest pain of 4 hours duration. Electrocardiographic examination revealed new Q wave with ST segment depression. He suffered to his illness within 24 hours of admission. The heart revealed presence of a transmural hemorrhagic area over the septum and anterior wall of the left ventricle. Light microscopic examination is most likely to reveal: *(AI 04)*
A. Edema in between normal myofibrils
B. Necrotic myofibrils with presence of neutrophils
C. Coagulative necrosis of the myocytes with presence of granulation tissue
D. Infiltration by histiocytes with hemosiderin laden macrophages

437. A myocardial infarct showing early granulation tissue has most likely occurred: *(AI 02)*
A. 1 hours old
B. 24 hours old
C. 1 week old
D. 1 month old

438. Most common cause of aortic aneurysm is: *(AI 98)*
A. Syphilis
B. Marfan's syndrome
C. Atherosclerosis
D. Congenital

439. Most common cause of Abdominal aneurysm is: *(AI 94)*
A. Atherosclerosis
B. Trauma
C. Marfan's syndrome
D. Congenital

440. In Marfan's syndrome, Aortic aneurysm occurs most commonly in: *(AI 95)*
A. Ascending aorta
B. Descending aorta
C. Abdominal aorta
D. Arch or aorta

441. Clinical finding in AV fistula is one of the following : *(AIIMS Nov 98)*
A. Pericarditis
B. Sinus tachycardia
C. Cardiac arrhythmia
D. Hypothermia

442. In gram negative septicemia, early findings setting before shock of florid is: *(AI 99)*
A. Cardiac output, Total peripheral resistance
B. Cardiac output, Total peripheral resistance
C. Cardiac output, Total peripheral resistance
D. Cardiac output, Total peripheral resistance

443. A 70 year old man develops pneumonia and septicemia. Patient goes into renal failure and has a BP of 70/50 mm of Hg. Drug that should be used to maintain BP is: *(AI 07)*
A. Adrenaline
B. Ephedrine
C. Phenylephrine
D. Nor epinephrine

444. Renal failure in patients with septic shock occurs primarily from:
A. Acute tubular mecrosis
B. Acute cortical necrosis
C. Acute clomerulonephritis
D. Acute papillary damage

445. Which of the following statements is true about High Attitude Pulmonary Edema (HAPE)? *(AIIMS Nov. 06)*
A. Not exacerbated by exercise
B. Associated with pulmonary vasoconstriction
C. Occurs only in unacclamatized individuals
D. Associated with low cardiac output

446. During cardiac imaging the phase of minimum motion of heart is: *(AI 2010)*
A. Late systole
B. Mid systole
C. Late diastole
D. Mid diastole

447. Cardiovascular complications of HIV infection include all of the following, Except *(AI 2009)*
A. Pericardial Effusion
B. Cardiac Tamponade
C. Cardiomyopathy
D. Aortic Aneurysm

ANSWERS, REFERENCES, EXPLANATIONS AND RELEVANT HIGH YIELD FACTS

Arterial Pulses

Pulsus Bisferiens

1. **Answer is D (Tetralogy of Fallot)**: *Harrison 18th/p 1824 Harrisons 17th / 1383, 1384; Harrisons 16th /1305; Hurst's 12th/ 245*

Pulsus Bisferiens is not associated with Tetralogy of fallot.

Pulsus Bisfenens

Characteristic Causes (Harrisons)	Other causes (Hurst)
• ***Aortic Refurgitation (AR)***[Q] • ***Aortic Regurgitation with Aortic Stenosis (AR+AS)***[Q] • ***Hypertrophic Cardiomyopathy***[Q]	Condition associated with rapid election of an increased stroke volume from the left ventricle • *Exercise* • *Fever* • *PDA*

Pulses alternans [Q]	Bisferiens pulse [Q]	Pulsus paradoxus [Q]	Dicrotic pulse [Q]
• Regular alteration of pressure in pulse with regular rhythm (single peak) • Seen in - LVF [Q] - may be seen in all conditions leading to LVF	• Two systolic peaks • Seen in - Aortic regurgitation[Q] ± AS - Hypertrophic cardiomyopathy [Q]	• Normal decrease in systolic pressure during inspiration is accentuated [Q] • Seen in - Pericardial tamponade [Q] - S.V.C. obstruction [Q] - COPD/Acute Severe Asthma - Constrictive pericarditis - Pulmonary embolism - Hypovolemic shock	• Has two palpable waves are in systole and one in diastole. • Seen in - dilated cardiomyopathy

2. **Answer is D (TOF)**: *Refer previous question*

Aortic Regurgitation alone or with Aortic stenosis and Hypertrophic cardiomyopathy are all associated with pulsus bisferiens

3. **Answer is C (Radial artery)**: *Harrison 18th/p 1824, 1825 Harrison 15th/ 1255, Harrison 16th/ 1305; Harrison 17th/1383, 1384*

Usually palpation of peripheral arterial pulses such as radial artery gives less information than examination of a more central pulse (Carotid pulse) regarding alterations in left ventricular ejection or Aortic valve function. However certain findings such as ***Bisferiens pulse of Aortic regurgitation or pulses alternans are more evident in peripheral arteries.*** *– Harrison*

Pulsus Paradoxus

4. **Answer is A (IPPV)**: *Harrison 18th/p 1824, 1825 Harrison 15th/ 1255, Harrison 16th/ 1305; Harrison 17th/ 1384*

Pulsus paradoxus is not a feature of IPPV.

Pulsus paradoxus may be seen in association with cardiac tamponade, constrictive pericarditis (infrequent) and COPD.

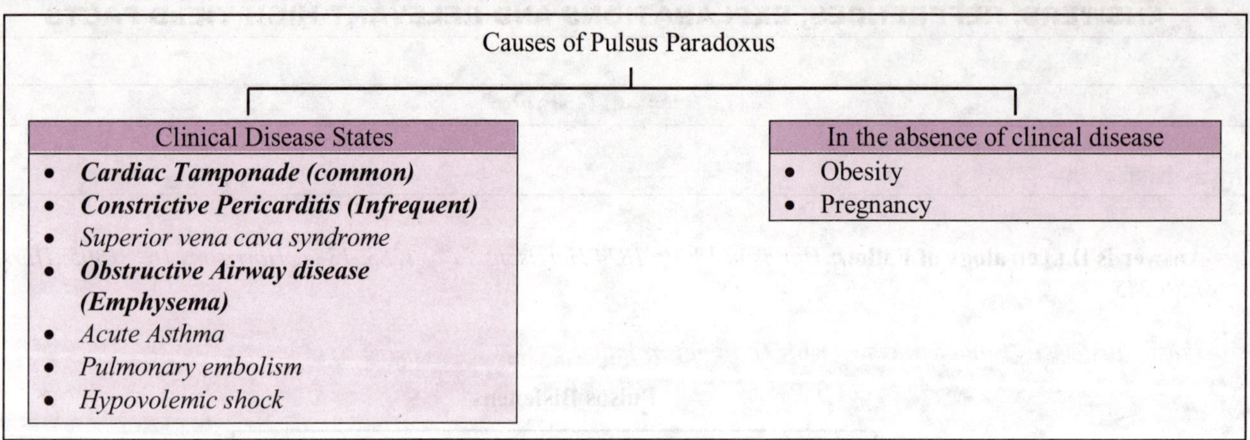

What is Pulsus Paradoxus

Normally the arterial pulse volume and arterial blood pressure decreases during inspiration and increases during expiration.

Pulsus paradoxus is an aggravation of a normal process and hence also called *pulses normalis aggregans.*

In pulses paradoxus the decrease in systolic arterial pressure during inspiration is accentuated.

What then in the paradox:

In patients with pericardial tamponade, airway obstruction or superior vena caval obstruction, the decrease in systolic arterial pressure may be so much that the peripheral pulse may completely disappear during inspiration.

The paradox is that the heart sounds may still be heard on auscultation over the apex at a time when no pulse is palpable at the radial artery.

5. **Answer is D (Hypertrophic cardiomyopathy):** *Harrison 18th/p 1824, 1825, 1975 Harrisons 17th/1384; 1491: Hurst 12th/241, 242, 245, 246 Braunwold 8th/133*

Pulsus paradoxus is not a feature of Hypertrophic cardiomyopathy.

Pulsus paradoxus may be associated with chronic obstructive pulmonary disease (emphysema), pulmonary embolism and Hypovolemic shock.

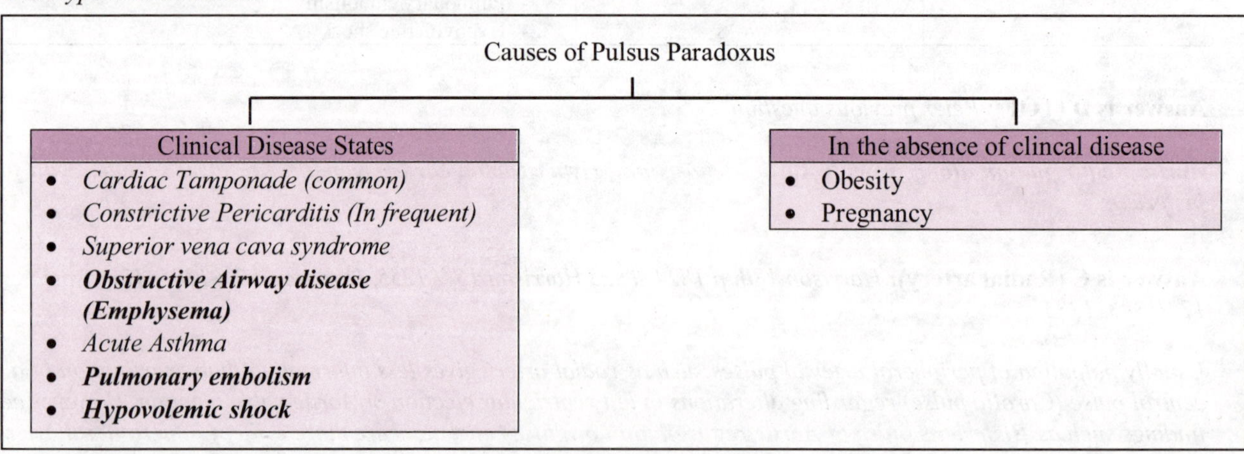

6. **Answer is C (Seen in constrictive pericarditis):** Harrison 18th/p 1975 *Harrisons 17th/1491*

Pulsus Paradoxus may be seen in constrictive pericarditis

'Pulsus paradoxus is charachteristic of cardiac tamponade but is also seen in about one- third of patients with constrictive pericarditis' - Harrisons

7. **Answer is A (Cardiac tamponade); B (Constrictive pericarditis); & E (Severe asthma):** Harrison 18th/p 1824, 1975 *Harrisons 17th/1384, 1491, Hurzt 12th/241, 242, 245, 246, Braunwald 8th/133*

Pulsus paradoxus is characteristic of cardiac tamponade but also seen in constrictive pericarditis and acute asthma

Pulsus alternans

8. Answer is D (MI): *Harrison 18th/p 1825 Harrisons 17th/1384, Hurst 12th/241*

Pulsus alternans indicates severe impairment in LV function and may be seen in conditions causing severe LV dysfunction such as Myocardial Infarction

Pulsus Alternans

- Pulsus alterans is charachterized by regular alteration of the pressure pulse amplitude despite a regular rhythm
- It is defined by beat to beat variation of the pulse amplitude but with a single peak and independent of the respiratory cycle.

In pulsus bigeminus there is also a regular beat to beat variation but it is caused by a premature ventricular contraction that follows each regular beat

- Pulsus alterans is charachteristically seen in Left ventricular failure and conditions causes LVF (including MI)

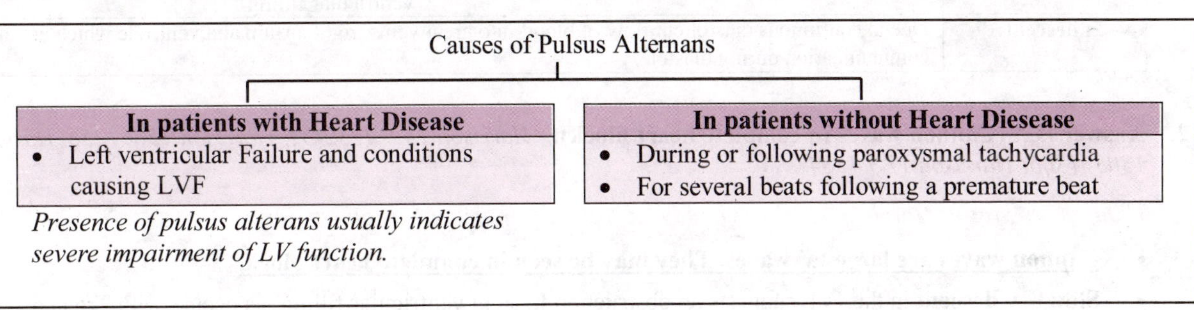

Miscellaneous Pulses

9. Answer is B (Aortic Regurgitation): Harrison 18th/p 1943, 1944 *Harrisons 17th/1476*

The Water hammer pulse or Corrigan's pulse is characterized by an abrupt and rapid carotid upstroke with a rapid fall off (collapsing pulse). It is characteristic of Aortic Regurgitation.

10. Answer is C (A.S): Harrison 18th/p 1939 *Harrisons 17th/1473*

Double Apical Impulse may be seen in Aortic Stenosis and Hypertrophic obstructive cardiomyopathy (HOCM)

Double Apical Impulse
• *Aortic Stenosis*[Q]
• *HOCM*[Q]

Jugular Venous Pulse (JVP)

11. Answer is A (c wave – onset of atrial systole): Harrison 18th/p 1823 *Harrison 15th/ 1256, Harrison 16th/ 1305, 1306; 17th/ 1384*

Onset of atrial systole is marked by production of a waves on JVP and not by c waves.

Jugular venous pulse : Review

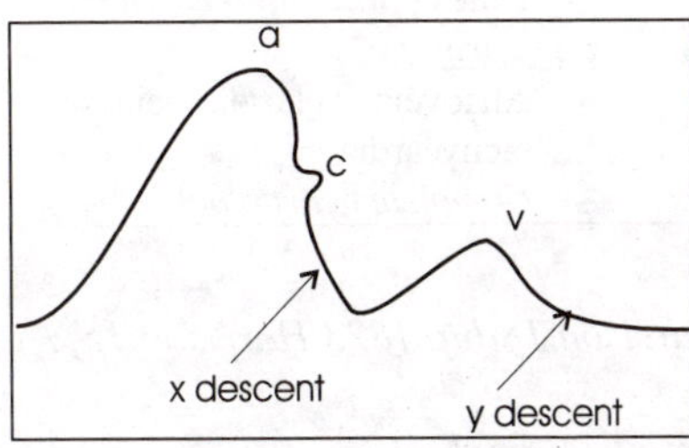

a waves :	Due to distention produced by rt. atrial contraction.	
c waves :	Are positive waves produced by bulging of tricuspid valve into right atrium during right ventricular isovolumetric contraction.	
v waves:	Due to increasing volume of blood in the right atrium during ventricular systole when the tricuspid valve is closed.	
a – x descent:	Due both to atrial relaxation and to the downward displacement of the tricuspid valve during ventricular systole.	
	Accentuated in	Reduced with
	- Constrictive pericarditis - Cardiac temponade - Restrictive cardiomyopathy	- Right ventricular dilatation Reversed with - Tricuspid Regurgitation
v – y descent:	By the opening of the tricuspid valve and the subsequent rapid inflow of blood into the right ventricle.	
	Accentuated in	Reduced with
	- Tricuspid regurgitation - Constrictive pericarditis	- Tricuspid stenosis - Right / Atrial Myxoma (Suggests obstruction to right ventricular filling)
y – a descent:	Due to continuous diastolic inflow of blood into great veins, right atrium and ventricle which are all in free communication during diastole.	

12. **Answer is A (Cannon waves in complete heart block):** *Harrison 14th/ 1232-34, Harrison 15th/ 1256, Harrison 16th/ 1305, 1306; Harrison 17th/ 1384*

Cannon a waves are large 'a' waves that may be seen in complete heart block.

- **<u>Cannon waves are large 'a' waves. They may be seen in complete heart block.</u>**
- **<u>Slow v-y descent</u>** in the JVP suggests an obstruction to right ventricular filling, as occurs with Tricuspid Stenosis or Right Atrial Myxoma.
  <u>Tricuspid Regurgitation</u> causes the v-waves to be prominent, when TR becomes severe, the combination of a prominent v-wave and obliteration of x-descent results in a single large positive systolic wave.
- **<u>Tricuspid stenosis is associated with large/giant 'a' waves and not large/giant c waves.</u>**
  <u>Tricuspid stenosis</u>- Positive presystolic a-wave is enlarged when the right atrium is contracting against an increased resistance.
- **<u>SVC obstruction</u>** causes raised JVP with absent pulsation (OHCM 5th/ 78)

Raised JVP ċ normal wave form	Raised JVP ċ absent pulsation
Fluid overload / Right heart failure	SVC obstruction

13. **Answer is C (Tricuspid Regurgitation):** Harrison 18th/p 1823 *Harrison 15th/ 1256, 1257, Harrison 16th/ 1306; Harrison 17th/ 1384*

Tricuspid stenosis (not Tricuspid regurgitation) is associated with large or 'a' giant waves.

<u>'a' waves in JVP:</u>
Are positive waves, due to distension produced by Right atrial contraction.
Large 'a' waves indicate atrium is contracting against increased resistance.

Large 'a' waves :	Cannon 'a' waves :	Absent 'a' waves :
• ***Tricuspid stenosis*** [Q] • Pulmonary stenosis [Q] • ***Pulmonary hypertension*** [Q]	• <u>Regularly</u> - During ***junctional rhythm*** [Q] • <u>Irregularly</u> - Atrioventricular dissociation with ventricular tachycardia - *Complete heart block* [Q]	*Atrial fibrillation* [Q]

14. **Answer is A (Atrial fibrillation):** *Harrison 18th/p 1823 Harrison 15th/ 1256, 1257, Harrison 16th/ 1306; Harrison 17th/ 1384*

Absent 'a' waves are characteristic of atrial fibrillation.

15. Answer is B (Tricuspid valve bulging into right atrium): Harrison 18th/p 1823 *Harrisons 17th /1384; Harrisons 16th/1305*

The 'C' Wave is a positive wave produced by the bulging of tricuspid valve into the right atrium *during right Ventricular isovolumetric systole and by impact of the carotid artery adjacent to the jugular vein. -Harrisons 17th /1384*

16. Answer is B (Bulging of Tricuspid valve): Harrison 18th/p 1823 *Harrison 17th/1384; Repeat*

The 'c' wave in JVP is a positive wave produced by the bulging of the tricuspid valve into the right atrium *during right ventricular isovolumetric systole and by the impact of the carotid artery adjacent to the jugular vein.*

17. Answer is A (Absent Y descent): *Harrison 18th/ 1972; Harrisons 17th/1490*

Cardiac tamponade is charachterized by jugular venous distension (↑ ed JVP) with a prominent X descent but an, absent Y descent *- Harrisons*

Feature	Tamponade	Constrictive pericarditis	Restrictive cordiomyopathy	RVMI
Prominent y descent	***Absent***	Usually present	Rare	*Rare*
Prominent x descent	Present	Usually present	Present	*Rare*

Pulse Pressure

18. Answer is C (Systolic – Diastolic B.P): *Ganong 21st / 589*

Pulse pressure is the difference between the systolic pressure and the diastolic pressure.

19. Answer is D (Congestive Heart Failure): *CPDT 16th/547*

Congestive Heart Failure is associated with a narrow pulse pressure

Pulse Pressure

Pulse pressure is the difference between systolic and diastolic blood pressure

Wide pulse pressure
(>50% systolic BP)

Common Causes

- *Aortic Regurgitation*
- *Patent Ductus Arteriosus*
- *Complete Heart Block*
- *Hyperthyroidism*
- *Beri Beri*
- *Pregnancy*
- *Fever /Hot weather*
- *Anemia*
- *Anxiety*
- *Paget's disease of bone (Extensive AV shunting through bone)*
- *Arteriovenous shunting*
- *Others (Life threatening increased ICP etc)*

Narrow Pulse Pressure
(<25% systolic BP)

Common causes

- *Congestive Heart Failure*
- *Aortic stenosis (severe)*
- *Cardioc Tamponade*
- *Dehydration*

Cardiac Auscultation: Heart Sounds and Murmurs

First Heart Sound (S1)

20. Answer is C (Heard at the end of ventricular systole): *Refer text below*

S1 is heard at the start of ventricular systole and not at the end.

S1 has a lower frequency (25-45 Hz) than S2 (50 Hz). It is caused by closure of mitral and tricuspid valves and is heard well with the diaphragm of stethoscope.

Heart Sounds :Review

Feature	1st heart sound	2nd heart sound	3rd heat sound	4th heart sound
Character	High pitched (lower than S_2) Slightly prolonged "lub"	High pitched (higher than S_1) Shorter "dup"	Soft low pitched weak rumbling	Low pitched heart sound
Duration	0.14 second	0.11 sec	0.1 sec	-
Frequency	25-45 Hz	50 Hz	-	***< 20 Hz***[Q]
Cause	Sudden closure of mitral & tricuspid valves	Closure of aortic & pulmonary valves	***Rapid ventricular filling***[Q] d/t inthrushing of blood from atria	***Ventricular filling***[Q] d/t atrial contraction causing inthrushing of blood
Timing	Start of ventricular systole	Just after end of ventricular systole	Begining of middle third of diastole	Immediately before 1st heart sound (presystolic)
Heard	Better heard with Diaphram	Better heard with Diaphram	***Better heard with the Bell***	***Better heard with the Bell***

S_3 & S_4 can often not be heard with a stethoscope (ear)[Q] and requirw phonocardiogram
S_3 often and S_4 sometimes can be recorded in phonocardiorgam

The first and second heart sounds and opening snaps are heard better with the diaphragm, and low-pitched sounds such as the third or fourth heart sound are beter heard with the bell of stethoscope – Hutchisons 20th/ 174

21. Answer is A (Short PR interval): Harrison 18th/p 1827 *Harrison 15th/ 1258, Harrison 16th/ 1307; Harrison 17th/ 1385*

Short PR interval is associated with a Loud S_1.
S_1 is produced as a result of closure of AV valves.
In short PR interval mitral leaflets are at a greater distance from neutral as decreased interval between atrial contraction and ventricular systole does not allow them to return towards neutral before the ventricular contraction arrives. This results in a louder S_1

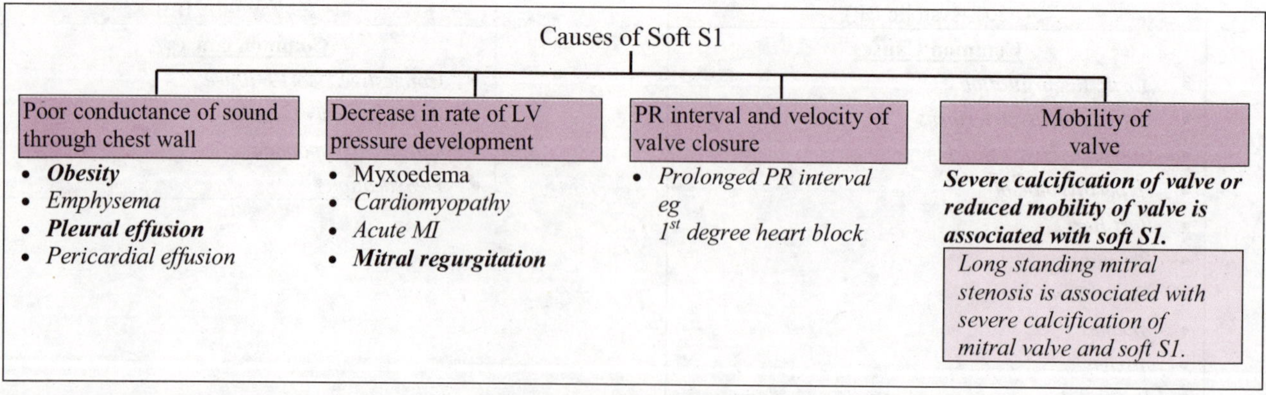

22. Answer is E (All of the above): Harrison 18th/p 1826 *Harrison 17th/1385; Hurst 12th/261*

Long standing severe M.S. (calcified mitral valve), obesity, mitral regurgitation and pleural effusions are all established causes of soft S1.

Factors that determine the intensity of S_1

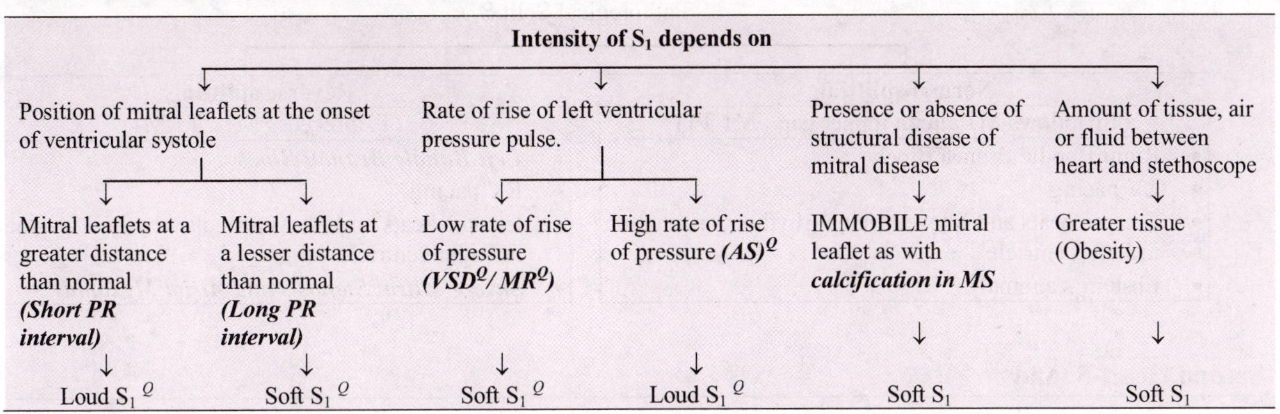

23. Answer is C (Short PR interval) and D (Tachycardia): Harrison 18th/826; *Harrison 17th 1385; Hurst 12th/260, 261*

Short PR interval and Tachycardia are associated with Loud S1.

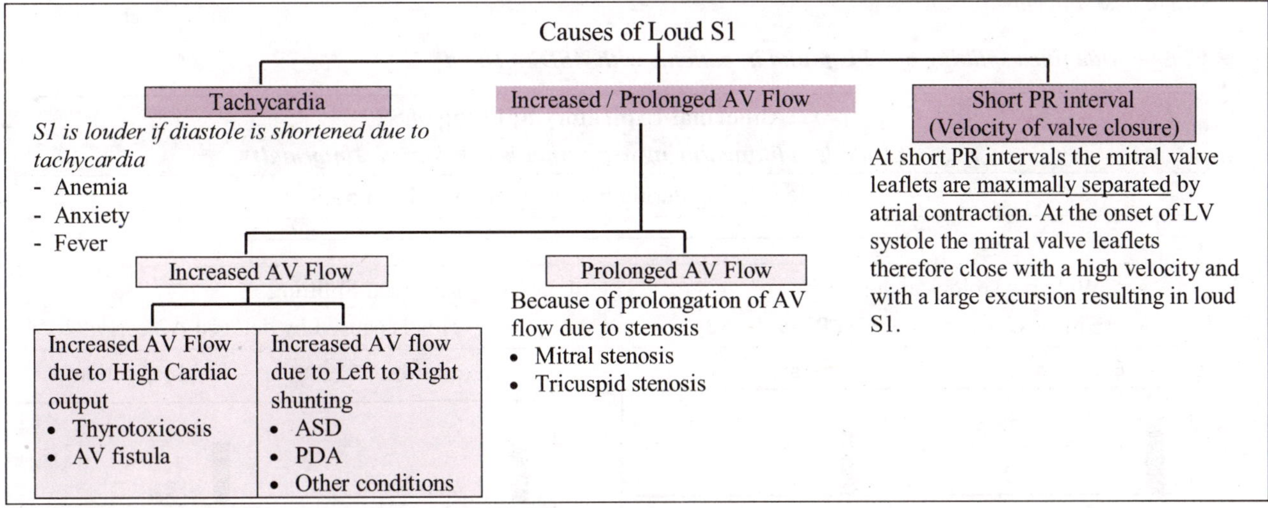

24. Answer is A (Prolonged flow through mitral valve): Harrison 18th/p 1826 *Harrison 17th/1385; Hurst 12th/260, 261;*

Refer previous question

Loud S1 in mitral stenosis results from prolonged AV flow through the mitral valve.

'S1 is louder if AV flow is prolonged because of mitral stenosis' – Harrison
Reduced mobility of valve (Immobility, calcification), and Prolonged PR interval (1st degree block) are all causes of soft S1.

Note:
First degree block is characterized by prolonged PR interval.

25. Answer is B (LBBB) and E (Atrial myxoma): Harrison 18th/p 1826 *Harrison's 17th/1385; Hurst's 10th/244, 242*

Left Bundle Branch Block, and Atrial myxoma are causes of reverse splitting of First Heart Sound (S1).

First heart Sound (S1) and Splitting

- First heart sound (M1T1) is produced by closure of Mitral valve (M1) and closure of Tricuspid valve (T1)
- The mitral valve closes slightly before the Tricuspid valve (M1 → T1)
  This normal splitting (physiological splitting) cannot be detected by auscultation because both components are low pitched and separated only by 20-30 ms.
- Therefore splitting of first heart sound, whenever audible is considered pathological.

Pathological Split S_1

Normal splitting (T1 follows M1 after a longer gap : M1 T1)	Reverse splitting (T1 precedes M1 : T1 M1)
• Right Bundle Branch Block	• ***Left Bundle Branch Block***
• LV pacing	• RV pacing
• Ectopic beats and Idioventricular rhythms originating in Left Ventricle	• Ectopic beats and Idioventricular rhythms originating in Right ventricle
• Ebstein's anomaly	• ***Severe Mitral Stenosis and Atrial Myxoma***

Second Heart Sound

26. Answer is C >A (ASD > VSD): Harrison 18th/p 1826 *Hurst's 12th / 266, 268; Harrisons 17th/ 1385*

Wide physiological splitting may be seen in both VSD and ASD but it is more characteristic of ASD. ASD is the single best anterior of choice.

Classic wide fixed splitting of S2 is found in patients with ASD' *– Hurst*

Abnormal Expiratory Splitting of S2
(Audible splitting during expiration is considered Abnormal)

Audible splitting during both expiration and inspiration

• Wide physiological splitting • This is caused by delayed P2/early A2	• Reversed Splitting • This is caused by delayed A2/early P2

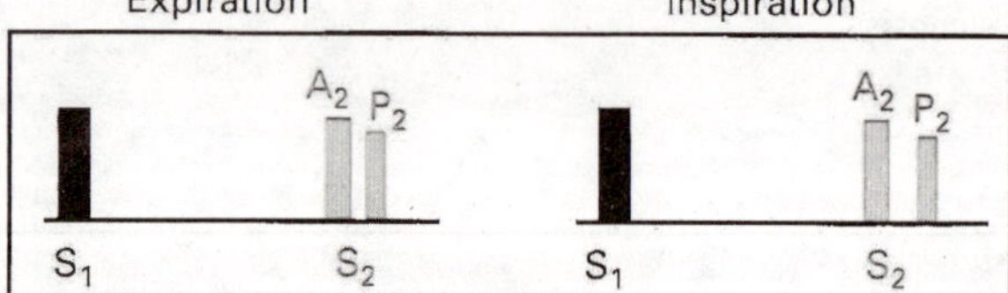

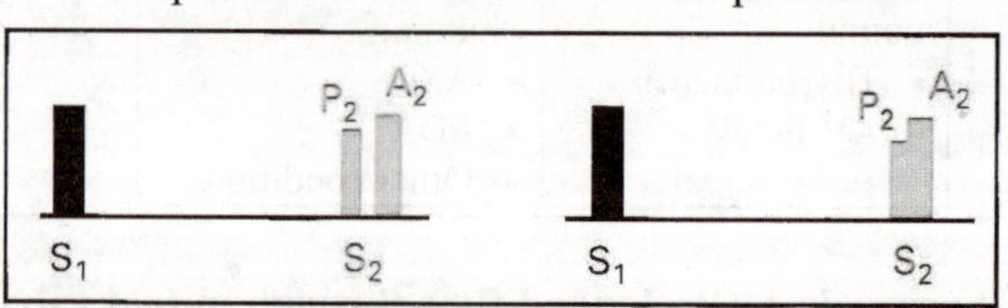

This is associated with Paradoxical movements i.e. P2 moves towards A2 with inspiration and hence splitting interval narrows with inspiration.

Wide Physiologic Splitting of the second Heart Sound	Reversed Splitting of the second Heart Sound
Delayed pulmonic closure	**Delayed aortic closure**
• Delayed electrical activation of the right ventricle	• Delayed electrical activation of the left ventricle
- Complete RBBB (proximal type)	- Complete LBBB (proximal type)
- Left ventricular paced beats	- Right ventricular paced beat
- Left ventricular ectopic beats	- Right ventricular ectopic beats
• Prolonged right ventricular mechanical systole	• Prolonged left ventricular mechanical systole
- Acute massive pulmonary embolus	- Complete LBBB (peripheral type)
- Pulmonary hypertension with right heart failure	- Left ventricular outflow tract obstruction
- Pulmonic stenosis with intact septum (moderate to severe)	- Hypertensive cardiovascular disease
	- Arteriosclerotic heart disease
	- Chronic ischemic heart disease
	- Angina pectoris

• Decreased impedence of the pulmonary vascular bed (increased hangout)	• Decreased impedance of the systemic vascular bed (increased hangout)
- Normotensive atrial septal defect - Idiopathic dilation of the pulmonary artery - Pulmonic stenosis (mild) - ***Atrial septal defect*** - Unexplained AES in normal subjects	- Poststenotic dilation of the aorta secondary to aortic stenosis or regurgitation - Patent ductus arteriosus
Early aortic closure	**Early pulmonic closure**
• Shortened LVET - ***Mitral regurgitation*** - ***Ventricular septal defect***	• Early electrical activation of the right ventricle - Wolff-Parkinson-White syndrome, type B

Normal Physiological Splitting	
No audible splitting on Expiration; Audible splitting present on Inspiration.	
• During expiration the Aortic sound (A2) and pulmonic sound (P2) are separated by less than 30 ms and are appreciated as a single sound • During inspiration the splitting interval widens and A2 and P2 are clearly separated into two distinctly audible sounds.	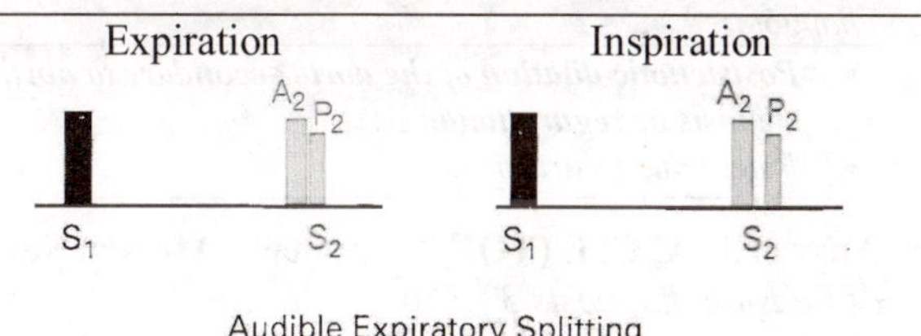

Note: Audible splitting during expiration is considered Abnormal

27. Answer is A, E (ASD, Pulmonary Stenosis): *Hurst 12th/268*

ASD and pulmonic stenosis are associated with wide splitting of second heart sound due to associated delayed closure of pulmonic valve.

28. Answer is A, B, D (ASD, MR, PS): *Hurst 12th/268*

ASD and PS are associated with wide split of second heart sound due to delayed pulmonic closure and MR is associated with wide split of second heart sound due to early aortic closure.

29. Answer is D (LBBB): *Hurst 12th /268; 'Cardiology' 3rd/6; Cleveland Clinic cardiology Board Rinen by Topol (2006)/33*

LBBB is associated with reversed or paradoxical spitting of S2 and not with fixed splitting.

Fixed splitting

Fixed splitting of S_2 is said to be present when the split does not vary with respiration and is present in both inspiration and expiration

This occurs due to minimum change in volume of right heart during inspiration and expiration

Causes of Fixed (wide) split
• ***ASD (Most characteristic cause for wide fixed splitting)***
• Pulmonic Stenosis
• *Acute Right Heart Failure (Pulmonary Embolism)*

30. Answer is B and C (WPW type A and LV pacing): *Hurst 12th/268*

WPW syndrome type A and LV pacing are not associated with reversed splitting.

WPW syndrome type B and RV pacing are associated with reversed splitting.

LBBB, Hypertensive heart disease (Hypertension) and post–stenotic dilatation in AS are all associated with reversed splitting due to associated delayed Aortic closure.

Reversed Splitting of the second Heart Sound

Delayed aortic closure	**Early pulmonic closure**
Delayed electrical activation of the left ventricle • *Complete LBBB (proximal type)* • ***Right ventricular paced beat*** • *Right ventricular ectopic beats*	*Early electrical activation of the right ventricle* ***Wolff-Parkinson-White syndrome, type B***
Prolonged left ventricular mechanical systole • ***Complete LBBB (peripheral type)*** • *Left ventricular outflow tract obstruction* • ***Hypertensive cardiovascular disease*** • *Arteriosclerotic heart disease* - *Chronic ischemic heart disease* - *Angina pectoris*	
Decreased impedance of the systemic vascular bed (increased hangout) • ***Poststenotic dilation of the aorta secondary to aortic stenosis or regurgitation*** • *Patent ductus arteriosus*	

31. Answer is A, C, E (TOF, Pulmonary Atresia, Severe Pulmonic stenosis): *Hurst 12th/269; Sapira's Art and Science of Bedside diagnosis 3rd/350*

TOF, Pulmonary Atresia and severe pulmonic stenosis are associated with single S_2 as one component of S2 is either absent or inaudible in these conditions.

Causes of single S_2

Conditions causing Delayed Aortic Closure	Conditions in which one component of S_2 is either absent or inaudible	Condition resulting in inability to hear the fainter of the two components of the sound (usually P_2)
All conditions associated with delayed A_2 can produce a single S_2 when the splitting interval becomes less than 30ms	Conditions in which one component of S_2 is either absent or in audible will produce a single S_2 • ***Severe TOF*** • Severe semilunor valve stenosis - severe AS - ***severe PS*** • ***Pulmonic valve atresia*** • Tricuspid valve atresia • Eisseminger syndrome	These conditions also produce a single S_2 • Emphysema • Obesity • Respiratory noise
Causes of Delayed A2 • Delayed electrical activation of the right ventricle - Complete RBBB (proximal type) - Left ventricular paced beats - Left ventricular ectopic beats • Prolonged right ventricular mechanical systole - Acute massive pulmonary embolus - Pulmonary hypertension with right heart failure - ***Pulmonic stenosis*** with intact septum (moderate to severe) • Decreased impedence of the pulmonary vascular bed (increased hangout) - Normotensive atrial septal defect - Idiopathic dilation of the pulmonary artery - ***Pulmonic stenosis*** (mild) - Atrial septal defect - Unexplained AES in normal subjects	Semilunar valves include Aortic valve, Pulmonary valve and trancal valves	

32. Answer is A and C (Pulmonary hypertension and Eisenmenger's syndrome): *Essential cardiology 2nd/108 Sapira's Art and science of Bed side diagnosis 3rd 1350*

Loud P_2 suggests the presence of pulmonary Arterial Hypertension.
Eisenmerger's syndrome is associated with pulmonary arterial hypertension and hence also causes a loud P_2.

Loud Pulmonary component of second Heart sound (Loud P_2)

- Loud Pulmonary component (P2) of the second heart sound signifies pulmonary arterial hypertension
  'Unless proved otherwise a loud P2 is considered to be caused by Pulmonary Hypertension' - 'Understanding Pediatric Heart sounds (2002)/97

- When a loud P_2 is described in the question, the most likely diagnosis is some form of pulmonary hypertension. Any etiological conditon leading to pulmonary hypertension may lead to a loud P2, including primary pulmonary hypertension, conditions of left side of heart (mitral stenosis), Eisenmenger's syndrome, or multiple pulmonary emboli.
- Eissenmenger's syndrome with Left to Right shunts leads to hyperkinetic pulmonary artery hypertension and may cause a loud P2

Eisemenger's syndrome (Left to Right shunt): Loud P2
ASD
VSD
PDA

Excluding other options

- TOF : Loud A2
- Pulmonic Stenosis : Soft P2
- Aortic Stenosis : Soft A2

Note:

- A loud P_2 is predictive of significant pulmonary hypertension
- *P_2 may appear louder than A_2 if the intensity of A_2 is decreased as in calcific or rheumatic aortic stenosis but this is not due to an abnormally increased intensity of P_2*

Third Heart Sound

33. Answer is B (Mitral stenosis): Harrison 18th/p 1827 *Harrison 15th/ 1259, Harrison 16th/ 1308; Harrison 17th/ 1386*

The left ventricular function is essentially normal in mitral stenosis and S_3 is not a presenting feature.

The third heart sound *(S_3) is a low pitched sound produced in the ventricle 0.14 to 0.16s after A_2, at the termination of rapid filling.*

Third Heart Sound (S3)

- *It is a low frequency sound*[Q]
- *It is a diastolic heart sound that occurs shortly after S2*[Q]
- *It occurs during rapid filling of the ventricles (termination of rapid filling)*[Q]
- *It is best heard at the apex in the left lateral position*[Q]
- *It is better heard with the bell of the stethoscope*[Q]

Third Heart Sound (S_3): Ventricular Diastolic Gallop, Protodiastolic Gallop, and Pericardial Knock

Physiologic S_3	Pathologic S_3

• Children
• High cardiac output
- ***Atheletes*** [Q]
- *Fever* [Q]
- *Pregnancy* [Q]
- *Thyrotoxicosis* [Q]
- *AV fistulas* [Q]
	• ***Ventricular dysfunction (LVF/RVF)*** – poor systolic function, increased end-diastolic and end-systolic volume, decreased ejection fraction, and high filling pressure.
	- Idiopathic dilated cardiomyopathy
	- *Ischemic heart disease*
	- Valvular heart disease
	- Congenital heart disease
	- Systemic and pulmonary hypertension
	• Excessively rapid early diastolic ventricular filling
	- Hyperkinetic states
	  - Anemia
	  - Thyrotoxicosis
	  - Arteriovenous fistula
	- Atrioventricular valve incompetence
	- ***Left to right shunts (VSD, PDA and ASD)***
	• Restrictive myocardial or pericardial disease
	• ***Constrictive pericarditis (pericardial knock)***
	• Restrictive cardiomyopathy
	• Hypertrophic cardiomyopathy.

***Pericardial knock is S_3** that occurs earlier (0.1 to 0.12 after A_2) and is higher pitched than normal. It often occurs in patients with constrictive pericarditis. Its presence depends upon the restrictive effect of the adherent pericardium, which halts diastolic filling abruptly. – Harrison*

34. Answer is A (Occurs due to rapid filling of the ventricles during atrial systole): Harrison 18th/p 1827 *Hurst 12th/270,271;Harrison 17th/1386*

Third heart sound occurs at the end of early rapid filling phase of the ventricle but not at the time of atrial systole.
The heart sound associated with ventricular filling during atrial systole is the fourth heart sound (S4)
Fourth Heart sound occurs in association with an effective atrial contraction[Q] (It is presumably caused by in-rush of blood into the ventricles when the atria contracts and hence it is also called the 'Atrial Heart Sound')

Pathological Third Heart Sound (S3) may be associated with ASD and VSD

*'A pathological S3 is often present in large left to right shunts due to high flow across the mitral valve with **VSD or patent ductus arteriosus** and with high flow across the tricuspid valve with **ASD**. The presence of this sound in these conditions does not imply congestive heart failure, and such patients may maintain normal myocardial contractility for years after the S3 is detected'- 'Hurst: The Heart' 11th/271*

Congenital Heart Diseases associated with Loud S3

- *Ventricular septal Defect (VSD)[Q]*
- *Patent Ductus Arteriosus (PDA)[Q]*
- *Atrial Septal Defect (ASD)[Q]*

Pathological Third Heart Sound (S3) may be associated with Constrictive Pericarditis
Constrictive pericarditis is characterixstically associated with pericardial knock which is a distinct form of third heart sound (S_3)
***'Pericardial knock is S_3 that occurs earlier** (0.1 to 0.12 after A2) and is higher pitched than normal. Its presence depends upon the restrictive effects of the adherent pericardium which halts diastolic filling abruptly' – Harrison*

35. Answer is C (Absent in MS): Harrison 18th/p 1827 *Hurst 12th/272, Harrisons 17th/1386; Refer previous question*

Third heart sound (S3) is commonly seen in association with ventricular dysfunction. Ventricular function is usually normal with MS and hence S3 is usually not a feature of MS.

Physiological S3 may be heard in athletes, while constrictive Pericarditis and ischaemic heart disease (MI) are established causes of pathological S3.

Fourth Heart Sound

36. Answer is C (Heard during ventricular filling): *Harrisons 16th/1308; Guyton 11th/270*

The fourth heart sound (S4) is a low pitched presystolic sound produced in ventricles during ventricular filling
– Harrison

Fourth Heart Sound (S4)

- Fourth Heart sound occurs in association with an *effective atrial contraction*[Q]
  (It is presumably caused by inrush of blood into the ventricles when the atria contracts and hence it is also called the 'Atrial Heart Sound')
- ***It is heard during the ventricular filling phase of the cardiac cycle (Presystolic[Q] heart sound)***
- ***It is low pitched (frequency usually 20 cycle/sec or less-(Guyton)***
- ***It is not audible to the unaided ear***
  Normally the fourth heart sound can almost never be heard even with a stethascope because of its weakness and low frequency *(Guyton)*

- S4 becomes audible when diminished ventricular compliance increases the resistance to normal filling
  When audible the S4 is *best heard with the bell of the stethescope*[Q]
- Pathologically may be seen in patients with

• Systemic Hypertension	• Ischaemic Heart Disease	• Pulmonic stenosis (Right S4)
• Aortic Stenosis	• Mitral Regurgitation	• Pulmonary H.T (Right S4)
• HOCM		

- Physiologically may be seen in patients with
  Increasing age
- Loudest (Best heard) at the Left ventricular Apex when the patient is in left Lateral position
- It is accentuated by mild isotonic or isometric exercises in the supine position

2

Cardiovascular System

37. Answer is C (Atrial Fibrillation): Harrison 18th/p 1827 *Hurtz 12th/281; Harrisons 17th/ 1386*

Atrial contraction must be present for production of S4. It is absent in atrial fibrillation.
Thyrotoxicosis. Acute MI, and Hypertrophic cardiomyopathy are all associated with pathological fourth Heart sound (S4).

Fourth Heart Sound (S4):
- *Low frequency sound (low pitched)*[Q]
- *It is a diastolic heart sound that occurs shortly before S1*[Q]
- *It occurs during the phase of ventricular filling and is associated with an effective atrial contraction Atrial contraction must be present for production of an S4*[Q]
- *It is best heard at the apex in the left lateral position*[Q]
- *It is better heard with the bell of the stethescope*[Q]

Causes of Pathological Fourth Heart sound

Fourth Hearth Sound (S4), Atrial Diastolic gallop, and Presystolic Gallop:

Decreased ventricular compliance

- Ventricular hypertrophy
  - Left or right ventricular outflow obstruction
  - Systemic or pulmonary hypertension
  - Hypertrophic cardiomyopathy
- Ischemic heart disease
  - Angina pectoris
  - Acute myocardial infarction
  - Old myocardial infarction
  - Ventricular aneurysm
- Idiopathic dilated cardiomyopathy

Excessively rapid late diastolic filling secondary to:

- Vigorous atrial systole
- Hyperkinetic states
  - Anemia
  - Thyrotoxicosis
- Arteriovenous fistula
- Acute atrioventricular valve incompetence

Arrhythmias

- Heart block

Physiologic S4 may be recordable, but is rarely audible

38. Answer is A (Ventricular aneurysm): Harrison 18th/p 1827 *Harrison 15th/ 1259, Harrison 16th/ 1386; Harrison 17th/ 1386*

In ventricular aneurysm the ventricle becomes more compliant than normal and offers lesser resistance to filling and hence no S_4 is heard. *S_4 is characteristically absent in ventricular aneurysm due to increased ventricular compliance.*

Fourth heart sound (S_4) :

- Is low pitched, presystolic sound, produced in ventricle during 2nd *rapid filling phase*.
- It is associated with *effective atrial contraction.*
- It occurs when there is increased resistance to ventricular filling due to *diminished ventricular compliance*

Common conditions producing S_4:	S_4 is absent in following conditions :
- ***Hypertension*** Q - *Aortic stenosis* Q - ***Hypertrophic cardiomyopathy*** Q - *Ischaemic heart disease* Q - ***Acute mitral regurgitation*** Q	- *Atrial fibrillation* - *Ventricular aneurysm*

Added Sound

39. Answer is C (Ejection click): Harrison 18th/p 1826, 1827 *Harrison 14th/ 1234, 1235, 1341, 1339, Harrison 16th/ 1308; Harrison 17th/ 1385, 1386*

Ejection click is a sharp high pitched sound Q ***that occurs immediately after First Heart Sound and not after the second.*** It occurs as a result of sudden opening of semilunar valves in conditions where this opening is delayed such as *Aortic valve stenosis* Q, *Pulmonary valve stenosis* Q, *Hypertension* Q.

Shortly after S1 Q	Shortly before S1 Q	Between S1 & S2 Q	Shortly after S2 Q
Ejection click	*Fourth heart sound*	*Midsystolic click*	*Opening snap / pericardial knock tumor plop / S3*

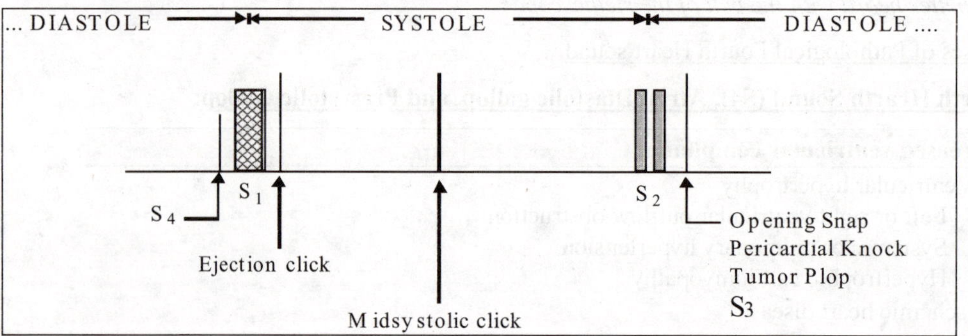

Ejection Click	Opening Snap	Pericardial knock	Tumor Plop
• *Sharp, High pitched sound* Q	• Brief, *High pitched sound* Q	• A third heart sound that is *higher pitched than normal* (S3 is low pitched).	• Tumor plop is a characteristic *low pitched sound* Q
• Audible during *early systole* Q *(immediately after S1)*	• Audible during *early diastole* Q *(between 0.04 to 0.12 sec after A2)*	• Audible during *early diastole* Q *(within 0.01 to 0.12 sec after A2)*	• Audible during *early or mid diastole* Q
• *Seen in Aortic stenosis* Q, *Pulmonary stenosis* Q, *Hypertension* Q *and is produced due to sudden opening of semilunar valves in conditions where this opening is delayed.*	• *Seen in stenosis of AV valves (Mitral stenosis* Q > Tricuspid stenosis)	• Seen in *constrictive pericarditis* Q and produced due to sudden deceleration of venticular filling because of restrictive effect of adherent pericardium.	• Seen in conditions like *atrial myxoma* Q and produced due to the tumor abruptly stopping as it strikes the ventricular wall

40. Answer is A (It is a high pitched diastolic sound): Harrison 18th/p 1930 *Harrison 15th/ 1259, Harrison 16th/ 1308, 1311; 17th/ 1466, 1467*

Opening snap is brief high pitched sound heard in early diastole.

Opening snap
- ***brief high pitched sound***   - *heard in early* ***diastole*** *(Ejection sound are heard in systole)*   - *It is usually due to* ***stenosis of an (A.V.)*** *most often mitral value.*   - *It* ***follows second heart sound,*** A_2 *by 0.05 to 0.12 sec.*   - *It is generally best heard at* ***lower left sternal border*** *and radiates well to the base of heart*   - *It is best heard during expiration*   - *The time interval between* A_2 *and* O_s *varies inversely with the severity of M.S.*   - *It is followed by low pitched rumbling diastolic murmur*

Note:

- O.S. may also be audible in tricuspid stenosis
- O.S. of tricuspid stenosis occurs later in diastole than the mitral O.S.

Opening snap indicates that :
- *M.S. is organic (and significant)* Q   - *Valve cusps are pliable* Q   - *High atroventricular pressure gradient is present* Q   - *Severe, AR, MR, AF, SABE are absent.* Q

41. Answer is D (Ejection click): Harrison 18th/p 1827 *Harrisons 17th /1385, 1386 Braunward 8th/136*

Ejection clicks are systolic sounds and not distolic sounds.
S3, S4 and opening snap are all diastolic sounds.

Added Heart Sounds

Diastolic sounds	Systolic sounds
• *Opening snap* Q	• *Ejection sound/click* Q
• *Third Heart sound (S3)* Q	• *Non ejection click/mid systolic click* Q
• *Fourth Heart sound (S4)* Q	
• *Pericardial knock* Q	
• *Tumor plop (Atrial myxoma)* Q	

42. Answer is D (Pink TOF): *Ghai 6th/385, 411; Moss & Adams Heart Disease in Infants, Children & Adolescents 7th/837; Pediatric Cardiology (2006) /59*

Pink TOF (Acyanotic TOF) is unlikely to be associated with a Left upper parasternal systolic thrill.

<u>Pink TOF is unlikely to be associated with a systolic thrill in 2nd & 3rd intercostal space</u>

Pink (Acyanotic) TOF is associated with only a mild degree of pulmonic stenosis.Such mild pulmonic stenosis is usually not associated with any thrill.

"When pulmonic stenosis is mild the precordium is quiet and a thrill is not present"

- Moss & Adams Heart Disease in Infants, Children and Adolescents 7th/837

Thrill is usually associated with a moderate to severe degree of stenosis   *When stenosis is mild a thrill is not present (Moss & Adams)*   *When stenosis is very severe (complete occlusion) thrill may be absent (Moss & Adams)*

Systolic thrill in Left 2nd & 3rd intercostals space will be present when the associated pulmonic stenosis is at least a moderate degree. Such cases are usually associated with cyanotic TOF.

<u>Systolic thrill in Left upper parasternal region is charachteristic of Pulmonic stenosis</u>

'A systolic thrill in the second or third left intercostal space near the sternum often occurs with pulmonic stenosis'.

– Hurst 12th/256

Systolic thrill is Left parasternal region may be seen in Ebstein anomaly

'A systolic thrill may be palpable at the left sternal border' - Ghai 6th/411

In Ebstein anomaly the septal leaflet of the tricuspid valve may be displaced into the RV outflow tract causing obstruction of antegrade flow into the pulmonary artery. ***This may produce a systolic thrill in the left parasternal region similar to Pulmonary stenosis (Upper Left parasternal area)***
Also presence of tricuspid regurgitation in patients with Ebstein's anomaly may produce a systolic thrill at the left lower sternal border

Systolic thrill in Left upper parasternal region may be present in sub pulmonic VSD

Subpulmonic VSD is a type of VSD where the defect is located in a more anterior portion in the ventricular septum such that *the VSD is closely related to the pulmonary artery.*
In subpulmonic VSD the left ventricle 'Ejects' directly into the pulmonary artery which may in turn produce a systolic thrill in the pulmonary area (Left 2nd & 3rd intercostals space)

Cardiac Murmur

43. Answer is D (Aortic stenosis): Harrison 18th/p 1827, 1828 *Harrison 15th/ 207, 208; Harrison 16th/1309, 1310; Harrison 17th/ 1387*

The murmur of Aortic Stenosis *is characteristically an* ***ejection systolic murmur*** *Q that occurs in* ***midsystole*** *(starts only shortly after S1 and never with S1) when the ventricular pressure becomes high enough to open the semilunar valve. The murmur increases in intensity as the velocity of ejection increases and as ejection declines it decreases. The murmur ends before ventricular pressure falls enough to permit closure of aortic or pulmonary leaflets.*

Systolic murmurs

Holosystolic /pan systolic murmurs	Midsystolic murmurs ejection systolic murmurs	Early systolic murmurs
Begin with S_1 and end after S_2 • VSD • Mitral Regurgitation • Tricuspid Regurgitation • Aortopulmonary shunts	***Starts shortly after S_1 and ends before S_2*** **Aortic**: Aortic stenosis; Coarctation; Aneurysm; PDA; High output states **Pulmonary**: P. stenosis; P. hypertension; P. artery dilatation; ASD; High output states	***Begin with first heart sound and end in midsystole*** • VSD - Large VSD with pulmonary hypertension - *V. small muscular VSD* • ***Tricuspid regurgitation*** in absence of Pul. Hypertension • Mitral regurgitation in a non compliant left atrium as in ***papillary muscle dysfunction***

Common condition producing acute MR include
- Rupture of chordae tendnae - ***Papillary muscle dysfunction*** or rupture following MI - Infective endocarditis

44. Answer is D (Pansystolic murmur): Harrison 18th/p 1944 *Harrisons 16th/ 1400; Harrison 17th/ 1476, 1475*

Murmur in AR : Harrison 16th/ 1400

Typical **diastolic murmur** of chronic AR	**Midsystolic** ejection murmur	Austin flint murmur (**diastolic**)
• High pitched, blowing, decrescendo diastolic murmur • Heard best in the third I.C.S. along the left sternal border Note: With marked post stenotic dilatation of aorta the murmur may be loudest in the 2nd or 3rd right interspace – API 7th/ 420	• Resembles murmur of AS but is higher pitched, shorter and less rasping • Heard best at the base of heart and is transmitted along the carotids	• Soft, low pitched rumbling middiastolic • Heard best at the apex • Produced by diastolic displacement of anterior leaflet of mitral valve by AR stream

45. Ans. Answer is A (Mitral Stenosis): *Harrison 17th /1467*

Mid diastolic murmur with with presystolic accentuation is typically seen in mitral stenosis.

'Mitral stenosis is associated with a low-pitched rumbling diastolic murmur heard best at the apex. The murmur typically peaks during mid-diastole and again immediately before the first heart sound ***(Pre-systolic accentuation)'***

- Evidence Based physical diagnosis (Elsevier) 2012/397

'Mitral stenosis is associated with a low-pitched rumbling diastolic murmur heard best at the apex with the patient in lateral decubitus position. In patients with sinus rhythm, the murmur often reappears or becomes louder during atrial systole ***(presystolic accentuation)'*** *- Harrison*

Mitral stenosis : Review

Mitral stenosis	
Auscultatory findings	**X Ray findings**
• S_1 : *accentuated.* • S_2 : *Normally split S_2 with accentuated P_2*[Q] • **Murmur :** *Low pitched*[Q]*, rumbling*[Q] *diastolic murmur*[Q] *with 'Pre-systolic accentuation' heard best at the apex in left lateral recumbent position*[Q]. • **Opening snap :** *brief, high pitched*[Q]*, early diastolic*[Q] *sound, best heard at the lower left sternal border*[Q].	• *Straightening of the left border of cardiac silhouette*[Q] • *Prominence of main pulmonary artery*[Q] • *Dilation of upper lobe pulmonary veins*[Q] • *Kerley B lines*[Q] • *Backward displacement of the esophagus*[Q]

46. Answer is D (HOCM): *Harrison 18th/1830; Harrison's 17th/1387; Current Diagnosis & Treatment in Cardiology 2nd/144*

Murmurs of HOCM are increased on Valsalva maneuver

Murmurs of VSD, MR and AS all decrease in intensity on Valsalva ***maneuver***

Differentiation of systolic murmurs base don changes in their intensity from physiologic maneuvers

Maneuver	HOCM	AS	MR/VSD	MVP	TR	Flow
Valsalva's maneuver	↑	↓	↓	↑	↓	↓
Stand	↑	-	-	↑	-	↓
Squat	↓	-	-	↓	-	↑
Handgrip/TAO	↓	-	↑	↑	-	↓
Inspiration	-	-	-	-	↑	- or ↑
Post-PVC	↑	↑	-	-	-	↑

AS= aortic stenosis; Flow = benign flow murmur; HOCM = hypertrophic obstructive cardiomyopathy; MR = mitral regurgitation; MVP = mitral valve prolapse; PVC = pressure ventricular contraction; TAO = transient arterial occlusion; TR = tricuspid regurgitation; VSD = ventriocular septal defect; ↑ = increased in murmur intensity; ↓ = decreased in murmur intensity; - = no predictable change

47. Answer is C (MVP): Harrison 18th/p 1830 *Harrison's 17th/1387; Current Diagnosis & Treatment in Cardiology 2nd/144*

Murmur of MVP increases both on hand grip and on Valsalva maneuver. Murmur of HOCM increases on valsalva, but decreases on handgrip.

Maneuver	HOCM	MVP
Valsalva's maneuver	↑	↑
Handgrip/TAO	↓	↑
Stand	↑	↑
Squat	↓	↓
Inspiration	-	-
Post-PVC	↑	-

48. Answer is B (HOCM): Harrison 18th/p 1830 *Harrison's 17th/1387; Braunwald 8th/ed 1663*

Murmur of HOCM typically increases with Valsalva maneuver.

'Most murmurs decrease in length and intensity with Valsalva Maneuver. Two exceptions are the systolic murmur of HOCM which usually becomes much louder and that of MVP which becomes longer and often louder' – Harrison

49. Answer is C (Associated with AR) : *Harrison 16th/1310; 17th/1387; API 8th/438; CMDT 06/405; 09/365;Ghai 6th/376*

Carey Coomb's murmur in a low pitched, delayed diastolic mitral murmur seen in rheumatic fever in association with Mitral Regurgitation. It is not associated with Aortic Regurgitation.

Carey Coomb's Murmur	Austin Flint Murmur
• Low pitched (soft) • Delayed diastolic (Middiastolis) • Mitral • Associated with Acute Rheumatic carditis	• Low pitched (soft) • Delayed diastolic (Middiastolic / Late diastolic) • Mitral • Associated with Aortic Regurgitation
Attributed to : • Inflammation of mitral valve cusps • Excessive left atrial blood flow as consequence of mitral regurgitation	**Attributed to :** • Anterior mitral valve leaflet when blood enters the left ventricle simultaneously from both the aortic route and the left atrium

"Carey Coomb's murmur is a delayed diastolic mitral murmur." *- Ghai 6th / 376*

Remember :

Low pitched, delayed diastolic mitral murmur in association with Rheumatic fever : Carey Coomb's murmur.
Low pitched, delayed diastolic mitral murmur is association with severe chronic AR : Austin Flint murmur.

50. Answer is B (Acute Rheumatic carditis): *Harrisons 17th/1387, Harrisons 16th/1310, API 8th/438,*

Carey coombs murmur is delayed diastolic murmur seen in acute rheumatic carditis and is attributed to excessive left atrial blood flow due to mitral regurgitation.
It is not seen in MR, AR or severe pulmonary Hypertension.

51. Answer is A (Mitral stenosis with Mitral Regurgitation): *Harrisons 17th/1388; Harrisons 16th/1311; Hurst's 12th/290*

Continuous murmur is not associated with mitral stenosis and mitral regurgitation.
Patent ductus arteriosus, Rupture of sinus of valsalva and systemic AV fistutas are all associated with continuous murmurs.

Causes of Continuous Murmur(Hurst)

Continuous Murmur caused by Blood flow	Continuous murmurs caused by high-to low-pressure shunts	Continuous murmurs secondary to localized arterial obstruction
• Venous hum • Mammary soufflé • Hemangioma • Hyperthyroidism • Acute alcoholic hepatitis • Hyperemia of neoplasm - hepatoma - renal cell carcinoma - paget disease	Systemic artery to pulmonary artery - Patient ductus arteriosus - Aortopulmonary window - Truncus arteriosus - Pulmonary atresia - Anamolous left coronary - Bronchiectasis - Sequestration of the lung Systemic artery to right heart - Ruptured sinus of Valsalva - Coronary artery fistula Left-to-right atrial shunting - Lutembacher syndrome - Mitral atresia plus atrial septal defect Venovenous shunts - Anomalous pulmonary veins - Portosystemic shunts Arteriovenous fistula (systemic or pulmonic)	• Coarctation of the aorta • Branch pulmonary stenosis • Carotid occlusion • Celiac mesenteric occlusion • Renal occlusion • Femoral occlusion • Coronary occlusion

52. Answer is D (Peripheral Pulmonary Stenosis): Harrison 18th/p 1829 *Harrison 16th/ 1310, 1311; Harrison 17th/ 1386*

The murmur of pulmonary stenosis is harsh systolic ejection murmur typically preceded by a systolic ejection sound. It is not a continuous murmur.

Continuous murmurs result from continuous flow between a high pressure and low pressure area that persists through the end of systole and beginning of diastole.

Common Causes of continuous murmurs
• ***Systemic arteriovenous fistula*** Q (congenital /acquired)
• ***Coronary arteriovenous fistula*** Q
• *Anomalous origin of Left coronary artery from pulmonary artery*
• ***Communication between sinus of valsalva and right side of heart*** Q ***(i.e. Ruptured sinus of valsalva*** Q ***into right side of heart)***
• ***Coarctation of Aorta : Continuous murmur in the back***
• ***Patent Ductus Arteriosus*** Q ***(PDA)***
• *Surgically created shunts e.g. Blalock-Tausig shunt*

53. Answer is A (Ventricular septal defect with Aortic Regurgitation): Harrison 18th/p 1829 *Harrisons 17th/1388; Refer previous question*

Ventricular septal defect with Aortic Requrgitation does not produce a continuous murmur

Patent Ductus Arteriosus produces a continuous murmur by the presence of a high to low pressure shunt
Coronary AV fistula also produces a continuous murmur by the presence of a high to low pressure shunt
Venous hum produces a continues murmur by rapid flow of blood
Venous hum is a continues murmur usually audible over the medial aspect of the right supraclavicular fossa with the patient upright (Harrison)

54. Answer is A and C (PDA and Shunt between pulmonary & subclavian artery): Harrison 18th/p 1829 *Hurzt 12th/290, Harrisons 17th/1388 Refer previous question*

Shunts between systemic artery and pulmonary artery (includes PDA and shunt between pulmonary artery and subclavian artery) are associated with continuous murmurs.

55. Answer is B (Systemic A V fistula); D (Aortopulmonary window) and E (Rupture of sinus valsalva): Harrison 18th/p 1829 *Harrisons 17th/1388: Hurst 12th/290*

Aortopulmonary window, systemic AV fistula and ruptured sinus of valsalva are associated with continuous murmurs caused by high to low pressure shunting of blood.

56. Answer is A (Complete heart block): Harrison 18th/p 1829 *CMDT 2008/323; CMDT 2009/321; 'Cardiology Secrets 2nd/113*

Complete heart block is not a cause for new onset systolic murmur after Acute Myocardial Infarction.

Cause of new systolic murmur after Acute Myocardial infarction
• *Papillary muscle dysfunction/rupture (causing severe mitral regurgitation)*
• *Rupture of interventricular septum*
• *Right ventricular infarction and tricuspid regurgitation*
• *Free wall rupture*
• *Left ventricular outflow tract obstruction*

Note:
Ischemic cardiomyopathy *is defined as dilated cardiomyopathy in a subject with history of MI. This may lead to papillary muscle dysfunction and hence produce a new onset systolic murmur.*

Cardiovascular Clubbing

57. Answer is D (Aortic Dissection): *Harrison 16th/211, 'Ultra Medicine' by Cockshoot and Monfredi (2005)/285*

Aortic Dissection is not a known cause for digital clubbing:
Digital clubbing results from long standing conditions that take months to develop. It is not associated with acute event like aortic dissection

Cardiovascular causes of Digital clubbing (Ultra medicine (2005)/285)

- *Subacute Bacterial Endocarditis(SBE)*
- *Cyanotic congenital Heart Disease*
  - *Tetralogy of Fallot (TOF)*
  - *Transposition of Great vessels (TGV)*
  - *Total Anomolous pulmonary venous circulation (TAPVC)*
  - *Ebstein's Anomaly*
  - ***Tricuspid Atresia***
- *Atrial Myxoma*
- *Arterio venous malformations (Brochial arteriovenous fistula)*
- *Axillary artery Aneurysms*

Clubbing is a feature of Subacute Bacterial Endocarditis (SBE) and is not seen in Acute Bacterial Endocarditis Acute endocarditis is a fulminant event while clubbing takes months to develop. Acute bacterial endocarditis is not associated with clubbing.

Electrocardiogram and Arrhythmias

General:

58. Answer is A (-30 to +90): *The EKG Handbook*

The normal axis flows down and towards the left lower aspect of the heart between -30 to +90

The Cardiac Axis

- The cardiac axis refers to the mean direction of the wave of ventricular depolarization in the vertical plane measured from a zero reference point
- The zero refrence point looks at the heart from the same view point as lead I
- An axis lying above this line is given a negative number while an axis lying below this line is given a positive number
- *Theoretically the cardiac axis may lie anywhere between +180 to -180*

Normal AXIS	Left Axis Deviation	Right Axis Deviation
Normal cardiac axis flows down and towards the left lower aspect of the heart between – 30 and +90	Cardiac axis flow is upward and towards the left upper half of the heart between -30 and -90	Cardiac axis flow is downwards and towards the right part of the heart between +90 and +/- 180

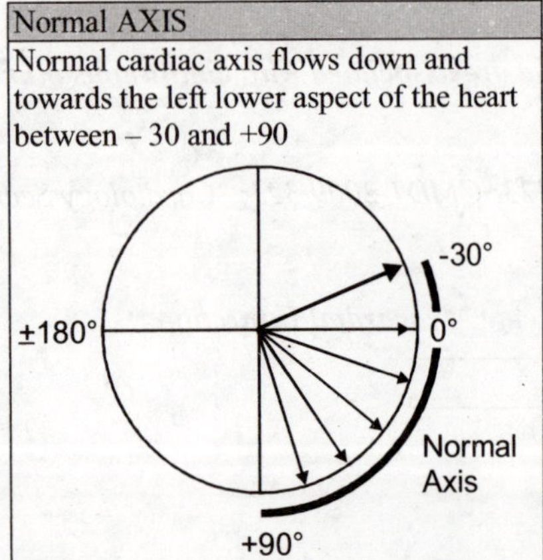

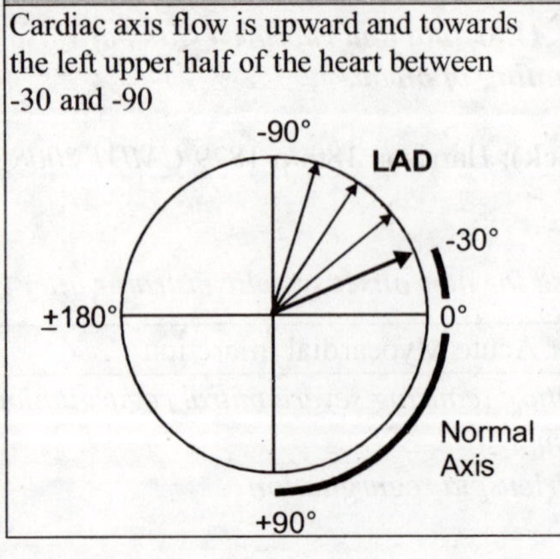

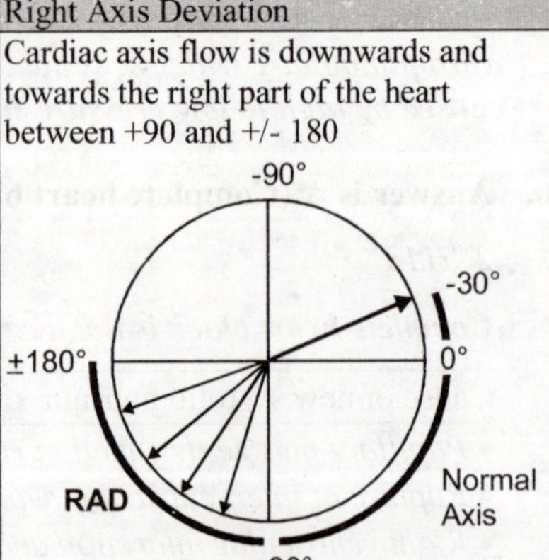

Extreme Right Axis Deviation
When flow of cardiac axis is upward and to the right between +/-180 and -90

- The standard cardiac axis is determined using Lead I and Lead II

Normal Axis	Left Axis Deviation	Right Axis Deviation
-30 to +90 Positive in Lead I Positive in Lead II	-30 to -90 Positive Lead I Negative in Lead II	+90 to ±180 Negative in Lead I Positive or Negative in Lead II

59. Answer is B (Positive in Lead I and Negative in Lead II) : *Harrison 17th /1764; Harrison's 18th/2312*

Left axis deviation is seen as positive deflexion in Lead I and a Negative deflection in Lead II.

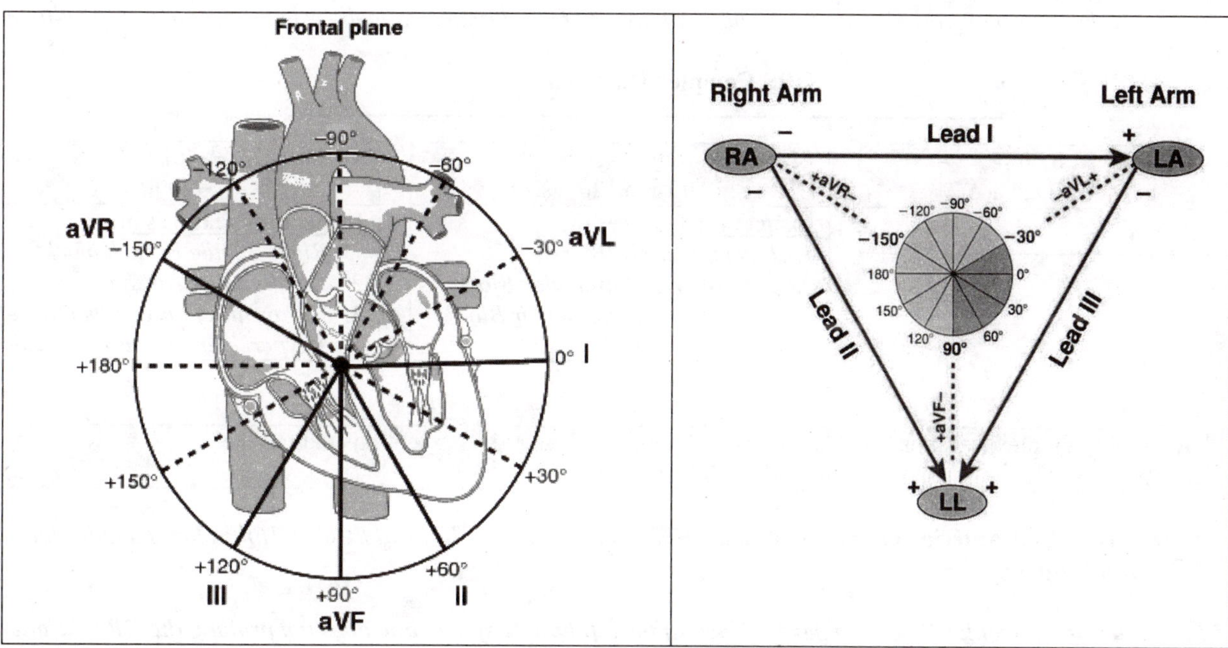

Calculating the cardiac axis:

	Normal Axis	Right axis deviation	Left axis deviation
Lead I	Positive	Negative	*Positive*
Lead II	Positive	Positive or negative	*Negative*
Lead III	Positive or negative	Positive	*Negative*

Note:
Lead I : POSITIVE BETWEEN -90 TO +90 (CLOCKWISE) Lead II : POSITIVE BETWEEN -30 TO +150 (CLOCKWISE) Lead III : POSITIVE BETWEEN +30 TO -150 (CLOCKWISE)

60. Ans. Answer is A (Atrial Depolarization): *Ganong 19th/526; Ganong 20th/532; Ganong 22nd/550, 551*

P wave is produced due to atrial depolarization.

(Table 28-2 Ganong 20th)

Intervals	Normal Duration (s)		Events in the Heart During Interval
	Average	Range	
PR interval	0.182	0.12-0.20	*Atrial depolarization and conduction through AV node*
QRS duration	0.08	to 0.10	*Ventricular depolarization and atrial repolarization*
QT interval	0.40	to 0.43	*Ventricular depolarization plus ventricular repolarization*
ST interval (QT minus QRS)	0.32	....	*Ventricular repolarization*
P wave			*Atrial depolarization*

61. Answer is D (Ventricular depolarisation): *Ganong 19th/526; Ganong 20th/532*

QRS complex is due to ventricular depolarization

62. Answer is D (Left Bundle Branch Block): *Cleveland Clinic Cardiology Board Review (Lippincott Williams) Harrison's 18th/1835*

Left Bundle Branch block is typically associated with a QRS duration greater than 120 milli seconds.

Partial Blocks (Fascicular or hemiblocks) in the left bundle system (left anterior or posterior fascicular blocks) generally do not prolong the QRS duration substantially and QRS duration typically remains less than 120 milliseconds.

QRS Complex Duration

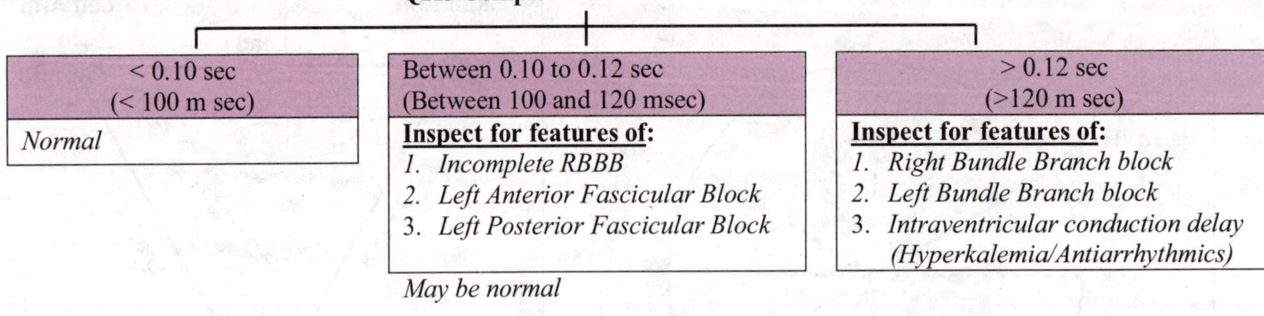

> Any QRS complex Duration > 0.12 seconds is abnormal. There are no exceptions to this rule
> (A QRS complex Duration < 0.12 seconds may be normal)

63. Answer is D (Left Anterior Fascicular Block): *Harrison 18th /1835; '12 Lead ECG by Holtz (Jones and Barlett) 2011/QRS Duration*

Left Anterior Fascicular Block is a partial block in the left bundle system and does not prolong the QRS duration significantly. Typically the QRS duration is slightly prolonged and remains between 0.10 to 0.12 seconds.

Causes of QRS Widening ≥ 0.12 seconds (in decreasing order of mortality)

- ***Hyperkalemia***
- ***Ventricular Tachycardia (Wide complex Tachycardia)***
- *Idioventricular Rhythm including heart blocks*

> *Wide QRS complex may be seen in Mobitz Type II second degree block and incomplete Third Degree Blocks but lacks certainity*

- *Drug effects and overdoses (especially Tricyclics)*
- ***Wolf Parkinson White syndrome***
- *LBBB; RBBB; Intraventricular conduction delay*
- *Ventricular premature contraction*
- *Aberrantly conducted complexes*

64. Ans. Answer is A (Bundle Branch blocks): *Harrison 18th /1835; 'ECG Interpretation: From Pathophysiology to clinical Application' by Kusmoto (Springer) 2009/219*

A wide QRS interval (Wide QRS complex) is most commonly caused due to abnormal conduction over the left or right blundle due to block or delay of ventricular activation (Bundle branch blocks).

> *Wide QRS complex may also be seen in mobitz type II block, but lacks certainity*

QRS complex: Wide or Narrow

- QRS complex represents ventricular depolarization and QRS interval represents the duration of ventricular depolarization.

The normal QRS interval (QRS duration) is less than 0.10 to 0.11 seconds.

- If the QRS complex is less than 0.12 second, ventricular depolarization is more or less occurring normally over the His-Purkinje system.
- There are several causes for a wide QRS complex, which result from abnormal activation of the ventricles.
- ***Most commonly, a wide QRS complex is due to abnormal conduction over the right or left bundle due to block or delay of ventricular activation.***
- Rarely, a wide QRS complex is observed because the ventricles are being activated via both the His-Purkinje system and an accessory pathway.
- With greater use of cardiac devices, a wide QRS complex will be observed in patients with pacemakers where the ventricle is being activated artificially from an electrical impulse delivered via a ventricular pacing lead.

Wide QRS complex with a nomtal rate: abnomtal ventricular activation

Condition	Pathophysiology	ECG findings
Bundle branch block	*Block in the right or left bundle leads to sequential activation of the right and left ventricles*	In right bundle branch block an rSR' will be seen in lead V_1 and in left bundle branch block a wide predominantly negative QRS complex will be seen
Accessory pathway	*The ventricles are activated by both the AV node and an accessory pathway*	The PR interval will be short due to early ventricular activation from the accessory pathway and the QRScomplex will be abnormal because of cell-to-cell activation of ventricular tissue
Hyperkalemia	*High levels of potassium lead to slow ventricular depolarization*	Prominent T waves will often be observed
Ventricular rhythm	*A site within the ventricles drives ventricular depolarization*	P waves will not precede the QRS complexes
Ventricular paced rhythm	*Similar to the ventricular rhythm*	A pacing artifact will be observed

65. Answer is D (Increased cardiac muscle mass)*: Ganong Review of Medical Physiology 22nd/550; Guyton 10th/127*

The normal voltage in the three standard leads as measured from the peak of R wave to the bottom of S wave is 0.5 – 2.0 millivolts. When the sum of *voltages of all the QRS complexes of the three standard leads is greater than 4 millivolts*, the ECG is considered **as *high voltage electrocardiogram.* Most often this is due to *increased cardiac muscle mass*[Q].**

66. Answer is B (Pericardial effusion): *'ECG Interpretation: From Pathophysiology to Clinical Interpretation (Springer) 2009/281; '150 Practice ECGs Interpretation & Review' by Taylor (John Wiley & Sons) 2003/48, 49*

Cardiac conditions associated with low QRS voltage on ECG include dilated cardiomyopathy, infiltrative cardiomyopathy, pericardial effusion and constrictive pericarditis' - 150 Practice ECG's

Low QRS voltage on ECG

- Diagnostic criteria for Low QRS voltage include QRS complex amplitude < 5mm in all limb leads (*when this is the case the amplitude in each of the precordial leads (V) is usually less than 10 mm, but this is not necessary for the diagnosis)*
- Low QRS voltage should be considered a description and not a diagnosis (it may be a normal variant)

Low QRS voltage or ECG
• *QRS amplitude <5 mm on all limb leads*
• *QRS amplitude < 10 mm on all precordial leads*

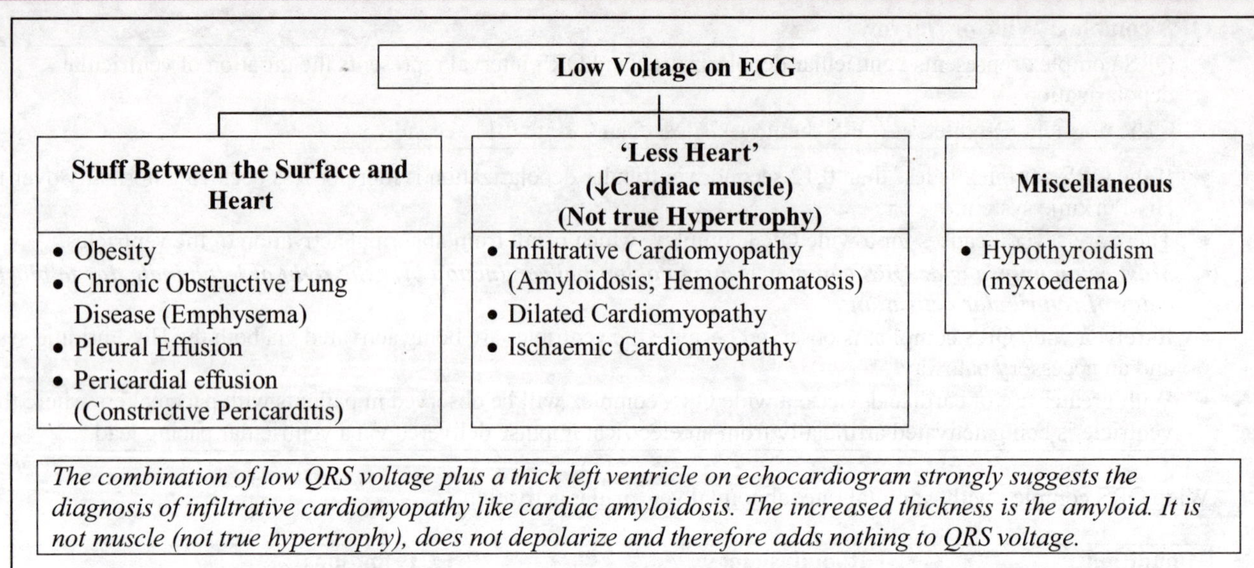

67. Answer is B (Cardiac Amyloidosis): *'150 Practice ECGs Interpretation and Review' by Taylor (John Wiley & Sons 2008/49)*

Low QRS voltage on ECG with left ventricular hypertrophy on Echocardiography suggests a diagnosis of infiltrative cardiomyopathy like amyloidosis.

The combination of low QRS voltage plus a thick left ventricle on echocardiogram strongly suggests the diagnosis of infiltrative cardiomyopathy like cardiac amyloidosis. The increased thickness is the amyloid. It is not muscle (not true hypertrophy), does not depolarize and therefore adds nothing to QRS voltage.

ST Segment

68. Answer is C (Constrictive pericarditis): *Harrison 15th/ 1371; Harrison 16th/1317; 17th/ 1394, 1395; Other texts*

ST segment elevation is seen in Acute pericarditis not constrictive pericarditis. Constrictive pericarditis is associated with flattening or inversion of T waves.

ECG findings of constrictive pericarditis include :

- *Low voltage QRS complexes in all leads*
- *Diffuse flattening or inversion of T waves.*

ST segment is measured from the end of QRS complex to the beginning of the T wave, and represents the time interval between ventricular depolarization and repolarization.

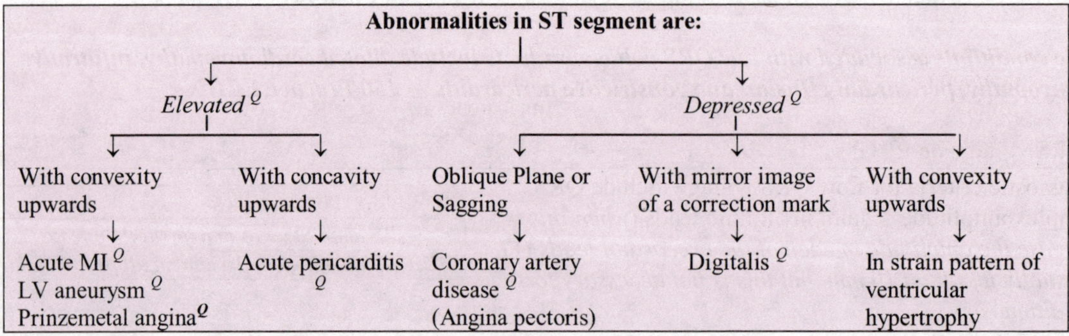

69. Answer is B (Constrictive pericarditis) : Harrison 18th/p 1837, 1838 *Harrison 16th/1318; Harrison 17th/ 1395; Previous question*

ST segment elevation is seen in acute pericarditis and not in constrictive pericarditis

Causes of ST segment elevation

Common causes	Rare causes
• Acute myocardial infarction • Prinzemetal angina (Non infarction transmural ischaemia) • Ventricular aneurysm (Post myocardial infarction) • Acute pericarditis • ***Normal variant ('early repolarization' pattern)*** • L.V. hypertrophy/ left bundle branch block	• Brugada syndrome • Class I C antiarrhythmic drugs • DC cardioversion • Hyperkalemia • Hypothermia (J wave / Osborn wave) • Myocardial injury (Myocarditis Trauma, Tumor invasion)

*Brugada syndrome shows RBBB like pattern with ST elevation) in right precordial leads**

70. Answer is C (ST segment elevation): Harrison 18th/p 1395 *Harrison 16th/ 1317; 17th/ 1393; Oxford handbook of clinical medicine 5th/88.*

E.C.G. changes in acute infarction

Early acute phase *(within hours)*	**Fully evolved phase**	**Old infarction** *(resolution phase)*
• *Elevation of ST segment* • *Tall wide (peaked) T wave*	• *Pathological Q wave* • *Elevated ST segment beings to resolve* • *T wave inverts*	• *Pathological Q wave* • *ST segment and T wave may be normal*

QT Interval

71. Answer is B (Digitalis toxity): Harrison 18th/p 1836 *Harrison 16th/ 1319; Harrison 17th/ 1395; Kundu II/ 89; Braunwald 8th/906*

QT interval is shortened in digitalis toxity and not prolonged

QT interval

- Is measured from the beginning of Q wave to the end of T wave Q
- It is the time taken for total ventricular events i.e. depolarization as well as repolarization Q
- Normal QT interval should not exceed 42 seconds

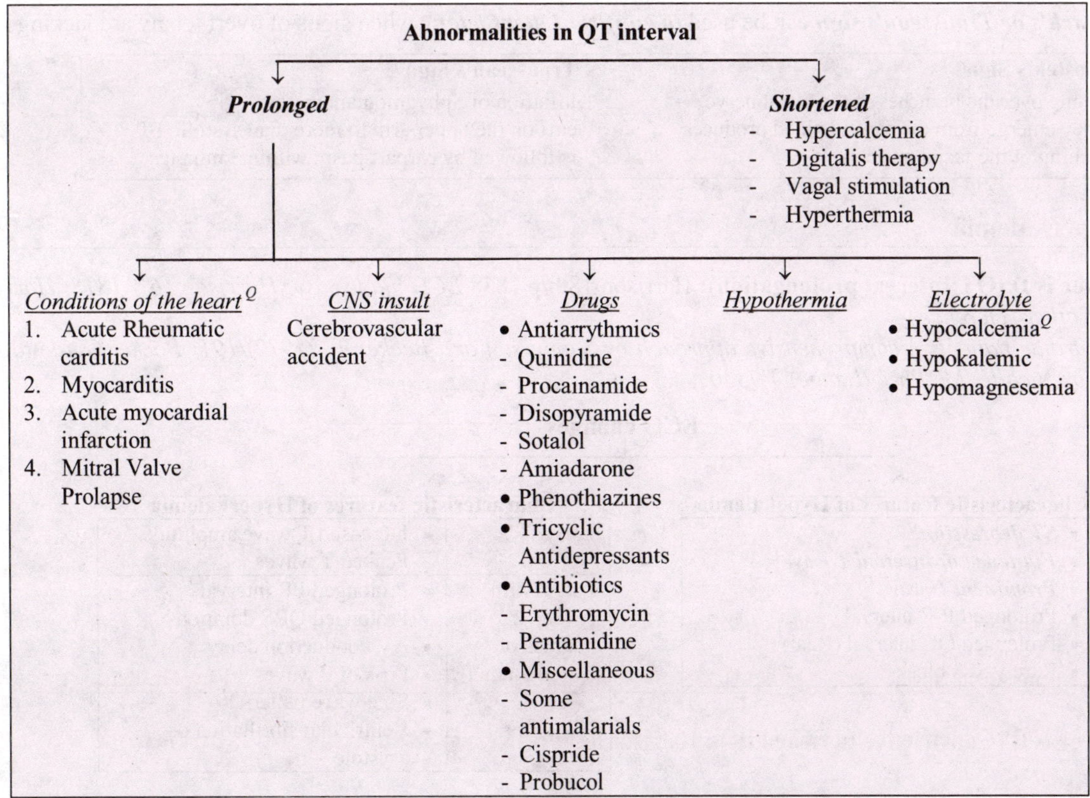

72. Answer is C (Hypercalcemia): Harrison 18th/p 1836 *Harrisons 17th/1395; Hurst 12th/312*

Hypercalcemia Shortens the QT interval

Causes of Short QT interval

Hypercalcemia
Digitalis glycosides
Hyperthermia (Hurst)
Some causes of hyperkalemia (Hurst)
Altered Autonomic tone (vagal stimulation)
Congenital short QT Syndrome

73. Answer is B (Decreased QT interval): Harrison 18th/p 1838 *Harrisons 17th/1395; Harrisons 16th/1318, 1319*

Hypercalcemia is characterized by a decreased QT interval.

74. Answer is C (Shortening of QT interval on ECG): Harrison 18th/p 1838 *Harrisons 17th/1395*

The QT interval on ECG is prolonged in hypocalcemia and shortened in hypercalcemia.

Manifestations of chronic hypocalcemia

Neuromuscular and Neurological	Mental changes	Miscellaneous	Cardiovascular
*Muscle spasms*Q *Carpopedal spasms*Q *Facial grimacing*Q *Laryngeal spasms*Q *Convulsions* Q *Circumoral tingling*Q	Irritability Depression Psychosis	Respiratory arrest *Increased ICT with papilloedema*Q Intestinal cramps Chronic malabsorption	Arrythmias *Prolonged QT interval*Q *Reduced effectiveness of digitalis*Q

Low serum calcium leads to increased excitability of peripheral nerves and hence ***hyperactive tendon reflexes*** is a distinctive finding.

Chrostek's or Trausseau's sign can be used ***to confirm Latent tetany*** when signs of overt tetany are lacking

Chvostek's SignQ	Trousseau's SignQ
Tapping over the branches of the facial nerve as they emerge from the parotid gland produces twitching of the facial muscles	Inflation of Sphygmomanometer cuff on the upper arm to more than systolic BP is followed by carpal spasm within 3 minutes

Hypo/Hyperkalemia

75. Answer is D (QT Interval prolongation): Harrison 18th/p 1838 *ECG made easy; Harrison 16th/ 1318; Harrison 17th/ 1395; other references*
The cardiac patient: A comprehensive approach by Sanderson and Becker 1st (1972)/191; Pocket Guide to Diagnostic Tests by Nicolle, Mc Phee (Lange) 4th/330

ECG changes

Characteristic features of Hypokalemia

- ***ST depression*** Q
- ***Flattened or inverted T wave*** Q
- ***Prominent U wave*** Q
- Prolonged P-R interval Q
- Prolonged QU interval (Real)
- Rarely S-A block

Characteristic features of Hyperkalemia

Early	• Increased T wave amplitude Q Peaked T waves
Later (with severe degrees of hyperkalemia)	• Prolonged PR interval Q • Prolonged QRS duration Q • AV conduction delay • Loss of P waves Q • Sine wave pattern Q • Ventricular fibrillation or asystole

Prominent U wave, ST segment sagging and T-wave flattening or inversion are characteristic features of Hypokalemia.

Hypokalemia may also present with a apparently prolonged QT interval on ECG. However this apparently prolonged QT interval is in reality the QU interval that mimics a prolonged QT interval due to fusion of T-U waves.
Prolonged QT interval is the single best answer of exclusion.

QT interval and Hypokalemia

- Hypokalemia causes an 'apparent' prolongation of the QT interval but the real QT interval remains 'normal'
- The apparent prolongation of QT interval is due to fusion of the T and U waves (T-U fusion)

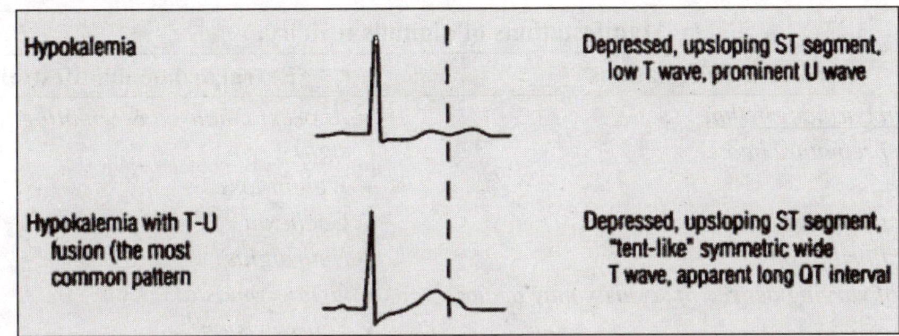

- The prolonged QT interval that is 'apparent' in hypokalemia is actually (in reality) a QU interval.
- Wgere T and U waves are separate and distinct, the QT interval is normal but the QU interval is prolonged.

76. Answer is A (Increased PR interval with ST depression): *Repeat*

Hypokalemia is associated with ST depression, prolonged PR interval, Flattened or Inverted T waves, Prominent U waves and rarely S - A block

Hypokalemia is associated with a prolonged QU interval and not a prolonged QT interval (Refer previous question)

Increased PR interval with ST depression therefore remains the single best answer of choice.

Note:

- *QT interval is prolonged in Hypocalcemia* [Q]
- *QT interval is decreased in Hypercalcemia* [Q]

77. Answer is B (Prolonged QT interval): *Refer text below*

Prolonged QT interval is a manifestation of hypocalcemia

An apparently prolonged QT interval may be associated with hypokalemia but is not a feature of hyperkalemia Prolonged PR interval, Sine wave pattern and loss of P waves may all be seen with hyperkalemia

ECG changes in hyperkalemia

Early	• *Increased T wave amplitude* [Q] *Peaked T waves*
Later (with severe degrees of hyperkalemia)	• *Prolonged PR interval* [Q] • *Prolonged QRS duration* [Q] • *AV conduction delay* • *Loss of P waves* [Q] • *Sine wave pattern* [Q] • *Ventricular fibrillation or asystole*

78. Answer is C (Prolonged QT interval): Harrison 18th/p 1838 *Harrison 16th /1318; Harrison 17th/ 1395;Refer previous question*

Prolonged QT interval is not a manifestation of hyperkalemia. Prolonged PR interval, prolonged QRS duration and ventricular asystole are all known manifestations of hyperkalemia. Prolonged QT interval is a manifestation of Hypocalcemia.

Digitalis Toxicity

79. Answer is C (Atrial flutter): Harrison 18th/p 1897 *Harrison 16th/ 1375; Harrison 15th/1327; Harrison 17th/ 1441*

"Digitalis is Profibrillatory but its administration does not cause Atrial Flutter"

Digitalis causes several disturbances in cardiac rhythm. Various manifestations seen are elaborated in the table below. Atrial Flutter has notably not been mentioned.

Manifestations of digitalis toxicity	
Cardiac manifestations	**Extracardiac manifestations**
Disturbance in cardiac rhythm • *Ventricular premature beats* • *Bigeminy* • *Ventricular tachycardia* • *Ventricular fibrillation* • *A.V. Block of varying degree of severity may occur.*	• *Anorexia, nausea & vomiting (earliest sign)* • *Weight loss* • *Cachexia* • *Neuralgias*[Q] • *Gynaecomastia*[Q] • *Yellow vision*[Q] • *Delirium*[Q]
Non paroxysmal atrial tachycardia with variable A.V. Block is characteristic of Digitalis intoxication	

Also remember : *Mobile type II block is not seen in digitalis intoxication* [Q]

Miscellaneous

80. Answer is A (Left axis deviation): *Diagnosis and treatment of diseases of the Respiratory tract by Iruvin Curley, Grossman (1997) / 236; Textbook of Cardiovascular medicine by Topol 3rd/988*

Left sided penumotharax is associated with right axis deviation and not left axis deviation

ECG Changes in left sided Pneumothorax

ECG changed in pneumothorax, specially on the left, are important as there may mimic ECG, changes of acute MI

These include

Right ward deviation of QRS axis (Right axis deviation)

Decreased/absent R waves in the precordial leads

T wave inversion in precordial leads

Pathological Q waves

Decreased QRS voltage

Electrical alternans (alternating QRS amplitude with each heart beat)

81. Answer is B (Left axis deviation): *See below*

A left sided pneumothorax will shift the axis of the heart towards the right leading to a right axis deviation rather than a left axis deviation.

Arrhythmias

AF and PSVT

82. Answer is B (Hypothroidism): Harrison 18th/p 1881 *Harrison 16th/1345; Harrisons 17th/1428; CMDT 2008/330; ; CMDT 2009/336; CEMDT (Emergency Medicine) 6th/582*

Atrial Fibrillation is associated with hyperthyroidism and not hypothyroidism

Important causes of Atrial Fibrillation

Cardiovascular causes of Atrial Fibrillation	Other Systemic Causes of AF
• ***Rheumatic Heart disease (Includes mitral stenosis and mitral regurgitation)*** • *Non Rheumatic Mitral valve disease* • *Chronic Hypertension* • ***Cardiomyopathy*** • *Myocarditis* • *Pericarditis* • *Congenital Heart Disease (eg ASD)* • *Coronary Heart Disease*	• ***Hyperthroidism*** • *Pulmonary embolism* • *Hypoxia* • *Excess consumption of alcohol (Also alcohol withdraw)* • *Excess consumption of Caffeine* • *May be seen in normal individuals* • *Particularly during emotional stress or following surgery, exercise or prominent surge of vagal tone (vasovagal response)*

AF often develops in patients with heart or lung disease who develop hypoxia, hypercapria or metabolic or hemodynamic derangements

Holiday Heart Syndrome: In predisposed individuals, AF may be precipitated by consumption of even small amounts of alcohol. This is called Holiday Syndrome and is usually transient and self limited

83. Answer is D (Atrial fibrillation): Harrison 18th/p 1881 *Harrison 15th/1360; Harrison 16th/1409, 1410; Harrison 17th/1428*

Atrial fibrillation is the most common arrhythmia appearing after a drinking binge. *Fibrillation is followed by atrial flutter and ventricular premature depolarization in frequency.*

Alcoholic Cardiotoxity may present as

Holiday heart syndrome	Dilated cardiomyopathy
• Typically appears after a drinking binge • Presents with arrhythmias without overt heart failure - Atrial fibrillation is seen most frequently - *Harrison* - Atrial flutter - Ventricular premature depolarization	• Seen with chronic consumption of large quantities of alcohol • Presents with heart failure.

84. Answer is C (Anticoagulation not required): Harrison 18th/p 1882, 1883 *CMDT 2008/331; CMDT 2009/338; Harrisons 17th/1428, 1429*

Anticoagulation is required in patients with Atrial fibrillation.

AF is associated with increased risk of Thromboembolism

Atrial fibrillation is associated risk with increased risk of thromboembolism as a result of stasis of blood and thrombus formation in left atrium

AF is thus an important risk factor for stroke and systemic embolism

Anticoagulation is required in patients with AF

Because of increased risk of stroke in association with AF, anticoagulation is of particular importance in patients who have known risk factors for AF.

Urgent Anticoagulation is achieved with Heparin.

Chronic anticoagulation is achieved with Warfarin.

Aspirin may be used as an alternative to Warfarin for some patients to achieve anticoagulation (Low risk patients)

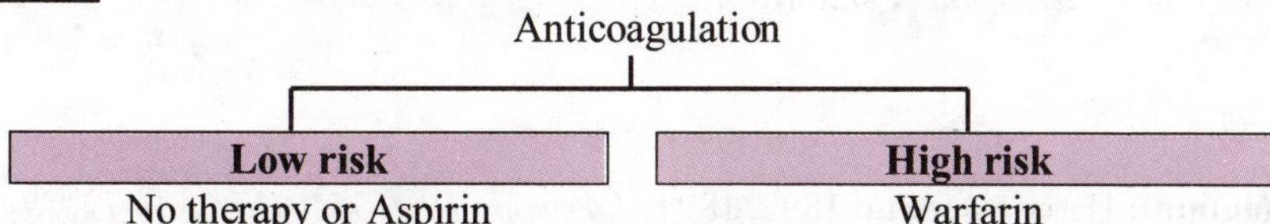

Evidence for Aspirin prophylaxis is weaker than that for warfarin

Digoxin is required for treatment of AF

Digoxin is indicated for control of ventricular rate in patient with AF.

85. Answer is A (Digitalis toxicity) : *Harrison 16th / 1345, 1375, 1394; CMDT 2008/347*

The patient in question has a complete heart block most likely from digitalis intoxication.
'If in the presence of atrial fibrillation the ventricular rhythm becomes slow and regular (30 - 60 / m) complete heart block is suggested. Digitalis intoxication is a common cause.' - Harrison

Approach to Patient in question :

- The patient in question is likely to be on digitalis for heart failure (due to MR) and to control ventricular rate from AF.
  'Digitalis is effective in patients with heart failure complicated by atrial flutter and fibrillation and a rapid ventricular rate, who benefit both from slowing of the ventricular rate and from positive inotropic effect'. -Harrison
- *The presence of a slow ventricular rate (30 - 60 / min) in presence of AF suggests complete AV block* and subsidiary ectopic pacemaker activity. *Syncope is likely to be a manifestation of complete heart block which in turn is a common complication of digitalis intoxication.*

86. Answer is B (Digitalis toxicity): *Harrison 15th/ 1295, Harrison 16th/ 1375*

"If in the presence of atrial fibrillation, the ventricular rhythm becomes regular and slow (30 to 60/m) complete heart block is suggested and if ventricular rhythm is regular and rapid > = 100/ min, a tachycardia arising in AV junction or ventricle should be suspected. Digitalis intoxication is a common cause of both phenomenon" – Harrison

The patient in question has a regular ventricular rate despite fibrillating atria (irregularly beating atria)

This indicates that

↓	↓
All supraventricular impulses are blocked from reaching the ventricle somewhere within the conducting system. - Complete A.V block	Ventricles are activated by a subsidery ectopic pacemaker situated either - In the A.V node below the level of block - Within the ventricles (Such a subsidery pacemaker is usually slow and fires at the rate of 30-60/sec.)

Digitalis toxicity is a common cause of such a presentation and hence has been picked up as the answer of choice. Infact "Non paroxysmal atrial tachycardia with AV block is characteristic of digitalis intoxication."

87. Answer is D (Adenosine): *Harrison 14th/ 1268; KDT 4th/ 516; Harrison 15th/ 1299; Harrison 16th/ 1347; 17th/ 1433*

Drug of choice for PSVT is Adenosine

Agents of First choice include	Agent of second choice are
Adenosine (Drug of choice) Verapamil	β *blockers* Q

Adenosine is preferred over Verapamil because of its extremely short half life, and lesser incidence of side effects Q
Thus DOC for PSVT is Adenosine. Q

88. Answer is C (Adenosine): *Harrison 14th/ 1268; KDT 4th/ 516; Harrison 15th/ 1299; Harrison 16th/ 1347; 17th/ 1433*

Drug of choice for PSVT is Adenosine.

89. Answer is A (Adenosine): *Repeat; Harrison 17th/ 1433*

Drug of choice to control supraventricular tachycardia is adenosine.

VT, VF and PVCs

90. Answer is B (Ventricular rate > 160/min): Harrison 18th/p 1892, 1893 *Harrisons 16th/1351; Harrison 17th/ 1437; CMDT 2002/ 416; CMDT 2009/342; Oxford handbook of medicine 5th/110*

In both ventricular and supraventricular tachycardia the ventricular rate is greater than 100/min, therefore ventricular rate > 160/min cannot be used to differentiate between ventricular & supraventricular tachycardia.

Ventricular tachycardia (Broad complex tachycardia)	**Supraventricular tachycardia** *(Narrow complex tachycardia)*
• Ventricular rate > 100 bpm • QRS duration > 0.12 sec. (>.14 sec.- Harrison)^{Q} • Cannot be relieved by carotid sinus massage. ^{Q}	• Ventricular rates > 100 bpm ^{Q} • QRS duration < 0.12 sec. • Can be relieved by carotid sinus message ^{Q}

Other features can be used to distinguish ventricular and supraventricular tachycardia.

- ***Variable First heart sound*** *is a features of ventricular tachycardia only.*
- *In ventricular tachycardia* ***QRS duration*** *is greater then 0.14 Sec, while in supra ventricular tachycardia it is less than 0.14 Sec.*
- *Supraventricular tachycardia can be relieved by* ***carotid sinus massage while ventricular tachycardia cannot.***

91. Answer is C (Typical right bundle branch block): *Harrisons 17th/ Braunwald 8th/898, Cardiology by 'Heger' 5th/52 Clevelend clinic cardiology board review (2006)/659 by Eric Topal ; Evidence based Medicine Guidelines (2005) / 112*

Wide complex tachycardia due to ventricular tachycardia (VT) is characterized by bizzare QRS pattern that does not mimic typical RBBB or LBBB QRS complexes

The presence of wide QRS complex tachycardia with typical RBBB or LBBB suggests supraventricular tachycardia with aberrant conduction.

Wide complex tachycardia (QRS duration >°12 seconds)

- Wide complex tachycardia is defined as tachyarrhythmia with a QRS duration greater than 0.12 seconds with a heart rate > 100/min
- Wide complex tachycardia may occurs as a result either from a ventricular (VT) or supraventricular mechanism (SVT with aberrancy)

Broad Complex Tachycardia

Ventricular Tachycardia	Supraventricular Tachycardia with abberancy
VT is the most common cause of Broad complex tachycardia accounting for >80% of cases	SVT with abberancy accounts for 15-20% cases of broad complex tachycardia Cause include • SVT with a bundle branch block either LBBB or RBBB • Atral flutter, Atrial fibrillation, AV reentrant tachycardia (AVRT) may also produce SVT with aberancy and result in wide complex tacycardia.

Distinguishing Features between Broad complex tachycardia due to VT and SVT with aberrancy

Differentiating features	Ventricular Tachycardia	Supraventricular Tachycardia with Abaerrancy
• *QRS duration*	*Broad complex Tachycardia with QRS duration usually greater that 0.14 seconds* *QRS ≥ 0.14 sec*	*Broad complex tachycardia with QRS duration usually between 0.12 sec to 0.14 seconds* *QRS ≤ 0.14 sec.*
• *Fusion Beats*	*Characteristic of VT*	*Absent*
• *Capture Beats*	*Characteristic of VT*	*Unusual*
• *AV dissociation*	*Characteristic of VT*	*Absent*
• *Independent P waves*	*May be seen* *Independent P waves when present are characteristic of VT. and indicate AV dissociation*	*Independent P work's are not seen* *P wave and QRS complex are linked to suggest that ventricular activation depends on atrial discharge*
• *QRS pattern*	*QRS pattern does not resemble /mimic typical LBBB or RBBB*	*QRS pattern often resembles /mimics typical LBBB or RBBB*
• *Axis (Frontal plane QRS)*	*Left axis deviation (< - 30°)*	*Normal or Right ward*
• *QRS morphology in V1*	*Monophasic or Biphasic*	*Triphasic*
• *R/S Ratio in V6*	*<1*	*>1*
• *Vagal manuvres*	*No effect*	*Slowing or termination of tachycardia by vagal manuvres*

92. Answer is A, B, C (Fusion beats; Capture beats and AV dissociation): *Refer previous question, Braunwald 8th/896, 897*

Presence of Fusion beats, capture beats and AV dissociation is charachteristic of ventricular tachycardia.

ECG feature that support a diagnosis of ventricular tachycardia (Vt) in patients with Wide Complex Tachycardia (Incomplete List)

- ***Presence of Fusion beats***
- ***Presence of capture beats***
- ***Presence of AV dissociation***

The presence of fusion beats and capture beats provides maximum support for the diagnosis of VT. AV dissociation also provides a strong support in favour of VT, but is less specific than fusion beats and capture. AV dissociation may uncommonly occur during supraventricular tachycardias and all cases of VT may not exhibit AV dissociation. Never the less presence of AV dissociation in cases of wide complex tachycardia is a strong presumptive evidence that tachycardia is of ventricular origin (VT).

Differentiating features	VT (Broad complex)	SVT with Aberrancy (Broad Complex)
Fusion beats	Characteristic	Absent
Capture beats	Characteristic	Unusual
AV dissociation	Characteristic	Absent
Effect of vagal manuvres	No effect	Slowing or termination of tachycardia
QRS morphology in V1	Monophasic or Biphasic	Triphasic

93. Answer is E (Typical RBBB QRS complex): Harrison 18th/p 1892 *Harrisons 17th/1437 Kelly's Essentials of Medicine 2nd/133*

Wide QRS complex, AV dissociation, capture beats, and fusion beats are characteristic features of ventricular tachycardia.

VT is characterized by bizarre QRS complexes that do not confirm to typical RBBB or LBBB QRS complexes

Ventricular Tachycardia (VT)

VT is defined as ≥ three consequtive premature ventricular complexes with a wide QRS complex of duration ≥0.12 sec (often ≥0.14 sec) and a heart rate between 100 to 240/minute. The QRS complexes are not preceded by atrial deflections.

Characteristic Features of Ventricular Tachycardia (VT)

- *AV dissociation* [Q]
- *Capture Beats* [Q]
- *Fusion Beats* [Q]
- *Compensatory Pause* [Q]
- *Wide QRS complex (>0.14 seconds)* [Q]
- *Bizarre QRS pattern that does not mimic typical RBBB or LBBB QRS complex* [Q]
- *Left axis deviation* [Q]

Additional features

- Heart Rate : The heart rate is >100/minute (usually >120/min
- Rhythm : Usually Regular
  May be irregular if there are sinus capture beats
- P:QRS : No fixed relation exists between the P wave & QRS complex
  - *P wave may not be visible at all*
  - *P wave may be dissociated from the QRS complex*

94. Answer is C (Prevalence decreases with age): *Braunwald 8th/895*

The presence of premature complexes increases with age *– Braunwald 8th/895*

Premature Ventricular Contractions or Premature Ventricular Complexes (VPC's)
(Ventricular Premature Beats, Ventricular Ectopic beats)

- Premature ventricular contractions / complexes are caused by an ectopic impulse that originates in the purkinje fibres distal to the bifurcation of the bundle of His, or in the working ventricular myocardium

- Such ectopic impulses arising from the ventricles do not enter the conducting pathway and hence do not depolarize both ventricles simultaneously but cause sequential depolarization of ventricles, one ventricle at a time
- Such sequential depolarization results in abnormal conduction of impulse and causes a wide bizarre QRS complex (> 0.12 sec)

Characteristics of PVC's (ECG)

- *The QRS complex is premature^Q^*
- ***The QRS complex is wide (>0.12 sec)^Q^ and BIZZARE^Q^ or distorted (notched)***
- *The QRS complex is not preceded by a P wave^Q^*
- *A' P' wave is not associated with the PVC^Q^*
- *The QRS complex is usually followed by a complete compensatory pause^Q^*
  *(The compensatory pause following PVC is frequently complete)^Q^*
- *The QRS complex may be monophasic or biphasic (Not Triphasic)^Q^*
- *The ST segment and T wave slope in the opposite direction from the main deflection of the QRS complex.^Q^*

Clinical features

- ***The prevalence of PVC increases with Age***
- They are associated with male gender (Male > Females)
- May occurs in patients with no cardiovascular abnormalities and in patients with underlying cardiovascular disease
- Majority of patients are asymptomatic
- *Presenting symptoms include* ***palpitations****, lightheadedness, fatigue, near syncope, syncope*

Prognosis

In presence of coronary artery disease (CAD) or history of MI, complex or frequent VPC's are associated with increased risk of sudden cardiac death.

95. Answer is D (Prolonged PR interval): Harrison 18th/p 1892 *Braunwald 8th/893-898, Harrisons 17th/1437, CMDT 2008/334, Cardiology' 5th/51,52*

PR interval does not characterize Ventricular Premature complexes because AV conduction is not involved.

Wide QRS complex, Absent P wave and a frequently Complete Compensatory Pause are all characteristic features of Premature ventricular complexes.

The basic ECG characteristics of PVCs include the following:

Rate	The underlying sinus rate is usually regular but is intermittently interrupted by the PVC. This results in an irregular and fluctuating heart rate.
Rhythm	The basic R-R interval is regular but is intemittently interrupted by the PVC. The R-R interval preceding the PVC is short due to the "prematurity" of the QRS complex and often the R-R interval after the PVC is longer due to a compenstory pause (Fig.2)
P wave	The premature QRS complex is not preceded by a conducted P wave (although in certain instances the PVC may coincidentally be preceded by a nonconducted sinus P wave)
PR interval	Not applicable because atrioventricular (AV) conduction is not involved.
QRS complex	*QRS complex is premature^Q^* *QRS complex is prolonged (>0.12 seconds)^Q^* *QRS complex is bizzare or distorted (notched)^Q^* *QRS complex is not proceeded by a P wave^Q^* *QRS complex is frequently followed by a complete compensatory pause^Q^*
ST segment and T wave	*The ST segment and T wave slope in the opposite direction from the main deflection of QRS complex^Q^*

Note

'AV dissociation' with 'capture beats' and 'fusion beats' are diagnostic criteria for ventricular tachycardia (VT) and not for PVC's.
However, VT is defined by the presence of three or more consecutive PVC and hence AV dissociation, capture beats and fusion beats may be said to be occasionally present in PVC's when they occur in consecutive bests.

96. Answer is D (Wide QRS complex): *Harrison 18th/p 1890Kelly's Essentials of Internal Medicine 2nd/133; Harrison 18th/p 1890 Harrison's 17th/1435, Braunward 8th/896, 897; CMDT 2009/341*

Wide QRS complex (>12sec) is characteristic of Premature ventricular beats

Presence of AV dissociation with fusion beats and capture beats is considered diagnostic for Ventricular Tachycardia and not PVC.

However, VT is defined by the presence of three or more than three ventricular premature beats (PVC) in succession and hence AV dissociation, Fusion beats and capture beats may be said to be present in PVC's also (provided PVCs occur in quick succession).

AV dissociation	Fusion Beats	Capture beats
The prevence of AV dissociation implies that atrial and ventricular activity are occurring in dependent of each other AV dissociation can occur in patients with ventricular tachycardia and retrograde conduction block The presence of AV dissociation favours a diagnosis of VT	• Fusion beats result from activation of ventricle by two foci, one supraventricular and the other ventricular • The presence of fusion beats supports a diagnosis of VT	• Capture beats indicate activation of the ventricle by a conducted supraventricular rhythm resulting in a shorter coupling interval and a QRS of normal morphology • The presence of capture beats favours a diagnosis of VT.

97. Answer is B (Narrow QRS complex): *Kelly's Essentials of Internal Medicine 2nd/133;* Harrison 18th/p 1890 *Harrison's 17th/1435, Braunward 8th/896, 897; CMDT 2009/341*

Premature Ventricular beats are characterized by a wide QRS Complex and not a narrow QRS complex.
AV dissociation, Fusion beats and capture beats may be observed when three or more than three PVC's occur in succession.

98. Answer is B (Myocardial Reperfusion): *ACS Essentials '2010' 3rd (2009) /132,* Harrison 18th/p 1890 *Harrisons 17th/1435, 1436; Hurst12th/ 1014; Braunwald 8th/-864-865-895-896-1278; 'Problem Oriented Approach in Interventional Cardiology' by Colombo (2007)/109*

Accelerated Idioventricular Rhythm is the most common arrhythmia seen after successful reperfusion of a blocked coronary vessel and hence is often also termed as a 'reperfusion rhythm or reperfusion arrhythmia'.

'Arrhythmias are common after reperfusion. The most common post reperfusion arrhythmia is Accelerated Idioventricular Rhythm (AIVR)' - Problem Oriented Approach in Interventional Cardiology

'Accelerated Idioventricular Rhythm is considered a reperfusion rhythm as it is often seen immediately after a successful reperfusion' - Washington manual of critical care /116

Myocardial Reperfusion, Dilated cardiomyopathy, Digitalis matoxication and Myocarditis *may all produce Accelerated Idioventricular Rhythms (AIVR), however AIVR is the most common arrhythmia seen after myocardial Reperfusion. AIVR is also the most charachteristic aryhythmia seen after reperfusion has begun and* ***hence Myocardial Reperfusion is the single best answer of choice.***

Accelerated Idioventricular Rhythm (AIVR)

- AIVR is an automatic rhythm originating within the ventricle with rates between 40 to 120 beats / min
- AIVR is believed to be caused by abnormal automaticity and is considered to be a brief self limiting arrhythmia , that does not usually require any specific treatment unless the patient is symptomatic
- The onset of this arrhythmia is gradual (non paroxysmal) and occurs when the rate of ventricular tachycardia exceeds the sinus rate because of sinus slowing or SA / AV block
- ***AIVR is a characteristic feature of myocardial reperfusion, and when it occurs in the setting of myocardial infarction and coronary reperfusion it is also called 'Reperfusion Arrhythmia' or 'Reperfusion Rhythm'.***

'It commonly occurs at the moment of reperfusion of an occluded coronaryartery' – Braunwald

- AIVR can be seen in the absence of any structural heart disease but is usually seen in patients who have an underlying structure heart disease.

Causes of Accelerated Idioventricular Rhythm (AIVR)

- Acute coronary syndromes
  -Acute Myocardial Infarction
  -***Myocardial Reperfusion***
- Cardiomyopathy
  -*Dilated cardiomyopathy*
  -Ischemic cardiomyopathy
- *Myocarditis* (Acute myocarditis)
- Rheumatic / Congenital Heart Disease
- **Digitalis Intoxication** (*AIVR is* **not** *the most common arrhythmia seen after Digitalis toxicity*)
- Cocaine Intoxication

'Arrhythmias are common after Reperfusion. The most common post reperfusion arrhythmia is Accelerated Idioventricular Rhythm'
- Interventional cardiology

Electocardiographic features of Accelerated Idioventricular Rhythm (similar to VT except ventricular rate)

• *Rate , 40 to 120 beats / min* • *Wide QRS complex (> 0.12 sec) (Bizzare)* • *Fusion beats* • *Capture beats* • *AV dissociation* • *Rhythm: Regular*	*Although the ventricular rate in AIVR by definition can be upto 120 beats / min, this is usually less than 100/min. A rate between 100 to 120 may represent VT and hence should be treated as VT.*

Treatment of Accelerated Idioventricular Rhythm

No specific treatment is usually required (No treatment in Asymptomatic patients)
Since the ventricular rate usually ranges the same as sinus rhythm, hemodynamic compromise does not occur Also the condition is self limiting and transient and does not appear to affect the patients clinical course or prognosis. Hence no specific treatment is required although these patients should be observed

Symptomatic patients with Hemodynamic compromise may require treatment
- Atropine or Atrial pacing may suppress the AIVR by simply increasing the sinus rate
- Lidocaine may be used for suppressive therapy

Torsades De Pointes

99. Answer is C (Prolonged QTc interval): Harrison 18th/p 1890 *Harrison 15th/1304, 16th/1353; 17th/1436; CMDT 2008/334; CMDT 2009/341*

'The ECG hallmark of torsades depoint's is marked QT prolongation'.

'Torsades de pointes' or 'twisting of the points' is a specific type of ventricular tachycardia

Characteristics of *Torsades de pointes*
- Polymorphic QRS complexes that change in amplitude
- Cycle length giving the appearance of oscillations around the baseline.
- Marked QT prolongation [Q]

100. Answer is B (polymorphic Ventricular Tachycardia): Harrison 18th/p 1891 *Hurst 12th/1082,1083*

Torsades de pointes is the hallmark arrythymia in the long QT syndrome *– Hurst 12th/1016*
Pylomorphic ventricular tachycardia is synonymous with Torsades de Pointes and the single best answer of choice.

Congenital long QT Syndrome is associated with reduced repolarization reserve. Reduced repolorization reserve. Reduced repolorization reserve predisposes patients with marked QT prolongation to develop Torsades de pointes.
- Hurst 12th/1082,1083

What is congenital long QT Syndrome
Congenital long QT Syndrome is a familial disorder characterized by a prolonged QT interval on Electrocardiogram Most forms of congenital long QT Syndromes are caused by Channelopathies created by mutations in one or more genes

Congenital long QT Syndrome	
Congenital long QT Syndrome with Associated Sensorineural Deafness	**Congenital long QT Syndrome with Normal Hearing**
Jervell and large Nielson Syndrome (Autosomal Recessive)	Romano- Ward Syndrome (Autosomal Dominant)

How do Patients with congenital long QT Syndrome present

- *May present with syncope due to* ***torsades de pointes***[Q]
- *May present with sudden death due to* ***ventricular fibrillation***[Q]

Note

Ventricular Tachyarrythmias commonly develop during periods of adrenergic stimulation such as fright or exertion but may also develop during sleep.

Most competitive sports are contraindicated for patients with congenital long QT syndrome

Clinical conditions that are associated with reduced repolarization reserve (Patient predisposed for marked QT prolongation and resultant Torsades-de pointes)

- *Congenital long QT Syndrome*
- *Acquired long QT Syndrome caused by a variety of drugs/ medications*
- *Bradycardia*
- *Female gender*
- *Ventricular Hypertrophy*
- *Electrolyte disturbances such as hypokalemia and hypomognesemia*

101. Answer is C (Hypomagnesemia): Harrison 18th/p 1891 *Hurst 12th/1082, 1083, 1016 Refer previous question*

Electrolyte disturbances including hypomagnesemia predispose patients for marked QT prolongation and Torsades – des – pointes as a result of reduced repolarization reserve.

Clinical conditions associated with reduced repolarization reserve
(Patients predisposed for marked QT prolongation and Torsades –de pointes)

- *Congenital long QT syndrome*
- *Acquired long QT syndrome (caused by variety of drugs /medications)*
- ***Electrolyte disturbances such as hypokalemia and hypomagnesemia***
- *Ventricular Hypertrophy*
- *Female gender*

WPW Syndrome

102. Answer is B (Right sided accessory pathway): *Refer text below*

Wolf Parkinson White syndrome is caused by the presence of on additional / accessory pathway (connection) between the atria and ventricle. The acessary pathway (called bundle of Kent) may be present as a connection between the left atrium and left ventricle (Left sided) or as a connection between the right atrium and right ventricle (Right sided).

Pre excitation resulting from left sided accessory pathways is called Type A Pre-excitation
Pre excitation resulting from right sided accessory pathway is called Type B Pre-excitation

The most common accessary pathways leading to pre-excitation syndromes (WPW) are left sided (connecting left atrium to left ventricle)[Q]

103. Answer is A (Left free wall): *Harrison 18th /1889; Braunwald Heart Diseases Review & Assessment' by Lilly (Elsevier) 2012/Q 249*

Left free wall accessory pathways are most common.

'Left free wall accessary pathways are most common followed by posteroseptal, right free wall and anteroseptal locations' - 'Braunwald Heart Diseases: Review & Assessment' by Lilly (2012)/Q249

'The most common accessary pathway connects the left atrium to the left ventricle followed by posterior septal, right free wall and anterior septal accessary pathways' – Harrison's 18th/1889

104. Answer is A (Orthodromic AV reentry): *Harrison 18th/1889*

The most common macro-reentrant tachycardia associated WPW syndrome is orthodromic AV reentry.

'The most common macro-reentrant tachycardia associated with WPW syndrome is referred to as Orthodromic AV reentry' – Harrison's 18th/1889

105. Answer is A (Narrow QRS complexes): Harrison 18th/p 1889 *Harrison 16th/1350, 17th/ 1434; ECG made easy by John R Hampton 8th*

WPW syndrome is characteristically associated with a wide QRS complex.

WPW Syndrome : Features

- *Wolf Parkinson White syndrome is caused by the presence of on additional / accessory pathway (connection) between the atria and ventricle.* Normally the AV node is the only pathway that allows electrical connection between atria and ventricles and allows some delay in conduction of impulses from atrial to ventricles.
  Accessory bundles do not have an AV node to delay conduction and form such a direct connection between atrium and ventricle – This constitutes WPW syndrome.
- A depolarization wave reaches the ventricle early and causes premature excitation of ventricles – *preexcitation.* Q
- *Paroxysmal tachycardias* Q *are produced as a result of such preexcitation.*
- *The acessary pathway (called bundle of Kent) may be present as a connection between the left atrium and left ventricle (Left sided) or as a connection between the right atrium and right ventricle (Right sided).*

Pre excitation resulting from left sided accessory pathways is called Type A Pre-excitation
Pre excitation resulting from right sided accessory pathway is called Type B Pre-excitation

- ***The most common accessary pathways leading to pre-excitation syndromes (WPW) are left sided (connecting left atrium to left ventricle)*** Q

Left free wall accessory pathways are most common.
'Left free wall accessary pathways are most common followed by posteroseptal, right free wall and anteroseptal locations' - 'Braunwald Heart Diseases: Review & Assessment' by Lilly (2012)/Q249

- ***The most common macro-reentrant tachycardia associated WPW syndrome is orthodromic AV reentry.***
  'The most common macro-reentrant tachycardia associated with WPW syndrome is referred to as Orthodromic AV reentry' – Harrison's 18th/1889

- ***WPW Syndrome has a charachteristic ECG Patern***

Typical ECG pattern includes

- *Short PR interval* Q
- *Slurred upstroke of QRS complex* Q *i.e. Delta wave.*
  The second part of QRS complex is normal as conduction through bundle of His catches up with preexcitation.
- *Wide QRS complex* Q

106. Answer is A, E (More common in females and Incidence is 0.3 to 0.7%): *Braunwald 8th/890, 884*

WPW syndrome is more common in males and the incidence varies from 0.1 to 3/1000 in apparently healthy subjects (i.e 0.01 to 0.3 percent)

WPW syndrome : Accessory AV Pathways

- WPW syndrome or 'Prexcitation syndrome' is charachterized by the presence of *tachyarrythmias*[Q] due to an *accessory conducting pathway*[Q] between atrium and ventricle
- WPW abnormality occurs when an impulse reaches the atria or ventricles earlier than would be expected if the impulse traveled by way of normal specialized conducting tissue *(Pre excitation)* [Q]

- When atrial impulse activates the entire or some part of ventricle
- When ventricular impulse activates the entire or some part of the atrium

Epidemiology

- ***Incidence varies from 0.1 to 3.0/1000 in apparently healthy subjects (Average = 1.5/1000)***
- It may be found in all ages (Neonates to Elderly)
- Prevalence decreases with age apparently because of loss of preexcitation
- ***It is more common in Males***
- Most adults with WPW syndrome have normal heart
  (However various acquired and congenital defects may be associated specially Ebstein's anomaly, MVP and cardiomyopathics)

Electrocardiographic features

Three basic features typify the ECG abnormalities with usual form of WPW syndrome

- Short PR interval (PR interval <120 ms during sinus rhythm)[Q]
- Wide QRS complex (>120 ms) with a slurred slowly rising upstroke (delta wave) [Q]
  The terminal portion of QRS complex is usually normal as conduction through bundle of His usually catches up with preexcitation
- Secondary ST-T changes[Q] that are generally directed to an opposite direction to the major Delta/ QRS vectors

Note

- **Fusion beats**: [Q] If the accessory pathway is capable of anteprade conduction, the typical QRS complex represents a 'Fusion beat' as a result of depolarization of the ventricle in part by the wave travelling from the accessory pathway and in part by wave travelling from normal AV nodal pathway
- **Normal p wave**[Q] – Since the atrial activation is normal, the P wave is usually normal

107. Answer is B (Procainamide): *Hurst 12th/981*

Intravenous Procainamide is recommended to restore sinus rhythm in patients with Atrial fibrillation associated with the WPW syndrome.
Procammide is the single best answer amongst the options provided.

Management of Atrial fibrillation with WPW Preexcitation Syndrome: Recommendations

1. Catheter ablation of the accessory pathway is recommended in symptomatic patients with AF who have WPW syndrome, particularly those *with syncope due to rapid heart rate or those with a short bypass tract refractory period.*
2. Immediate direct-current cardioversion is recommended to prevent ventricular fibrillation in patients with a *short anterograde bypass tract refractory period in whom AF occurs with a rapid ventricular response associated with hemodynamic instability.*
3. **Intravenous procainamide or ibutilide** is recommended to restore sinus rhythm *in patients with WPW in whom AF occurs without hemodynamic instability in association with a wide QRS complex on the electrocardiogram* (ECG) (greater than or equal to 120-ms duration) or with a rapid preexcited ventricular response.

108. Answer is C (WPW): *Harrison 15th/ 1308, Harrison 16th/ 1351;* Harrison 18th/p 1889, 1890 *Harrison 17th/ 1415, 1434, 1435*

'Ablation of bypass tract offers a permanent cure of supraventricular tachycardias.
The advent of radiofrequency catheter ablation has virtually eliminated the need for surgery.' *– Harrisons*

Heart block and Conduction Disturbance

109. Answer is A (Constant PR interval): *Refer text below*

Mobitz Type I block (second degree: Wenchebach type) is characterized by a variable PR interval, (PR interval is not constant). PR interval in type I block characteristically gets longer until a QRS complex is dropped

First Degree AV Block

First degree AV block is charachterized by a delay in conduction across the conducting tissue (prolonged PR interval)

Features

- *PR interval is prolonged (>0.20 seconds)*[Q]
- *PR interval is constant (at the prolonged duration)*[Q]
- *Rhythm is regular*[Q]
- *Each P wave is followed by a QRS complex*[Q]
- *QRS complex morphology / duration is usually normal*[Q]

Second Degree AV Block

Second degree AV block is characterized by intermittent failure of conduction from atria to ventricles

Type I (Mobitz) / Wenchebeck Type

This is charachterized by progressive prolongation of PR interval prior to a non conducted P wave

Features

- *Atrial Rhythm regular*[Q]
- *Ventricular Rhythm irregular*[Q]
- *Atrial rate exceeds ventricular rate*[Q]
- *PR internal varies*[Q]
- *PR progressively gets longer until a QRS is dropped*[Q]
- *QRS morphology is often normal*[Q]

Type II (Mobitz)

This is characterized by constant PR interval prior to a non conducted P wave

Features

- *Atrial Rhythm regular*[Q]
- *Ventricular Rhythm Regular (unless conduction rations vary)*[Q]
- *Atrial Rate exceeds ventricular rate*[Q]
- *PR interval is constant*[Q]
  PR interval does not get progressively longer and a QRS is dropped suddenly
- *QRS morphology is usually abnormal*[Q] *(rarely normal)*

Third Degree AV Block: Complete AV Block

Third degree AV block or complete AV block is charachterized by complete failure of conduction from atria to ventricles. (Atria and ventricles are under the control of separate pacemakers).

Features

- *Atrial Rhythm regular*[Q]
- *Ventricular Rhythm regular*[Q]
- *Atrial rate exceeds ventricular rate*[Q] *(The inherent rate of ventricular pacemaker is slower)*
- *PR interval varies*[Q] *(variable)*
- *P waves have no constant relationship to QRS complexes*[Q] *(AV dissocation)*
- *QRS complex morphology may be abnormal*[Q]

110. Answer is A, C (First –Degree block and Second Degree Mobitz type II): *Refer text below*

First degree Heart block and second degree Mobitz type II block are associated with constant PR interval.

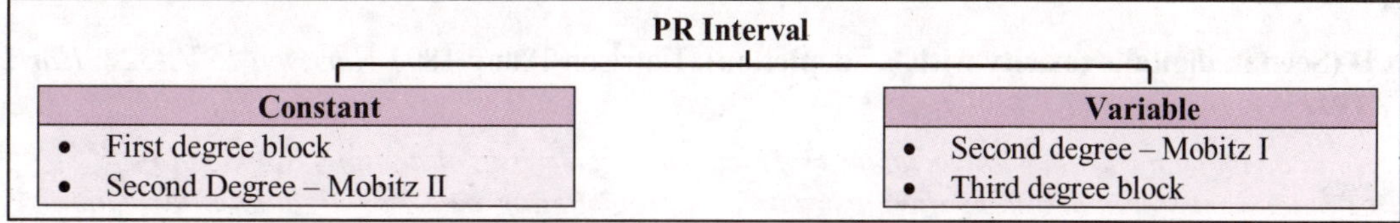

PR constant (First-degree) (First-degree)	PR varies (Second-degree, Mobitz 1)
PR constant	*PR varies*
PR prolonged	*PR progressively gets longer until a QRS is dropped*
Regular atrial rhythm; Regular ventricular rhythm	*Regular atrial rhythm; Irregular ventricular rhythm*
(Second –degree, Mobitz II)	**(Third- degree)**
PR constant	*PR varies*
PR normal or prolonged Two or three P waves (possibly more) to each QRS	*P waves have no constant relationship to QRS (found hidden in QRS complexes and T waves)*
Regular atrial rhythm; Regular ventricular rhythm (unless conduction ratios vary)	*Regular atrial rhythm; Rgular ventricular rhythm*

111. Answer is A, B, and C: *Hurst 12th/1029, 1030; ECG Workbook by Huff 5th/155*

Second degree AV block (Type I and /or Type II) may be associated with prolonged conduction time (prolonged PR interval), Atrial rate more than ventricular rate and change in QRS complex morphology (Type II).

Name	Rhythm	Rate (beats/minute)	P waves (lead II)	PR Interval	QRS complex
First-degree atrio-ventricular (AV) block	Regular	That of underlying sinus rhythm; both atrial and ventricular rates will be the same	***Sinus origin; one P wave to each QRS complex***	Prolonged (more than 0.20 second); remains constant	Normal (0.10 second or less)
Second-degree AV block, Mobitz I	Atrial: regular Ventricular: irregular	Atrial: that of underlying sinus rhythm Ventricular: depends on number of impulses conducted through AV node: ***will be less than atrial rate***	Sinus origin	Varies; progressively lengthens until a P wave isn't conducted (P wave occurs without the QRS cmplex); a pause follows the dropped QRS complex	Normal (0.10 second or less)
Second-degree AV block, Mobitz II	Atrial: regular ventricular: usually regular, but may be irregular if conductions ratios vary	Atrial: that of underlying sinus rhythm Ventricular: depends on number of Impulses conducted through AV node; will be ***less than atrial rate***	Sinus origin: two or three P waves (sometimes more) before each QRS complex	Normal or prolonged; remains constant	Normal if block at level of bundle of His; ***Wide if block in bundle branches***
Third-degree AV block	Atrial: regular Ventricular: regular	Atrial: that of underlying sinus rhythm Ventricular:40 to 60 if paced by AV junction; 30 to 40 (sometimes less) if paced by ventricles; will be less than atrial rate	Sinus P waves with ***no constant relationship to the QRS complex***; P waves found hidden in QRS complexes and T waves	Varies greatly	Normal if block at level of AV node or bundle of His; wide if block in bundle branches

No constant Relationship between P wave and QRS complex is a feature of Third degree or complete heart block.
One P wave to each QRS complex is a feature of First degree block

112. Answer is D (Seen in digitalis toxicity with K^+ depletion): Harrison 18th/p 1897 *Harrison 15th/ 1327; Harrison 16th/ 1375; 17th/ 1441*

Nonparoxysmal atrial tachycardia with variable AV block is characteristic of digitalis intoxication.
Depletion of potassium stores is one of the most common precipitating cause of digitalis intoxication. Presence of potassium depletion in association with digitalis is thus likely to result in manifestations of digitalis toxicity.

113. Answer is D (Diltiazem): Harrison 18th/p 1867, 1874 *Harrison 16th/1348, 1339; Harrison 17th/ 1416-1422*

Diltiazem is used in the treatment of tachyarhythmias and not in the treatment of bradyarrhythmias.

Diltiazem is a class IV antiarrhythmogenic drug, used in atrial fibrillation/flutter and supraventricular tachycardias (tachycardias) to slow the ventricular rate, by decreasing conduction velocity and increasing refractoriness in the AV nodal tissue. ***Atropine, Isoproterenol and pacemakers are all useful in the management of bradycardia.***

- ***Atropine*** and ***isoproterenol*** are useful in increasing heart rate and decreasing symptoms in patients with sinus ***bradycardia*** or AV block localized to AV node.' - *Harrison 16th/1339*
- Long term therapy of brady arrhythmias is best accomplished by ***pacemakers***. - *Harrison 16th/1339*

Management of Bradycardias : Oxford hand book of Medicine : *6th/126*

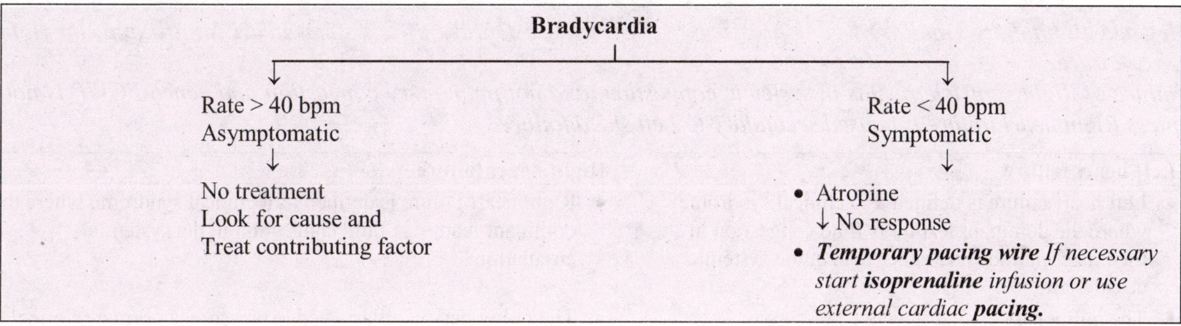

Miscellaneous

114. Answer is A (Increased amplitude of QRS complex): *'The 5 Minute Sports Medicine Consult' (2001) /378*

Increased amplitude voltage of QRS complex is a frequent finding in Athletic Heart Syndrome

Athletic Heart Syndrome

- Athletic Heart Syndrome is a benign condition consisting of physiologic adaptations to the increased cardiac workload of exercise in trained athletes
- It represents a constellation of clinical findings that are the result of normal physiologic adaptation to strenuous physical activity
- In response to the increased physical demand, the left ventricles dilates and wall thickness increases. The mass to volume ratio however does not change

Physical examination

- *Decreased body fat and increased muscle mass (generally very physically fit)*
- *Pulse slow and often irregular (sinus bradycardia or bradycardia with first-and second-degree blocks)*
- *Grade I or II mid-systolic murmurs (benign functional ejection murmur resolves with valsalva maneuver)*
- *Third and fourth heart sounds very common benign filling sounds)*
- *Blood pressure typically remains normal*

Electrocardiogram rhythm

- Rhythm
  - ***Sinus bradycardia*** of 40 to 55 beats /min while at rest
  - Sinus pauses of more than 2.0 seconds due to increased vagal tone
  - Wandering atrial pacemaker, found only in dynamic athletes
  - First degree atrioventricular block present only at rest; P-R interval normalizes with exercise
  - Second degree atrioventricular block present only at rest: Mobitz I (wenckebach block) common in marathon runners; Mobitz II rare in athlete's heart.
- ***Voltage: ↑QRS voltage (Amplitude)***
  - Left ventricular hypertrophy found in 85% of olympic marathon runners
  - Right ventricular hypertrophy common in dynamic athletes but rarely seen in sedentary controls and static athletes sedentary control and static athletes

- Repolarization
  - S-T segment elevation with peaked T waves, normalizes with exertion
  - S-T segment depression may be rarely found in athletes
  - T-wave inversion in lateral leads associated with interventricular septal hypertrophy in static athletes (can be normal finding in dynamic athletes)

Chest radiography

- Heart is globular in appearance, particularly in endurance athletes.
- Cardiomegaly (cardiothoracic ratio >0.50)

Congestive Heart Failure and PCWP

115. Answer is A (Increased PCWP): *Hurst 12th/692, 'Heart failure' 1st/163, 164; Refer text below*

Elevated Pulmonary capillary wedge pressure (↑ PCWP) is a feature of left sided heart failure and not right sided heart failure.

Failure of Right ventricle results in systemic congestion, and not pulmonary congestion and hence PCWP is not raised unless Right heart failure is caused secondary to Left sided failure.

Left heart failure	Right heart failure
• Left heart failure is defined as a clinical syndrome where the dominant feature is fluid congestion in the lungs (pulmonary) rather than in the systemic circulation • The pulmonary capillary wedge pressure is typically elevated (↑PCWP) • Predominant symptoms are related to passive congestion of lungs and pulmonary edema • Dyspnea • Orthopnea • Paroxysmal Nocturnal Dyspnea (PND) • Cough with Pink Frothy Sputum • Rales / Crackles	• Right heart failure is defined as a clinical syndrome where the dominant feature is fluid congestion in the systemic circulation. • The pulmonary capillary wedge pressure is normal (Normal PCWP) unless Right heart failure is caused secondary to left sided heart failure (↑ed PCWP) ***(PCWP is not elevated in isolated Right heart failure)*** • Predominant symptoms are related to passive systemic congestion • Peripheral Edema • Ascitis • Congestive hepatomegaly (may be pulsatile) • Congestive splenomegaly • Weight gain • Nocturia • Raised JVP • Positive Hepatojugular reflex

116. Answer is D (Normal JVP): *Hurst 72th/692; 'Heart failure' 1st/163*

Right ventricular infarcts will cause failure of Right Ventricle resulting in systemic congestion and a Raised JVP.

Right heart failure
• Right heart failure is defined as a clinical syndrome where the dominant feature is fluid congestion in the systemic circulation. • The pulmonary capillary wedge pressure is normal (Normal PCWP) unless Right heart failure is caused secondary to left sided heart failure (↑ed PCWP) ***(PCWP is not elevated in isolated Right heart failure)*** Predominant symptoms are related to passive systemic congestion • Peripheral Edema • ***Ascitis*** • Congestive hepatomegaly (may be pulsatile) • Congestive splenomegaly • Weight gain • ***Nocturia*** • ***Raised JVP*** • Positive Hepatojugular reflex

117. Answer is D (Hepatomegaly): *Harrison 15th/1323 (not a new edition); Family Medicine (Lange) 4th/450*

Hepatomegaly is a minor Framingham criterion in CHF.

The Framingham Heart Study Criteria:

Major Criteria	Minor Criteria
• Paroxysmal nocturnal dyspnea • Neck vein distension • Rates • Cardiomegaly • Acute pulmonary edema • S3 gallop • Increased venous pressure (> 16 cm) • Circulation time ≥ 25s • Hepatojugular reflux positive	• Ankle edema • Night cough • Hepatomegaly • Pleural effusion • Vital capacity reduced by one third from predicted • Tachycardia (≥ 120)
Major or minor criterion	
• Weight loss of more than 4.5 kg over 5 days in response to treatment	
Definite CHF	
• Two major criteria or one major and two minor criteria.	

118. Answer is A (Mitral Stenosis): Harrison 18th/p 1931 *Harrisons 17th/-1467*

Isolated Mitral Stenosis is not associated with Left Ventricular Hypertrophy

Isolated Mitral Stenosis is not associated with Left ventricular Hypertrophy

The burden of Mitral Stenosis (from obstruction of flow across the mitral valve) is received by the left atrium followed by pulmonary circulation, right ventricle and right atrium in that sequence

Left ventricle is off loaded and neither receives pressure overload nor volume overload and hence does not show any hypertrophy

Pathophysiological overload features from Mitral Stenosis may results in

- *Left Atrial Hypertrophy (↑left Atrial pressure)*
- *Pulmonary Hypertension (Dilatation of pulmonary vessels)*
- *Right ventricular Hypertrophy (Secondary to pulmonary Hypertension)*
- *Right Atrial Hypertrophy (May be seen with severe M.S. secondary to Pulmonary Hypertension*

Aortic Stenosis, Aortic Regurgitation and Mitral Regurgitation may all lead to Left Ventricular Hypertrophy

Left Ventricular Hypertrophy may result from either pressure overload (e,g AS) or volume overload (MR, AR etc) of the left ventricle

Left Ventricular Hypertrophy

Pressure Overload	Volume Overload
• Occurs when heart is forced to pump against increased resistance such as - Systemic ***Hypertension***Q - Aortic ***stenosis***Q • These conditions cause ***systolic overload***Q • This causes ***concentric Hypertrophy***Q of left ventricle. (ventricular wall thickens in relation to ventricular cavity) Systolic overload on ECG is characterized by : - ↑QRS voltage - Depressed ST segment - Inverted T waves } in left precordial Lead	• Occurs when end diastolic wall stress is such as valvular regurgitation • Aortic Regurgitation • Mitral Regurgitation • These conditions cause ***diastolic overload***Q • This causes ***Eccenteric hypertrophy***Q of Left ventricle (Ventricular wall thickness remains normal in relation to chamber dilatation Diastolic overload on ECG is characterized by - Tall Late 'R' waves in V_5 & V_6

119. Answer is B (Serum Sodium) : Harrison 18th/p 1906, 1907 *Harrison 16th/255, 1366; Harrison 17th/1447,1448; CMDT 2008/343; CMDT 2009/350*

Congestive Cardiac failure is associated with Hyponatremia or Decreased Serum Sodium levels. – Hari. 16th / 255

- **Heart failure is associated with Hyponatremia. -** *CMDT / Harrison*
  Mechanism of hyponatremia is primary Na^+ gain exceeded by secondary water gain.
  In heart failure total body sodium is increased, yet effective circulating volume is sensed as inadequate by baroceptors. Increased ADH and Aldosterone results which causes retention of water and sodium. Secondary water gain exceeds primary sodium gain resulting in hyponatremia.
- **Elevated serum urea levels may be seen.**
- *Biochemical studies in heart failure may show renal insufficiency. Renal functions tests also determine whether cardiac failure is associated with prerenal azotemia.*
- **Right atrial mean pressure is increased congestive heart failure.**
  In heart failure one or the other ventricle fails to discharge its contents or fails to fill normally.
  As a result the pressure in the atrium and venous system behind (upstream) the failing ventricle rise.
  - Harrison
- **In patients will heart failure the levels of circulating norepinephrine may be markedly elevated** *reflecting the increased activity of the adrenergic nervous system. - Harrison*

120. Answer is C (Decreased after load): Harrison 18th/p 1823 *Harrison 17th/1384; 'Textbook of Cardiovascular Medicine' by Topol 3rd/200*

Hepatojugular reflux results from an increase in preload and afterload to the right atrium and ventricle (and not by a decrease in after load).

Hepatojugular reflux is a characteristic feature of Right ventricular failure. Tricuspid regurgitation and Pulmonic stenosis are both causes of right ventricular failure and may hence produce a positive hepatojugular reflux.

Hepatojugular Reflux

Hepatojugular Reflux test is a helpful test in patients with suspected Right ventricular failure with a normal resting CVP (This test can be used to detect latent right heart failure)

Hepatojugular Reflux

With the patient in semirecumbant position (45° position) continuous pressure is applied with the palm of examiner over the abdomen / Liver for 10 seconds or more.

In patients with compromised Right Ventricular Function	In patients with adequate Right ventricular Function
Abnormal Hepatojugular Reflux Three is rapid elevation in JVP that remains persistently elevated by 4cm or more during the entire 10 seconds when pressure is maintained followed by a drop in pressure on release of compression.	Normal Hepatojugular Reflux There may be a transient increase in JVP however the increase in JVP is not sustained for the entire '10' seconds when pressure is maintained and pressure rapidly returns to or near the baseline in less than 10 seconds even when pressure is still maintained.

Pathophysiology

- During abdominal compression with increased abdominal pressure, there is an increased venous return to the right atrium and right ventricle (Increased preload)
  Concurrently there is an increase in right ventricular after load owing to upward movement of diaphragm which reduces the intrathoracic volume capacity.
- The normal functioning right ventricle handles this increase in preload and after load and systemic venous pressure remains normal.
- The dysfunctioning right ventricle however fails to accept this increase in preload and after load and hence systemic venous pressure remains persistently elevated.

121. Answer is D (Decreased After-load): *Harrisons 18th/1823, 1824, 1948; Textbook of Cardiovascular Medicine by Topal 3rd/200; Congestive Heart Failure by Greenberg (Lippincott) 2006 (3rd)/561*

Positive Hepatojugular Reflux represents decreased compliance of the right ventricle and right atrium. This may result from an increase in preload and/or afterload to the right atrium and/or right ventricle.
Decrease in after-load does not cause a Positive Hepatojugular Reflux

Hepatojugular Reflux

Hepatojugular Reflux test is a helpful test in patients with suspected Right ventricular failure with a normal resting CVP (This test can be used to detect latent right heart failure)

Hepatojugular Reflux

With the patient in semirecumbant position (45° position) continuous pressure is applied with the palm of examiner over the abdomen / Liver for 10 seconds or more.

In patients with compromised Right Ventricular Function	In patients with adequate Right ventricular Function
Abnormal Hepatojugular Reflux Three is rapid elevation in JVP that remains persistently elevated by 4cm or more during the entire 10 seconds when pressure is maintained followed by a drop in pressure on release of compression.	Normal Hepatojugular Reflux There may be a transient increase in JVP however the increase in JVP is not sustained for the entire '10' seconds when pressure is maintained and pressure rapidly returns to or near the baseline in less than 10 seconds even when pressure is still maintained.

Pathophysiology

- During abdominal compression with increased abdominal pressure, there is an increased venous return to the right atrium and right ventricle (Increased preload)
  Concurrently there is an increase in right ventricular after load owing to upward movement of diaphragm which reduces the intrathoracic volume capacity.
- The normal functioning right ventricle handles this increase in preload and after load and systemic venous pressure remains normal.
- The dysfunctioning right ventricle however fails to accept this increase in preload and after load and hence systemic venous pressure remains persistently elevated.

Causes of Positive Hepatojugular Reflux

Left Heart Failure	Right Heart Failure
The most common cause of Positive Hepatojugular Reflux in adults in Left Heart failure due to Dilated Cardiomyopathy (Constrictive Pericarditis and Restrictive cardiomyopathy may also cause a positive Hepatojugular Reflux).	Positive Hepatojugular Reflux may also be observed in patients with Right atrial or Right ventricular failure • ***Tricuspid stenosis*** • ***Tricuspid Regurgitation*** • ***Pulmonary Hypertension*** • ***Right ventricular infarction***

122. Answer is A (Tricuspid Regurgitation (TR): *Harrisons 18th/1948*

Hepatomegaly (Enlarged liver) with systolic pulsations (of the liver) and ascitis are typically seen in Tricuspid Regurgitation.

Tricuspid Regurgutation

The clinical features of Tricuspid Regurgitation result primarily from *systemic venous congestion and reduction in cardiac output.*

Typical Physical Examination Findings in Tricuspid Regurgitation
• *Gross Fluid Retention* - *Significant Peripheral Edema* - ***Ascitis*** - *Pleural Effusion* • ***Hepatomegaly with a Pulsatile liver (Enlarged tender liver with systolic pulsations)*** • *Positive hepatojugular reflux* • *Dilated Jugular veins with prominent 'v' waves and rapid 'y' decent* • *Blowing Holosystolic murmur along lower left sternal margin that increases with inspiration* • *Prominent RV Pulsations (Parasternal Heaves) over left parasternal region.*

123. Answer is A (Pulmonary Capillary Pressure): *Hurst 12th/494*

Pulmonary Capillary Wedge Pressure (PCWP) Closely approximates Left Atrial (LA)Pressure- *Hurst 12th / 494.*

124. Answer is A (Narcotic overdose): Harrison 18th/p 281 *Harrison 16th/ 1592,204 Harrison 17th /224; API 7th/1240*

Pulmonary edema with normal pulmonary capillary wedge pressure suggests a diagnosis of ARDS or non cardiogenic pulmonary edema. ***Narcotic overdose is the only non cardiogenic cause for pulmonary edema (ARDS) amongst the options provided and hence the answer here.***

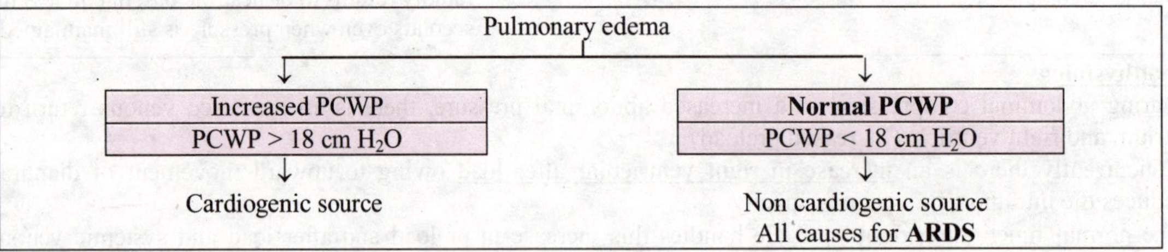

Causes of Pulmonary Edema with Normal Pulmonary Capillary Wedge pressure (PCWP=Normal)

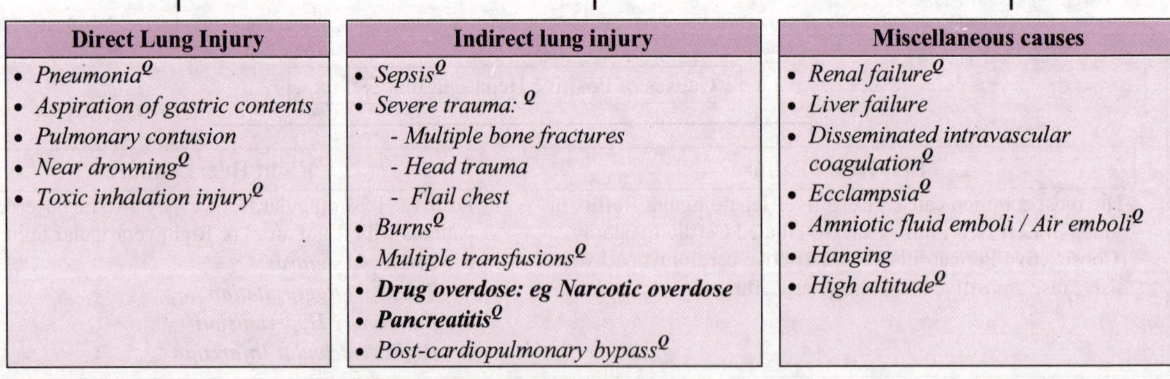

Direct Lung Injury	Indirect lung injury	Miscellaneous causes
• *Pneumonia*[Q] • *Aspiration of gastric contents* • *Pulmonary contusion* • *Near drowning*[Q] • *Toxic inhalation injury*[Q]	• *Sepsis*[Q] • *Severe trauma:* [Q] - *Multiple bone fractures* - *Head trauma* - *Flail chest* • *Burns*[Q] • *Multiple transfusions*[Q] • ***Drug overdose: eg Narcotic overdose*** • ***Pancreatitis***[Q] • *Post-cardiopulmonary bypass*[Q]	• *Renal failure*[Q] • *Liver failure* • *Disseminated intravascular coagulation*[Q] • *Ecclampsia*[Q] • *Amniotic fluid emboli / Air emboli*[Q] • *Hanging* • *High altitude*[Q]

125. Answer is B (High Altitude): Harrison 18th/p 2205 *Harrison's 16th/ 1592; Harrison 17th/ 1680; API 7th/ 1240*

Pulmonary edema with normal pulmonary capillary wedge pressure suggests a diagnosis of ARDS or non cardiogenic pulmonary edema.

High altitude has been grouped as one of the miscellaneous causes for ARDS, reflecting pulmonary oedema with a normal PCWP *- API 7th/ 1240*

Some miscellaneous causes for ARDS
• Renal failure • Liver failure • Disseminated intravascular coagulation

- Ecclampsia
- Amniotic fluid emboli / Air emboli
- Hanging
- High altitude

126. Answer is D (Bilateral Renal Artery Stenosis)): Repeat

Bilateral Renal Artery Stenosis is not a cause for pulmonary edema with normal PCWP
High Altitude, narcotic overdose (Cocaine overdose),and cardiopulmonary bypass are all know causes for pulmonary edema with normal PCWP.

127. Answer is B (Drug induced cardiac toxicity): *Harrison 16th / 584; 17th / H-e 91, CMDT 2008 / 1418, 1675*

Features of cardiac failure in a patient on doxorubicin suggests the possibility of Anthracycline induced cardiac toxity. *Risk of Anthracyclinc induced cardiac toxicity is increased with concomitent radiation and cyclophosphamide. Cardiac failure after 6 months of chemotherapy with doxorubicin (anthracycline) and cyclophosphamide, is consistent with a diagnosis of drug induced cardiac toxity which is the single best answer of choice.*

Anthracycline Induced Cardiac toxity
• Most anthracyclines damage the heart muscle • The problem is greater with doxorubicin because it has a major role and is used in repeated doses. o Change in cardiac dynamics occur in most patients by the time they have received 300mg/m^2 of doxorubicin. o Patient should not receive a total dose in excess of 450 ml/m^2 o Toxicity may be irreversible at dosage level > 550 mg/m^2 (CHF) (About 5% of patient who receive > 550 mg/m^2 of doxorubicin will develop CHF). • Anthracyline induced CHF is not readily reversible and mortality is as high as 50%.Thus prevention is the best approach - Harrison • Risk of cardiotoxicity increase with radiation, cyclophosphamide – CMDT

Anthracycline Antibiotics
• Doxorubicin • Daunomyocin • Idarubicin
Mitoxantrone (Similar drug)

128. Answer is A (Digoxin): *Harrison 18th/2236, 2237; Kumar & Clarke 7th/343; European Society of Cardiology Guidelines; Modern Management of cardiogenic Pulmonary Edema (Emergency Medicine Clinics of North America); Americal College of Cardiology/Americal Heart Practice Guidelines*

Digoxin has no definitive role in the management of Acute Pulmonary Edema

'Digitalis is not the initial drug of choice for management of patients with acute severe pulmonary edema (severe heart failure) because of its mild inotropic effect and because of the delay in time to peak action. It should not be used in the management of acute cases, in the absence of atrial arrhythmias as its use may complicate an already difficult management problem. Digoxin is only recommended if the patient is in atrial fibrillation and this is contributing to the cardiac failure – 'Circulation' Journal of American Heart Association

'Digoxin is not recommended in acute pulmonary edema unless there is associated rapid atrial fibrillation. Rapid atrial fibrillation in this situation is better treated with urgent cardioversion' – 'Coronary care manual' by Thompson (Elsevier) 2nd/508

'Digoxin has no definitive role in the management of acute congestive heart failure (acute pulmonary edema)'
– Clinical Emergency Medicine (Cambridge University Press) 2005/499

'Once a mainstay of treatment because of their positive inotropic action digitalis glycosides are rarely used at present. However they may be useful for control of ventricular rate in patient with rapid atrial fibrillation or flutter with LV dysfunction' – Harrison 18th/2237

Initial Management of Acute Pulmonary Edema (Acute Heart Failure)
• *Oxygentation* with face mask or ***Positive Pressure Ventilation (Non invasive)*** • ***Vasodilatation by Nitrates (or Nitroprusside)*** • ***Diuretic therapy by Furosemide (or other loop diuretics)*** • *Morphine* for relief of physical psychological stress and to improve haemodynamics.
Inotropes should be used based on clinical and haemodynamic parameters of the patient who does not respond to initial treatment.

Acute Pulmonary Edema

Oxygen and Ventilatory Support	Morphine	Vasodilators	Diuretics	Inotropic Agents
• **Supplemental oxygen** The maintenance of SaO2 within normal limits (95-98%) is important to maximize oxygen delivery to tissues • **Non invasive ventilation** (without endotrachial intubation) *CPAP or Non invasive positive Pressure Ventilation (NIPPV)* *The use of CPAP and NIPPV in Acute Cardiogenic Pulmonary Edema is associated with a significant reduction in the need of tracheal intubation and mechanical ventilation.*	*Morphine* diminishes anxiety and decreases sympathetic outflow, thereby reducing both venous and arterial vasoconstriction resulting in decreases in ventricular preload and after load. • *Morphine is recommended for the treatment of Acute severe pulmonary edema especially if associated with restlessness and dyspnea* (effectively ameliorates symptoms)	*Vasodilators* are indicated in most patients with acute pulmonary edema (AHF) as first line therapy if associated with adequate blood pressure and signs of congestion with low diuresis to open the peripheral circulation and to lower preload. • Nitrates (sublingual/Intravenous) (Agent of choice) • Nitroprusside (Associated Hypertensive Crisis) • Nesiritide	*Diuretics* are recommended for initial management of acute severe pulmonary edema especially in the presence of symptoms secondary to fluid retension (Reduce Alveolar Edema) • Intravenous administration of Loop Diuretics (Furosemide, Bumetonide or Torasemide) is the preferred choice due to their strong and brisk diuretics effect.	*Inotropic agents* are indicated in the management of Acute pulmonary edema in the presence of peripheral hypoperfusion (hypotension/reduced renal function) with or without congestion or pulmonary edema refractory to diuretics and vasodilators at optimal doses. • Dobutamine/Dopamine • Phosphodiesterase Inhibitors (Milrinone / Enoximone) • Levosimenden • Norepinephrine/ Epinephrine

Digoxin is not recommended as on inotrope for the management of Acute pulmonary Edema *because of its mild inotropic effect and delay in time to peak action (slow action). Digoxin may be selectively considered for patients with Atrial Fibrillation where AF is contributing to cardiac failure / pulmonary edema.*

129. Answer is D (Trimetazidine): *Harrison 18th/1907-12; KDT 6th/534, 535, 502; Harrisons 17th/ 1449, 1450, 1451, 1452*

Trimetazidine is not used in the management of congestive heart failure.

Trimetazidine *is a novel anti-ischemic agent used for the treatment of coronary conditions like angina. Although it's exact mechanism of action is not known, it is believed to act by improving cellular tolerance to ischemia unlike other conventional antianginal agents.*

Spironoloactone, Nitrates and Nesritide may all be used in the managed of congestive Heart Failure

- Nestritide and nitrates are vasodilatory that help CHF by lowering left ventricular filling pressures (by decreasing preload)
- Spironolactone is an aldosterone antagonist that helps in CHF by antagonizone tha effects of aldosterone.

Drugs Used in Heart Failure

Drugs which help in relieving congestive / low output symptoms and restoring cardiac performance	Drugs which help in arresting / reversing disease progression and prolonging survival
• **Diuretics** - *Furosemide Torsemide / Bumetanide / Hydrochlorthiaizide / Metazolone* • **Vasodilators** - **Nitrates** - Nisoprusside - **Nesiritide** • **Inotropes** - *Digoxin* - *Dopamine / Dobutamine* - *Mitrinone* - *Levasimendan* • **Vasoconstrictors** (to maintain blood pressure) - *Dopamine for Hypotension* - *Epinephrine / Phenylephrine* - *Vasopressin*	• **ACE Inhibitors** - *Captopril / Enalapril / Lisinopril / Ramipril etc* • **Angiotension Receptor Blockers** - *Losartan / Valsartan / Irbesartan etc* • **Beta Blockers** - *Carvedilol / Bisoprolol / Metoprolol* • **Aldosterone Antagonist** - ***Spironolactone***

130. Answer is A (They should be initiated at the effective doses): Harrison 18th/p 1909 *Harrison's 17th/1450, 51; KDT 6th/505, 506; Goodman & Gillman's Manual of Pharmacology (2007)/570*

Beta blocker should be initiated at lower than effective doses in CHF

Beta blockers should be initiated at lower than effective doses in CHF and be

*'Beta blockers **should be initiated at low doses** followed by gradual increments in the dose if lower doses have been well tolerated. The dose of beta blockers should be increased until the doses used are similar to those that have been reported **effective** in clinical trials. The titration of beta blockers should proceed no more rapidly than at 2 week intervals because the initiation and / or increased dosing of these agents may lead to worsening fluid retention' – Harrison's 17th/1450*

Special precaution should be taken in NYHA class III & IV

'Although data suggests that patients with NYHA class IIIB and IV CHF may tolerate beta blockers and benefit from their use, this group of patients should be approached with considerable caution'

–Goodman & Gillman's Manual of Pharmacology (2007)/570

Carvedilol and Metoprolol are the preferred beta blockers in CHF

*'Non selective third generation beta blockers (Bucindolol, **Carvedilol**) as well a the Beta-1 selective agent (**Metoprolol**) are generally well tolerated by patients with CHF'.*

-'Current Diagnosis & Treatment in Cardiology' 3rd/217

131. Answer is D (Digoxin): *CMDT 2003/384, 385, 386;* Harrison 18th/p 1906, 1908, 1909 *Harrison 16th/1375; Harrison 17th/1448-1451; CMDT 2009/354*

'Digitalis does not improve survival in patients with heart failure and sinus rhythm.' – Harrison 16th/ 1375

It reduces symptoms of heart failure and need for hospitalization. ACE inhibitors (Corvedilol and enalapril) and Betablockers (Metaprolol) prolong life.

'ACE inhibitors improve symptoms and prolong life' – *Oxford handbook 5th/ 122*
ACE inhibitors – Harrison 16th

Patients with LV dysfunction without HF	Patients with HF/ After Acute MI / with vascular disease
Prevents or retards development of H.F.	• Reduces symptoms • Enhances exercise performance • *Reduces long term mortality*

Beta blockers : 'Recent randomized trials show that β blockers decrease mortality in heart failure'-*Oxford handbook 5th/ 122*

Administration of gradually escalating doses of β-blockers has shown to: (Harrison)
• Improve symptoms of HF • *Reduce all – cause death:* - Cardiovascular death - Sudden death - Pump failure death • Reduce rehospitalization for HF

132. Answer is C (Actively metabolized in Liver): *KDT 5th/ 461, 462*

Digoxin is excreted unchanged by the Kidney, mainly by Glomerular filtration. *It is not metabolized by liver.* ***Dose of digoxin need not to be changed in Liver failure.***

Do not confuse digoxin with digitoxin :

- *The most lipid soluble cardiac glycoside is = Digitoxin* Q
- *The most rapidly absorbed oral glycoside is = Digitoxin* Q
- Digitoxin *is primarily metabolized by the liver* Q
- *Dose of digitoxin needs to be reduced in liver failure.* Q

133. Answer is D (Hepatic dysfunction): *KDT 4th/ 498, KDT 5th/ 463*

Digoxin toxicity is enhanced by *renal failure* as it is excreted through kidneys where as **digitoxin toxicity** is enhanced by liver failure because it is eliminated by hepatic metabolism. Hepatic dysfunction does not affect digoxin elemination.

Reduced tolerance to digoxin may be seen in :
• Advanced age Q • Acute myocardial infarction Q / ischaemia / hypoxemia • Magnesium depletion Q • Hypercalcemia Q • Hypothyroidism Q • Renal insufficiency Q • Electrical cardioversion.
The administration of following drugs raises the serum concentration of digoxin : *(by reducing both the renal and nonrenal elimination of digoxin and by reducing its volume of distribution)*
• *Quinidine* Q • *Verapamil* Q • *Amiodarone* Q • *Propafenone* Q

134. Answer is A (Hypocalcemia): *KDT 4th/ 449, 448, KDT 5th/ 463, 464; Harrison 14th/1295, 16th/ 1375; CMDT 2008/347*

Calcium synergizes with digitalis and precipitates its toxicity. Thus digitalis toxicity is associated with hypercalcemia and not hypocalcemia

Also Remember:

• ***Digitalis does not cause Hypokalemia Q but Hypokalemia enhances digitalis toxicity Q*** - Digitalis toxicity causes Hyperkalemia Q - *Harrisons* - Hypokalemia enhances digitalis toxicity (by increasing its binding to Na+/K+ ATPase Q

- ***Both Hyperthyroidism and Hypothyroidism enhance digitalis toxicity***
  - Thyrotoxicosis : patients are more prone to develop digitalis arrhythmia. Q
  - Myxoedema : enhances responsiveness. These patients eliminate digoxin more slowly. Q
- ***Magnesium depletion (hypomagnesimia) may reduce tolerance to digitalis*** Q - *Harrison 16th / 1375*

135. Answer is D (Hemodialysis): *Harrison 15th/ 1327; Harrison 16th/ 1375; CMDT 2008/347; KDT; CMDT 2009/354*

Hemodialysis has no role in treatment of digoxin overdose.

Management of digitalis overdose includes:

- Withdrawl of drug Q
- *Potassium*Q: administer *cautiously and by oral route* whenever possible if hypokalemia is present. Potassium must not be employed in the presence of A-V block or hyperkalemia
- *Phenyloin/β blocker or Lidocaine* Q: Lidocaine is effective in treatment of digitalis induced ventricular tachyarrhythmias.
- *Cardiac pacemaker* : may be required in digitalis induced A-V block
- *Electrical conversion* : may be life saving in digitalis induced ventricular fibrillation
- *FAB fragments/digitalis antibodies* Q : are potentially life saving in severe intoxication.

Hemodialysis is not useful in poisonings due to:
• *Digoxin* Q
• *Kerosene* Q
• *Benzodiazepines* Q
• *Organophosphates* Q

136. Answer is D (Haemodialysis): *Harrisons 16th/1375, KDT 6th/498,499; Refer previous question*

Hemodialysis is not useful in digitalis poisoning.

Haemodialysis is not useful in poisoning due to
Digoxin
Kerosene
Benzodiazepines
Organophosphates

137. Answer is B (Prominent lower lobe vessels): Harrison 18th/p 1914 *Harrison 17th/ 1447, 1454; Read text below*

Congestive cardiac failure or corpulmonale are associated with prominence of upper lobe vessels and not lower lobe vessels.

Features of Congestive Cardiac Failure(CCF / CHF) include :
1. ***Enlarged cardiac silhouette / Cardiac shadow on chest X-ray*** Q
2. Ground glass appearance of pulmonary edema Q
3. ***'Kerley B' lines*** Q
4. ***Prominence of upper lobe blood vessels*** Q *(not lower lobe veins)*
5. *Pleural effusion, usually bilateral* Q

'Kerley B' lines'**, also known as **'Septal lines'**, represent dilated lymphatics and distended interlobular septa. They occur **most commonly in pulmonary edema as a result of chronic pulmonary venous hypertension (in CCF).

Kerley 'A' lines stand for Apex, 'B' for Base, and 'C' for Central region.

B lines are most commonly seen Q. ***Infact they have a relation with left atrial pressure*** Q *: They are invariably present if LA pressure goes above 20 mmHg.* Q

Valvular Heart Diseases

Mitral Stenosis

138. Answer is C (4-6 cm^2): *Braunwald 6th/378,1643,1673*

The normal area of mitral valve is 4-6 cm^2.

Mitral Valve & pathology	Area
Normal Mitral Valve	*4-6 cm^2*[Q]
Mild Mitral Valve	*< 2 cm^2*
Severe Mitral Stenosis	*< 1.3 cm^2*[Q]
Critical Mitral Stenosis	*< 1 cm^2*[Q]
Aortic Valve & pathology	*Area*
Normal Aortic Valve	*2.6 – 3.5 cm^2*[Q]
Mild Aortic Stenosis	*1.5 – 2 cm^2*
Moderate Aortic Stenosis	*1 – 1.5 cm^2*
Severe Aortic Stenosis	*< 0.8cm^2*

139. Answer is A (Right ventricular hypertrophy): Harrison 18th/p 1931 *Harrison 15th/1343, Harrison 16th/ 1390; Harrison 17th/ 1467*

Mitral stenosis is associated with right ventricular hypertrophy.

Left ventricular diastolic pressure is normal in isolated MS – Harrison 16th/ 1390

Mitral stenosis : Features

- left atrial pressure is increased
- pulmonary arterial pressure is increased
- Increased right ventricular after load impedes the emptying of this chamber and Right ventricular end diastolic pressure and volume increase.
- Right ventricular hypertrophy occurs.

140. Answer is A (Mitral Stenosis): *Harrison 17th /1467*

Mid diastolic murmur with with presystolic accentuation is typically seen in mitral stenosis.

*'Mitral stenosis is associated with a low pitched rumbling diastolic murmur heard best at the apex. The murmur typically peaks during middiastole and again immediately before the first heart sound **(Pre-systolic accentuation)**'*

- Evidence Based physical diagnosis (Elsevier) 2012/397

*'Mitral stenosis is associated with a low pitched rumbling diastolic murmur heard best at the apex with the patient in lateral decubitus position. In patients with sinus rhythm, the murmur often reappears or becomes louder during atrial systole **(presystolic accentuation)'** - Harrison*

Mitral stenosis : Review

Mitral stenosis

Auscultatory findings

- **S_1 :** *accentuated.*
- **S_2 :** *Normally split S_2 with accentuated P_2*[Q]
- **Murmur :** *Low pitched*[Q]*, rumbling*[Q] *diastolic murmur*[Q] *with 'Pre-systolic accentuation' heard best at the apex in left lateral recumbent position*[Q].
- **Opening snap:** *brief, high pitched*[Q]*, early diastolic*[Q] *sound, best heard at the lower left sternal border*[Q].

X Ray findings

- *Straightening of the left border of cardiac silhouette*[Q]
- *Prominence of main pulmonary artery*[Q]
- *Dilation of upper lobe pulmonary veins*[Q]
- *Kerley B lines*[Q]
- *Backward displacement of the esophagus*[Q]

141. Answer is C (Opening snap delayed from S2): *Harrison 17th /1467*

The interval between opening snap and S2 is shortened (reduced) as severity of mitral stenosis increases.

'The opening snap generally follows the sound of Aortic valve closure (A2, S2) by 0.5 – 0.12 seconds. The time interval between S2 and OS varies inversely with the severity of MS'- Harrison 18th/1930

Features suggesting severe M.S.
• *Proximity of S2-OS gap* Q
• *Longer Duration of mid –diastolic murmur* Q

Atrial Fibrillation may be seen in severe Mitral stenosis
Mitral stenosis and mitral regurgitation are common causes of Left atrial enlargement which predisposes to AF. The probability of AF increases as severily of MS increases.

'The irregularly irregular pulse of AF usually means severe mitral stenosis except in elderly patients when AF can occur with mild mitral stenosis' - 'Clinical Methods in cardiology' by Raju (Orient Blackswan) 2003/201

Pulsatile liver may be seen in severe Mitral Stenosis
*Enlarged Pulsatile Liver is essentially a feature of Tricuspid Regurgitation*Q. *Patients with severe MS have pulmonary hypertension that may cause Tricuspid Regurgitation and result in a pulsatile liver.*
- 'Specialist Training in Cardiology' by Rao (Elsvier, India) 2007/339

142. Answer is B (Length of murmur): *Harrison 18th/p 1930, 1931; Harrison 14th/ 1313, Harrison 15th/ 1344-45, Harrison 16th/ 1391; 17th/ 1467*

'The duration of murmur correlates with the severity of stenosis - Harrison

Features suggesting severe MS are :
1. *Proximity of S2 - O.S. gap* Q, *and*
2. *Longer duration of mid-diastolic murmur* Q

143. Answer is B and C (S_2 – OS gap and Prolonged Diastolic murmur): Harrison 18th/p 1930, 1931 *Harrisons 17th/1467; Harrisons 16th/1391*

The severity of mitral stenosis may be clinically judged by the gap between the opening snap (OS) and the aortic component of second heart sound (S_2) and by the duration of diastolic murmur.

Features suggesting severe M.S.
• *Proximity of S2-OS gap* Q
• *Longer Duration of mid –diastolic murmur* Q

Mitral Regurgitation

144. Answer is C (Left Ventricular S_3) : *' The Art and Science of Cardiac Physical Examination' by Ranganathan & Value 1st/243*

The severity of Mitral Regurgitation may be judged clinically by the presence of left ventricular dilatation and the presence of third heart sound (Left Ventricular S_3). These features indicate a more severe disease

'A third heart sound (S_3) in chronic mitral regurgitation is usually indicative of severe regurgitation'

Severity of Mitral Regurgitation : Features indicating increased severity:
• ***Presence of Left ventricular S_3 or an inflow rumble at the apex***
• *Harsh Decrescendo murmur with lot of low and medium frequencies*
• *Wide split S_2 due to early A_2 (not caused by P_2 delay) in presence of MR*

Severity of Mitral Regurgitation:

1. If the murmur is harsher and has a lot of low and medium frequencies. It usually indicates a lot of flow and therefore will imply significant regurgitation.
   A harsh decrescendo mitral regurgitation murmur is usually indicative of severe regurgitation because the decrscendo effect is caused by early buildup of a very high v wave pressure in the left atrium resulting from a severe degree of regurgitation. Thus decreasing the gradient in late systole
   (If the murmur, on the other hand, is all pure high frequency and confined only to late systole. Then it must indicate a high pressure difference between the left ventricle and the left atrium and therefore only mild regurgitation).
2. When the mitral regurgitation is severe, the volume overload on the left ventricle will be high, resulting in an enlarged left ventricle. This may be reflected in a displaced hyperdynamic wide –area left ventricular apical impulse. In addition, the hyperdynamic left ventricle will have rapid ejection. This will make the A2 occur early. Resulting in a wide-split S2. Thus, a wide –split S2 in the presence of mitral regurgitation is a sign of severe regurgitation if the wide split is not caused by P2 delay.
3. In addition, severe regurgitation because of the volume load effect will have a torrential inflow through the mitral valve during diastole. This will set up the necessary conditions for the production of an S3 or a mid –diastolic inflow rumble. The presence of an S3 or an inflow rumble at the apex will, therefore, be a sign of significant mitral regurgitation as well.

<u>Note</u>

Loudness and duration of Mitral regurgitation murmur does not always correlate with the severity of the regurgitation

145. Answer is None or D (Intensity of systolic murmur across mitral valve): *References with individual options; O.P. Ghai Pediatrics 5th/ 279, 280, 281;* Harrison 18th/p 1935 *Harrison 17th/ 1470*

Intensity of Mitral regurgitation murmur does not always correlate with the severity of the regurgitation.

Probably all features mentioned in the option may suggest severe MR. The presence of systolic mumur of at least grade III/VI suggests severe MR, but no where does any text suggest that intensity of this murmur shall increase with the severity of MR. Therefore this may probably be the single best answer of exclusion.

<u>Features suggesting severe MR:</u>

• LV enlargement:	'The degree of LV enlargement usually reflects the severity of regurgitation' – *CMDT 2005/ 233*
• Wide split of S_2:	'In patients with severe MR, the aortic valve may close prematurely resulting in wide splitting of S_2' – *Harrison 16th/ 1394*
• Third heart sound 'S_3':	'A third heart sound is an important auscultatory feature of severe MR' – *Harrison 16th/ 1394*
• Fourth heart sound 'S_4':	A fourth heart sound is often audible in patients with acute severe MR of recent onset who are in sinus rhythm.
• Systolic murmur:	'A systolic murmur of at least grade III/VI intensity is the most characteristic auscultatory finding in severe MR' – *Harrison 16th/ 1394*
• Diastolic murmur:	'With severe mitral regurgitation, a delayed diastolic mitral murmur starting with the third heart sound is audible' – ***Ghai 6th/ 381*** The delayed diastolic murmur is secondary to a large flow across the mitral valve during diastole.
• Pulmonary hypertension:	Presence of features of pulmonary arterial hypertension in a patient having pure mitral regurgitations suggests, severe MR, acute MR or a failing myocardium' – *Ghai 5th/ 380*

From the above texts it is clear that all features mentioned as options may suggest severe MR. However if we focus on the option of systolic murmur which does not state merely the 'presence of a systolic murmur' but the 'intensity of systolic murmur across the mitral valve' as a reflection of the severity of MR. We may have our doubts. The presence of systolic murmur of at least grade III/VI suggests severe MR, but nowhere does any text suggest that intensity of murmur shall increase with the severity of MR..

146. Answer is A (Mitral valve repair or replacement) : Harrison 18th/p 1936 *Harrisons 16th/ 139538.5; Harrison 17th/ 1471*

"Surgical treatment of severe MR should be considered even in asymptomatic patients or those with mild symptoms whose LV dysfunction is progressive with LV ejection fraction declining below 60%" - Harrisons

Indications of surgical management :

Symptomatic patient	Asymptomatic patient	
Patients with severe MR whose limitations do not allow full time employment or the performance of normal household activities despite optimum medical management.	Asymptomatic patients when LV dysfunction is progressive	
	LVEF	Declining below 60%
	Endosystolic cavity dimension on Echo	Rising above 45mm

Mitral Valve Prolapse (MVP)

147. Answer is A (Myxomatous degeneration): Harrison 18th/p 1937 *Harrison's 17th/1472*

Presence of midsystolic click in an asymptomatic female suggests a diagnosis of Mitral Valve Prolapse (MVP). MVP is associated with myxomatous degeneration of the mitral valves.

Ruptured chordae tendinae may be seen in MVP but these patients are usually symptomatic with significant Regurgitation (MR).

Mitral Valve Prolapse Review

- Also known as *'Barlow's syndrome'* Q or *'Billowing mitral valve'* Q or *'Floppy valve syndrome'* Q.
- It is most common in *females* Q
  Most commonly seen in young adults (15 to 50 years)
  (MVP may be seen in older individuals > 50 yrs. When seen in older individuals most patients are males and MR is more common and severe and requires surgical treatment)
- Inheritance in familial cases is *autosomal dominant* Q.
- Clinical course is usually benign
  - Patients are *usually asymptomatic* Q
  - Patients may present with *non specific chest pain, dyspnea, fatigue and palpitations.* Q
- Auscultatory findings are characteristic and most important :
  - Characteristic *mid systolic* Q or late systolic *non ejection* Q *clicks* Q which may be *multiple* Q
  - Late systolic ejection murmur (Often but not always)
  - Accentuation of findings by *Valsalva and standing.* Q
  - Diminished by *squatting and isometric exercises.* Q
- Diagnosis :
  - *Investigation of choice is echocardiography.* Q
  - *ECG in most cases is normal.* Q
- Pathological Findings:
  - ***Myxomatous degeneration of mitral valve (less commonly in tricuspid and aortic valves)***
  - Elongated, Redudant or Ruptured chordae tendinae
    (patients with ruptured chordae tendinae are usually symptomatic with significant regurgitation – MR)
  - Dysfunction and ischaemia of papillary muscles
  - Progressive dilatation and calcification of mitral valve annulus
- Complications :
  - *M.R* Q.
  - *Arrythmias* Q
  - *Sudden death* Q
  - *Transient ischemic attack* Q
  - *Infective endocarditis* Q

148. Answer is B (Most patients are symptomatic): Harrison 18th/p 1937 *Harrisons 17th/1472; Harrisons 16th/1395,1396*

Most patients are asymptomatic and remain so for their entire lives- *Harrisons 17th/1972*

149. Answer is B (Mostly Symptomatic): Harrison 18th/p 1937 *Harrisons 17th/1472: Harrisons 16th/1395,1396*

Most patients are asymptamatic and remain so for their entire lives)-*Harrisons 17th/1472*

150. Answer is B (Majority of the case present with features of mitral regurgitation): Harrison 18th/p 1937 *Harrison 16th/1395, 2330; CMDT 2006/330, 331*

Majority of patients with MVP are asymptomatic *but may present with non specific chest pain, dyspnea, fatigue or palpitation. MVP has distinct auscultatory presentation in the form of mid or late non ejection systolic clicks. Mitral regurgitation is seen only as a complication of MVP resulting from rupture of chordae tendinae or failure of papillary muscles.* ***Thus although features of mitral regurgitation may be associated in cases of MVP, these are definitely not the presenting features in the majority.***

- ***Valve leaflets show myxomatous degeneration***
  'In most patients with MVP, however **myxomatous degeneration** is confined to the mitral or less commonly the tricuspid or aortic valves without other clinical or pathologic manifestations of disease' – Harrison 16th/1395
- ***Autosomal dominant inheritance***
  There is an increased familial incidence suggesting an **autosomal dominant form of inheritance'**– Harrison 16th/1395
- ***The disease is one of the common cardiovascular system manifestations of Marfans syndrome***
  'Cardiovascular abnormalities are the major source of morbidity and mortality *(in patients with Marfan's syndrome). Mitral valve prolapse develops early in life and in one quarter of patients progresses to mitral valve regurgitation of increasing severity' – Harrison 16th/2330*

151. Answer is C (Echocardiography): Harrison 18th/p 1937 *Harrison 14th/ 1317, Harrison 15th/ 1348; 16th/ 1395, 1396; Harrison 17th/ 1472*

The history suggests the diagnosis of 'Mitral valve prolapse'(MVP). Investigation of choice for MVP is Echocardiography.

152. Answer is A (Echocardiography): Harrison 18th/p 1937 *Harrison 16th/ 1396; Harrison 17th/ 1472*

The investigation of choice in MVP is echocardiography.

Two dimensional echocardiography is particularly effective in identifying the abnormal position and prolapse of mitral valve leaflets.

Aortic Stenosis

153. Answer is B (Aortic stenosis): Harrison 18th/p 1939 *Harrison 14th/ 1318, Harrison 16th/ 1397; Harrison 17th/ 1472*

Angina pectoris and Syncope are characteristic features of Aortic stenosis.

Aortic stenosis is characterized by three cardinal symptoms:
- ***Dyspnea*** Q
- ***Angina pectoris*** Q
- *Exertional syncope* Q

Aortic stenosis :

Dyspnea	*Angina pectoris*	*Syncope*
Results primarily from elevation of the pulmonary capillary pressure caused by elevation of LV diastolic pressure secondary to reduced compliance.	Reflects an imbalance between the augmented myocardial oxygen requirement (increased myocardial mass) and reduced oxygen requirement (compression of coronary vessels by hypertrophied myocardium)	Results from a decline in arterial pressure caused by vasodilation in the exercising muscles and inadequate vasoconstriction in non exercising muscles in the face of a fixed CO or from a sudden fall in CO produced by an arrhythmia.

154. Answer is C (Aortic stenosis): *Harrison 18th/p 1939 Harrisons 16th/1397; 17th/ 1473; CMDT 2006/333; CMDT 2009/302; OHCM 6th/136*

'Angina pectoris, Exertional syncope, and dyspnea (LV failure) represent the charactristic clinical triad of Aortic stenosis.' *- Harrison 16th/1397*

'Patients present with LV failure, angina pectoris or syncope *all occurring with exertion.' - CMDT 2006/ 333*

Symptoms of Aortic Stenosis

Dyspnea[Q]	**Angina Pectoris**[Q]	**Syncope (Exertional)**[Q]
• Results primarily from elevation of pulmonary capillary pressure secondary to LV failure *LVF and RVF may occur independently or together as* ***'congestive cardiac failure'****. Aortic stenosis leads to chronic excessive after load and results in LVF followed by RVF, thus presenting as CCF*	• Results from imbalance between - increased myocardial oxygen requirement from increased myocardial mass and intraventricular pressure (and) - reduced oxygen availability	Syncope occurs due to stimulation of reflex baroceptors. With exertion, the LV pressure rise stimulating these baroceptors to peripherally vasodilate. *This results in an attempt to further increase cardiac output. Syncope occurs when the stenotic valve does not allow an adequate increase in cardiac output and systemic BP falls.*

155. Answer is C (ST segment changes in ECG): Harrison 18th/p 1939 *Harrison 17th/ 1473, 1474; O.P. Ghai 5th/ 311-312, O.P. Ghai 6th/ 418*

'ST and T wave changes on ECG favour severe aortic stenosis' *– Ghai*

Thus ST segment changes in ECG is the answer of choice.

- ***Ejection click*** *is not used to assess the severity of stenosis. The later having* ***the peak of ejection systolic murmur,*** *the more severe is the stenosis.*
- ***Cardiac size*** usually remains normal and so the apex though is not shifted outwards usually.
- ***S_2*** does not show much variation in intensity. With increasing severity the S_2 follows the following order normal split → single → paradoxical split

The clinical assessment of severity of aortic stenosis depends on the following: Ghai 6th/ 418

- ***Presence of Symptoms : Symptomatic patients*** *have severe Aortic stenosis however if the patient is asymptomatic it does not rule out severe Aortic stenosis.*
- *Pulse pressure :* Narrower the pulse pressure, the more sever the stenosis
- *Systolic thrill*

Only in the suprasternal notch not at the second Rt. interspace	**Systolic thrill at the second Rt. interspace**	**Disappearance of an earlier existent thrill**
Mild or critical aortic stenosis	*Severe aortic stenosis*	*Very severe aortic stenosis*

- *Peak of the ejection systolic murmur :* The later the peak of the ejection systolic murmur, the more severe is the *stenosis*
- *S_2 Split*

Normal split	**Closely split/ Normal/ Single**	**Paradoxical split**
Mild	*Moderate*	*Severe*

- *Presence of S4*
- *Presence of S3 indicates severe aortic stenosis with congestive cardiac failure.*
- *ECG changes : ST & T wave changes in ECG*
- *X Ray chest: Cardiac enlargement*
- *Doppler echo:* Quantitative gradient

156. Answer is D (Delayed peak of systolic murmur): Harrison 18th/p 1939 *Harrison 17th/ 1474; Ghai 4th/ 255, Ghai 5th/ 312, Ghai 6th/ 417*

The ejection systolic murmur starts after the ejection click reaches a peak in midsystole.
With increasing severity of aortic stenosis the peak gets delayed so that the maximum intensity of the murmur is closer to the end rather than being midsystolic *– Ghai*

157. Answer is C (Aortic stenosis): Harrison 18th/p 2004 *Harrison 15th/ 1407; Harrison 17th/ 1519; CMDT 2005/ 330*

"Many of the traditional contraindications such as recent myocardial infarction or congestive heart failure are no longer considered if the patient is stable and ambulatory but Aortic Stenosis remains a contraindication" *- CMDT 2005 / 333*

Contraindications to exercise stress testing: *Harrisons 15th/1402*
1. Acute myocardial infarction (< 4 - 5 days)
2. Rest angina < 48 hours
3. Unstable rhythm
4. Severe Aortic Stenosis
5. Acute Myocarditis
6. Uncontrolled heart failure
7. Active infective endocarditis

Exercise testing should also not be done during an episode of unstable angina and its presence in the options confuses the issue. However, going with what CMDT has to say, aortic stenosis remains the answer of choice.

Exercise testing in unstable angina : Unstable angina is a term used to describe patients who present with rapidly worsening angina, severe angina at rest or prolonged or ischaemia chest pain without ECG or enzyme evidence of MI.

Unstable angina episode → Admit, Bed Rest, Aspirin, β blockers → Exercise Tolerance test

Exercise testing is indicated in unstable angina once the plaque has stabilized and is arranged later, in order to assess the patients need for coronary angiography if the test is positive at low work load. – Davidsons 17th / 256

158. Answer is A (Aortic Stenosis) : *Harrison's 15th / 1350*

Aortic calcification is most commonly associated with Aortic stenosis

Aortic Calcification in Aortic stenosis is usually apparent on fluoroscopic examination with an image intensifier or by echocardiography.

The absence of aortic calcification in an adult suggests that severe valvular Aortic stenosis is not present.– Harrison's

159. Answer is B > D (Aortic valve replacement > Observation) : *ACC/AHA guidelines; European Cardiology Society Guidelines;* http://circ.ahajournals.org/content/122/17/1734.full.pdf+html; http://circ.ahajournals.org/content/122/17/1734.full.pdf+html

The patient in question has asymptomatic aortic stenosis but develops symptoms on exercise (abnormal/positive exercise test). Also the presence of mean pressure gradient of 60mm Hg put this patient into the category of 'Very Severe Aortic Stenosis' or 'Critical Aortic Stenosis'.

Optimal management of asymptomatic severe Aortic Stenosis continues to be a source of ongoing clinical controversy*. Surgical Aortic Valve Replacement and Watchfull waiting with frequent reassessments (observation), both continue to be legitimate though debatable treatment options.*

Since the patient in question has 'Very Severe AS' and 'Abnormal Stress Testing' he should be considered for surgical intervention in the form of Aortic Valve Replacement (AVR).

50-year-old patient with Asymptomatic Severe Aortic Stenosis

Positive Exercise Stress Test

Symptoms during exercise such as dyspnea, angina, and syncope or near syncope constitute positive criteria indicating an abnormal stress test in patients with asymptomatic aortic stenosis.

'Severe Aortic Stenosis with an abnormal response to exercise is considered a Class IIb indication for Aortic Valve Replacement according to the ACC/AHA Guidelines.'

'Severe Aortic Stenosis with an abnormal response to exercise is considered a Class IC indication for Aortic Valve Replacement according to European Cardiology Society Guidelines (ECS Guidelines)'

Mean Pressure Gradient ≥ 60 mm Hg

Mean pressure gradient > 60 mm Hg and/or Aortic valve area < 0.6 cm^2 and /or Aortic Jet velocity > 5.0 m per second is classified as '*Extremely Severe Aortic Stenosis'* (Critical Aortic Stenosis)

'Extremely Severe Aortic Stenosis (mean gradient ≥ 60 mm Hg) is considered a class IIb indication for Aortic Valve Replacement according to the ACC/AHA Guidelines.'

Indications of AVR in Asymptomatic Severe Aortic Stenosis

Class I	Class IIb
• Patients undergoing cardiac surgery for other indications (Coronary artery bypass graft surgery or aortic surgery) • Left ventricular ejection fraction <= 50 %	• ***Abnormal Hemodynamic Response to Exercise*** (Symptoms or asymptomatic hypotension) • High Probability of rapid progression (Age, Calcification, Concomitant CAD) • ***Asymptomatic 'very severe AS'*** (*Transaortic jet velocity >=5m/s, mean gradient >=50mm Hg, aortic valve ara <=0.6 cm2*) when operative mortality is < 1%

Taken from American College of Cardiology/American Heart Association Guidelines

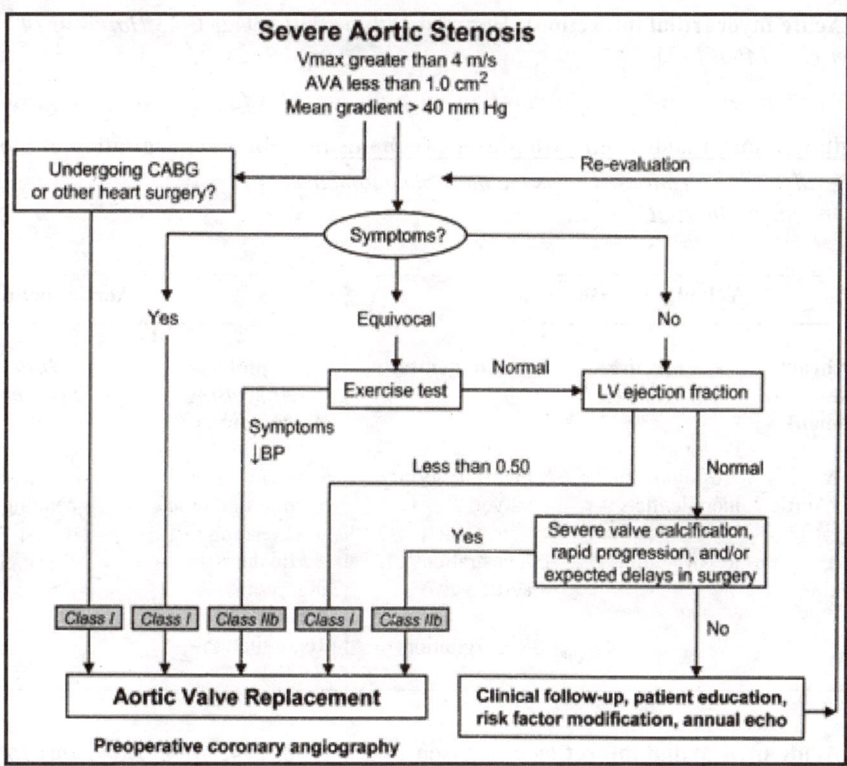

Recent studies supporting AVR in 'VERY SEVER AS':

Study	*Conclusion*
1. *'Clinical outcomes in non-surgically managed patients with very severe versus severe aortic stenosis'* *(Heart doi:0. 1136/heartjnl-2011-300137; Valvular heart disease; Original article)*	***'Surgery should always be considered in very severe AS regardless of symptoms, and particular attention needs to be paid to their extremely poor outcomes.'***
2. *'Early Surgery Versus Conventional Treatment in Asymptomatic Very Severe Aortic Stenosis'* ('Circulation': 2010; 121: 1502-1509; Valvular heart disease; Original article)	***'Compared with the conventional treatment strategy, early surgery is associated with improved survival by effectively decreasing cardiac mortality and sudden cardiac death in patients with very severe AS****. This result suggests that early surgery can be a therapeutic option to further improve clinical outcome in asymptomatic patients with very severe AS and low operative risk.'*

Classification of Aortic Valve Stenosis Severity

Severity	*Valve Area (cm2)*	*Maximum Aortic Velocity (m/sec))*	*Mean Pressure Gradient (mm Hg)*
Mild	*1.5 – 2.0*	*2.5 – 3.0*	*<25*
Moderate	*1.0 – 1.5*	*3.0-4.0*	*25-40*
Severe	*0.6-1.0*	*>4.0*	*>40*
Critical (Extremely Severe)	*<0.6*	*>5.0*	*>50-60*

2

Aortic Regurgitation

160. Answer is B (Acute myocardial infarction): Harrison 18th/p 1930, 1942, 1943 *Harrison 14th/ 1320, Harrisons 16th/ 1399; Harrison 17th/ 1466, 1475*

All options other than acute myocardial infarction are known causes for acute aortic regurgitation.

Aortic regurgitation may result from Two Major Mechanisms : allow regurgitation of blood back into LV.

1. *By causing valvular deformities. This is the most common cause*
2. *By deforming the aortic root.*

Valvular disease			Aortic root disease		
Rheumatic heart disease (most common)	***Infective endocarditis*** Q	**Congenital**	**Syphilis & *Ankylosing Spondylitis*** Q	***Marfan's Syndrome*** Q	**Idiopathic dilatation of aorta.**
- Thickening, deformation & shortening of Aortic valve cusps ↓ Regurgitation	Perforation or erosion of one or more leaflets ↓ Regurgitation	- Congenital bicuspid aortic valve - congenital fenestrations of aortic valve ↓ Regurgitation	Cellular infarction and scarring of 'media' of thoracic aorta leading to Aortic dilatation, aneurysm formation & Regurgitation	Cystic necrosis of media of the ascending aorta ↓ Dilatation ↓ Regurgitation	Osteogenesis imperfecta, & Severe hypertension ↓ widened aortic annulus ↓ Regurgitation

161. Answer is A (Acute myocardial infarction): Harrison 18th/p 1930, 1942, 1943 *Harrisons 16th/ 1399; Harrison 17th/ 1466, 1477; See previous question.*

Amongst the options provided Acute MI is most unlikely to produce Aortic regurgitation.
Acute MI is the single best answer of exclusion.

162. Answer is D (Pansystolic murmur): Harrison 18th/p 1944 *Harrisons 16th/ 1400; Harrison 17th/ 1476, 1475*

Murmur in AR : Harrison 16th/ 1400

Typical **diastolic murmur** of chronic AR	**Midsystolic** ejection murmur	Austin flint murmur (**diastolic**)
• High pitched, blowing, decrescendo diastolic murmur • Heard best in the third I.C.S. along the left sternal border Note: With marked post stenotic dilatation of aorta the murmur may be loudest in the 2nd or 3rd right interspace – API 7th/ 420	• Resembles murmur of AS but is higher pitched, shorter and less rasping • Heard best at the base of heart and is transmitted along the carotids	• Soft, low pitched rumbling middiastolic • Heard best at the apex • Produced by diastolic displacement of anterior leaflet of mitral valve by AR stream

163. Answer is A (A.R.): Harrison 18th/p 1943, 1944, 3212 *Harrison 16th/ 1399, 1400, 2329, 2330; 17th/ 1475, 1476, 1477, 1499t, 2468*

Arm span greater than height is suggestive of Marfan's syndrome. *Aortic regurgitation (A.R.) is a feature associated with Marfans as well as consistent with a diastolic murmur is second right intercostal space.*

Marfan Syndrome: Review

Marfan's syndrome is a genetic disorder of the connective tissue of the body manifested principally by changes in the skeleton, eye and cardiovascular system

Mutation in the fibrillary gene Q (15 q 21.1) Q

↓

Loss of fibrillary fibre base for deposition of elastin

↓

Altération in connective tissue in various parts of the body particularly in

Skeletal changes of marfans syndrome:	Cardiovascular changes Q	Ocular changes Q
- *Patients are usually tall* Q - *Have long limbs* Q - *The ratio of upper segment to lower segment is usually* ***2 SDs below*** *the mean for age, race &sex* - *Arachnodactyly (fingers are long and slender, spider like in appearance)* Q - *Pectus Excavation, Pectum Carinatum.* Q - *Scoliosis, Kyphosis* Q	- *Dmitral valve prolapse &* Q - *Mitral valve progresses to* ***Mitral valve Regurgitation*** - *Aortic aneurysm occurs it can leads to* ***Aortic Regurgitation.*** • **Associated changes** - *Spontaneous pneumothorax* Q - *Inguinal & incisional hernias* - *Striae may occur over the shoulders & buttocks.*	- *Dislocation of the lens* Q - *Elongation of globe (Myopia)* Q - *Retinal detachment.* Q

164. Answer is C (A.R.): Harrison 18th/p 1943, 1944, 3212 *Harrison 17th/ 1475, 1476, 1477, 2468; See previous question*

A diastolic murmur in second right intercostals space in a patient of Marfan's syndrome suggests a diagnosis of Aortic Regurgitation.

165. Answer is C (Aortic incompetance): *Harrison 15th/ 1351, 1343, Harrison 16th/ 1399; 17th/ 1476; other references.*

Aortic regurgitation is associated with LV dilatation, LV hypertrophy and LV failure

AR	The total volume ejected by the ventricle (forward stroke + volume of blood that regurgitates back into L.V.) is increased in ***A.R.*** Also, here, the entire L.V. stoke volume is ejected into a high pressure zone, the Aorta. This leads to dilatation of LV, followed by deterioration of LV function i.e. LVF; Considerable thickening of LV wall (LV hypertrophy) also occurs with chronic AR. - *Harrison 14th / 1321*
M.S.	The left ventricular diastolic pressure is *normal* in isolated ***Mitral Stenosis***. Mitral stenosis leads to elevated left atrial pressure, elevated pulmonary venous and capillary pressures, with resultant increase in right ventricular after load and ultimately RV failure. - *Harrison 14th / 1312*
ASD	An ***ASD*** allows shunting of blood from LA to RA and then to RV. It is Rt side of the heart that is primarily involved. No haemodynamic effects are seen on L.V.
Carcinoid syndrome	***Carcinoid syndrome*** may cause valvular heart disease by causing endocardial fibrosis. However it is the right side of the heart that is usually involved. Q Proximal side Q of tricuspid and pulmonary valves are involved, leading to tricuspid insufficiency or pulmonary stenosis and thereby secondary 'Right sided heart failure'. Q - *Harrison 14th / 586, 15th/597*

Pulmonic Stenosis

166. Answer is D (All of the above) : *Ghai 4th / 258, 5th/315*

Pulmonic stenosis may occur at valvular, supravalvular and subvalvular level.

Anatomically, Pulmonary stenosis may be located at:
1. Valvular level
2. Subvalvular level : This is also called *Infundibular pulmonary stenosis.*
3. Supravalvular level : This is also called *Peripheral pulmonary stenosis..*

167. Answer is C and E (William syndrome and Rubella) : *Harrisons 16th/1382, 1383; Fundamentals of Diagnostic Radiology 3rd/645*

Peripheral pulmonic stenosis is often associated with various congenital and acquired conditions including Rubella and williams syndrome.

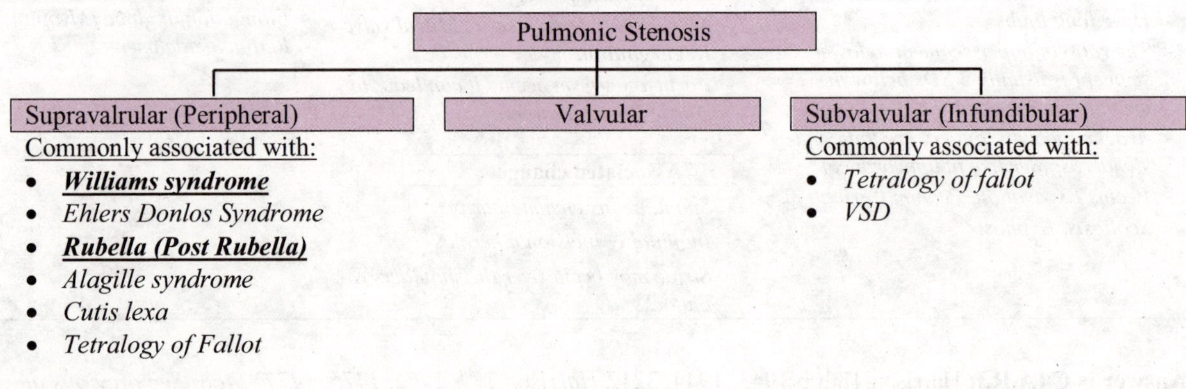

Tricuspid Regurgitation

168. Answer is B (Dilatation of right ventricle): Harrison 18th/p 1948 *Harrison 17th/1479 ; 16th/1402*

"Most commonly Tricuspid Regurgitation is functional and secondary to marked dilatation of RV and the tricuspid annulus" *– Harrisons*

169. Answer is A (Tricuspid Regurgitation): Harrison 18th/p 1948 *Harrison 17th/1479*

Systolic pulsations of the liver and marked hepatomegaly are characteristic features of Tricuspid Regurgitation.

'Hepatic pulsation in Tricuspid Regurgitation are caused by reversed systolic blood flow in the great veins' – 'Synopsis of Cardiac Physical Diagnosis 2nd/266'

'In about 2/3rd of patients with Tricuspid Regurgitation there is associated systolicpulsations of liver which may be considerably enlarged and tender' – Oxford Textbook of Medicine 4th/1012.

Ischemic Heart Disease and Atherosclerosis

Risk Factors / Atherosclerosis:

170. Answer is C (Decreased fibrinogen levels): Harrison 18th/p 1987 *Harrison 16th/1430, 1432; Harrison 17th/ 1505 http://www.ncbi.nlm.nih.gov/entrez/query.fcgi?cmd=Retrieve&db=PubMed&list_uids=1998650&dopt=Abstract*

Increased levels of fibrinogen (and not decreased fibrinogen levels) are associated with increased risk of atherosclerosis.

- ***Fibrinogen Levels***
  'Fibrinogen levels correlate with coronary risk and provide information regarding coronary risk independent of lipoprotein profile. Elevated fibrinogen levels might promote a thrombotic diathesis'. - Harrison 16th/1432
- ***Waist Hip Ratio :*** This refers to a characteristic 'male' distribution of adipose tissue i.e. excess of fat in the abdomen compared with that in hips.
  'An elevated waist/hip ratio has been associated with symptomatic cardiovascular disease and cerebrovascular disease in both men and women. *- Pubmed (NCBI - website)*
- ***Hyperhomocysteinemia and low HDL levels*** are known risk factors for Atherosclerosis (as depicted in the following table).

Major risk Factors for Atherosclerosis - *Harrisons 16th/1430*
• *Cigarette smoking*
• *Hypertension (BP > 140/90mm/hg) or (on Antihypertensive medication)*
• ***Low HDL cholesterol***
• Diabetes mellitus
• Family history of CHD
• Age (Men > 45 years; Women ≥ 55 years)
• Life style risk factors
Obeity (BMI > 30 kg/m²)
Physical inactivity
Atherogenic diet
Emerging risk factors
• Lipoprotein (a)
• ***Homocystine***
• Prothrombotic factors (Fibrinogen)
• Pro inflammatory factors
• Impaired fasting glucose
• Subclinical atherogenesis

171. Answer is A (hs CRP): *Braunwald's 8th/1013, 1014*

hs CRP which is a serum marker of systemic inflammation has emerged as a major risk factor marker for future cardiovascular events

CRP and Future risk of cardiovascular events

- *CRP when measured by high sensitivity assays (hs CRP) strongly and independently predicts risk of Myocardial Infarction, Stroke, Peripheral Arterial disease and Sudden Cardiac Death among healthy individuals*
- hs CRP adds prognostic information at all levels of LDL cholesterol and at all levels of risk as determined by the Framingham risk score
- ***hs CRP is a better predictor of cardiovascular risk than lipoprotein 'a', homocysteine or interleukin 6 and an elevated hs CRP carries a significantly higher relative risk of future cardiovascular events than any of the other individual factors***
- Infact hs CRP may be a better predictor of cardiovascular risk than elevated LDL cholesterol levels
  'Absolute vascular risk is higher in individuals with elevated hs CRP levels and low levels of LDL cholesterol than in those with elevated levels of LDL cholesterol but low levels of hs CRP'
- hs CRP interpretation

Hs CRP levels	Risk
<1 mg/l	Low
1 – 3 mg/l	Moderate
> - 3 mg/l	High

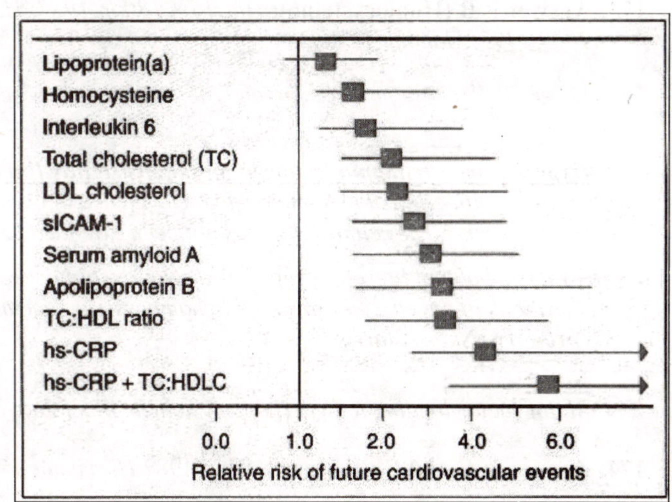

hsCRP, high reactivity C-reactive protein;
siCAM-1, soluble intercellular adhesion molecule-1;
HDLC, high density lipoprotein cholesterol

172. Answer is A (hs CRP): *Braunwald's 8th/1013, 1014*

hs CRP which is a serum marker of systemic inflammation has emerged as a major risk factor marker for future cardiovascular events

CRP and Future risk of cardiovascular events

- *CRP when measured by high sensitivity assays (hs CRP) strongly and independently predicts risk of Myocardial Infarction, Stroke, Peripheral Arterial disease and Sudden Cardiac Death among healthy individuals.*
- *hs CRP* adds prognostic information at all levels of LDL cholesterol and at all levels of risk as determined by the Framingham risk score
- ***hs CRP is a better predictor of cardiovascular risk than lipoprotein 'a', homocysteine or interleukin 6 and an elevated hs CRP carries a significantly higher relative risk of future cardiovascular events than any of the other individual factors***
- Infact hs CRP may be a better predictor of cardiovascular risk than elevated LDL cholesterol levels
  '*Absolute vascular risk is higher in individuals with elevated* hs CRP *levels and low levels of LDL cholesterol than in those with elevated levels of LDL cholesterol but low levels of hs CRP*'
- hs CRP interpretation

Hs CRP levels	Risk
<1 mg/l	Low
1 – 3 mg/l	Moderate
> - 3 mg/l	High

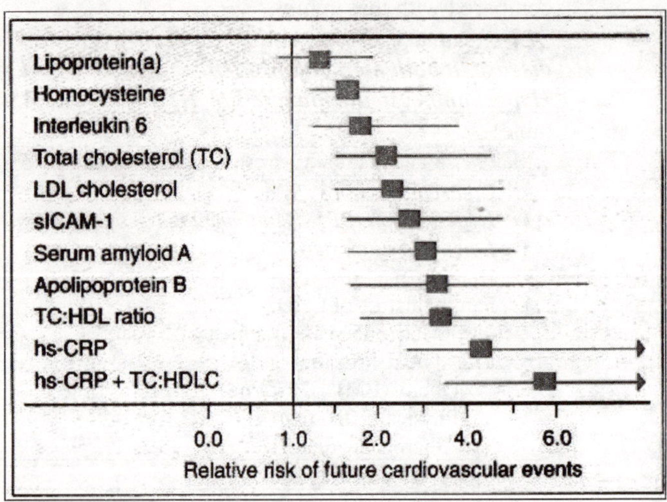

hsCRP, high reactivity C-reactive protein;
siCAM-1, soluble intercellular adhesion molecule-1;
HDLC, high density lipoprotein cholesterol

173. Answer is B (Homocysteine): *Harrison 18th/p 1987; Harrison 16th/1430,1432; 17th/1505; CMDT 2006/1706; 2009/1497; Ganong 22nd/623*

'There is a strong positive correlation between atherosclerosis and circulating levels of Homocysteine'

- Ganong 22nd/623

Hyperhomocysteinemia has been most consistently linked with atherosclerosis and coronary thrombotic events

"Patient with clinical and angiographic evidence of coronary artery disease tend to have higher levels of plasma homocysteine. The relationship has not been extended to cerebrovascular and peripheral vascular disease"- CMDT

"A large body of literature suggests a relationship between ***hyperhomocysteinemia and coronary events.*** *Several mutations in the enzymes involved in homocysteine accumulation correlate to* ***thrombosis*** *and (in some studies)* ***coronary risk"*** *-. Harrison*

Note :
Major factor leading to hyperhomocysteinemia is folate deficiency – CMDT

174. Answer is C and E : Harrison 18th/p 1987 *Harrisons 17th/1505 : Harrisons 16th/1430, 1432*

Increased homocysteine levels and increased lipoprotein (a) levels are risk factors for cornonary artery disease

Increased risk of coronary artery disease is also associated with:

- *High LDL (not low LDL)*
- *Low HDL (not high HDL)*
- *Increased Fibrinogen levels (not decreased fibrinogen levels)*

175. Answer is B (↑ Lipoprotein B): *Robbin's illustrated 7/e, p 520; Harrison's 16/e, p 1430-1433*

Predisposing factors for coronary artery disease include an increased lipoprotein 'a' and not lipoprotein 'b'.

176. Answer is C (Atherosclerosis): Harrison 18th/p 1987 *Harrison 17th; Ganong 20th/600*

Raised levels of lipoprotein a is a risk factor for Atherosclerosis

'In addition to a high cholesterol level there is a positive correlation between atherosclerosis of coronary artery and other arteries and circulating levels of lipoprotein-(a)".
Lp(a) interferes with fibrinolysis by down regulating plasmin generation and thus contibutes to atherosclerosis.

177. Answer is C (Nephrotic syndrome) : *Read text below*

Nephrotic syndrome is associated with hyperlipidemia with an increased level of LDL and cholesterol in most patients. This hyperlipidemia may accelerate atherosclerosis and increase the susceptibility to coronary artery disease

Type V hyperlipoprotenemia is associated with normal / low levels of LDL and does not appear to increase the risk of CHD.

Hyperlipidemia in Nephrotic syndrome may accelerate Atherosclerosis

- Hyperlipidemia is part of the clinical complex of Nehrotic syndrome

Nephrotic syndrome is a clinical complex characterized by -
Proteinuria
Hypoalbuminemia
Edema
Hyperlipidemia / Lipiduria

- Hyperlipedemia in Nephrotic syndrome is a consequence of increased hepatic lipoprotein synthesis
Low density lipoproteins and cholesterol are increased in majority of patients
This Hyper lipidemia ***may accelerate atherosclerosis*** and progression of Renal disease - *Harrison's*

Hyperlipidemia in Type B hyperlipoprotenemia does not appear to increase risk of CHD

- *This disorder does not appear to increase risk of CHD* either because large trylyceride rich lipoproteins are not atherogenic or because only normal amount of LDL can be generated - *Harrison's*

Condition	Risk Of Coronary Artery Disease
Type I (Familial Hyper Chylomicronemia)	*Not increased*
Type II A (Familial Hyper Cholesterolemia)	Accelerated
Type II B (Familial Combined Hyperlipidemia)	Accelerated
Type III (Familial Dysbetalipoprotenemia	Accelerated
Type IV (Familial Hyper Triglyceredemia)	Accelerated
Type V (Familial Mixed Hypertriglyceredemia)	***Not increased***

- *Hyperlipidemia in type V hyperlipoprotenemia is not associated with increased LDL*

Type V hyper liprotenemia :
VLDL and Chylomicrons are increased
LDL is normal or decreased

178. Answer is A (LDL/HDL Ratio): *Braunwald 8th/1008*

LDH/HDL Ratio is the strongest predictor of risk of cardiovascular disease amongst the options provided

The ratio of either LDL cholesterol to HDL Cholesteral or Total cholesterol to HDL cholesterol is highly predictive of CHD in elderly people – Essential Cardiology 2nd/6

Risk Factors for atherosclerosis and cardiovascular complications (Braunwald)

- Abnormalities in plasma lipoproteins and derangement in lipid metabolism rank as the most firmly established risk factors for atherosclerosis.
- Adusted relative risk for future cardiovascular events for selected lipid fractions and lipid ratios in decreasing order are given in the following table.

Relative risk for future cardio vascular events	Lipid Fractions and Lipid Ratios
Decreasing Predictivity of Risk	• *Total chotesterol: HDL Cholestrol Ratio (TC: HDLC)* • *Apopratein B100: HDL Cholesterol Ratio (APo B100: HDLC)* • *LDL Cholesteral : HDL Cholesterol Ratio (LDLC: HDLC)* • *Apoprotein B100: Apoprotein A-1 (APO B100: APO A1)* • *Non HDL Cholesterol fraction* • *Apolipoprotein B-1 Fraction* • *HDL cholesterol Fraction* • *Total cholesterol Fraction* • *Apolipoprotein A1 Fraction* • *LDL cholesterol Fraction*

179. Answer is D (LDL/HDL): *Braunwald 8th/1008; Essential Cardiology 2nd/ 6; Refer previous quetion*

LDL / HDL ratio is the strongest predictor of risk of cardiovascular disease, amongst the options provided

'The ratio of either LDL cholesterol to HDL cholesterol (LDH / HDL ratio) or Total cholesterol to HDL cholesterol (TC /HDL ratio) is highly predictive of coronary heart disease' – Essential cardiology 2nd/6

180. Answer is D (Avoid Alcohol): *Braunwald 8th/1110, 1112, 1114; 'Clinical Lipidology:Companion to Brounwald's Heart Disease' 1st(2009)/203-204*

Avoidance of alcohol is not part of dietary recommendation in patients with CHD.

'Moderate alcohol consumption is strongly and consistently associated with lower risk of CHD than either abstention or higher in takes. Current recommendations from AHA (American Heart Association) and the U.S. Dietary Guidelines Advisory committee are that men who drink alcohol may consume upto two alcoholic beverages per day, and women no more than one per day' – Braunwald 8th/1110

Saturated fats should be limited to < 7% of total calories

Recent guidelines from AHA recommend consumption of < 7% of calories as saturated fat'-*Braunwald 8th/1112*

NCEP – ATP III Guidelines (National Cholesterol Education Programme-Adult Treatment Panel)

The NCEP – ATP III guidelines have placed major emphasis on *Therapeutic Lifestyle change (TLC)* as an essential modality in clinical management of patients at risk of CHD.
The '*Therapeutic Lifestyle Change'* Diet is designed to achieve risk reduction and makes recommendations regarding nutrient compositions in diet to reduce LDL levels and metabolic syndrome

Nutrient Composition of the Therapeutic Lifestyle Changes Diet

Nutrient	Recommended Intake
Saturated fat	<7% of total calories
Polyunsaturated fat	Up to 10% of total calories
Carbohydrate	Up to 20% of total calories
Fiber	20-30 g/d
Protein	Approximately 15% of total calories
Cholesterol	<200 mg/d
Total Calories	Balance energy intake expenditure to maintain desirable body weight/prevent weight gain

AHA recommends limiting salt intake to < 6gm/day to reduce risk of CHD

'Available data support the current AHA guideline of limiting salt intake to 6 gm/day, the equivalent of 100 mmol of sodium (2400 mg) per day' - Braunwald 8th/1114

LDL cholesterol < 100 mg/dl is recommended for patients with high risk of CHD

'The goal of LDL-lowering therapy in high risk patients is an LDL cholesterol level of < 100 mg/dl'

- 'Clinical Lipidology: A companion to Braunwald's Heart Disease' 1st (2009) /203

NCEP – ATP III Guidelines (National Cholesterol Education Programme-Adult Treatment Panel)

According to NCEP-ATP III Guidelines persons are categorized *into three risk categories* depending or the presence of established CHD and risk factors. *Patients with established coronary heart disease (CHD) and CHD risk equivalents are considered high risk.*

CHD risk equivalent's include non coronary forms of clinical at atherosclerotic disease, diabetes and multiple risk factors with 10 year risk of CHD > 20%

The goal for LDL levels is determined by the risk category as detailed in the table below.

For high risk patients with established CHD or CHD risk equivalents the LDL levels are targeted at < 100 mg/dl.

Three categories of Risk that modify Low Density Lipoprotein Cholesterol Goals	
Risk category	LDL Goal (mg/dl)
CHD and CHD risk equivalents	<100
Multiple (2+) risk factors	<130
0-1 risk factors	<160

Major risk factors (Exclusive of LDL Cholesterol) that modify LDL Goals
• Cigarette smoking
• Hypertension (blood pressure ≥140/90 mmHg or on antihypertensive medication)
• Low HDL cholesterol (<40 mg/dL)
• Family history of premature CHD (CHD in male first-degree relative <55 years; CHD in female first-degree relative <65 years)
• Age (men ≥ 45 years; women ≥ 55 years)

181. Answer is D (Omega 3 Polyunsaturated Fatty Acids); *American Heart Association (AHA) Dietry Guidelines (2000)/http://csre.aha journals.org/cgl/content/full/02/18/2284; Braunnwald 8th/1108 http://circ.ahajournals.org/cgl/content/full/02/18*

Consumption of Omega 3 PUFA is associated with reduced total mortality and sudden cardiac death in patients with ischemic heart disease

***A number of studies have reported that consumption of Omega 3 fatty acids confers protection from ischaemic heart disease and that this relationship is particulary strong for coronary heart disease mortality and sudden cardiac de**ath*

– Branuwald 8th/1108

High fibre diet: *Fibre supplements may reduce levels of total cholesterol and LDL Cholesteral, and may cause a reduction in coronary heart disease. However use of high fibre diet has not shown any benefit in overall mortality from CHD and has not yet been recommended for risk reduction in CHD by the American Heart Association (AHA)*

Sterol Esters: Sterol esters containing food have been documented to decrease Total Cholesterol levels and LDL cholesterol levels. They may be recommended in selected individual with hypercholesterolemia for lowering of total and LDL cholesterol levels and for secondary prevention after an atherosclerotic event.

However the use of these agents require further monitoring as concerns have been raised regarding their tendency to decrease B cortene (vitamin A) and α-tocopherol (vit-E) levels. A clear benefit in reduction of mortality has not been documented

Omega 3 PUFA: Omega 3 PUFA have been documented to decrease total mortality and sudden death in patients with ischaemic heart disease. Benefit are most prominently reported with Omega 3 PUFA's derived from marine sources, namely Eicosopentanoic acid (EPA) and ducosahexanoic acid (DHA)

The supplemental use of Omega 3 Fatty acids (EPA plus DHA) has been recommended by the American Heart Association (Braunwald 8th/1108).

Pottassium Supplements: *These agents have not been recommended by the American heart association for risk reduction in patients with coronary heart disease.*

Beneficial cardiovascular effects of selected dietry components
Preventive Cardiology by Wong, Black, and Gordon/320

• *Omega 3 Fatty, Acids*	*↓↓Triglycerides, ↓ Platelet Aggregation*
• *High Fibre Diet*	*↓Total cholesterol, ↓ LDL Cholesterol*
• *Sterol esters (Phytosterols)*	*↓ Total cholesterol, ↓ LDL Cholesterol*
• *Soy protein*	*↓Triglycerides, ↓ LDL Cholesterol*
• *Vitamin E*	*↓LDL oxidative susceptibility*
• *Vitamin C*	*Recycles vitamin E*
• *Folic Acid/Vitamin B6*	*↓Homocystine Levels*
• *Moderate Alcohol Consumption*	*↑HDL Cholesterol* *↓Blood clotting coagulation*

182. Answer is C (Increased LDL and Decreased total cholesterol)
Comprehensive management of high tisk cardiovascular patients by cotte Toth and braunwald (2006)/367; Brawnwald 8th/1108

The major effect of Omega -3-polyunsaturated Fatty Acids on plasma lipids is to decrease serum triglyceride levels. They do not have a consistent effect on total cholesterol and LDL cholesterol however most studies have reported a rise in LDL cholesterol and a decreased in total cholesterol.

Increased LDL and Decreased total cholesterol is the single best answer of choice

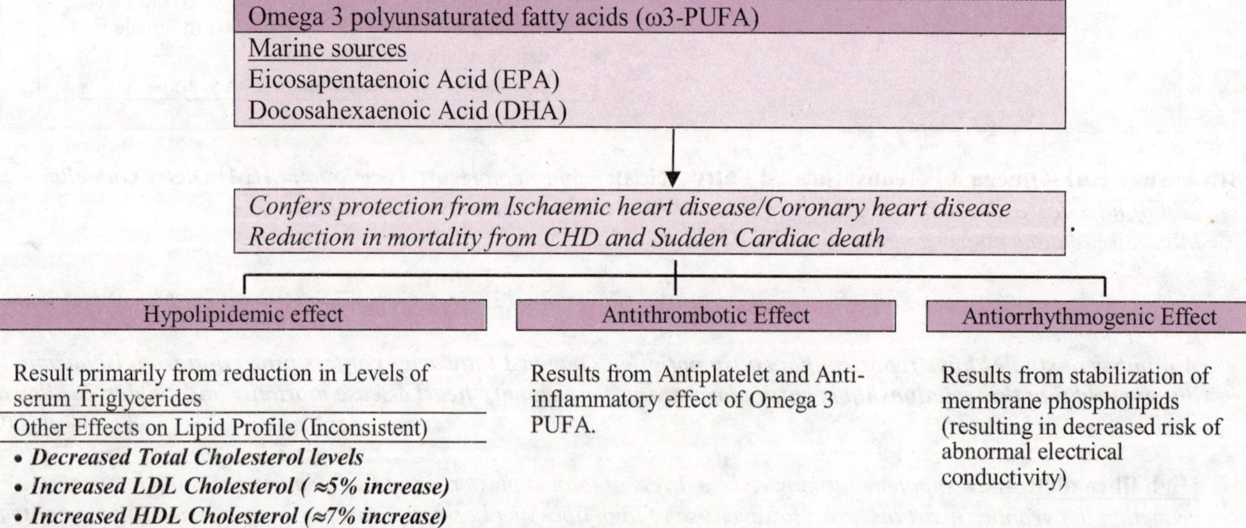

Effect of omega 3 fatty acids on LDL levels
(Atherothrombosis and coronary Artery Disease by Fuste, Topel and Nobel /41)

- *In patients with high triglycerides omega 3 PUFA cause on increase in LDL cholesterol*
- *In patients with normal triglycarides omega 3 PUFA do not decrease LDL cholesterol*
- *When omega 3 PUFA are used in place of saturated fatty Acids LDL cholesterol levels decline (but this effect is same as that found with use of other types of PUFA).*

183. Answer is A (Intake of Unsaturated Fatty Acids is associated with decreased risk): *Reference with text*

Intake of Unsaturated Fatty Acids (PUFA > MUFA) is associated with decreased risk of Atherosclerosis.

The maximal benefit is observed with Omega 3 Poly-unsaturated Fatty Acids, however Mono-unsaturated Fatty Acids also have consistent anti-atherosclerotic benefits and both Poly-unsaturated Fatty Acids (PUFA) and Mono-unsaturated Fatty Acids (MUFA) are considered Cardioprotective Fatty Acids.

Hypercholestoremia alone may increase the risk of Atherosclerosis

'Hyperlipidemia and more specifically hypercholesterolemia is a major risk factor for atherosclerosis. Even in the absence of other factors, hypercholesterolemia is sufficient to stimulate lesion development'. – Robbins 8th/497

Extent of Athrosclerosis is more severe in arteries than in veins

Atherosclerosis is always severe in areas where pressure and velocity are high (as in arteries) in contrast to areas where pressure and velocity are low (as in veins).

'Overall atherosclerosis is more severe in high-pressure arteries than in pulmonary arteries with lower blood pressure. It is least severe in veins where pressure and velocity are lowest' – 'Pan – Vascular Medicine' by Topol (2002)/90

Abdominal Aorta is more commonly involved than Thoracic Aorta

'Abdominal Aorta is more commonly involved than Thoracic Aorta. Within the abdominal aorta lesions tend to be more prominent around the ostia' – 'Med Essentials' (Kaplan Publishing) 2007/249

'In the systemic circulation severity is accentuated in the abdominal aorta and large arteries of the lower limb where pulse wave reflection and summation effect elevate the pulse and systolic pressures. The disease is more severe in large rather than small vessels indicating the importance of mural tension and Reynolds number both of which are proportional to radius increasing the likelihood and severity of effects of blood flow disturbance at arterial forks, junctions and curvatures'.- 'Pan Vascular Medicine' by Topal (2002)/90

Myocardial Infarction / Angina

184. Answer is D (Three times increase in Troponin levels after Coronary Artery Bypass Grafting (CABG): *'Universal Definition of Myocardial Infarction': Expert Consensus Document Circulation 2007 (American Heart Association Journals); 'ECS-ACCF-AHA-WHF Universal Definition of Myocardial Infarction'; http://circ.ahajournals.org/content/116/22/2634.full.pdf*

Myocardial Infarction associated with CABG is defined by an increase in cardiac biomarkers to more than 5 times normal (> 5 times above the 99th percentile).

Universal Defination of Myocardial infarction

Myocardial infarction related to ischemia due to primary coronary event (plaque rupture) ***or imbalace between oxygen demand and supply*** (coronary spasm, hypotension etc)	***Myocardial Infarction related Sudden Cardiac Death*** (Death occuring before blood samples could be obtained, or at a time before the appearance of cardiac biomarkers in the blood.)	***Myocardial Infarction associated with PCI*** (in patients with normal baseline troponin values)	***Myocardial infarction associated with CABG*** (in patients with normal baseline troponin values,)
Detection of rise and/or fall of cardiac biomarkers (preferably troponin) with at least one value above the 99th percentile of the upper reference limit (URL) together with evidence of myocardial ischaemia with at least one of the following: • Symptoms of ischaemia • ECG changes indicative of new ischaemia [new ST-T changes or new left bundle branch block (LBBB)] • Development of pathological Q waves in the ECG • Imaging evidence of new loss of viable myocardium or new regional wall motion abnormality.	*Sudden, unexpected cardiac death, involving cardiac arrest, often with :* • ***Symptoms suggestive of myocardial ischaemia***, and accompanied by • New ST elevation, or new LBBB, and/or • Evidence of fresh thrombus by coronary angiography and/or at autopsy,	• ***By convention, increases of biomarkers greater than 3 x 99th percentile*** *URL have been designated as defining PCI-related myocardial infarction.*	• ***By convention, increases of biomarkers greater than 5 x 99th percentile*** URL plus either new pathological Q waves or new LBBB, or angiographically documented new graft or native artery occlusion, or imaging evidence of new loss of viable myocardium have been designated as defining CABG-related myocardial infarction.

Universal Definition of Myocardial Infarction:

Criteria for acute myocardial infarction

The term myocardial infarction should be used when there is evidence of myocardial necrosis in a clinical setting consistent with myocardial ischaemia.

Under these conditions any one of the following criteria meets the diagnosis for myocardial infarction.

- Detection of rise and/or fall of cardiac biomarkers (preferably troponin) with at least one value above the 99th percentile of the upper reference limit (URL) together with evidence of myocardial ischaemia with at least one of the following:
  - Symptoms of ischaemia
  - ECG changes indicative of new ischaemia [new ST-T changes or new left bundle branch block (LBBB)]
  - Development of pathological Q waves in the ECG
  - Imaging evidence of new loss of viable myocardium or new regional wall motion abnormality.
- *Sudden, unexpected cardiac death*, involving cardiac arrest, often with symptoms suggestive of myocardial ischaemia, and accompanied by presumably new ST elevation, or new LBBB, and/or evidence of fresh thrombus by coronary angiography and/or at autopsy, but death occuring before blood samples could be obtained, or at a time before the appearance of cardiac biomarkers in the blood.
- *For percutaneous coronary interventions (PCI)* in patients with normal baseline troponin values, elevations of cardiac biomarkers above the 99th percentile URL are indicative of peri-procedural myocardial necrosis. By convention, increases of biomarkers greater than 3 x 99th percentile URL have been designated as defining PCI-related myocardial infarction. A subtype related to a documented stent thrombosis is recognized.
- *For Coronary Artery Bypass Grafting (CABG)* in patients with normal baseline troponin values, elevations of cardiac biomarkers above the 99th percentile URL are indicative of peri-procedural myocardial necrosis. By convention, increases of biomarkers greater than 5 x 99th percentile URL plus either new pathological Q waves or new LBBB, or angiographically documented new graft or native artery occlusion, or imaging evidence of new loss of viable myocardium have been designated as defining CABG-related myocardial infarction.
- *Pathological findings* of an acute myocardial infarction

Criteria for prior myocardial infarction

Any one of the following criteria meets the diagnosis for prior myocardial infarction

- Development of new pathological Q waves with or without symptoms
- Imaging evidence of a region of loss of viable myocardium that is thinned and fails to contract, in the absence of a non-ischaemic cause.
- Pathological findings of a healed or healing myocardial infarction.

Taken from :Expert Consensus Document Circulation 2007 (American Heart Association Journals); 'ECS-ACCF-AHA-WHF Universal Definition of Myocardial Infarction'; http://circ.ahajournals.org/content/116/22/2634.full.pdf

185. Answer is A (Anterior wall of left ventricle) : *Robbins 6th/557*

The most common site of myocardial infarction is the anterior wall of the left ventricle.

The frequency of critical narrowing of arterial trunks and corresponding sites of myocordial lesions are as follows :

Left anterior discending (LAD) (br. of LCA)	40 to 50% (Most common)	Anterior wall of L.V. near apex Anterior portion of ventricular septum
Right coronary artery (RCA)	30 to 40%	Inferior/Posterior wall of L.V Post. portion of ventricular septum Inferior/posterior right ventricular free wall in some cases
Left circumflex (br. of LCA)	15 to 20%	Lateral wall of left ventricle except the apex.

186. Answer is B (Left ventricle) : *Robbins 6th / 557*

The most common site of myocardial infarction is the anterior wall of Left ventricle.

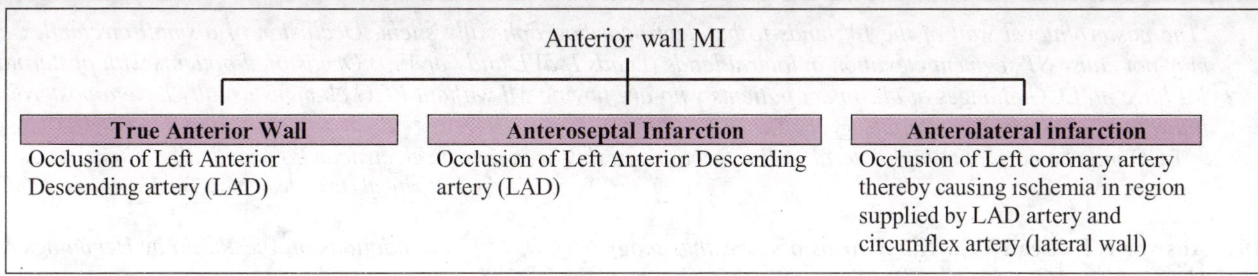

187. Answer is A (Anterior wall): *Repeat*

The most common site of myocardial infarction is the anterior wall of left ventricle.

188. Answer is D (Marginal artery): *Robbin's 7th/577-578; Snell's 7th/117-119*

Marginal branches are not commonly involved.

The frequency of critical narrowing of arterial trunks

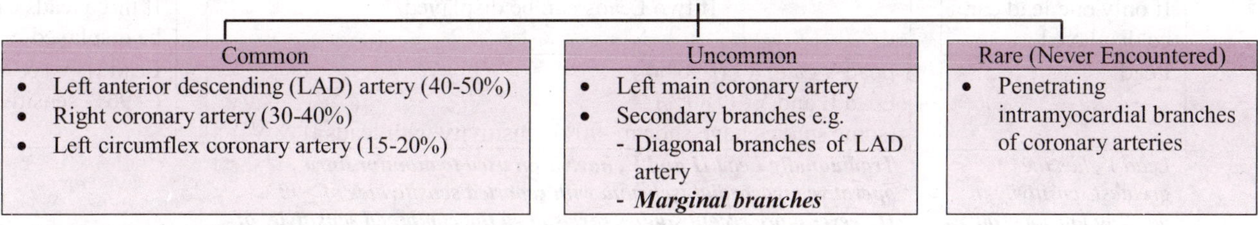

189. Answer is C (Tall T waves with increased amplitude): *Harrison 18th /1836*

Acute myocardial infarction is associated with 'ST segment' elevation and tall, positive, hyperacute T waves (increased amplitude of T waves).

'When the acute ischemia is transmural, the ST vector usually is shifted in the direction of outer layers (epicardial), producing ST elevation and sometimes in the earliest stages of ischemia, tall, positive so called hyperacute T waves over the ischemic zone'- Harrison's 18th / 1836

E.C.G. changes in acute infarction

Early acute phase *(within hours)*	**Fully evolved phase**	**Old infarction** *(resolution phase)*
• *Elevation of ST segment* • ***Tall wide (peaked) T wave***	• *Pathological Q wave* • *Elevated ST segment beings to resolve* • *T wave inverts*	• *Pathological Q wave* • *ST segment and T wave may be normal*

190. Answer is B (Left Circumflex (LCx)): *References with text*

Ischemia in the distribution of Left Circumflex Artery is difficult to detect on standard 12 lead ECG

'Circumflex distribution ischemia is notoriously silent on an ECG as the posterolateral wall is under-represented on a conventional 12 lead ECG' – 'Manual of cardiovascular medicine' by Griffin 3rd/528

'A normal ECG does not exclude acute MI especially when the Left circumflex is the culprit vessel because most of the area supplied by the LCx is not represented in the standard 12 lead ECG'

– 'Basic and Bedside Electrocardiography' by Baltazar (Lippincott Williams, 2009) 1st /344

'Acute Myocardial Infarctions in the distribution of the circumflex artery are likely to have non diagnostic ECG'

– 'Management of Acute Coronary Syndromes' by Cannon (2003) /213

There are areas of the heart that are difficult to 'see' with the ECG particularly in the left circumflex distribution Small areas of ischemia may be missed altogether – 'Cardiovascular Biomarkers' by Morrow (2006)/182

'The posterolateral wall of the LV tends to be electrocardiographically silent. Occlusion of a small circumflex artery may not cause ST segment elevation in lateral leads (Leads I, aVL and / or V_{5-6}).Occasional patients with posterolateral MI have no ECG changes at all. Infact patients who are having MI without ECG changes usually have a posterolateral infarction' – Primary Care Cardiology' by Taylor 2nd/139

'ECG *may be normal in high lateral wall infarctions as this area may be electrocardiographically 'Silent'*

– 'Critical care Medicine : The Essentials' (2009)/385

191. Answer is E (Lead V_5): *Yao & Artusio's Anesthesiology 6th/149, 150; Foundations of Anesthesia by Hemmings & Hopkins 2nd/ 160, 161; Cardiac Surgery in the Adult by Cohn 3rd/285*

The most sensitive lead in detecting intraoperative myocardial ischemia is lead V_5

'If only one lead can be displayed V5 should be used because V5 has the greatest sensitivity: 75% intraoperatively and 89% during exercise treadmill testing'-Yao & Artusio's Anesthesiology: Problem Oriented Patient Management 6th/-150

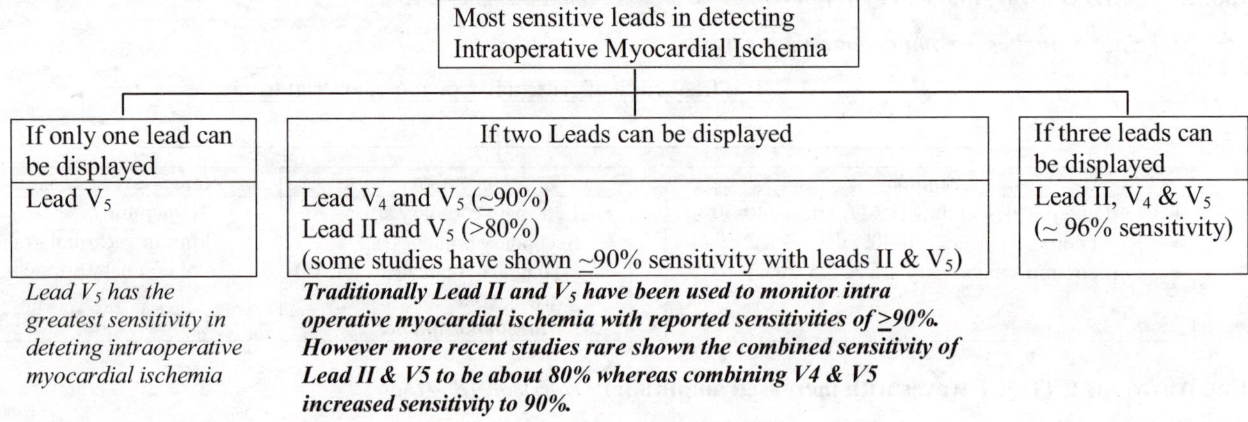

192. Answer is A (Anterolateral wall): *Chandrasoma Taylor 3rd/ 361; Robbins illustrated 6th/ 557; 7th/578*

Occlusion of anterior descending branch of left coronary artery leads to infarction of anterior wall of LV with or without involvement of the septum *– Chandrasoma Taylor 3rd/ 361*

The site of involvement of Arteries and the corresponding sites of myocardial lesions:

Left anterior descending artery (40-50%)	Right coronary artery (30-40%)	Left circumflex artery (15-20%)
• *Anterior wall of left ventricle near apex*Q • *Ant. portion of ventricular septum*Q • *Apex Circumferentially*Q	• *Inf. post. wall of left ventricle*Q • *Post. portion of ventricular septae*Q • *Inf. post. right ventricular free wall in some cases*Q	• *Lateral wall of left ventricle except at apex*Q

193. Answer is A (An ECG): *Harrison 18th/p 2001; Harrison 16th/1449-1450; Harrison 17th/ 1517*

The patient in question may well be suffering from an acute myocardial infarction. An ECG to exculde an acute MI should be the initial Investigation.

'Presence of Epigastric pain in association with breathlessness and evidence of parasympathetic overactivity (bradycardia and hypotension) suggests the diagnosis of an acute (inferior) MI.' ECG therefore should be done as an initial investigation to exclude / confirm a diagnosis of acute MI.'

The following lines from Harrison give away the answer to the question :

- 'Typically the pain involves the central portion of chest and / or epigastrum'.
- 'The frequent location of the pain beneath the xiphoid and patients denial that they may be suffering a heart attack are chiefly responsible for the common mistaken impression of indigestion.
- In the elderly, MI may present with sudden onset breathlessness.
- Although many patients have a normal pulse and blood pressure about one fourth of patients with anterior infarction have manifestations of sympathetic nervous system hyperactivity (tachycardia and / or hypertension) ***and upto one half with inferior infarction show evidence of parasympathetic hyperactivity (bradycardia and / or hypotension)***.

194. Answer is D (The levels of cardiac markers remain unchanged): *Harrison's 15th/ 1401; Harrison 16th/1444; Chandrasoma Taylor 3rd/ 366*

Necrotic myocardial fibres release a variety of enzymes into blood stream.
In stable angina necrosis of the cell does not occur so there is no elevation of serum enzymes.

Stable angina	Unstable angina	Variant angina (Prinzemetal angina)
• Chest pain or arm discomfort on effort that is - relieved within 5' – 10 minutes by rest and or sublingual nitroglycerine. - Reproduced by physical exertion or stress • No elevation of cardiac enzymes	• Anginal pain or discomfort when - it occurs at rest usually lasting > 10 min - it becomes distinctly more severe, prolonged or frequent (crescendo pattern) • No elevation in cardiac enzymes	• Anginal pain that occurs at rest, not related to excretion, with transient ST elevation and is produced due to focal spasm of an epicardial coronary artery leading to severe myocardial ischaemia. • Small elevations of cardiac enzymes may occur.

When a patient with unstable angina develops elevated cardiac biomarkers a diagnosis of Non ST-elevation MI is established.

195. Answer is C (ST segment elevation): Harrison 18th/p 2023 *Harrison 17th/ 1533; Read text below; Repeat*

E.C.G. changes in acute infarction

Early acute phase *(within hours)*	Fully evolved phase	Old infarction *(resolution phase)*
• *Elevation of ST segment* • *Tall wide (peaked) T wave*	• *Pathological Q wave* • *Elevated ST segment beings to resolve* • *T wave inverts*	• *Pathological Q wave* • *ST segment and T wave may be normal*

196. Answer is A (Anterolateral wall MI) : Harrison 18th/p 1836 *Harrisons 17th/1393 Braunwald 8th/176*

Acute transmural Anterolateral wall ischaemia is associated with changes in one or more of the precordial leads (V1 through V6) and in leads I and aVL

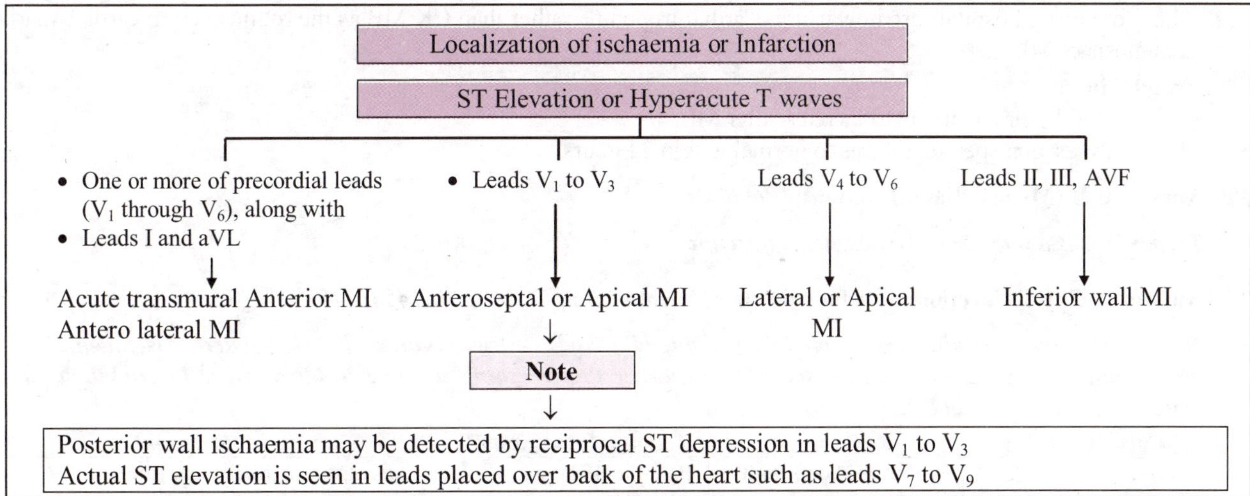

197. Answer is C (Creatinine phosphokinase): *Chandrasoma Taylor IIIrd / 365;*

Creatinine phosphokinase is seen at 2-4 hours, peaks at 24 hours and return to normal by 72 hours.

Enzyme	Seen at	Peaks at	Returns to Normal
CPKMB	2-4 hrs[Q]	24 hr[Q]	72 hr[Q]
LDH	24 hr	4-5 days	After 10 days[Q]
AST or SGOT	Within 12 hr	48 hrs	4-5 days[Q]

LDH and AST are non specific and there use now is limited

Other features

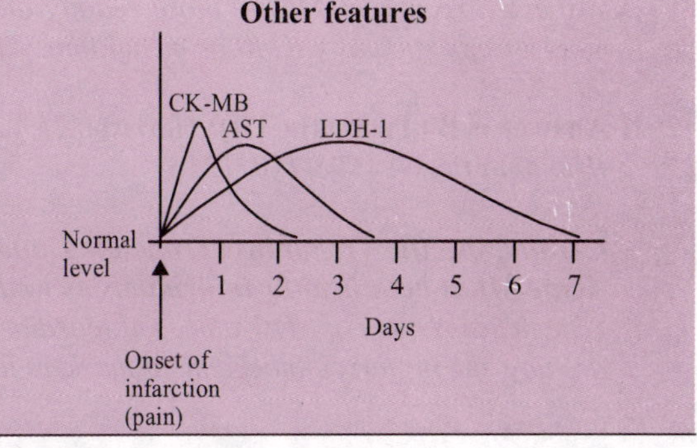

Creatinine phosphokinase MB (CPKMB)

- **Very sensitive** (*CPK MB isoenzyme increases the specificity)*
- *'Absence in change in levels of CPK and CPKMB during the 1st 2 days essentially excludes the diagnosis of MI' – Chandrasoma*
- *CK elevation used to be test of* **choice** *in First 24 hours.***('Cardiac troponins are now preferred').**
- *CKMB is still the test of choice for detecting recurrent ischaemic event.*

198. Answer is B (Cardiac troponins): Harrison 18th/p 2016, 2023, 2024 *Harrison 16th/ 1451; Harrison 17th/ 1528, 1534*

***'Cardiac troponins are now the preferred biochemical markers for MI'** – Harrison's 16th/ 1450*

Cardiac troponins

- Cardiac specific troponin T and cardiac specific troponin I are now the preferred biochemical markers for MI – Harrisons 16th/ 1451
- Many hospitals are now using cTnT or cTnI rather than CkmB as routine serum cardiac marker for diagnosis of AMI.
- They are not normally detectable in blood of a healthy individual but may increase after myocardial infarction to levels over 20 times higher
- They are particularly valuable where there is clinical suspicion of either skeletal muscle injury or a small myocardial infarction that may be below the detection limit of CK and CKMB.

Marker	Rise	Remains elevated for
Troponin I	Within 4-8 hours	7-10 days
Troponin T	Within 4-8 hours	10-14 days

Creatinine phosphokinase:

- 'CK-MB' was until recently considered the test of choice in diagnosis of acute MI in first 24 hours.
- The CK-MB isoenzyme may be elevated following cardiac surgery, myocarditis, and electrical cardioversion and therefore many hospitals are now using. Cardial troponins rather than CK MB as the routine serum cardiac marker for diagnosis of MI.

Myoglobin

- It is one of the first markers to increase after MI.
- It is however non specific returns to normal within 24 hours.

199. Answer is D (Myocardial infarction): *Robbin's 7th/557*

Troponin T is a marker of Myocardial infarction.

200. Answer is C (Reinfarction after four days): *Harrison 18th/p 2024; 16th/ 1450, 1451; 17th/ 1534*

Because cardiac troponins are elevated for prolonged periods (> 1 week) an episode of recurrent ischaemia after four days would be more readily diagnosed with a marker that remains elevated in blood more briefly such as cKMB which returns to normal levels by 72 hours.

Cardiac Marker	Seen	Returns to Normal	Features
CK MB	Within 2-4 hours with	By 24 to 48 hours	Quiet specific (MB isoenzyme)
Troponin - I	Within 4-8 hours	After 7 to 10 days	Cardiac specific
Troponin- T	Within 4-8 hours	After 10 to 14 days	Not detectable in blood of normal individuals

Limitation of troponin measurements :

Because these markers remain elevated for prolonged periods (> 1 week) episodes of recurrent ischemic discomfort and suspected recurrent MI are more readily diagnosed with a serum cardiac marker that remains elevated in the blood more briefly such as CKMB or myoglobin. – Harrison 16th/ 1451

201. Answer is B (Troponin T/I): *Harrison 18th/2023, 2024; 'Point-f-Care Testing' 2nd/305; 'Cardiac Markers' by Wu (Humana Press) 1998/120, 121*

Cardiac specific Troponins (Troponin T and Troponin I) are the biochemical markers of choice for detection of Acute MI in both healthy individuals as well as atheletes.

'The measurement of cTnT and cTnI (cardiac specific Troponin T & I) is of considerable diagnostic usefulness and they are now the preferred biochemical markers for MI' – Harrison's 18th/2023

CK-MB isoenzyme is not a sensitive marker for AMI in Athletes

- The MB isoenzyme of CK has the advantage over total CK that it is not present in significant concentration in extracardiac tissue and therefore is considerably more specific. CK-MB rises within 4-8 hr after Acute MI and elevated *CK-MB is accepted as a sensitive marker for diagnosis of Acute Myocardial Infarction in healthy individuals*.
- *Individuals who train for long distance races (Athletes like marathan runners) however have been observed to have very high resting concentration of CK-MB in skeletal muscles*. This may be owing to an adaptation by the athelete to produce a higher relative content of CKMB within skeletal muscles themselves.
- *Studies of CK-MB levels in trained marathan runners have reveaked that total CK and percentage of MB isoenzyme is asymptomatic runners have been comparable to levels of CK and CKMB in patients with myocardial Infarction.*

> *'Because of nonspecificity of CKMB fraction in runners (atheles) the measurement of this isoenzyme is of little value in making an early diagnosis of myocardial injury in athelets. A measurement of troponin I is much better because it is specific for cardiac injury' – 'Point-of-Care Testing' 2nd/305*

Enzyme	Seen at	Peaks at	Returns to Normal
CPKMB	4-8 hrs[Q] ***(H 18th/2024)***	24 hr[Q]	72 hr[Q]
LDH	24 hr	4-5 days	After 10 days[Q]
AST or SGOT	Within 12 hr	48 hrs	4-5 days[Q]

LDH and AST are non specific and their use now is limited

Cardiac Marker	Seen	Returns to Normal
CK MB	Within 4-8 hours	By 24 to 48 hours
Troponin - I	Within 4-8 hours	After 7 to 10 days
Troponin- T	Within 4-8 hours	After 10 to 14 days

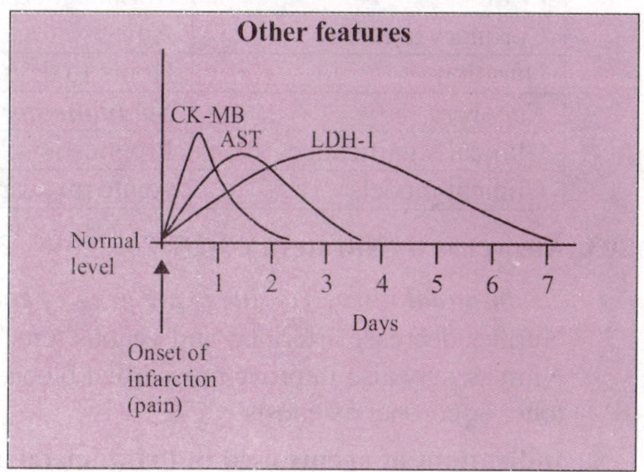

202. Answer is B (Hibernating Myocardium): *'Panvascular Medicine' by Topal (Springer) 2002/735; 'Ischemic Heart Disease' by Falk (Manson Publishing)/2010/46, 47; 'Stress Echocardiography' by Picano (Springer) 5th/274*

The contractile function of Hibernating Myocardium can be completely restored after reperfusion.

'Hibernating Myocardium is a reversible state of contractile dysfunction observed in the course of chronic ischemia associated with reduction of coronary blood flow without major evidence of irreversible myocardial damage (viable myocardium). The contractile function of the hibernating myocardium can be almost completely restored after reperfusion (revascularization)' – 'Panvascular Medicine' by Topal (Springer) 2002/735

Stunned Myocardium	Hibernating Myocardium
• 'Stunned Myocardium refers to a state of post-ischemic '*reversible*' myocardial contractile dysfunction ***that persists despite myocardial reperfusion.*** • Myocardial stunning essentially describes the post-ischemic metabolic and contractile compromise in viable myocardium after a transient coronary occlusion (i.e. post successful reperfusion in AMI). • In stunned myocardium contraction does not return to baseline for a prolonged period of time after restoration of blood supply and the eventual recovery of contractile dysfunction is believed to be 'spontaneous'. • Stunned myocardium is typified by a normal or near normal regional blood flow and represents a mismatch between flow and function.	• Hibernating myocardium refers to a state of ischemic (chronic) *reversible* myocardial contractile dysfunction ***that is almost completely restored after myocardial reperfusion.*** • Myocardial Hibernation essentially describes a chronic state of contractile dysfunction at rest in non-infarcted viable myocardium as a result of persistently reduced blood flow, which has the potential to improve function after restoration of myocardial blood supply. • In Hibernating myocardium the eventual return of contractile dysfunction is believed to be directly related to myocardial reperfusion/revascularization. • Hibernating myocardium is typified by reduced regional blood flow and reduced flow matches contractile dysfunction.

Conceptual model of myocardial stunning	Conceptual model of hibernating myocardium
Acute coronary occlusion ↓ Ischemic ventricular dysfunction ↓ *Early reperfusion* ↓ *Persistent ventricular Dysfunction* —(Inotropic Stimulation)→ Improved ventricular function ↓ Delayed spontaneous recovery of ventricular function	**Chronic** severe coronary stenosis ↓ Chronic reduction in blood flow and ischemia ↓ Myocardial metabolic adaptation ↓ Chronic contractile dysfunction —(Inotropic Stimulation)→ Improved Contractile function ↓ Revascularization Improved contractile function

Features	Stunned Myocardium	Hibernated Myocardium
Resting function	Depressed	Depressed
Flow	*Normal/Increased*	*Decreased/Normal*
Coronary anatomy	Any	Severe stenosis or occlusion
Duration	Hours to days	Days to months
Recovery	***Spontaneous***	***After revascularization***
Clinical significance	Prognostic	Therapeutic
Clinical models	Acute myocardial infarction	Ischemic cardiomyopathy

203. Answer is B (Nitrates): *CMDT 2002/ 392; 2008/ 307; CMDT 2009/316; Harrison's 16th/ 1448; Harrison 17th/ 1531*

"Sublingual nitroglycerine is the drug of choice" *– CMDT*

Nitrates decrease arteriolar and venous tone, reduce preload and afterload, and reduce the oxygen demand of the heart. Nitrates may also improve myocardial blood flow by dilating collateral channels in the presence of increased vasomotor tone, or coronary stenosis.

Indications of agents used in Prinzemetal angina :

Sublingual nitroglycerine	:	Abolish episodes of variant angina promptly
Long acting nitrates	:	Useful in preventing recurrences.
Calcium channel blockers	:	Extremely effective in prevention of coronary artery spasms of prinzemetal angina.
Beta blockers	:	Response is variable

204. Answer is C (Early Primary coronary intervention): Harrison 18th/p 2027; *17th/1537; Braunwald 8th/1233 to 1333*

Streptokinose (Thrombolysis) is a form of Reperfusion therapy that is indicated for only ST Elevation MI (STEMI). Its use is contraindicated in cases of Non ST Elevation MI (NSTEMI)

Early Primary Coronary Intervention (Early PCI) can be used as a form of Reperfusion therapy for both STEMI and NSTEMI. Early Primary Caronary Intervention is therefore the single best answer of choice amongst the options provided.

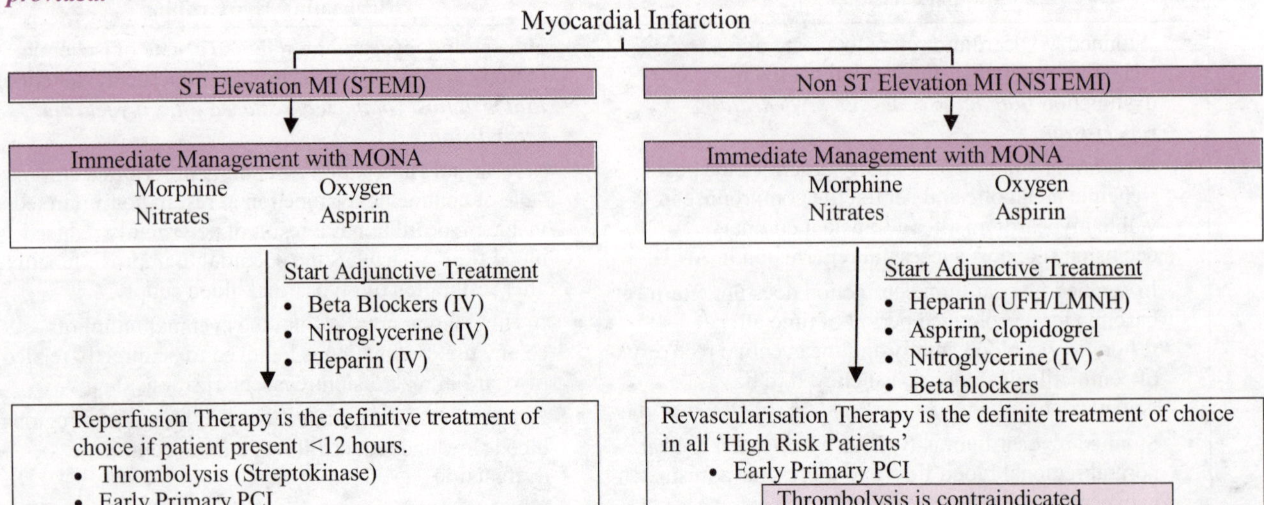

205. Answer is B (Early Revascularization with PCI): *Refer text below*

The patient presenting as a case of NSTE M I to the emergency department.

The presence of elevated cardiac troponins and history of previous PCI place the patient into a high 'risk category'.

The Patient in question is thus a 'high risk' patient with NSTEMI
Such patients are candidates for early invasive management with PCI/CABG.

Management of NSTEMI

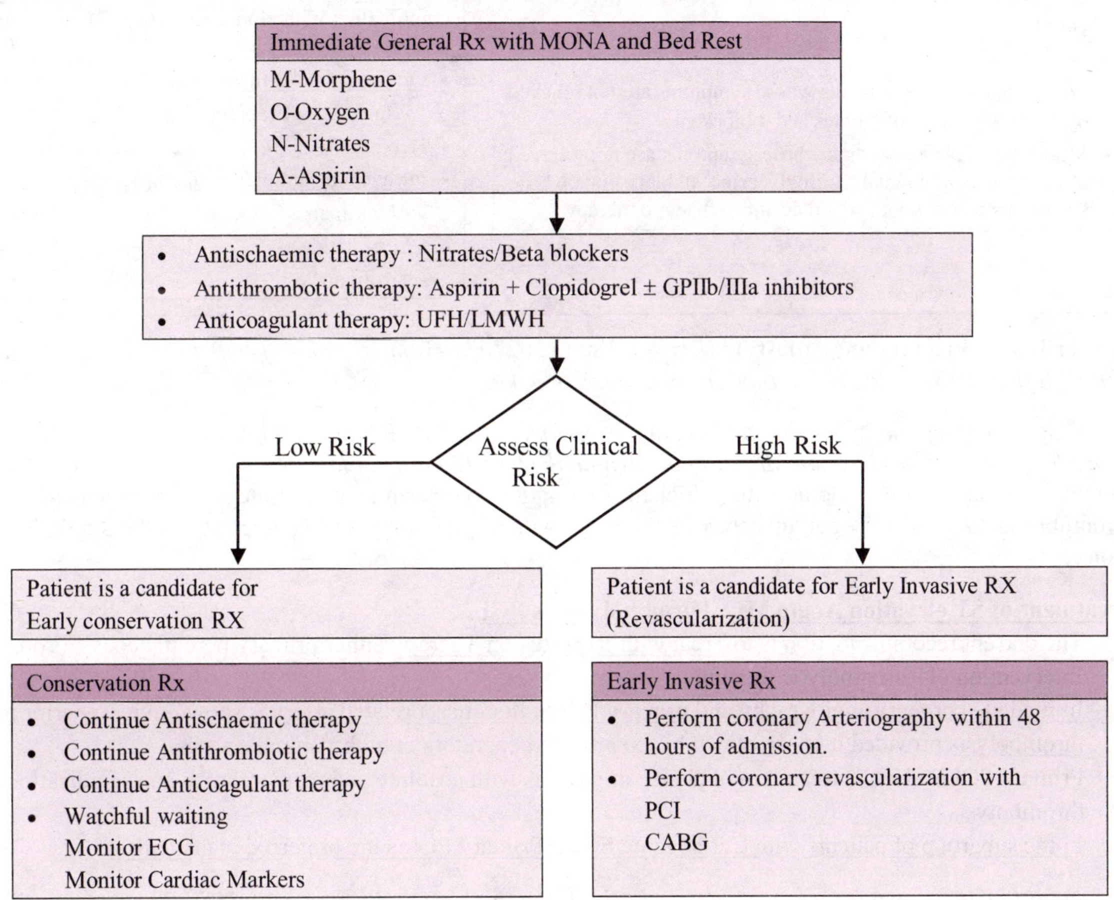

206. Answer is D (Lidocaine by Bolus infusion): Harrison 18th/p 2016-2020 *Harrison's 15th/ 1408, 16th/ 1446, 1447; 17th/ 1529, 1530, 1531*

This patient with several risk factors for ischaemic heart disease and chronic exertional dyspnea now develops 'several daily' episodes of chest pain and 'pain at rest' suggesting a diagnosis of U.A (or NSTEMI). While nitrate are recommended as the initial antiischaemic treatment, aspirin and heparin form part of antithrombotic treatment. Lidocaine is not indicated.

Unstable angina is defined as angina pectoris or equivalent ischaemic discomfort with at least one of three features :

1.	it occurs at rest or with minimal exertion usually lasting > 10 min.
2.	it is severe and of new onset (i.e. within the prior 4-6 weeks)
3.	it becomes distinctly more severe prolonged or frequent then previously i.e. crescendo pattern.

Non ST elevation MI: If a patient with clinical features of unstable angina develops evidence of myocardial necrosis (elevated cardiac enzymes) a diagnosis of NSTEMI is established.

Management of unstable angina/ NSTEMI

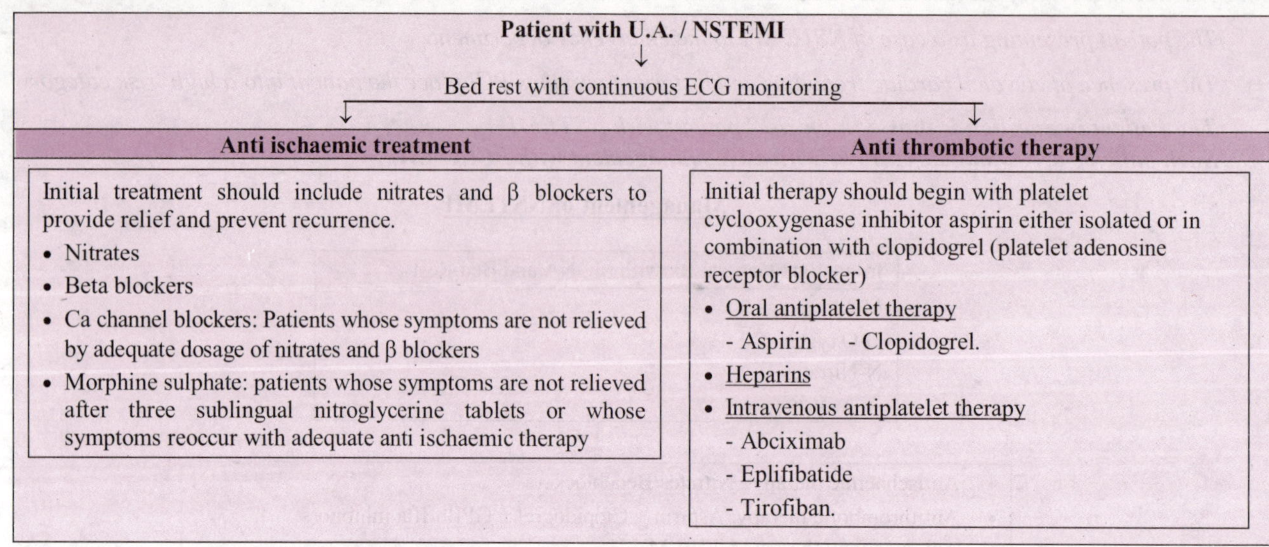

207. Answer is a D (Primary angioplasty) : Harrison 18th/p 2027 *Harrison 16th/1453, 1460; 17th/ 1537;CMDT 2006 / 38 360; CMDT 2009/314; ALS resusci-tation council UK 5th / 4*

Immediate coronary angiography and primary percutaneous intervention (angioplasty stenting) is the treatment of choice for patient of ST elevation MI presenting within the first 12 hours of MI.

The question does not provide us with sufficient information to determine best strategy of management. Presuming all favourable factors, primary percutaneous intervention with angiography and angioplasty is the single best answer of choice.

Treatment of ST elevation Acute MI : Thrombolysis vs PCI

- The current recommendation is to Treat with Reperfusion Therapy either primary percutaneous Coronary Intervention of Thrombolytic therapy.
- Immediate coronary angiography and primary PCI of the infarct related artery is shown to be superior to thrombolysis provided it is performed by experienced operators in high volume centres.
- Primary PCI is also the treatment of choice in patients with absolute and many relative contraindications to thrombolysis.
- In the subgroup of patients with Cardiogenic Shock Primary PCI is the preferred management.

The patient in question has an acute anterior wall infarction along and is presenting with hypotension (? Cordiogenic shock). Angiography will primary PCI (Angiopathy) is the recommended / ideal immediate modality of treatment.

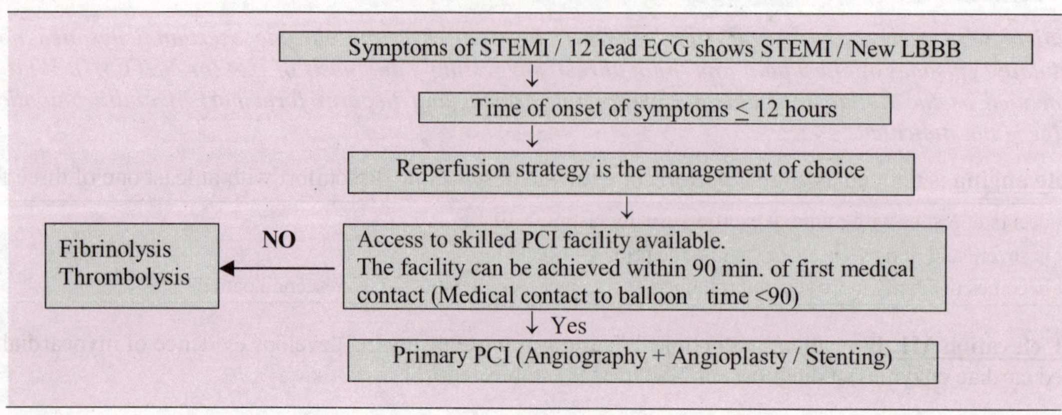

208. Answer is D (Streptokinase): *Refer previous question*

The patient is presenting as a case of Non ST Elevation MI (NSTEMI).
Thrombolytic therapy is reserved for patient with STEMI and is not indicated in NSTEMI.

209. Answer is A (Aspirin): Harrison 18th/p 2025, 2029 *Harrison 17th/1535,1538; Hurst 12th/1378*

Aspirin decreases mortality in myocardial infarction and should be administered as early as possible and in patients with Acute coronary syndromes including STEMI*-Hurst*

Althrough reperfusion therapy (Thrombolytic therapy) forms the main goal of management in STEMI, administration of Aspirin should not be delayed while patient is being assessed for suitability of thrombolysis. Aspirin has been shown to offer nearly as great an advanteage as that of streptokenose alone in certain trials. Aspirin should be administered as soon as a patient presents with any suspected Acute coronary syndrome including STEMI (As soon as possible)

210. Answer is D (Calcium channel blockers): Harrison 18th/p 2026 *Harrison 15th/1389, 1390; 16th/1455; 17th/1536; CMDT 2004/ 344*

'Results of multiple trials of different calcium antagonists have failed to establish a role for these agents in the treatment of most patients with MI, in contrast to the more consistent data that exist for other drugs eg. beta blockers, aspirin and fibrinolytic agents. The routine use of calcium channel blockers can not be recommended'
– Harrisons 16th/ 1455.

Management of acute MI

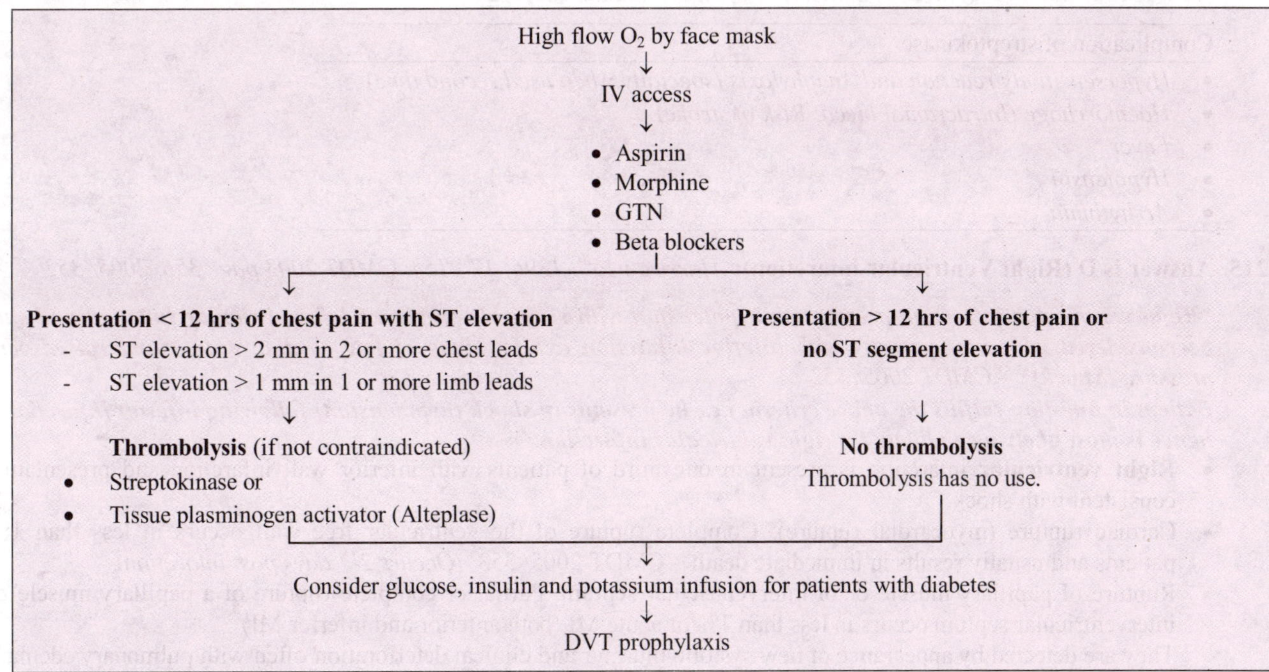

211. Answer is B (Plasminogen activator inhibitor): *Harrison 17th/1536; CMDT 2008/317*

Plaminogen Activators are used in MI and not inhibitors of Plasminogen activators.
The management of MI requires fibrinolysis, which is achieved by Plasminogen activators and not by Plasminogen inhibitor.

212. Answer is D (Warfarin): Harrison 18th/p 2030 *Harrison 17th/1539; CMDT 2008/317, 318, 320*

Warfarin is not indicated in the immediate management of Acute myocardial infarction.
Warfarin is the single best answer of exclusion.

Aspirin and Heparin *are used in early treatment of Acute Myocardial infarction to prevent thrombosis.*
Alteplase or Tissue Plasminogen Activator *is a thrombolystic agent and is indicated early in the treatment of STEMI.*

213. Answer is A (Intracranial malignancy): *Braunwald's 8th/1237*

Malignant Intracranial Neoplasm is an absolute contraindication for Thrombolysis (Streptokinase / Urokinase).

Contraindications and Cautions for Fibrinolytic Use in STEMI:

Absolute Contraindications	Relative Contraindications
• Any prior intracranial hemorrhage • Known structural cerebral vascular lesion (e.g., arteriovenous malformation) • ***Known malignant intracranial neoplasm (primary or metastatic)*** • Ischemic stroke within 3 months (Except acute inschemic stroke within 3 hr.) • Suspected aortic dissection • Active bleeding diathesis (excluding menses) • Significant closed head or facial trauma within 3 mo.	• History of chronic severe poorly controlled hypertension • Severe uncontrolled hypertension on presentation (SBP > 180 Hg or DBP > 110 Hg) • History of prior ischemic stroke > 3 months, dementia, or known intracranial pathology not covered in contraindications • Traumatic or prolonged (>10 min) CPR or major surgery (<3 wk) • Recent (within 2-4 week) internal bleeding • Non compressible vascular punctures • For streptokinase/anistreplase: prior exposure (>5 days ago) or prior allergic reaction to these agents • Pregnancy • Active peptic ulcer • Current use of anticoagulants (the higher the INR, the higher the risk of bleeding)

214. Answer is A (Joint Pain): Harrison 18th/p 2028 *KDT 6th/606; Harrison 17th/1538*

Joint pain is not a recognized complication of streptokinase usage.

Complication of streptokinase
• *Hypersensitivity reaction and Anaphylaxis (specially when used second time)*
• *Haemorrhage (Intracranial bleed: Risk of stroke)*
• *Fever*
• *Hypotensin*
• *Arrhythmia*

215. Answer is D (Right Ventricular infarction): *Harrison 15th/ 1396; 17th/154, CMDT 2003 page 356, 2005/ 352*

"Right ventricular infraction presents as hypotension with relatively preserved left ventricular function and should be considered whenever patients with inferior infarction exhibit signs of low cardiac output and raised venous pressure (Shock)" *– CMDT 2005/ 352*

Patient in question fulfills the above criteria i.e., he presents in shock (hypotension) following inferior infarction and hence is most likely a candidate for right ventricular infarction.

- **Right ventricular** infarction is present in one third of patients with inferior wall infarction and presentation is consistent with shock.
- Cardiac rupture (myocardial rupture): Complete rupture of the ventricular free wall occurs in less than 1% of patients and usually results in immediate death – CMDT 2005/ 353 *(Occurs 2-7 days post infarction)*
- Rupture of papillary muscle or of interventricular septum: Partial or complete rupture of a papillary muscle or of interventricular septum occurs in less than 1% of acute MI (both anterior and inferior MI)
  They are detected by appearance of new systolic murmur and clinical deterioration often with pulmonary edema.

216. Answer is A (Fluids): Harrison 18th/p 2032 *Harrison 17th/1541; Harrison pretest based on Q. 32 15th/e*

The man in question has a right ventricular infarction as indicated by signs of low cardiac output and shock following an inferior MI. The fact that right atrial pressure is elevated out of proportion to left atrial pressure almost confirms the diagnosis. Therapy consists of volume expansion or fluid loading to maintain adequate RV preload.

Pulmonary Artery pressure	22/4 mmHg	Represent Right Atrial pressure
Pulmonary Capillary Wedge pressure	4 mmHg	Represents Left Atrial pressure

Cardiac output is depressed due to an insufficient left heart filling pressure. The best treatment consists of administration of fluids.

217. Answer is A (I.V. fluids): *Harrison 14th/ 1361; Harrison 16th/1456; Harrison 17th/1541* Harrison 18th/p 2032

Inferior wall MI suggests that the patient has right ventricular infarction. Therapy usually consists of volume expansion or fluid loading to maintain adequate R.V. preload.

218. Answer is A (I.V. fluids): *Harrison 14th/ 1361, Harrison 15th/ 1396; Harrison 17th/1541;* Harrison 18th/p 2031 *CMDT 2005/ 352*

Inferior wall MI suggests that the patient has right ventricular infarction.
R.V. infarction should be considered whenever a patient with inferior wall infarction exhibits signs of low cardiac output and raised venous pressure with or without hypotension.
Therapy essentially consists of volume expansion or fluid loading to maintain adequate R.V preload, and efforts to improve left ventricular performance with a tendent reduction in PCWP and pulmonary arterial pressure.

2

219. Answer is C (Right Ventricular infarction): Harrison 18th/p 2031 *Harrison 17th/1541; CMDT 2005/352; Repeat*

'Right ventricular infarction should be considered whenever a patient with inferior infarction exhibits signs of low cardiac output and raised venous pressure' *– CMDT*
Mitral regurgitation, decreased ejection fraction and septal defect are features of anterior wall MI.

220. Answer is B (Mitral regurgitation): *Harrison 14th/ 1362; Harrison 15th/ 1396; Harrison 16th/ 1450; 17th/ 1533* Harrison 18th/p 2022

The most common valvular lesion seen in MI is mitral regurgitation.
The reported incidence of these murmurs of MR during first few days of onset of MI varies widely from 10 to 50 percent of patients – Harrison 14th

- Dysfunction of mitral valve apparatus with a transient midsystolic or late systolic apical systolic murmur (regurgitant murmur) may be present as part of the physical findings of MI – Harrison 16th/7
- The most common cause of MR following MI is dysfunction of mitral valve due to ischaemia or infarction.

221. Answer is D (External cardiac rupture): *Harrison 14th/1362; 15th/1396; 16th/not elaborated in text. 17th/1491, 1492*

Typical symptoms of sudden decrease in B.P. and electromechanical disassociation seen in the first week of M.I., point to the diagnosis of External cardiac rupture.

Risk factors	Clinical presentation
1. Increasing age 2. History of hypertension 3. First infraction 4. No history of angina 5. Large Q wave infarct 6. Presentation during first week following MI.	Sudden loss of pulse. BP consciousness while ECG continues to show sinus rhythm i.e. ***electromechanical dissociation.***

The patient in question fulfills most diagnostic features leading us to a diagnosis of Myocardial free wall rupture.

222. Answer is A (Complete heart block): *CMDT 2008/323; 'Cardiology Secrets 2nd/113*

Complete heart block is not a cause for new onset systolic murmur after Acute Myocardial Infarction.

Cause of new systolic murmur after Acute Myocardial infarction
• *Papillary muscle dysfunction/rupture (causing severe mitral regurgitation)* • *Rupture of interventricular septum* • *Right ventricular infarction and tricuspid regurgitation* • *Free wall rupture* • *Left ventricular outflow tract obstruction*

Note:
Ischemic cardiomyopathy *is defined as dilated cardiomyopathy in a subject with history of MI. This may lead to papillary muscle dysfunction and hence produce a new onset systolic murmur.*

223. Answer is A (Occurs with in hours after myocardial infarction): D. Responds well to salicylates *Robbin's illustrated 7th/ 557*
Dressler's syndrome develops after an interval of 1 to 4 weeks (or even month) following cardiac injury (MI) and not within hours.

Dressler's syndrome / Post Cardiac Injury Syndrome
• *Dressler's syndrome refers to an acute form of pericarditis that develops after myocardial infarction* • ***The pericarditis typically develops 1 to 4 weeks following cardiac injury / MI but may appear after several months*** • ***Recurrence may be seen sometimes upto 2 years or more after MI / Injury*** • *Pathological pericarditis may be of the fibrinous variety* • *The mechanism is not certain but they are believed to result from a hypersensitivity reaction in which the antigen originates from the injured myocardial tissue.* • *Circulating antibodies to myocardium occur frequently.* • ***The principal symptom is 'chest pain' of acute pericarditis.*** • *Leukocytosis, ↑ESR and ECG changes of acute Pericarditis may also occur.* • ***The pericarditis is usually resolves in 1 to 2 weeks and often no treatment is necessary apart from aspirin, NSAIDS or analgesics.*** • ***Therepy with NSAIDS or corticosteroids is usually effective.***

224. Answer is B (Thallium scan): Harrison 18th/p 2024 *Harrison 17th/1534, Pathophysiology of Heart Disease br 'Lilly' 4th/68*

Reversible Myocardial Ischemia can be detected by myocardial perfusion imaging using compounds labeled with thallium- 201 (Thallium Scan)

What is Reversible Myocardial Ischemia: Role of Thallium scanning
• Reversible myocardial ischemia refers to areas of myocardium that become ischemic on stress /exercise, but region viability / circulation on resting and do not progress to infarction • Such areas of myocardium can be detected by myocardial perfusion imaging using the Thallium scan. • Thallium scan can thus help in distinguishing between on ischemic area (reversible) and an infracted / scarred area of myocardium (irreversible)

Thallium Scanning

Thallium ~201 (T_1^{201}) is injected intravenously while patient is exercising on Trade mill or stationary bicycle.

- Thallium enters myocytes depending on vascular supply (perfusion) and membrane function (tissue viability)
- The intracellular concentration of thallium is estimated by the density of image

Normal Myocardium

Shows homogeneous distribution of thallium in the myocardial tissue and appears dark on the scan

Ischemic / Infracted (scarved) Myocardium

Do not accumulate as much thallium as normal myocardium and appear as 'light' or 'cold spots' on the scan.

Thallium accumulation does not remain fixed in myocytes. Rather continuous redistribution of the isotope occurs across the cell membrane over time, and after few hours all viable myocytes accumulate more isotope and redistribution causes all viable myocytes to have equal concentration of T_1^{201}

To differentiate between reversible myocardial ischemia and irreversible myocardial ischemia (infarction) another set of images are taken when patient is resting (acquired after several hours)

Delayed Thallium Scan (After 3-4 hours) (Redistribution Imaging)

Reversible Ischemia

Defects seen on initial films that have resolved suggest Reversible ischemia (cold spot disappears)

Irreversible Ischemia (Infarction / scarring

Defects seen on initial film that persist as cold spots suggest irreversible ischemia or infracted /scarred myocardium

225. Answer is C (Thallium scan): Harrison 18th/p 2024 *Harrison 15th/ 1276; Harrison 16th/ 1324; Harrison 17th/ 1534; Refer previous question*

Reversible Myocardial Ischemia can be detected by myocardial perfusion imaging using compounds labeled with thallium- 201 (Thallium Scan).

226. Answer is A (Rofecoxib): *Harrison 18th/47; Goodman & Gillman 12th/974; 'Drug-Induced Diseases' 2nd/406*

Rofecoxib (selective COX-2 inhibitor) induces a Prothrombotic state and has been linked to increased incidence of thrombotic events including myocardial infarction, stroke and venous thrombosis.

'*Selective COX-2 inhibitor Rofecoxib increases the risk of myocardial infarctions*' – Harrison 18th/47

'*Placebo controlled trials with three structurally distinct COX-2 inhibitors – Celecoxib, valdecoxib (withdrawn) and rofecoxib (withdrawn) revealed an increase in the incidence of myocardial infarction, stroke and thrombosis*'.

– Goodman & Gillman 12th/974

Rofecoxib and Valdecoxib were withdrawn from the market in 2004 and 2005 respectively due to increased risk of thrombogenic cardiovascular events (myocardial infarction, stroke and thrombosis)

Mechanisms of Drug-Induced Myocardial Ischemia and Acute Coronary Syndrome

Mechanism	Examples
Increased Myocardial Oxygen Demand	
• Increased heart rate	Directly: Cocaine, adrenergic adrenergic β-agonists, sympathomimetics, withdrawal of β-antagonists Indirectly: potent vasodilators (Nifedipine, minoxidil, hydralazine)
• Increased myocardial contractility	Directly: Cocaine, adrenergic β-agonist, sympathomimetics, withdrawal of β-antagonists Indirectly: potent vasodilators (Nifedipine, minoxidil, hydralazine)
• Increased left ventricular systolic wall tension	Cocaine, phenylephrine
Decreased Myocardial Oxygen Supply (temporary, non-total occlusion)	
• Increased coronary vascular resistance (vasospasm, thrombosis)	Cocaine, anti-migraine agents (ergot alkaloids, triptans)
• Decreased coronary diastolic perfusion pressure	Enalapril, nifedipine, minoxidil, hydralazine, nitroprusside, adenosine, dipyridamole
Drug-Induced Acute Coronary Syndromes	
• **Acute coronary syndrome associated with acute drug therapy**	
- Coronary artery thrombosis, superimposed on a damaged atherosclerotic plaque	Cocaine, oral contraceptives, estrogens, ***COX-2 inhibitors***, NSAIDs
- Coronary artery vasospasm (with or without a superimposed coronary artery thrombosis)	Cocaine, anti-migraine agent (ergot alkaloids, triptans)
• **Acute coronary syndrome associated with chronic drug therapy** (Increased cardiovascular risk)	Cocaine, estrogens, ***COX-2 inhibitors***, NSAIDs, HIV agents/protease inhibitors, oral contraceptives, rosiglitazone

227. Answer is B (Left ventricular ejection fraction): Harrison 18th/p 2024, 2031, 2034 *Harrison 15th/ 1313, 16th/ 1456, 1362; 17th/ 1534, 1535, 1540, 1543*

Pump failure is now the primary cause of in hospital death following MI. The degree of pump failure relates well with mortality.

The most sensitive index of cardiac function amongst the options provided is 'ejection fraction' i.e. the ratio of stroke volume to end diastolic volume. This is thus the best indicator of mortality & morbidity following MI.

Cardiomyopathy/HOCM

228. Answer is D (Alkaptonuria): *Harrison 16th /1408; Harrison 17th/1481 (table 231-1); 1410; Harrison 18th/ 1959, 1965*

Friedreich's ataxia, Glycogen storage diseases and Muscular dystrophies are known to cause of cardiomyopathy. Alkaptonuria has not been mentioned to cause cardiomyopathy.

Primary myocardial involvement	
Idiopathic (D,R,H) Failmilial (D,R,H) Eosinophilic endomyocardial disease (R) Endomyocardial fibrosis (R)	
Secondary Myocardial involvement	
Infective (D) • Viral myocarditis • Bacterial myocarditis • Fungal myocarditis • PRotozoal myocarditis • Metazoal myocarditis • Spirochetal • Rickettsial *Metabolic (D)* *Familial storage disease (D,R)* • ***Glycogen storage disease*** • Mucopolysaccharidoses • Hemochromatosis • Fabry's disease *Deficiency (D)* • Electrolytes • Nutritional	*Connective tissue disorder (D)* • Systemic lupus erythematosus • Polyarteritis nodosa • Rheumatoid arthritis • Progressive systemic sclerosis • Dermatomyositis *Infiltratiions and granulomas (R,D)* • Amyloidosis • Sarcoidosis • Malignancy *Neuromuscular (D)* • ***Muscular dystrophy*** • Myotonic dystrophy • ***Friedreich's ataxia (H,D)*** *Sensitivity and toxic reactions (D)* • Alcohol • Radiation • Drugs *Peripartum heart disease (D)*

229. Answer is A (Dilated cardiomyopathy): *Harrison 18th /1952*

Contractile dysfunction (systolic failure) is the dominant feature of dilated cardiomyopathy.

'An enlarged left ventricle with decreased systolic function (contractile dysfunction) as measured by left ventricular ejection fraction charachterizes diated cardiomyopathy. Systolic failure is more marked than the frequently accompanying diastolic dysfunction'- Harrison's 18th/ 1952

230. Answer is C (Amyloidosis) : *Harrison 16th/1412; 17th/ 1485, 1486;* Harrison 18th/p 1965 *CMDT 2003 /395, 396; 2005/391; 2008/357*

Although all options mentioned in the question other than alcohol have been listed as causes for restrictive cardiomyopathy, amyloidosis appears to be the commonest cause amongst them.

- *'The most frequent causes of restrictive cardiomyopathy are amyloidosis, radiation and myocardial fibrosis fter open heart surgery' – CMDT 2005 / 391*
- 'Myocardial involvement with amyloid is a common cause of secondary restrictive cardiomyopathy' – Harrison 16th/

Causes include: *(Harrison 16th/ 1412)*	
1. Amyloidosis.	6. Fabry's disease
2. Hemochromatosis	7. Eosinophilia
3. Glycogen deposition	8. Scleroderma
4. Endomyocardial fibrosis	9. Transplanted heart
5. Sarcoidosis	10. Mediastinal irradiation
	11. Neoplastic irradiation

231. Answer is A (HOCM) : *Harrisons 16th /1410, 1411, API textbook of Medicine 8th/575*

Syncope and sudden death following competitive sports in young individuals is characteristic of Hypertrophic Obstructive Cardiomyopathy (HOCM). The presence of Left ventricular Hypertrophy predominantly affecting the Septum, on autopsy confirms the suspected diagnosis of HOCM.

'Syncope and sudden death following competitive sports warrants early diagnosis of this condition in suspected families, Echocardiography should be done to screen their asymptomatic relatives' – API

'Left ventricular Hypertrophy predominantly affecting the septum and anterolateral wall is the diagnostic feature'- API

Distinctive Pathophysiological features include

Heterogeneous hypertrophy of LV

Septal Hypertrophy	Dynamic LV outflow obstruction
• Pattern of hypertrophy is distinctive • ***Asymmetrical septal hypertrophy*** is characteristic • Thickness of ventricular septum is disproportionately increased when compared with the free wall	• Dynamic LV outflow obstruction: it is related to narrowing of the subaortic area as a consequence of opposition of anterior mitral valve leaflet against the hypertrophied septum in midsystole. The concept is termed ***systolic anterior motion (SAM)*** of mitral valve. • Dystolic dysfunction: The ubiquitous pathophysiological abnormality is not systolic but rather ***diastolic dysfunction*** - *Harrison*

Clinical spectrum of HOCM

Asymptomatic patient Q	Sudden death Q	Symptomatic patient
many patients are asymptomatic	Sudden death may be first clinical manifestation of disease (commonly seen in young adults after competitive sports)	

Symptomatic patient:

Symptoms	Signs		
• Dyspnea Q is the commonest symptom • Angina pectoris/chest pain Q • Fatigue Q • Syncope Q	• **Double or triple precardial impulse** Q • **Brisk carotid upstroke** Q (Rapidly rising carotid pulse)	• **Fourth heart sound** Q	**Systolic murmur** (Hallmark of disease) • Harsh Q • Diamond shaped (crescendo decrescendo) Q • Best heard at lower left sternal border as well as at apex Q

232. Answer is A. (HOCM): *Harrison's 16th/1410-1411, API Textbook of medicine 8th/575; Harrison's 17th/1484-1485* Harrison 18th/p 1968, 1970

Sudden death following competitive sports in young individuals is characteristic of hypertrophic obstructive cardiomyopathy (HOCM). The presence of chamber and septal hypertrophy on autopsy confirms the suspected diagnosis of HOCM

233. Answer is A (β agonists are useful): *Harrison 14th 15th/ 1351, 1343; 16th/ 1399; 17th/ 1485;* Harrison 18th/p 1969 *other references.*

β blockers should be used as the initial drug in symptomatic individuals. β agonists are contraindicated.

- Hypertrophic obstructive cardiomyopathy is characterized by hypertrophy of left ventricle in the absence of an obvious cause such as hypertension or aortic stenosis.

Distinctive Pathophysiological features include:

Heterogeneous hypertrophy of LV	Dynamic LV outflow obstruction
• Pattern of hypertrophy is distinctive • ***Asymmetrical septal hypertrophy*** is characteristic mainly affecting the IV septum and anterolateral wall • Thickness of ventricular septum is disproportionately increased when compared with the free wall	• The LV outflow obstruction is dynamic i.e. it is related to narrowing of the subaortic area as a consequence of opposition of anterior mitral valve leaflet against the hypertrophied septum in midsystole. The concept is termed ***systolic anterior motion (SAM)*** of mitral valve.

- The obstruction in HOCM is dynamic and is caused by the opposition of mitral valve leaflet against the hypertrophied septum during systole. Increase in volume of blood in LV will move the muscular obstruction away from the opposite wall and decrease the obstructing agent as well as the intensity of murmur. Passive leg raising augments venous return, increases the volume of blood in LV, decreases the obstruction and hence decreases the murmur.
- Increase in myocardial contractility worsens the obstruction by moving the opposing walls closer to each other. β agonists (increase myocardial contractility) would thus increase the obstruction and should not be used. β blockers on the other hand are the agent of choice as these decrease myocardial contractility and hence relieve the obstruction by moving the opposing walls away from each other.

Remember

Clinical Features:
- Most common complaint in symptomatic patient -- Dyspnoea. [Q]
- Sudden Death [Q] may be the first manifestation.
- The Hallmark of HOCM is a *systolic murmur* [Q] most often due to MR. [Q]
- Double - Triple Apical impulse may be seen. [Q]

Diagnosis: The mainstay of diagnosis is *Echocardiography* [Q] which demonstrates :
- Asymmetrical LV hypertrophy. [Q]
- Systolic anterior motion of mitral valve. [Q]

Treatment:
- **β blockers should be the initial drug** [Q] *in symptomatic* individuals.
- *Ca*$^{++}$ *channel blockers may be given.* [Q]

Avoid [Q]:
- Digitalis [Q]
- Nitrates [Q]
- Diuretics [Q]
- β agonists [Q]

234. Answer is B (Murmur radiating to neck): *Harrison 16th/ 1411; Harrison 17th/ 1484, 1485*Harrison 18th/p 1968

Hypertrophic cardiomyopathy is characterized by a harsh systolic diamond shaped (crescendo-decrescendo) murmur best heard at lower left sternal border as well as at apex. Murmur does not radiate to the neck. Other features mentioned are consistent with the diagnosis

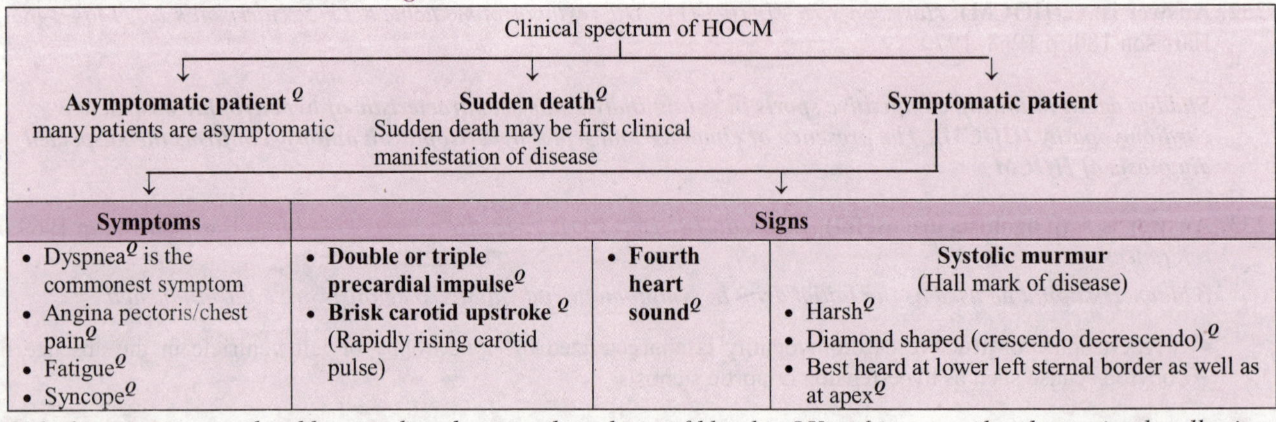

Symptoms	Signs		
• Dyspnea[Q] is the commonest symptom • Angina pectoris/chest pain[Q] • Fatigue[Q] • Syncope[Q]	• **Double or triple precardial impulse**[Q] • **Brisk carotid upstroke** [Q] (Rapidly rising carotid pulse)	• **Fourth heart sound**[Q]	**Systolic murmur** (Hall mark of disease) • Harsh[Q] • Diamond shaped (crescendo decrescendo) [Q] • Best heard at lower left sternal border as well as at apex[Q]

Valsalva maneuver and sudden standing decrease the volume of blood in LV and increase the obstruction by allowing better opposition between the hypertrophied septum of the mitral valve leaflet. Thus these will also increase the intensity of the murmur

235. Answer is A (Systolic dysfunction): *Harrison 16th/1410; Harrison 17th/ 1484; Harrison 18th/p 1968*

'The ubiquitous pathophysiological abnormality in hypertrophic obstructive cardiomyopathy is not systolic but rather diastolic dysfunction' *– Harrisons*

Note: It has now been demonstrated that systolic dysfunction characterized by an outflow tract pressure gradient is present only in about one quarter of patients with HCM. The pathophysiological abnormality that has now been demonstrated is diastolic dysfunction characterized by increased stiffness of the hypertrophied muscle.

236. Answer is A (Supine position): *Harrison 15th/ 1362, Harrison 16th/ 1411; Harrison 17th/ 1484; Harrison 18th/p 1968*

Condition which increase obstruction & intensity of murmur	Conditions which decrease obstruction & intensity of murmur
Factors that increase myocardial contractility • *Exercise*[Q] • *Sympathomimetic Amines*[Q] • *Digitalis Glycosides*[Q] **Factors which decrease Ventricular volume** • *Valsalva maneuver*[Q] • *Sudden standing*[Q] • *Nitroglycerine*[Q] • *Amyl nitrite*[Q] • *Tachycardia*[Q] **Decreased aortic impedance & afterload:**	**Factors that decrease myocardial contractility** • β blockers • calcium channel blockers **Factors which increase Ventricular volume** • *Augmentation of venous return by passive leg raising*[Q] • *Expansion of Blood Volume*[Q] • *Supine* ***Position***[Q] **Increased aortic impedance & afterload:** • *Elevation of Arterial pressure by phenylephrine*[Q] • *Sustained hand grip*[Q] • *Squatting*

237. Answer is B (Decrease of murmur with handgrip): *Harrison 15th/ 1361 & 1362, Harrison 16th/ 1411; Harrison 17th/ 1484;* Harrison 18th/p 1968 *(Q.No 36 C.V.S Harrison pretest for medicine, 15/e)*

The murmur decreases with increase in ventricular volume during isometric exercise (handgrip)

Echocardiographic evidence of disproportionately thickened ventricular septum and systolic anterior motion (SAM) of mitral valve strongly suggests Idiopathic hypertrophic Subaortic stenosis. ***The Typical harsh systolic murmur does not radiate to carotid arteries and decreases with increase in ventricular volume during isometric exercise (handgrip).***

Congestive heart failure often occurs because of reduced ventricular compliance despite normal ventricular systolic function. The carotid upstroke is brisk and often bifid.

238. Answer is C (Digoxin): *Harrison 17th /1764; Harrison's 18th/2312*

Digitalis is contraindicated in hypertrophic obstructive cardiomyopathy (HOCM).

Digitalis causes an increase in myocardial contractility, which increases the degree of obstruction in HOCM and worsens the condition.

Drugs Contraindicated in HOCM are

Drugs that increase myocardial Contractility	Drugs which decrease ventricular volume (preload)
• *Digitalis* [Q] • *Sympathomimetic amines* [Q] • *β agonist*	• *Nitrates* [Q] • *Diuretics* [Q]

Any increase in myocardial contractility or decrease in ventricular volume (preload) increase the degree of obstruction in HOCM[Q]

239. Answer is C (Propranolol): *Harrison 15th/ 1361, Harrison 16th/ 1410; Harrison 17th/ 1485* Harrison 18th/p 1969, 1970

The symptoms of the patient and echocardiographic finding of asymmetrical septal hypertrophy almost confirms the diagnosis of Hypertrophic cardiomyopathy. Beta Blockers should be the initial drug [Q] ***in symptomatic individuals***

Management of HOCM

- Avoidance of strenuous physical activity
- **Beta Blockers** should be the initial drug Q in symptomatic individuals. They reduce:
  - *Heart rate*
  - *Blood pressure*
  - *Stiffness of left ventricle*
  - *Fatal arrythmias*
- **Calcium channel Blockers**Q (verapamil and diltiazem) are alternative drugs.
  - They reduce-stiffness of ventricle
  - Elevated diastolic pressures
- **Amiadarone** may be used to reduce arrythmias.
- **Surgical myomectomy**

240. Answer is D (Idiopathic Hypertrophic Sub Aortic Stenosis): *Harrison 15th/ 1362, 16th/ 1411; 17th/ 1484, 1485 Harrison 18th/p 1968, 1969, 1970*

Idiopathic hypertrophic subaortic stenosis (HOCM) is a dynamic outflow obstruction which is increased by any mechanism decreasing the preload. ***Nitrates decrease the preload, & the volume of blood in LV & thereby increase the dynamic obstruction & symptoms of angina.***

241. Answer is B (Hypertrophic obstructive cardiomyopathy): *Harrison 15th/ 1362; Harrison 16th/1411; 17th/ 1484, 1485*

Harrison 18th/p 1968-1970

Family history of the disease and aggravation of symptoms with the intake of Nitroglycerine (Nitrates) sugget the diagnosis of Hypertrophic obstructive cardiomyopathy.

242. Answer is A (Digitalis is useful): *Harrison 17th/ 1485; Repeat*

Digitalis is contraindicated in hypertrophic obstructive cardiomyopathy (HOCM).

Digitalis causes an increase in myocardial contractility which increases the degree of obstruction in HOCM and worsens the condition.

Drugs Contraindicated in HOCM are

Drugs that increase myocardial Contractility	Drugs which decrease ventricular volume (preload)
• *Digitalis* Q	• *Nitrates* Q
• *Sympathomimetic amines* Q	• *Diuretics* Q
• *β agonist*	

*Any increase in myocardial contractility or decrease in ventricular volume (preload) increase the degree of obstruction in HOCM*Q

Pericardial Disease

Cardiac Tamponade

243. Answer is D (Kussmaul's sign): *Harrison 15th/ 1367, Harrison 16th/ 1416; Harrison 17th/ 1490, 1491; Repeat* Harrison 18th/p 1975

Pulsus paradoxus clinically, electrical alternans on ECG and RVDC on Echocardiography are chracteristic features of Cardiac tamponade.

A positive Kussmaul's sign is rare in cardiac tamponade. Its presence suggests that an organizing process and epicardial constriction are present in addition to effusion' – Harrisons

Characteristic	Tamponade	Constrictive Pericarditis	Restrictive Cardiomyopathy	RVMI
Clinical				
Pulsus paradoxus	**Common**	**Usually absent**	**Rare**	**Rare**
Jugular veins				
Prominent y descent	Absent	Usually present	Rare	Rare
Prominent x descent	Present	Usually present	Present	Rare
Kussmaul's sign	**Absent** (Rare)^Q	**Present**	**Present**	**Present**
Third heart sound	Absent	Absent	Rare	May be present
Pericardial knock	Absent	Often present	Absent	Absent
Electrocardiogram				
Low ECG voltage	May be present	May be present	May be present	Absent
Electrical alternans	**May be present**	**Absent**	**Absent**	**Absent**
Echocardiography				
Thickened pericardium	Absent	Present	Absent	Absent
Pericardial calcification	Absent	Often present	Absent	Absent
Pericardial effusion	Present	Absent	Absent	Absent
RV size	Usually small	Usually normal	Usually normal	Enlarged
Myocardial thickness	Normal	Normal	Usually increased	Normal
Right atrial collapse and RVDC	**Present**	**Absent**	**Absent**	**Absent**
Increased early filling, ↑ mitral flow velocity	Absent	Present	Present	May be present
Exaggerated respiratory variation in flow velocity	Present	Present	Absent	Absent
CT/MRI				
Thickened/calcific pericardium	Absent	Present	Absent	Absent
Cardiac catheterization Equalization of diastolic procedures	Usually present	Usually present	Usually absent	Absent or present
Cardiac biopsy helpful?	No	No	Sometimes	No

*RV, right ventricle; RVMI, right ventricular myocardial infarction; RVDC, right ventricular diastolic collapse; ECG, electrocardiograph.

Note:

*'A positive Kussmaul's sign is rare in cardiac tamponade. Its presence suggests that an organizing process and epicardial constriction are present in addition to effusion' – Harrisons 16th/ 1416

244. Answer is A (Kussmaul's sign): *Harrison 16th/1416; Harrison 17th/ 1490, 1491; Repeat* Harrison 18th/p 1975

Pulsus paradoxus clinically, electrical alternans on ECG and RVDC on Echocardiography are chracteristic features of Cardiac tamponade.

245. Answer is C (Rapid y descent): *Harrison 15th/ 1357, Harrison 16th/ 1416; Harrison 17th/ 1490* Harrison 18th/p 1972

***Cardiac tamponade is characterized by elevation of JVP with a prominent x descent and a diminutive or absent 'y' descent** – Harrison 16th/ 1416*

Rapid 'y' descent is seen in constrictive pericarditis.

Kussumaul sign is a feature of constrictive pericarditis and not cardiac tamponade. It can however be seen (rare) in tamponade. *Its presence suggests that an organizing process and epicardial constriction are present in addition to effusion – Harrison 16th/ 1416*

Clinical	Tamponade	Constrictive Pericarditis
• Pulsus parodoxus^Q	**Common**	Usually absent
• Jugular veins		
- Raised JVP	Present	Present
- *Prominent Y descent*^{Q}	**Absent**	Usually Present
- *Prominent X descent*^{Q}	Present	Usually present
• Kussumaul's sign^Q	**Absent (Rare)**	Present

246. Answer is B (Cardiac Tamponade): Harrison 18th/p 1975 *Harrisons 17th/1491, Hurst 12th/246,1966*

Pulsus Paradoxus is most characteristic of cardiac tamponade amongst the options provided.

Feature	Cardiac Tamponade	Constrictive Pericarditis	Restrictive Cardiomyopathy	RVMI
Pulsus paradoxus	Common	Usually Absent	Rare	Rare

Pulsus Paradoxus is much more common with cardiac tamponade than with constrictive pericarditis of paradoxical pulse is considered more characterstic of cardiac tamponade than constrictive pericarditis.
Presence of paradoxical pulse is however not a specific feature of cardiac tamponade

247. Answer is B (Cardiac Tamponade): Harrison 18th/p 1972 *Harrison's 17th/1490*

Beck's triad is a feature of cardiac tamponade.

Beck's triad of Cardiac tamponade

- *Hypotension*Q
- *Soft or Absent Heart Sounds*Q
- *Jugular venous distension*Q *(↑JVP with a prominent x descent but absent y descent)*

248. Answer is D (Tachycardia): Harrison 18th/p 1972 *Harrisons 17th/1490*

The three principle features of Beck's triad are hypotension, soft or absent heart sounds and increased JVP

Beck's Triad of Cardiac Tamponade

- *Hypotension*Q
- *Soft or absent Heart sounds (Silent Heart)* Q
- *Increased JVP (with a prominent x descent but absent y descent)*Q

249. Answer is A, B, D: Harrison 18th/p 1972 *Harrisons 17th/1490*

The principle features of Beck's triad are Hypotension, Reduced or Absent Heart sounds (Silent Heart) and elevated JVP (Neck vein distension)

250. Answer is C (Cardiac Temponade): *Harrison 14th/ 1336, 15th/ 1367, 16th / 1416; Harrison 17th/ 1490, 1491 Harrison 18th/p 1975, 1972*

Cardiac Tamponade should be suspected in any patient who has a rapid down hill course and exhibits the features of rising venous pressure and falling arterial pressure following blunt injury to the chest.

The triad of cardiac tamponade :

1. Rising systemic venous pressure
2. Falling Arterial pressure
3. Quiet heart (distant heart sounds)

We are often given a set of findings and asked to distinguish between cardiac temponade and constrictive pericarditis. Few guidelines to answer these kind of questions :

Guidelines :

If the question talks about any of the following, mark your answer as 'Cardiac Temponade'	If the question talks about any of these, mark your answer as 'Constrictive Pericarditis'.
a. Elevated J.V.P. with a ***prominent x-descent*** (y-descent is diminutive or negative)	a. Elevated J.V.P. with a ***prominent y-descent*** (along with a prominent x-descent)
b. ***Electrical Alternans***	***b. Kussumaul's sign***, which is rare in cardiac temponade
c. ***Pulses paradoxus:*** *Hallmark of cardiac Temponade.*	***c. Pericardial knock***, which is rare in cardiac temponade

251. Answer is B (Urgent pericardial tap): *Harrison 15th/ 1367, 1368, 1369; Harrison 17th/ 1490, 1491, 1492 Harrison 18th/p 1972, 1974*

'If manifestations of pericardial tamponade appear pericardiocentesis must be carried out at once; since relief of intrapericardial pressure may be life saving' *– Harrison 16th/ 1417*

- This patient is a case of acute tamponade as seen after cardiac trauma as suggested by the classical findings of :

  - *Falling arterial pressure*
  - *Increased venous pressure and*
  - *Faint heart sounds*

In case of tamponade pericardiocentesis (pericardial tap) should be carried out at once, as the release of intrapericardial pressure is life saving.

- Rapid **blood transfusion** though essential will be effective only once pericardial tap decompresses the pericardium and enables the heart to pump normally.
- **Intercostal tube drainage** is not indicated as air entry is adequate in both lung fileds.
- **Fixation of femur and repair of femoral artery** is not the immediate priority. Weak femoral pulsation may be a manifestation of falling arterial pressure due to cardiac tamponade and need to be explored only if patient fails to improve after pericardial tap and blood transfusion.

252. Answer is D (Cardiac tamponade): *Harrison 15th/ 1364, Harrison 16th/ 1416; 17th/ 1490* Harrison 18th/p 1972

Features of rising pressure, falling arterial pressure and pulsus paradoxus following surgery on the heart leads us to the diagnosis of cardiac tamponade.

253. Answer is C (Cardiac tamponade) most probably: *Harrison 16th/1416; Harrison 17th/1490, 1491;* Harrison 18th/p 1975 *Braunwald 8th/130*

Kussmaul's sign is absent in cardiac tamponade.

Presence of Kussmaul's sign in cardiac tamponade suggests an organizing process and presence of epicardial constriction (constrictive pericarditis) in addition to effusion. ***Kussmaul's sign is not a feature of isolated cardiac tamponade.***

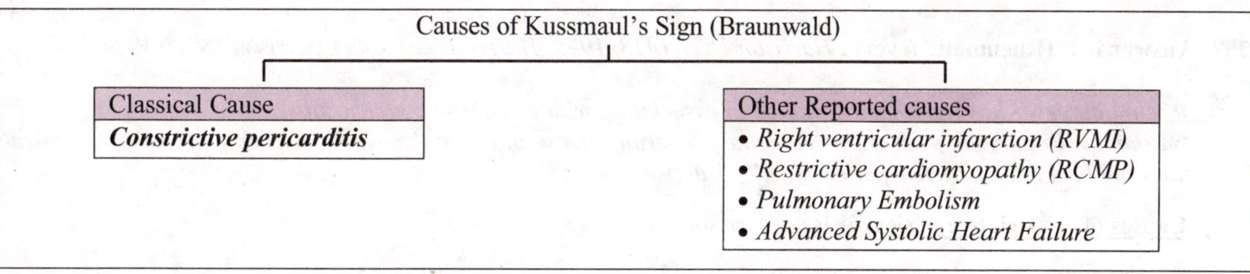

Kussmaul's sign is absent inisolated cardiac tamponade

- *It is frequent with constrictive pericarditis and R.V.M.I.*
- *Not so frequent in R.C.M.P. but definitely present*
- *Rare (absent) in Cardiac Tamponade*

254. Answer is B (Low ECG voltage): Harrison 18th/p 1975 *Harrison 17th/1491*

The patient is presenting with characteristic features of Cardiac Tamponade.

'Low ECG voltage' is a feature of cardiac tamponade and the single best answer of choice amongst the options provided.

Presence of raised JVP and inspiratory decline in systolic arterial pressure of > 10mm Hg suggests a diagnosis of acute tamponade.

An important clue to the diagnosis of cardiac tamponade is the presence of greater than nonrmal (10mm Hg) inspiratory decline in systolic arterial pressure – Harrison 17th/1491

Kussmaul's sign, prominent y descent and thickened pericardium are not seen in cardiac tamponade.

Features	Cardiac Tamponade
Kussmaul's sign	*Absent*
Prominent y descent	*Absent*
Thickened Pericardium	*Absent*
Low ECG voltage	*May be present*

255. Answer is A (Cardiac tamponade): *Harrison 14th/ 1336, Harrison 15th/ 1270, 1367; Harrison 17th/ 1396* Harrison 18th/p 1839, 1975

Electrical alternans refers to a beat-to-beat alteration in one or more components of the ECG signal.
Total electrical alternans (P-QRS-T) with sinus tachycardia is a relatively specific sign for pericardial effusion, often with cardiac tamponade. *– Harrison 16th / 1319*

Feature	Cardiac Tamponade	Constrictive Pericarditis	Restrictive Cardiomyopathy	RVMI
Electrical Alternans	*May be present*	Absent	Absent	Absent

Constrictive Pericarditis

256. Answer is D (Constrictive pericarditis): *Robbins 7th/601, 602; Robbins Patho Illustrated 6th/ 589*

Constrictive pericarditis is not haemorrhagic

Causes of haemorrhagic pericarditis: *Robbins 7th/601, 602*
Bacterial infections: infective endocarditis
Tuberculosis
Bleeding diathesis
Following cardiac surgery
Ruptured MI
Ruptured aortic dissection
Traumatic perforation

The latter four conditions are mentioned as causes of haemorrhagic pericardial effusion or hemopericardium.

257. Answer is D (Rheumatic fever) : *Harrison 16th / 1418, 1978; Harrison 17th/ 1493* Harrison 18th/p 1976

Rheumatic fever has not been mentioned in association with constrictive pericarditis.
"Although Rheumatic pericarditis can cause a serous effusion, fibrin deposits and even pericardial calcification, it does not lead to constrictive pericarditis." - Harrison 16th/1978

Causes of constrictive pericarditis : *- Harrison 16th / 1418*

- Trauma
- ***Cardiac operation of any type***
- Mediastinal irradiation
- ***Purulent infection (Staph. effusion)***
- ***Histoplasmosis / Tuberculosis***
- Neoplastic disease especially breast cancer, lung cancer and lymp
- Acute viral pericarditis
- Rheumatoid arthritis, SLE
- Chronic renal failure with uremia treated by chronic dialysis
- Idiopathic

In the past ***Tuberculosis*** *was the most common cause but the process not more often occurs after radiation therapy.* ***Cardiac surgery*** *or viral pericarditis. Histoplasmosis is another uncommon cause. - CMDT 2006/409*

258. Answer is A (Commonest cause in India is 'Idiopathic'): Harrison 18th/p 1975, 1976 *Harrisons 17th/ 1493 Kelly's Essentials of Medicine 2nd/119*

The commonest cause of constrictive pericarditis in developing countries including India is tuberculosis

Commonest cause of constrictive pericarditis in India is Tuberculosis

Commonest cause of contrictive pericarditis in developing countries is tuberculosis.

Commonest cause of constrictive pericarditis in North America is 'Idiopathic' – Kelly's Essentials of Medicine 2nd /119

Commonest cause of constrictive pericarditis

Developed Nations	Developing Nations
• ***Post viral pericarditis or Idiopathic pericarditis*** • *Previous cardiac surgery* • *Chest Radiation therapy*	***Tuberculosis***

Kussmaul's sign is positive in constrictive pericarditis (Harrisons 17th/1491)

Feature	Tamponade	Constrictive pericarditis	Restrictive cardiomyopathy	RVMI
Kussmaul's sign	*Absent (Rare)*	***Present***	*Present*	*Present*

Ascitis in constrictive pericarditis is out of proportion to peripheral Edema *(CMDT 2007/419)*

'Ascitis often seems out of proportion to degree of peripheral edema (CMDT)

Right ventricular End Diastolic pressure is raised in constrictive Pericarditis

'In constrictive pericarditis ventricular end diastolic volume and stroke volume are reduced and the end diastolic pressures in both ventricles are elevated' - Harrison

259. Answer is D (Acute Pulmonary Edema): Harrison 18th/p 1976 *Harrisons 17th/1493*

Acute Pulmonary Edema is not a usual feature of constrictive pericarditis.

Constrictive Pericarditis represents a chronic process of fibrosis, scarring and calcification that continues for months or years. Acute left ventricular failure or Acute Pulmonary Edema is very uncommon in constrictive pericarditis.

Ascites is a common presenting feature of constrictive pericarditis

Ascites is common and is usually more prominent than dependent edema

Ascites often seems out of proportion to peripheral edema (CMDT)

Apex beat in constrictive Pericarditis may be Retractile

The Apical pulse is reduced and may retract during systolic (Broad bent's sign) – Harrisons 17th/1994

Inward motion of the apex beat called Apical Retraction suggests constrictive Pericarditis

Pericardial knock is a charachteristic feature of constrictive Pericarditis

Pericardial knock is produced as a result of abrupt cessation of ventricular filling as a result of fibrotic and thickened pericardium.

Feature	Tamponade	Constrictive pericarditis	Restrictive cardiomyopathy	RVMI
Pericardial knock	*Absent*	***Often present***	*Absent*	*Absent*

260. Answer is D (Constrictive pericarditis): Harrison 18th/p 1976 *Harrisons 17th/1493; Current Diagnosis & Treatment in Cardiology 2nd/ 214, 215 CMDT 2007/419*

Square Root sign is a characteristic (but not pathognomic) feature of constrictive pericarditis.

Square root sign : Dip and Plateau wave form

- 'The square root sign' describes the diastolic pressure waveform observed during ventricular pressure tracings on cardiac catheterization
- The wave form is called 'square root sign' as it is charachterized by an early diastolic dip followed by a high diastolic plateau with an elevated end diastolic pressure resembling the 'square root sign'.
  (It results from early rapid diastolc filling with sudden cessation as the pericardium reaches its compliance limit)
- This sign is also called 'dip and plateau' sign
- The square root sign is charachtristic of constrictive pericarditis but it is not pathonognomic of constrictive pericarditis.
  The square root sign may also be found in restrictive cardiomyopathy

Square Root sign
Constrictive Pericarditis (More Prominent)
Restrictive cardiomyopathy (Less prominent)
Square root sign is more prominent in constrictive pericarditis than restrictive cardiomyopathy

2

Cardiovascular System

261. Answer is A and C (Diastolic Pressure are equalized; Thick pericardium is present): Harrison 18th/p 1975 *Harrisons 17th/1491; Refer previous table*

Diastolic pressure are equalized in constrictive pericarditis but not in Restrictive cardiomyopathy
Thickenned pericardium is seen in constrictive pericarditis but not in Restrictive cardiomyopathy

Right ventricular size is usually normal in both and pericardial effusion is usually absent in both, RV size and pericardial effusion, therefore can not distinguish between constrictive pericarditis and Restrictive cardiomyopathy

Feature	Constrictive Pericarditis	Restrictive Cardiomyopathy
• Thickenned pericardium	*Present*	*Absent*
• Pericardial Effusion	*Absent*	*Absent*
• RV size	*Usually Normal*	*Usually Normal*
• Equalization of diastolic pressure	*Usually present*	*Usually Absent*

262. Answer is C (RVMI) : Harrison 18th/p 1975 *Harrisons 17th/1491*

Rapid 'x' descent is rare in RVMI

Feature	Tamponade	Constrictive Pericaditis	Restrictive Cardiomyopathy	RVMI
Prominent x descent	Present	Usually present	Present	***Rare***
Prominent y descent	Absent	Usually present	Rare	Rare

Hypertension

General

263. Answer is C (Diet modification, exercise & drugs): *Harrison 18th /2054*

Management of uncomplicated essential hypertension includes health promoting lifestyle modifications (includes dietry modification & exercise) and pharmacological therapy (drugs).

Management of Uncomplicated Essential Hypertension

Lifestyle modification

Weight reduction	Attain and maintain BMI <25 kg/m^2
Dietary salt reduction	<6 g NaCl/d
Adapt DASH-type dietary plan	Diet rich in fruits, vegetables, and low-fat dairy products with reduced content of saturated and total fat
Moderation of alcohol consumption	For those who drink alcohol, consume 2 drinks/day in men and 1 drink/day in women
Physical activity	Regular aerobic activity, e.g., brisk walking for 30 min/d

Pharmacological Therapy

- In uncomplicated essential hypertension the treatment is started with a low-dose thiazide (hydrochlorothiazide 12.5-25 mg per day), an ACE inhibitor or a beta-blocker.
- Calcium-channel blocker can be used as the first-line treatment if the systolic pressure is high.
- Angiotensin-II receptor antagonists should be considered when the adverse effects of ACE inhibitors or other drugs have proven problematic.
- If no response is achieved, or adverse effects emerge, a product of another drug group should be prescribed.
- Combination therapy is started if desired blood pressure reduction is not achieved with monotherapy.
- The reasons behind poor response must be established.

264. Answer is A (ACE inhibitors and Beta blockers): *API 6th/537: Harrisons 16th/1479*

Combination therapy involving ACE inhibitors and Beta blocker is not recommended.

Drug combination in Hypertension

Useful Combinations	Undesirable Combinations
ACE inhibitor and calcium blocker (A+C)	Low dose diuretic and calcium blocker
ACE inhibitor (or AII receptor antagonist) and diuretic (A+D)	Beta-blocker and verapamil/diltiazem
Beta-blocker and Calcium blocker (amlodipine) (B+C)	Beta-blocker and ACE inhibitor
Diuretic and beta-blocker (B+D)	Two drugs from the same class

Combination Therapy *(Harrisons 16th/1479)*

For Medium to high risk patients strongly consider low dose combination therapy as initial therapy

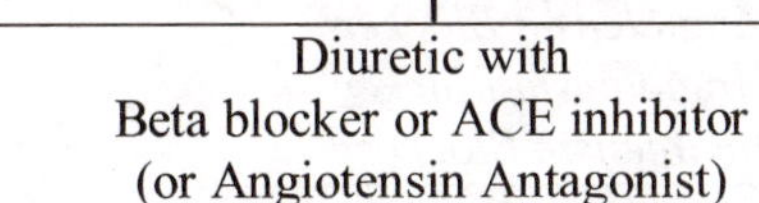

Calcium channel blocker with
ACE inhibitor or Beta blocker

Rational Combination therapies : Step-wise approach (API textbooks)

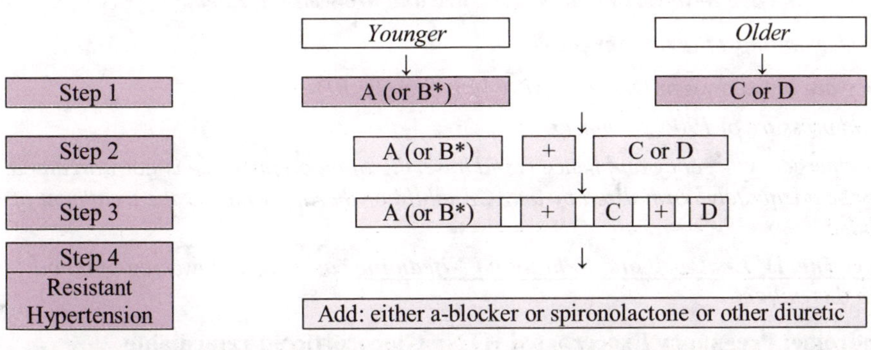

A : ACE inhibitor or angiotensin receptor blocker B: β-blocker
C : Calcium channel blocker D : Diuretic (thiazide)

265. Answer is A (Beta Blockers): *Evidence Based Medicine Guidelines (John Wiley & Sons) 2005/4.26; 'Hypertension: A companion to Braunwald's Heart Disease (Elsevier) 2007/335*

Beta-blockers are the first line drugs of choice for treatment of hypertension in patients with coronary artery disease & stable angina

'Beta blockers are the first line choice when treating hypertension in a patient with coronary artery disease' – Evidence Based Medicine Guidelines (John Wiley & Sons)

'Beta blockers reduce angina symptoms, improve mortality and lower BP, and they should be the drugs of first choice in hypertensive patients with CAD and stable angina' – 'Hypertension: A companion to Braunwald's Heart Disease'

266. Answer is C (Enalaprilat): *Harrisons 16th/1478,1479*

The presence of proteinuria in this diabetic patient suggest a diagnosis of diabetic nephropathy.

The drugs of choice for management of hypertension in patients with diabetes are ACE inhibitors
Enalapril is an ACE inhibitor and the drug of choice for management of hypertension in patients with diabetic nephropathy.

ACE inhibitors or Angiotensin blockers should be the first line therapy in hypertensive individuals with type 2 Diabetes. They have no known adverse effect on glucose or lipid metabolism and minimize the development of diabetic nephropathy by reducing renal vascular resistance and renal perfusion pressure- Harrison

Indication		Treatment of choice
Hypertensive patient with protenuria[Q]	-	*ACE inhibitors or Angiolensin Blocker*
Hypertensive patient with Diabetes[Q]	-	*ACE inhibitors or Angiotensin Blocker*
Hypertensive patient with diabetic Nephropathy[Q]	-	*ACE inhibitor or Angiotensin Blocker*

ACE inhibitors have become the drug of choice for chronic renal disease whether diabetic or non diabetic in origin.
– Braunwald 8th/1063.

267. Answer is C (Enalapril): *Refer previous question*

ACE inhibitors (Enalapril) are the agents of choice for treatment of hypertension in diabetic patients with proteinuria.

Indication		Treatment of choice
Hypertensive patient with protenuria[Q]	-	*ACE inhibitors or Angiolensin Blocker*
Hypertensive patient with Diabetes[Q]	-	*ACE inhibitors or Angiotensin Blocker*
Hypertensive patient with diabetic Nephropathy[Q]	-	*ACE inhibitor or Angiotensin Blocker*

268. Answer is C (Oral Enalapril): *API 8th/532, 537*

Oral Enalapril (ACE inhibitors) are effective in lowering blood pressure and are well tolerated.

Oral Enalapril is the agent of choice amongst the options provided.

Hypertensive emergencies/urgency are defined when Diastolic BP> 120; Systolic BP>220.

The patient in question has a blood pressure of 190/120 mmHg.

This is not a case of hypertensive emergency/urgency and hence rapid lowering of blood pressure is not warranted. Blood pressure in such cases may be adequately normalized by an ACE inhibitor therapy which is the treatment of choice amongst the options provided

IV Nitroglycerine, Oral Nitroglycerine, IV Enalapril and Sublingual Nifedipine *cause rapid lowering of blood pressure which is not indicated in this patient.*

269. Answer is B,C,E (Gordon's syndrome; Pregnancy Exacerbated HTN; Glucocorticoid-remediable hyperaldosteronism): *Harrison 17th/1557*

Rare monogenic forms of hypertension that are inherited as Autosoma l Dominant traits include Gordon's syndrome, Pregnancy Exacerbated HTN and Glucocorticoid-remediable hyperaldosteronism
17- α Hydroxylase deficiency ay also present as a rare form of monogenic hypertension but this is inherited as an Autosomal Recessive trait

Monogenic form of hypertension Mandelian Forms of Hypertension (Rare)	
Autosomal dominant	Autosomal recessive
• *Glucocorticoid-remediable hyperaldosteronism* • *Liddle's syndrome* • *Pseudohypoaldosteronism type II (Gordon's syndrome)* • *Hypertension exacerbated in pregnancy (apparent mineralocorticoid excess syndrome)* • *Polycystic kidney disease* • *Pheochromocytoma*	• *17α-hydroxylase deficiency* • *11 β -hydroxylase deficiency* • *11 β -hydroxysteroid dehydrogenase deficiency*

Hypertensive Crisis

270. Answer is D (All of the above): *Braunwald 8th/1045*

Acute Aortic Dissection, Hypertensive Encephalopathy and Intracerbral haemorrhage are all hypertensive emergenices that require rapid reduction of blood pressure

Indications for rapid reduction of BP

- Rapid reduction of blood pressure is indicated in hypertensive emergencies and hypertensive urgencies(Braunwald)
- Hypertensive emergencies require very rapid reduction or immediate reduction in blood pressure preferably within minutes (within 1 hour) Hypertensive urgencies also require rapid reduction but, reduction required is not immediate and can be achieved more slowly over hours (or over days)

Clinical Circumstances requiring rapid reduction of BP (Braunwald 8th/1045) (Hypertensive Emergencies and Hypertensive Urgencies)
• Accelerated-malignant hypertension with papilledema • Cerebrovascular - Hypertensive encephalopathy - Atherothrombotic brain infarction with severe hypertension - Intracerebral hemorrhage - Subarachnoid hemorrhage • Cardiac - Acute aortic dissection - Acute left ventricular failure - Acute or impending myocardial infarction - After coronary bypass surgery • Renal - Acute glomerulonephritis - Renal cries from collagen-vascular diseases - Severe hypertension after kidney transplantation • Excessive circulating catecholamines - Pheochromocytoma crisis - Food or drug interactions with monoaime oxidase inhibitors - Sympathomimetic drug use (cocaine) - Rebound hypertension after sudden cessation of antihypertensive drugs • Eclampsia • Surgical - Severe hypertension in patients requiring immediate surgery - Postoperative hypertension - Postoperative bleeding from vascular suture lines • Severe body burns • Severe epistaxis • Thrombotic thrombocytopenic purpura

271. Answer is A (Hypertensive urgency is characterized by marked elevation of blood pressure and rapidly evolving end organ damage): *Braunwald 8th/1045; Harrisons 17th/1561,1562; Hurst 12th/1625*

Rapidly evolving end organ damage is a feature of hypertensive emergency and not hypertensive urgency.

Hypertensive urgency is defined by a markedly elevated blood pressure usually in the same range as seen in hypertensive emergencies but without the rapid progression of target organ damage.-Hurst 12th/1625

Hypertensive Crisis

Hypertensive Emergencies	**Hypertensive urgencies**
• Marked elevation of Blood pressure with rapidly evolving end organ damage. • No fixed Blood pressure cut off values are defined but, in general the blood pressure values are as follows. Diastolic BP> 120; Systolic BP>220 • Rapid /Immediate reduction of blood pressure is indicated in these patients • Blood pressure should be controlled within hours (Preferably within 1 hours) • Intensive monitoring in a critical care setting is mandatory	• Marked elevation of blood pressure without rapidly evolving end organ damage • No fixed blood pressure cut off values are defined but in general the blood pressure values may approach the same range as seen in hypertensive emergencies • Lowering of blood pressure is essential but immediate very rapid reduction is often not required • Blood pressure should be controlled over a period of hours or days (Preferably within 24 hours) • Intensive monitoring in a critical care setting is not always required *If the patient is asymptomatic or clinically stable the patient can be managed as an outpatient with dose follow up within days without an intensive monitoring setting usually with oval medications – Hurst 12th/1625*

272. Answer is C (Indapamide): *Braunwald 8th/1066; API 8th/538; KDT 6th/115; Hurst 12th/1626*

Indapamide is a mild diuretic that may be used for treatment of mild to moderate hypertension. It is not effective in the treatment of hypertensive urgencies or emergencies.

Commonly used Drugs in the Management of Hypertensive Crisis

Common Intravenous Agents **(Used for Hypertensive Emergencies)**	Common Oral Agents **(Used for Hypertensive Urgencies)**
Diuretics *Furosemide* **Vosodilators** *Sodium Nitroprusside* *Nitroglycerine* *Fenoldapam* *Nicardipine* *Hydralazine* *Enolaprilant* **Adrenergic Inhibitors** *Phentolamine* *Esmolol* *Metaprolol* *Labetolol* *Urapidil*	*Nifedipine (Not Recommended now)* *Nicardipine* *Israpidine* *Clonidine* *Coptopril* *Labetolol* *Hydralazine* *Nitroglycerine*

**** Nifedipine should be used with great caution 'if at all' according to the US F.D.A.'***

273. Answer is B (Labetalol): *Harrison 17th /1561, 1562; Hurst 12th/1625*

Symptomatic Hypertension with diastolic pressure of 120 suggest a diagnosis of Hypertensive Emergency. Labetalol (intravenous) is the drug of choice for management of Hypertensive Emergencies (amongst the options provided).

Hypertensive Crisis

Hypertensive Emergencies	Hypertensive urgencies
• Marked elevation of Blood pressure with rapidly evolving end organ damage. • No fixed Blood pressure cut off values are defined but, in general the blood pressure values are as follows. Diastolic BP> 120; Systolic BP>220 • Rapid /Immediate reduction of blood pressure is indicated in these patients • Blood pressure should be controlled within hours (Preferably within 1 hours) • Intensive monitoring in a critical care setting is mandatory	• Marked elevation of blood pressure without rapidly evolving end organ damage • No fixed blood pressure cut off values are defined but in general the blood pressure values may approach the same range as seen in hypertensive emergencies • Lowering of blood pressure is essential but immediate very rapid reduction is often not required • Blood pressure should be controlled over a period of hours or days (Preferably within 24 hours) • Intensive monitoring in a critical care setting is not always required *If the patient is asymptomatic or clinically stable the patient can be managed as an outpatient with follow up within days without an intensive monitoring setting usually with oral medications – Hurst 12th/1625*

Commonly used Drugs in the Management of Hypertensive Crisis

Common Intravenous Agents **(Used for Hypertensive Emergencies)**	Common Oral Agents **(Used for Hypertensive Urgencies)**
Diuretics *Furosemide* **Vosodilators** *Sodium Nitroprusside* *Nitroglycerine* *Fenoldapam* *Nicardipine* *Hydralazine* ***Enolaprilat*** **Adrenergic Inhibitors** *Phentolamine* *Esmolol* *Metaprolol* ***Labetolol*** *Urapidil*	*Nifedipine (Not Recommended now)* *Nicardipine* *Israpidine* *Clonidine* *Coptopril* *Labetolol* *Hydralazine* *Nitroglycerine*

274. Answer is D (Indapamide): *KDT 6th/115,342 : API 8th/538; Hurst 12th/1626; Braunwald 8th/1066*

Indapamide is a mild diuretic that may be used for treatment of mild to moderate hypertension It is not effective for the treatment of hypertensive urgencies or emergencies where rapid reduction of blood pressure is required. Indapamide is the single best answer of exclusion.

Trimethophan (KDT 6th/115)

Trimethophan is an ultrashort acting ganglion blocker

IT has been occasionally used in treatment of hypertensive emergencies due to Aortic dissecton (KDT)

Nifedipine (KDT 6th/554)

Nifedipine may be employed for rapid reduction of BP in hypertensive urgencies although its use is not recommended
Nifedipine was once one of the most popular drugs used hypertensive urgencies

Hydralazine

Hydralazine is an effective agent for the management of hypertensive urgencies and emergencies.

275. Answer is D (Clonidine): *Braunwald 8th/1066; API 8th/538; Hurst 12th/1626; 'Koda-kimble and young's manual of Therapeutics: Clinical use of Drugs' (Lippincott William) 2012/525*

Clonidine is a central Alfa-agonist that is recommended for the management of severe hypertension, that is not accompanied by evidence of end organ damage. However clonidine is not recommended for true hypertensive emergencies (crisis) where the goal is to reduce the blood pressure within minutes (preferably in less than one hour)

Fenoldapam, Nitroglycerine and Nitroprusside may all be used intravenously for rapid reduction of Blood Pressure in patients with true Hypertensive emergencies.

Commonly used Drugs in the Management of Hypertensive Crisis

Common Intravenous Agents **(Used for Hypertensive Emergencies)**	Common Oral Agents **(Used for Hypertensive Urgencies)**
Diuretics *Furosemide* **Vosodilators** *Sodium Nitroprusside* *Nitroglycerine* *Fenoldapam* *Nicardipine* *Hydralazine* *Enolaprilant* **Adrenergic Inhibitors** *Phentolamine* *Esmolol* *Metaprolol* *Labetolol* *Urapidil*	*Nifedipine (Not Recommended now)* *Nicardipine* *Israpidine* *Clonidine* *Coptopril* *Labetolol* *Hydralazine* *Nitroglycerine*

**** Nifedipine should be used with great caution 'if at all' according to the US F.D.A.'***

276. Answer is D (Nifedipine): *KDT 6th/554; Harrisons 16th/1475; Cardiac drug therapy by Gabriel Khan 7th/128,129; Kidney and hypertension by Bakris (2004)/146*

Nifedipine is used as an oral/sublingual agent. It is not available for intravenous administration.

Nifedipine in Hypertensive Urgencies

- Nifedipine is a short acting Dihydropyridene calcium channel blocker
- Nifedipine may be employed for rapid reduction of blood pressure in hypertensive urgencies but it is not recommended for such use because it has been reported to increase the incidence of acute coronary events.
- According to the US Food and Drug administration Nifedipine should be used with great caution 'if at all'
- ***Nifedipine is available for oral administration only and cannot be administered intravenously***

***Urapidil** (Cardiac drug therapy by Gabriel khan 7th/128,129)*

- Urapidil is a selective alpha 1 adrenoceptor antagonist effective in the treatment of hypertensive emergencies.
- It may be administerd intravenously and is also available for oral administration

Fenoldopam *(Hurst 12th/1626)*

- Fenoldopam is a selective dopamine -1 Receptor Agonist effective in the treatment of hypertensive emergencies
- It is available for intravenous administration.

Enalaprilat

- Enalaprilat is an ACE inhibitor effective in the treatment of hypertensive emergencies
  (Enalaprilat is the active of Enalapril that is available for intravenous administration. Enalapril can only be administered orally).

277. Answer is A, C and E (Nifedipine, Phenoxybenzomine, Labetalol) : *Refer text below*

A blood pressure recording of 200/120 with symptoms of headache and sweating suggests a diagnosis of Hypertensive crisis (urgency / Emergency). ***Nifedipine, Methyl Dopa and Phenoxybenzamine arenot preferred in the treatment of Hypertensive crisis***

Nifidipine, Methyl Dopa and phenoxybenzamine are not preferred for treatment of Hypertensive crisis

- **Nifedipine** was once one of the most popular drugs used in hypertensive urgencies, but its use is no longer recommended since it has been reported to increase the risk of acute coronary events.
  'Short acting nifedipine has no role in the treatment of hypertension' – Harrison
  'Nifedipine should be used with great caution 'if at all' according to the USFDA'

- **Methyl Dopa** has a relatively slow onset of action. It is not a preferred agent for treatment of hypertensive crisis owing to its adverse effect profile and because of its relatively slow action . It is now usually reserved for the treatment of hypertension in pregnancy

Preferred Agents for Treatment of Hypertensive Crisis of Pregnancy
Hydralizene, Labetalol, Nicardipine

- **Phenoxybenzomine is a long acting alpha adrenergic blocker that can produce a 'Chemical sympathethectomy'**

  Phenoxybenzamine is primarily used to control episodes of hypertension in patients with pheochromocytoma and in preoperative management of hypertension in patients with pheochromocytoma, who are being prepared for surgery. *It has a relatively slow onset of action is and is not preferred for the management of hypertensive crisis even in patients with pheochromocytoma*

Preferred Agents for Treatment of Hypertensive crisis in pheochromocytoma (Adrenergic / catecholamine crisis)
Phentolamine, Nitroprusside, Labetalol

Sodium Nitropnesside and Labetalol are preferred agents for treatment of Hypertensive Crisis

Preferred parenteral drugs for selected hypertensive emergencies	
Hypertensive encephalopathy	***Nitroprusside***, nicardipine, ***labetalol***
Malignant hypertension (when IV therapy is indicated)	***Labetalol***, nicardipine, ***nitroprusside***, enalaprilat
Stroke	Nicardipine, **labetalol**, *nitroprusside*
Myocardial infarction/unstable angina	Nitroglycerin, nicardipine, ***labetalol***, esmolol
Acute left ventricular failure	Nitroglycerin, enalaprilat, loop diuretics
Aortic dissection	***Nitroprusside***, esmolol, labetalol
Adrenergic crisis	Phentolamine, ***nitroprusside***
Postoperative hypertension	Nitroglycerin, ***nitroprusside, labetalol***, nicardipine
Preeclampsia/eclampsia of pregnancy	Hydralazine, ***labetalol,*** nicardipine

278. Answer is D (Metabolic Alkalosis): *Harrison 17th/293; Harrison 16th/268; Therapy of Renal Disease and Related disorders 2nd/169*

Accelerated Hypertension is associated with metabolic alkalosis.

Accelerated Hypertension is a state in which there is renal underperfusion, high renin and increased aldosterone. This may result in hypokalemia and metabolic alkalosis.

Renovascular Hypertension

279. Answer is B (CT Angiography): *Harrison 16th/1470; Braunwald 8th/1040; The Cleveland Clinic Cardiology Board Review (Lippincott Williams) 1st/514*

Spiral CT scan with intravenous contrast (CT angiography) is the most sensitive and specific test amongst the options provided.

Note:

Magnetic Resonance Angiography (MRA) has now emerged as the diagnostic test of choice at several centres with a sensitivity and specificity similar or even better than CT Angiography.

However as MRA has not been provided amongst the options, CT Angiography remains the single best answer of choice.

*MRA is also more likely to be used more widely **(preferred)** because it reduces the possibility of contrast induced nephrotoxicity and avoids exposure to ionizing radiations.*

Renovascular Hypertension

Screening Test of Choice	Gold Standard Diagnostic Test
Magnetic Resonance Angiography (MRA) Spiral CT or Angiography (CTA)	Renal Angiography / Arteriography (conventional)

MRA is now emerging as the screening test of choice

280. Answer is A (Magnetic Resonance Angiography (MRA): *'The Clevland Clinic Board Review' (Lippincott Williams) 1st/514; Harrison 16th/1470; Cardiovascular Therapeutic 3rd*

Magnetic Resonance Angiography (MRA) has now emerged as the most sensitive and specific screening test for Renovascular hypertension.

Note:

Harrison 16th edition (old) mentions Spiral CT scan as the most sensitive and specific screening test for Renovascular Hypertension, however most recent textbooks now prefer MRA as the screening test of choice with similar or even better sensitivity and specificity than spiral CT Angiography.

Renovascular Hypertension

Screening Test

Test	Sensitivity (%)	Specificity (%)
Magnetic resonance angiography (MRA)	100	96
Spiral computerized tomography	98	94
Captopril renogram	70-93	95
Duplex Doppler ultrasonography	69-96	86-90
IVP	~75	~85

Gold Standard / Diagnostic Test

Test	Sensitivity	Specificity
Conventional Renal Angiography	>99%	>99%

281. Answer is C (Condition is nearly always bilateral): Harrison 18th/p 2375, 2376 *Harrisons 17th/- 1811-1812*

*Presence of hypertension (BP = 160 / 110) and bruit in bilateral flanks suggest a diagnosis of Bilateral Renal Artery Stenosis in this patient. **Renal Artery Stenosis is bilateral in 50% of cases and is not nearly always bilateral***

ACE inhibitors (eg Enalapril) may deteriorate renal function in patients with Bilateral Renal Artery Stenosis

ACE inhibitors (eg Enalapril) are the agents of choice for treatment of hypertension in patients with unilateral renal artery stenosis, but *are **contraindicated in patients with bilateral disease***. The presence of bruit in both flanks suggest *bilateral disease in this patient and hence enalapril should not be used*

Contrast Enhanced Arteriography (Angiography) is the most definitive diagnostic procedure for the diagnosis of Renal Artery stenosis while Magnetic Resonance Angiography (MRA) is the most sensitive and specific non invasive test (screening test) for its diagnosis.

Fibromuscular dysplasia is the most common cause of Renal Artery stenosis in young women while Atherosclerotic disease is the most common cause in middle aged/ elderly patients. *The patient in question is a young female (20 years) and hence the most likely cause of Renal Artery stenosis in this patient is fibromuscular dysplasia*

Surgical Intervention may be required in patients with Bilateral Renal Artery Stenosis

Surgical intervention in the form of angioplasty and stent placement is indicated when medical therapy has failed to control BP or resulted in > 30% increase in serum creatinine.

Renal Artery Stenosis: Review
• Renal Artery stenosis is an important cause of Renovascular Hypertension • ***Bilateral involvement is seen in half of the affected cases (50%)***
Etiology
• Atherosclerotic disease : This is the most common cause in middle aged /elderly patients • Fibromuscular Dysplasia : ***This is the most important cause in young females***
Presentation
• Hypertension - Abrupt onset of hypertension - Acceleration of previously well controlled hypertension - Refractory Hypertension • Features of increased sympathetic neural activity (which is associated with Renovascular disease) - Flushing - Loss of nocturnal BP decrease - Putonomic instability - Rapid BP swings • Progressive Renal failure / Azotemia
Diagnosis
Magnetic Resonance Angiography (MRA): MRA is the most sensitive (>90%) and specific (95%) non invasive test for the diagnosis of RAS **Contrast Enhanced Arteriography**: Contrast enhanced angiography is the most definitive (but invasive) diagnostic procedure for diagnosis of RAS
Management
Medical Therapy with ACE Inhibitors or Angiotensin Receptor Blockers
Indications — **Unilateral Renal artery Stenosis** - With hypertension & normal renal function (more effective than other antihypertensives) - With hypertension & abnormal renal function (beneficial effect on survival without affecting renal function) - With hypertension, diabetes, proteinuria and normal or abnormal renal function (effective antihypertensives)
Contra indications — **Bilateral Renal Artery stenosis** ACE inhibitors or Angiotensin receptor blockers are contraindicated in patients with Bilateral renal artery stenosis or stenosis in a solitary kidney as their use in such patients leads to worsening of renal failure (These patients are especially sensitive to decline in intraglomerular pressure)
Note ***Acute Renal Failure / Worsening of Renal Failure with Angiotension Receptor Inhibitors is a diagnostic clue to the diagnosis of renal artery stenosis (indicates bilateral disease)***
Surgical Therapy with Angioplasty + Stent placement
Should be considered only after optimal medical therapy has failed to achieve goal BP or resulted in a > 30% increase in serum creatinine

282. Answer is B (Non specific aorto-arteritis): *Disease of kidney and urinary tract 8th/1279; Tropical Neurology 1st (2003)/440; Surgical Neuroangigraphy 2nd/115*

The most common cause of renal artery stenosis in young adults in India is Non specific aorto-arteritis.

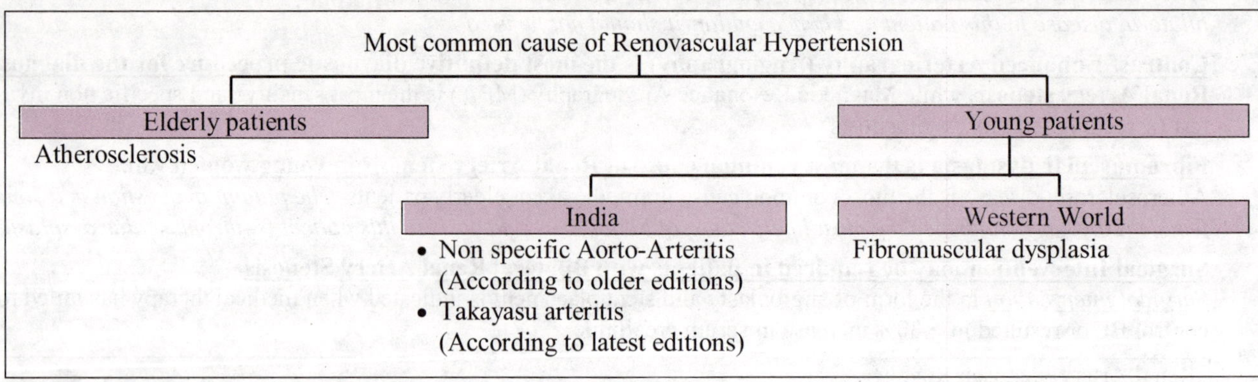

The non specific aorto-arteritis causing renal artery stenosis is now believed to be Aorto-arteritis secondary to Takayasu arteritis

Aorto-arteritis/Takayasu arteritis is the most common cause of renovascular hypertension in India

Non specific Aorto-arteritis is the most common cause of renovascular hypertension in India and China – Tropical Neurology 1st (2003)/440

Takayasu arteritis (Aorto-arteritis) is the most common cause of renovascular hypertension in India and China.' – Diseases of kidney and Urinary Tract 8th/1279

In India, China, Korea, Japan and other South East Asian countries, Takayasu arteritis is the most common cause of renovaascular hypertension.' – Surgical Neuroangiography 2nd/115

Note:
The non specific aorto-arteritis causing renal artery stenosis is now believed to be Aorto-arteritis secondary to Takayasu arteritis

283. Answer is D (Polyarteritis nodosa): *Harrison 16th/1707,2007,2009; CMDT'06,460, API 8th.541; References alongside explanation*

Amongst the options provided renal artery stenosis is least likely to be seen in association with Polyarteritis nodosa.

- **Atherosclerosis and Fibromuscular disease**
  - Renal artery stenosis is produced predominantly by atherosclerotic occlusive disease (80% to 90% of patients) or fibromuscular dysplasia (10-15% of patients).- *CMDT'06 p 460*
  - The common cause of renal artery stenosis ***in the middle aged and elderly*** is an atheromatous plaque at origin of renal artery. *Harrison*
  - ***In younger women*** stenosis is due to intrinsic structural abnormalities of the arterial wall caused by a heterogenous group of lesions called 'fibromuscular dysplasia'. - *Harrison 16th/1707*
- **PAN or Takayasu arteritis ?**

  Harrison, CMDT do not mention PAN or Takayasu arteritis as a cause for renal artery stenosis.
  However, Takayasu arteritis is certainly a more common cause of renal artery stenosis than PAN.
  Takayasu arteritis (Aorto-arteritis) *is beleiveds to be the most common of renovascular hypertension in India and China. – Diseases of Kidney and Urinary Tract 8th/1279*

A number of research publications, however show Takayasu arteritis as a cause for renal artery stenosis.

Takayasu Arteritis	PAN
Takayasu arteritis (Aorto-arteritis) is the most common cause of renovascular hypertension in India and China.' – Diseases of kidney and Urinary Tract 8th/1279	Renal artery stenosis in a Case of PAN has only been described as an unusual association and published as a rare case report (single case) ***Reference :*** "PAN with renal Artery Stenosis": Indian Pediatrics Volume 41-Jan.17, 2004.

PAN
Although renal involvement is seen in upto 60% of patients with PAN its pathology does not involve renal artery stenosis.

The pathology involves arteritis without glomerulonephritis and is characterised by aneurysms of small and medium sized arteries. **Stenosis of main renal artery is an unusual association'.**

-Research paper, www. Indian paediatrics. net/Jan 2004/86.pdf

Causes of Renal artery stenosis : *API 8th/541; Renal Artery Stenosis : Diagnosis and Management - IHJ : May-June 2002, Vol. 54/No. 3*
1. Atherosclerosis
2. Fibromuscular dysplasia
3. Non specific Aorto arteritis
4. Takayasu arteritis and giant cell arteritis (Takayasu > Giant cell)
5. Antiphospholipid syndrome
6. Transplant renal artery stenosis
7. Renal artery embolism
8. Dissecting aneurysm of aorta
9. Radiation arteritis

Pulmonary Hypertension

284. Answer is A (Bone morphogenic Receptor Protein II): Harrison 18th/p 2077 *Harrisons 16th/1405; Harrisons 17th/1577; Robbins 7th /743,744*

Gene coding the type II bone morhphogenetic protein receptor II (BMPR II) is associated with familial cases of primary pulmonary hypertension and designated as the PPH I gene.

Bone morphogenic protein receptor II (BMPRII) and pulmonary Hypertension

- BMPRII is a cell surface protein receptor belonging to the TGF-β receptor superfamily (located on chromosome 2q31)
- BMP-BMPRII signaling plays an important role in embryogenesis, apoptosis, cell proliferation and differentiation.
- In vascular smooth muscles normal BMPR2 signalling causes inhibition of proliferation and favour apoptosis, thereby protecting the vessels from narrowing and development of hypertension
- Primary pulmonary hypertension is believed to be caused by a mutation in the gene coding for the BMPR II signaling pathway (PPH-1 gene/BMPRII gene)
- ***Mutation in the BMPR II gene (PPH-1gene) predisposes the cells to undergo proliferation rather than apoptosis and results in development of pulmonary hypertension.***

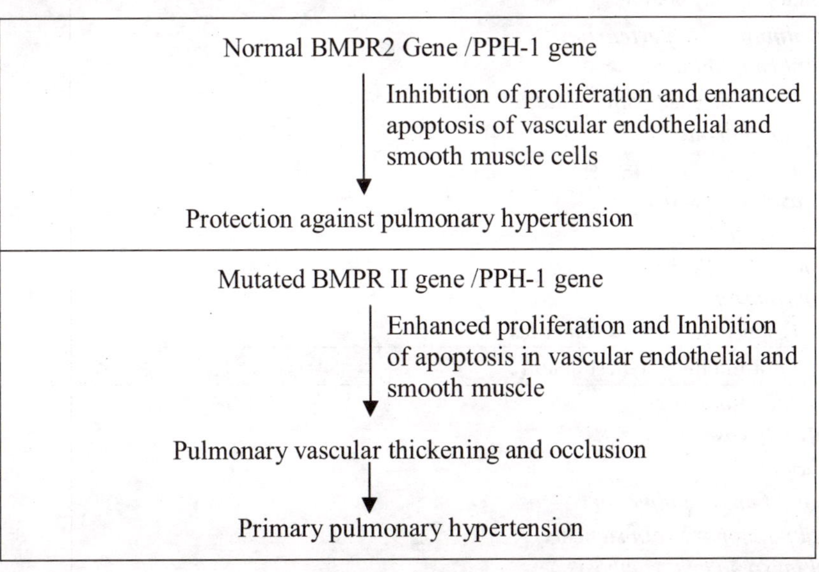

285. Answer is D (↑ Pulmonary wedge pressure): *Internal Medicine 5th/293*

↑ pulomary wedge pressure is not a feature of Precapillary Pulmonary hypertension.

In precapillary pulmonary hypertension the abnormality that leads to elevated pulmonary pressure is located in the pulmonary artery or arterioles. The Left atrial pressure or Pulmonary capillary wedge pressure is essentially normal.

Features	Precapillary	Passive (Post-capillary)
Pathophysiology	Abnormality that leads to elevated pulmonary artery pressure is located in the pulmoanry artery or arterioles.	Abnormalities that lead to elevated pulmonary artery pressure are located beyond the pulmonary arteries. These are caused by diseases that lead to increased pulmonary venous pressure that in turn produces secondary elevation in pulmonary arterial pressure.
Pulmonary artery mean pressure	↑/↑↑	↑
Left Atrial Pressure (PCWP)	***Normal***	↑
PA left Atrial Pressure Gradient	> 12mm	<12mm Hg
Conditions/Causes	• *Primary pulmonary hypertension* • *Disorders of ventilation* • *Congenital heart disease with pulmonary vascular disease* • *Pulmonary embolism* • *Schistosmiasis* • *Collagen vascular disease* • *Pulmonary vasculitis* • *Sickle hemoglobinopathies* • *Portal hypertension* • *Ingestion of drugs and herbal remedies*	• *Left ventricular failure* • *Mitral valve disease* • *Cor triatriatum* • *Obstruction of major pulmonary veins* • *Congenital pulmonary vein stenosis* • *Left atrial myxoma or thrombosis*

286. Answer is A (Mitral stenosis): *Internal Medicine* 5th*/293*

Mitral stenosis is a cause of post-capillary pulmonary hypertension or passive pulmonary hypertension.

Causes of pulmonary hypertension:

Precapillary pulmonary hypertension

- ***Primary pulmonary hypertension***
- *Disorders of ventilation*
- *Congenital heart disease with pulmonary vascular disease*
- ***Pulmonary embolism***
- *Schistosmiasis*
- *Collagen vascular disease*
- ***Pulmonary vasculitis***
- *Sickle hemoglobinopathies*
- *Portal hypertension*
- *Ingestion of drugs and herbal remedies*

Passive (Post-capillary) pulmonary hypertension

- *Left ventricular failure*
- ***Mitral valve disease***
- *Cor triatriatum*
- *Obstruction of major pulmonary veins*
- *Congenital pulmonary vein stenosis*
- *Left atrial myxoma or thrombosis*

Reactive pulmonary hypertension

- *Some patients with mitral valve disease*
- *Rarely, other cause of pulmonary venous hypertension, including pulmonary veno-occlusive disease*

287. Answer is A (Hyperventilation): Harrison 18th/p 2078, 2080 *Harrisons 17th/1577,1579*

Pulmonary hypertension may be caused by hypoventilation but not by hyperventilation.

Chronic exposure to high altitude sleep disordered breathing due to obesity and anorexic agents including fenfluramine are known causes of pulmonary hypertension.

Clinical Classification of Pulmonary Hypertension

1. **Pulmonary arterial hypertension (PAH)**
   - Idiopathic (IPAH)(formerly PPH)
   - Familial (FPAH)
   - Associated with (APAH)
     - *Collagen vascular disease*
     - *Congenital systemic-to-pulmonary shunts*
     - *Portal hypertension*
     - *HIV infection*
     - *Drugs and toxins (including fenfluramine)*
     - *Other (thyroid disorders, glycogen storage disease, Gaucher disease, hereditary hemorrhagic telangiectasia, hemoglobinopathies, myeloproliferative, disorders, splenectomy)*
   - Associated with significant venous or capillary involvement
     - *Pulmonary veno-occlusive disease (PVOD)*
     - *Pulmonary capillary hemangiomatosis (PCH)*
     - *Persistent pulmonary hypertension of the newborn*
2. **Pulmonary hypertension with left heart disease**
   - *Left-sided atrial or ventricular heart disease*
   - *Left-sided valvular heart disease*
3. **Pulmonary hypertension associated with lung diseases and/or hypoxemia**
   - *Chronic obstructive pulmonary disease*
   - *Interstitial lung disease*
   - ***Sleep-disordered breathing***
   - *Alveolar hypoventilation disorders*
   - ***Chronic exposure to high altitude***
   - *Developmental abnormalities*
4. **Pulmonary hypertension due to chronic thrombotic and/or embolic disease**
   - *Thromboembolic obstruction of proximal pulmonary arteries*
   - *Thromboembolic obstruction of distal pulmonary arteries*
   - *Nonthombotic pulmonary embolism (tumor, parasites, foreign material)*
5. **Miscellaneous**
   Sarcoidosis, histiocytosis X, lymphangiomatosis, compression of pulmonary vessels (adenopathy, tumor, fibrosing mediastinitis)

A causal relationship has been established between exposure to several anorexigens including aminorex and the ***fenfluramines*** *and the development of PAH-Harrison*

288. Answer is D (Argemone mexicana poisoning): Harrison 18th/p 2082 *Reference with text*

Argemone mexicana poisoning has not been mentioned as a cause for pulmonary hypertension. It is the single best answer of exclusion.

Toxic oil syndrome is associated with pulmonary Hypertension *(Goldrank's Toxicological Emergencies 7th/25)*
Toxic oil syndrome also called toxic epidemic syndrome is a multi system disorder characterized by pneumonitis, eosinophilia, ***pulmonary hypertension***, scleroderma like feature and neuromuscular changes
Toxic oil syndrome has first observed as an epidemic in spain due to consumption of 'Rapeseed oil' as cooking oil.

Sickle cell anemia is associated with pulmonary hypertension(H17th/1581)
Cardiovascular abnormalities including pulmonary hypertension are prominent abnormalities in the clinical spectrum of sickle cell disease-H17th/1581

Systemic sclerosis is associated with pulmonary hypertension
All collagen vascular diseases including systemic sclerosis may be associated with pulmonary hypertension.(H17th/1579)

289. Answer is D (Bronchoconstriction): Harrison 18th/p 2081 *Harrison 17th/1580*

Bronchoconstriction is not a cause for Pulmonary Hypertension

Pulmonary Hypertension in COPD has been attributed to multiple factors including:

- ***Hypoxia***
- ***Pulmonary vasoconstriction (secondary to hypoxia)***
- *Acidemia*
- *Hypercapnia*
- *Mechanical effect of* ***high lung volume*** *on pulmonary vessels*
- *Loss of small vessels in vascular bed*
- *Regions of emphysematous lung destruction*

Aortic Dissection

290. Answer is A (Acute Aortic dissection): *Harrison 16th/1483; API 7th/512; Harrison 17th/1565, 1566; 18th/ 2064*

Chest pain radiating to the back and interscapular region, with shock in presence of risk factors such as hypertension suggest a diagnosis of acute aortic dissection. *Loss of pulses occurs when vessel orifices are obstructed by mobile intimal flaps and pulses may well be preserved if such obstruction does not occur. A pleural effusion (left sided) may also be present. – Harrison & API*

- A ***pleural effusion*** (usually left sided) may also be present. The effusion is typically serosanguinous and does not indicate rupture unless accompanied by hypotension and falling haematocrit. – *Harrison 16th*
- ***Pain*** may be localized to the front back of the chest, often in the interscapular region and typically migrates with propagation of the lesion.
  'Severe pain from onset differentiates it from myocardial infarction' – *API7th/512*
  Sudden onset pain, severe, tearing associated with diaphoresis.
- ***Pulse deficits*** may be produced obstruction of the branches by compression of the true lumen by distended false lumen or by obstruction of the vessels orfice by mobile intimal flag. Peripheral pulses thus may be normal if the pathologic process does not compromise their orifices.
- ***Risk factor*** include old age (50-70 yrs), ***hypertension***, females sex, pregnancy bicuspid or unicuspid aortic valve, Noonan or Turner's syndrome, cocaine abuse or connective tissue disorders such as Marfan's Ehler's Danlos syndrome, or arteritis such as Takayasu's or giant cell arteritis.

291. Answer is C (MR): Harrison 18th/p 2064 *Harrison 17th/1566*

Mitral Regurgitation is not a feature of Aortic dissection

Aortic Regurgitation and Pericardial Tamponade may be seen in proximal dissection

Hemopericardium and cardiac tamponade may complicate a dissection involving the ascending aorta (type A lesion with retrograde dissection): H17th/1566

Acute Aortic Regurgitation (AR) is an important and common complication of proximal dissection – H 17th/1566

Acute Myocardial Ischemia may be associated with Aortic dissection

'Bowel Ischemia, hematuria and myocardial Ischemia have all benn observed with Aortic dissection' – H 17th/1566

292. Answer is C (In Ist trimester pregnancy): *Harrison 17th/1656*

Aortic dissection is predisposed during Third trimester of pregnancy and not during the first trimester of pregnancy

Risk factors / Predisposing factors for Aortic Dissection

- ***Systemic Hypertension and cystic medial necrosis***
- Connective Tissue Disorders
  - ***Marfan's Syndrome***
  - Ehler's Danlos Syndrome
- Inflammatory Aortititis
  - ***Takayasu arteritis***
  - Giant cell arteritis
- Congenital Aortic Valve abnormalities
  - Bicuspid Aortic Valve
- ***Coarctation of Aorta***
- Aortic trauma
- ***Third trimester of pregnancy***

293. Answer is B and D (Diazoxide and Hydralazine): Harrison 18th/p 2064 *Harrison 17th/1566*

Diazoxide and Hydralazine are direct vasodilators and isolated use of direct vasodilators is contraindicated in Aortic dissection because these agents may propagate dissection by increasing hydraulic shear.

'Isolated use of direct vasodilators such as diazoxide and hydralazine is contraindicated because these agents can increase hydraulic shear and may propogate dissection'- H17th/1566

Agents recommended in treatment of Aortic Dissection

- ***Beta Adrenergic blockers (propanolol/metoprolols/esmolol) intravenously***
- ***Sodium Nitroprusside***
- ***Labetolol (may be used)***
- *Calcium channel blockers (Verepamil/Diltiazam)*
  (May be used if Beta blockers or Nitroprusside cannot be employed)

Cardiopulmonary Resuscitation

294. Answer is A (Ventricular Tachycardia): Harrison 18th/p 2239, 2244 *Harrisons 17th/1712,1708*

Defibrillation is indicated when cardiac arrest occurs secondary to ventricular fibrillation or pulseless ventricular tachycardia (shockable rhythms)

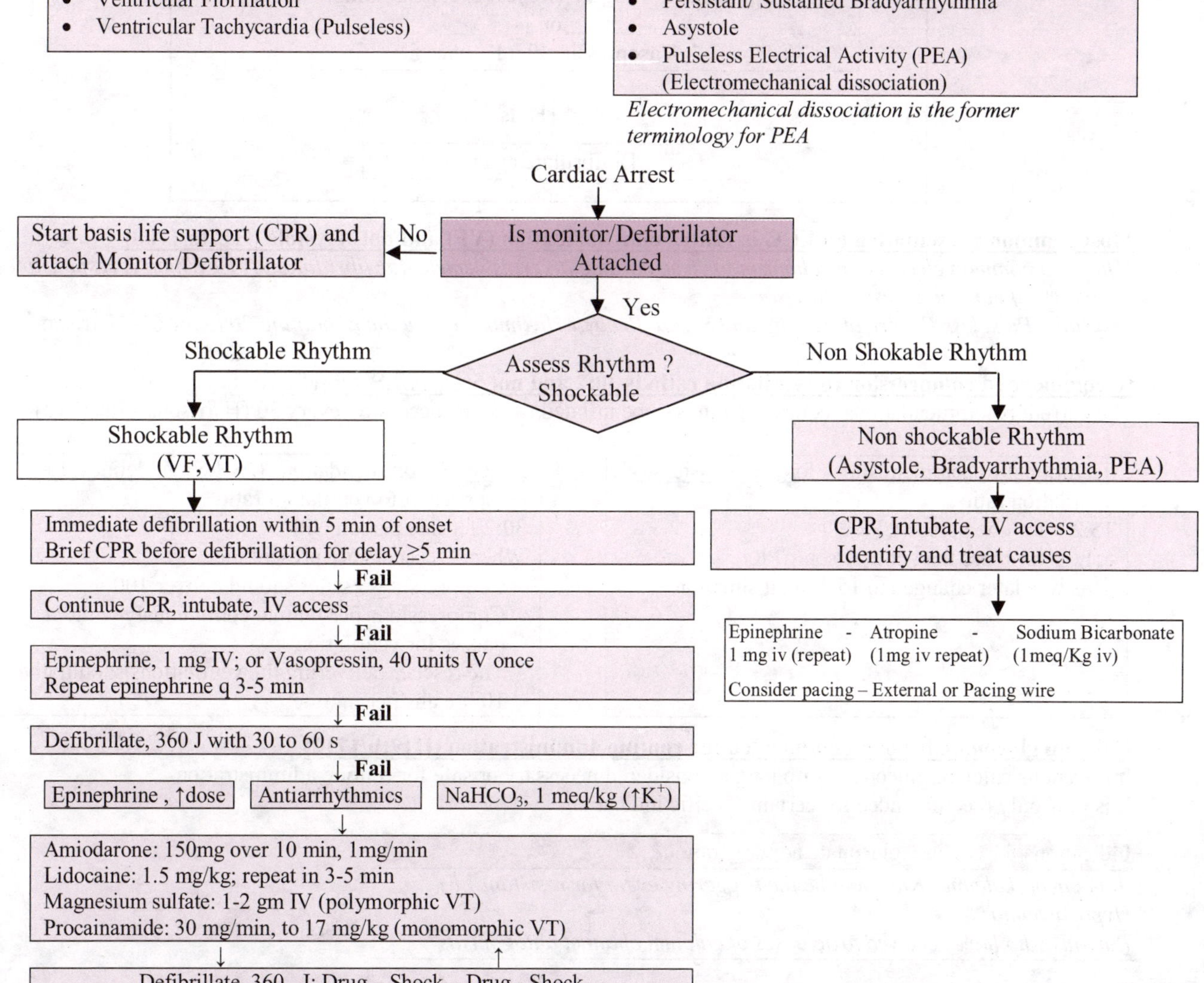

295. Answer is C (Adrenaline is given if cardioversion fails): Harrison 18th/p 2239, 2243, 2244 *Harrisons 17th/1708,1711,1712; Harrisons 16th/1622,1623*

During cardiopulmonary rescuscitation (CPR), administration of Adrenaline is recommended only after attempts at cardioversion fail.

<u>Adrenaline (Epinephrine) is given if cardioversion fails. (H17th/1712)</u>

Cardioversion is a brief procedure where an electric shock is given to the heart to convert an abnormal heart rhythm back to a normal rhythm (Defibrillation)
Cardioversion/Defibrillation is recommended as the immediate step during cardiopulmonary resuscitation.
Adrenalene/Epinerphrine is recommended only after failed defibrillation/cardioversion
'Epinephrine 1 mg intravenously is given after failed defibrillation' –H17th/1712

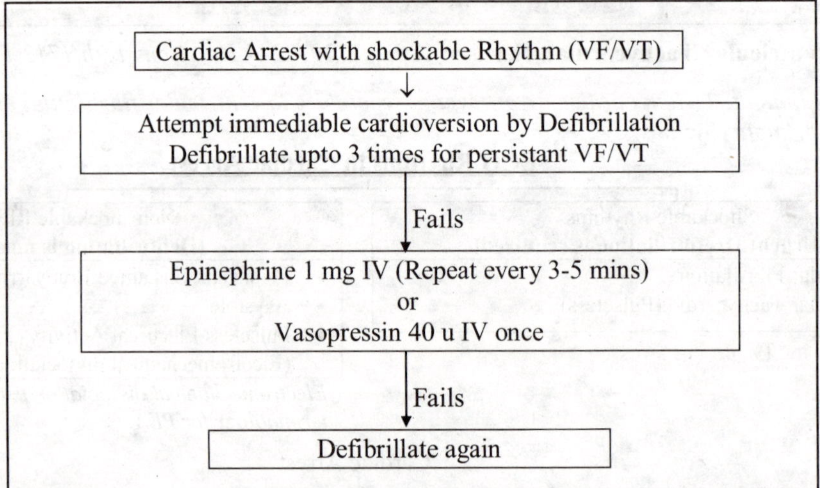

<u>Most common presentation on ECG is ventricular fibrillation (VF) and not Asystole (H17th/1708)</u>
'The most common electrical mechanism for true cardiac arrest is ventricular fibrillation (VF) Which is responsible for 65 to 80% of cardiac arrest'– Harrison
'Asystole, Pulseless Electrical Activity and Severe Bradyarrhythmias cause the remaining 20 to 30%' - Harrison

<u>Recommended compression to ventilation ratio is 30:2 and not 5:1 (ACLS guidelines)</u>
The current recommendations require the lungs to be inflated twice in succession every 30 (Harrisons 17th/1712)

<u>Traditional Recommendations for compression to ventilation ratio</u>	<u>Recent Recommendations (ACLS) guidelines) for compression to ventilation ratio</u>
15:2 for one person CPR 5:1 for more than one person CPR This was later changed to 15:2 in all situation	30:2 for one person CPR When 2 rescuers are present the - Compressing rescuer should deliver 100 Compressions per minute continuously without pauses for ventilation - The rescuer delivering the ventilations should give 8-10 breaths per minute

<u>Calcium gluconate is not recommended for routine administration (H17th/1712)</u>
Intravenous calcium gluconate is no longer considered necessary or safe for routine administration
It is now only recommended for certain specific indications

Indications for calcium gluconate administration
Acute hyperkalemia (Known to be the triggering event for resistant VF)
Hypocalcemia[Q]
Patients who have received toxic doses of calcium channel antagonists[Q]

296. Answer is A & B (Atropine) & (External cardiac pacing): Harrison 18th/p 2239, 2244 *Harrison's 17th/-1712, 1708, Advanced cardiac Life support (ACLS) Manual Irwin & Rippe's Intensive care medicine 6th/332*

Atropine and External cardiac pacing may be used in cardiac arrest following non shockable rhythms like Asystole but they have no role in the management of cardiac arrest with shockable rhythms like VF

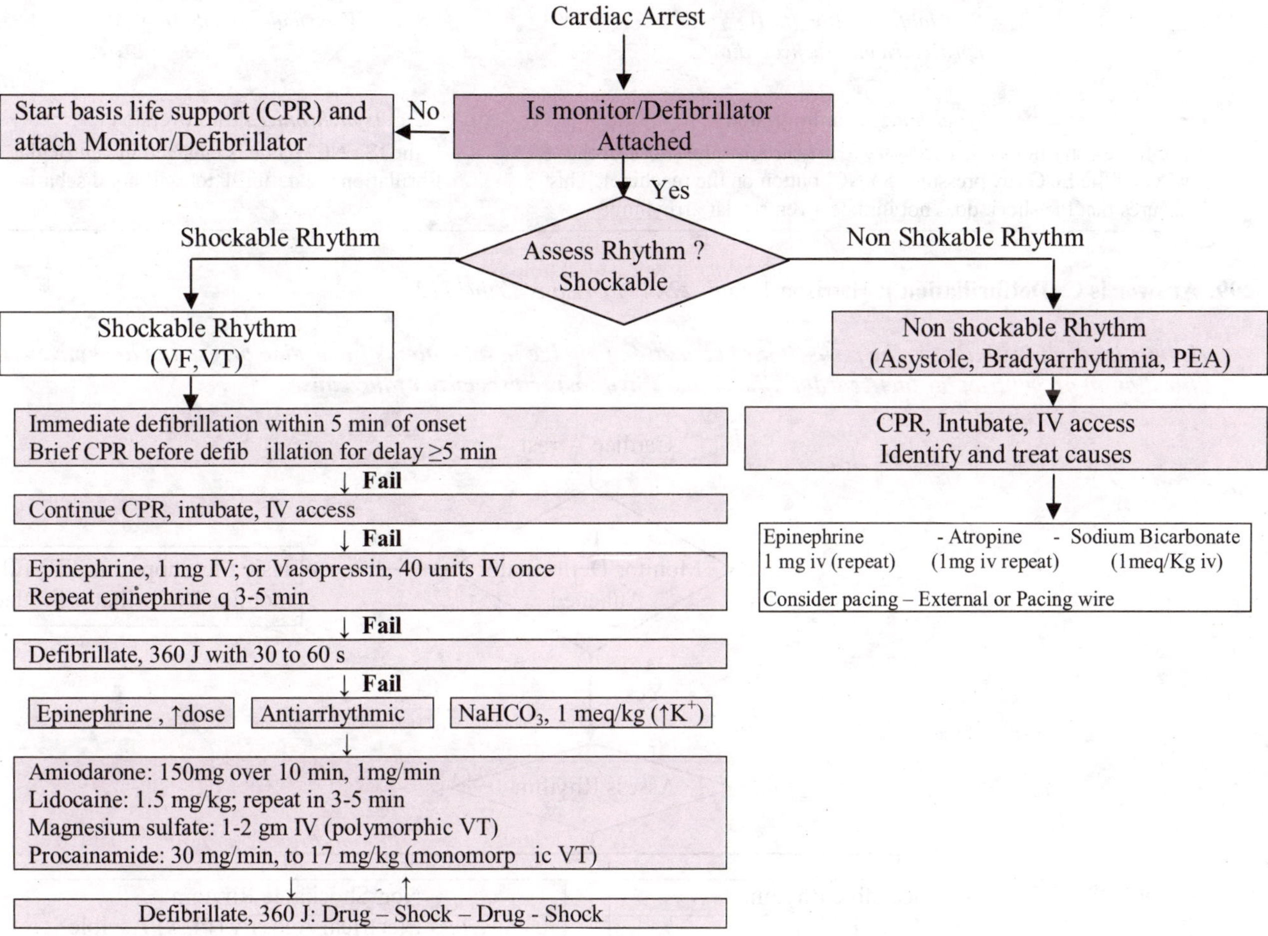

Role of vasopressin

Vasopressin has recently emerged as a potential agent for use in patients with cardiac arrest unresponsive to epinephrine and defibrillation 'Revised guidelines for ACLS recommend vasopressin as an alternative to epinephrine for the treatment of adult shock refractory ventricular fibrillations'- *Irwin & Rippe's Intensive care medicine 6th/-332*

297. Answer is C (Adrenaline is given if cardioversion fails): Harrison 18th/p 2244 *Harrisons 17th/1711, 1712*

Cardioversion is a brief procedure where an electric shock is given to the heart to convert an abnormal heart rhythm back to a normal rhythm.

Cardioversion / Defibrillation is recommended as the immediate step during cardiopulmonary resuscitation. Adrenaline (Epinephrine) is recommended only after failed defibrillation / cardioversion

'Epinephrine 1mg intravenously is given after failed defibrillation / cardioversion' - Harrison

298. Answer is B (Ventricular fibrillation): *Oxford handbook of Medicine 5th/712.*

Asynchronous cardioversion is the most reliable method for terminating V.F.

Electrical cardioversion and defibrillation are the most reliable methods for termination of arrhythmias. These methods depolarize all or at least a large portion of excitable myocardium in a near homogenous fashion. Thereby interrupting reequitant rhythms.

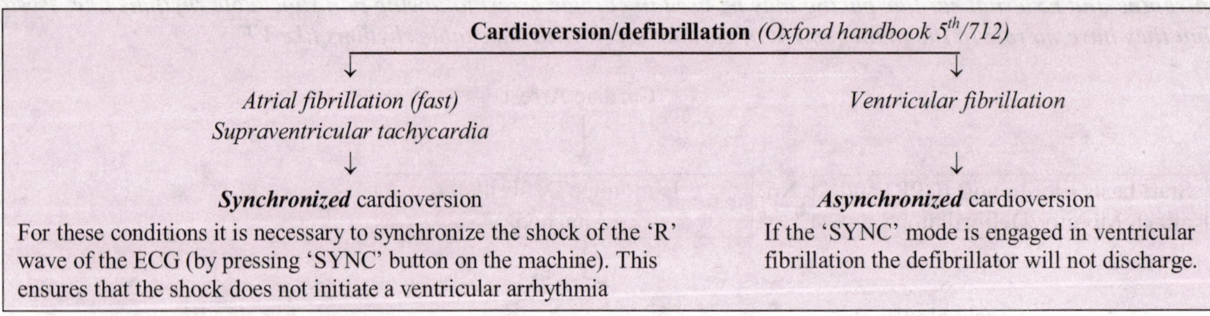

299. Answer is C (Defibrillation): Harrison 18th/p 2244 *Harrisons 17th/1712*

Immediate Defibrillation is the resuscitative measure of choice in all patients in cardiac arrest due to ventricular fibrillation on ventricular tachycardia (Shockable Rhythms) irrespective of the cause.

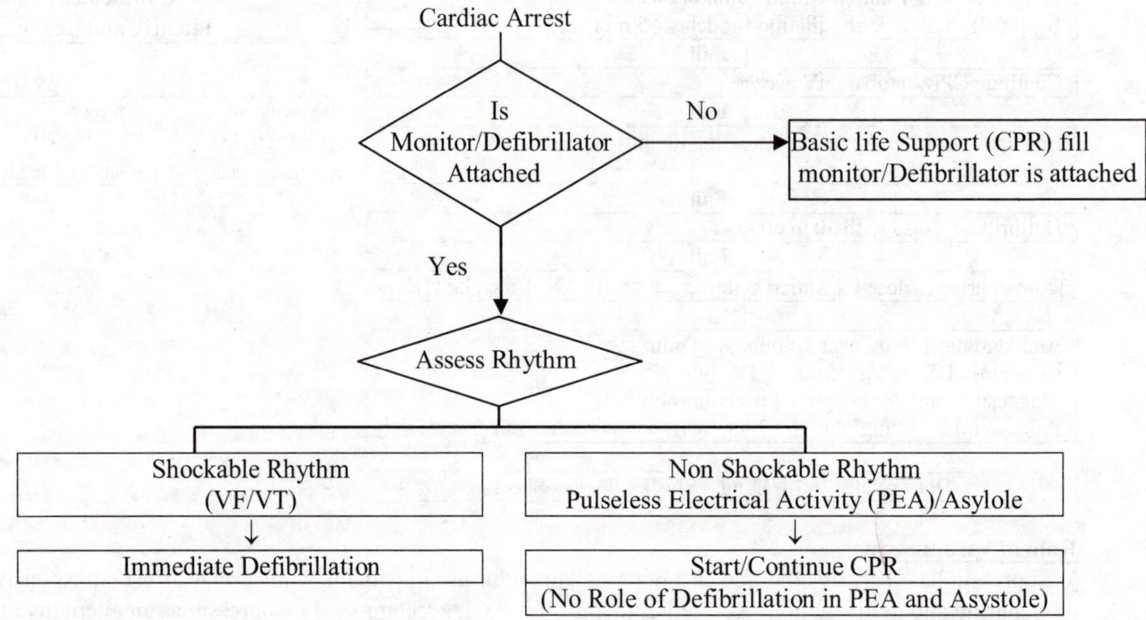

Note

- *The speed with which defibrillation /cardioversion is carried out is the most important determinant for the success of resuscitation.*
- *Defibrillation should be carried out immediately (as early as possible), even before intubation or insertion of an intravenous device.*

300. Answer is A (Ventricular Tachycardia): Harrison 18th/p 2243 *Harrisons 17th/1711*

The outcome after cardiac arrest is best if the mechanism is ventricular tachycardia- *Harrisons 17th/1711*

Outcome after cardiac arrest in decreasing order of success
Ventricular tachycardia (Best)
Ventricular fibrillation (Second Best)
Asystole
Pulseless Electrical activity (Electromechanical dissociation)

301. Answer is B (Hyperkalemia) : Harrison 18th/p 2244 *Harrisons 17th/1712*

Calcium gluconate is indicated in Hyperkalemia and not in hypokalemia

Calcium gluconate in Cardiopulmonary Resuscitation

Intravenous calcium gluconate is no longer considered necessary or safe for routine administration during cardiopulmonary resusciatation

Calcium gluconate may however be recommended for certain specific indications during CPR These include

Indications for Intervenous calcium gluconate during CPR
Hyperkalemia (When Acute hyperkalemia is known to be the triggering event for resistant VF) Q *Hypocalcemia*Q *Calcium channel anatagonist toxity*Q

Cardiac Tumors

302. Answer is A (Myxoma) : *Harrison 14th/1341, 15th/1373;Robbins 6th/589*

The most common primary cardiac tumor is Myxoma.

Remember
• The most frequent cardiac tumor for all age groups is - ***Metastasis***. • The most frequent primary cardiac tumor for age groups is - ***Myxoma***. • The most frequent primary cardiac tumor in infants and children is - ***Rhabdomyoma***.

303. Answer is A (Myxoma): *Repeat*

The commonest tumor of myocardium is a myxoma.

304. Answer is A (Most common in Left Atrium): *Harrison 14th/ 1341; 15th/ 1373; 16th/ 1421; 17th/ 1495, 1496*

Cardiac Myxomas are usually located in the atria, most common in the left.

Cardiac myxomas :

- Are the most common type of primary cardiac tumors. Q
- Occur at *all ages* and show ***no sex preference (mixes equally with both sexes)*** Q
- ***Most cardiac myxomas are sporadic***, while some may be familial

Sporadic myxomas :	Familial myxomas :
• Are solitary Q • Located in Atria, most commonly in the left Q • Unlikely to have post-op recurrence Q • Occur in younger individuals Q	• Are multiple Q • More likely to have post op recurrence Q

- ***Myxomas are benign tumors and therefore distant metastasis are not seen.***Q

305. Answer is D (Most myxomas are fmilial): *Previous question*

Most cardiac myxomas are sporadic while some may be familial.

306. Answer is C (Hypertension): *Harrison 14th/ 1341, 16th/ 1421; 17th/ 1495, 1496; Repeat* Harrison 18th/p 1979

All options other than hypertension are mentioned as features of atrial myxoma.

Atrial Myxoma : Clinical Presentation:

Presentation is highly dependent on position of tumour and hence it is intermittent and sudden in onset. *(as a result of changes in tumor position with gravity).*

Cardiac signs and symptoms	Non cardiac signs and symptoms
- Picture of Mitral valve disease - Characterised by low pitched sound– 'tumor plop' Q (audible during early or mid diastole).	- **Peripheral or pulmonary emboli** Q - **Fever** : Prolonged pyrexia of unknown origin Q - **Clubbing** Q - Raynaud's Phenomenon Q - Anemia/polycythemia or thrombocytopenia / thrombocytosis Leucocytosis - Elevated ESR Q - Rash Q - Weight loss, cachexia, malaise, arthralgia

307. Answer is A (Commonest site is LA): *Harrison 14th/ 1341; 15th/ 1373; 16th/ 1421; 17th/ 1495, 1496; 18th/p 1979*

Cardiac Myxomas are usually located in the atria, most common in the left.

Cardiac myxomas :

- Are the most common type of primary cardiac tumors. Q
- Occur at *all ages* and show *no sex preference* (mixes equally with both sexes) Q
- Most cardiac myxomas are sporadic, while some may be familial

Sporadic myxomas :	Familial myxomas :
• Are solitary Q • Located in Atria, most commonly in the left Q • Unlikely to have post-op recurrence Q • Occur in younger individuals Q	• Are multiple Q • More likely to have post op recurrence Q

- *Myxomas are benign tumors and therefore distant metastasis are not seen.* Q

308. Answer is C (Left atrial myxoma): *Harrison 15th/ 1279; 16th/1421; Harrison 17th/ 1496* Harrison 18th/p 1979

An increased gradient during diastole is suggestive of an obstructive lesion between Left atrium and Left ventricle that is not allowing pressures to normalize between the atria and ventricle such as atrial myxoma.

Pulmonary artery wedge pressure represents Left atrial pressure.

Left ventricular end diastolic pressure represents Left ventricular pressure.

Gradient between Left atrial pressure (PCWP) and Left ventricular pressure during diastole:

Normally there is no gradient during diastole as both pressures are equal.

An increased gradient during diastole is suggestive of an obstructive lesion between Left atrium and Left ventricle that is not allowing pressures to normalize between the atria and ventricle.

This may thus be seen in obstructive lesions between Left atria and ventricle such as :

1. Mitral stenosis
2. Atrial myxomas

Rheumatic Fever

309. Answer is C (Fever): *Harrison 16th / 1978; Harrison 17th/2095* Harrison 18th/p 2755

Fever is a Minor Jones Criteria for diagnosis of Rheumatic fever.

The Jones Criteria

Jones criteria were first proposed in 1944.

The most recent modification of the Jones criteria was published in 1992 and these were termed updated Jones criteria.

Updated Jones Criteria for Rheumatic fever

Major Criteria	Minor Criteria
• Carditis • Migratory polyarthritis • Sydenham's chorea • Subcutaneous nodules • Erythema marginatum	• ***Fever (clinical)*** • Arthralgia (clinical) • Elevated acute phase reactions (LAB) • Prolonged PR internal (LAB / ECG)

Essential Criteria
Supporting evidence of recent group A streptococcal infection. • Positive throat culture or rapid antigen detection test and / or • Elevated or increasing streptococcal antibody test.

To fulfill the Jones Criteria,

Two major criteria or One major criteria And Two minor criteria

PLUS

Essential criteria are required.

310. Answer is C (Fever): *Harrison 16th / 1978*

Fever is a Minor Jones Criteria for diagnosis of Rheumatic fever.

The Jones Criteria

Jones criteria were first proposed in 1944.
The most recent modification of the Jones criteria was published in 1992 and these were termed updated Jones criteria.

Updated Jones Criteria for Rheumatic fever

Major Criteria	Minor Criteria
• Carditis • Migratory polyartbritis • Sydenham's chorea • Subcutaneous nodules • Erythema marginatum	• ***Fever (clinical)*** • Arthralgia (clinical) • Elevated acute phase reactions (LAB) • Prolonged PR internal (LAB / ECG)

Essential Criteria
Supporting evidence of recent group A streptococcal infection. • Positive throat culture or rapid antigen detection test and / or • Elevated or increasing streptococcal antibody test.

To fulfill the Jones Criteria,
Two major criteria or One major criteria And Two minor criteria
PLUS
Essential criteria are required.

311. Answer is D (High ESR): Harrison 18th/p 2755 *Harrison's 17th/2095*

Elevated (High) ESR is a minor criterion and not a major criterion (Jones criteria)

World Health Criteria for the diagnosis of Rheumatic fever and rheumatic heart disease	
Major manifestations	• *Carditis* • *Polyarthritis* • *Chorea* • *Erythema marginatum* • *Subcutaneous nodules*
Minor manifestations	• Clinical: fever, polyarthralgia • Laboratory: elevated erythrocyte sedimentation rate or leukocyte count • Electrocardiogram: prolonged P-R interval *@1992 Revised Jones criteria do not include elevated leucocyte count as a laboratory minor manifestation (but do include elevated C-reactive protein)*
Supporting evidence of a preceding streptococcal infection within the last 45 days	• Elevated or rising anti-streptolysin O or other streptococcal antibody, or • A positive throat culture, or • Rapid antigen test for group A streptococcus, or • Recent scarlet fever *@1992 Revised Jones criteria do not include recent scarlet fever as supporting evidence of a recent streptococcal infection*

Diagnostic Categories	Criteria
Primary episode of rheumatic fever	*Two major or one major two minor manifestations plus evidence of preceding group A streptococcal infection*
Recurrent attack of rheumatic fever in a patient without established rheumatic heart disease	*Two major or one minor manifestations plus evidence of preceding group A streptococcal infection*
Recurrent attack of rheumatic fever in a patient with established rheumatic heart disease	*Two minor manifestations plus evidence of preceding group A streptococcal infection*

312. Answer is A, C and E (Chorea, Arthritis and carditis): *Harrisons 17th / 2095; Harrisons 16th / 1978; Nelsons 18th /1141* Harrison 18th/p 2755

Chorea, Arthritis and Carditis are major criteria for diagnosis of Rheumatic fever
Fever is a minor criteria
Erythema Marginatum is a major criteria and not Erythema nodosum.

313. Answer is A, C, E (Chrorea, Arthritis, Carditis) : *Refer text below*

Chorea, Arthritis and Carditis are major criteria for diagnosis of Acute Rheumatic fever
Acute Rheumatic fever is associated with Erythema marginatum and not Erythema nodosum
Acute Rheumtic fever is associated with Antecedent Group A streptococcal infection and not with antecedent α - hemolytic streptococcal infection.

314. Answer is D (Pancarditis) : *Robbins 7th /593*

Rheumatic fever is characterized by Pancarditis.

During Acute Rheumatic fever, diffuse inflammation and Aschoff bodies may be found in any of the three layers of heart - pericardium, myocardium or endocardium, hence the lesion is called pancarditis. – Robbin's 7th/593

315. Answer is B (Rupture of Chordae tendinae) : *Pathologic basis by Robbins 5th / 547; 6th/322*

Rupture of chordae temdinae is not a feature of Acute rheumatic fever

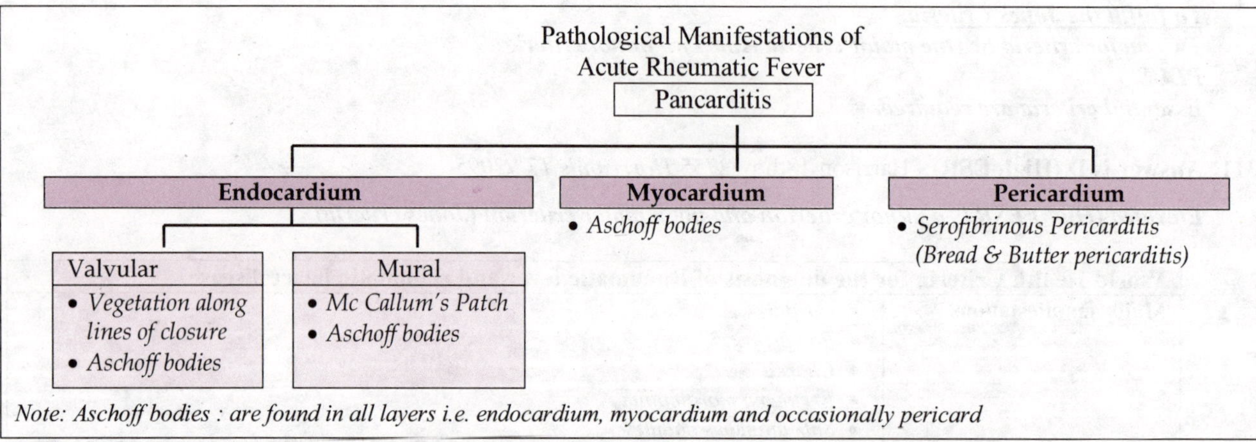

Note: Aschoff bodies : are found in all layers i.e. endocardium, myocardium and occasionally pericard

316. Answer is A (Aschoff's nodule) : *Robbins 5th / 549*

"Aschoff's body is pathognomic of Rheumatic fever" *- Robbins*

Aschoff's bodies *are focal inflammatory lesions, that may be found in any of the three layers of the heart - Pericardium, Myocardium and Endocardium, during acute Rheumatic fever.*

Aschoff bodies consist of foci of swollen eosinophillic collagen surrounded by
• Lymphocytes (primarily T cells) • Occasional plasma cells • Aschoff giant cells (macrophages of rheumatic fever) • Antitschkow cells *(Antischkow cells are modified macrophages with abundant cytoplasm and central round to ovoid nuclei in which the chromatin is disposed in the central, slender wavy ribbon like pattern – caterpillar cells)*

317. Answer is C (Rheumatic carditis): *Robbins 7th/ 593; (Repeat)*

Aschoff bodies are characteristic focal inflammatory lesions of acute rheumatic fever found in any of the three layers of the heart.

"Aschoff's body is pathognomic of Rheumatic fever" - Robbins

Aschoff bodies:

- Aschoff bodies are focal inflammatory lesions seen during acute rheumatic fever
- During acute RF, Aschoff bodies may be found in any of the three layers of the heart – pericardium, myocardium and endocardium.
- *Aschoff's body is pathognomic of Rheumatic fever*

318. Answer is B (Rheumatic endocarditis) : *Harsh Mohan 4th / 304*

Mac Callum's Patch is a feature of mural endocarditis in Rheumatic fever.

Mac Callum's Patch

- '*Mc.Callum's patch*' is the region of endocardial surface *in the posterior wall*[Q] of left atrium just above the posterior leaflet of mitral valve.
- It appears as a 'map like' area of thickened, roughened, and wrinkled part of endocardium.
- It is perhaps produced as a result of regurgitant jets.

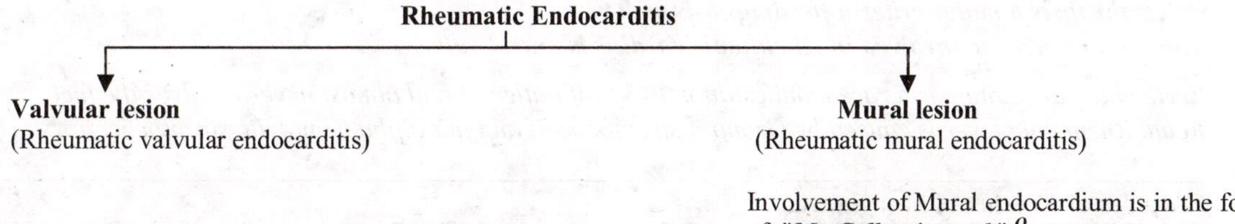

Involvement of Mural endocardium is in the form of ***"Mc.Callum's patch"*** [Q]

319. Answer is C (Communicable disease): Harrison 18th/p 2752, 2753 *Harrison 17th/2092, 2093; Nelson 16th/ 806*

Rheumatic fever is not a communicable disease. *Rheumatic fever occurs as a result of immunological hypersensitivity*[Q] *to streptococcal antigens.*

- *Group A β hemolytic streptococii is the causative agent.*
- *The major risk factor for development of acute rheumatic fever is a group A streptococcal pharyngitis (upper respiratory tract infection).*
- *Group A streptococcal impetigo (slum infection) does not result in acute rheumatic fever.*
- *[Post streptococcal glomerulonephritis however may be caused following both, an upper respiratory tract infection as well as infection of slum.]*
- *Rheumatic fever is most frequently observed in the age group of 5-15 years.*
- *The incidence* of rheumatic fever has declined in developed countries while in developing countries (poor socioeconomic groups) it remains a significant problem.

320. Answer is A (Chorea is aggrevated during pregnancy): Harrison 18th/p 2754 *Harrisons 17th/2094 Recent advances in Pediatrics 23rd/12*
The 5 minute Neurology Consult (2003) /394, Oxford textbook of Medicine 4th/1052: Nelsons 18th/1142.

Sydenham's chorea may be aggravated by pregnancy.

'Patient's with sydenham's chorea may have chorea during pregnancy (chorea gravidarum) and are at higher risk of chorea induced by phenytoin or oral contraceptives' - The 5- Minute Neurology consult (2003) /399

Sydenhom's chorea usually occurs in isolation and is not associated with arthritis usually. Subcutaneous nodules are typically non tender. Rheumatic fever is associated with Erythema marginatum and not Erythema multiforme

Featues of Sydenham's chorea in Rheumatic Fever (10-15% of patients)

- *It usually occurs after a prolonged latent period after group A streptococcus*
- *It usually occurs in the absence of other manifestation (usually not associated with arthritis or carditis)*
- *It usually occurs in females*
- *Presents as rapid, jerkey, involuntary movements (choreiform movements) affecting predominantly the Head /Face and Upper limbs*

- *May be generalized or restricted to one side / asymmetrical*
- *Typical signs include*
  - *Milk maid Grip*
  - *Spooning of extended hands*
  - *Darting of the protruded tongue*
  - *Pronator signs*
- *Typically associated with excessive emotional lability and personality changes*
- *It is a self limiting condition and eventually resolves completely, usually within 6 weeks.*
- *Recurrence of chorea may be seen late after complete resolution*
  Factors inducing Recurrence
  - *Pregnancy (Chorea gravidorum)*
  - *Re infection with streptocossus / non specific infections*
  - *Use of oral contraceptives*

321. Answer is A and D (Polyarthritis and MC valve involvement is Mitral): Harrison 18th/p 2753, 2754, 2755 *Harrisons 17th/2093, 2094, Ghai 6th/376-378*

Polyarthritis is a major criteria for diagnosis of RF.
Most common valve involved in Rheumatic carditis is mitral valve.

Erythema marginatum is a rare manifestation (<3% of patients) and almost never involves the face.
Acute Rheumatic fever is caused by Group A streptococcii and not alpha hemolytic streptococcii

Features of Erythema Marginatum

- ***Erythema marginatum is rare (< 3% of patients with Acute Rheumatic fever)***
- *Erythema marginatum is charachteristic / classic rash of Acute Rheumatic fever (Rare but charachteristic)*
- ***Typically occurs on the trunk or the proximal limbs (Never on the Face)***
- *Appears as ring that extends contrifugally (marginatum) while the skin in the centre of the ring returns to normal*
- *Rash is evanescent, pink to red*
- *Rash is non pruiritic*
- ***Rash occurs commonly in assoication with carditis (usually occurs only in patients with carditis)***
- *Rash leaves no induration and no scarring.*

322. Answer is D (usually associated with carditis) : Harrison 18th/p 2754 *Harrisons 17th/2094; Nelson's 18th/1142; Mayo clinic Cardiology / 3rd /551*

Erythema marginatum and sub cutaneous nodules are usually associated with carditis manifestation
Erythema marginatum is a rare (< 3%) manifestation of Acute Rheumatic fever. Rash is charachteristically non pruiritic and almost never involves the face.

323. Answer is A & C (Non tender; Present on extensor surfaces):*Harrison 18th/2754; 17th/2094; Nelson's 18th/1142-43*

Subcutaneosis nodules in Rheumatic fever are non tender and commonly located on extensor surfaces

These are a rare manifestation of Rheumatic fever and are commonly associated with carditis

Features of Subcutaneous nodules in Rheumatic Fever

- *Rare manifestation (≤ 1% of patients with acute Rheumatic fever)*
- *Delayed manifestation (appearing 2-3 weeks after onset of disease)*
- *Located commonly along the extensor surfaces of tendons near bony prominences (particularly hands, feet, elbows, occiput / occasionally vertebra)*
- *Painless (Non tender)*
- *Mobile*
- *Small in size (0.5 – 2cm)*
- *Commonly assoicated with carditis*
- *Nodules last for just a few days to upto 3 weeks*

324. Answer is A (Mitral Regurgitaion): *Harrison 18th/p 2753 Harrisons 17th/2094*

The most common valvular lesion is Acute Rheumative fever a mitral Regurgitation.
Mitral valve is the most commonly involved valve in Rheumatic fever
The most common valvular abnormality secondary to Rheumatic fever is mitral stenosis, however mitral stenosis is seen as a chronic manifestation of Rheumatic heart disease and is not a manifestation of Acute Rheumatic fever
Early valvular damage leads to mitral regurgitation which is the commonet lesion seen in Acute Rheumatic fever.

Congenital Heart Disease

General:

325. Answer is D (Multifactorial): Harrison 18th/p 1920 *Harrison 17th/1458; Robbins 6th/ 592; Robbins 5th/ 571*

Congenital heart disease is the most common type of heart disease among children. Q
Multifactorial Genetic and Environmental factors account for the majority of cases. *– Robbins*

Remember :

Extracardiac Lesion	Most likely congenital cardiac lesion
Down's syndrome Q	ASD Q of endocardial cushion type
Turner's Syndrome Q	Coarctation Of Aorta Q Pulmonic Q Stenosis (*in Noonan Syndrome*) Aortic Stenosis
Holt Oram Syndrome Q	Familial ASD Q (ASD with Bony Abnormalities)
Marfan's Syndrome Q	Aortic or Pulmonary Artery Dilatation Mitral Q or Aortic Regurgitation Q
Ellis Van Crevald Syndrome Q	ASD Q + Single Atrium
Rubella Q	PDA Q (Most Common), Pulmonary Stenosis Q *VSD* Q (according to CPDT/ Ghai)

Remember :

- The strongest familial (genetic) tendency is known in 'Holt Oram Syndrome' Q
- The strongest environmental factor known is : High altitude Q
- There is higher incidence of patient ductus arteriosus and arterial septal defects in children born at high altitudes. (Memo : Increased oxygen tension is responsible for closure of ductus arteriosus.) Q

326. Answer is C (Pulmonary stenosis): *CPDT 15th/ 933, Nelson 17th/ 1925*

Pulmonary stenosis is the most common cardiac abnormality in Noonan's syndrome.

Turner's syndrome	Noonan's syndrome
Most common cardiac defect associated is • Coarctation of aorta • Bicuspid aortic valve	*Most common cardiac defect associated is* • *Pulmonary valvular stenosis (most common)* • *Hypertrophic cardiomyopathy* • *ASD*

327. Answer is C (PDA): Harrison 18th/p 1924 *Harrison 17th/1461; Ghai 6th/; Chandrasoma Taylor 3rd/ 342; Read text below*

Differential cyanosis is a characteristic feature of Patent ductus arteriosus

328. Answer is D (Supravalvular Aortic stenosis): *'The Art and Science of Cardiac Physical Examination' by Ranganathan and Vohe 1st/53*

In supravalvular aortic stenosis the direction of jet of flow tends to be directly directed into the innominate artery. This often results in the direct impact pressure of the central jet being transmitted to right arm, thus making the right arm pressure higher than the left *- 'The Art and Science of Cardiac Physical Examination' by Ranganathan and Vohe 1st/53.*

329. Answer is C and E (Ebstein's anomaly and Single ventricle with pulmonic stenosis) : *Harrisons 16th/1384*

Ebstein's anomaly and single ventricle with pulmonic stenosis are associated with normal or decreased pulmonary blood flow.

Truncus Arteriosus, complete TGA and TAPVC are associated with increased pulmonary blood flow.

Cyanotic Congenital Heart Disease

Increased pulmonary blood flow	Normal or decreased pulmonary blood flow
1. Complete transposition of the great arteries	*1. Tricuspid atresia*
2. Double- outlet right ventricle of the Taussing- Bing type	***2. Ebstein's anomaly with right- to-let arterial shunt***
3. Truncus arteriosus	*3. Pulmonary atresia with intact ventricular septum*
4. Total anomalous pulmonary venous connection	*4. Pulmonic stenosis or atresia with ventricular septal defect (tetralogy of Fallot)*
5. Single ventricle without pulmonic stenosis	*5. Pulmonic stenosis with Right – to – Left arterial shunt*
6. Common atrium	*6. Complete transposition of the great arteries with pulmonic stenosis*
7. Tetralogy of Fallot with pulmonary atresia and increased collateral arterial flow	*7. Double – Outlet right ventricle with pulmonic stenosis*
8. Tricuspid atresia with large ventricular septal defect and no pulmonic stenosis	***8. Single Ventricle with pulmonic Stenosis***
9. Hypoplastic left heart (aortic atresia, itral atresia)	*9. Pulmonary arteriovenous fistula*
	10. Vena Caval to left arterial communication

330. Answer is B (PDA) : *Harrisons 16th/1384*

Patent Ductus Arteriosus is not classified as a cyanotic congenital heart disease.

PDA is an Acyanotic Heart disease with Left to Right shunt

Cyanotic congenital Heart Diseases

Increased Pulmonary Blood Flow

1. Complete transposition of the great arteries
2. Double- outlet right ventricle of the Taussing- Bing type
3. Truncus arteriosus
4. Total anomalous pulmonary venous connection
5. Single ventricle without pulmonic stenosis
6. Common atrium
7. Tetralogy of Fallot with pulmonary atresia and increased collateral arterial flow
8. Tricuspid atresia with large ventricular septal defect and no pulmonic stenosis
9. Hypoplastic left heart (aortic atresia, itral atresia)

Normal or Decreased Pulmonary Blood Flow

1. Tricuspid atresia
2. Ebstein's anomaly with right- to-left arterial shunt
3. Pulmonary atresia with intact ventricular septum
4. Pulmonic stenosis or atresia with ventricular septal defect (Tetralogy of Fallot)
5. Pulmonic stenosis with right – to – Left arterial shunt
6. Complete transposition of the great arteries with pulmonic stenosis
7. Double – Outlet right ventricle with pulmonic stenosis
8. Single Ventricle with pulmonic Stenosis
9. Pulmonary arteriovenous fistula
10. Vena Caval to left arterial communication

331. Answer is C (TOF): *Ghai 6th/406 – 409; Harrisons 16th/399*

ASD, LVF and VSD are all associated with pulmonary congestion and hence predispose to pulmonary infections. TOF is associated with reduced pulmonary blood flow (oligenic lung fields) due to right ventricular outflow obstruction and hence does not predispose to recurrent pulmonary infections.

Tetralogy of Fallot

332. Answer is C (ASD): *Ghai 6th/406*

ASD is not part of the four constituents that characterize the tetralogy of fallot

Tetralogy of Fallot: *Ghai 6th/406*
1. Ventricular Septal Defect
2. Right ventricular outflow tract obstruction (Infundibular stenosis / Pulmonic Stenosis)
3. Overriding or dextroposed aorta
4. Right Ventricular Hypertrophy

333. Answer is A (Valvular Stenosis): *CMDT 2007 / 328*

Valvular stenosis is not an essential criteria for Tetralogy of Fallot according to CMDT

'Patients with Tetralogy of Fallot have a VSD, RV infundibular stenosis, RV hypertrophy and dilated (overriding) aorta. There may or may not be pulmonary valve stenosis (valvular stenosis) as well' - CMDT

Essential Criteria for Tetralogy of Fallot

- Ventricular septal Defect
- Right ventricular out flow tract obstruction (RV OT obstruction)
  The most common cause of RVOT obstruction is infundibular stenosis
  Pulmonary valvular stenosis is less common and may or may not be present
- Right ventricular Hypertrophy
- Dilated (Overriding) Aorta

334. Answer is A (ASD): *Dorland's Medical Dictionary 28th/1253, 1746; Stedman's Medical Dictionary 28th/1452*

Pentalogy of Fallot encompasses the four defects included in Tetralogy of Fallot together with patent foramen ovale or atrial septal defect.

- **Tetralogy of Fallot:** *Ghai 6th*

Tetralogy of Fallot

- *Ventricular septal defect*[Q]
- *RVOT (Infundibular stenosis > Pulmonic Stenosis)*
- *Overriding or Dextroposed Aorta*[Q]
- *Right Ventricular Hypertrophy*[Q]

- **Pentalogy of Fallot** *(Dorland's 28th/1253; Stedman's 28th/1452)*

Association of four defects occurring in Tetralogy of Fallot with either ASD or Patent Foramen Ovale.

Pantalogy of Fallot	=	Tetralogy of Fallot	+	Atrial Septal Defect (ASD) OR Patent Foramen Ovale

- **Trilogy of Fallot:** *Dorland's 28th/1746; Stedman's 28th/2033*

Applied to the combination of Pulmonic Stenosis, ASD and Right Ventricular Hypertrophy

Trilogy of Fallot

- *Pulmonic Stenosis*
- *Atrial Septal Defect (ASD)*
- *Right Ventricular Hypertrophy*

335. Answer is D (First Heart Sound is soft) : *Ghai 6th/408*

First heart sound (S1) is normal in Tetralogy of Fallot.

Physical Examination in Tetralogy of fallot

General Examination
- *Cyanosis present[Q]*
- *Clubbing present[Q]*
- *Normal Arterial pulse[Q]*
- *Normal JVP[Q] (a wave may be slightly prominent)*

Auscultation

Heart Sounds
- *S1 : Normal[Q]*
- *S2 : Single[Q]*

Only A_2 Heard
P_2 is soft, delayed and inaudible

Heart murmur

Shunt murmur (VSD) Absent
Flow Murmur : *Pulmonory ejection systolic murmur located in left third intercostal space present*

The murmur in tetralogy of Fallot relates to the degree of right ventricular outflow obstruction (pulmonic stenosis). It is a harsh ejection systolic murmur resulting from turbulent flow across the stenotic pulmonic valve
The shunt murmur is absent because the shunt operates at a low pressure difference

336. Answer is C (Predominantly left to right shunt): *Ghai 6th/406-409*

Tetralogy of fallot is associated with a predominant Right to left shunt

Tetralogy of fallot is associated with a predominant Right to left shunt
Tetralogy of fallot is associated with Right ventricular out flow tract obstruction due to Pulmonic Stenosis
This results in flow of blood from right to left across the VSD into the aorta – ***Predominant Right to left shunt***

When the ductus arteriosus in patent i.e In the presence of patent Ductus Arteriosus	When the ductus arteriosus closes after birth In the absence of patent ductus Arteriosus
↓	↓
Unoxygenated blood can flow through the PDA into the lungs and become oxygenated	Unoxygenated blood is transmitted to the systemic circulation and the infant becomes cyanotic

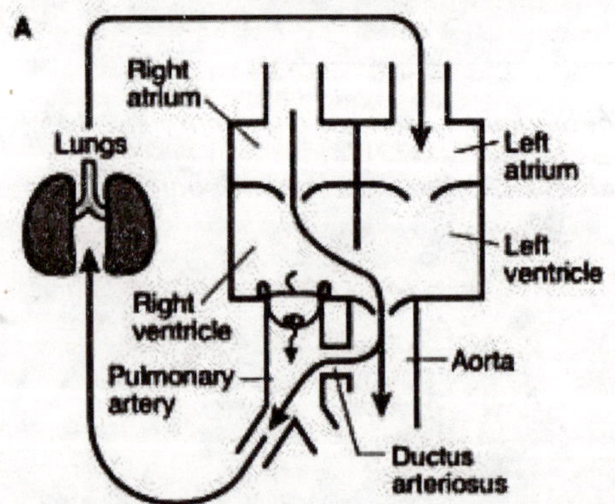

In the presence of a patent ductus arteriosus (PDA), unoxygenated blood can flow through the PDA to the lungs and become oxygenated.

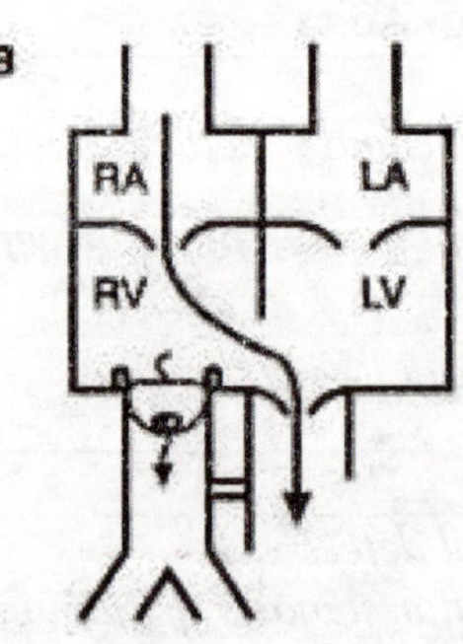

When the ductus arteriosus closes after birth, unoxygenated blood is transmitted to the systemic circulation and the infant becomes cyanotic

Diagram shows the four cardiac chambers, the stenotic pulmonic valve, the perimembranous ventricular septal defect, and the overriding aorta.

337. Answer is D (Tetralogy of Fallot) : *Ghai 5th /303*

'Coeur en Sabot' refers to the radialogical appearance of heart in a patient with Tetralogy of Fallot.
The cardiac silhouette resembles that of a'boot' or *Wooden shoe in 'Coeur en Sabot' [boot shaped heart[Q]].*

338. Answer is A (Aorta to Pulmonary Artery): *Ghai 6th/409 Nelson 17th*

Blalock Taussig shunt consists of subclavian artery (br. of aorta) and pulmonary artery anastamosis. This inturn actually establishes a shunt between the aorta (Via the subclavian artery) and the pulmonary artery.

The concept is to anastamose a systemic artery to the pulmonary artery to increase the blood flowing through the lungs and thus increase the amount of oxygenated blood reaching the systemic circulation. Amongst the options provided the single best answer is the anastomosis between aorta and pulmonary artery.

Surgical management of Tetralogy of fallot

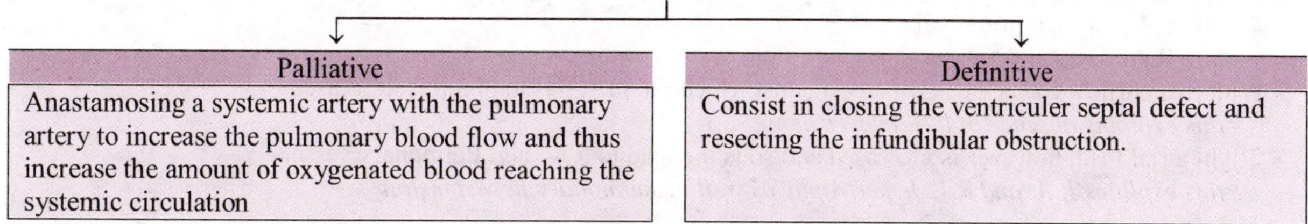

Palliative	Definitive
Anastamosing a systemic artery with the pulmonary artery to increase the pulmonary blood flow and thus increase the amount of oxygenated blood reaching the systemic circulation	Consist in closing the ventriculer septal defect and resecting the infundibular obstruction.

Shunt		Anastomosis
Blalock-Taussig shunt	:	Subclavian artery- Pulmonary artery
Pott's shunt	:	Descending aorta- Pulmonary artery
Waterson shunt	:	Ascending aorta- Palmonary artery

339. Answer is B (Descending aorta with left pulmonary artery) : *Sabiston 15th/2023-4*

Pott's shunt involves anastomosis between descending aorta and pulmonary artery

Palliative treatment in Fallot's Tetralogy consists of anastamosing a systemic artery with the pulmonary artery to increase the pulmonary blood flow and thus increase the amount of oxygenated blood reaching the systemic circulation. These palliative procedures prolong life and increase exercise tolerance.

There are three such systemic - pulmonary anastamosis:

1. *Ballock Tausigg shunt*[Q] : Anastamosis between subclavian artery and pulmonary artery. [Q]
2. **Potts shunt**[Q] **:** Anastamosis between descending aorta and pulmonary artery.[Q]
3. Waterson shunt : Anastamosis between ascending aorta and right pulmonary artery.

340. Answer is C and D (VSD and Blalock taussig shunt ...): *Ghai 6th/406-409*

Ventricular septal Defect is a constituent of Tetralogy of Fallot
Blalock Taussig shunt consists of subclavian artery – Pulmonary artery anastomosis

Tetralogy of Fallot is associated wit Right axis deviation
Tetralogy of Fallot is associated with right ventricular Hypertrophy
Morphine is indicated in the management of Anoxic Spells

Atrial Septal Defect

341. Answer is C (Ostium primum atrial septal defect): Harrison 18th/p 1921, 1922 *Harrison 17th/1459, 1460; O.P. Ghai 6th/ 401*

Wide fixed splitting of S_2 with ejection systolic murmur in left 2nd intercostal space points towards the diagnosis of Atrial septal defect.. Presence of left axis deviation indicates an ostium primum ASD.

Clinical picture in ASD : *Ghai 6th/ 401*

Sounds	Murmur	ECG
• S_1 *Accentuated (Loud)* [Q] • *S2 wide* fixed split [Q]	• *Shunt murmur : is absent i.e. there is no murmur as a result of shunt* • *Flow murmurs:* murmurs present are due to increased flow of blood through respective valves Tricuspid valve: — Delayed diastolic Pulmonary valve — Ejection systolic	Ostium [Q] primum — Left axis deviation Ostium [Q] secundum — Right axis deviation + RVH

342. Answer is B (Left aterial hypertrophy): Harrison 18th/p 1921, 1922 *Harrison 17th/1459, 1460; Ghai 5th/ 296, Ghai 6th/ 400, 401; Read text below*

ASD is associated with RA and RV hypertrophy but not LA hypertrophy.

Left Atrium has two outflow tracts in ASD
- into L.V. through mitral valve
- into R.A. through ASD

- With two outflow tracts the resistance against which the L.A. has to pump is decreased
  - *this explains absence of L.A. hypertrophy*
- Right atrial load, however is increased and so is the load to R.V. and Pulmonary vessels
  - *this explains R.A. and R.V. hypertrophy as well as pulmonary hypertension*

Remember :

- Most common form of ASD is : Ostium secundum Q
- Lutembacher syndrome is : ASD + Mitral stenosis Q
- Patients with ASD are generally asymptomatic Q
- Congestive cardiac failure is rare in patients with ASD (it almost never occurs in patients with T.O.F.) Q
- Infective endocarditis is very rare in patients with ASD (because pressure gradient is very less) Q
- In ASD pulmonary flow is greater than systemic flow (Hilar dance and pulmonary plethora are seen) Q
- High incidence of ASD is seen in patients with Down's syndrome. Q

343. Answer is B (Left parasternal heeve is due to increased pulmonary artery flow) : *Ghai 5th/296*

In ASD large volume of blood reaches the left atrium, right atrium, right ventricle and Pulmonary circulation.

Consequently ***there is enlargement of LA, RV as well as of the pulmonary artery and its branches, and this may contribute to the left parasternal haeve.***

ASD is a defect in atrial septum and not in patent foramen ovale. Q

S_2 is wide and fixed (not variable). P2 is accentuated. Q

Systolic murmur in ASD is not caused by rapid flow of blood across the shunt.

There is only a minor difference of pressure between the left and the right atrium. The shunt murmurs is therefore absent. Q

Murmurs present are flow murmurs and not shunt murmurs :
- Delayed diastolic murmurs : due to increased flow across the tricuspid valve
- Ejection systolic : due to increased flow across the pulmonary valve

344. Answer is C (Ostium primum with floppy mitral valve): *'Pediatrics: A concise Text' by Kabra & Srivastava (Elsevier, India) 2010/135, Instant Pediatrics' by Agarwal (Ane Books)2008/86*

'Presence of a pansystolic murmur of mitral regurgitation with left axis deviation in a patient with ASD suggests the presence of ostium primum defect with a cleft mitral valve leaflet or a floppy mitral valve with mitral valve prolapse'

- Pediatrics: A concise Text (Elsevier)2010/135

Presence of Pansystolic Murmur in a patient with ASD suggests.
• *Ostium Primum Defect* • *Floppy mitral valve* • *Cleft mitral valve* • *Associated Rheumatic Mitral Regurgitation*

ASD type	ECG
Ostium Primum	*Left Axis Deviation*
Ostium Secondum	*Right Axis Deviation*

345. Answer is B (ASD): *Ghai 6th/400*

ASD is associated with an enlarged right atrium & right ventricle to accommodate large volume of blood. *The left atrium is not enlarged because it decompresses itself by shunting blood to the right atrium at a minor difference in pressure.* ***The left atrium may enlarge once Eisen menger's syndrome develops and a reversal of shunt is seen across the defect.***

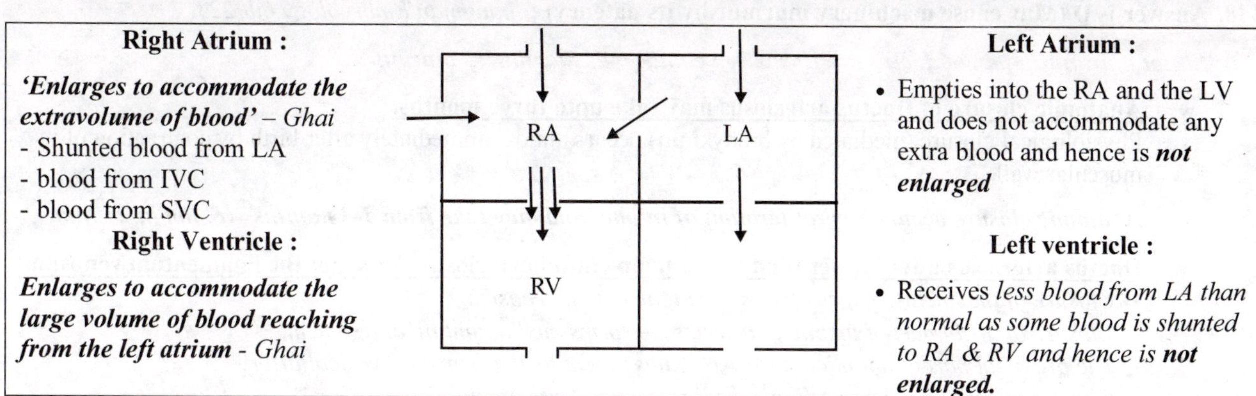

Ventricular Septal Defect (VSD)

346. Answer is D (Pulmonary oligemia in X ray chest): *Ghai 5th/ 298, 299, Ghai 6th/ 402, 403*

V.S.D. is characterized by pulmonary plethora and not pulmonary oligemia.
***Pulmonary vasculature is increased** – Ghai 6th/403*

- **Chest X-ray in VSD does not show pulmonary oligemia.**
  A ventricular septal defect results in shunting of oxygenated blood from left ventricle to the right ventricle. This left to right shunt therefore streams the blood to the pulmonary artery and then to the lungs. *The pulmonary vasculature is thus increased and pulmonary plethora is seen.*
- **Small holes in VSD may close spontaneously**
  Disappearance of ventricular defects is called spontaneous closure. *Almost 70-80 percent of all ventricular defects become smaller in size or disappear entirely*
- **Defect in VSD is usually in membranous part.**
  90% defects are located in the membranous part – Ghai 6th/402
- **Endocarditis is commonest complication of VSD.**
  VSD is the *commonest congenital lesion complicated by infective endocarditis – Ghai 6th/404.*

Patent Ductus Arteriosus (PDA)

347. Answer is C (PDA): *Harrison 18th/1924; 17th/1461; Ghai 6th/; Chandrasoma Taylor 3rd/ 342; Read text below*

Differential cyanosis is a characteristic feature of Patent ductus arteriosus

Cyanosis is bluish discoloration of skin and mucus membranes caused by increased amount of reduced hemoglobin in arterial blood.

In congenital heart disease, cyanosis is caused by right to left shunt, which allows unoxygenated venous blood to bypass the lungs and enter systemic circulation.

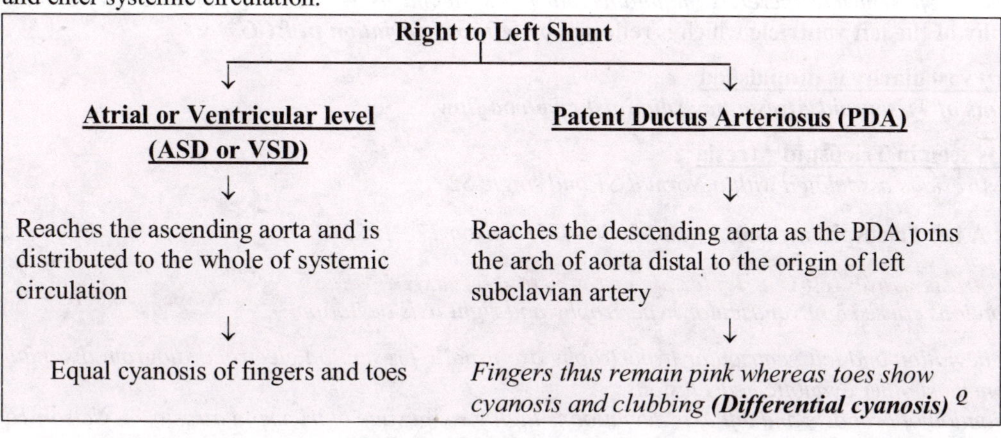

348. Answer is D (May cause machinery murmur by its patency) : *Langman Embryology 6th/223*

Shunt murmur in patent ductus arteriosus is a continuous machinery murmur.

- **Anatomic closure of Ductus arteriosus may take upto three months.**
  Physiological closure (mediated by bradykinin) occurs almost immediately after birth by contraction of its muscular wall.

  Anatomic closure occurs by proliferation of intima, and may take from 1-3 months*[Q] *(& not in 24 hrs).

- **Ductus arteriosus after obliteration forms ligamentum arteriosum.[Q] (& not the ligamentum venosum)**
  - *Closure of the ductus venosus forms the Ligamentum venosum.*
  - *Closure of distal part of umbilical arteries →forms medial umbilical ligament.* [Q]
  - *The proximal part of umbilical artery remains patent as the "superior vesical artery".* [Q]
  - *Closure of umbilical vein →forms the ligamentum teres hepatis.* [Q]

- **Prostaglandins maintain patency of ductus arteriosus, and do not induce it to close**
  "In neonates with congenital heart defects, till surgery is undertaken, PGE_1 (Alprostadil) is used to maintain patency of ductus arteriosus".- KDT4th/219
  Prostaglandins maintains patency of ductus arteriosus
  NSAIDs - help in early closure of ducts arteriosus

- **Ductus arteriosus may cause a machinary murmur by its patency.**
  "Shunt murmur is a continuous machinery murmur". - Ghai 5th/301
  The murmur is best heard at the 2nd left intercostal space and is also well heard below the left clavicle, where it maintains its continuous machinery character.

349. Answer is A and B (CCF and Infective Endocarditis) : *Harrisons 16th/1386*

The leading causes of death in adults with patient ductus are cardiac failure and infective endocarditis.

-Harrisons 16th /1386

Tricuspid Atresia

350. Answer is D (Splliting of S_2): *Ghai 6th/408, 410, 414-415; Nelson 17th/1531*

Tricuspid Atresia is associated with a single S2 and not a split S2

Tricuspid Atresia is associated with Right Ventricular hypoplasia.
Atresia of the tricuspid valve results in the absence of a communication between the right atrium and right ventricle therefore the **right ventricle is underdeveloped the inflow portion being absent.**
Tricuspid Atresia is associated with Left ventricular hypertrophy and Left Axis Deviation
The only exit for systemic venous blood coming to the right atrium is by way of *Atrial Septal defect.* Through this the blood goes to left atrium from where it enters left ventricle.
A *ventricular septal defect* provides communication between the left ventricle and the outflow portion of the right ventricle. The *left ventricle therefore maintain both the systemic as well as the pulmonary circulation* thus there is **hypertrophy of the left ventricle** which is reflected by ***left axis deviation in ECG*.***

Pulmonary vascularity is diminished
90% patients of Triscuspid Atresia have diminished blood flow.

Single S2 is seen in Tricuspid Atresia
Tricuspid Atresia is associated with a Normal S1 and single S2.

351. Answer is A i.e. Tricuspid atresia: *Ghai 6th/408-415; Nelson 17th/1531*

Tricuspid atresia causes left ventricular hypertrophy and left axis deviation.
All other options cause right ventricular hypertrophy and right axis deviation.

"Left axis deviation and left ventricular hypertrophy are usually present on electrocardiogram distinguishing tricuspid atresia from most other cyanotic heart lesions.
The combination of cyanosis and left axis deviation is highly suggestive of tricuspid atresia." - Nelson 16th/1391

352. Answer is B (Tricuspid Atresia): *Ghai 5th/304*

Presence of Left Ventricular hypertrophy and left axis deviation on ECG in a child suggests a diagnosis of Trocuspid atresia.

Tricuspid Atresia

Congenital absence of tricuspid valve is called tricuspid atresia.

Haemodynamics:
- *The inflow portion of R.V. is hypoplastic*[Q]
- *The systemic venous blood coming to R.A. exits by way of a patent foramen ovale or an ASD.*[Q]
- *A VSD provides communication between L.V. and outflow portion of R.V.*[Q]
  The L.V. thus maintains both the systemic and pulmonary circulation.[Q]
- *The saturation of blood in the pulmonary artery and aorta is identical.*[Q]
- *The pulmonary blood flow is dependent on size of VSD*[Q]
- *The VSD in tricuspid atresia is always a muscular defect.*[Q]

Features suggestive of tricuspid atresia :
- ***L.V. type of apical impulse***[Q]
- *Prominent large 'a' waves*[Q]
- *Enlarged liver with presystolic pulsations (a waves)*[Q]
- ***ECG characterised by Left axis deviation and Left ventricular hypertrophy.***[Q]

Clinical features : (are similar to Fallot's tetralogy[Q])
- *Child is cyanotic from birth*[Q]
- *Anoxic spells and squatting may be present*[Q]

353. Answer is B (Tricuspid Atresia): *Ghai 6th/410*

Tricuspid Atresia is associated with Left Axis deviation and not Right Axis deviation.
Symptoms and signs of Tricuspid Atresia are similar to those of Tetralogy of Fallot.

Features suggesting Tricuspid Atresia are
- Left ventricular type of apical impulse
- Prominent large 'a' waves in JVP
- Enlarged liver and presystolic pulsations (a waves)
- Left axis deviation and left ventricular hypertrophy on ECG

Coarctation of Aorta

354. Answer is D (Coarctation of aorta): Harrison 18th/p 1925 *Harrison 14th/ 306, Harrison 15th/ 1337, Harrison 16th/ 1387; Harrison 17th/1462*

Intermittent claudication, dizziness and headache are all suggestive of coarctation of aorta

Coarctation of Aorta: Review

Clinical presentation :
- Most patients are asymptomatic[Q]
- Symptomatic patients usually present with :
  - *Headache, dizziness,*[Q]
  - Epistaxis
  - *Cold extremities, and weakness in the legs*[Q]
  - ***Claudication with exercise***[Q]
- Hypertension in upper extremities with marked diminution of pulsation in lower extremities.[Q]
- Mid systolic or continuous murmur over anterior part of chest and back[Q]
- Enlarged and pulsatile collateral vessels in intercostal spaces anteriorly in axilla or posteriorly in interscapular area[Q]
- Upper extremity and thorax may be more developed than lower extremities.[Q]

Investigations :
• ECG: shows L.V. Hypertrophy Q • Radiography : - *Indentation of aorta at site of coarctation and '3 sign' on paramediastinal shaddon are almost pathogenic.* Q - *Notching* (erosion) of inferior surfaces of ribs. Q
Complications :
• Cerebral aneurysms and haemorrhage Q • Rupture of aorta • Left ventricular failure Q • Infective endocarditis Q
Treatment :
• Is surgical *resection* Q of 'coarctation' and end to end anastomosis *Remember that HT may not be corrected even after surgical correction of the 'coarctation'.* Q
Few other questions : *Most common site* Q of coarctation of aorta : *distal to origin of left subclavian artery.* Q *Most common associated cardiac anomaly* Q : *bicuspid aortic valve.* Q *May be associated with* Q : *Turner's syndrome.* Q

355. Answer is B (Coarctation of aorta): *Ghai 6th/419*

Feeble femoral pulsations compared to strong brachial pulsations suggests the diagnosis of coarctation of aorta. *Hypertension and strong pulsations in the upper extremities and absence, marked dimunition or delay in pulsations in the femoral artery are characteristic in coarctation. Also failure to thrive and congestive heart failure are consistent with the diagnosis of congestive heart failure.*

Coarctation of Aorta: *Ghai*

- *'Physical examination shows delayed and weak or impalpable femorals compared to strong brochial arteries'-Ghai*
- *'Coarctation may result in congestive heart failure in infancy'-Ghai*
  (in congestive failure does not occur in infancy it is unlikely to occur throughout the pediatric age group unless complicated by infective endocarditis or anemia)
- *Failure to thrive is a manifestation of congestive heart failure.*

Remember:

- *Differential cyanosis is a manifestation of PDA*Q
- *Differential pulses/Blood pressure is a manifestation of Coarctation*Q

356. Answer is C (Coarctation of aorta): *Harrison 18th/1925 Harrison 16th/e 1387; Harrison 17th/1462; Previous questions*

Hypertension in upper extremity with absence, dimunition or delay in pulsations in lower extremity suggests the diagnosis of coarctation of aorta. *Other options have been explained in the previous questions.*

Murmurs in coarctation of aorta:

Murmur due to the narrowing or coarctation	Flow murmur across collaterals
Midsystolic or continuous mumur over the anterior part of chest, back and spinous processes due to narrowing of lumen and resultant high velocity jet	Systolic or continuous mumur over lateral thoracic wall due to increased flow through dilated and tortuous collateral vessels.

357. Answer is B (Coarctation of aorta): *Harrison 18th/1925; 15th/ 1337; Harrison 16th/1387; Harrison 17th/1462*

Hypertension in the upper extremities and absence, marked diminution or delayed pulsations in the femoral arteries are on physical examination are characteristic in coarctation of aorta *– Harrison 16th/ 1387*
Associated notching of ribs along the lower border leaves no doubt as regards the correct diagnosis.

358. Answer is D (Coarctation of Aorta): *SOAP for Cardiology (2006) /100, 101; Moss and Adam's 7th/1288; Nelson's 18th/1900, 1901; Hurst 11th/ed 1809; Oski's Pediatrics 2nd/714; 'Pediatrics' Board Review Series 2nd/341*

Isolated upper extremity hypertension (200 / 140 mm Hg), together with absent/ diminished femoral pulses is a characteristic feature of coarctation of aorta.
Although coarctation of aorta does not commonly present with seizures, these may be seen as a consequence of severe hypertension (BP = 200/140) or complications like intracranial haemorrhage (from Berry aneurysms which are more common in patients with coarctation.

Coarctation of Aorta is the most likely diagnosis: Approach *(Nelson/Hurst)*

- The classic sign of coarctation of aorta is a disparity in pulsations and blood pressure in arms and legs. *The femoral, popliteal, posterior tibial and dorsalis pedis pulses are weak (or absent in upto 40% of patients) in contrast to bounding pulses in the arms and carotid vessels.*
- The blood pressure is the legs is lower than in the arms and *90% of patients with coarctation have hypertension in an upper extremity* greater than 95th perecentile for age

Age (yrs)	95th percentile (mm Hg)
> 1 yrs	*110 / 60*
1 – 5 yrs	*115 /75*
6 – 10 yrs	*125 /85*
11 – 18 yrs	*140 /90*

- *Severe hypertension* may be seen as a consequence of persistant hypertension in an individual who has not undergone corrective surgery for coarctation, and this usually *appears in the second or third decade of life (Hurst)*

A blood pressure of 200 /140 mm Hg in a 10 year old boy suggests severe hypertension (95th percentile at 10 years – 125/85)

- ***Children with severe / malignant hypertension may develop headaches, seizures and stroke (haemorrhage from Berry aneurysms which are more common in patients with coarctation).***

Takayasu Aortoarteritis may also present with severe hypertension and absent femoral pulses due to acquired midaortic coarctation but this is an uncommon presentation in Takayasu aortoarteritis (and hence not the single best answer of choice)

Takayasu arteritis (or non specific aortoarteritis) is a chronic vasculitis disease of medium and large sized arteries with a strong predilection for aortic arch and its branches.
This may lead to stenosis of the involved vessels and hence a picture of acquired coarctation. It may thus produce a clinical picture similar to that of coarctation with disparity in pulsations and blood pressure in arms & legs with hypertension depending on the site of the acquired stenosis.

However, this condition is *more common in women* and most *commonly affects the subclavican artery*. Hence it ***more commonly presents with*** claudication, along with unequal and ***reduced pulses / BP in the upper extremity*** than the lower extremity. Also *systemic symptoms are more common* is Takayasu than in coarctation. *Nevertheless Takayasu arteritis may affect the Thoracic or Abdominal aorta and present with absent lower limb pulses and upper extremity hypertension like coarctation of aorta.*
Takayasu arteritis can be picked as the answer if Coarctation of aorta is not provided amongst the options

Coarctation	Takayasu
• More common condition	• Less common condition
• More common in boys	• More common in girls (8 : 1 = F:M)
• Upper extremity hypertension	• Absent or decreased upper limb pulses (brachial / radial) and blood pressure difference between left and right arm is characteristic *('Reverse coarctation': Oski's Essential Pediatrics)*
• Bounding pulses in with arms and diminished / absent lower limb pulsations is characteristic	**Note** *Clinical picture similar to coarctation with absent lower limb pulsations and upper extremity hypertension may be seen if site of lesion is in the thoracic aorta / abdominal aorta (But this is not charachteristic).*
• Hypertension is frequent	• Hypertension is frequent

Renal Parenchymal Disease and Grandmal seizures do not present with isolated upper extremity hypertension and absent femoral pulses.

359. Answer is D (Coarctation of aorta): *Harrison 14th /1306 (Repeat), 15th/1337*

The child is presenting with characteristic features of coarctation of aorta.

360. Answer is C (Coarctation of aorta): Harrison 18th/p 1925, 1926 *Harrison 17th/1462; Refer text below*

Classical clinical presentation with characteristic notching of ribs is diagnostic of coarctation of aorta.

Remember:
- *Rib signs are unusual before 10 yrs of age*
- *Notching affects inferior surface of ribs*
- *Unilateral and right sided ribs are affected if the coarctation is proximal to the left subclavian artery*

361. Answer is C (Inability to augment cardiac output with exercise): *Harrison 15th/ 1337 Q 22 (CVS) pre test based on Harrison 15th/, Harrison 16th/ 1387; Harrison 17th/1462, 1463* Harrison 18th/p 1925

In coarctation of aorta unless the hypertension is very severe or left ventricular failure has ensued, cardiac output responds normally to exercise.
- *Usually a systolic ejection murmur is heard anteriorly and over the back. If the obstruction is very severe a continuous murmur would be heard. Coarctation of aorta is commonly accompanied by a bicuspid aortic valve, which can produce the diastolic murmur of aortic regurgitation.*
- Coarctation of the Aorta usually occurs just distal to the origin of the left subclavian artery. If it arises above the left subclavian, Arterial blood pressure elevation may be evident only in the right arm.
- In coarctation of aorta unless the hypertension is very severe or left ventricular failure has ensued, cardiac output responds normally to exercise.
- Hypertension is the major clinical problem and may persist even after complete surgical correction.

362. Answer is A (Most common site is distal to the origin of left subclavian artery) : *Harrison 14th/ 1306; Harrison 15th/1337; Nelson 15th / 1302*

The most common site of coarctation of aorta is distal to the origin of left subclavian artery.

Notching occurs on Inferior surface and not on the superior surface.
L.V. Hypertrophy is prominent and not RV hypertrophy.
It is the L.V. which is subjected to increased afterload because of the coarctation, and therefore L.V. Hypertrophy is the prominent finding. *Q*
Most common age of presentation in coarctation of aorta is during infancy or early childhood
Only about 20 percent of patients with mild disease present during adolescence and adulthood

363. Answer is B (Bicuspid Aortic Valve): Harrison 18th/p 1925 *Harrison's 17th /1462.*

The most common associated cardiac anomaly with coarctation of aorta is bicuspid aortic valve (Harrison's 17th /1462)
Coarctation of aorta is associated with a bicuspid aortic valve in more than 70% of cases - (Nelson 18th /1900)

Associated anomalies with coarctation of Aorta Q
• **Bicuspid Aortic valve**Q **(commonest)** • PDAQ • VSDQ • Tubular hypoplasia of aortic archQ • Aortic stenosisQ (valvular / subvalvular)
Other Associated lesions that have been asked previously
• Mitral valve abnormalities (Subvalvular mitral ring /parachute mitral valve) • Turner's syndromeQ

Shone complexQ
Coarctation of Aorta + Left sided obstructive lesions *(Mitral valve abnormalities and subaortic stenosis)*

364. Answer is A (Bicuspid Aortic valve): *Harrison 18th/p 1925 Harrison's 17th /1462.*

The most common associated cardiac anomaly with coarctation of aorta is bicuspid aortic valve *-Harrison's 17th /1462*
Coarctation of aorta is associated with a bicuspid aortic valve in more than 70% of cases - (Nelson 18th /1900)

Associated anomalies with coarctation of Aorta [Q]
• ***Bicuspid Aortic valve[Q] (commonest)***   • *PDA[Q]*   • *VSD[Q]*   • *Tubular hypoplasia of aortic arch[Q]*   • *Aortic stenosis[Q] (valvular / subvalvular)*   *Other Associated lesions that have been asked previously*   • *Mitral valve abnormalities (Subvalvular mitral ring /parachute mitral valve)*   • *Turner's syndrome[Q]*

Shone complex[Q]
Coarctation of Aorta   +   Left sided obstructive lesions   *(Mitral valve abnormalities and subaortic stenosis)*

365. Answer is C (Pulmonary stenosis): Harrison 18th/p 1925 *Harrison 17th/1462; CPDT 15th/ 498*

Coarctation of aorta is not associated with Pulmonary stenosis.

Coarctation Syndrome
• Coarctation of aorta   • Patent ductus arteriosus   • Bicuspid aortic valve   • Tubular hypoplasia of aortic isthumus   • VSD

Coarctation of aorta is also seen in Turner's syndrome – Harrison

Turner's Syndrome	• Coarctation • Bicuspid valve / stenosis

366. Answer is C (Renal artery stenosis): *Harrison 18th/p 1925 Harrison 15th/ 1332; 16th / 1383; 17th/1462; Ghai 6th /419*

Renal artery stenosis is not associated with any form of congenital heart disease. *In young it is usually a result of fibromuscular dysplasia and in elderly due to atheromatous plaques secondary to hypertension and diabetes.*

- ***Turner's syndrome*** is associated with coarctation of aorta and bicuspid valve. - *Harrison 14th / 1302*
- *Most common associated congenital cardiac anomaly with coarctation of aorta* is bicuspid aortic valve-*Harrison 14th / 1306, 15th /1337*
- *PDA may be associated.*

367. Answer is B (Turner's syndrome): *Nelson 16th / 1747*

Turner's syndrome is commonly associated with coarctation of aorta.

Congenital Syndromes	Cardiac anomaly
Turner's syndrome	***Coarctation of Aorta*** [Q] *Pulmonic stenosis* [Q] *Aortic stenosis* [Q]
Down's syndrome	*ASD* [Q] - endocardial cushion type
Noonan's syndrome *(Nelson 6th / 1747)*	*Pulmonary stenosis* [Q] ASD Hypertrophic cardiomyopathy

368. Answer is D (Neurofibromatosis) : *Radiology by Wolfgang Dahnert 5th/ 19; Grainger & Allison's 5th / 551*

Neurofibromatosis is associated with superior rib notching

Inferior rib notching is characteristically seen in coarctation of Aorta and may also be seen in Superior vena cava obstruction and a Blalock-Taussig shunt[Q] operation

Rib-Signs in Coarctation of aorta:

- ***Inferior rib notching[Q]*** is characteristic, and is believed to be due to *pressure erosion by intercostal arteries.*
- ***Inferior rib notching[Q]*** takes several years to develop and is ***rarely seen before the age of 8 years.***[Q]
- ***'3' sign[Q]*** may be seen due to enlargement of *left subclavian artery* above the coarctation

- ***Usually spares fist two ribs***[Q] where intercostal arteries arise from costocervical trunk which is proximal to the usual site of CA. *Mostly commonly affected ribs are the 4th to 8th ribs.*
- ***Usually bilateral but asymmetrical.***

Unilater left notching (absent on right side)	**U/L right notching** (absent on left side)
• *Anomalous origin of right subclavian artery distal to coarctation*	• *Stenosed / occluded left subclavian artery* • *Coarctation is proximal to left subclavian.*

Causes of Rib notching:

Superior R.N.	Inferior R.N.
Poliomyelitis Osteogenesis imperfecta Restrictive lung disease ***Neurofibromatosis***[Q] *Marfan's syndrome* Connective tissue disease - Rheumatoid Arthritis (RA) - *Systemic Lupus Erythematosis (SLE)* - Scleroderma - Sjogren's syndrome - Hyperparathyroidism	**Arterial** ***Coarctation of Aorta***[Q] *Aortic thrombosis*[Q] ***Blalock-Taussig shunt***[Q] (Subclavian obstruction) Pulmonary – oligemia / A-V malformation Pulmonary stenosis Tetralogy of fallot Absent pulmonary artery **Venous** AV malformation of chest wall ***Superior vena cava obstruction*** **Neurogenic** Intercostal neuroma Neurofibromatosis type 1 Poliomyelitis/quadriplegia/paraplegia **Osseous** Hyperparathyrpoidism Thalassemia Melnick-Needle Syndrome

369. Answer is C (Coarctation of Aorta): *Radiology and imaging by Bhaduri/112*

Rib notching and double bulge sign are characteristic radiological signs of coarcation of aorta.

Signs in coarctation of aorta

Abnormal Aortic arch

Commonest finding[Q]
Site of narrowing may be seen as an identation. [Q]
Classic '3 sign'[Q] or *double bulge sign'* [Q] on left border of aortic shadow is formed by (above downwards)
- prestenotic dilatation
- coarctation itself (indentation)
- poststenotic dilatation

Inferior Rib notching

Is a frequent sign in adults. It is not seen until late childhood.
It is seen on the inferior margin of posterior halves of ribs from 3rd or 4th ribs downwards.
Rib notching is *due to enlargement of intercostal arteries which act as collateral vessels.*
These collateral vessels produce indentation, on the ribs at the above sites.

370. Answer is D (Anterior MI): *CMDT 2008/282, CSDT / 426*

Myocardial Infarction has not been listed as a hazard /cause of death in coarctation of Aorta

Causes of death in coarctation of Aorta (CSDT / CMDT)

- *Congestive Heart Failure*
- *Endo carditis*
- *Aortic Rupture*
- *Intracranial Hemorrhage* } *Hypertension*
- *Aortic dissection* }

Death is most frequently caused by complication of Hypertension such as stroke or aortic dissection. Other causes include endocarditis and congestive heart failure - Hurst 11th/1867

Total Anomalous Pulmonary Venous Connection (TAPVC)

371. Answer is A (Supracardiac): *Schwartz 8th/ 622*

***Type I** TAPVC with anomalous connection at the **supracardiac level** is the most common type accounting for about 45% of all cases.*

Total anomalous pulmonary venous connection (TAPVC) is characterized by abnormal drainage of pulmonary veins into the right heart either by direct connection into the right atrium or into its tributaries.

According to the site or level of connection of the pulmonary veins to the systemic venous system TAPVC has been classified into four types:

Type 1 (45%)	:	Anomalous connection at ***supracardiac level*** (Pulmonary veins drain into left innominate vein or right SVC)
Type II (25%)	:	Anomalous connection at cardiac level (Pulmonary veins joint the coronary sinus or enter right atrium directly)
Type III (25%)	:	Anomalous connection at infracardiac level (Pulmonary veins drain into the portal vein)
Type IV (5%)	:	Anomalous connection at multiple levels

372. Answer is B (Always associated with VSD): *Ghai 5th*

TAPVC is not always associated with a VSD.
Communication between the left and the right heart, is either via ASD or a Patent Foramen Ovale.

TAPVC: is an uncommon congenital cyanotic heart disease.[Q]

Defect
All pulmonary veins are connected anomolously and reach the right Atrium directly or indirectly instead of reaching the left atrium. This may occur through the following ways (Anatomic classification):
Anatomical Classification :
Supracardiac : Pulmonary veins join together to form a common pulmonary vein which may drain either into the left brachiocephalic vein or Superior venacava to reach Rt Atrium. Cardiac : The veins join the coronary sinus. Infracardiac : The common pulmonary veins drain into portal vein. *Remember : TheTAPVC of the infracardiac type is always obstructive, while cardiac and supracardiac types, may or may not have pulmonary venous obstruction.* [Q]
Hemodynamics :
The blood flow to the left atrium is the Rt to Left shunt via a patent foramen ovale or an ASD. ***Because mixing of blood occurs in Rt atrium, the oxygen saturation of blood in the pulmonary artery is identical or even higher to that in the aorta.*** [Q]
Presentation :
Obstructive type: presents with marked cyanosis and CHF within the first 1 - 2 weeks of life. *Non obstructive type:* presents with cyanosis and CHF but presentation is delayed to around 4 to 10 weeks of age.
X-ray chest
Snowman or figure of '8' configuration [Q] *Ground glass appearance :* (Characteristic of *Obstructive TAPVC.* [Q])

Transposition of Great Vessels(TGV)

373. Answer is B (Transposition of great vessels) : *Read text below*

Transposition of Great vessels is a condition chracterized by aorta arising from the right ventricle and pulmonary artery from the left ventricle.

This results in complete separation of systemic and pulmonary circulation. Since systemic and pulmonary circulations are separate, survival depends on mixing of oxygenated pulmonary blood and deoxygenated *systemic blood which can occur:*

At Atrial level	:	*Through ASD*
At Ventricle level	:	*Through VSD*
At Great vessel level	:	*Through Patent ductus arteriosus*

Oxygenation is normal in foetus but after birth as ductus arteriosus closes severe hypoxia occurs and in the absence of V.S.D, or ASD child presents with cyanosis and tachypnea at birth.

<u>Management of patients with transposition of great vessels</u>:

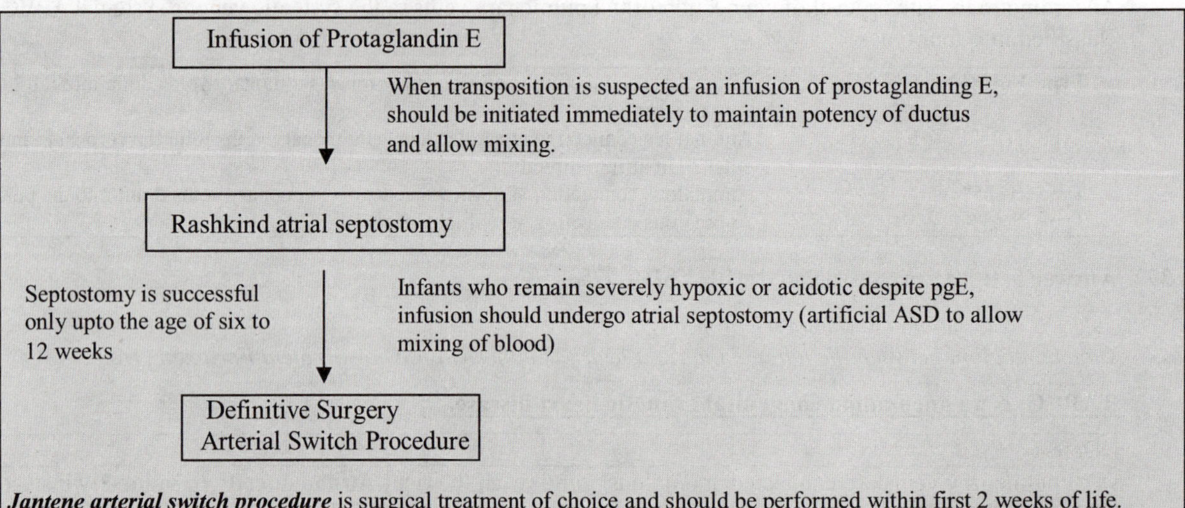

Jantene arterial switch procedure is surgical treatment of choice and should be performed within first 2 weeks of life.

- Aorta and pulmonary artery are divided just above the sinuses and reanastomosed in correct anatomical positions.
- The coronary arteries are then removed from old aortic root along with a button of aortic wall and reimplanted in the old pulmonary root.

Other operations available : Arterial switch operation by Mustard and Senning[Q].

Anamolous Coronary Artery

374. Answer is D (Anomalous coronary artery) : *Nelson 15th/1308, Nelson 16th/1406*

Characteristic symptoms of restlessness, irritability and diaphoresis on feeding and an increased risk of MI suggests a diagnosis of Anomalous Coronary artery.

<u>Anomalous origin of the coronary arteries : anomalous origin of the left coronary artery from the pulmonary artery:</u>

In this anomaly the blood supply of the left ventricular myocardium is severely compromised. Soon after birth (Neonate) as the pulmonary arterial pressure falls, perfusion pressure to the left coronary artery becomes inadequate. ***Myocardial infarction and fibrosis may result.***

<u>Clinical manifestion</u> :

- Congestive heart failure becomes manifest within first few month of life and is often precipitated by respiratory infection.
- Recurrent attacks of discomfot, ***restlessness, irritability, diaphoresis***, dyspnea and pallor with or without cyanosis occur-could be caused by angina pectoris.
- Cardiac enlargement is moderate to massive
- ***Murmurs*** may be present.

Eissenmerger's Syndrome

375. Answer is A (Return of left ventricle and right ventricle to normal size): *Ghai 6th/415; Braunwald 7th/1498*

Eisenminger syndrome is associated with severe pulmonary arterial hypertension and right ventricular hypertrophy. The right ventricular size will certainly not return to normal once eisenminger syndrome develops.

- ***Dilated central pulmonary arteries and rapid tapering of the peripheral pulmonary vasculature (pruning)** are the radiographic hallmarks of Eisenminger's syndrome' – Braunwald.*
  'The hilar (central) area suggests pulmonary plethora whereas the peripheral lung fields suggets pulmonary oligemia' – Ghai 6th/415
- 'Pulmonary hypertension develops due to pulmonary vascular obstructive disease affecting the 'pulmonary ***arteries***'. ***'Pulmonary vein'** will not be distended.*

Miscellaneous

376. Answer is A (ASD): *see below ; Q.202 / AI 2002*

ASD is the single best answer of exclusion.

Cardiac anomalies in congenital rubella are mentioned differently in different books !

According to GHAI	: PDA > PS> VSD
According to CPDT	: PDA > PS> VSD
According to Harrison	: PDA > PS> ASD
According to Nelson	: PDA > PS (ASD & VSD not mentioned)

We have chosen ASD as the one to be excluded as both GHAI & CPDT mention VSD as a finding is cases of congenital rubella. Nevertheless Harrison mentions ASD as well, and so you are on your own, if you wish to differ.
The commonest congenital cardiac anomaly is Congenital Rubella is PDA.

377. Answer is C (Renal Parenchymatous disease): *Refer text below*

Sustained severe hypertension in children is most commonly caused by Renal parenchymatous disease.

378. Answer is C (Assessment of child for presence of Heart disease): *Ghai 5th / 294*

NADA's criteria are used for assessment of child for presence of heart disease.

The assessment of a child for the presence or absence of heart disease can be done with the help of some guidelines suggested by NADA. These guidelines are called NADA's criteria.

Major	Minor
• Systolic murmur, grade III or more, especially with a thrill	• Systolic murmur < grade III
• Diastolic murmur	• Abnormal 2nd heart sound • Abnormal ECG
• Cyanosis	• Abnormal X Ray
• Congestive cardiac failure	• Abnormal BP

Presence of one major and two minor criteria are essential for indicating the presence of heart disease.

Endocarditis

379. Answer is C (Raised ESR): *Harrison 18th /1055*

Raised ESR is not part of diagnostic criterion for infective endocarditis. Positive Rheumatoid Factor (immunogenic phenomen) is a minor criteria while positive blood culture and positive echocardiogram are both major criterion for diagnosis of Infective Endocarditis.

The Duke Criteria for the Clinical Diagnosis of Infective Endocarditis:

Major Criteria
1. Positive blood culture
• Typical microorganism for infective endocarditis from two separate blood cultures • Viridans streptococci, *Streptococcus gallolyticus*, HACEK group, *Staphylococcus aureus*, *or* • Community-acquired enterococci in the absence of a primary focus, *or* • Persistently positive blood culture, defined as recovery of a microorganism consistent with infective endocarditis from: • Blood cultures drawn >12 h apart; *or* • All of 3 or a majority of 4 separate blood cultures, with first and last drawn at least 1 h apart • Single positive blood culture for *Coxiella burnetii* or phase I IgG antibody titer of >1:800
2. Evidence of endocardial involvement
• ***Positive echocardiogram***[b] • Oscillating intracardiac mass on valve or supporting structures or in the path of regurgitant jets or in implanted material, in the absence of an alternative anatomic explanation, *or* • Abscess, *or* • New partial dehiscence of prosthetic valve, *or* • New valvular regurgitation (increase or change in preexisting murmur not sufficient)
Minor Criteria
1. Predisposition: predisposing heart condition or injection drug use 2. Fever 38.0°C (100.4°F) 3. Vascular phenomena: major arterial emboli, septic pulmonary infarcts, mycotic aneurysm, intracranial hemorrhage, conjunctival hemorrhages, Janeway lesions 4. Immunologic phenomena: glomerulonephritis, Osler's nodes, Roth's spots, ***rheumatoid factor*** 5. Microbiologic evidence: positive blood culture but not meeting major criterion as noted previously[c] or serologic evidence of active infection with organism consistent with infective endocarditis

[a]Definite endocarditis is defined by documentation of two major criteria, of one major criterion and three minor criteria, or of five minor criteria.

[b] Transesophageal echocardiography is recommended for assessing possible prosthetic valve endocarditis or complicated endocarditis.

[c]Excluding single positive cultures for coagulase-negative staphylococci and diphtheroids, which are common culture contaminants, and organisms that do not cause endocarditis frequently, such as gram-negative bacilli.

Note: HACEK, *Haemophilus* spp., *Aggregatibacter actinomycetemcomitans*, *Cardiobacterium hominis*, *Eikenella corrodens*, *Kingella* spp.

380. Answer is A (ASD): *Harrison 14th/ 786, 16th/ (not elaborated); Harrison 17th/1460; API 8th/500; Harrison 18th/p 1923*

Endocarditis is unusual in sites with a small pressure gradient as in – ASD *– Harrison*

Endocarditis tends to occur in

- High pressure areas (left side of heart)
- Downstream from sites where blood flow at a high velocity through a narrow orifice from a high to a low pressure chamber (distal to constriction in coarctation of aorta)
- Endocarditis occurs more frequently in patients with valvular incompetance than in those with pure stenosis.

Risk of infective endocarditis in various lesions :

High Risk	Moderate Risk	Low Risk
• *Prosthetic heart value* • *Tetralogy of fallot* • *PDA* • *A regurgitation* • *A stenosis* • *Coarctation of Aorta* • *VSD* • *Mitral regurgitation*	• *MVP + M.R.* • *T. stenosis* • *T. Regurgitation* • *P. Stenosis* • *M. Stenosis*	• *ASD* • *MVP without MR*

381. Answer is A (Small ASD): *Harrison 18th/1863; Harrison 17th/1460; API 8th/500*

Endocarditis is unusual in sites with a small pressure gradient as in – ASD *– Harrison*

Risk of infective endocarditis in various lesions

High Risk	Moderate Risk	Low Risk
• *Prosthetic heart valve* • *Tetralogy of fallot* • *PDA* • *A regurgitation* • *A stenosis* • *Coarctation of Aorta* • *VSD* • *Mitral regurgitation*	• *MVP + M.R.* • *T. Stenosis* • *T. Regurgitation* • *P. Stenosis* • *M. Stenosis*	• *ASD* • *MVP without MR*

Endocarditis tends to occur in
- High pressure areas (left side of heart)
- Downstream from sites where blood flow at a high velocity through a narrow orifice from a high to a low pressure chamber (distal to constriction in coarctation of aorta)
- Endocarditis occurs more frequently in patients with valvularincompetance than in those with pure stenosis.

382. Answer is D (Ostium Secondum ASD): *API 8th/500; Harrisons 16th/739; Repeat*

Endocarditis is unusual in sites with a small pressure gradient as in ASD
ASD is low risk lesion for the development of infective endocarditis and the single best answer amongst the options provided

383. Answer is D (ASD) : *API 8th/500; Harrisons 16th/739; Repeat copy above Answer 289*

Endocarditis is unusual in sites with a small pressure gradient as in ASD
ASD is low risk lesion for the development of infective endocarditis and the single best answer amongst the options provided

384. Answer is D (ASD): *API 8th/500; Harrisons 16th/739*

Endocarditis is unusual in sites with a small pressure gradient as in ASD
ASD is low risk lesion for the development of infective endocarditis and the single best answer amongst the options provided.

385. Answer is D (ASD) : *API 8th/500; Harrisons 16th/739; Repeat*

Vegetations of infective endocarditis are least common with ASD amongst the options provided

386. Answer is A (ASD) : *API 8th/500; Harrsions 16th/739: Repeat*

Endocarditis is unusual in sites with a small pressure gradient as in ASD
ASD is low risk lesion for the development of infective endocarditis and the single best answer amongst the options provided

387. Answer is B (VSD): *Ghai 6th/ 404*

VSD is the most common congenital lesion to be complicated by infective endocarditis – Ghai 6th/ 404

388. Answer is B (Mitral regurgitation): *See previous question*

Amongst the choices provided only mitral regurgitation has been grouped as one with a high risk. All others are grouped as conditions carrying only a moderate risk.

389. Answer is A (Lung): *Read text below*

Mitral valve vegetation would obviously not go to the lung, as that would involve a 'backward flow'.

390. Answer is D (Tricuspid valve): *Harrison 15th/ 811; 16th / 734; 17th/791* Harrison 18th/p 1055

Most common heart valve involved in IV drug layers is tricuspid valve. *'In almost 50% of patients who have endocarditis associated with injection drug use, infection is limited to the tricuspid valve' – Harrisons 16th/ 734*

Endocarditis in drug abusers:

- most *common age of patients affected – young males*[Q]
- *most often source of infecting microorganisms is: skin*[Q]
- *most common agent is staphylococcus aureus*
- *most common valve involved is Tricuspid valve.*
- *tricuspid valve (50%) > aortic valve (25%) > mitral valve (20%) > multiple valves (rest)*
- *murmurs are* frequently absent[Q]

Cardiac murmurs are almost always present in infective endocarditis except in patients with:
- early acute endocarditis
- ***intravenous drug abuse with tricuspid valve infection***

391. Answer is A (Septic Infarcts to lung): *See previous question*

Septic infarcts from the right side of the heart will first reach the lungs via the pulmonary artery due to normal forward flow.

392. Answer is C (Tip of palms and soles): *Harrison 17th/791; Read text below* Harrison 18th/p 1054, 1055

Oster's nodes are painful tender nodules in the pulp of fingers and soles, seen in patient of infective endocarditis.

Lesions seen in infective endocarditis that merit attention are :

- **Osler's nodes** :
  - *Painful*[Q] tender pea size erythematous nodules *in the pulp of finger and sole.*
  - Occur in crops and
  - Indicate either an immunological phenomenon or emboli to distal digital arteries.
- **Janeway lesions**[Q] **:**
  - *Small maculopapular erythematous or hemorrhagic nontender*[Q] *lesions.*
  - *Commonly seen in palms and soles*[Q]
- **Roth's lesions**[Q] **:**
  - *Oval, retinal haemorrhages with a clear pale centre.*
- **Splinter hemorrhages**[Q] **:**
  - *Linear subungual dark red streaks*
  - *Commonly seen in fingers; less commonly in toes*[Q]

393. Answer is A (Infective Endocarditis): *Harrison 17th /791; Macleod's Clinical Examination 12th/327*

Roth's spots (lesions) are oval retinal haemorrhages with a clear pale center that are typically seen in patients with subacute bacterial endocarditis. They are believed to be caused by immune complex deposition and are included as a minor criterion amongst Duke's criteria for clinical diagnosis of Infective Endocarditis.

Typical Named Lesions
Minor criteria for diagnosis of Infective Endo carditis (Duke's)

Vascular Phenomenon	Immunologic Phenomenon
• *Janeway's lesions* Small maculopapular erythematous or hemorrhagic **non tender**[Q] lesions typically seen in palms & soles	• *Oster's nodes* Painful[Q], tender[Q], pea size erythematous nodules in the pulp of fingers & soles • *Roth's spots* Oval retinal haemorrhages with a clear pale center (flame shaped haemorrhages with a central cotton wool spot)

394. Answer is C (Thrombus in left atria): *Harrison 15th/ 811; Robbins 5th/ 552, Robbins 6th/ 574*

Infective endocarditis does not lead to formation of thrombi within the left atrial. It may however lead to formation of friable vegetations that may embolize to the systemic circulation as infective emboli.

Infective endocarditis is characterized by colonization or invasion of the heart valves or mural endocardium by a microbiological agent, leading to the formation of bulky, friable vegetations laden with organisms

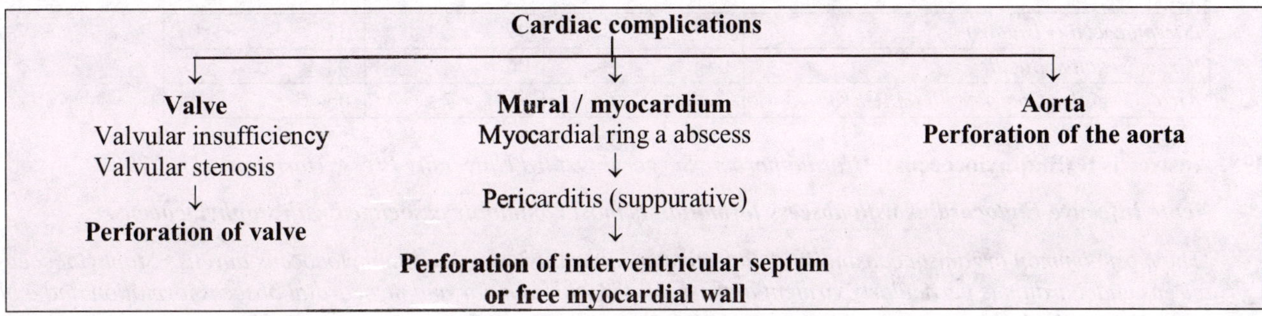

395. Answer is C (Salmonella Typhi): *Harrison 16th/732, 820, 830, 891, 899; Ananthnarayanan 7th/192, 200, 204, 212, http://www.ncbi.nlm.nih.gov/entrez/query.fcgi?cmd=Retrieve&db=PubMed&list_uids=1998650&dopt=Abstract*

Endocarditis is common with staphylococcus albus, streptococcus fecalis and pseudomonas aeruginosa.
Endocarditis has only been mentioned as rare complication of salmonella typhi infection. – *Harrison 16th/899*

The least likely organism to infective endocarditis amongst the options provided is salmonella typhi.

Other options

Staphylococcus albus (Staph. epidermis) (Coagulase Negative staph.)	**Streptococcus fecalis (Enterococci)**	**Pseudomonas Aeroginosa Gram negative bacilli**
• S. epidermis (albus) is the most Common coagulase negative staphylococii • Coagulase negative staph (S. epidermidis/alba) are the *most common cause of 'Prosthetic valve endocarditis'*	• Streptococci fecalis is the *most common cause of enterococcal infective endocarditis* • These organism account for 10 - 20% of cases of bacterial endocarditis	• *Common agent in endocarditis among infection drug users* • P. aerug inosa infects the native heart valves of intravenous drug users as well as prosthetic heart valves

396. Answer is C (Staphylococcus Aureus): *Harrison 18th/p 1053 Harrisons 17th/790, Harrisons 16th/732*

The most common cause for infective endocarditis overvall is staphylococcus aureus

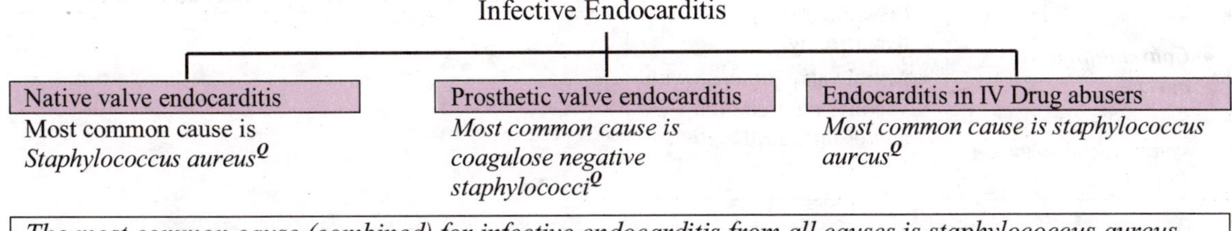

The most common cause (combined) for infective endocarditis from all causes is staphylococcus aureus

397. Answer is B (Staphylococcus Epidermidis): *Harrison's 17th/ 790*

The most common causative organisms of infective endocarditic within the first 12 months after valve surgery are Coagulase Negative Staphylococci. ***Staphylococcus Epidermidis is a coagulase negative staphylococcus and the single best answer of choice.***

Organism	Prothetic Valve endocarditis (% of cases) Time of onset after valve surgery		
	< 2 months	2-12 months	> 12 months
Coagulase Negative Staphylococcus	**33**	**32**	11
Staphylococcus Aureus	22	12	18
Enterococcii	08	12	11
Streptococcii (Viridans)	01	09	***31***
Gram Negative Bacilli	05	06	08
Gram Negative Coccobacilii (HACEK)	-	-	06

398. Answer is B (Staphylococcus): *'Cardiothorocic Surgery' Oxford University Press; Harrison's 17th/ 790*

Acute Infective Endocarditis with abscess formation is most commonly associated with staphylococcus.

'The most common organism causing acute infective endocarditis overall is staphylococcus aureus. Staphylococcus aureus endocarditis is particularly virulent and associated with annular and myocardial abscess formation and a higher mortality' – 'Cardiothorocic surgery' Oxford 2012/80

> *Paravalvular abscesses in patients with acute infective endocarditis is especially seen in association with virulent organisms like staphylococci and enterococcii. Such abscesses may also be seen in association with some virulent strains of streptococcal endocarditis.* ***Staphylococcus however are the most common organisms associated with such abscesses.***

399. Answer is D (Coarctation of Aorta) : *Harrisons 16th/739*

Coarctation of Aorta is a high risk cardiac lesion for the development of infective endocarditis and an indication for antibiotic prophyloxis.

Prophylaxis for infective Endocarditis

Cardiac lesion for which Endocarditis Prophylaxis is advised (moderate/High risk lesions)	
High Risk	Moderate Risk
• Prosthetic heart valves • Prior bacterial endocarditis • Complex cyanotic congenital heart disease; other complex congenital lesion after correction (see text) • Patient ductus arteriosus • ***Coarctation of the aorta*** • Surgically constructed systemic-pulmonary shunts	• Congenital cardiac malformations (other than high -/low-risk lesions), ventricular septal defect, bicuspid aortic valve • Acquired aortic and mitral valve dysfunction • Hypertrophic cardiomyopathy (asymmetric septal hypertrophy) • Mitral valve prolapse with valvular regurgitation and/or thickened leaflets

Cardiac lesion for which Endocarditis Prophylaxis is not advised (Low risk lesions)
• Isolated secundum ASD • Surgically repaired ASD, VSD, PDA (without residual defect, >6 months after repair) • Prior coronary artery bypass graft • Mitral valve prolapse without regurgitation or thickened leaflets • Physiologic or functional murmur • Prior Kawasaki disease or acute rheumatic fever without valve dysfunction • Cardiac pacemakers or implanted defibrillators

400. Answer is A (Amoxycillin): *Harrisons 16th/739*

Amoxycillin is the standard drug of choice for antibiotic prophyloxis for oral cavity procedures in adults at moderate or high risk of infective endocarditis.

Antibiotic Regimen for Prophylaxis of endocarditis in adults (Moderate/high risk)

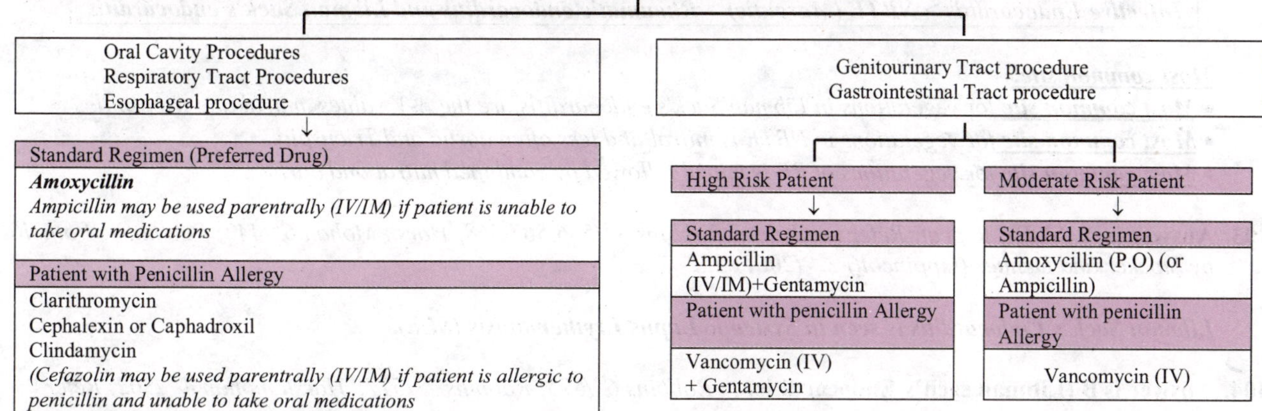

401. Answer is A (Infective endocarditis): *Repeat; Refer text below: Robbins 8th/566,567,568; Harsh Mohan 6th/447; Paediatric Pathology by Stocker and Dehner (Lippincott) 2nd (2001)/552*

Most friable vegetations with the highest risk of embolization are seen in infective endocarditis.

Friability of Vegetation and risk of embolization
Infective Endocarditis > NBTE (Marantic) > Rheumatic endocarditis and Libman Sack's endocarditis

Rheumatic Fever	**Non bacterial Thrombotic (Marantic Endocarditis)**	**Libman Sack's Endocarditis (SLE)**	**Infective Endocarditis**
• Small • Warty, verrucous • Usually Firm May be friable (but less than those of NBTE) (embolization rare)	• Small (but larger than those of rheumatic) • Friable (embolization common)	• Medium sized(small) • Flat, Verrucous,Irregular • Usually Firm; occasionally friable (embolization rare)	• Large, Bulky • Irregular • Friable *(most friable)*[Q] (embolization common)
• Along lines of closure	• Along lines of closure	• On surface of cusps Both surfaces may be involved most common being the undersurface, less often on mural endocardium • In pockets of valves	• Irregular vegetations on valve cusps that can extend onto the chordae. • Less often on mural endocardium
• Sterile (no organisms)	• Sterile	• Sterile	• Non-sterile (bacteria)
• Non destructive Valve perforation : no Mural involvement: rare	• Non destructive Valve perforation : no Mural involvement: rare	• Destructive Valve perforation : no Mural involvement: common	• Destructive Ulcerates or perforates underlying valve (or myocardium)
• Seen in Rheumatic fever	• Seen in hyper coagulable states e.g. cancer, promyelocytic leukemia increased estrogenic state	• Seen in SLE	• Seen in Infective endocarditis

Most common site:

- ***Most common site*** *for vegetations in Libman Sack's endocarditis are the A-V values, mitral and tricuspid.*
- ***Most common site*** *for vegetations in NBTE is mitral and less often aortic and Tricuspid.*
- ***Most common site*** *for vegetations of RF is mitral followed by combined mitral and aortic.*

402. Answer is A (Infective endocarditis): *Repeat; Refer text below: Robbins 8th/566,567,568; Harsh Mohan 6th/447; Paediatric Pathology by Stocker and Dehner (Lippincott) 2nd (2001)/552*

Most friable vegetations with the highest risk of embolization are seen in infective endocarditis.

Friability of Vegetation and risk of embolization
Infective Endocarditis > NBTE (Marantic) > Rheumatic endocarditis and Libman Sack's endocarditis

Most common site:

- ***Most common site*** *for vegetations in Libman Sack's endocarditis are the A-V values, mitral and tricuspid.*
- ***Most common site*** *for vegetations in NBTE is mitral and less often aortic and Tricuspid.*
- ***Most common site*** *for vegetations of RF is mitral followed by combined mitral and aortic.*

403. Answer is A (SLE): *Repeat; Refer text below: Robbins 8th/566,567,568; Harsh Mohan 6th/447; Paediatric Pathology by Stocker and Dehner (Lippincott) 2nd (2001)/552*

Libman Sack's Endocarditis is seen in Systemic Lupus Erythematosis (SLE).

404. Answer is B (Libman sach's Endocarditis) : *Robbins 6th/575; Robbins 7th/517; Harsh mohan 4th /302; Refer previous question*

Flat vegetation in pockets of valves are charachteristic of Libman sach's endocarditis

405. Answer is A (Along line of closure of valves) : *Robbins 7th/597*

Rheumatic heart disease is charachterized by vegetations along lines of closure of valves

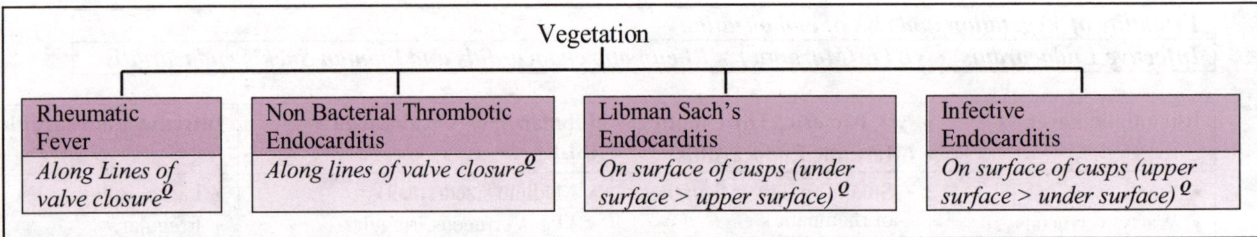

406. Answer is A (Rheumatic Heart Disease) : *Robbins 6th/ 575; Robbins 7th /597; Harshmohan 4th/302*

Firm warty vegetations along lines of closure of valves are charachteristic of Rheumatic Heart disease

Cardiac Involvement in Carcinoid Syndrome

407. Answer is A (Pulmonary valve): Harrison 18th/p 3062 *Harrison 17th/2351*

Carcinoid syndrome most frequently involves the ventricular aspect of the tricuspid valve.

Cardiac manifestations of carcinoid syndrome

- Cardiac disease is due to involvement of endocardium by dense fibrous deposits
- Cardiac disease primarily involves the right side (although left side lesions may also occur)
- The most commonly involved valve is tricuspid valve (ventricular surface/under surface)
- The second most commonly involved valve is pulmonary valve
- Predominant vavular lesion due to involvement of tricuspid valve is tricuspid regurgitation (valve is fixed open)
- Predominant valvular lesion due to involvement of pulmonary valve is pulmonic stenosis (valve is constricted)
- Most patients with cardiac lesion develop heart failure (80%)

408. Answer is A (Fibrous endocardial thickening of Right ventricle, Tricuspid valve & Pulmonary valve): *Robbins 7th/599, Braunwald 8th/297, Hurst 11th/2092; 'Pathology Pre test' 11th/211*

Fibrous enodocardial thickening involving the right ventricle, tricuspid valve and pulmonic valve is the charachteristic pathological finding in carcinoid heart disease.

Carcinoid Heart Disease

- Carcinoid heart disease is the cardiac manifestation of systemic syndrome caused by carcinoid tumors and results primarily from the bioactive products elaborated by carcinoid tumors at other sites.
- *Cardiac involvement predominantly **affects the endocardium and valves on the right side of heart**[Q] (because bioactive tumor substances are inactivated by the lung) and **usually occurs in patients with hepatic metastasis**[Q] (This bypasses the inactivation by the liver & exposes right heart to high levels of bioactive products)*
- This consists of firm plaque like (endocardial) fibrous thickening of the right ventricle tricuspid and pulmonic valves composed predominantly of ***smooth muscle cells and sparse collagen fibres***[Q], embedded in an acid mucopolysacharide rich matrix material. ***Elastic fibres are not present.***
- **Right sided cardiac lesions** are common and include involvement of the tricuspid valve, pulmoary valve and the right ventricular endocardium.

Charachteristic Cardiac Lesions in Carcinoid Heart Disease (Right side of Heart)	
• Tricuspid valve thickening	***Tricuspid Regurgitation is the primary lesion*** ***Tricuspid stenosis is minimal***
• Pulmonic valve thickenning	*Pulmonic Regurgitation (variable degree)* *Pulmonic stenosis (variable degree)*
• Right ventricular endocardial thickening	*Restrictive cardiomyopathy may be seen*

- **Left sided cardiac lesions** are uncommon but may be seen when blood containing the responsible mediator enters the left heart in certain specific circumstances.
  - Incomplete inactivation in lung due to very high blood levels
  - Incomplete inactivation due to '*right to left*' intra-cardiac shunt from a patent foramen ovale
  - Pulmonary carcinoid /pulmonary metastasis

Note:
Endocardial thickening of Tricuspid valve with Tricuspid stenosis may be seen, but is not a charachteristic feature of carcinoid heart disease. The charachteristic valvular pathology affective the tricuspid valve is tricuspid valve regurgitation.
'Tricuspid stenosis is usually minimal'- Braunwald 8th/297; 'Pure tricuspid stenosis is rare' – Essentials of Anatomic Pathology 2nd/21-8

409. Answer is B (Tricuspid valve): *Harrison 17th/235*

The most commonly involved valve in carcinoid syndrome is tricuspid valve.

410. Answer is B (Inflow tract of RV): Harrison 18th/p 3062 *Harrison 17th/2351; Refere previous question*

The most commonly involved valve in carcinoid syndrome is tricuspid valve which forms the inflow tract of Right ventricle.

Most commonly involved part of heart	: Inflow tract of RV (Tricuspid valve)
Second most commonly involved part of heart	: Outflow tract of RV (Pulmonic valve)

Sudden Cardiac Death

411. Answer is D (Ventricular septal defect): *Harrison 16th/1619; Harrison The Eisenmenger Syndrome in Adults': http"//www.annals.org/cig/content/full/128/9/745 May 1998/Volume 128 Issue 9/Pages 745-755*

Amongst the options provided ventricular septal defect is the least likely diagnosis to result in sudden cardiac death.

- **Hypertrophic and Dilated Cardiomyopathy :**
  The cardiomyopathies (Hypertrophic and Dilated) are the second most common category of diseases associated with risk of 'Sudden cardiac death'.- *Harrison 16th/1620*
- **Eisenmenger's Syndrome :**
  "Most patients with the Eisenmenger's syndrome die of 'sudden cardiac death', probably from a ventricular arrythmia." The Eisenmenger Syndrome in Adults':http"//www.annals. org/cig/content/full/128/9/745 May 1998/Volume 128 Issue 9/Pages 745-755

- **Ventricular septal defect :**
  The occurance of sudden cardiac death in cases of isolated ventricular septal defect has not been emphasized in literature. Sudden death may probably be seen in early childhood but only isolated case reports have been documented. ***VSD therefore is the least likely diagnosis and hence the answer of exclusion.*** *-J Paediatr Child Health. 1994 Oct;30(5):439-40*

Caridac Arrest and Sudden Cardiac Death

Structural Causes	Functional Contributing Factors
I. Coronary heart disease	I. Alterations of coronary blood flow
A. Coronary artery abnormalities	A. Transient ischemia
1. Chronic atherosclerotic lesions	B. Reperfusion after ischemia
2. Acute (active) lesions (plague fissuring, platelet aggregation, acute thrombosis)	II. Low cardiac output states
3. Anomalous coronary artery anatomy	A. Heart failure
B. Myocardial infarction	1. Chronic
1. Healed	2. Acute decompensation
2. Acute	B. Shock
II. Myocardial hypertrophy	III. Systemic metabolic abnormalities
A. Secondary	A. Electrolyte imbalance (e.g., hypokalemia)
B. ***Hypertrophic cardiomyopathy***	B. Hypoxemia, acidosis
1. Obstructive	IV. Neurophysiologic disturbances
2. Nonobstructive	A. Autonomic fluctuations: central, neural, humoral
III. ***Dilated cardiomyopathy – primary muscle disease***	B. Receptor function
IV. Inflammatory and infiltrative disorders	V. Toxic responses
A. Myocarditis	A. Proarrhythmic durg effects
B. Noninfectious inflammatory diseases	B. Cardiac toxins (e.g. cocaine, digitalis intoxication)
C. Infiltrative diseases	C. Drug interactions
D. Right ventricular dysplasia	
V. Valvular heart disease	
VI. Electrophysiologic abnormalities, structural	
A. Anomalous pathways in Wolff-Parkinson-White syndrome	
B. Conducting system disease	
VII. Inherited disorders of molecular structure associated with electrophysiologic abnormalities (e.g., congenital long QT syndromes, Brugada syndrome)	

Miscellaneous

412. Answer is D (Generates impulses at the highest rate): *Ganong 22nd/547; 21st/ 549; Guyton 10th/ 111*

"The sinus node controls the beat of the heart because its rate of discharge is greater than that of any other part of the heart. Therefore the sinus node is the pacemaker of the heart" - Guyton

Although the AV node and Purkinje fibres are also capable of generating impulses spontaneously, it is the sinus node which controls the hearts rhythmicity and acts as the pacemaker of the heart.

This is attributed to the fact that the discharge rate of the SA node is considerably faster than the natural self excitatory discharge of either the AV node or the Purkinje fibres. Each time the sinus node discharges its impulse is conducted into both, the AV node and Purkinje fibres and discharges their excitable membranes. Then these tissues as well as the sinus node recover and start almost at the same time, but the sinus node discharges again much more rapidly and discharges the AV node & Purkinje fibres again before they can reach their own threshold for self excitation.

Rhythmicity of Heart

Tissue	Rate of impulse generation
SA node	**70-80/minutes** *(Highest)*Q
AV node	**40-60/minutes**
Bundle of His	**40/minutes**
Purkinje system	**24/minutes**

Rate of impulse generation to decreasing order:
*SA node*Q **> AV node > Bundle of His >** *purkinje system*Q

AV node **and** ***purkinje fibres*** **are also capable of generating impulses spontaneously but SA node discharges most rapidly (70-80/min) & depolarizes the AV node and purkinje fibres before they can reach their own threshold for self excitation.**

413. Answer is A (SA Node): *Refer previous question; Ganong 22nd/549; Gyuton 10th/111*

The rate of impulse generation/rate of discharge is highest in the SA node.

Note:		
Highest Rate of impulse generation in seen in	:	SA Node^{Q}
Highest Rate of conduction is seen in	:	Purkinje System^{Q}

414. Answer is D (Purkinje System) : *Ganong 20th / 530 (table 28-1)*

Purkinje system has the highest conduction speed in cardiac tissue.

The conduction rate of various cardiac tissues:

Tissue	**Conduction rate (m/s)**	**Relative value**
S A node	**0.05**	*2nd least* ^{Q}
AV node	**0.02 – 0.05**	*Least* ^{Q}
Atrial pathway	**1**	
Bundle of His	**1**	
Ventricular muscle	**1**	
Purkinje system	4^{Q}	*Highest*^{Q}

415. Answer is D (Purkinje System): *Ganong 22nd/549*

Purkinje fibers has fastest conduction^{Q}

416. Answer is A (AV node): *Ganong 22nd/547-549; NMS Physio 4th/139*

Minimum conduction velocity is seen in AV node.

Conduction Rate in decreasing order:
Purkinje fibers ^{Q} **> Bundle of His = Ventricular muscle = Atrial pathway> SA node** > *AV node*^{Q}

Tissue	**Conduction rate (m/s)**	**Relative value**
S A node	**0.05**	*2nd least* ^{Q}
AV node	**0.02 – 0.05**	*Least* ^{Q}
Atrial pathway	**1**	
Bundle of His	**1**	
Ventricular muscle	**1**	
Purkinje system	4^{Q}	*Highest*^{Q}

417. A i.e. Septum – Endocardium – Epicardium: *Ganong 22nd/ 549, 550*

Activation preads from septum to endocardium to epicardium

Order of Activation of Ventricular Muscle

First the ***Purkinje system*** inside the ***septum***^{Q}

↓

Entire ***Endocardium***^{Q} of ventricle

↓ *through ventricular muscle*

Epicardium^{Q}

418. Answer is D (Right bundle branch) : *Snell's 7th/119-120*

Right bundle is supplied by the Left coronary artery.
Right coronary artery supplies the SA node (in 65% cases), AV node, AV bundle or Bundle of His and part of left bundle branch(LBB)
Left cronoary artery supplies the right bundle branch (RBB, part of LBB and sometimes the SA node (in 35% cases),

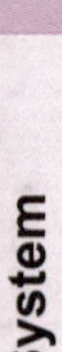

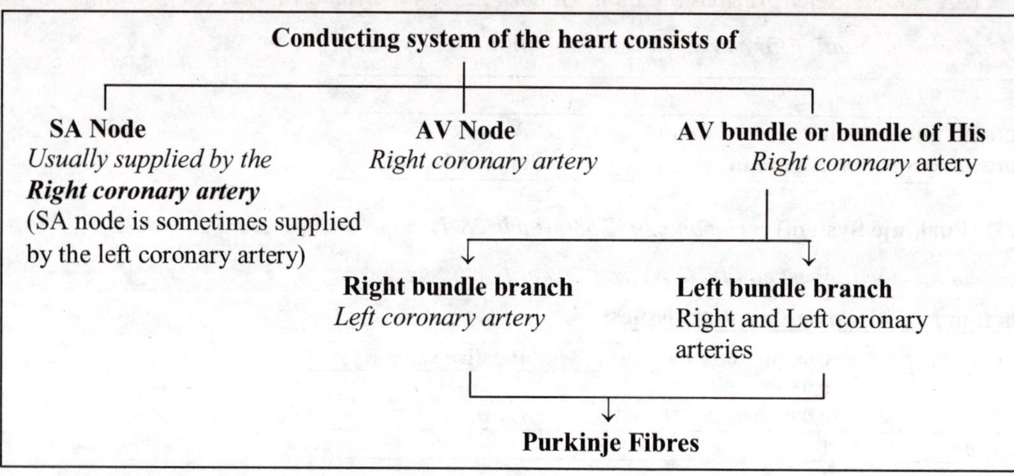

419. Answer is B (Left dominance): *Snell's 8th/113-114; BDC 4th Vol I/251*

When the posterior interventricular artery is derived from the circumflex artery (br. of left coronary artery) the circulation is described as 'left dominant'

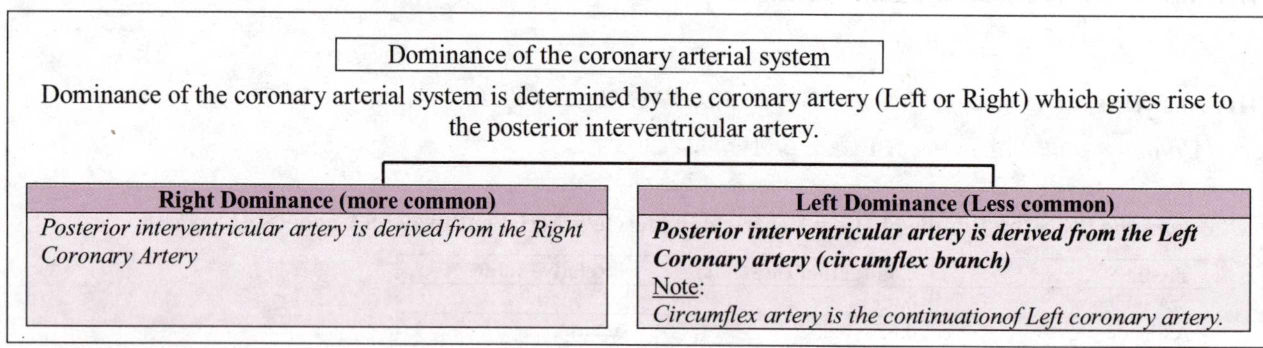

420. Answer is B (End of isovolumetric contraction) : *Guyton 10th / 99*

The Aortic valve opens at the end of isovolumic contraction.

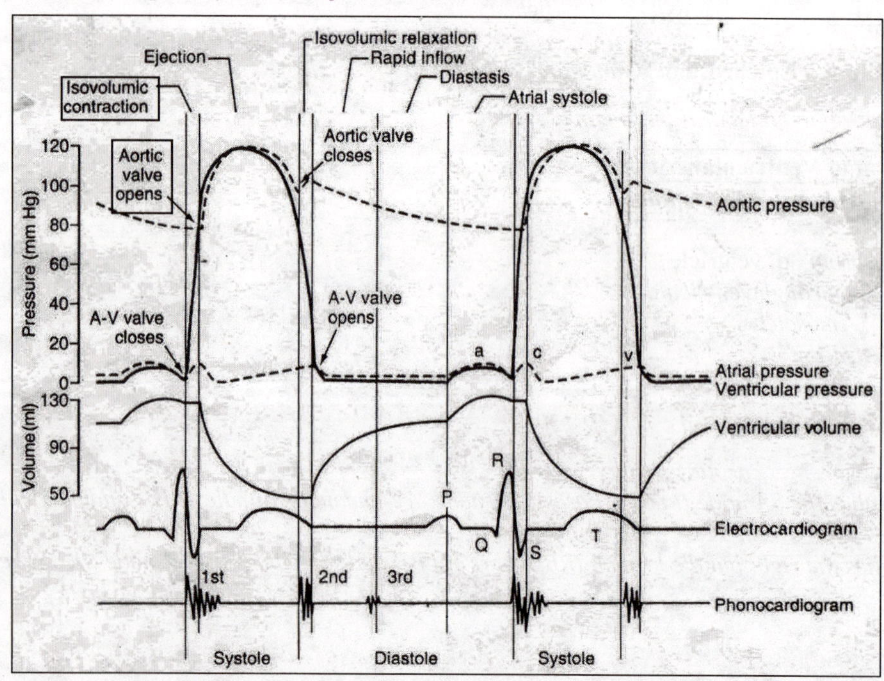

The period of isovolumetric contraction *is when ventricle contracts as a closed chamber with both the semilunar and AV valves closed.*
The total period of isovolumetric contraction lasts about .05 sec until the pressure in the left and right ventricle exceeds the pressure in the aorta and the aortic and pulmonary valves open.

Note from figure above :

Beginning of systole[Q]	AV valves close
End of isovolumetric contraction[Q]	Semilunar valves open
End of diastole[Q]	AV valves close
End of diastasis[Q]	AV valves are open and semilunar valves are closed

421. Answer is A (Atrio-ventricular valves open): *Guyton 10th/99; Refer previous question*

AV valves open at the end of isovolumetric relaxation.

AV valves open:
At the end of iso-volumetric relaxation phase, AV valves open, so as to allow blood to flow rapidly into ventricles (ventricular filling phase).
AV valves close:
AV valves close at the begining of iso-volumetric relaxation.
Peak of C wave on JVP:
Peak of 'c' wave corresponds to the end of iso-volumetric contraction.
T wave in JVP
'T' waves in ECG begin slightly before the end of ventricular contraction and end with the end of iso-volumetric relaxation phase.

422. Answer is C (Both valves are closed)

During isovolumetric contraction the ventricle contracts as a closed chamber with both the semilunar and AV valves closed (All valves are closed)

423. Answer is B (Opening of A-V valves): *Ganong Review of Medical Physiology 22/e P- 565-666; Chaudhuri Concise Medical Physiology 5/e P- 176; Sembulingum Essentials of Medical Physiology 3/e P- 436; Repeat*

Isovolumetric Relaxation phase ends with opening of the Av valves *(Refer figure)*

Valvular event (valves)	Cardiac events	ECG	JVP (Jugular venous Pressure curve)
Opening of AV valve[Q]	***End of isovolumic relaxation phase[Q]***	***End of T wave[Q] (phase b/w T wave and new p wave)***	***V-Y descent[Q]***
Closure of AV valve	- End of diastole - Beginning of isovolumic contraction	Later half of R wave	End of 'x' descent
Opening of semilunar valve	*End of isovolumic contraction[Q]*	ST segment	Peak of 'C' wave
Closure of semilunar valve	- Beginning of isovolumic relaxation phase - Beginning of diastole	Later half of T wave	

424. Answer is B (3.2): *Ganong 20th/550; Guyton 10th/210*

The cardiac index in a normal person is approximately 3.2 L/min/m²

$$\textbf{Cardiac Index} = \frac{\text{Cardiac Output}}{\text{Body Surface Area}} = \frac{5}{1.7} = 3\text{L / min /m}^2$$

425. Answer is B (Mean Stroke Volume) : *Ganong 20th / 550; Guyton 10th / 210*

Mean stroke volume is the amount of blood pumped out of each ventricle per beat. It is calculated as the cardiac output in L/min divided by the heart rate.

$$\text{Mean Stroke Volume} = \frac{\text{Cardiac Output}}{\text{Hear Rate}}$$

Parameter	Definition	Value
Cardiac output	The output of the heart per unit time	*5L/min*^Q
Stroke volume	The amount of blood pumped out of each ventricle per beat. ***Mean stroke volume***^Q ***= Cardiac output/Heart rate***	*70 ml*^Q
Cardiac Index	*Cardiac output/ body surface area*^Q	*3.2L/min/m*^{2}^Q

426. Answer is D (Diastole + 1/3rd Pulse pressure) : *Chaudhary 2nd / 244; Chaudhary 5th/244*

Mean arterial pressure can be measured as Diatolic BP + 1/3 Pulse Pressure

Mean arterial pressure is the 'weighted' mean pressure of the blood.
In a cardiac cycle, the systole lasts for about 0.3 sec and diastole for about 0.5 sec. Therefore in a subject having a cardiac cycle of 0.8 sec, the mean BP cannot be taken as (systole + diastole)/2 mmHg but instead a weighed mean (in which duration of systole and diastole are taken care of) is required.

Calculations for Mean Blood Pressure
Mean BP = Diastolic BP + 1/3rd Pulse pressure^Q
Mean BP = Diastolic BP + 1/3rd (Systolic BP – Diastolic BP)^Q
Mean BP = $\frac{1}{3}$ ***(Systolic BP + 2 Diastolic BP)***

427. Answer is A (SBP + 2DBP)/3: *Chaudhary 2nd / 244; Chaudhary 5th/244*

Mean arterial pressure can be measured as (SBP+2DBP/3)

428. D i.e. Peripheral resistance x cardiac output: *Ganong 22nd/590*

Blood pressure is defined as the product of cardiac output and peripheral resistance.

Blood pressure =	**Cardiac output x peripheral resistance**^Q **or Blood flow (Q) x resistance (R)**

429. Answer is C (kP$_a$): *Taber's Cyclopedic Medical Dictionary / 2216 ; Ganong 18th / 54*

Pressure in SI units is measured in Pascal [Pa]
Blood pressure in SI units is measured in kPa.

430. Answer is B (Is higher than intraarterial pressure): *Ganong 22nd/ 590 , Medicine for Anaesthetists 4th/ 285 Screening for Diseases by Snow (2004) /135]*

Blood pressure measured by Sphygmomanometer with a standard cuff tend to overestimate 'true' arterial pressures as measured by arterial cannulation, especially in the elderly and the obese – Ganong.

Blood pressure Measurement with Sphygmomanometers

- Sphygmomanometer is a device that measures blood pressures indirectly.

External pressure is applied with a sphygmomanometer cuff to the overlying tissues and the pressure required to occlude the artery is assumed to be equal to the intra arterial pressure.

- The sphygmomanometer will give accurate readings only if no pressure (zero mm. of mercury) is dissipated in compressing the soft tissues overlying the artery.

However in practice, some pressure is always dissipated in compressing the blanket of soft tissues overlying the artery and hence ***blood pressure measured by the sphygmomanometer are slightly higher than true intra arterial pressures.***

- The amount by which the sphygmomanometer overestimates the true blood pressure is influenced by the amount of overlying fat and the compressibility of the vessles.

Sources of Error
Blood Pressure measured by Sphygmomanometer

Overlying Soft tissue Blanket	Compressibility of vessels	Size of Cuff
• Thick overlying soft tissue blanket leads to overestimation of blood pressure • *Obese individuals*[Q] have a thick blanket of fat which dissibates cuff pressure. Hence Blood pressure is likely to be overestimated when measured by sphygmomanometer and a standard cuff.	• Vessels that are difficult to compress lead to overestimation of blood pressure • Blood pressure measured in such individuals with sphygmomanometer will result in over estimation of blood pressure (Pseudohypertension) • Such Patients include *Elderly individuals, diabetics*[Q] *and patients who* may have rigid sclerotic vessels that are difficult to compress (*Mokenberg's asteriosclerosis*).	• *Small (Narrow) cuff*[Q] leads to falsely high blood pressure recordings (overestimation) *Large (wide) cuff*[Q] leads to falsely lower blood pressure recordings (under estimation) • If the standard arm cuff is used to measure blood pressure in the thigh falsely high blood pressure values will be obtained (due to relatively smaller cuff size and greater soft tissue blanket). • If the standard arm cuff is used on the forearm falsely lower blood pressure values may be recorded.

Note
- *More accurate pressure can be recorded in obese individuals by using a wider cuff size*[Q]
- *More accurate pressure can be recorded in the thigh by using a wider cuff size*[Q]

431. Answer is B (Diastolic BP is indicated by 4th Kovotkoff's sound): *Ganong 22/ 589-90;Snow Screening for disease (2004) /135; Medicine for anesthesia 4th/285; Guyton 11th/166-67,175-76*

Diastolic blood pressure is indicated by the 5th fourth Korotkoff sound (not by fourth Korotkoff sound).

Diastolic blood pressure is best indicated by fifth Korotkoff sound

Korotkoff sounds are produced by turbulent flow in artery

1.	Faint, clear, tapping sounds	It indicates ***systolic BP***[Q]
2.	Murmur / swishing sounds	
3.	More intense, crisper sounds	
4.	Distinct abrupt muffled f sounds	*Indicates diastolic BP in children.*
5.	No sound	***Best correlates with diastolic BP in normal adults***[Q].

Cuff width should be 40% of arm circumference

Appropriate Cuff size

- Ratio of width of compression cavity of cuff (bladder) to circumference of extremity is of critical importance.

According to American Heart Association

Bladder **width** ***should be 40% of circumference or 1.2 times of diameter of extremity***[Q]

Bladder **length** should be ***80% of arm circumference***[Q]

Length to width ratio is 2 : 1

Small cuff measures spuriously elevated Diastolic blood pressure and Monkenberg sclerosis causes pseudohypertension

False High values are found in	False low values are found in
Thick overlying Soft tissue blanket • *Obese individuals*[Q] **Limited Compressibility of vessels** • *Elderly* • *Atherosclerosis* • *Diabetics* • *Mokenberg's arteriosclerosis* **Size of cuff** • Small narrow cuff	Large (wide) cuff eg standard arm cuff used in forearm. Too fast Deflation rate leads to too low systolic pressure. Improper interpretation of Auscultatory gap It is the interval of pressure where Korotkoff's sounds indicating true systolic pressure fade away and reappear at a lower pressure. The improper interpretation of this gap may l/t errors made in falsely low recording of systolic BP. It usually occurs at high pressures, when there is silence at pressures greater than systolic BP, except that the pulse can still be palpated.

432. Answer is A (Auscultatory gap): *Ganong 22nd/590; Chaudhuri Concise Medical Physiology 5th/210*

Sources of error (Spuriously high BP)

Thick overlying Soft tissue blanket	Limited Compressibility of vessels	Size of cuff
Obese individuals[Q] have a thick blanket of fat which dissibates cuff pressure. Hence Blood pressure is likely to be overestimated when measured by sphygmomanometer and a standard cuff.	- Elderly - Atherosclerosis - Diabetics - Mokenberg's arteriosclerosis	• *Small (Narrow) cuff*[Q] leads to falsely high blood pressure recordings (overestimation)

433. The Answer is B (more than intravascular pressure) : *Ganong 22nd/ 590 , Medicine for Anaesthetists 4th/ 285 Screening for Diseases by Snow (2004) /135; Bijlani 1st / 189 ; Ganong / 20th 568*

Blood pressure measured by Sphygmomanometer with a standard cuff tend to overestimate 'true' arterial pressures as measured by arterial cannulation, especially in the elderly and the obese – *Ganong*

434. Answer is D (These may result in aneurysm): *Robbins 7th/575*

Ventricular aneurysms result from transmural infarcts, which involve the whole thickness of myocardium from epicardium to endocardium. ***Subendocardial infarcts being limited to only the inner one third or at most one half of the ventricular wall do not cause ventricular aneurysms.***
Aneurysm of the ventricular wall most commonly results from a large transmural anteroseptal infarct'- Robbins

Transmural infarcts	Subendocardial infarcts
• Ischaemic necrosis involves the full or nearly full thickness of ventricular wall. (Myocardium from epicardium to endocardium is involved) • Associated with coronary atherosclerosis acute plaque change and superimposed thrombosis. • Usually limited to the distribution of a single coronary artery and hence unifocal.	• Ischaemic necrosis involves the inner one third or at most one half of the ventricular wall. (Epicardium is not involved) • Associated either with atherosclerosis, plaque changes and thrombosis 'or' from prolonged and severe reduction in systemic blood pressure as in shock. • Usually multifocal (may be unifocal) - Limited to distribution of a single coronary artery when it results from plaque disruption & thrombosis - Usually multifocal as it most often results from reduction in perfusion (The subendocardial region is the least well perfused region of myocardium and is most vulnerable to any reduction in coronary flow.)

A transmural infarct involves the full thickness of the myocardial wall and is usually caused by acute plaque disruption with superimposed occlusive thrombosis.

A subendocardial infarct is in area of normally diminished perfusion – the inner one-third to one-half of the ventricular wall. These infarcts are typically a result of global atherosclerosis that leads to global borderline perfusion. The critical point is reached by increased oxygen demand, vasospasm, or hypotension without superimposed thrombosis. The myocardial injury is therefore ***multifocal***' - *Unstable Angina and NSTEMI': Journal of emergency medicine.*

435. Answer is C (Neutrophilic infiltration Surrounding Coagulative necrosis) : *Robbins 7th ; Hurst 11th / 122*

The patient in question succumbed to Myocardial infarction after four days of its onset. Charachteristic morphological changes evolve in the heart of patients with MI depend on the duration since the attack.

After four days the microscopic examination is most likely to reveal large number of PMNs (Neutrophils) at borders of coagulative necrosis

Granulation tissue *first appears about 6 – 7 days after MI*

Collagenous tissue *first appears about 10 days after MI*

Evolution of MI (Table from 'Hurst')

Time of Occlusion	Gross	Histologic
12 h	No change / pallor	Wavy fibers
24 – 48 h	Pallor – yellow, soft	Hypereosinophilic fibers, PMNs at borders
3 – 5 days	Yellow center, hyperemic borders	***Large number of PMNs at border, coagulation necrosis loss of nuclei***
6 – 10 days	Yellow, depressed central infarct, tanred margins	***Mummified fibers in center, macrophage phagocytosis + granulation tissue at borders***
10 – 14 days	Gray red borders, infiltrating central tan-yellow infarct if large	***Marked granulation tissue, collagen deposition,***
2 – 8 weeks	Gelatinuous to gray white scar, greater healing at border zone	Collagen deposition with prominent large capillaries.

Evolution of MI (Table From Robbins)

Time	Gross Features	Light Microscope
Reversible Injury		
0 to ½ hr	None	None
Irreversible injury		
½ - 4 hr	None	Usually none; variable waviness of fibres at border
4-12 hr	Occassionally dark mottling	Beginning coagulation necrosis; edema; hemorrhage
12-24 hr	Dark mottling	Ongoing coagulation necrosis; pyknosis of nuclei; myocyte hypereosinophilia; marginal contraction band necrosis; beginning neutrophilic infiltrate
1-3 days	Mottling with yellow-tan infarct center	***Coagulation necrosis, with loss of nuclei and striations; interstitial infiltrate of neutrophils***
3-7 days	Hypermic border; central yellow-tan softening	Beginnig disintegration of dead myofibers, with dying neutrophils; early phagocytosis of dead cells by macrophages at infarct border
7-10 days	Maximally yellow tan and soft, with depressed red-tan margins	Well-developed phagocytosis of dead ells; ***early formation of fibrovascular granulation tissue at margins***
10-14 days	Red-gray depressed infarct borders	Well-established granulation tissue with new blood vessels and collagen deposition
2-8 wks	Gray-white scar, progressive from border toward core of infarct	Increased collagen deposition, with decreased cellularity
> 2 mo	Scarring complete	Dense collagen scar

436. Answer is B (Necrotic myofibres with presence of neutrophils): *Robbins 6th/558*

The patient in question succumbed to myocardial infarction after about 24 hours of the attack. Characteristic morphological changes evolve in the heart of patients with MI depending on duration since the attack.

After twenty four hours of the attack light microscope shows coagulative necrosis of myofibrils with loss of nuclei and striations along with an interstitial infiltrate of neutrophils.

Evolution of morphologic changes in myocardial infarction

Time	Gross Features	Light Microscope	Electron Microscope
Reversible Injury			
0 to ½ hr	None	None	Relaxation of myofibrils; glycogen loss; mitochondrial swelling
Irreversible injury			
½ - 4 hr	None	Usually none; variable waviness of fibres at border	Sarcolemmal disruption; mitochondrial amorphous densities
4-12 hr	Occassionally dark mottling	Beginning coagulation necrosis; edema; hemorrhage	
12-24 hr	Dark mottling	Ongoing coagulation necrosis; pyknosis of nuclei; myocyte hypereosinophilia; marginal contraction band necrosis; beginning neutrophilic infiltrate	
1-3 days	Mottling with yellow-tan infarct center	***Coagulation necrosis, with loss of nuclei and striations; interstitial infiltrate of neutrophils***	
3-7 days	Hypermic border; central yellow-tan softening	Beginnig disintegration of dead myofibers, with dying neutrophils; early phagocytosis of dead cells by macrophages at infarct border	
7-10 days	Maximally yellow tan and soft, with depressed red-tan margins	Well-developed phagocytosis of dead ells; ***early formation of fibrovascular granulation tissue at margins***	
10-14 days	Red-gray depressed infarct borders	Well-established granulation tissue with new blood vessels and collagen deposition	
2-8 wks	Gray-white scar, progressive from border toward core of infarct	Increased collagen deposition, with decreased cellularity	
>2 mo	Scarring complete	Dense collagen scar	

437. Answer is C (1 week old): *Chandrasoma Taylor 3ed/364: Refer previous question*

Early formationof granulation tissue is seen about 7-10 days after myocardial infarction.

438. Answer is C (Atherosclerosis) : *Harrison 14th/1394*

'***The most common pathologic condition associated with aortic aneurysm is Atherosclerosis***': *H14th/1394*

439. Answer is A (Atherosclerosis) : *Robbins 6th / 525, 526*

Atherosclerosis is the major etiological factor in abdominal[Q] aortic aneurysm – *Robbins*

Remember:

- *Atherosclerotic aneurysms most frequently occur in the Abdominal aorta.[Q]*
- *Most common site of abdominal aortic aneurysm is above the bifurcation of aorta and below the renal arteries.[Q]*
- *Most common age group for abdominal aortic aneurysm depends is elderly (> 50 years).* [Q]
- *Risk[Q] of rupture of an abdominal aortic aneurysm depends upon its size[Q] (aneurysm larger than 5 cm are classified as dangerous[Q])*
- Most common source of infection in a Mycotic abdominal aortic aneurysm is Bacteremia [Q] from a p*rimary Salmonella gastro-enteritis.[Q]*
  (Mycotic aneurysm are abdominal aortic aneurysm that have become infected by lodgment of circulating organisms in the wall)

440. Answer is A (Ascending Aorta) : *Robbins 6th/141*

Aortic aneurysms in Marfan's syndrome occur most frequently in the ascending aorta.

Cardiovascular lesions in Marfan's syndrome

Cardiovascular lesions are the most life threatening features of Marfan's syndrome.

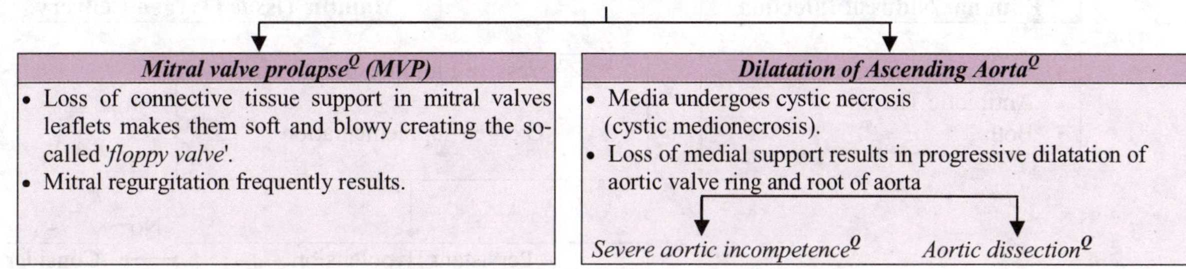

441. Answer is B (Sinus tachycardia): *Read text below*

AV fistulas cause short circuiting of blood from an artery to a vein thereby increasing the pulse rate (sinus tachycardia) & cardiac output.

Sinus tachycardia **:**
It is a regular rhythm with SA node discharging in excess of 100 times/ minute (usually 100-160/min)

Common causes include:

Physiological	Pathological
• High altitude	• Thyrotoxicosis
• Exercise	• Anxiety states
• Excitement	• Fever and infections
• Pregnancy	• Cardiac failure
• Pain	• Pulmonary embolism
	• AV fistulae.

442. Answer is B (↑cardiac output, ↓ total P.R.) : *Harrison 16th/1608; 14th / 778, 15th/226-27*

Septic shock is characterized by normal or increased cardiac output and decreased systemic vascular resistance.

***Septic Shock* :** Usually results from a severe decrease in systemic vascular resistance, besides various other features. *Cardiac output is initially normal or even elevated.*

Infact, *normal or increased cardiac output and decreased systemic vascular resistance characterize septic shock* (as in Gram negative septicemia here) and distinguish it from cardiogenic, extra-cardiac, obstructive and hypovolumic shock.

443. Answer is D (Norepinephrine) : *Harrisons 16th / 1605, 1611; Harrisons 14th / 221, 222 (Detailed in H14th)*

The patient in question is presenting with features of septic shock. Dopamine is the initial recommended vasopressor agent to maintain blood pressure but is not provided amongst the options. Patients who remain hypotensive despite dopamine should be adminstered norepinephrine and hence norepinephrine is the single best answer of choice here.

Harrison 14th / 221 Treatment of septic shock

If fluid therapy alone fails to restore adequate arterial pressure and organ perfusion , therapy with vaso pressor agent should be intitiated. For the persistantly hypotensive patient dopamine frequently raises arterial pressure and maintains or enhances blood flow to the renal and splanchnic circulation. ***Patients who remain hypotensive despite dopamine require nor epinephrine, a more potent vasopressor.***

Once hypotension, has been corrected to optimize oxygen delivery to tissues, raising a low cardiac index with dobutamine can be useful - Harrisons 14th / 221, 222

Harrisons 16th / 605 : Treatment of septic shock

In the presence of sepsis, augmentation of cardiac output may require inotropic support with dopamine, nore pinephrine or vaso pressin in the presence of hypotension or with dobutamine if arterial pressure is normal

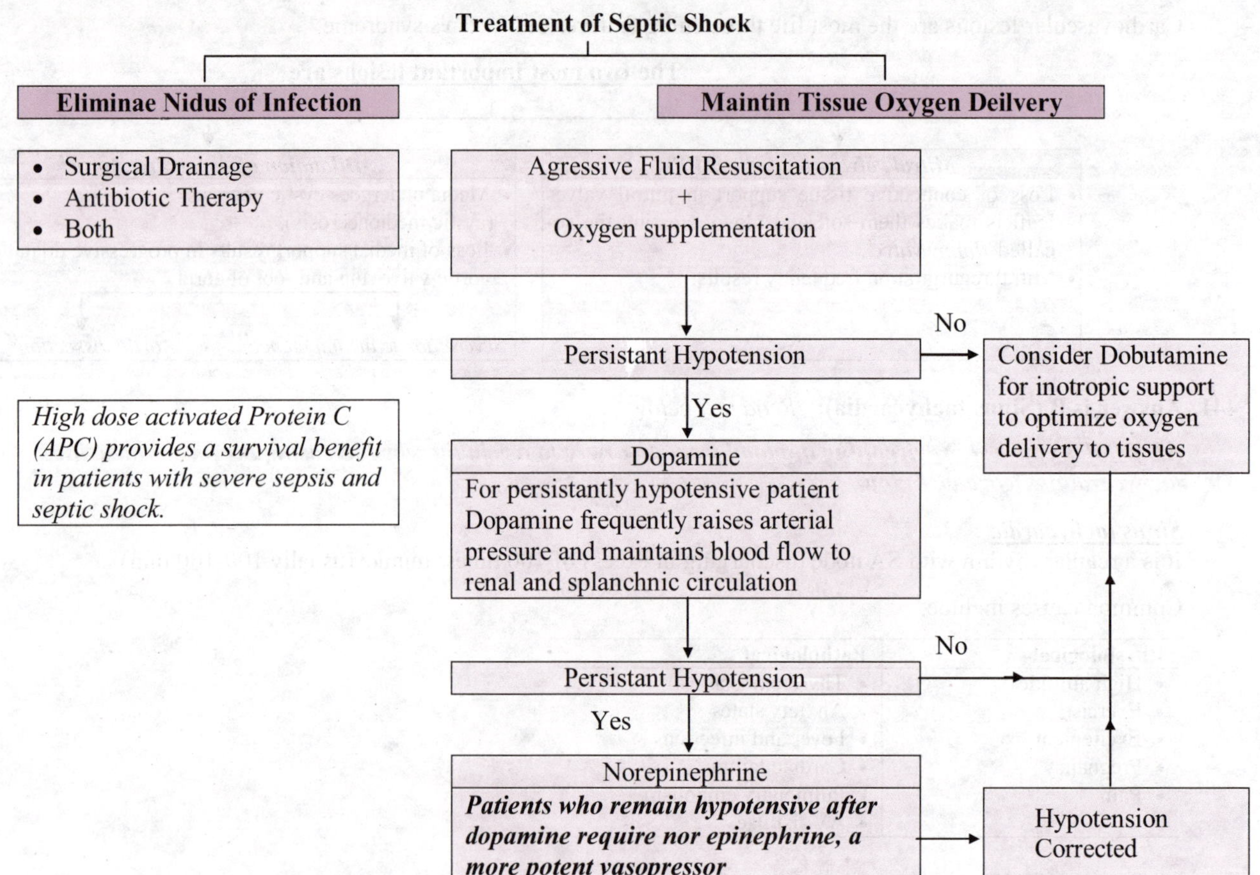

444. Answer is A (Acute Tubular necrosis): Harrison 18th/p 2227 *Harrisons 17th/1699*

Most common cause of renal failure in patients with septic shock is Acute tubular necrosis

Most renal failure is due to acute tubular necrosis induced by hypotension or capillary injury although some patients also have glomerulonephritis, renal cortical necrosis or interstitial nephritis-Harrison's 17th/1699

445. Answer is B (Associated with pulmonary vasoconstriction) : Harrison 18th/p 280 *Harrison 16th / 205; 17th / 224*

Although the mechanism of high altitude pulmonary edema remains obscure most studies suggest pulmonary vasoconstriction (venconstriction or arteriolar constriction) as the prime mechanism.

HAPE : High Altitude Pulmonary Edema

This is a serious complication usually occruing at exposure to high altitude (>300m) in association with severe physical exercise and is classically seen in unacclametized healthy individuals.

Pulmonary vasoconstriction has been suggested as the prime mechanism.

"Studies have been conflicting, some suggesting pulmonary venous constriction and other indicating pulmonary arteriolar constriction as the prime mechanism."- Harrison

May occur in both acclamatized and unacclamatized individuals

"Well recognized in unacclamatized yet otherwise healthy persons."

"***Acclamatized high altitude natives also develop this syndrome*** upon return to high altitude after a relatively brief sojourn at low altitudes." - *Harrison*

HAPE is exacerbated by exercise and is associated with high cardiac output.

Increased cardiac output and pulmonary arterial pressures with exercise combined with hypoxic pulmonary arteriolar constriction which is more prominent in young persons may combine to make this an example of prearteriolar high pressure pulmonary edema.

446. Answer is D (Mid diastole): *Harrison's Advances in Cardiology 'by Braunwald (2002/227); 'Multislice CT' by Becker 3rd/ 197; MD CT: A Practical Approach (2006) / 213; MD CT: From Protocols to Practice (2008) / 213; Computed Tomography of the Cardiovascular System (2007) / 110*

Mid Diastolic phase of the cardiac cycle is associated with the lowest mean motion of the heart

'Imaging for electron beam tomography (EBT) is performed during mid- diastole when the heart motion is at minimum'
- Harrison's Advances in Cardiology (2002) / 227

'The period in which heart has the least motion is usually (but not always) in mid- diastole'
- 'MDCT: A practical approach by Saini, Rubin & Kalra (2006) / 213

Minimum Cardiac Motion and its Application

- Early detection of coronary artery disease is possible with the use of Computed Tomography (CT) and Magnetic Resonance Imaging (MRI)
- The application of these tools to cardiac imaging is however severely limited by motion artifacts as the heart is constantly in motion completing an entire cycle of contraction and relaxation in about 1 second.
- *Application of these tools to cardiac imaging requires a 'Window' where cardiac motion is minimum to reduce motion artifacts and achieve meaningful images.*
- The optimal trigger point for such imaging is the phase of the cardiac cycle when cardiac motion is minimum. This period where cardiac motion is minimum is usually (but not always) the mid diastolic phase of cardiac cycle, just before atrial systole.

Diastole consists of four distinct phase: isometric relaxation, early rapid filling, diastasis and atrial systole. Of these four phases diastasis has the least mean cardiac motion.

- The phase of minimum cardiac motion is however variable and depends on several factors especially the heart rate

Mid –diastole represents the phase of minimum cardiac motion only in patients with low / intermediate heart rates

As heart rate increases the duration of diastole is shortened and the minimum mid- diastolic motion increases. In contrast the duration of systole is less affected by changes in heart rate. The late systolic phase provides another window where cardiac motion is low and at high heart rates the lowest motion may be recorded in late systole rather than during mid – diastole.

Note
Optimum phase for imaging coronary vessels (minimum cardiac motion) at low/intermediate heart rates is Mid- diastolic phase *Optimum phase for imaging coronary vessels (minimum cardiac motion) at high rates is variable and may occur in late systole.*

- This phase of minimum cardiac motion also varies on whether the Left Atrium. Right Atrium, Left Ventricle and Right Ventricle are being specifically imaged.

Phases of Relatively Rapid Cardiac motion	Phase of Relatively minimal cardiac motion
• Early systole • Mid systole • Early diastole (during rapid filling) • Late diastole (Atrial systole)	• ***Mid diastole (diastasis)*** • *Early diastole (During Isovolumetric relaxation)* • *Late systole*

447. Answer is D (Aortic Aneurysm) : *Harrison's 17th/1172, Hurst's 12th/2119; Braunwald' 8th/1794, 1795*

Aortic Aneurysm has not been mentioned as a complication of HIV infection

Although accelerated atherosclerosis and vasculitis have been mentioned as complications of HIV infection, an increased incidence of Aortic Aneurysm has not been listed as a complication in any standard textbook.

Aortic aneurysm is thus the most unlikely complication amongst the options provided and the single best answer of exclusion

Pericardial effusion and cardiac tamponade may be seen in HIV infection

'HIV infection should be suspected whenever young patients present wth pericardial effusion or tamponade'
– Braunwald's 8th/1798

Asymptomatic Pericardial Effusion is common in HIV patients and occurs in about 11% of AIDS patients (*Braunwald*)
Pericardial Tamponade is an uncommon / rare manifestation in HIV patients but may be seen (*Harrison / Braunwald*)

Cardiomyopathy may be seen in HIV infection

Dilated cardiomyopathy associated with congestive heart failure (HIV cardiomyopathy) is the most common clinically significant cardiac finding as a primary consequence to HIV infection (Harrison's)

Cardiac Manifestation of HIV/AIDS	
Pericardial Effusion *(Rarely **pericardial tamponade**)*	• Idiopathic • Infectious (viral, bacterial especially tuberculous, and fungal) • Neoplastic (Kaposi sarcoma and non-Hodgkin lymphoma)
Heart muscle disease	• Myocarditis (idiopathic/lymphocytic, specific infections, toxins) • Dilated ***cardiomyopathy*** & LV dysfunction
Endocarditis	• Marantic (non bacterial thrombotic endocarditis) • Infective
Tumors	• Kaposi sarcoma • Lymphoma
Right ventricular dysfunction & Pulmonary hypertension	• Primary • Secondary (recurrent chest infections, thromboembolism)
Premature atherosclerosis & coronary artery disease	
Adverse drug effects	• Hyperlipidemia • Proarrhythmia
Vasculitis and Lipodystrophy	• Drug Therapy : Protease inhibitors
Autonomic dysfunction	• Drug therapy, CNS disease Prolonged immunodeficiency, malnutrition

***

Respiratory System

ESSENTIAL REVISION NOTES

Respiratory failure

Respiratory failure *is defined as a disorder wherein, lung function is inadequate to meet the metabolic demands of the individual and is unable to maintain normal arterial gas levels in the blood.*

It is of two types:

Type I Respiratory failure	Type II Respiratory failure
Represents failure of oxygenation and is characterized by a low PaO_2 with normal or low $PaCO_2$. PaO_2 : Low (< 60 mm Hg) $PaCO_2$: Normal or low (≤ 49 mm Hg) $P_{A-a}O_2$: Increased	Represents a defect in ventilation (hypoventilation) and is characterized by decreased PaO_2 with increase $PaCO_2$. PaO_2 : Decreased (< 60 mm Hg) $PaCO_2$: Increased (> 49 mm Hg) $P_{A-a}O_2$: Normal
Causes :	**Causes :**
This type is caused by conditions which affect oxygenation, like: • Parenchymal diseases (V-Q mismatch) • Diseases of vasculature/shunts Examples: - *Pneumonia* Q - *ARDS* Q - *Emphysema* Q - *Right to left shunts* Q	This type is caused by conditions causing hypoventilation as in: • Obstructive lung disease: *COPD, F. body* • Decreased central respiratory drive *e.g. CNS disorders like : Brain injury, Meningitis* • Weakness of respiratory muscle e.g. - *Peripheral N.S. disorders like: M. gravis.* - *Interstitial lung disease.* Q - *MS disorders like polymyositis.* - *Rib cage disorders : Kyphoscoliosis.*

Type I Respiratory failure	Type II Respiratory failure
Hypoxemia with decreased $PaCO_2$	*Hypoxemia with increased $PaCO_2$*

Approach to patient with Hypoxia (Hypoxemia)

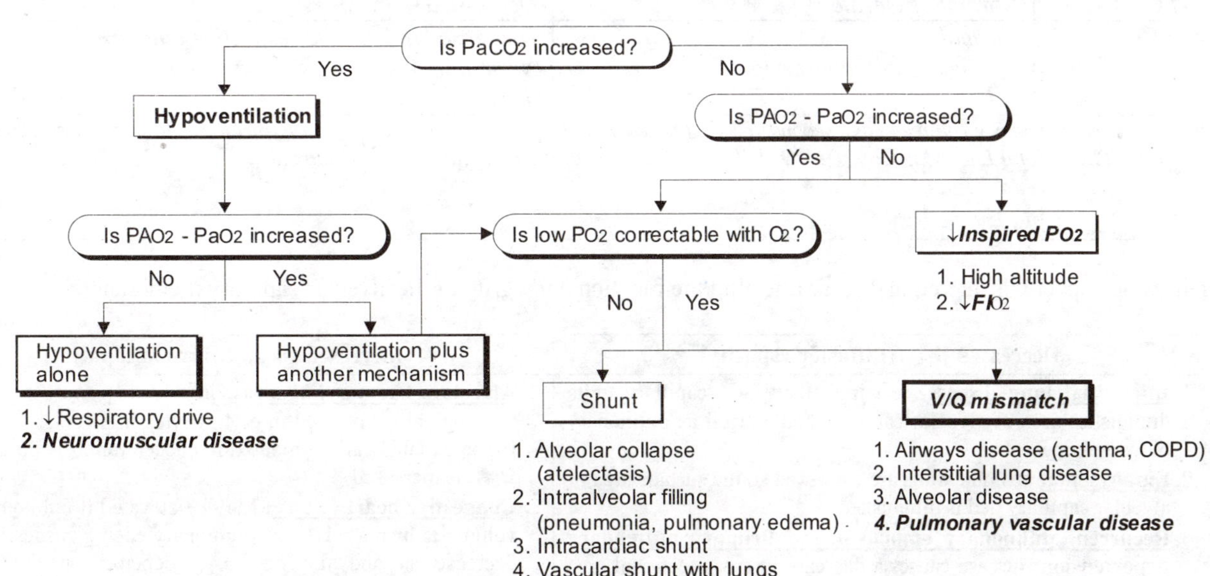

Obstructive versus Restrictive Respiratory Diseases

Classification of Respiratory Disorders

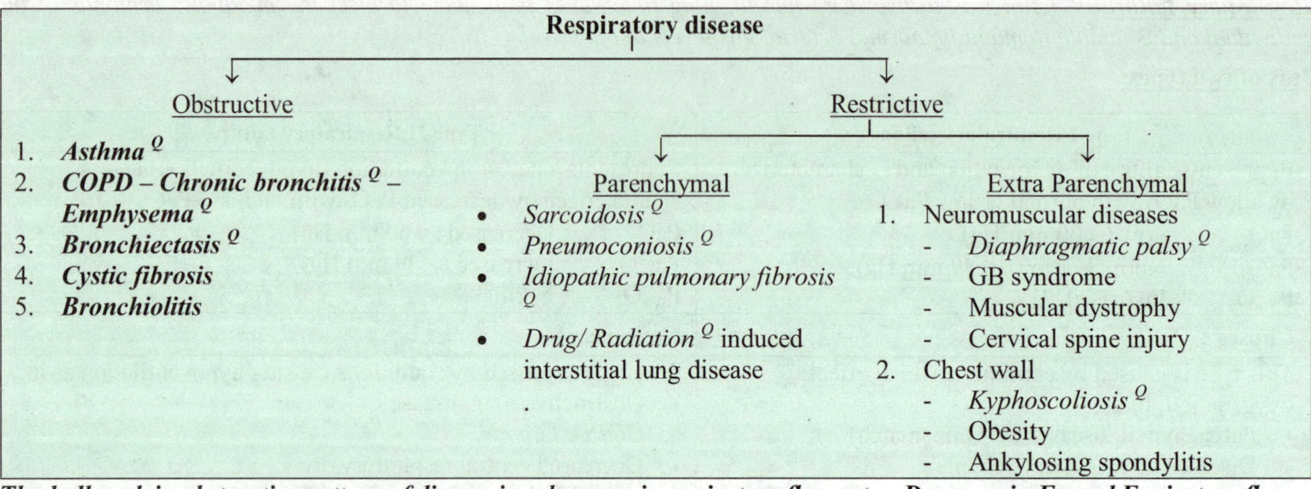

The hallmark in obstructive pattern of disease is a decrease in expiratory flow rates. Decrease in Forced Expiratory flow rate (FEF_{25-75}) and FEV_1/FVC are characteristic.

Differences between Obstructive and Restrictive Respiratory Diseases

PFT Result	Obstructive Pattern	Restrictive Pattern
FEV_1	*Decreased (<80% predicted)* *(Decreased out of proportion to FVC)*	*Decreased (May be preserved)* *(Decreased in proportion to FVC)*
FVC	*Decreased (May be preserved)*	*Decreased (<80% predicted)*
FEV_1/FVC (FEV_1%)	*Decreased (<0.7)*	*Normal or Increased (>0.7)*
FEF_{25-75}	*<50% predicted*	*Decreased in proportion to loss of lung volume*
TLC	*Normal or elevated*	*Decreased*
DLCO	*Normal* *Decreased in Emphysema*	*Decreased in intrinsic restrictive lung disease.* *Normal in neuromuscular or musculoskeletal restrictive disease*

__FEV_1__=forced expiratory volume in one second; __FVC__=Forced Vital Capacity; __FEF_{25-75}__=Forced Expiratory Flow at 25%=75% vital capacity; __TLC__= Total Lung Capacity; __DLCO__=Diffusion Capacity of the Lung for Carbon monoxide.

Diffusion capacity of Lung for carbon monoxie (DLCO)

Diffusion capacity is altered in disease affecting the functional integrity of the alveolar capillary membrane.

Decreased D_{LCO} (Diffusion capacity)	Increased D_{LCO} (Diffusion capacity)
1. **Interstitial lung disease**: scarring of alveolar capillary units diminishes area of alveolar capillary bed as well as pulmonary blood volume 2. **Emphysema:** alveolar walls are destroyed so the surface area of alveolar capillary bed is diminished 3. **Recurrent pulmonary embolism and Primary pulmonary hypertension:** disease causes a decrease in cross sectional area and volume of pulmonary vasculature	1. **Alveolar haemorrhage:** as in Good pasture's syndrome: haemoglobin contained in erythrocytes in alveolar lumen binds Co so exhaled carbon monoxide concentration is diminished & D_{LCO} is increased 2. **Congestive heart failure:** May be elevated if pulmonary blood volume is increased. Once pulmonary edema ensues D_{LCO} may decrease as and the net D_{LCO} depends on the opposing influences.

Three main categories are associated with lowered DLCO

- *Emphysema* [Q]
- *Interstitial Lung Disease* [Q]
- *Pulmonary vascular disease (Recurrent Pulmonary emboli or Primary Pulmonary Hypertension)* [Q]

Alveolar arterial difference in oxygen

Increased $PaO_2 – PaO_2$
(Alveolar arterial difference in oxygen)

Correctible with oxygen
V/Q Mismatch

Not correctible with oxygen
Shunt

V/Q Mismatch:
- Airway disease (Asthma, COPD) - Interstitial lung disease - Alveolar disease - Pulmonary vascular disease

Shunt:

- Alveolar collapse
- Intra alveolar filling
  - Pneumonia
  - Pulm edema
- Intracardiac shunt
- Vascular shunt within lung

Bronchial Asthma

Features of Asthma: Chronic inflammatory disorder

Features of Asthma

- ***Chronic inflammatory disorder***
- ***Hyperresponsiveness of airways (AHR)***
- *Airway epithelial shedding*
- *Subepithelial fibrosis and thickening of basement membrane*
- *Hypertrophy and Hyperplasia of airway smooth muscle*
- *Increased mucosal blood flow (vascular congestion)*
- *Microvascular leakage resulting in* ***airway edema*** *and plasma exudation into airway lumen*
- ***Mucus Hypersecretion*** *and formation of viscid mucus plugs that occlude airways*
- *Airway remodelling*
- *Defects in autonomic neural control*

Charachterisitc microscopically identifiable features described in sputum of Bronchial Asthma Patients

The microscopically identifiable features described in sputum are three 'C's
Charcot Leyden crystals: Derived from granules of eosnophils and found only in Asthma
Curshmann spirals: Curiously twisted casts of airways : Whorls of shed epethelium
Creola bodies: Clumps of cells or isolated metaplastic cells

Classification of Bronchial Asthma

Asthma

Extrinsic Asthma / Allergic Asthma	**Intrinsic Asthma /Idiosyncratic Asthma**
• History of Atopy is present	• No history of Atopy (Concomitant nasal polyps are usually present and patients may be aspirin sensitive)
• Attacks related to environmental exposures	• Attacks not related to environmental exposures: Occur without provocation
• IgE antibody levels are ↑ ed	• IgE antibody levels are normal
• Early onset of disease (young)	• Delayed onset of disease (Adult onset Asthma)
• Usually is less severe, intermittent Asthma that may however progress to severe persistent Asthma	• Usually have more severe persistent Asthma

Features of Intrinsic Asthma

Features of Intrinsic Asthma
(Nonatopic asthma- Approximately 10% of asthmatic patients are intrinsic)

- ***Negative Family History of allergy***
- ***Negative skin test to common inhalant allergens (Not primarily caused by allergy)***
- *Normal serum concentration of IgE.*
- *Concomitant nasal polyps (Common)*
- *Sensitivity to aspirin and related chemicals*
- *Later onset of disease (adult-onset asthma)*
- *More servere, persistent disease/asthma.*

Classification of severity of asthma execrbations:

	Mild	Moderate	Severe	Impending Respiratory Failure
Symptoms				
Breathlessness	With activity	With talking	At rest	At rest
Speech	Sentences	Phrases	Words	Mute
Signs				
Body position	Able to recline	Prefers sitting	Unable to recline	Unable to recline
Respiratory rate	Increased	Increased	Often > 30/min	> 30/min
Use of accessory respiratory muscle	Usually not	Commonly	Usually	Paradoxical thoracoabdominal movement
Breath sounds	***Moderate wheezing at mid-to-end-expiration***	***Loud wheezes throughout expiration***	***Loud inspiratory and expiratory wheezes***	***Little air movement without wheezes (silent chest)***
Hear rate (beats/min)	<100	100-120	***>120***	Relative bradycardia
Pulsus paradoxus (mm Hg)	< 10	10-25	***Often > 25***	Often absent
Mental status	May be agitated	Usually agitated	Usually agitated	Confused or drowsy
Functional assessment				
PEF (% predicted)	> 80	50-80	***< 50***	< 50
Sao_2 (%, room air)	> 95	91-95	< 91	< 91
Pao_2 (mm Hg, room air)	Normal	> 60	< 60	<60
$Paco_2$ (mm Hg)	< 42	< 42	≥ 42 ***(Respiratory acidosis)***	≥ 42

Panacinar emphysema and Centriacinar emphysema

There are two types of emphysema that cause clinically significant airflow obstruction:

Panacinar emphysema	Centriacinar emphysema
• Acini are uniformly involved from level of respiratory bronchiole to terminal blind alveoli. Q • Lesions are more common in lower zone and bases Q • Occurs in association with α_1 antitrypsin deficiency Q	• Central or proximal parts of acini formed by respiratory bronchioles are affected whereas distal alveoli are spared Q • Lesions are more severe and common in Upper lobes Q • Occurs predominantly in smokers Q • Is the commonest pattern Q

Idiopathic Interstitial Lung Diseases / Idiopathic Interstitial Pneumonias

- Idiopathic Interstitial Pneumonias are *interstitial lung diseases of unknown etiology* that *share similar clinical and radiological features* and are *distinguished primarily by the histopathological pattern on lung biopsy*

Histologic Name	Clinical Syndrome	Salient Pathological Features
Usual Interstitial Pneumonia (UIP)	*Idiopathic pulmonary fibrosis (Cryptogenic fibrosing alveolitis)*	*Temporally and spatially heterogeneous pattern with areas of normal lung, fibroblastic foci, and patchy sub-pleural fibrosis*
Desquamative Interstitial Pneumonia (DIP)	*Desquamative interstitial pneumonia*	*Homogenous intra-alveolar macrophage accumulation. Mild alveolar septal thickening*
Acute Interstitial Pneumonia (AIP)	*Acute interstitial pneumonia (Hamman-Rich syndrome)*	*Homogenous, diffuse lung injury with hyaline membranes, fibroblast proliferation*
Bronchiolitis Obliterans Organizing pneumonia (BOOP)	*Cryptogenic organizing pneumonia, (Idiopathic BOOP)*	*Multifocal organizing pneumonia, with granulation tissue and polyps in alveolar ducts and bronchioles*
Non-Specific Interstitial Pneumonia (NSIP)	*Nonspecific interstitial pneumonia*	*Temporally and spatially homogenous cellular inflammation with mild fibrosis*
Respiratory Bronchiolitis Associated Lung Disease(RBILD)	*Respiratory Bronchiolitis Associated Interstitial Lung Disease*	

- Detailed Histopathological features are often required to distinguish various forms of Idiopathic Interstitial Pneumonias and hence these have been listed in a tabular form in the following table.

Pathologic features of Idiopathic Interstitial Pneumonias							
Feature	***AIP***	***BOOP***	***DIP***	***RBILD***	***UIP***	***NSIP-Cellular***	***NSIP-Fibrosing***
Distribution	*Diffuse*	*Certrilobular*	*Diffuse*	*Mild, focal*	**Patchy**, *Sub-pleural*	*Diffuse*	*Diffuse/panacinar*
Temporal appearance	*Homogenous*	*Homogenous*	*Homogenous*	*Homogenous*	***Herterogenous (Variegated)***	*Homogenous*	*Homogenous*
Septal Inflammation	Scant	Scant	Scant	None	Scant, patchy	Prominent	Scant. diffuse
Collagen fibrosis	Absent	Scant	Variable Diffuse	Scant Patchy	***Characterisitc Patchy***	Absent	Diffuse
Fibroblast proliferation	*Diffuse (interstitial)*	*Diffuse (intralumiral)*	*Absent*	*Absent*	***Fibroblastic Foci prominent***	*Absent*	***Fibroblastic Foci Rare***
Honey-combing	Absent	Absent	Absent	Absent	Characteristic	Absent	Rare
Alveolar macrophage	Absent	Absent	Diffuse	Peribonchiolar	Occasional	Occasional	Occasional
Hyaline membranes	Occasional	Absent	Absent	Absent	Absent	Absent	Absent

Asbestos Related Lung Disease

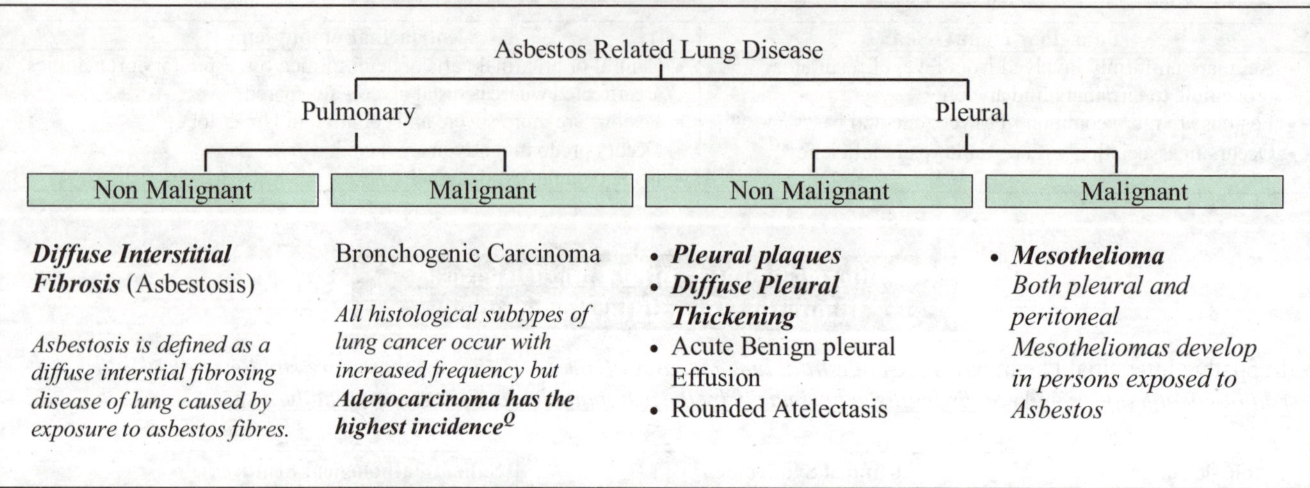

Idiopathic Pulmonary Hemosiderosis (IPH)

IPH is a disorder of unknown etiology characterized by recurrent episodes of Diffuse Alveolar Hemorrhage (DAH)

It has been classically characterized by the triad of iron deficiency anemia, hemoptysis and alveolar infiltrates on chest radiographs.

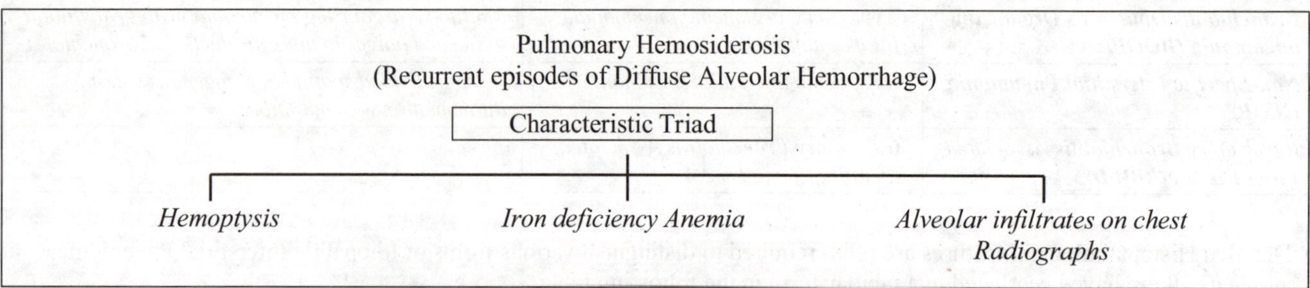

Pulmonary Infiltrates with Eosinophilia (Pulmonary eosiniophilic pneumonia)

Differential Diagnosis of Pulmonary Infiltrates with Eosinophilia

Pulmonary infiltrates with eosinophilia: (PIE, eosinophilic pneumonias). Constituted by distinct individual syndromes characterized by eosinophilic pulmonary infiltrates and ***peripheral blood eosinophilia.***

Pulmonary Infiltrates with Eosinophilia (Pulmonary eosiniophilic pneumonia)

Etiology Known	Idiopathic
Allergic bronchopulmonary mycoses	*Loeffler's syndrome*
Parastitic infestations	*Acute eosinophilic pneumonia*
Drug reactions	*Chronic eosinophilic pneumonia*
Eosinophilia-myalgia syndrome	*Allergic granulomatosis of Churg and Strauss*
	Hypereosinophilic syndrome

Allergic Bronchopulmonary Aspergillosis

Allergic bronchopulmonary aspergillosis is a pulmonary hypersensitivity disorder caused by allergy to fungal antigens that colonize the tracheobronchial tree. It most commonly occurs in atopic asthmatic individuals in response to antigen of aspergillus species.

Main diagnostic criteria	Secondary diagnostic criteria
1. *Clinical history of Asthma* Q	1. *History of brownish plugs in sputum*
2. *Pulmonary infiltrates (transient / fleeting or fixed)* Q	2. *Indentification / culture of A. fumigatus from sputum*
3. *Peripheral eosinophilia (> 1000 /μL)* Q	3. *Late skin reactivity to aspergillus antigen – CMDT*
4. *Immediate skin reactivity to Aspergillus antigen (wheal and flare response)*	4. *Elevated IgE (and IgG) class antibodies specific for A. fumigatus – Harrisons*
5. *Serum precipitins to A. fumigatus*	
6. *Elevated serum IgE levels* Q *(>1000ng/ml)*	
7. *Central / proximal bronchiectasis* Q	

Note

Elevated IgE (and IgG) class antibodies specific for A. fumigatus has been mentioned as a secondary diagnostic criteria in Harrison's textbook while Fishman's textbook includes this as a main/major diagnostic criteria.

Criteria for the Diagnosis of ABPA Primary

Primary
• *Episodic bronchial obstruction (asthma)*
• *Peripheral blood eosinophilia (>1000/mm^3)*
• *Elevated serum IgE concentrations (>1000ng/ml)*
• *Immediately type skin reactivity to Aspergillus antigens*
• *Precipitating serum antibodies (precipitants) against Aspergillus antigens*
• *Elevated serum IgE and/or IgG antibodies specific to A. fumigatus**
• *History of pulmonary infiltrates (transient/ fleeting or fixed) on chest radiographs or CT scans*
• *Central proximal bronchiectasis on chest CT*
Secondary
• *A. fumigatus in sputum (by repeated culture or microscopic examination)*
• *History of expectoration of brown plugs or flecks*
• *Arthus reactivity (late skin reactivity) to Aspergillus antigen*

**Elevated IgE (and IgG) class antibodies specific for A. fumigatus has been mentioned as a secondary diagnostic criteria in Harrison's textbook while Fishman's textbook includes this as a main/major diagnostic criteria.*

Aspergillus fumigatus is a known cause for bronchopulmonary Aspergillosis

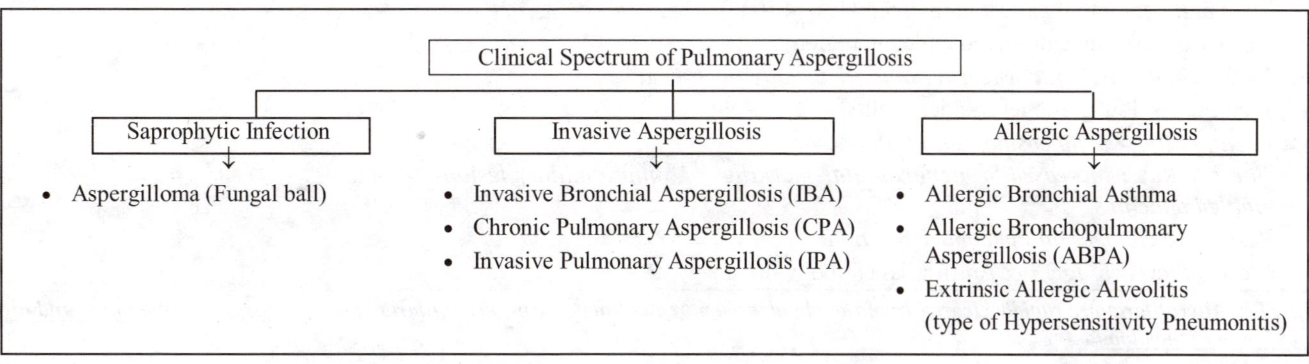

Hypersensitivity Reaction to Aspergillus

Hypersensitivity Reaction to Aspergillus

Hypersensitivity Lung diseases that result from exposure to A. Fumigatus allergens include Bronchial Asthma, ABPA and Extrinsic Allergic Alveolitis (Hypersensitivity Pneumonitis)

In Atopic Individual	In Non atopic Individuals
Allergic Bronchial Asthma and ABPA	*Extrinsic Allergic Alveolitis (Hypersensitivity penumonitis)*
Allergic Bronchial Asthma and ABPA are seen in atopic individuals and immune response is IgE mediated	Extrinsic Allergic Alveolitis or Hypersensitivity penumonitis is seen in non atopic individuals and immune response is not IgE mediated. Immune response may involve cell mediated (type IV) or immune complex (Type III) reactions.

Differentiating features: Bronchial Asthma, ABPA and Extrinsic Allergic Alveolitis

Features	***Asthma***	***ABPA***	***Extrinsic allergic alveolitis (Hypersensitive pneumonitis)***
Pathology	*Hypertrophied mucus glands*	*Colonization of airways, viscid mucoid impaction, tissue eosinophilia*	*Lymphocytic infiltration of interstitium, noncaseating granuloma*
Radiological features			
Early	*Normal, hyperinflation*	*Migratory peripheral infiltrates, atelectasis, bronchiectasis*	*Diffuse alveolar-interstitial infiltrates*
Late	*Normal, hyperinflation*	*Fibrosis*	*Reticulonodular interstitial opacities*
Skin test reactions to Aspergilus antigens			
Immediate	*Positive*	*Positive*	*Positive*
Delayed	*Negative*	*Positive*	*Positive*
Peripheral eosinophilia	*Negative*	*Positive*	*Negative*
IgG Aspergillus precipitins	*Positive (upt o 25%)*	*Positive*	*Positive*
Serum IgE levels	*Normal or mildly elevated*	*Marked deviation*	*Normal*

Tropical Pulmonary Eosinophilia

Tropical Pulmonary Eosinophilia (TPE) is a distinct syndrome that develops in individuals infected with Lymphatic filarial species.

Clinical symptoms result from allergic and inflammatory reaction elicited by the cleared parasites.

Features of Tropical Pulmonary eosinophilia (TPE) :

- Male more commonly affected than females (4 : 1)
- History of resistance in filarial endemic region
- ***Paroxysmal cough and wheezing that are usually nocturnal***[Q]
- Weight loss, low grade fever, adenopathy
- ***Eosinophilia > 3000 eosinophilia / μL*** [Q]
- ***Chest X-Ray : increased bronchovascular markings*** [Q] , *diffuse miliary lesions* [Q] , or ***mottled opacities***.
- *Restrictive changes on Pulmonary function test* [Q]
- *Elevated levels of IgE* [Q] & Antifilarial antibody titers.

In TPE, Microfilaria are rapidly cleared from the blood stream by the lungs. Thus, microfilariae are sequestrated in the lungs and are not found in the blood.

Typical Air Space Pneumonias and Atypical Pneumonias

AIR Space Penumonia (Typical Pneumonia)	Interstitial Pneumonia (Atypical Pneumonia)
Exudate in alveoli i.e. consolidation	No exudate, alveoli are air filled i.e. no consolidation (Infiltrate in interstitium)
Infiltrate is primarily of neutrophills (PMN)	Infiltrate is primarily lymphocytic
Agents responsible are extracellular	Agents responsible are intracellular
Cough is productive of purulent sputum	Cough is dry
Chest X-ray shows alveolar pattern	Chest X-ray shows interstitial pattern
Causes of Typical pneumonias • *Staphylococcal* • *Pneumococcal (Streptococcus Pneumoniae)* • *Kleibsella* • *Pseudomonas* • *Anaerobic Bacteria* • *Other Bacterial* Pneumoniae	**Causes of Atypical pneumonias** • *Mycoplasma pneumonias* • *Viral pneumonias –* *Influenza, RSVAdenovirus, Rhinovirus, Rubeola, Varicilla, Corona* • *Chlamydia pneumonia* • *Coxiella burnetti* • *Pneumocystis carinii* • *Legionella*

Typical Bacterial Pneumonias associated with cavitation

Bacterial Pneumonas associated with cavitation: Review
• *Staphylococcus*[Q] • *Kleibsella*[Q] • *Pseudomonas*[Q] • *Anaerobic bacteria*

Characteristic Feature of Stapylococcal Pneumonias

Bacterial Pneumonas associated with cavitation: Review
• *Cavitation*[Q] *(single or Multiple thick walled cavities) (may be Bilateral)* • *Pneumatoceles*[Q] *(Thin walled cystic spaces that may contain air fluid levels)* • *Pleural Effusion*[Q] */ Empyema*[Q] *with or without bronchopleural fistulas (Pyopneumothorax)* • *Abscess formation*[Q]

Classic Histopathology in atypical pneumonia caused by Pneumocystis Pneumonia

Classic Histopathology in Pneumocystis Pneumonia

Intra- Alveolar Changes	Interstitial Changes
Prominent Eosinophilic foamy, vacuolated intraalveolar exudate (HE staining) • Intra alveolar exudate contains the organisms, which can be identified in various stages of development (trophozoite and cystic stage) by the use of special stains such as - Methamine silver / Toluidine stain - Wright Giemsa stain - Papanicolaou's stain • Intraalveolar exudate also contains host serum proteins, debris, & surfactant proteins Alveolar macrophages are present but not prominent in phagocytosis of organism. • The principle host effector cells against pneumocystis are alveolar macrophages which ingest & kill the organism	Mild interstitial Pneumonitis • Mononuclear interstitial cell infiltrate (mild) • Damaged type I Pneumocytes • Hypertrophy /proliferation of type II pneumocytis (Reparative response) *Pneumocystis attaches to, and damages type I pneumocytes. There is associated compensatory hypertrophy of type II pneumocytes.* Note: *Most compromised hosts display a mild mononuclear interstitial cell infiltrate however malnourished children display an intense interstitial plasma cell infiltrate which was responsible for the diseases early name of interstitial plasma cell pneumonia'*

Legionnaire's disease:

- Legionnaires disease presents as an '***atypical pneumonia***'^{Q} where a gram stained smear of sputum does not show organisms (Caused by *Legionella).*

Legionella
• ***Legionella*** *is a gram negative* ^{Q}, *motile* ^{Q}, *non-encapsulated bacilli* ^{Q}, *classified under a miscellaneous group* • *Man-to-Man transmission does not occur with Legionella.* ^{Q} • *No animal reservoirs occur.* ^{Q} • *Disease is limited to humans.* ^{Q} *Legionella survive and multiply inside free-living amoeba and protozoa, distributed in natural reservoirs such as stagnant waters* ^{Q}, *mud and hot spring.*

- Human infection is typically acquired by *inhalation of aerosols, which form the only source of infection.*^{Q}
- Smoking and immunocompromised status are known risk factors.
- The disease occurs with *unusual frequency among patients with hairy cell leukemia* but not among patients with other types of leukemia

Common Risk factors for Legionnaires disease

• *Advancing age*
• *Immunocompromised patients:*
  - *Transplant recipients, HIV, Glucocorticoid recipients*
  - *Hairy cell leukaemia (monocyte deficiency and dysfunction)*
• *Chronic lung disease*
• *Smokers*
• *Diabetes mellitus (Javetz)*

- Presents as mild cough slightly productive sputum, sometimes streaked with blood, along with high fever and nonspecific symptoms such as malaise, fatigue, anorexia & headache.

Think about the diagnosis as Legionaire's disease whenever the question talks about a pneumonia like picture along with any of the these :
a. *Occurrence of illness in immunocompromised* ^{Q}, *smokers* ^{Q} *or those with chronic lung disease* ^{Q}, *or* b. *Occurance of illness in an environment where potable water supply is known to be contaminated with Legionella* c. *Onset of symptoms within 10 days of discharge from a hospital (I.P. 2 to 10 day), or* d. *High fever,* ^{Q} *or* e. *Gastrointestinal difficulties like diarrhea,* ^{Q} *or* f. *Neurological abnormalities like confusion or altered Sensorium,* ^{Q} *or* g. *Numerous neutrophils but no organisms revealed by gram staining of respiratory secretions, or* h. *Hyponatremia* ^{Q} *is more common in Legionnaire's, than in any other form of pneumonia, or* i. *Failure to respond to β-lactam drugs* ^{Q} *(penicillin or cephalosporins) and aminoglycosids antibiotics.*

- ***Azithromycin and Respiratory Quinolones are the drugs of choice for Legionnaire's disease***

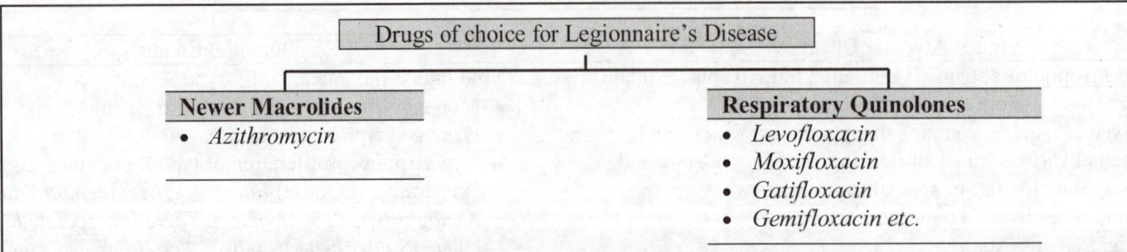

Tuberculosis: Congenital Tuberculosis and Primary Tuberculosis

Congenital Tuberculosis

- *True congenital Tuberculosis is defined as tuberculosis occurring in infants as a result of infection with M. Tuberculosis during intrauterine life.*
- Three modes of fetal infection have been proposed
  a. Transplacental (Hematogenous infection via the umbilical vein)
  b. Fetal aspiration of infected amniotic fluid
  c. Fetal ingestion of infected amniotic fluid

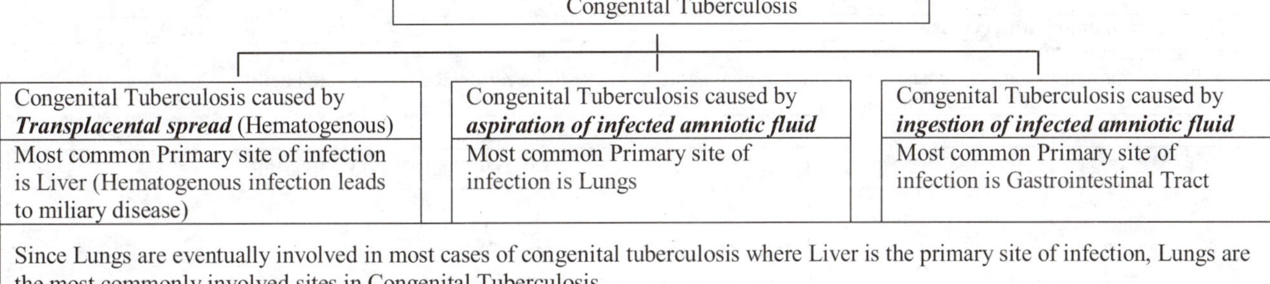

- When infection enters the fetus through the umbilical veins, the primary tubercular lesions (primary complex) develop in the liver. *(Lesions may also develop in the lungs suggesting further passage of bacilli through the ductus venosus)*

> ***'The only lesion in the neonate that is unquestionably associated with congenital infection is a primary complex in the liver; all others may be acquired congenitally or postnatally***

- When infection enters the fetus through the aspiration / inhalation of infected amniotic fluid the primary lesions (primary complex) develops in the lungs.

  Tuberculous involvement of Lungs without associated hepatic lesions indicates aspiration of infected ammotic fluid on inhalation of tubercle bacilli.

> ***Lungs are the most common organs involved in congenital tuberculosis being involved almost all cases***

- *Congenital Tuberculosis is charachterized by a nonimmune, non-reactive response with abundant caseation and an unsually large number of bacilli. There may be multiple foci of infection within the primary site and the distribution is usually miliary.*

Diagnostic Criteria for Congenital Tuberculosis

Beitzke' Criteria (1935)	Revised Criteria by Cantwell (1994)
i. Bacteriological Proof of Tuberculosis ***ii. Primary complex in Liver*** iii. If primary complex is lacking in Liver then tuberculosis can be considered congenital only if: a. Tuberculous lesions present in fetus or newborn are only few days old b. Or in an older infant extrauterine infection can be excluded with certainity	i. Lesion in first week of life ***ii. A primary hepatic complex or caseating hepatic granuloma*** iii. Tuberculous infection of placenta or maternal genital tract iv. Exclusion of possibility of postratal transmission by a thorough investigation of contacts including the infant's hospital attendants or birth attendants

Primary tuberculosis:

- *It is the first infection with tubercle bacilli in individuals who have not been previously exposed to the organisms*
- *Seen in children* [Q]
- Primary complex is characteristic

Primary (Ghon) complex
• Unilateral enlarged hilar lymph nodes [Q] • Ghon focus [Q]: Epitheloid-cell granulomatous inflammation (consolidation) at site of parenchymal infection. Usually small and subpleural most commonly located under pleura in lower part of upper lobe

- Usually a symptomatic [Q] or manifested by a mild flu like illness at time of tuberculin conversion
- Lesion heal by fibrosis [Q] and may calcify [Q]
- Radiological evidence of healed primary infection may or may not be present [Q]

Effects of primary tuberculosis
• Tuberculin positivity [Q] • Partial immunity to tuberculosis[Q]: individual requires a higher dose to be reinfected by tubercle bacilli • Presence of dormant tubercle bacilli

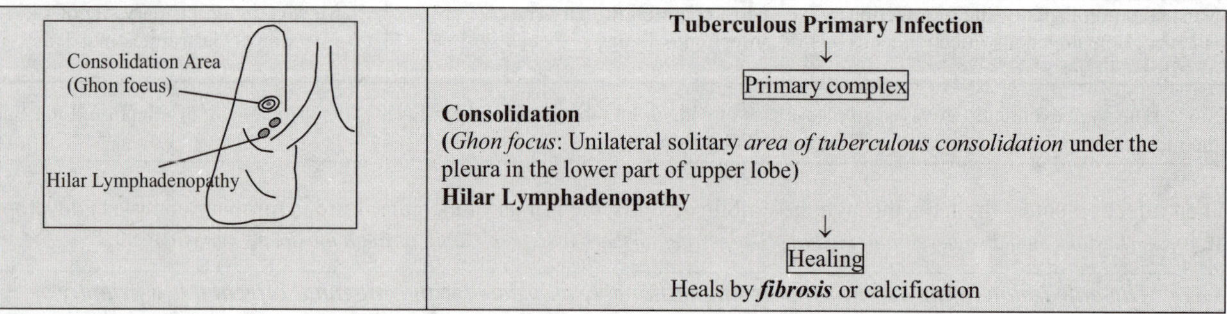

Montoux test

Montoux test is carried out by injecting one tuberculin unit (1TU) of PPD in 0.1 ml on the flexor surface of forearm (PPD RT 23 with Tween 80)

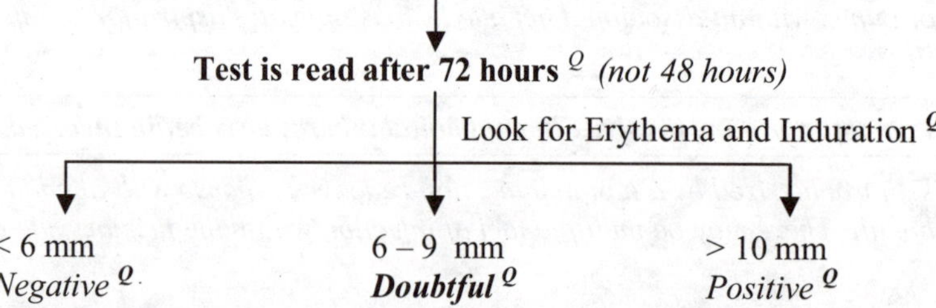

- ***A positive test indicates that patient is infected with M. tuberculosis. It does not however prove that the person is 'suffering' from the disease*** – *Park*
- ***Studies indicate that 92% of new cases occur in persons who already are tuberculin reactors.*** – *Park*
- ***6-9 mm induration does not indicate high chances of developing tuberculosis.*** Infact patients with 25 mm induration have more chances of developing tuberculosis than those with 6-9 mm induration - *Park*

Causes of False Negative Tuberculin Tests (Anergy)

False negative tuberculin tests (Anergy) may occur in situations such as :
• *Miliary tuberculosis* [Q] • Convalescence from some viral infections like *Measles* [Q] • Lymphoreticular malignancy • *Sarcoidosis* [Q] • *Severe malnutrition* [Q] • *Immunosuppressive therapy* [Q] • *Defective cell mediated immunity* [Q]

Sources of Bleeding in Hemoptysis

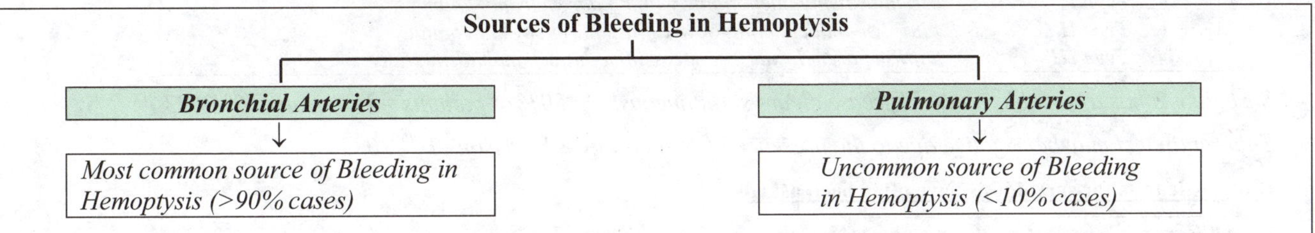

A pulmonary arterial source should be considered in addition to the more common systemic source (bronchial artery) in the setting of destructive lung lesion such as cavitatory tuberculosis. However the vascular structure that should be evaluated first is the bronchial artery.

Remember: Ramussen Aneurysm

- Ramussen aneurysm is a rare cause of bleeding in cavitatory tuberculosis and results from erosion of tuberculous cavity into a pulmonary artery branch.
- *The most common source of bleeding in Remussen aneurysm is the pulmonary artery*[Q].

Facts to Remember about Hemoptysis

The most common cause of Hemoptysis	*Bronchitis and Bronchogenic CA*[Q] *(Bronchitis > Bronchogenic CA)*[Q]
The most common causes of Hemoptysis in India	*Tuberculosis*[Q]
The most common cause of Massive Haemoptysis	*Bronchectasis (World wide)*[Q] *Tuberculosis(India)*[Q]

Sarcoidosis

- Sarcoidosis is a chronic multisystem disorder of unknown cause characterized by accumulation of T lymphocytes and mononuclear phagocytes in various tissues of body
- The inflammatory process in sarcoidosis is characterized by formation of sarcoid granulomas in various organs.
- Giant Cells within granulomas can be of '*Langerhan's or Foreign body variety*' and often contain inclusions bodies

Inclusions seen in giant cells in sarcoidosis. (Remember as **SAR**coidosis)
- ***S**chaumann bodies*[Q]
- ***A**steroid bodies*[Q]
- ***R**esidual bodies*[Q]

- Non-caseating **SAR**coid granulomas can affect several organ or organ systems

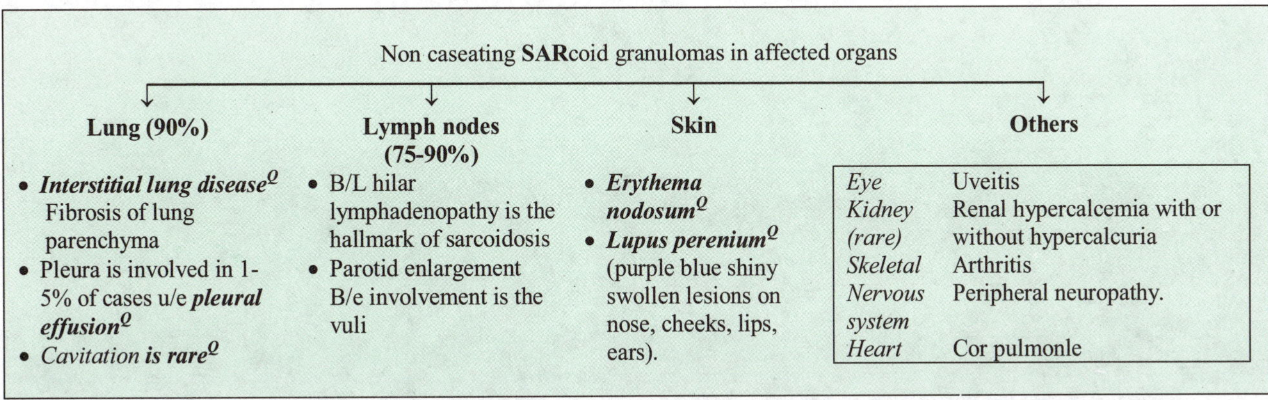

- ***Bilateral hilar lymphadenopathy is the hallmark of disease***

The three classic x-ray pattern of pulmonary sarcoidosis are		
• ***Type I***	:	*B/L hilar lymphadenopathy with no parenchymal changes*
• ***Type II***	:	*B/L hilar lymphadenopathy with diffuse parenchymal changes*
• ***Type III***	:	*Diffuse parenchymal change with no hilar lymphadenopathy.*

- *Sarcoidosis has a variable course. Disease clears spontaneously in 50% of patients – Harrisons 16th/2023*
- *Tuberculin test may be negative due to the presence of skin anergy – Harrisons 16th/2023*

Diagnostic tests for sarcoidosis have often been asked

Ancillary	*Confirmatory*
• Blood: ***ACE***Q • ***X ray chest***Q • ***Skin test for anergy***Q • ***Gallium 67 etc.***Q	• Biopsy

X-Ray chest:	• Bilateral hilar lymphadenopathy is the hallmark of disease • Parenchymal involvement may or may not be present ***(clear lung fields)***Q • ***Egg shell calcification of hilar nodes may be seen***Q
Kveim siltzbach testQ**:** ***Skin test***Q:	• Intradermal injection of a heat treated suspension of a sarcoidosis spleen extract.
Angiotensin converting enzyme (ACE) in bloodQ:	• ACE is elevated in 2/3 of patients with sarcoidosis Q (60%) Q • ACE levels indicate activity of diseaseQ • ACE levels provide an important method of monitoring the course of disease.Q *(The cells in granuloma release angiotensin converting enzyme into the serum)*
Gallium 67 scan:	• Gallium 67 lung scan is usually abnormal showing a pattern of diffuse uptake
Bronchoalveolar lavage	• Lavage fluid is characterized by *-increase in Lymphocytes*Q *-high CD4 / CD8 cell ratio*Q
Biopsy:	• Biopsy is mandatory to make a definitive diagnosis of sarcoidosis • Characteristic finding is a typical non casseating granulomaQ
Lung function	• Typical for interstitial lung disease.

Acute/Adult Respiratory Distress syndrome (ARDS)

Synonyms used for Acute/Adult Respiratory Distress syndrome.

Synonym: for ARDS *(Taken from 'Pathology of Lung')*

- *Shock lung*
- *Blast lung*
- *Traumatic wet lung*
- *Congestive Atelectasis*
- *DoNang Lung*
- *Noncardiogenic Pulmonary Edema*
- *Diffuse Alveolar Damage*

Clinical disorders associated with lung injury/ ARDS

Direct lung injury	Indirect lung injury
• Pneumonia • Aspiration of gastric contents • Pulmonary contusion • Near drowning • Toxic inhalation injury	• Sepsis • Severe trauma: - Multiple bone fractures - Head trauma - Flail chest • Burns • Multiple transfusions • Drug overdose: eg Narcotic overdose • Pancreatitis • Post-cardiopulmonary bypass

Miscellaneous causes for ARDS
• *Renal failure* • *Liver failure* • *Disseminated intravascular coagulation* • *Ecclampsia* • *Amniotic fluid emboli / Air emboli* • *Hanging* • *High altitude*

Pathophysiology features and diagnostic criteria for ARDS

ARDS is an acute form of lung injury characterized by:

- Increased permeability of alveolar capillary membrane.
- ***Diffuse alveolar damage.***
- Accumulation of proteinaceous pulmonary edema (non cardiogenic pulmonary edema [Q])

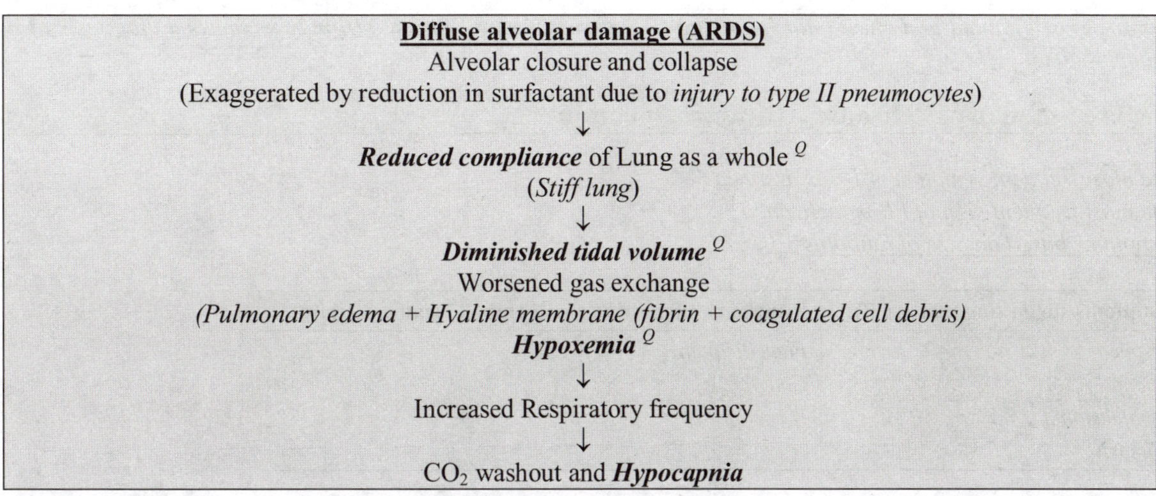

Diffuse alveolar damage (ARDS)
Alveolar closure and collapse
(Exaggerated by reduction in surfactant due to *injury to type II pneumocytes*)
↓
Reduced compliance of Lung as a whole [Q]
(*Stiff lung*)
↓
Diminished tidal volume [Q]
Worsened gas exchange
(Pulmonary edema + Hyaline membrane (fibrin + coagulated cell debris)
Hypoxemia [Q]
↓
Increased Respiratory frequency
↓
CO_2 washout and ***Hypocapnia***

Features of ARDS

Clinical /Physiological
• Clinical history of insult known to cause ARDS • Clinical exclusion of chronic lung disease and Left ventricular failure • ***Diffuse alveolar damage.*** • *Reduced surfactant (Injury to type II pneumocytes)* • Increased permeability of alveolar capillary membrane. • Accumulation of *proteinaceous pulmonary edema* (non cardiogenic pulmonary edema [Q]) • Pulmonary edema + ***Hyaline membrane*** (fibrin + coagulated cell debris) • ***Reduced compliance*** *(stiff lung)* • ***Diminished tidal volume*** [Q] • ***Hypoxemia*** [Q] (Worsened gas exchange d/t ***pulmonary shunting***) • ***Hypocapnia*** [Q](CO_2 washout)

Diagnostic Criteria (ARDS)	
PaO_2/FiO_2	*≤200 mm Hg*
Onset	*Acute*
Chest Radiograph	*Bilateral Alveolar or Interstitial infiltrates*
Absence of Left Atrial Hypertension	• *PCWP≤18 mmHg* • *No clinical evidence of increased left atrial pressure*

Differentiating Features between Acute Lung Injury (ALI) and ARDS

Acute Lung Injury (ALI) is a less severe disorder than ARDS but has the potential to evolve into ARDS. ALI can be differentiated from ARDS by the arterial PO_2/FiO_2 (Inspiratory O_2 fraction) ratio.

Diagnostic Criteria	ALI	ARDS
PaO_2/FiO_2	*≤300 mm Hg*	*≤200 mm Hg*
Onset	*Acute*	*Acute*
Chest Radiograph	*Bilateral Alveolar or Interstitial infiltrates*	*Bilateral Alveolar or Interstitial infiltrates*
Absence of Left Atrial Hypertension	• *PCWP≤ 18 mmHg* • *No Clinical evidence of increased left atrial pressure*	• *PCWP≤18 mmHg* • *No clinical evidence of increased left atrial pressure*

Pulmonary Thromboembolism

Sudden onset of dyspnea and chest pain following surgery or immobilization, strongly suggests a diagnosis of pulmonary thromboembolism.

Classic Presentation of Pulmonary Thromboembolism

- *The most frequent symptom of PE is dyspnea* [Q]
- *The most frequent sign of PE is tachypnea* [Q]
- *Symptoms based on Size of Embolus*

Symptoms suggesting massive PE	Symptoms suggesting small emboli located distally
Dyspnea *Syncope* *Hypotension* *Cyanosis*	*Pleuritic pain* *Cough* *Haemoptysis*

Classic Abnormalities on ECG in pulmonary Embolism

- *Sinus Tachycardia (Commonest : OHCM)*
- *Right ventricular strain pattern (T wave inversion in leads V1 to V4 perhaps most frequent - Harrison)*
- *S_I Q_{III} T_{III} Pattern : (Classic pattern but rare (OHCM))*

> - Deeps S waves in lead I
> - Q wave
> - Inverted T wave in lead III

- *New onset Atrial Fibrillation / Atrial Flutter.*
- *Right Axis Deviation / RBBB.*

Diagnostic Strategy in cases of suspected Pulmonary Thromboembolism

Most definitive / specific test for PE [Q]
Pulmonary angiography [Q]

Best initial imaging test for diagnosis of PE [Q]
CT scan with intravenous contrast [Q] *(Preferred choice, against a lung V-Q scan)*

Clinical Assessment and Estimate Clinical Likelihood of Pulmonary Embolism

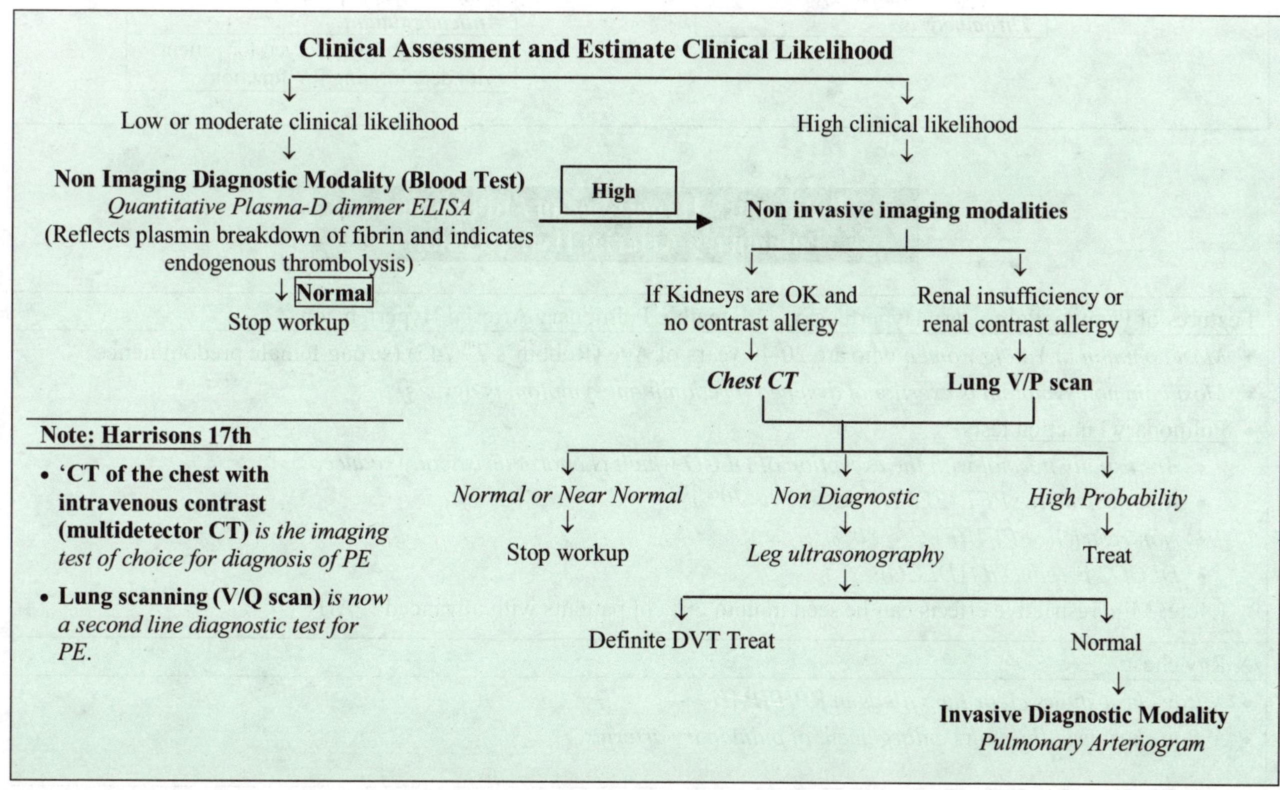

Respiratory System

3

Treatment of Patients with Pulmonary Embolism based on Risk Stratification

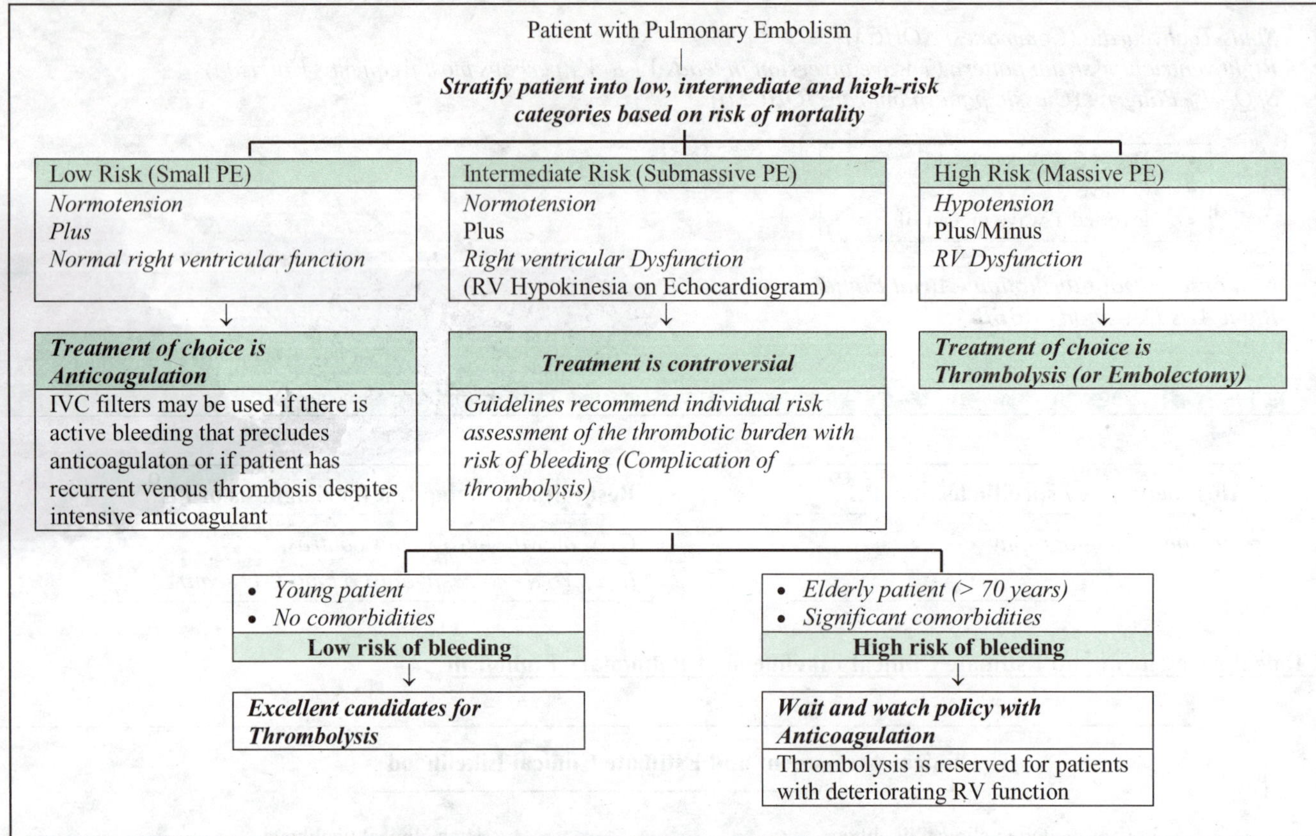

Pulmonary Hypertension / Idiopathic Pulmonary Arterial Hypertension

Features of Primary Pulmonary Hypertension / Idiopathic Pulmonary Arterial Hypertension

- *Most common in Young women* who are 20-40 years of Age (Robbin's 7th/745) (strong female predominance)
- *Most common symptom is exertional dyspnea (predominant symptom is dysnea)*
- Pulmonary Function tests
  - *Are usually normal with the exception of DLCO which is characteristically reduced.*
  - *Non obstructive PFT (FEV1/FVC>0.7 or 70%)*
  - *Non restrictive PFT (FVC > 80%)*
  - *DLCO2 is reduced (↓DLCO)*

  (Note: Mild restrictive effects can be seen in upto 20% of patients with advanced IPAH)

X Ray chest

- *X Ray chest shows clear lung fileds in PPH/IPAH*
- *X Ray chest usually shows enlargement of pulmonary arteries*

Exercise tolerance

- *Exercise tolerance is markedly reduced*

  (The exercise capacity of these patients appears to be limited by a low cardiac output because of a decrease in the functional pulmonary vascular bed)

Cor-Pulmonale

The most common cause of chronic cor pulmonale is chronic obstructive pulmonary disease - *Rubin's pathology*

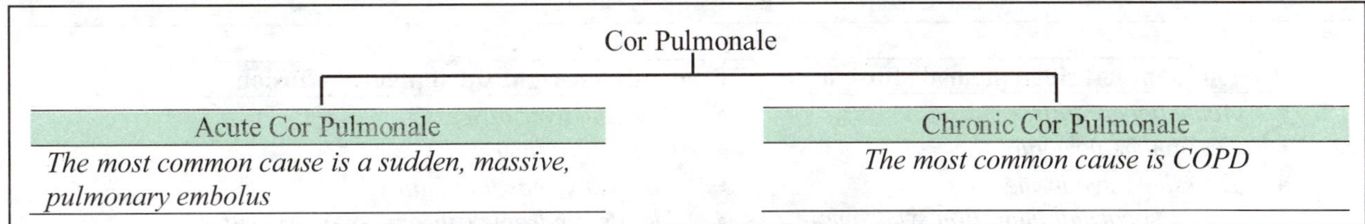

Bronchial Breath Sounds

The bronchial breath sound originates in the larger airways and are transmitted directly to the chest wall without passing through the alveoli. The sound passing through the lung tissue is not modified and auscultated like bronchial sounds from the chest walls. This sound resembles the sound obtained by listening over the trachea (directly placing a stethoscope on the trachea).

The characteristics of these sounds are:

1. Duration of expiration is equal to or longer than that of inspiration.
2. Intensity of expiration is more than that of inspiration.
3. There is a definite gap between inspiration and expiration.
4. Sounds are harsh or aspirate in nature.
5. They are high-pitched with frequencies above 600Hz.

Types of Bronchial Breath Sounds

Bronchial breath sounds are of three types: tubular, cavernous, and amphoric.

Bronchial Breath Sounds

Tubular Bronchial Breath sound	Caveronous Bonchial Breath sound	Amphoric Bronchial Breath sound
The tubular bronchial breath sound is a high pitched sound resulting from the passage of vibrations produced in the small bronchi directly to the chest wall through a solid lung tissue. This is seen when the lung parenchyma becomes a solid mass, as in consolidation.	The cavernous bronchial breath sounds is a low pitched bronchial breath sound heard over a cavity, which is situated superficially and communicated to a patent bronchus. The size of the cavity should be more than 2 cm in diameter to produce a cavernous breath sound.	The amphoric bronchial breath sounds is a high pitched bronchial sound that resembles the sound produced by blowing air into a wide-mouthed bottle. This is heard over a very large cavity communicating pneumothorax. It is also seen in large pulmonary cysts having communication with a patent bronchus.

Clinical Distinguishing Features on Clinical Examination

	Tracheal deviation (Mediastinal shift)	Chest expansion	Percussion note ↓ Duller ↑ Hyper-resonant	Breath sounds ↑ Louder ↓ Softer	Added sounds	Vocal resonance
Consolidation	No	Normal, or↓	Normal, or↓	↑ (Bronchial)	Coarse crackles +/- rub	↑ Whispering Pectoriloquy
Lobar collapse	Yes (Towards collapse)	↓	↓	↓	No	↓
Pleural effusion	No	↓	↓ (Stony dull)	↓	Occasional rub	↓
Pneumothorax	Yes (Specially with tension)	Normal or↓	↑	↓	Occasional click	↓

Pleural Effusion

Differential Diagnosis of Pleural Effusion based on predominant side of involvement

Predominant left sided pleural effusion

- *Acute pancreatitis*
- *Oesophageal rupture*
- *Dressler's syndrome (postmyocardial infarction syndrome)*

Predominant right sided pleural effusion

- *Amoebic liver abscess*
- *Cirhosis of liver*
- *Congestive cardiac failure*
- *Meig's syndrome (fibroma of ovary with ascites ad pleural effusion)*

Differential Diagnosis of Pleural Effusion based on pleual fluid biochemical findings

Pleural Fluid with decreased glucose

Conditions associated with Decreased Glucose (<60mg/dl) in pleural fluid

- ***Malignant Effusion***[Q] *(Also mentioned in Harrisons)*
- ***Rheumatoid Effusion***[Q] *(Also mentioned in Harrisons)*
- ***Parapneumonic Effusion***[Q] *(Bacterial Infections as mentioned in Harrisons)*
- *Tuberculous Effusion*[Q] *(Also mentioned in CMDT)*
- *Hemothorax*
- *Paragonimiasis*
- *Churg-Strauss Syndrome*

Pleural effusion with low glucose (< 60 mg/dl)
1. Malignancy
2. Bacterial infections
3. Rheumatoid pleuritis

Pleural Fluid with High Amylase

High amylase level in pleural fluid suggests

- *Esophageal rupture*[Q]
- *Pancreatic pleural effusion*[Q] *(Pancreatitis/Pancreaticpseudo cyst)*
- *Malignancy*[Q] (Adenocarcinoma of lung/pancreas)

Pleural Fluid with Cholesterol Crystals

Pleural effusion with cholesterol crystals

- *Hypothyroidism (myxoedema)*
- *T.B.*
- *Rheumatoid arthritis*

Characteristics of Tuberculous effusion

Characteristics of Tuberculous effusion

- *Exudative*
- *Proteins increased (Pleural fluid protein / Serum protein > 0.5)*
- *Pleural fluid LDH increased (P. Fluid LDH/ Serum LDH > 0.6*
- *Haemorrhagic*
- *Glucose: equal to serum levels; occasionally < 60 mg/dl*
- *WBC count increased: predominantly small lymphocytes*
- *High levels of TB markers in pleural fluid*

  Adenosine deaminase > 45 IU/L

  Interferon V > 140 pg/ml

  Positive PCR for tubercular DNA

Pneumothorax

Primary Spontaneous Pneumothorax (Primary pneumothorax)

- ***Primary spontaneous penumothorax occurs in persons with no clinical evidence of lung disease and often without an obvious precipitating event***
- Most of these patients have occult lung disease (sub clinical lung disease) in the form of subpleural apical blebs (recognized on CT scan)
- *Characteristic risk factors include a positive family history and history of smoking (occurs almost exclusively in smokers according to Harrisons)*
- *Characteristically affects tall, thin boys and men between the age of 10 and 30 years*
- *Left-sided pneumothorax is associated with right axis deviation.*

Primary Spontancous pneumothorax
• *No clinical evidence of pre existing lung disease*[Q]
• *Rupture of apical subpleural blebs*[Q]
• *Positive family history*[Q]
• *History of smoking*[Q]
• *Tall and thin individual* [Q]
• *Young adults (10 to 30 years of age)* [Q]
• *Male gender*[Q]

Iatrogenic Pneumothorax

Common Causes of Iatrogenic Pneumothorax

Common causes of Iatrogenic Pneumothorax (Decreasing order of frequency)
• *Transthoracic Needle Lung Biopsy*
• ***Subclavian vein cannulation***
• *Thoracocentesis*
• *Pleural Biopsy*
• *Positive Pressure ventilation*

Presentation of iatrogenic Pneumothorax

Iatrogenic Pneumothorax

History
• History of Procedure known to cause iatrogenic pneumothorax (subclavian vein cannulation)
• Sudden onset Breathlessness
• Chest discomfort / chest pain

Examination
Inspection/ palpatum
• Reduced movements over affected side • Mediastinal shift to opposite side • Decreased vocal fremitus
Percussion
Hyper-resonant
Auscultation
Diminished or absent breath sound

Sleep Apnea

Sleep Apnea

- Sleep Apnea is defined as an intermittent cessation of airflow at the nose and mouth during sleep
- ***By definition/convention breath cessation for at least 10 seconds is termed Apnea***

By convention sleep apnea is defined by breath cessation for at least 10 seconds. Most patients with sleep apneas have cessation for 20-30 seconds. The duration of breath cessation may be as long as 2-3 minutes.

- Sleep apneas can be central or obstructive

Central sleep Apnea	Obstructive sleep Apnea
Sleep apnea occurs due to transient cessation of neural drive to all respiratory muscles	Sleep Apnea occurs due to transient occlusion of the orapharyngeal airway despite continued respiratory drive

Primary pulmonary hypoventilation

Characterized by:
Impaired chemoreception resulting in decreased ventilatory drive. Chronic hypercapnia and hypoxemia in the absence of identifiable neuromuscular disease or mechanical ventilatory impairment.
Presentation :
Occurs in all age groups but majority of cases have been reported in males aged 20-50 years. Early: lethargy, fagtigue, daytime somnolence, disturbed sleep and morning headache. Late: Cyanosis polycythemia, pulmonary hypertension, congestive heart failure. Note : Dyspnea is uncommon despite severe arterial blood gas derangements because of impaired chemotherapy.
Diagnosis :
The key diagnostic feature is respiratory acidosis in the absence of respiratory muscle weaknesses or impaired ventilatory mechanics.

Bronchogenic Carcinoma: Lung Cancer

Histological type	Frequency (Worldwide)	
Adenocarcinoma	*32%*	• ***Most common Bronchogenic Carcinoma in India is squamous cell carcinoma***
Squamous cell ca	*29%*	
Small cell carcinoma	*18%*	• ***Most common Bronchogenic Carcinoma worldwide is Adenocarcinoma***
Large cell carcinoma	*9%*	
Carcinoid	*1%*	

Facts to remember about Bronchogenic Carcinomas

Q *Most frequent histological type*	*: Adenocarcinoma*
Q *Most frequent histological type in India*	*: Squamous cell carcinoma*
Q *Most common histological variety in life time non-smokers*	*: Adenocarcinoma*
Q *Most common histological variety in young patients.*	*: Adenocarcinoma*
Q *Most common histological variety in females*	*: Adenocarcinoma*
Q *Most common site for metastasis from Ca lung*	*: Liver (page 521/H)*
Q *Most common endocrine organ to be involved by metastasis from Ca lung*	*: Adrenals.*
Q *Ca lung which metastizes to opposite lung*	*: Adenocarcinoma.*
Q *Commonest tumor to metastise to heart*	*: Ca lung (Bronchogenic Ca)*
Q *Histological varieties that cavitate*	*: Squamous cell and large cell.*
Q *Histological varieties that are central in distribution*	*: Squamous cell and small cell.*
Q *Histological varieties that are peripheral in distribution*	*: Adenocarcinoma.*
Q *Pancoost tumor is histologically*	*: Squamous cell.*
Q *Most common variety associated with paraneoplatic syndrome*	*: Small cell variety.*
Q *Most common variety associated with hypokalemia*	*: Small cell (presumably d/t ACTH)*
Q *Most common variety associated with hypercalcemia*	*: Squamous cell (presumably d/t PTH)*
Q *Histological variety most responsive to chemotherapy*	*: Small cell*
Q *Histological variety response to Radiotherapy*	*: Small cell*
Q *Histological variety associated with best prognosis*	*: Squamous cell*

Small-Cell Carcinoma versus Non-Small-Cell Carcinoma

Property	<u>**Small cell carcinoma**</u> • *Oat cell Carcinoma*	<u>**Non small cell Carcinoma**</u> • *Squamous cell carcinoma* • *Adenocarcinoma* • *Large cell carcinoma* • *Bronchoalveolar carcinoma*
Location	• ***Central location***	• *Peripheral location*
	Central location[Q] • *Squammous cell*[Q] • *Small cell*[Q]	**Peripheral location**[Q] • *Adenocarcinoma*[Q] • *Large cell variant*[Q]
Cavitation	• ***Rare***	• *Common in Squamous Cell* • *Also seen in Large Cell*
	Cavitatory variant • *Squammous cell (most common)* • *Large cell*	**Non cavitatory variants** • *Small cell* • *Adeno carcinoma*
Metastasis	• ***Highly metastatic lesion*** with widespread metastasis at time of diagnosis • Common site of metastasis include brain, bone, Liver and adrenals	Less metastatic than small cell carcinomas
Paraneoplastic syndrome	• *ACTH* • *AVP (Vasopressin)* • *Calcitonin* • *ANF* • *Gastrin Releasing peptide*	• ***PTH***
Response to chemotherapy	<u>***Superior Response***</u> ***Overall regression rate is 90%*** Rate of complete regression is 30%	<u>Inferior Response</u> *Objective shrinkage in 30-50%* Complete response : uncommon
Response to Radiotherapy	<u>***Superior Response***</u> *Objective Shrinkage in 80-90%* *Complete response: Often*	<u>Inferior Response</u> *Objective shrinkage in 30-50%* *Complete response: Uncommon*
Primary management	*Managed primarily with Chemotherapy with or without Radiotherapy*	*Management primarily with Surgery or Radiotherapy (localized lesions)*
	• *Small cell lung carcinomas behave as systemic disease.* • Most small cell carcinomas have already spread at the time of presentation beyond the bounds of surgery and they are *managed primarily by chemotherapy with or without radiotherapy.* ***Small cell carcinomas are highly chemosensitive with an overall 90% regression rate with chemotherapy.***	*For non small cell carcinomas the primary modality depends on the extent of disease* • <u>**Localized diseases**</u>**: (Stage I & II)** Primary modality of treatment is surgery – **pulmonary resection.** • <u>**Advanced disease**</u>**:** **Radiotherapy with curative intent** is advocated (± chemotherapy) • <u>**Metastatic disease**</u> **(Stage IV)** symptomatic/supportive

<u>**Cavitation is a feature of squammous cell and large cell variants and not of oat cell/small cell variant**</u>

'In contrast to squammous cell carcinoma in which central cavitation is noted in 10-20% of cases, small cell cancer rarely cavitates' - *Clinical Hematology & Oncology (2003)/945*

<u>**Adenocarcinomas present as peripheral masses and not as central masses**</u>

'Squammous and small cell cancers usually present as central masses while adenocarcinoma and large cell cancers tend to present as peripheral nodule and masses' – Harrison

Presenting Symptoms of Bronchogenic Carcinoma

The most common presenting symptom of lung cancer is cough – *Robbins*

Common presenting symptoms of lung cancer (Robbins)
Cough (75%-Commonest)
Weight loss (40%)
Chest pain (40%)
Dyspnea (20%)

Common presenting symptoms of lung cancer (*General Thoracic Surgery*) In decreasing order of frequency.
Cough (commonest)
Hemoptysis
Chest pain
Dyspnea
Wheezing or strider
Hoarseness
Pleural effusion
Superior vena caval syndrome
Pancoast tumour
Dysphagia
Phrenic palsy

Superior vena caval syndrome (SVC syndrome)

- SVC syndrome results from an impedance in outflow from superior vena cava due to external compression
- *The most common cause of SVC syndrome is external compression by a malignant tumour*[Q]
- *The most common malignant tumor causing SVC syndrome is bronchogenic carcinoma*[Q]
- *The most common histological type of bronchogenic carcinoma causing SVC syndrome is small cell carcinoma*[Q]

Etiologies of Superior Vena Cava Obstruction:

Malignancy	**95%**
Lung Cancer	*65%*
Lymphoma	*15%*
Breast cancer	*5%*
Germ-cell	*2%*
Thymic cancer	*2%*
Other cancer	*4%*
Benign	**5%**
Central venous device related	*1%*
Mediastinal fibrosis	*3%*

- **Clinical manifestations of obstruction to SVC :**

Symptoms	Signs
• ***Swelling around neck & face*** especially around the eyes • ***Dyspnea*** • Cough • Others: Hoarseness / Headache / Tongue Swelling / Nasal congestion / Epistaxis Haemoptysis / Dysphagia / Pain / Dizziness / Syncope	• Dilated neck veins • ***Increased number of collateral veins over anterior chest wall*** • Cyanosis • Edema of face, arms & chest • Proptosis, glossal and Laryngeal edema and obtundation in severe cases

Symptoms are aggrevated by bending forwards and lying down.

Cystic Fibrosis

Charachteristic Classical Manifestations of Cystic Fibrosis
(Typical System Involvement)

Respiratory system (Sinopulmonary disease)

- Pulmonary infection
  Persistant colonization/infection with typical cystic fibrosis pathogens, including Staphylococcus aureus, nontypeable, Hemophilus influenzae, ***mucoid and nonmucoid Pseudomonas aeruginosa***, Burkholderia cepase
- Chronic obstructive Pulmonary Disease
- Bronchiectasis is typical
- Airway obstruction manifested by wheezing and air trapping
- Chronic cough & sputum production
- Digital clubbing
- Persistent chest radiograph abnormalities (eg. Bronchiectasis, atelectasis, infiltrates, hyperinflation)
- Nasal Polyps
  Radiographic or computed tomographic abnormalities of paranasal sinuses

Gastrointestinal System (Intestinal; Hepatobiliary; Pancreatic)

Intestinal
meconium ileus, distal intestinal obstruction syndrome, rectal prolapse.
Pancreatic
Pancreatic exocrine deficiency
Hepatobiliary
Hepatic disease manifested by clinical or histologic evidence of focal biliary ***cirrhosis***, or multilobular ***cirrhosis***
Nutritional
Failure to thrive (protein-calorie malnutrition), hypoproteinemia, edema, complications secondary to fat-soluble vitamin deficiency

Genitourinary System (Male Infertility)

Male urogenital abnormalites resulting in obstructive zoospermia are typical

Metabolic Abnormalities are typically charachterized by **salt depletion syndrome**, *(Hyponatremia, Hypocholeremia and Hypokalemic Metabolic Alkalosis)*

Pulmonary Infection in Cystic Fibrosis

- *The most common cause of Pulmonary infection in cystic fibrosis in children is staphylococcus aureus*[Q]
- *The most common cause of Pulmonary infection in cytic fibrosis in adolescents and adults is Pseudomonas Aeroginosa.*
- *The two most common cause of pulmonary infection in cystic fibrosis are staphylococcus aureus and Pseudomonas Aeroginosa*

  Overall (all agegroups) Pseudomonas Aeroginosa is marginally more common than staphylococcus aureus as a cause of pulmonary infection in cystic fibrosis.

- *The most* common organism causing chronic lung disease in patients with cystic fibrosis is pseudomonas aeroginosa

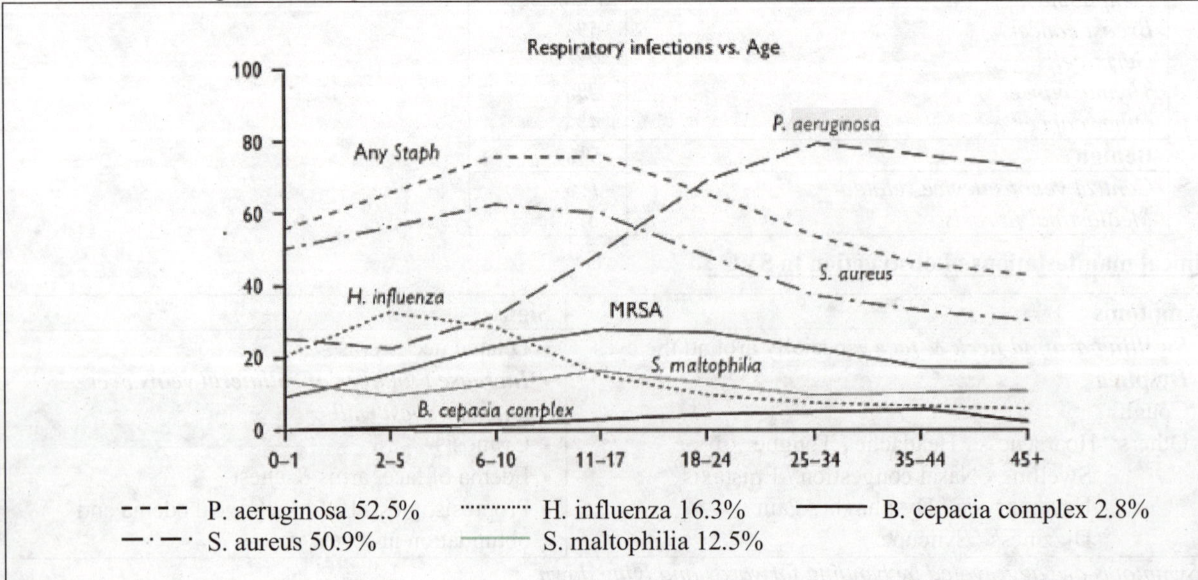

Kartagener's syndrome

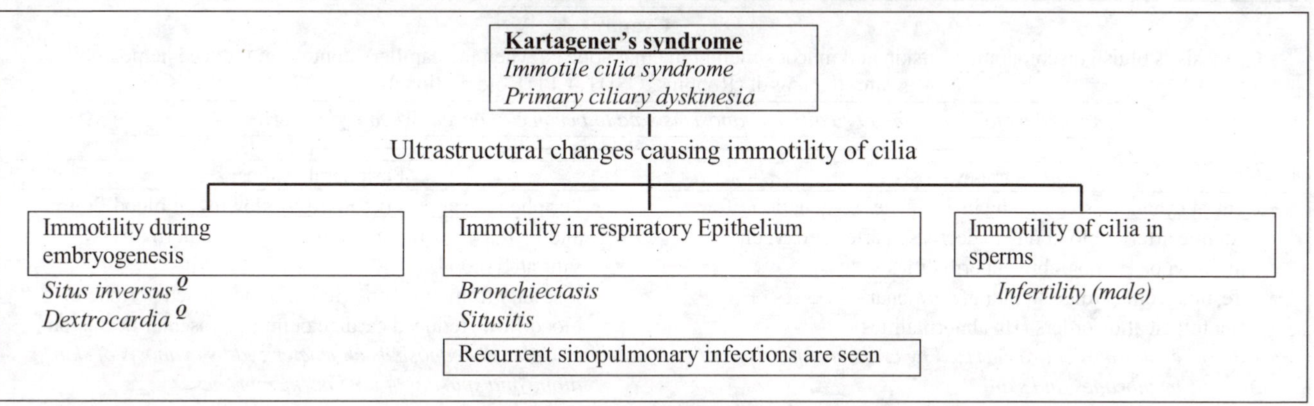

Syndrome	Major cardiac Anomaly	Major non cardiac anomaly
Kartagener's syndrome *(Immotile cilia syndrome)* *(Primary ciliary dyskinesia)*	*Dextrocardia*[Q]	• *Situs inversus* [Q] • *Sinusitis* [Q] • *Bronchiectasis* [Q] • *Infertility* [Q]

Note

Situs inversus refers to perfect mirror image of normal physiologic position of visceral organs with preservation of their A-P relationship. Situs inversus is usually associated with dextrocardia (Heart on Right Side of chest).

Goodpasture's Syndrome

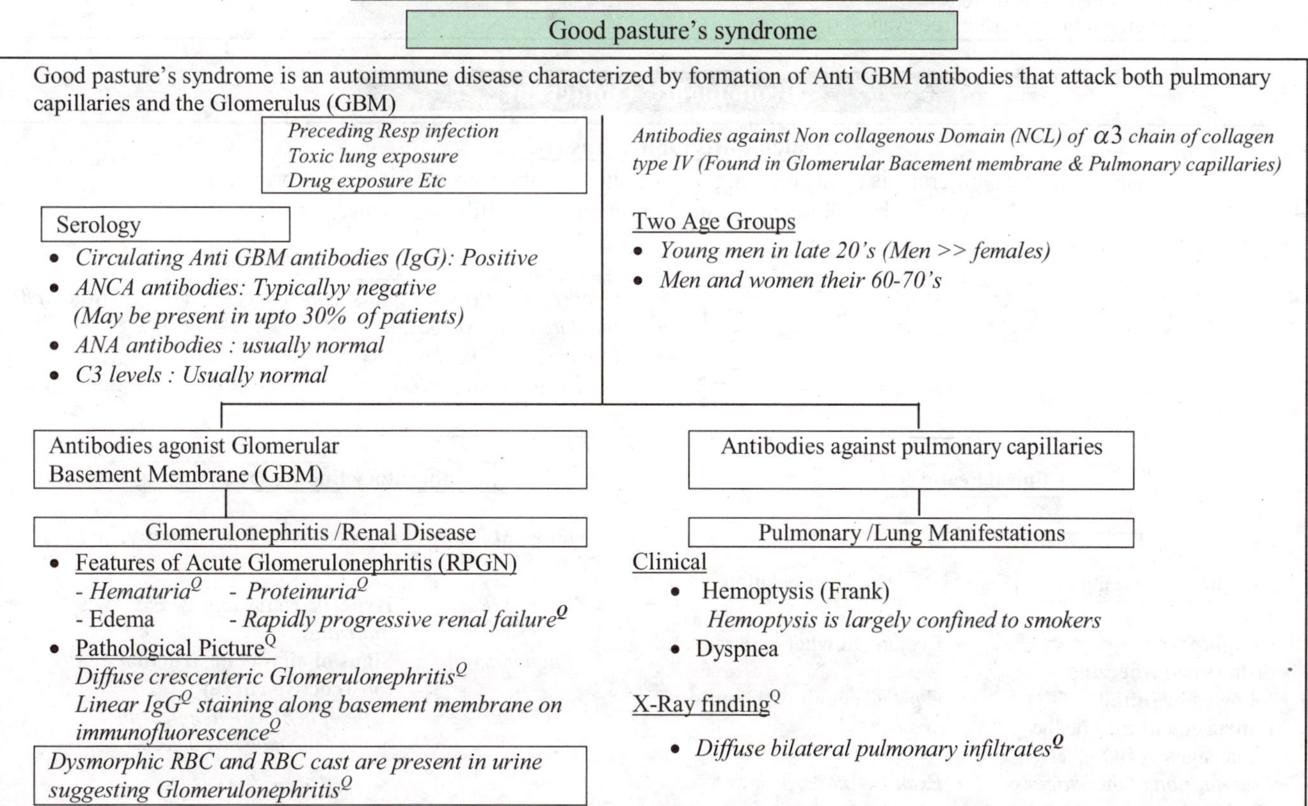

3

Cyanosis

Cyanosis

Cyanosis is bluish discolouration of skin and mucous membrane that appears when the capillary content of reduced hemoglobin is greater than 5g/dl (Robbins, CSDT, CPDT old editions)

According to Harrisons 17th edition cyanosis is said to become apparent when reduced Hb > 4g/dl

Central cyanosis

- Central cyanosis is caused by in adequate oxygenation of systemic arterial blood due to decreased arterial oxygen saturation or Hemoglobin abnormalities
- It results from cardiac shunting, pulmonary diseases or hematological disorders (Hb abnormalities)
- *Central cyanosis is charachterized by cyanosis affective both mucous membranes and skin*

Causes

Decreased arterial oxygen saturation

- Decreased atmospheric pressure – high altitude
- Impaired pulmonary function
  - ***Alveolar hyoventilation***
  - ***Uneven relationships between pulmonary ventilation and perfusion*** (perfusion of hypoventilated alveoli)
  - Impaired oxygen diffusion
- Anatomic shunts
  - Certain types of congenital heart disease
  - Pulmonary arteriovenous fistulas
  - Multiple small intrapulmonary shunts
- Hemoglobin with low affinity for oxygen

Hemoglobin abnormalities

- ***Methemoglobinemia – hereditary, acquired***
- Sulfhemoglobinema – acquired
- Carboxyhemoglobinemia (not true cyanosis)

Peripheral cyanosis

- Peripheral cyanosis is caused by slowing of blood flow and increased extraction of oxygen from normally saturated blood
- It results from vasoconstriction or decreased peripheral blood flow, reduced cardiac output or vascular occlusion
- *Peripheral cyanosis is characterized by cyanosis of skin alone and sparing of mucous membranes*

Causes

- Vascular occlusion
  - Arterial obstruction
  - Venous obstruction
- Reduced cardiac output
- Cold exposure
- Redistribution of blood flow from extremities

Bronchiolitis Obliterans

Bronchiolitis Obliterans (BO)

Bronchiolitis Obliterans is a chronic lung disease that results from obstruction of bronchii, bronchioles and smaller airways from fibrous tissue.

Obstruction by fibrous tissue may be a sequelle to: (Etiology)

- *Respiratory infections : Most common is Adenovirus*[Q] *(Rudolph)*
- *Inhalation of toxic gases*
- *Connective tissue disorders*
- Transplant recipients[Q]

Clinical Features

Initial Presentation

Cough, fever respiratory distress and **wheezing** followed by **initial improvement** may be the initial signs of BO –Nelson

Presentation at this stage is similar to pneumonia, bronchitis, acute bronchiolitis

Later Presentation

- **Prolonged wheeze (stridor)**
- *Chronic* **cough with sputum** *production*
- *Exercise intolerance (dyspnea)*

Laboratory findings and imaging

(Suggest Features of Obstructive Lung disease)

Chest X-Ray	:	**Hyperluscency** *and Patchy infiltrates*
Pulmonary	:	**Signs of airway obstruction (obstructive curve)**
V-Q scan	:	*Typical moth eaten appearance of multiple matched defects*

QUESTIONS

Respiratory failure & Disturbance in Respiratory Functions

1. False statement about type I respiratory failure is: *(AI 2001)*
   A. Decreased PaO_2
   B. Decreased $PaCO_2$
   C. Normal $PaCO_2$
   D. Normal A-a gradient
2. In type - II respiratory failure, there is : *(AIIMS Nov 02)*
   A. Low pO2 and low pCO_2
   B. Low pO2 and high pCO_2
   C. Normal pO2 and high pCO_2.
   D. Low pO2 and normal pCO_2.
3. A patient with salicylic acid poisoning has the following arterial blood gas analysis report : pH = 7.12 : pCO_2 = 18mmHg; HCO_3 = 12mmol/L. The resulting acid base abnormality can be best labeled as: *(AIIMS Nov 03)*
   A. Metabolic acidosis with compensatory respiratory alkalosis
   B. Metabolic acidosis with compensatory respiratory alkalosis
   C. Respiratory acidosis with metabolic alkalosis
   D. Metabolic acidosis
4. In a patient PO_2 is 85 mmHg, PCO_2 – 50mmHg, pH is 7.2 and HCO_3 is 32 meq/l is suffering from :
   A. Respiratory acidosis with compensatory metabolic alkalosis *(AIIMS June 2000)*
   B. Respiratory acidosis with compensatory metabolic acidosis
   C. Metabolic acidosis
   D. Metabolic alkalosis
5. A patient presents with following parameters pH 7.5, p CO_2 30 mmHg, pO_2 102 mmHg and HCO_3 16 meq/l. Which of the following correctly describes the compensatory mechanism: *(AI 2010)*
   A. Respiratory Alkalosis
   B. Metabolic Alkalosis
   C. Respiratory Acidosis
   D. Metabolic Acidosis
6. The acid base status of a patient reveals a p^H = 7.46 and pCO_2=30 mm Hg. The patient has a partially compensated primary: *(AI 2011)*
   A. Metabolic acidosis
   B. Metabolic alkalosis
   C. Respiratory alkalosis
   D. Respiratory acidosis
7. Arterial blood gas analysis of a patient reveals pH 7.2, HCO_3 36mmol/L, pCO_2 60mm of Hg. The abnormality is : *(AIIMS June 99)*
   A. Respiratory acidosis with compensatory metabolic alkalosis *(AI 1996)*
   B. Respiratory acidosis
   C. Respiratory alkalosis with compensatory metabolic acidosis
   D. Respiratory acidosis with compensatory metabolic acidosis
8. A 40 year old male develops excessive hyperventilation. ABG reveals pH- 7.5, PCO_2 24 mmHg, PO_2 88 mm of Hg. Treatment is : *(AIIMS June 1999)*
   A. Respiratory alkalosis
   B. Metabolic alkalosis
   C. Respiratory acidosis
   D. Metabolic acidosis
9. An ABG analysis shows : pH 7.2, raised pCO_2, decreased HCO_3; diagnosis is : *(AIIMS June 97)*
   A. Respiratory acidosis
   B. Compensated metabolic acidosis
   C. Respiratory and metabolic acidosis
   D. Respiratory alkalosis
10. A 10 year old boy with short stature presents with polyuria & polydipsia. Laboratory values reveal a pH of 7.4; HCO^3 of 17; Na^+ 140; pCO2 32; K^+ 4.9; Cl^- 112. Likely acid base abnormality is:
    A. Metabolic Alkalosis *(AIIMS Nov 2010)*
    B. Non-Anion gap Metabolic Acidosis
    C. Anion gap Metabolic Acidosis
    D. Respiratory Acidosis
11. Blood gas measurements of a patient shows the following values pH 7.2, pCO2 80 mm Hg, pO2 46 mm Hg. Which of the following could be the most probable diagnosis: *(AIIMS Nov 2000)*
    A. Acute asthma
    B. Acute exacerbation of COPD
    C. ARDS
    D. Severe pneumonia
12. The blood gas parameters: pH 7.58, pC02 23 mm Hg pO2 300 mm Hg and oxygen saturation 60% are most consistent with- *(AI 03)*
    A. Carbon monoxide poisoning
    B. Ventilatory malfunction
    C. Voluntary hyperventilation
    D. Methyl alcohol poisoning

Obstructive / Restrictive Pulmonary Diseases

Pulmonary Function Test

13. All the following are true about Chronic Obstructive lung disease *except:*
    A. Decreased FeV_1 *(AI 1994)*
    B. Decreased MEFR *(AIIMS June 97)*
    C. Increased RV
    D. Decreased diffusion capacity

14. All of the following are characteristic feature of obstructive pulmonary disease, except:
A. Normal Residual Volume *(DNB June 2010)*
B. Decreased FEV_1
C. Normal Vital Capacity
D. Decreased FCV_1/FVC

15. FEV_1/FVC is reduced in case of :
A. Pleural effusion *(AIIMS May 95)*
B. Lung fibrosis
C. Asthma
D. All of the above

16. Pulmonary function changes in acute bronchial asthma in untreated patient - *(PGI June 03)*
A. ↑ ed peak expiratory flow
B. ↓ ed TLC
C. ↑ ed FVC
D. ↑ ed RV
E. ↑ ed FEV

17. Features of restrictive lung disease is *(AIIMS June 98)*
A. FEV_1/FVC decreases and compliance decreases
B. FEV_1/FVC increases and compliance increases
C. FEV_1/FVC decreases and compliance increases
D. FEV_1/FVC increases and compliance decreases

18. The abnormal preoperative pulmonary function test in a patient with severe kyphoscoliosis includes:
A. Reduced RV/TLC *(AI 05)*
B. Reduced FEV1/FVC.
C. Reduced FEV25-75
D. Increased FRC

19. A 28 years old woman having limited cutaneous scleroderma for the last 10 years comaplins of shortness of breath for last one month. Her pulmonary functions tests (PFT) are as follows :

PFT	Observed	Predicted
FVC	2.63	2.82
$FEV_{1\%}$	88%	80%
DLCO	5.26	16.3

What is the most likely diagnosis in this case ?
A. Intestitial lung disease *(AI 06)*
B. Pulmonary artery hypertension
C. Congestive heart failure
D. Bronchiectasis

20. A 28 years old woman having limited cutaneous scleroderma for the last 10 years complains of shortness of breath for last one month. Her pulmonary functions tests (PFT) are as follows:

PFT	Observed	Predicted
FVC	2.63	2.82
$FEV_{1\%}$	88%	80%
DLCO	5.26	16.3

What is the most likely diagnosis in this case?
A. Interstitial lung disease *(AIIMS Nov 09)*
B. Pulmonary artery hypertension
C. Congestive heart failure
D. Bronchiectasis

21. A patient presents with decreased vital capacity and total lung volume. What is the most probable diagnosis? *(AI 2007)*
A. Bronchiectasis
B. Sarcoidosis
C. Cystic fibrosis
D. Asthma

22. All are decreased in infiltrative lung disease, *except*:
A. Vital capacity *(AIIMS Feb 97)*
B. Alveolar arterial difference in PaO_2
C. Total lung capacity
D. Lung compliance

23. Carbon monoxide diffusion capacity decreases in all, *except* : *(AIIMS Feb 97) (AI-2003)*
A. Emphysema
B. Primary pulmonary hypertension
C. Alveolar haemorrhage
D. Infiltrative lung disease

24. Diffusion capacity for carbon monoxide is decreased in all of the following Except: *(AIIMS May 94)*
A. Chronic Bronchitis
B. Emphysema
C. Interstitial lung disease
D. Pulmonary embolism

25. Decreased maximum mid-expiratory flow rate indicates obstruction in : *(AI 1994)*
A. Small airways *(AIIMS May 95)*
B. Trachea
C. Large airways
D. Trachea & Bronchi both

Bronchial Asthma

26. All of the following are true about intrinsic Asthma, Except: *(PGI Dec 04)*
A. Increasing Incidence
B. Allergic Asthma is more common in young patients
C. Idiosyncratic Asthma is more common older patients
D. IgE is increased in Idiosyncratic Asthma
E. IgE is increased in Extrinsic Asthma

27. All of the following statements about intrinsic allergic Asthma are true, Except: *(PGI 2009)*
A. Nasal polyp
B. Normal IgE
C. Family history Positive
D. More aggressive
E. Allergic in nature

28. Aspirin-sensitive asthma is associated with:
A. Obesity *(AI 1995)*
B. Urticaria
C. Nasal polyp
D. Extrinsic asthma

29. Bronchial Asthma is characterized by all of the following, Except: *(PGI June 05)*
    A. Inflammatory disease of airway
    B. Allergic disease of airway
    C. Hyporesponsive ness of airway
    D. Hyperresponsiveness of airway
    E. Treatment is mostly inhaled steroid
30. All of the following are true about Asthma, Except:
    A. Charcol Leydin crystals may be seen in sputum
    B. Reversible Airflow obstruction is a characteristic feature
    C. Large airways are involved
    D. Small airways are not involved
    E. Intermittent Asthma responds better to bronchodilator therapy than persistant Asthma
31. True about Asthma except: *(PGI 05)*
    A. Inflammatory disease
    B. Hyperresponsive airways
    C. Necrosis of airways
    D. Mucous plug formation
    E. Airway edema
32. Feature of Acute severe Asthma include all of the following, Except:
    A. Tachycardia > 120/min
    B. Pulsus paradoxus
    C. Respiratory acidosis
    D. PEFR < 50%
    E. None (All are Features of Acute severe Asthma)
33. In a patient with bronchial asthma silent chest signifies *(DNB 2010)*
    A. Good Prognosis
    B. Bad Prognosis
    C. Grave Prognosis
    D. Not a Prognostic sign
34. Universal finding in Asthma is *(PGI June 02)*
    A. Hypoxia
    B. Hypercarbia
    C. Respiratory acidosis
    D. Metabolic Acidosis
35. Bronchial Asthma is best diagnosed by: *(PGI Dec 01)*
    A. Wheeze
    B. Dyspnea and cough
    C. FEV_1 values
    D. Demonstration of Reversible obstruction
    E. Normal FEV_1
36. Anti-inflammatory action on airways is seen with (Mark two correct option): *(PGI June 05)*
    A. Fluticasone
    B. Iprotropium bromide
    C. Budesonide
    D. Theophylline
    E. Tebutaline
37. All are used in bronchial asthma, *except* :
    A. Salbutamol *(AIIMS June 97)*
    B. Morphine
    C. Aminophylline
    D. Steroid
38. All of the following drugs useful in the treatment of a patient with acute bronchial asthma *except :*
    A. Ipratropium *(AIIMS Nov 03)*
    B. Salbutamol
    C. Montelukast
    D. Hydrocortisone
39. All of the following statements about Leukotriene modifiers in the management of bronchial asthma are true except : *(AIIMS May 1996)*
    A. May be used for acute asthma
    B. May be used for exercise induced asthma
    C. Zileuton is Leukotriene modifier
    D. May uncover Churg strauss syndrome
40. The most predictive and dangerous side effect of propranolol that makes it to be avoided in known patient of COPD is induction of : *(AIIMS Nov 01)*
    A. Respiratory failure
    B. Acute asthmatic attack
    C. Glaucoma
    D. Pleural effusion
41. A drug is to be delivered by a nebuliser. The size of a droplet for its humidification is :
    A. $< 5\ \mu$ *(AI 2000)*
    B. 5-10
    C. 10-15
    D. 15-20

Chronic Bronchitis

42. Increased Reid Index is used to characterized:
    A. Chronic Bronchitis *(AI 2012)*
    B. Bronchiectasis
    C. Bronchial Asthma
    D. Emphysema

Emphysema

43. α_1 Antitrypsin deficiency is associated with :
    A. Centriaciner emphysema *(AI 1999)*
    B. Panaciner-emphysema
    C. Irregular emphysema
    D. Paraseptal-emphysema
44. All of the following statements about Emphysema are true, Except: *(PGI Dec 04)*
    A. Breathlessness is the charachteristic presenting symptom
    B. Diffusion rate of carbon monoxide is reduced
    C. Restrictive pattern on pulmonary function test is seen
    D. Long term bronchadilater therapy does not improve lung function

45. Lung functions in Emphysema reveal all of the following , Except (PGI – Dec –01)
 A. Decreased vital capacity
 B. Increased diffusion capacity for carbon monoxide (DLCO)
 C. Increased Total Lung capacity
 D. Decreased FEV_1
 E. Decreased FEV_1 / FVC ratio
46. In an emphysematous patient with bullous lesions, which is the best investigation to measure lung volume: (AIIMS Nov 08)
 A. Body Plethysmography
 B. Gas dilution
 C. Transdiaphragmatic pressure
 D. DLco

Bronchiectasis

47. Bronchiectasis is most common in which lobe: (AIIMS May 95)
 A. Right upper lobe
 B. Right middle lobe
 C. Left upper lobe
 D. Left lower lobe
48. Which of the following is NOT a complication of bronchiectasis : (AIIMS Sept 96) (AI 1998)
 A. Lung abscess
 B. Lung cancer
 C. Amylodosis
 D. Empyema
49. Rampal, 45 yr old man presents with history of recurrent hemoptysis and purulent sputum. His chest X-Ray is normal, which of the following will be the next best investigation for him? (AIIMS Nov 01)
 A. HRCT
 B. CT guided angiography
 C. Angiography
 D. Spiral CT

Interstitial Lung Disease

50. All are true about Interstitial Fibrosis, Except (PGI – June 03)
 A. FVC < 80% Predicted
 B. FEV1/FVC < 0.7
 C. DLCO is decreased
 D. TLC is decreased
51. All of the following are true about interstitial lung disease, Except: (PGI June 07)
 A. Decreased FVC
 B. Decreased FEV1
 C. Decreased FEV1/FVC
 D. Decreased Diffusion capacity
52. A 40 year old female presents with progressive dyspnea for one year. Physical examination reveals bibasilar end-inspiratory crepitations. All of the following statements about her condition are true, Except:
 A. May be associated with connective tissue disease
 B. Residual volume is increased
 C. Total Lung capacity is decreased
 D. HRCT is a useful diagnostic test
53. A female presents with history of progressive breathlessness. Histology shows heterogenous patchy fibrosis with several fibroblastic foci. The most likely diagnosis is: (AI 2010)
 A. Cryptogenic Organizing Pneumonia
 B. Non Specific Interstitial pneumonia
 C. Usual Interstitial Pneumonia
 D. Desquamative Interstitial Pneumonia
54. Investigation of choice for interstitial disease is: (AIPGMEE 08)
 A. Chest X-ray
 B. HRCT
 C. Gallium-67 DTPA scan
 D. MRI
55. Which of the following is characteristically not associated with the development of interstitial lung disease? (AI 2002)
 A. Coal dust
 B. Sulfur dioxide
 C. Thermophilic actenomycetes
 D. Tobacco smokes
56. Caplan Syndrome is Pneumoconiosis with
 A. Lymphadenopathy
 B. Congestive Cardiac Failure
 C. Rheumatoid Arthritis
 D. HIV
57. All of the following features are seen in asbestosis except- (AIIMS Nov 02)
 A. Diffuse pulmonary interstitial fibrosis
 B. Fibrous pleural thickening
 C. Emphysema
 D. Calcific pleural plaques
58. True statements about asbestosis – (PGI Dec 04)
 A. Causes Lung Ca
 B. Pleural mesothelioma
 C. Peritoneal mesothelioma
 D. Pulmonary fibrosis
 E. All of the above
59. All of the following statements about silicosis are true, Except (PGI Dec 04)
 A. Pleural plaques
 B. Prediliction for upper lobes
 C. Calcific Hilar Lymphadenopathy
 D. Associated with tuberculosis
60. Not seen idiopathic pulmonary hemosiderosis (AI 2009)
 A. Eosinopenia
 B. Iron deficiency anemia
 C. Diffuse alveolar hemorrhage
 D. Hemoptysis
61. All of the following are true about Idiopathic Pulmonary Hemosiderosis Except:
 A. Hypoxemia
 B. Alveolar capillary constriction

C. Hyperplasia of type II Pneumocytes
D. Hemosiderin laden macrophages

62. All of the following are associated with pulmonary eosinophillic pneumonia, Except: *(PGI 2009)*
A. ABPA
B. Loeffler's pneumonia
C. Churg Strauss Syndrome
D. Tropical pulmonary eosinophilia
E. Wegener's granulomatosis

Allergic Bronchopulmonary Aspergillosis (ABPA)

63. Diagnostic features of allergic bronchopulmonary aspergillosis (ABPA) include all of the following *except*: *(AI 2003)*
A. Changing pulmonary infiltrates
B. Peripheral eosinophilia
C. Serum precipitins against Aspergillosis fumigants
D. Occurrence in patients with old cavitatory lesions.

64. Diagnostic criteria for Allergic Bronchopulmonary Aspergillosis include all, except *(PGI-Dec05)*
A. Peripheral eosinophilia (>$0.1\times 10^9/mm^3$)
B. Central bronchiectasis
C. Episodic Asthma
D. Detection of Aspergillus in sputum
E. ↑ IgG antibodies specific to A. Fumigatus

65. A 40 year old man presented with repeated episodes of bronchospasm and hemoptysis. Chest X-ray revealed perihilar bronchiectasis. The most likely diagnosis is : *(AI 2002)*
A. Sarcoidosis
B. Idiopathic pulmonary fibrosis
C. Extrinsic allergic alveolitis
D. Bronchopulmonary aspergillosis

66. All the following are true about bronchopulmonary aspergillosis *except*: *(AI 1995)*
A. Central bronchiectasis
B. Pleural effusion
C. Asthma
D. Eosinophilia

67. True statements about ABPA include all of the following, Except: *(PGI Dec 04)*
A. Serum IgE > 1000 ng/ml
B. Eosinophils > $1000/mm^3$
C. Elevated IgG antibodies
D. Proximal Bronchiectasis
E. Lower lobe predominance

68. Which is not true about aspergillosis-
A. Aspergillus Niger is the cause of fungal otitis externa
B. It is highly contagious
C. Aspergilloma is common in preexisting TB, or cystic disease
D. Aspergillus fumigatus is a cause of bronchial aspergillosis

69. 40 year old patient with history of prolonged exposure to Aspergillus presents with repeated episodes of breathlessness. Chest X-ray shows diffuse pulmonary infiltrates. Skin hypersensitivity test is positive for Aspergillus antigen Peripheral blood picture shows normal eosinophil count and serum IgE levels are normal The most likely diagnosis is
A. Allergic bronchial Asthma
B. Allergic Bronchopulmonary Aspergillosis (ABPA)
C. Extrinsic Allergic Alveolitis
D. Invasive Pulmonary Aspergillosis

70. All the following are features of Tropical pulmonary Eosinophilia except-
A. Eosinophilia > 3000/mm3
B. Microfilaria in blood
C. Paroxysmal cough and wheeze
D. Bilateral chest mottling and increased bronchovascular markings

71. All the following diseases are associated with peripheral blood eosinophilia *except* :
A. Allergic bronchopulmonary aspergillosis (ABPA). *(AIIMS Nov 02)*
B. Loffler's syndrome.
C. Pulmonary eosinophilic granuloma.
D. Chrug-Strauss syndrome.

72. A 54 year old smoker man comes with severe hemoptysis weight loss and oligoarthritis. Serial skiagram shows fleeting opacities. What is the diagnosis? *(AIIMS Nov 08)*
A. Allergic bronchopulmonary aspergillosis
B. Ca lung
C. Tb
D. Wegener's granulomatosis

Pneumonias and Tuberculosis

Bacterial Pneumonia

73. The most common causative organism for lobar pneumonia is :
A. Staphylococcus aureus
B. Streptococcus pyogenes
C. Streptococcus pheumoniae
D. Haemophilus influenzae

74. Nosocomial pneumonia is most commonly caused by:
A. Gram -ve bacilli *(AI 1998)*
B. Gram +ve bacilli
C. Gram -ve cocci
D. Mycoplasma

75. Predisposing factors for Pneumococcal Pneumonia include all of the following Except: *(PGI June 01)*
A. CRF

B. Lymphoma
C. Old Age
D. Thalassemia
E. Sickle cell disease

76. Cavitatory lesions in lung are seen in: *(AI 2010)*
A. Primary pulmonary Tuberculosis
B. Staphylococcal pneumonia
C. Preumoconiosis
D. Interstitial Lung disease

77. Devi, a 28 year female, has diarrhoea, confusion, high grade fever with bilateral pneumonitis. The diagnosis is : *(AI 2000)*
A. Legionella
B. Neisseria meningitis
C. Streptococcus pneumoniae
D. H. influenzae

78. A 30 year old male presents with pneumonia and diarrhea five days after discharge from a hospital. The drug of choice for treating him is:
A. Vancomycin
B. Ciprofloxacin
C. Azithromycin
D. Gentamycin
E. Tetracycline

79. An elderly male admitted for Pneumonia presents with diarrhea and gripping abdominal pain five days after discharge from the hospital. Drug which is likely to benefit is. *(DNB June 2009)*
A. Imodium
B. Metranidozole
C. Diphenoxylate
D. Levofloxacin

80. Which is not true about legionnaire pneumonia:
A. Seen mainly in immunocompromised person
B. Erythromycin is drug of choice *(AIIMS May 95)*
C. Common in patients with hairy cell leukemia
D. Smoking and alcohol are risk factor.

81. Fever persisting even after treatment of pneumonia likely diagnosis is : *(AIIMS June 97)*
A. Empyema
B. Fungal lesion
C. Carcinoma bronchus
D. Any of the above

82. Most common cause of empyema is:
A. Bronchopleural fistula *(AIIMS Dec 97)*
B. Tubercular pneumonia
C. Bacterial pneumonia
D. Pleurisy

Atypical Pneumonia

83. Atypical pneumonia can be caused by the following microbial agents *except*? *(AI 2005)*
A. Mycoplasma pneumoniae.
B. Legionella pemmophila.
C. Human Corona virus.
D. Klebsiella pneumoniae.

84. All of the following features are seen in the viral pneumonia *except* : *(AI 2005)*
A. Presence of interstitial inflammation.
B. Predominance of alveolar exudates.
C. Bronchiolitis.
D. Multinucleate giant cells in the bronchiolar wall.

85. Features of pneumocystic carini pneumonia are:
A. Interstial pneumonitis *(PGI Dec 98)*
B. Eosinophilic exudate
C. Damage to type I pneumocytes
D. Hypertrophy of type II pneumocytes
E. All of the above

86. A 45 year old, HIV positive patient presents with features of pneumonia. Characteristic histopathological features suggesting pneumocystis carinii pneumonia is: *(PGI-Dec-2000)*
A. Prominent Interstitial Pneumonitis
B. Eosinophilic Alveolar Exudates
C. Prominent mononuclear cells in Alveolar exudates
D. Neutrophilic infiltration of alveolar interstitium
E. Hypertrophy of type I pneumocytes

87. A truck driver presented with history of fever since four weeks, and dry cough. He also gives a history of weight loss of about 10 kg. X-ray shows bilateral reticulonodular infiltrates. The most likely diagnosis is: *(AI 2010)*
A. Tuberculosis
B. Pneumocystis carinii Pneumonia
C. Pneumococcal pneumonia
D. Interstitial Lung Disease

88. All of the following statements about Pneumocystis Jiroveci are true Except: *(AI 2008)*
A. Usually associated with CMV infection
B. May be associated with Pneumatocele
C. Usually diagnosed by sputum examination
D. Causes disease only in the immunocompromised host

89. True Statement about Pneumocystic Jiroveci is:
A. Often associated with CMV infection
B. Usually diagnosed by sputum examination
C. Infection occurs only in immunocompromised patients
D. Always associated with Pneumatocele

90. Indication for prophylaxis in pneumocystis carini pneumonia include (choose two best option)
A. CD_4 count < 200 /µl
B. Tuberculosis
C. Viral load > 25,000 copies/ml
D. Oral candidiasis

91. All the following are used in the treatment of *Pneumocystis carinii except:* *(AI 1994)*
A. Pentamidine
B. Dapsone
C. Cotrimoxazole
D. Fluoroquinolones

92. Drug of choice for *Mycoplasma pneumoniae* is : *(AIIMS Dec 94, May 94)*
A. Penicillin
B. Tetracycline
C. Cefuroxime
D. Erythromycin

93. In mycoplasma pneumonia, following are seen except *(PGI-Dec-97)*
A. Diffuse infiltration of lungs
B. Cannot be cultured routinely
C. Cefotaxime is the drug of choice
D. Serology is useful in diagnosis

94. Treatment of chlamydia pneumonia is : *(AIIMS Sept 96)*
A. Erythromycin
B. Ceftriaxone
C. Penicillin
D. Sulphonamide

95. Commonest sign of aspiration pneumonitis is : *(AIIMS Dec 94)*
A. Cyanosis
B. Tachypnea
C. Crepitations
D. Rhonchi

Tuberculosis

96. True regarding presentation of primary T.B. is :
A. B/L pleural effusion with negative Tuberculin test. *(AIIMS Dec 98)*
B. U/L hilar lymphadenopathy
C. Sustained chronic pyrexia
D. B/L pleural effusion with positive tuberculin test.

97. All of the following statements about primary Tuberculosis are true, Except:
A. Cavitatory lesion
B. Pleural effusion
C. Fibrocasseous lesion
D. Phlyctenular conjunctivitis

98. All are features of primary tuberculosis; *except* : *(AIIMS June 98)*
A. Pleural effusion
B. Consolidation
C. Pulmonary fibrosis
D. Lymphadenopathy

99. Primary Tuberculosis most commonly involves *(DNB 2012)*
A. Lungs
B. Liver
C. Brain
D. Intestine

100. Primary complex in which of the following sites suggest congenital tuberculosis *(DNB 2011)*
A. Lungs
B. Liver
C. Lymph nodes
D. Skin

101. Most common site of primary infection in congenital tuberculosis is *(DNB 2012)*
A. Lungs
B. Liver
C. Lymph nodes
D. Skin

102. Most commonly involved organ in congenital tuberculosis is *(DNB 2010)*
A. Lungs
B. Liver
C. Lymph nodes
D. Skin

103. All of the following statements about Miliary Tuberculosis are true Except:
A. May occur following primary infection
B. May occur following secondary reactivation
C. Sputum microscopy is usually negative
D. Montoux is always positive
E. Liver, kidney and spleen are common sites of involvement

104. The following statement stands *true* for Mantoux test *(AI 1996)*
A. Test is read before 48 hrs
B. 6-9 mm induration shows maximum chances of developing TB
C. A positive test does not indicate that the person is suffering from disease.
D. New cases are more likely to occur in tuberculin negative person than those who already are tuberculin reactors

105. False-negative tuberculin test is seen in *all except:* *(AI 1996)*
A. After 4-6 weeks of measles attack
B. Immunodeficiency state
C. Miliary tuberculosis
D. Atypical mycobacterial infection

106. Investigations in a clinically suspected case of tuberculosis – *(PGI June 07)*
A. Mantoux (in children)
B. Sputum AFB
C. PCR
D. Bactec
E. All of the above

107. A man presents with fever, wt loss and cough; Mantoux reads an induration of 17 x 19 mm; Sputum cytology is negative for AFB. Most likely diagnosis is: *AI 2001)*
A. Pulm tuberculosis
B. Fungal infection
C. Viral infection
D. Pneumonia

108. A 25 year old man presented with fever, cough, expectoration and breathlessness of 2 months duration. Contrast enhanced computed tomography of the chest showed bilateral upper lobe fibrotic lesions and mediastinum had enlarged necrotic nodes with peripheral rim enhancement. Which one of the following is the most probable diagnosis: *(AI 03)*
A. Sarcoidosis
B. Tuberculosis
C. Lymphoma
D. Silicosis

109. A 25 year old man presented with fever and cough, expectoration and breathlessness of 2 months

duration. Contrast enhanced computed tomography of the chest showed bilateral upper lobe fibrotic lesions and mediastinum had enlarged necrotic nodes with peripheral rim enhancement. Which one of the following is the most probable diagnosis:
A. Sarcoidosis (AIIMS May 04)
B. Tuberculosis
C. Lymphoma
D. Silicosis

110. Rasmussen's aneurysm arises from
A. Bronchial artery
B. Pulmonary artery
C. Vertebral artery
D. Posterior intercostals artery

111. Multidrug Resistance Tuberculosis (MDR-TB) should be considered in patients with:
A. Contact with a known case of MDR TB
B. Clinical Deterioration (PGI-Dec-05)
C. Sputum smear positive at 5 months of treatment
D. All of the above

112. A young man with tuberculosis presents with massive recurrent hemoptysis. For angiographic treatment which vascular structure should be evaluated first-
A. Pulmonary artery (AIIMS May 03)
B. Bronchial artery
C. Pulomary vein
D. Superior vena cava

Sarcoidosis

113. B/L hilar lymphadenopathy, along with non caseating granulomas is a characteristic feature of: (AI 1997)
A. Sarcoidosis
B. Scleroderma
C. SLE
D. Stein-leventhal syndrome

114. All are correct regarding sarcoidosis *except* :
A. Often cavitate (AIIMS Dec 98)
B. Spontancous remission is usual
C. Tuberculine test is negative
D. B/L hilar lymphadenopathy.

115. A woman is admitted with complains of low-grade fever of 6 weeks duration. Chest radiograph reveals bihilar adenopathy with clear lung fields. All of the following investigations will be useful in differential diagnosis *except* : (AI 2004)
A. CD4/CD8 counts in the blood
B. Serum ACE levels
C. CECT of chest
D. Gallium scan

Adult Respiratory Distress Syndrome (ARDS)

116. Shock Lung is better known as: (DNB 2010)
A. Alveolar Proteinosis
B. Alveolar Haemorrhage
C. Pulmonary edema
D. ARDS

117. Acute lung injury in caused by all of the following *except* : (AIIMS May 02)
A. Aspiration
B. Toxic gas inhalation
C. Cardiopulmonary bypass with heart lung machine.
D. Lung contusion.

118. Normal PCWP with pulmonary oedema is seen in :
A. Left atrial myxoma (AIIMS June 98)
B. High altitude
C. Pulmonary vein obstruction
D. Pulmonary artery obstruction.

119. ARDS is associated with (PGI Dec-04)
A. Acute pancreatitis
B. Trauma
C. Severe Falciparum malaria
D. All of the above

120. A patient comes with sudden respiratory distress, on examination, bilateral basal crepts are present over chest suggestive of pulmonary edema with normal alveolar wedge pressure. The likely cause is
A. Narcotic overdose (AIIMS June 2000)
B. Congestive heart failure
C. Myocardial infarction
D. Cardiogenic shock

121. Which of the following is the most characteristic feature of Adult Respiratory Distress Syndrome (ARDS): (AI 2012)
A. Diffuse Alveolar Damage
B. Hypoxemia and Hypoxia
C. Surfactant Deficiency
D. Hypocapnia

122. All are seen in ARDS, *except* : (AIIMS May 95)
A. Pulmonary edema
B. Decreased tidal volume.
C. Hypercapnia
D. Decreased compliance

123. All of the following features can seen in ARDS except:
A. Pulmonary Shunting
B. Reduced compliance
C. Hypoxemia
D. Hypercapnia

124. Which of the following is not seen in ARDS:
A. Pulmonary edema (AI 1996)
B. Hypoxemia
C. Stiff lung
D. Hypercapnia

125. Which of the following is not seen in ARDS
A. Hypoxemia (DNB 2012)
B. Hypercapnia
C. Pulmonary edema
D. Stiff lung

126. In ARDS, not true is – (PGI June 99)
A. Decreased pulmonary compliance
B. Increased pulmonary artery pressure

C. Increased left atrial pressure
D. Severe hypoxemia

127. Feature of shock lung is- *(AIIMS Nov 07)*
A. Diffuse alveolar damage
B. Usual interstitial penumonitis
C. Organizing pneumonia
D. Bronchilolitis

128. Acute Lung Injury (ALI) is characterized by all except
A. $PaO_2/FiO_2 < 200$mm Hg
B. Bilateral interstitial infiltrates
C. PCWP <18 mm Hg
D. Normal Left atrial pressure

129. Acute Lung injury is characterized by all, Except:
A. Alveolar infiltrates *(PGI Dec 04)*
B. Hypoxemia
C. Pulmonary shunting
D. $PaO_2/FIO_2 <200$mm of Hg
E. None of the above

Pulmonary Thromboembolism

130. A patient with fracture pelvis is admitted in ICU after surgery. Post operatively he develops sudden dyspnea and chest pain. The likely cause is :
A. Pulmonary thromboembolism *(AIIMS Nov 99)*
B. Shock
C. Respiratory infection
D. ARDS

131. All are true about pulmonary embolism, except :
A. Chest pain is the most common symptom
B. Most commonly presents within 2 weeks
C. More is the survival time, more is the chance of recovery *(AIIMS May 94)*
D. Arises from leg veins

132. The most common cause of preventable Hospital Death is *(DNB 2009)*
A. Acute Pulmonary Embolism
B. Heart Failure
C. Myocardial Infarction
D. Cancer

133. The most common cause of Pulmonary thromboembolism *(DNB 2009)*
A. DIC
B. Coagulation Disorder
C. DVT
D. Venous Hypertension

134. The most common source of pulmonary embolism is:
A. Amniotic fluid embolism *(AIIMS May 95)*
B. Calf vein thrombi
C. Large veins of leg
D. Cardio thoracic surgery

135. All of the following conditions may predispose to pulmonary embolism except: *(AI 2003)*
A. Protein S deficiency
B. Malignancy
C. Obesity
D. Progesterone therapy

136. In acute pulmonary embolism, the most frequent ECG finding is :
A. S1Q3T3 pattern *(AIIMS May' 06)*
B. P. pulmonale
C. Sinus tachycardia
D. Right axis deviation

137. D-Dimer values may be increased in all of the following Except
A. Myocardial infarction
B. Pneumonia
C. Anticoagulant therapy
D. Pregnancy

138. D-dimer is the most sensitive diagnostic test for –
A. Pulmonary embolism *AIIMS May 05)*
B. Acute pulmonary oedema
C. Cardiac tamponade
D. Acute myocardial infarction

139. D-Dimer is the most sensitive test for
A. DVT
B. Pulmonary Embolism
C. Acute Pulmonary adema
D. Acute myocardial infarction

140. Best investigation when there is clinical suspicion of pulmonary embolism in a patient is-
A. D-Dimmer Assay
B. Multidetector CT angiography
C. Doppler ultrasound
D. Catheter angiography

141. A 55 year old man who has been on bed rest for the past 10 days, complains of breathlessness and chest pain. The chest X-ray is normal. The next investigation should be: *(AI 2003) (AI 2004)*
A. Lung ventilation-perfusion scan
B. Pulmonary arteriography
C. Pulmonary venous angiography
D. Echocardiography

142. The most definitive method of diagnosing pulmonary embolism is : *(AIIMS Nov. 05)*
A. Pulmonary aterigraphy
B. Radioisotope perfusion pulmonary scintigraphy
C. EKG
D. Venography

143. A young patient presents to the Emergency with Acute pulmonary embolism. Patient's blood pressure is normal but echocardiography reveals Right ventricular hypokinesia and compromised cardiac output.
The treatment of choice in this patient is:
A. Thrombolytic therapy *(AIIMS Nov 2001)*
B. Anticoagulation with low molecular weight heparin
C. Anticoagulation with warfarin
D. Inferior vena cora filters

3

Respiratory System

Pulmonary Hypertension

144. In primary pulmonary hypertension basic abnormality in gene lies in: *(AIIMS May 07)*
   A. Bone morphogenic protein receptor II
   B. Endothelin
   C. Homebox gene
   D. PAX – 11
145. Not seen in pre capillary pulmonary hypertension: *(PGI June 98)*
   A. ↑ pressure in pulm. circulation
   B. ↑ capillary pressure
   C. Rt-vent.hypertrophy
   D. ↑ Pulmonary wedge pressure
146. Precapillary Pulmonary hypertension is caused by all Except: *(PGI June 03)*
   A. Mitral stenosis
   B. Pulmonary vasculitis
   C. Primary pulmonary hypertension
   D. Thromboembolism
147. All are causes of pulmonary hypertension except- *(AIIMS Nov 07)*
   A. Hyperventilation
   B. Morbid obesity
   C. High altitude
   D. Fenfluramine
148. Pulmonary hypertension may occur in all of the following conditions except- *(AIIMS Nov 06)*
   A. Toxic oil syndrome
   B. Progressive systemic sclerosis
   C. Sickle cell anemia
   D. Argemone mexicana poisoning
149. Pulmonary hypertension in COPD is due to all, Except: *(PGI Dec 97)*
   A. Hypoxia
   B. Pulmonary vasoconstriction
   C. High lung volume
   D. Bronchoconstriction
150. A 29 year old unmarried female presents with progressive dyspnea. Her X ray chest shows clear lung fields. Pulmonary function testing reveals in FVC of 92%; FEV1/FVC of 89%; and dlCO of 59%. On exercise testing her oxygen saturation drops from 92% to 86%. What is the likely diagnosis: *(AIIMS Nov 2008)*
   A. Alveolar hypoventilation
   B. Primary pulmonary hypertension
   C. Interstitial lung disease
   D. Anxiety
151. A 29 year old anxious lady presents with a history of progressive breathlessness and exercise intolerance since four months. Her FVC is 90% and FEV1 / FVC is 86%. Oxygen saturation after exercise was observed to drop from 92% to 86%. What is the likely diagnosis : *(AI 2010)*
   A. Primary alveolar hypoventilation
   B. Primary pulmonary hypertension
   C. Anxiety disorder
   D. Interstitial lung disease
152. Chronic Cor pulmonale is seen in all except: *(PGI-Dec-04)*
   A. Pulmonary embolization
   B. COPD
   C. Cystic fibrosis
   D. Primary pulmonary hypertension
153. The most common cause for chronic cor pulmonale is: *PGI Dec 04)*
   A. Recurrent pulmonary embolization
   B. COPD
   C. Cystic fibrosis
   D. Bronchial Asthma
   E. Airway foreign body
154. The most common cause of acute cor pulmonale is: *(AIIMS Nov 02)*
   A. Pneumonia.
   B. Pulmonary thromboembolism.
   C. Chronic obstructive pulmonary disease.
   D. Primary spontaneous pneumothorax.
155. All the following are radiological features of Chronic Cor pulmonale except-
   A. Kerley B lines
   B. Prominent lower lobe vessels
   C. Pleural effusion
   D. Cardiomegaly

Pleural Diseases

Pleural Effusion

156. Which one of the following conditions may lead to exudative pleural effusion *(AI 2003)*
   A. Cirrhosis
   B. Nephrotic syndrome
   C. Congestive heart failure
   D. Bronchogenic carcinoma
157. All of the following are causes of Transdative pleural effusion Except: *(PGI-June-02)*
   A. Nephrotic syndrome
   B. Rheumatoid arthritis
   C. Constrictive pericarditis
   D. Myxedema
   E. Pulmonary embolism
158. Left –sided pleural effusion seen in *(PGI- June- 02)*
   A. Pancreatitis
   B. Rheumatoid arthritis
   C. Hypoproteinemia
   D. CCF
   E. Esophageal rupture
159. All of the following are true about pleural effusion, Except: (select two options)
   A. Horizontal fluid level
   B. Decreased lung volume
   C. Decreased heart sounds
   D. Decreased chest movement
   E. Succussion splash

160. Tuberculous pleural effusion is characterised by all of the following features *except* effusion :
A. Harmorrhagic effusion *(AI 1997)*
B. Pleural fluid LDH more than 60% that of serum LDH.
C. Increased deaminase
D. Increased mesothelial cells

161. Pleural fluid having low glucose is seen in all, except-
A. Tuberculosis *(AIIMS May 93)*
B. Empyema
C. Mesothelioma
D. Rheumatoid arthritis

162. All of the following show low glucose in pleural fluid, EXCEPT- *(AIIMS Dec 94)*
A. Empyema
B. Malignant pleural effusion
C. Rheumatoid arthritis
D. Dressler's syndrome

163. Low glucose in pleural effusion is seen in all, *except*
A. Dressler syndrome *(AIIMS May 94)*
B. Empyema
C. Malignant pleural effusion
D. Rheumatoid arthritis

164. Decreased Glucose in pleural effusion is seen in: (Select best two correct options) *(PGI June 99)*
A. Rheumatoid arthritis
B. SLE
C. Pneumococcal infection
D. P.carinii infection

165. A high amylase level in pleural fluid suggests a diagnosis of *(AIIMS May 03)*
A. Tuberculosis
B. Malignancy
C. Rheumatoid arthritis
D. Pulmonary infarction

166. Amylase increased in pleural fluid is seen in following except: *(PGI June 2000)*
A. Rheumatoid arthritis
B. Esophageal perforation
C. Malignancy
D. Gall stone pancreatitis

167. Presence of cholesterol crystal in pleural effusion is a feature of : *(AIIMS June 97)*
A. Myxoedema
B. Hypertriglyceridemia
C. Hyperthyroidism
D. Sarcoidosis

168. In an adult patient with plural effusion, the most appropriate site for plurisentesis done by inserting a needle is in: *(AI 2002)*
A. 5th intercostals space in midclevicular line
B. 7th intercostal space in mid axillary's bone
C. 2nd intercostals space adjacent to the sternum
D. 10th intercostal space adjacent to the vertebral column

Pneumothorax

169. Pneumothorax is seen in all, except-
A. Marfan syndrome *(AIIMS May 94)*
B. Assisted ventilation
C. Eosinophilic granuloma
D. Bronchopulmonary Aspergillosis

170. While inserting a central venous catheter, a patient develops respiratory distress. The most likely cause is: *(AI 2002)*
A. Hemothorax
B. Pneumothorax
C. Pleural effusion
D. Hypovolumia

171. All of the following are characteristic features of primary spontaneous penumotharax Except
A. Male gender *(AIIMS 92)*
B. Old age
C. Tall stature
D. History of smoking

172. Spontaneous pneumothorax is commonly seen in:
A. Smokers *(PGI June 02)*
B. Young females
C. Old age
D. Short statured men

173. Which of the following statements about pneumothorax is true: *(AIIMS Dec 94)*
A. Breath sounds are increased
B. Percussion note is decreased
C. Always needs chest tube insertion
D. Often needs chest tube insertion

174. A 30 year old female comes acute breathlessness, neck vein distention, and absent breath sounds and nediastinal shift. Which of the following should be done immediately? *(PGI June 2008)*
A. HRCT is the investigation of choice
B. ABG analysis should be done
C. CXR
D. Large bore needle puncture of pleura

175. In left sided massive pneumothorax, ECG shows all, *except :* *(AIIMS May 94)*
A. Left axis deviation
B. Absent R wave
C. Peaked P wave
D. Precordial T wave inversion

176. IPPV can cause all of the following *except*:
A. Barotrauma *(AI 2001)*
B. Pleural effusion
C. Missing
D. None of the above

Disorders of Ventilation and Mediastinitis

177. "Sleep apnoea", is defined as a temporary pause in breathing during sleep lasting at least-
A. 40 seconds *(AIIMS May 03)*

B. 30 seconds
C. 20 seconds
D. 10 seconds

178. True about primary pulmonary hypoventilation is:
A. Does not respond to chemical stimuli
B. Hypocapnoea and normal PaO_2
C. Common in children (AIIMS Feb 97)
D. Respiratory alkalosis is diagnostic

179. All are true about bilateral diaphragmatic paralysis, *except*: (AIIMS May 95)
A. Sniff test is positive
B. Causes normocapnic failure
C. Diaphragmatic pacing is useful if any nerve is intact
D. None of the above

180. Most common cause of Mediastinitis is:
A. Tracheal rupture (AIIMS 97)
B. Esophageal rupture
C. Drugs
D. Idiopathic

Lung (Bronchogenic) Tumors

Bronchogenic carcinoma

181. Most common bronchogenic carcinoma is
A. Small cell carcinoma (AIIMS June 2000)
B. Squamous cell carcinoma
C. Mixed cell carcinoma
D. Adenocarcinoma

182. Most common type of carcinoma lung is-
A. Small cell carcinoma (AIIMS May 93)
B. Adenocarcinoma
C. Squamous cell carcinoma
D. Large cell carcinoma

183. All of the following are true regarding oat cell carcinoma of lung, *except*: (AIIMS June 99)
A. Varient of large cell anaplastic CA
B. Chemotherapy is effective
C. Paraneoplastic syndrome may be present
D. Causes SIADH

184. All of the following statements about small cell carcinomas are true, Except (PGI-June- 06)
A. Commonest Malignancy of lung
B. Associated with parancoplastic syndrome
C. Cause SVC obstruction
D. Chemosensitive
E. Commonly metaslistre to brain

185. Which of the following statements about small cell carcinoma is true? (AI 2009)
A. Bone metastasis is uncommon
B. Peripheral in location
C. Chemosensitive tumor
D. Paraneoplastic syndrome with ↑PTH is common

186. All of the following statements about Non Small Cell Carcinoma of Lung (NSCCL) are true, Except:
A. Contralateral mediastinal nodes are a contraindication to surgical resection (AI 2012)
B. Single Agent Chemotherapy is preferred for patient > 70 years with advanced disease
C. Squammous Cell Carcinoma is the most common NSCCL amongst Asian population
D. Gefitinib is most effective for female smokers with adenocarcinoma on histology

187. In a chronic smoker, a highly malignant aggressive and metastatic lung carcinoma is :
A. Squamous cell Carcinoma (AIIMS May 01)
B. Small cell Carcinoma
C. Adenocarcinoma
D. Large cell carcinoma

188. Following hormonal levels are increased in small cell carcinoma of lung *except*: (AI 1997)
A. ACTH
B. Growth hormone
C. ANF
D. AVP

189. Type of lung carcinoma producing superior vena cava syndrome: (AIIMS June 97)
A. Squamous cell carcinoma
B. Adenocarcinoma
C. Small cell carcinoma
D. Anaplastic carcinoma

190. Carcinoma lung responding best to chemotherapy-
A. Squamous cell type
B. Oat cell type
C. Adenocarcinoma
D. All respond equally

191. Clubbing is least common in: (AIIMS Dec 97)
A. Squamous cell carcinoma
B. Adenocarcinoma
C. Small cell carcinoma of lung
D. Mesothelioma

192. A 60 year old man presents with non productive cough and haemoptysis for 4 weeks; He has grade III clubbing, and a lesion in the apical lobe on x ray. Most likely diagnosis here is :
A. Small cell ca (AI 2001) (AIIMS June 2000)
B. Non small cell ca
C. Fungal infection
D. Tuberculosis

193. What is TRUE regarding adenocarcinoma lung
A. Causes 50% of lung cancers (AIIMS Dec 94)
B. Unlikely histological variant in young patients
C. Associated with subcutaneous angiomyolipoma
D. Peripheral location

194. True statement about adenocarcinoma lung are (Choose two best options): (PGI June 05)
A. Common in females
B. Not associated with smoking

C. Central cavitation is a charachteristic feature
D. Peripheral involvement is common
E. Upper lobe involvement is common

195. Commonest type of lung carcinoma in nonsmokers is
A. Squamous cell carcinoma *(AIIMS Dec 94)*
B. Adenocarcinoma
C. Alveolar cell carcinoma
D. Small cell carcinoma

196. Lung to lung metastasis is seen in-
A. Adenocarcinoma of lung
B. Squamous cell carcinoma
C. Small cell carcinoma
D. Neuroendocrine tumor of lung

197. A patient presents with secondaries to the adrenals. The most common site of primary is :
A. Lung *(AI 2000)*
B. Kidney
C. Breast
D. Stomach

198. Which of the following statements about lung carcinoma is true *(AI 2010)*
A. Squammous cell variant accounts for 70% of all lung cancers
B. Oat cell variant typically present with cavitation
C. Oat cell variant is typically associated with hilar adenopathy
D. Adenocarcinoma variant is typically central in location

199. Most common symptom of lung carcinoma
A. Cough *(AIIMS 90)*
B. Dyspnoea
C. Weight loss
D. Chest pain

200. The commonest intrabronchial cause of haemopysis is
A. Carcinoma lung *(AIIMS May 95)*
B. Adenoma lung
C. Emphysema
D. Bronchiectasis

201. A 60 years old chronic smoker presents with complaints of hemoptysis. Her chest X-ray appears to be normal. What is the next best investigation:
A. Bronchoscopy *(AIIMS Nov. 2000)*
B. High resolution CT
C. Sputum cytology
D. Pulmonary function test

202. A 60 year old man is suspected of having bronchogenic ca: TB has been ruled out in this pt. What should be the next investigation- *(AI 01)*
A. CT guided FNAC
B. Bronchoscopy and biopsy
C. Sputum cytology
D.. X-Ray chest

203. A 60 yr old man is suspected of having bronchogenic ca; TB has been ruled out in this pt.What should be the next investigation :
A. CT guided FNAC *(AI 2001)*
B. Bronchoscopy and biopsy
C. Sputum cytology
D. X-Ray chest.

204. A patient presents with a cavitatory lesion in right upper lobe of lung. The best investigation is –
A. Branchoscopy, lavage and brushing *(AI 2000)*
B. C.T. Scan
C. X ray
D. FNAC

205. A patient presents with a cavitatory lesion in right upper lobe of lung. The best investigation is-
A. Branchoscopy, lavage and brushing *(AI 2000)*
B. C.T. Scan
C. X ray
D. FNAC

206. Serum ACE may be raised in all of the following *except* : *(AI 2005)*
A. Sarcoidosis
B. Silicosis
C. Berylliosis
D. Bronchogenic carcinoma

207. A 60 year old male was diagnosed as carcinoma right lung. On CECT chest there was a tumor of 5x5 cm in upper lobe and another 2x2 cm size tumor nodule in middle lobe. The primary modality of treatment is :
A. Radiotherapy *(AI 2004)*
B. Chemotherapy
C. Surgery
D. Supportive treatment

208. Ramesh 40 yrs male patient presenting with polyuria, pain abdomen, nausea, vomiting, altered sensorium was found to have bronchogenic carcinoma. The electrolyte abnormality seen in him would be:
A. Hypokalemia *(AIIMS May 02)*
B. Hyperkalemia
C. Hypocalcaemia
D. Hypercalcemia

209. A 60 year old male presented to the emergency with breathlessness, facial swelling and dilated veins on the chest wall. The most common cause is: *(AI 2003)*
A. Thymoma
B. Lung cancer
C. Hodgkin's lymphoma
D. Superior vena caval obstruction

210. Which of the following tumor is most commonly associated with superior vena cava syndrome:
A. Lymphoma *(AI 2011)*
B. Small cell carcinoma
C. Non small cell carcinoma
D. Metastasis

Cystic Fibrosis

211. Which of the following systems is least likely to be affected in cystic fibrosis *(DNB June 2010)*
   A. Respiratory
   B. Genitourinary
   C. Hepatobiliary
   D. Endocrine
212. The most common cause of pulmonary infection in cystic fibrosis is
   A. Pseudomonas Aeroginosa
   B. Staphylococcus Aureus
   C. Bukholderia cenocapacea
   D. Nontuberculous mycobacteria
213. Most common pathogen causing, pulmonary infection in cystic fibrosis in infants & young children is
   A. Staphylococcus Aureus
   B. Pseudomonas Aeroginosa
   C. Bukholderia Cenocapacea
   D. Nontubercular mycobacteria

Bronchial Ademoma and Bronchial Cysts

214. Bronchial adenoma commonly present as :
   A. Recurrent hemoptysis
   B. Cough
   C. Dysponea
   D. Chest pain
215. Which of the following statements about Branchial cysts is true: *(AI 1993)*
   A. 50-70% are seen in lungs
   B. Most common site is mediastinum
   C. They are premalignant lesions
   D. Infection is uncommon in Pulmonary bronchogenic cysts

Kartagener's Syndrome

216. All of the following are true about Kartagener's syndrome, Except *(PGI-Dec-04)*
   A. Dextrocardia
   B. Infertility
   C. Mental retardation
   D. Bronchiectasis
217. Kartagener's syndrome includes all of the following, Except : *(PGI June 01)*
   A. Situs inversus
   B. Bronchiectasis
   C. Sinusitis
   D. Male infertility
   E. Cystic fibrosis

Pulmonary Renal Syndrome

218. Causes of pulmonary renal syndrome: *(PGI June 07)*
   A. Leptospirosis
   B. Hanta virus
   C. Paraquat poisoning
   D. All of the above
219. A patient presents with hemoptysis and hematuria few weeks after a respiratory tract infection. ANCA antibodies are present. Likely diagnosis is:
   A. Goodpasture's syndrome *(AI 1995)*
   B. IgA Nephropathy
   C. Nephrotic syndrome
   D. PSGN
220. Rama, a 20 year old smoker, presents with hemoptysis and hematuria. Likely diagnosis is:
   A. Good pasture's syndrome *(AI 1997)*
   B. Nephrotic syndrome
   C. Gullian Barre syndrome
   D. IgA Nephropathy

Neonate Alveolar Proteinosis

221. A male born at term after an uncomplicated pregnancy, labor and delivery develops severe respiratory distress within a few hours of birth. Results of routine culture were negative. The chest roengogram reveals a normal heart shadow and fine reticulonodular infiltrates radiating from the hilum. ECHO findings reveal no abnormality. Family history reveals similar clinical course and death of a male and female sibling at 1 month and 2 months of age respectively. The most likely diagnosis is: *(AI 2008)*
   A. Neonatal Alveolar Proteinosis
   B. Total Anomalous Pulmonary Venous Circulation (TAPVC)
   C. Meconium Aspiration Syndrome
   D. Diffuse Herpes simplex infection
222. 3.5 kg term male baby, born of uncomplicated pregnancy, developed respiratory distress at birth, not responded to surfactant, ECHO finding revealed nothing abnormal, X-ray showed ground glass appearance and culture negative. Apgars 4 and 5 at 1 and 5 minutes. History of one month female sibling died before. What is the diagnosis? *(AIIMS Nov 07)*
   A. TAPVC
   B. Meconium aspiration
   C. Neonatal pulmonary alveolar proteinosis
   D. Diffuse herpes simplex infection

Symptoms and Signs of Respiratory Disease

223. Which of the following is least likely cause of hemoptysis *(PGI June 07)*
 A. Pneumonia
 B. Empyema
 C. Bronchiectasis
 D. Metral stenosis

224. Cavernous Respiration is seen in: *(DNB 2012)*
 A. Cavity
 B. Consolidation
 C. Fibrosis
 D. Interstitial Inflammation

225. Which of the following is not a feature of consolidation *(DNB 2010)*
 A. Increased vocal resonance
 B. Dull Percussion note
 C. Bronchial Breath sounds
 D. Tracheal shift to side of consolidation

226. A patient presents with sudden onset of breathlessness after a subclavian vein cannulation. On examination, breath sounds are absent while the chest is hyper-resonant on percussion on one side. Most likely cause is: *(AI 2012)*
 A. Iatrogenic Pneumothorax
 B. Subclavian Vein air embolus
 C. Malposition of cannula
 D. Cardiac Arrhythmia

227. The most common site of bleeding in Hemoptysis is *(DNB)*
 A. Tracheobronchial tree
 B. Pulmonary Parenchyma
 C. Pleural Disease
 D. All of the above

228. The artery most frequently responsible for bleeding in massive hemoptysis is *(DNB 2009)*
 A. Bronchial Artery
 B. Pulmonary Artery
 C. Intersegmental Artery
 D. Intercostal Artery

229. All of the following statements about central cyanosis are true Except:
 A. Central cyanosis becomes evident when reduced haemoglobin < 5g/dl
 B. Chronic Asthma may cause central cyanosis
 C. Alveolar Hypoventilation causes central cyanosis
 D. Methemoglobinemia causes central cyanosis

230. Cause of central cyanosis include all of the following, Except
 A. Chronic Asthma
 B. Congenital Pulmonary stenosis
 C. Congestive heart failure
 D. Alveolar hypoventilation

231. Cyanosis NOT improving with 100% oxygen in case of: *(AIIMS May 93)*
 A. Cardiac Asthma
 B. Interstitial lung disease
 C. Bronchial asthma
 D. Tetralogy of Fallot (TOF)

232. One of the following condition is not associated with clubbing : *(AIIMS Dec 98)*
 A. Primary biliary cirrhosis
 B. Chronic bronchitis
 C. Cryptogenic fibrosing alveolitis
 D. Central bronchiectasis

233. Causes of unilateral clubbing include all of the following, Except *(PGI June 05)*
 A. Congenital cyanotic heart disease
 B. Panicoast tumor
 C. Aortic Aneurym
 D. Brachial AV fistulas

234. Hypoxemia seen in: *(PGI June 02)*
 A. Hypoventilation
 B. Decreased Fio_2
 C. Myasthenia gravis
 D. Pulmonary emboli
 E. All of the above

235. Platypnea may be seen in all of the following conditions, except *(PGI June 05)*
 A. Bilateral Diaphragmatic palsy
 B. Pleural effusion
 C. Pulmonary embolism
 D. Cirrhosis
 E. COPD

236. Homogenous opacification of right hemithorax with right sided shift of mediastinum may be caused by *(PGI June 97)*
 A. Collapse of Right lung
 B. Consolidation of Right lung
 C. Right sided hemothorax
 D. Left sided hydrothorax
 E. All of the above

237. A child develops acute respiratory distress, stridor, hyperinflation on one side of chest with decreased breath sound on that side. Most likely cause is : *(AIIMS June 2000)*
 A. Asthma
 B. Aspiration pneumonia
 C. Foreign body aspiration
 D. Pleural effusion

Miscellaneous

238. Bilateral Rhonchii may be seen in all of the following Except *(PGI June 08)*
 A. Pulmonary Edema
 B. Bronchiectasis
 C. Pulmonary Embolism
 D. Emphysema

239. Static compliance is decreased in all of the following except: *(PGI 2000)*
 A. ARDS
 B. Pulmonary edema
 C. Interstial fibrosis
 D. Fibrosing alveolitis
 E. Emphysema

240. Pulmonary Compliance is decreased in all of the following conditions, Except: *(AI 2011)*
A. Pulmonary Congestion
B. COPD
C. Decreased Surfactant
D. Pulmonary Fibrosis

241. Thickening of pulmonary alveolar – capillary membrane is seen in : *(PGI June 07)*
A. Asthma
B. Bronchitis
C. Pulmonary fibrosis
D. Emphysema

242. Smoking is generally not associated as a risk factor with- *(AI 06)*
A. Small cell carcinoma
B. Respiratory bronchiolitis
C. Emphysema
D. Bronchiolitis obliterans organizing pneumonia

243. All are cavitating lesions in the lungs, except-
A. Caplan's syndrome *(AIIMS May 94)*
B. Hamartoma
C. Wegner's granuloma
D. Squamous cell carcinoma

244. Which of the following statements is true about High Attitude Pulmonary Edema (HAPE)?
A. Not exacerbated by exercise *(AIIMS Nov. 06)*
B. Associated with pulmonary vasoconstriction
C. Occurs only in unacclamatized individuals
D. Associated with low cardiac output

245. Bronchial hyperplasia may be caused by all except-
A. Smoking
B. Theophylline
C. Prematurity
D. Allergy

246. Most common cause of amoebic lung abscess is :
A. Aspiration *(AI 1997)*
B. Direct spread from liver
C. Hematogenous spread from liver
D. Hematogenous spread from gut

247. Measurements of intravacular pressure by a pulmonary artery catheter should be done: *(AI 2002)*
A. At end expiration
B. At peak of inspiration
C. During mid inspiration
D. During mid expiration

248. A 62 years old man with carcinoma of lung presented to emergency department with respiratory distress. His EKG showed electrical alternans. The most likely diagnosis is : *(AIIMS May 03)*
A. Pneumothorax.
B. Pleural effusion.
C. Cardiac tamponade.
D. Constrictive pericarditis.

249. The most common fetal response to acute hypoxia is:
A. Tachycardia *(AI 2009)*
B. Tachypnea
C. Bradycardia
D. Ventricular Arrhythmia

250. Hypersensitivity Pneumonitis is classically described as a: *(AI 2009)*
A. Type I hypersensitivity reaction
B. Tye II hypersensitivity reaction
C. Type III (Immune complex) Hypersensitivity
D. Type IV (Cell mediated) Hypersensitivity

251. A child presented with severe respiratory distress two days after birth.On examination he was observed to have a scaphoid abdomen and decreased breath sounds on the left side. He was managed by prompt Endotracheal intubation .After ET tube placement the maximal cardiac impulse shifted further to the right side. What should be the next step in management?
A. Confirm the position of endotracheal tube by chest X ray *(AI 2008)*
B. Remove tube and reattempt intubation
C. Nasogastric tube insertion & decompress the bowel
D. Chest X ray to confirm diagnosis

252. A child presented with severe respiratory distress two days after birth. On examination he was observed to have a scaphoid abdomen and decreased breath sounds on the left side. He was managed by prompt Endotracheal intubation. After ET tube placement the maximal cardiac impulse shifted further to the right side. What should be the next step in management?
A. Confirm the position of endotracheal tube by chest X ray *(AI 2008)*
B. Emergency surgery
C. Nasogastric tube insertion & decompress the bowel
D. Chest X ray to confirm diagnosis

253. A $7_{1/2}$ months old child with cough, mild stridor is started on oral antibiotics. The child showed initial improvement but later developed wheeze, productive cough, and mild fever. X–ray shows hyperlucency and PFT shows an obstructive curve. The most probable diagnosis is, *(AI 2008)*
A. Bronchiolitis obliterans
B. Post viral syndrome
C. Pulmonary alveolar microlithiasis
D. Follicular bronchitis

254. Respiratory centre depression is caused by all of the following, Except: *(AIIMS Nov 2010)*
A. Opium
B. Strychnine
C. Barbiturates
D. Gelsemium

ANSWERS, REFERENCES, EXPLANATIONS AND RELEVANT HIGH YIELD FACTS

Respiratory failure & Disturbance in Respiratory Functions

1. Answer is D (Normal A-a gradient): *Harrison 16th/1583,1584; 17th/1590; API 8th/1286; Refer previous question*

Type I Respiratory failure is characterized by an increase in alveolar arterial O_2 gradient.

Respiratory failure *is defined as a disorder wherein, lung function is inadequate to meet the metabolic demands of the individual and is unable to maintain normal arterial gas levels in the blood.*

It is of two types:

Type I Respiratory failure	Type II Respiratory failure
Represents failure of oxygenation and is characterized by a low PaO_2 with normal or low $PaCO_2$. PaO_2 : Low (< 60 mm Hg) $PaCO_2$: Normal or low (≤.49 mm Hg) $P_{A\text{-}a}O_2$: Increased	Represents a defect in ventilation (hypoventilation) and is characterized by decreased PaO_2 with increase $PaCO_2$. PaO_2 : Decreased (< 60 mm Hg) $PaCO_2$: Increased (> 49 mm Hg) $P_{A\text{-}a}O_2$: Normal
Causes :	**Causes :**
This type is caused by conditions which affect oxygenation, like: • Parenchymal diseases (V-Q mismatch) • Diseases of vasculature/shunts Examples: - Pneumonia Q - ARDS Q - Emphysema Q - Right to left shunts Q	This type is caused by conditions causing hypoventilation as in: • Obstructive lung disease: COPD, F. body • Decreased central respiratory drive e.g. CNS disorders like : Brain injury, Meningitis • Weakness of respiratory muscle e.g. - Peripheral N.S. disorders like: M. gravis. - Interstitial lung disease. Q - MS disorders like polymyositis. - Rib cage disorders : Kyphoscoliosis.

2. Answer is B (Low PO_2 and high PCO_2): *Harrison 18th/p 2200 Harrison 17th/1676; API Medicine 6th/ 278; 8th/1287*

Type II respiratory failure (or pump failure) *is characterized by* ***decreased PaO_2 and increased $PaCO_2$*** *as a result of alveolar hypoventilation. There is a fall in minute ventilation which causes a rise in $PaCO_2$ and fall in PaO_2.* ***The alveolar arterial gradient (PaO_2 is normal).***

Type I Respiratory failure	Type II Respiratory failure
Hypoxemia with decreased $PaCO_2$	Hypoxemia with increased $PaCO_2$

3. Answer is A (Metabolic acidosis with compensatory respiratory alkalosis): *Harrison 17th/1590; Oxford handbook of Medicine 5th/684*

With pH < 7.35 (7.12) acidosis is confirmed. Abbnormal CO_2 with change in opposite to expected. (acidosis should have increased CO_2) indicates that the change in compensatory (compensatory respiratory alkalosis), Decreased bicarbonates with change in keeping with change in pH suggests that the problem is metabolic. Thus the whole picture respresents metabolic acidosis with compensatory respiratory alkalosis.

Explanation :

Acid base disorders needlessly, confuse many people, but if a few simple rules are applied then interpretation and diagnosis are easy.

pH < 7.35 is acidosis ; pH > 7.45 is alkalosis
1° change in HCO_3^- is termed as metabolic
if change in HCO_3^- is in keeping with the pH (i.e. if there is acidosis and HCO_3^- decreased) the problem is a Metabolic one. If change in HCO_3^- is opposite with the pH (if there is acidosis and HCO_3^- is increased or normal) the problem is compensatory metabolic.
1° change is CO_2 is termed as respiratory
If change in CO_2 is in keeping with the pH (if in acidosis CO_2 is raised) the problem is termed respiratory If change in CO_2 is opposite with the pH (if there is acidosis and CO_2 is decreased or normal) problem is termed as compensatory respiratory.

STEP 1 : What is the pH.

Normal pH	pH of patient	Inference	Acidosis
7.35 – 7.45	7.12	pH is decreased	Acidosis

STEP II : Is it a metabolic or respiratory change

Parameter	Inference	Is change towards acidosis or alkalosis	Is change in keeping with change in pH	Final Inference
pCO_2 = 18mm Hg (Respiratory component)	pCO_2 is decreased	Alkalosis	No	Respiratory component is compensatory
HCO_3- = 12 mmol/1 (Metabolic component)	HCO_3^- is decreased	Acidosis	Yes	Metabolic component is primary

STEP III : Final deduction

Because metabolic component is primary and respiratory component is compensatory the acid base disorder is Metabolic acidosis with compensatory Respiratory alkalosis.

4. **Answer is A (Respiratory acidosis with compensatory metabolic alkalosis) :** *Harrison 18th/p 363, 364 Harrison 17th/1590, 288, 289; Read text below*

Because primary respiratory component is causing acidosis and metabolic component is compensatory by producing alkaosis, the acid base disorder is Respiratory acidosis with compensatory metabolic alkalosis.

STEP 1 : What is the pH.

Normal pH	pH of patient	Inference	Is it acidosis or alkalosis
7.35 – 7.45	7.2	Decreased pH	Acidosis

STEP II : What component is primary and what is compensatory

Parameter	Inference	Is change towards acidosis or alkalosis	Is change in keeping with change in pH	Final Inference
pCO_2 = 50mm Hg (Respiratory component)	increased	acidosis	Yes (pH=7.2 = Acidosis)	Primary component is respiratory (acidosis)
HCO_3^- = 32 mmHg (metabolic component)	increased	Alkalosis	No (pH=7.2 = Acidosis)	Metabolic component is compensatory (alkalotic)

STEP III : Final deduction

Because the primary component is respiratory and the metabolic component is compensatory the acid base disorder is respiratory acidosis with compensatory metabolic alkalosis.

5. **Answer is D (Metabolic Acidosis):** *Textbelow; Oxford Hand book of Medicine 5th/684*

The patient in question has a primary respiratory alkalosis with compensatory metabolic acidosis (↓HCO_3^-). Since the question specifically asks about the compensatory mechanism, metabolic acidosis is the single best answer

The confusing part in the question is the fact that the primary acid base disorder has not been asked. On the contrary the examiner wants to know the compensatory mechanism involved. The compensatory mechanism here is metabolic acidosis which is the single best answer of choice.

PH	Primary Disorder & Parameter	Compensatory mechanism and parameter	Compensatory Mechanism
↓ed	*Metabolic Acidosis (↓HCO_3^-)*	*Respiratory Alkalosis (↓PCO_2)*	*Hyperventilation*
↑ed	*Metabolic Alkalosis (↑HCO_3^-)*	*Respiratory Acidosis (↑PCO_2)*	*Hypoventilation*
↓ed	*Respiratory Acidosis (↑PCO_2)*	*Metabolic Alkalosis (↑HCO_3^-)*	*↑ HCO_3^- reabsorption by kidneys*
↑ed	*Respiratory Alkalosis (↓PCO_2)*	*Metabolic Acidosis (↓HCO_3^-)*	*↓HCO_3^- reabsorption by kidneys*

How we approached the above question : (Refer subsequent explanation)

With pH of 7.5 (> 7.45) alkalosis is confirmed as the primary disorder.
Since change in PCO_2 (↓ed) is in keeping with the change in pH (alkalosis) the primary disorder is Respiratory (Respiratory Alkalosis).
Since change in (↓HCO_3^-) is opposite with the pH (There is alkalosis and HCO_3^- is reduced), the metabolic component (HCO_3^-) is compensatory.
The patient therefore has primary Respiratory Alkalosis with Compensatory Metabolic Acidosis

Step by Step Approach for such questions

Remember : Acidosis is inkeeping with Decreased HCO_3 and Raised pCO2
Remember : Alkalosis is inkeeping with Increased HCO_3 and Decreased pCO2

pH < 7.35 is acidosis ; pH > 7.45 is alkalosis
1° change in HCO_3^- is termed as metabolic (Normal HCO3- = 22 – 30 meq/l)
if change in HCO_3^- is in keeping with the pH (i.e. if there is acidosis and HCO_3^- decreased) the problem is a Metabolic one.
If change in HCO_3^- is opposite with the pH (if there is acidosis and HCO_3^- is increased or normal) the problem is compensatory metabolic.
1° change is CO_2 is termed as respiratory (Normal pCO2 = 35 – 45 mmHg)
If change in CO_2 is in keeping with the pH (if in acidosis CO_2 is raised) the problem is termed respiratory
If change in CO_2 is opposite with the pH (if there is acidosis and CO_2 is decreased or normal) problem is termed as compensatory respiratory.

STEP 1 : What is the pH.

Normal pH	pH of patient	Inference	Primary disorder (Acidosis/Alkalosis)
7.35 – 7.45	7.5	pH is increased	Alkalosis

STEP II : Is it a metabolic or respiratory change

Parameter	Inference	Is change towards acidosis or alkalosis	Is change in keeping with change in pH	Final Inference
pCO_2 = 30mm Hg (Respiratory component)	pCO_2 is decreased	Alkalosis	Yes (pH=7.5 = Alkalosis)	Respiratory component is Primary
HCO_3- = 18 meq/l (Metabolic component)	HCO_3^- is decreased	Acidosis	No (pH=7.5 = Alkalosis)	Metabolic component is Compensatory

STEP III : Final deduction

*Because Respiratory component is primary and metabolic component is compensatory the acid base disorder in this patient is Primary Respiratory Alkalosis with **compensatory Metabolic Acidosis. The compensatory mechanism in this patent therefore is Metabolic Acidosis.***

6. **Answer is C (Respiratory alkalosis):** *Repeat*

A pH of 7.46 (alkalosis) and a reduced pCO2 (30 mmHg) suggests a diagnosis Respiratory alkalosis.
The change in CO2 (alkalosis) is in-keeping with the pH change (alkalosis) thereby suggesting a primary diagnosis of Respiratory alkalosis.

Rules to acid base disorders: Review

pH < 7.35 is acidosis ; pH > 7.45 is alkalosis
1° change in HCO_3^- is termed as metabolic (Normal HCO3- = 22 – 30 meq/l)
if change in HCO_3^- is in keeping with the pH (i.e. if there is acidosis and HCO_3^- decreased) the problem is a Metabolic one.
If change in HCO_3^- is opposite with the pH (if there is acidosis and HCO_3^- is increased or normal) the problem is compensatory metabolic.
1° change is CO_2 is termed as respiratory (Normal pCO2 = 35 – 45 mmHg)
If change in CO_2 is in keeping with the pH (if in alkalosis CO_2 is reduced) the problem is termed respiratory
If change in CO_2 is opposite with the pH (if there is alkalosis and CO_2 is raised) problem is termed as compensatory respiratory.

Stap 1 : What is the pH

Normal pH	pH of patient	Inference	Acid / Base disorder
7.35 – 7.45	7.46	pH is increased	Alkalosis

Step II : Is it metabolic or Respiratory

CO_2 parameter (Normal)	pCO_2 of patient	Inference	Is change towards acidosis or alkalosis	Is change in keeping with pH change
pCO_2 35-45 mm Hg	30 mm Hg	pCO_2 decreased	Alkalosis	Yes

If change in pCO_2 is inkeeping with pH (if in alkalosis pCO_2 is reduced) the primary acid base abnormality is respiratory.

The patient in question thus has primary respiratory alkalosis which may have been partially compensated (data On HCO_3^- values to assess the extent of compensation is not provided in the question).

7. **Answer B (Respiratory acidosis)** *Harrison 18th/p 363, 364 Harrison 17th/1590, 288, 289; Refer previous question*

8. **Answer A (Respiratory alkalosis)** *Harrison 18th/p 363, 364 Harrison 17th/1590, 288, 289;Refer previous questions*

There is alkalosis (pH = 7.5) and CO2 is low (alkalosis). Change in CO2 is in keeping with change in pH and thus the primary cause is respiratory. The acid base disturbance is thus primary respiratory alkalosis.

9. **Answer is C (Respiratory and metabolic acidosis)** *Harrison 18th/p363, 364 Harrison 17th/1590, 288, 289; See text below; Refer previous questions*

The acid base disorder is therefore both respiratory and metabolic acidosis.

- There is ***acidosis*** (pH < 7.35).
- Raised PCO_2 (acidosis) indicates that change in CO_2 is in keeping with change in pH. The ***respiratory component is therefore primary***.
- Decreased HCO_3 (acidosis) indicates that ***change in HCO_3 is also primary***.

The acid base disorder is therefore both respiratory and metabolic acidosis.

10. **Answer is B (Non Anion Gap Metabolic Acidosis):** *Refer text below*

The patient in question has metabolic acidosis with a normal anion gap

The Acid base abnormality is Metabolic Acidosis

The change in HCO^3 (↓) is in keeping with the change in pH (acidosis); therefore the primary acid base abnormality is metabolic (acidosis)

Normal pH	pH of patient	Inference	Acid-Base abnormality
7.35-7.45	7.34	pH is ↓ed	Acidosis

Normal Paremeter	Patient Parameter	Deviation	Direction of change	Inkeeping with pH	Final Inference
HCO_3^- (22-30)	17	Decreased	Acidosis	Yes (ph=Acidosis)	Primary mechanism metabolic
pCO2 (35-45)	32	Decreased	Alkalosis	No (ph=Acidosis)	Compensatory mechanism Respiratory

The patient in question therefore has Primary Metabolic Acidosis with Compensatory Respiratory Alkalosis

Is this metabolic acidosis associated with a normal or increased Anion Gap

Anion Gap is Normal in this case of Metabolic Acidosis *(as calculated in the following text)*

Anion Gap is calculated by subtracting the measured anions from cations. *Anion Gap = (Na+ K+) – (HCO_3^- + Cl⁻)* ***Normal anion gap is about 12-16 meq/l)***
For the patient in question with HCO^3 of 17; Na^+ 140; pCO2 32; K^+ 4.9; Cl^- 112 *Anion Gap = (140 + 4.9) – (17+112)* *Anion Gap = 15.9*
Inference for the patient in question *The anion gap (15.9) is close to the normal range, hence this is a normal anion gap metabolic acidosis*

11. Answer is B (Acute exacerbation of COPD): Refer textbelow

The patient in question is presenting with type II Respiratory failure (Decreased PaO2 and increased $PaCO_2$) which indicates an obstructive lung disease. Amongst the options provided Asthma and COPD, both are examples of obstructive lung diseases. Obstructive lung disease with elevated PCO_2 is more characteristic and common in acute exacerbations of COPD than in Acute Asthma and hence acute exacerbation of COPD is the single best answer of choice.

Parameter	Normal	Patient	Inference	
pH	7.38-7.44	7.2	Acidosis	
Pco2	40 mm/hg	80mm	Increased	Type II respiratory failure
Pco2	100 mm/hg	46mm	Decreased	

Acute Asthma and COPD are both examples of Obstructive lung diseases.

Both conditions may present with the above picture but an elevated PCO_2 is more characteristic of COPD than asthma

In acute episodes of Asthma most patients increase total ventilation sufficiently to maintain arterial PCO_2 in or below the normal range until a late stage while in cases of COPD persistent elevation of PCO_2 is characteristic

Disease	PaO_2	$PaCO_2$
Acute Exacerbation of COPD	Decreased/Hypoxemia	***Increased/Hypercarbia***
Acute Episode of Asthma	Decreased/Hypoxemia	***Normal or Decreased due to hyperventilation*** *May be elevated/increase at a late stage when respiratory muscles become tired*

ARDS and Pneumonia are conditions that lead to a primary defect in oxygenation. These are associated with normal or reduced levels of $PaCO_2$ and cause type I respiratory failure

Disease	PaO_2	$PaCO_2$
ARDS	Decreased/Hypoxemia	*Normal or Reduced*
Pneumonia	Decreased/Hypoxemia	*Normal or Reduced*

12. Answer is B (Ventilatory malfunction) : *Refer text below*

Ventilatory malfunction is the single best answer of exclusion

The patient has a blood pH of 7.58 indicating alkalosis, decreased oxygen saturation, a low PCO_2 and a high PO_2.

Parameter	Normal	Patient	Inference
pH	7.38 to 7.44	7.58	Alkalosis
P_{CO2}	35 to 45 mmHg	23 mmHg	Decreased
P_{O2}	80 to 100 mmHg	300 mmHg	Increased
Oxygen saturation	97%	60%	Decreased

This is consistent with a diagnosis of ventilatory mal function.

None of the other three condition satisfy the given parameters of the patients. The answer of exclusion therefore is some form of ventilatory malfunction.

- In **carbon monoxide poisoning** ABG analysis would reveal acidosis and normal PO_2
- In **voluntary hyperventilation** oxygen saturation would be normal.
- In **methyl alcohol poisoning** ABG would reveal acidosis and not alkalosis.

Obstructive / Restrictive Pulmonary Diseases

Pulmonary Function Test

13. Answer is D (Decreased diffusing capacity) : *Harrison 18th/ 2092; 15th/ 1448; 16th/ 1500; 17th /1588, 1587, 1637*

Diffusion capacity is not affected in Obstructive lung diseases [Q] (acute or chronic). It is decreased in restrictive lung disease. [Q]

- Decreased in expiratory flow rate is a hallmark of obstructive lung disease. (↓MEFR)
- Residual volume is increased & *FEV_1/FVC is decreased (FEV_1 is also decreased).*

PFT Result	Obstructive Pattern	Restrictive Pattern
FEV_1	***Decreased (<80% predicted)*** *(Decreased out of proportion to FVC)*	*Decreased (May be preserved)* *(Decreased in proportion to FVC)*
FVC	*Decreased (May be preserved)*	***Decreased (<80% predicted)***
FEV_1/FVC (FEV_1%)	***Decreased (<0.7)***	***Normal or Increased (>0.7)***
FEF_{25-75}	*<50% predicted*	*Normal / Decreased in proportion to loss of lung volume*
TLC	*Normal or elevated*	*Decreased*
RV	*Increased*	*Decreased*
DLCO	*Normal* *Decreased in Emphysema*	*Decreased in intrinsic restrictive lung disease.* *Normal in neuromuscular or musculoskeletal restrictive disease*

FEV_1=forced expiratory volume in one second; **FVC**=Forced Vital Capacity; **FEF_{25-75}**=Forced Expiratory Flow at 25%=75% vital capacity; **TLC**= Total Lung Capacity; **DLCO**=Diffusion Capacity of the Lung for Carbon monoxide.

14. Answer is A (Residual volume Normal): *Harrison 17th /1588*

Obstructive Lung disease is typically associated with an Increased Residual volume

Disease Pattern	TLC	RV	Vital Capacity	FEV1/FVC	FEF 25-75
Obstructive Lung Dusease	N or ↑ed	↑ed	↓ed or Normal	↓ed	↓ed

Taken from Harrison 17th/1588

The hallmark of obstructive Lung Disease is decreased expiratory flow rate such the FEF_{25-75} is reduced and FEV_1 is typically reduced out of proportion to the Forced Vital Capacity (↓FEV_1/FVC). ***The Residual volume is typically increased.*** The vital capacity (FVC) may be normal or decreased while Total Lung capacity may be normal or increased.

The hallmark of Restrictive Lung Disease is a decrease in lung volume typically TLC and vital capacity. Flow rates are preserved and hence FEF_{25-75} is generally normal. Also, when FEV_1 is considered as a percentage of FVC, (FEV_1/ FVC), the flow rates are often supranormal i.e. disporoportionately high relative to the size of lungs. ***Residual volume is also generally decreased.***

15. Answer is C (Asthma): *Harrisons 16th/ 1500, 1501; Harrison 17th/1587, 1588, 1589; Harrison 18th/2092*

Reduction in FEV_1/FVC is the hallmark of obstructive lung diseases. Amongst the options provided, Asthma is the only obstructive disease and thus the answer of choice.

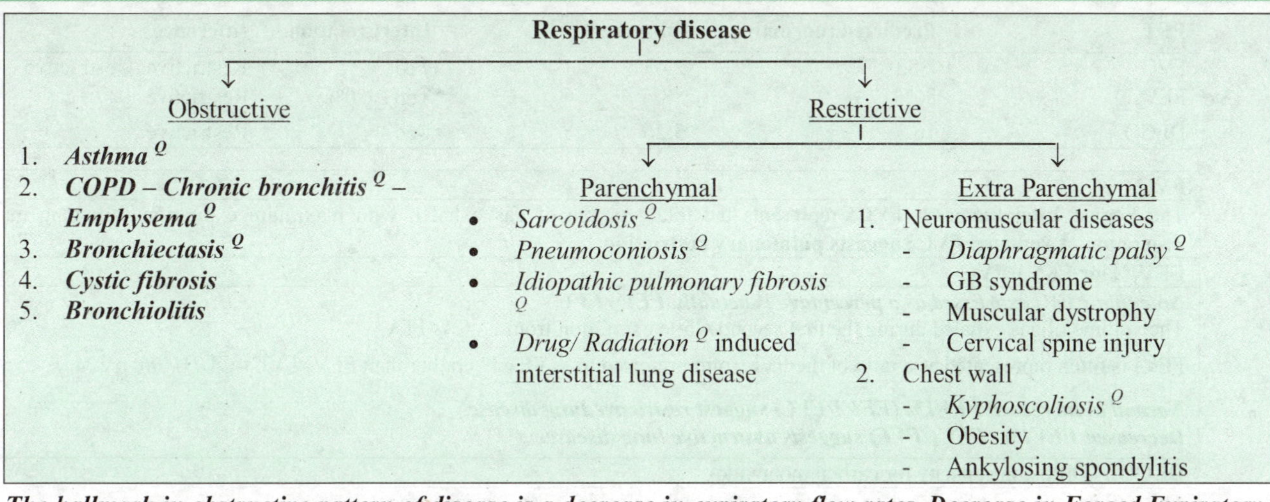

The hallmark in obstructive pattern of disease is a decrease in expiratory flow rates. Decrease in Forced Expiratory flow rate (FEF_{25-75}) and FEV_1/FVC are characteristic.

16. Answer is D (↑ ed Residual Volume): *Repeat*

Bronchial Asthma presents with an obstructive pattern on Pulmonary function Testing and is associated with an increased Residual volume.

17. Answer is D (FEV_1/FVC increase and compliance decreases): *Harrison 15th/ 1449; 16th/ 1500; 17th/ 1588*

Restrictive lung diseases are characterized by decreased compliance and increased FEV_1/FVC

FEV_1 & FVC	FEV_1 / FVC
Forced Vital Capacity (FVC) is decreased Forced expiratory flow rates are relatively preserved (FEV_1 is preserved)	When FEV_1 is considered as a percentage of FVC, the flow rates tend to become supranormal or disproportionately high relative to size of lungs.
FEV_1 is preserved and FVC is decreased so FEV_1/FVC is increased	

The hallmark of restrictive lung diseases is a decrease in lung volumes primarily TLC and V.C.' (FVC is decreased)- Harrison

Compliance *decreases in restrictive lung disease. Compliance is usually unaffected in obstructive lung diseases except in emphysema where it is increased.*

18. Answer is A (Reduced RV/TLC): *Harrisons 16th/ 1500, 1501*

Severe kyphoscoliosis is a restrictive extra-parenchymal disease and presents with decreased RV & decreased TLC on pulmonary function tests.

	Obstructive lung disease	Restrictive lung disease
Total lung capacity	***Normal to Increase*** Q	***Decrease*** Q
Residual volume	***Increase*** Q	***Decrease*** Q
Vital capacity	***Decrease*** Q *(May be normal)*	***Decrease*** Q
FEV_1/FVC	***Decrease*** Q ***(< 0.7)***	***Normal to Increase*** Q ***(>0.7)***
FEF 25-75% (Forced expiratory flow rate)	↓	***Normal***
Diffusion capacity	***Normal (↓ in emphysema)***	***Decreased***

19. Answer is A (Interstitial lung disease): *Harrison 16th/1500, 1556; 17th/1587-1589, 1643; CMDT 06th/223*

'Presence of long standing scleroderma together with a 'restrictive pattern' on pulmonary function tests suggests a diagnosis of interstitial lung disease. *Interstitial lung diseases produce a restrictive defect. FEV_1 and FVC are reduced, but the FEV_1/FVC ratio is usually normal or increased.* ***Note that FEV expressed as a percentage is actually FEV_1 /FVC.*** *Scleroderma or systemic sclerosis is a known cause for interstitial lung disease.*

PFT	Predicted (normal)	Observed	Interpretation	Inference
FVC	2.82	2.63	↓ed	Restrictive /Obstructive
$FEV_{1\%}$	80%	88%	↑ed (>80%)	Restrictive
DLCO	16.3	5.26	↓ed	Restrictive

FVC

The Forced Vital Capacity (FVC) represents the total volume of gas exhaled with maximum expiration following maximal inspiration. **A reduced FVC suggests pulmonary restriction.**

FEV_1% or FEV1/FVC

Note that FEV_1 exprEssed as a percentage is actually FEV_1/FVC.

The volume of gas exhaled during the first second while expiration from FVC is FEV_1.

FEV_1 is often represented as a ratio of the FVC (often referred to as FEV1% rather than FEV_1/FVC)-*CMDT'06, p 223*

Normal to increased FEV1% (FEV1/FVC) suggest restrictive lung disease
Decreased FEV1% (FEV_1/FVC) suggests obstructive lung disease.

DLCO : (Diffusion capacity for carbon monoxide)

This reflects the ability of lungs to transfer gas across the alveolar - capillary interface.

Decreased DLCO is consistent with a diagnosis of :

- ***Interstitial lung disease***
- *Emphysema*
- *Pulmonary hypertension*

Parameter	Obstructive lung disease	Restrictive lung disease
Total lung capacity	***Normal to Increase*** Q	***Decrease*** Q
Residual volume	***Increase*** Q	***Decrease*** Q
Vital capacity	***Decrease*** Q *(May be normal)*	***Decrease*** Q
FEV_1/FVC (FEV_1%)	***Decrease*** Q	***Normal to Increase*** Q
FEF 25-75% (Forced expiratory flow rate)	↓	***Normal***
Diffusion capacity	***Normal (↓ in emphysema)***	***Decreased***

20. Answer is A (Interstitial lung disease): *Refer previous question; Harrison 16th/1500, 1556; 17th/1587-89,1643; CMDT 6th/223b*

'Presence of long standing scleroderma together with a 'restrictive pattern' on pulmonary function tests suggests a diagnosis of interstitial lung disease. *Interstitial lung diseases produce a restrictive defect. FEV_1 and FVC are reduced, but the FEV_1/FVC ratio is usually normal or increased.* ***Note that FEV expressed as a percentage is actually FEV_1 /FVC.*** *Scleroderma or systemic sclerosis is a known cause for interstitial lung disease.*

21. Answers is B (Sarcoidosis) : *Harrison 16th / 1500-1501; Harrison 17th/1588, 1589*

Decreased Vital capacity and Decreased Total Lung Volume suggests a Restrictive Lung Disease picture. Amongst the options provided Sarcoidosis is the only Restrictive Lung Disease and hence the answer of choice.

22. Answer is B (Alveolar arterial difference in PaO_2): *Harrison 15th/ 1452; 16th/ 1500, 1504; 17th/ 1588, 1590, 1591*

If the gas exchange at alveolar capillary level occurs normally, the alveolar arterial difference in PaO_2 is not elevated. ***In infiltrative lung disease the alveolar capillary bed is damaged and there is a decrease in diffusion capacity. This results in an increase in alveolar arterial differences in PaO_2.***

Increased PaO_2 – PaO_2
(Alveolar arterial difference in oxygen)

↓ Correctible with oxygen — V/Q Mismatch

↓ Not correctible with oxygen — Shunt

V/Q Mismatch:
- Airway disease (Asthma, COPD)
- Interstitial lung disease
- Alveolar disease
- Pulmonary vascular disease

Shunt:
- Alveolar collapse
- Intra alveolar filling
  - Pneumonia
  - Pulm edema
- Intracardiac shunt
- Vascular shunt within lung

23. Answer is C (Alveolar hemorrhage): *Harrison 15th/ 1453; 16th/ 1504, 1505; 17th/ 1591, 1592 Harrison 18th/p 2092*

An elevated D_{LCO} is characteristic of alveolar haemorrhage as in Good pastures syndrome. *Hemoglobin contained in erythrocytes in alveolar lumen binds carbon monoxide, so that exhaled CO concentration is diminished and the measured D_{LCO} is increased.*

Diffusion capacity

This is measured by estimating D_{LCO} (carbon monoxide diffusion).
It is most useful in assessing disease affecting the
Alveolar capillary bed (interstitial lung disease, emphysema)
Pulmonary vasculature (pulmonary embolism or prim. pul. hypertension)

Decreased D_{LCO} (Diffusion capacity)	Increased D_{LCO} (Diffusion capacity)
1. **Interstitial lung disease**: scarring of alveolar capillary units diminishes area of alveolar capillary bed as well as pulmonary blood volume 2. **Emphysema:** alveolar walls are destroyed so the surface area of alveolar capillary bed is diminished 3. **Recurrent pulmonary embolism and Primary pulmonary hypertension:** disease causes a decrease in cross sectional area and volume of pulmonary vasculature	1. **Alveolar haemorrhage:** as in Good pasture's syndrome: haemoglobin contained in erythrocytes in alveolar lumen binds Co so exhaled carbon monoxide concentration is diminished & D_{LCO} is increased 2. **Congestive heart failure:** May be elevated if pulmonary blood volume is increased. Once pulmonary edema ensues D_{LCO} may decrease as and the net D_{LCO} depends on the opposing influences.

24. Answer is A (Chronic Bronchitis): *Harrisons 17th/ 1592 Harrison 18th/p 2092*

Diffusion capacity for carbon monoxide (DLCO) is usually normal in chronic bronchitis and other obstructive lung diseases with the exception of Emphysema where it is decreased.

Diffusion capacity for carbon monoxie (DLCO)
Diffusion capacity is altered in disease affecting the functional integrity of the alveolar capillary membrane.
In Emphysema, alveolar walls are destroyed, so the *surface area of alveolar–capillary bed is diminished resulting in diminished DLCO.*

Three main categories are associated with lowered DLCO

- *Emphysema* Q
- *Interstitial Lung Disease* Q
- *Pulmonary vascular disease (Recurrent Pulmonary emboli or Primary Pulmonary Hypertension)* Q

25. Answer is A (Small airways): *Harrison 15th/ 1446, 1448; Harrisons 16th/ 1500; Harrison 17th/ 1588*

Maximum mid-expiratory flow rate (MMFR) **is the average expiratory flow rate during the middle 50% of the vital capacity, i.e. forced expiratory flow rate between 25 and 75% of the vital capacity.**
MEFR is considered a more sensitive measurement of early airflow obstruction particularly in small airways.
'With obstructive disease only in the small airways, the only abnormality noted on routine testing of pulmonary function may be a depression in FEF_{25-75} and an abnormal terminal portion of forced expiratory flow volume curve. FEV_1/FVC may be normal' – Harrisons.

Bronchial Asthma

26. Answer is D (IgE is increased in Extrinsic Asthma): *Harrisons 17th/1596, Clinical Anaesthesiology by Morgan 4th/573 Harrison 18th/p 2102*

Idiosyncratic Asthma (Intrinsic Asthma) is associated with normal IgE levels.

Asthma

Extrinsic Asthma / Allergic Asthma	Intrinsic Asthma /Idiosyncratic Asthma
• History of Atopy is present	• No history of Atopy (Concomitant nasal polyps are usually present and patients may be aspirin sensitive)
• Attacks related to environmental exposures	• Attacks not related to environmental exposures: Occur without provocation
• IgE antibody levels are ↑ ed	• IgE antibody levels are normal
• Early onset of disease (young)	• Delayed onset of disease (Adult onset Asthma)
• Usually is less severe, intermittent Asthma that may however progress to severe persistent Asthma	• Usually have more severe persistent Asthma

The incidence of Asthma is increasing

There is a rising incidence of Asthma in developing countries – Harrisons 17th/1596

27. Answer is C, E (Family history +ve; Allergic in nature): *Harrison 17th/1596 Harrison 18th/p 2102*

Intrinsic Asthma by defination is not allergic in nature and is not associated with a positive family history of allergy

Features of Intrinsic Asthma
(Nonatopic asthma- Approximately 10% of asthmatic patients are intrinsic)

- ***Negative Family History of allergy***
- ***Negative skin test to common inhalant allergens (Not primarily caused by allergy)***
- *Normal serum concentration of IgE.*
- *Concomitant nasal polyps (Common)*
- *Sensitivity to aspirin and related chemicals*
- *Later onset of disease (adult-onset asthma)*
- *More servere, persistent disease/asthma.*

28. Answer is C (Nasal polyp): *Harrison's 14th/ 1421; Harrison's 15th/ 1458; 16th/ 1510; 17th/ 1596, 1606 Harrison 18th/p 2102, 2115*

'Aspirin associated Asthma usually begins with perennial vasomotor rhinitis that is followed by a hyperplastic rhinosinusitis with nasal polyps' *– Harrisons*

Aspirin associated Asthma:

- Primarily affects adults, although the condition may occur in childhood.
- Usually begins with perennial vasomotor rhinitis that is followed by hyperplastic rhinosinusitis with nasal polyps. Progressive asthma then appears.
- On exposure to even very small quantities of aspirin affected individual typically develop ocular and nasal congestion and acute, often severe episodes of airways obstruction.
- Death may follow ingestion of aspirin.

29. Answer is C (Hyporesponsiveness of airway): *CMDT 2008 / 206; 2009/210; Harrisons 17th/1598, 1601, 1603 Harrison 18th/p 2104, 2108, 2111*

Asthma is characterized by Hyperresponsiveness of airways and not hyporesponsivenes

Asthma is an inflammatory disorder of the airways

Asthma is a chronic inflammatory disorder of the airways – CMDT-2009/210

Asthma is an allergic disease of the airways

The pattern of inflammation in Asthma is characteristic of allergic disease' – Harrison 17th/1598

The strongest identifiable predisposing factor for Asthma is Atopy.

*Exposure of sensitive patients to **'allergans'** increases airway inflammation airway hyper responsiveness and symptoms - CMDT 2009/210*

Asthma is associated with hyper responsiveness of airways (AHR)

Airway hyperresponsiveness (AHR) is the characteristic physiologic abnormality of Asthma

AHR describes the excessive bronchoconstricter response to multiple inhaled triggers that would have no effect on normal airways- Harrison 17th/1601

Inhaled corticosteroids are the mainstay of treatment

Inhaled corticosteroids are by far the most effective controllers for Asthma and their early use has revolutionized asthma therapy.

Inhaled corticosteroids are now given as first line therapy to patients with persistent Asthma - Harrisons 17th/1603

30. **Answer is D (Small airways are not involved):** *Refernces alongwith text*

Asthma involves both large and small airways but alveoli are not involved

Charcot Leyden crystals may be seen in sputum: *Robbins 7th/726 Pathology by woolf 1st (1998)/434*

Sputum from Asthmatics show certain characteristic features, including charcot leydencrystas

The microscopically identifiable features described in sputum are three 'C's	
Charcot Leyden crystals	*: Derived from granules of eosnophils and found only in Asthma*
Curshmann spirals	*: Curiously twisted casts of airways : Whorls of shed epethelium*
Creola bodies	*: Clumps of cells or isolated metaplastic cells*

Reversible Airflow obstruction is a charachteristic feature (Davidsons 18th/55, 326)

Reversible Bronchoconstriction is the hallmark of Asthma

The charachteristic feature of Asthma is Intermittent and Reversible airflow obstruction.

Narrowing of airways is usually reversible, but in some patients with chronic asthma there may be an element of irreversible air flow obstruction

Asthma involves both large and small airways

Asthma involves Large and small airways but not alveoli - 'Allergic Diseases: Diagnosis Treatment' 3rd/ 120

The large and small airways are both involved in Asthma -'Childhood Asthma: Diagnosis, Treatment & Management' 1st/15

Intermittent Asthma responds better to bronchodilator therapy than persistant Asthma

Bronchodilators are effective drugs for the treatment of acute exacerbations or intermittent episodes of Asthma but they are not sufficient to control asthma in patients with persistant symptoms (persistant asthma)

'Bronchodilators are not sufficient to control Asthma in patients with persistant symptoms' – Harrisons 17th/1602

31. **Answer is C (Necrosis of airways):** *Harrison 18th/p 2107 Harrisons 17th/1600*

Necrosis of Airways is not a feature of Bronchial Asthma

Features of Asthma: Chronic inflammatory disorder

- ***Chronic inflammatory disorder***
- ***Hyperresponsiveness of airways (AHR)***
- *Airway epithelial shedding*
- *Subepithelial fibrosis and thickening of basement membrane*
- *Hypertrophy and Hyperplasia of airway smooth muscle*
- *Increased mucosal blood flow (vascular congestion)*
- *Microvascular leakage resulting in **airway edema** and plasma exudation into airway lumen*
- ***Mucus Hypersecretion** and formation of viscid mucus plugs that occlude airways*
- *Airway remodelling*
- *Defects in autonomic neural control*

32. **Answer is E (None: All are Features of Acute severe Asthma) :** *CMDT 2008/207; 2009/211*

Tachycardia (HR>120/min). PEFR < 50%, Pulsus paradoxus and Respiratory Acidosis are all features of Acute severe Asthma.

Classification of severity of asthma execrbations:

	Mild	Moderate	Severe	Impending Respiratory Failure
Symptoms				
Breathlessness	With activity	With talking	At rest	At rest
Speech	Sentences	Phrases	Words	Mute
Signs				
Body position	Able to recline	Prefers sitting	Unable to recline	Unable to recline
Respiratory rate	Increased	Increased	Often > 30/min	> 30/min
Use of accessory respiratory muscle	Usually not	Commonly	Usually	Paradoxical thoracoabdominal movement
Breath sounds	Moderate wheezing at mid-to-end-expiration	Loud wheezes throughout expiration	Loud inspiratory and expiratory wheezes	Little air movement without wheezes
Hear rate (beats/min)	<100	100-120	***>120***	Relative bradycardia
Pulsus paradoxus (mm Hg)	< 10	10-25	***Often > 25***	Often absent
Mental status	May be agitated	Usually agitated	Usually agitated	Confused or drowsy
Functional assessment				
PEF (% predicted)	> 80	50-80	***< 50***	< 50
Sao_2 (%, room air)	> 95	91-95	< 91	< 91
Pao_2 (mm Hg, room air)	Normal	> 60	< 60	<60
$Paco_2$ (mm Hg)	< 42	< 42	≥ 42 ***(Respiratory acidosis)***	≥ 42

33. Answer is C (Grave Prognosis): *'CMDT 2013; Branchial Asthma' by Gershin (Springer) 2012/181*

Silent chest (Little/no air movement without wheezes in Bronchial Asthma suggests a grave prognosis/ impending respiratory failure (Life threatening Asthma).

'Signs of impending respiratory failure include drowsiness or confusion, diaphoresis, bradycardia, paradoxical thoracoabdominal movement ***and a silent chest*** *and should prompt preparation for intubation and mechanical ventilation' - 'Bronchial Asthma' (Springer) 2012/181*

'Features of life threatening asthma that indicate respiratory failure (impending arrest) include confusion and drowsiness, ***silent chest****, PEFR < 33% predicted, paradoxical thoracoabdominal excursions (outward abdominal and inward chest movement during inspiration), bradycardia, hypotension, pulsus paradoxus and hypercapnea (hypoxemia)'- Acute & Critical Care Medicine at a Glance' by Leach (John Wiley & Sons) 2010/75*

34. Answer is A (Hypoxia): *Harrison 18th/ 2109; Harrisons 11th/1062 (Not elaborated in new edition.)*

Hypoxia is a universal finding during acute exacerbation's *– Harrisons 11th/1062*

Hypoxia is a universal finding during acute exacerbations. Most Asthmatics have hypocapnia and respiratory alkalosis.
- Harrison

Hypoxia is the universal finding in Asthma

Hypocapnia and respiratory alkalosis is seen in most asthmatic patients

Hypercarbia and Respiratory acidosis *are very late features of Asthma and signify severe obstruction and respiratory failure. These are not universal findings in Asthma.*

Metabolic acidosis *is not a feature of Asthma.*

35. Answer is D (Demonstration of Reversible obstruction): *Harrison 18th/p 2109 Harrisons 17th/ 1602*

The diagnosis of asthma is usually apparent from the symptoms (Wheezing, dyspnea, cough) but is confirmed by objective measurement of lung function and demonstration of reversibility

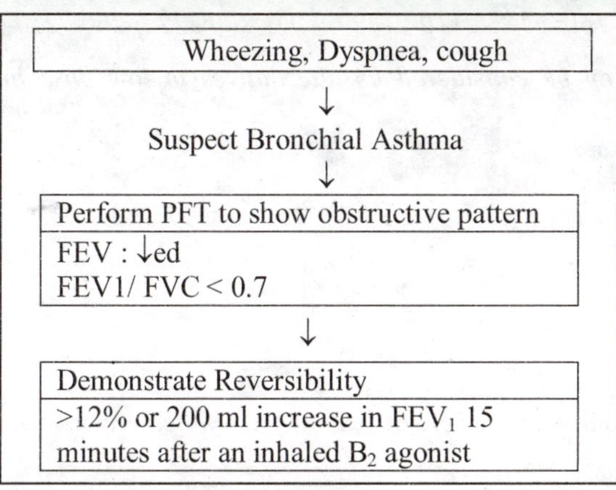

36. Answer is A and C (Fluticasone and Budesonide): *Ref. Text below*

Fluticasone and Budesonide are inhaled corticosteroids and potent anti-inflammatory medications in Asthma

Medications in Bronchial Asthma

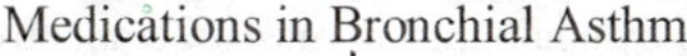

Bronchodilators	Anti-inflammatory (Controllers)
Beta 2 Sympathomimetics	Corticosteroids (Inhalational)
• *Salbutamol*	• *Beclomethasone*
• *Terbutaline*	• *Budesunide*
• *Bambuterol*	• *Fluticasone*
• *Salmeterol*	• *Flunisolide*
• *Formeterol*	• *Ciclesonide*
• *Ephedrine*	Corticosteroids (systemic)
Methylxonthines	• *Prednisolone, Hydrocortisone e/c*
• *Theophylline*	Mast cell stabilizers
• *Aminophylline*	• *Sodium cromoglycate (Nedoevil sodium)*
Articholinergics	• *Ketotifen*
• *Ipratropium bromide*	Leukotriene antogonist
• *Tiotropium bromide*	• *Montelukast*
	• *Zafirlukast etc*

37. Answer is B (Morphine): *Harrison 17th/ 1605; KDT 5th/ 423*

Morphine is contraindicated in asthma because it causes constriction of bronchial muscle by causing histamine release.

Management of Acute Bronchial Asthma:

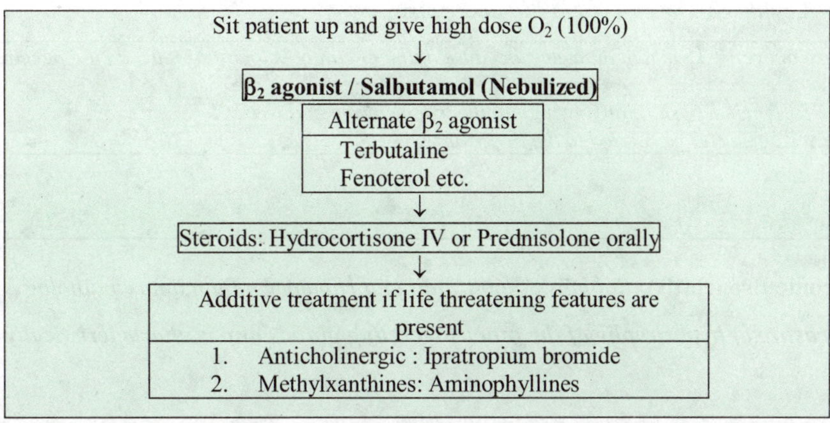

38. Answer is C (Montelukast): *Harrison's 16th/1514; 17th/ 1602-1604; 18th/2110-2112 CMDT 2009/222; 2008/210-213*

'Leukotriene modifiers (eg. Monteleukast, Zafirulukast) may be considered as alternatives to low dose inhaled corticosteroids in patients with mild persistent asthma' *– CMDT*
They have no role in aborting an attack of acute severe asthma.

39. Answer is A (May be used for acute asthma): *Harrison's 16th/ 1514; 17th/ 1604; 18th/2112; CMDT 2009/ 222; 2008/212*

Leukotriene modifiers have no role in aborting an attack of bronchial Asthma.

Leukotriene Modifiers:

These are new group of agents used for asthma and act by modifying the role of leukotrienes which are critical in the pathway of generating features of asthma.

Action	
Leukotrienes are responsible for many of the critical elements of asthma Leukotriene modifiers act by two mechanisms to disable the deleterious effects of leukotrenes	
Reduce synthesis of all Leukotrienes by inhibiting enzyme involved in their formation i.e. 5 Lipooxygenase	Competitive blockage of principal leukotriene (LTD 4)
Zileuton	Montelukast or Zafirulukast
Uses	
1. Used as alternative to low dose inhaled corticosteroids in patients with mild persistent asthma - reduces asthma morbidity - diminishes nocturnal symptoms 2. Used for protection against exercise induced Asthma.	
Side effects: Leukotriene blockers have been associated with Churg-Strauss Syndrome [Q]	

40. Answer is B (Acute Asthmatic Attack): *KDT 5th/ 127, 4th/ 141; KDT 5th / 1207*

" Propanalol worsens chronic obstructive lung disease. It can precipitate life threatening attack of Bronchial Asthma as it increases Bronchial resistance by Blocking $_2$ receptors" *– KDT*

Drugs most commonly associated with the induction of acute episodes of Asthma
1. Aspirin [Q]
2. Beta adrenergic blockers [Q]
3. Colouring agents such as tartrazine
4. Sulfiting agents.

41. Answer is A (< 5 μ): *Harrison 18th/p 2122; Harrison 14th/ 1489, 15th/ 1530; 17th/ 1612;*

'Particles of size < 2.5 mm can be carried to the lower airways.

- *'Particles with size above 10-15 mm in diameter, because of their settling velocities in air, do not penetrate beyond the upper airways'*
- *'Particle of size 2.5-10 mm deposit relatively high in the tracheobronchial tree.'*
- *'Particles of size < 2.5 mm can be carried to the lower airways.'*

Chronic Bronchitis

42. Answer is A (Chronic Bronchitis): *Robbins 8th/668; Bail and Hammer's Pulmonary pathology 3rd/866*

Reid Index is a measure of hypertrophy of the mucus secreting glands and is characteristically increased in Chronic Bronchitis.

Reid Index: Measures Hypertrophy of mucus glands
• Chronic Bronchitis is assoicated with hypertrophy of the mucus secreting glands of the submucusa in the cartilaginous airways.   *The histologic correlate of chronic bronchitis is the presence of mucus gland hyperplasia.*   • This manifests as an increased percentage of bronchial wall occupied by submucosal mucus glands (*This is classically defined by the 'Reid Index'.*)   • ***<u>Reid Index</u> is the ratio of the thickness of the mucous gland layer to the thickness of the bronchial wall*** (between basal lamina of mucosa and inner perichondrium)   • *The normal Reid Index is less than 0.4*   *Reid index > 0.4 (typically > 0.5) suggests mucous gland hyperplasia*   • The Reid index is increased in chronic bronchitis usually in proportion to the severity and duration of disease.   *There is a direct correlation between the value of Reid Index and the volume of daily sputum production by the patient.*

3

Respiratory System

Emphysema

43. Answer is B (Panacinar emphysema): *Robbins 5th/685; Robbins 7th/718*

Panacinar emphysema is associated with α_1 antitrypsin deficiency. *– Robbins 7th/ 718*

<u>There are two types of emphysema that cause clinically significant airflow obstruction:</u>

Panacinar emphysema	Centriacinar emphysema
• Acini are uniformly involved from level of respiratory bronchiole to terminal blind alveoli. Q • Lesions are more common in lower zone and bases Q • Occurs in association with α_1 antitrypsin deficiency Q	• Central or proximal parts of acini formed by respiratory bronchioles are affected whereas distal alveoli are spared Q • Lesions are more severe and common in Upper lobes Q • Occurs predominantly in smokers Q • Is the commonest pattern Q

44. Answer is C (Restrictive pattern on pulmonary function test is seen): *Harrison 18th/2156 Harrisons 17th/1640 CMDT 2008/219; 09/230*

The hallmark of Emphysema is air flow obstruction and pulmonary function tests show an obstructive pattern

<u>Breathlessness (Dyspnea) is a charachteristic presenting symptom</u>

The three most common symptoms in COPD (emphysema) are cough, sputum production and ***exertional dyspnea***

<u>Obstructive (and not Restrictive) pattern is seen on PFT</u>

The hallmark of Emphysema (COPD) is airflow obstruction.

PFT shows airflow obstruction with a reduction in FEV_1/FVC (< 0.7)

<u>Diffusion of carbon monoxide is Reduced (↓DLCO)</u>

Three main categories of disease with Reduced DLCO are:
Interstial Lung disease   ***Emphysema***   *Pulmonary vascular Disease*

<u>Long term bronchodilater therapy does not improve lung function</u>

'Bronchodilators do not alter the inexorable decline in lung function that is a hallmark of the disease' -CMDT 2008/219

The only drug therapy that is documented to improve the natural history (lung function) of COPD patients is supplemental oxygen in those patients with resting hypoxemia -CMDT 09/230

The only three interventions that influence the natural history of COPD patients
Smoking cessation   *Oxygen therapy in chronically hypoxemic patients*   *Lung volume reduction surgery in selected patients with emphysema*

45. Answer is B (Increased diffusion capacity for carbon monoxide (DLCO)): *Harrison 18th/2092; 17th/1592*

Emphysema is associated with a decreased diffusion capacity for carbon monoxide

Lung Function Tests in Emphysema		
TLC	:	*Normal or Increased*
FEV_1	:	*Decreased (< 80% predicted) (Decreased out of proportion to FVC)*
FVC	:	*Decreased*
FEV1 / FVC	:	*Decreased (< 0.7)*
FEF_{25-75}	:	*Decreased (<50% predicted)*
DLCO	:	*Decreased*

Note that DLCO is normal in other obstructive lung diseases like chronic bronchitis

Diffusion capacity for carbon monoxie (DLCO)
Diffusion capacity is altered in disease affecting the functional integrity of the alveolar capillary membrane.
In Emphysema, alveolar walls are destroyed, so the *surface area of alveolar–capillary bed is diminished resulting in diminished DLCO.*

Three main disoders are associated with lowerd DLCO

- *Emphysema*[Q]
- *Interstitial Lung Disease*[Q]
- *Pulmonary vascular disease (Recurrent Pulmonary emboli or Primary Pulmonary Hypertension)*[Q]

46. Answer is A (Body Plethysmography): *Harrison's 7th/1587; Pulmonary / Respiratory Therapy Secrets 2nd/45*

Body Plethysmography is the investigation of choice for estimating lung volumes in the setting of COPD with bullous lesions (trapped air)

Estimating Lung Volumes

Gas Dilution Technique
(Helium / Nitrogen Dilution Method)

- Gas dilution methods are *fairly accurate in measurement of lung volumes in restrictive lung diseases*, but *not so in obstructive lung diseases with trapped air in bullae*.
- *Gas dilution methods tend to under-estimate lung volumes in patients with emphysema with ballous lesions as they do not measure the volume of trapped gas or bullae.*

Body Plethysmography

- Body Plethysmography is *fairly accurate in measurement of lung volumes in both restrictive lung diseases and obstructive lung diseases even with trapped air in bullae*
- *Body Plethysmography also measures the volume of any gas containing space in the thorax, including bullae.*

The difference between Lung volume measurements by Body Plethysmography and gas dilution technique reflects the amount of gas trapped in bullae.

Bronchiectasis

47. Answer is D (Left lower lobe): *API Medicine 6th/ 236, API 7th/ 306*

"Bronchiectasis is commonly affects lower lobe bronchi, the left side being affected more frequently than right"
– API 7th

Right middle lobe and lingual are next in frequency of involvement.

48. Answer is B (Lung cancer): *API 6th/ 238, API 7th/ 306, 308; API 8th / 374, 375; CMDT 2003/ 243; 09/234*

Bronchiectasis is not a premalignant condition.

Complications of Bronchiectasis:
- Massive hemoptysis.
- Empyema with or without bronchopleural fistula.
- Purulent pericarditis.
- Respiratory failure with chronic cor pulmonale.
- Metastatic abscesses in brain and bones.
- Secondary amyloidosis with nephrotic syndrome.
- Lung abscess: Bronchiectasis is a predisposing factor for Lung abscess API 7th/ 308.

49. Answer is A (HRCT) : *Harrison 15th/206; Harrisons 16th/208; Harrison 17th/ 1630 Harrison 18th/p 2143*

Presence of purulent sputum with recurrent haemoptysis suggests a diagnosis of **bronchiectasis**. ***HRCT is now the diagnostic procedure of choice having replaced bronchiography***. *– Harrison 16th/208*

Interstitial Lung Disease

50. Answer is B (FEV1/FVC < 0.7): *Harrison 18th/p 2154, 2155, 2156 Harrisons 17th/1587, 1588, 1638, 1639, 1640; Harrisons 16th/1499, 1500, 1550, 1551, 1501*

Interstitial lung disease like interstial fibrosis are characterized by a normal or elevated FEV_1/FVC ratio which is characteristically > 0.7.

PFT results comparing obstructive and restrictive disease
(may not be applicable for all forms of lung (disease)

PFT Result	Obstructive Pattern	Restrictive Pattern
FEV_1	***Decreased (<80% predicted)*** *(Decreased out of proportion to FVC)*	*Decreased (May be preserved) (Decreased in proportion to FVC)*
FVC	*Decreased (May be preserved)*	***Decreased (<80% predicted)***
FEV_1/FVC (FEV_1%)	***Decreased (<0.7)***	***Normal or Increased (>0.7)***
FEF_{25-75}	*<50% predicted*	*Decreased in proportion to loss of lung volume*
TLC	*Normal or elevated*	*Decreased*
DLCO	*Normal* *Decreased in Emphysema*	*Decreased in intrinsic restrictive lung disease.* *Normal in neuromuscular or musculoskeletal restrictive disease*

FEV_1=forced expiratory volume in one second; **FVC**=Forced Vital Capacity; **FEF_{25-75}**=Forced Expiratory Flow at 25%=75% vital capacity; **TLC**= Total Lung Capacity; **DLCO**=Diffusion Capacity of the Lung for Carbon monoxide.

51. Answer is C (Decreased FEV1/FVC): *Repeat : Refer previous question*

Interstial lung diseases produce a restrictive pattern on Pulmonary function testing and are characterized by a normal or elevated FEV_1/FVC ratio which is greater than 0.7
FEV_1 and FVC are both reduced in interstitial lung disease but the decrease in FEV1 is in proportion to decrease in FVC and hence the FEV1/FVC ratio is normal (or increased)

52. Answer is B (Residual volume is increased): *Harrison 18th/p 2160-2164 Harrison's 17th/1643-1646*

Residual volume is decreased in patients with Interstitial Lung Disease

Progressive dyspnea and presence of bibasilar end-inspiratory crepitations suggests a diagnosis of interstitial lung disease

'Dyspnea is a common and prominent complaint in patients with Interstitial Lung Disease(ILD)'-Harrison 17th/1645

'Most commonly, physical examination reveals tachypnea and bibasilar end – inspiratory dry crackles which are common in most forms of ILD' – Harrison 17th/1645

Interstitial Lung Disease (ILD) may be associated with connective tissue diseases

'ILDs have been difficult to classify because > 200 known individual disease are characterized by diffuse parenchymal lung involvement either as primary condition or as a significant part of a multiorgan process, as may occur in connective tissue disorders (CTD's)'- Harrison 17th/1643

Interstial Lung disease produce a restrictive effect on Pulmonary Function Testing

*'Most forms of ILD produce a restrictive defect with **reduced total lung capacity (↓TLC)**, functional residual capacity and **residual volume (↓RV).** Forced expiratory volume in one second (FEV1) and forced vital capacity (FVC) are reduced; but, the FEV1/FVC ratio is normal or increased' – Harrison 17th/1646*

HRCT is a useful test for ILD

HRCT is the investigation of choice for Interstitial Lung Disease.

53. Answer is C (Usual Interstitial Pneumonia): *Harrison 18th/p 2165 Harrisons 17th/1647; Robbins 8th/; Diffuse Lung Diseases (Springer) 1st (2006)/223; 'Imaging in Diffuse Lung Diseases' by Lynch & Lee (2000)/61*

Presence of heterogenous, patchy fibrosis with fibroblastic foci is characteristic of Usual Interstitial Pneumonia

*'The histologic hallmark and chief diagnostic criterion of **UIP** is a **heterogenous appearance**, interstitial inflammation, foci of proliferating fibroblasts (**fibroblastic foci**) dense collagen fibrosis and honey-comb changes. The interstitial **inflammation is usually patchy** and the histopathological changes affect the peripheral sub-pleural parenchyma most severely' – Harrisons 17th/1647*

Usual Interstitial Pneumonia (UIP) is the histopathologic pattern of Idiopathic Pulmonary Fibrosis (IPF), a chronic fibrosing interstitial lung disease of unknown etiology (idiopathic)

Idiopathic Interstitial Lung Diseases / Idiopathic Interstitial Pneumonias

- Idiopathic Interstitial Pneumonias are *interstitial lung diseases of unknown etiology* that *share similar clinical and radiological features* and are *distinguished primarily by the histopathological pattern on lung biopsy.*

Histologic Name	Clinical Syndrome	Salient Pathological Features
Usual Interstitial Pneumonia (UIP)	*Idiopathic pulmonary fibrosis (Cryptogenic fibrosing alveolitis)*	*Temporally and spatially heterogeneous pattern with areas of normal lung, fibroblastic foci, and patchy sub-pleural fibrosis*
Desquamative Interstitial Pneumonia (DIP)	*Desquamative interstitial pneumonia*	*Homogenous intra-alveolar macrophage accumulation. Mild alveolar septal thickening*
Acute Interstitial Pneumonia (AIP)	*Acute interstitial pneumonia (Hamman-Rich syndrome)*	*Homogenous, diffuse lung injury with hyaline membranes, fibroblast proliferation*
Bronchiolitis Obliterans Organizing pneumonia (BOOP)	*Cryptogenic organizing pneumonia, (Idiopathic BOOP)*	*Multifocal organizing pneumonia, with granulation tissue and polyps in alveolar ducts and bronchioles*
Non-Specific Interstitial Pneumonia (NSIP)	*Nonspecific interstitial pneumonia*	*Temporally and spatially homogenous cellular inflammation with mild fibrosis*
Respiratory Bronchiolitis Associated Lung Disease(RBILD)	*Respiratory Bronchiolitis Associated Interstitial Lung Disease*	

- Detailed Histopathological features are often required to distinguish various forms of Idiopathic Interstitial Pneumonias and hence these have been listed in a tabular form in the following table.

Pathologic features of Idiopathic Interstitial Pneumonias							
Feature	***AIP***	***BOOP***	***DIP***	***RBILD***	***UIP***	***NSIP-Cellular***	***NSIP-Fibrosing***
Distribution	*Diffuse*	*Certrilobular*	*Diffuse*	*Mild, focal*	***Patchy**, Sub-pleural*	*Diffuse*	*Diffuse/panacinar*
Temporal appearance	*Homogenous*	*Homogenous*	*Homogenous*	*Homogenous*	***Herterogenous (Variegated)***	*Homogenous*	*Homogenous*
Septal Inflammation	Scant	Scant	Scant	None	Scant, patchy	Prominent	Scant. diffuse
Collagen fibrosis	Absent	Scant	Variable Diffuse	Scant Patchy	***Characterisitc Patchy***	Absent	Diffuse
Fibroblast proliferation	*Diffuse (interstitial)*	*Diffuse (intralumiral)*	*Absent*	*Absent*	***Fibroblastic Foci prominent***	*Absent*	***Fibroblastic Foci Rare***
Honey-combing	Absent	Absent	Absent	Absent	Characteristic	Absent	Rare
Alveolar macrophage	Absent	Absent	Diffuse	Peribonchiolar	Occasional	Occasional	Occasional
Hyaline membranes	Occasional	Absent	Absent	Absent	Absent	Absent	Absent

54. Answer is B (HRCT): *Grainger 4th/278, 279; Sutton 7th/33; Haga CT and MRI of the whole body 4th/838*

High Resolution CT (HRCT) is investigation of choice for interstitial lung disease and bronchiectasis as it can delineate the lung parenchyma upto the level of secondary pulmonary lobule.

55. Answer is D (Tobacco smoke): *Harrison 17th/ 1643; Robbins Basis 6th/ 729t*

- Coal dust & Sulphur dioxide are mentioned as a cause Interstitial Lung Disease in the table.
- Thermophilic actinomycite is a well known cause
- ***So tobacco smoke is the answer of exclusion.***

56. Answer is C (Rheumatoid Arthritis): *Harrison's 18th/2739-2125*

Caplan's syndrome refers to the association of Pneumoconiosis and Rheumatoid Arthritis.

Caplan's Syndrome is a rare subset of pulmonary nodulosis characterized by the development of nodules and pneumoconiosis following *silica exposure* in patients with *Rheumatoid Arthritis*.

Caplan's Syndrome first described in coal miners but subsequently found in patients with silicosis includes ***seropositive Rheumatoid arthritis with charachteristic pneumoconiotic nodules***. Silica has immunoadjuvant properties and is often present in anthractic coal dust.

Felty's syndrome[Q] *is defined by the clinical triad of Neutropenia, Splenomegaly and Nodular RA, typically seen in late stages of severe Rheumatoid Arthritis - Harrison's 18th/2740*

57. Answer is C (Emphysema): *Robbins 7th/736; Harrison 18th/p2161; Harrisons 17th/1612,1613; Fishman's pulmonary Diseases 4th/943*

Emphysema has not been mentioned as a feature of Asbestos related lung disease.

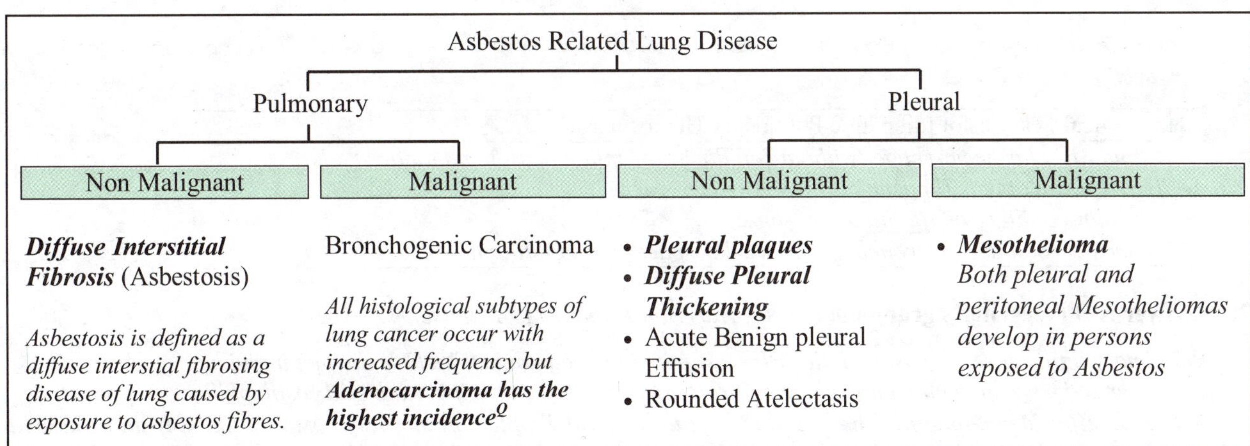

58. Answer is E (All of the above) : *Refer previous question*

Asbestosis may be associated with Bronchogenic carcinoma, Mesotheliomas (pleural and peritoneal) and Pulmonary fibrosis.

59. Answer is A (Pleural plaques): *Harrison 18th/p 2123, 2024; Harrisons 17th/1614*

Pleural plaques are characteristically associated with Asbestosis and not silicosis

Silicosis has predilection for upper lobes

'Radiographs typically show fine nodularity in the upper zones of the lung' –Robbins 7th/735
'Rounded opacities appear in the upper lobes on chest radiograph' – Harrison 17th/1614

Silicosis is associated with calcific Hilar Adenopathy

Calcification of hilar lymph nodes may occur in as many as 20% of cases and produce a charachteristic "egg shell" pattern.

Silicosis is associated with Tuberculosis

'Because silica is cytotoxic to alveolar macrophages, patients with silicosis are at greater risk of acquiring lung infections that involve these cells as a primary defense including mycobacterium tuberculosis, atypical mycobacteria and fungi' – H17th/1614

60. Answer is A (Eosinopenia): *Nelson 18th/1824*

Eosinopenia is not a feature of Idiopathic Pulmonary Hemosiderosis

Idiopathic Pulmonary Hemosiderosis (IPH)

IPH is a disorder of unknown etiology characterized by recurrent episodes of Diffuse Alveolar Hemorrhage (DAH)

It has been classically characterized by the triad of iron deficiency anemia, hemoptysis and alveolar infiltrates on chest radiographs.

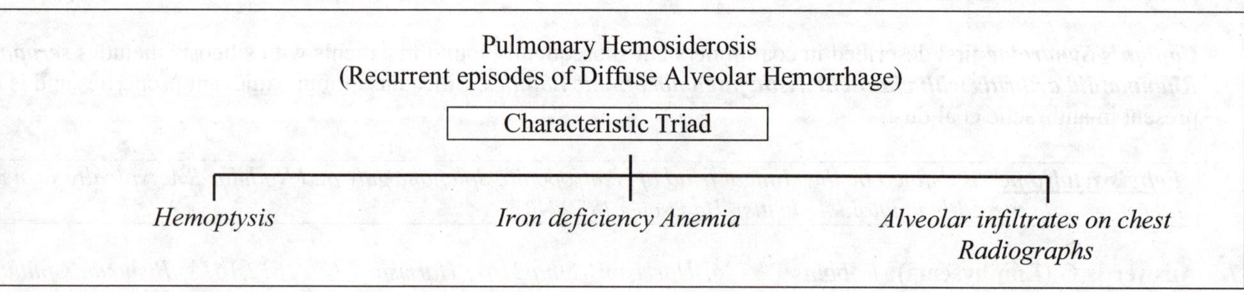

61. Answer is B (Alveolar capillary constriction): *Crofton and Douglas 5th/1333; Color Atlas & Text of Pulmonary Pathology 1st/265*

Idiopathic Pulmonary Hemosiderosis is associated with alveolar capillary dilatation and not alveolar capillary constriction.

Pathological Features of Idiopathic Pulmonary Hemosiderosis
• *Bland Alveolar hemorrhage (without capillaritis or inflammation of blood vessels)*
• *Hyperplasia of type II pneumocytes*
• *Alveolar capillary **dilatation** and tortuosity*
• *Hemosiderin laden macrophages in alveolar spaces of interstitium*

62. Answer is D (Wegener's granulomatosis) : *Harrison 18th/p 2119 Harrison 17th/1610*

Pulmonary infiltrates with eosinophilia (PIE, eosinophilic pneumonias) include distinct individual syndromes characterized by eosinophilic pulmonary infiltrates and commonly, peripheral blood eosinophilia

ABPA, Loeffler's pneumonia, Churg Strauss Syndrome and Tropical pulmonary eosinophilia may all be associated with Eosinophillic Pulmonary Infiltrates (Pulmonary Eosinophilic Pneumonias)

Pulmonary Infiltrates with Eosinophilia (Pulmonary eosiniophilic pneumonia)

Etiology Known	Idiopathic
Allergic bronchopulmonary mycoses	*Loeffler's syndrome*
Parastitic infestations	*Acute eosinophilic pneumonia*
Drug reactions	*Chronic eosinophilic pneumonia*
Eosinophilia-myalgia syndrome	*Allergic granulomatosis of Churg and Strauss*
	Hypereosinophilic syndrome

Allergic Bronchopulmonary Aspergillosis (ABPA)

63. Answer is D (Occurrence in patients with old cavitatory lesions): *Harrison's 15th/ 1466; 16th/ 296; 17th / 1610 Harrison 18th/p 2120*

Definitive major and minor diagnostic criteria have been defined for diagnosis of Allergic bronchopulmonary aspergillosis. Occurance in patients with old cavitatory lesion is not a part of either of these.

Allergic bronchopulmonary aspergillosis is a pulmonary hypersensitivity disorder caused by allergy to fungal antigens that colonize the tracheobronchial tree. It most commonly occurs in atopic asthmatic individuals in response to antigen of aspergillus species.

Main diagnostic criteria	Secondary diagnostic criteria
1. *Clinical history of Asthma* [Q]	1. *History of brownish plugs in sputum*
2. *Pulmonary infiltrates (transient / fleeting or fixed)* [Q]	2. *Indentification / culture of A. fumigatus from sputum*
3. *Peripheral eosinophilia (> 1000 /μL)* [Q]	3. *Late skin reactivity to aspergillus antigen – CMDT*
4. *Immediate skin reactivity to Aspergillus antigen (wheal and flare response)*	4. *Elevated IgE (and IgG) class antibodies specific for A. fumigatus – Harrisons*
5. *Serum precipitins to A. fumigatus*	
6. *Elevated serum IgE levels* [Q] *(>1000ng/ml)*	
7. *Central / proximal bronchiectasis* [Q]	

Note

Elevated IgE (and IgG) class antibodies specific for A. fumigatus has been mentioned as a secondary diagnostic criteria in Harrison's textbook while Fishman's textbook includes this as a main/major diagnostic criteria.

64. Answer is A (Peripheral eosinophilia ($>0.1\times 10^9/mm^3$)): *Fishman's Pulmonary Diseases and Disorders 4th/2299; Harrison 18th/p 2120 Harrison 17th/1610*

Peripheral blood eosinophilia with eosinophil count $>1000/mm^3$ is included in the primary diagnostic criteria (and not an eosinophil count $> 0.1\times 10^9/mm^3$)

Criteria for the Diagnosis of ABPA Primary

Primary
• *Episodic bronchial obstruction (asthma)*
• *Peripheral blood eosinophilia ($>1000/mm^3$)*
• *Elevated serum IgE concentrations (>1000ng/ml)*
• *Immediately type skin reactivity to Aspergillus antigens*
• *Precipitating serum antibodies (precipitants) against Aspergillus antigens*
• *Elevated serum IgE and/or IgG antibodies specific to A. fumigatus**
• *History of pulmonary infiltrates (transient/ fleeting or fixed) on chest radiographs or CT scans*
• *Central proximal bronchiectasis on chest CT*
Secondary
• *A. fumigatus in sputum (by repeated culture or microscopic examination)*
• *History of expectoration of brown plugs or flecks*
• *Arthus reactivity (late skin reactivity) to Aspergillus antigen*

**Elevated IgE (and IgG) class antibodies specific for A. fumigatus has been mentioned as a secondary diagnostic criteria in Harrison's textbook while Fishman's textbook includes this as a main/major diagnostic criteria.*

65. Answer is D (Bronchopulmonary Aspergillosis): *Harrison 18th/2120; 17th/ 1610; CMDT 2002/ 296; 2008/222; 2009/234*

Coexistence of repeated of bronchospasm (asthma), Central (perihilar) bronchiectasis and haemoptysis suggest a diagnosis of allergic bronchopulmonary aspergillosis.

The questions gives us three leads : bronchospasm, hemoptysis, bronchiectasis.

- Presence of repeated episodes of bronchospasm indicates towards a possible existence of asthma.
- Hemoptysis, central bronchiectasis are well known complications of Allergic Broncho Pulmonary Aspergillosis.

All three of these features are consistent with the diagnosis of ABPA.

66. Answer is B (Pleural effusion): *Harrison's 16th/ 1188; 17th/ 1610; API 8th / 392 Harrison 18th/p 2119, 2120*

Pleural effusion is not seen as part of allergic bronchopulmonary Aspergillosis

- ABPA occurs in patients with preexisting ***asthma*** and cystic fibrosis. – Harrisons
- ABPA causes intermittent episodes of wheezing, pulmonary infiltrates, sputum and ***blood eosinophilia***, low grade fever and brownish or greenish flecks in the sputum.
- Patients with repeated exacerbations develop ***central bronchiectasis*** and progressive loss of pulmonary function.

67. Answer is E (Lower lobe predominance): *Fishman's Pulmonary diseases 4th/2296*

ABPA predominant involves the upper lobes and not lower lobes

Upper Lobe Predominance
'ABPA Lesions are either focal or bilateral and tend to occur more frequently in Upper lobes' - Fishman's 4th/2296

Proximal (central) Branchiectasis is a charachteristic feature
'Presence of proximal (central) bronchiectasis which is charachterized by normal filling of bronchii distal to the saccular bronchial lesion is considered a hallmark for diagnosis of ABPA' - Fishman's 4th/2296

IgE > 1000 ng/ml, Eosinophils >1000/mm^3 and elevated IgG/IgM antibodies are all criteria for diagnosis of ABPA

68. Answer is B (It is highly contagious): *Current Diagnosis and Treatment in Infectious Diseases (CIDT) 1st/751; Harrisons 17th/1257,1256 Harrison 18th/p 1655, 1656*

Human Aspergillosis mostly results from inhalation of conidia and is not a contagious disease. Person to person transmission does not occur – *Current diagnosis and Treatment in Infections Disease*

Aspergillosis is not a contagious disease (CIDT/751; Harrison 17th/1257)
- It is not a contagious disease and person to person transmission does not occur
- Routes of transmission include
  - Inhalation of conidia(major route)-Environmental Exposure
  - Direct inoculation into skin
  - Direct inoculation into blood amongst drug abusers
- Nosocomial infection may occur amongst hospitalized, immunocompromised patients

Aspergillosis is common in preexisting tuberculosis and cystic disease
'Patient with chronic pulmonary aspergillosis have a wide spectrum of underlying pulmonary disease including tuberculosis and sarcoidosis' – Harrisons
'Preexisting cavitatory lesions predispose to the formation of Aspergilloma or fungal ball' (CIDT)

Aspergillus fumigatus is a known cause for bronchopulmonary Aspergillosis

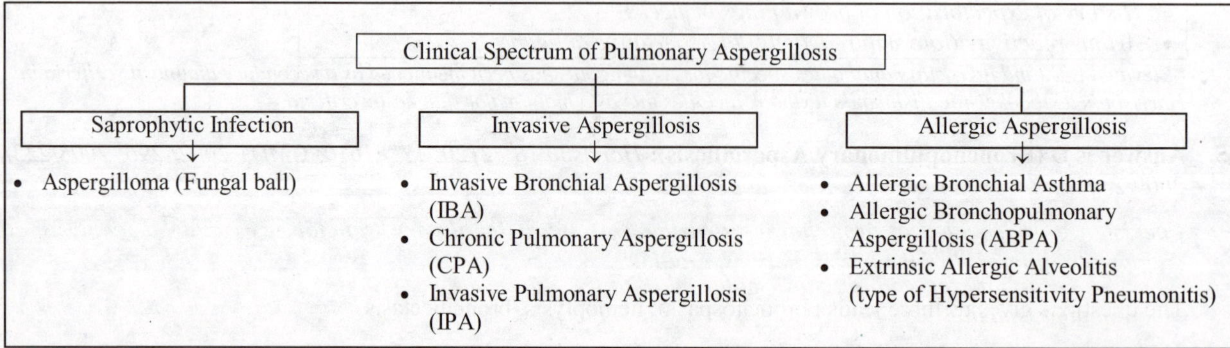

Aspergillus niger more commonly colonizes the upper respiratory tract and causes otitis externa *(Harrison)*

The most common species of Aspergillosis causing pulmonary infections is Aspergillus Fumigatus.
The most common species of Aspergillosis causing otitis externa is Aspergillus niger.

69. Answer is C (Extrinsic Allergic Alveolitis) : *Fishman's pulmonary diseases and disorders 4th/2295*

Diffuse pulmonary infiltrates on X-Ray with normal levels of IgE and absence of peripheral eosinophilia is characteristic of Extrinsic Allergic Alveolitis.

Hypersensitivity Reaction to Aspergillus

Hypersensitivity Lung diseases that result from exposure to A. Fumigatus allergens include Bronchial Asthma, ABPA and Extrinsic Allergic Alveolitis (Hypersensitivity Pneumonitis)

In Atopic Individual	In Non atopic Individuals
Allergic Bronchial Asthma and ABPA	*Extrinsic Allergic Alveolitis (Hypersensitivity penumonitis)*
Allergic Bronchial Asthma and ABPA are seen in atopic individuals and immune response is IgE mediated	Extrinsic Allergic Alveolitis or Hypersensitivity penumonitis is seen in non atopic individuals and immune response is not IgE mediated. Immune response may involve cell mediated (type IV) or immune complex (Type III) reactions.

	Asthma	ABPA	Extrinsic allergic alveolitis
Pathology	Hypertrophied mucus glands	Colonization of airways, viscid mucoid impaction, tissue eosinophilia	Lymphocytic infiltration of interstitium, noncaseating granuloma
Radiological features Early	Normal, hyperinflation	Migratory peripheral infiltrates, atelectasis, bronchiectasis	Diffuse alveolar-interstitial infiltrates
Late	Normal, hyperinflation	Fibrosis	Reticulonodular interstitial opacities
Skin test reactions to Aspergilus antigens Immediate	Positive	Positive	Positive
Delayed	Negative	Positive	Positive
Peripheral eosinophilia	Negative	Positive	Negative
IgG Aspergillus precipitins	Positive (upt o 25%)	Positive	Positive
Serum IgE levels	Normal or mildly elevated	Marked deviation	Normal

70. Answer is B (Microfilaria in blood) : *Harrison 16th/1263; 15th/1240; CMDT 2002/1520; 2009/1353-1354*

In TPE, Microfilaria are rapidly cleared from the blood stream by the lungs. Thus, microfilariae <u>are sequestrated in the lungs and are not found in the blood.</u>

<u>Tropical Pulmonary Eosinophilia</u>

Tropical Pulmonary Eosinophilia (TPE) is a distinct syndrome that develops in individuals infected with Lymphatic filarial species.

Clinical symptoms result from allergic and inflammatory reaction elicited by the cleared parasites.

Features of Tropical Pulmonary eosinophilia (TPE) :

- Male more commonly affected than females (4 : 1)
- History of resistance in filarial endemic region
- ***Paroxysmal cough and wheezing that are usually nocturnal***[Q]
- Weight loss, low grade fever, adenopathy
- ***Eosinophilia > 3000 eosinophilia / μL***[Q]
- ***Chest X-Ray : increased bronchovascular markings***[Q], *diffuse miliary lesions*[Q], or ***mottled opacities***.
- *Restrictive changes on Pulmonary function test*[Q]
- *Elevated levels of IgE*[Q] & Antifilarial antibody titers.

In TPE, Microfilaria are rapidly cleared from the blood stream by the lungs. Thus, microfilariae <u>are sequestrated in the lungs and are not found in the blood.</u>

71. Answer is C (Pulmonary eosinophilic granuloma) : *CMDT 2002/ 296; 2005/ 243; API 8th / 391, 392, 393*

All options mentioned in the question other than pulmonary eosinophilic granuloma are classified under this group of disorders termed 'pulmonary infiltrates with eosinophilia'.

Pulmonary infiltrates with eosinophilia: (PIE, eosinophilic pneumonias). Constituted by distinct individual syndromes characterized by eosinophilic pulmonary infiltrates and ***peripheral blood eosinophilia.***

These include:

Etiology known	Idiopathic
• ***Allergic bronchopulmonary mycosis***	• ***Loeffler's syndrome***
• *Parasitic infestations*	• *Acute eosinophilic pneumonia*
• *Drug reactions*	• *Chronic eosinophilic pneumonia*
• *Eosinophilia myalgia syndrome*	• ***Allergic granulomatosis of Churg & Strauss Hypereosinophilic syndrome.***

72. Answer is D>A (Wegener's granulomatosis > Allergic bronchopulmonary aspergillosis): *Current Rheumatology Diagnosis and Treatment 2nd/276, 279; Bronchial Asthma 4th/350*

The presence of fleeting opacities on serial skiagrams is consistant with a diagnosis of Allergic bronchopulmonary Aspergillosis and Wegner's granulomatosis. Associated Oligoarthritis however favours a diagnosis of Wegener's granulomatosis which is the single best answer of choice.

Oligoarticular Arthritis is a feature of Wegner's granulomatosis and is not mentioned as a feature of ABPA.

'Pauciarticular (oligoarticular) or Polyarticular arthritis may be seen in Wegner's granulomatosis'.

– Current Rheumatology 2nd/276, 279

Presence of fleeting opacities may be seen in ABPA and Wegner's granulomatosis

Fleeting opacities in ABPA	Fleeting opacities in Wegner's
'Patients with ABPA typically have fleeting infiltrates on chest X-ray' – Crofton and Douglas Respiratory Diseases 5th/803	'Focal infiltrates which may be fleeting are seen' – Radiology of Chest Disease 3rd/103

	ABPA	Wegner's
Age of Presentation	Most of the Age range is 20-40 years	Mean age at diagnosis is 50 years
Fever, weight loss Hemoptysis	May be seen	May be seen
Oligoarthritis	Not associated	Pauciarticular (oligoarticular), or Polyarticular arthritis may be seen
Fleeting opacities	May be seen	May be seen

The presence of Oligoarticular arthritis and age of presentation favour a diagnosis of Wegener's granulomatosis.

Fleeting opacities are not associated with CA lung, and tuberculosis

Pneumonias and Tuberculosis

Bacterial Pneumonia

73. Answer is C (Stretptococcus pneumonia) : *Robbins 7th /748*

'Streptococcus pneumonia or pneumococcus is the most common cause of community acquired acute pneumonia *– Robbins 7th/748*

Lobar pneumonia refers to an acute bacterial infection that results in consolidation of a large portion of a lobe or an entire lobe. Streptococcus pneumonia produces a picture of lobar pneumonia.

74. Answer is A (Gram –ve bacilli): *Harrison 16th/ 1539; 17th/ 1625-1628; Ananthnarayan 6th/ 588*

'Nosocomial pneumonias are common in immunocompromised patients and are characterized by colorization of the nasopharynx by ***'Gram negative bacilli'*** followed by trickling of upper airway secretions into lower airways, resulting in pneumonia' – *API 7th/ 304*

*'In a national survey in United States, 64% of all microorganisms isolated from the lungs of patients with nosocomial pneumonias were **gram negative bacilli'** – Harrison 16th/ 1539.*

Remember: Changing trend:

S. aureus (gram positive cocci) is the most common cause of nosocomial pneumonia in the United States - Harrison 16th/1539

*Thus while overall gram negative bacilli are the most common of cumulative agents for nosocomial pneumonias, **Staph aureus is the most common individual etiological agent.***

75. Answer is D (Thalassemia): *Harrisons 17th/866*

Thalassemia has not been mentioned in the list of conditions that commonly predispose to pneumococcal infection Thalassemia is the single best answer of exclusion.

Conditions that commonly predispose to pneumococcal infection:

Increased risk of exposure
- *Day care centres*
- *Military training camps*
- *Prisons*
- *Shelters for the homeless*

Respiratory infection, inflammation
- *Influenza, other viral respiratory infections*
- *Air pollution*
- *Allergies*
- *Cigarette smoking*
- *Chronic obstructive pulmonary disease*
- *Other cause of chronic pulmonary inflammation of obstruction*

Anatomical disruption of meninges (dural tear)

Defective antibody formation
- Common variable hypogammaglobulinemia
- Selective IgG subclass deficiency
- Multiple myeloma
- Chronic lymphocytic leukemia
- ***Lymphoma***

Defective complement function

Defective bacterial clearance
- *Congenital asplenia, hyposplenia*
- *Splenectomy*
- ***Sickle cell disease***

Multifactorial conditions
- ***Infancy and aging***
- *Chronic disease*
- *Prior hospitalization*
- *Alcoholism*
- *Malnutrition*
- *HIV infection*
- *Chronic lung disease*
- *Glucocorticoid treatment*
- *Cirrhosis of liver*
- *Renal insufficiency*
- *Diabetes mellitus*
- *Anemia*
- *Coronary artery disease*
- *Fatigue, stress, and/or exposure to cold*

76. Answer is B (Staphylococcal pneumonia): *Robbins 7th/ed 383, 385; Oxford Hand book of Medicine 6th/ed 174; Differential Diagnosis is conventional Radiology 3rd/ 574*

Cavitatory lesions and /or Pneumatoceles are characteristic of staphylococcal pneumonias

Primary Pulmonary tuberculosis does not usually present with cavitatory lesions. Cavitatory lesions are a feature of post-primary or secondary tuberculosis

Cavitation is characteristic of Staphylococcal Pneumonia

Cavitation suggests aggressive bacterial infections by bacteria such as Staph.aureus (and gram negative bacilli)

Characteristic Feature of Stapylococcal Pneumonias
• *Cavitation^Q (single or Multiple thick walled cavities) (may be Bilateral)*
• *Pneumatoceles^Q (Thin walled cystic spaces that may contain air fluid levels)*
• *Pleural Effusion^Q / Empyema^Q with or without bronchopleural fistulas (Pyopneumothorax)*
• *Abscess formation^Q*

Bacterial Pneumonas associated with cavitation: Review

- *Staphylococcus*[Q]
- *Kleibsella*[Q]
- *Pseudomonas*[Q]
- *Anaerobic bacteria*

Cavitation is a feature of secondary / Post- primary Tuberculosis and not Primary Pulmonary Tuberculsis

The chorachteristic lesion in primary Tuberculosis is the fibrocasseous Ghon focus which presents as an area of consolidation on Radiographs

Cavitation is rare in primary tuberculosis (although it may be seen)

'Cavitation may be seen in primary tuberculosis but it is a rare feature' – Robbins

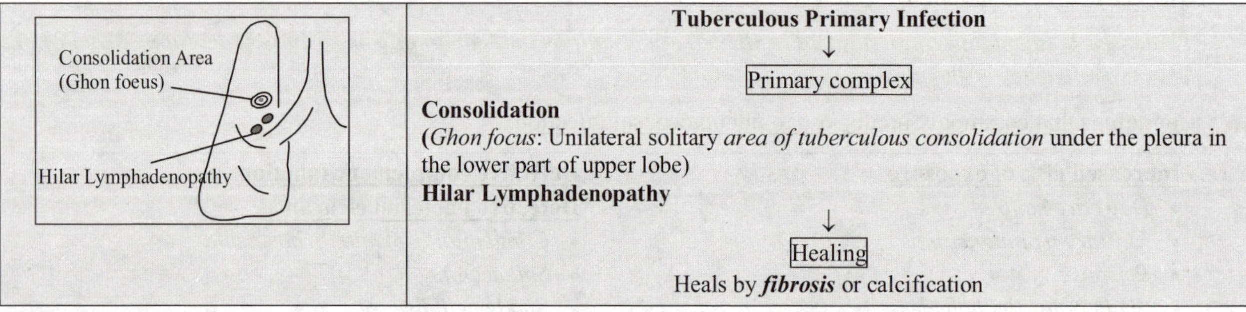

Interstitial lung diseases / Pneumoconiosis do not present with cavitatory lesions

77. Answer is A (Legionella): *Harrison 18th/1237, 1238; 14th/ 930, 15th/ 945; 16th/ 872; 17th/ 930; Ananthnarayan / 377*

Pneumonia in association with clinical clues in the form of high grade fever, confusion and diarrhea suggests a diagnosis of Legionnaire's pneumonia

Legionnaire's disease :

- Legionnaires disease presents as an '***atypical pneumonia***'[Q] where a gram stained smear of sputum does not show organisms (Caused by *Legionella).*

Legionella
• **Legionella** is a gram negative [Q], motile [Q], non-encapsulated bacilli [Q], classified under a miscellaneous group • Man to Man transmission does not occur with Legionella. [Q] • No animal reservoirs occur. [Q] • Disease is limited to humans. [Q]
Legionella survive and multiply inside free living amoeba and protozoa, distributed in natural reservoirs such as stagnant waters [Q], mud and hot spring.

- Human infection is typically acquired by inhalation of aerosols, which form the only source of infection.[Q]
- Smoking and immunocompromised status are known risk factors.
- The disease occurs with unusual frequency among patients with hairy cell leukemia but not among patients with other types of leukemia

Common Risk factors for Legionnaires disease

• Advancing age
• Immunocompromised patients:
  - Transplant recipients, HIV, Glucocorticoid recipients
  - Hairy cell leukaemia (monocyte deficiency and dysfunction)
• Chronic lung disease
• Smokers
• Diabetes mellitus (Javetz)

- Presents as mild cough slightly productive sputum, sometimes streaked with blood, along with high fever and nonspecific symptoms such as malaise, fatigue, anorexia & headache.

Think about the diagnosis as Legionaire's disease whenever the question talks about a pneumonia like picture along with any of the these :

a. Occurrence of illness in immunocompromised [Q], smokers [Q] or those with chronic lung disease [Q], or
b. Occurance of illness in an environment where potable water supply is known to be contaminated with Legionella
c. Onset of symptoms within 10 days of discharge from a hospital (I.P. 2 to 10 day), or
d. High fever, [Q] or
e. Gastrointestinal difficulties like diarrhea, [Q] or
f. Neurological abnormalities like confusion or altered Sensorium, [Q] or
g. Numerous neutrophils but no organisms revealed by gram staining of respiratory secretions, or
h. Hyponatremia [Q] is more common in Legionnaire's, than in any other form of pneumonia, or
i. Failure to respond to β-lactam drugs [Q] (penicillin or cephalosporins) and aminoglycosids antibiotics.

- Azithromycin and Respiratory Quinolones are the drugs of choice for Legionnaire's disease

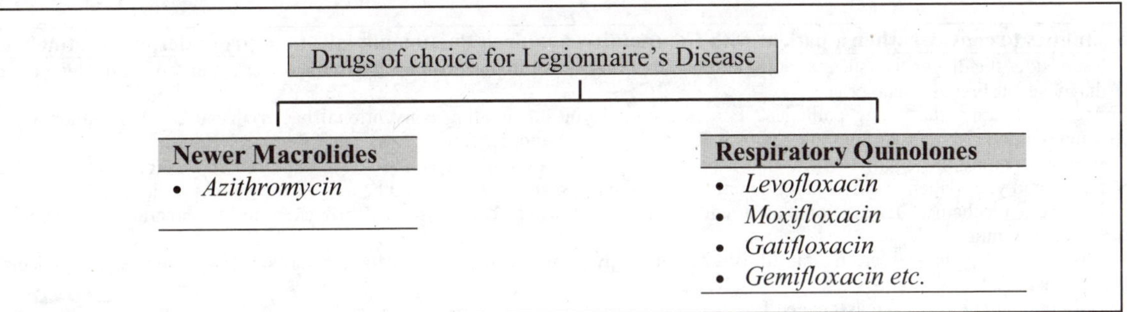

78. Answer is C (Azithromycin): *Harrison 18th/p 1238, 1239, 1240 Harrison's 17th/930, 932*

Azithromycin and Respiratory Quinolones are the drugs of choice for Legionnaire's disease

Development of pneumonia and diarrhea within 10 days after discharge from hospital hints to a possible diagnosis of Legionnaire's disease. ***The drugs of choice for Legionnaire's disease include Azithromycin and Respiratory Fluoroquinolones such as Levofloxacin, Gatifloxacin, Gemifloxacin and Moxifloxacin.***

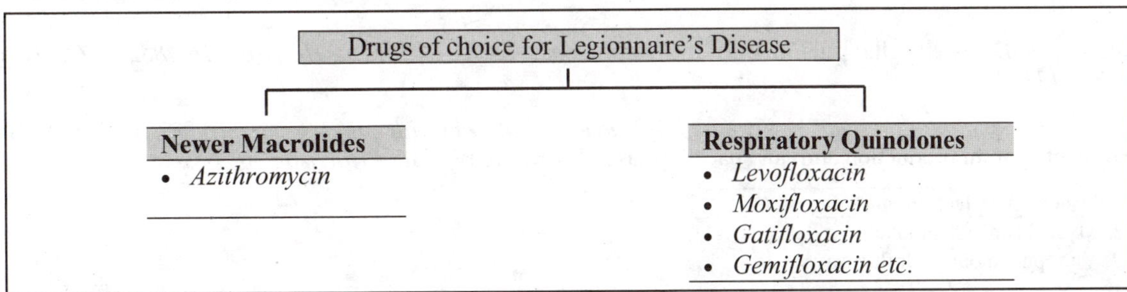

Think about the diagnosis as Legionaire's disease whenever the question talks about a pneumonia like picture with onset of symptoms within 10 days of discharge from a hospital along with gastrointestinal difficulties like diarrhea (Refer previous question)

79. Answer is D (Levofloxacin): *Harrison 17th /930, 932*

Development of pneumonia and gastrointestinal symptoms (diarrhea & gripping abdominal pain) within 10 days after discharge from hospital hints to a possible diagnosis of Legionnaire's disease. ***The drugs of choice for Legionnaire's disease include Azithromycin and Respiratory Fluoroquinolones such as Levofloxacin, Gatifloxacin, Gemifloxacin and Moxifloxacin.***

80. Answer is B (Erythromycin is the drug of choice): *Harrison 18th/p 1238, 1239 CMDT 2005/ 1373;2009/1278; Harrison 16th/ 871, 872; 17th / 929-932 Goodman Gillmons 10th/ 1154; Jawetz 23rd/ 313*

'Azithromycin, Clarithromycin or a fluoroquinolone (eg Levofloxacin) ***and not erythromycin*** *is the drug of choice for treatment legionellosis because of their excellent intracellular penetration and in vitro activity as well as desirable pharmacokinetic properties that permit oral administration and once or twice daily dosing - CMDT2005/1373; 09/1278*

Agent	Disease	First choice	Second choice	Third choice
Legionella penumophilia	Legionnaire's disease	Azithromycin Fluoroquinolone	Erythromycin	• Trimethoprim sulfomethoxazole • Doxycycline

3

81. Answer is D (Any of the above): *Harrison 18th/p 2136 Harrisons 16th/ 1536; 17th/1624, 1658, 1659; API 7th 308*

Fever persisting even after treatment of pneumonia indicates treatment failure. All of the options mentioned should be considered when a patient with pneumonia fail to improve despite treatment.

Possibilities to consider when a patient with Community-Acquired Pneumonia fails to improve despite treatment
1. Reconsider the diagnosis. Is this another illness presentinga pneumonia? Collagen vascular diseases involving the lung are frequently diagnosed at first as pneumonia.
2. Are you treating the wrong pathogen? For example, if you are treating conventional bacterial causes of pneumonia, is this case actually due to Mycobacterium tuberculosis, Pneumocystis, or another **fungus**?
3. Are you treating the right pathogen with the wrong drug? For example, if you are using nafcillin or claxacillin to treat Staphyloccos aureas and your patient is infected with methicillin resistant S. aureus you should be using vancomycin or linezolid.
4. Is there a mechanical reason for the patient's failure to improve (e.g. obstructed bronchus due to **carcinoma** or seqestation of a segment of lung?
5. Have you over looked an undrained or metastatic pyogenic focus(e.g.**empyema**, brain abscess, endocarditis, splenic, abscess, osteomyelitis?
6. Does the patient have drug associated fever?

Respiratory System

82. Answer is C (Bacterial pneumonia): *API 7th/ 308; Harrisons 16th/ 1566; 17th/1658, 1659 Harrison 18th/p 2179*

Empyema thoracic is collection of pus in pleural space and is synonymous with grossly purulent exudative parapneumonic effusions.

'In the pre antibiotic era aerobic bacteria (pneumococci and streptococci) were the most frequent causes but anaerobic bacteria are the most common causes now' *– API*

Atypical Pneumonia

83. Answer is D (Kleibsella pneumonia) : *Chandrasoma Taylor 3rd /516; Harrison 16th/882; 17th/ 1620 Harrison 18th/p2131*

Kleibsella pneumonia presents as a typical 'air space' pneumonia with cough productive of purulent sputum.
'Purulent sputum production and 'air space' diseases X Ray are typical' – *Harrison 16th/882*

Causes of Atypical pneumonias
1. Mycoplasma pneumonias
2. Viral pneumonias - Influenza - RSV - Adenovirus - Rhinovirus - Rubeola - Varicilla - Corona virus
3. Chlamydia pneumonia
4. Coxiella burnetti
5. Pneumocystis carinii
6. Legionella

Corona virus is an infrequent cause of pneumonia.
SARS associated corona virus *(SARS - CoV) caused epidemic of pneumonia from Nov 2002 to July 2003 - Harrison*

84. Answer is B (Predominance of alveolar exudates) : *Robbins 7th/751*

Viral pneumonias are an example of 'atypical pneumonias' and are characterized by inflammatory reaction predominantly restricted within the walls of alveoli within the intertitium. The alveoli may be free from exudates – *Robbins.*
The alveolar septa are widened and edematous and usually have a mononuclear inflammatory infiltrate. *Alveoli may be free from exudates* but in many patients there is *accumulation of intraalveolar proteinaceous matrial*[Q], a cellular exudates and characteristically pink hyaline membranes. These changes reflect alveolar damage similar to that seen diffusely in ARDS.

AIR Space Penumonia (Typical Pneumonia)	Interstitial Pneumonia (Atypical Pneumonia)
Exudate in alveoli i.e. consolidation	No exudate, alveoli are air filled i.e. no consolidation (infiltrate in interstitium)
Infiltrate is primarily of neutrophills (PMN)	Infiltrate is primarily lymphatic
Agents responsible are extracellular	Agents responsible are intracellular
Cough is productive of purulent sputum	Cough is dry
Chest X-ray shows alveolar pattern	Chest X-ray shows interstitial pattern

85. Answer is E (All of the above): *Fishman's pulmonary diseases 4th/2362, Harrisons 17th/1267, 1268, 1269, Harrisons 11th/797 (old edition) Harrison 18th/p 1671, 1672, 1673*

Pneumocytic carinii pneumonia is charachterized by a prominent eosinophilic exudate and mild interstitial pneumonitis. These is damage to type I pneumocytes and associated compensatory hypertrophy of type II pneumocytes.

Classic Histopathology in Pneumocystis Pneumonia

Intra- Alveolar Changes	Interstitial Changes
Prominent Eosinophilic foamy, vacuolated intraalveolar exudate (HE staining) • Intra alveolar exudate contains the organisms, which can be identified in various stages of development (trophozoite and cystic stage) by the use of special stains such as - Methamine silver / Toluidine stain - Wright Giemsa stain - Papanicolaou's stain • Intraalveolar exudate also contains host serum proteins, debris, & surfactant proteins Alveolar macrophages are present but not prominent in phagocytosis of organism. • The principle host effector cells against pneumocystis are alveolar macrophages which ingest & kill the organism	Mild interstitial Pneumonitis • Mononuclear interstitial cell infiltrate (mild) • Damaged type I Pneumocytes • Hypertrophy /proliferation of type II pneumocytis (Reparative response) *Pneumocystis attaches to, and damages type I pneumocytes. There is associated compensatory hypertrophy of type II pneumocytes.* Note: *Most compromised hosts display a mild mononuclear interstitial cell infiltrate however malnourished children display an intense interstitial plasma cell infiltrate which was responsible for the diseases early name of interstitial plasma cell pneumonia'*

86. Answer is B (Eosinophilic Alveolar Exudate): *Fishman's Pulmonary Diseases 4th /2362, Harrisons 17th/1267, 1268, 1269 Harriosns 11th/ 797 (old edition); Refer previous question Harrison 18th/p 1671, 1672, 1673*

The most characteristic histopathological feature of pneumocystis carinii pneumonia in adults is predominantly alveolar, foamy vacuoloted, eosinophilic exudates.

Interstitial pneumonitis is usually mild and shows infiltration with PML and mononuclear cells.

Note

Pneumocystic Pneumonia in Adults	Pneumocystis Pneumonia in molnourished infants
In adults the disease appears to be predominantly alveolar *Air spaces (alveoli) are filled with a foamy, eosinophilic exudate and appear honey coombed* *The intra-alveolar exudate consists of organisms, surface glycoprotein exudate and debri of macrophages and inflammatory cells.*	***In infants the disease has a predominant interstitial component*** *The interstitium is filled with fluid plasma cells and lymphocytes.* *These formed elements seem to overflow into air spaces which are filled with a frothy eosinophilic exudates.*

Respiratory System

3

87. Answer is B (Pneumocystis carinii Pneumonia): *Harrison 18th/ p1671,1672 Harrison's 17th/1267, 1268; Textbook of Pulmonary Medicines by Behera 2nd/ 413; Fishman's Pulmonary Diseases & Disorders 4th/ 1108, 2353, 2356, 2358*

Presence of prolonged fever, weight loss and bilateral reticulonodular infiltrates in a person at increased risk of HIV (Long distance Truck drivers in India) suggests a diagnosis of Atypical pneumonia due to pneumocystis carinii infection.

Pneumocystic pneumonia is one of the most common AIDS – defining opportunistic infections and should be considered in any patient presenting with atypical pneumonia who is at increased risk of acquiring HIV (eg Professional sex workers, Homosexuals men, Intravenous drug users and Long distance Truck drivers in India)

Presentation of patient is consistant with diagnosis of Pneumocystic Pneumonia

- Pneumocystis carinii is an important cause of Atypical Pneumonia in immunocompromised states especially AIDS
- Pneumocystic Pneumonia is recognized as one of the most common AIDS defining oppostunistic infections.

'A diagnosis of Pneumocystic pneumonia should be considered in any patient presenting with sings / symptoms of Atypical Pneumonia in a patient who is at increased risk of acquiring HIV infection'

Long Distance Truck Drivers in India are considered a high risk population for contracting the HIV virus *(Nag, 1996)*

- Charachteristic clinical manifestations include significant weight loss, fever, non productive cough and dysponea

Clinical Manifestations *(Textbook of Pulmonary Medicine' by Behera 2nd/413)*
- *Profound **weight loss** (~100%)*
- ***Fever** (~ 97%)*
- *Dyspnea (~ 63%)*
- ***Non Productive cough** (~ 75%)*

- The most charachteristic finding an chest X-Ray is bilateral diffuse infiltrates beginning in the perihilar region although various atypical manifestations including nodular lesions, cavitatory lesions etc have also been reported

The classic finding on chest radiography consists of bilateral diffuse infiltrates beginning in the perihilar region

However no radiographic pattern is pathognomic for pneumocystic pneumonia.

Tuberculosis is *unlikely* *as it usually present with productive cough* and the patient in question has a non productive dry cough. Also, *bilateral diffuse reticulonodular infiltrates are not charachteristic of Tuberculosis.*

Interstitial Lung Diseases is *unlikely* *as these disorders usually do not present with fever and weight loss*, although bilateral reticulonodular infiltrates may be seen on chest x-Ray.

'With most interstitial lung diseases, constitutional symptoms like fevers, chills and weight loss are absent'

– Fishman's Pulmonary Diseases 4th/1108

Note: Patients with Acute Interstitial Pneumonias (Type of ILD) may present with the a similar clinical and radiological picture, but these disorders constitute only a small fraction of Interstitial Lung Diseases (< 1%).

Pneumococcal Pneumonia *is unlikely as it presents with typical features of pneumonia including productive cough and consolidation on chest x-rays.* The patient in question has a form of *atypical pneumonia.*

AIR Space Penumonia (Typical Pneumonia)	Interstitial Pneumonia (Atypical Pneumonia)
Exudate in alveoli i.e. ***consolidation***	No exudate, alveoli are air filled i.e. ***no consolidation*** (infiltrate in interstitium)
Infiltrate is primarily of neutrophills (PMN)	Infiltrate is primarily lymphatic
Agents responsible are extracellular	Agents responsible are intracellular
Cough is productive of purulent sputum	***Cough is dry***
Chest X-ray shows alveolar pattern	Chest X-ray shows interstitial pattern

88. Answer is A (Usually associated with CMV infection): *Washington manual of Pulmonary Medicine (2006)/ 104 Harriosns 16th/ 1194, 1195; Jawetz 24th/ 648, 649; 'Pneumocystic Pneumonia' by Wolzer & Cushion 3rd/418; CT scan of the body by Mathias /362*

Pneumocystis Jiroveci may be associated with CMV infection but it is not usually associated with CMV infection.

Pneumocystis Jiroveci is the new nomenclature for human infection with Pneumocystic carini (which is now used for organisms found in rats)

Pneumocystis infection in Humans : P. Jiroveci

Pneumocystis infection in Rats : P. Carini

- ***Pneumocystic Jiroveci disease and immunosupression***
  'Pneumocystis Jiroveci does not cause disease in the absence of immuno supression' – Jawetz 24th/648

  Note
  Pneumocystic Jiroveci may infect immunocompetent hosts but the disease (pneumocystis pneumonia) occurs only when the host is immunosupressed
  Most individuals are infected in early childhood But pneumonia occurs in immunocompromised patients only either due to reactivation or new infection.

  Persons at risk for Pneumocystic disease (Pneumocystosis)
  - Acquired *Immunodeficiency* Disease (eg AIDS)
  - Patients Recieving *Immunosupressive* therapy (especially Glucocorticoids) for cancer, organ transplantation etc.
  - Children with primary *immunodeficiency* diseases
  - Premature malnourished infants (*immunodeficient*)

- ***Pneumocystic Pneumonia : Diagnosis***
  Diagnosis of Pneumocystic Pneumonia is based on specific identification of organism in respiratory specimen with appropriate histological staining
  - *Pneumocystis infection is usually diagnosed by sputum examination*
    Sputum samples should always be obtained by induction (with hypertonic saline)
    Routine sputum specimen is often inadequate (Washington manual of Pulmonary medicine)
  - *BAL forms the mainstay of diagnosis for Pneumocystic Pneumonia*
    If organisms are not seen on induced sputum examination a Bronchoalveolar lavage specimen should be obtained. BAL forms the mainstay of diagnosis for Pneumocystic Pneumonia - Harrisons 16th

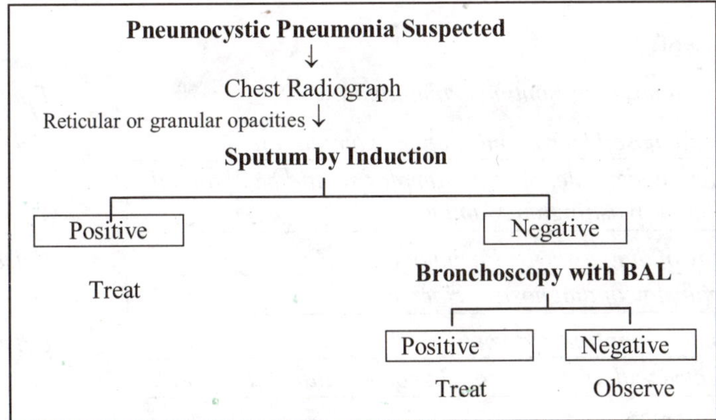

- ***Pneumocystic Pneumonia and CMV infection*** ('Pneumocystic Pneumonia' by Wolzer & Cushion 3rd/418)
  'Several studies have indicated that CMV is a risk factor for Pneumocystis Pneumonia in Renal transplant patients
  These is however no convincing evidence to show a direct effect of the CMV virion on Pneumocystis'

  > Thus we conclude
  > Pneumocystic ***may be associated*** with CMV infection but in a few selected cases and special circumstances like Renal tansplantation. CMV is ***not usually associated*** with pneumocystic pneumonia.

- ***Pneumocystis Pneumonia and Pneumatocele***
  Pneumocystic Pneumonia ***may be associated*** with pneumotocele formation but Pneumatoceles are ***not associated in all cases*** of Pneumocystic pneumonia

  Pneumatocele: Differential Diagnosis *(CT scan of the body by Mathias /362)*
  - *Post infectious (Staphylococcal*[Q] and other bacterial infections)
  - ***Pneumocystic***[Q]
  - Post traumatic (Laceration)
  - After treatment of metastasis (rare)

89. Answer is B (Usually diagnosed by Sputum examination) : Refer previous question

Pneumocystis Jiroveci is usually diagnosed by sputum examination. This is the single best answer of choice amongst the options provided.

- **Pneumocystic infection is usually diagnosed by sputum examination although mainstay of diagnosis for pneumocystic infection is Bronchoscopy with BAL**

  Sputum examination is the initial procedure of choice to confirm the presence of Pneumocystic Jiroveci infection

P. Jiroveci infection is usually diagnosed by histopathological staining of an induced sputum specimen BUT ⇓ BUT *Sputum examination is not the mainstay of diagnosis of P. Jiroveci infection.* Fibreoptic *Bronchoscopy with BAL which is more sensitive than sputum examination remains the mainstay of Pneumocystis diagnosis – Harrison 17th/1195*

- **Pneumocystis infection may occur in healthy individuals but disease due to Pneumocystic infection does not occur in the absence of Immunosupression**

'Serological endence suggests that most individuals are infected in early childhood' – Jawetz 24th/648 *'Most healthy children have been exposed to the organism by 3 to 4 years of age' – Harrisons 16th/1194* BUT ⇓ BUT *'In the absence of immunosupression P. Jiroveci does not casue disease' – Jawetz 24th/ 648*

- **Pneumocystic Jiroveci infection may be associated with CMV infection and may present with Pneumatocele (Not always)** (Refer previous question)

Remember : Facts: Confusing statements

- *Pneumocystis infection is usually diagnosed by sputum examination.* : *True*
- *Pneumocystis infection is usually diagnosed by routine sputum examination* : *False*

Routine sputum specimen are often inadequate. Sputum samples should be obtained by induction with hypertonic saline - Washington Manual

- *Sputum examination is the mainstay of diagnosis for Pneumocystis* : *False*

Bronchoscopy with BAL is the mainstay of diagnosis – Harrison

- *Pneumocystis infects only the immunocompromised host* : *False*

Most healthy individuals are infected with pneumocystis in early childhood – Jawetz

- *Pneumocystic pneumonia occurs only in the immunocompromised host* : *True*

P. Jiroveci does not cause disease in the absence of immunsupression – Jawetz

90. Answer is A and D (CD_4 count <200 ml and oral condidiasis): *Harrisons 17th/1269 Harrison 18th/p 1672, 1673*

CD_4 count <200 and Oropharyngeal candidiasis are indications for prophylaxis against pneumocystis carini pneumonia.

Indications for prophylaxis against Pneumocystic carinii
• An absolute CD_4 count <200/μL (CD_4 percentage <20%) (Primary prophylaxis) • Oropharyngeal candidiasis (Primary prophylaxis) • *Prior Pneumocystic carinii pneumonia (Secondary prophylaxis)*

Remember

Criteria for discontinuing primary prophylaxis
CD_4 + Tcell count > 200 for ≥ 3 months

The drug of choice for primary and secondary prophylaxis is TMP- SMX

91. Answer is D (Fluoroquinolones): *Harrison 15th/ 1184; 17th/ 1268, 1269; Goodman Gillman's pharmacology 10th/ 1156. Harrison 18th/p 1672, 1673*

Fluoroquinolones are not used in the treatment of P. carinii infection

Drugs used for treatment of *Pneumocystis carinii* infection include :

Agent	Disease	First choice drug	Second choice	Third choice
Pneumocystis carinii	Mild to moderate pneumonia	Trimethoprim Sulfamethoxazole	Trimethoprim – Dapsone Clindamycin – Primaquine	Atovaquone
	Sever pneumonia	Trimethoprim Sulfamethoxazole	Pentamidene Clindamycin-Primaquine	Trimetroxate

Drug of choice for all forms of pneumocystosis : *Trimethoprim-Sulfamethoxazole (Cotrimoxazole)*

92. Answer is D (Erythromycin): *Harrison 18th/p 1419 Harrison 16th/ 1010; 17th/ 1068, 1069;KDT 5th/ 688; CMDT 2009/238(t 9-9);2005/246*

***Erythromycin is used as a first choice drug for atypical pneumonia caused by mycoplasma pneumoniae**-KDT*

According to CMDT:

Agent / organism	Preferred:	Alternative: Antimicrobial therapy
Mycoplasma pneumoniae	Erythromycin or Doxycycline	Clarithromycin; Azithromycin, Fluoroquinolone

93. Answer is C (Cefotaxime is the drug of choice): *CMDT- 2008/1125; 2009/238(t 9-9)*

The drugs of choice for mycoplasma are Erythromycin and Doxycycline and not Cefotaxime.

Etiologic Agent	Drugs of First choice	Alternative Drugs
Mycoplasmas	*Erythromycin or Doxycycline*	*Clarithromycin, Azithromycine Fluoroquinolones*

94. Answer is A (Erythromycin): *Harrison 18th/p 1430 Harrison 17th /1078; CMDT 2005/ 246; 2009/238(t 9-9)*

Erythromycin is the answer of choice here as Doxycycline has been not provided in the options.

Drugs used for treatment of Chlamydia pneumonia :

According to CMDT:

Preferred agent	Alternative agent
Doxycycline	Erythromycin Clarithromycin Azithromycin Fluoroquinolone

According to Goodman & Gillman's :

First choice drug	Second choice drug
Doxycycline Azithromycin or Clarithromycin or Erythromycin	Fluoroquinolone

95. Answer is B (Tachyapnea): *Harrison 16th/ 1538; Clinical/Anesthesiology 3rd/ 250*

***Aspiration pneumonitis** is characterized by an acute onset of dyspnea, tachypnea, bronchospasm and cyanosis with a chest radiograph often showing diffuse opacities. – Harrisons*

Dyspnea & tachypnea are certainly the earliest manifestations to appear following aspiration of any material. The commonest and the earliest 'sign' of aspiration pneumonitis thus would be tachypnea.

Tuberculosis

96. Answer is B (Unilateral hilar lymphadenopathy): *Harrison 15th/ 1027*

Unilateral hilar lymphadenopathy as part of the primary complex is a characteristic feature of primary tuberculosis

Primary tuberculosis:

- It is the first infection with tubercle bacilli in individuals who have not been previously exposed to the organisms
- Seen in children [Q]
- Primary complex is characteristic

Primary (Ghon) complex
• Unilateral enlarged hilar lymph nodes [Q] • Ghon focus [Q]: Epitheloid-cell granulomatous inflammation (consolidation) at site of parenchymal infection. Usually small and subpleural most commonly located under pleura in lower part of upper lobe

- Usually a symptomatic [Q] or manifested by a mild flu like illness at time of tuberculin conversion
- Lesion heal by fibrosis [Q] and may calcify [Q]
- Radiological evidence of healed primary infection may or may not be present [Q]

Effects of primary tuberculosis
• Tuberculin positivity [Q] • Partial immunity to tuberculosis[Q]: individual requires a higher dose to be reinfected by tubercle bacilli • Presence of dormant tubercle bacilli

97. Answer is A (Cavitatory lesion): *Harrisons 17th/1008-1011, Robbins 7th/383-385*

Cavitatory lesions are a feature of post primary or secondary tuberculosis and not primary tuberculosis cases
Cavitation is rare in primary tuberculosis
Cavitation is a feature of secondary Tuberculosis (Robbins)

Cavitation occurs readily in the secondary form.
Indeed cavitation is almost inevitable in neglected secondary tuberculosis.
Cavitation may be seen in primary tuberculosis but it is a rare feature. *- Robbins*

Fibrocasseous lesion are charachteristic in primary Tuberculosis
The charachteristic pulmonary lesion in primary tuberculosis is a Ghon's focus, which is in fact a fibrocasseous lesion showing marked granulomatous inflammatory reaction with casseous necrosis.

Phlectenular conjunctivitis is a feature of primary tuberculosis
Phlyctenular conjunctivits is a hypersensitivity reaction in the eye to the presence of TB bacilli elsewhere in the body. It is commonly seen in children with primary tuberculosis

The onset of tubercular infection may be accompanied by erythema nodosum or phlyctenular conjunctivitis which are regarded as hypersensitivity reactions to mycobacteria. These lesions reflect tuberculin conversion in primary tuberculosis

Hallmarks indicating Hypersensitivity to Mycobacteria in Primary pulmonary TB
• *Erythema nodosum* • *Phlyctenular conjunctivitis*

Pleural effusion is common in primary tuberculosis
'Pleural effusion is found in upto 2/3 of cases of primary tuberculosis and results from penetration of bacilli into the pleural space from an adjacent subpleural focus' - Harrison

98. Answer is None (All may be seen): *Harrison 18th/1343-1346;17th/1008-11, Robbins 7th/383-85;API Medicine 7th/ 310*

All features mentioned may be seen in the normal course of a primary tuberculous infection.

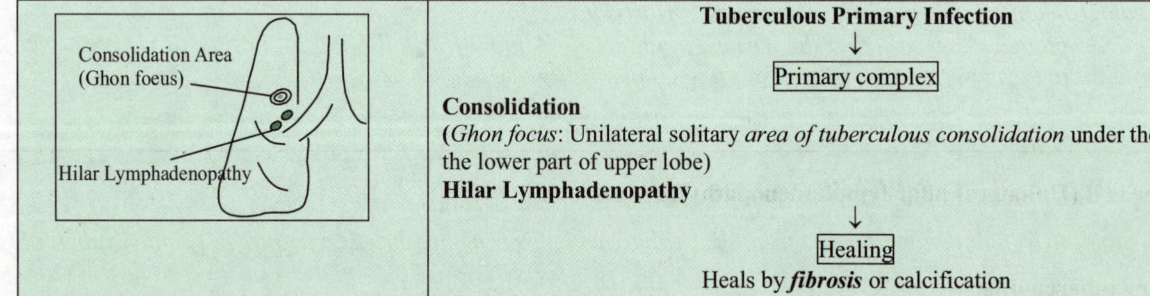

Pleural effusion may be seen in primary tuberculosis
'Pleural effusion is found in upto 2/3 of cases of primary tuberculosis and results from penetration of bacilli into the pleural space from an adjacent subpleural focus' - Harrison

99. Answer is A (Lungs): *Robbins 8th/chap 8; Oski's Pediatrics 4th/1144, Principles of Pulmonary Medicine (Elsevier) 5th/307*

The most common primary site for primary tuberculosis is the Lung.

'Primary site is the Lung in upto 95% of cases' - Oski's Pediatrics

'For both primary and reactivation tuberculosis the lungs are the most commonly affected site.'

- Principles of Pulmonary Medicine (Elsevier) 5th/107

Most common primary site for Primary Tuberculosis is Lungs[Q] *Most common site for Post-Primary Reactivation Tuberculosis is Lung*[Q]
Most common primary site for congenital tuberculosis is Liver[Q] *Most common site /organ involved in congenital tuberculosis in Lung*[Q]

Primary tuberculosis:

- It is the first infection with tubercle bacilli in individuals who have not been previously exposed to the organisms
- Seen in children [Q]
- Primary complex is characteristic

Primary (Ghon) complex
• Unilateral enlarged hilar lymph nodes [Q] • Ghon focus [Q]: Epitheloid-cell granulomatous inflammation (consolidation) at site of parenchymal infection. Usually small and subpleural most commonly located under pleura in lower part of upper lobe

- Usually a symptomatic [Q] or manifested by a mild flu like illness at time of tuberculin conversion
- Lesion heal by fibrosis [Q] and may calcify [Q]
- Radiological evidence of healed primary infection may or may not be present [Q]

Effects of primary tuberculosis
• Tuberculin positivity [Q] • Partial immunity to tuberculosis[Q]: individual requires a higher dose to be reinfected by tubercle bacilli • Presence of dormant tubercle bacilli

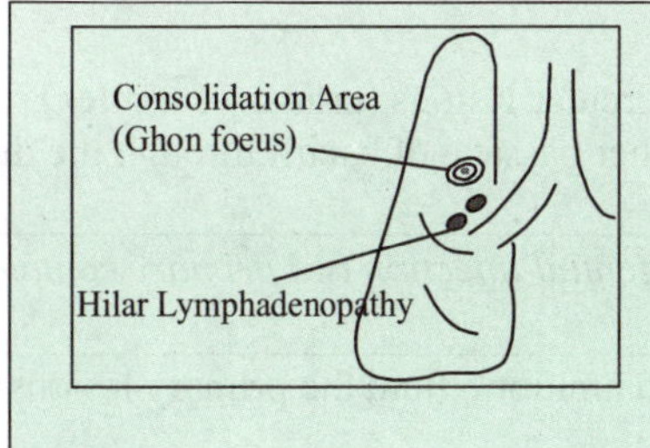

Tuberculous Primary Infection

↓

Primary complex

Consolidation

(*Ghon focus*: Unilateral solitary *area of tuberculous consolidation* under the pleura in the lower part of upper lobe)

Hilar Lymphadenopathy

↓

Healing

Heals by ***fibrosis*** or calcification

100. Answer is B (Liver): *'Avery's Diseases of the Newborn' (Elseiver 2005)8th/544; Essentias of Tuberculosis in Children by Seth & Kabro (Jaypee) 2006/299,300*

Primary Complex in the Liver suggests congenital tuberculosis.

'The only lesion in a neonate that is unquestionably associated with congenital infection is a primary complex in the liver; all others may be acquired congenitally or postnatally'- Avery's Diseases of the New born

Diagnostic Criteria for Congenital Tuberculosis

Beitzke' Criteria (1935)	**Revised Criteria by Cantwell (1994)**
i. Bacteriological Proof of Tuberculosis ***ii. Primary complex in Liver*** iii. If primary complex is lacking in Liver then tuberculosis can be considered congenital only if: a. Tuberculous lesions present in fetus or newborn are only few days old b. Or in an older infant extrauterine infection can be excluded with certainity	i. Lesion in first week of life ***ii. A primary hepatic complex or caseating hepatic granuloma*** iii. Tuberculous infection of placenta or maternal genital tract iv. Exclusion of possibility of postnatal transmission by a thorough investigation of contacts including the infant's hospital attendants or birth attendants

101. Ans. Answer is B (Liver): *Thurlbeck's Pathology of the Lung (Thieme)2005/223; Avery's Diseases of the Newborn/ (Lippincott)8th/543, 543, 544, 545; Oski's Pediatrics 4/h/1151; Liver Disease in Children (Cambridge University Press 2007/876)*

The most common primary site for, true congenital tuberculosis (primary complex in congenital tuberculosis) is Liver (followed by Lungs).

Congenital Tuberculosis

Congenital Tuberculosis caused by ***Transplacental spread*** (Hematogenous)	Congenital Tuberculosis caused by ***aspiration of infected amniotic fluid***	Congenital Tuberculosis caused by ***ingestion of infected amniotic fluid***
Most common Primary site of infection is Liver (Hematogenous infection leads to miliary disease)	*Most common Primary site of infection is Lungs*	*Most common Primary site of infection is Gastrointestinal Tract*
Since Lungs are eventually involved in most cases of congenital tuberculosis where Liver is the primary site of infection, Lungs are the most commonly involved sites in Congenital Tuberculosis		

Congenital Tuberculosis

- True congenital Tuberculosis is defined as tuberculosis occurring in infants as a result of infection with M. Tuberculosis during intrauterine life.
- Three modes of fetal infection have been proposed
  a. Transplacental (Hematogenous infection via the umbilical vein)
  b. Fetal aspiration of infected amniotic fluid
  c. Fetal ingestion of infected amniotic fluid
- When infection enters the fetus through the umbilical veins, the primary tubercular lesions (primary complex) develops in the liver. (Lesions may also develop in the lungs suggesting further passage of bacilli through the ductus venosus)

  'The only lesion in the neonate that is unquestionably associated with congenital infection is a primary complex in the liver; all others may be acquired congenitally or postnatally
- When infection enters the fetus through the aspiration / inhalation of infected amniotic fluid the primary lesions (primary complex) develops in the lungs.

  Tuberculous involvement of Lungs without associated hepatic lesions indicates aspiration of infected ammotic fluid on inhalation of tubercle bacilli.

  Lungs are the most common organs involved in congenital tuberculosis being involved almost all cases.
- Congenital Tuberculosis is charachterized by a nonimmune, non reactive response with abundant caseation and an unsually large number of bacilli. There may be multiple foci of infection within the primary site and the distribution is usually miliary.

102. Ans. Answer is A (Lungs): *Textbook of Pulmonary Medicine by Behera' 2nd/495*

The most common organ involved in congenital tuberculosis are the Lungs followed by Liver.

'The form of disease is usually miliary with multiple organ involvement. Lungs are involved in almost all cases. Other sites frequently involved are liver, spleen, lymph nodes, the gastrointestinal tract and kidney'.

-Textbook of Pulmonary Medicine by Behera 2nd/495

103. Answer is D (Monotoux is always positive): *Harrison 18th/p1349 Harrisons 17th/1013 Harrisons 11th/629*

Montoux test is not always positive in cases of Miliary Tuberculosis.

It may be negative /non reactive as a result of anergy.

Miliary Tuberculosis may occur following primary infection and secondary reactivation

Miliary tuberculosis is due to hematogenous dissemination of tubercle bacilli.
'Classically miliary tuberculosis develops following hematogenous dissemination at the time of primary infection' - *Harrisons 11th/629*

'In adults miliary tuberculosis may be due to reactivation of old disseminated foci (secondary reactivation)'
- Harrisons 17th/1013

Sputum microscopy is usually negative (Harrisons 17th/1013)
'Sputum smear microscopy is negative in 80% of cases' – Harrison 17th/1013
Montoux test is negative in 20-30% of patients with Miliary Tuberculosis
'The Tuberculn skin Test (montoux) may be non reactive due to anergy' -Nelson 5th/567

'Tubercular anergy is common in Miliary Tuberculosis and a negative skin test should not be a deterrant to the consideration of this diagnosis' - Harrison 11th/629

'Upto 30% of children have a negative tuberculin skin test' - 'Tuberculosis : Current concepts and Treatment' 2nd/201

Liver, kidney and spleen are common sites of involvement along with other sites
Almost every organ in the body may be involved. Miliary tuberculosis is most prominent in Liver, spleen, kidney and other organs including bone marrow, adrenals, meninges, fallopian tubes and epididymis - Robbins 7th/386

104. Answer is C (A positive test does not ......): *Park*

***A positive test indicates that patient is infected with M. tuberculosis. It does not however prove that the person is 'suffering' from the disease** – Park*

Montoux test
Montoux test is carried out by injecting one tuberculin unit (1TU) of PPD in 0.1 ml on the flexor surface of forearm (PPD RT 23 with Tween 80)

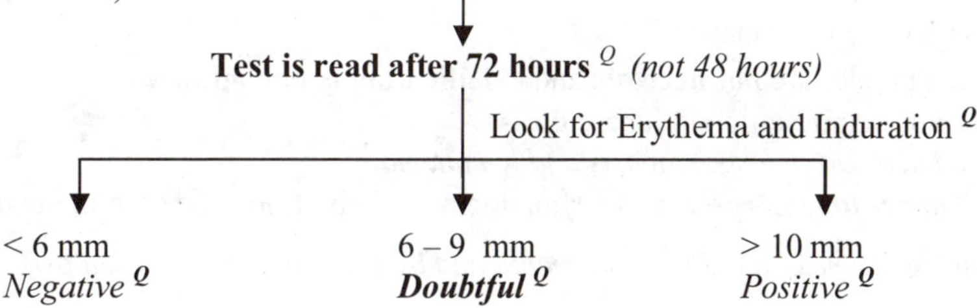

- ***A positive test indicates that patient is infected with M. tuberculosis. It does not however prove that the person is 'suffering' from the disease** – Park*
- ***Studies indicate that 92% of new cases occur in persons who already are tuberculin reactors**.– Park*
- ***6-9 mm induration does not indicate high chances of developing tuberculosis.*** Infact patients with 25 mm induration have more chances of developing tuberculosis than those with 6-9 mm induration - *Park*

105. Answer is D (Atypical mycobacterial infection): *Ananthnarayan 6th / 333; Park 18th/150*

Infection with atypical mycobacteria or other related mycobacteria are associated with false positive reactions and not false negative tests.

False negative tuberculin tests (Anergy) may occur in situations such as :

- *Miliary tuberculosis* [Q]
- Convalescence from some viral infections like *Measles* [Q]
- Lymphoreticular malignancy
- *Sarcoidosis* [Q]
- *Severe malnutrition* [Q]
- *Immunosuppressive therapy* [Q]
- *Defective cell mediated immunity* [Q]

106. Answer is E (All of the above): *Harrison 18th/p 1350, 1351 Harrisons 17th/1014,1015*

Montoux testing, sputum for AFB, PCR and BACTEC (culture method) may all be used fo establish the diagnosis of Tuberculosis.

107. Answer is A (Pulmonary tuberculosis): *CMDT 2005/ 254; 2009/246*

All features mentioned in this question are in favour of pulmonary tuberculosis and the only feature that troubles is a 'negative sputum cytology'. A negative sputum cytology however does not rule out pulmonary tuberculosis.
'A negative sputum cytology does not rule out pulmonary tuberculosis'*- CMDT*

'There is a definite set for patients of 'suspected TB with negative sputum smears'. These patients are usually investigated by bronchoscopy as the next diagnostic step. Bronchial washings and transbronchial lung biopsies are specially helpful and increase the diagnostic yield'. – CMDT

Definitive diagnosis of TB :
Does* not depend on sputum cytology** but, ***it depends on recovery of Mycobacterium TB in cultures or identification of organism by DNA probe.

Remember: "***demonstration of acid fast bacilli on sputum smears does not confirm a diagnosis of TB***".

Since saphrophytic and non tuberculous mycobacteria make colonize the airways or cause pulmonary disease.
It is sputum culture with demonstration of M. TB that is diagnostic.

108. Answer is B (Tuberculosis) : *Harrison 17th/2020, 1523, 956; 15th/1969, 1470, 1024, 1025, 1027*

Most common cause of necrotic lymph nodes with peripheral rim enhancement is tuberculosis.

- **Peripheral rim enhancement is seen in most granulomatous lymphadenopathies.**
  Most common cause of necrotic lymph nodes with peripheral rim enhancement is Tuberculosis
  - In tuberculosis affected lymph nodes show relatively low attenuation of their central region and peripheral rim enhancement after I.V. contrast material
  - In Sarcoidosis lymph nodes are **not necrotic** and **calcification is uncommon**
- ***Expectoration*** is a major manifestation in tuberculosis.
  It is usually not associated sarcoidosis, silicosis and lymphoma.
- ***Cough and bilateral upper lobe fibrosis*** makes lymphoma unlikely. It may be seen in the other conditions.

The only condition satisfying all the clinical features mentioned in the question is tuberculosis and hence is the answer of choice.

109. Answer is B (Tuberculosis) : *Refer previous question*

Most common cause of necrotic lymph nodes with peripheral rim enhancement is Tuberculosis.

110. Answer is B (Pulmonary Artery): *'Churchill Livingstone Medical Dictionary' by Brooker 16th/410; 'Step by Step Computed Tomography' by Karthikeyan & Chegu (Jaypee) 2004 /134*

Rasmussen's aneurysm refers to an aneurysm of the pulmonary artery within/adjacent to a tuberculous cavity

Rasmussen's aneurysm

- This is an aneurysm *arising from the pulmonary artery*
- This is typically a *'pseudoaneurysm'* resulting from inflammatory necrosis of the vessel wall, by *direct invasion* of the pulmonary arterial wall by adjacent tuberculous infection
- Typically the vessel injury occurs in the *upper lobes* of sites of pulmonary tuberculosis
- Rupture of these aneurysms results in *hemoptysis and pulmonary hemorrhage*

111. Answer is E (All of the above): *'Infection Control In The community' by Lawrence & May 1st (2003)*

All of the options require consideration for a diagnosis of MDR – TB.

Mult Drug Resistant Tuberculosis (MDR TB)

MDR-TB is defined by the presence of resistance to both Rifampicin and Isoniazid with or without other resistance

MDR TB should be considered in patients with:

- *Previous drug treatment for tuberculosis*
- *Contact with a case of known MDRTB*
- *HIV infection*
- *Failure of clinical response on treatment*
- *Prolonged sputum smear or culture positive while on treatment (smear positivity at 4 months or culture positivity at 5 months)*

112. Answer is B (Bronchial Artery): *Harrison 18th/p 284 Harrisons 17th/227; Harrisons 16th/207; Diagnosis and treatment of symptoms of Respiratory; Vascular and Interventional Radiology by bakal (2002)/158*

Hemoptysis usually arises from the bronchial arteries. Pulmonary arteries are a rare source of hemorrhage. The vascular structure that should be evaluated first for angiographic treatment are therefore bronchial arteries.

'Majority of cases of hemoptysis represent bleeding from the bronchial arteries, therefore bronchial angiography is usually the initial angiographic procedure'-Diagnosis and Treatment of symptoms of the Respiratory Tract (2007)/177

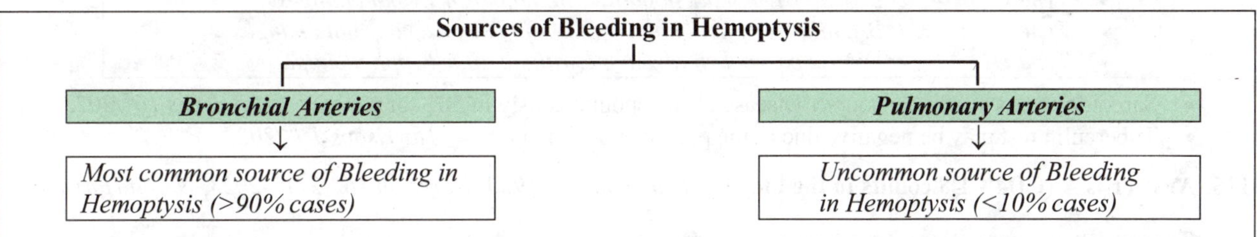

A pulmonary arterial source should be considered in addition to the more common systemic source (bronchial artery) in the setting of destructive lung lesion such as cavitatory tuberculosis. However the vascular structure that should be evaluated first is the bronchial artery.

Remember : Ramussen Aneurysm

- Ramussen aneurysm is a rare cause of bleeding in cavitatory tuberculosis and results from erosion of tuberculous cavity into a pulmonary artery branch.
- *The most common source of bleeding in Remussen aneurysm is the pulmonary artery*[Q].

Sarcoidosis

113. Answer is A (Sarcoidosis): *Harrison 18th/p 2806, 2807, 2808 Harrison 14th/1927, 1923, 15th/1971, 1969; Harrisons 16th/ 2017, 2018, 2023; Harrison 17th/2136, 2137*

The presence of non-caseating granuloma, along with bilateral hilar lymphadenopathy, goes strongly in favour of a diagnosis of Sarcoidosis'.

Sarcoidosis: *Review*

Sarcoidosis is a chronic multisystem disorder of unknown cause characterized by accumulation of T lymphocytes and mononuclear phagocytes in various tissues of body

Non caseating **SAR**coid granulomas in affected organs

Lung (90%)	Lymph nodes (75-90%)	Skin	Others	
• ***Interstitial lung disease***[Q] - Fibrosis of lung parenchyma • Pleura is involved in 1-5% of cases u/e ***pleural effusion***[Q] • *Cavitation* ***is rare***[Q]	• B/L hilar lymphadenopathy is the hallmark of sarcoidosis • Parotid enlargement B/e involvement is the vuli	• ***Erythema nodosum***[Q] • ***Lupus perenium***[Q] (purple blue shiny swollen lesions on nose, cheeks, lips, ears).	Eye	Uveitis
			Kidney (rare)	Renal hypercalcemia with or without hypercalcuria
			Skeletal	Arthritis
			Nervous system	Peripheral neuropathy.
			Heart	Cor pulmonle

Sarcoid granulomas: The inflammatory process in sarcoidosis is characterized by formation of sarcoid granulomas in various organs. – *Harrisons 16th/ 2018*

Giant Cells within granulomas can be of Langerhan's or Foreign body variety and often contain inclusions bodies:

Inclusions seen in giant cells in sarcoidosis. (Remember as **SAR**coidosis)
- ***S**chaumann bodies*[Q]
- ***A**steroid bodies*[Q]
- ***R**esidual bodies*[Q]

114. Answer is A (Often cavitate) : *Harrison 18th/2807; 15th/1971; Harrison 16th/2020, 2023; Harrison 17th/2136, 2137*

Cavitation is uncommon seen only in less than 5% of patients with sarcoidosis.

- Of individuals with **sarcoidosis** 90% have abnormal findings on chest x ray Sarcoidosis of the lung is primarily an interstitial lung disease in which the inflammatory process involves the alveoli, small bronchi and small blood vessels. **Cavitation is seen in <5% patients with sarcoidosis**.- Harrisons 16th-2020
- B/e hilar lymphadenopathy is the hallmark of disease – Harrisons 16th/2023

The three classic x-ray pattern of pulmonary sarcoidosis are		
• ***Type I***	:	*B/L hilar lymphadenopathy with no parenchymal changes*
• ***Type II***	:	*B/L hilar lymphadenopathy with diffuse parenchymal changes*
• ***Type III***	:	*Diffuse parenchymal change with no hilar lymphadenopathy.*

- Sarcoidosis has a variable course. Disease clears spontaneously in 50% of patients – *Harrisons 16th/2023*
- Tuberculin test may be negative due to the presence of skin anergy – *Harrisons 16th/2023*

115. Answer is A (CD4/CD8 counts in the blood): *Harrison 15th/1970; Harrison 16th/2017-2023; Not in Harrison 17th*

The patient in question is suffering from sarcoidosis.

'***While there is marked enhancement of no. of TH cells at the sites of disease the number of TH cells in the blood are normal***' – *Harrison*

'*Where as TH cells in the involved organs are proliferating at an enhanced rate the T cells in other sites such as blood are quiescent*' - *Harrison*

It is the CD4 / CD8 counts in the affected organs which is an important ancillary aid in established the diagnosis of sarcoidosis and not the CD4 / CD8 count in the blood as specifically asked in the question.

Active sarcoidosis results from an exaggerated cellular immune response resulting in accumulation of large no. of T4 cells in the affected organs, where the ratio of CD4 to CD8 cells may be as high as 10:1.

Although CT of chest is also only rarely helpful, it may identify early fibrosis and active alveolitis and thus contribute to a diagnosis of sarcoidosis.

Diagnostic tests for sarcoidosis have often been asked

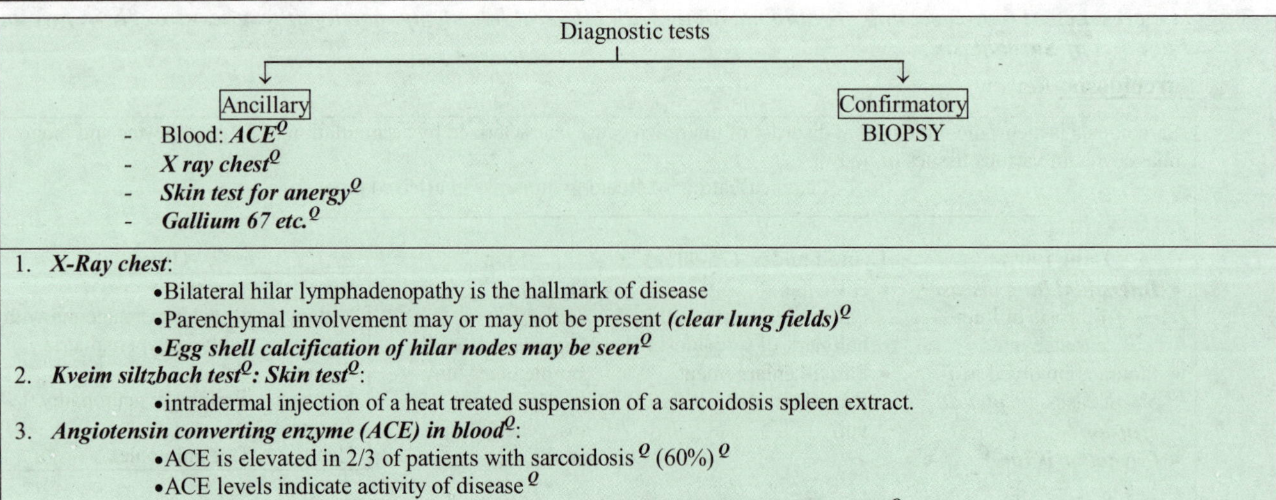

1. ***X-Ray chest***:
   - Bilateral hilar lymphadenopathy is the hallmark of disease
   - Parenchymal involvement may or may not be present *(clear lung fields)*[Q]
   - ***Egg shell calcification of hilar nodes may be seen***[Q]
2. ***Kveim siltzbach test[Q]: Skin test[Q]***:
   - intradermal injection of a heat treated suspension of a sarcoidosis spleen extract.
3. ***Angiotensin converting enzyme (ACE) in blood[Q]***:
   - ACE is elevated in 2/3 of patients with sarcoidosis [Q] (60%) [Q]
   - ACE levels indicate activity of disease [Q]
   - ACE levels provide an important method of monitoring the course of disease.[Q]

   (The cells in granuloma release angiotensin converting enzyme into the serum)

4. ***Gallium 67 scan***: Gallium 67 lung scan is usually abnormal showing a pattern of diffuse uptake
5. ***Bronchoalveolar large:*** Lavage fluid is characterized by
   - increase in Lymphocytes[Q]
   - high CD4 / CD8 cell ratio[Q]
6. ***Biopsy***:
   - Biopsy is mandatory to make a definitive diagnosis of sarcoidosis
   - Characteristic finding is a typical non casseating granuloma[Q]
7. ***Lung function abnormalities***: Typical for interstitial lung disease.

Adult Respiratory Distress Syndrome (ARDS)

116. Answer is D (ARDS): *Harrison 17th /1680; Robbins 7th/715*

Shock lung is a synonym used for Acute/Adult Respiratory Distress syndrome.

Synonym: for ARDS *(Taken from 'Pathology of Lung')*

- *Shock lung*
- *Blast lung*
- *Traumatic wet lung*
- *Congestive Atelectasis*
- *DoNang Lung*
- *Noncardiogenic Pulmonary Edema*
- *Diffuse Alveolar Damage*

117. Answer is None or C (Cardiopulmonary bypass with heart lung machine): *Harrison 18th/p 2205 Harrison 16th/1592; 17th /1680 API 7th/1240*

Cardiopulmonary bypass is a cause for indirect lung injury while the rest three cause direct injury to lungs. Although all four options may cause acute lung injury, the single best answer of exclusion would be cardiopulmonary bypass.

Clinical disorders associated with lung injury/ ARDS

Direct lung injury	Indirect lung injury
• Pneumonia • Aspiration of gastric contents • Pulmonary contusion • Near drowning • Toxic inhalation injury	• Sepsis • Severe trauma: - Multiple bone fractures - Head trauma - Flail chest • Burns • Multiple transfusions • Drug overdose: eg Narcotic overdose • Pancreatitis • Post-cardiopulmonary bypass

118. Answer is B (High Altitude): *Harrison's 16th/ 1592; Harrison 17th/ 1680; API 7th/ 1240*

Pulmonary edema with normal pulmonary capillary wedge pressure suggests a diagnosis of ARDS or non cardiogenic pulmonary edema.

High altitude has been grouped as one of the miscellaneous causes for ARDS, reflecting pulmonary oedema with a normal PCWP - *API 7th/ 1240*

Some miscellaneous causes for ARDS
• Renal failure • Liver failure • Disseminated intravascular coagulation • Ecclampsia • Amniotic fluid emboli / Air emboli • Hanging • High altitude

119. Answer is D (All of the above): *Harrison 18th/p 2205 Harrisons 17th/1680; 16th/1592*

Acute Pancreatitis, Trauma and severe Falciparum malaria may all lead to ARDS

120. Answer is A (Narcotic overdose): *Read text below*

Pulmonary edema with normal pulmonary capillary wedge pressure suggests a diagnosis of ARDS or non cardiogenic pulmonary edema. ***Narcotic overdose is the only non cardiogenic cause for pulmonary edema (ARDS) amongst the options provided and hence the answer here.***

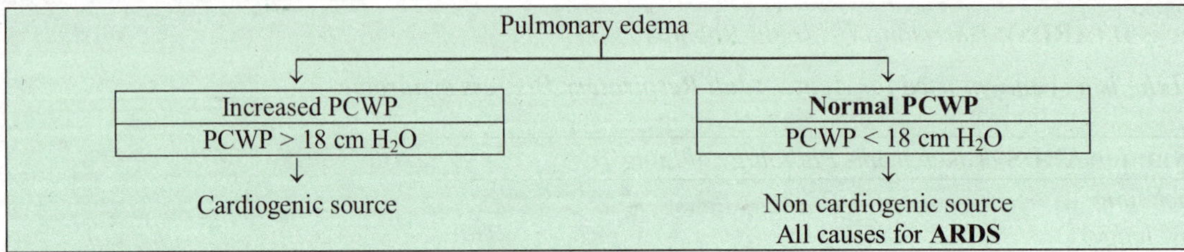

121. Answer is A (Diffuse Alveolar Damage): *Harrison 18th/2205, 2206, 2207*

Diffuse Alveolar Damage (DAD) is the histopathological hallmark of Acute Respiratory Distress Syndrome (ARDS) and the most characteristic feature amongst the options provided. Diffuse Alveolar Damage is often used as a synonym for ARDS.

'The pathological hallmark of ARDS is Diffuse Alveolar Damage'
– Thoracic Imaging (Thieme) 2010/Case 78

'The histological hallmark of ARDS is Diffuse Alveolar Damage'
– 'Intensive Critical Care Medicine' (Springer) 2009/210

Synonyms for ARDS
• ***Diffuse Alveolar Damage*** • *Shock Lung* • *Blast Lung* • *Traumatic Wet Lung* • *Congestive Atelectasis* • *Do Nang Lung* • *Noncardiogenic Pulmonary Edema*
Taken from 'Pathology of the Lung'

ARDS (Acute Respiratory Distress Syndrome)

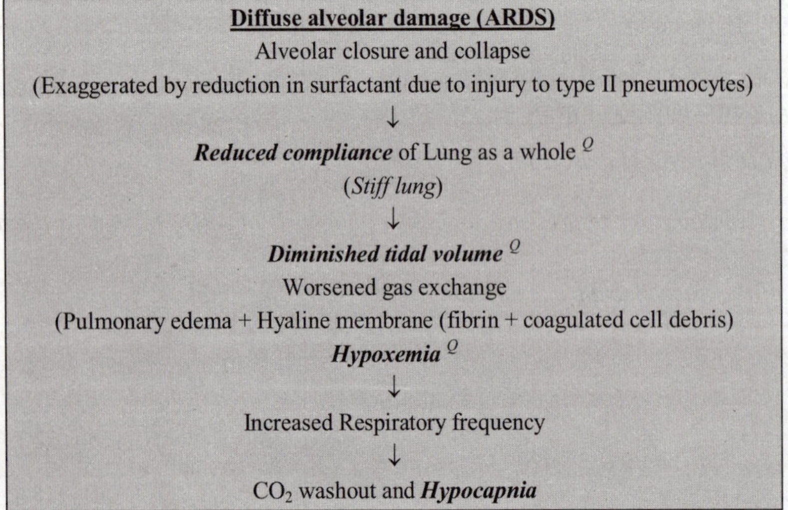

ARDS is an acute form of lung injury characterized by:
• Increased permeability of alveolar capillary membrane. • ***Diffuse alveolar damage.*** • Accumulation of proteinaceous pulmonary edema (non cardiogenic pulmonary edema Q)

Features of ARDS

Clinical /Physiological
• Clinical history of insult known to cause ARDS • Clinical exclusion of chronic lung disease and Left ventricular failure • ***Diffuse alveolar damage.*** • *Reduced surfactant (Injury to type II pneumocytes)* • Increased permeability of alveolar capillary membrane. • Accumulation of *proteinaceous pulmonary edema* (non cardiogenic pulmonary edema [Q]) • Pulmonary edema + ***Hyaline membrane*** (fibrin + coagulated cell debris) • ***Reduced compliance*** (*stiff lung*) • ***Diminished tidal volume*** [Q] • ***Hypoxemia*** [Q] (Worsened gas exchange d/t ***pulmonary shunting***) • ***Hypocapnia*** [Q](CO_2 washout)

Diagnostic Criteria (ARDS)	
PaO_2/FiO_2	*≤200 mm Hg*
Onset	*Acute*
Chest Radiograph	*Bilateral Alveolar or Interstitial infiltrates*
Absence of Left Atrial Hypertension	• *PCWP≤18 mmHg* • *No clinical evidence of increased left atrial pressure*

122. Answer is C (Hypercapnia): *Harrison 18th/p 2205, 2206, 2207; Harrison 15th/ 1524; Harrison 16th/ 1592; Harrison 17th/ 1680, 1681*

ARDS results in Type I Respiratory failure and is characterized by normal or low $PaCO_2$ (Hypocapnia) and not Hypercapnia *(see previous explanation on types of respiratory failure).*

ARDS (Acute Respiratory distress syndrome)

ARDS is an acute form of lung injury characterized by:
- Increased permeability of alveolar capillary membrane.
- Diffuse alveolar damage.
- Accumulation of proteinaceous pulmonary edema (non cardiogenic pulmonary edema [Q])

Diffuse alveolar damage (ARDS)
Alveolar closure and collapse
(exaggerated by reduction in surfactant due to injury to type II pneumocytes)
↓
Reduced compliance of Lung as a whole [Q]
(*stiff lung*)
↓
Diminished tidal volume [Q]
Worsened gas exchange
(pulmonary edema + Hyaline membrane (fibrin + coagulated cell debris)
Hypoxemia [Q]
↓
Increased Respiratory frequency
↓
CO_2 washout and ***Hypocapnia*** [Q]

123. Answer is D (Hypercapnia): *Refer previous question*

ARDS results in type I Respiratory failure and is characterized by normal or low $PaCO_2$ (Hypocapnia) and not hypercapnia.

Pulmonary Shunting: Significant shunt occurs in ARDS where pulmonary arterial blood shunts past flooded and collapsed Alveoli into pulmonary veins. Shunting of the poorly oxygenated venous blood into arterial circulation significantly contributes to arterial hypoxemia.

Reduced compliance: Reduced lung compliance and stiff lung are characteristic features of ARDS

Hypoxemia: Arterial hypoxemia is a characteristic feature of ARDS and may be caused by reduced lung compliance and pulmonary shunting.

Features of ARDS

Clinical /Physiological
• Clinical history of insult known to cause ARDS • Clinical exclusion of chronic lung disease and Left ventricular failure • ***Diffuse alveolar damage.*** • *Reduced surfactant (Injury to type II pneumocytes)* • Increased permeability of alveolar capillary membrane. • Accumulation of *proteinaceous pulmonary edema* (non cardiogenic pulmonary edema [Q]) • Pulmonary edema + ***Hyaline membrane*** (fibrin + coagulated cell debris) • ***Reduced compliance*** (*stiff lung*) • ***Diminished tidal volume*** [Q] • ***Hypoxemia*** [Q] (Worsened gas exchange d/t ***pulmonary shunting***) • ***Hypocapnia*** [Q](CO_2 washout)

Diagnostic Criteria (ARDS)	
PaO_2/FiO_2	*≤200 mm Hg*
Onset	*Acute*
Chest Radiograph	*Bilateral Alveolar or Interstitial infiltrates*
Absence of Left Atrial Hypertension	• *PCWP≤18 mmHg* • *No clinical evidence of increased left atrial pressure*

124. Answer is D (Hypercapnia): *Harrison 18th/2205; Harrison 16th/1592; 17th/ 1680, 1681API 7th/1240; Refer question on Respiratory failure*

ARDS or Adult respiratory distress syndrome is a condition characterized by Acute Hypoxemic Type I Respiratory failure due to pulmonary edema caused by increased permeability of the alveolar capillary barrier. *It is thus* ***associated with Hypoxemia but not with Hypercapnia***.*(Refer question on respiratory failure)*

125. Answer is B (Hypercapnia): *Harrison 17th /1680, 1681*

ARDS results in Type I Respiratory failure and is characterized by normal or low $PaCO_2$ (Hypocapnia) and not Hypercapnia *(see previous explanation on types of respiratory failure).*

ARDS (Acute Respiratory distress syndrome)

ARDS is an acute form of lung injury characterized by:

- Increased permeability of alveolar capillary membrane.
- Diffuse alveolar damage.
- Accumulation of proteinaceous pulmonary edema (non cardiogenic pulmonary edema [Q])

Diffuse alveolar damage (ARDS)

Noncardiogenic Pulmonary Edema

Alveolar closure and collapse

(exaggerated by reduction in surfactant due to injury to type II pneumocytes)

↓

Reduced compliance of Lung as a whole [Q]

(stiff lung)

↓

Diminished tidal volume [Q]

Worsened gas exchange

Pulmonary edema *(non cardiogenic)* + Hyaline membrane *(fibrin + coagulated cell debris)*

↓

Hypoxemia [Q]

↓

Increased Respiratory frequency

↓

CO_2 washout and ***Hypocapnia*** [Q]

Features of ARDS

Clinical /Physiological
• Clinical history of insult known to cause ARDS • Clinical exclusion of chronic lung disease and Left ventricular failure • ***Diffuse alveolar damage.*** • *Reduced surfactant (Injury to type II pneumocytes)* • Increased permeability of alveolar capillary membrane. • Accumulation of *proteinaceous* ***pulmonary edema*** (non cardiogenic pulmonary edema [Q]) • Pulmonary edema + ***Hyaline membrane*** (fibrin + coagulated cell debris) • ***Reduced compliance (stiff lung)*** • ***Diminished tidal volume*** [Q] • ***Hypoxemia*** [Q] (Worsened gas exchange d/t ***pulmonary shunting***) • ***Hypocapnia*** [Q](CO_2 washout)

Diagnostic Criteria (ARDS)	
PaO_2/FiO_2	*≤200 mm Hg*
Onset	*Acute*
Chest Radiograph	*Bilateral Alveolar or Interstitial infiltrates*
Absence of Left Atrial Hypertension	• *PCWP≤18 mmHg* • *No clinical evidence of increased left atrial pressure*

126. Answer is C (Increased Left atrial pressure): *Repeat; Refer previous question*

ARDS is characterized by a PCWP of ≤ 18mm Hg with no clinical evidence of increased left atrial pressure.

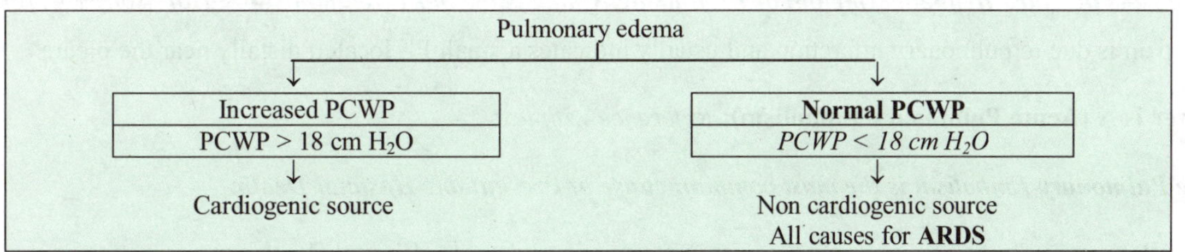

127. Answer is A (Diffuse Alveolar Damage): *Harrison 18th/p 2205 Robbins 7th/715; Harrisons 17th/1680*

'Shock lung' is a synonym used for Acute Respiratory Distress Syndrome.
Diffuse alveolar damage is a characteristic feature of ARDS/Shock lung and is also often used as a synonym for ARDS.

128. Answer is A (PaO_2/FiO2)>200 mmHg): *Harrison 18th/p 2205 Harrisons 17th/1680*

'Acute Lung Injury' is a milder disorder than ARDS and is characterized by PaO_2/FiO_2 of less than 300 mm Hg.

Diagnostic Criteria	ALI	ARDS
PaO_2/FiO_2	*≤300 mm Hg*	*≤200 mm Hg*
Onset	*Acute*	*Acute*
Chest Radiograph	*Bilateral Alveolar or Interstitial infiltrates*	*Bilateral Alveolar or Interstitial infiltrates*
Absence of Left Atrial Hypertension	• *PCWP≤ 18 mmHg* • *No Clinical evidence of increased left atrial pressure*	• *PCWP≤18 mmHg* • *No clinical evidence of increased left atrial pressure*

ALI is a less severe disorders than ARDS but has the potential to evolve into ARDS. ALI can be differentiated from ARDS by the arterial PO_2/FiO_2 (Inspiratory O_2 fraction) ratio.

129. Answer is D (PaO2/FIO2 ≤ 200): *Harrison 18th/2207; 17th/1681; Harrisons 16th/1592; Ref. Previous question*

ALI is associated with a PaO2/FIO2 ≤ 300 and not PaO2/FIO2 ≤ 200
Bilateral alveolar interstial infiltrates on Radiographs along with, hypoxemia and pulmonary shunting due to intra alveolar filling are characteristic features of both ALI and ARDS.

Pulmonary Thromboembolism

130. Answer is A (Pulmonary thromboembolism): *Harrison 18th/p 2172 Harrison 15th/ 1508, Harrison 16th/ 1561; Harrison 17th/ 1651, 1652*

Sudden onset of dyspnea and chest pain following surgery or immobilization, strongly suggests a diagnosis of pulmonary thromboembolism.

Remember:
- The most frequent symptom of PE is dyspnea Q
- The most frequent sign of PE is tachypnea Q.

Symptoms suggesting massive PE	Symptoms suggesting small emboli located distally
Dyspnea Syncope Hypotension Cyanosis	Pleuritic pain Cough Haemoptysis

131. Answer is A (Chest pain is the most common symptom): *Harrison 18th/p 2172 Harrison 15th/ 1509; 16th/ 1561; 17th/ 1651, 1652*

'Dyspnea is the most frequent symptom of PE and tachypnea is the most frequent sign'–*Harrisons 16th/1561*

Chest pain is due to pulmonary infarction and usually indicates a small PE located distally near the pleura.

132. Answer is A (Acute Pulmonary Embolism): *Reference with text*

Acute Pulmonary Embolism is the most common cause of Preventable Hospital Death.

'Acute Pulmonary Embolism is the most common cause of preventable Hospital Death'
- 'The 5 minute ICU consult / Lippincott Williams/2012/384

'Pulmonary embolism is the most common preventable cause of death in the hospital'.
- 'Comprehensive Hospital Medicine: An Evidence based approach (Elsevier) 2007/89

- *Acute Pulmonary Embolism is the third most common cause of hospital death in the united states after heart failure and cancer*
- *Acute Pulmonary Embolism is the most common cause of preventable hospital death*Q
- *Acute Pulmonary Embolism is the most common cause of death after surgery in a surgical patient*Q

133. Answer is C (DVT): *Harrison 17th /1651; 'Peripheral Vascular Disease Basic Diagnostic and Therepeutic Approaches' by Abela (Lippincott Williams) 2004*

The most common cause of pulmonary thromboembolism is Deep Vein Thrombosis.

'A deep vein thrombosis is the most common source of pulmonary embolism' - Peripheral vascular Disease

About half the patients with pelvic vein thrombosis or proximal leg deep vein thrombosis have pulmonary thromboembolism. Isolated calf vein thrombosis pose a lower risk of pulmonary embolism *– Harrisons*

'The most common source of pulmonary embolism is deep vein thrombosis of Proximal veins of lower extremity (above knee thrombi). Below the knee thrombi (calf vein thrombosis) by themselves are infrequently associated with embolism unless they extend proximally to the papliteal vein or above' - Peripheral Vascular Disease

Remember:

- **Most common site for deep vein thrombosis:** Calf vein (tendency to embolize is less)
- **Most common *source for pulmonary emboli :*** *Proximal vein of lower extremity* (Pelvic or femoral veins) (tendency to embolize is high)

134. Answer is C (Large veins of leg): *Harrison 18th/p 2171 Harrison 15th/ 1509, 16th/ 1561; 17th/ 1651; Bailey and love 24th/866*

About half the patients with pelvic vein thrombosis or proximal leg deep vein thrombosis have pulmonary thromboembolism. Isolated calf vein thrombosis pose a lower risk of pulmonary embolism *– Harrisons*

Remember:

- **Most common site for deep vein thrombosis:** Calf vein (tendency to embolize is less)
- **Most common *source for pulmonary emboli :*** *Proximal vein of lower extremity* (Pelvic or femoral veins) (tendency to embolize is high)

135. Answer is D (Progesterone therapy): *Bailey 23rd/263; CMDT 2002 /233; 2009/260-261*

"Oestrogen predisposes to thrombosis and not progesterone" *- Dutta 4th; Bailey 23rd/263*
'Pulmonary embolism and deep vein thrombosis are two manifestations of the same disease. The risk factors for pulmonary emboli are the risk factors for thrombus formation.'- CMDT 09/260

Inherited disorders predisposing to thrombosis

Defective Inhibition of Coagulation Factors	Impaired clot lysis
Factors V Leiden resistance (Resistance to activated protein C)	- Dysfibrogenemia
Antithrombin III Deficiency	- Plasminogen deficiency[Q]
Protein C Deficiency	- TPA deficiency
Protein S deficiency	- Uncertain Mechanism
Prothrombin gene mutation (G40210A)	- Homocystinuria[Q]
Antiphospholipid antibody or lupus anticoagulant	

Risk factors for vernous throboembolism / Pulmonary thrmoboembolism

Age (Increasing age) [Q]	Surgery / Trauma[Q] : Specially of pelvis hip or lower limb
Obesity[Q]	Malignancy[Q]: Specially pelvis, abdominal, metastatic
Immobility (bed rest > 4 days) [Q]	Heart failure[Q] / Recent myocardial infarction
Pregnancy[Q]	Nephrotic syndrome[Q]
Puerperium[Q]	Inflammatory bowel disease
High dose oestrogen therapy[Q]	Polycythemia
Varicose veins[Q]	PNH or Lupus anticoagulant[Q]
Inherited disorders as detailed above	Behcet's syndrome[Q]
	Homocytinuria[Q]
	Paralysis of Lower Limnbs
	Infection

136. Answer is C (Sinus Tachycardia) : *Harrison 18th/p 2172 Harrison 17th/ 1653; Oxford Handbook of Clinical Medicine(OHCM) 5th / 88*

Sinus tachycardia is the commonest ECG abnormality in pulmonary embolism *- OHCM 5th / 88*

Classic Abnormalities on ECG in pulmonary Embolism

- Sinus Tachycardia (*Commonest : OHCM*)
- Right ventricular strain pattern (*T wave inversion in leads V1 to V4 perhaps most frequent - Harrison*)
- S_I Q_{III} T_{III} Pattern :(*Classic pattern but rare (OHCM)*)

  - Deeps S waves in lead I
  - Q wave
  - Inverted T wave in lead III

- New onset Atrial Fibrillation / Atrial Flutter.
- Right Axis Deviation / RBBB.

137. Answer is C (Anticoagulant therapy): *Harrison 18th/p2172 Harrisons 17th/1653; Clinical Hematology 4th/359*

D-Dimer values are falsely decreased in patients receiving anticoagulant therapy *–Clinical Hematology*

Myocardial infarction, pneumonia and pregnancy are all established causes for false positive (Elevated) D-Dimer values

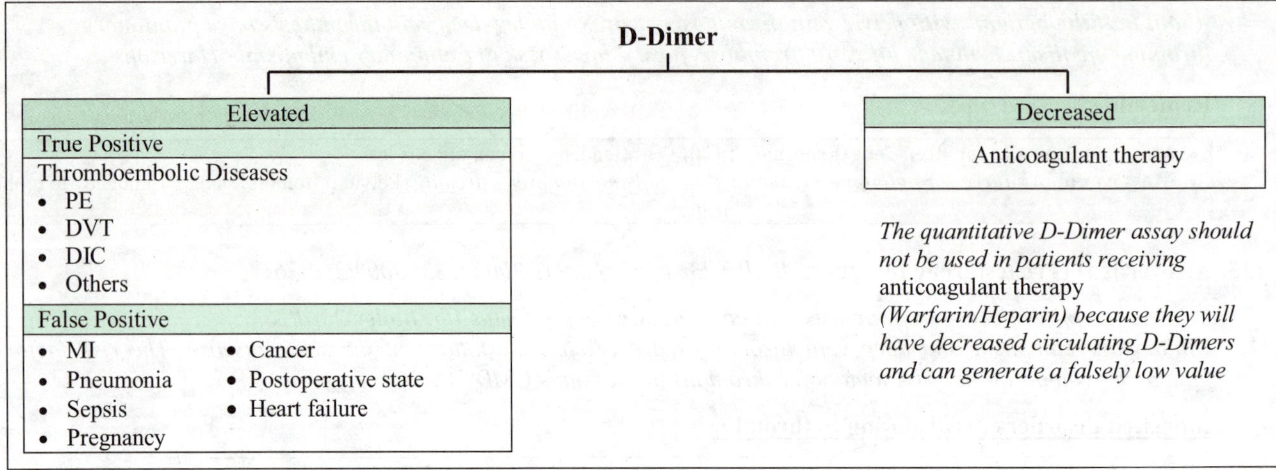

138. Answer is A (Pulmonary Embolism): *Harrison 18th/p 2172 Harrisons 17th/1653*

The D-dimer assay is most sensitive for pulmonary embolism with a sensitivity of greater than 95%.

Dimmer Assay in P.E (and DVT):

- D-Dimmer is a specific fragment generated from two cross linked fibrin molecules after a clot has formed
- D-Dimer fragments reach circulation when the fibrin clot is degraded by the action of plasmin (D-Dimer is a fibrin degradation product)
- Elevation of D-Dimer thus indicates that a coagulation fibrinolytic process is taking place.
- Elevation indicates endogenous and often clinically ineffective thrombolysis
- D-Dimer assays are highly sensitive for presence of Thromboembolic Disease
- D-Dimer test is useful as a 'test for exclusion' or a 'rule out test' and is not a diagnostic test.

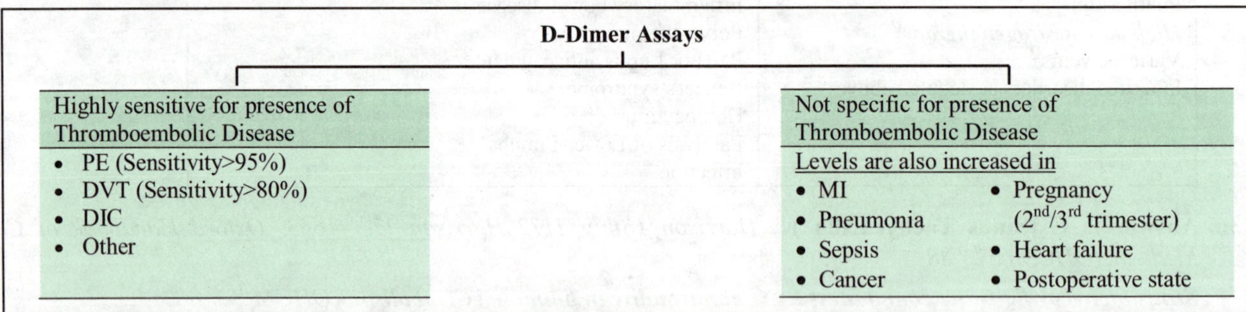

139. Answer is B (Pulmonary Embolism): *Harrison 18th/p 2172 Harrisons 17th/1653*

D-Dimer test is a sensitive test for detection of DVT and PE.
Amongst DVT and PE, the D-Dimer test is less sensitive for DVT than PE. (More sensitive for PE)

The sensitivity of the D-Dimer assay is greater than 80% for DVT and greater than 95% for PE. The D-Dimer test is less sensitive for DVT than PE because the DVT thrombus size is smaller-Harrison 17th/1653

140. Answer is B (Multidetector CT Angiography): *Harrison 18th/p 2172 Harrison 17th/1652*

For patients with strong clinical suspicions/high likehood of DVT. Imaging tests are obligatory.

CT scan with intravenous contrast (Multidetector CT Angiography) is the test of choice for the diagnosis of PE.

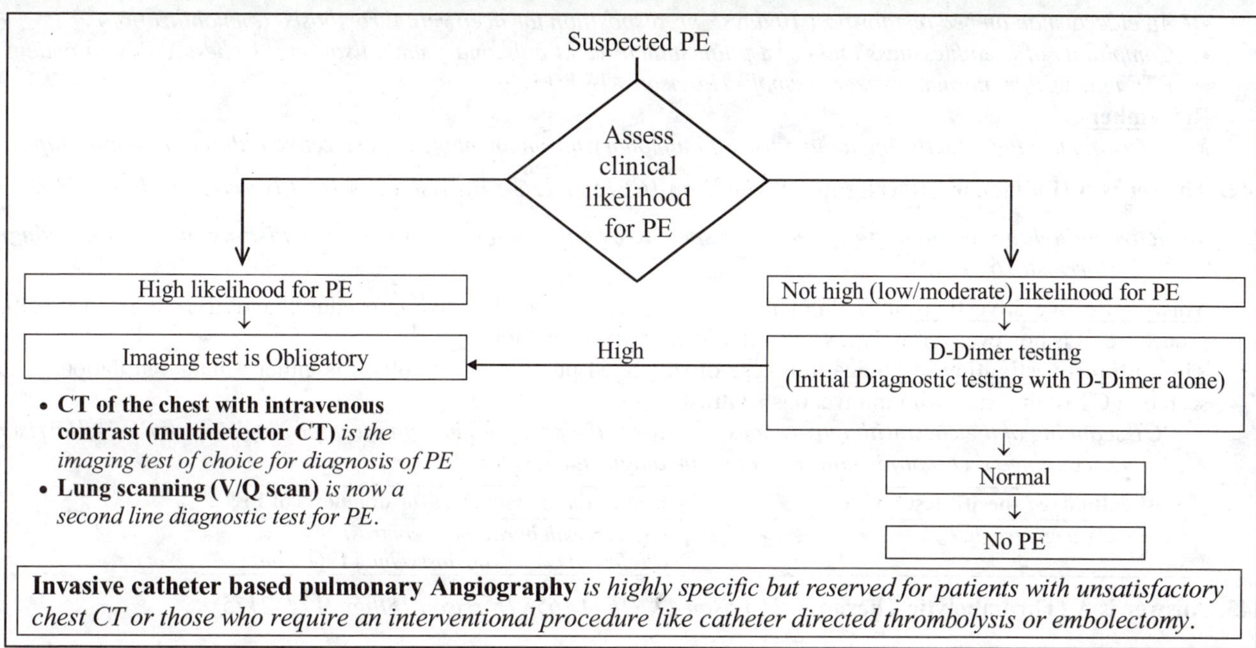

141. Answer is A (Lung perfusion – ventilation scan): *Ref: Harrison 15th/ 1510, 1511, 16th/ 1562, 1563; 17th/ 1652, 1663 Harrison 18th/p 2171, 2173*

The clinical picture depicted in the question is suggestive of a ***case of pulmonary thromboembolism.***

As the patient has a high clinical likelihood, the first investigation should be a non invasive imaging modality in accordance with the diagnostic strategy for PTE outlined in Harrison's textbook.CT of the chest with intravenous contrast (Multidetector CT) is the imaging test of choice but it has not been provided amongst the options.

As CT scan of the chest is not provided amongst the options, a Lung Ventilation Perfusion Scan is the modality of choice.

Diagnostic Strategy in cases of suspected Pulmonary Thromboembolism

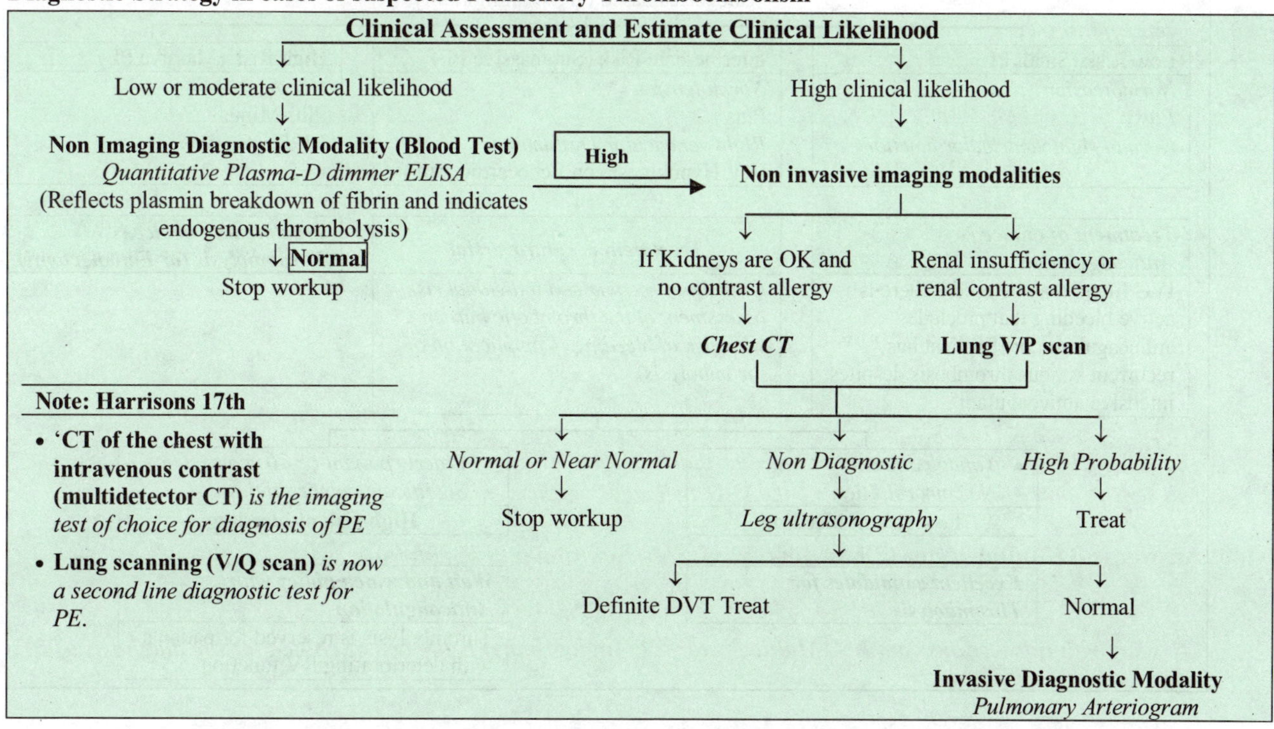

- *An elderly man on bed rest for past 10 days: predisposition for deep vein thrombosis. (immobilization)*
- *Complaints of breathlessness and chest pain: indicative of pulmonary embolisation. (A chest X-Ray in patient with PTE may well be normal or near normal - Harrison's 15th/1510)*

Remember-

*Most specific test for establishing a diagnosis of pulmonary thromboembolism is **selective pulmonary angiography**[Q]*

142. Answer is A (Pulmonary arterigraphy): *Harrison 16th/1563-1564; Harrison 17th/1654 Harrison 18th/p 2173, 2174*

***'Selective pulmonary angiography is the most specific examination available for establishing the definitive diagnosis of PE.'**- Harriosn 16th/1563*

Most definitive investigation : Pulmonary angiography is an invasive procedure, and it is the most definitive procedure. It is however certainly not the initial investigation of choice.

The initial investigation of choice in a case of suspected pulmonary embolism is either a lung ventilation perfusion scan or a CT of the chest with intravenous contrast.

'CT scanning of the chest with intravenous contrast is the principal imaging test for diagnosis of PE.' - Harrison
'Lung scanning (V/Q scan) is now a second line diagnostic test for PE'

Most definitive / specific test for PE [Q]
Pulmonary angiography[Q]

Best initial imaging test for diagnosis of PE[Q]
CT scan with intravenous contrast [Q] *(Preferred choice, against a lung V-Q scan)*

143. Answer is A (Thrombolytic Therapy): *Harrison 17th/1654,1655 Harrison 18th/p 2174, 2175*

*Normotension with Right ventricular hypokinesia suggests a diagnosis of submassive pulmonary embolism and stratifies the patient into an intermediate risk category. Treatment for intermediate risk patients with submassive PE is controversial. Guidelines recommend individual risk assessment for the thrombotic burden versus risk of bleeding. **According to Harrisons textbook young patients without any comorbidities that fall into the intermediate risk category are excellent candidates for thrombolysis.*** The patient in question is a young 20 years old patient and the question makes no mention of any comorbidities, hence thrombolysis is the single best answer of choice

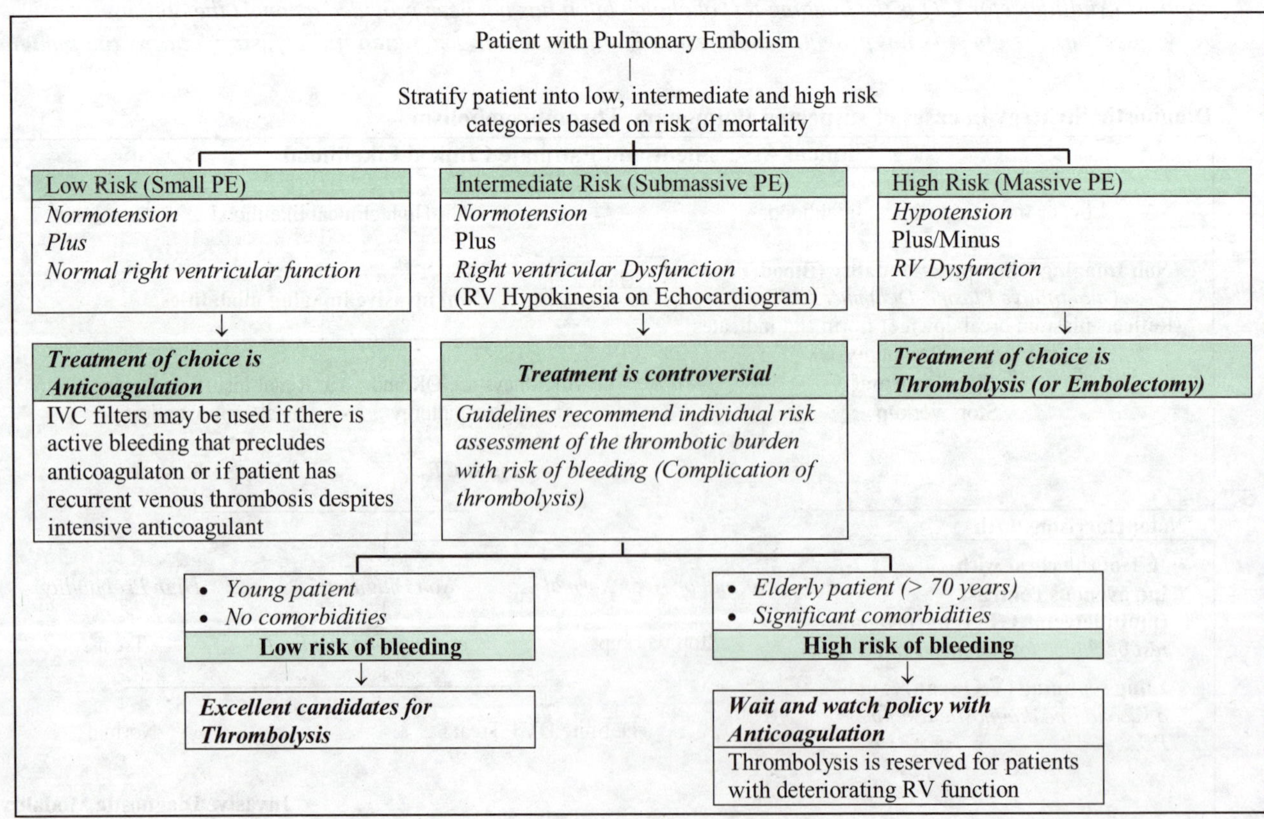

Pulmonary Hypertension

144. Answer is A (Bone morphogenic Receptor Protein II): *Harrisons 16th/1405; Harrisons 17th/1577; Robbins 7th /743,744 Harrison 18th/p 2077*

Gene coding the type II bone morhphogenetic protein receptor II (BMPR II) is associated with familial cases of primary pulmonary hypertension and designated as the PPH I gene.

Bone morphogenic protein receptor II (BMPRII) and pulmonary Hypertension

- BMPRII is a cell surface protein receptor belonging to the TGF-β receptor superfamily (located on chromosome 2q31)
- BMP-BMPRII signaling plays an important role in embryogenesis, apoptosis, cell proliferation and differentiation.
- In vascular smooth muscles normal BMPR2 signalling causes inhibition of proliferation and favour apoptosis, thereby protecting the vessels from narrowing and development of hypertension
- Primary pulmonary hypertension is believed to be caused by a mutation in the gene coding for the BMPR II signaling pathway (PPH-1 gene/BMPRII gene).
- ***Mutation in the BMPR II gene (PPH-1gene) predisposes the cells to undergo proliferation rather than apoptosis and results in development of pulmonary hypertension.***

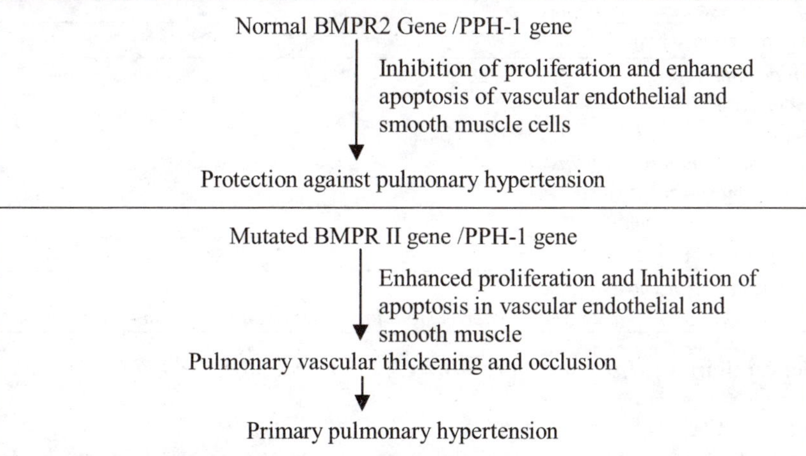

145. Answer is D (↑ Pulmonary wedge pressure): *Internal Medicine 5th/293*

↑ pulomary wedge pressure is not a feature of Precapillary Pulmonary hypertension.

In precapillary pulmonary hypertension the abnormality that leads to elevated pulmonary pressure is located in the pulmonary artery or arterioles. The Left atrial pressure or Pulmonary capillary wedge pressure is essentially normal.

Features	Precapillary	Passive (Post-capillary)
Pathophysiology	Abnormality that leads to elevated pulmonary artery pressure is located in the pulmoanry artery or arterioles.	Abnormalities that lead to elevated pulmonary artery pressure are located beyond the pulmonary arteries. These are caused by diseases that lead to increased pulmonary venous pressure that in turn produces secondary elevation in pulmonary arterial pressure.
Pulmonary artery mean pressure	↑/↑↑	↑
Left Atrial Pressure (PCWP)	***Normal***	↑
PA left Atrial Pressure Gradient	> 12mm	<12mm Hg
Conditions/Causes	• *Primary pulmonary hypertension* • *Disorders of ventilation* • *Congenital heart disease with pulmonary vascular disease* • *Pulmonary embolism* • *Schistosmiasis* • *Collagen vascular disease* • *Pulmonary vasculitis* • *Sickle hemoglobinopathies* • *Portal hypertension* • *Ingestion of drugs and herbal remedies*	• *Left ventricular failure* • *Mitral valve disease* • *Cor triatriatum* • *Obstruction of major pulmonary veins* • *Congenital pulmonary vein stenosis* • *Left atrial myxoma or thrombosis*

146. Answer is A (Mitral stenosis): *Internal Medicine 5th/293*

Mitral stenosis is a cause of post-capillary pulmonary hypertension or passive pulmonary hypertension.

Causes of pulmonary hypertension:

Precapillary pulmonary hypertension
• ***Primary pulmonary hypertension*** • *Disorders of ventilation* • *Congenital heart disease with pulmonary vascular disease* • ***Pulmonary embolism*** • *Schistosmiasis* • *Collagen vascular disease* • ***Pulmonary vasculitis*** • *Sickle hemoglobinopathies* • *Portal hypertension* • *Ingestion of drugs and herbal remedies*
Passive (Post-capillary) pulmonary hypertension
• *Left ventricular failure* • ***Mitral valve disease*** • *Cor triatriatum* • *Obstruction of major pulmonary veins* • *Congenital pulmonary vein stenosis* • *Left atrial myxoma or thrombosis*
Reactive pulmonary hypertension
• *Some patients with mitral valve disease* • *Rarely, other cause of pulmonary venous hypertension, including pulmonary veno-occlusive disease*

147. Answer is A (Hyperventilation): *Harrison 18th/p 2078, 2080 Harrisons 17th/1577,1579*

Pulmonary hypertension may be caused by hypoventilation but not by hyperventilation.

Chronic exposure to high altitude sleep disordered breathing due to obesity and anorexic agents including fenfluramine are known causes of pulmonary hypertension.

Clinical Classification of Pulmonary Hypertension

1. **Pulmonary arterial hypertension (PAH)**
   - Idiopathic (IPAH)(formerly PPH)
   - Familial (FPAH)
   - Associated with (APAH)
     - *Collagen vascular disease*
     - *Congenital systemic-to-pulmonary shunts*
     - *Portal hypertension*
     - *HIV infection*
     - *Drugs and toxins (including fenfluramine)*
     - *Other (thyroid disorders, glycogen storage disease, Gaucher disease, hereditary hemorrhagic telangiectasia, hemoglobinopathies, myeloproliferative, disorders, splenectomy)*
   - Associated with significant venous or capillary involvement
     - *Pulmonary veno-occlusive disease (PVOD)*
     - *Pulmonary capillary hemangiomatosis (PCH)*
     - *Persistent pulmonary hypertension of the newborn*
2. **Pulmonary hypertension with left heart disease**
   - *Left-sided atrial or ventricular heart disease*
   - *Left-sided valvular heart disease*
3. **Pulmonary hypertension associated with lung diseases and/or hypoxemia**
   - *Chronic obstructive pulmonary disease*
   - *Interstitial lung disease*
   - ***Sleep-disordered breathing***
   - *Alveolar hypoventilation disorders*
   - ***Chronic exposure to high altitude***
   - *Developmental abnormalities*
4. **Pulmonary hypertension due to chronic thrombotic and/or embolic disease**
   - *Thromboembolic obstruction of proximal pulmonary arteries*
   - *Thromboembolic obstruction of distal pulmonary arteries*
   - *Nonthrombotic pulmonary embolism (tumor, parasites, foreign material)*
5. **Miscellaneous**
   Sarcoidosis, histiocytosis X, lymphangiomatosis, compression of pulmonary vessels (adenopathy, tumor, fibrosing mediastinitis)

A causal relationship has been established between exposure to several anorexigens including aminorex and the ***fenfluramines*** *and the development of PAH-Harrison*

148. Answer is D (Argemone mexicana poisoning): *Harrison 18th/p 2082 Reference with text*

Argemone mexicana poisoning has not been mentioned as a cause for pulmonary hypertension. It is the single best answer of exclusion.

Toxic oil syndrome is associated with pulmonary Hypertension *(Goldrank's Toxicological Emergencies 7th/25)*
Toxic oil syndrome also called toxic epidemic syndrome is a multi system disorder characterized by pneumonitis, eosinophilia, ***pulmonary hypertension***, scleroderma like feature and neuromuscular changes
Toxic oil syndrome has first observed as an epidemic in spain due to consumption of 'Rapeseed oil' as cooking oil.

Sickle cell anemia is associated with pulmonary hypertension(H17th/1581)
Cardiovascular abnormalities including pulmonary hypertension are prominent abnormalities in the clinical spectrum of sickle cell disease-H17th/1581

Systemic sclerosis is associated with pulmonary hypertension
All collagen vascular diseases including systemic sclerosis may be associated with pulmonary hypertension.(H17th/1579)

149. Answer is D (Bronchoconstriction): *Harrison 18th/p2081 Harrison 17th/1580*

Bronchoconstriction is not a cause for Pulmonary Hypertension

Pulmonary Hypertension in COPD has been attributed to multiple factors including:

- ***Hypoxia***
- ***Pulmonary vasoconstriction (secondary to hypoxia)***
- *Acidemia*
- *Hypercapnia*
- *Mechanical effect of* ***high lung volume*** *on pulmonary vessels*
- *Loss of small vessels in vascular bed*
- *Regions of emphysematous lung destruction*

150. Answer is B (Primary Pulmonary Hypertension): *Harrison 18th/p 2076 Harrisons 17th/1577; Robbins 7th/745; Textbook of Cardiovascular Medicine by Topol 3rd/468; Pulmonary vascular disease 1st (2006)/192*

Isolated reduction in diffusion capacity (DLCO) with nearly normal flow volumes (FVC; FEV1/FVC) in a young female with progressive dyspnea is characteristic of Primary Pulmonary Hypertension.

Features of Primary Pulmonary Hypertension / Idiopathic Pulmonary Arterial Hypertension

- *Most common in Young women* who are 20-40 years of Age (Robbin's 7th/745) (strong female predominance)
- *Most common symptom is exertional dyspnea (predominant symptom is dysnea)*
- Pulmonary Function tests
  - *Are usually normal with the exception of DLCO which is characteristically reduced.*
  - *Non obstructive PFT (FEV1/FVC>0.7 or 70%)*
  - *Non restrictive PFT (FVC > 80%)*
  - *DLCO2 is reduced (↓DLCO)*

  (Note: Mild restrictive effects can be seen in upto 20% of patients with advanced IPAH)

X Ray chest

- *X Ray chest shows clear lung fileds in PPH/IPAH*
- *X Ray chest usually shows enlargement of pulmonary arteries*

Exercise tolerance

Exercise tolerance is markedly reduced
(The exercise capacity of these patients appears to be limited by a low cardiac output because of a decrease in the functional pulmonary vascular bed)

Understanding the PFT results of the patient in question
The patient in question has an almost normal PFT with the exception of a reduced DLCO.

The patient in question does not have a restrictive disease as FVC >80%

Severity of restrictive disease is based on the assessment of FVC.

FVC < 80%	Mild restriction
FVC < 70%	Moderate Testriction
FVC < 50%	Severe Restriction

Patient in question with an FVC of 92% is not a case of restrictive pulmonary disease

The patient in question does not have a obstructive lung disease as FEV_1/FVC > 0.7 (70%)

Severity of obstruction is based on FEV1 and FEV/FVC ratio

FEV1/FVC ≤ 70; FEV_1 ≥80%	Mild obstruction
FEV1/FVC ≤ 70; FEV_1 ≥ 30%	Moderate obstruction
FEV1/FVC ≤70; FEV_1 ≤ 30%	Severe obstruction

Patients in question has FEV1/FVC > 70% and hence does not have an obstructive lung disease.

151. Answer is B (Primary pulmonary hypertension): *Harrison 17th/1587-1589, 1576, 1576, 1662; 'Spiral manual of pulmonary medicine (Lippincott's)' 6th/444*

Reduced exercise tolerance and drop in oxygen saturation from 92% to 86% on exercise with a normal FVC and FEV_1/FVC is consistent with a diagnosis of Primary Pulmonary Hypertension.

Primary Pulmonary Hypertension characteristically presents with exertional dyspnea, exercise intolerance and a normal FVC; FEV1 /FVC ratio

The most common symptom attributable to pulmonary hypertension is exertional dyspnea and reduced exercise capacity – Harrison

Primary pulmonary hypertension is neither a restrictive nor obstructive pulmonary disease, and hence spirometry results are essentially normal with both FVC and FEV1 / FVC ratio > 80% of predicted

Obstructive disease	Restrictive disease
FEV1 / FVC is characteristically < 80% of predicted	FVC is characteristically < 80% of predicted

Interstitial lung disease does not present with a normal FVC

Interstitial lung disease should present with a *restrictive pattern on 'pulmonary function tests'* with a *reduced FVC to values less than 80% of predicted.* A forced vital capacity of 90% (FVC = 90%) is normal and hence makes a diagnosis of interstitial lung disease unlikely

Primary Alveolar Hypoventilation does not present with dyspnea and exercise intolerance

Patients with primary pulmonary hypoventilation may have normal pulmonary function test with a normal FEV1 and normal FVC/FEV1. However, ***dyspnea or shortness of breath is remarkably absent or extremely uncommon*** despite severe arterial blood gas derangements presumably because of impaired chemoreceptor and ventilatory drive. Also *exacerbation of hypoxemia or* ***drop in oxygen saturation is characteristically seen during sleep*** *and not on exercise.*

'Despite severe arterial blood gas derangements is uncommon' – Harrison

'Dyspnea is remarkably absent' – Spiral Manual of pulmonary Medicine (Lippincott) 6th/444

Anxiety disorder: Hyperventilation does not present with exercise intolerance

Patients with Anxiety associated Hyperventilation may also present with normal spirometry results with a normal FVC and FEV1/FVC. Dyspnea may also be a presenting feature; however such ***patients do not show features of exercise intolerance.***

'Patients with psychogenic hyperventilation typically complain of dyspnea at rest, but not during mild exercise. During mild or moderate exercise their hyperventilation tends to disappear' - Harrison

152. Answer is None or A (None or Pulmonary embolization): *Harrison 18th/p 1914 Harrisons 17th/1454*

Recurrent pulmonary embolization leads to chronic cor pulmonale, but the question does not mention 'Recurrent' and hence this is the single best answer of exclusion

COPD, Cystic Fibrosis and Bronchiectasis may all progress to chronic cor pulmonale

Etiology of Chronic Cor Pulmonale

Diseases Leading to Hypoxic Vasoconstriction	Disease That Casue Occlusion of the Pulmonary Vascular Bed	Diseases That Lead to Parenchymal Disease
Chronic bronchitis	***Recurrent pulmonary thromboembolism***	*Chronic bronchitis*
Chronic obstructive pulmonary disease	***Primary pulmonary hypertension***	*Chronic obstructive pulmonary disease*
Cystic fibrosis	*Venocclusive disease*	*Bronchiectasis*
Chronic hypoventilation	*Collagen vascular disease*	*Cystic fibrosis*
Obsity	*Drug-induced lung disease*	*Pneumoconiosis*
Neuromuscular disease		*Sarcoid*
Chest wall dysfunction		*Idiopathic pulmonary fibrosis*
Living at high altitudes		

153. Answer is B (COPD): *Rubin's pathology 5th/231*

The most common cause of chronic cor pulmonale is chronic obstructive pulmonary disease *- Rubin's pathology*

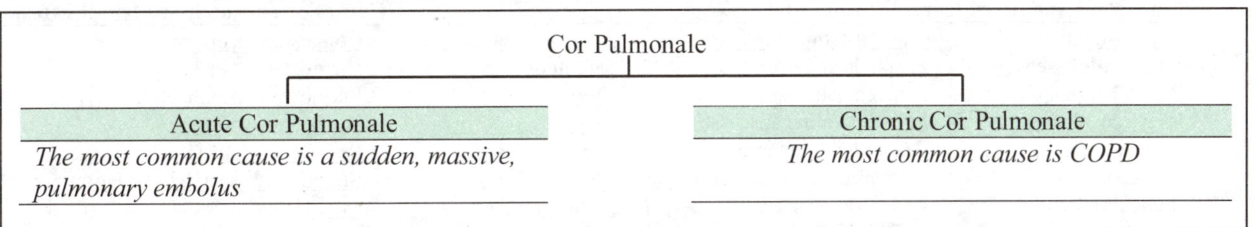

154. Answer is B (Pulmonary thromboembolism): *Ref: Harrison 15th/ 1355; Harrison 17th/ 1454 Harrison 18th/p 1914*

Most common causes of acute cor pulmonale is Pulmonary thromboembolism

Most common cause of chronic cor pulmonale is Severe COPD.

155. Answer is B (Prominent lower lobe vessels) :

Chronic Cor Pulmonale is associated with prominence of upper lobe and not lower lobe veins.

Features of Congestive Cardiac Failure(CCF / CHF) include :

1. ***Enlarged cardiac silhouette / Cardiac shadow on chest X-ray*** Q
2. Ground glass appearance of pulmonary edema Q
3. ***'Kerley B' lines*** Q
4. ***Prominence of upper lobe blood vessels*** Q *(not lower lobe veins)*
5. *Pleural effusion, usually bilateral* Q

- ***'Kerley B' lines'***, also known as ***'Septal lines'***, represent dilated lymphatics and distended interlobular septa. They occur ***most commonly in pulmonary edema as a result of chronic pulmonary venous hypertension (in CCF).*** Kerley 'A' lines stand for Apex, 'B' for Base, and 'C' for Central region.
  B lines are most commonly seen Q. ***Infact they have a relation with left atrial pressure*** Q : *They are invariably present if LA pressure goes above 20 mmHg.* Q
- Small bilateral ***pleural effusions*** are frequently seen in acute LVF. Large effusion may be present in long standing cases of congestive heart failure.

Pleural Diseases

Pleural Effusion

156. Answer is D (Bronchogenic Carcinoma): *Harrison 15th/ 1513, 1514; 16th/1567; 17th/ 1660; (table 257.1) Harrison 18th/p 2180 (Table 263.1)*

Malignant pleural effusions secondary to metastatic disease are exudative in nature. The three tumors that cause approx. 75% of all malignant pleural effusions are lung carcinoma, breast carcinoma, and Lymphoma.

Exudative pleural effusion			Transudative pleural effusion
Exudative pleural effusion occurs when ***local factors*** that influence the formation and absorbtion of pleural fluid are altered.			Transudative pleural effusion occurs when ***systemic factors*** that influence the formation and absorbtion of pleural fluid are altered.
Distinguishing Laboratory features :			
• Total serum protein > 3 gm /dL • *Pleural fluid protein / Serum protein > 0.5* • *Pleural fluid LDH / Serum LDH > 0.6* • *Pleural fluid LDH >2/3 upper limit of serum*			Total serum protein < 3 gm /dL *Pleural fluid protein / Serum protein < 0.5* *Pleural fluid LDH / Serum LDH < 0.6* *Pleural fluid LDH<2/3 upper limit of serum*
Causes of Exudative Pleural Effusion:			**Causes of Tansudative Pleural Effusion:**
• Neoplastic diseases Metastatic disease Mesothelioma • Infectious diseases Bacterial infections Tuberculosis Fungal infections Tuberculosis Viral infections Parasitic infections • Collagen-vascular diseases Rheumatoid pleuritis SLE Drug-induced lupus Sjogren's syndrome Wegner's granulomatosis Churg-Strauss syndrome	• Gastrointestinal disease Esophageal perforation Pancreatic disease Intraabdominal abscesses Diaphragmatic hernia After abdominal surgery Endoscopy variceal sclerotherapy • After liver transplant • Post-coronary artery bypass surgery • Drug-induced pleural disease Nitrofurantoin Dantrolene Methylsergide Bromocriptine Procarbazine Amiodarone	• Pulmonary embolism • Sarcoidosis • Uremia • Asbestos exposure • Meig's syndrome • Yellow nail syndrome • Trapped lung • Radiation therapy • Post-cardiac injury syndrome • Hemothorax • Iatrogenic injury • Ovarian hyperstimulation syndrome • Pericardial disease • Chylothorax	1. Congestive heart failure 2. Cirrhosis 3. Pulmonary embolization 4. Hephrotic syndrome 5. Peritoneal dialysis 6. Superior vena cava obstruction 7. Myxedema 8. Urinothorax

157. Answer is B (Rheumatoid arthritis): *Harrison 18th/p 2178, 2179, 2180 Harrisons 17th/1658, 1659, 1660 (±)*

Rheumatoid Arthritis is a cause for exudative pleural effusion

158. Answer is A and E (Pancreatitis and Esophageal rupture): *Kundu 3rd/ 52*

Predominantly left side effusion is a feature of Pancreatic effusion and effusion secondary to esophageal rupture.

Pleural Effusion

Predominant left sided pleural effusion	Predominant right sided pleural effusion
• *Acute pancreatitis* • *Oesophageal rupture* • *Dressler's syndrome (postmyocardial infarction syndrome)*	• *Amoebic liver abscess* • *Cirhosis of liver* • *Congestive cardiac failure* • *Meig's syndrome (fibroma of ovary with ascites ad pleural effusion)*

159. Answer is A and E (Horizontal fluid level and succussion splash): *Refer text below*

Succussion splash & horizontal fluid levels are features of hydropneumothorax & not pleural effusion.
Pleural efusions are associated with decreased chest movements, decreased lung volumes and may be associated with diminished heart sounds
Fluid level is typically concave & succession splash is not demonstable

Succussion splash is a feature of Hydropneumothorax and not pleural Effusion
Fluid movement in a cavity devoid of air is silent. When the cavity contains both air and fluid, body movements cause a splash audible to the patient and examiner – *succussion splash*

- A succussion splash in the thorax suggests a hydropneumothorax
- A succussion splash in the thorax may also result from a fluid filled stomach herniating into the thorax through a diaphragmatic hernia
- A succussion splash in the thorax in theory might be produced by a lung abscess, but in practice this almost never occurs because the pus is so thick that it does not splash.

Horizontal Fluid level is a feature of Hydropneumothorax
Pleural effusion presents with a concave fluid level (concave upper edge)
Presence of horizontal fluid level indicates the presence of associated air in the pleural cavity and suggests a diagnosis of Hydropneumthorax

160. Answer is D (Increased Mesothelial cells): *Harrison 14th/ 1474; 15th/ 1514; 16th/1567; 17th/ 1658, 1659 Harrison 18th/p 2178, 2179*

Presence of Mesothelial cells > 5% make diagnosis of Tubercular effusion unlikely *– CMDT 2009/277 t 9-23*

Characteristics of Tuberculous effusion
• Exudative • Proteins increased (Pleural fluid protein / Serum protein > 0.5) • Pleural fluid LDH increased (P. Fluid LDH/ Serum LDH > 0.6 • Haemorrhagic • Glucose: equal to serum levels; occasionally < 60 mg/dl • WBC count increased: predominantly small lymphocytes • High levels of TB markers in pleural fluid Adenosine deominase > 45 IU/L Interferon V > 140 pg/ml Positive PCR for tubercular DNA

Eosinophils > 10% or mesothelial cells > 5% make diagnosis of tubercular effusion unlikely.

161. Answer is None>A (None>Tuberculosis): *Harrison 18th/p 2179 Harrisons 17th/1658; Fishman's textbook of pulmonary Diseases and Disorder's 4th/1488; CMDT 2008/269; 2009/277 t 9-23*

Parapneumonic effusions (bacterial infections), Rheumatoid effusions, Malignant effusions (Mesothelioma) and Tuberculous effusions are all established causes that may present with low glucose (<60 mg/dl) in pleural fluid.
Although tuberculosis may present with low glucose levels and is included in the differential diagnosis for conditions with low glucose in pleural fluid, the glucose levels in Tuberculosis is more often equal to serum levels. Tuberculosis is therefore the single best answer of exclusion amongst the options provided.

Glucose levels in TB are usually equal to serum levels but Tuberculosis may present occasionally with Glucose < 60mg/dl- CMDT 09/277

According to Fishman's textbook on pulmonary disease, the presence of pleural fluid glucose below 60 mg/dl narrows the diagnostic possibilities to seven conditions.

Conditions associated with Decreased Glucose (<60mg/dl) in pleural fluid
• *Malignant Effusion[Q] (Also mentioned in Harrisons)* • *Rheumatoid Effusion[Q] (Also mentioned in Harrisons)* • *Parapneumonic Effusion[Q] (Bacterial Infections as mentioned in Harrisons)* • *Tuberculous Effusion[Q] (Also mentioned in CMDT)* • *Hemothorax* • *Paragonimiasis* • *Churg-Strauss Syndrome*

162. Answer is D (Dressler's Syndrome): *Harrison 18th/p 2178 Harrisons 17th/1658; Fishman's Pulmonary Diseases and Disorders 4th/1488*

Dressler's Syndrome is not associated with low glucose in pleural fluid.

Rheumatoid Arthritis, Malignancy and Empyema (Bacterial infections) are all established causes of pleural effusion with low glucose.

Pleural effusion with low glucose (< 60 mg/dl)
1. Malignancy
2. Bacterial infections
3. Rheumatoid pleuritis

163. Answer is A (Dressler syndrome): *Harrison 18th/p 2178 Harrison 15th/ 1513; Harrison 16th/ 1566; Harrison 17th/ 1658 (Fig. 257.1)*

Dressler's Syndrome is not associated with low glucose in pleural fluid.

Rheumatoid Arthritis, Malignancy and Empyema (Bacterial infections) are all established causes of pleural effusion with low glucose.

164. Answer *is A and C (Rheumatoid arthritis and Pneumococcal infection)* *Refer Previous question*

Rheumatoid Effusion and effusion secondary to bacterial infections (pneumococcus) are established causes for decreased glucose in pleural fluid.

165. Answer is B (Malignancy): *Harrison 15th/ 1513, 1514; 16th/ 1566; 17th/ 1658; (Fig. 257.1); CMDT 2009/ 276 Harrison 18th/p 2178*

Malignancy is associated with high levels of amylase in pleural fluid

High amylase level in pleural fluid suggests
Esophageal rupture[Q]
Pancreatic pleural effusion[Q] (Pancreatitis/Pancreaticpseudo cyst)
Malignancy[Q] (Adenocarcinoma of lung/pancreas)

166. Answer is A (Rheumatoid arthritis): *Refer previous question*

Rheumatoid Arthritis is not associated with increased amylase in pleural fluid.

Conditions with High Amylase in pleural Fluid
• *Esophageal Rupture* [Q]
• *Pancreatic effusion* [Q]
• *Malignancy* [Q]

167. Answer is A (Myxoedema): *See text below*

Pleural effusion secondary to Myxoedema (Hypothyroidism) is associated with presence of cholesterol crystals.

Pleural effusion with cholesterol crystals
• *Hypothyroidism (myxoedema)*
• *T.B.*
• *Rheumatoid arthritis*

168. Answer is B (7th Intercostal space in mid axillary line): *Pretest Anatomy; P.J. Mehta 13th/361*

Site of pleural effusion drainage is seventh intercostal space in mid-axillary line.

Pneumothorax

169. Answer is D (Bronchopulmonary Aspergillosis)

Bronchopulmonary Aspergillosis has not been mentioned as a cause for penumothorax.
Artificial ventilation is an established cause for iatrogenic pneumothorax while Marfan's syndrome and Eosinophilic granuloma are established causes for secondary spontaneous pneumothorax.

Pneumothorax

Spontaneous Pneumothorax

Primary Spontaneous Pneumothorax
- Occur in persons with No clinical evidence of lung disease and without precipitating event
- Most of these patients have occult lung disease (sub clinical) with subpleural blebs on CT scan

Characteristics of affected people are
- *Tall, thin, males*[Q]
- *Smokers*[Q]
- *Subpleural blebs*[Q] *on lungs*

Secondary spontaneous pneumothorax
- Occurs in persons with an underlying lung disease as a complication of the underlying disease process

Traumatic Pneumothorax
(Non spontaneous Pneumothorax)
- These penumothoroces occur as a result of:
  - Blunt trauma or
  - Penetrating trauma
- Iatrogenic penumotharax is subcategory of Traumatic Pneumothorax

Causes of Iatrogenic Pneumothorax
- Thoracocentesis
- Insertion of central venous catheter
- ***Mechanical ventilation*** (IPPV, Assisted ventilation etc)
- Surgery

Etiology of Secondary Pneumothorax

Obstructive Lung Disease	Malignancy
Chronic obstructive lung disease (COPD) *Asthma*	*Primary lung carcinoma* *Pulmonary metastasis (especially sarcomas)* *Complications of chemotherapy*
Interstitial lung disease	**Connective tissue disease**
Idiopathic pulmonary fibrosis (usual interstitial pneumonitis (UIP)) *Non-specific interstitial pneumonitis* ***Eosinophillic granuloma*** *Lymphangioleimyomatosis* *Sarcoidosis* *Langerhans cell granulomatosis* *Radiation pneumonitis of fibrosis* *Histocytosis X*	*Rheumatoid arthritis* *Ankylosing spondylitis* ***Marfan's syndrome*** *Ehlers-Danlos syndrome* *Polymyositis/dermatomyositis* *Scleroderma*
Infection	**Other**
P. jerovici pneumonia *Tuberculosis* *Coccidioodomycosis* *Acute bacterial pneumonia (i.e. staphylococcus)*	*Catamenial pneumothorax* *Pulmonary infarction* *Pulmonary hemorrhage* *Pulmonary alveolar proteinosis* *Tuberous sclerosis* *Von Recklinghausen's disease* *Wegner's granulomatosis*

170. Answer is B (Pneumothorax): *Handbook Of Critical Care By Paul Ellis Marik / 469*

Pneumothorax and/or less commonly hemothorax occurs due to injury to pleura and underlying Lung
– Critical care handbook.

171. Answer is B (Old age): *Harrison 18th/p 2181 Harrisons 17th/1660; CMDT 2008/271; 2009/278*

Primary spontaneous pneumothorax is characteristically affects young individuals and not elderly individuals.

Primary Spontaneous Pneumothorax (Primary pneumothorax)

- ***Primary spontaneous penumothorax occurs in persons with no clinical evidence of lung disease and often without an obvious precipitating event***
- Most of these patients have occult lung disease (sub clinical lung disease) in the form of subpleural apical blebs (recognized on CT scan)
- *Characteristic risk factors include a positive family history and history of smoking (occurs almost exclusively in smokers according to Harrisons)*
- *Characteristically affects tall, thin boys and men between the age of 10 and 30 years*

Primary Spontaneous pneumothorax
• *No clinical evidence of pre existing lung disease*[Q]
• *Rupture of apical subpleural blebs*[Q]
• *Positive family history*[Q]
• *History of smoking*[Q]
• *Tall and thin individual* [Q]
• *Young adults (10 to 30 years of age)* [Q]
• *Male gender*[Q]

172. Answer is A (smokers): *Repeat*

Spontaneous pneumothorax is common in smokers.

Spontaneous pneumothorax characteristically affect young, tall and thin men/boys (male gender).

173. Answer is D (Often need chest tube insertion): *CMDT 2008/272; 2009/279*

Pneumothorax is associated with decreased breath sounds, hyperresonant (increased) percussion note. Chest tube drainage is often required but is not necessary in all cases.

Many small pneumothoraces resolve spontaneously as air is reabsorbed from the pleural space. In reliable patients with small stable pneumothorax observation alone may be appropriate

174. Answer is D (Large Bore needle puncture of pleura): *Harrison 18th/p 2181 Harrisons 17th/1660*

Acute breathlessness absent breath sounds, neck vein distension and mediastinal shift suggests a diagnosis of Tension Pneumothorax.

Tension pneumothorax must be treated as a medical emergency and therapeutic intervention should not be delayed while waiting for investigations. Immediate puncture of pleura with a large bore needle through the second intercostal space is the treatment of choice.

175. Answer is A (Left axis deviation): *Repeat*

Left-sided pneumothorax is associated with right axis deviation.

176. Answer is B (Pleural effusion): *Harrison 14th/ 1489, 15th/ 1530; Harrison 17th/ 1688 Harrison 18th/p 2213, 2215*

Pleural effusion has not been mentioned as a complication of IPPV.

Complications of endotracheal intubation and positive pressure mechanical ventilation include :

Pulmonary complications:	Gastrointestinal complications:	Others:
1. ***Barotrauma***	1. *Stress ulceration* [Q]	1. Malnutrition
2. Nosocomial pneumonia	2. Mild to moderate *cholestasis* [Q]	2. *Decubitus ulcers* [Q]
3. *Oxygen toxicity* [Q]		3. *Venous thrombosis* [Q]
4. *Tracheal stenosis* [Q]		4. *Depression* [Q]
5. Deconditioning of respiratory muscles		

Disorders of Ventilation and Mediastinitis

177. Answer is D (10 seconds): *Harrison 18th/p2186, 2187 Harrisons 17th/1665,1666; Harrisons 16th/1573,1574; CMDT 2008/273; 2009/280*

Sleep Apnea is defined as temporary cessation of breathing for at least 10 seconds (CMDT)

Sleep Apnea: Review

- Sleep Apnea is defined as an intermittent cessation of airflow at the nose and mouth during sleep
- ***By definition/convention breath cessation for at least 10 seconds is termed Apnea***

By convention sleep apnea is defined by breath cessation for at least 10 seconds. Most patients with sleep apneas have cessation for 20-30 seconds. The duration of breath cessation may be as long as 2-3 minutes.

- Sleep apneas can be central or obstructive

Central sleep Apnea	Obstructive sleep Apnea
Sleep apnea occurs due to transient cessation of neural drive to all respiratory muscles	Sleep Apnea occurs due to transient occlusion of the orapharyngeal airway despite continued respiratory drive

178. Answer is A (Does not respond to chemical stimuli): *Harrison 18th/p 2183; 15th/ 1518; 16th/1570; 17th/ 1663*

Ventilatory responses to chemical stimuli are reduced or absent *– Harrison 16th/1570*

Primary pulmonary hypoventilation

Characterized by:
Impaired chemoreception resulting in decreased ventilatory drive. Chronic hypercapnia and hypoxemia in the absence of identifiable neuromuscular disease or mechanical ventilatory impairment.
Presentation :
Occurs in all age groups but majority of cases have been reported in males aged 20-50 years. Early: lethargy, fagtigue, daytime somnolence, disturbed sleep and morning headache. Late: Cyanosis polycythemia, pulmonary hypertension, congestive heart failure. Note : Dyspnea is uncommon despite severe arterial blood gas derangements because of impaired chemotherapy.
Diagnosis :
The key diagnostic feature is respiratory acidosis in the absence of respiratory muscle weaknesses or impaired ventilatory mechanics.

179. Answer is B (Causes normocapnic failure): *Harrisons 15th/1516; Harrison 16th/1569; Harrison 17th/221, 1663*

"Most patients with severe diaphragmatic weakness present with hypercapnic respiratory failure" *-Harrison*

- **Sniff test** is a confirmatory test of ***unilateral diaphragmatic paralysis***. *Whether sniff test is also useful for bilateral diaphragmatic paralysis is unconfirmed,* although it could show a paradoxical diaphragm movement on both sides. (The person is asked to sniff and is observed with fluoroscopy. The paralyzed diaphragm moves paradoxically upwards during inhalation due to negative intrathoracic pressure.)
- **Diaphragmatic pacing** may be a viable alternative if the nerve to the diaphragm is intact.
  Treatment of choice for Bilateral Diaphragmatic Paralysis is assisted ventilation

Note:

1. Unilateral paralysis occurs due to more local cause e.g. nerve invasion from bronchogenic carcinoma. Patients are usually asymptomatic.
2. Bilateral paralysis occurs due to more central or generalized causes e.g. high spinal cord injury, muscular dystrophy chest trauma.
   Patients present with hypercapnic respiratory failure, frequently complicated by cor-pulmonale, right ventricular failure (because of hypoxemic vasoconstriction in the lungs) pneumonia and atelectasis.

180. Answer is B (Esophageal rupture): *Ref: Harrison 14th/ 1475; 15th/ 1516; 16th/1568; 17th/ 1660, 1661; 18th/p 2182*

Most cases of acute mediastinitis are due to esophageal perforation or occur after median sternotomy for cardiac surgery *– Harrison*

Acute Mediastinitis	Chronic Mediastinitis
1. Esophageal rupture [Q] 2. Median sternotomy for cardiac surgery	1. Tuberculosis / Histoplasmosis (most cases) [Q] 2. Sarcoidosis, silicosis [Q] 3. Other fungal diseases

Bronchogenic carcinoma

181. Answer is D (Adenocarcinoma): *Ref: Harrison 15th/ 562; Harrison 16th/ 506; Harrison 17th/ 552 Harrison 18th/p 738*

Most common Bronchogenic Ca in world is Adenocarcinoma

Most common Bronchogenic Ca in India is Squamous ca

Histological type	Frequency
Adenocarcinoma	32%
Squamous cell ca	29%
Small cell carcinoma	18%
Large cell carcinoma	9%
Carcinoid	1%

Facts to remember

Q Most frequent histological type	*: Adenocarcinoma*
Q Most frequent histological type in India	*: Squamous cell carcinoma*
Q Most common histological variety in life time non-smokers	*: Adenocarcinoma*
Q Most common histological variety in young patients.	*: Adenocarcinoma*
Q Most common histological variety in females	*: Adenocarcinoma*
Q Most common site for metastasis from Ca lung	*: liver (page 521/H)*
Q Most common endocrine organ to be involved by metastasis from Ca lung	*: Adrenals.*
Q Ca lung which metastizes to opposite lung	*: Adenocarcinoma.*
Q Commonest tumor to metastise to heart	*: Ca lung (Bronchogenic Ca)*
Q Histological varieties that cavitate	*: squamous cell and large cell.*
Q Histological varieties that are central in distribution	*: squamous cell and small cell.*
Q Histological varieties that are peripheral in distribution	*: Adenocarcinoma.*
Q Pancoost tumor is histologically	*: squamous cell.*
Q Most common variety associated with paraneoplatic syndrome	*: small cell variety.*
Q Most common variety associated with hypokalemia	*: Small cell (presumably d/t ACTH)*
Q Most common variety associated with hypercalcemia	*: Squamous cell (presumably d/t PTH)*
Q Histological variety most responsive to chemotherapy	*: Small cell*
Q Histological variety response to Radiotherapy	*: Small cell*
Q Histological variety associated with best prognosis	*: Squamous cell*

182. Answer is B (Adenocarcinoma): *Harrison 18th/p 738 Harrisons 17th/551*

The most common type of lung cancer is Adenocarcinoma

Fact to remember:

The most common histological type of lung cancer in India is squamous cell carcinoma.

183. Answer is A (Variant of large cell Anaplastic Carcinoma): *Harrison 16th/562-509; Harrison 17th/ 554, 555*

Oat cell carcinomas are synonymous with small cell carcinomas of lung. Large cell anaplastic carcinoma constitutes an entirely different entity.

Characteristic of Small cell carcinoma lung:

- Usually present as central masses
- Cigarette smoking is an important risk factor and association of smoking with small cell carcinoma lung is high.
- Associated with release of ACTH, AVO, calcitonin, ANF and Gastrin releasing peptide and thus may manifest with hypokalemia (ectopic ACTH).
- Highly malignant tumors with least five year survival rates.
- Highly metastatic lesions with widespread disease at time of diagnosis.
- Management is primarily with chemotherapy with or without radiotherapy
- 90% regression with chemotherapy
- Objective shrinkage in 80% to 90% patients with radiotherapy.
- Surgery is unlikely to be curative because disease is usually widespread at presentation.

184. Answer is A (Commonest Malignancy of lung): *Harrison 18th/p 738 Harrisons 17th/551, 552*

The commonest malignancy of lung is Adenocarcinoma and not small cell carcinoma

The most common malignancy of lung is Adenocarcinoma (overall/ world wide)
Most common lung cancer worldwide is Adenocarcinoma
Most common lung cancer in India is squammous cell carcinoma
Most common lung cancer in women is adenocarcinoma
Most common lung cancer in smokers is squammous cell carcinoma
Most common lung cancer in nonsmokers is adenocarcinoma
Most common lung cancer in young patients is adenocarcinoma
Most common lung cancer to metastasize is small cell carcinoma

Small cell carcinomas are associated with paraneoplastic syndromes

Small cell carcinomas are the most common type associated with ectopic hormone production – Robbins 7th/762

Ectopic hormones produced by small cell carcinoms	Paraneoplastic syndrome
• *ACTH*	*Cushing's syndrome*
• *SIADH/ANP*	*Hyponatremia*
• *Calcitonin*	*Hypocalcemia*
• *Gonadotropins*	*Gynaecomastia*

Small cell carcinomas are an established cause for SVC obstruction
The most common type of Lung cancer associated with SVC syndrome is small cell carcinoma – Schwartz 8th/562

Small cell carcinomas are chemosensitive
'Small cell carcinomas are particularly sensitive to radiation and chemotherapy' -Robbins 7th/763

Small cell carcinomas commonly present with metastasis to brain (Harrison 16th/508)
Small cell carcinomas are aggressive tumors that metastisize widely (>95% patients).
Common sites of metastasis include Brain, Bone Liver and Adrenals

185. Answer is C (Chemosensitive tumor): *Harrison 18th/749, 750, 751, 752; Harrison's 17th/ 551,552,553,554; Harrisons 16th/506,507*

Small cell carcinomas are highly chemosensitive with an overall 90% regression rate with chemotherapy.

Property	Small cell Carcinoma	Non small cell Carcinoma
Location	• ***Central location***	*Peripheral location*
Metastasis	• ***Highly metastatic lesion*** with widespread metastasis at time of diagnosis • Common site of metastasis include brain, bone, Liver and adrenals	Less metastatic than small cell carcinomas
Paraneoplastic syndrome	• *ACTH* • *AVP (Vasopressin)* • *Calcitonin* • *ANF* • *Gastrin Releasing peptide*	• ***PTH***
Response to chemotherapy	Superior Response ***Overall regression rate is 90%*** Rate of complete regression is 30%	Inferior Response *Objective shrinkage in 30-50%* Complete response : uncommon

186. Answer is D (Gefitinib is most effective for female smokers with adenocarcinoma on histology): *Harrison 18th/751; Fishman's Pulmonary Diseases and Disorders 4th/1877; Davidson's 21st/703*

Gefitinib is an oral 'small molecule Tyrosine kinase Inhibitor' (that inhibit signalling via EGFR) approved for the treatment of patients with NSCCL. Data to support the use of Gefitinib in NSCCL are however diminishing and ***Gefitinib is most effective in females who have never smoked with adenocarcinoma on histology.***

Single agent cgemotherapy is prefered for elderly patients (> 70 years)

American Society of Clinical Oncology (ASCO) recommends the use of single agent chemotherapy for elderly patients (> 70 years) with a poor performance status (2003 Guidelines)

It has however now been stressed (2009 Guidelines) that age alone should not be used to select chemotherapy for patients with advanced NSCLC. Physiological Age (not chronological age) and performance status should be considered when selecting the chemotherapy regimen.

Chemotherapy for Advanced (Stage IV) NSCLC

Young patient Good performance status (PS < 2)	**Elderly patient** Poor performance status (PS ≥ 2)
• ***Double agent chemotherapy is preferred for first line therapy*** • Platinum based combinations are preferred over non platinum based combinations	• ***Single Agent Chemotherapy is preferred to reduce potential toxicity from chemotherapeutic agents.*** • Vinorelbine or docetexal are often used for single agent chemotherapy in the elderly with a poor PS.

Gefitinib is most effective for females with adenocarcinoma histology who have never smoked

Gefitinib is an acceptable second line agent for treatment of patients with advanced NSCLC with adequate performance status when the disease has progressed during or after first line platinum based chemotherapy.

Clinical Features that correlate with responsiveness to Gefitinib *(Harrison)*
• ***Female Sex*** • ***Never smoking status*** • ***Adenocarcinoma Histology*** • ***Asian Ethinicity***

Contralateral Mediastinal nodes are a contraindication to Surgical Resection

Contraindication to surgical resection in NSCLC (Davidson)
• *Distant metastasis (M1)* • *Invasion of central mediastinal structures including heart, great vessels. trachea and oesophagus (T4)* • *Malignant pleural effusion (T4)* • ***Contralateral mediastinal nodes (N3)*** • *FEV, < 0.8L* • *Severe or unstable cardiac or other medical condition*

N.B. In otherwise fit individual, direct extension of tumour into the chest wall, diaphragm, mediastinal pleura or pericardium or to within 2 cm of the main carina does not exclude surgery. Though surgically resectable, patients with N2 (ipsilateral mediastinal) nodes may require neoadjuvant or adjuvant therapy.

Squammous Cell Carcinoma is the most common histological subtype of Lung Cancer in Asia (Including India)

Most common lung cancer worldwide is adenocarcinoma
Most common lung cancer in India (Asia) is squammous cell carcinoma
Most common lung cancer in women is adenocarcinoma
Most common lung cancer in smokers is squammous cell carcinoma
Most common lung cancer in nonsmokers is adenocarcinoma
Most common lung cancer in young patients is adenocarcinoma
Most common lung cancer to metastasize is small cell carcinoma

187. Answer is B (Small cell carcinoma): *Ref: Harrison 16th/ 506, 507; Harrison 17th/ 552, 554 Harrison 18th/p 738*

Cigarette smoking is most strongly associated with squamous cell ca and small cell carcinoma and less commonly with adenocarcinoma.

Out of squamous cell and small cell carcinomas, the small cell variant is more malignant and metasizes early.

Thus the option of choice as regards a 'highly malignant' and metastatic lung carcinoma in a chronic smoker is a small cell carcinoma

Histological type	Association with smokers	5 years survival
Squamous cell carcinoma	High	15
Small cell carcinoma	High	5 (more malignant)
Adenocarcinoma	Low	17
Large cell carcinoma	Low	11

188. Answer is B (Growth Hormone): *Ref: Harrison 14th/ 554, 15th/ 564-5; Harrison 16th/507*

Hormones produced by Small Cell variant	*Hormone produced by non small cell variants*
1. ACTH Q 2. AVP (Vasopressin) Q 3. Calcitonin Q 4. ANF Q 5. Gastrin releasing peptide Q	PTH Q

189. Answer is C (Small cell carcinoma): *Schwartz 8th 562; Current critical care Diagnosis and treatment 3rd/465*

The incidence of superior vena caval syndrome is highest with small cell carcinoma.

Superior vena caval syndrome (SVC syndrome)

- SVC syndrome results from an impedance in outflow from superior vena cava due to external compression
- *The most common cause of SVC syndrome is external compression by a malignant tumour* Q
- *The most common malignant tumor causing SVC syndrome is bronchogenic carcinoma* Q
- *The most common histological type of bronchogenic carcinoma causing SVC syndrome is small cell carcinoma* Q

190. Answer is B (Oat cell carcinoma): *Harrisons 16th/506, 507; Harrisons 17th/Limited information*

Oat cell carcinoma is the other name for small cell carcinoma. Small cells carcinoma respond best to chemotherapy, and they are managed primarily by chemotherapy with or without Radiotherapy.

Non small cell carcinomas do not respond as well to chemotherapy as small cell cancers-Harrisons
Small Cell Lung cancer (SCLC) is a chemotherapy sensitive disease-H 17th/561

Property	**Small cell carcinoma**	**Non small cell carcinoma**
	Also called oat cell carcinoma	• *Squamous cell carcinoma* • *Adenocarcinoma* • *Large cell carcinoma* • *Bronchoalveolar carcinoma*
Response to Chemotherapy	***Superior Response*** *Overall Regression rate is 90%* *Rate of complete regression is 30%*	Inferior Response *Overall Regression rate is 40 to 60%* *Rate of complete regression 5%*
Response to Radiotherapy	***Superior Response*** *Objective Shrinkage in 80-90%* *Complete response: Often*	Inferior Response *Objective shrinkage in 30-50%* *Complete response: Uncommon*
Primary management	*Managed primarily with Chemotherapy with or without Radiotherapy*	*Management primarily with Surgery or Radiotherapy (localized lesions)*

191. Answer is C (Small cell Ca of Lung): *Harrison 16th/ 509; Harrison 17th/ 554 Harrison 18th/p 743*

'Skeletal connective tissue syndromes including clubbing is usually seen in no n small cell carcinomas'*H-16th*
Clubbing is thus least common with small cell carcinoma of lung

192. Answer is B (non small cell carcinoma): *Read text below: Harrison 16th/ 506-510; 17th/ 552-554; 18th/742, 743*

Presence of non productive cough, haemoptysis, clubbing and an apical lobe lesion in a sixty year old male suggests a diagnosis of carcinoma lung.

Association with clubbing and a peripheral location lead us to a diagnosis of non small cell variant.

Most common histological variant associated with clubbing : non small cell carcinoma
Most common histological variant presenting at peripheral location : non small cell carcinoma

Tuberculosis although, may present with such symptomatology, the age of the patient and non productive nature of cough go against its diagnosis.

193. Answer is D (Peripheral location): *Harrison15th/562,563;16th/506;17th/551,552;18th/738 Robbins7th/760; Chandrasoma Taylor 3rd/549*

'Adenocarcinomas are usually more peripherally located' *– Robbins 7th/ 760.*

- Squamous and small cell carcinomas usually present as central masses with endobronchial growths, while adenocarcinomas and large cell cancers tend to present as peripheral nodules or masses frequently with pleural involvement. – *Harrisons 16th/ 507*
- Adenocarcinomas constitute 32% of all lung cancers.
- Adenocarcinomas are the most common form of lung cancer arising in young patients (< 45 years).

Adenocarcinomas of lungs:
• Most common histological variant of Bronchogenic carcinoma in the world
• Most common histological variant of Bronchogenic carcinoma in females
• Most common histological variant of Bronchogenic carcinoma in nonsmokers
• Most common histological variant of Bronchogenic carcinoma in young patients

194. Answer is A and D (More common in females; Peripheral involvement is common): *Harrison 18th/p 738 Harrisons 17th/552; Robbins 7th/760*

Adenocarcinoma is the most common form of lung cancer in women and Adenocarcinoma usually presents as a peripheral lesion.

Adenocarcinoma is common in females

Adenocarcinoma is the most common type of lung cancer in women

Adenocarcinoma is associated with smoking, but may be seen in nonsmokers

'All histological types of lung cancer are associated with smoking' - Harrison

However *lung cancer can also occur in individuals who have never smoked and the most common type of lung cancer in life time non smokers is adenocarcinoma*

Adenocarcinomas are usually more peripherally located (Robbins 7th/760)

'Squamous and small cell carcinomas usually present as central masses while adenocarcinoma and large cell cancers tend to present as peripheral nodules or masses' - Harrison

195. Answer is B (Adenocarcinoma): *Ref: Harrison 15th/ 562; Harrison 16th/507; Harrison 17th/551 Harrison 18th/p 738*

'The most common lung carcinoma arising in life time non smokers in Adenocarcinoma'*-Harrisons 16th/507*

196. Answer is A (Adenocarcinoma): *Harrisons 17th/554*

197. Answer is A (Lung): *Ref: Harrison 14th/ 520; Not elaborated in Harrison 16th; Not elaborated in Harrison 17th*

The most common site of primary in a patient presenting with secondries to adrenals is Melanoma. Lung and bladder are the second most frequent sites of primary.

Amongst the options provided Lung is the single best answer.

Most common sites of spread to Adrenals:

Primary	Metastatic site (% involvement)
Melanoma	48%
Lung	35%
Bladder	35%
Cervix	31%
Colorectum	31%
Breast	31%
Kidney	20%
Ovary	20%
Prostate	17%

198. Answer is C (Oat cell variant is typically associated with hilar adenopathy): *Harrisons 17th/551, 552; 18th /738*

Oat cell variant (small cell carcinoma) is typically associated with hilar adenopathy in most cases.

Hilar lymphadenopathy is a typical feature of small cell (oat cell) variant

'Small cell (oat cell) carcinoma usually occurs in central bronchi with associated mediastinal and hilar adenopathy being a common presentation at time of diagnosis' - Thoracic Imaging: A practical Approach (1998)/72

'Small cell (oat cell) carcinoma is associated with significant degrees of mediastinal and hilar adnopathy in most cases'
– 'Essential Radiology' by Gunderman (1998)/164

'Bilateral bulky hilar adenopathy is typical of oat cell carcinoma'
– Clinical Imaging: An Atlas of Differental Diagnosis by Eisenberg (2009)/96 (f)

Squammous cell carcinoma accounts for about 30% of lung cancers

Adenocarcinoma is the most frequent histological variant of Lung cancer world wide[Q]

Histological subtype	Approximate Frequency
Adenocarcinoma	*≃ 32%*
Squammous cell carcinoma	*≃ 29%*
Small cell carcinoma	*≃ 18%*
Large cell carcinoma	*≃ 9%*

Cavitation is a feature of squammous cell and large cell variants and not of oat cell/small cell variant

'In contrast to squammous cell carcinoma in which central cavitation is noted in 10-20% of cases, small cell cancer rarely cavitates' - Clinical Hematology & Oncology (2003)/945

Cavitatory variant	Non cavitatory variants
• *Squammous cell (most common)*	• *Small cell*
• *Large cell*	• *Adeno carcinoma*

Adenocarcinomas present as peripheral masses and not as central masses

'Squammous and small cell cancers usually present as central masses while adenocarcinoma and large cell cancers tend to present as peripheral nodule and masses' – Harrison

Central location[Q]	Peripheral location[Q]
• *Squammous cell[Q]*	• *Adenocarcinoma[Q]*
• *Small cell[Q]*	• *Large cell variant[Q]*

199. Answer is A (Cough): *Robbins 7th/763; General Therosis Surgery 6th/1508*

The most common presenting symptom of lung cancer is cough *– Robbins*

Common presenting symptoms of lung cancer (Robbins)
Cough (75%-Commonest)
Weight loss (40%)
Chest pain (40%)
Dyspnea (20%)

Common presenting symptoms of lung cancer (General Thoracic Surgery) In decreasing order of frequency.
Cough (commonest)
Hemoptysis
Chest pain
Dyspnea
Wheezing or strider
Hoarseness
Pleural effusion
Superior vena caval syndrome
Pancoast tumour
Dysphagia
Phrenic palsy

200. Answer is A (Carcinoma lung): *Harrison 18th/p 284 Harrison 17th/227*

The two most common causes for hemoptysis are bronchitis and bronchogenic carcinoma. Bronchitis is not provided amongst the options and hence bronchogenic carcinoma is the single best answer of choice.

'Although the relative frequency of the different etiologies of hemoptysis varies from series to series, most recent studies indicate that bronchitis and bronchogenic carcinoma are the two most common causes (in the United States)'- Harrisons

Facts to Remember		
The most common cause of Hemoptysis	:	*Bronchitis and Bronchogenic CA*[Q] *(Bronchitis > Bronchogenic CA)*[Q]
The most common causes of Hemoptysis in India	:	*Tuberculosis*[Q]
The most common cause of Massive Haemoptysis	:	*Bronchectasis (World wide)*[Q] *Tuberculosis (India)*[Q]

201. Answer is A (Bronchoscopy) : *Harrison 15th/206; Harrison 16th/208; Harrison 17th/ 228 Harrison 18th/p 286*

The patient presents a case of hemoptysis with normal X-ray but with risk factors for cancer (Age and history of smoking). Bronchoscopy together with a bronchial or transbronchial biopy is the investigation of choice as indicated in the following algorithm from harrisons text.

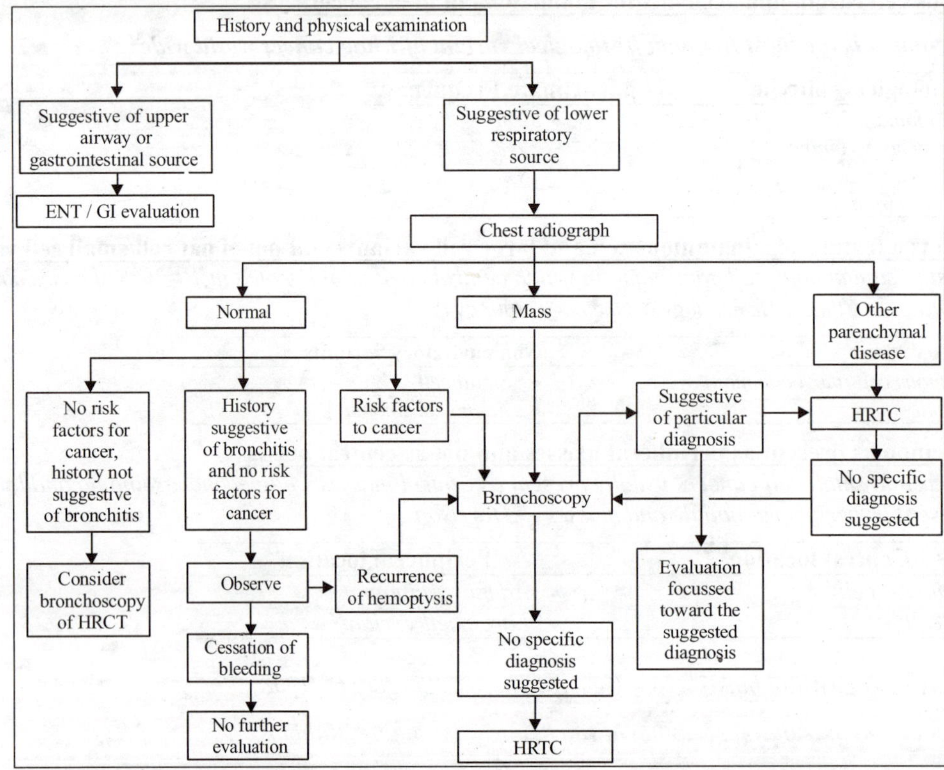

Algorithm in Harrisons 16th/208 does not elaborate the distinction between bronchoscopy and HRTC and thus reference to previous editions is recommended.

202. Answer is B (Bronchoscopy and biopsy) : *Harrison 14th/555, 198; 15th/206; 16th/208*

Fibreoptic bronchoscopy with a brochial or transbronchial biopsy is the better option here as it also allows direct visualization of the tumor mass

'The screening of lung cancer by means of sputum cytology & chest radiographs is not very effective'-H14th/255

Once signs/symptoms or screening studies suggest a diagnosis of bronchogenic carcinoma it is necessary to establish a tissue diagnosis of malignancy. From the options provided tumor tissues can be obtained by a bronchial or transbronchial biopsy during fibreoptic bronchoscopy or CT guided FNAC. Fibreoptic bronchoscopy is the preferred initial investigation to obtain a tissue diagnosis.

Approach to diagnosis

- *The first investigation while investigating a case of haemoptysis*: should be 'X-Ray chest'.
- *Once X-Ray chest suggests bronchogenic carcinoma (i.e. suspected mass)* the next investigation should be Bronchoscopy
- *An HR-CT should be done only if bronchoscopy is negative.*

In this question we already suspect the diagnosis of bronchogenic carcinoma. The investigation protocol, therefore expects us to proceed further from this point, hence a bronchoscopy should be the next investigation.

HRCT and guided FNAC is done only if bronchoscopy is negative.

As TB has already been ruled out sputum cytology is not the investigation to be done.

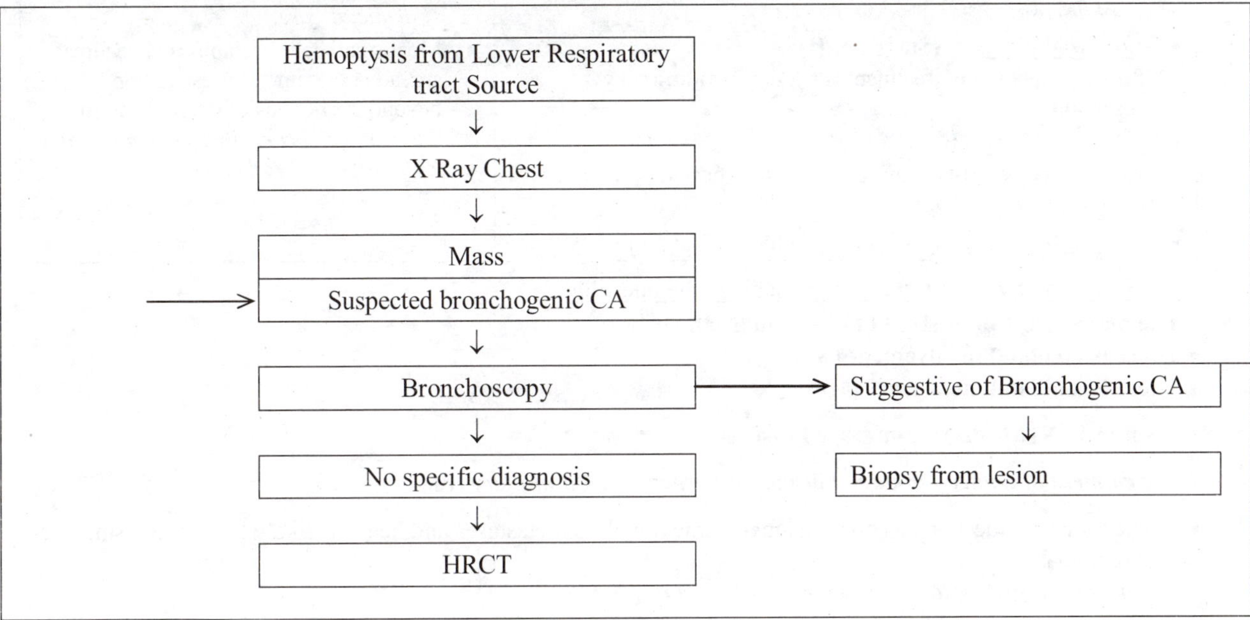

203. Answer is B (Bronchoscopy and biopsy): *Harrison 14th/555,198; 15th/206; 16th/208; 17th/554,555; Refer algorithm previous question*

This patient represents a case of suspected bronchogenic carcinoma. ***Fibreoptic bronchoscopy and biopsy is the investigation of choice*** *as it allows direct visualization of the tumor mass and provides a means of obtaining tumor tissue for histological diagnosis.*

HRCT is the alternate investigation but should be done if no specific diagnosis is suggested on bronchoscopy.

204. Answer is A (Bronchoscopy, lavage and brushing) : *16th/1507; Repeat*

The bascic idea is to obtain a tissue biopsy. FNAC could be used, however it would certainly not be the best. Bronchoscopy would allow, both, direct visualization and biopsy, and so is the best option here.

205. Answer is A (Bronchoscopy, lavage and brushing) : *Harrison 16th/1507*

The basic idea is to obtain a tissue biopsy. FNAC could be used, however it would certainly not be the best. Bronchoscopy would allow, both, direct visualization and biopsy, and so is the best option here.

206. Answer is D (Bronchogenic carcinoma) : *Harrison 16th/2023; Harrison 17th /2140 Harrison 18th/p 2810*

ACE levels are not elevated in Bronchogenic carcinoma

Serum levels of ACE may be increased in :	
Sarcoidosis	Hypersensitivity pneumonitis
Aesbestosis	Leprosy
Silicosis	Lymphoma
Berthosis	Tuberculosis
Fungal infection	
Granulomatous hepatitis	

207. Answer is C (surgery): *Harrison's 15th/565; Oxford text book of surgery IInd/2480, Schwartz 7th/753*

The baffling aspect of the question is that it does not mention whether it is a small cell carcinoma or a non small cell carcinoma as this histological distinction is the bases of the primary modality of treatment.

Non small cell carcinomas	Small cell carcinomas
For non small cell carcinomas the primary modality depends on the extent of disease • **<u>Localized diseases</u>: (Stage I & II)** Primary modality of treatment is surgery – **pulmonary resection.** • **<u>Advanced disease</u>:** **Radiotherapy with curative intent** is advocated (± chemotherapy) • **<u>Metastatic disease</u> (Stage IV)** symptomatic/supportive	• *Small cell lung carcinomas behave as systemic disease.* • Most small cell carcinomas have already spread at the time of presentation beyond the bounds of surgery and they are *managed primarily by chemotherapy with or without radiotherapy.*

<u>If we were to go by the information available in the question,</u>

- **The maximum tumor size (T) is = 5 cm (≥ 3), i.e. T_2**
- **There is no nodal involvement (No)**
- **There is no distal metastases (Mo)**

Thus it is T_2 N_0 M_0 disease or stage I disease

The treatment of choice for stage I disease is surgery i.e. Pulmonary resection

- The tumor in question has no nodal involvement and no metastases and hence is likely to be a non small cell carcinoma.
  Further, according to oxford textbook of surgery 2nd/2480
- "Recent data suggest that staging small cell lung cancer using TNM system employed for non small cell carcinomas may be helpful. For patients with stage I disease surgical resection and postoperative adjuvant chemotherapy provides a better prognoses than non surgical therapy".

Thus within the limits of information provided the primary modality of treatment here should be surgery.

		5 Year Survival Rate, %	
Stage	**TNM Descriptors**	**Clinical Stage**	**Surgical Pathologic Stage**
IA	T1 N0 M0	61	67
IB	T2 N0 M0	38	57
IIA	T1 N1 M0	34	55
IIB	T2 N1 M0	24	39
IIB	T3 N0 M0	22	38
IIIA	T3 N1 M0 T1-2-3 N2 M0	9 13	25 23
IIIB	T4 N0-1-2 M0 T1-2-3-4 N3 M0	7 3	<5 <3
IV	Any T any N M1	1	<1

Tumor (T) status descriptor	
T0	No evidence of a primary tumor
TX	Primary tumor cannot be assesed, or tumor proven by the presence of malignant cells in sputum or bronchial washings but not visualized by imaging or bronchoscopy.
TIS	Carcinoma is situ
T1	Tumor > 3 cm in greatest dimension, surrounded by lung or visceral pleura, without bronchoscopic evidence of invasion more proximal than lobar bronchus (i.e. not in main bronchus)
T2	Tumor with any of following: > 3 cm in greatest dimension: inolves main bronchus, >= 2 cm distal to the carina: invades visceral pleura; associated with atelectasis or obstructive pneumonitis extending to hilum but does not involve entire lung.
T3	Tumor of any size that directly invades any of the following: chest wall (including superior sulcus tumors), diaphragm, mediastinal pleura, parietal pericardium; or tumor in main bronchus < 2 cm distal to carina but without involvement of carina; or associated atelectasis or obstructive pneumonitis of entire lung.
T4	Tumor of any size that invades any of the following: mediastinum, heart, great vessels, trachea, esophagus, vertebral body, carina or tumor with a malignant pleural or paericardial effusion, or with satellite tumor nodule(s) within the ipsilateral primary-tumor lobe of the lung.

Lymph node (N) involvement of descriptor	
NX	Regional lymph nodes cannot be assessed
N0	No regional lymph node metastasis
N1	Metastasis to ipsilateral peribronchial and/or ipsilateral hilar lymph nodes, and intrapulmonary nodes involved by direct extension of the primary tumor.
N2	Metastasis to ipsilateral mediatinal, contralateral lymph node(s)
N3	Metastasis to contralateral mediastinal, contralateral hilar, ipsilateral or contralateral scalene, or supraclavicular lymph node(s)

Distant metastasis (M) descriptor	
MX	Presence of distant metastasis cannot be assessed
M0	No distant metastasis
M1	distant metastasis present

208. Answer is D (Hypercalcemia): *Ref: Harrison 15th/ 2209, 280; Harrison 2252, 2257; Harrison 17th/ 2380, 554 Harrison 18th/p 3100, 743*

Presence of polyuria, abdominal pain, and general symptoms such as nausea, vomiting and altered sensorium in a patient with bronchogenic carcinoma suggest a diagnosis of hypercalcemia secondary to paraneoplastic syndrome from PTH related peptide production.

The symptomatic profile of this patient matches with that of hypercalcemia

Manifestations of Hypercalcemia

General	Renal feature	Bones	Abdomen	Cardiac	Calcification
• Anorexia • Nausea • Vomiting • Fatigue • Mental confusion (≅ altered sensorium)	• Polyuria* & Nocturia • Renal colic from stones	• Bone pain • When cause is hyperparathyroidism • Bone cysts • Brown tumors	• Abdominal pain (peptic ulceration) • Constipation	• Short QT interval in ECG & in some patients cardiac arrythmias	Ectopic calcification & chondrocalcinosis

* **Polyuria** results from effect of hypercalcemia on renal tubules reducing there concentrating ability a form of nephrogenic diabetes insipidus

209. Answer is D (Superior Vena cava obsrtuction) : *Read text below; Harrison's 15th/642*

The patient in question is presenting with classical signs and symptoms of superior mediastinal syndrome or Superior vena caval syndrome.

Lung cancer is the commonest cause of superior vana caval syndrome or SVC obstruction. As the options provided include superior vena caval obstruction as a distinct entity, it is the option of choice.

Clinical manifestations of obstruction to SVC :

Symptoms	Signs
• ***Swelling around neck & face*** especially around the eyes • ***Dyspnea*** • Cough • Others: Hoarseness / Headache / Tongue swelling / Nasal congestion / Epistaxis Haemoptysis / Dysphagia / Pain / Dizziness / Syncope	• Dilated neck veins • ***Increased number of collateral veins over*** • ***anterior chest wall*** • Cyanosis • Edema of face, arms & chest • Proptosis, glossal and Laryngeal edema and obtundation in severe cases

Symptoms are aggrevated by bending forwards and lying down.

210. Answer is B (Small cell carcinoma): *'Clinical Hematology and Oncology' by Furie (2003) 1st/99; Schwartz 8th/562; Current Critical Care Diagnosis & Treatment 3rd /465*

The incidence of superior vena caval syndrome is highest with small cell carcinoma.

Superior vena caval syndrome (SVC syndrome)

- SVC syndrome results from an impedance in outflow from superior vena cava due to external compression
- *The most common cause of SVC syndrome is external compression by a malignant tumour*[Q]
- *The most common malignant tumor causing SVC syndrome is bronchogenic carcinoma*[Q]
- *The most common histological type of bronchogenic carcinoma causing SVC syndrome is small cell carcinoma*[Q]

Etiologies of Superior Vena Cava Obstruction:

Malignancy	**95%**
Lung Cancer	*65%*
Lymphoma	*15%*
Breast cancer	*5%*
Germ-cell	*2%*
Thymic cancer	*2%*
Other cancer	*4%*
Benign	**5%**
Central venous device related	*1%*
Mediastinal fibrosis	*3%*

Cystic Fibrosis

211. Answer is D (Endocrine): *Refere text below*

Cystic fibrosis is typically charachterized by Exocrine Pancreatic insufficiency.
Endocrine Pancreatic insufficiency is not seen as a tyical manifestation of cystic fibrosis.

Charachteristic Classical Manifestations of Cystic Fibrosis
(Typical System Involvement)

Respiratory system (Sinopulmonary disease)

- Pulmonary infection
  Persistant colonization/infection with typical cystic fibrosis pathogens, including Staphylococcus aureus, nontypeable, Hemophilus influenzae, ***mucoid and nonmucoid Pseudomonas aeruginosa***, Burkholderia cepase
- Chronic obstructive Pulmonary Disease
- Bronchiectasis is typical
- Airway obstruction manifested by wheezing and air trapping
- Chronic cough & sputum production
- Digital clubbing
- Persistent chest radiograph abnormalities (eg. Bronchiectasis, atelectasis, infiltrates, hyperinflation)
- Nasal Polyps
  radiographic or computed tomographic abnormalities of paranasal sinuses

Gastrointestinal System (Intestinal; Hepatobiliary; Pancreatic)

Intestinal
meconium ileus, distal intestinal obstruction syndrome, rectal prolapse.

Pancreatic
Pancreatic exocrine deficiency

Hepatobiliary
Hepatic disease manifested by clinical or histologic evidence of focal biliary ***cirrhosis***, or multilobular ***cirrhosis***

Nutritional
Failure to thrive (protein-calorie malnutrition), hypoproteinemia, edema, complications secondary to fat-soluble vitamin deficiency

Genitourinary System (Male Infertility)

Male urogenital abnormalites resulting in obstructive azoospermia are typical

Metabolic Abnormalities are typically charachterized by **salt depletion syndrome,**
(Hyponatremia, Hypocholeremia and Hypokalemic Metabolic Alkalosis)

212. Ans. Answer is A (Pseudomonas Aeroginosa): *Cystic Fibrosis' (Oxford University Press)2000/31*

The most common cause of Pulmonary infections in cystic fibrosis is Pseudomonas aeroginosa

'The most common pathogen in CF is Pseudomonas Aeroginosa followed by Staphylococcus'
- 'Pseudomonsa:Gemmu & Molecular Biology' (Harizon Scientific Press)2008/160

Pulmonary Infection in Cystic Fibrosis

- *The most common cause of Pulmonary infection in cystic fibrosis in children is staphylococcus aureus*[Q]
- *The most common cause of Pulmonary infection in cytic fibrosis in adolescents and adults is Pseudomonas Aeroginosa.*
- The two most common cause of pulmonary infection in cystic fibrosis are staphylococcus aureus and Pseudomonas Aeroginosa.

Overall (all age groups) Pseudomonas Aeroginosa is marginally more common than staphylococcus aureus as a cause of pulmonary infection in cystic fibrosis.

- *The most common organism causing chronic lung disease in patients with cystic fibrosis is pseudomonas aeroginosa*

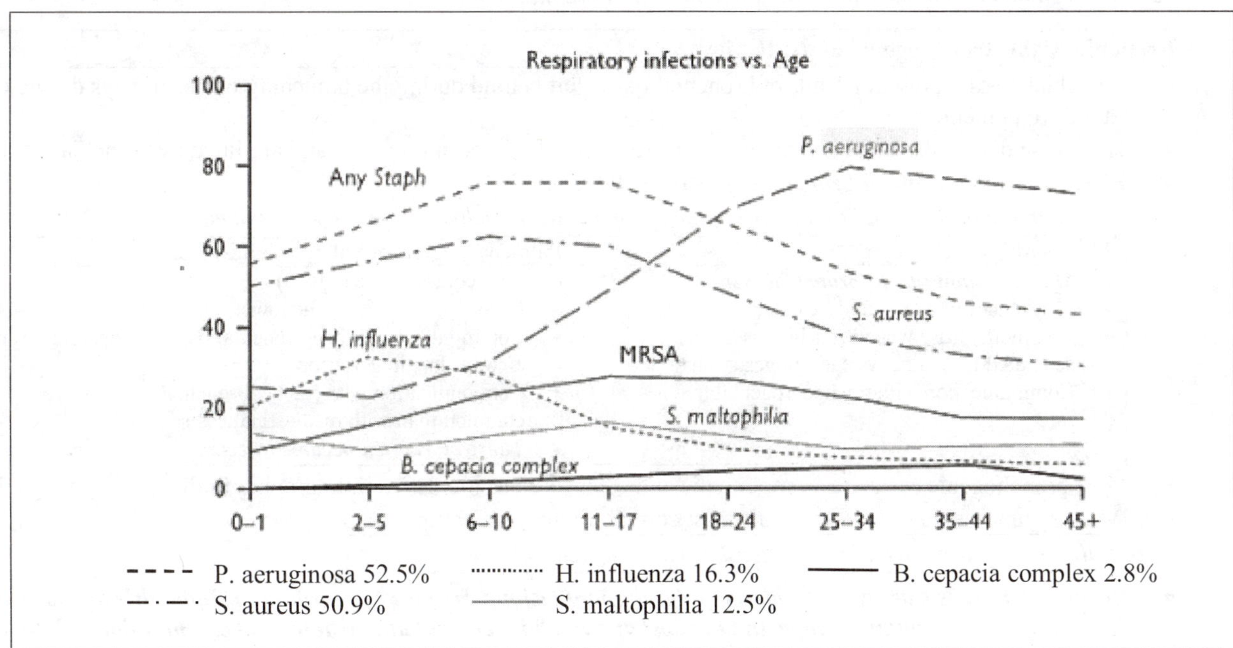

213. Ans. Answer is A (Staphylococcus Aureus): *Imaging in Pediatric Pulmonology (Springer) 2012/313*

Staphylococcus Aureus (Methicillin sensitive) are the most common pathogen isolated in sputum of children with cystic fibrosis during the first decade.

'The most prevalent pathogen to cause pulmonary infection in cystic fibrous during childhood is staphylococcus aureus. Pseudomonas aeroginosa becomes the most common organism in adolescents and adults. Hemophilus influenza is also seen in early life (2-5 years) and its frequency decreases with age. Bukholderia capacia is also infrequent but its incidence increase with age. Stenotrophomonos is an infrequent organism seen at any age.
– USMLE Step III: Review/Q1 Case 7

'The most common cause of pneumonia in a patient with cystic fibroses is Pseudomonas aeroginosa, but initial infection is most often due to staphylococcus aureus'- Microbiology: Pearls of Wisdom' by Booth (Jones & Barlett) 2000/203

Bronchial Ademoma and Bronchial Cysts

214. Answer is A (Recurrent haemoptysis): *Harrison 14th/561; 15th/570-71; 16th/515; 17th/ 562; Harrison 18th/p 753*

Bronchial adenomas are hypervascular, and can bleed profusely. Recurrent haemoptysis is the most common manifestations.

Bronchial adenomas include:
Carcinoids : 80-90%
Adenocystic tumors (cylindromas): 10 to 15%)
Mucoepidermoid tumors : 2-3%

Broncheal adenomas are hypervascular, and can bleed profusely. Recurrent haemoptysis is the most common manifestations. Others being, chronic cough, obstruction with atelectasis, lobar collapse, pneumonitis and abscess formation.

215. Answer is B (Most common site is mediastinum): *Rudolph's Fundamentals of Pediatrics 3rd/716*

Most common site of bronchial/bronchogenic cysts is mediastinum. Only about 15% of bronchogenic cysts occur in the lungs (pulmonary bronchial cysts). Pulmonary bronchogenic cysts often become infected. Bronchogenic cysts are benign lesion and do not have malignant potential (not premalignant).

Bronchial Cyst/Bronchogenic cysts: Review

- Bronchial cysts represent islands of bronchial tissue left behind during the branching of the airways during early fetal development.
- They arise due to abnormal budding of the tracheobronchial tree and foregut and are lined by bronchial epithelium.
- ***The most common site of bronchial cysts is mediastinum.***
- *The other site of bronchial cyst is within the pulmonary parenchyma (lung) (Less common site – 15%)*

Mediastinal bronchial cyst	Pulmonary parenchymal cyst (lungs)
• ***Most common site for bronchial cysts***	• Less common site (- 15%)
• Most common site is middle mediastinum	• Most common site is the lower lobes
• Commonly arise when bronchial tissue is separated from airways early in gestation	• Commonly arise when bronchial tissue is separated from airways late in gestation
• Communication with tracheobronchial tree is rare	• Communication with tracheobronchial tree is more common than with mediastinal cysts.
	• ***These cysts often become infected.***

- Most bronchogenic cysts are asymptomatic and discovered as incidental radiographic findings in a young adult.
- When symptoms do occur they result most commonly from infection.

Pulmonary parenchymal cysts often become infected *– Rudolph*

- ***Bronchogenic cysts are not considered premalignant lesions. However according to Rudolph's textbook there is a small risk of malignant change and the best approach is removal and histological examination.***

Kartagener's Syndrome

216. Answer is C (Mental retardation): *Robbins 7th/727; Harrisons (old edition) 11th/940, 1082*

Mental Retardation is not a feature of Kartagener's syndrome.

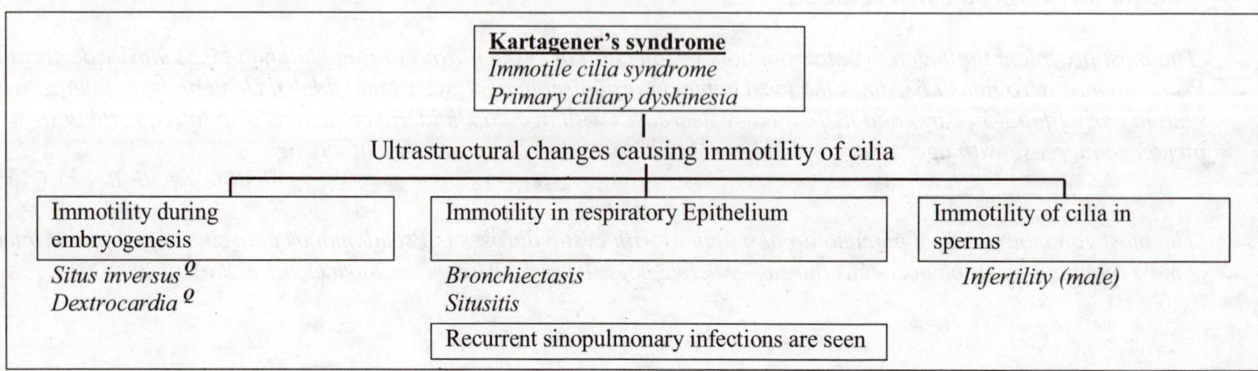

217. Answer is E (Cystic fibrosis): *Harrisons 17th/1629 (not eloborated): Harrison 11th/1082, 940 Robbins 7th/727*

Kartagener's syndrome is associated with situs inversus, sinusitis, infertility and bronchiectasis

Syndrome	Major cardiac Anomaly	Major non cardiac anomaly
Kartagener's syndrome *(Immotile cilia syndrome)* *(Primary ciliary dyskinesia)*	*Dextrocardia*Q	• *Situs inversus* Q • *Sinusitis* Q • *Bronchiectasis* Q • *Infertility* Q

Note

Situs inversus refers to perfect mirror image of normal physiologic position of visceral organs with preservation of their A-P relationship. Situs inversus is usually associated with dextrocardia (Heart on Right Side of chest).

Pulmonary Renal Syndrome

218. Answer is D (All of the above): *Acute Renal failure in Practice' 1st/345; Oxford Testbook of clinical Nephrology 3rd/582*

Laptosporiasis, hanta virus infection and Paraquat poisoning may all cause Pulmonary Renal syndrome

Differential diagnosis of the "pulmonary- renal syndrome"

Lung haemorrhage and glomerulonephritis

- *ANCA-associated vasculitis*
  - *Wegener's granulomatosis*
  - *Microscopic polyarteritis*
  - *Churg Strauss Syndrome*
  - *Renal Limited vasculitis*
- *Anti-GBM disease – Good posture's syndrome*
- *Cryoglobulinemic vasculitis*
- *Henoch-Schonlein purpura*
- *Bechet's syndrome*
- *Systemic lupus erythematosus, RA, systemic sclerosis, Polymyositis and other connective tissue disorders*

Pulmonary infections with renal failure

- *Any severe pneumonia with ATN*
- *Legionella*
- *Hantavirus*
- *Leptospirosis*

Severe pulmonary oedema associated with renal failure of any cause

- *RPGN*
- *Idiopathic immune complex GN*

Pulmonary emboli with IVC thrombosis

Paraquat poisoning

219. Answer is A (Goodpasture's syndrome): *Refer text below; Current Diagnosis and Treatment in Pulmonary Medicine 1st (2003)/211*

Association of hematuria and hemoptysis suggest a diagnosis of Goodpasture's syndrome. *ANCA antibodies are usually negative but may be present in upto 30% of patients*

Good pasture's syndrome

Good pasture's syndrome is an autoimmune disease characterized by formation of Anti GBM antibodies that attack both pulmonary capillaries and the Glomerulus (GBM)

Preceding Resp infection
Toxic lung exposure
Drug exposure Etc

Antibodies against Non collagenous Domain (NCL) of $\alpha 3$ chain of collagen type IV
(Found in Glomerular Bacement membrane & Pulmonary capillaries)

Serology

- *Circulating Anti GBM antibodies (IgG): Positive*
- *ANCA antibodies: Typicallyy negative (May be present in upto 30% of patients)*
- *ANA antibodies : usually normal*
- *C3 levels : Usually normal*

Two Age Groups

- *Young men in late 20's (Men >> females)*
- *Men and women their 60-70's*

Antibodies agonist Glomerular Basement Membrane (GBM)

Glomerulonephritis /Renal Disease

- Features of Acute Glomerulonephritis (RPGN)
  *Hematuria*Q
  *Proteinuria*Q
  Edema
  *Rapidly progressive renal failure*Q
- Pathological PictureQ
  *Diffuse crescenteric Glomerulonephritis*Q
  *Linear IgG*Q *staining along basement membrane on immunofluorescence*Q

*Dysmorphic RBC and RBC cast are present in urine suggesting Glomerulonephritis*Q

Antibodies against pulmonary capillaries

Pulmonary /Lung Manifestations

Clinical

- Hemoptysis (Frank)
  Hemoptysis is largely confined to smokers
- Dyspnea

X-Ray findingQ

- *Diffuse bilateral pulmonary infiltrates*Q

Goodpasture's syndrome and ANCA

ANCA is typically negative in Goodpastures syndrome and it is classified as an ANCA negative vasculitis
Nevertheless
ANCA seropositivity may occur in upto 30 percent of patients with Goodpasture's syndrome.These patients with ANCA have subtle signs of a systemic vasculitis and represent an overlap between goodpastures and either Wegener's granulomatosis (WG) or Microscopic polyangitis(MPA)-Current Diagnosis and Treatment in Pulmonary Medicine 1st (2003)/211

220. Answer is A (Good pasture's syndrome): *Current critical cace diagnosis & Treatment 3rd*

Association of hematuria and hemoptysis suggests a diagnosis of Goodpasture's syndrome

Good pasture's syndrome is an autimmune disease charachterized by formation of Anti GBM antibodies, that attack both the pulmonary capillaries (hemoptysis) and the glomerulus (hematuria).
The classical presentation is that of a young male smoker with signs of acute glomerulonephritis (hematuria, proteinuria & RBC cast) and hemoptysis associated with bilateral pulmonary infiltrates.

Neonate Alveolar Proteinosis

221. Answer is A (Neonatal Alveolar Proteinosis): *Nelsons 18th/ 1821; Pediatric Imaging by Siegel and Coley (2005)/101*

The child in question is presenting with characteristic features of Neonatal Pulmonary Alveolar Proteinosis (PAP).
Familial cases of Neonatal Pulmonary Alveolar Proteinosis have been observed and a genetic basis has been suggested.
None of the other options have a familial basis and hence neonatal PAP is the single best answer of choice.
TAPVC is unlikely as ECHO is unremarkable and TAPVC does not have a familial basis.
Meconium aspiration syndrome is unlikely as it does not have a familial basis and the question provides no other clinical clues to suggest meconium aspiration such as meconium staining
Congenital Herpes infection has an entirely different mode of presentation and can be safely excluded.

Pulmonary Alveolar Proteinosis (PAP)

- PAP is a disorder characterized by the intra-alveolar accumulation of pulmonary surfactant proteins

Etiology
• Defect in surfactant proteins (SP) (SP –B & SP –C) • Defect in colony stimulating factor receptor (GM –CSF) gene • Defect in ATP – binding cassette transporter Gene (ABCA3

- ***It may present in neonates*** (Neonatal PAP) and in older infants, children and adults

Neonatal (Congenital PAP)
This has a fulminant course and is often fatal

PAP in older children and Adults (Adult PAP)
This has a gradually progressive course

(Note that the neonatal and adult forms are distinct entities and have different etiologies and manifestations)

- ***Familial cases have been observed and a genetic basis (****Autosomal recessive****) has been suggested for neonatal congenital PAP.***
  No Gender difference in frequency has been observed.
- *Neonatal PAP presents with severe* ***respiratory distress in the neonatal period.***
- ***Radiological features resemble those of hyaline membrane disease and may show fine reticulonodular infiltrates radiating from the hilum.***
- *It* ***has a fulminant course and leads to death from rapidly developing respiratory failure****.*

222. Answer is C (Neonatal pulmonary alveolar proteinosis): *Repeat. Refer previous question*

Symptoms and Signs of Respiratory Disease

223. Answer is B (Empyema): *Harrisons 16th/208; Harrisons 17th/227 Harrison 18th/p 284, 285*

Empyema by itself is not a cause for hemoptysis.

Pneumonia, Mitral stenosis and Bronchiectasis are established causess for hemoptysis.

Differential Diagnosis of hemoptysis

Tracheobronchial source	Pulmonary parenchymal source
• Neoplasm (branchogenic carcinoma, endobronchial metastatic tumor, Kaposi's sarcoma, bronchial carcinoid) • Bronchitis (acute or chronic) • ***Bronchiectasis*** • Broncholithiasis • Airway trauma • Foreign body	• Lung abscess • ***Pneumonia*** • Tuberculosis • Mycetoma ("fungus ball") • Goodpasture's syndrome • Idiopathic pulmonary hemosiderosis • Wegener's granulomatosis • Lupus pneumonitis • Lung contusion
Primary vascular source	**Miscellaneous/rare causes**
• Arterivenous malformation • Pulmonary embolism • ***Elevated pulmonary venous pressure (esp. mitral stenosis)*** • Pulmonary artery rupture secondary to balloon- tip pulmonary artery catheter manipulation	• Pulmonary endometriosis (catamenial hemoptysis) • Systemic coagulopathy or use of anticoagulants or thrombolytic agents

224. Answer is A (Cavity): '*Textbook of practical physiology' by Pal (Orient Longman) 2001/171*

Cavernous Respiration (Cavernous Breathing) is a low pitched bronchial breath sound heard over a cavity which is situated superficially and communicates with a patent bronchus.

Bronchial breath sounds

The bronchial breath sound originates in the larger airways and are transmitted directly to the chest wall without passing through the alveoli. The sound passing through the lung tissue is not modified and auscultated like bronchial sounds from the chest walls. This sound resembles the sound obtained by listening over the trachea (directly placing a stethoscope on the trachea).

The characteristics of these sounds are:

1. Duration of expiration is equal to or longer than that of inspiration.
2. Intensity of expiration is more than that of inspiration.
3. There is a definite gap between inspiration and expiration.
4. Sounds are harsh or aspirate in nature.
5. They are high-pitched with frequencies above 600Hz.

Bronchial Breath Sounds

Bronchial breath sounds are of three types: tubular, cavernous, and amphoric.

Tubular Bronchial Breath sound	Cavernous Bonchial Breath sound	Amphoric Bronchial Breath sound
The tubular bronchial breath sound is a high pitched sound resulting from the passage of vibrations produced in the small bronchi directly to the chest wall through a solid lung tissue. This is seen when the lung parenchyma becomes a solid mass, as in consolidation.	The cavernous bronchial breath sounds is a low pitched bronchial breath sound heard over a cavity, which is situated superficially and communicated to a patent bronchus. The size of the cavity should be more than 2 cm in diameter to produce a cavernous breath sound.	The amphoric bronchial breath sounds is a high pitched bronchial sound that resembles the sound produced by blowing air into a wide-mouthed bottle. This is heard over a very large cavity communicating pneumothorax. It is also seen in large pulmonary cysts having communication with a patent bronchus.

225. Ans. Answer is D (Tracheal shift to side of consolidation): *Text below*

Trachea stays in midline in consolidation (no mediastinal shift).

Consolidation is usually caused by pneumonia. In this situation alveoli are full of inflammatory exudates but the size of the lung is unaffected so the trachea remains in its normal midline position.

	Tracheal deviation (Mediastinal shift)	Chest expansion	Percussion note ↓ Duller ↑ Hyper-resonant	Breath sounds ↑ Louder ↓ Softer	Added sounds	Vocal resonance
Consolidation	No	Normal, or↓	Normal, or↓	↑ (Bronchial)	Coarse crackles +/- rub	↑ Whispering Pectoriloquy
Lobar collapse	Yes (Towards collapse)	↓	↓	↓	No	↓
Pleural effusion	No	↓	↓ (Stony dull)	↓	Occasional rub	↓
Pneumothorax	Yes (Specially with tension)	Normal or↓	↑	↓	Occasional click	↓

226. Answer is A (Iatrogenic Pneumothorax): *Refer text below; 'Complications in Anesthesiology' by Kirby (2007)/169*

Subclavian vein cannulation is an important cause of iatrogenic pneumothorax. Absence of breath sounds and Hyper-resonance of chest wall on percussion alongwith sudden breathlessness after attempted subclavian vein cannulation suggests a diagnosis of Iatrogenic Pneumothorax.

Common causes of Iatrogenic Pneumothorax (Decreasing order of frequency)
Transthoracic Needle Lung Biopsy
Subclavian vein cannulation
Thoracocentesis
Pleural Biopsy
Positive Pressure ventilation

Iatrogenic Pneumothorax

History
• History of Procedure known to cause iatrogenic pneumothorax (subclavian vein cannulation) • Sudden onset Breathlessness • Chest discomfort / chest pain

Examination
Inspection/ palpatum
• Reduced movements over affected side • Mediastinal shift to opposite side • Decreased vocal fremitus
Percussion
Hyper-resonant
Auscultation
Diminished or absent breath sound

	Tracheal deviation (Mediastinal shift)	Chest expansion	Percussion note ↓ Duller ↑ Hyper-resonant	Breath sounds ↑ Louder ↓ Softer	Added sounds	Vocal resonance
Consolidation	No	Normal, or↓	Normal, or↓	↑ (Bronchial)	Coarse crackles +/- rub	↑ Whispering Pectoriloquy
Lobar collapse	Yes (Towards collapse)	↓	↓	↓	No	↓
Pleural effusion	No	↓	↓ (Stony dull)	↓	Occasional rub	↓
Pneumothorax	Yes (Specially with tension)	Normal or↓	↑	↓	Occasional click	↓

227. Answer is A (Tracheobronchial tree): *Harrison 17th /227*

The most common source of hemoptysis is the tracheobronchial tree.
The most common site of hemoptysis within the tracheobronchial tree are small to medium sized airways.

'The most common site of bleeding is the tracheobronchial tree'Q - Harrison's 17th/227 *'The most common site of hemoptysis is bleeding from the small to medium sized airways'Q - Harrison's 18th/284*

228. Answer is A (Bronchial Artery): *Harrison 17th /227; Harrison's 18th/285*

The most common source of bleeding in massive hemoptysis are the Bronchial arteries which are part of the high pressure systemic circulation

'The most common source of bleeding in hemoptysis is the tracheobronchial tree which can be affected by inflammation (bronchitis, bronchiectasis) or neoplasm (bronchiogenic carcinoma, endobronchial metastatic carcinoma or bronchial carcinoid tumor). The bronchial arteries which originate from either the aorta or from intercostal arteries, and are therefore part of the high pressure systemic circulation are the source of bleeding in bronchitis, bronchiectasis or with endobronchial tumors' - Harrison's 17th/227

'While alveolar haemorrhages arise from capillaries that are part of the low pressure pulmonary circulation, bronchial bleeding is generally from bronchial arteries which are under systemic pressure and therefore predisposed to large volume bleeding' - Harrison's 18th/284

229. Answer is A (Central cyanosis becomes evident when reduced Hb < 5g/dl): *Harrison 18th/p 288, 289 Harrisons 17th/230*

Cyanosis (both central and peripheral) become evident when the amount of reduced Hb exceeds 5g/dl (becomes >5gm/dl) and not when reduced Hb is less than 5g/dl.

Cyanosis becomes evident when Reduced Hb exceeds 4-5g/dl

'Cyanosis becomes evident when reduced Hb exceeds 5g/dl'- Wintrobe's 6th/ 194; CSDT 3rd/19; Guyton 6th/535

'Cyanosis becomes evident when reduced Hb exceeds 4g/dl'- Harrisons 17th/230

Pulmonary diseases such as chronic Asthma, Alveolar hypoventilation and Hemoglobin disorders like methemoglobinemia all cause central cyanosis

Cyanosis

Cyanosis is bluish discolouration of skin and mucous membrane that appears when the capillary content of reduced hemoglobin is greater than 5g/dl (Robbins, CSDT, CPDT old editions)

According to Harrisons 17th edition cyanosis is said to become apparent when reduced Hb > 4g/dl

Central cyanosis

- Central cyanosis is caused by in adequate oxygenation of systemic arterial blood due to decreased arterial oxygen saturation or Hemoglobin abnormalities
- It results from cardiac shunting, pulmonary diseases or hematological disorders (Hb abnormalities)
- *Central cyanosis is charachterized by cyanosis affective both mucous membranes and skin*

Causes

Decreased arterial oxygen saturation

- Decreased atmospheric pressure – high altitude
- Impaired pulmonary function
  - ***Alveolar hyoventilation***
  - ***Uneven relationships between pulmonary ventilation and perfusion*** (perfusion of hypoventilated alveoli)
  - Impaired oxygen diffusion
- Anatomic shunts
  - Certain types of congenital heart disease
  - Pulmonary arteriovenous fistulas
  - Multiple small intrapulmonary shunts
- Hemoglobin with low affinity for oxygen

Hemoglobin abnormalities

- ***Methemoglobinemia – hereditary, acquired***
- Sulfhemoglobinema – acquired
- Carboxyhemoglobinemia (not true cyanosis)

Peripheral cyanosis

- Peripheral cyanosis is caused by slowing of blood flow and increased extraction of oxygen from normally saturated blood
- It results from vasoconstriction or decreased peripheral blood flow, reduced cardiac output or vascular occlusion
- *Peripheral cyanosis is characterized by cyanosis of skin alone and sparing of mucous membranes*

Causes

- Vascular occlusion
  - Arterial obstruction
  - Venous obstruction
- Reduced cardiac output
- Cold exposure
- Redistribution of blood flow from extremities

230. Answer is C (Congestive heart failure): *Harrison 18th/p288 Harrisons 17th/231 Refer previous question*

Congestive Heart Failure is a cause for Peripheral cyanosis and not central cyanosis

Cyanosis when present in Asthma, pulmonic stenosis and alveolar hypoventilation is of the central type.

231. Answer is D (Tetralogy of Fallot (TOF): *Harrisons 16th/1504; Harrisons 17th/1592; Nelsons 16th/1886*

Presence of cyanosis that does not improve with supplemental oxygen suggest true pathological cardiac or pulmonary shunting of blood.

Presence of a cyanotic heart disease with an active right to left shunt (Tetralogy of Fallot) is a characteristic cause for failure of improvement with 100% oxygen supplementation. This occurs because desaturated blood in TOF shunts directly from the right (deoxygenated) side of the heart to the left side (systemic) of the heart by passing the lungs where oxygenation occurs.

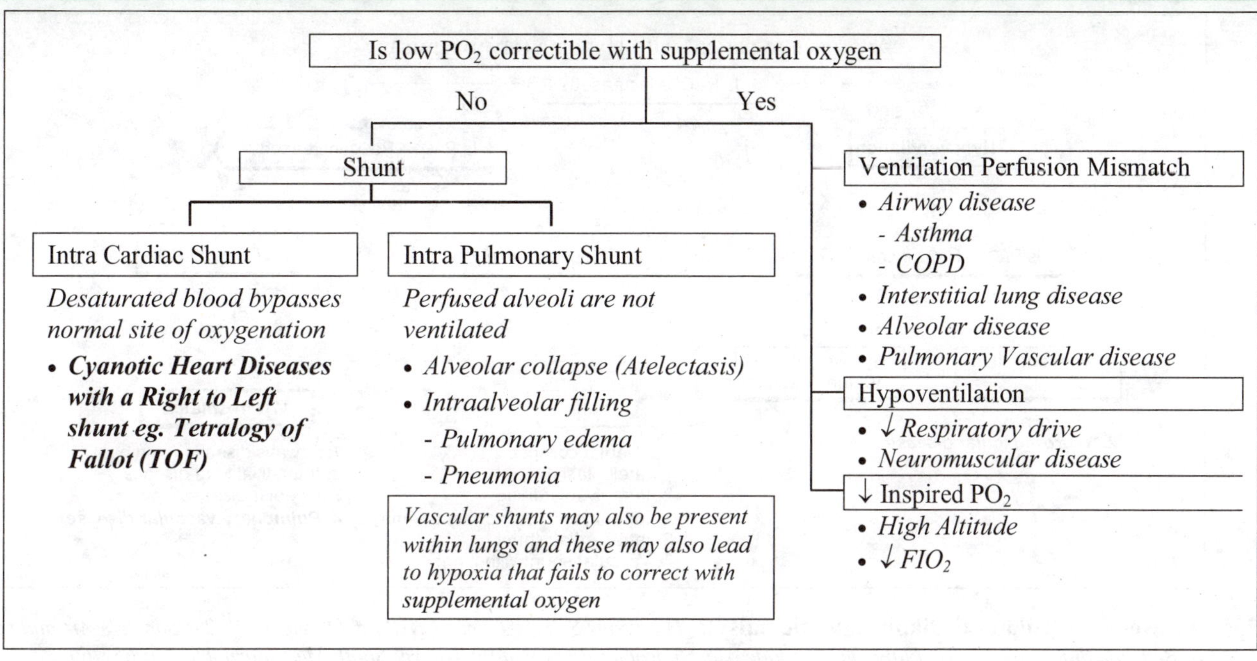

232. Answer is B (Chronic bronchitis): *Kumar Clarke 5th/ 845; Harrisons 16th/ 210; 17th/ 231; API 8th /348 Harrison 18th/p290*

Chronic bronchitis does not cause clubbing

Some causes of finger clubbing	
Respiratory	**Cardiovascular**
Bronchial carcinoma, especially epidermoid (squamous cell) type (major cause) Chronic suppurative lung disese **Bronchiectasis** Lung abscess Empyema Pulmonary fibrosis (e.g. cryptogenic fibrosing alveolitis) Pleural and mediastinal tumours (e.g. mesothelioma) **Cryptogenic organizing pneumonia**	Cyanotic heart disease Subacute infective endocarditis **Miscellaneous** Congenital – no disease Cirrhosis Inflammatory bowel disease **Primary billiary cirrhosis**

233. Answer is A (Congenital Cyanotic Heart Disease) : *Harrisons 17th/2982; Sapira's Art and Science of Bed side Diagnosis 3rd /159; PJ Mehta 15th/14; Physical Diagnosis : PreTest 6th/28 (Q-29)*

Congenital cyanotic heart disease is a cause for bilateral clubbing

Causes of Unilateral Clubbing
• *Aneurysm of Aorta, innonimate artery, subclavian artery or axillary artery*
• *Brachial AV fistulas / malformations*
• *Infected arterial grafts*
• *Pancoast tumors*
• *Unilateral Erythromelalgia*

234. Answer is E (All of the above): *Harrisons 17th/1591*

The four basic mechanisms of hypoxemia are a decrease in inspired PO_2 (Decreased FiO_2), hypoventilation (as in Myaesthenia gravis), VQ mismatch (as in pulmonary emboli) and shunting

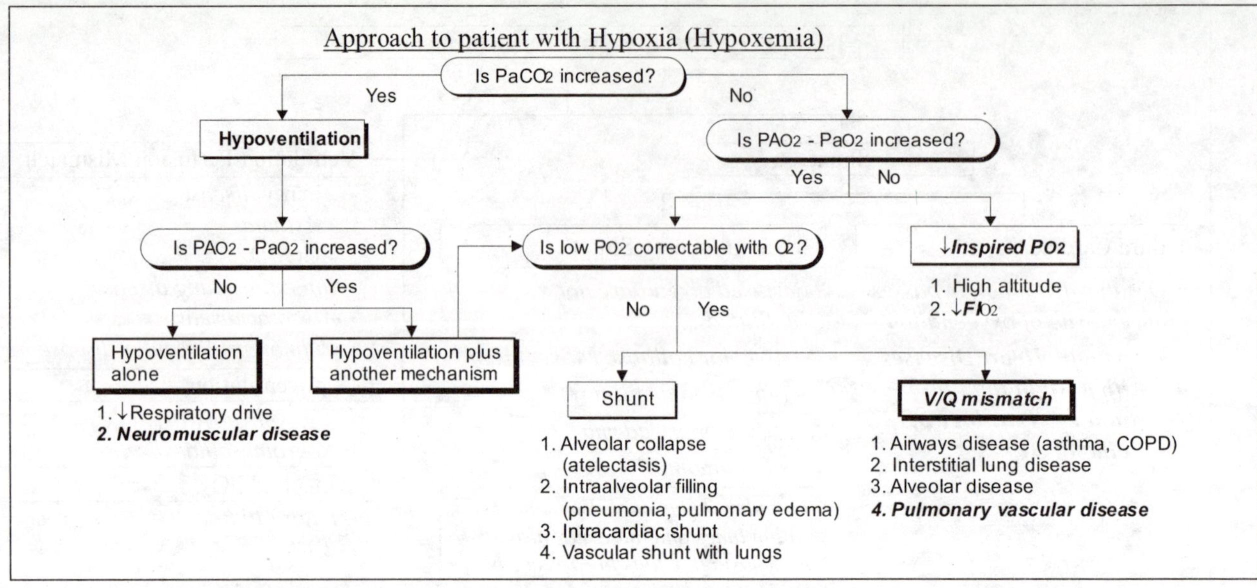

235. Answer is A (Bilateral Diaphragmatic palsy): *Harrisons Self Assessment & Board Review 17th/29; Sapira's Art and science of Bed side diagnosis 3rd /97; Platypnea Orthodeoxia syndrome: Review of Literature; South Med.Journal 97(7); 657-662*

Bilateral diaphragmatic palsy is associated with orthopnea and not platypnea. It has not been mentioned as a cause for platypnea

Severe COPD, pleural effusion and pulmonary embolism may present with either orthopnea or platypnea depending on the pathophysilogy.

Cirrhosis is an established cause for platypnea

Platypnea	Orthodeoxia

Platypnea refers to an increase in dyspnea / breathlessness in the upright position

Orthodeoxia refers to decrease in oxygen saturation in the erect posture

Platypnea is usually accompanied by orthodeoxia Platypnea-Orthodeoxia syndrome:

Causes of Platypnea – Orthodeoxia Syndrome

Pulmonary disease

In any pulmonary disease that affects primarily the basal segments of the lungs, the assumption of an erect posture increases the ventilation perfusion mismatch and causes platypnea-orthodeoxia

Various forms of severe pulmonary disease
- Severe /Necrotizing Pneumonia
- Pleural effusions
- Basal Tuberculosis
- ARDS
- Severe parenchymal lung disease including interstial fibrosis and COPD (infrequently)
- Multiple Recurrent pulmonary emboli
- Post Pneumonectomy

AV malformations
- Congenital
- Cirrhosis
- Microvascular shunts due to hepatopulmonary syndrome

Cardiac Disease

Right to left intracardiac shunts
- ASD
- Patent foramen ovale
- Fenestrated atrial septal aneurysm

Right to left shunts in association with
- Pericardial effusion
- Constrictive pericarditis
- Eosinophlic endomyocardial disease

Clinical states associated with the platypnea –orthodeoxia syndrome -	
Cardiac	*Pulmonary disease*
• Patent foramen ovale	• ***Chronic obstructive pulmonary disease***
• Atrial septal defect	• ***Pulmonary embolism***
• Atrial septal aneurysm	• ***Pleural effusion***
• Persistent eustachian valve	• Pulmonary emphysema
• Aortic aneurysm	• Pneumonectomy
• ***Pericardial effusion***	• Lobectomy
• Constrictive pericarditis	• Severe/Necrotizing pneumonias
• Eosinophilic endomyocardial disease	- Staphylococcal pneumonea
Abdominal	- Bibasilar pneumonia with pneumatocele
• Hepatic cirrhosis	• Acute respiratory distress syndrome
• Ileus	• Hepatopulmonary syndrme
Miscellaneous	• Amiodarone toxicity
• Autonomic neuropathy	
• Kyphoscoliosis	

Footnote

Platypnea-orthodeoxia is a clinical syndrome characterized by dyspnea and deoxygenation accompanying a change to a sitting or standing position from a recumbent one. Two conditions must coexist to cause platypnea- orthodeoxia: An anatomic component in the form of an interatrial communication and a functional component that produces a deformity in the atrial septum and results in a redirection of shunt flow with the assumption of an upright posture. The anatomic defect can be an atrial septal defect, a patent foramen ovale, or a fenstrated atrial septal aneurysm. The functional component may be cardiac, such as pericardial effusion or constrictive pericarditis; pulmonary, such as emphysema, arteriovenous malformation, pneumonectomy, or amiodarone toxicity, abdominal, such as cirrhosis of the liver or illeus or vascular, such as aortic aneurysm.

236. Answer is A (Collapse of Right lung): *Refer text below*

Collapse of Right lung may present with homogeneous opacification of right hemithorax and ipsilateral mediastinal Shift.

Condition		Findings
• *Consolidation*	:	*Ipsilateral Hamogenous opacification & No mediastinal shift*
• *Collapse*	:	*Ipsilateral Homogenous opacification & Ipsilateral mediastinal shift*
• *Hemothorax*	:	*Ipsilateral homogenous opacification & Contralateral shift*
• *Hydrothorax*	:	*Ipsilateral homogenous opacification & Contralateral shift*

237. Answer is C (Foreign Body Aspiration): *O.P. Ghai Pediatrics 5th/ 340*

Foreign Body Aspiration is an important cause of stridor in children. Obstruction leads to hyperinflation, chest wall hyperresonance and decreased breath sounds.

All the other choices mentioned in the question do not cause stridor.

Miscellaneous

238. Answer is C (Pulmonary Embolism): *Harrison's 17th/1584*

Pulmonary Embolism is not associated with rhonchi

Rhonchi

- Rhonchi are defined as *low pitched continuous sound's longer than 250 ms*
- These sounds are usually produced by presence of free liquid or mucus in the airways but may also be caused by vibration of larger airways at point of closure. They may also be produced by narrowing of lumen by foreign bodies or tumor

Common causes of Rhonchi include:
• *Bronchial Asthma*
• *COPD – Chronic bronchitis, Bronchiectasis, Emphysema*
• *Cardiac Asthma (Pulmonary Edema)*
• *Foreign body* (Fixed monomorphic rhonchi - localized)
• *Tumor* (Fixed monomorrphic rhonchi – localized.)

239. Answer is E (Emphysema): *Principles of Medical Physiology by Sircar 1st (2008)/320; Current Diagnosis & Treatment in Pulmonary Medicine 1st (2003)/5*

Emphysema is associated with an increased static compliance but decreased dynamic compliance.

'The effect of emphysema on compliance is unique in that it results in an increase in static compliance but a decrease in dynamic compliance.

Static compliance increases due to destruction of elastic tissues in the alveolar walls. The reduction in elastic tissue makes it easier for the lung to expand in response to distending pressure, However the loss of elastic tissue in the walls of smaller airways makes them vulnerable to dynamic airway compression. This increases the airway resistance with consequent decrease in dynamic compliance - 'Principles of Medical physiology' by Sircar 1st (2008)/320

Compliance

Compliance is a measure of 'distensibility' and is measured as a change in lung volume per unit change in pressure.

Static Complianc	Dynamic Compliance
• Static compliance indicates compliance when the lungs are at rest • Static compliance values reflect true lung compliance alone • Static compliance reflects elasticity of the lung and is not affected by airway resistance because there is no flow	• Dynamic compliance indicates compliance when air flow is occurring • Dynamic compliance values reflect lung compliance along with airway resistance • Dynamic compliance is affected by both elasticity of the lung and airway resistance
Reduced static compliance indicates rigid lung tissue	Reduced Dynamic compliance (without change in static compliance) indicates ↑ed airway resistance
• Interstitial fibrosis (Fibrosing alveolitis) • Atelectosis • Pulmonary edema • Pneumonia • ARDS	• Obstruction • Bronchospasm (Allergic Asthma) • Collapse of small airways etc
Reduced static compliance is usually also associated with a decreased dynamic compliance due to associated airway resistance	Reduced Dynamic compliance with reduced static compliance *Most conditions where static compliance is reduced are also associated with reduced dynamic compliance due to associated increase in airway resistance*
Increased static compliance indicates easily expandible lung • Emphysema *Emphysema is associated with an increased static compliance but decreased dynamic compliance due to associated increased airway resistance.*	

240. Answer is B (COPD) : *Ref. Text below; Harrison; Ganong*

Pulmonary Compliance is increased in Emphysema (COPD)

Pulmonary Congestion, decreased surfactant and pulmonary fibrosis are all associated with reduced pulmonary Compliance.

Pulmonary Compliance

- Pulmonary Compliance expresses the distensibility (expansibility) of the lung and chest well
- *'Compliance'* refers to the change in lung volume (V) per unit change in trans pulmonary pressure

(*Compliance in inversely proportional to lung Elastance*)

Decreased Lung Compliance	**Increased Lung Compliance**
Decreased lung compliance may be caused by conditions where lung is difficult to distend or surface tension is increased • *Pulmonary fibrosis* • *Atelectasis / pneumonia* • *Pulmonary edema* • *ARDS* • *Pleural effusion / Empyema* • *Pneumothorax* • *Decreased surfactant (↑ surface tension)*	Increased compliance may be caused by loss of elastic recoil of lungs or decreased surface tension • *Emphysema (COPD)* • *Ageing* • *Increased surfactant (↓ surface tension)*

241. Answer is C (Pulmonary fibrosis): *Refer text below*

Pulmonary Alveolar – capillary membrane thickening is a characteristic feature of interstitial lung disease like pulmonary fibrosis

Characteristic Pathological Changes in Lungs

Thickening of Bronchial Epethelial basement membrane	Thickening of Alveolar Capillary Membrane
• *Asthma (diffuse and hyaline)* • *Chronic bronchitis (focal & variable)* • *Other parenchymal chronic inflammatory diseases (Associated with normal DLCO)*	***Charachteristic of interstial lung disease*** (Associated with Decreased DLCO)

Emphysema causes a decrease in DLCO due to reduced surface area of alveolar capillary bed and not due to thickenning of alveolar capillary membrane.

242. Answer is D (Bronchiolitis obliterans organizing pneumonia): *Harrison 16th/1495*

Bronchialitis obliterans organizing pneumonia has not been mentioned in association with smoking. All other options have been mentioned in relation to smoking in Harrison's text.

***'Even though chronic obstructive lung disease and neoplasia** are two most important respiratory complications of smoking, other respiratory disorders (spontaneous pneumothorax, **respiratory broncholitis**- interstitial lung disease, eosinophilic granuloma of the lung and pulmonary haemorrhage with Good pasture's syndrome) are also associated with smoking.' – Harrison 16th/1495*

Respiratory disease linked to Smoking

Significant associations	Less significant associations
• **Chronic obstructive pulmonary disease** - ***Emphysema*** - Chronic bronchitis • **Lung cancer (Bronchial carcinoma)** *Best documented associations is with squamous cell carcinoma, but may also be present with other histological subtypes* ***(eg. small cell)*** *(87% of lung carcinoma occur in active smokers those who have recently stopped smoking.)*	• Spontaneous pneumothorax • Interstitial lung diseases - ***Respiratory bronchilitis*** - DIP (Desquammative interstitial pneumonia) - PLCH

243. Answer is B (Hamartoma): *Sutton 7th/138,140,123; Harrisons 15th/1448*

Hamartomas produce non cavitating popcorn calcifications.

Malignant lesions (squamous cell carcinoma) and granulomatous lesions (Wegener's granulomatosis, Caplan's syndrome) are established causes of cavitatory lesions.

244. Answer is B (Associated with pulmonary vasoconstriction) : *Harrison 16th / 205; 17th/ 224 Harrison 18th/p 281*

Although the mechanism of high altitude pulmonary edema remains obscure most studies suggest pulmonary vasoconstriction (venconstriction or arteriolar constriction) as the prime mechanism.

HAPE : High Altitude Pulmonary Edema

This is a serious complication usually occruing at exposure to high altitude (>300m) in association with severe physical exercise and is classically seen in unacclametized healthy individuals.

Pulmonary vasoconstriction has been suggested as the prime mechanism.

"Studies have been conflicting, some suggesting pulmonary venous constriction and other indicating pulmonary arteriolar constriction as the prime mechanism."- Harrison

May occur in both acclamatized and unacclamatized individuals

"*Well recognized in unacclamatized yet otherwise healthy persons.*"

"***Acclamatized high altitude natives also develop this syndrome*** upon return to high altitude after a relatively brief sojourn at low altitudes." - *Harrison*

HAPE is exacerbated by exercise and is associated with high cardiac output.

Increased cardiac output and pulmonary arterial pressures with exercise combined with hypoxic pulmonary arteriolar constriction which is more prominent in young persons may combine to make this an example of prearteriolar high pressure pulmonary edema.

245. Answer is B (Theophylline): *Read text below*

***Theophylline** relaxes the tone of bronchial smooth muscles, thereby causing bronchodilation*
It may be used in the treatment of bronchial hyperplasia, it certainly does not contribute to bronchial hyperplasia.

Smoking and other irritants cause the *hypertrophy of mucus glands*[Q] within the brochial wall, and contributes to narrowing of bronchioles by a variety of factors.

Prematurity *may be associated with bronchopulmonary dysplasia*[Q] *and bronchial hyperplasia*[Q]

246. Answer is B (Direct spread from liver): *Read below*

An *amoebic lung abscess is almost always secondary to spread from the liver.*

Extraintestinal infection by E. histolytica most often involves the liver. Further involvement most commonly leads to Amoebic lung abscess.

Infact pleuropulmonary involvement (Lung): is the most frequent complication of Amoebic liver abscess.

Remember:

Most common cause of a lung abscess is - 'Aspiration'. *However this holds true* ***for pyogenic (bacterial lung abscess)***

247. Answer is A (At end expiration): *Schwartz Pre-Test / Q.20*

The changes in intrathoracic pressure that occur during different phases of respiration influence measurement of intravascular pressure. These changes are minimal at end expiration which therefore is the best phase for measurement of intravascular pressure.

248. Answer is C (Cardiac tamponade): *Harrison 14th/1336; 15th/1270, 1367; 16th/1319, 1416; 17th/ 1490, 1491 Harrison 18th/p 1972, 1973*

Electrical alternans refers to a beat-to-beat alteration in one or more components of the ECG signal.
Total electrical alternans (P-QRS-T) with sinus tachycardia is a relatively specific sign for pericardial effusion, often with cardiac tamponade. *– Harrison 15th /1270*

Feature	Cardiac Tamponade	Constrictive Pericarditis	Restrictive Cardiomyopathy	RVMI
Electrical Alternans	*May be present*	Absent	Absent	Absent

Note: Pleural effusion and pneumothorax both are potential complications of carcinoma lung that present with respiratory distress but electrical alternans is not associated.

249. Answer is C (Bradycardia): *'Rudolph's Pediatrics" 21st/71; Fetal and Neonatal Neurology' 4th/493*

The most common fetal response to acute hypoxia is Bradycardia

'The initial response of the normal fetus to acute hypoxia or asphyxia is bradycardia. Bradycardia results from chemoreceptor stimulation of vagal nerve' - Rudolph 21st/71

250. Answer is C > D (Immune complex > cell mediated) : *Harrison 18th/p 2116 Harrison's 17th /1607;Rubin's Pathology 5th / 524,Robbins 7th / 739*

Hypersensitivity pneumonitis is an immunologically mediated response to an extrinsic antigen that involves both immune complex (Type III) and cell mediated (Type IV) hypersensitivity reactions.

Classically however, Hypersensitivity pneumonitis was believed to be a immune complex (Type III) mediated hypersensitivity response which is therefore the better answer amongst the options provided.
However in strict terminology both option C and D should be correct.

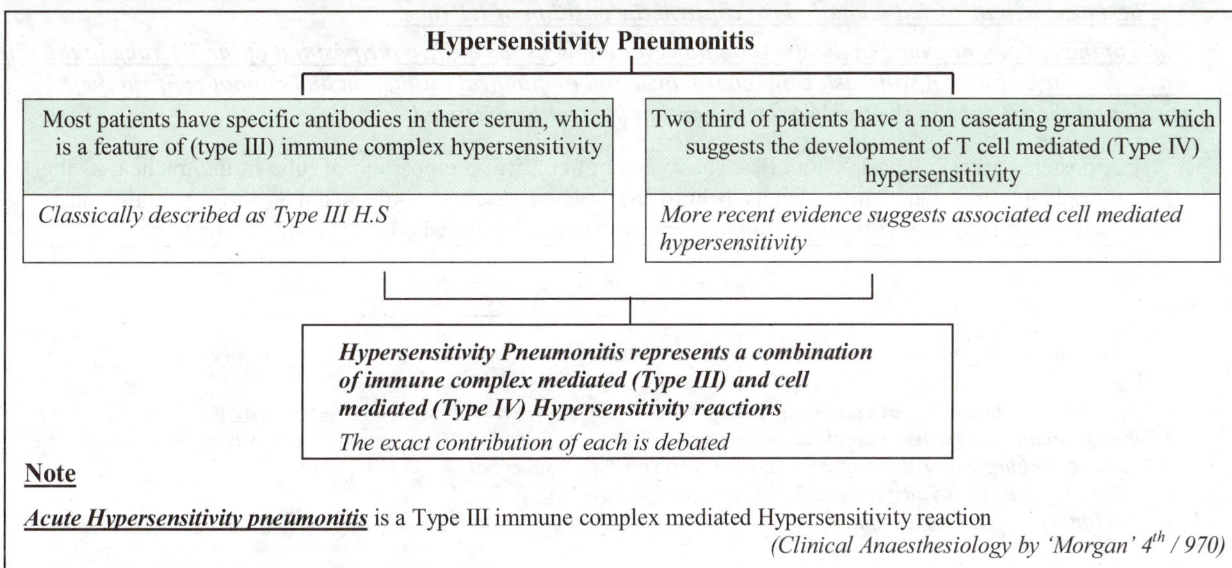

Types of Hypersensitivity Reactions: Review

Type I Hypersensitivity (IgE)[Q]	**Type II Hypersensitivity (IgG & IgM)**[Q] **Cytotoxic, complement mediated lysis**[Q]
Includes: • Local: Eczema, Hay fever, Asthma (Atopy).[Q] • Systemic: Anaphylaxis. <u>*Examples based on type I.H.S*</u>[Q]*:* • *Theoblad Smith phenomenon:*[Q] *This is anaphylaxis in guinea pigs.* • *PK reaction (Prusnitz Kunster):*[Q] *Demonstrate that IgE is homocytotropic i.e. species specific.* • *Casoni's test: Immediate type (IgE) H.S*	*Includes:* • Complement mediated lysis.[Q] • Antibody dependent cell mediated toxicity (formerly classified as type I).[Q] • Changes in cellular function (former type V).[Q] - Increased function: Grave's disease.[Q] - Decreased function: M. Gravis.[Q] • Phagocytosis.[Q] <u>*Examples includes:*</u> • *Those with Ag on RBC.* *- Blood transfusion reaction.*[Q] *- Hemolytic anemia e.g. with I.M. and mycoplasma.*[Q] • *Those with Ag on Neutrophils: Agranulocytosis.*[Q] • *Those with Ag on platelets: e.g. ITP.*[Q] • *Those with Ag on basement membrane: Goodpasture's*[Q]
Type III Immune complex (IgM & IgG)	**Type IV Delayed hypersensitivity (cellular immunity)**
Includes: • Local: Arthus reaction.[Q] • Systemic: Serum sickness.[Q] <u>*Examples:*</u> • *Shick's test.*[Q] • *Post streptococcal G.N.*[Q] • *Detected by RAJI Assay.*[Q]	<u>*Includes:*</u> • *Tuberculin test.*[Q] • *Lepromin test.*[Q] • *Contact dermatitis.*[Q] • *Jones-Mote reaction (cutaneous basophilic hypersensitivity).*[Q] • *Graft rejection (chronic).*[Q]
Hyprsensitivity Pneumonitis is associated with both Type III and Type IV Hypersensitivity	

251. Answer is B (Remove tube and Reattempt intubation): *Lee synopsis of Anaesthesia 13th/215*

The ideal next step is to confirm the position of ET tube and / or Remove the tube and reattempt intubation, if the tube is not in the trachea.As none of the options provided in the question can confirm the true position of the ET tube in the trachea the best course of action is to remove the tube and reattempt intubation.

The patient in question is presenting with characteristic features of left sided diaphragmatic hernia.
<u>Incorrect placement of the tube into the esophagus (Esophageal intubation) will result in</u> distension of stomach and bowel loops in the left hemithorax which would inturn shift the mediastinum and apical impulse to the right.

The apical cardiac impulse in this patient has been observed to shift further to the right after attempted ET intubation.This raises doubt about the correct positioning of ET tube in the trachea and suggests the possibility of improper placement of the ET tube into the esophagus.

The best next step in such a scenario is to confirm the position of ET tube.

None of the options provided in the question however allow us to confirm the position of the ET tube in the trachea
An X- ray chest cannot distinguish between tracheal and esophageal intubation and cannot confirm the position of the ET tube in the trachea. Hence option (A) can be excluded.

A postero- anterior chest X-Ray (PA chest) can not confirm the position of tube in the trachea, as the oesophagus is situated immediately behind the trachea. A chest x-ray taken following intubation is done to confirm correct length of the tube rather than to find out whether it is sited in the trachea.

Methods to confirm tracheal intubation

Tests which suggest tracheal placement (Not confirmatory)

- *Symmetrical bilateral chest movements when reservoir bag is squeezed*
- *Equal Breath sounds over lung fields when reservoir bag is squeezed*
- *Absence of gurgle over the epigastrium when reservoir bag is squeezed*
- *Misting of the tube (Water vaour deposition) during expiration*
- *Feeling of correct lung compliance and refilling of bag during expiration*

Confirmatory tests

- *Capnography*
  Measures End tidal CO_2 in expired gas
- *Esophageal detector device*

This leaves us still in doubt regarding the correct position of the ET tube and when in doubt, the best course of action is to remove the tube and reattempt intubation.

'When in doubt take it out'. It is easy to wrongly intubate the esophagus. This must be recognized immediately. If the clinical state of the patient deteriorates after intubation or if there is any doubt about tube placement, the tube should be removed' – Lee

252. Answer is C (Nasogastric tube insertion) : *Refer previous question*

The ideal next step is to confirm the position of ET tube and / or Remove the tube and reattempt intubation, if the tube is not in the trachea. 'Removal of tube and reattempting intubation' is not provided amongst the option and position of the ET tube cannot be confirmed by chest X-ray. As both these possibilities are not provided in the list of options, the next best step is to decompress the bowel by nasogastric tube insertion and aspiration. This would help in relieving some respiratory distress and is therefore the single best answer of choice amongst the options provided.
X-Ray chest should be next step after nasogastric tube insertion to confirm the diagnosis, followed by surgery once the patient has been resuscitated, investigated and stabilized.

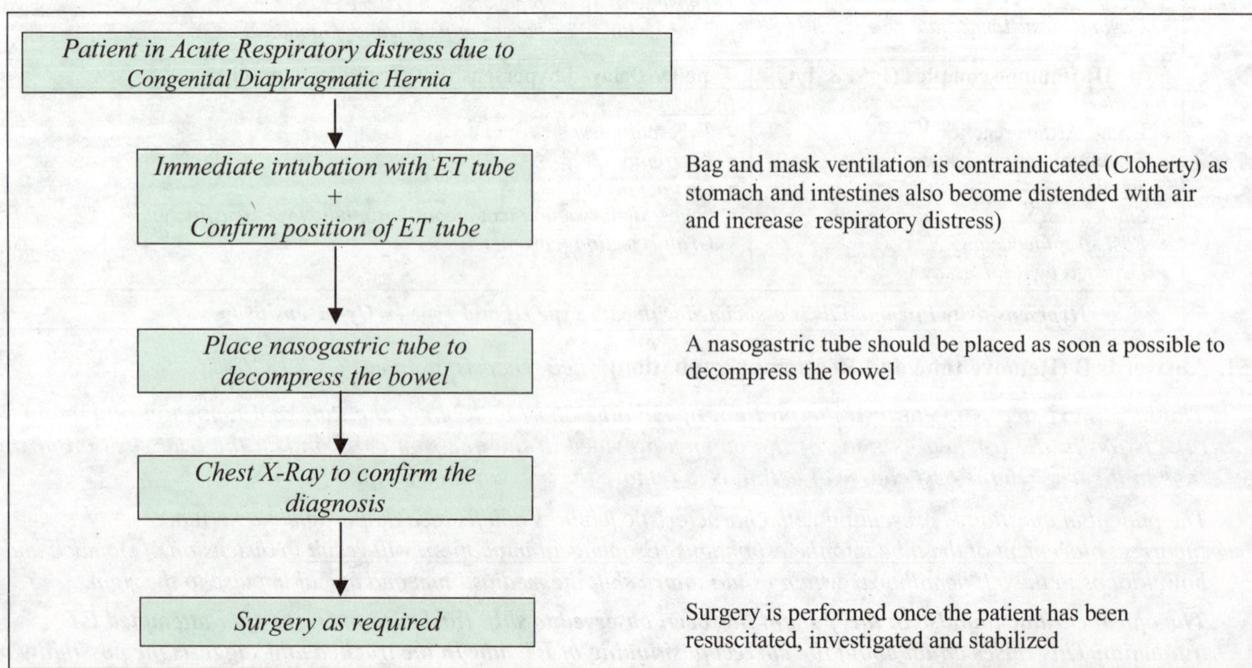

253. Answer is A (Bronchiolitis obliterans): *Nelson 18th /1782.*

The patient in question is presenting with charachteristic features of bronchiolitis obliterans.

Fever, cough, and wheeze are common clinical features of bronchiolitis obliterans and a period of initial improvement may well be seen in cases of bronchiolitis obliterans (Initial sign of B.O).
Hyperluscency or chest X-Ray and obstructive curve on pulmonary function tests furthur suggest the diagnosis of bronchiolitis obliterans.

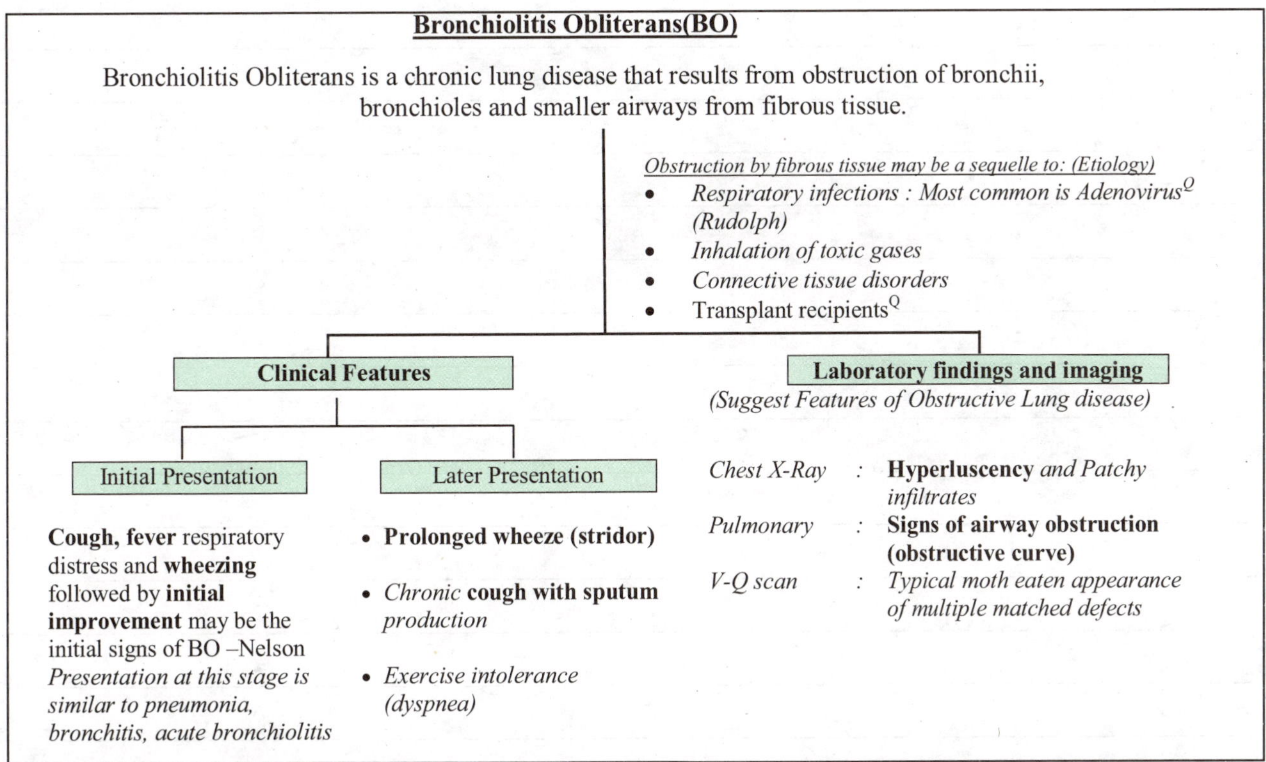

254. Answer is B (Strychnine): *KDT 6th/454, 391; Encyclopedia of poisons and Antidotes 3rd/112*

Strychnine is a CNS stimulant. It does not cause respiratory depression

Gelsemium causes Respiratory Depression

Gelsemium (ergot type alkaloid) is a CNS depressant.
*'Symptoms of toxicity include difficulty in the use of voluntary muscles, muscle rigidity and weakness, dizziness, dry mouth, visual disturbances, tremor of extremities, sweating, conrulsions and **respiratory depression**. With large doses, paralysis and **death from respiratory failure can occur**' - 'The Encyclopedia of poisons and Antidotes' 3rd/112*

Opium and Barbiturates are known to cause Respiratory Depression.

Barbiturates cause respiratory depression in high doses (KDT6th/391) (Barbiturates are CNS Depressants)
Opiates depress respiratory centre in a dose dependant manner (KDT 6th/454)

NOTES

Kidney and Urinary Tract

ESSENTIAL REVISION NOTES

Urinary casts

Urinary casts are formed when proteins and other organic matter solidify in the renal tubule. The presence of casts in urine is indicative of disease of the nephron.

Casts may contain:

Proteins	*Erythrocytes*	*Leucocytes*	*Epethelial cells*
Hyaline casts	Red cell casts	WBC cast	Epithelial casts

Clinical significance of different casts:

a. ***Hyaline casts*** :	• This is a *normal constituent* [Q] of urine and has *no attached significance* [Q]. • *Tom Horsfall protein* [Q] is protein *secreted by epithelial cells of loop of henle* [Q]. • *This protein may be excreted as Hyaline cast.* [Q]
b. ***RBC cast*** :	• Are suggestive of *glomerular injury* [Q].
c. ***White cell casts*** :	• Are suggestive of *interstitial injury* and may be seen in *interstitial nephritis* [Q] *WBC cast with bacteria indicate pyelonephritis* [Q].
d. ***Broad granular casts*** :	• Are *seen in CRF* [Q] and suggests interstitial fibrosis and dilatation of tubules.
e. ***Pigmented muddy brown granular casts*** :	• Are suggestive of *ischaemic or nephrotoxic injury* [Q] i.e. *Tubular Necrosis* [Q].

Presence of β_2 microgloobulin *in urine indicates tubular injury and not glomerular injury.*

Tomm Harsfall Protein in urine is a feature of tubular proteinuria

Tomm Harsfall protein is synthesized in the tubular cells of ascending limb of loop of henle and distal tubule and is secreted into urine. Under conditions of tubulo interstitial injury (tubular proteinuria) increased Tomm Harsfall protein may be secreted in urine from injured tubular cells.

Glomerular proteinuria is associated with an increase Albumin: β2 microglobulin, ratio usually > 1000:1

Feature	Normal value	Glomerular proteinuria	Tubular proteinuria
Albumin: β2 microglobulin ratio	Usually 50:1 to 200:1	Usually >1000 : 1	Usually < 10:1

Colour and Appearance of Urine

Red Urine
- *Beet ingestion (Betacyanin excretion)*
- *Phenolpthaline (in Laxatives)*
- *Vegetable dye ingestion*
- *Myoglobinuria*
- *Haemoglobinuria*
- *Seoratia Marcescens bacteria can cause the Red diaper' syndrome*

Reddish Brown / Brown
- ***Nitrofurantoin*** *(Brown)*
- *L-Dopa*
- *Alpha Methyl Dopa*
- *Metronidazole*

Orange /yellow orange
- ***Rifampicin*** *(yellow orange)*
- ***Pyridium*** *(orange) (Phenazopyridine)*

Renal Function Tests

Renal Function Test

Estimation of Glomerular Function
- ***Creatinine Clearance Tests*** [Q]
- ***Inulin Clearance test*** [Q] *(used to assess Glomerular Filtration Rate- GFR)*

Estimation of tubular function
- ***Water Deprivation Test*** *(used to assess Distal Tubular Function)*

Estimation of Renal Blood Flow/ Renal Plasma Flow
- ***Paraaminohippurate (PAH) clearance****(used to assess Renal Plasma Flow -RPF)*

Renal Failure & Tubulointerstitial Diseases

Urine Diagnostic Indices: Differentiation of Prerenal and Intrinsic Renal failure.

Acute tubular necrosis is a cause of Intrinsic ARF. ^{Q}

Differentiating features between Pre-renal and Intrinsic ARF

- Prerenal Azotemia is the most common form of ARF and is caused by renal hypoperfusion either from generalized hypovolemia or from altered renal hemodynamics resulting in hypoperfusion
- ***By definition Renal parenchymal tissue is not damaged in prerenal ARF and prerenal ARF is rapidly reversible upon correction of the primary hemodynamic abnormality***
- Analysis of urine and blood biochemistry provides several useful 'Renal failure Indices' to distinguish prerenal ARF from intrinsic ARF (Ischemic /Nephrotoxic ARF)

Urine Diagnostic Indices: Differentiation of Prerenal and Intrinsic Renal failure.

Diagnostic index	Prerenal ARF	Intrinsic renal ARF
Fractional Excretion of Na ^{Q} (%)	<1	>1
Urine Sodium Concentration (mmol/L) ^{Q}	<10 mmol/L	>20 mmol/L
Urine Sodium concentration (meq/L) ^{Q}	< 20meq/L	> 40 meq/L ^{Q}
Urine Creatinine To Plasma Creatinine ratio ^{Q}	>40	<20
Urine specific gravity ^{Q}	>1.020	~1.010
Urine osmolality ^{Q} (mosmol/kg H_2O)	> 500	< 350
Renal failure Index ^{Q} $U_{Na}/(U_{CR}/P_{CR})$	<1	>1
Urine urea Nitrogen to plasma urea Nitrogen ^{Q}	> 8	<3
Plasma BUN/Creatinine Ratio ^{Q}	>20	<10-15
Urinary sediment ^{Q}	Hyaline Casts	Muddy Brown Granular Cast

Renal papillary Necrosis

Renal Papillary Necrosis

- Renal papillary necrosis is typically caused by ischaemic necrosis and sloughing of Renal Papllae (The papillary tip is the apex of renal pyramid)
- It is clinically charachterized by

  Loin Pain
  Hematuria
  Variable degree of renal impairment

Etiology / Predisposing factors

- ***Diabetes and analgesic abuse (NSAIDS) are the most common predisposing factors***
- The Acronym POST CARD is traditionally used to enlist the causes of papillary necrosis but it does not put the causes in a useful order of incidence

P	Pyelonephritis
O	Obstruction
S	Sickle –cell disease
T	Tuberculosis
C	Cirrhosis
A	Analgesic abuse/Alcohol
R	Renal vein thrombosis
D	Diabetes

POSTCARD – causes of papillary necrosis

Stages of Chronic Renal Failure (CRF)

Stages	Pathophysiologic factors
Stage I: **Dimninished renal reserve**	Residual renal function is 50% of the normal kidney function. • *Excretory and regulatory renal functions are intact.* • *Renal laboratory studies are asymptomatic (BUN and serum creatinine are normal).* • *At least a 50-60% loss of renal function is required before signs of renal failure are evident.* • *No symptoms are evident until there is a loss of at least 80% renal function.*
Stage II: **Renal insufficiency**	Residual renal function is 20-40% of the normal kidney function. • *There is a decrease in the glomerular filtration rate (GFR), solute clearance, ability to concentrate urine, and hormone secretion.* • *Renal laboratory studies reveal a rising BUN and serum creatinine, mild azotemia, polyuria, nocturia, and anemia.* • *Signs and symptoms become more severe if the kidneys are stressed. i.e., fluid volume depletion or exposure to a nephrotic substance.*
Stage III: **Renal failure**	Residual renal function is 10-20% of the normal kidney function. • *There is an inability of the kidneys to regulate volume and solute composition.* • *Renal laboratory studies reveal an increased BUN and serum creatinine, azotemla, anemia, and metabolic acidosis. Signs and symptoms of renal failure are present.*
Stage IV: **End – stage renal disease (ESRD)**	Residual renal function is <10% of the normal kidney function. • *Excretory, regulatory, and hormonal renal functions are severely impaired and unable to maintain homeostasis.* • *Renal laboratory studies and physical symptoms reveal markedly elevated BUN and serum creatinine levels.* • *Anemia, hyperphosphatemia, hypocalcemia, metabolic acidosis, hyperuricemia, hyperkalemia, fluid overload, usually oliguric, and urine osmolality similar to serum osmolality.* • *A uremic syndrome develops and all body systems are affected by renal failure.* • *Mortality rate is 100% if peritoneal dialysis, hemodialysis, or renal transplant is not implemented.*

Electrolyte Disturbaces in Uremia

Electrolyte disturbances in Uremia: - *Harrison*
Hyponatremia (Hypernatremia may also be seen)
Hyperkalemia (Hypokalemia may also be seen)
Hyperphosphatemia
Hypocalcemia
Hyperuricemia

Management of Hyperkalemia

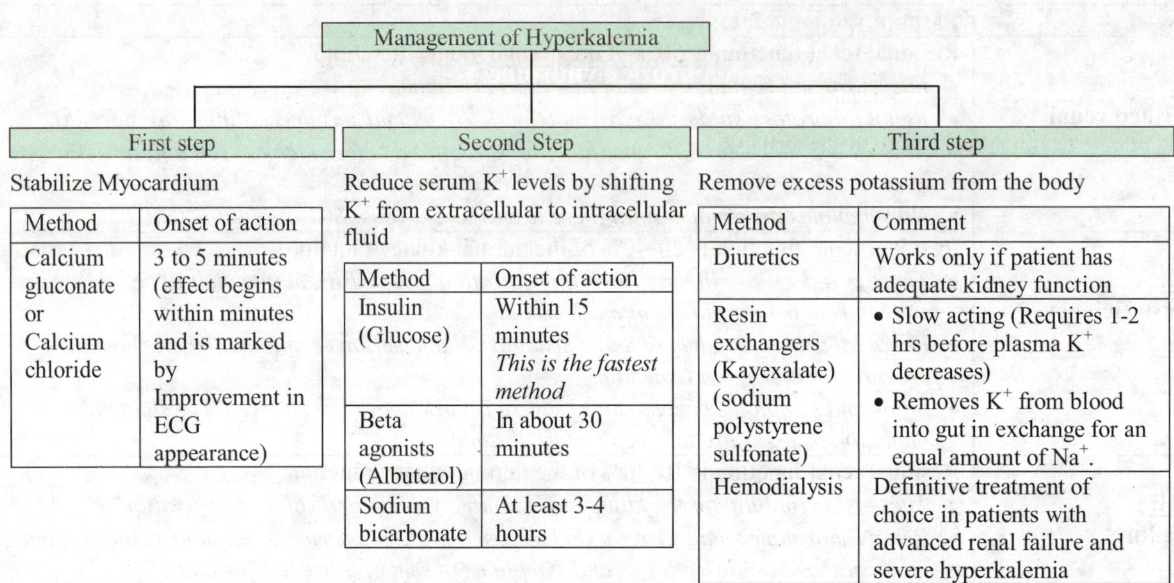

Management of Hyperkalemia

First step

Stabilize Myocardium

Method	Onset of action
Calcium gluconate or Calcium chloride	3 to 5 minutes (effect begins within minutes and is marked by Improvement in ECG appearance)

Second Step

Reduce serum K^+ levels by shifting K^+ from extracellular to intracellular fluid

Method	Onset of action
Insulin (Glucose)	Within 15 minutes *This is the fastest method*
Beta agonists (Albuterol)	In about 30 minutes
Sodium bicarbonate	At least 3-4 hours

Third step

Remove excess potassium from the body

Method	Comment
Diuretics	Works only if patient has adequate kidney function
Resin exchangers (Kayexalate) (sodium polystyrene sulfonate)	• Slow acting (Requires 1-2 hrs before plasma K^+ decreases) • Removes K^+ from blood into gut in exchange for an equal amount of Na^+.
Hemodialysis	Definitive treatment of choice in patients with advanced renal failure and severe hyperkalemia

Advanced Life Support Guidelines for Treatment of Hyperkalemia

Advanced Life Support Guidelines for Treatment of Hyperkalemia

Mild elevation (5.5-6 mmol/L)	**Moderate / severe elevation without ECG changes (>6 mmol/l)**	**Moderate / severe elevation With toxic ECG changes (>6 mmol/l)**
Remove K+ from body ▪ Cation exchange resins ▪ Diuretics ▪ Consider dialysis	Remove K+ from body ▪ Dextrose / insulin infusion (+/-) ▪ Nebulized salbutamol ▪ Intravenous NaHCO3 (+) ▪ strategies as for mild elevation	First stabilize the heart / Antagonize the toxic effects of Hyperkalemia. Calcium gluconate (+) Other strategies

Glomerular Diseases

Nephrotic Syndrome

'Essentials' in the diagnosis of nephrotic syndrome:

'Essentials' in the diagnosis of nephrotic syndrome :

1. Proteinuria : excretion > 3.5g/1.73 m2 per 24 hrs. [Q]
2. Hypoalbunemia : albumin < 3g/dl. [Q]
3. Peripheral edema. [Q]

Hyperlipidemia[Q] occurs in 50% of those with early nephrotic syndrome and is much more common in patients who excrete larger amounts of protein per day.

Features of Nephrotic Syndrome

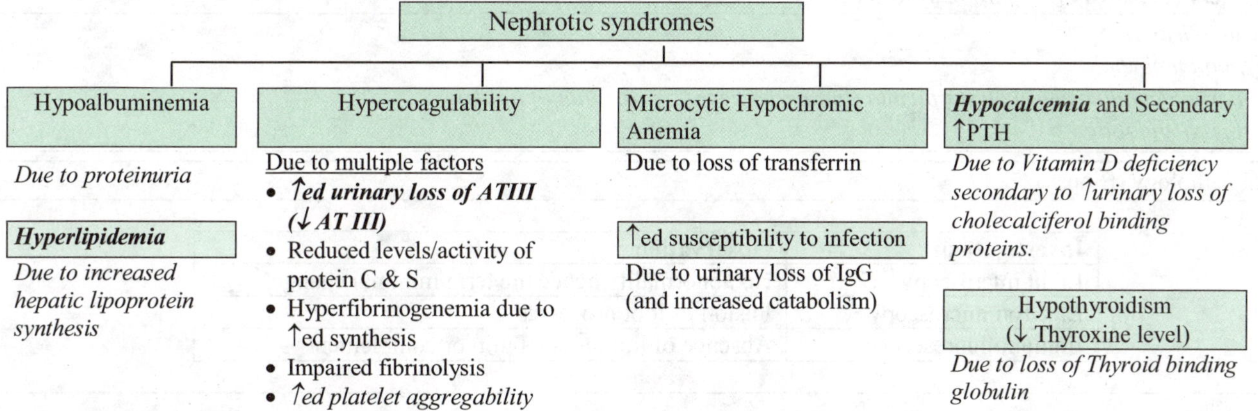

Lipid Profile in Nephrotic Syndrome

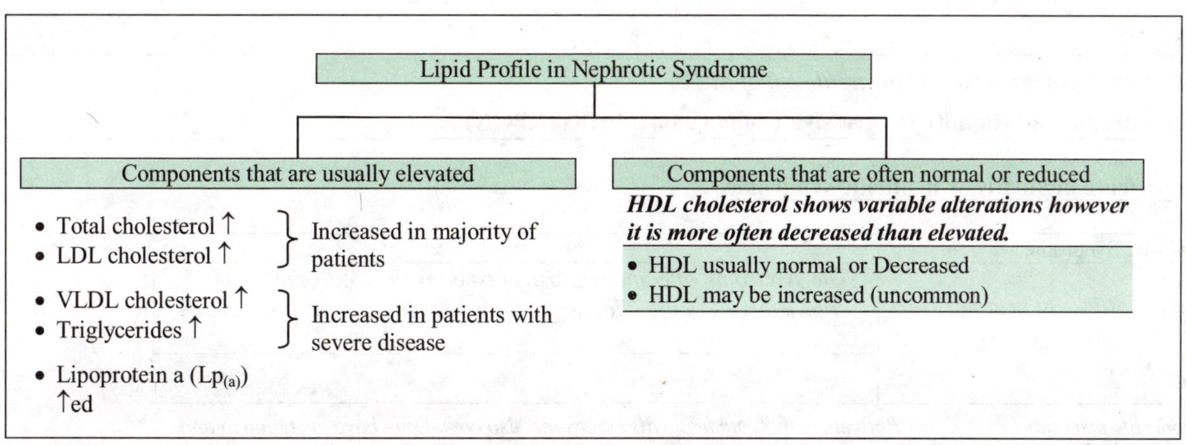

Minimal Change Disease

Minimal Change Disease

- Most common cause of Nephrotic syndrome in children (80% in children; 20% in adults)
- Peak Age of onset is between 6-8 years of Age (usually < 10 years)
- Type of onset : Insiduous

Clinical features

- Peripheral Edema: Presenting Feature

Nephrotic syndrome is the typical presentation
Peripheral edema is the hallmark of Nephrotic syndrome occurring when serum albumin levels become less than 3g/dl
Initially dependent Edema $\xrightarrow{\text{Later}}$ Generalized edema
May develop Pleural effusion, pulmonary edema, ascitis

- Hematuria : 20-30%
- Hypertension : V. Rare
- Renal failure : Does not usually progress to renal failure

Laboratory (Features of Nephrotic syndrome)

- *Proteinuria*
- *Hypoalbuminemia*
- *Hyperlipidemia/Hyper cholesterolemia (Increased hepatic prduction of lipids)*
- *Hypercoagulability*

Renal pathology (Biopsy)

Investigation	Observation
Light microscopy [Q]	No abnormality hence the term minimal change
Electron microscopy [Q]	Fusion of foot processes
Immunofluorescence [Q]	Absence of immunoglobulin or complement

Prognosis

- *Prognosis is Good*
- *Response to steroids is Excellent*
- *Does not progress to Renal Failure*

Treatments

- *Corticosteroids form the mainstay for treatment of MCD*

Nephritic Syndrome and Rapidly Progressive Glomerulonephritis (RPGN)

Syndrome of acute nephritis or nephritic syndrome

Acute Nephritic Syndrome	
Hypertension [Q] *Hematuria with RBC cast in urine* [Q] *Oliguria* [Q] *Pyuria* [Q] *Azotemia* [Q]	*The syndrome of acute nephritis or nephritic syndrome characterizes acute Glomerulonephritis clinically.*
Mild to moderate proteinuria [Q] *Edema* [Q]	*Patients with Acute nephritis syndrome also commonly have proteinuria and edema but these are not as severe as those encountered in nephrotic syndrome.*

Rapidly Progressive Glomerulonephritis (RPGN) or Crescenteric Glomerulonephritis

Types of Crescenteric Glomerulonephritis (RPGN)

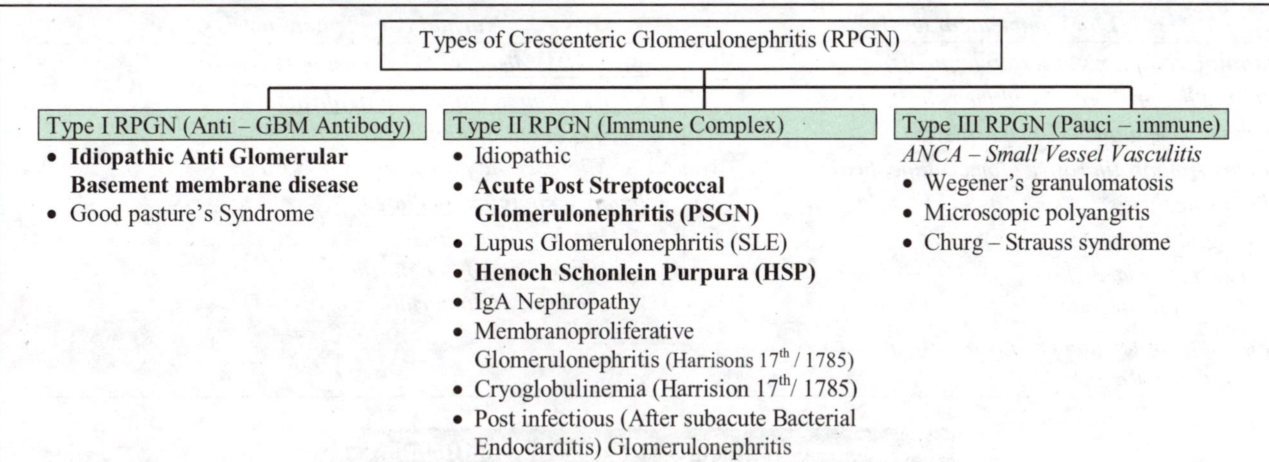

Features of RPGN

RPGN is characterized by a Subacute glomerular inflammation with:

- *Nephritic urinary sediment, i.e. RBC casts, WBC casts*
- *Sub-**nephrotic non-selective proteinuria*** (proteinuria < 3.5 g/24 hr) *(selective proteinuria is a feature of minimal change disease)*
- *Oliguria and Edema*
- *Hypertension*
- *Presence **of crescents** pathologically*

Differential Diagnosis of Glomerulonephritis based on Proliferative changes

Proliferative changes in Glomerulonephritis *(Refer: Chandrsoma Taylor 3rd /702, 708)*

- *Glomerulus contains Endothelial cells, Epethelial cells, and Mesangial cells. Any of the three cell types may undergo proliferation in different types of Proliferativ Glomerulonephritis.*
- *Proliferative changes are not limited to Membranoproliferative and Mesangioproliferative Glomerulonephritis, but may be seen in several other forms of Glomerulonephritis*

Glomerulonephritis and Proliferative changes

Glomerulonephritis without proliferative changes

Glomerulonephritis	*Proliferative changes*
Minimal change Disease	*- (Absent)*
Membranous Glomerulonephritis	*- (Absent)*
Diabetic Nephropathy	*- (Absent)*
Amyloidosis	*- (Absent)*
Focal segmental Glomerulosclerosis	± Variants with proliferative lesions have been described including cellular lesions with endocapillary hypercellularity- (Harrisons)

Glomerulonephritis with proliferative changes

Glomerulonephritis	*Proliferative changes*
Post streptococcal GN	*+ (Crescents)*
Antibasement membrane disease (Good – pasture's syndrome)	*+ (Crescents)*
IgA Nephropathy (Berger's)	*+ (Mesangial)*
Henoch Schonlein Purpura	*+ (Mesangial)*
Mesangioproliferative GN	*+ (Mesangial)*
Membranoproliferative GN **(Mesangiocapillary GN)**	*+ (Endothelial & Mesangial)*
Focal Glomerulonephritis	*+ (Focal)*
Secondary Glomerulonephritis SLE / PAN	*+ Variable*

Note : Crescents represent proliferation of epethelial cells

Differential diagnosis of Nephritic syndromes based on complement levels

Low complement levels	*Normal complement levels*
(Immune complex glonerulonephritis) • *Idiopathic proliferative glomerulonephritis* • *Crescentric glomenelonephritis* • *Membranoproliferative glomerulonephritis* • *Lupus nephritis* • *Cryoglobulinemia* • *Bacterial endocarditis* • *Shunt nephritis* • *Post infectious glomerulonephritis (post streptococcal)*	• ***Anti GBM disease:*** *Good posture's syndrome* • ***Pauci*** *immune* ***glomenulonephritis*** - *Wegeners granulomatoses* - *Microscopic polyarteritis nodosa* • *Immune* ***complex mediated*** - *IgA Nephropathy* - *Henoch schonlein purpura* - *Fibrillary Glomerulonephritis*

Recurrent episodes of gross haematuria

Recurrent Gross Haematuria should be distinguished from isolated episodes of gross hematuria, as it is a charachteristic feature of some specific disorders

Charachteristic Causes of Recurrent Gross Haematuria (Nelson 18th/2169)	
1. IgA Nephropathy *2. Alports syndrome* *3. Thin Glomerular basement membrane disease*	*Isolated Glomerular diseases with recurrent Gross haematuria*
4. Hypercalciuria *5. Urolithiasis*	

Hematuria following Respiratory Tract Infection: Approach

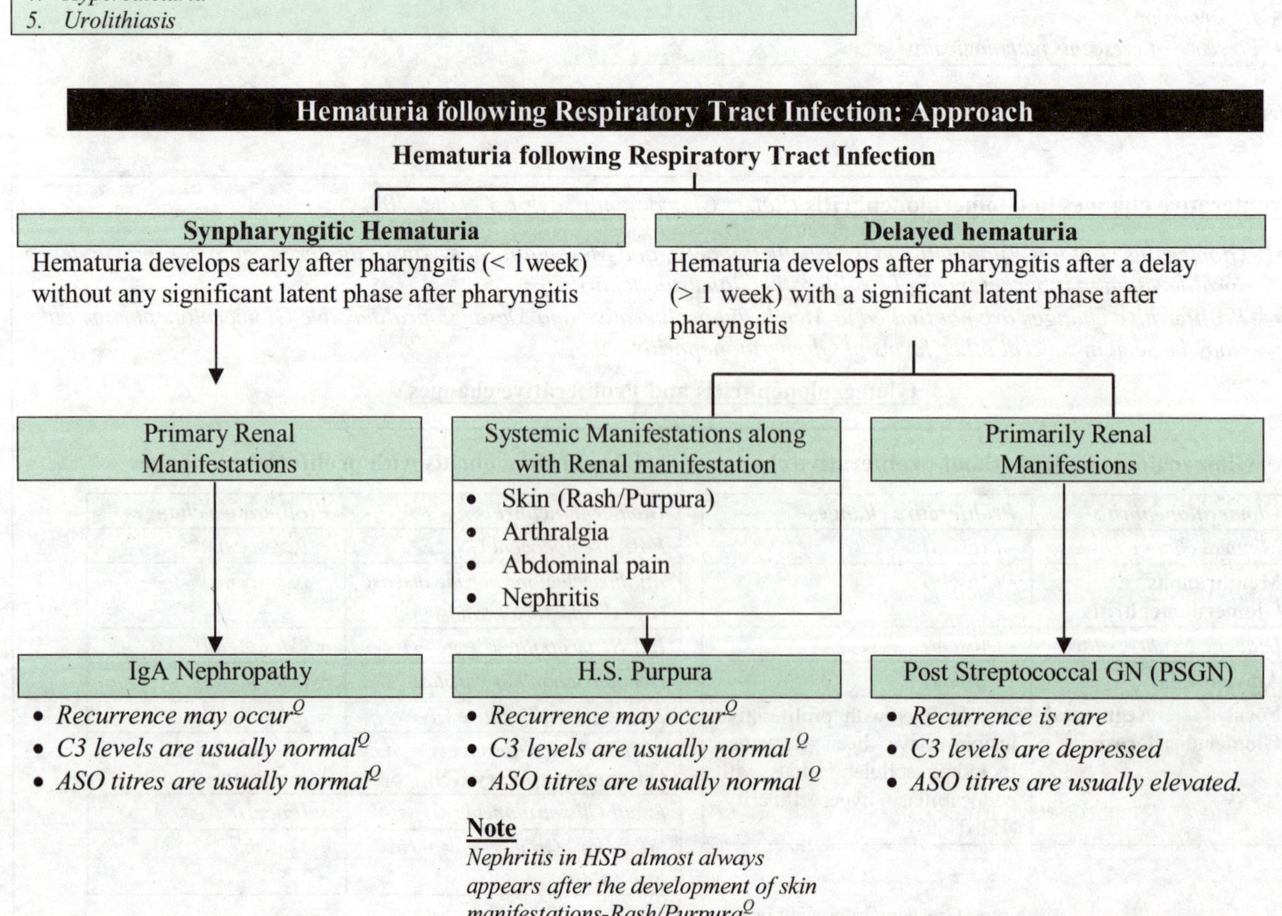

Differentiating IgA Nephropathy from Post-streptococcal Glomeulonephritis

IgA Nephropathy	Post streptococcal Glomerulonephritis
• **Synpharygitic Hematuria** *Hematuria develops usually within 2-4 days of Pharyngitis /URTI* *This is called synpharygitis hematuria since there is no significant latent period between development of hematuria and pharyngitis*	• Delayed Haematuria Hematuria develops 1-3 weeks after pharyngitis /URTI *This is called delayed Hematuria since there s a significant latent period between development of hematuria and pharyngitis*
• **Recurrence is common** *'Hematuria occuring in IgA nephropathy typically lasts for several days and then subsides, only to return every few months'* Recurrent Gross Hematuria	• Recurrence is rare *'Complete Recovery occurs in more than 95% of patients with PSGN. One attack confers life long immunity and recurrences are extremely rare*
• **Serum complement C3 levels are Normal** C3 levels Normal	• **Serum levels of complement C3 are reduced** C3 levels depressed in > 90%
• **Antistreptolysin O titres are usually normal**	• **Antistreptotysin O titres are usually elevated** *'Increased ASO titres are associated with Acute PSGN rather than IgA Nephropathy'*

Laboratory Feature of Renal vasculitis in children due to HSP	
• *Serum IgA levels*	*Elevated (60% of patients have an elevated serum IgA)*
• *Antinuclear Antibody (ANA)*	*Negative*
• *Antineutrophil cytoplasmic Antibodies (ANCA)*	*Negative*
• *Complement (C3, C4)*	*Normal (Even though immune complexes containing IgA are essential to the pathophysiology of HSP, serum complement levels are usually normal*
• *Cryoglobulins*	*Negative*

Berger's Disease/IgA Nephropathy

Aetiopathogenesis

Respiratory or gastrointestinal exposure to environmental agents (viruses, bacteria etc.)

↓

Genetic or acquired abnormality of immune regulation resulting in *increased mucosal IgA synthesis*[Q]

↓

Formation of circulating *IgA immune complexes*[Q], which are entrapped *in mesangium.* [Q]

Microscopic Pathology[Q]	Immunofluorescence	Electron Microscope
Mesangioproliferative *(diffuse) glomerulonephritis >* ***Segmental*** *proliferation confined to some glomeruli (**focal** proliferative glomerulonephritis)>* *Overt crescentric glomerulonephritis (rare)*	*Mesangial deposition of IgA often with C3 and properidin*[Q] *(IgG is present in 50% of cases)* [Q]	*Electron dense deposits in mesangium*[Q]. mesangial hypercellularity, sclerosis

Clinical

Haematuria : Most common presentation is with ***gross haematuria*** *24 to 48 hrs after a pharyngeal / gastrointestinal infection*[Q] / vaccination or strenuous exercise.

Microscopic haematuria[Q] detected during routine physical examination may be the presentation.

Proteinuria (Nephrotic syndrome) : *may or may not be present* [Q] *- Robbins*

Hypertension (20-30%) is *unusual at presentation.* [Q]

Goodpasture's Syndrome

Good pasture's syndrome

Good pasture's syndrome is an autoimmune disease characterized by formation of Anti GBM antibodies that attack both pulmonary capillaries and the Glomerulus (GBM)

Preceding Resp infection
Toxic lung exposure
Drug exposure Etc

Antibodies against Non collagenous Domain (NCL) of $\alpha3$ chain of collagen type IV
(Found in Glomerular Bacement membrane & Pulmonary capillaries)

Serology
- *Circulating Anti GBM antibodies (IgG): Positive*
- *ANCA antibodies: Typically Negative (May be present in upto 30%)*
- *ANA antibodies : usually normal*
- *C3 levels : Usually normal*

<u>Two Age Groups</u>
- *Young men in late 20's (Men >> females)*
- *Men and women their 60-70's*

Antibodies agonist Glomerular Basement Membrane (GBM)

Antibodies against pulmonary capillaries

Glomerulonephritis /Renal Disease
- <u>Features of Acute Glomerulonephritis (RPGN)</u>
  Hematuria[Q]
  Proteinuria[Q]
  Edema
  Rapidly progressive renal failure[Q]
- <u>Pathological Picture</u>[Q]
  Diffuse crescenteric Glomerulonephritis[Q]
  Linear IgG[Q] *staining along basement membrane on immunofluorescence*[Q]

Dysmorphic RBC and RBC cast are present in urine suggesting Glomerulonephritis[Q]

Pulmonary /Lung Manifestations

<u>Clinical</u>
- Hemoptysis (Frank)
  Hemoptysis is largely confined to smokers
- Dyspnea

<u>X-Ray finding</u>[Q]
- *Diffuse bilateral pulmonary infiltrates*[Q]

Goodpasture's syndrome and ANCA

ANCA is typically negative in Goodpastures syndrome and it is classified as an ANCA negative vasculitis
<u>Nevertheless</u>
ANCA seropositivity may occur in upto 30 percent of patients with Goodpasture's syndrome.These patients with ANCA have subtle signs of a systemic vasculitis and represent an overlap between goodpastures and either Wegener's granulomatosis (WG) or Microscopic polyangitis(MPA)-Current Diagnosis and Treatment in Pulmonary Medicine 1st (2003)/211

Triad of Goodpasture's syndrome (*Ferri's Color Atlas & Text of Clinical Medicine*)
- *Glomerulonephritis*[Q] *(RPGN; crescents)*
- *Pulmonary Haemorrhage*[Q] *(Diffuse Alveolar Haemorrhage)*
- *Antibodies to basement membrane antigens*[Q] *(Anti-GBM antibodies)*

Alport's Syndrome

Alport's Syndrome
Alport's syndrome is an inherited disorder charachterized by hereditary nephritis, senserineural deafness and ocular abnormalities. *Alport's syndrome is the most common hereditary nephritis*[Q]
Genetic defect, Pathology
• Primary pathology in Alport's syndrome is an abnormality in type IV collagen (Type IV collagen is the predominant collagen in basement membrane) • ***The most common form of Alport's syndrome is due to mutation of the COLA4A5 ($\alpha - 5$ Chain) gene located on the X chromosome***[Q]**.** • The most common inheritance pattern for Alport's syndrome is X Linked – *Classic Alport's syndrome* *Alport's syndrome may be inherited as X-Linked, Autosomal recessive, or Autosomal dominant disorder but classic Alport's syndrome in inherited as an X linked disorder.*
Clinical Triad
Alport's Syndrome **Nephrosis / Kidney**: • *Hematuria (Micro /Macro)* • *Proteinuria* • *Progressive **Renal Failure*** **Otological (Ears) Symptoms**: • *Sensorineural hearing loss* (Labyrinthine hearing loss particularly in high frequency) **Ocular (Eye)**: • ***Lenticonus*** is characteristic • *Cataract (lens opacity)* • *Corneal erosions* • *Keratoconus* *Myopia induced by Lenticonus & keratoconus*
Pathological Findings in kidney
• *Nephritis (Hematuria, Proteinuria, Progressive renal insufficiency)* • *Sensorineural deafness* • *Ocular abnormalities (Lenticonus > Recurrent corneal erosisons, corneal opacipies)* • *Irregular thickening and thinning of Basement membrane* • *GBM may appear normal or diffusely thin* • *Splitting of Lamina and micro granulation's may be seen*
Treatment and Prognosis
• *No specific treatment to slow the progress of this condition.* • *Patients are good candidates for Renal transplantation.* • *Recurrence of disease in renal transplant is rare.*

Clinical Manifestation of Alport's Syndrome (Triad)

Because it is inherited as an Xlinked disorder, women are usually less severely affected than men.

Most common inheritance: X Linked (Recessive)
Most common defect : Alpha 5 chain of collagen IV

Nephritis	Sensorineural Deafness	Ocular Abnormalities
• Hematuria is the classic presenting feature and occurs early in life • Proteinuria often develops but its development is usually noticed years after hematuria is first observed (delayed) • Chronic Renal Failure develops in most individuals and is often observed in late teens or early 20's	• Sensorineural deafness is the most common extrarenal manifestation in Alport's syndrome • Primarily in the high tone range • Frequently detectable only by an audiogram • Usually not progressive (Harrison) *According to Clinical Pediatric Nephrlogy, hearing loss is progressive*	• Anterior Lenticonus is charachteristic (often bilateral) • Recurrent corneal erosisns and lens opacities are often associated *Lenticonus together with hematuria is considered pathognomic of classic AS*

Diabetic Renal Disease

Microalbuminuria and Diabetic Renal Disease

- *Microalbuminuria is the first clinically detectable sign of diabetic nephropathy*
- Microalbuminuria refers to excretion of albumin in the urine in amounts that are abnormal but below the limit of detection of conventional urine dipsticks[Q]

Microalbuminuria is defined as excretion of 30-300 mg of albumin/day in a 24 hour collection[Q] or 30-300µg/mg[Q] creatinine in a spot collection.

- The presence of albumin in the urine in the range of microalbuminuria is *best determined by a urinary Albumin/Creatinine ratio in a spot voided urine (Prefered method for delecting microalbuminuria)*[Q]
- *Microalbuminuria is best detected by Sensitive Radioimmuneassays*[Q]
- The recognition of microalbuminuria in patients with diabetes mellitus allows identification of diabetic nephropathy and institution of treatment to reduce the risk of progressive kidney disease at an earlier stage than would be possible with conventional urine dip-sticks

There is clear evidence that the detection of early diabetic nephropathy manifested by microalbuminuria is responsive to antihypertensive therapy in particular the use of ACE Inhibitors or Angiotensin Receptor Blockers.

Stages of Diabetic Nephropathy according to Mogensen:

Stage	Duration of diabetes	Clinical, biological and pathological signs related to renal disease
1	At diagnosis	• *No clinical or biological signs of renal injury* • *Hypertrophy of the kidneys* • *Glomerular hyperfiltration*
2	2-5 years	*Clinically and biologically 'silent' nephropathy*
3	5-10 years	**Early nephropathy:** • ***Microalbuminuria*** • *High blood pressure* • *Normal GFR*
4	10-20 years	**Established diabetic nephropathy:** • ***Macroalbuminuria*** • *High blood pressure* • *Decreasing GFR* • *Pathology: mesangial expansion; GBM thickening; and glomerular sclerosis*
5	>20 years	**End-stage renal disease** • *Pathology: advanced fibrosis of the kidneys* Need for: • *Renal transplant (± pancreas)* • *Peritoneal dialysis* • *Hemodialysis*

Glomerular Lesions in Diabetes

Diffuse glomerulosclerosis :	Nodular glomerulosclerosis
• Is the ***most common pattern of involvement***[Q] • The most common pathological change is ***thickening of glomerular basement membrane***[Q] which occurs virtually in all diabetics and is part and parcel of diabetic microangiopathy • Various exudative lesions such as capsular hyaline drops or 'fibrin caps' may be present • ***Capsular drop***[Q]: is an eosinophilic thickening of parietal layer of Bowman's capsule and bulges into glomerular space • ***Fibrin caps***[Q] : is a homogeneous eosinophilic material appearing on the wall of a peripheral capillary of a lobule	• Is virtually ***pathognomic***[Q] ***of diabetes mellitus*** • Is also called ***Kimmelstiel-Wilson lesion*** or ***Intercapillary glomerulosclerosis***[Q] • The pathological change consist of one or more nodules in a few or many glomeruli • Uninvolved lobules and glomeruli all show striking diffuse glomerulosclerosis

Capillary basement membrane thickening

"The earliest morphological abnormality in diabetic nephropathy is thickening of basement membrane" (and expansion of mesangium due to accumulation of extracellular matrix)

Glomerular Lesions in SLE (Wire Loop Lesions)

Wire loop lesions:

- Wire loop lesions represent local PAS – Positive thickening of glomerular capillary walls and are characteristically seen in Lupus Nephritis (SLE)
- These lesions result from subendothelial deposits between endothelium and basement membrane. When extensive and confluent, these subendothelial deposits create a homogenous thickening of the capillary wall which can be seen in light microscopy as 'Wire loop lesion'
- Wire loop lesions are most characteristic of Lupus Nephritis Class IV or Diffuse Lupus Nephritis
  These may however also be seen in Class III (Focal Lupus Nephritis) and Class V (membranous) Lupus Nephritis.

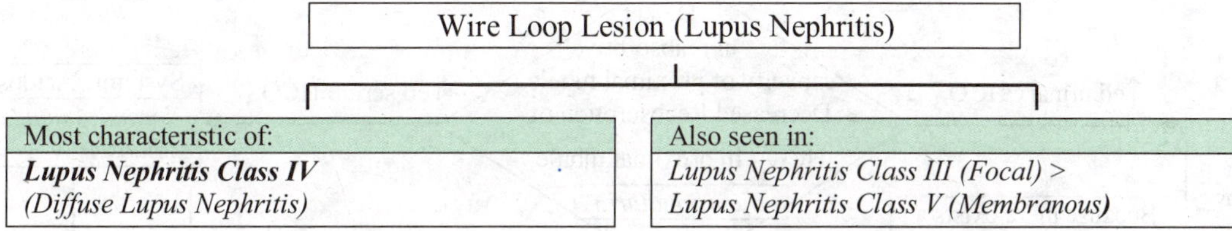

Glomerular Lesions in HIV

The most charachteristic Glomerulopathy in HIV is focal segmental Glomerulosclerosis (FSGS), which typically reveals collapse of the glomerular capillary tuft called collapsing glomerulopathy

Hepatitis C infection and Glomerular lesions

Three clinicopathologic glomerular syndromes associated with hepatitis C are:
• *Secondary MPGN* • *Cryoglobulinemic Glomerulopathy* • *Membranous nephropathy*

MPGN is the most common lesion*. These patients typically have haematuria, hypertension, proteinuria and anemia. Hypocomplementemia is very common with C4 typically more reduced than C3.*

Renal Lesions in Leprosy

'Chronic renal failure in leprosy is commonly due to proliferative glomerulonephritis, interstitial nephritis and renal amyloidosis and is a common cause of death' *– Rooks*
Remember however that most other infectious causes lead to membranous glomerulonephritis rather than MPGN.

Renal Tubular Acidosis

Proximal Renal Tubular Acidosis (Type II RTA)

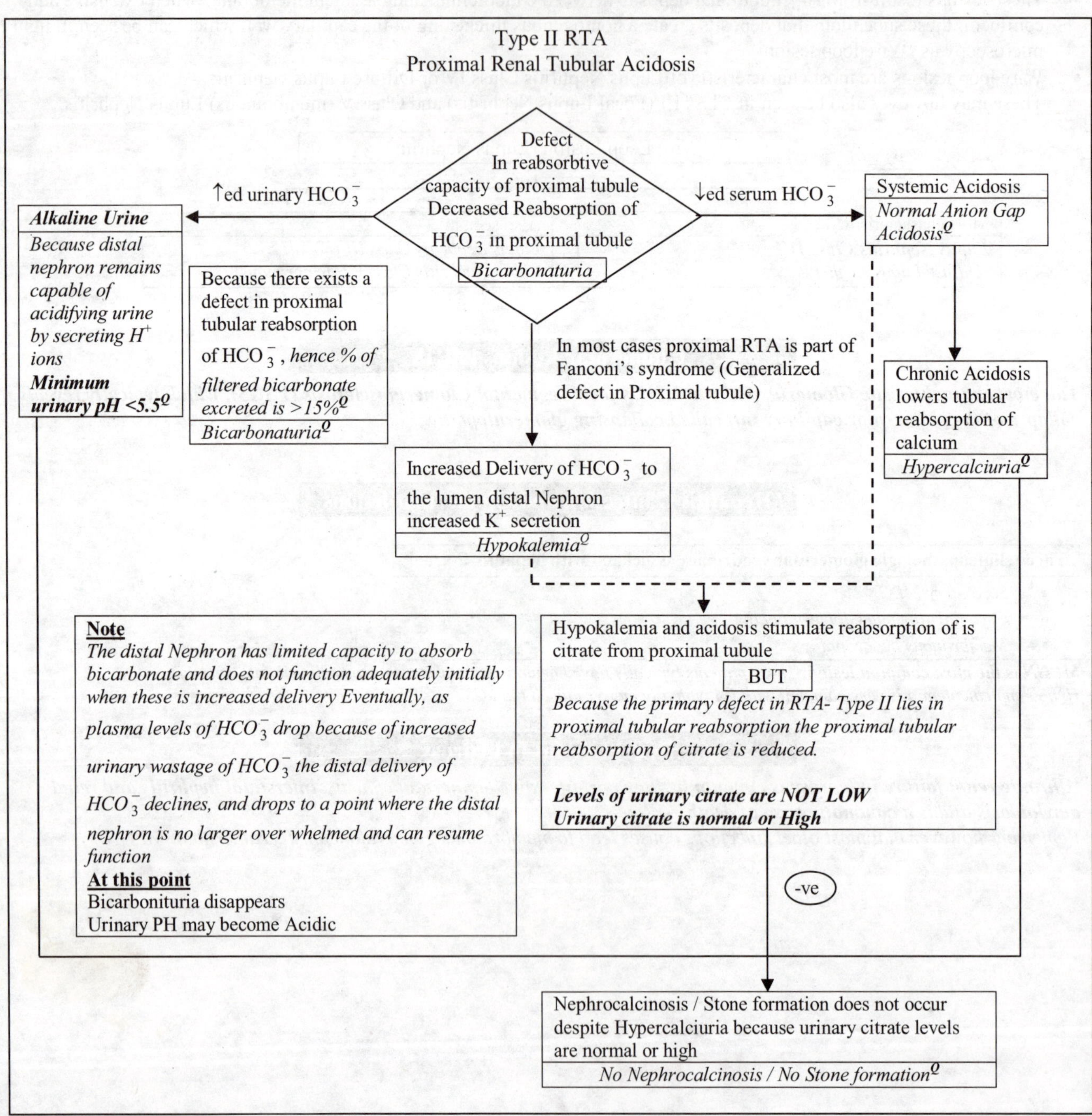

Distal Renal Tubular Acidosis (Type I RTA)

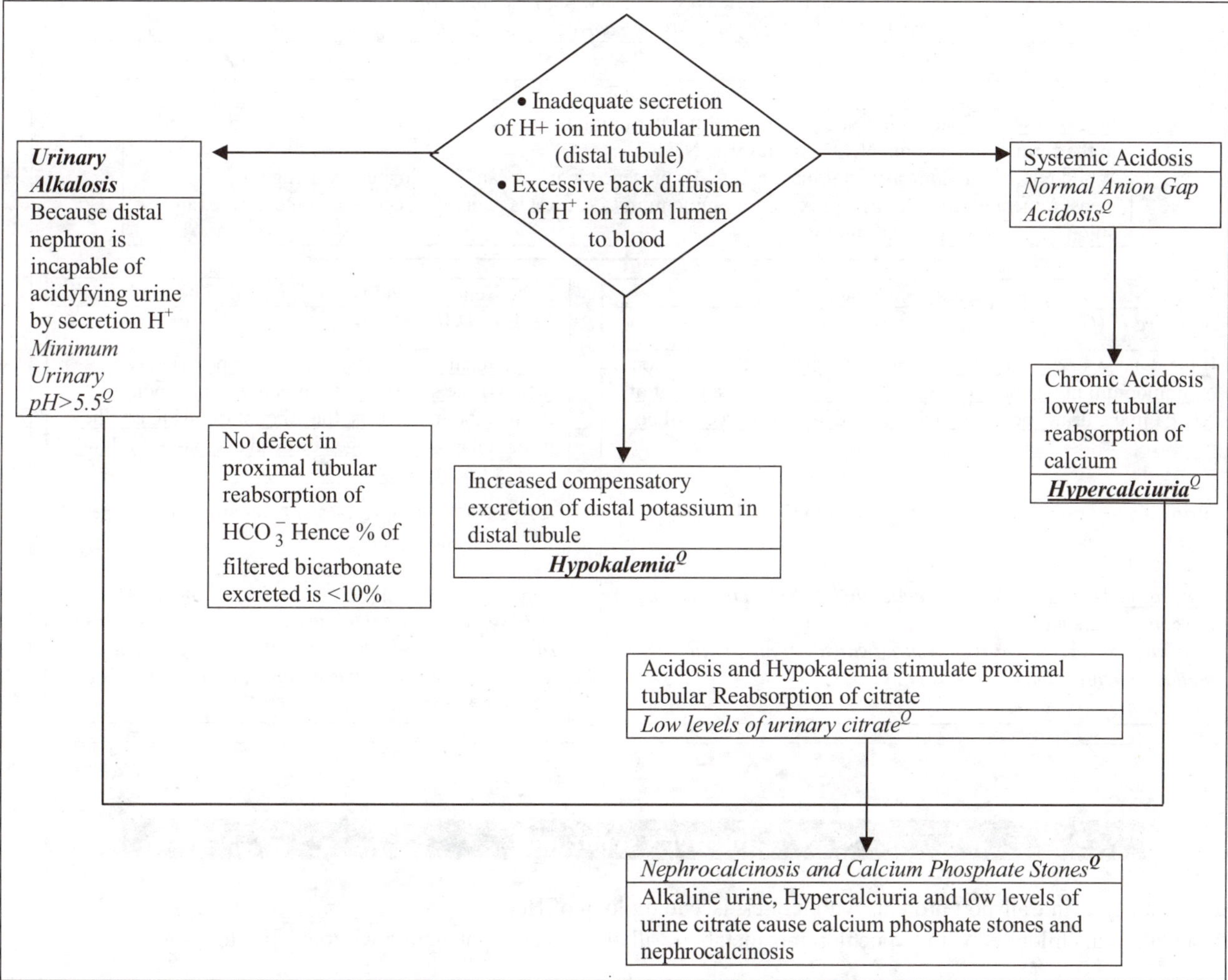

Type I (Distal) RTA is associated with Hyperkalemia, failure to acidify urine to a pH of <5 and an increased risk of urinary stones

Distinguishing Features of Various Types of Renal Tubular Acidosis

Feature	Type I	Type II	Type IV
Normal anion gap	*Yes*	*Yes*	*Yes*
Minimum urine pH	***> 5.5***	*< 5.5*	*< 5.5*
% Filtered bicarbonate excreted	*< 10*	*> 15*	*< 10*
Serum potassium	***Low***	***Low***	***High***
Fanconi syndrome	*No*	*Yes*	*No*
Stones / Nephrocalcinosis	***Yes***	*No*	***No***
Daily acid excretion	*Low*	*Normal*	*Low*
Urinary anion gap	*Positive*	*Positive*	*Positive*

Type I RTA is associated with failure to acidify urine to a pH <5 because distal nephron is incapable of acidyfying urine by secretion of H^+ (Minimum Urinary pH>5.5[Q])

Urinary Anion Gap

Urinary Anion Gap

Urinary Anion Gap (UAG) is defined by the difference between major urinary cations and major urinary anion

UAG = (Urine Na+ + Urine K+) – Urine Cl-

Normally / Typically the UAG is nearly zero or slightly positive

Response to Metabolic Acidosis

In response to a metabolic acidosis, a normally functioning renal system is able to secrete additional acid in the form of ammonium NH_4^+, generally as NH4Cl.

While NH_4^+ is an unmeasured urinary cation, its presence in urine can be estimated by using the measurement of urine Cl^- as a proxy since ammonium (a cation) is generally secreted with chloride (an anion) to maintain electroneutrality

With a Normally Functioning Renal System ***Negative UAG***	If the Renal System is not functioning normally ***Positive UAG***
If the renal system is able to appropriately increase the secretion of ammonium in response to a metabolic acidosis, the amount of NH_4Cl in the urine increases and the UAG or net charge will be negative: (urine Na^+ + urine K^+) – (a larger amount of urine Cl-)= a negative number. ***A negative UAG*** *suggests that renal tubular dysfunction is not the cause of the metabolic acidosis.* ***This may be seen in Gastrointestinal causes of metabolic acidosis such as diarrhea***	If, the renal system is not able to appropriately increase the secretion of ammonium in response to the metabolic acidosis, the amount of NH4Cl in the urine remains unchanged or even decreases, and the UAG or net charge will be positive: (urine Na^+ + urine K^+)- (a smaller amount of urine Cl^-) = a positive number ***A positive UAG*** *suggests that there is impaired renal acid secretion and that the renal system is the cause of, or at least contributing to, the metabolic acidosis.* ***This may seen in Distal Renal Tubular Acidosis or chronic kidney disease***

Bartter's syndrome

- Inherited defect in transport proteins within thick ascending loop of Henle.
- Presentation in childhood with hypochloremic metabolic alkalosis and hypokalemia without hypertension

Metabolic Alkalosis[Q]
Hypokalemia[Q]
Absence of Hypertension: BP is normal or low[Q]

- Other metabolic defects /Electrolyte defects include hypercalciuria, hypomagnesemia and increased urinary prostaglandiN secretion

  - *Hypercalciuria with nephrocalcinosis*
  - *Hypomagnesemia*
  - *↑ urinary PGE2*

- Clinical presentation includes polyuria, polydypsia, salt craving and growth retardation or failure to thrive.

  - *Polyurea, polydipsia, salt craving*
  (Fetal polyurea in antenatal period may cause polyhydramnios and premature labor)
  - *Growth retardation or failure to thrive*
  - *Fever, vomiting & diarrhea may occur due to PGE2 over production*

- Patients who survive early childhood may develop chronic renal failure

CRF is a known complication

Hemolytic Uremic Syndrome

It is a vessel wall disorder charactarized by deposition of localized platelet and thrombi within the renal vasculature

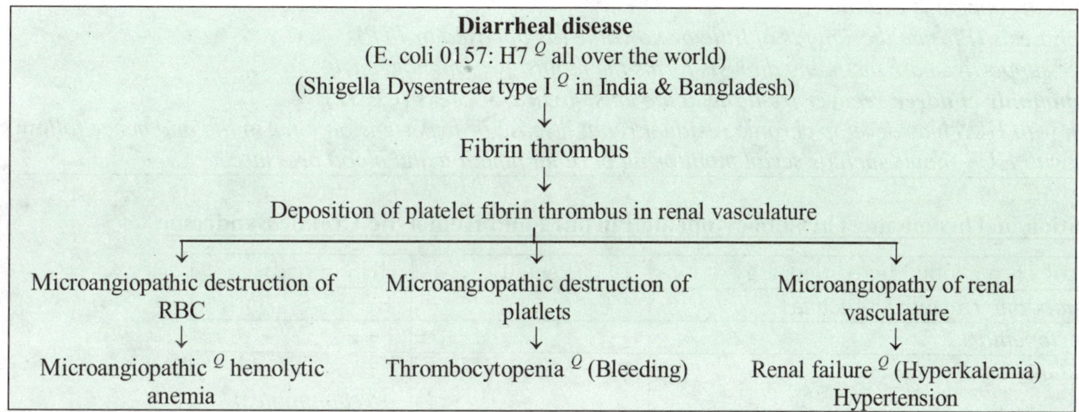

Essentials of Diagnosis for Hemolytic Uremic Syndrome (HUS):

HUS should be strongly suspected in any child, who presents with:
- *Anemia,* Q
- *Bleeding* Q *(which is due to thrombocytopenia),* Q *or*
- *Renal failure* Q *(as indicated here by decreased urine output)* Q

Especially so, if it occurs after a diarrheal illness Q (due to infection with E. coli, Shigella or Salmonella)Q.

Essentials of diagnosis as mentioned in CMDT :
- Microangiopathic hemolytic anemia
- Thrombocytopenia
- Renal failure
- Elevated serum LDH
- Normal coagulation tests
- *Absence of Neurological abnormality*

There are no neurological manifestations other than those due to uraemia – CMDT
Neurological symptoms other than those associated with uremia are uncommon – Harrison
Nevertheless, confusion does prevail as Nelson confuses the issue – Extra renal manifestations may include CNS manifestations – Nelson

Laboratory Findings in Hemolytic Uremic Syndrome (HUS):

Laboratory findings in HUS – *CMDT 2002 / 556*
1. Anemia: Microangiopathic hemolytic
   Red blood cell fragmentation on peripheral smear
   Helmet cells / Burr cells
2. Thrombocytopenia
3. WBC counts rise (Nelson 16th/ 1587)
4. LDH levels are elevated out of proportion to degree of hemolysis
5. *Coomb's test is negative*
6. Tests of coagulation are normal (exclude DIC) with the exception of – elevated fibrin degradation products (explains hypofibrinogenemia)

Treatment of Hemolytic Uremic Syndrome:

- **Hemolytic Uremic Syndrome is often a self-limiting condition**
  '***Typical HUS (D+ HUS) is often a self limiting condition****, although many children need extensive supportive care including dialysis, for a period of time' – 'Chronic Complex Diseases of Childhood' (Universal Publishers) 2011/363*
- ***The treatment of typical HUS (D+ HUS) is essentially supportive.***
- *No specific treatment is available.*
- *Plasmapharesis (Plasma therapy) is of little or no value (as opposed to TTP)*
- *Extensive supportive care including dialysis forms the mainstay of management*
- ***Most commonly children recover from the acute episode in 2-3 weeks (CPDT)***
- *Children with HUS may develop chronic residual renal disease or hypertension later in life and hence follow up of patients with HUS should include serial monitoring of renal function and blood pressure.*

Differentiation of Thrombotic Thrombocytopenic Purpura and Hemolytic Uremic Syndrome

PENTAD of Thrombotic Microangiopathy	TTP (Pentad)	HUS (Triad)
Microangiopathic Hemolytic Anemia	+++	+++
Thrombocytopenia	+++	+++
Renal Dysfunction	+++	+++ *(Predominates)*
Fever	**+++**	***+/- (Uncommon)***
Neurological Dysfunction	+++	*+/- (Uncommon)*

Fever in Hemolytic Uremic Syndrome is usually mild or absent

'Fever is typically mild or absent' – Hoffman's Hematology (2009)/2106

'HUS often presents without fever or neurological dysfunction'

– Washington Manual of Hematology and Oncology Subspecialty Consult (2003)/53

Hemolytic Uremic syndrome usually follows Haemorrhagic Colitis

Typical Hemolytic Uremic syndrome is diarrheal associated disease triggered by intestinal infection with Shiga toxin or Shiga like toxin producing bacteria (This is termed as D (+) HUS).

These cases of HUS are typically preceded by episodes of bloody diarrhea or Haemorrhagic colitis (Most common presenting features)

Typical HUS; D (+) HUS	Atypical HUS; D (-) HUS
• *Shiga producing toxin is implicated in pathogenesis* • *Usually preceded or associated with bloody diarrhea (Hemorrhagic colitis)*	• *Shiga producing toxin is not implicated in pathogenesis* • *Neither preceded nor associated with bloody diarrhea*

Serotoxin/Shiga Like Toxin/ShigellaVerotoxin (VT) is the most common toxin implicated in the pathogenesis of HUS

Typical Hemolytic Uremic Syndrome is a diarrhea-associated condition triggered by intestinal infection with *serotoxin/shiga like toxin producing bacteria*

- *ShigellaDysentreas type I, producing Shiga Toxin is the most common organism in India & Bangladesh*
- *Shiga like toxin (serotoxin) producing E. coli (EHEC 0157:H7) is the most common implicated agent worldwide.*

Nephrosclerosis

Benign Nephrosclerosis	***Malignant Nephrosclerosis***
This term is used to describe the changes in kidney associated with benign phase of hypertension	*This term is used to describe the changes in kidney associated with malignant or accelerated hypertension.*
Gross	*Gross*
• Kidney *size is either* normal[Q] *or may be moderately* reduced[Q]	• Kidney size *is* variable[Q] *May be* smaller in size[Q] *(when superimposed on benign nephrosclerosis) or Larger in* size *(enlarged)*[Q] *than normal (patients who develop malignant hypertension in pure form)*
• Grain leather appearance[Q] *: The cortical surface has a fine even granularity*	• Flea bitten appearance[Q]: ***The cortical surface*** *may show multiple small* ***peticheal haemorrhages***[Q] *from rupture of arterioles or glomerular capillaries.*
Microscopic (Vascular Changes & Parenchymal Changes)	*Microscopic (Vascular Changes & Parenchymal Changes)*
• **Hyaline Arteriosclerosis** [Q] *Narrowing of the lumens of arterioles and small arteries caused by thickenning and hyalnization of the walls*	• **Fibrinoid necrosis of arterioles**[Q] **(Necrotizing arteriolitis**[Q]**)** *The vessel wall shows fibrinoid necrosis. Represents an acute event and necrosis is usually not accompanied by intense inflammation*
• Fibroelastic Hyperplasia[Q]*: in the intima (intimal thickenning*[Q]*), duplication of elastic lamina and hypertrophy of the 'media'*	• **Hyperplastic intimal sclerosis**[Q] / Onion – Skinning[Q] **Concentric laminae** *of proliferated smooth muscle cells, collagen and basement membrane* **(producing intimal thickenning)**
• *Parenchymal changes (due to ischaemic) Variable degree of Atrophy of parenchyma due to ischaemia*	• *Parenchymal changes (due to ischaemia) Variable degree of atrophy of paranchyma due to ischaemia. Infarction necrosis distal to abnormal vessels may be seen*

Causes of Contracted Kidneys

Causes of Contracted Kidneys
• *Chronic Glomerulonephritis (Bilateral)*
• *Nephrosclerosis because of systemic hypertension (Bilateral)*
• *Chronic pyelonephritis (Usually unilateral)*
• *Global renal infarction (Unilateral)*
• *Radiation nephritis (Unilateral)*
• *Renal artery stenosis (Unilateral)*
• *Post obstructive atrophy (Unilateral)*

Note that Acute Glomerulonephritis, and acute pyelonephritis are associated with enlarged kidneys but chronic cases are associated with contracted kidneys

Renal Artery Stenosis

Renal Artery Stenosis: Review

- Renal Artery stenosis is an important cause of Renovascular Hypertension
- ***Bilateral involvement is seen in half of the affected cases (50%)***

Etiology

- Atherosclerotic disease : This is the most common cause in middle aged /elderly patients
- Fibromuscular Dysplasia : ***This is the most important cause in young females***

Presentation

- Hypertension
  - Abrupt onset of hypertension
  - Acceleration of previously well controlled hypertension
  - Refractory Hypertension
- Features of increased sympathetic neural activity (which is associated with Renovascular disease)
  - Flushing
  - Loss of nocturnal BP decrease
  - Putonomic instability
  - Rapid BP swings
- Progressive Renal failure / Azotemia

Diagnosis

Magnetic Resonance Angiography (MRA)	Contrast Enhanced Arteriography
MRA is the most sensitive (>90%) and specific (95%) non invasive test for the diagnosis of RAS	Contrast enhanced angiography is the most definitive (but invasive) diagnostic procedure for diagnosis of RAS

Management

Medical Therapy with ACE Inhibitors or Angiotensin Receptor Blockers

Indications	Contra indications
Unilateral Renal artery Stenosis - With hypertension & normal renal function (more effective than other antihypertensives) - With hypertension & abnormal renal function (beneficial effect on survival without affecting renal function) - With hypertension, diabetes, proteinuria and normal or abnormal renal function (effective antihypertensives)	**Bilateral Renal Artery stenosis** ACE inhibitors or Angiotensin receptor blockers are contraindicated in patients with Bilateral renal artery stenosis or stenosis in a solitary kidney as their use in such patients leads to worsening of renal failure (These patients are especially sensitive to decline in intraglomerular pressure)

Note

Acute Renal Failure / Worsening of Renal Failure with Angiotension Receptor Inhibitors is a diagnostic clue to the diagnosis of renal artery stenosis (indicates bilateral disease)

Surgical Therapy with Angioplasty + Stent placement

Should be considered only after optimal medical therapy has failed to achieve goal BP or resulted in a > 30% increase in serum creatinine

Renal Vein Thrombosis

Causes of Renal Vein Thrombosis:

Causes of Renal Vein Thrombosis

Primary	Secondary
• Dehydration Dehydration is the most common cause of primary RVT in Newborns • Nephrotic syndrome Nephrotic syndrome is the most common cause of primary RVT in adults.	• Trauma • Extrinsic compression (Lymphnode, tumor, aortic aneurysm) • Invasion by Renal cell carcinoma • Pregnancy or oral contraceptives

Common Renal pathologies causing Renal Vein Thrombosis:

Nephrotic Syndrome: Common Renal pathologies causing Renal Vein Thrombosis
• *Membranous Glomerulonephritis (strongest association)*
• *Membranoproliferative Glomerulonephritis*
• *Amyloidosis*
• *Lupus Nephritis (Thrombosis & hemorrhage 3rd/724)*

Nephrotic syndrome due to diabetic mellitus, minimal change disease and focal segmental sclerosis are rarely associated with renal vein thrombosis

Nephrolithiasis and Nephrocalcinosis

Renal Calculi: Composition and Features

Stone Type	X Ray finding	Predisposing features	Comments
Oxalate stones (calcium oxalates)	***Radiopaque***	*Hypercalciuria* *Hyperoxaluria*	*Most common types of Renal Calculi*
Phosphate Stones - *Calcium phosphate* - *Magnesium Ammonium Phosphate (Struvite)*	*Radiopaque*	• ***Excess Alkali consumption*** • ***Alkaline urine*** • *Infection with urease splitting organisms eg. Proteus*	*Struvite stones are often solitary* *Struvite stones form staghorn calculi*
Cystine Stones	*Radiopaque*	*Inherited cystinuria*	• ***Form in acidic urine***[Q] • *Extremely hard stones*[Q] • *Relatively resistant*[Q] *to fragmentation with ESWL*
Uric acid stones	*Radioluscent*	*Gout* *Hyperuricemia*	• *Form in acidic urine* • ***Most responsive to lithotripsy***
Xanthine stones	*Radioluscent*	*Deficiency of xanthine oxidase*	-

Lithotripsy and Renal Calculi Composition

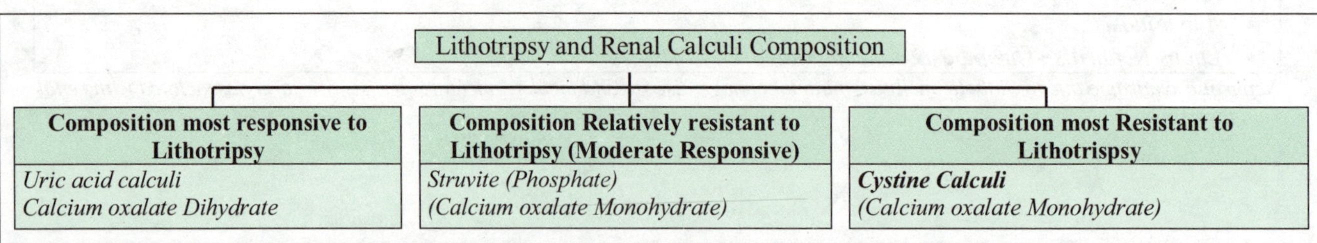

Cystine stones are most resiatnt to Lithotripsy.
Uric acid stones are infact most responsive to Lithotripsy along with calcium oxalate dehydrate stones

Radio-opacity and Renal Calculi Composition

Renal Stones

Radiopaque	Radioluscent

• *Oxalate Stones*
  - *Calcium Oxalate*
• *Phosphate Stones*
  - *Calcium phosphate*
  - *Magnesium ammonium phosphate (struvite)*
• *Cystine stones*
	• *Uric Acid Calculi*
	• *Xanthine Calculi*
	• *Indinavir Calculi (complication of Indinavir use-Proteinase inhibitor)*
	• *Triametrene calculi (complication of Triamterene use-Antihypertensive)*

Triple-Phosphate Stones

Triple Phosphate Stones (Phosphate stones)

- *Triple phosphate stones are composed predominantly of magnesium ammonium phosphate (strurite) with variable amounts of calcium phosphate.*
- *They form in the presence of high urinary concentration of ammonia (bicarbonate and carbonate)*
- *They form in cases of UTI when urine is infected with urea splitting bacteria i.e. Proteus, Kleibsella and Pseudomonas*
- *They form in urine with an alkaline pH.*

Urea splitting organisms split urea to ammonia there by providing an alkaline pH which facilitates precipitation of phosphate crystals.

Location of Ureteric colic (pain)

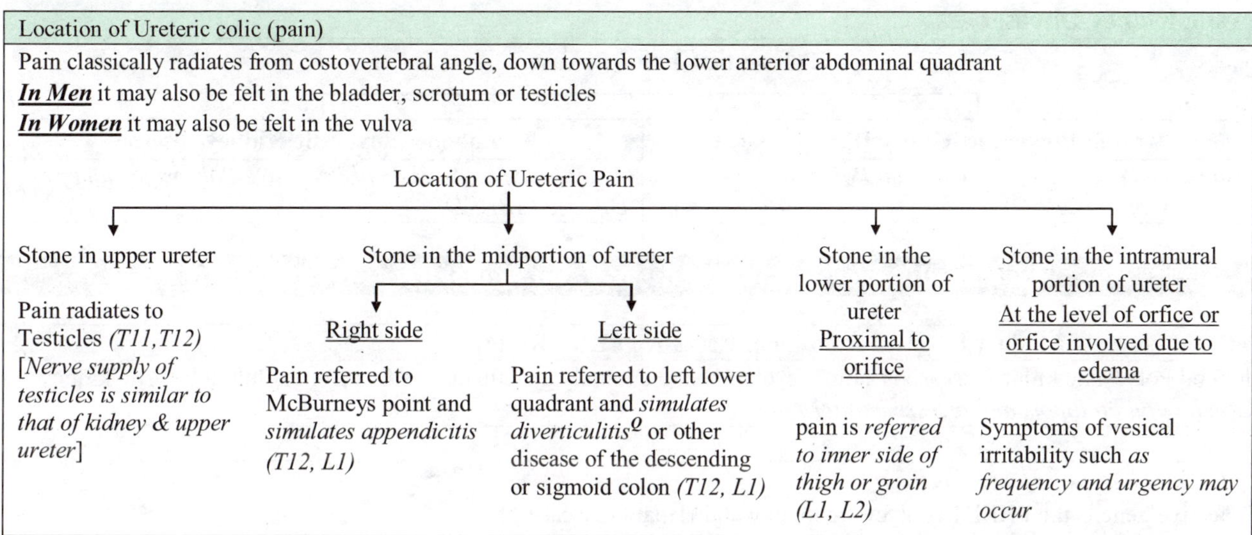

Indications and methods for removal of stone

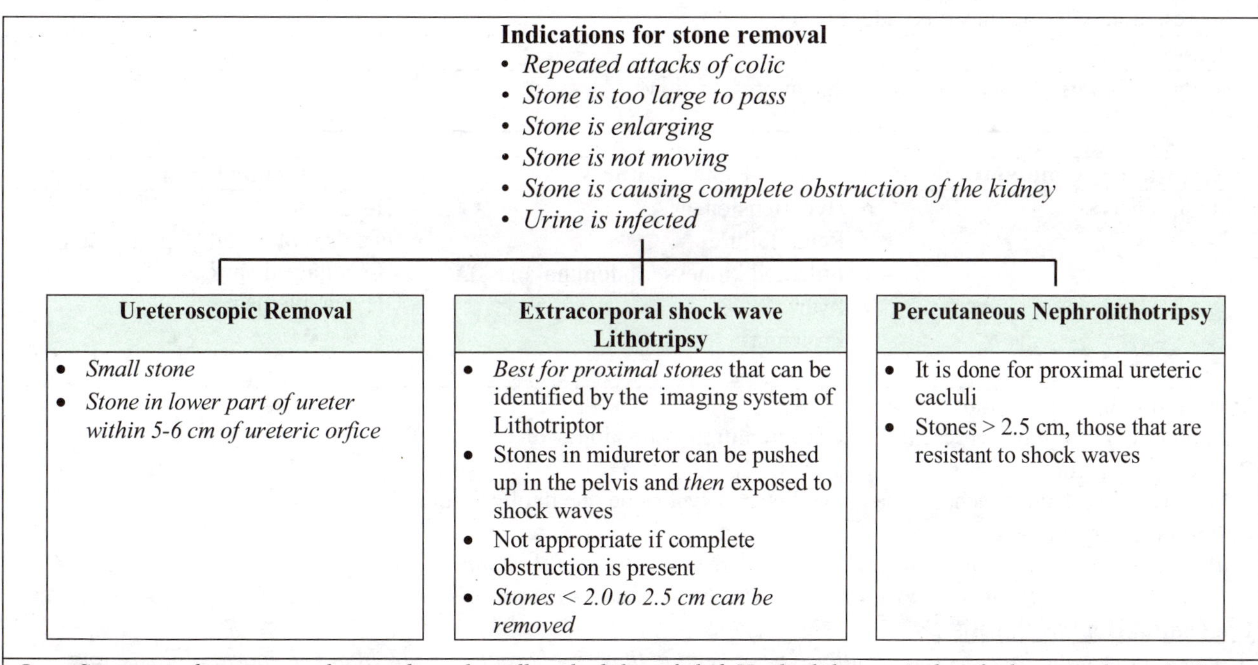

Congenital Diseases of the Kidney

Polycystic Kidney Disease

Polycystic Kidney Disease

Adult Polycystic Kidney Disease	Childhood Polycystic Kidney Disease
Also termed as Autosomal Dominant Polycystic kidney disease (ADPKD)	*Also termed as Autosomal Recessive Polycystic kidney Disease (ARPKD)*

Childhood Polycystic kidney Disease / Autosomal Recessive PKD

Childhood Polycystic kidney Disease / Autosomal Recessive PKD : Review

Childhood Polycystic kidney disease is a rare developmental anomaly genetically distinct from Adult polycystic kidney Disease ***having an autosomal recessive inheritance***

Genetics

- *Autosomal Recessive inheritance*
- Defective gene is the PKHD1 (Polycystic kidney and Hepatic Disease 1)
- PKHD1 gene codes for a protein 'Fibrocystin' (defective protein in ARPKD)[Q]

Epidemiology

- Majority of patients present during infancy (first year of life)
- May present later in life (in young adults)

Presentation

- Presentation is variable and depends on age at presentation

Respiratory Symptoms	Renal Features	Hepatic Features
Respiratory distress	• Hypertension • Renal failure • Enlarged kidneys (abdominal mass) • Pyuria • Proteinuria	• Hepatomegaly • Features of portal Hypertension -Esophageal varices -Hypersplenism

Associations

- **Maternal Oligohydramnios**
  Oligohydramnios may be present due to severe intrauterine kidney disease
- **Potter's syndrome**
  Most severely affected neonates may have Potter's syndrome due to oligohydramnios
- **Pulmonary Hypoplasia**
  Pulmonary hypoplasia may result from severe oligohydramnios and as part of Potter's sequence
  'About 50% of affected neonates die of pulmonary hypoplasia' - Harrison's
- **Congenital Hepatic fibrosis**
  Congenital Hepatic Fibrosis is a peculiar type of hepatic fibrosis characterized by bland periportal fibrosis, and proliferation of well differentiated biliary ductules
  Hepatic cysts may be seen (In almost all cases liver has cysts with portal fibrosis - Robbins)
- **Biliary Ductal Atresia**
  ARPKP is invariably associated with congenital hepatic fibrosis and various degrees of biliary ductal Atresia

Renal Pathology

- Kidney's are enlarged (invariably Bilateral)
- Numerous small cysts are present in kidney which give it ' Sponge like appearance'
- Cysts are primarily located in distal tubule and collecting duct
- ***Cysts may be discovered prenatally, at birth or later in life***

Adult Polycystic kidney: Autosomal Dominant PKD

Inheritance : Autosomal Dominant

Pathology:

- Kidneys are grossly enlarged with multiple cysts
- Cyst are distributed uniformly throughout cortex and medulla
- Cysts contain straw coloured fluid that may become haemorrhagic

Presentation: usually occurs in IIIrd / IVth decade

Renal	Extra renal manifestation
1. Pain: due to infection (Pyelonephritis) / obstruction / sudden haemorrhage 2. Haematuria ^{Q} 3. Nocturia: due to impaired concentrating ability 4. Nephrolithiasis (15-20%) ^{Q} 5. Hypertension (75% adults and 25% children) : due to activation of rennin angiotensin system. ^{Q} 6. Progressive decline in renal function – CRF	1. Cysts: Liver (most common) Spleen, pancreas and ovaries 2. Intracranial aneurysms 3. Colonic diverticular disease 4. Cardiac: Mitral valve prolapse / AR / TR

Cystic Disease of Renal Medulla

Cystic Disease of Renal Medulla

Nephrophtysis – Medullary cystic kidney

Both these conditions may progress to end stage Renal disease and present with similar clinical features.

Nephrophthysis	Medullary Cystic kidney
• Autosomal Recessive	Autosomal dominant
• Age of onset in 1st decade (Juvenile)	Age of onset in 3rd or 4th decade (Adult)
• Progression to ESRD occurs <20 years of age	• Progression to ESRD occurs >20 years to age
• Growth Retardation is present as it affects growing children	• Growth retardation is usually not associated as it affects adults
• Extra renal abnormalities are frequent and include *Retinitis pigmentosa* *Cerebellar Ataxia* *Hepatic fibrosis* *Skeletal abnormalities*	• Extra renal abnormalities are absent.

Medullary Sponge kidney

This is a relatively benign condition

Juvenile Nephronophthisis

Juvenile Nephronophthisis

Chronic Tubulo-interstitial Nephritis which uniformly progresses to End stage Renal Disease.

Extrarenal Abnormalities[Q]
Ritinitis Pigmentosa
Cerebellar Ataxia
Hepatic Fibrosis
Skeletal Anomalies

Autosomal Recessive disease[Q]

Pathology Triad
- Tubular Basement Membrane Disintegration
- Tubular cyst formation (Medullary Cyst)
- Tubulo interstitial inflammation

Kidney size is normal or Reduced (shrunken)[Q]

Loss of Urinary Concentrating Ability

Polyurea[Q], *Polydipsia*[Q] — *Nocturnal Enuresis*[Q]

Low urinary osmolarity which does not increase after desmopressin administration

Salt wasting

- *Hyponatremia*[Q]
- *Hypovolumia (dehydration)*[Q]
- *Hypotension (low BP)*[Q]

Progressive Renal failure

Because of loss of urinary concentrating ability and salt wasting, typical symptoms of renal failure do not occur until late in disease

Edema, Hypertension, Hematuria and proteinuria do not occur until late in disease

- *Anemia*[Q]
- *Growth Retardation*[Q]
- *Elevated BUN/creatinine*[Q]

Renal Tumours

Renal Neoplasms

Classification of epithelial neoplasms arising from the kidney

Carcinoma Type	Cell of Origin	Cytogenetics
Clear cell	Proximal tubule	3p deletions (3p-), VHL gene mutations, 5q gains
Papillary	Proximal tubule	Trisomy of chromosome 7 and 17 (+7, +17) Loss of Y chromosome (-Y)
Chromophobe	***Cortical collecting duct***	***Hypodiploid / Monosomy*** ***Loss of multiple chromosomes 1, 2, 6, 10, 13, 17, 21 & Y***
Oncocytic	Cortical collecting duct	Undetermined Either karyotypically normal or contain limited number of karyotypic abnormalities including -1, -Y and translocations involving chromosme II
Collecting duct	Medullary collecting duct	Undetermined Losses of multiple chromosomes 1, 6, 14, 15 & 22

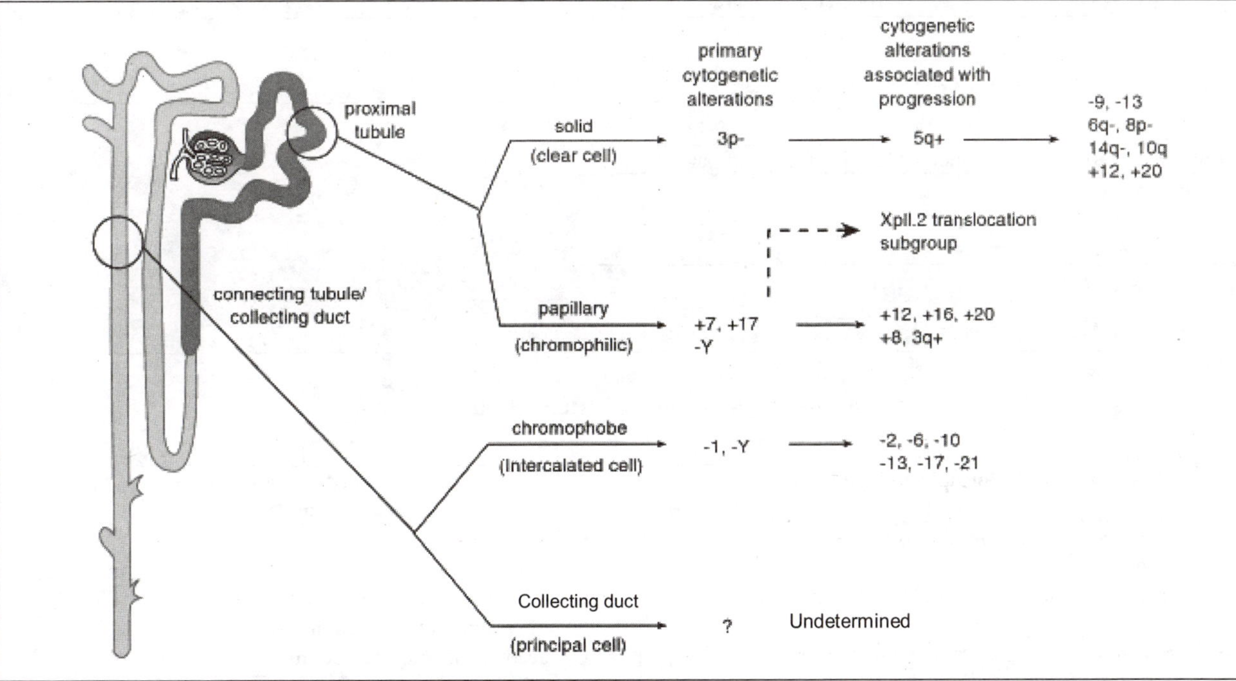

Features of three major histological variants of renal call carcinoma:

Features of three major histological variants of renal call carcinoma:

Clear cell carcinoma (Non papillary)	Papillary carcinoma	Chromophobe renal carcinoma
• Most common Q type Q (70-80%) • Cells have clear Q or granular cytoplasm and are non papillary • Defect lies in chromosomes 3 Q	• Second most common type (10-15%) • Papillary Q growth pattern is characteristic (clear cell not seen) • Psammoma bodies may be present • Most common cytogenetic abnormality are - trisomy of chromosome 7, 16 & 17 and loss of Y in male patients in sporadic form - trisomy 7 in familial form • Q Striking characteristic of tumor is: **Tendency to invade the renal vein** and grow as a solid column of cells within the vessels. Extension may produce a continuous cord of tumor in IVC and even in the right side of heart.	• Least common (5%) • Pale eosinophilic cytoplasm • Multiple chromosomal losses and extreme haploploidy

Classic Triad of Renal cell carcinoma

Classic Triad of Renal cell carcinoma (seen in 10-20% of patients)
• *Hematuria (Gross)*
• *Pain (Abdominal / Flank)*
• *Mass (Abdominal / Flank)*

Paraneoplastic Syndromes is Renal Cell Carcinoma

Paraneoplastic Syndromes is Renal Cell Carcinoma

Characteristic Paraneoplastic Syndromes (common)	Other Paraneoplastic Syndromes (Less common / Not characteristic)
• ***Erythrocytes/Polycythemia*** (due to ↑ed erythropoietin) • ***Hypercalcemia*** (due to ↑ed parathyroid related peptide) • ***Hypertension*** (due to ↑ed rennin production) • *Non metastatic Hepatic Dysfunction (Stauffer syndrome)* (due to ↑ed granulocyte-macrophage colony stimulating factor)	• Cushing's syndrome (due to ↑ ACTH production) • Galactorrhea (due to ↑ed prolactin production) • Hypoglycemia (due to ↑ed Insulin) • Gynaecomastia & decreased libido (due to ↑ gonadotropins) • Hirsuitism, amenorrhea and male pattern balding (due to ↑ gonadotropins) • Amyloidosis • Leukemoid Reaction and Eosinophilia • Dysfibrinogenemia

Note that while Harison's textbook does not include Cushing's syndrome in the list of paraneoplastic syndromes associated with Renal cell carcinoma, this condition is clearly mentioned as an associated paraneoplastic syndrome in other standard textbooks like Robbin's and Smith's Urology.

Wilm's Tumor

Typical Congenital Malformations seen in association with Wilm's Tumor:

Wilm's Tumor

The risk of Wilm's tumor is increased in associations with at least three recognizable groups of congenital malformations associated with distinct chromosomal loci

WAGR syndrome

Characterized by:
- *Wilm's tumor*
- ***Aniridia***
- *Genital Anomalies*
- *Retardation (Mental)*

Denys Drash Syndrome

Characterized by:
- *Gonadal Dysgenesis* ***(male pseudohermaphroditism)***
- *Early onset nephropathy (diffuse mesangial sclerosis/renal failure)*

Beckwith Wiedemann Syndrome

Characterized by:
- *Organomegaly*
- *Macroglossia*
- ***Hemihypertrophy***
- *Omphalocele*
- *Adrenal cytomegaly (Abnormal large cells in Adrenal cortex)*

Staging Systems used for the staging of Wilm's Tumor

Two Staging Systems are currently being used for the staging of Wilm's Tumor

Pre-chemotherapy Staging System

- *Developed by the National Wilm's Tumor staging Group (NWTSG) (NWTSG – Staging system)*
- This staging system is widely used in North America and Canada
- *'NWTSG' approach involves employment of 'primary Surgery'. Chemotherapy with or without Radiation therapy is given after surgery*
- ***Staging is done at time of surgery (Pre – chemotherapy)***
- Primary advantage is more accurate staging

Post-chemotherapy Staging System

- *Developed by the International Society of Pediatric Oncology (SIOP) (SIOP – Staging system)*
- This staging system is widely used in Europe
- 'SIOP' Approach involves employment of preoperative chemotherapy without histological confirmation of Wilm's tumor. (Primary chemotherapy for all patients regardless of extent)
- ***Staging is done at time of surgery (Post-chemotherapy)***
- Primary advantage is easier surgical removal of tumor with decreased tumor rupture due to shrinkage of tumor by preoperative chemotherapy

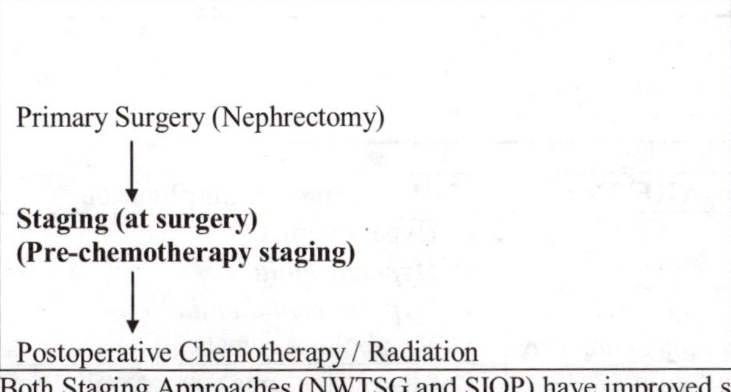

Primary Chemotherapy (Preoperative)
↓
Surgery (Nephrectomy)
↓
Staging (at surgery)
(Post-chemotherapy staging)
↓
Postoperative chemotherapy / Radiation

Both Staging Approaches (NWTSG and SIOP) have improved survival for patients with Wilm's tumor Success rates of treatment with both approaches are comparable

Rhabdomyolysis /Crush Syndrome

Rhabdomyolysis

Rhabdomyolysis

Clinical Triad
- Myalgias/Tender muscles
- Weakness (often proximal)
- Dark urine

Release of cellular content of muscle into ECF
- ↑ K+ → Hyperkalemia (cardiac arrhythmias)
- ↑ P → Hyperphospatemia
- ↑ Uric acid → Hyperuricemia
- ↑ Lactic acid → Metabolic Acidosis
- ↑ Thromboplastin → DIC
- ↑ Myoglobin → Myoglobinuria
- ↑ Creatine/↑ Creatine kinase

Uptake of ECF and other substances into the muscle
- ↓ ECF
  Movement of large amount of ECF into muscle induces ECF contraction and swelling of muscle predisposing to compartment syndrome.
- ↓Albumin (Hypoalbuminemia)
  Hypoalbuminemia may occur from leakage of plasma albumin across injured capillaries into muscle.

Hypocalcemia[Q]
Hyperphosphatemia promotes deposition of calcium phosphate in injured muscle thereby contributing to Hypocalcemia

Cardiac Arrhythmias
These may develop due to hyperkalemia

Renal failure & pigment nephropathy[Q]
↑ed Myoglobin, ECF contraction and systemic acidosis contribute to pigment nephropathy
- ↑ Blood urea
- ↑ Creatinine
- Tubular cast formation

Classical Triad of Crush Syndrome

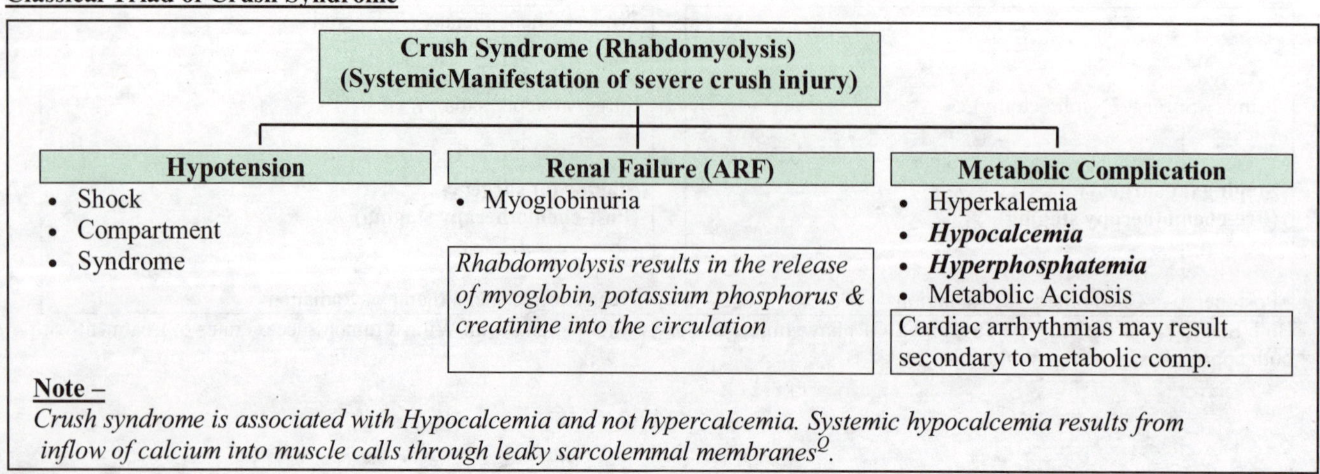

Crush Syndrome (Rhabdomyolysis)
(SystemicManifestation of severe crush injury)

Hypotension
- Shock
- Compartment
- Syndrome

Renal Failure (ARF)
- Myoglobinuria

Rhabdomyolysis results in the release of myoglobin, potassium phosphorus & creatinine into the circulation

Metabolic Complication
- Hyperkalemia
- ***Hypocalcemia***
- ***Hyperphosphatemia***
- Metabolic Acidosis

Cardiac arrhythmias may result secondary to metabolic comp.

Note –
Crush syndrome is associated with Hypocalcemia and not hypercalcemia. Systemic hypocalcemia results from inflow of calcium into muscle calls through leaky sarcolemmal membranes[Q].

Ureteropelvic Junction Obstruction (UPJ Obstruction)

Ureteropelvic Junction Obstruction (UPJ Obstruction)

- UPJ obstruction is the *most common obstructive lesion in childhood*[Q] and is the *most common cause of hydronephrosis found on prenatal and early postnatal ultrasonography*[Q].
- It is most commonly caused by intrinsic stenosis of a segment of ureter which is usually localized to the region of pelviureteric junction. Other causes include ureteric folds & extrinsic obstruction by crossing lower pole vessels.

Presentation

- ***Hydronephrosis*** revealed by maternal USG ***(Dilated renal pelvis but normal ureter)***
- Palpable Renal Mass in new borns or infants
- ***Abdominal flank or Back pain typically*** exacerbated by drinking large volumes of liquid
- UTI / Haematuria after minimal trauma

Epidemiology

- Left side more commonly involved than right (Bilateral = 10%)
- Male more commonly involved than females (M:F= 2:1)

Initial Diagnosis by Ultrasonography

- ***Hydronephrosis with dilated renal pelvis***
- Ureter if visualized is of normal caliber (not delated)

Renal Differential function

Nuclear Renography is used to determine Renal Differential function

- ***A differential function of <40% is considered significant and often an indication for surgical management***
- *Differential function of < 10% is often considered an arbitrary cut off for nephrectomy*

Management of PUJ

Conservative

Differential Renal function > 40% is usually managed conservatively especially when AP diameter of PUJ < 30 mm

Surgical

- Differential Renal Function < 40% is usually an indication of surgical management especially if AP diameter of PUJ > 30 mm
- Deteriorating Renal function (a decrease in differential function by more than 10% on follow up USS).
- Persistant symptoms of pain, UTI
- Concern that the function of kidney will decline if it is left untreated (AP diameter of renal pelvis may indicate this).

Procedure of choice

Pyeloplasty is the surgical procedure of choice

- ***Open pyeloplasty is considered the traditional gold standard***
- Laporascopic pyeloplasty is gaining growing acceptance

Other procedures

- External Drainage (Nephrostomy)
- Endopyelotomy
- Nephrectomy

External Drainage (Nephrostomy)

This is used to provide temporary drainage particularly when children present with pyonephrosis or ***when differential renal function is <10-15%*** to assess potential recovery of function before considering definitive surgery.

Endopyelotomy

Endopyelotomy involves incising the UPJ junction by either a retrograde or antegrade route, by a minimally invasive approach. ***The success rate is inferior to open pyeloplasty. A large hydronephrosis and differential renal function <20% are considered relative contraindications for Endopyelotomy.***

Nephrectomy

Nephrectomy may be considered when renal differential function is very low and the likelihood of functionl recovery is minimal. ***Most pediatric urologists consider an arbitrary cut off for differential function in the range of 10-15%.*** However a reconstructive procedure (pyeloplasty) should always be considered as the procedure of choice to salvage the kidney.

Hepatorenal Syndrome

Hepatorenal syndrome

- Hepatorenal syndrome is defined as a state of functional renal failure (Reduced GFR) in patients with severe liver disease
- ***Structurally /Histologically the kidneys are normal and recover function after successful liver transplantation.***
- The pathogenetic hallmark of hepatorenal syndrome is intense renal vasoconstriction with coexistent systemic vasodilatation
- The diagnosis of hepatorenal syndrome is considered in accordance with the following diagnostic criteria.

Diagnostic of Hepatorenal Syndrome
Major criteria
• *Low glomerular filtration rate, as indicated by serum creatinine > 1.5 mg/dL or 24-hr creatinine clearance < 40 mL/min*
• *Absence of shock, ongoing bacterial infection, fluid losses, and current treatment with nephrotoxic drugs*
• *No sustained improvement in renal function (decrease in serum creatinine to 1.5 mg/dL or increase in creatinine clearance to 40 mL/min) after diuretic withdrawal and expansion of plasma volume with 1.5L of a plasma expander*
• *Proteinuria <500 mg/dL and no ultrasonographic evidence of obstructive uropathy or parenchymal renal disease*
Additional criteria
• *Urine volume < 500 mL/d*
• *Urine sodium < 10 meq/L*
• *Urine osmolality greater than plasma osmolality*
• *Urine red blood cells <50/high- power field*
• *Serum sodium concentration < 130 mEqL*
Note: All major criteria must be present for the diagnosis of hepatorenal syndrome. Additional criteria are not necessary for the diagnosis but provide supportive evidence.

QUESTIONS

Urinalysis

1. Urinalysis shows RBC casts; likely source is : *(AI 2001)*
   A. Kidney
   B. Ureter
   C. Bladder
   D. Urethra
2. Presence of which of the following in the urine is diagnostic of glomerular injury: *(AIIMS- June 99)*
   A. Bright red cells
   B. 20% dysmorphic RBC's
   C. 100 RBC per high power field
   D. beta 2 micro globulin
3. Feature of glomerular haematuria (select two options): *PGI June 05)*
   A. Dysmorphic R.B.C
   B. Fragmented R.B.C.
   C. Full of R.B.C.
   D. Gross haematuria
   E. R.B.C. cast
4. Presence of which of the following in the urine is diagnostic of glomerular injury: *(AIIMS June 99)*
   A. Bright red cells
   B. 20% dysmorphic RBC's
   C. 100 RBC per high power field
   D. Beta 2 micro globulin
5. In hematuria of glomerular origin the urine is characterized by the presence of all of the following *except*: *(AI 2004)*
   A. Red cell casts
   B. Acanthocytes
   C. Crenated red cells
   D. Dysmorphic red cells
6. Recurrent gross hematuria is seen in (select two best options): *(PGI Dec 2000)*
   A. Alports's syndrome
   B. IgA nephropathy
   C: Focal segmental glomerulosclerosis
   D. Membranous nephropathy
7. Presence of which of the following correlates best with renal pathology *(AIIMS June 2000)*
   A. Hyaline cast
   B. Coarse granular cast
   C. Broad cast
   D. Epithelial cast
8. Which of the following is indicative of renal tubular disease *(AIIMS May 01)*
   A. Hyaline casts
   B. Coarse granular casts
   C. Cystine Oxalate cells
   D. White cell casts
9. A boy is suffering from acute pyelonephritis. Most specific urinary finding will be- *(AIIMS May 07)*
   A. W.B.C. casts
   B. Leucocyte esterase test
   C. Nitrite test
   D. Bacteria in gram stain
10. Acute pyelonephritis and uncomplicated UTI may be differentiated by all of the following Except : *(AI 2008)*
    A. WBC cast
    B. Concentrating defect
    C. Organisms in excess of 100,000 cfu/ml
    D. Antibody to Tomm Horsfall protein
11. In differentiating Glomerular proteinuria from Tubular proteinuria, Glomerular proteinuria is indicated by: *(PGI June 05)*
    A. Proteinuria >3.0 – 3.5 g/day
    B. Globulin > Albumin
    C. Albumin to β2 microglobulin ratio of 100:1
    D. Tomm Harsfall protein
12. Which of the following statements about orthostatic proteinuria is true: *(PGI Dec 2000)*
    A. Seen in recumbent position
    B. Is benign
    C. Future risk of nephrotic syndrome
    D. < 300 mg/day
13. Bence Jones proteins are derived from: *(AI 2010)*
    A. Alpha Globulins
    B. Beta Globulins
    C. Gamma Globulins
    D. Delta Globulins
14. Bence Jones proteinuria may be seen in: *(AI 2010)*
    A. Alpha heavy chain disease
    B. Gamma heavy chain disease
    C. 'Mu' heavy chain disease
    D. Epsilon heavy chain disease
15. In a child, non-functioning kidney is best diagnosed by: *AI 2005)*
    A. Ultrasonography.
    B. IVU.
    C. DTPA renogram.
    D. Creatinine clearance.
16. A patient presented with ARF with complete anuria, but a normal ultrasound. Next investigation is: *(AI 99)*
    A. IVP
    B. Antegrade pyelography
    C. Retrograde pyelography
    D. Radio renogram
17. A patient presents with acute renal failure with normal ultrasound abdomen report. Next most useful investigation is : *(AIIMS June 99)*
    A. Intravenous pyelography

B. DTPA scan
C. Retrograde pyelography
D. X-ray abdomen and CT scan.

18. In urinary system disease, GI symptoms appears because of : *(AIIMS June 98)*
A. Chemical reaction
B. Renogastric reflex
C. Peritoneal reaction
D. Reflux phenomenon

19. Which of the following best methods of urine collection is associated with least contamination : *(AI 2008)*
A. Suprapubic aspiration
B. Mid stream collection
C. Catheterization
D. Urine Bag specimen

20. Coloured urine is not seen in : *(AI 2008)*
A. Quinine
B. Rifampcin
C. Nitrofurantoin
D. Pyridium

21. Creatinine Clearance test is used to assess:
A. Glomerular Filtration
B. Proximal Tubulr Function
C. Distal Tubular Function
D. Renal Plasma Flow

22. Which of the following is the most accurate method to assess decline in GFR during initial stages of Renal insufficiency *(DNB / NEET June 2009)*
A. Serum creatinine
B. Creatinine Clearance
C. Serum BUN
D. Serum Urea

23. Which of the following statements about creatinine clearance test is true: *(DNB June 2009)*
A. Creatinine clearance test is the most accurate / gold standard test for assessing GFR
B. Creatinine clearance may overestimate the actual GFR as renal function declines
C. Creatinine clearance may underestimate the actual GFR as renal function declines
D. Creatinine clearance is more accurate than Inulin clearance in estimating GFR

24. Water Deprivation Test is used to assess *(DNB/NEET)*
A. Glomerular Function
B. Proximal Tubular Function
C. Distal Tubular Function
D. Renal Plasma Flow

Renal Failure & Tubulointerstitial Diseases

Acute Renal Failure:

25. Most unlikely cause of acute tubular necrosis amongst the following is : *(AI 1999)*
A. Severe-bacterial-infection
B. Massive burn
C. Severe crush injury in the foot
D. Rupture of aortic aneurysm

26. Causes of Acute Tubular necrosis include: *(PGI June 07)*
A. Radiocontrast agents
B. Psrsproteins
C. Amphoterecin B
D. Abruptio placentae
E. All of the above

27. Which of the following values are suggestive of acute tubular necrosis : *(AIIMS Nov. 2000)*
A. Urine osmolality>500
B. Urine sodium>40
C. Blood urea nitrogen/plasma creatinine>20
D. Urine creatinine /plasma creatinine>40

28. Fractional excretion of sodium <1 is seen in *(AIIMS Nov- 07)*
A. Prerenal azotemia
B. Acute tubular necrosis
C. Acute ureteral obstruction
D. Interstitial nephritis

29. Pre-renal azotemia is associated with one of the following characteristic feature : *(AIIMS Nov. 2000)*
A. Urinary $Na^+ < 10$ mmol/L
B. Renal failure index > 1
C. Osmolality < 500
D. Urinary creatinine / P. creatinine ratio < 20

30. Pre-Renal Azotemia is characterized by all of the following. Except : *(AI 2010)*
A. Fractional Excretion of Na < 1%
B. Urinary osmolality > 500 mosm/kg
C. Urinary sodium concentration > 40 meq/l
D. Reversible with replacement fluids

31. Plasma urea / creatinine ratio of 20:1 may be seen in : *(AI 2010)*
A. Rhabdomyolysis
B. Ureteric calculi
C. Pre-renal failure
D. Chronic Glomerulonephritis

32. Prerenal and renal azotemia is differentiated on the basis of: *(PGI Dec 99)*
A. Creatinine clearance
B. Serum creatinine level
C. Sodium fraction excretion
D. Urine bicarbonate level

33. In tubular necrosis, ratio of urine to plasma creatinine is: *(PGI Dec 99)*
A. 20
B. 40
C. 20-30
D. 30-40

34. Which of the following is true about Acute Tubular Necrosis *(PGI June 07)*
A. Urine specific gravity > 1.020
B. Urine osmolality >350 mosmol/kg
C. Urine Na < 10meq/L
D. Blood urea : creatinine ratio < 20

35. All of the following are true about Prerenal Azotemia, Except: *(PGI June 05)*
A. Urinary Cr/Plasma Cr >40
B. FE_{Na} < 1
C. Urinary output < 400ml/day
D. Plasma BUN/Creatinine ratio <20
E. Urinary sodium concentration < 20meq/l

36. Which differentiating prerenal azotemia with ATN features favouring pre-renal azotemia (select two options): *(PGI Dec 2002)*
A. Urine osmolality > 500 mosmol/kg
B. Sodium <10 mmol/l
C. Plasma transferrin/Ig ratio
D. Fractional excretion of sodium >1
E. Plasma BUN/creatinine ratio < 20

37. All of the following are true about Oliguric ARF
A. Anemia *(AI-1993)*
B. Metabolic Acidosis
C. Uremia
D. Hypercalcemia

38. Oliguric phase of renal failure, all are TRUE, EXCEPT: *(AIIMS May 93)*
A. Hypercalcemia
B. Hyponatremia
C. Anaemia
D. Hyperkalemia

39. Non Oliguric Acute Renal Failure is typically associated with *(DNB / NEET Dec 2011)*
A. Aminoglycoside toxicity
B. Contrast Induced Nephrotoxity
C. Hemolytic Uremic syndrome
D. Glomerulonephritis

40. All of the following are seen in oliguric phase of Acute Tubular necrosis, Except: *(AI 1992)*
A. Hypernatremia
B. Hypermagnesemia
C. Hyper uricemia
D. Hyper phosphatemia

41. Hypophosphatemia is seen in all except :
A. Acute renal failure *(AI 2007)*
B. Resolving phases of diabetic ketocidosis
C. Respiratory alkalosis / COPD
D. Chronic alcoholism

Chronic Renal Failure

42. Feature of CRF include all, except: *(PGI June 05)*
A. Impotence
B. Restless legs
C. Isothenuria
D. Broad cast in urine
E. All of the above

43. Decrease in GFR is apparent in which of the following stages of Chronic Kidney Disease
A. Stage I *(DNB / NEET)*
B. Stage II
C. Stage III
D. Stage IV

44. Signs and symptoms of a Renal Failure are evident when Renal function deteriorates by more than:
A. 40% *(DNB / NEET)*
B. 50%
C. 60%
D. 80%

45. Overt symptoms of Renal failure become evident when Renal Function Deteriorates by more than
A. 40-50% *(DNB / NEET)*
B. 50-60%
C. 70-80%
D. >90%

46. Restless leg syndrome (RLS) is seen in: *(AI 2009)*
A. Hypercalcemia
B. Hyperphosphatemia
C. Chronic renal failure
D. Hyperkalemia

47. Central nervous system manifestation in chronic renal failure are result of all of the following, *except*:
A. Hyperosmolarity *(AI 2003)*
B. Hypocalcemia
C. Acidosis
D. Hyponatremia

48. Chronic Renal Diseases / failure is commonly associated with *(DNB / NEET)*
A. Metabolic Acidosis
B. Metabolic Acidosis
C. Respiratory Acidosis
D. Respiratory Acidosis

49. Metabolic complication in CRF include all of the following *except* : *(AI 1998)*
A. Hyperkalemia
B. Hypophosphatemia
C. Hypocalcemia
D. Hypokalemia

50. Which of the following metabolic complications is not seen in Chronic Renal Failure: *(DNB Dec 2010)*
A. Hyperkalemia
B. Hyponatremia
C. Hypercalcemia
D. Hyperphosphatemia

51. Renal osteodystropy differs from nutritional and genetic forms of osesteomalacia in having :
A. Hypocalcaemia *(AI 2002)*
B. Hypercalcemia
C. Hypophostaemia
D. Hyperphosphatemia

52. Which of the following types of glomerulonephritis is least likely to cause CRF: *(AI 1999)*
A. Post streptococcal glomerulonephritis
B. Membranous GN
C. Membrano proliferative GN
D. Focal segmental glomerulosclerosis

4

Kidney and Urinary Tract

53. Nail and half nail sign, seen in uremia is
A. Due to melanin deposition (AIIMS May- 07)
B. Increased capillary density at the distal half of nails
C. Hypoproteinemia
D. Circulating toxin

54. All improves after dialysis except: (AIIMS Nov 08)
A. Pericarditis
B. Peripheral neuropathy
C. Metabolic acidosis
D. Seizure

55. A girl aged 8 years has been admitted for dialysis. She has serum K of 7.5 meq/l, which is the fastest way to reduce the hyperkalemia? (AI 2009)
A. Kayexalate enema
B. Infusion of insulin + glucose
C. IV calcium gluconate
D. IV $NaHCO_3$

56. A patient in Chronic renal failure presents with tall peaked T waves on ECG. Management includes: (select two options) (PGI June 05)
A. IV K-bicarbonate
B. KCl
C. $CaCl_2$
D. Sodium bicarbonate

57. All of the following are used for treatment of hyperkalaemia except : (AIIMS May' 06)
A. Calcium gluconate
B. Sodium bicarbonate
C. Intravenous infusion of glucose with insulin
D. Beta blockers

Tubulointestinal Disease

58. Interstitial nephritis is seen with all except:
A. Beta lactam inhibitors (AIIMS May 07)
B. INH
C. Diuretics
D. Allopurinol

59. Salt losing nephritis is a feature of : (AI 2000)
A. Interstitial nephritis (AIIMS 95)
B. Renal Amyloidosis (AIIMS May 94)
C. Lupus nephritis
D. Post Streptococcal Glomerulonephritis

60. Necrotizing papilities is seen in all of the following except: (AIIMS May 02)
A. Salicylate poisoning
B. Renal vascular thrombosis
C. PNH
D. Diabetes mellitus

61. Necrotizing pappillitis may be seen in all of the following conditions *except* : (AI 2002)
A. Sickle cell disease
B. Tuberculous pyelonephritis
C. Diabetes mellitus
D. Analgesic nephropathy

62. Necrotizing pappillitis is seen in : (AIIMS 2002)
A. Salicylate poisoning
B. Glomerulonephritis
C. PNH
D. Diabetes insipidus

63. Necrotizing pappillitis is seen in all of the following *except* : (AIIMS May 02)
A. Salicylate poisoning
B. Renal vascular thrombosis
C. PNH
D. Diabetes mellitus

64. Renal papillary necrosis is almost always associated with one of the following conditions :
A. Diabetes-mellitus (AI 99)
B. Analgesic-nephropathy
C. Chronic pyelonephritis
D. Post streptococcal GN

65. Which of the following is associated with Renal Papillary Necrosis
A. Alcohol
B. Heroine
C. Morphine
D. Tramadol

Glomerular Diseases

Nephrotic Syndrome

66. All are true of Nephrotic syndrome, *except* :
A. RBC casts in urine (AI 2000)
B. Hypo-proteinemia
C. Oedema
D. Hyperlipidemia

67. All of the following are decreased in Nephrotic syndrome *except* : (AI 1997)
A. Transferrin
B. Ceruloplasmin
C. Albumin
D. Fibrinogen

68. All of the following proteins are decreased in Nephrotic syndrome. Except (PGI 2012)
A. Transferrin
B. Fibrinogen
C. Albumin
D. Thyroxine Binding Globulin

69. All of the following are decreased in nephrotic syndrome *except* : (AIIMS 1998)
A. Serum transferrin
B. Serum fibrinogen
C. Serum ceruloplasmin
D. Serum albumin

70. Hypercoagulation in Nephrotic syndrome is caused by: (AI 2010)
A. Loss of Antithrombin III
B. Decreased Fibrinogen
C. Decreased Metabolism of Vitamin K
D. Increase in protein C

71. Which is seen in nephrotic syndrome (select two options): (PGI June 99)
   A. Low serum calcium
   B. Raised AT – III
   C. Low lipid
   D. Platelet activation
72. Nephrotic syndrome may be associated with:
   A. ↓ Total cholesterol (PGI 2000)
   B. ↓ LDL cholesterol
   C. ↓ VLDL cholesterol
   D. ↓ Triglycerides
   E. ↓ HDL cholesterol
73. Most common cause of nephrotic range proteinuria in an adult is: (AI 2007)
   A. Diabetes Mellitus
   B. Amyloidosis
   C. Hypertensive nephropathy
   D. Wegner's Granulomatosis
74. The Finnish type of congenital nephrotic syndrome occurs due to gene mutations the following protein:
   A. Podocin (AI 2009, 08)
   B. Alpha – actinin
   C. Nephrin
   D. CD2 activated protein
75. A patient with nephrotic syndrome on longstanding corticosteroid therapy may develop all the following *except*: (AI 2002)
   A. Hyperglycemia
   B. Hypertrophy of muscle
   C. Neuropsychiatric symptoms
   D. Suppression of the pituitary adrenal axis

Nephritic Syndrome and RPGN

76. Following are features of Acute GN except:
   A. Polyuria (PGI June 97)
   B. Hematuria
   C. Red cell cast
   D. Oliguria
77. Post-infective glomerulonephritis present as:
   A. ARF (AI 1996)
   B. Nephrotic syndrome
   C. Nephritic syndrome
   D. Asymptomatic hematuria
78. Cresentirc Glomerulonephritis may be seen in all of the following Except? (AI 2008)
   A. Post Streptococcal Glomerulonephritis (PSGN)
   B. Henoch Schonlein Purpura (HSP)
   C. Anti Basement Membrane Disease
   D. Alport syndrome
79. Crescent formation is characteristic of the following glomerular disease: (AI-2002)
   A. Minimal change disease
   B. Rapidly progressive glomerulonephritis
   C. Focal and segmental glomerulonephritis
   D. Rapidly non progressive glomerulonephritis
80. All can cause R.P.G.N., *except* : (AIIMS June 97)
   A. Minimal change glomerulonephritis
   B. Poststreptococcal glomerulonephritis
   C. Wegener granulomatosis
   D. S.L.E.
81. RPGN occurs in A/E: (AIIMS Sep 96)
   A. SLE
   B. Post streptococcal glomerulonephritis
   C. Diabetic nephropathy
   D. Good pastures syndromes
82. Which of the following conditions are assoiciated with pauci – immune crescenteric glomerulonephritis:
   A. Henoch – Schonlein Nephritis (AI 2009)
   B. Lupus Nephritis (SLE)
   C. Microscopic polyangitis
   D. Nephritis in Alport's syndrome
83. All are features of RPGN *except*
   A. Rapid recovery (AIIMS June 1997)
   B. Crescent formation
   C. Hypertension
   D. Non-selective proteinuria
84. The prognosis of rapidly prolifeating glomerulonephritis (Crescentric GN) depends upon –
   A. Number of crescents (AIIMS Nov 01)
   B. Size of crescents
   C. Shape of crescents
   D. Cellularity of crescents
85. Non –proliferative Glomerulonephritis include all of the following, Except: (AI 2008)
   A. Focal Segmental Glomerulonephritis (FSGS)
   B. Mesangiocapillary Glomerulonephritis
   C. Membranous Glomerulonephritis
   D. Amyloidosis
86. A 30-year-old man presents with generalized edema and hypertension. Urine examination shows subnephrotic proteinuria (< 2gm) and microscopic hematuria. Serum complement levels are decreased and he is positive for anti-hepatitis C antibodies. The most likely diagnosis is: (AI 2012)
   A. Post streptococcal Glomerulonephritis (PSGN)
   B. Cryoglobulinemia
   C. Membranoproliferative Glomerulonephritis (MPGN)
   D. Focal Segmental Glomerular Sclerosis (FSGS)
87. A 60-year-old woman presents with generalized edema, skin ulceration and hypertension. Urine examination shows subnephrotic proteinuria (<2gm) and microscopic haematuria. Serum complement levels are decreased and she is positive for anti-hepatitis C antibodies. The likely diagnosis is: (AI 2012)
   A. Post-streptococcal Glomerulonephritis
   B. Essential Mixed Cryoglobulinemia
   C. Membranoproliferative Glomerulonephritis (MPGN)
   D. Focal SegmentalGlomerulosclerosis (FSGS)

IgA Nephropathy and PSGN

88. Which of the following is not true about Berger's disease? *(AI / AIIMS)*
   A. The pathological changes are proliferative and usually confined to mesangial cells; usually focal and segmental
   B. Hematuria may be gross or microscopic
   C. On immunofluorescence deposits contain both IgA and IgG
   D. Absence of associated proteinuria is pathognomonic

89. IgA-nephropathy is seen in: *(AIIMS June 2000)*
   A. Membranous glomerulonephritis
   B. Mesangioproliferative glomerulonephritis
   C. Focal glomerulonephritis
   D. Cresentic glomerulonephritis

90. Increased IgA deposits are seen in:
   A. Henoch Schonlein Purpura *(AIIMS June 2000)*
   B. Minimal Change Glomemlonephritis
   C. Chronic Pyelonephritis
   D. Haemolytic Uremic Syndrome

91. A 6 yr child presents with recurrent episodes of gross hematuria for 2 yrs. He is likely to have: *(AI 2008)*
   A. IgA nephropathy
   B. Wilm's tumour
   C. Henoch Schonlein Purpura (HSP)
   D. Neuroblastoma

92. A feature of Renal vaculitis in children is -
   A. IgA raised *(AIIMS- Sep- 96)*
   B. Antinuclear antibody in serum
   C. Low complement level
   D. Cytoplasmic antinuclear Ab in serum

93. Marker for the renal vasculitis in children is –
   A. Increased IgA level *(AI 98)*
   B. Low complement level
   C. ↑ Antineutrophilic cytoplasmic antibody titre
   D. Increase antinuclear antibody

94. 12 years old Shyam presented with gross hematuria with 80% dysmorphic RBC's 2 days after a attack of upper respiratory tract infection. Diagnosis is –
   A. Microangiopathic thrombotic anaemia
   B. IgA Nephropathy *(AIIMS Nov- 01)*
   C. PSGN
   D. H.S. purpura

95. A six year old male baby presents to a hospital with recurrent gross hematuria for 2 years. There is no h/o burning micturition or pyuria. Urine routine examination demonstrated no pus cells and urine culture was sterile. Serum C3 levels were normal. What is the most probable diagnosis –
   A. Wilm's tumour *(AIPGMEE-08)*
   B. IgA nephropathy
   C. Post –streptococcal glomerulonephritis
   D. Urinary tract infection

96. A young man develops gross heamaturia 3 days after an attack of URTI; likely renal pathology is: *(AI 2001)*
   A. Acute glomerulonephritis
   B. Minimal change disease
   C. IgA nephropathy
   D. Membranous glomerulonephritis.

97. A female patient Nandini presents with upper respiratory tract infection. After 15 days, she develops hematuria. Probable diagnosis is:
   A. IgA nephropathy *(AIIMS June 99)*
   B. Wegener's granulomatosis
   C. Henoch scholein purpura
   D. Post streptococcal glomerulonephritis.

98. True about Post-Streptococcal Glomerulonephritis is:
   A. 50% of cases occur after pharyngitis
   B. Early treatment of Pharyngitis eliminates the risk of P.S.G.N. *(AI 2000)*
   C. Glomerulonephritis, secondary to skin infection, is more common in summer
   D. Recurrence is seen

Goodpasture's Syndrome

99. A patient presents with hemoptysis and hematuria few weeks after a respiratory tract infection. ANCA antibodies are present. Likely diagnosis is:
   A. Goodpasture's syndrome *(AI 1995)*
   B. IgA Nephropathy
   C. Nephrotic syndrome
   D. PSGN

100. Rama, a 20 year old smoker, presents with hemoptysis and hematuria. Likely diagnosis is:
   A. Good pasture's syndrome *(AI 1997)*
   B. Nephrotic syndrome
   C. Gullian Barre syndrome
   D. IgA Nephropathy

101. Good pasture's syndrome is charachterized by:
   A. Anti-GBM antibodies *(PGI June 99)*
   B. Crescenteric glomerulonephritis
   C. Diffuse alveolar haemorrhage
   D. All of the above

102. Good pasture's syndrome is characterized by all of the following, except: *(AIIMS May 08)*
   A. Glomerulonephritis
   B. Leucocytoclastic Vasculitis
   C. Diffuse alveolar haemorrhage
   D. Presence of antibodies to Basement Membrane

Alport's Syndrome

103. Association of deafness & nephritis is seen in –
   A. Pickwickian syndrome *(AIIMS May 93)*
   B. Alport's syndrome
   C. Fabry's disease
   D. Lawrence Moon Biedl syndrome

104. A 25 year old boy presents with renal failure. His uncle died of renal failure three years ago. Slit lamp examination reveals Lenticonus / Keratoconus. The likely diagnosis is: *(AIIMS Nov 2010)*
   A. Autosomal Dominant Polycystic Kidney (ADPCKD)
   B. Autosomal Recessive polycystic kidney (ARPCKD)
   C. Alport's syndrome
   D. Denysh-Drash Syndrome
105. Mutation in alpha 5 chain of collagen 4. The diagnosis – *(AIIMS Nov- 06)*
   A. Alport's syndrome
   B. Thin membrane disease
   C. Nodular glomerulosclerosis
   D. Good pasture syndrome
106. Presenting manifestation of Alport syndrome is :
   A. Haematuria *(AIIMS Feb 97)*
   B. Proteinuria
   C. Oliguria
   D. Sensorineural deafness
107. Disease, does not recur in the kidney after renal transplant is : *(AIIMS Feb 97)*
   A. Alport syndrome
   B. Amyloidosis
   C. Good Pasteur's syndrome
   D. Diabetic nephropathy

Minimal Change Nephropathy

108. A 7 year old boy presented with generalized edema. Urine examination revealed marked albuminuria. Serum biochemical examinations showed hypoalbuminaemia with hyperlipidemia. Kidney biopsy was undertaken. On light microscopic examination, the kidney appeared normal. Electron microscopic examination is most likely to reveal –
   A. Fusion of foot processes of the glomerular epithelial cells *(AIIMS Nov-03)*
   B. Rarefaction of glomerular basement membrane
   C. Deposition of electron dense material in the basement membrane
   D. Thin basement membrane
109. A 7 year old girl is brought with complaints of generalized swelling of the body. Urinary examination reveals Grade 3 proteinuria and the presence of hyaline and fatty casts. She has no history of Hematuria. Which of the following statements about her condition is true: *(AI 2009)*
   A. No IgG deposits or C3 deposition on Renal biopsy
   B. Her C3 levels will be low
   C. IgA Nephropathy is the likely diagnosis
   D. Alport's syndrome is the likely diagnosis
110. True about light microscopy in minimal change disease is: *(AIIMS 2001)*
   A. Loss of foot process seen
   B. Anti GBM Abs seen
   C. IgA deposits seen
   D. No change seen
111. True about Light microscopic changes in Minimal Change Glomerulonephritis is: *(AI 95)*
   A. No abnormality
   B. Fusion of foot process
   C. Absence of Immunoglobulins
   D. Absence of complement
112. True about Minimal change disease is : *(AII Inida)*
   A. Appears normal under light microscopy but electron microscope shows loss of foot processes.
   B. Mesangial deposits
   C. Tram Track appearance
   D. Gross haematuria
113. A child presents with hematuria and nephrotic syndrome. A diagnosis of minimal change disease was made. Which of the following statements about the diagnosis is true: *(All India)*
   A. Glomerular function is lost due to loss of polyanions around the foot processes
   B. Foot processes of podocytes in the Glomerular membrane are normal
   C. Glomerular function is lost due to deposition of IgA on the glomerular membrane
   D. Focal segmental changes are observed
114. Typical features of Lipoid nephrosis include:
   A. Normal light microscopy *(PGI 2009)*
   B. FSGS
   C. Glomerular tuft sclerosis
   D. Effacement of foot processes
   E. Tubular sclerosis
115. Clinical features of minimal change : glomerulonephritis are *all except* *(AI 1996)*
   A. Hypertension
   B. Edema
   C. Selective proteinuria
   D. Fever
116. Minimal change glomerulopathy may be seen in association with all of the following except :
   A. Hepatitis B *(AIIMS Nov. 05)*
   B. HIV
   C. Drug - induced interstitial nephritis
   D. Hodgkin's disease
117. All are steroid resistant *except:* *(AI 96)*
   A. Post-streptococcal glomerulonephritis
   B. Minimal change glomerulonephritis
   C. RPGN
   D. Recurrent hematuria

Diabetic Glomerulopathy

118. Most common pathological features in diabetes mellitus is : *(AI 1998)*
   A. Papillary necrosis
   B. Diffuse glomerulosclerosing
   C. Renal atherosclerosis
   D. Chronic pyelonephritis
119. Which of the following is the first clinically detectable sign of diabetic nephropathy
   A. Serum creatinine
   B. Creatinine clearance
   C. Microalbuminuria
   D. Macroalbuminuria
120. Preferred method for determining microalbuminuria is:
   A. Urinary dipsticks
   B. 24 hour urinary protein collection
   C. Urinary A/C Ratio in a spot voided sample
   D. Urinary A/C Ratio in a 24 hour collection
121. Pathological changes of diabetic nephropathy are *all except:* *(AI 1995)*
   A. Fibrin caps and capsular drops
   B. Intercapillary glomerulosclerosis
   C. Focal sclerosis
   D. Capillary basement membrane thickening
122. The Recommended treatment of early diabetic nephropathy manifested by microalbuminuria is
   A. Strict glycemic control
   B. Low protein Diet
   C. Strict glycemic control and Low Protein Diet
   D. Strict glycemic control, Low protein Diet and ACE Inhibitors

HIV Glomerulopathy

123. Most characteristic GN in HIV is: *(PGI Dec99)*
   A. FSGN
   B. MPGN
   C. MCD
   D. RPGN
124. HIV associated nephropathy is a type of:
   A. Membranous glomerulonephritis *(AIIMS Nov 04)*
   B. Immunotaetoid glomerulopathy
   C. Collapsing glomerulopathy
   D. Fibrillary glomerulopathy
125. Collapsing glomerulopathy, features –
   A. Tuft necrosis
   B. Mesangiolysis
   C. Proliferation of parietal epithelium cells
   D. Hypertrophy of visceral epithelium cells

Lupus nephritis

126. In Lupus nephritis, characteristic kidney lesion is:
   A. Mesangial proliferation *(PGI Dec 98)*
   B. Tubular fibrin deposits
   C. Wire loop lesions
   D. IgG deposits
127. Wire loop lesions are often characteristic for the following class of lupus nephritis: *(AIIMS May 04)*
   A. Mesangial proliferative glomerulonephritis(WHO class II)
   B. Focal proliferative glomerulonephritis (WHO class III)
   C. Diffuse proliferative glomerulonephritis (WHO class IV)
   D. Membranous glomerulonephritis (WHO class V)
128. All of the following factors are associated with adverse prognosis and high risk of Renal progression in Lupus Nephritis, Except: *(PGI Dec 03)*
   A. High levels of Anti-ds DNA
   B. Persistant proteinuria (Nephrotic range > 3gm/day)
   C. Hypocomplementenemia
   D. Anti LA (SSB)

Amyloid Nephropathy

129. A patient who has been diagnosed with bronchiectasis 5 years ago presents with edema on legs and proteinuria. The most likely finding in his kidney will be: (AI 2012)
   A. Minimal Change Disease
   B. Amyloid Nephropathy
   C. Rapidly Progressive Glomerulonephritis (RPGN)
   D. Crescenteric Glomerulonephritis

Leprotic Glomerulopathy

130. In Leprosy most common renal lesion seen is:
   A. MGN *(AI 1999)*
   B. MPGN
   C. Focal glomeruloselerosis
   D. Diffuse glomerulosclerosis

Miscellaneous Glomerulonephritis

131. Reflux Nephropathy with protenuria in the nephrotic range may be seen in patients with : *(AIIMS Nov 06)*
   A. Membranous glomerulonephritis
   B. Focal segmental Glomerulosclerosis
   C. Nodular glomerulosclerosis
   D. Crescenteric glomerulonephritis
132. A 30 year old man presents with generalized edema and hypertension. Urine examination shows subnephrotic proteinuria (< 2gm) and microscopic hematuria. Serum complement levels are decreased and he is positive for antihepatitis C antibodies. The most likely diagnosis is : *(AI 2007)*
   A. Post streptococcal Glomerulonephritis (PSGN)
   B. Mixed cryoglobulinemia
   C. Membranoproliferative glomerulonephritis (MPGN)
   D. Focal symentat Glomerular sclerosis (FSGS)

133. A 60 year old woman presents with generalized edema, skin ulceration and hypertension. Urine examination shows subnephrotic proteinuria (<2gm) and microscopic haematuria. Serum complement levels are decreased and she is positive for anti-hepatitis C antibodies. The likely diagnosis is : *(AI 2007)*
A. PSGN
B. Essential mixed cryoglobulinemia
C. Membrano proliferative glomerulonephritis
D. Focal segmental glomerulosclerosis

134. Serum C3 is persistently low in the following except: *(AI / AIIMS)*
A. Post streptococcal glomerulonephritis
B. Membranoproliferative glomerulonephritis
C. Lupus nephritis
D. Glomerulonephritis related to bacterial endocarditis

135. All of the following are associated with low complement levels *except*: *(AII India)*
A. Lupus nephritis
B. Mesangio capillary glomerulonephritis
C. Diarrhea-associated hemolytic uremic syndrome
D. Post-infections glomerulonephritis

136. Hypocomplementemia is seen (select three options): *(PGI June 2008)*
A. PSGN
B. Membranous GN
C. Focal segmental DN
D. MPGN
E. Infective endocarditis.

137. Non –proliferative Glomerulonephritis include all of the following, Except: *(AI 2008)*
A. Focal Segmental Glomerulonephritis (FSGS)
B. Mesangiocapillary Glomerulonephritis
C. Membranous Glomerulonephritis
D. Amyloidosis

138. Proliferative glomerular deposits in kidney are found in *(AI-2000)*
A. Amyloidosis
B. Diabetes mellitus
C. IgA nephropathy
D. Membranous glomerulonephritis

Renal Tubular Acidosis

139. Type II RTA is associated with all of the following, EXCEPT *(AI-1990)*
A. Normal Anion Gap Acidosis
B. Hyper calciuria
C. Decreased urinary citrate
D. Minimum urinary pH < 5.5

140. Type IRTA is associated with all of the following, Except: *(AI 1993)*
A. Urinary PH > 5.5
B. Normal Anion Gap Acidosis
C. ↑ urinary calcium
D. ↑ urinary citrate

141. Which of the statements about Renal Tubular Acidosis type I (Type I RTA) is not true: *(AI 2012)*
A. Failure to acidify urine to a pH < 5
B. Associated with increased risk of urinary stones
C. Associated with Hyperkalemia
D. Treatment involves alkali replacement as bicarbonate

142. Proximal & distal renal tubular acidosis is differentiated by all, except: *(AIIMS June 98)*
A. Stones in kidney
B. Hypokalemia
C. Daily acid secretion
D. Presence of Fanconi syndrome

143. All are features of renal tubular acidosis type I, except : *(AIIMS Sept 96)*
A. Stone in kidney
B. No anion gap
C. Hypokalemia
D. Fanconi syndrome

144. Positive Urinary Anion Gap helps to establish the diagnosis of : *(AI 2009)*
A. Alcoholic ketoacidosis
B. Diabetic ketoacidosis
C. Renal tubular Acidosis
D. Acidosis in Diarrhea

Disorders of Renal Vasculature

HUS

145. An 8 yrs old boy presents to casualty with history of diarrhoea, followed by decreased urine output. Blood examination shows thrombocytes 90,000/cm^3. Diagnosis is : *(AI 2000)*
A. Hemolytic Uremic Syndrome.
B. Disseminated Intravascular Coagulation
C. Hemophilia
D. Idiopathic Thrombocytopenic Purpura

146. Which of the following statements about Hemolytic Uremic Syndrome is least correct: *(AI 2012)*
A. Usually follows Haemorrhagic colitis
B. Often self-limited
C. Fever is usually mild or absent
D. Serotoxin has no role in pathogenesis

147. All are features of haemolytic uremic syndrome, *except*: *(AIIMS Dec 95)*
A. Hyperkalemia
B. Anaemia
C. Renal microthrombi
D. Neuropsychiatric disturbances

148. All of the following statements are true about Hemolytic uremic syndrome *except* : *(AI 1997)*
A. Uraemia
B. Hypofibrinogenemia
C. Thrombocytopenia
D. Positive coomb's test

149. A 20 year old male presents with features of acute renal failure 5 days after an episode of diarrhea. Blood examination shows thrombocytopenia and Hb-10 gm%. Likely cause is: *(AIIMS June 99)*
   A. Haemolytic uremic syndrome
   B. Hereditary spherocytosis
   C. Haemolytic crises
   D. Chronic glomerulonephritis

Benign /Malignant Hypertension

150. Which of the following changes does not occur in malignant hypertension : *(AI 2008)*
   A. Peticheal Haemorrhages on cortical surface
   B. Fibrinoid necrosis of arterioles
   C. Intimal concentric thickening
   D. Hyaline arteriosclerosis
151. Commonest histoloical finding in Benign Hypertension is: *(AI 2009)*
   A. Proliferative endarteritis
   B. Necrotizing arteriolitis
   C. Hyaline arteriosclerosis
   D. Cystic Medial Necrosis
152. Which characteristic feature is seen in the kidney in Malignant hypertension: *(AI 1994)*
   A. Hyaline necrosis
   B. Fibrinoid necrosis
   C. Medial wall hyperplasia
   D. Micro-aneurysm
153. Common pathological changes seen in kidney in benign hypertension are: *(AI 97)*
   A. Fibronoid necrosis
   B. Microaneurysm
   C. Hyaline arteriosclerosis
   D. Thining of walls

Renovascular Hypertension

154. Which of the following is the most specific and sensitive screening test for Renovascular Hypertension. *(AIIMS May 01)*
   A. HRCT
   B. CT Angiography
   C. Captopril enhanced radionucleatide scan
   D. MRI
155. Which of the following is the most specific screening test for renovascular hypertension: *(PGI 2008)*
   A. Magnetic Resonance Angiography (MRA)
   B. Spiral Computed Tomographic Angiography (CT Angiography)
   C. Captopril induced Radionucleotide Scan (Captopril Renogram)
   D. Duplex Doppler Ultrasonography
156. Most common cause of renal artery stenosis in young adults in India is: *(AIIMS Dec 97)*
   A. Atherosclerosis
   B. Non specific aorto-arteritis
   C. Fibro muscular dysplasia
   D. None of the above
157. Renal artery stenosis may occur in all of the following except: *(AI 2006)*
   A. Atherosclerosis
   B. Fibromuscular dysplasia
   C. Takayasu's arteritis
   D. Polyarteritis nodosa
158. A 20 year old female presents with a blood pressure of 160/110 mm Hg. Clinical examination reveals a bruit in both flanks. Which of the following statements about this patient is not true (select one option) *(PGI 09)*
   A. Enalapril may deteriorate renal function
   B. Most definitive diagnostic procedure is contrast enhanced angiography
   C. Condition is nearly always bilateral
   D. Surgical intervention may be used
   E. Fibromuscular dysplasia is the likely cause in this patient

Renal Vein Thrombosis

159. Renal vein thrombosis is most commonly associated with : *(AI 2002)*
   A. Diabetic nephropathy
   B. Membranous glomerulopathy
   C. Minimal change disease
   D. Mesangio-proliferative glomerulonephritis
160. Renal vein thrombosis (RVT) may be seen in : *(PGI 2009)*
   A. Trauma
   B. Renal Cell Ca
   C. Pregnancy
   D. Nephrotic Syndrome
   E. Dehydration
161. Renal vein thrombosis is most commonly associated with: *(AI 2001)*
   A. Diabetic nephropathy
   B. Membranous glomerulopathy
   C. Minimal change disease
   D. Membrano-proliferative glomerulonephritis
162. All of the following are causes of Renal Vein Thrombosis, Except: *(PGI Dec 01)*
   A. Membranous Nephropathy
   B. Membranoproliferative glomerulonephritis
   C. Lupus Nephritis
   D. Renal Amyloidosis
   E. Post streptococcal Glomerulonephritis (PSGN)
163. A 10 year old child develops hematuria after 2 days of diarhoea. Blood film shows fragmented RBCs & thrombocytopenia. Ultrasound shows marked enlargement of both kidneys. The likely diagnosis is: *(AIIMS June 99)*
   A. Acute pyelonephritis
   B. Disseminated intravascular coagulopathy
   C. Haemolytic uremic syndrome
   D. Renal vein thrombosis

Nephrolithiasis and Nephrocalcinosis

Nephrolithiasis (Renal/Ureteric Stones)

164. All of the following statement about Renal Calculi are true, Except: *(AI 1993)*
   A. Cystine stones form in acidic urine
   B. Struvite stones form in alkaline urine
   C. Oxalate stones are radiopaque
   D. Uric acid stones are resistant to ESWL
165. Stone which is resistant to lithotripsy: *(AIIMS May 07)*
   A. Calcium oxalate
   B. Triple phosphate stone
   C. Cystine stone
   D. Uric acid stone
166. Which of the following stones is hard to break by ESWL: *(AI 2010)*
   A. Calcium Oxalate Monohydrate
   B. Calcium Oxalate Dihydrate
   C. Uric acid
   D. Struvite
167. All of the follwing types of Renal Stones are Radiopaque, Except: *(AIIMS June 2000)*
   A. Oxalate
   B. Uric Acid
   C. Cystine
   D. Mixed
168. Renal Calculi associated with proteus infection: *(AI 2009)*
   A. Uric Acid
   B. Triple Phosphate
   C. Calcium oxalate
   D. Xanthine
169. Commonest type of Renal stone seen in cases of UTI is: *(AIIMS Nov 1997)*
   A. Phosphate
   B. Oxalate
   C. Urate
   D. Cysteine
170. Ureteric colic due to stone is caused by: *(AI 2008)*
   A. Stretching of renal capsule due to back pressure
   B. Increased peristalsis of ureter to overcome the obstruction
   C. Irriation of intramural ureter
   D. Extravasation of urine.
171. Locate the renal stone with pain radiating to medial side of thigh and perineum due to slipping of stone in males: *(AIIMS June 2000)*
   A. At pelvic brim
   B. Intramural opening of ureter
   C. Junction of ureter and renal pelvis
   D. At crossing of gonadal vessels and ureter
172. Referred pain from ureteric colic is felt in the groin due to involvement of the following nerve: *(AI 2003)*
   A. Subcostal
   B. Iliohypogastric
   C. Ilioinguinal
   D. Genitofemoral
173. A 10-mm calculus in the right lower ureter associated with proximal hydroureteronephrosis is best treated with: *(AI 2003)*
   A. Extracorporeal shockwave lithotripsy
   B. Antegrade percutaneous access
   C. Open ureterolithotomy
   D. Ureteroscopic retrieval
174. A child presents with abdominal colic and hematuria. On ultrasonography a stone 2.0 cm in diameter is seen in the renal pelvis. The next step in management of this case is - *(AIIMS Nov 2000)*
   A. Pyelolithotomy
   B. Nephroureterostomy
   C. Conservative
   D. ESWL
175. T/t used for lower ureteric stone is: *(AIIMS June 98)*
   A. Endoscopic removal
   B. Diuretics
   C. Drug dissolution
   D. Laser
176. Chandu, a 45 yrs male shows calcification on the Rt side of his abdomen in an AP view. In lateral view the calcification is seen to overlie the spine. Most likely diagnosis is: *(AI 2001)*
   A. Gallstones
   B. Calcified mesenteric nodes
   C. Renal stones
   D. Calcified rib

Nephrocalcinosis

177. Nephrocalcinosis is seen in all except– *(AIIMS May 07)*
   A. Sarcoidosis
   B. Distal RTA
   C. Milk alkali syndrome
   D. Medullary cystic kidney
178. Nephrocalcinosis is a feature of A/E: *(PGI June 2000)*
   A. Primary hyperparathyroidism
   B. Medullary sponge kidney
   C. Vitamin D intoxication
   D. Pseudo hypoparathyroidism
179. Nephrocalcinosis is seen in (select two options): *(PGI Dec 05)*
   A. Medullary sponge disease
   B. Acute pyelonephritis
   C. Acute glomerulonephritis
   D. Chronic pyelonephritis
   E. Hyper parathyroidism
180. A patient is known to have calcium nephrocalcinosis for the post 10 years. All of the following dietary recommendations should be suggested, Except: *(AIIMS Nov 2010)*
   A. Protein Restriction
   B. Calcium Restriction
   C. Salt Restriction
   D. All of the above

Congenital Diseases of the Kidney

181. Adult polycystic kidney is inherited as : *(AI 1997)*
   A. Autosomal-co-dominant
   B. Autosomal dominant
   C. Autosomal recessive
   D. X-linked dominant
182. True about adult polycystic kidney disease is all. except: *(AIIMS 2001)*
   A. Autosomal dominant inheritance
   B. Hypertension is rare
   C. Can be associated with cysts in liver, lungs and pancreas
   D. Pyelonephritis is common
183. Which of the following is associated with adult polycystic kidney disease? *(AIIMS 2001)*
   A. Berry Aneurysm in Circle of Willis
   B. Saccular aneurysms of aorta
   C. Fusiform aneurysms of aorta
   D. Leutic aneurysms
184. Polycystic disease of the kidney may have cysts in all of the following organs *except :* *(AI 2004)*
   A. Lung
   B. Liver
   C. Pancreas
   D. Spleen
185. Which of the following is the common extrarenal involvement in autosomal dominant polycystic kidney disease – *(AIIMS Nov 04)*
   A. Mitral valve prolapse
   B. Hepatic cysts
   C. Splenic cysts
   D. Colonic diverticulosis
186. Which one of the following statements is wrong regarding adult polycystic kidney disease *(AIIMS May 04)*
   A. Kidneys are enlarged in size
   B. The presentation is unilateral
   C. Intracranial aneurysms may be associated
   D. Typically manifests in the 3rd decade
187. All of the following are true about Childhood Polycystic Kidney Disease, Except. *(AI 2009)*
   A. Autosomal Dominant
   B. Pulmonary Hypoplasia may be seen
   C. Renal cysts are present at birth
   D. Congenital Hepatic fibrosis may be seen
188. Which of the following is the most common renal cystic disease in infants is? *(AI 2005)*
   A. Polycystic kidney.
   B. Simple renal cyst.
   C. Unilateral renal dysplasia.
   D. Calyceal cyst.
189. A 12- year –old boy is referred for evaluation of nocturnal enuresis and short stature. The blood pressure is normal. The blood urea is 112 mg/dl, creatinine 6 mg/dl, sodium 119 mEq/1, potassium 4 mEq/1, calcium 7mg/dl, phosphate 6mg/dl and alkaline phosphatase 400 U/l.Urinalysis shows trace proteinuria with hyaline casts; no red and white cells are seen. Ultrasound shows bilateral small kidneys and the micturating cystourethrogram is normal. The most likely diagnosis is: *(AIIMS Nov 03)*
   A. Alport's syndrome
   B. Medullary sponge kidney
   C. Chronic glomerulonephritis
   D. Nephronophthisis
190. An 8 year old child suffering from recurrent attacks of polyurea since childhood presents to the paediatrics OPD. On examination the child is short statured. Vitals and B.P. are normal. Serum Creatinine – 6 mg%, HCO3 – 16 meg, Na-134, K^+ 4.2. On USG bilateral small kidneys are seen. Diagnosis is – *(AIIMS May 01)*
   A. Reflux Nephropathy
   B. Nephronophthisis
   C. Polycystic kidney disease
   D. Medullary cystic kidney disease
191. Medullary cystic disease of the kidney is best diagnosed by: *(AI 2002)*
   A. Ultrasound
   B. Nuclear scan
   C. Urography
   D. Biopsy
192. The most common cause of renal scarring in a 3 year old child is: *(AI 2005)*
   A. Trauma.
   B. Tuberculosis.
   C. Vesicoureteral reflux induced pyelonephritis.
   D. Interstitial nephritis.
193. The neonatal kidney achieves concentrating ability equivalent to adult's kidney by: *(AI 2004)*
   A. One year of age
   B. Eighteen months of age
   C. Three to six months of age
   D. Just before puberty

Renal Tumours

Renal Cell Carcinoma (RCC)

194. The most common histological variant of renal cell carcinoma is: *(AIIMS Nov 2005)*
   A. Clear cell type
   B. Chromophobe type
   C. Papillary type
   D. Tubular type
195. Chromophobe variant of Renal cell carcinoma is associated with : *(AI 2010)*
   A. VHL gene mutations
   B. Trisomy of 7 and 17 (+7, +17)
   C. 3 p deletions (3p-)
   D. Monosomy of 1 and Y (-1, -Y)
196. A 40 year old man presented with painless hematuria Bimanual examination revealed a ballotable mass over the right flank. Subsequently right nephrectomy

was done and mass was seen to be composed of cells with clear cytoplasm. Areas of hemorrhage and necrosis were frequent. Cytogenic analysis of this mass is likely to reveal an abnormality of: *(AI 2004)*
A. Chromosome 1
B. Chromosome 3
C. Chromosome 11
D. Chromosome 17

197. Which of the following statement about Renal Cell Carcinoma (Hypernephroma) is false:*(AIIMS Nov 93)*
A. Originate in the cortex
B. Histologically are usually Adenocarcinomas
C. May present with varicocele
D. Radiosensitive

198. Not correct regarding Renal cell carcinoma:
A. May be associated with varicocele
B. May invade renal vein *(AIIMS Dec 94)*
C. More common in female
D. Arises from proximal convoluted tubule

199. Classic triad inRenal cell carcinoma includes all of the following, Except: *(AI 1991)*
A. Hematuria
B. Hypertension
C. Flank mass
D. Abdominal Pain

200. All can be seen in hypernephroma, Except:
A. Polycythemia *(AIIMS Nov 93)*
B. Renal vein thrombosis
C. Hypertension
D. Hematuria

201. Paraneoplastic syndroime associated with RCC are all of the following except: *(AI 2009)*
A. Polycythemia
B. Hypercalcemia
C. Malignant hypertension
D. Cushing syndrome

202. Most common site for secondary metastasis in a case of Hypernephroma: *(AIIMS Feb 1997)*
A. Adrenal
B. Lungs
C. Brain
D. Bones

203. A pt. presented with renal cell carcinoma invadving IVC and the renal vein. False statement is:
A. Preop biopsy is not necessary
B. IVC involvement indicates inoperability
C. Pre op radiotherapy is not essential
D. Chest x-ray should be done to rule out pulmonary metastasis.

Wilm's Tumor

204. All are associated with Wilm's tumor except: one:
A. Anirida *(AIIMS Feb 1997)*
B. Male pseudohermaphrodite
C. Arthogryposis multiplex congenital
D. Hemihypertrophy

205. Commonest presentation of Wilm's Tumor is:
A. Hematuria *(AIIMS Nov 95)*
B. Abdominallump
C. Hydronephrosis
D. Pain in abdomen

206. Whichof the following statements about Wilm's tumor is true: *(AIIMS Nov 92)*
A. Always Unilateral
B. Associated with poor prognosis
C. Most common site of metastasis is bone
D. Radiosensitive

207. The most important determinant of prognosis in Wilms tumor: *(AI 2006)*
A. Stage of disease
B. Loss of heterozygosity of chromsome 1p
C. Histology
D. Age less than one year at presentation

208. Which of the following is the Post – Chemotherapy based staging system in Wilm's tumor: *(AI 2009)*
A. National Wilm's Tumor staging System (NWTSG)
B. International Society of Pediatric Oncology (SIOP)
C. AJCC TNM
D. Chadwick

Hepatorenal Syndrome

209. Features of Hepatorenal syndrome are (select two options): *(PGI June 06)*
A. Urine sodium < 10 meq/l
B. Normal renal histology
C. Renal function abnormal even after liver become normal
D. Proteinuria < 500 mg/day

210. Which of the following statements is incorrect with regard to Hepatorenal syndrome in a patient with cirrhosis
A. Createnine clearance < 40 ml/min *(AI 2003)*
B. Urinary sodium < 10mq/L
C. Urine osmolality lower than plasma osmolality
D. No sustained improvement in renal function after volume expansion.

211. Which of the following statements is incorrect with regard to heptorenal syndrome in a patient with cirrhosis
A. The creatinine clearance is > 40 ml/min
B. The urinary sodium is less than 10 mmol/L
C. The urine osmolality is lower than the plasma osmolality *(AIIMS Nov 2004)*
D. There is poor response to volume expansion

Rhabdomyolysis

212. A 28 year old boy met with on accident and sustained severe crush injury. He is most likely to develop:
A. Acute Renal Failure *(AIIMS Nov 09)*
B. Hypophosphatemia
C. Hypercalcemia
D. Acute Myocardial Infarction

213. All of the following are causes of Rhabdomyolysis, Except: *(PGI June 99)*
A. Cocaine Intoxication
B. Hyperphosphatemia
C. Hypokalemia
D. Crush injury

214. Rhabdomyolysis and Myoglobinuria may be seen in: *(PGI June 02)*
A. Viperbite
B. Multiple Hornet Stings
C. Clostridium Perfringes
D. Streptococcus
E. All of the above

215. All of the following are causes of Rhabdomyolysis and myoglobinuria, Except: *(PGI Dec 06)*
A. Hyperpyrexia
B. Viper snake venom
C. Hyperthyroidism
D. Multiple Hornet Stings
E. All of the above

216. All of the following are true about Rhabdomyolysis, Except: *(PGI Dec 04)*
A. Hyperuricemia
B. Hyperphosphatemia
C. Hypercalcemia
D. ↑ Creatine kinase

217. Features of Rhabdomyolysis include all of the following, Except: *(PGI Dec 04)*
A. Acute muscular weakness
B. Myoglobinuria
C. Hemoglobinuria
D. Acute Renal Failure

Miscellaneous

218. A 65 year old male smoker presents with gross total painless hematuria. The most likely diagnosis is: *(AI 2003)*
A. Carcinoma of urinary bladder
B. Benign prostatic hyperplasia
C. Carcinoma prostate
D. Cystolithiasis

219. An elderly male presents with one episode of gross haematuria. All of the following investigations are recommended for investigating this patient except: *(AI 2007)*
A. Cystoscopy
B. Urine microscopy for malignant cells
C. Urine tumor markers
D. Intravenous Pyelogram

220. A 60 yr old smoker came with a history of painless gross hematuria for one day. Most logical investigation would be: *(AI 2007)*
A. Urine routine
B. Plain X ray KUB
C. USG KUB
D. Urine microscopy for malignant cytology

221. A seven year old asymptomatic girl is found to have persistant hypertension. There is no significant history and urine examination is normal. Which of the following is the most likely cause: *(AI 2010)*
A. Essential Hypertension
B. Renal Parenchymal Disease
C. Polycystic Kidney Disease
D. Coarctation of Aorta

222. A child presented with intermittent episodes of left sided flank pain. Ultrasonography reveals a large hydronephrosis with dilated renal pelvis and cortical thinning with a normal ureter. Kidney differential function was observed to be 19% which of the following is the best management: *(AI 2010)*
A. Nephrectomy
B. Pyeloplasty
C. External Drainage
D. Endopylostomy

223. Not a cause of granular contracted kidney- *(AIIMS Dec 94)*
A. Diabetes mellitis
B. Chronic pyelonephritis
C. Benign nephrosclerosis
D. Chronic glomerulonephritis

224. All of the following are causes of granular contracted kidney except: *(AI 1997)*
A. Benign nephrosclerosis
B. Chronic pylonephritis
C. Diabetes mellitus
D. Chronic glomerulonephritis

225. All of the following are features of Bartter's syndrome, Except.
A. Hypokalemia
B. Hypermagnesemia
C. Hyperprostaglaridine
D. Hyper calciurea

226. Urinary K^+ excretion is increased in: *(AIIMS Nov-04)*
A. Bronchiectasis
B. Meningitis
C. Osteomyelitis
D. Hepatitis

227. Renal damage due to amphotericin B are all, *except* *(AIIMS Nov 01)*
A. Azotemia
B. Renal tubular acidosis
C. Glomerulonephritis
D. Hypokalemia

228. Which of the following drugs is not a part of the 'Triple Therapy' immunosuppression for post-renal transplant patients? *(AI 2006)*
A. Cyclosporine
B. Azathioprine
C. FK 506
D. Prednisolone

ANSWERS, REFERENCES, EXPLANATIONS AND RELEVANT HIGH YIELD FACTS

Urinalysis

1. **Answer is A (Kidney):** *Chandrasoma Taylor 2nd/ 127; Harrison 16th /251, 248; Harrison 17th/ 270-273, 1758 Harrison 18th/p 336-339, 2301*

RBC casts are suggestive of glomerular (Kidney) injury.

Urinary casts are formed when proteins and other organic matter solidify in the renal tubule. The presence of casts in urine is indicative of disease of the nephron.

Casts may contain:

Proteins	*Erythrocytes*	*Leucocytes*	*Epethelial cells*
Hyaline casts	Red cell casts	WBC cast	Epithelial casts

Clinical significance of different casts:

a. ***Hyaline casts*** :	• This is a *normal constituent* Q of urine and has *no attached significance* Q. • *Tom Horsfall protein* Q is protein *secreted by epithelial cells of loop of henle* Q. • *This protein may be excreted as Hyaline cast.* Q
b. ***RBC cast*** :	• are suggestive of *glomerular injury* Q.
c. ***White cell casts*** :	• are suggestive of *interstitial injury* and may be seen in *interstitial nephritis* Q *WBC cast with bacteria indicate pyelonephritis* Q.
d. ***Broad granular casts*** :	• are *seen in CRF* Q and suggests interstitial fibrosis and dilatation of tubules.
e. ***Pigmented muddy brown granular casts*** :	• are suggestive of *ischaemic or nephrotoxic injury* Q i.e. *Tubular Necrosis* Q.

2. **Answer is B (20% Dysmorphic RBC) :** *Harrison 18th/p 339, 340 Harrison 17th/272, 273 Harrison 16th/251*

Presence of Dysmorphic RBC's cast suggests hematuria of glomerular origin.

Presence of Bright Red RBC's and 100 RBC per HPG suggest gross hematuria but do not indicate glomerular origin of hematuria.

Presence of β_2 microgloobulin in urine indicates tubular injury and not glomerular injury.

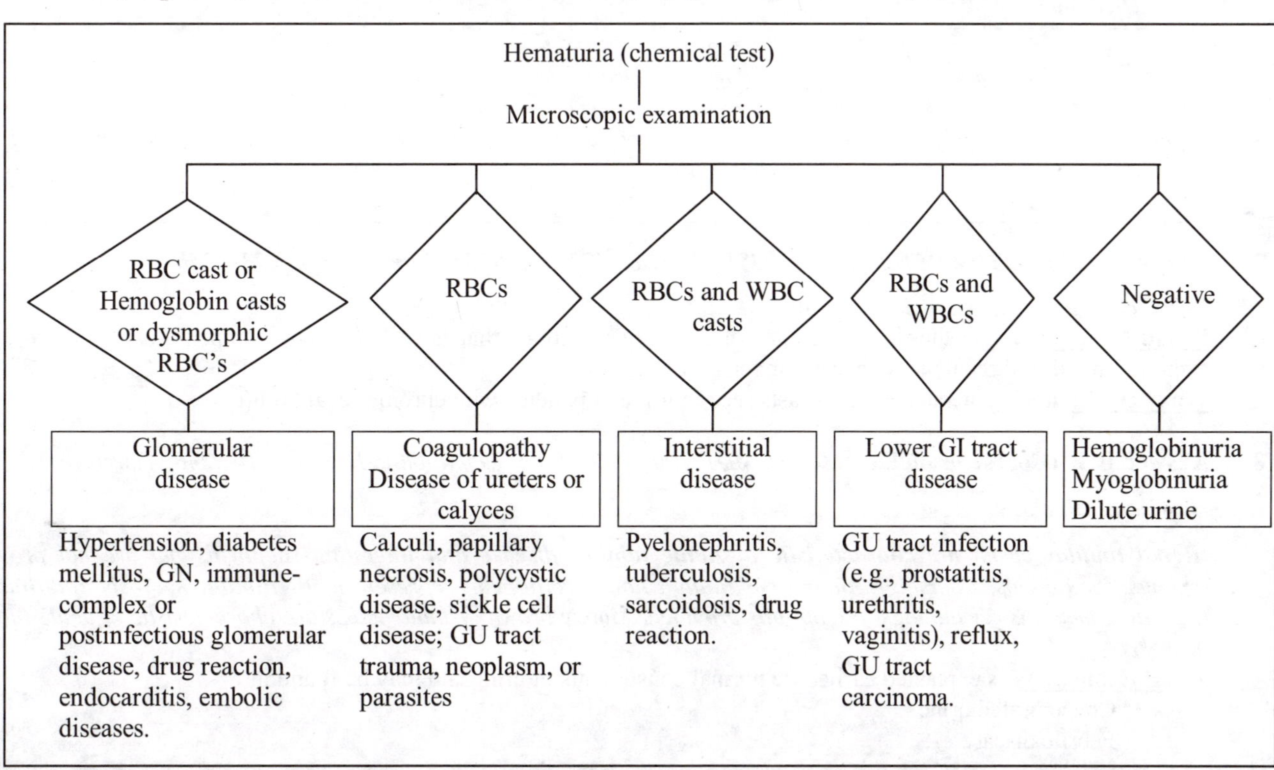

3. **Answer is A and E (Dysmorphic R.B.C and R.B.C. cast):** *Harrison 18th/p 339 Harrisons 17th/ 272, 273; 16th/251; Refer previous question*

Presence of Dysmorphic RBC and RBC cast suggests hematuria of glomerular origin or a glomerular disease.

4. **Answer is B (20% Dysmorphic RBC's):** *Harrison 15th/267; 16th/251; Harrison 17th/ 273 Harrison 18th/p 339*

'The RBC's of Glomerular origin are often Dysmorphic when examined by Phase contrast microscopy'. 'Hematuria with Dysmorphic RBC's cast and protein excretion > 500 mg/d is virtually diagnostic of Glomerulonephritis.'
- Harrisons 17th/273

5. **Answer is B (Acanthocytes):** *Harrison 15th/ 681; 16th/615; Harrison 17th/ 652, 1786 Harrison 18th/p 2340, 2301*

Acanthocytes are erythrocytes characterized by multiple spiny cytoplasmic protections (spur cells).
These are seen as a consequence of abnormal lipid metabolism such as in severe liver disease and are not a feature of glomerular (renal disease).
Haematuria with dysmorphic RBC's cast are a characteristic feature of glomeulonephritis.
(crenated RBC are a type of dysmorphic RBC's).

6. **Answer is A and B (Alports's syndrome and IgA nephrotpathy):** *Nelsons 18th/2169, 2170-2173; Rudolph Pediatrics 21st /1682*

Alports's syndrome and IgA nephropathy are characterized by recurrent episodes of gross hematuria.

<u>Recurrent episodes of gross haematuria</u>
Recurrent Gross Haematuria should be distinguished from isolated episodes of gross hematuria, as it is a charachteristic feature of some specific disorders

Charachteristic Causes of Recurrent Gross Haematuria (Nelson 18th/2169)	
1. IgA Nephropathy	Isolated Glomerular diseases with recurrent Gross haematuria (1–3)
2. Alports syndrome	
3. Thin Glomerular basement membrane disease	
4. Hypercalciuria	
5. Urolithiasis	

<u>Recurrent Gross Haematuria must be distinguished from Urethrorrhagea.</u>
Urethrorrhagia refers to urethral bleeding in the absence of urine.It is associated with dysuria and blood spots on underwear after voiding .It often occurs in prepubertal boys at intervals, several months apart over a period of many years, and has a benign self limiting cause.

7. **Answer is C (Broad Cast):** *Harrison 16th/251; Harrison 17th/ 273, 1758 Harrison 18th/p 339, 340*

Broad casts are characteristic of Chronic Renal failure.
<u>Broad Casts :</u> arise in the dilated tubules of enlarged nephrons, that have undergone compensatory hypertrophy in response to reduced renal mass i.e. chronic renal failure.
<u>Waxy casts :</u> are degenerated cellular casts seen in urine of patients with chronic renal failure.

8. **Answer is B (Coarse granular casts):** *CMDT 2002/ 920; 2009/795 (table); Harrison 16th/248; Harrison 17th/ 273 Harrison 18th/p 339*

***'Renal tubular casts' are characteristic of Acute tubular disease and interstitial nephritis** but are not provided amongst the options. **Coarse granular casts though non specific, can represent acute tubular necrosis and thus are the single best answer amongst the options provided.** Muddy brown granular casts are characteristic of acute tubular necrosis.*

- **<u>Hyaline casts</u>** as explained earlier are normal constituents of urine and may be found in
  - Concentrated urine
  - Febrile disease

- After strenuous exercise
- In the course of diuretic therapy

They are thus not indicative of any form of renal disease.

- **White cell casts** indicate an interstitial type of renal disease such as interstitial nephritis and infective diseases like pyelonephritis but not a renal tubular disease.
- **Cystein oxalate cell casts** are specific entities present only when excretion of these are raised and do not indicate a tubular disorder.

9. **Answer is A (W.B.C):** *Harrisons 16th/251, 248, 17th/ 272, 273, Harrison 18th/p 339 Chandrasoma Taylor 2nd/127*

Presence of W.B.C cast in urine of patients with suspected pyelonephritis is considered pathognomic.

'Leucocyte casts (W.B.C cast) are present in the urine of some patients with Pylonephritis and the detection of these is considered pathognomic' – Harrisons 16th/1717

10. **Answer is C (Organisms in excess of 100,000 (CFU/ml):** *Heptinstall's Pathology of the kidney 6th/994; Diagnosis of Genitourinary disease by Resnick and Older 2nd /275, 276, 277*

Although acute pyelonephritis is usually associated with organisms in excess of 100,000 CFU/ml, this test cannot be utilized to localize the infection to kidney as such high counts may well be seen in cases of uncomplicated infections of the lower urinary tract.

- ***White Blood cell casts :***
'Presence of white blood cell casts in urine suggest that inflammation is taking in the kidney itself' - Heptinstall
'Leucocyte casts (WBC casts) are present in urine of some patients with Acute pyelonephritis and the detection of these casts is pathognomic' – Harrisons 16th/1717
- ***Antibody to Tomm Horsfall Protein***
Tomm Horsfall protein is exclusively produced by cells in the ascending limb of loop of Henle and is normally found in urine. In conditions such as pyelonephritis *(secondary to conditions such as obstructive renal disease or severe vesico- uretric reflux)* this protein gets deposited in renal interstitium and bowman's space where it stimulates antibody fermation. **Antibodies to Tomm Horsfall proteins suggest infection of the upper renal tract (pyelonephritis) - Diagnosis of Genitourinary disease**
- ***Tests for impaiment of concentrations of urine*** may be used to differentiates acute pyelonephritis and infection confined to lower urinary tract – Heptinstall

Test to localize bacteria to Kidney (Pyelonephritis)
(Complicated vs Uncomplicated UTI)

Invasive (Gold standard)	Non Invasive tests (Suggestive)
Bacterial growth in urine collected by direct ureteral catheterization	• ***White blood cell casts in urine*** • ***Raised serum antibody levels to Tomm Horsfall proteins*** • Elevated levels of beta – 2 microglobulins in urine • Urinary enzyme estimation for LDH • The presence of antibody coated organisms in urine • Raised serum levels of C reactive proteins • ***Determination of maximum urinary concentrating ability*** • **Imaging tests:** USG, IVU, DMSA, CTscan *'The DMSA scintography provides the most reliable test at the present time for the diagnosis of acute Pyelonephritis'*

11. **Answer is A (Proteinuria >3.0 – 3.5 g/day):** *'Manual of Nephrology 7th/141, 142; Diseases of Kidney and Urinary Tract 8th/317, 318*

Nephrotic range proteinuria (> 3.0 – 3.5 g/day) is characteristic of Glomerular proteinuria.

Tomm Harsfall Protein in urine is a feature of tubular proteinuria

Tomm Harsfall protein is synthesized in the tubular cells of ascending limb of loop of henle and distal tubule and is secreted into urine. Under conditions of tubulo interstitial injury (tubular proteinuria) increased Tomm Harsfall protein may be secreted in urine from injured tubular cells.

Glomerular proteinuria is associated with an increase Albumin: β2 microglobulin, ratio usually > 1000:1

Feature	Normal value	Glomerular proteinuria	Tubular proteinuria
Albumin: β2 microglobulin ratio	Usually 50:1 to 200:1	Usually >1000 : 1	Usually < 10:1

Glomerular proteinuria is associated with Albumin > Globulin

Albuminuria is the hallmark of glomerular proteinuria

Albumin > Globulin

Feature	Glomerular Proteinuria	Tubular proteinuria
Pathology	Defect in glomerular filtration barrier resulting in increased filtration of normal proteins	Defect in tubular reabsorption resulting from damage to renal tubulointestitial region
Total protein excretion per day	Usually > 2.0 g/day Proteinuria may reach nephrotic range > 3.5 g/day	Usually < 2.0 g/day Proteinuria never reaches nephrotic range.
Protein type	• *Albuminuria is the hallmark of Glomerular proteinuria.* • **Proteinuria chiefly consists of albumin** • Other low molecular weight proteins, may be present • Globulin may be present when proteinuria is not selective. • **Albumin is usually greater than globulins** (Albumin >Globulin)	• *Low molecular weight proteinuria is the hallmark of tubular proteinuria.* • Proteinuria chiefly consists of Low molecular weight proteins (alpha and beta microglobulins). Albumin is invariably present • Albumin is invariably present
Albumin/ β2 microglobulin ratio	• Albumin is significantly greater than other low molecular weight proteins eg. β2 microglobulin • Albumin :β2 microglobulin ratio usually exceeds 1000:1	• Albumin microglobulin ratio is reduced as increased amount of β2 microglobulin is excreted. • Albumin: β2 microglobulin ratio is usually less than 10:1
Tomm Harsfall Protein	Tomm Harsfall proteins are not increased as there is no injury to tubular cells	Tomm Harsfall protein secretion may be increased by injured tubular cells of ascending loop of henle & distal tubule.
• N Acetyl glucosamine • Lysozyme	Normal	May be increased (Increased in case of tubular cell injury)

12. Answer is B (Is benign): *Rudolph Pediatrics 21st/1664*

Orthostatic proteinuria is believed to be benign condition and long term studies have shown that it is not associated with any renal disease.

Orthostatic proteinuria
• *Orthostatic proteinuria is defined as proteinuria occurring only in the upright position* • *It is most commonly seen in children and young adults and its prevalence decreases with age* • *Orthostatic proteinuria does not typically exceed 1gm/day (<1.0 gm/day)* • *Orthostatic proteinuria is a benign condition and may resolve spontaneously* • *Orthostatic proteinuria is not associated with increase risk of any renal disease.*

13. Answer is C (Gamma Globulins): *Harrison's 16th/657; Primer on kidney diseases 4th/256; clinical Laboratory medicine 6th/350*

Bence Jones proteins are composed of light chains of the type found in normal or pathological gamma globulins

Bence Jones proteins: Review

- Bence Jones Proteins are abnormal proteins charachteristically found in the urine of patients with multiple myeloma (and other paraprotenemias)
- These proteins have been shown to be composed of only of immunoglobulin light chains (Normal complete immunoglobulins comprise of both heavy chains and light chains and hence Bence one Proteins are believed to represent Incompete Immunoglobulins
- Since Bence Jones proteins respresent light chains found in normal immunoglobulins, these proteins also belong to the category of gamma globulins like normal immunoglobulins
- In multiple myelma (and some other paraproteinemisa) there is excessive production of light chains over heavy chains. These light chains are eliminated in urine as Bence Jones proteins
- Bence ones proteins can be detected in urine by a charachteristic *heat coagulability test*[Q] due to their very distinctive chemical character.
  'These proteins (Bence Jones / Light chains) precipitate when heated to between 40°C and 60°C, dissoive an boiling (90°C- 100°C) and reprecipitate when cooled back to between 40°C and 60°C'

This unusual heat solubility property of Bence Jones protein is used as a screening test for the presence of urinary Bence Jones proteins.

14. Answer is C (Mu heavy chain disease): *Harrison's 17th/707, Refer text below*

Bence Jones Proteinuria may be seen in 'Mu' heavy chain disease due to excretion of kappa light chains in urine

Bence Jones proteins (free light chains) are characteristically absent in alpha and gamma light chain diseases but may be seen in mu heavy chain disease. The presence of Bence Jones light chains in urine particularly kappa light chains is a distinguishing feature to identify mu heavy chain disease.

*'The only features that may distinguish patients with mu heavy chain disease are the presence of vacuoles in malignant lymphocytes and excretion of **kappa light chains in urine**' – Harrison*

'Bence Jones Protein is absent in alpha and gamma light chain diseases but has been reported in mu heavy chain disease' - Clinical Biochemistry (Churchill- Livingstone) 1st (1995) / 502

'Although mu chain is not found in the urine of patients with mu heavy chain disease, Bence Jones light chains are commonly (50%) found in urine particularly kappa chains. The latter while still produced in mu heavy chain disease are not assimilated because of heavy chain gene aberrancies leading to truncated forms'- Pathology and Genetics of Tumors of Haemopoetic and Lymphoid Tissue (WHO classification of Tumors) 2001/155

Heavy chain diseases *are rare lymphoplasmacytic malignancies that exclusively produce monoclonal heavy chains and no light chains. Heavy chains diseases are classified as Alpha, Gamma and Mu heavy chain diseases based on the defect in synthesis of alpha, gamma or mu heavy chains, respectively (Delta and Epsilon heavy chain diseases are extremely rare and have not been reported). The diagnosis of heavy chain diseases depends on demonstration of the specific monoclonal heavy chain in serum or tissues by electrophoresis, immunoelectrophoresis or immunofixation techniques*

15. Answer is C (DTPA renogram) :*Principles And Practice Of Paediatric Nephrology by Nammalwar and Vijay Kumar/85*

Now the most convenient method of estimating renal function is by isotope renography- *Nammalwar /85*

DYNAMIC RENAL SCAN (RENOGRAM, DTPA scan or a Mag3)	STATIC RENAL SCAN (DMSA SCAN)
• DTPA and Mag3 are rapidly excreted by the kidney and are therefore used as radiopharmaceutical agents for a dynamic scan • The patient is given a small and simple intravenous injection and a *series of images* of the kidneys are taken immediately thereafter with the help of a gamma camera - Angiographic phase - Parenchymal phase - Drainage phase • This scan is preferred for information about the blood flow to the kidneys ,how well each kidney is functioning for the production of urine and if there is any obstructions in urine output.	• DMSA is an agent that concentrates in the renal parenchyma for a long time and is therefore used for a static scan • The patient is given a small and simple injection into a vein. After *this the patient may leave but will be given a time to return about three hours later*. The patient will then be required to lie on a scanning table and images will be taken with the help of a gamma camera. • This scan is preferred for information about the size, shape and position of the kidneys. • The test also shows if there are there are scars on the kidney from a previous infection.

Remember :

- **Renogram, MAG3 or DTPA** is primarily used to study the ***function of kidneys.***
- **Static Renal Scan ,DMSA scan** is primarily used to look at the ***structure of kidneys.***

16. Answer is D (Radio-Renogram i.e. DTPA Scan) : *Ghai 4th / 364 ; Bhaduri / 343*

Radiorenogram is the next best investigation of choice.

The next step would be to assess Renal function and the possible site of obstruction if that is the cause for anuria. The choice lies between an IVP or a Radio-Renogram. Out of these two a Radio Renogram is a distinctly better option. Imaging of the kidney and urinary tract have been greatly simplified by introduction of Radio nucleotide methods. These are now fast Replacing radiocontrast studies like IVP.
Radionucleotide procedures are non invasive, highly sensitive and expose patients to less radiation.

17. Answer is B (DTPA scan): *Repeat; Refer previous question*

The next step would be to assess Renal function which is best achieved by DTPA scan amongst the options provided.

18. Answer is B (Renogastric Reflex): *S. Das Surgery 4th/ 410*

Afferent stimuli from renal capsule or musculature of pelvis may produce reflex spasm of the pylorus through the Renogastric reflex. This explains GI symptoms in Renal disease.

Renal disease often presents with various GIT manifestation such as – abdominal distension, tenderness, pain, vomiting.

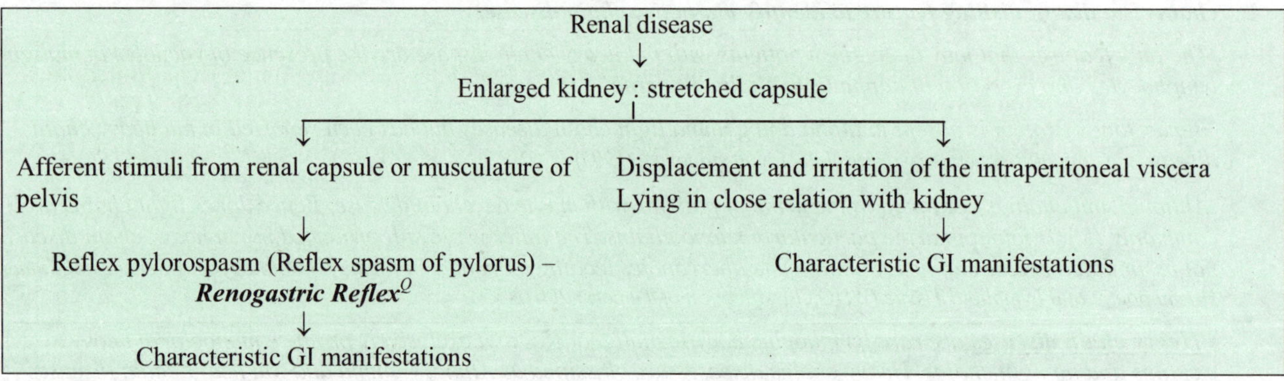

19. Answer is A (Suprapubic aspiration): *Smiths Urology 16th/46, 47, 205; Diseases of the Kidney & Urinary tract 8th/832*

Urine obtained from suprapubic aspiration is least likely to be contaminated–*Diseases of the kidney & urinary tract 8th/832*

Contamination with different methods of urine collection

Sample from Urine bag > Voiding sample (Mid stream) > Sample from Urinary catheter > Sample from Suprapubic aspiration

Suprapubic aspiration avoids potential contamination but is rarely used because of its invasiveness
It may be indicated in children[Q] (and selected other patients)

Desirable properties of a voided sample

1. It is best to collect a clean voided mid stream urine sample
   (First 15-30 ml are discarded and the next 50- 100 ml are collected)
   The midstream clean catch method reduces the likelihood of contamination with meatal or urethral secretions
2. Freshly voided specimen should be tested (Within one hour of voiding)
3. Urine specimen should not be collected immediately after the patient has eaten
   (Should be obtained a few hours after the patient has eaten)
4. First voided morning specimen should be obtained for qualitative protein testing
   (Patients with possible orthostatic proteinuria) and for specific gravity testing.

20. Answer is A (Quinine): *Smith's Urology 17th/47*

Quinine is not associated with discoloured urine.

Colour and Appearance of Urine

Urine is often coloured owing to drugs and other causes

Red Urine	Reddish Brown / Brown	Orange /yellow orange
• *Beet ingestion (Betacyanin excretion)* • *Phenolpthaline (in Laxatives)* • *Vegetable dye ingestion* • *Myoglobinuria* • *Haemoglobinuria* • *Seoratia Marcescens bacteria can cause the Red diaper' syndrome*	• ***Nitrofurantoin*** *(Brown)* • *L-Dopa* • *Alpha Methyl Dopa* • *Metronidazole*	• ***Rifampicin*** *(yellow orange)* • ***Pyridium*** *(orange) (Phenazopyridine)*

21. Answer is A (Glomerular Filtaration): *Essentials of Nephrology 2nd/32, 33*

Creatinine Clearance is used to assess Glomerular function or the Glomerular Filtration Rate.

***Creatinine** in serum is the end product of endogenous muscle breakdown. Creatinine is comptetely filtered by the glomerulus and neither significantly absorbed nor significantly secreted into the tubules and hence for clinical purpose creatinine clearance is the most commonly used test to assess Glomerular function.*

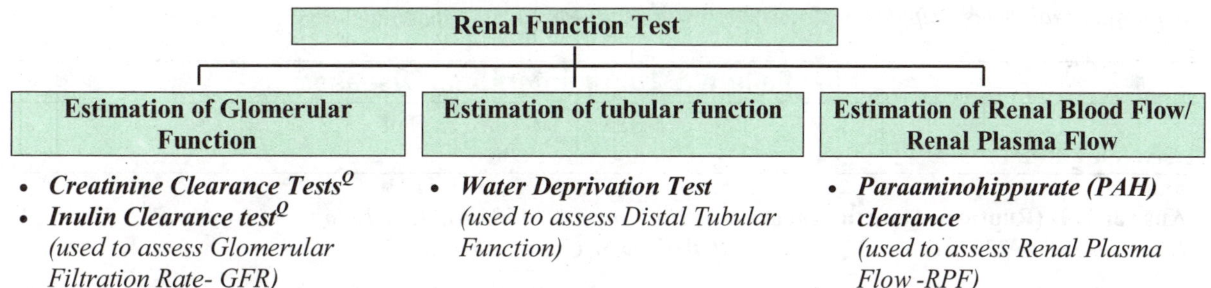

22. Answer is B (Creatinine Clearance): *Diseases of Kidney and Urinary Tract 8th (Lippincott Williams) / 2059; 'Applied Physiology in Intensive Care Medicine 2nd (Springer) / 94*

Creatinine clearance is the most accurate estimation of decline in GFR amongst the option provided.

Creatinine clearance is the most accurate endogenous marker for estimation of GFR to assess renal function

- *'Assessment of GFR is the single most important test of renal function in clinical practice'-Diseases of Kidney & Urinary Tract*
- *Creatinine clearance is the most accurate **endogenous marker** for estimation of GFR to assess renal function.*

> ***Inulin** is an **exogenous marker** that is freely filtered by the kidneys without undergoing any metabolism, tubular secretion and /or reabsorption. Inulin is thus rapidly excreted in urine by glomerular filtration and 'Inulin clearance' has remained the Gold standard for estimation of GFR.*

- *Estimation of serum creatinine is the most widely used measure to assess renal function but is not the most accurate.*

> ***Serum creatinine is not an accurate enough measure of renal function and can be normal in initial stages of renal failure.***
>
> *'In early renal disease, however GFR can decrease substantially without changes in serum creatinine. The serum creatinine does not significantly change until the creatinine clearance is less than 70 ml/min /1.73m^2'.*
>
> *– The Chemotherapy Source Book 4th (Lippincott Williams) / 224*

- *Serum creatinine estimation is more accurate than estimation of serum urea or serum BUN in assessing renal function*

23. Answer is B (Creatinine clearance may overestimate the actual GFR as renal function declines)

Creatinine clearance may overestimate the GFR as renal function declines, since secretion of creatinine from tubular cells is increased as renal function declines (when GFR decreases).

Creatinine is an endogenous metabolite that is freely filtered by the glomerulus but is also actively secreted by the proximal tubular cells into the renal tubules in very small amounts. In the steady state such 'Secretion' of creatinine into the tubules is minimal, however as GFR falls creatinine secretion is increased. Creatinine clearance thus over estimates the actual GFR especially in conditions with mild to moderate reductions in GFR.

> ***Inulin is still considered the 'Gold standard' test for assessing GFR.***
> *Inulin clearance is more accurate than creatinine clearance as Inulin is not secreted by tubular cells.*

24. Answer is C (Distal Tubular Function): *Essentials of Nephrology 2nd/33*

Water Deprivation Test is used to assess Distal Tubular Function.

Water Deprivation Test

Water deprivation test is used to assess the tubule's ability to concentrate urine. When a normal person is deprived of water, ADH secretion occurs, which acts on the ***distal tubule and collecting ducts****, making them freely permeable to water, allowing reabsorption of water from these segments, thereby producing concentrated urine. Inability to concentrate urine during the water deprivation test thereby suggests dysfunction of distal tubules and helps to identify nephrogenic diabetes insipidus.*

Renal Failure & Tubulointerstitial Diseases

Acute Renal Failure:

25. Answer is D (Rupture of Aortic Aneurysm): *Harrison 14th/ 1505 (t); 15th/ 1546 t; 16th/1648; 17th/1753 (table 273.1); Harrison 18th/p 2294 (Table: 279-1) Renal Pathology by Craig Tisher 2nd/ 770;*

Rupture of Aortic Aneurysm is the most unlikely cause of ATN amongst the following. It would rather result in instant death.

Causes of Acute Tubular Necrosis

Ischemic
- *Hypovolemia* Q
- *Low cardiac output* Q
- *Renal vascular occlusion.* Q i.e. Renal vasoconstriction, DIC, Thrombotic microangiopathy (HUS, TTP, Malignant Hypertension, Vasculitis)

Toxins

Endogenous Toxins
- *Rhabdomyolysis or Crush Syndrome (myoglobins)* Q
- *Hemolysis (hemoglobins)* Q
- *Uric acid, Oxalate* Q
- *Plasma cell dyscrasias (Paraproteinemias e.g. myeloma)* Q
- *Massive burns* Q

Exogenous Toxins
- *Radiocontrast agents* Q
- *Cyclosporine* Q
- *Antibiotics (e.g. Aminoglycosides, Amphoterein B)* Q
- *Chemotherapy (eg. Cisplatin)* Q
- *Organic Solvents (e.g. Ethylene Glycol)* Q
- *Paracetamol* Q
- *Illegal Abortifacients*

26. Answer is E (All of the above): *Harrison 18th/2294; Harrison 17th/1753*

All of the options provided can lead to Acute Tubular Necrosis and are listed in the table in the previous question. *Abruptio placentae is an established cause of DIC and may thus cause ATN.*

27. Answer is B (Urine sodium > 40): *Harrison 15th/1547; 16th/1649; Harrison 17th/ 271, 1758 Harrison 18th/p 337, 2301*

Urinary sodium excretion of more than 20mmol/L suggests intrinsic renal failure such as ATN.

Urine Diagnostic Indices: Differentiation of Prerenal and Intrinsic Renal failure.

Diagnostic index	Prerenal ARF	Intrinsic renal ARF
Fractional Excretion of Na [Q] (%)	<1	>1
Urine Sodium Concentration (mmol/L) [Q]	<10 mmol/L	>20 mmol/L
Urine Sodium concentration (meq/L) [Q]	< 20meq/L	> 40 meq/L [Q]
Urine Creatinine To Plasma Creatinine ratio [Q]	>40	<20
Urine specific gravity [Q]	>1.020	~1.010
Urine osmolality [Q] (mosmol/kg H_2O)	> 500	< 350
Renal failure Index [Q] $U_{Na}/(U_{CR}/P_{CR})$	<1	>1
Urine urea Nitrogen to plasma urea Nitrogen [Q]	> 8	<3
Plasma BUN/Creatinine Ratio [Q]	>20	<10-15
Urinary sediment [Q]	Hyaline Casts	Muddy Brown Granular Cast

Acute tubular necrosis is a cause of Intrinsic ARF. [Q]

28. **Answer is A (Prerenal Azolemia):** *Harrison 18th/p 2302 Harrisons 17th 1758; Harrisons 16th/1649*

Fractional Excretion of Na^+ < 1 is a charachteristic of Prerenal Azotemia

Diagnostic Index	Prerenal ARF	Intrinsic Renal ARF
Fractional Excretion of Na^+	< 1	> 1

29. **Answer is A (Urinary Na^+ < 10 mmol/litre):** *Harrison 16th/1649; Harrison 17th/271, 1758 Harrison 18th/p337, 2302*

Prerenal azotemia is associated with a urinary sodium excretion of less than 10 mmol/L.

30. **Answer is C (Urinary sodium concentration > 40 meq/l):** *Harrison 18th/p 337, 2302 Harrisons 17th/271, 1758*

Prerenal Azotemia (Prerenal ARF) is associated with a urinary sodium concentration < 20 meq/l. A urinary sodium concentration > 40 meq /l suggests intrinsic type of ARF.

Differentiating features between Pre-renal and Intrinsic ARF

- Prerenal Azotemia is the most common form of ARF and is caused by renal hypoperfusion either from generalized hypovolemia or from altered renal hemodynamics resulting in hypoperfusion
- ***By definition Renal parenchymal tissue is not damaged in prerenal ARF and prerenal ARF is rapidly reversible upon correction of the primary hemodynamic abnormality***
- Analysis of urine and blood biochemistry provides several useful 'Renal failure Indices' to distinguish prerenal ARF from intrinsic ARF (Ischemic /Nephrotoxic ARF)

Urine Diagnostic Indices: Differentiation of Prerenal and Intrinsic Renal failure.

Diagnostic index	Prerenal ARF	Intrinsic renal ARF
Fractional Excretion of Na [Q] (%)	<1	>1
Urine Sodium Concentration (mmol/L) [Q]	<10 mmol/L	>20 mmol/L
Urine Sodium concentration (meq/L) [Q]	< 20meq/L	> 40 meq/L [Q]
Urine Creatinine To Plasma Creatinine ratio [Q]	>40	<20
Urine specific gravity [Q]	>1.020	~1.010
Urine osmolality [Q] (mosmol/kg H_2O)	> 500	< 350
Renal failure Index [Q] $U_{Na}/(U_{CR}/P_{CR})$	<1	>1
Urine urea Nitrogen to plasma urea Nitrogen [Q]	> 8	<3
Plasma BUN/Creatinine Ratio [Q]	>20	<10-15
Urinary sediment [Q]	Hyaline Casts	Muddy Brown Granular Cast

31. **Answer is C (Pre-renal failure):** *Harrison 18th/p 337, 2302 Harrisons 17th/271, 1758, 1753 (1)*

Plasma urea / creatinine ratio of 20:1 is characteristic of prerenal ARF
Rhabdomyolysis and chronic glomerulonephritis are causes of Intrinsic ARF and are associated with a plasma urea / creatinine ratio of < 10-15. Ureteric calculi are associated with post-renal ARF

Indices	Pre-renal ARF	Intrinsic Renal ARF
Plasma Urea / Creatinine Ratio	> 20	< 10-15

32. Answer is C (Sodium Fraction Excretion): *Harrison 18th/p 337, 2302 Harrison 17th/271, 1758; Harrison 16th/1649*

Fractional Excretion of Na can distinguish Pre renal ARF from Renal ARF.

Indices	Prerenal ARF	Renal ARF
Fractional Excretion of Na (FE_{Na})	< 1	> 1

33. Answer is A (20): *Harrison 18th/p337 Harrison 17th/217; Harrison 16th/1649*

The urinary creatinine to plasma createnine ratio in Intrinsic renal failure (Acute Tubular Necrosis) is less than 20.

Indices	Prerenal ARF	Renal ARF (ATN)
Urine creatinine/Plasma Creatinine (U_{cr}/P_{cr})	>40	<20

34. Answer is D (Blood urea creatinine ratio < 20): *Harrison 18th/p 337 Harrison 17th/271; Harrison 16th/1649*

Intrinsic Renal Failure (ATN) is associated with a Blood Urea Creatinine ratio of <10-15 : 1. BUN creatinine ratio < 20 is thus the single best answer of choice.

Index	Acute Tubular Necrosis
Urine specific gravity	< 1.020 (~1.010)
Urine osmolality	< 350 mosmol/kg
Urine sodium excretion	> 20 mmol/L or > 40 meq/L
BUN/creatinine ratio	<10-15 : 1

35. Answer is D (Plasma BUN/Creatinine ratio <20): *Harrison 18th/337; Harrison 17th/271; Harrison 16th/1649*

Prereanl Azotemia is characterized by Plasma BUN/creatinine ratio of >20:1

Oliguria (urine output <400) is a feature of prerenal Azotemia that cannot be used to differentiate Prerenal Azotemia from Intrinsic Renal failure (ATN)

Urine output <500 may be seen in both Prerenal and Renal Azotemia.

Decreased urine output represents oliguric renal failure and may be seen in both prerenal and renal azotemia.

Ucr/Pcr >40; FE_{Na} < 1 and U_{NA} < 20 meq/l are features of Prerenal Azotemia that may be used to distinguish Prerenal Azotemia from Intrinsic Renal Azotemia.

36. Answer is A and B (urine Osmolality > 500 and sodium excretion <10 mmol/L): *Harrison 17th/271; Harrison 16th/1649*

Prerenal Azotemia is associated with sodium excretion <10mmol/L and a urine osmolality >500 mosmol/kg
Fractional excretion of Na > 1 and plasma BUN/creatinine ratio <20 favours a diagnosis of Intrinsic Renal Azotemia or ATN.

37. Answer is D (Hypercalcemia): *Harrison 18th/ 2303, 2306; Harrisons 17th/1754, 1759, 1760*

Oliguric ARF is associated with hypocalcemia and not hypercalcemia.

Hypocalcemia is caused by metastatic deposition of calcium phosphate, tissue resistance to PTH and reduced levels of active vitamin D.

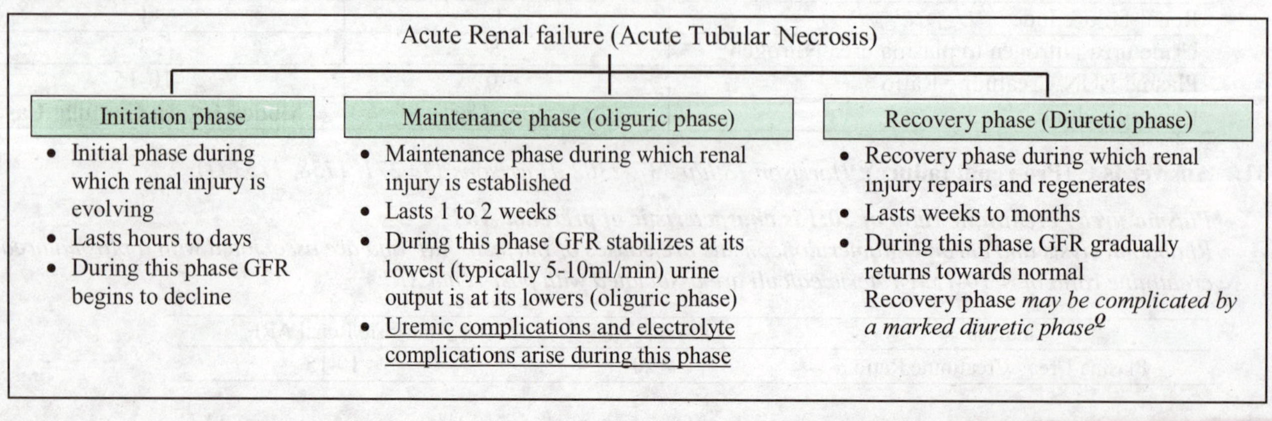

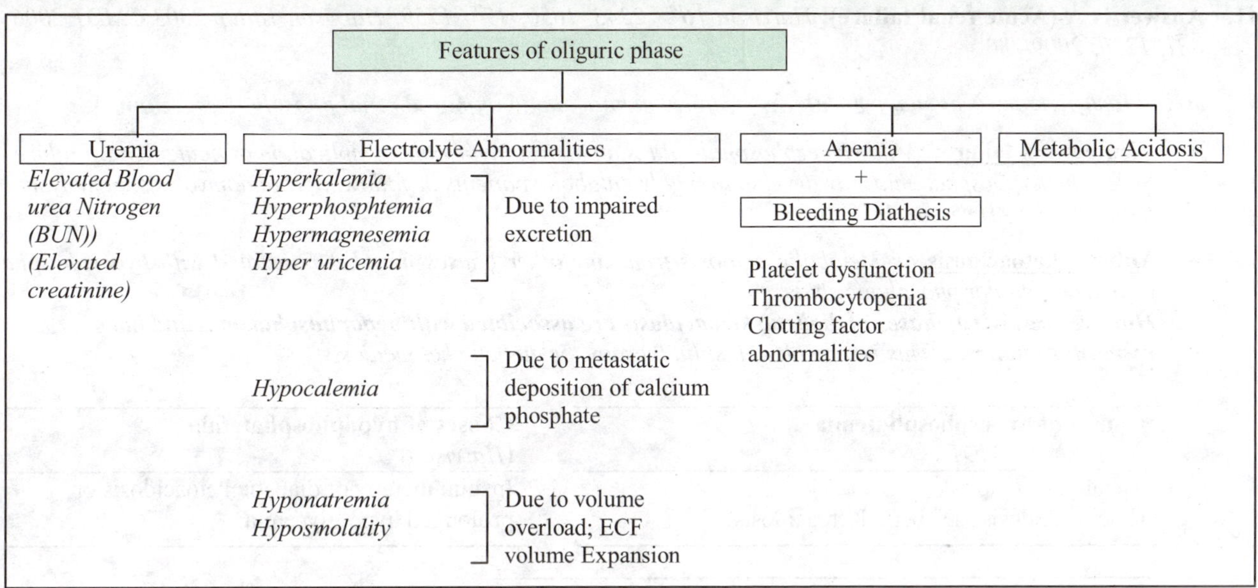

38. Answer is A (Hypercalcemia): *Harrison 18th/p 2303, 2306 Harrisons 17th/1754, 1759, 1760*

The oliguric phase of acute renal failure is associated with hypocalcemia and not hypercalcemia

The oliguric phase (maintenance phase) of acute renal failure is associated with uremic and electrolyte complications. Metastatic deposition of calcium phosphate leads to hypocalcemia. Other factors that lead to hypocalcemia include tissue resistance to the actions of parathyroid hormone and reduced levels of vitamin D.

39. Answer is A (Hypernatremia): *Harrison 18th/p 2303, 2306 Harrisons 17th/ 1754, 1759, 1760, Harrisons 16th/1650, Refer Previous question.*

Oliguric phase of ATN is asociated with Hyponatremia and not hypernatremia

Hyponatremia results from expansion of ECF volume due to dimnished water excretion and excessive administration of free water (volume overload)

40. Answer is A (Aminoglycoside toxicity): *Harrison 18th /2298; Management of Acute Kidney Problems (Springer) 2010 / 321; References with Text; Pediatric Nephrology (Lippincott Williams) 2004 /1235*

Non-Oliguric Renal Failure is typically associated with Aminoglycoside toxicity.

'Aminoglycoside nephrotoxicity typically is associated with non-oliguric renal failure'

– Management of Acute Kidney Problems

'Non-Oliguric renal failure is a common expression of aminoglycoside nephrotoxity and may reflect a direct inhibitory effect on solute transport along the thick ascending loop of Hence or possibly tubulointerstitial cell injury.

- Diseases of Kidney and Urinary Tract 8th/1035

'Non-Oliguric Acute Kidney Injury accompanies 10-30% of courses of aminoglycosides even when plasm levels are in therapeutic range'- Harrison 18th/ 2298

'The Acute Kidney Injury of Aminoglycoside toxicity is characteristically non-oliguric and reversible with a low mortality' - 'Renal and Electrolyte Disorders' by Shriev (Lippincott Williams) 2010/357-358

Cause of ARF	Aminoglycoside Toxicity	Contrast Associated Nephritoxicity	Glumerulonephritis	HUS
Urine output	*Typically Non-Oligouric*	*Oliguric more than Non-oliguric*	*Usually Oliguric*	*Usually Oliguric*

Non-Oliguric renal failure may also be associated with contrast induced nephropathy, however it is most typical /characteristic of Aminoglycoside toxity.

41. Answer is A (Acute renal failure): *Harrison 16th / 2243, 1650; 17th/ 1759; Harrison 18th/p 2303 CMDT 2006 / 882, 881, 1230; 2009/780*

Renal insufficiency is associated with hyperphosphatemia due to impaired renal phosphate excretion.

- **Acute renal failure:** *'Mild Hyperphosphatemia is an almost invariable complication of Acute Renal Failure. Severe hyperphosphatemia may develop in highly catabolic patients or following rhabdomyolysis, hemolysin or tumor lysis.' – Harrison 16th / 1650*
- **Dibetic ketoacidosis** *or Metabolic acidosis from any other causes may be associated with hyperphosphatemia from transcellular phosphatic shifts.*
  However resolving phases of diabetic ketoacidosis are associated with hypophosphatemia and not hyperphosphatemia. *This is a result of insulin therapy for diabetic ketoacidosis.*

Causes of hyperphosphatemia (*Harrison / CMDT*)
Metabolic acidosis (Lactic acidosis / Diabetic Ketoacidosis)

Causes of hypophosphatemia (*Harrison*)
Insulin therapy of diabetic ketoacidosis or prolonged hyperglycemia.

Laboratory values in DKA / Harrison 6th / 323 - 324
Phosphate values are : decreased *(large changes occurs during treatment of DKA*

Also note that total body stores of phosphorus (Also potassium, sodium, chloride, magnesium) are reduced in DKA, but are not accurately reflected by their levels (serum values may be increased) because of dehydration and hyperglycemia. – Harrison

- **Respiratory alkalosis** is associated with ***hypophosphatemia*** by causing intracellular shift of phosphorus into cells.

Hypophosphatemia	Hyperphosphatemia
• Metalbolic alkalosis • Respiratory alkalosis	• Metabolic acidosis • Respiratory acidosis

- **Chronic alcoholism / Alcoholism** *is known to cause* ***hypophosphatemia****. – Harrison 16th / 881*
  Severe hypophosphatemia is common and multifactorial in alcoholic patients.
  Chronic alcohol use results in a decrease in the renal threshold of phosphate excretion.' – CMDT 09/780
- **Patients with COPD and Asthma** *commonly have* ***hypophosphatemia****.*
  This is attributed to xanthine derivatives causing shifts of phosphate intracellularly and the phosphaturic effects of beta – adrenergic agonists , loop diuretics , xanthine derivatives and corticosteroids. – CMDT 2006 / 88; 09/780

Chronic Renal Failure

42. Answer is E (All of the above): *CMDT 2008/793*

Isothenuria and Broadcast sediment are common in chronic renal failure. Impotence and Restless legs are features of uremia seen in chronic renal failure.

Essentials of Diagnosis of CRF:
Progressive Azotemia over months to years
Symptoms and signs of uremia when nearing endstage disease
Hypertension in the majority
Isothenuria and broad casts in urinary sediment are common
Bilateral small kidneys on ultrasound are diagnostic.

Symptoms and Signs of Uremia:

Organ System	Symptoms	Signs
General	Fatigue, weakness	Sallow appearing, chronically ill
Skin	Pruritus, easy bruisability	Pallor, ecchymoses, excoriations, edema, xerosis
ENT	Metallic taste in mouth, epistaxis	Urinous breath
Eye		Pale conjunctiva
Pulmonary	Shortness of breath	Rales, pleural effusion
Cardiovascular	Dyspnea on exertion, retrosternal pain on inspiration (pericarditis)	Hypertension, cardiomegaly, friction rub
Gastrointestinal	Anorexia, nausea, vomiting, hiccups	
Genitourinary	Nocturia, ***impotence***	***Isosthenuria***
Neuromuscular	***Restless legs,*** numbness and cramps in legs	
Neurologic	Generalized irritability and inability to concentrate, decreased libido.	Stupor, asterixis, myoclonus, peripheral neuropathy

43. Answer is B (Stage II): *Harrison 18th /2319*

Kidney damage with mild decrease in GFR is classified as stage II of chronic Kidney Disease.

Clinical Action Plan			
Stage	**Description**	**GFR, mL/min per 1.73 m^2**	**Action**
1	*Kidney damage with normal or ↑GFR*	90	Diagnosis and treatment, treatment of comorbid conditions, slowing progression, cardiovascular disease (CVD) risk reduction
2	***Kidney damage with mild ↓GFR***	60–89	Estimating progression
3	*Moderate ↓GFR*	30–59	Evaluating and treating complications
4	*Severe ↓GFR*	15–29	Preparation for kidney replacement therapy
5	*Kidney failure*	<15 (or dialysis)	Kidney replacement (if uremia present)

44. Answer is C (>60%): *'Fluid Electrolytes with Clinical Applications' 7th (Cengage Learning) 2004*

Signs of renal failure become apparent when renal function deteriorates by more than 60% while overt symptoms usually develop only after renal function has deteriorated by >75 – 80%.
Since the question specifically asks about both signs and symptoms of Renal failure, deterioration of Renal function by more than 60% is the single best answer of choice.

Stages of CRF:

Stages	Pathophysiologic factors
Stage I: dimninished renal reserve	Residual renal function is 50% of the normal kidney function. • *Excretory and regulatory renal functions are intact.* • *Renal laboratory studies are asymptomatic (BUN and serum creatinine are normal).* • *At least a 50-60% loss of renal function is required before signs of renal failure are evident.* • *No symptoms are evident until there is a loss of at least 80% renal function.*
Stage II: renal insufficiency	Residual renal function is 20-40% of the normal kidney function. • *There is a decrease in the glomerular filtration rate (GFR), solute clearance, ability to concentrate urine, and hormone secretion.* • *Renal laboratory studies reveal a rising BUN and serum creatinine, mild azotemia, polyuria, nocturia, and anemia.* • *Signs and symptoms become more severe if the kidneys are stressed. i.e., fluid volume depletion or exposure to a nephrotic substance.*
Stage III: Renal failure	Residual renal function is 10-20% of the normal kidney function. • *There is an inability of the kidneys to regulate volume and solute composition.* • *Renal laboratory studies reveal an increased BUN and serum creatinine, azotemla, anemia, and metabolic acidosis. Signs and symptoms of renal failure are present.*

Stage IV: end – stage renal disease (ESRD)	Residual renal function is <10% of the normal kidney function. • *Excretory, regulatory, and hormonal renal functions are severely impaired and unable to maintain homeostasis.* • *Renal laboratory studies and physical symptoms reveal markedly elevated BUN and serum creatinine levels.* • *Anemia, hyperphosphatemia, hypocalcemia, metabolic acidosis, hyperuricemia, hyperkalemia, fluid overload, usually oliguric, and urine osmolality similar to serum osmolality.* • *A uremic syndrome develops and all body systems are affected by renal failure.* • *Mortality rate is 100% if peritoneal dialysis, hemodialysis, or renal transplant is not implemented.*

45. Answer is C (70-80%): *Refer previous question*

46. Answer is C (Chronic Renal Failure): *Harrison 18th/218, 2317; Harrison 17th/176, 1768; The 5 minute Clinical Consult (2007)/1494*

Iron deficiency and chronic renal failure may cause Restless leg syndrome *– Harrison 17th/176*

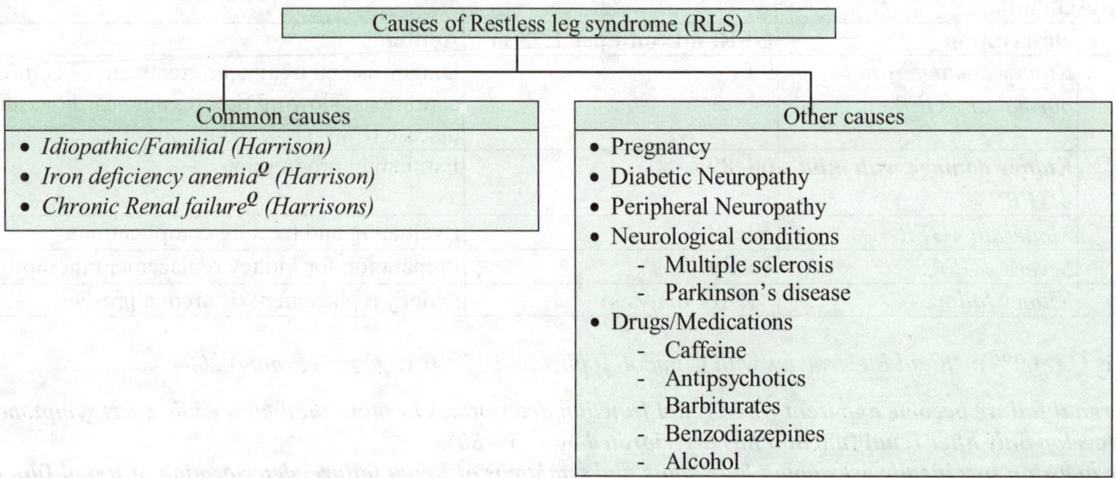

47. Answer is B (Hypocalcemia): *Harrison 15th/ 1555, 16th/1656; 17th / 1764, 1768; Harrison 18th/2317; Adam's 8th / 970*

'The total plasma calcium concentration in CRF patient is significantly low. ***Patient with chronic renal disease tolerate the hypocalcemia quite well and rarely is a patient symptomatic from the decreased calcium concentration.*** This may be partly due to concomitant acidosis.' - *Harrison*

Hyponatremia, acidosis and hyper osmolarity can lead to various CNS manifestation as lethargy, altered mentation, seizure, coma, and paralysis etc.

48. Answer is A (Metabolic Acidosis): *Harrison 17th /1764; Harrison's 18th/2312*

Chronic Renal Disease / Failure is commonly associated with metabolic acidosis.

'Metabolic acidosis is a common disturbance in advanced chronic Renal Disease' - Harrison's 18th/2312

49. Answer is B (Hypophosphatemia): *Harrison 14th/ 1516; 15th/ 1553 t; 16th/1655; 17th/ 1763 (t. 274.31); Harrison 18th/p 2311 (Table: 280.4)*

Hypophosphatemia has not been mentioned as a manifestation in Uremia

Electrolyte disturbances in Uremia: - *Harrison*
Hyponatremia (Hypernatremia may also be seen)
Hyperkalemia (Hypokalemia may also be seen)
Hyperphosphatemia
Hypocalcemia
Hyperuricemia

50. Answer is C (Hypercalcemia): *Harrison 14th/ 1516; 15th/ 1553 t; 16th/1655; 17th/ 1763 (t. 274.31)*

Chronic Renal Failure is associated with Hypocalcemia and not hypercalcemia.

51. Answer is D (Hyperphosphatemia): *CMDT*

Serum phosphorus in renal osteodystrophy is either high or normal.

The disorders of calcium, phosphorus and bone in chronic renal failure are referred to as Renal Osteodystrophy. In CRF as GFR decreases below 25% of normal, phosphorus excretion is impaired leading to hyperphosphatemia which in turn leads to hypocalcemia, which stimulates secretion of Parathormone, which has a phosphaturic effect and normalizes serum phosphorus. ***Thus serum phosphorus in renal osteodystrophy is either high or normal.***
While in Osteomalacia there is hypophosphatemia *(CMDT 09/781).*

52. Answer is A (Post streptococcal GN): *Robbins 6th/ 951; API / 652, 656; Harrison 16th/1680; Harrison 17th / 1787 Harrison 18th/p 2340*

Acute post streptococcal GN is a cause of acute Renal failure and not Chronic Renal Failure. The other types of GN listed in the question are causes of CRF.
In Post Streptococcal Gn *(Acute GN): 95% of the affected children recover. The remaining of who do not recover, develop a Rapidly Progressive form of Glomerulonephritis and land up in ACUTE RENAL FAILURE.*

53. Answer is B (Increased capillary density at distal half of nails): *Oxford Textbook of clinical Nephrology 3rd/1883*

The increase in capillary density of nail bed accounts for the band of discolouration *–Oxford Text book of Clinical Nephrology*

Half and Half Nail: Typical nail sign in Uraemia

- In half-and half nail, two portions can be distinguished separated almost horizontally by a clear line of demarcation.
- Proximally the nail has a dull whitish ground glass appearance Distally the nail bed, is red, pink or brown (occupies 20-60% of total nail length)
- When pressure is applied, the discolouration does not fade completely
- Change can affect single nails or all nails of the hands, feet or both

Pathology /Histology

- *The disorder is believed to result from increase in capillary density of the nail bed*
- *The number of capillaries under the nail plate is increased, with remarkable thickening of the capillary walls*
- *The histology of the nail plate itself shows no change and it contains no melanin.*

54. Answer is B or D (Peripheral Neuropathy or Seizures): *Harrison 17th/1763 Harrison 18th/p 2310, 3311*

The response to dialysis in Peripheral Neuropathy and seizures is variable.
These abnormalities may persist even after initiation of dialysis.

Effect of dialysis and related therapy:

(I) denotes an abnormality that usually improves after dialysis and related therapy
(P) denotes an abnormality that tends to persist or even progress after dialysis and related therapy
(D) denotes an abnormality that usually develops after dialysis and related therapy

Fluid and electrolyte disturbances	**Neuromuscular disturbances**	**Dermatologic disturbances**
Volume expansion (I)	Fatigue (I)	Pallor (P)
Hyponatremia (I)	Sleep disorders (P)	Hyperpigmentation (I, P or D)
Hyperkalemia (I)	Headache (P)	Pruritus (P)
Hyperphosphatemia (I)	Impaired mentation (I)	Ecchymoses (I)
Endocrine metabolic disturbances	Lethargy (I)	Nephrogenic fibrosing dermopathy (D)
Secondary hyperparathyroidism (I or P)	Asterixis (I)	Uremic frost (I)
Adynamic bone (D)	Muscular irritability	**Gastrointestinal disturbances**
Vitamin D deficient osteomalacia (I)	Peripheral neuropathy (I or P)	Anorexia (I)
Carbohydrate resistance (I)	Restless leg syndrome (I or P)	Nausea and vomiting (I)
Hyperuricemia (I or P)	Myoclonus (I)	Gastroenteritis (I)

Hypertriglyceridemia (I or P) Increased Lp(a) level (P) Deacreased high density lipoprotein level (P) Proteinenergy malnutrition (I or P) Impaired growth and development (P) Infertility and sexual dysfunction (P) Amenorrhea (I/P) β2-Microglobulin associated amyloidosis (P or D)	Seizures (I or P) Coma (I) Muscle cramps (P or D) Dialysis disequilibrium syndrome (D) Myopathy (P or D) **Cardiovascular and pulmonary disturbances** Arterial hypertension (I or P) Congestive heart failure or pulmonary edema (I) Pericarditis (I) Hypertrophic or dilated cardiomyopathy (I, P or D) Uremic lung (I) Accelerated atherosclerosis (P or D) Hypotension and arrhythmias (D) Vascular calcification (P or D)	Peptic ulcer (I or P) Gastrointestinal bleeding (I, P or D) Idiopathic ascites (D) Peritonitis (D) **Hematologic and immunologic disturbances** Anemia (I) Lymphocytopenia (P) Bleeding diathesis (I or D) Increased susceptibility to infection (I or P) Leucopenia (D) Thrombocytopenia (D)

55. Answer is B (Infusion of insulin and glucose): *Harrison 18th/p 358, 359 Harrison 17th/284; Primer on kidney disease 4th/118*

'Intravenous insulin is the fastest way to lower serum potassium levels' *– Primer on Kidney Diseases 4th/118*

Management of Hyperkalemia

First step

Stabilize Myocardium

Method	Onset of action
Calcium gluconate or Calcium chloride	3 to 5 minutes (effect begins within minutes and is marked by Improvement in ECG appearance)

Second Step

Reduce serum K^+ levels by shifting K^+ from extracellular to intracellular fluid

Method	Onset of action
Insulin (Glucose)	Within 15 minutes *This is the fastest method*
Beta agonists (Albuterol)	In about 30 minutes
Sodium bicarbonate	At least 3-4 hours

Third step

Remove excess potassium from the body

Method	Comment
Diuretics	Works only if patient has adequate kidney function
Resin exchangers (Kayexalate) (sodium polystyrene sulfonate)	• Slow acting (Requires 1-2 hrs before plasma K^+ decreases) • Removes K^+ from blood into gut in exchange for an equal amount of Na^+.
Hemodialysis	Definitive treatment of choice in patients with advanced renal failure and severe hyperkalemia

56. Answer is C and D (Calcium chloride and sodium bicarbonate): *ALS manual of Resuscitation Council UK 5th*

Tall Peaked T waves on ECG indicate cardiac toxicity secondary to severe hyperkalemia. Management includes immediate administration of ***<u>Calcium salts</u>*** *(Calcium gluconate or Calcium chloride) to counteract the myocardial effects of hyperkalemia*

<u>Sodium bicarbonate</u> *helps reduce serum potassium concentration by redistributing potassium and shifting K^+ into cells.*

57. Answer is D (Beta blocker) : *Harrison 16th / 262-263; 17th / 284; Harrison 18th/p 358, 359 ALS Manual:Resuscitation council UK; 5th edition*

Beta blockers have no role in management of hyperkalemia

Parenteral or Nebulrized Beta 2 agonist may be useful by promoting cellular uptake of K^+.***Calcium gluconate*** *provides cardiac protection by decreasing membrane excitability, white* ***Insulin and Sodium bicarbonate*** *decrease plasma K^+ concentration by shifting K^+ into cells.*

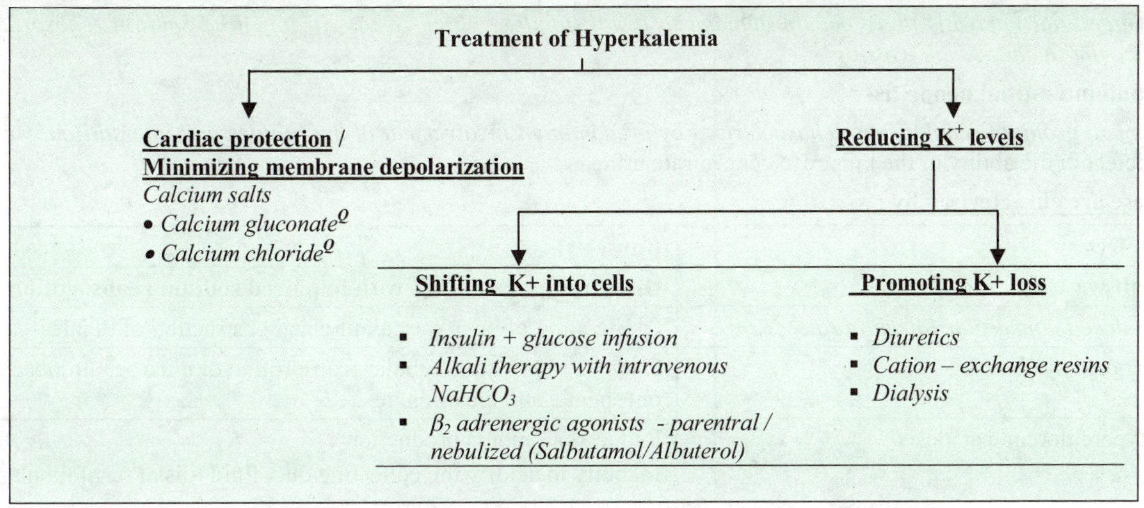

Advanced Life Support Guidelines for Treatment of Hyperkalemia

Mild elevation (5.5-6 mmol/L)	**Moderate / severe elevation without ECG changes (>6 mmol/l)**	**Moderate / severe elevation With toxic ECG changes (>6 mmol/l)**
Remove K+ from body ▪ Cation exchange resins ▪ Diuretics ▪ Consider dialysis	Remove K+ from body ▪ Dextrose / insulin infusion (+/-) ▪ Nebulized salbutamol ▪ Intravenous NaHCO3 (+) ▪ strategies as for mild elevation	First stabilize the heart / Antagonize the toxic effects of Hyperkalemia. Calcium gluconate (+) Other strategies

Tubulointestinal Disease

58. Answer is B (INH): *Harrison 18th/p 2367 Harrisons 17th/ 1807 Harrisons 16th/1702*

INH is not associated with interstitial nephritis

Beta Lactom antibiotics, Diuretics and Allopurinol may all be associated with interstitial nephritis

Drugs causing interstitial Nephritis

Antibiotics	NSAIDS	Diuretics	Anticonvulsants	Miscellaneous
• Antibiotics (β-lactams, sulfnamides, quinolones, vancomycin, erythromycin, minocycline, rifampin, ethambutol, acyclovir) • Nosteroidal anti-inflammatory drugs • Cyclooxygenase 2 inhibitors	• Bacteria (streptococcus, Staphylococcus, legionella, Salmonella, Brucella, Yersinia, Corynebacterium diphtheriae) • Viruses (Epstein-Barr virus, cytomegalovirus, Hantavirus, polymavirus, (HIV)	Diuretics (thiazides, furosemide, triamterene)	Anticonvulsants (phenytoin, phenobarbital, carbamazepine, valporic acid)	Miscellaneous (captopril, H2 receptor blockers, proton pumpinhibitors, mesalazine, indinavir, allopurinol)

59. Answer is A (Interstitial Nephritis): *Harrison 16th/1703; 17th/1806, 1807; (t-279.2) Harrison 18th/p 2367 Robbin's illustrated 6th/971*

In interstitial nephritis there occurs damage to distal tubules, which results in impaired sodium reabsorption and hence the so called 'salt wasting'.

Tubulointerstitial nephritis-

This is a group of renal disease characterized by predominant involvement of the ***tubules*** *and* ***interstitium*** which leads to defect in the ability of the kidney to concentrate urine.

These are chracterised by :

Defect	Causes(s)
Salt wasting	**Distal tubular damage with impaired sodium reabsorption**
Reduced glomerular filtration rate	Obliteration of microvasculature and obstruction of tubules
Fanconi syndrome	Damage to proximal tubular reabsorption of glucose, aminoacids, phosphate, and bicarbonate
Hyperchloremic acidosis	Reduced ammonia production Inability to acidify the collecting duct fluid (distal renal tubular acidosis) Proximal bicarbonate wasting
Tubular or small-molecular weight preoteinuria	Failure of proximal tubule protein reabsorption
Polyuria, isothenuria	Damage to medullary tubules and vasculature
Hyperkalemia	Potassium secretory defects including aldosterone resistance

60. Answer is C (PNH): *Fundamentals of Uroradiology (1999) /64; 20 common problems in urology (2001)/156 Harrisons 17th*

PNH is not associated with necrotizing papillitis or papillary necrosis

Diabetes milletus, analgesic abuse (salicylate poisoning) and Renal vein thrombosis are documented causes for renal papillary necrosis

Renal Papillary Necrosis
• Renal papillary necrosis is typically caused by ischaemic necrosis and sloughing of Renal Papllae (The papillary tip is the apex of renal pyramid) • <u>It is clinically charachterized by</u> *Loin Pain* *Hematuria* *Variable degree of renal impairment*
Etiology / Predisposing factors
• Diabetes and analgesic abuse (NSAIDS) are the most common predisposing factors • The Acronym POST CARD is traditionally used to enlist the causes of papillary necrosis but it does not put the causes in a useful order of incidence

P	Pyelonephritis
O	Obstruction
S	Sickle –cell disease
T	Tuberculosis
C	Cirrhosis
A	Analgesic abuse/Alcohol
R	Renal vein thrombosis
D	Diabetes

POSTCARD – causes of papillary necrosis

61. Answer is B (Tuberculous Pyelonephritis): *Harrison 18th/2367; Harrison 17th/1807, 1825, 1826; Robbins 7th/1000, 1003, 1004, 1011*

Tuberculosis is the least important/common cause of necrotizing papillitis amongst the options provided.

Causes of Renal Papillary Necrosis /Necrotizing Papillitis

- *Analgesic Abuse Nephropathy (NSAIDs)*
- *Diabetes Mellitus*
- *Sickle cell Disease*
- *Obstruction in association with infection (pyeloneplíritis)*
- *Chronic Alcoholism*
- *Vascular Renal Diseases (Renal vein thrombosis)*

Dibetese Mellitus and Analgesic abuse are the most frequent causes of Renal Papillary Necrosis

62. Answer is A (Salicylate poisoning): *Harrison 15th/ 1625, 1607; 16th/1703; 17th/1807; Robbins 7th /1003, 1004*

'Salicylate poisoning' or analgesic abuse nephropathy is one of the most common causes of necrotizing papillitis.

63. Answer is C (PNH): *Harrison 17th/ 1807, 1825, 1826; Refer previous question for references*

All causes other than PNH are known causes of necrotizing papillitis

64. Answer is A (Diabetes Mellitus): *Dorland's Illustrated Medical Dictionary 28th/ 1104*

'Renal papillary necrosis, an accompaniment of acute pyelonephritis is most often seen in diabetics and is characterised by necrosis of renal papillae of one or both kidneys with sharped demarcation between necrotic and living tissue' *– Dorlands*
Thus while papillary necrosis is a feature of more than one conditions mentioned in the question, it is most commonly seen with diabetes mellitus.

65. Answer is A (Alcohol): *Harrison 17th /1825*

Chronic Alcoholism is an established cause of Renal Papillary Necrosis.

Glomerular Diseases

Nephrotic Syndrome

66. Answer is A (RBC cast in urine): *CMDT 2005/885, 890; Harrison 17th/1785, Harrison 18th/p 2337 CMDT 2003/891; 2009/794*

RBC cast in urine is a feature of Nephritic Syndrome and not nephrotic syndrome,

The other 3 points mentioned are <u>'essentials' in the diagnosis of nephrotic syndrome</u> :

1. Proteinuria : excretion > 3.5g/1.73 m2 per 24 hrs. ^{Q}
2. Hypoalbunemia : albumin < 3g/dl. ^{Q}
3. Peripheral edema. ^{Q}

Hyperlipidemia ^{Q} occurs in 50% of those with early nephrotic syndrome and is much more common in patients who excrete larger amounts of protein per day.

67. Answer is D (Fibrinogen): *Harrison 16th/1684, 1685; 17th / 1789, 1790 Harrison 18th/p 2345*

Nephrotic syndrome is characteristically associated with increased fibrinogen levels – Hyper fibrinogenemia.

- ***Nephrotic syndrome is characteristically associated with increased fibrinogen levels – Hyper fibrinogenemia.*** *This is due to increase hepatic synthesis, impaired fibrinolysis, and increased platelet aggregability. It is an important factor responsible for hypercoagulability seen in Nephrotic syndrome.* ***<u>Patient of nephrotic syndrome can develop spontaneous peripheral arterial or venous thrombosis.</u>***
  - Renal vein thrombosis ^{Q}
  - Pulmonary embolisms.
- ***Serum albumin*** *is decreased* due to proteinuria ^{Q}. Hypoalbumnimia is compounded by increased renal catabolism and inadequate albeit increased hepatic synthesis of albumin.

- ***Transferrin*** loss in urine leads to decreased levels of serum transferrin. This is responsible for *iron resistant microcytic hypochromic anemia.* [Q]
- ***Ceruloplasmin level**, too are decrease* on account of its loss in urine. [Q]

68. Answer is B (Fibrinogen): *Harrison 16th/1684, 1685; Harrison 17th/ 1789, 1790*

Nephrotic syndrome is characteristically associated with increased fibrinogen levels – Hyper fibrinogenemia.

Proteins increased in nephrotic syndrome
1. Fibrinogen
2. Lipoproteins: due to increased synthesis

Most proteins are however decreased in Nephrotic Syndrome.

Proteins decreased	Consequence
Albumin	Oedema due to hypoalbunimia [Q]
Transferrin	Fe resistant microcytic anemia [Q]
Cholecalciferol binding protein	Hypocalcemia [Q]
Thyroxine binding globulin	Decreased thyroxin (Hypothyroid state)

69. Answer is B (Serum Fibrinogen): *Harrison 16th/1684, 1685; Harrison 17th/ 1789, 1790 Harrison 18th/p 2345*

Nephrotic syndrome is characteristically associated with increased fibrinogen levels – Hyper fibrinogenemia.

Proteins increased in nephrotic syndrome
1. Fibrinogen
2. Lipoproteins: due to increased synthesis

Most proteins are however decreased in Nephrotic Syndrome.

Proteins decreased	Consequence
Albumin	Oedema due to hypoalbunimia [Q]
Transferrin	Fe resistant microcytic anemia [Q]
Cholecalciferol binding protein	Hypocalcemia [Q]
Thyroxine binding globulin	Decreased thyroxin (Hypothyroid state)

70. Answer is A (Loss of Antithrombin III): *Harrisons 17th/272*

Loss of Antithrombin III contributes to the hypercoagulable state in Nephrotic syndrome

*'A hypercoagulable state frequently accompanies severe nephrotic syndrome **<u>due to urinary losses of antithrmbin III</u>**, reduced serum levels of protein C and S, hyperfibrinogenemia and enhanced platelet aggregation' – Harrison 17th/272*

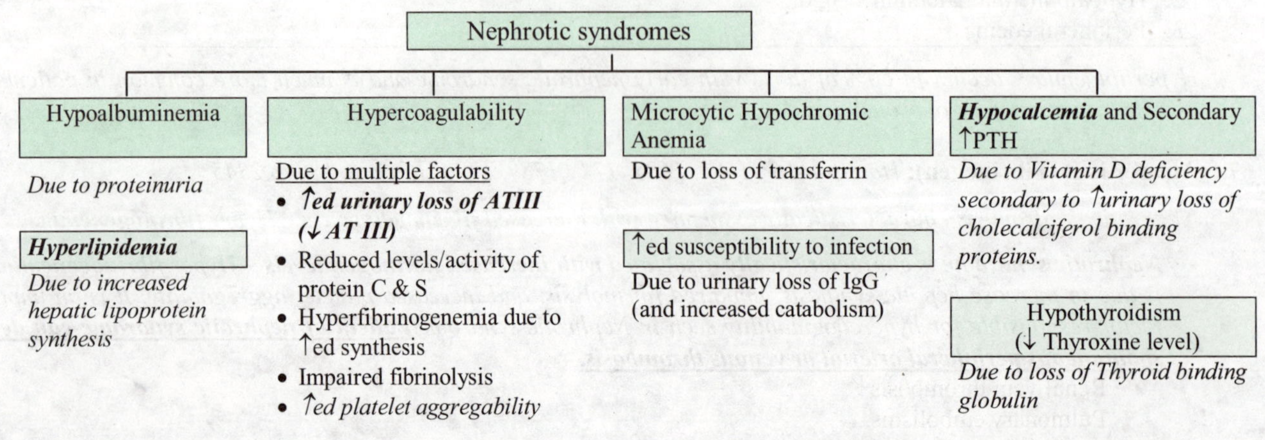

71. Answer is A and D (Low serum calcium and Platelet activation): *Harrison 16th/1684; 17th/272 Harrison 18th/p 339*

Nephrotic syndrome is associated with hypocalcemia and increased platelet activity (↑ed platelet aggregability)

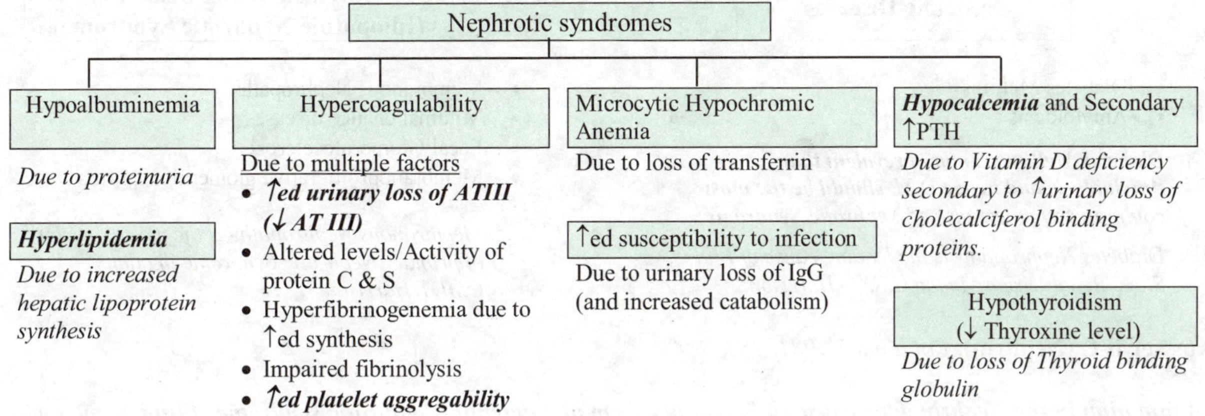

72. Answer is E (↓ HDL cholesterol): *Harrison 16th/1684; Harrison 17th; Clinical Pediatric Nephrology 2nd/173*

HDL levels are more often decreased in Nephrotic syndrome although they may be normal or elevated but still ↓HDL is the single best answer of choice

'The lipid profile in Nephrotic syndrome is characterized by elevations in total plasma cholesterol, very low density lipoproteins (VLDL) and low density lipoproteins (LDL) and often triglycerides levels as well as variable alterations (more often decreased) in high density lipoproteins (HDL)' – Clinical pediatric nephrology 2nd/173

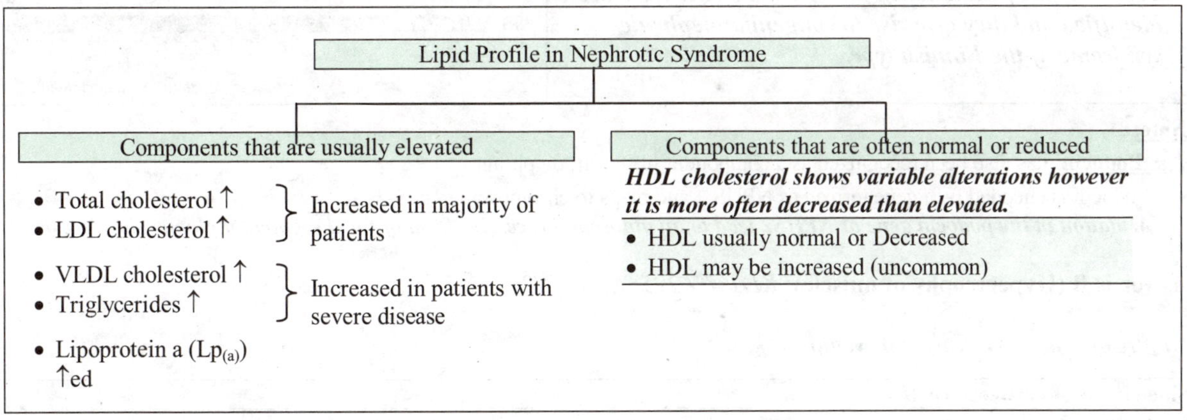

73. Answer is A (Diabetes Mellitus): *CMDT 2007/941; 2009/818; Harrison 16th/1684*

The most common cause of primary Nephrotic Syndrome in adult is Membranous Nephropathy but this is not provided amongst the options.

The most common systemic Renal Diseases associated with Nephrotic Syndrome are Diabetic Mellitus, Amyloidosis and Systemic Lupus Erythematosis (CMDT)

As per the prevalence of Diabetes Mellitus is much higher than Amyloidosis, Diabetes Mellitus is the single best answer of choice amongst the options provided.

There is no direct reference, quoting Diabetes Mellitus as the most common systemic disease associated with Nephrotic Syndrome. Neverthless, the text from both Harrison and CMDT supports this presumption.

Most common causes of Nephrotic Syndrome (Harrison)

Systemic Diseases	**Intrinsic Renal Diseases (Idiopathic Nephrotic Syndrome)**
• Diabetes Mellitus • Amyloidosis ***Diabetes Mellitus is more prevalent than Amyloidosis and hence D.M. should be the most common systemic cause of Nephrotic Syndrome*** *Diabetes Nephropathy is the leading cause of End Stage Renal Disease in the U.S.* Q *– Harrison*	• Membranous Nephropathy • Minimal change disease • Focal Glomerulosclerosis • Membranoproliferative glomerulonephritis *Membranous Nephropathy is the most common* Q *cause of primary Nephrotic Syndrome in adults – CMDT/Harrison*

74. Answer is C (Nephrin): *Robbin's 7th/981, 983, 984*

"***A mutation in the Nephrin gene causes a hereditary form of congenital Nephrotic syndrome (Finnish type) with minimal change glomerular morphology***"*- Robbins 7th/981*

Nephrin

- Nephrin is a key component of the slit diaphragm
- It is a zipper like structure between podocyte foot processes that might control glomerular permeability
- The Nephrin gene maps to chromosome 19q13 and is termed as NPHS1.
- ***Several type of Mutations of the NPHS1 gene have been identified and they give rise to congenital nephritic syndrome of the Finnish type.***

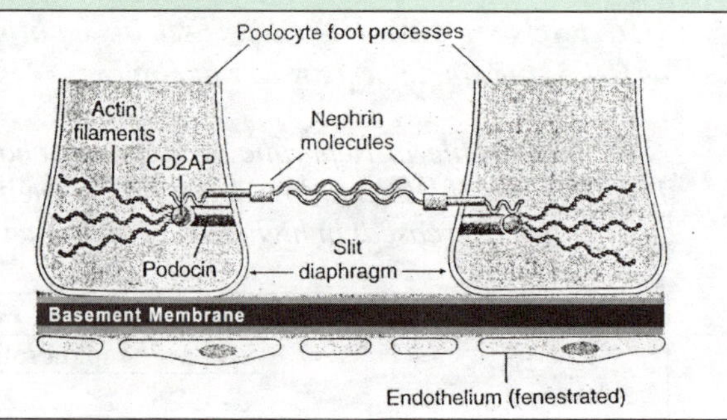

Note:

- **'Podocin'** has also been recognized as a component of the slit diaphragm
- Podocin is encoded by a gene termed as NPHS 2 and maps to chromosome 1q25-31
  Mutation in the podocin gene or NPHS2 lead to an autosomal recessive form of focal segmental glomerulosclerosis

75. Answer is B (Hypertrophy of muscle): *KDT 4th/ 295; KDT 5th/264, 265*

Atrophy of muscles / muscular weakness is seen.

Side effects of corticosteroids:	
- *Cushing's habitus* Q	- *Fragile skin, purple striae* Q
- ***Hyperglycemia*** Q	- *Muscular weakness* Q
- *Susceptibility to infection*	- *Delayed wound healing* Q
- *Peptic ulceration* Q	- *Osteoporosis* Q
- *Posterior subcapsular cataract* Q	- *Glaucoma* Q
- *Growth retardation*	- ***Psychiatric disturbances*** Q
- ***Suppression of hypothalamo-pituitary-adrenal axis***	

Nephritic Syndrome and RPGN

76. Answer is A (Polyuria): *Harrison 18th/p 2337, 2340 Harrison 17th/1785, 1786; Robbins 7th/973, 974*

Polyuria is not a feature of acute glomerulonephritis

Acute Glomerulonephritis is characterized clinically by the syndrome of acute nephritis or nephritic syndrome.

Acute Nephritic Syndrome	
Hypertension[Q] *Hematuria with RBC cast in urine*[Q] *Oliguria*[Q] *Pyuria*[Q] *Azotemia*[Q]	
Mild to moderate proteinuria[Q] *Edema*[Q]	*Patients with Acute nephritis syndrome also commonly have proteinuria and edema but these are not as severe as those encountered in nephrotic syndrome.*

77. Answer is C (Nephritic syndrome): *Robbins 6th / 935; Robbins 7th*

Post infective glomerulonephritis are acute glomerulonephritis that usually present with Acute Nephrotic syndrome.

It is the classic presentation of Post-Streptococcal or Post-Infective glomerulonephritis. *– Robbins 6th/935*

78. Answer is D (Alports syndrome): *Robbins 7th/ 977 Harrison 17th/1785 Harrison 18th/p 2338*

Alports syndrome is not associated with Rapidly Progressive Glomerulonephritis or Crescentric Glomerulonephritis
-Harrison 17th /1785

Rapidly progressive Glomerulonephritis (RPGN) / Crescentric Glomerulonephritis

Crescentric Glomerulonephritis is a histopathological diagnosis based upon the presence of 'crescents' in most of the Glomeruli. This type of histopathological picture (crescents) is seen in cases of Rapidly Progressive Glomerulonephritis (RPGN) and hence *RPGN and Crescentric Glomerulo–nephritis are often used synonymously.*

Causes of Crescenteric Glomerulonephritis (RPGN)

Type I RPGN (Anti – GBM Antibody)

- ***Idiopathic Anti Glomerular Basement membrane disease***
- *Good pasture's Syndrome*

Type II RPGN (Immune Complex)

- *Idiopathic*
- ***Acute Post Streptococcal Glomerulonephritis (PSGN)***
- *Lupus Glomerulonephritis (SLE)*
- ***Henoch Schonlein Purpura (HSP)***
- *IgA Nephropathy*
- *Membranoproliferative Glomerulonephritis (Harrisons 17th / 1785)*
- *Cryoglobulinemia (Harrision 17th/ 1785)*
- *Post infectious (After subacute Bacterial Endocarditis) Glomerulonephritis*

Type III RPGN (Pauci – immune)

- ANCA – Small Vessel Vasculitis
- *Wegener's granulomatosis*
- *Microscopic polyangitis*
- *Churg – Strauss syndrome*

Renal disease in Alport's syndrome (Harrisons 17th /1794)

Patients with Alport's syndrome develop *thinning and splitting of Glomerular basement membrane*[Q]*, and chronic glomerulosclerosis*[Q], leading to renal failure. *(Clinically present with hematuria & proteinuria)*
Rapidly progressive Glomerulonephritis or crescentric glomerulonephritis is not associated with Alport's syndrome.

79. Answer is B (Rapidly progressive glomerulonephritis): *Robbins 6th/ 452; 7th/977; Harrison 16th/1674; 17th / 1785 Harrison 18th/p 2337*
Rapidly progressive glomerulonephritis also known as Crescentic glomerulonephritis is characterized by the presence of crescents is most of the glomeruli.

Crescents are produced by
Proliferation of the *parietal epithelial cells* Q of Bowman's capsule Infiltration of *monocytes* Q and macrophages.

80. Answer is A (Minimal change disease): *Chandrasoma Taylor, 3rd/ 711; Robbins 7th/977; Harrison 16th/1679; 17th/1786, 1787, 1789 Harrison 18th/p 2337, 2341*

Minimal change disease is not associated with rapidly progressive glomerulonephritis (RPGN)

Rapidly progressive glomerulonephritis is a syndrome associated with severe glomerular injury.

It does not denote a specific etiologic form of glomerulonephritis.

RPGN is defined by 2 criteria.- Chandrasoma Taylor
Presence of *epithelial crescents* in more than 70% of glomeruli Q Occurrence of rapidly progressive renal failure.

End stage disease occurs within months.

Causes of rapidly progressive glomerulonephritis *table 48.4 Chandrasoma Taylor 3rd*

Post infections	Multisystem disease	Drugs	Idiopathic
• *Post-streptococcal Glomerulonephriti* Q • *Non streptococcal G.N.* • *Infective endocarditis* Q	• *Good pasture's syndrome* Q • *SLE* Q • *H. S. purpura* Q • *Berger's disease* Q *(IgA Nephropathy)* • *PAN* Q • *Wegener's granulomatosis* Q • *Membrano-proliferative glomerulonephritis*	• *Pencillamine* Q	• *Type I – with Anti GBM Ab* Q(*(20 %)* • *Type II-with immune complexes* Q *(30 %)* • *Type-III pauci immune (50%)* Q

81. Answer is C (Diabetic Nephropathy): *Robbins 7th/977; Harrison 18th/p 2338; 17th/ 1785; Refer previous question*

Diabetic Nephropathy is not associated with rapidy progressive Glomerulonephritis (RPGN).

Acute post streptococcal GN, SLE and Good pasture's syndrome are all associated with Rapidly progressive Glomerulonephritis.

82. Answer is C (Microscopic polyangitis): *Robbins 7th / 977*

Pauci – immune crescenteric glomerulonephritis (Type III RPGN) is charachteristic of Microscopic Polyangitis

Henoch Schonlein Nephritis and Lupus Nephritis are examples of Immune complex mediated crescenteric nephritis (Type II RPGN)

Nephritis in Alports syndrome is not associated with crescenteric glomerulonephritis or RPGN

Pauci – Immune Crescenteric Glomerulonephritis : Type III RPGN

- Pauci – Immune crescenteric glomerulonephrits represents those cases of RPGN in which glomerular immunoglobulin deposits, either linear or granular are absent
  (Immunoflorescence and electron microscopy in these cases charachteristically show absence of Anti GBM antibodies and immune complexes)
- Most patients with Pauci – immune crescenteric G.N are positive for ANCA (upto 90% of patients), and hence this group is often called ANCA associated RPGN

Pauci – Immune crescenteric Glomerulonephritis includes
• *Idiopathic RPGN* Q • *Wegener's Granulomatosis* Q • *Microscopic polyangitis (Microscopic PAN)* Q

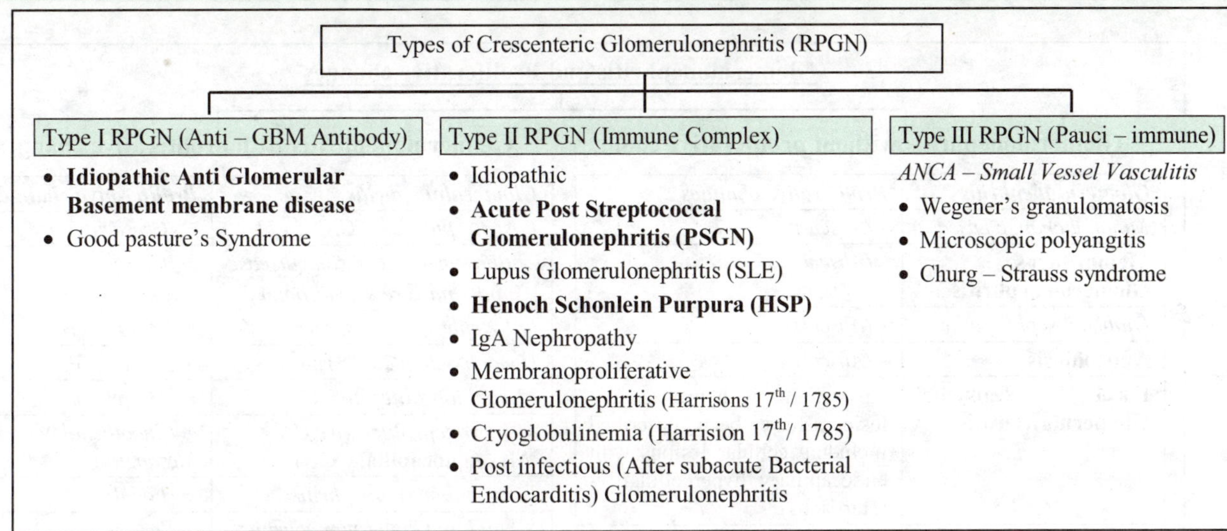

83. Answer is A (Rapid recovery) : *Harrison 14th / 1536 ; 15th / 1581; 16th/1679; API 8th / 747; CMDT 2008/803; Causes of RPGN*

RPGN is characterised by rapidly progressive renal disease which culminates in End stage renal disease (ESRF) within months after onset. Recovery is rare.

RPGN is characterized by a Subacute glomerular inflammation with :

- *Nephritic urinary sediment, i.e. RBC casts, WBC casts*
- *Sub-**nephrotic non-selective proteinuria*** (proteinuria < 3.5 g/24 hr) *(selective proteinuria is a feature of minimal change disease)*
- *Oliguria and Edema*
- *Hypertension*
- *Presence **of crescents** pathologically*

84. Answer is A (Number of crescents): *Robbins 6th /453*

The prognosis of crescentric glomerulonephritis relates to the number of crescents

'Prognosis can be roughly related to the number of crescents' - Robbins

85. Answer is B (Mesangiocapillary Glomerulonephritis) : *Harrison 18th/p 2334 Harrisons 17th /1789, Chandrasoma Taylor 3rd /708*

Mesangiocapillary Glomerulonephritis is the other name for Membranoproliferative glomerulonephritis. It is a type of proliferative Glomerulonephritis. *(Harrisons 17th /1789)*

Proliferative changes in Glomerulonephritis *(Refer: Chandrsoma Taylor 3rd /702, 708)*

- *Glomerulus contains Endothelial cells, Epethelial cells, and Mesangial cells. Any of the three cell types may undergo proliferation in different types of Proliferativ Glomerulonephritis.*
- *Proliferative changes are not limited to Membranoproliferative and Mesangioproliferative Glomerulonephritis, but may be seen in several other forms of Glomerulonephritis*

Glomerulonephritis and Proliferative changes

Glomerulonephritis without proliferative changes

Glomerulonephritis	*Proliferative changes*
Minimal change Disease	*- (Absent)*
Membranous Glomerulonephritis	*- (Absent)*
Diabetic Nephropathy	*- (Absent)*
Amyloidosis	*- (Absent)*
Focal segmental Glomerulosclerosis	± Variants with proliferative lesions have been described including cellular lesions with endocapillary hypercellularity- (Harrisons)

Glomerulonephritis with proliferative changes

Glomerulonephritis	*Proliferative changes*
Post streptococcal GN	*+ (Crescents)*
Antibasement membrane disease (Good – pasture's syndrome)	*+ (Crescents)*
IgA Nephropathy (Berger's)	*+ (Mesangial)*
Henoch Schonlein Purpura	*+ (Mesangial)*
Mesangioproliferative GN	*+ (Mesangial)*
Membranoproliferative GN **(Mesangiocapillary GN)**	*+ (Endothelial & Mesangial)*
Focal Glomerulonephritis	*+ (Focal)*
Secondary Glomerulonephritis SLE / PAN	*+ Variable*

Note : Crescents represent proliferation of epethelial cells

86. Answer is C >B (Membranoproliferative Glomerulonephritis > Cryoglobulinemia): *Harrison 16th / 1682. 2012; CMDT 2006 / 925*

The association of generalized edema, hypertension, proteinuria, hematuria along with hypocomplimentemia and positive anti-hepatitis C antibodies may be seen in both Membranoproliferative Glomerulonephritis and Mixed Cryoglobulinemia.

With the limited information provided in question MPGN appears to be a better option in comparison to Essential Mixed Cryoglobulinemia for the following reasons:

- *Cryoglobulinemic Glomerulopathy is most common with the Mixed Cryoglobuliinemias Type II and III that are most common in females and begin in the sixth decade. – Harrison 16tth / 1682*

  The patient in question is a male in the 4th decade of life (30years)

- *Most patients with cryoglobulinemia present with variable combination of stress ulceration, arthralgia, fatigue and Raynaud's phenomenon other than renal manifestations. The fundamental finding is presence of circulating cryoprecipitates.*

  The patient in question is not presenting with any of the above features to favour Mixed Cryoglobulinemia over MPGN.

- ***Membranoproliferative glomerulonephritis is responsible for 80% of all Renal lesions in Essential Mixed Cryoglobunemia.*** *-Harrison 16th / 2012*

Hepatitis C infection and Glomerular lesions (CMDT 924)
Three clinicopathologic glomerular syndromes associated with hepatitis C are: • ***Secondary MPGN*** • ***Cryoglobulinemic Glomerulopathy*** • *Membranous nephropathy*
MPGN is the most common lesion. *These patients typically have haematuria, hypertension, proteinuria and anemia. Hypocomplementemia is very common with C4 typically more reduced than C3.*

Low complement level nephritis syndromes
(Immune complex glonerulonephritis) • *Idiopathic proliferative glomerulonephritis* • *Crescentric glomenelonephritis* • ***Membranoproliferative glomerulonephritis*** • *Lupus nephritis* • ***Cryoglobulinemia*** • *Bacterial endocarditis* • *Shunt nephritis* • *Post infectious glomerulonephritis (post streptococcal)*

87. Answer is B > C (Essential mixed cryoglobulinemia): *Refer Previous question*

The presence of skin ulceration on clinical examination in a female patient around the 6th decade favors a diagnosis of Essential Mixed Cryoglobulinemia over MPGN.
Nevertheless if Essential Mixed Cryoglobulinemia were not amongst the options MPGN would be the single best answer of choice. ***Membranoproliferative glomerulonephritis is a responsible for 80% of all renal lesions in essential mixed cryoglobulinemia.***

IgA Nephropathy and PSGN

88. Answer is D (Absence of associated proteinuria is pathognomic) : *Robbins 6th/962; Robbins 7th/988; Harrison's 15th/1589; Harrison 16th/1690; Harrison 17th / 1788, 1789, Harrison 18th/p 2342, 2343 Chandrasoma Taylor 3rd/7110*

"Proteinuria may or may not be associated" *- above references*

Berger's Disease/IgA Nephropathy

Aetiopathogenesis		
Respiratory or gastrointestinal exposure to environmental agents (viruses, bacteria etc.) ↓ Genetic or acquired abnormality of immune regulation resulting in *increased mucosal IgA synthesis*[Q] ↓ Formation of circulating *IgA immune complexes*[Q] which are entrapped *in mesangium.*[Q]		
Microscopic Pathology[Q]	**Immunofluorescence**	**Electron Microscope**
Mesangioproliferative *(diffuse) glomerulonephritis > **Segmental** proliferation confined to some glomeruli (**focal** proliferative glomerulonephritis)> Overt crescentric glomerulonephritis (rare)*	*Mesangial deposition of IgA often with C3 and properidin*[Q] *(IgG is present in 50% of cases.)*[Q]	*Electron dense deposits in mesangium*[Q]. mesangial hypercellularity, sclerosis
Clinical		
Haematuria : Most common presentation is with ***gross haematuria*** *24 to 48 hrs after a pharyngeal / gastrointestinal infection*[Q] / vaccination or strenuous exercise. ***Microscopic haematuria***[Q] detected during routine physical examination may be the presentation. ***Proteinuria*** (Nephrotic syndrome) : *may or may not be present*[Q] *- Robbins* ***Hypertension*** (20-30%) is *unusual at presentation.*[Q]		

89. Answer is B (Mesangioproliferative glomerulonephritis): *Harrison 16th/1675; 17th/1788,1790; Harrison 18th/p 2342, 2343 Chandrasoma Taylor 3rd/711;*

IgA Nephropathy is a type of mesangioproliferative glomerulonephritis with IgA deposition in the mesangium

Mesangioproliferative Glomerulonephritis:

Causes	Typical pathological findings	Typical clinical presentation
IgA Nephropathy Henoch Schonlein Purpura	Proliferation of mesangial cells and deposition of IgA in matrix	Haematuria Proteinuria Hypertension

90. The Answer is A (Henoch schonlein purpura) : *Harrison 18th/p 2342, 2343 Harrison 17th/1788, 1789;Robbins 6th / 965; 7th/990; Chandrasoma Taylor 3rd /712*

Renal manifestations in henoch schonlein purpura are very similar to those in IgA nephropathy. IgA is deposited in the glomerular mesangium in a distribution similar to IgA nephropathy.

Renal manifestations of Henoch Schonlein Purpura include:

Haematuria (gross or microscopic), proteinuria, and nephrotic syndrome.
Rapidly progressive G.N. may be seen.
The difficulty in isolating cases of Henoch schonlein purpura from those of Ig A nephropathy has led to the notion that these are spectra of the same disease.

91. Answer is A (IgA Nephropathy) : *Nelsons 18th/2169, 2170-2173; Rudolph Pediatrics 21st /1682*

Recurrent episodes of painless gross haematuria represent the classic clinical presentation of IgA nephropathy.
- Rudolph's Pediatrics 21st/1682

Recurrent episodes of gross haematuria

Recurrent Gross Haematuria should be distinguished from isolated episodes of gross hematuria, as it is a charachteristic feature of some specific disorders

Charachteristic Causes of Recurrent Gross Haematuria (Nelson 18th/2169)	
1. IgA Nephropathy 2. Alports syndrome 3. Thin Glomerular basement membrane disease	*Isolated Glomerular diseases with recurrent Gross haematuria*
4. Hypercalciuria 5. Urolithiasis	

Recurrent Gross Haematuria must be distinguished from Urethrorrhagea.

Urethrorrhagia refers to urethral bleeding in the absence of urine.It is associated with dysuria and blood spots on underwear after voiding .It often occurs in prepubertal boys at intervals, several months apart over a period of many years, and has a benign self limiting cause.

- ***Recurrent episodes of gross hematuria is a charachteristic feature of IgA Nephropathy***

  IgA nephropathy is the most frequent glomerular disease in the world (Rudolph)
  It presents most commonly in children (patient in question is 6 year old) and young adults.

  Recurrent episodes of painless gross (macroscopic) haematuria is the classical presentation of IgA Nephropathy.

  Patients classically present with gross haematuria within 1 – 2 days after the onset of an upper respiratory tract infection that typically resolves within 5 days

  IgA Nephropathy is the single best answer amongst the options provided

- ***Gross Haematuria is an uncommon presentation in Wilm's tumor*** *(CPDT 18th/905)*

  Wilm's tumor is unlikely to present with recurrent gross haematuria.

- ***Gross Haematuria is not a feature of Neuroblastoma***

- ***Henoch Schonlein Purpura*** *may present with Gross haematuria in 20 –30% of cases, Gross haematuria however is not as common in H.S. Purpura as in IgA nephropathy and H.S purpura is not listed in the list of suggested diagnosis in a child presently with recurrent Gross Haematuria*

92. Answer is A (IgA Raised): *Current Rheumatology Diagnosis & Treatment 2nd/319, Robbins 7th/990; Chandrsoma Taylor 3rd/712*

The most common systemic vasculitis in children is Henoch Schonlein Purpura, and the most common primary glomerular disease is IgA Nephropathy. H.S purpura and IgA nephropathy may actually represent spectra of same disease and both are associated with elevated levels of IgA which is the single best answer of choice.

Antinuclear Antibodies (ANA) and Antineutrophilic Cytoplasmic Antibodies (ANCA) are characteristicaly Negative and serum complement levels are typically normal.

Laboratory Feature of Renal vasculitis in children due to HSP	
• *Serum IgA levels*	*Elevated (60% of patients have an elevated serum IgA)*
• *Antinuclear Antibody (ANA)*	*Negative*
• *Antineutrophil cytoplasmic Antibodies (ANCA)*	*Negative*
• *Complement (C3, C4)*	*Normal* *Even though immune complexes containing IgA are essential to the pathophysiology of HSP, serum complement levels are usually normal*
• *Cryoglobulins*	*Negative*

93. Answer is A (Increased IgA levels): *Current Rheumatology Diagnosis and Treatment 2nd/319, Robbins 7th/990; Chandrasoma 3rd/712*

The most common systemic vasculitis in children is Henoch Schonlein Purpura, and the most common primary of glomerular disease is IgA Nephropathy. H.S purpura and IgA nephropathy may actually represent spectra of same disease and both are associated with elevated levels of IgA which is the single best answer of choice.

94. Answer is B (IgA Nephropathy): *CMDT 2007/939; 2009/813-14; Harrisons 17th/1788; 16th/1690; Harrison 18th/p 2342, 2343 Refer Previous question.*

Presence of synpharyngitic hematuria (No significant latent phase between hematuria and pharyngitis) suggests a diagnosis of IgA Nephropathy

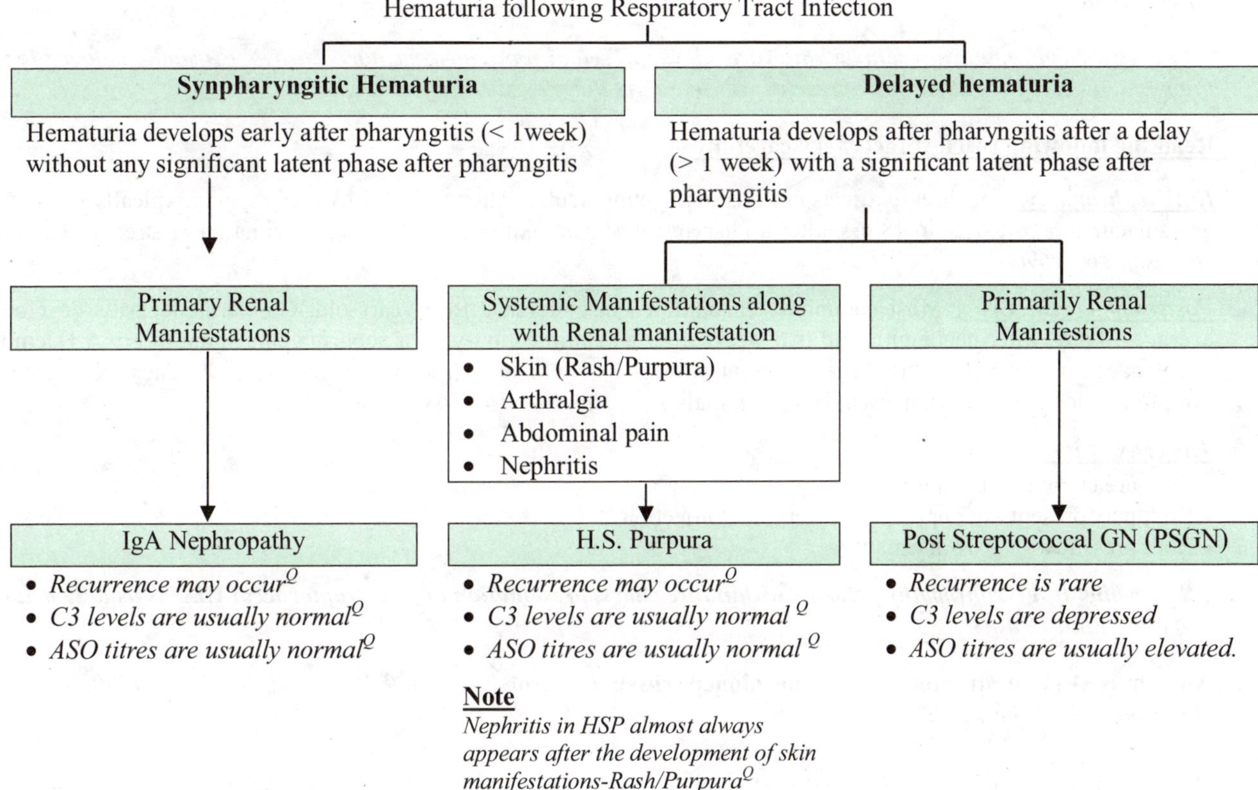

95. Answer is B (IgA Nephropathy): *Harrison 18th/p 2342, 2343; 17th/1789, 1788; 16th/1690, Nelsons 17th/1737, 1738.*

Recurrent Gross hematuria is a charachteristic feature of IgA Nephropathy A diagnosis of IgA Nephropathy is further supported by the presence of normal complement C3 levels.

IgA Nephropathy	Post streptococcal Glomerulonephritis
• **Synpharygitic Hematuria** *Hematuria develops usually within 2-4 days of Pharyngitis /URTI* *This is called synpharygitis hematuria since there is no significant latent period between development of hematuria and pharyngitis*	• Delayed Haematuria Hematuria develops 1-3 weeks after pharyngitis /URTI *This is called delayed Hematuria since there s a significant latent period between development of hematuria and pharyngitis*

- **Recurrence is common**
  'Hematuria occuring in IgA nephropathy typically lasts for several days and then subsides, only to return every few months'
  Recurrent Gross Hematuria
- **Serum complement C3 levels are Normal**
  C3 levels Normal
- **Antistreptolysin O titres are usually normal**

- Recurrence is rare
  'Complete Recovery occurs in more than 95% of patients with PSGN. One attack confers life long immunity and recurrences are extremely rare
- **Serum levels of complement C3 are reduced**
  C3 levels depressed in > 90%
- **Antistreptotysin O titres are usually elevated**
  'Increased ASO titres are associated with Acute PSGN rather than IgA Nephropathy'

96. Answer is C (IgA Nephropathy): *Harrison 16th/1690, 1680; 17th / 1786, 1788; Harrison 18th/p2340, 2342 Nelson 17th / 1737, 1738*

While, IgA Nephrapathy presents within three days, presentation of poststreptococcal GN is usually delayed to more than 10 days'. As the patient here presents within 3 days diagnosis is IgA nephropathy.

Read the following two text facts very carefully

IgA Nephropathy: The disease affects children and young adults. Patients with IgA nephropathy typically present with gross haematura, often 24 to 48 hrs. after a Pharyngeal or gastrointestinal infection, vaccination or strenous exercise. – *Harrison 16th/1690*

Poststreptococcal GN : Most commonly encountered in children 2 to 6 years old. Glomerulonephritis develops on average 10 days after pharangitis and two weeks after a skin infection with a nephritogenic strain of gp. A Haemolytic streptococci. Those with overt disease present with gross haematuria (red or smokes urine) headache and generalise symptoms such as anorexia, nausea, vomiting, malaise. – *Harrison 16th/1680*

The crux of it is :
- Both are common in children
- Both may present after upper respiratory tract infection.
- Both present with gross haematuria,

'But while, IgA Nephropathy presents within three days, presentation of poststraptococcal GLN is usually delayed to more than 10 days'.

97. Answer is D (Post streptococcal glomerulonephritis): *Harrison 15th/ 1589; Harrison 16th/1680, 1690; 17th / 1786 Harrison 18th/p 2340, 2342*

While, IgA Nephropathy presents within three days, presentation of poststreptococcal GN is usually delayed to more than 10 days'.

Heamaturia after 10-14 days of URTI	Heamaturia within 3 day of URTI
Post streptococcal GN [Q]	IgA nephropathy [Q]

98. Answer is C (Glomerulonephritis secondary to skin infection is more common in Summer): *Harrison 15th/ 1582; Nelson 15th/ 1487; Harrison 17th/*

'During cold weather post streptococcal glomerulonephritis commonly follows streptococcal pharyngitis; whereas during warm weather, the G.N. generally follows streptococcal skin infection or pyoderma'. *- Nelson 15th/1487*

- *"Early systemicantibiotic therapy of Streptococcal throat and skin infection will NOT eliminate the risk of glomerulonephritis". Nelson 15th / 1488*
- *"Recurrence are extremely rare"* Nelson 15th / 1488 ......Immunity to strains causing G.N. is type-specific and long-lasting, and hence repeated infection and nephritis are rare.
- Post streptococcal glomerulonephritis may follow either pharyngitis or, skin infection (pyoderma) with a nephritogenic strain of *group A beta haemolytic streptococci*.

- I could not however, find what percentage of PSGN cases follow pharyngitis and what percentage follow skin infections. [*I looked in Harrison, Robbins, Nelson, CMDT, Ananth Narayan as well as Chandrasoma Taylor*]. All I could gather was that these incidences are relative, depending upon the climatic conditions of the area concerned such that in the tropics, skin infection is more important than pharyngitis as a cause.
  The epidemic forms, *on the other hand,* ***are seen in children of 2-6 years of age, and are secondary to pharyngitis.*** Thus no exact demarcation in terms of percentages can be made.

Goodpasture's Syndrome

99. Answer is A (Goodpasture's syndrome): *Refer text below; Current Diagnosis and Treatment in Pulmonary Medicine 1st (2003)/211*

Association of hematuria and hemoptysis suggest a diagnosis of Goodpasture's syndrome.

Good pasture's syndrome

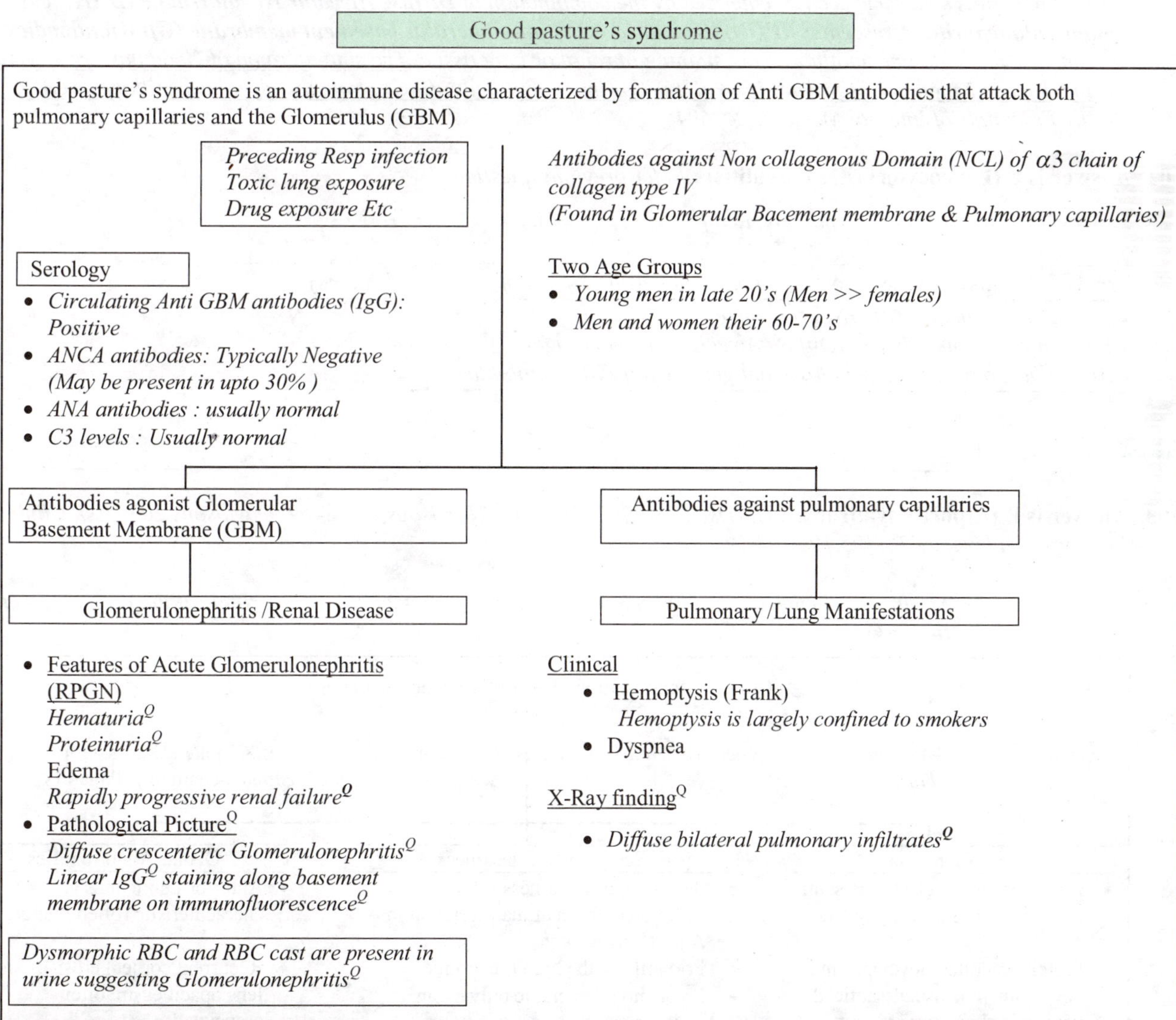

Goodpasture's syndrome and ANCA

ANCA is typically negative in Goodpastures syndrome and it is classified as an ANCA negative vasculitis
Nevertheless
ANCA seropositivity may occur in upto 30 percent of patients with Goodpasture's syndrome. These patients with ANCA have subtle signs of a systemic vasculitis and represent an overlap between goodpastures and either Wegener's granulomatosis (WG) or Microscopic polyangitis(MPA)-Current Diagnosis and Treatment in Pulmonary Medicine 1st (2003)/211

100. Answer is A (Good pasture's syndrome): *Current critical case diagnosis & Treatment 3rd*

Association of hematuria and hemoptysis suggests a diagnosis of Goodpasture's syndrome

Good pasture's syndrome is an autimmune disease charachterized by formation of Anti GBM antibodies, that attack both the pulmonary capillaries (hemoptysis) and the glomerulus (hematuria).
The classical presentation is that of a young male smoker with signs of acute glomerulonephritis (hematuria, proteinuria & RBC cast) and hemoptysis associated with bilateral pulmonary infiltrates.

101. Answer is D (All of the above): *Kelly's textbook of Internal Medicine 2nd/694; Harrison 18th/p 2351 Harrison's 17th/1788; Robbins 7th/745, 746; Current Diagnosis &Treatment in Pulmonary Medicine (2003)/211*

Good pasture's syndrome is typically associated with anti-GBM antibodies, crescenteric glomerulonephritis (RPGN) and diffuse alveolar haemorrhage

'Good pasture's syndrome is charachterized by the combination of ***Diffuse Alveolar Haemorrhage (DAH)*** *and* ***glomerulonephritis (Crescents; RPGN)*** *associated with* ***anti-gomerular basement membrane (GBM)antibodies*** *in serum or evident on immunofluorescent staining of renal or lung tissue. The sine-qua-non of Good pasture's syndrome is the demonstration of linear deposition of Ig -G – immunoglobulin (IgG) along the alveolar capillary or GBM.' - Kelly Essentials of Internal Medicine 2nd/694*

102. Answer is B (Leucocytoclastic Vasculitis) : *Refer previous question*

Leucocytoclastic vasculitis is not a typical feature of Good pasture's syndrome

Triad of Goodpasture's syndrome (*Ferri's Color Atlas & Text of Clinical Medicine*)
• *Glomerulonephritis^Q (RPGN; crescents)* • *Pulmonary Haemorrhage^Q (Diffuse Alveolar Haemorrhage)* • *Antibodies to basement membrane antigens^Q (Anti-GBM antibodies)*

Alport's Syndrome

103. Answer is B (Alport's syndrome): *Harrison 18th/p 2351, 3213 Harrisons 17th/2469, Davidsons 20th /504, Clinical Pediatric Nephrology 2nd/195,196,197,198*

Alport's syndrome is an inherited disorder characterized by hereditary nephritis, sensorineural deafness and ocular abnormalities particularly lenticonus.

Clinical Manifestation of Alport's Syndrome (Triad)

Because it is inherited as an Xlinked disorder, women are usually less severely affected than men.

Most common inheritance: X Linked (Recessive)
Most common defect : Alpha 5 chain of collagen IV

Nephritis	Sensorineural Deafness	Ocular Abnormalities
• Hematuria is the classic presenting feature and occurs early in life • Proteinuria often develops but its development is usually noticed years after hematuria is first observed (delayed) • Chronic Renal Failure develops in most individuals and is often observed in late teens or early 20's	• Sensorineural deafness is the most common extrarenal manifestation in Alport's syndrome • Primarily in the high tone range • Frequently detectable only by an audiogram • Usually not progressive (Harrison) *According to Clinical Pediatric Nephrlogy, hearing loss is progressive*	• Anterior Lenticonus is charachteristic (often bilateral) • Recurrent corneal erosisns and lens opacities are often associated *Lenticonus together with hematuria is considered pathognomic of classic AS*

104. Answer is C (Alport's syndrome): *Harrison 18th/p 2351, 3213 Harrison's 17th/1794, 2469, Differential Diagnosis in Internal Medicine: From Symptom to Diagnosis by Siegenthaler (Thieme) 2007/877*

Association of Renal failure with Lenticonus / Keratoconus with a positive family history suggests a diagnosis of Alport's syndrome.

Alport's Syndrome

Nephrosis / Kidney	Otological (Ears) Symptoms	Ocular (Eye)
• *Hematuria (Micro /Macro)* • *Proteinuria* • *Progressive **Renal Failure***	• *Sensorineural hearing loss* (Labyrinthine hearing loss particularly in high frequency)	• ***Lenticonus*** is characteristic • *Cataract (lens opacity)* • *Corneal erosions* • *Keratoconus* *Myopia induced by Lenticonus & keratoconus*

105. Answer is A (Alport's syndrome): *Harrison 18th/p 3213 Davidsons 20th/503, 504, Harrisons 17th/2469 Clinical Pediatric Nephrology 2nd/195, 196, 197, 198*

Most cases of Alport's syndrome arise from a mutation or deletion of the COL4/A5 gene located on the X chromosome which codes for alpha 5 chain of type IV collagen *- Davidson*

Alport's syndrome

Alport's syndrome is an inherited disorder charachterized by hereditary nephritis, senserineural deafness and ocular abnormalities.

Alport's syndrome is the most common hereditary nephritis[Q]

Genetic defect, Pathology

- Primary pathology in Alport's syndrome is an abnormality in type IV collagen (Type IV collagen is the predominant collagen in basement membrane)

Type IV collagen consists of six different α chains $\alpha1(IV)$ *to* $\alpha6(IV)$ $\alpha4(IV)$			
α1and α2 : Located on chromosome 13	:	Genes COLA4A1, COLA4A2	α3, α4 and α5 chain form a callogen network present in • Glomerular Basement membrane (GBM) • Cochlea • Lens capsule
α3 and α4: Located on chromosome 2	:	Genes COLA4A3, COLA4A2	
α5 and α6 : Located on X chromosome	:	Genes COLA4A5, COLA4A6	

- ***The most common form of Alport's syndrome is due to mutation of the COLA4A5 ($\alpha-5$ Chain) gene located on the X chromosome***[Q].
- The most common inheritance pattern for Alport's syndrome is X Linked – *Classic Alport's syndrome*

Alport's syndrome may be inherited as X-Linked, Autosomal recessive, or Autosomal dominant disorder but classic Alport's syndrome in inherited as an X linked disorder.

Clinical Triad

- *Nephritis (Hematuria, Proteinuria, Progressive renal insufficiency)*
- *Sensorineural deafness*
- *Ocular abnormalities (Lenticonus > Recurrent corneal erosisons, corneal opacipies)*

Pathological Findings in kidney

- *Irregular thickening and thinning of Basement membrane*
- *GBM may appear normal or diffusely thin*
- *Splitting of Lamina and micro granulation's may be seen*

Treatment and Prognosis

No specific treatment to slow the progress of this condition.
Patients are good candidates for Renal transplantation.
Recurrence of disease in renal transplant is rare.

106. Answer is A (Haematuria): *Harrisons 15th/ 1595, 2300; 16th/1691, 2331; 17th/1794, 2469 Harrison 18th/p 2351, 3213*

Most patients with Alports syndrome present with haematuria.

Alport syndrome is the 'most common hereditary nephritis' and it is characterized by haematuria – Harrison

Manifestations

Renal manifestations	Extrarenal manifestations
- Microscopic haematuria - Proteinuria (nephrotic range – 30%) - Progressive renal insufficiency	- Sensorineural hearing loss - Bilateral anterior lenticonus (15 to 30%) - Recurrent corneal erosions

- **Sensorineural deafness** is primarily in the high tone range and can frequently be detected only by an audiogram. It is thus unlikely to be a presenting symptom. (It is usually non progressive)
- **Proteinuria** by itself is again unlikely to be a presenting symptom.
- **Oliguria** would develop with progressively increasing renal insufficiency

107. Answer is A (Alport's syndrome): *API 6th/ 666*

Alport is syndrome has not been mentioned to recur in kidney after a renal tansplant.

Disease associated with significant though varying recurrence rates in the graft include

Glomerulonephritis	Metabolic
- Membranoproliferative type II - IgA nephropathy - Anti GBM disease (Good pastures) - Focal segmental glomerulosclerosis (FSGS) - Haematytic uraemic syndrome	- Type I Diabetes - Amyloidosis - Oxalosis - Cystinosis

Minimal Change Nephropathy

108. Answer is A (Fusion of foot processes of the glomerular epithelial cells): *CMDT 2007/942; 2009/818; NMS medicine 6th/256, Harrison 18th/p 2345 Harrisons 17th/1790, Harrisons 16th/1684, 1685, Nelsons 17th/1754; Chandrasoma Tayler 3rd/705; Robbins 6th/956*

The presence of generalized edema is a 7 year old boy with proteinuria suggests a diagnosis of Nephrotic syndrome. This child is likely to have. Minimal change disease as this is the most common cause of Nephrotic syndrome in children and is associated with normal findings on Light microscopy

Patients with minimal change disease characteristically show fusion of foot processes of the glomerular epethelial cells on electron microscopy.

Minimal change Disease: Review
• Most common cause of Nephrotic syndrome in children (80% in children; 20% in adults) • Peak Age of onset is between 6-8 years of Age (usually < 10 years) • Type of onset : Insiduous
Clinical features
Peripheral Edema: Presenting Feature
Nephrotic syndrome is the typical presentation Peripheral edema is the hallmark of Nephrotic syndrome occurring when serum albumin levels become less than 3g/dl Initially dependent Edema —Later→ Generalized edema May develop Pleural effusion, pulmonary edema, ascitis
• Hematuria : 20-30% • Hypertension : V. Rare • Renal failure : Does not usually progress to renal failure
Laboratory (Features of Nephrotic syndrome)
• *Proteinuria* • *Hypoalbuminemia* • *Hyperlipidemia/Hyper cholesterolemia (Increased hepatic prduction of lipids)* • *Hypercoagulability*

Renal pathology (Biopsy)	
Investigation	**Observation**
Light microscopy [Q]	No abnormality hence the term minimal change
Electron microscopy [Q]	Fusion of foot processes
Immunofluorescence [Q]	Absence of immunoglobulin or complement

Prognosis
• *Prognosis is Good*   • *Response to steroids is Excellent*   • *Does not progress to Renal Failure*

Treatments
• *Corticosteroids form the mainstay for treatment of MCD*

109. Answer is A (No IgG Deposits or C3 deposition on Renal biopsy)

The presence of generalized edema significant proteinuria and absence of hematuria in a young (7 year old) girl suggests a diagnosis of Nephrotic syndrome. Minimal change disease (Lipoid nephrosis) is the commonest cause of Nephrotic syndrome in children and is the most likely diagnosis of the patient in question.

***Minimal change disease** is characterized by absence of IgG deposits and / or complement on immunofluorescence (biopsy specimen) and is therefore the single best answer of choice.*

IgA Nephropathy and Alport's syndrome characteristically present with an Acute Nephritic syndrome with recurrent gross hematuria. The patient in question has no hematuria and hence these diagnosis can be excluded.
Serum complement C3 levels are characteristically normal in Minimal change disease

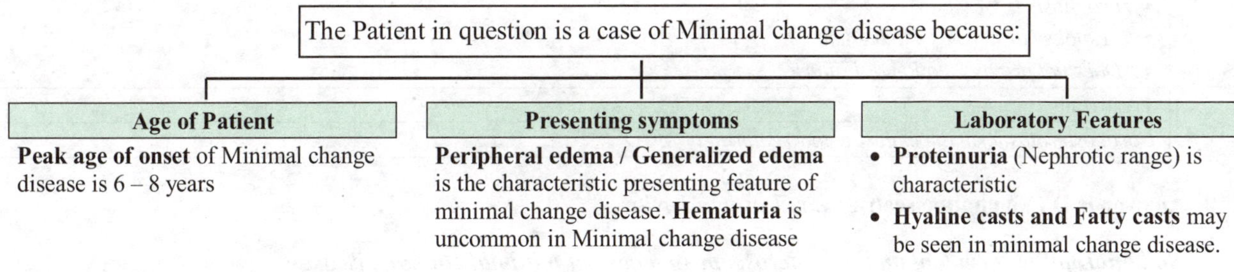

Occasional Hyaline casts and Fatty casts may be seen in Minimal change disease

- Clinical Laboratory Medicine' by Ravel 6th /156

Hyaline Casts	Fatty Casts
• Hyaline casts are composed almost exclusively of protein alone and they pass almost unchanged down the urinary tract	• Fatty casts are a special type of cellular cast associated with fatty degeneration of tubular epithelium
• Small number of ***these casts may be seen in normal urine and in*** any condition associated with proteinuria (including Minimal change disease)	• These casts are composed of fatty droplets and protein
• These casts carry no attached significance and do not necessarily imply an underlying renal disease	• ***Presence of these casts suggests a disease associated with nephrotic syndrome such as primary lipoid nephrosis*** (minimal change) or nephrosis secondary to Diabetes, SLE, amyloidosis etc.

Minimal change Disease: Review

- Most common cause of Nephrotic syndrome in children (80% in children; 20% in adults)
- Peak Age of onset is between 6-8 years of Age (usually < 10 years)
- Type of onset : Insidious

Clinical features

- ***Peripheral Edema: Presenting Feature***

Nephrotic syndrome is the typical presentation
Peripheral edema is the hallmark of Nephrotic syndrome occurring when serum albumin levels become less than 3g/dl
Initially dependent Edema —Later→ Generalized edema
May develop Pleural effusion, pulmonary edema, ascitis

- ***Hematuria*** : ***Uncommon*** (may be seen in 20-30% of patients)
- Hypertension : V. Rare

Laboratory (Features of Nephrotic syndrome)

- *Proteinuria*
- *Hypoalbuminemia*
- *Hyperlipidemia/Hyper cholesterolemia (Increased hepatic production of lipids)*
- *Hypercoagulability*

Serum Complement 'C3' levels are Normal

Renal pathology (Biopsy)

Investigation	Observation
Light microscopy [Q]	***No abnormality*** hence the term minimal change
Electron microscopy [Q]	Fusion of foot processes
Immunofluorescence [Q]	***Absence of immunoglobulin or complement***

No immunoglobulin deposit (IgG) are seen as Renal biopsy

Prognosis

- *Prognosis is Good*
- *Response to steroids is Excellent*
- *Does not progress to Renal Failure*

Treatments

Corticosteroids form the mainstay for treatment of MCD

110. Answer is D (No change seen): *Chandrasoma Taylor 3rd/ 705*

No abnormality is evident on light microscopy in a case of minimal change disease.

Investigation	Observation
Light microscopy [Q]	*No abnormality hence the term minimal change*
Electron microscopy [Q]	*Fusion of foot processes*
Immunofluorescence [Q]	*Absence of immunoglobulin or complement*

111. Answer is A (No abnormality): *Chandrasoma Taylor 3rd/705; Harrison 18th/p 2345 Harrisons 17th/1790; Harrisons 16th/1684, Nelsons 17th/1754*

Light microscopy shows no abnormality in Minimal change Disease

Investigation	Observation
Light microscopy [Q]	*No abnormality hence the term minimal change*
Electron microscopy [Q]	*Fusion of foot processes / Effacement of foot process*
Immunofluorescence [Q]	*Absence of immunoglobulin or complement*

112. Answer is A (Appears normal under light microscope but Electron microscope shows loss of foot processes) - *Robbins 6th/ 954 Refer previous question; Robbins 7th/981*

- ***It is characterised by diffuse loss of foot processes of epithelial cells, which however, is detectable by electron microscopy only; Glomeruli appear normal by Light microscopy.***
- No electron dense deposits are seen in minimal change disease. Mesangial deposits are a feature of mesangio-proliferative G.N. eg. Ig A nephropathy.
- Tram-track appearance is a feature of membrano-proliferative G.N.
- Haematuria is not a feature of minimal change disease. Gross haematuria is seen in glomerulonephritis that cause acute nephritic syndrome eg. post streptococcal G.N. and IgA G.N.

113. Answer is A (Glomerular function is lost due to loss of polyanions around the foot processes) : *Heptinstall's pathology of kidney 6th/128, Clinical Pediatric Nephrology 2nd/6 ; Harrison 18th/p 2345 Harrisons 17th.1790: Harrisons 16th/1684, 1685*

Loss of polyanionic charge is believed to be the main cause for loss of glomerular function (albuminuria) in minimal change disease

Loss of polyanions is believed to result in effacement of foot processes and development of proteinuria in minimal change disease

Mechanism of Proteinuria in Minimal change Disease (MCD) (Heptinstall's)

Effacement of foot process (Earlier called fusion of foot process) is believed to play an important role in causes proteinuria in MCD.

The mechanisms responsible for fusion /effacement of foot processes include:

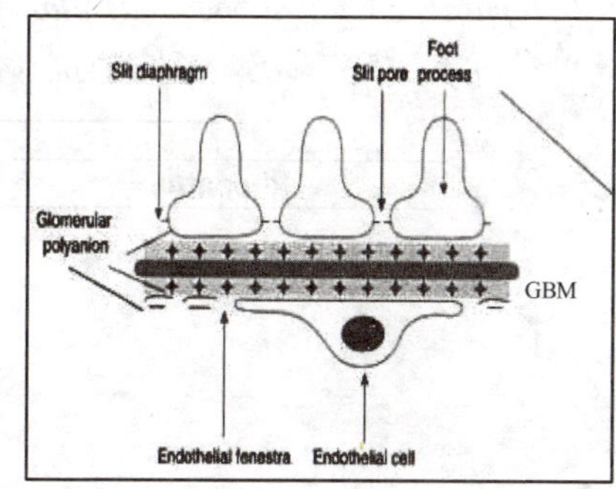

- ***Loss of negative charge (Loss of Polyanions)***
- *Disruption of components of slit diaphragm*
  (Demonstrated in congenital nephrotic syndrome of the Finnish type)
- *Loss of actin cytoskeleton*
- *Detachment of the podocyte from the GBM.*

Note

Minimal change disease is characterized by diffuse effacement of foot process 'diffuse effacement of foot process is synonymous with fusion of foot processes.

114. Answer is A, D (Normal light microscopy; Effacement of foot process): *Harrison 18th/p 2345 Harrison 17th /1790*

Minimal Change Disease or Lipoid Nephrosis is typically charachterized by a normal light microscopy and effacement of foot processes on electron microscopy

'MCD on renal biopsy ***shows no obvious glomerular lesion by light microscopy*** *and is negative for deposits by immunofluorescent microscopy, or occasionally shows small amounts of IgM in the mesangium.* ***Electron microscopy, however consistently demonstrates an effacement of the foot process*** *supporting the epithelial podocytes with weakening of slit-pore membranes.'- Harrison's 17th / 1790*

FSGS may be seen in the small subset of patients with steroid resistance but its presence is not a typical feature of Lipoid Nephrosis

'Patients with steroid resistance can develop FSGS on repeat biopsy'- Harrison's 17th/ 1790

115. Answer is A (Hypertension): *Harrison 18th/p 2345 Harrison 17th/, 1790; Ghai 5th / 370; Ghai 6th/451*

Hypertension is not a feature of nephrotic syndrome and is rare in Minimal change disease.

Edema and *Selective proteinuria are features of nephrotic syndrome. Fever may be present on account of increased susceptibility to infection.*

Minimal Change Disease *is the most common cause of Nephrotic syndrome in children.*

Hypertension is not a feature of nephrotic syndrome and is rare in Minimal change disease.

Features	Minimal Change Disease
Light Microscopy	Minimal Change / No significant abnormalities
Electron microscopy	Obliteration of epithelial foot processes
Immunofluorescence	No deposits of immune reactants
Serum complements	*Levels are normal* Q
Age of onset	*Mainly below 6 years* Q
Type of Onset	*Insidious* Q
Hematuria	*Rare* Q
Hypertension	***Rare*** Q
Edema	*Presenting feature*Q
Proteinuria	*Present (mainly Albumin)* Q
Response to steroids	*Excellent (Abolition of proteinuria)* Q
Prognosis	*Good* Q

116. Answer is A (Hepatitis B): *Harrison 16th/1685 (Tab. 264-3); Harrison 17th/ 1790 Harrison 18th/p 2345*

'Hepatitis B' has not been mentioned to have any association with minimal change disease'.

Major Causes of Minimal Change Disease / (Nil) disease / Lipoid Nephrosis

Idiopathic	In association with systemic diseases or drugsQ
	HIV infectionQ
	Hodgkins diseaseQ and other Lymphoproliferative malignancies
	Drug induced Interstitial NephritisQ
	NSAIDS
	Rifampicin
	Interferon α

117. Answer is B (Minimal Change Glomerulonephritis) : *See above*

Steroids produce on excellent response in minimal change disease and remission has been found to occur in 75% pediatric patients. *(Judged as an abolition of proteinuria) – Ghai 5th / 370*

Diabetic Glomerulopathy

118. Answer is B (Diffuse glomerulosclerosis): *Robbins 6th/ 966; 7th/991; Harsh Mohan Pathology 5th/701*

Diffuse glomerular lesions are the most common *– Harsh Mohan*

The morphological changes in Glomeruli is diabetic glomerulosclerosis include:

Capillary basement membrane thickening	Diffuse glomerulo sclerosis	Nodular glomerulo sclerosis
"The earliest morphological abnormality in diabetic nephropathy is thickening of basement membrane" (and expansion of mesangium due to accumulation of extracellular matrix)	"Diffuse glomerular lesions are the most common". *– Harsh Mohan 7th/701*	also called intercapillary glomerulosclerosis or kimmetstiel – Wilson disease. Are virtually pathognomic of diabetes (most specific) *- Robbins 6th/ 967.*

119. Answer is C (Microalbuminuria): *Harrison 17th /2288; 'Hypertenson primer' by Tzzo (Lippincott Williams & Wilkins) 2008 4th/384; 'Starnberg's Diagnostic surgical pathology 4th/1890; 'General Surgery Principles and International practice' (Springer) 2008/322*

The first clinically detectable sign of diabetic nephropathy is microalbuminuria.

'The first clinically detectable sign of diabetic nephropathy is microalbuminuria'.
- General Surgery Principles & International Practice 2008/522

'The first sign of diabetic renal disease is microalbumin in the urine'- 'Management of Diabetic Mellitus' 6th (Springer)/359

Microalbuminuria and Diabetic Renal Disease

- *Microalbuminuria is the first clinically detectable sign of diabetic nephropathy*
- Microalbuminuria refers to excretion of albumin in the urine in amounts that are abnormal but below the limit of detection of conventional urine dipsticks[Q]

Microalbuminuria is defined as excretion of 30-300 mg of albumin/day in a 24 hour collection[Q] or 30-300µg/mg[Q] creatinine in a spot collection.

- The presence of albumin in the urine in the range of microalbuminuria is *best determined by a urinary Albumin/Creatinine ratio in a spot voided urine (Prefered method for delecting microalbuminuria)*[Q]
- *Microalbuminuria is best detected by Sensitive Radioimmuneassays*[Q]
- The recognition of microalbuminuria in patients with diabetes mellitus allows identification of diabetic nephropathy and institution of treatment to reduce the risk of progressive kidney disease at an earlier stage than would be possible with conventional urine dip-sticks

There is clear evidence that the detection of early diabetic nephropathy manifested by microalbuminuria is responsive to antihypertensive therapy in particular the use of ACE Inhibitors or Angiotensin Receptor Blockers.

Stages of Diabetic Nephropathy according to Mogensen:

Stage	Duration of diabetes	Clinical, biological and pathological signs related to renal disease
1	At diagnosis	• *No clinical or biological signs of renal injury* • *Hypertrophy of the kidneys* • *Glomerular hyperfiltration*
2	2-5 years	*Clinically and biologically 'silent' nephropathy*
3	5-10 years	**Early nephropathy:** • ***Microalbuminuria*** • *High blood pressure* • *Normal GFR*
4	10-20 years	**Established diabetic nephropathy:** • ***Macroalbuminuria*** • *High blood pressure* • *Decreasing GFR* • *Pathology: mesangial expansion; GBM thickening; and glomerular sclerosis*
5	>20 years	**End-stage renal disease** • *Pathology: advanced fibrosis of the kidneys* Need for: • *Renal transplant (± pancreas)* • *Peritoneal dialysis* • *Hemodialysis*

120. Answer is C (Urinary A/C Ratio in a spot voided sample): *'Hypertension Primer' 4th/384*

The preferred method to establish microalbuminuria is to determine Albuma / Creatinine Ratio (A/C Ratio) in a spot voided urine sample.

'The presence of albumin in the urine in the range of microalbuminuria is best determined by a urinary A /C Ratio in a spot voided sample. The A/C ratio correlates closely with 24 hour urine albumin estimation and this measure has the advantage of avoiding in accuracies in urine collection and the unpleasentness of having to store urine during the collection process'- Hypertension Primer' 4th/384

121. Answer is C (Focal sclerosis): *Harsh Mohan 4th / 662*

Focal sclerosis has not been mentioned as a characteristic feature of Diabetic Nephropathy.

Glomerular Lesions in Diabetes	
Diffuse glomerulosclerosis:	**Nodular glomerulosclerosis**
• Is the ***most common pattern of involvement***[Q] • The most common pathological change is ***thickening of glomerular basement membrane***[Q] which occurs virtually in all diabetics and is part and parcel of diabetic microangiopathy • Various exudative lesions such as capsular hyaline drops or 'fibrin caps' may be present • ***Capsular drop***[Q]: is an eosinophilic thickening of parietal layer of Bowman's capsule and bulges into glomerular space • ***Fibrin caps***[Q] : is a homogeneous eosinophilic material appearing on the wall of a peripheral capillary of a lobule	• Is virtually ***pathognomic***[Q] ***of diabetes mellitus*** • Is also called ***Kimmelstiel-Wilson lesion*** *or* ***Intercapillary glomerulosclerosis***[Q] • The pathological change consist of one or more nodules in a few or many glomeruli • Uninvolved lobules and glomeruli all show striking diffuse glomerulosclerosis *Focal sclerosis has not been mentioned in the entire description on diabetic nephropathy and therefore is the answer of exclusion.*

122. Answer is C (Strict glycemic control, Low protein Diet, ACE Inhibitors): *Harrison 17th /2288*

Recommended intervention for early diabetic nephropathy manifested by microalbuminuria include glycemic control, strict blood pressure control, ACE Inhibitors/ARB and low protein diet.

The Recommendation for treatment of early diabetic nephropathy manifested by microalbuminuria is to delay the progression from microalbuminuria to macroalbuminuria

Effective Recommended Interventions in diabetic patients with microalbuminuria

- *Immproved Glycemic control (Normalization of glycemia)*
- *Strict Blood Pressure Control (Blood pressure aim < 125/75)*
- *ACE Inhibitors and/or Angiotensin Receptor Blockers*
  (Provide drug specific benefit independent of blood pressure control)
- *Modest Reduction in Protein Intake (0.8g/kg /day)*

HIV Glomerulopathy

123. Answer is A (FSGN): *Harrison 18th/p 2353 Harrisons 17th/ 1796*

The most charachteristic Glomerulopathy in HIV is focal segmental Glomerulosclerosis (FSGS) which typically reveals collapse of the glomerular capillary tuft called collapsing glomerulopathy.

HIV associated Nephropathy is severe rapidly progressive collapsing form of FSGS

124. Answer is C (Collapsing glomerulopathy): *Harrison 18th/p 2353 Harrisons 17th/1796*

The most charachteristic glomerulonephritis in HIV is focal segmental Glomerulosclerosis (FSGS). The FSGS characteristically reveals collapse of glomerular capillary tuft and is called collapsing glomerulopathy.

125. Answer is D (Hypertrophy of visceral epithelium cells) : *Robbins 7th/983 Pediatric Nephrology (2003)/486*

The charachteristic feature of collapsing glomerulopathy are collapse of glomerular tuft and proliferation and hyperplasia of glomerular visceral epethelial cells. Amongst the options provided Hypertrophy of visceral epethelial cells is the single best answer of choice.

'A charachteristic feature of collapsing glomerulopathy is proliferation and hypertrophy of visceral epithelial cells'
- Robbins 7th/983

According to working Classification of FSGS (Pediatric Nephrology)

Type of FSGS	Key Histological Feature	Prognosis
Collapsing FSGS	*Collapse of Tuft* *Glomerular visceral Epethelial cell Hyperplasia (GVEC hyperplasia)*	Poor

Option A in question mentions 'tuft necrosis' and not collapse of tuft hence option D becomes the single best answer of choice.

Lupus nephritis

126. Answer is C (Wire loop lesions): *Robbin's 7th/232; Harrison 18th/p 2727 Harrison 17th/2077; Fundamentals of Renal Pathology (2006) 1st/85*

Wire loop lesions are characteristic of Lupus nephritis.

Wire loop lesions:

- Wire loop lesions represent local PAS – Positive thickening of glomerular capillary walls and are characteristically seen in Lupus Nephritis (SLE)
- These lesions result from subendothelial deposits between endothelium and basement membrane. When extensive and confluent, these subendothelial deposits create a homogenous thickening of the capillary wall which can be seen in light microscopy as 'Wire loop lesion'
- Wire loop lesions are most characteristic of Lupus Nephritis Class IV or Diffuse Lupus Nephritis
  These may however also be seen in Class III (Focal Lupus Nephritis) and Class V (membranous) Lupus Nephritis.

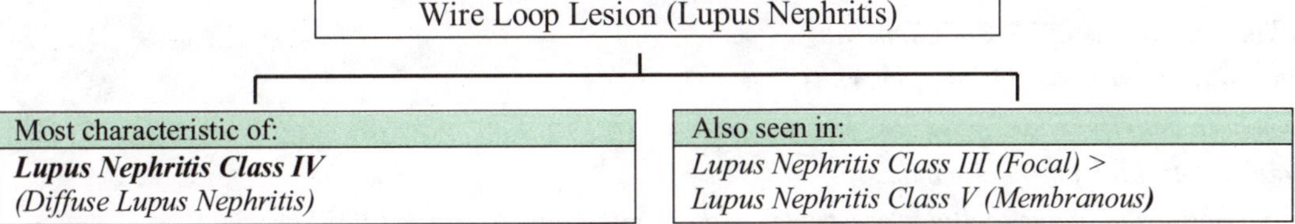

127. Answer is C (Diffuse Proliferative Glomerutonephritis); *Sternberg's Diagnostic surgical pathology 4th/1910,1911*

Heptinstall's Pathology of the kidney 6th/546,547; Diseases of the kidney and Urinary Tract 8th/1688; Harrison 18th/p 2727 Harrisons 17th/2076, 2077, 2078; Harrisons 16th/1961,1963

Wire loop lesions are most charachteristic of diffuse proliferative glomerulonephritis (Class IV WHO) but may also be seen in focal proliferative glomerulonephritis (Class III WHO).

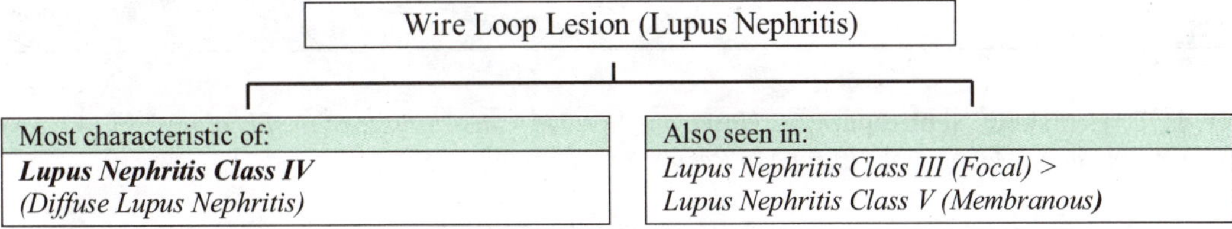

128. Answer is D (Anti – LA (SSB)): *Samter's Immunologic disease 6th/497; 'Systemic Lupus Erythematosis' 4th/894*

Presence of Anti – LA (SSB) in SLE suggests concomitant Sjogren's syndrome. In SLE, patients with concomitant Sjogren's syndrome have a lower frequency of glomerulonephritis and a relatively good prognosis – Samter's Immunologic Diseases 6th/497

Factors associated with Adevrse Prognosis and High Risk of Renal Progression in Lupus Nephritis
Demographic *Black race* *Hispanic ethnicity* *Male gender* *Extremes of age at onset of SLE* *Limited access to health care* Clinical *Hypertension* *Severe extrarenal (especially neuropsychiatric) lupus activity* *Failure to achieve remission or marked delay to renal remission* *Pregnancy*

Laboratory

Nephritic urinary sediment
Azotemia
Anemia
Thrombocytopanea
Thrombotic microangiography (with or without anti-phospholipid antibodies)
Hypocomplementemia (especially falling levels)
High anti- ds DNA (especially rising titres)
Persistent severe nephritic syndrome (artherosclerotic and thrombotic diathesis)

Renal pathology

Contracted kidney size
Proliferative glomerulonephritis (WHO class III, IV)
Mixed membranous (V) and proliferative (III-IV) glomerulonephritis
Cellular crescents (>25% of glomeruli)
Fibrinoid necrosis (>25% of glomeruli)
Very high activity index
Moderate-to-high chronicity index
Combinations of active (cellular crescents) and chronic features (interstitial fibrosis)
Extensive subendothelial deposits

Note:
The presence of Anti-RO or Anti-La antibodies in a pregnant woman is associated with a chance of 'neonatal lupus' developing in the infant (1-5%)
This may present in the fetus as a congenital heart block or neonatal lupus rash.

Amyloid Nephropathy

129. Answer is B (Amyloid Nephropathy): *Harrison 18th/945; 'Essentials of Nephrology' by Visveswaran 2nd/330; European Respiratory Monograph (European Respiratory Society) 2011/156*

Secondary / Reactive Amyloidosis is an established typical complication of chronic conditions like bronchiectasis. Secondary amyloidosis is typically distributed in solid abdominal viscera like the kidney, liver, spleen and adrenals. *Kidneys are the most frequently affected organs.* ***Renal Amyloidosis is an established cause of secondary glomerular disease from chronic conditions like bronchiectasis and presence of edema on legs and proteinuria in a patient with chronic bronchiectasis should auggests the possibility of secondary/reactive renal amyloidosis.***

'Renal Amyloidosis is usually manifested as proteinuria, often in the nephrotic range and associated with significant hypoalbuminemia, and edema or anasarca' – Harrison 18th/947

Bronchiectasis is the most common respiratory disease underlying AA Amylodosis in the UK.

Leprotic Glomerulopathy

130. Answer is B (MPGN): *Rooks Dermatology 5th/ 1073;*

'Chronic renal failure in leprosy is commonly due to proliferative glomerulonephritis, interstitial nephritis and renal amyloidosis and is a common cause of death' *– Rooks*
Remember however that most other infectious causes lead to membranous glomerulonephritis rather than MPGN.

Miscellaneous Glomerulonephritis

131. Answer is B (Focal segmental Glomerulosclerosis): *Harrison 16th/1686,1679; Midline References Robbins 7th/973, 1000*

Focal segmental glomerulosclerosis may develop following acquired loss of nephrons from reflux nephropathy. Proteinuria is nonselective in most cases and may be in subnephrotic range (nephritic range < 3.0 g/24h) or nephrotic range. *- Harrison*

Association of Reflux Nephropathy and proteinuria suggests an irreversible glomerular lesion most commonly focal segmental glomerulosclerosis : Medline

Association of Reflux Nephropathy / Focal Segmental Glomerulosclerosis and Proteinuria

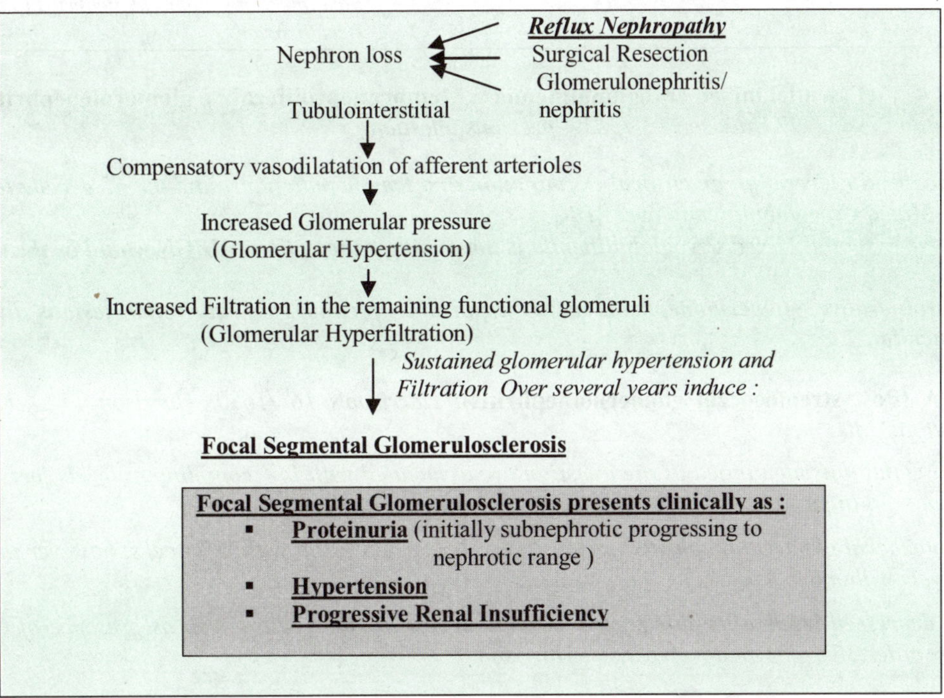

132. Answer is C >B (Membranoproliferative Glomerulonephritis > Mixed cryogloulinemia):
-Harrison 16th / 1682. 2012; 17th/2129; Harrison 18th/p 2798, 2799 CMDT 2006 / 925; 2009/821

The association of generalized edema, hypertension ,proteinuria, hematuria along with hypocomplimentemia and positive anti-hepatitis C antibodies may be seen in both Membranoproliferative Glomerulonephritis and Mixed Cryoglobulinemia. ***With the limited information provided in question MPGN appears to be a better option in comparison to Essential Mixed Cryoglobulinemia for the following reasons:***

- *Cryoglobulinemic Glomerulopathy is most common with the Mixed Cryoglobuliinemias Type II and III which are most common in females and begin in the sixth decade. – Harrison 16tth / 1682*
  The patient in question is a male in the 4th decade of life (30 years)
- *Most patients with cryoglobulinemia present with variable combination of stress ulceration, arthralgia, fatigue and Raynaud's phenomenon other than renal manifestations. The fundamental finding is presence of circulating cryoprecipitates.*

  The patient in question is not presenting with any of the above features to favour Mixed Cryoglobulinemia over MPGN.
- ***Membranoproliferative glomerulonephritis is responsible for 80% of all Renal lesions in Essential Mixed Cryoglobunemia.*** *-Harrison 16th / 2012*

Hepatitis C infection and Glomerular lesions (CMDT 06/924)
<u>Three clinicopathologic glomerular syndromes associated with hepatitis C are</u> : • *Secondary MPGN* • *Cryoglobulinemic Glomerulopathy* • *Membranous nephropathy*
***MPGN is the most common lesion**. These patients typically have haematuria, hypertension, proteinuria and anemia. Hypocomplementemia is very common with C4 typically more reduced than C3.*

Low complement level nephritis syndromes
(Immune complex glonerulonephritis) • *Idiopathic proliferative glomerulonephritis* • *Crescentric glomenelonephritis* • *Membranoproliferative glomerulonephritis* • *Lupus nephritis* • *Cryoglobulinemia* • *Bacterial endocarditis* • *Shunt nephritis* • *Post infectious glomerulonephritis (post streptococcal)*

133. Answer is B > C (Essential mixed cryoglobulinemia > Membranoproliferative glomerulonephritis)
Harrison 18th/p 2798, 2799 Harrison 17th/2129; previous question

The presence of skin ulceration on clinical examination in a female patient around the 6th decade favors a diagnosis of Essential Mixed Cryoglobulinemia over MPGN.
Nevertheless if Essential Mixed Cryoglobulinemia is not amongst the options MPGN would be the single best answer of choice.
Membranoproliferative glomerulonephritis is a responsible for 80% of all renal lesions in essential mixed cryoglobulinemia.

134. Answer is A (Post streptococcal glomerulonephritis): *Harrison's 16th/1680; Harrison 17th / 1786, 1787; not et Harrison 18th/p 2340*

Although all conditions mentioned in the question are associated with low compliment levels 'persistently depressed levels' are not seen in post streptococcal glomerulonephritis.

***In post streptococcal glomerulonephritis:** serum C_3 levels are depressed within 2 weeks, however these usually return to normal levels within 6 to 8 weeks*

***Persistently depressed levels after this period should suggest another cause** such as presence of C_3 nephritic factor (Membranoproliferative glomenulonephritis) – Harrison*

<u>Differential diagnosis of Nephritic syndromes based on complement levels</u>

Low complement levels	*Normal complement levels*
(Immune complex glonerulonephritis) • *Idiopathic proliferative glomerulonephritis* • *Crescentric glomenelonephritis* • *Membranoproliferative glomerulonephritis* • *Lupus nephritis* • *Cryoglobulinemia* • *Bacterial endocarditis* • *Shunt nephritis* • *Post infectious glomerulonephritis (post streptococcal)*	• ***<u>Anti GBM disease:</u>** Good posture's syndrome* • *<u>**Pauci** immune **glomenulonephritis**</u>* - *Wegeners granulomatoses* - *Microscopic polyarteritis nodosa* • *<u>Immune **complex mediated**</u>* - *IgA Nephropathy* - *Henoch schonlein purpura* - *Fibrillary Glomerulonephritis*

135. Answer is C (Diarrhea associated hemolytic uremic syndrome): *Refer previous question; Harrison 16th/1680*

Lupus Nephritis, post streptococcal glomerulonephritis and membrano proliferative glomerulonephritis are all associated with low complement levels as depicted in the table in the previous question. ***Depressed complement levels are not seen in HUS***
<u>Hemolytic uraemic syndrome</u> is characterized by microangiopathic hemolytic anemia, thrombocytopenia and renal failure due to microangiopathy.

Depressed complement levels are not seen and laboratory features include:
- Thrombocytopenia
- Normal tests of coagulation with exception of elevated fibrin degradation products
- Microangiopathic hemolytic anemia: striking red blood cell fragmentation on peripheral blood smear
- *LDH elevation, out of proportion to degree of hemolysis.*

136. Answer is A, D and E (PSGN, MPGN and Infective endocarditis): *Refer previous question*

PSGN, MPGN and Infective endocarditis are associated with depressed complement levels or Hypocomplementemia.

137. Answer is B (Mesangiocapillary Glomerulonephritis) : *Harrison 18th/p 2344 Harrisons 17th /1789, Chandrasoma Taylor 3rd /708*

Mesangiocapillary Glomerulonephritis is the other name for Membranoproliferative glomerulonephritis. It is a type of proliferative Glomerulonephritis. *(Harrisons 17th /1789)*

Proliferative changes in Glomerulonephritis *(Refer: Chandrsoma Taylor 3rd /702, 708)*

- Glomerulus contains Endothelial cells, Epithelial cells, and Mesangial cells. Any of the three cell types may undergo proliferation in different types of Proliferativ Glomerulonephritis.
- Proliferative changes are not limited to Membranoproliferative and Mesangioproliferative Glomerulonephritis, but may be seen in several other forms of Glomerulonephritis

Glomerulonephritis and Proliferative changes

Glomerulonephritis without proliferative changes

Glomerulonephritis	*Proliferative changes*
Minimal change Disease	- (Absent)
Membranous Glomerulonephritis	- (Absent)
Diabetic Nephropathy	- (Absent)
Amyloidosis	- (Absent)
Focal segmental Glomerulosclerosis	*± Variants with proliferative lesions have been described including cellular lesions with endocapillary hypercellularity- (Harrisons)*

Glomerulonephritis with proliferative changes

Glomerulonephritis	*Proliferative changes*
Post streptococcal GN	*+ (Crescents)*
Antibasement membrane disease (Good – pasture's syndrome)	*+ (Crescents)*
IgA Nephropathy (Berger's)	*+ (Mesangial)*
Henoch Schonlein Purpura	*+ (Mesangial)*
Mesangioproliferative GN	*+ (Mesangial)*
Membranoproliferative GN **(Mesangiocapillary GN)**	*+ (Endothelial & Mesangial)*
Focal Glomerulonephritis	*+ (Focal)*
Secondary Glomerulonephritis SLE / PAN	*+ Variable*

Note : Crescents represent proliferation of epethelial cells

138. Answer is C (IgA Nephropathy): *Chandrasoma Taylor 2nd/703*

Proliferative glomerular deposits are characteristic of IgA nephropathy.

Diabetes, Amyloidosis and membranous glomerulonephritis are not associated with proliferative changes.

Type	**Proliferative**	**Membranous**	**Diffuse/Focal**
IgA Nephropathy (Mesangial)	+ve	-ve	Diffuse
Membranous GN	-ve	+ve	Diffuse
Diabetic Nephropathy	-ve (Focal sclerosis)	+ve	Diffuse/Focal
Amyloidosis	-ve	+ve	Diffuse

Renal Tubular Acidosis

139. Answer is C (Decreased Urinary citrate): *Harrisons 16th/1699*

Type II RTA is associated with normal or increased urinary citrate

'Urine citrate levels are normal or high because of reduced proximal tubular reabsorption of citrate' – Harrisons

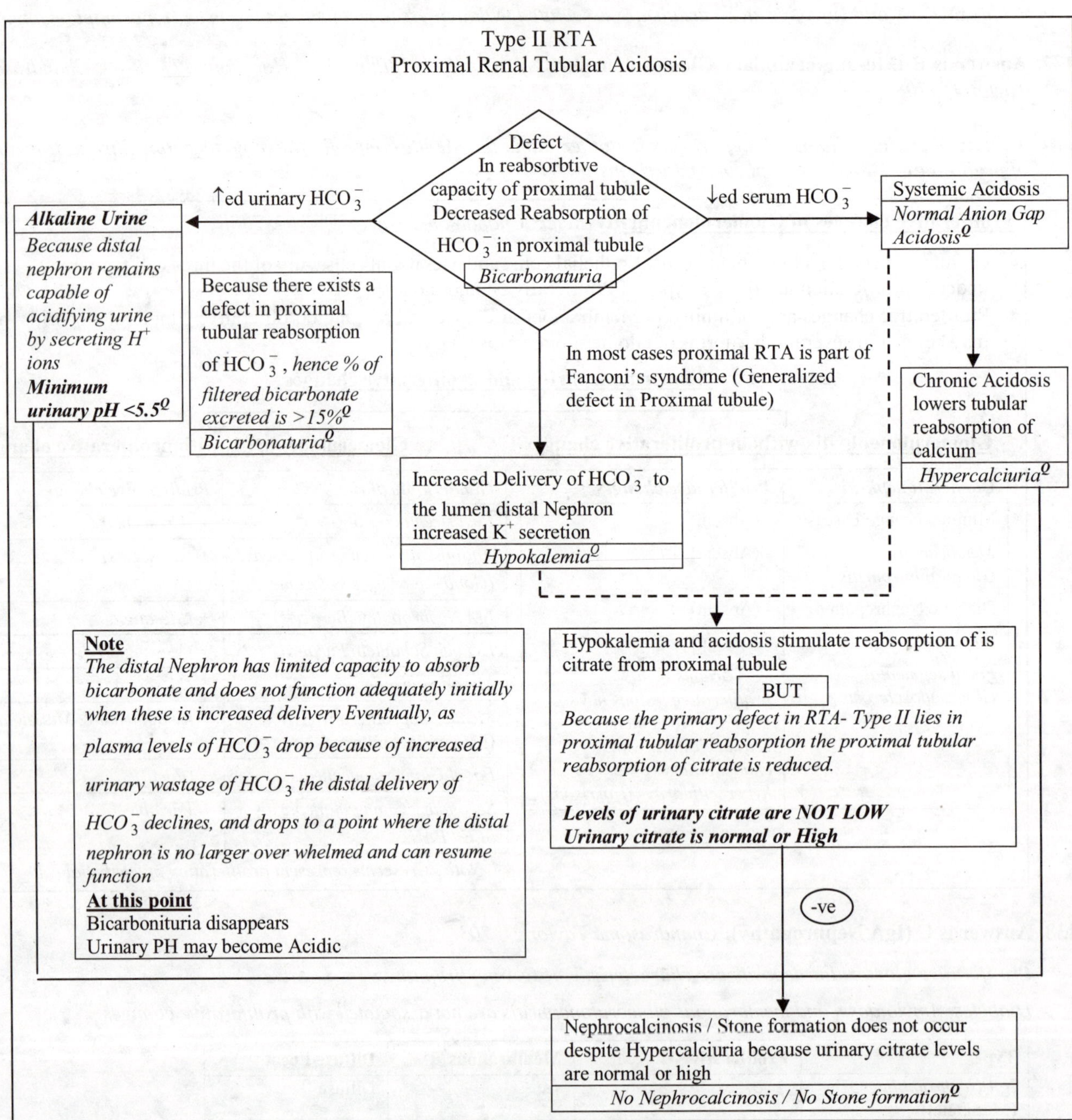

140. Answer is D (↑ Urinary citrate): *Harrisons 16th/1698, 1699*

Type I Renal Tubular Acidosis is associated with low levels of urinary citrate

Urinary citrate excretion is low as hypokalemia and acidosis stimulate proxmal tubular reabsorption of citrate.

Type I RTA
Distal Renal Tubular Acidosis

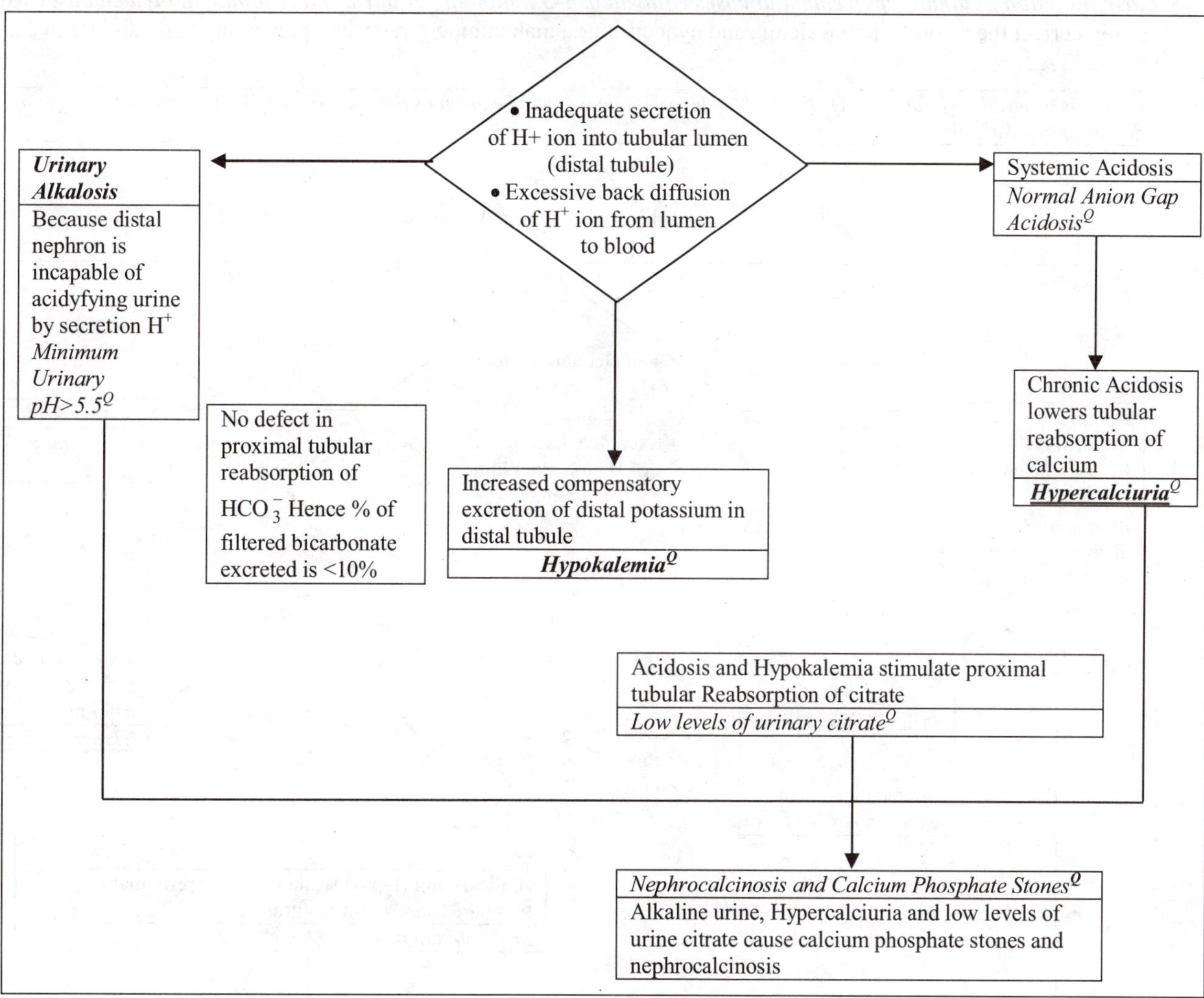

141. Answer is C (Associated with Hyperkalemia): *Harrison 18th/2364*

Type I RTA is associated with Hypokalemia and not Hyperkalemia.

Type I and Type II RTA are both associated with hypokalemia. Hyperkalemia is a feature of Type IV Renal Tubular Acidosis.

Type I (Distal) RTA is associated with Hyperkalemia, failure to acidify urine to a pH of <5 and an increased risk of urinary stones

Feature	Type I	Type II	Type IV
Normal anion gap	*Yes*	*Yes*	*Yes*
Minimum urine pH	***> 5.5***	*< 5.5*	*< 5.5*
% Filtered bicarbonate excreted	*< 10*	*> 15*	*< 10*
Serum potassium	***Low***	***Low***	***High***
Fanconi syndrome	*No*	*Yes*	*No*
Stones / Nephrocalcinosis	***Yes***	*No*	***No***
Daily acid excretion	*Low*	*Normal*	*Low*
Urinary anion gap	*Positive*	*Positive*	*Positive*

Type I RTA is associated with failure to acidify urine to a pH <5 because distal nephron is incapable of acidyfying urine by secretion of H+ (Minimum Urinary pH>5.5Q)

Treatment of Type I (Distal) RTA involves alkali replacement with bicarbonate

Early initiation of alkali replacement at doses equivalent 1-3 mmol/kg per day of bicarbonate in divided doses will usually correct the acidosis, hypokalemia and hypocitraturia maintaining growth and preventing bone disease in early onset dRTA.

Citrate is generally tolerated better than sodium bicarbonate and can be given as the potassium or sodium salt depending on degree of hypokalemia.

Type I RTA
Distal Renal Tubular Acidosis

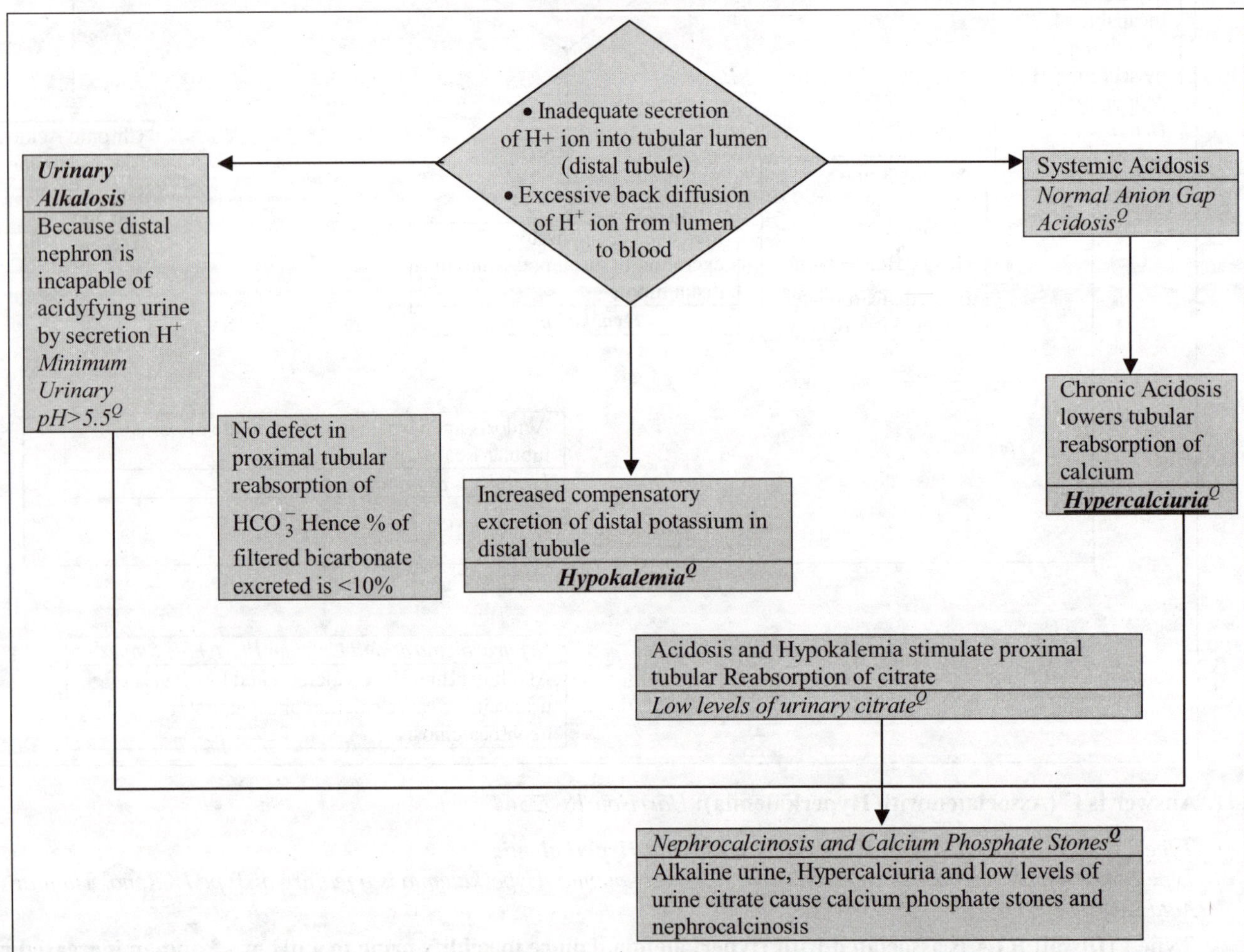

142. Answer is B (Hypokalemia): *Harrison 16th/1699; Harrison 17th/1805; Harrison 18th/p 2364, 2365*

Both type I and type II RTA, are associated with Hypokalemia. Hypokalemia therefore cannot be used to differentiate between Type I and Type II RTA.

Feature	Type I	Type II	Type IV
Normal anion gap	*Yes*	*Yes*	*Yes*
Minimum urine pH	*> 5.5*	*< 5.5*	*< 5.5*
% filtered bicarbonate excreted	*< 10*	*> 15*	*< 10*
Serum potassium	***Low***	***Low***	*High*
Fanconi syndrome	***No***	***Yes***	*No*
Stones / Nephrocalcinosis	***Yes***	***No***	***No***
Daily acid excretion	***Low***	***Normal***	*Low*
Urinary anion gap	*Positive*	*Positive*	*Positive*

143. Aswer is D (Fanconi syndrome): *See previous question; Harrison 16th/1699,267; 17th/1805; 18th/p 2364, 2365 Kumar & Clarke 5th/1116*

Fanconi syndrome occurs in renal tubular acidosis type II.

Feature	Type I RTA	Type II RTA	Type IV RTA
Fanconi syndrome	No	Yes	No

Fanconis Syndrome *is an entity characterized by defective tubular reabsorption of most amino acids, glucose. urate, phosphate and bicarbonate. Defective tubular absorption of bicarbonate, with failure to transport hydrogen ions* ***causes a renal tubular acidosis*** *producing hyperchloremic acidosis.*

Proximal RTA (RTA type II) *is most often due to generalized proximal tubular dysfunction manifested by glycosuria aminoaciduria and phosphaturia (Fanconi's Syndrome) – Harrisons*

144. Answer is C (Renal Tubular Acidosis): *Harrison 18th/368, 369; 17th/292; Washington Manual of Critical Care (2007)/182*

Positive Urinary Anion gap helps in establishing a diagnosis of Renal Tubular Acidosis

Urinary Anion Gap (UAG) can be used to estimate renal ammonium production and distinguish Renal Tubular Acidosis (Positive UAG) from G1 bicarbonate loss (Negative UAG)- Harrisons

Urinary Anion Gap (UAG)

- Urinary Anion Gap (UAG) calculation is useful in cases of *Normal Anion Gap (Hyperchloremic) Metabolic Acidosis*
- Normal Anion Gap Acidosis may result from excessive bicarbonate losses from either the gastrointestinal tract (eg diarrhea) or renal sources (eg Renal Tubular Acidosis)
- *Urinary Anion Gap Estimation helps to distinguish Renal bicarbonate loss from Gastrointestinal bicarbonate loss thereby helping in establishing the cause of normal anion gap metabolic acidosis*

Positive Urinary Anion Gap: Implies Renal loss of Bicarbonate and the diagnosis is usually distal RTA
Negative Urinary Anion Gap: Implies Gastrointestinal loss of Bicarbonate

Note

In type II (Proximal RTA) the kidney has defective HCO3- reabsorption leading to increased HCO3- excretion rather than decreased NH4Cl excretion. Thus the urinary anion gap is often negative

Urinary Anion Gap

Urinary Anion Gap (UAG) is defined by the difference between major urinary cations and major urinary anion

UAG = (Urine Na+ + Urine K+) – Urine Cl-

Normally / Typically the UAG is nearly zero or slightly positive

Response to Metabolic Acidosis

In response to a metabolic acidosis, a normally functioning renal system is able to secrete additional acid in the form of ammonium NH_4^+, generally as NH4Cl.

While NH_4^+ is an unmeasured urinary cation, its presence in urine can be estimated by using the measurement of urine Cl^- as a proxy since ammonium (a cation) is generally secreted with chloride (an anion) to maintain electroneutrality

With a Normally Functioning Renal System	If the Renal System is not functioning normally
Negative UAG	***Positive UAG***
If the renal system is able to appropriately increase the secretion of ammonium in response to a metabolic acidosis, the amount of NH_4Cl in the urine increases and the UAG or net charge will be negative: (urine Na^+ + urine K^+) – (a larger amount of urine Cl-)= a negative number. ***A negative UAG*** *suggests that renal tubular dysfunction is not the cause of the metabolic acidosis.* ***This may be seen in Gastrointestinal causes of metabolic acidosis such as diarrhea***	If, the renal system is not able to appropriately increase the secretion of ammonium in response to the metabolic acidosis, the amount of NH4Cl in the urine remains unchanged or even decreases, and the UAG or net charge will be positive: (urine Na^+ + urine K^+)- (a smaller amount of urine Cl^-) = a positive number ***A positive UAG*** *suggests that there is impaired renal acid secretion and that the renal system is the cause of, or at least contributing to, the metabolic acidosis.* ***This may seen in Distal Renal Tubular Acidosis or chronic kidney disease***

Disorders of Renal Vasculature

HUS

145. Answer is A (HUS): *CMDT 2005 / 504*

The child in question presents with thrombocytopenia and evidence of renal failure following a diarrheal disease. This suggests a diagnosis of HUS.

HUS should be strongly suspected in any child, who presents with:
• Anemia, [Q] • Bleeding [Q] (which is due to thrombocytopenia), [Q] or • Renal failure [Q] (as indicated here by decreased urine output) [Q]
Specially so, if it occurs after a diarrheal illness [Q] (due to infection with E. coli, Shigella or Salmonella) [Q].

<u>**HUS**</u> - It is a vessel wall disorder charactarized by deposition of localized platelet and thrombi within the renal vasculature

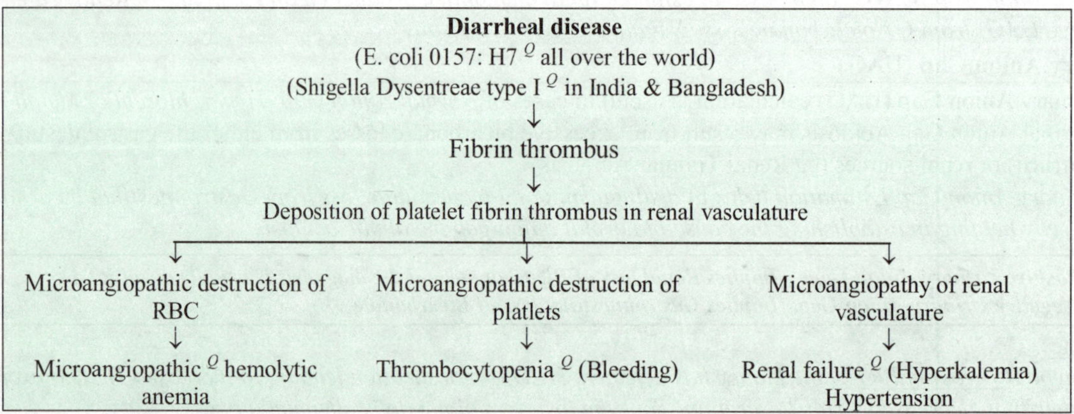

146. Answer is D (Serotoxin has no role in pathogenesis): *Hoffman's Hematology (2009)/2106; Wintrobe's Hematology 12th/1319, 1320; Harrison's 18th/970; CPDT 20th/685; Chronic Complex Disease of Childhood (Universal Publishers) 2011/365*

Serotoxins also known as Shiga like toxin (SLT; STx) or Verotoxin (VT) are the most commonly implicated toxins in the pathogenesis of Hemolytic Uremic Syndrome.

<u>**Serotoxin/Shiga Like Toxin/ShigellaVerotoxin (VT) is the most common toxin implicated in the pathogenesis of HUS**</u>

Typical Hemolytic Uremic Syndrome is a diarrhea-associated condition triggered by intestinal infection with *serotoxin/shiga like toxin producing bacteria*

- *ShigellaDysentreas type I, producing Shiga Toxin is the most common organism in India & Bangladesh*
- *Shiga like toxin (serotoxin) producing E. coli (EHEC 0157:H7) is the most common implicated agent worldwide.*

Hemolytic Uremic syndrome usually follows Haemorrhagic Colitis

Typical Hemolytic Uremic syndrome is diarrheal associated disease triggered by intestinal infection with Shiga toxin or Shiga like toxin producing bacteria (This is termed as D (+) HUS).

These cases of HUS are typically preceded by episodes of bloody diarrhea or Haemorrhagic colitis

(Most common presenting features)

Typical HUS; D (+) HUS	Atypical HUS; D (-) HUS
• *Shiga producing toxin is implicated in pathogenesis* • *Usually preceded or associated with bloody diarrhea (Hemorrhagic colitis)*	• *Shiga producing toxin is not implicated in pathogenesis* • *Neither preceded nor associated with bloody diarrhea*

Fever in Hemolytic Uremic Syndrome is usually mild or absent

'Fever is typically mild or absent' – Hoffman's Hematology (2009)/2106

'HUS often presents without fever or neurological dysfunction'

– Washington Manual of Hematology and Oncology Subspecialty Consult (2003)/53

PENTAD of Thrombotic Microangiopathy	TTP (Pentad)	HUS (Triad)
Microangiopathic Hemolytic Anemia	+++	+++
Thrombocytopenia	+++	+++
Renal Dysfunction	+++	+++ *(Predominates)*
Fever	**+++**	***+/- (Uncommon)***
Neurological Dysfunction	+++	*+/- (Uncommon)*

Hemolytic Uremic Syndrome is often a self-limiting condition

*'**Typical HUS (D+ HUS) is often a self limiting condition**, although many children need extensive supportive care including dialysis, for a period of time' – 'Chronic Complex Diseases of Childhood' (Universal Publishers) 2011/363*

- ***The treatment of typical HUS (D+ HUS) is essentially supportive.***
- *No specific treatment is available.*
- *Plasmapharesis (Plasma therapy) is of little or no value (as opposed to TTP)*
- *Extensive supportive care including dialysis forms the mainstay of management*
- ***Most commonly children recover from the acute episode in 2-3 weeks (CPDT)***
- *Children with HUS may develop chronic residual renal disease or hypertension later in life and hence follow up of patients with HUS should include serial monitoring of renal function and blood pressure.*

147. Answer is D (Neuropsychiatric manifestations): *CMDT 2005 / 504*

Absence of neurological manifestations has been termed as a chracteristic essential diagnoistic feature for HUS in CMDT text. *Hyperkalemia is a manifestation of Renal failure and hence appears justified.*

Essentials of diagnosis as mentioned in CMDT :

- Microangiopathic hemolytic anemia
- Thrombocytopenia
- Renal failure
- Elevated serum LDH
- Normal coagulation tests
- ***Absence of Neurological abnormality***

There are no neurological manifestations other than those due to uraemia – CMDT
Neurological symptoms other than those associated with uremia are uncommon – Harrison
Nevertheless, confusion does prevail as Nelson confuses the issue – Extra renal manifestations may include CNS manifestations – Nelson

148. Answer is D (Positive coomb's test): *CMDT 2005 /504; Nelson 16th/1587*

Coomb's test is negative in HUS

Laboratory findings in HUS – *CMDT 2002 / 556*

1. Anemia: Microangiopathic hemolytic
   Red blood cell fragmentation on peripheral smear
   Helmet cells / Burr cells
2. Thrombocytopenia
3. WBC counts rise (Nelson 16th/ 1587)
4. LDH levels are elevated out of proportion to degree of hemolysis
5. ***Coomb's test is negative***
6. Tests of coagulation are normal (exclude DIC) with the exception of – elevated fibrin degradation products (explains hypofibrinogenemia)

149. Answer is A (Hemolytic uremic syndrome): *Harrisons 15th/ 750; Harrison 17th/723 Harrison 18th/p 970*

Patient presents with Renal failure 5 days after an episode of diarrhea. He has associated Anemia and Thrombocytopenia and thus qualifies the triad of HUS i.e.

- Anemia
- Thrombocytopenia
- Renal failure

Remember

- *In contrast to TTP, the* ***HUS*** *remains localized to the kidney, where hdyaline thrombi are seen in the afferent arterioles and glomerular capillaries. Such thrombi are not present in other vessels and* ***neurologic symptoms, other than those associated with uremia are uncommon****.*
- DIC is not seen in both TTP & HUS

Benign /Malignant Hypertension

150. Answer is D (Hyaline Arteriosclerosis) : *Robbins 7th /1006, 1007, 1008, Harsh Mohan 5th/ 711, 712, 713*

Hyaline arteriosclerosis is a feature of Benign Nephrosclerosis associated with benign phase of Hypertension. It is not a feature of Malignant Hypertension.

Benign Nephrosclerosis	***Malignant Nephrosclerosis***
This term is used to describe the changes in kidney associated with benign phase of hypertension	*This term is used to describe the changes in kidney associated with malignant or accelerated hypertension*
Gross	*Gross*
• Kidney *size is either* normal[Q] *or may be moderately* reduced[Q]	• Kidney size *is* variable[Q] *May be* smaller in size[Q] *(when superimposed on benign nephrosclerosis) or Larger in* size *(enlarged)*[Q] *than normal (patients who develop malignant hypertension in pure form)*
• Grain leather appearance[Q] *: The cortical surface has a fine even granularity*	• Flea bitten appearance[Q]: ***The cortical surface*** *may show multiple small* ***peticheal haemorrhages***[Q] *from rupture of arterioles or glomerular capillaries.*
Microscopic (Vascular Changes & Parenchymal Changes)	*Microscopic (Vascular Changes & Parenchymal Changes)*
• **Hyaline Arteriosclerosis** [Q] *Narrowing of the lumens of arterioles and small arteries caused by thickenning and hyalnization of the walls*	• **Fibrinoid necrosis of arterioles**[Q] **(Necrotizing arteriolitis**[Q]**)** *The vessel wall shows fibrinoid necrosis. Represents an acute event and necrosis is usually not accompanied by intense inflammation*
• Fibroelastic Hyperplasia[Q]*: in the intima (intimal thickenning*[Q]*), duplication of elastic lamina and hypertrophy of the 'media'*	• **Hyperplastic intimal sclerosis**[Q] / Onion – Skinning[Q] **Concentric laminae** *of proliferated smooth muscle cells, collagen and basement membrane* **(producing intimal thickenning)**
• *Parenchymal changes (due to ischaemic) Variable degree of Atrophy of parenchyma due to ischaemia*	• *Parenchymal changes (due to ischaemia) Variable degree of atrophy of paranchyma due to ischaemia. Infarction necrosis distal to abnormal vessels may be seen*

151. Answer is C (Hyaline Arteriosclerosis) : *Robbins 7th / 1006, 1007, 1008, Harsh mohan 5th / 711, 712, 713*

The charachteristic histological finding in Benign Hypertension is Hyaline arteriosclerosis

Benign Nephrosclerosis	***Malignant Nephrosclerosis***
This term is used to describe the changes in kidney associated with benign phase of hypertension	*This term is used to describe the changes in kidney associated with malignant or accelerated hypertension*
Gross	*Gross*
• Kidney *size is either* normal[Q] *or may be moderately* reduced[Q]	• *Kidney size is variable*[Q] May be smaller in size[Q] (when superimposed on benign nephrosclerosis) or Larger in size (enlarged)[Q] than normal (patients who develop malignant hypertension in pure form)
• Grain leather appearance[Q] *: The cortical surface has a fine even granularity*	• *Flea bitten appearance*[Q]*:* **The cortical surface** may show multiple small **peticheal haemorrhages**[Q] from rupture of arterioles or glomerular capillaries.

Microscopic (Vascular Changes & Parenchymal Changes)	*Microscopic (Vascular Changes & Parenchymal Changes)*
• **Hyaline Arteriosclerosis** [Q]	• **Fibrinoid necrosis of arterioles**[Q] **(Necrotizing arteriolitis**[Q]**)**
• *Narrowing of the lumens of arterioles and small arteries caused by thickenning and hyalnization of the walls*	*The vessel wall shows fibrinoid necrosis. Represents an acute event and necrosis is usually not accompanied by intense inflammation*
	• **Hyperplastic intimal sclerosis**[Q] / Onion – Skinning[Q]
• Fibroelastic Hyperplasia[Q]*: in the intima (intimal thickenning*[Q]*), duplication of elastic lamina and hypertrophy of the 'media'*	**Concentric laminae** *of proliferated smooth muscle cells, collagen and basement membrane* (**producing intimal thickenning)**
• *Parenchymal changes (due to ischaemic) Variable degree of Atrophy of parenchyma due to ischaemia*	• *Parenchymal changes (due to ischaemia)* *Variable degree of atrophy of parenchyma due to ischaemia. Infarction necrosis distal to abnormal vessels may be seen*

152. Answer is B (Fibrinoid necrosis): *Refer previous question*

Malignant hypertension is characterized by Fibrinoid necrosis** (Necrotizing arteriolitis*[Q]*) **of arterioles.

153. Answer is C (Hyaline Arteriosclerosis): *Robbins 7th /1006-1008, Harsh Mohan 5th/ 711, 712, 713; Refer previous question*

Benign hypertension is characterized by hyaline arteriosclerosis.

Renovascular Hypertension

154. Answer is B (CT Angiography): *Harrison 16th/1470; Braunwald 8th/1040; The Cleveland Clinic Cardiology Board Review (Lippincott Williams) 1st/514*

Spiral CT scan with intravenous contrast (CT angiography) is the most sensitive and specific test amongst the options provided.

Note:
Magnetic Resonance Angiography (MRA) has now emerged as the diagnostic test of choice at several centres with a sensitivity and specificity similar or even better than CT Angiography.
However as MRA has not been provided amongst the options, CT Angiography remains the single best answer of choice.
*MRA is also more likely to be used more widely **(preferred)** because it reduces the possibility of contrast induced nephrotoxicity and avoids exposure to ionizing radiations.*

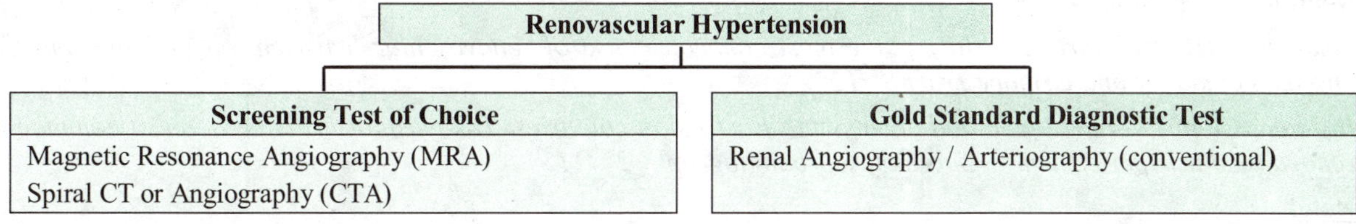

Renovascular Hypertension

Screening Test of Choice	Gold Standard Diagnostic Test
Magnetic Resonance Angiography (MRA) Spiral CT or Angiography (CTA)	Renal Angiography / Arteriography (conventional)

MRA is now emerging as the screening test of choice

155. Answer is A (Magnetic Resonance Angiography (MRA): *'The Clevland Clinic Board Review' (Lippincott Williams) 1st/514; Harrison 16th/1470; Cardiovascular Therapeutic 3rd*

Magnetic Resonance Angiography (MRA) has now emerged as the most sensitive and specific screening test for Renovascular hypertension.

Note:

Harrison 16th edition (old) mentions Spiral CT scan as the most sensitive and specific screening test for Renovascular Hypertension, however most recent textbooks now prefer MRA as the screening test of choice with similar or even better sensitivity and specificity than spiral CT Angiography.

Renovascular Hypertension

Screening Test

Test	Sensitivity (%)	Specificity (%)
Magnetic resonance angiography (MRA)	100	96
Spiral computerized tomography	98	94
Captopril renogram	70-93	95
Duplex Doppler ultrasonography	69-96	86-90
IVP	~75	~85

Gold Standard / Diagnostic Test

Test	Sensitivity	Specificity
Conventional Renal Angiography	>99%	>99%

156. Answer is B (Non specific aorto-arteritis): *Disease of kidney and urinary tract 8th/1279; Tropical Neurology 1st (2003)/440; Surgical Neuroangigraphy 2nd/115*

The most common cause of renal artery stenosis in young adults in India is Non specific aorto-arteritis.

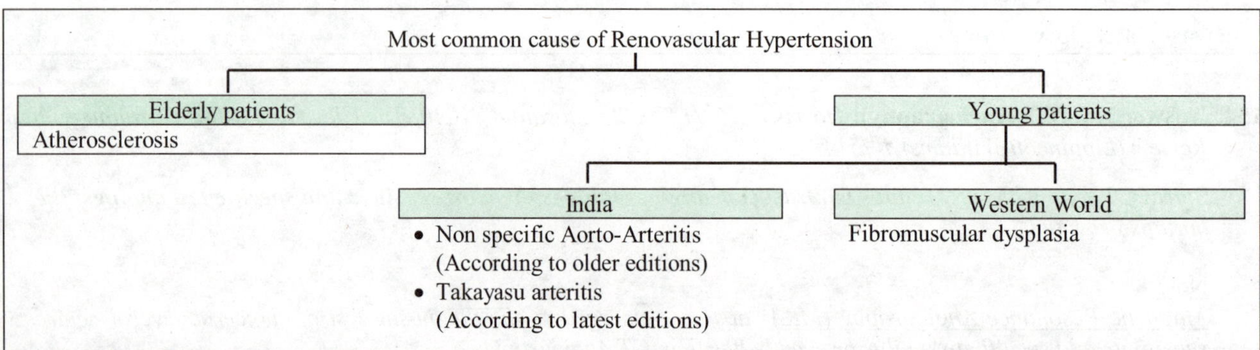

The non specific aorto-arteritis causing renal artery stenosis is now believed to be Aorto-arteritis secondary to Takayasu arteritis

Aorto-arteritis/Takayasu arteritis is the most common cause of renovascular hypertension in India

Non specific Aorto-arteritis is the most common cause of renovascular hypertension in India and China – Tropical Neurology 1st (2003)/440

Takayasu arteritis (Aorto-arteritis) is the most common cause of renovascular hypertension in India and China.' – Diseases of kidney and Urinary Tract 8th/1279

In India, China, Korea, Japan and other South East Asian countries, Takayasu arteritis is the most common cause of renovaascular hypertension.' – Surgical Neuroangiography 2nd/115

Note:
The non specific aorto-arteritis causing renal artery stenosis is now believed to be Aorto-arteritis secondary to Takayasu arteritis

157. Answer is D (Polyarteritis nodosa): *Harrison 16th/1707,2007,2009; CMDT'09/810; API 8th.541; References alongside explanation*

Amongst the options provided renal artery stenosis is least likely to be seen in association with Polyarteritis nodosa.

- **Atherosclerosis and Fibromuscular disease**
  - Renal artery stenosis is produced predominantly by atherosclerotic occlusive disease (80% to 90% of patients) or fibromuscular dysplasia (10-15% of patients).- *CMDT'09 p 810*
  - The common cause of renal artery stenosis ***in the middle aged and elderly*** is an atheromatous plaque at origin of renal artery. *Harrison*
  - ***In younger women*** stenosis is due to intrinsic structural abnormalities of the arterial wall caused by a heterogenous group of lesions called 'fibromuscular dysplasia'. - *Harrison 16th/1707*

- **PAN or Takayasu arteritis ?**

  Harrison, CMDT do not mention PAN or Takayasu arteritis as a cause for renal artery stenosis.
  However, Takayasu arteritis is certainly a more common cause of renal artery stenosis than PAN.
  Takayasu arteritis (Aorto-arteritis) *is beleiveds to be the most common of renovascular hypertension in India and China. – Diseases of Kidney and Urinary Tract 8th/1279*

A number of research publications, however show Takayasu arteritis as a cause for renal artery stenosis.

Takayasu Arteritis	**PAN**
Takayasu arteritis (Aorto-arteritis) is the most common cause of renovascular hypertension in India and China.' – Diseases of kidney and Urinary Tract 8th/1279	Renal artery stenosis in a Case of PAN has only been described as an unusual association and published as a rare case report (single case) ***Reference :*** "PAN with renal Artery Stenosis": Indian Pediatrics Volume 41-Jan.17, 2004.

PAN

Although renal involvement is seen in upto 60% of patients with PAN its pathology does not involve renal artery stenosis.

The pathology involves arteritis without glomerulonephritis and is characterised by aneurysms of small and medium sized arteries. **Stenosis of main renal artery is an unusual association'.**

-Research paper, www. Indian paediatrics. net/Jan 2004/86.pdf

Causes of Renal artery stenosis : *API 8th/541; Renal Artery Stenosis : Diagnosis and Management - IHJ : May-June 2002, Vol. 54/No. 3*
1. Atherosclerosis
2. Fibromuscular dysplasia
3. Non specific Aorto arteritis
4. Takayasu arteritis and giant cell arteritis (Takayasu > Giant cell)
5. Antiphospholipid syndrome
6. Transplant renal artery stenosis
7. Renal artery embolism
8. Dissecting aneurysm of aorta
9. Radiation arteritis

158. Answer is C (Condition is nearly always bilateral): *Harrison 18th/p 2375, 2376 Harrisons 17th/- 1811-1812*

Presence of hypertension (BP = 160 / 110) and bruit in bilateral flanks suggest a diagnosis of Bilateral Renal Artery Stenosis in this patient. ***Renal Artery Stenosis is bilateral in 50% of cases and is not nearly always bilateral***

ACE inhibitors (eg Enalapril) may deteriorate renal function in patients with Bilateral Renal Artery Stenosis
ACE inhibitors (eg Enalapril) are the agents of choice for treatment of hypertension in patients with unilateral renal artery stenosis, but *are* ***contraindicated in patients with bilateral disease***. The presence of bruit in both flanks suggest *bilateral disease in this patient and hence enalapril should not be used*

Contrast Enhanced Arteriography (Angiography) is the most definitive diagnostic procedure for the diagnosis of Renal Artery stenosis while Magnetic Resonance Angiography (MRA) is the most sensitive and specific non invasive test (screening test) for its diagnosis.

Fibromuscular dysplasia is the most common cause of Renal Artery stenosis in young women while Atherosclerotic disease is the most common cause in middle aged/ elderly patients. *The patient in question is a young female (20 years) and hence the most likely cause of Renal Artery stenosis in this patient is fibromuscular dysplasia*

Surgical Intervention may be required in patients with Bilateral Renal Artery Stenosis
Surgical intervention in the form of angioplasty and stent placement is indicated when medical therapy has failed to control BP or resulted in > 30% increase in serum creatinine.

Renal Artery Stenosis: Review

- Renal Artery stenosis is an important cause of Renovascular Hypertension
- ***Bilateral involvement is seen in half of the affected cases (50%)***

Etiology

- Atherosclerotic disease : This is the most common cause in middle aged /elderly patients
- Fibromuscular Dysplasia : ***This is the most important cause in young females***

Presentation

- Hypertension
  - Abrupt onset of hypertension
  - Acceleration of previously well controlled hypertension
  - Refractory Hypertension
- Features of increased sympathetic neural activity (which is associated with Renovascular disease)
  - Flushing
  - Loss of nocturnal BP decrease
  - Putonomic instability
  - Rapid BP swings
- Progressive Renal failure / Azotemia

Diagnosis

Magnetic Resonance Angiography (MRA)	Contrast Enhanced Arteriography
MRA is the most sensitive (>90%) and specific (95%) non invasive test for the diagnosis of RAS	Contrast enhanced angiography is the most definitive (but invasive) diagnostic procedure for diagnosis of RAS

Management

<u>Medical Therapy with ACE Inhibitors or Angiotensin Receptor Blockers</u>

Indications	Contra indications
Unilateral Renal artery Stenosis - With hypertension & normal renal function (more effective than other antihypertensives) - With hypertension & abnormal renal function (beneficial effect on survival without affecting renal function) - With hypertension, diabetes, proteinuria and normal or abnormal renal function (effective antihypertensives)	**Bilateral Renal Artery stenosis** ACE inhibitors or Angiotensin receptor blockers are contraindicated in patients with Bilateral renal artery stenosis or stenosis in a solitary kidney as their use in such patients leads to worsening of renal failure (These patients are especially sensitive to decline in intraglomerular pressure)

Note

Acute Renal Failure / Worsening of Renal Failure with Angiotension Receptor Inhibitors is a diagnostic clue to the diagnosis of renal artery stenosis (indicates bilateral disease)

Surgical Therapy with Angioplasty + Stent placement

Should be considered only after optimal medical therapy has failed to achieve goal BP or resulted in a > 30% increase in serum creatinine

Renal Vein Thrombosis

159. Answer is B (Membranous Glomerulopathy): *Thrombosis Hemorrhage 3rd/724; Harrison 14th/ 1559; 16th/1684; 17th/1790 Harrison 18th/p 2345*

Membranous glomerulonephritis has the strongest association with development of thrombisis in Renal veins.

- Thrombosis & Hemorrhage 3rd/724

<u>Nephrotic Syndrome</u> accompanying <u>membranous glomerulopathy</u> and certain carcinomas predisposes to Development of Renal vein thrombosis (which occurs in 10-50% of patients with these disorders) *-Harrison*

Nephrotic Syndrome: Common Renal pathologies causing Renal Vein Thrombosis

- *Membranous Glomerulonephritis (strongest association)*
- *Membranoproliferative Glomerulonephritis*
- *Amyloidosis*
- *Lupus Nephritis (Thrombosis & hemorrhage 3rd/724)*

Nephrotic syndrome due to diabetic mellitus, minimal change disease and focal segmental sclerosis are rarely associated with renal vein thrombosis

Causes of Renal Vein Thrombosis

Primary	Secondary
• Dehydration Dehydration is the most common cause of primary RVT in Newborns • Nephrotic syndrome Nephrotic syndrome is the most common cause of primary RVT in adults.	• Trauma • Extrinsic compression (Lymphnode, tumor, aortic aneurysm) • Invasion by Renal cell carcinoma • Pregnancy or oral contraceptives

160. Answer is A,B,C,D,E (All of the above) : *Harrison 18th/p 2382 Harrison 17th/1815*

Trauma, Renal Cell Ca, Pregnancy, Nephrotic Syndrome and Dehydration can all be associated with Renal Vein Thrombosis

Conditions associated with Renal Vein Thrombosis : *Harrison 17th/1815*
Trauma
Extrinsic compression (lymph nodes, aortic aneurysm, tumor)
Invasion by renal cell carcinoma
Dehydration (infants)
Nephrotic syndrome
Pregnancy or oral contraceptives

161. Answer is B (Membranous Glomerulopathy): *Harrison 16th /1684; 15th /1584 - 85; Harrison 14th / 1559; Thrombosis and Hemorrhage 3rd/724*

Renal vein thrombosis is most commonly associated with nephrotic syndrome secondary to membranous glomerulopathy.

'Amongst kidney pathologies causing nephritic syndrome, membranous glomerulopathy has the strongest association with the development of thrombosis in the Renal vein. – Thrombosis & Hemorrhage 3rd/724

*'Nephrotic Syndrome accompanying **membranous glomerulopathy** and certain carcinomas predisposes to development of Renal vein thrombosis (which occurs in 10-50 % of patients with these disorders)' - Harrison*

162. Answer is E (PSGN): *Harrison 16th/1684, 1707; Thrombosis & Hemorrhage 3rd/724*

Post streptococcal Glomerulonephritis has not been mentioned as a cause of Renal Vein thrombosis

Nephrotic Syndrome: Common Renal pathologies causing Renal Vein Thrombosis

- *Membranous Glomerulonephritis (strongest association)*
- *Membranoproliferative Glomerulonephritis*
- *Amyloidosis*
- *Lupus Nephritis (Thrombosis & hemorrhage 3rd/724)*

Nephrotic syndrome due to diabetic mellitus, minimal change disease and focal segmental sclerosis are rarely associated with renal vein thrombosis

163. Answer is D (Renal vein thrombosis): *Nelson 16th/ 1589*

Although presentation of patient is similar to that of hemolytic uremic syndrome the presence of marked enlargement of both kidneys takes the whole diagnosis in favour of renal vein thrombosis.

Note : *Nelson 16th – 1587 :*

Patients who have bilateral renal vein thrombosis may be difficult to distinguish from those with the hemolytic uraemic syndrome.
- Both disorders may be preceded by gastroenteritis and in both children may present with dehydration, pallor and evidence of microangiopathic hemolytic anemia, thrombocytopenia and acute renal failure. - The marked enlargement of kidneys of a child with renal vein thrombosis helps to distinguish the disorder. - Doppler flow study or angiography of IVC may be necessary to confirm the diagnosis.

Patient in question has marked enlargement of both kidneys which takes the whole diagnosis in favour of renal vein thrombosis.

Nephrolithiasis and Nephrocalcinosis

Nephrolithiasis (Renal/Ureteric Stones)

164. Answer is D (Uric acid stones are resistant to ESWL): *Schwartz 8th/1547; Bailey 24th/1319; Clinical Pediatric Urology 4th/1238*

Uric acid stones are not resistant to ESWL.

Uric acid stones are infact most responsive to Lithotripsy along with calcium oxalate dehydrate stones.

Stone Type	X Ray finding	Predisposing features	Comments
Oxalate stones (calcium oxalates)	***Radiopaque***	*Hypercalciuria* *Hyperoxaluria*	*Most common types of Renal Calculi*
Phosphate Stones - *Calcium phosphate* - *Magnesium Ammonium Phosphate (Struvite)*	*Radiopaque*	• ***Excess Alkali consumption*** • ***Alkaline urine*** • *Infection with urease splitting organisms eg. Proteus*	*Struvite stones are often solitary* *Struvite stones form staghorn calculi*
Cystine Stones	*Radiopaque*	*Inherited cystinuria*	• ***Form in acidic urine***[Q] • *Extremely hard stones*[Q] • *Relatively resistant*[Q] *to fragmentation with E5WL*
Uric acid stones	*Radioluscent*	*Gout* *Hyperuricemia*	• *Form in acidic urine* • ***Most responsive to lithotripsy***
Xanthine stones	*Radioluscent*	*Deficiency of xanthine oxidase*	-

165. Answer is C (Cystine stones): *Schwartz 8th/1547; Bailey & Love 24th/1319; Clinical Pediatric Urology 4th/1238; Washington Manual of Ambulatory Therapeutics 1st (2002)/449*

Cystine stones are most resiatnt to Lithotripsy.

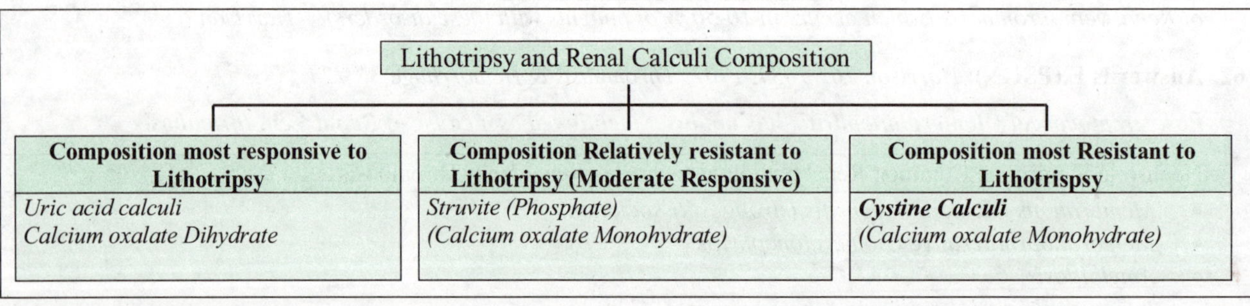

Lithotripsy and Renal Calculi Composition

Composition most responsive to Lithotripsy	Composition Relatively resistant to Lithotripsy (Moderate Responsive)	Composition most Resistant to Lithotrispy
Uric acid calculi *Calcium oxalate Dihydrate*	*Struvite (Phosphate)* *(Calcium oxalate Monohydrate)*	***Cystine Calculi*** *(Calcium oxalate Monohydrate)*

166. Answer is A (Calcium Oxalate Monohydrate): *Smith's textbook of Endourology 1st (2007)/143*

Calcium Oxalate Monohydrate Stones (and cysteine) stones are very hard to break by ESWL.

'Very hard stones such as cysteine or calcium oxalate monohydrate are more likely to fail ESWL'.

– Smith's Textbook of Endourology 1st/143

'Likelihood of fragmentation with ESWL depends on stone composition. Less effective for stones composed of cystine or calcium oxalate monohydrate (very hard)' – Oxford handbook of urology (2005)/366

'Softer stones (calcium oxalate dehydrate, uric acid, apatite, and struvite) are more easily fragmented with SWL than are harder stones (calcium oxalate monohydrate, brushite, and cystine) - Therapy in Nephrology & Hypertension (Sanders) 2nd/406

167. Answer is B (Uric Acid): *Bailey and Love 24th/1317; Smith's Urology 16th/262; 'Beat the Boards' 1st (2006)/214*

Uric acid stones are characteristically Radiolucent

Renal Stones

Radiopaque		Radioluscent
• *Oxalate Stones* - *Calcium Oxalate* • *Phosphate Stones* - *Calcium phosphate* - *Magnesium ammonium phosphate (struvite)* • *Cystine stones*		• *Uric Acid Calculi* • *Xanthine Calculi* • *Indinavir Calculi* *(complication of Indinavir use-Proteinase inhibitor)* • *Triametrene calculi* *(complication of Triamterene use-Antihypertensive)*

168. Answer is B (Triple phosphate): *Bailey 24th/1316. 1319; Smith's Urology 16th/262; Schwartz 8th/1547; Clinical Pediatric Urology 4th/1238*

Phosphate stones (Triple phosphate stones) form in the presence of high concentration of ammonia which essentially means that they form when the urine is infected (UTI) with Urea splitting organisms (eg. Proteus, Kleibsella, Pseudomonas sp.)

Triple Phosphate Stones (Phosphate stones)

- *Triple phosphate stones are composed predominantly of magnesium ammonium phosphate (struvite) with variable amounts of calcium phosphate.*
- *They form in the presence of high urinary concentration of ammonia (bicarbonate and carbonate)*
- *They form in cases of UTI when urine is infected with urea splitting bacteria i.e. Proteus, Kleibsella and Pseudomonas*
- *They form in urine with an alkaline pH.*

Urea splitting organisms split urea to ammonia there by providing an alkaline pH which facilitates precipitation of phosphate crystals.

Stone Type	X Ray finding	Predisposing features	Comments
Oxalate stones (calcium oxalates)	***Radiopaque***	*Hypercalciuria* *Hyperoxaluria*	*Most common types of Renal Calculi*
Phosphate Stones - *Calcium phosphate* - *Magnesium Ammonium Phosphate (Struvite)*	*Radiopaque*	• ***Excess Alkali consumption*** • ***Alkaline urine*** • *Infection with urease splitting organisms eg. Proteus*	*Struvite stones are often solitary* *Struvite stones form staghorn calculi*
Cystine Stones	*Radiopaque*	*Inherited cystinuria*	• ***Form in acidic urine***[Q] • *Extremely hard stones*[Q] • *Relatively resistant*[Q] *to fragmentation with E5WL*
Uric acid stones	*Radioluscent*	*Gout* *Hyperuricemia*	• *Form in acidic urine* • ***Most responsive to lithotripsy***
Xanthine stones	*Radioluscent*	*Deficiency of xanthine oxidase*	-

169. Answer is A (Phosphate): *Bailey 24th/1316; Smith's Urology 16th/262; Beat the Boards 1st (2006)/214*

Phosphate stones (Triple phosphate stones) form in the presence of high concentration of ammonia which essentially means that they form when the urine is infected (UTI) with Urea splitting organisms (eg. Proteus, Kleibsella, Pseudomonas sp.)

Triple Phosphate Stones (Phosphate stones)

- *Triple phosphate stones are composed predominantly of magnesium ammonium phosphate (strurite) with variable amounts of calcium phosphate.*
- *They form in the presence of high urinary concentration of ammonia (bicarbonate and carbonate)*
- *They form in cases of UTI when urine is infected with urea splitting bacteria i.e. Proteus, Kleibsella and Pseudomonas*
- *They form in urine with an alkaline pH.*

> *Urea splitting organisms split urea to ammonia there by providing an alkaline pH which facilitates precipitation of phosphate crystals.*

170. Answer is B (Increased peristalsis of the ureter to overcome obstruction) : *Smiths Urology 17th /31*

***The severity and colicky nature of ureteric colic pain are caused by the hyperperistasis and spasm of smooth muscles of the ureter as it attempts to rid itself of a foreign body or to overcome obstruction** – Smith*

Pain from Acute obstruction of Ureter
(Stone or Blood clot)

Back Pain	Severe Colicky Pain
This results from renal capsular distention	This results from renal, pelvic and ureteral muscle spasm. The severity and ***colicky nature of this pain are caused by the hyperperistalsis and spasm of this smooth muscle organ (ureter) as it attempts to rid itself of a foreign body or to overcome obstruction.***

171. Answer is A (At pelvic brim): *S. Das 4th/408; Bailey & Love, 24th/1317; Smith's Urology 17th/31*

Pain radiating to medial side of thigh and perineum suggetsts a stone in lower portion of ureter (proximal to orifice) or at pelvic brim.

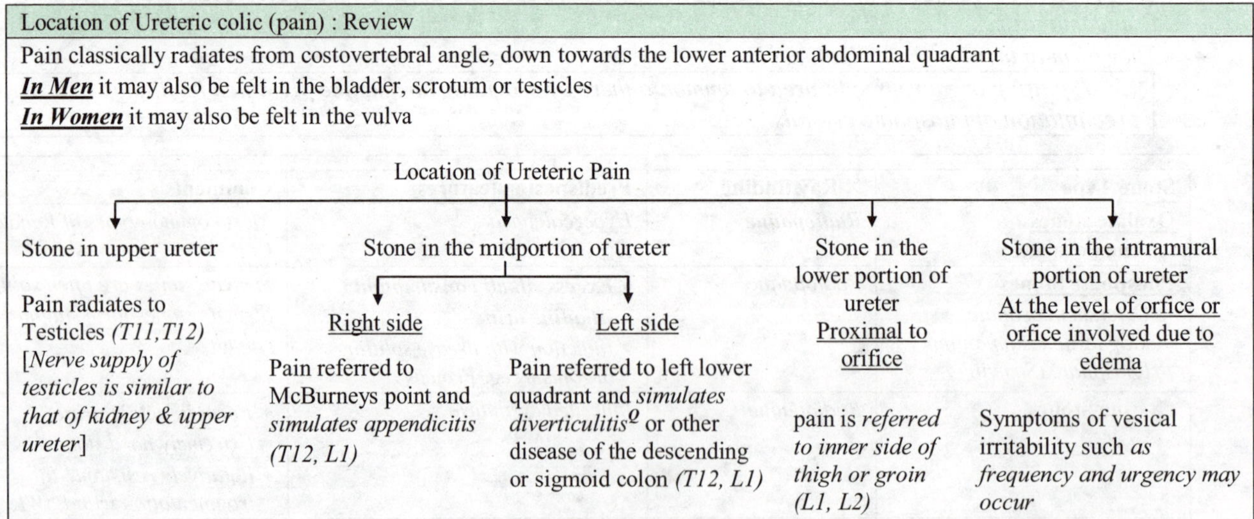

172. Answer is D (Genitofemoral nerve): *Gray's Anatomy 38th/18*

Pain of uerteric colic is refered to the proximal anterior aspect of thigh (groin) via supply of the genitofemoral nerve (L1)

173. Answer is D (Ureteroscopic Retrieval) : *Bailey Love 23rd/1189; Smith's general urology 15th/308, 309*

The patient in question has a small calculus (1.0 cm) in size, which is located in the distal ureter and hence is amenable to ureteroscopic removal. The presence of proximal hydroureteronephrosis indicates obstruction and forms the indication for stone removal.

Indications and methods for removal of stone

Indications for stone removal
- *Repeated attacks of colic*
- *Stone is too large to pass*
- *Stone is enlarging*
- *Stone is not moving*
- *Stone is causing complete obstruction of the kidney*
- *Urine is infected*

Ureteroscopic Removal	Extracorporal shock wave Lithotripsy	Percutaneous Nephrolithotripsy
• *Small stone* • *Stone in lower part of ureter within 5-6 cm of ureteric orfice*	• *Best for proximal stones* that can be identified by the imaging system of Lithotriptor • Stones in miduretor can be pushed up in the pelvis and *then* exposed to shock waves • Not appropriate if complete obstruction is present • *Stones < 2.0 to 2.5 cm can be removed*	• It is done for proximal ureteric cacluli • Stones > 2.5 cm, those that are resistant to shock waves

Open Surgery *is done very rarely nowadays when all methods have failed, Urethrolithotomy is done for long standing calculi not accessible by instruments and ESWL.*

174. Answer is D (ESWL): *Refer previous question*

The patient in question has a small calculus (< 2.5 cm) located in the proximal portion of the renal tract (pelvis). Such stones are easily amenable to ESWL which is the management of choice.

175. Answer is A (Endoscopic removal): *Refer previous question*

Stones in the lower part of ureter within 5-6 cm of ureteric orifice (that are small in size) are best managed by Ureteroscopic (Endoscopic) removal.

176. Answer is C (Renal stone): *Clinical Surgery by S. Das*

Calcification on the right side of the abdomen on an AP view and calcification overlying the spine on lateral view is consistent with diagnosis of renal stones.

Characteristics of a Renal stone that aid in the diagnosis :
- *In lateral view the* **Renal stone lies superimposed on shadow of vertebral column** *while gall stones are seen well infront of the vertebral bodies.*
- *Renal calculii moves with respiration*[Q] which can be verified with two exposures, one in full inspiration & other in full expiration.
- Density of a Renal stone is uniform, while a gall stone is less dense in the centre.
- *Renal stone take the shape of the Renal pelvis*[Q] & calyces while a solitary *gallstone* is usually round and *multiple ones are multifaceted*[Q].
- *Majority of Renal calculi are Radioopaque*[Q] except *pure uric acid stones* which *are Radiolucent*[Q].

A renal calculus has to be differentiated from
1. Gallstone[Q]
2. Calcified Lymphnode[Q]
3. Calcified costal cartilage[Q]
4. Calcified aneurysm of the abdominal aorta[Q]

Nephrocalcinosis

177. Answer is D (Medullary cystic kidney): *Harrison 18th/p 2382, 2383 Harrisons 17th/1815, 1816; Ultrasound of the Urogenital system' by Baxter (2006) /32, 33*

Nephrocalcinosis is a fracture of medullary sponge kidney disease but is not a feature of Medullary cystic kidney disease or Nephronophthysis.

Distal RTA, Sarcoidosis and Milk Alkali syndrome are established causes for Nephrocalcinosis.

Nephrocalcinosis

Nephrocalcinosis is a broad term that refers to pathological deposition of calcium in the renal parenchyma
Nephrocalcinosis may present as medullary nephrocalcinosis or cortical nephrocalcinosis

Causes of nephrocalcinosis

Medullary
(common form of Nephrocalcinosis)

- Renal tubular acidosis (distal or Type I)
- Oxalosis
- Papillary necrosis
- Medullary sponge kidney
- Frusemide abuse
- Bartter Syndrome
- Hypercalcemia
  - Primary hyperparathyroidism
  - Sarcoidosis
  - Vitamin D excess
  - Hypercalcemia of malignancy
  - Cushing disease
  - Milk-alkali syndrome

Cortical
(Uncommon /Unusual with incidence <5%)

Renal cortical necrosis
Chronic glomerulo nephritis
Transplant rejection
Tuberculosis
Oxalosis

Oxalosis typically causes both cortical and medullary nephrocalcinosis

178. Answer is D (Pseudohypoparathyroidism): *Refer previous question*

Pseudohypoparathyroidism is not associated with nephrocalcinosis

Primary hyperparathyroidism. Medullary Sponge Kidney and Vitamin D excess are established causes for nephrocalcinosis.

179. Answer is A & E (Medullary sponge kidney & Hyperparathyroidism): *Refer previous question*

Medullary sponge kidney and Hyperparathyroidism are established causes of Nephrocalcinosis.

180. Answer is B (*Calcium Restriction*): *'The Washington Manual Nephrology Subspecialty Consult' 2nd/245*

Low protein, Low sodium and Normal Calcium diet is recommended for patients with calcium nephrolithiasis

Dietry Intervention in patients with Calcium Nephrolithiasis

*'Dietary intervention plays a cardinal role in the preventive treatment of calcium nephrolithiasis. Studies have shown that a **low protein, low salt diet significantly reduces nephrolithiasis** recurrence rates in patients with idiopathic hypercalciuria. Long term dietary compliance with a low protein, low salt diet has been shown to be superior to a low calcium diet in prevention of nephrolithiasis. **A low calcium diet may increase the intestinal absorption of oxalate reducing the effectiveness of this therapy. Therefore low calcium diets are not recommended.** Diets containing 700 to 800 mg of calcium are adequate for patients with idiopathic hypercalciuria. Low protein diets reduce purine intake, resulting in reduced systemic acid and uric acid loads. Low sodium diets reduce the amount of calcium in urine'*

- The Washington Manual Nephrology Subspecialty Consult' 2nd/245

Congenital Diseases of the Kidney

181. Answer is B (Autosomal dominant): *Harrison 14th/ 380; 15th/386; 16th/1694; 17th/1797; Harrison 18th/p 2355 Robbins 7th/962, 963*

***Adult polycystic kidney disease is inherited as autosomal dominant trait** -Harrison 16th/1694*

Remember:

Autosomal dominant disorders:	Autosomal recessive disorders:	X-Linked disorders:
Familial hypercholesterolemia	Deafness	Hemophilia A [Q] (recessive)
Hereditary nonpolyposis colon cancer	Albinism [Q]	G6PD deficiency [Q] (recessive)
Polyposis of the colon [Q]	Wilson's disease [Q]	Ducchene/Becker muscular dystrophy [Q] (recessive)
BRCA1 and BRCA2 breast cancer	Hemochromatosis [Q]	Fabry's disease
Hereditary hemorrhagic telengiectasia	Sickle cell anemia [Q]	Ocular albinism
Marfan's syndrome [Q]	β thalassemia [Q]	Testicular feminization
Hereditary spherocytosis [Q]	Cystic fibrosis [Q]	Chronic granulomatous disease
Adult polycystic kidney disease [Q]	Hereditary emphysema (α_1 antitrypsin deficiency)	Hypophosphatemic rickets [Q] (dominant)
Huntington's chorea [Q]	Homocystinuria [Q]	Fragile-X syndrome [Q] (recessive)
Acute intermittent porphyria [Q]	Freidrich's ataxia [Q]	Color blindness [Q]
Osteogenesis imperfecta tarda [Q]	Phenylketonuria [Q]	
von Willebrand's disease [Q]	Fanconi's Syndrome -[*H 14th/ 2201*]	
Myotonic dystrophy [Q]	Gaucher's Disease - [*H 14th/ 2174*]	
Familial hypertrophic cardiomyopathy		
Neurofibromatosis [Q]		
Tuberous sclerosis [Q]		
Otospongiosis [Q]		
Achondroplasia [Q]		

182. Answer is B (Hypertension is rare): *Harrison 15th/1598, 1599; 16th/1694; 17th/1797,1798; Harrison 18th/p 2355, 2356 Robbins 7th /962, 963*

***Hypertension is common in patients with autosomal dominant polycystic kidney disease. It is found in 75% of adults and 20 to 30% of children** – Harrison 16th/1694*

Adult Polycystic kidney:

<table>
<tr><td colspan="2">Inheritance : Autosomal Dominant</td></tr>
<tr><td colspan="2">Pathology:</td></tr>
<tr><td colspan="2">- Kidneys are grossly enlarged with multiple cysts
- Cyst are distributed uniformly throughout cortex and medulla
- Cysts contain straw coloured fluid that may become haemorrhagic</td></tr>
<tr><td colspan="2">Presentation: usually occurs in IIIrd / IVth decade</td></tr>
<tr><td>Renal</td><td>Extra renal manifestation</td></tr>
<tr><td>1. Pain: due to infection (Pyelonephritis) / obstruction / sudden haemorrhage
2. Haematuria [Q]
3. Nocturia: due to impaired concentrating ability
4. Nephrolithiasis (15-20%) [Q]
5. Hypertension (75% adults and 25% children) : due to activation of rennin angiotensin system. [Q]
6. Progressive decline in renal function – CRF</td><td>1. Cysts: Liver (most common)
Spleen, pancreas and ovaries
2. Intracranial aneurysms
3. Colonic diverticular disease
4. Cardiac: Mitral valve prolapse / AR / TR</td></tr>
</table>

183. Answer is A (Berry Aneurysm in Circle of Willis): *Harrison 15th/1600; 16th/1696; 17th/1798; Harrison 18th/p 2356 Chandrasoma Taylor3rd/700*

Intracranial Berry aneurysms are important extrarenal associations of adult polycystic kidney disease.

Extra renal anomalies seen in patients with adult polycystic kidney disease.

GIT	CNS	Cardiac
• Cysts in Liver, Spleen, Pancreas • Colonic diverticular disease	• Intracranial aneurysms (Berry)	• Mitral valve prolapse Q • Aortic and tricuspid insufficiency

Cysts may also be seen in the ovary.

184. Answer is A (Lung): *Harrison 15th/ 1600; Harrison 16th/1696; 17th/1798; Harrison 18th/p 2356 Robbins 7th/964*

Cysts in lung are not associated with PCKD

Cysts in polycystic kidney disease may be seen in :

- Liver : Hepatic cysts (50 – 70 %)
- Spleen
- Pancreas
- Ovaries

- *Most common extrarenal sites of cyst formation is the Liver* Q
- *Hepatic cysts occur in 50 – 70% of cases* Q
- *Cysts are generally asymptomatic and liver function is normal.* Q

185. Answer is B (Hepatic cysts) : *Urology secrets 3rd/134 Clinical pedicatric urology (2002)/ 657; Refer text below*

Hepatic cysts are the most common extra renal manifestations of Adult polycystic kidney Disease–*Urology secrets 3rd/134*

Confusion on the most common extra renal manifestation of APCKD

Most standard text books mention Liver cysts as the most common extrarenal manifestation of Adult polycystic kidney disease

Urology secrets 3rd/134;
Adult and Pediatric Urology 4th/831
'Clinical Pediatric Urology'(2002) / 657
'Liver disease: Diagnosis & 'Management' (2000)/322

Few standard tetxbooks including Old edition of Harrisons (not mentioned in new editions) mention Colonic diverticular disease as the most common extrarenal manifestation of APCKD.

Harrisons 15th/1600 (Not in new edition)
First AID for USMLE STEP 1 (2006)/281

186. Answer is B (Presentation is Unilateral): *Harrison 16th/ 1696; 17th/1797, 1798, Harrison 18th/p 2355, 2356 Robbins 7th/962, 963;Bailey 24th/1307*

- ***The presentation in Polycystic disease of kidney is characteristically bilateral***
  - *The bilateral enlargement can hardly be mistaken on routine examination – Bailey*
  - *USG and CT show multiple cysts in both kidneys - Bailey*
- The disease may present at any age but *the most common age of presentation is in the 3rd or 4th decade.*
- **Both the kidney are grossly enlarged and situated with multiple cysts.**
- Intracranial berry aneurysms are seen in 5-10 % of patients.

187. Answer is A (Autosomal Dominant) : *Nelson's 18th / 1706, Robbins 7th / 964; Harrison's 17th / 1799, Harrison 18th/p 2358, 2359 Clinical Pediatric Nephrology 2nd / 262*

Childhood Polycystic Kidney Disease is synonymously used for Autosomal Recessive Kidney Disease.

Polycystic Kidney Disease

Adult Polycystic Kidney Disease	Childhood Polycystic Kidney Disease
Also termed as Autosomal Dominant Polycystic kidney disease (ADPKD)	*Also termed as Autosomal Recessive Polycystic kidney Disease (ARPKD)*

Childhood Polycystic kidney Disease / Autosomal Recessive PKD : Review

Childhood Polycystic kidney disease is a rare developmental anomaly genetically distinct from Adult polycystic kidney Disease ***having an autosomal recessive inheritance***

Genetics

- *Autosomal Recessive inheritance*
- Defective gene is the PKHD1 (Polycystic kidney and Hepatic Disease 1)
- PKHD1 gene codes for a protein 'Fibrocystin' (defective protein in ARPKD)[Q]

Epidemiology

- Majority of patients present during infancy (first year of life)
- May present later in life (in young adults)

Presentation

- Presentation is variable and depends on age at presentation

Respiratory Symptoms	Renal Features	Hepatic Features
Respiratory distress	• Hypertension • Renal failure • Enlarged kidneys (abdominal mass) • Pyuria • Proteinuria	• Hepatomegaly • Features of portal Hypertension -Esophageal varices -Hypersplenism

Associations

- **Maternal Oligohydramnios**
  Oligohydramnios may be present due to severe intrauterine kidney disease
- **Potter's syndrome**
  Most severely affected neonates may have Potter's syndrome due to oligohydramnios
- **Pulmonary Hypoplasia**
  Pulmonary hypoplasia may result from severe oligohydramnios and as part of Potter's sequence
  'About 50% of affected neonates die of pulmonary hypoplasia' - Harrison's
- **Congenital Hepatic fibrosis**
  Congenital Hepatic Fibrosis is a peculiar type of hepatic fibrosis characterized by bland periportal fibrosis, and proliferation of well differentiated biliary ductules
  Hepatic cysts may be seen (In almost all cases liver has cysts with portal fibrosis - Robbins)
- **Biliary Ductal Atresia**
  ARPKP is invariably associated with congenital hepatic fibrosis and various degrees of biliary ductal Atresia

Renal Pathology

- Kidney's are enlarged (invariably Bilateral)
- Numerous small cysts are present in kidney which give it ' Sponge like appearance'
- Cysts are primarily located in distal tubule and collecting duct
- ***Cysts may be discovered prenatally, at birth or later in life***

188. Answer is C (Unilateral renal dysplasia): *Sutton's Radiology 6th/ 1105; Nelson 17th/ 1784*

*The multicystic **dysplastic kidney** is the commonest form of **congenital cystic renal dysplasia**, and is due to complete uretric obstruction in fetal life. The condition is **usually unilateral**; bilateral disease is lethal.*

Cystic diseases of kidney in infants
• Dysplastic kidney (multicystic) • Polycystic kidney (Autosomal Recessive; Autosomal dominant) • Multilocular cystic nephroma

Renal dysplasia. Multicystic kidney:

'It is the commonest cause of renal mass in infants' – Ghai 6th/ 467

189. Answer is D (Nephronopthisis) : Refer previous question

Presence of nocturnal enuresis, growth retardation (short stature) and renal failure (elevated urea and creatinine) without hematuria, edema or hypertension and the presence of small sized shrunken kidneys suggest the diagnosis of Nephronophthysis.

The diagnosis of Nephronophthysis should be considered if a child presents with:

- *Polyuria (or nocturnal enuresis), Polydypsia and Urinary sodium loss (hyponotremia)*
- *Growth retardation (short stature), and anemia*
- *Renal insufficiency (elevated BUN/creatinine) without hematuria, proteinuria, edema or hypertension*
- *Normal or small sized kidney on USG*

Diagnostic Clues in the question

- Age = 12years (Juvenile Age group)
- Biochemical parameters

Parameter	Normal value	Value in child	Inference
Urea	10-40mg/dl	112mg/dl	Elevated (Renal failure)
Creatinine	<1.5 mg/dl	6mg/dl	Elevated (Renal failure)
Sodium	136-146 meq/dl	119 meq/dl	Hyponatremia (salt wasting)

- Symptoms: Nocturia (polyurea) and short stature (Growth Retardation)
- **Features of Renal Failure :** No Hematuria, No Hypertension, No significant proteinuria
- USG: Bilateral small kidneys.

The presence of Nocturia, Growth retardation and onset of Renal feature at an age <20 years without hematuria, hypertension, and edema along with shrunken kidney on USG suggests – the diagnosis of Nephronophysis.

Cystic Disease of Renal Medulla

Nephrophtysis – Medullary cystic kidney		Medullary Sponge kidney
Both these conditions may progress to end stage Renal disease and present with similar clinical features.		This is a relatively benign condition
Nephrophthysis	**Medullary Cystic kidney**	
• Autosomal Recessive	Autosomal dominant	
• Age of onset in 1st decade (Juvenile)	Age of onset in 3rd or 4th decade (Adult)	
• Progression to ESRD occurs <20 years of age	• Progression to ESRD occurs >20 years to age	
• Growth Retardation is present as it affects growing children	• Growth retardation is usually not associated as it affects adults	
• Extra renal abnormalities are frequent and include *Retinitis pigmentosa*, *Cerebellar Ataxia*, *Hepatic fibrosis*, *Skeletal abnormalities*	• Extra renal abnormalities are absent.	

190. Answer is B (Nephronophthisis): *Harrison 18th/p 2359 Harrisons 17th/1799*

Repeated attacks of polyurea, salt wasting (hyponatremia), evidence of renal failure (elevated creatinine) and small size of kidneys suggests a diagnosis of Nephropthisis or Medulary cystic disease.

The presence of this condition in juvenile age group (8 years) favours a diagnosis of Nephrophthisis which is the single best answer of choice. (Medullary cystic kidney disease presents in adults in 3rd or 4th decade).

Juvenile Nephronophthisis

Chronic Tubulo interstitial Nephritis which uniformly progresses to End stage Renal Disease.

Extrarenal Abnormalities[Q]
Ritinitis Pigmentosa
Cerebellar Ataxia
Hepatic Fibrosis
Skeletal Anomalies

Autosomal Recessive disease[Q]

Pathology Triad
- Tubular Basement Membrane Disintegration
- Tubular cyst formation (Medullary Cyst)
- Tubulo interstitial inflammation

Kidney size is normal or Reduced (shrunken)[Q]

Loss of Urinary Concentrating Ability

Polyurea[Q], *Polydipsia*[Q] — *Nocturnal Enuresis*[Q]

Low urinary osmolarity which does not increase after desmopressin administration

Salt wasting

- *Hyponatremia*[Q]
- *Hypovolumia (dehydration)*[Q]
- *Hypotension (low BP)*[Q]

Progressive Renal failure

Because of loss of urinary concentrating ability and salt wasting, typical symptoms of renal failure do not occur until late in disease

Edema, Hypertension, Hematuria and proteinuria do not occur until late in disease

- *Anemia*[Q]
- *Growth Retardation*[Q]
- *Elevated BUN/creatinine*[Q]

191. Answer is D (Biopsy): *Harrison 17th/1800; CMDT 2005/899*

Although ultrasonography and CT scan can be useful in making a diagnosis of medullary cystic disease, an open renal biopsy that ensures recovery of tissue from the corticomedullary junction is definitive.

192. Answer is C (Vesicouretrial reflux induced pyelonephritis): *Pediatr Nephrol. 1993 Aug;7(4):361-4 The small scarred kidney in childhood ;. Risdon RA.*

*Renal scarring is most commonly a result of chronic pyogenic infection of the kidney or chronic pyelonephritis. Chronic pyelonephritis occurs only in patients with major anatomic abnormalities, such as obstructive uropathy, struvite calculi, or, **most commonly, VUR (in 30 to 45% of young children with symptomatic UTI).** - Mercks manual (http://www.merck.com/mrkshared/mmanual/section17/chapter227/227a.jsp)*

***'In children < 10 yr, about 30 to 50% of UTIs are associated with vesicoureteral reflux (VUR) which can lead to** renal scarring **and renal insufficiency if not treated'** – Merck's manual*

Remember *: Renal tuberculosis is always secondary to some primary focus elsewhere in body and occurs later in life then other forms (commonly around 20-40 years age group.)*

193. Answer is A (One year of age) : *Paediatrics Urology, Gear Heart / 16*

"Normal adult kidney can produce urine with an osmolality of greater than 1000 m Osm/kg water. The healthy new born infant, subject to water deprivation for 10-14 hours can achieve an osmolality of only 500-700 m osm / kg. ***This value increases gradually during the first few months and approximates to the adult value by about one year of age."***

Renal Tumours

194. Answer is A (Clear cell type): *Harrison 17th/592; Robbins 7th/1016*

Clear cell carcinomas are the most common histological type of Renal cell carcinoma

Carcinoma Type	Frequency	Place of origin	Cell of origin	Cytogenetics	Growth Pattern
Clear cell	***60%***	***Cortex***	***Proximal tubule***	*3p-*	Acinar or sarcomatoid
Papillary	5-15%	Cortex	Proximal tubule	*+7, +17, -Y*	Papillary or sarcomatoid
Chromophobic	5-10%	Cortex	Cortical collecting duct	***Hypodiploid***	Solid, tubular, or sarcomatoid
Oncocytic	5-10%	Cortex	Cortical collecting duct	Undetermined	Tumor nests
Collecting duct	< 1%	Medulla	Medullary collecting duct	Undetermined	Papillary or sarcomatoid

195. Answer is (Monosomy of 1 and y): *Harrison's 17th/592, Urological Surgical Pathology' by Bostwick & Chang 2nd/96, 'The kidney' by Vize, Woolf & Bard 1st (2003)/454, 'Renal cell carcinoma' by Campbell & Rini 1st (2009)/42,43*

Chromophobe variants of renal cell carcinoma are charachterized by widespread / extensive chromosomal losses resulting in monosomy or hypodiploid DNA index. This includes loss of chromosome 1 and Y.

'The abnormalities most consistently observed have been multiple losses of whole chromosomes, most frequently 1, 2, 6, 10, 13, 17, 21 and the Y chromosome' – *Urological Surgical Pathology*

Classification of epithelial neoplasms arising from the kidney

Carcinoma Type	Cell of Origin	Cytogenetics
Clear cell	Proximal tubule	3p deletions (3p-), VHL gene mutations, 5q gains
Papillary	Proximal tubule	Trisomy of chromosome 7 and 17 (+7, +17) Loss of Y chromosome (-Y)
Chromophobe	***Cortical collecting duct***	***Hypodiploid / Monosomy*** ***Loss of multiple chromosomes 1, 2, 6, 10, 13, 17, 21 & Y***
Oncocytic	Cortical collecting duct	Undetermined Either karyotypically normal or contain limited number of karyotypic abnormalities including -1, -Y and translocations involving chromosme II
Collecting duct	Medullary collecting duct	Undetermined Losses of multiple chromosomes 1, 6, 14, 15 & 22

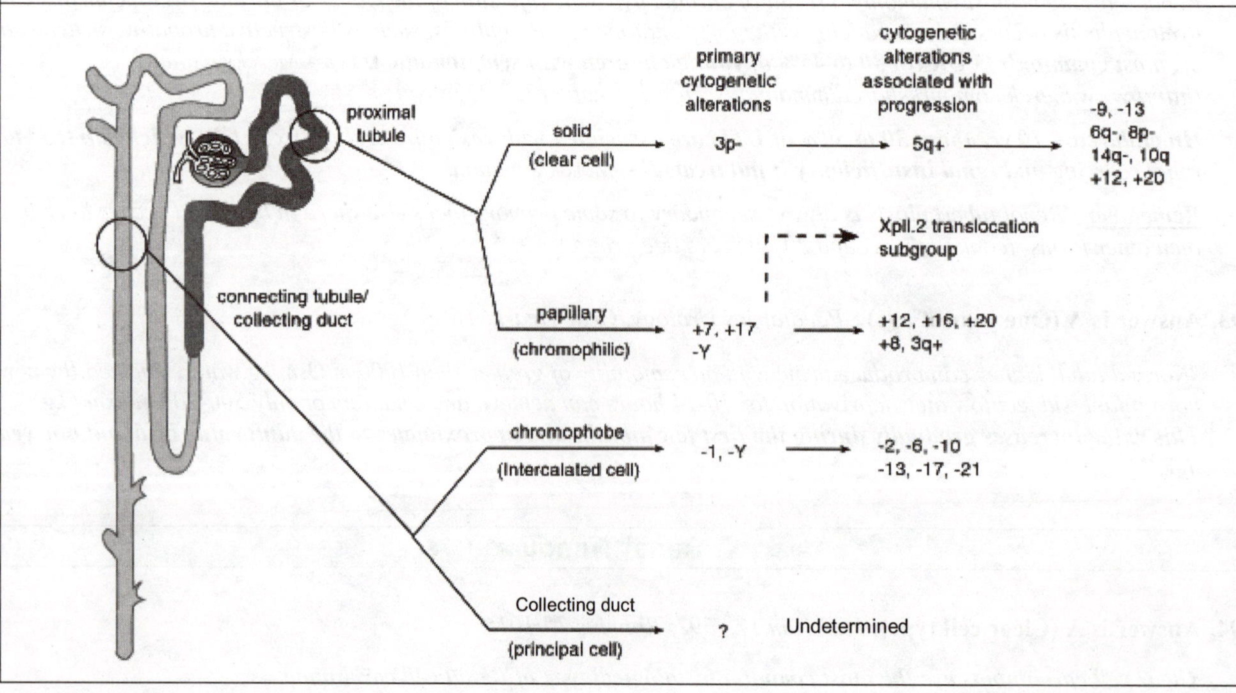

196. Answer is B (Chromosome-3): *Harrison 15th/ 607; Harrison 17th/ 592 Harrison 18th/p 793 Robbins 6th/ 993*

Presence of painless haematuria with balottable mass in right flank in this forty years old male suggests diagnosis of renal cell carcinoma. The most common histological variant 'clear cell carcinome' is associated with a defect in chromosome 3.

Features of three major histological variants of renal call carcinoma:

Clear cell carcinoma (Non papillary)	**Papillary carcinoma**	**Chromophobe renal carcinoma**
• Most common [Q] type [Q] (70-80%) • Cells have clear [Q] or granular cytoplasm and are non papillary • Defect lies in chromosomes 3 [Q]	• Second most common type (10-15%) • Papillary [Q] growth pattern is characteristic (clear cell not seen) • Psammoma bodies may be present • Most common cytogenetic abnormality are - trisomy of chromosome 7, 16 & 17 and loss of Y in male patients in sporadic form - trisomy 7 in familial form • [Q] Striking characteristic of tumor is: **Tendency to invade the renal vein** and grow as a solid column of cells within the vessels. Extension may produce a continuous cord of tumor in IVC and even in the right side of heart.	• Least common (5%) • Pale eosinophilic cytoplasm • Multiple chromosomal losses and extreme haplopoidy

197. Answer is D (Radiosensitive): *Harrison 17th/592, 593; Harrison 18th/p 793 CMDT 2008/1430, 1437; 2009/1463-1464; Robbins 7th/1016-1018; Smith's Urology 16th/357, 349; Bailey 24th/1332*

Renal cell carcinoma is a relatively radioresistant tumor.

<u>**Renal cell carcinoma originates in the Renal cortex**</u>
'Renal cell carcinoma originates in the Renal cortex and tends to grow out into perinephric tissue causing the typical bulge or mass effect that aids in their detection by diagnostic imaging studies' – Smith's Urology

<u>**Renal Cell carcinoma are adenocarcinomas**</u> *(Robbins 7th/1016)*
Histologically Renal cell carcinoma is most often a mixed adenocarcinoma – Smith's Urology

<u>**Renal cell carcinomas may present with varicocele**</u>
'Renal cell carcinomas may present with Rapidly developing varicocele. Varicocele is usually observed on the left side. This occurs because left gonadal vein is obstructed where it joins the left renal vein.

<u>**Renal cell carcinomas are Relatively Radioresistant tumors**</u>
Renal cell carcinomas are generally considered radioresistant tumors
<u>Role of Radiotherapy in renal Cell carcinoma</u>

- *Preoperative Radiation has shown no impact on survival*
- Postoperative Radiation has also shown no evidence of improved survival but may be used as it shows improvement in local control.
- *Palliative Radiotherapy has been shown to be effective in metastatic disease to brain, bone and lungs.*

198. Answer is C (More common in female): *Harrison 18th/p 793 Harrison 17th/592*

Renal cell carcinoma is more common in males.

<u>**Renal cell carcinoma is more common in males**</u>
The male to female ratio of RCC is 2:1

<u>**Renal cell carcinoma arises from the proximal tubule**</u>
'RCC arise form the proximal tubular epithelium as evidenced by electron microscopy' – Smith's Urology 16th/349

- *RCC arise most commonly from Renal cortex*
- *RCC originates most commonly from proximal renal tubular epithelium*
- *RCC more often arises from the 'poles' particularly the upper pole*

Renal cell carcinoma may invade the Renal vein

Renal cell carcinoma may extend directly into the renal vein and inferior vena acav

Stage III A Disease	Tumor invades main renal vein or IVC

Renal cell carcinoma present with varicocele

'Renal cell carcinomas may present with Rapidly developing varicocele. Varicocele is usually observed on the left side. This occurs because left gonadal vein is obstructed where it joins the left renal vein.

199. Answer is B (Hypertension): *Harrison 18th/p 793 Harrison 17th/592*

Hypertension may be seen in patients with Renal cell carcinoma but it does not form part of the classically described triad.

Classic Triad of Renal cell carcinoma (seen in 10-20% of patients)
• *Hematuria (Gross)* • *Pain (Abdominal / Flank)* • *Mass (Abdominal / Flank)*

200. Answer is None (All may be seen): *Harrison 18th/p 793, 2382 Harrison 17th/592; 1815*

Renal cell carcinoma may present with Polycythemia (Erythrocytosis), Hypertension, Hematuria and Renal vein thrombosis.

Polycythemia (Erythrocytosis), Hypertension, Hematuria are signs of Renal Cell Carcinoma. *(Harrison 17th/592)*

Signs and symptoms in patients with renal cell cancer

Presenting Sign or Symptom	Incidence, %
Classic triad: hematuria, flank pain, flank mass	10-20
Hematuria	40
Flank pain	40
Palpable mass	25
Weight mass	33
Anemia	33
Fever	20
Hypertension	20
Abnormal liver function	15
Hypercalcemia	5
Erythrocytosis	3
Neuromyopathy	3
Amyloidosis	2
Increased erythrocyte sedimentation rate	55

Secondary Renal Vein Thrombosis may be seen due to invasion by Renal Cell Carcinoma *(Harrison 17th/1815)*

Causes of Renal Vein Thrombosis

- *Trauma*
- *Extrinsic compression (Lymphnode, tumor, aortic aneurysm)*
- ***Invasion by Renal cell carcinoma***
- *Dehydration*
- *Nephrotic syndrome*
- *Pregnancy or oral contraceptives*

201. Answer is None or D (None or Cushing;s syndrome): *Harrison 18th/p 793 Harrison 17th/592; Robbin's 7th/1018; Smith's Urology 16th/351*

Amongst the options provided, Cushing's syndrome is the least common paraneoplastic syndrome associated with Renal cell carcinoma, and hence the single best answer of exclusion.

Note that while Harison's textbook does not include Cushing's syndrome in the list of paraneoplastic syndromes associated with Renal cell carcinoma, this condition is clearly mentioned as an associated paraneoplastic syndrome in other standard textbooks like Robbin's and Smith's Urology.

Paraneoplastic Syndromes is Renal Cell Carcinoma

Characteristic Paraneoplastic Syndromes (common)	Other Paraneoplastic Syndromes (Less common / Not characteristic)
• ***Erythrocytes/Polycythemia*** (due to ↑ed erythropoietin) • ***Hypercalcemia*** (due to ↑ed parathyroid related peptide) • ***Hypertension*** (due to ↑ed rennin production) • *Non metastatic Hepatic Dysfunction (Stauffer syndrome)* (due to ↑ed granulocyte-macrophage colony stimulating factor)	• Cushing's syndrome (due to ↑ ACTH production) • Galactorrhea (due to ↑ed prolactin production) • Hypoglycemia (due to ↑ed Insulin) • Gynaecomastia & decreased libido (due to ↑ gonadotropins) • Hirsuitism, amenorrhea and male pattern balding (due to ↑ gonadotropins) • Amyloidosis • Leukemoid Reaction and Eosinophilia • Dysfibrinogenemia

202. Answer is B (Lungs): *Smith's Urology 16th/349*

'The most common site of distant metastasis (in RCC) is the lung' – *Smith's Urology 16th/349*

203. Answer is B (IVC involvement indicates inoperability): *Harrison 16th/542; Harrison 17th/593 Harrison 18th/p 795*

Extension of tumor into IVC does not indicate inoperability.

'Extension into renal vein or inferior vena cava ***does not preclude resection*** *even if cardiopulmonary bypass is required. Half of these patients have prolonged survival' - Harrison*

204. Answer is C (Arthogryposis multiplex congenita): *Robbin's 7th/604, 605; Ghai 6th/574*

Arthrogryposis multiplex congenita is not associated with Wilm's tumor.

Wilm's Tumor

The risk of Wilm's tumor is increased in associations with at least three recognizable groups of congenital malformations associated with distinct chromosomal loci

WAGR syndrome	Denys Drash Syndrome	Beckwith Wiedemann Syndrome
Characterized by: • *Wilm's tumor* • ***Aniridia*** • *Genital Anomalies* • *Retardation (Mental)*	Characterized by: • *Gonadal Dysgenesis* ***(male pseudohermaphroditism)*** • *Early onset nephropathy (diffuse mesangial sclerosis/renal failure)*	Characterized by: • *Organomegaly* • *Macroglossia* • ***Hemihypertrophy*** • *Omphalocele* • *Adrenal cytomegaly (Abnormal large cells in Adrenal cortex)*

205. Answer is B (Abdominal lump): *Robbin's 7th/506; Ghai 6th/574*

Most common presentation of Wilm's tumor is an asymptomatic Abdominal Mass.

206. Answer is D (Radiosensitive): *Bailey 23rd/1196; Nelson 18th/2142; Ghai 6th/574, 575; Robbin's 7th/506*

Wilm's tumor is both chemosensitive and Radiosensitive *(unlike renal cell carcinoma which is considered radioresistant and chemoresistant)*

Wilm's tumor is associated with a good prognosis

The prognosis of Wilm's tumor is currently very good and excellent results are obtained with a combination of chemotherapy & nephrectomy.

Most common site of Metastasis in Wilm's Tumor is Lungs

Metastasis occurs early, mainly by the blood stream to the lungs.
Liver and bone metastasis are rare and brain metastasis even more so.

Wilm's tumor may be bilateral (not always unilateral)

Wilm's tumor may arise in one or both kidneys.
The incidence of bilateral Wilm's tumor is 7% - Nelson

207. Answer is C > A (Histology > Stage of disease): *Devita 6th/2177*

Both stage of the tumor and the histological grade have been described as the most important determination of prognosis, in different texts. If we have to choose a single best option, 'Histology' is the single best answer.
'The histology of Wilm's tumor was identified as the most important determinant of prognosis'- Devita 6th/2177

208. Answer is B (International Society of Pediatric Oncology-SIOP) : *Devita's 8th / 2051 , Schwartz 8th / 1509*

The post-chemotherapy based staging system is the 'SIOP' staging system developed by the International society of pediatric oncology.

Two Staging Systems are currently being used for the staging of Wilm's Tumor

Pre-chemotherapy Staging System	Post-chemotherapy Staging System
• *Developed by the National Wilm's Tumor staging Group (NWTSG) (NWTSG – Staging system)*	• *Developed by the International Society of Pediatric Oncology (SIOP) (SIOP – Staging system)*
• This staging system is widely used in North America and Canada	• This staging system is widely used in Europe
• *'NWTSG' approach involves employment of 'primary Surgery'. Chemotherapy with or without Radiation therapy is given after surgery*	• 'SIOP' Approach involves employment of preoperative chemotherapy without histological confirmation of Wilm's tumor. (Primary chemotherapy for all patients regardless of extent)
• ***Staging is done at time of surgery (Pre – chemotherapy)***	• ***Staging is done at time of surgery (Post-chemotherapy)***
• Primary advantage is more accurate staging	• Primary advantage is easier surgical removal of tumor with decreased tumor rupture due to shrinkage of tumor by preoperative chemotherapy

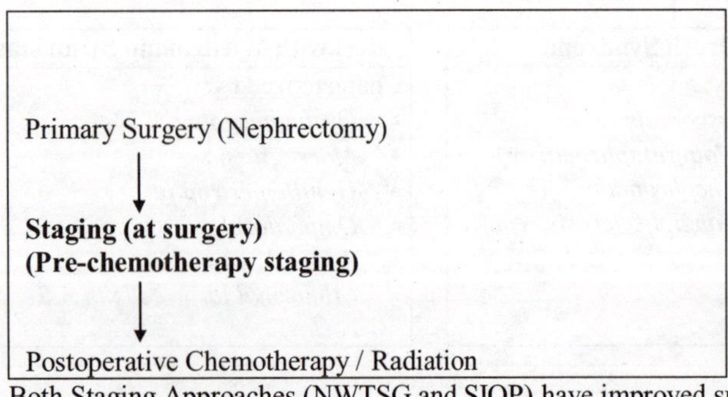

Primary Chemotherapy (Preoperative)
↓
Surgery (Nephrectomy)
↓
Staging (at surgery)
(Post-chemotherapy staging)
↓
Postoperative chemotherapy / Radiation

Both Staging Approaches (NWTSG and SIOP) have improved survival for patients with Wilm's tumor Success rates of treatment with both approaches are comparable

Hepatorenal Syndrome

209. Answer is A & B (urine Na < 10 meq/l and Normal Renal Histology): *Walker's Pediatric Gastrointestinal Disease 5th/1140*

Hepatorenal syndrome is associated with normal renal histology and supported by a urine sodium excretion < 10meq/L

Hepatorenal syndrome

- Hepatorenal syndrome is defined as a state of functional renal failure (Reduced GFR) in patients with severe liver disease
- ***Structurally /Histologically the kidneys are normal and recover function after successful liver transplantation.***
- The pathogenetic hallmark of hepatorenal syndrome is intense renal vasoconstriction with coexistent systemic vasodilatation
- The diagnosis of hepatorenal syndrome is considered in accordance with the following diagnostic criteria.

Diagnostic of Hepatorenal Syndrome
Major criteria
• *Low glomerular filtration rate, as indicated by serum creatinine > 1.5 mg/dL or 24-hr creatinine clearance < 40 mL/min*
• *Absence of shock, ongoing bacterial infection, fluid losses, and current treatment with nephrotoxic drugs*
• *No sustained improvement in renal function (decrease in serum creatinine to 1.5 mg/dL or increase in creatinine clearance to 40 mL/min) after diuretic withdrawal and expansion of plasma volume with 1.5L of a plasma expander*
• *Proteinuria <500 mg/dL and no ultrasonographic evidence of obstructive uropathy or parenchymal renal disease*
Additional criteria
• *Urine volume < 500 mL/d*
• *Urine sodium < 10 meq/L*
• *Urine osmolality greater than plasma osmolality*
• *Urine red blood cells <50/high- power field*
• *Serum sodium concentration < 130 mEqL*
Note: All major criteria must be present for the diagnosis of hepatorenal syndrome. Additional criteria are not necessary for the diagnosis but provide supportive evidence.

210. Answer is C (Urine osmolality is lower than plasma osmolality): *Washington manual of Medical Therapeutics 32nd/506*

Hepatorenal syndrome is associated with urine osmolality greater than plasma osmolality (and not lower than plasma osmolality)

Creatinine clearance < 40 ml/minute and poor response to volume expansion are major diagnostic features of hepatorenal syndrome while urinary sodium of less than 10 mmol/L is an additional criteria that provides supportive evidence.

Diagnostic of Hepatorenal Syndrome
Major criteria
• *Low glomerular filtration rate, as indicated by serum creatinine > 1.5 mg/dL or 24-hr creatinine clearance < 40 mL/min*
• *Absence of shock, ongoing bacterial infection, fluid losses, and current treatment with nephrotoxic drugs*
• *No sustained improvement in renal function (decrease in serum creatinine to 1.5 mg/dL or increase in creatinine clearance to 40 mL/min) after diuretic withdrawal and expansion of plasma volume with 1.5L of a plasma expander*
• *Proteinuria <500 mg/dL and no ultrasonographic evidence of obstructive uropathy or parenchymal renal disease*
Additional criteria
• *Urine volume < 500 mL/d*
• *Urine sodium < 10 meq/L*
• *Urine osmolality greater than plasma osmolality*
• *Urine red blood cells <50/high- power field*
• *Serum sodium concentration < 130 mEqL*
Note: All major criteria must be present for the diagnosis of hepatorenal syndrome. Additional criteria are not necessary for the diagnosis but provide supportive evidence.

211. Answer is A > C (The creatinine clearance is > 40 ml/min) : *Washington Manual of medical Therapeutics 32nd/506, Refer previous question.*

Hepatorenal syndrome is associated with creatinine clearance < 40 ml/min which is a major criteria in the diagnsis of hepatorenal syndrome and the single best answer of choice

Hepatorenal syndrome is also associated with a urine osmolaity that is higher (and not lower) than plasma osmolality. However this is an additional or supportive criteria that is not necessary for diagnosis and hence this is not the answer of choice.

Rhabdomyolysis

212. Answer is A (Acute Renal Failure): *Refer text below*

Acute Renal failure is an established complication of crush syndrome.

Acute Renal Failure is usually caused by a combination of hypovolemia and release of nephrotoxic substances into the circulation such as myoglobin

Crush syndrome is associated with hypocalcemia and hyperphosphatemia

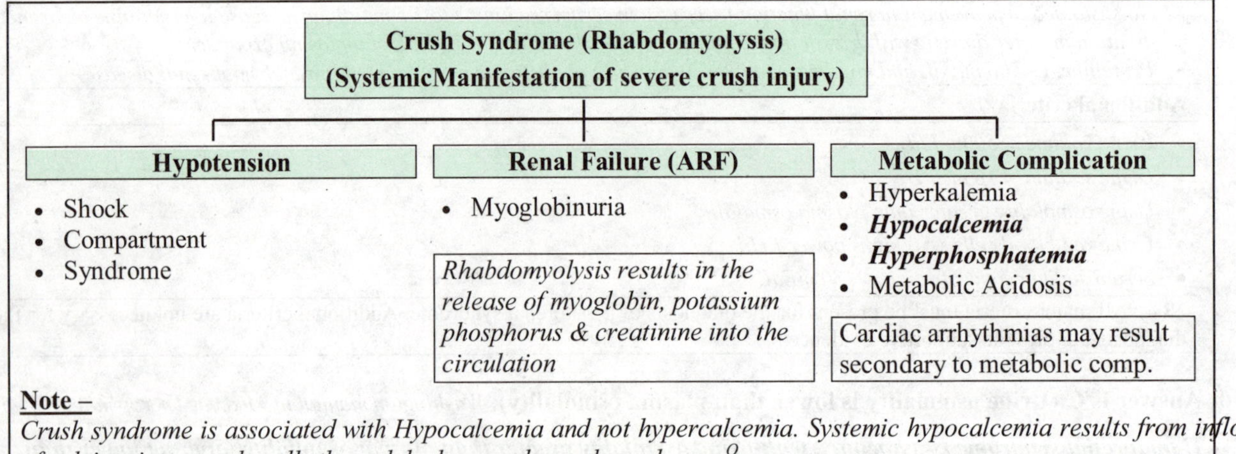

213. Answer is B (Hyperphosphatemia): *Current Critical Care Diagnosis and Treatment 3rd/326; Diseases of Kidney & urinary Tract 8th/1185*

Rhabdomyolysis may be caused by hypophosphatemia and not by hyperphosphatemia.

'When severe and sustained hypophosphatemia can cause severe myopathy and rhabdomyolysis'.

– Current Diagnosis and Treatment in Neurology 1st/373

Selected Causes of Rhabdomyolysis (Incomplete list):

Physical Trauma	Anoxic injury
• Crush injury	• Arterial occlusion
• Heat stress	• Seizures
• Electrocution	• Tetanus
• Exercise	• Compartment syndrome
• Hypothermia	• Delirium tremens
• Malignant hyperthermia	**Toxins**
• Neuroleptic malignant syndrome	• Ethanol
• Severe burns	• Heroin
• Contact sports	• Barbiturates
• Direct muscle trauma	

Metabolic
• Hypokalemia • Hypophosphatemia • Diabetic ketaoacidosis • Diabetic hyperosmolar non ketotic coma • Myxedemia • Carnitine deficiency • Hereditary muscle enzyme deficiency -Phosphorylase deficiency (McArdle's disease) -Phosphofructokinase deficiency -α-Glucosidase deficiency -Carnitine palmityltransferase deficiency -Amylo-1,6-glucosidase deficiency
Infections
Inflammation
• Polymyositis • Dermatomyositis
Poisons
• Snake, spider and insect venoms

- Cocaine
- Amphetamine
- Benzodiazepines
- Phencyclidine
- HMG-CoA reductase inhibitors (statins)
- Fibric acid derivatives (clofibrate, gemfibrozil)
- Hemlock
- Salicylates
- Carbon monoxide
- Ethylene glycol
- Isopropyl alcohol
- Snake and insect venoms
- Succinylcholine
- Colchicine
- Propofol
- Para-phenylenediamine
- Colchicum autumnale (autumn crocus)
- Monensin

214. Answer is E (All of the above): *'Clinical Infectious Disease' by Schlossberg 1st (2008)/492, 493*

Bacterial infections from clostridium species and streptococcus and envenomations from Russel Viper and Hornet may all cause rhabdomyolysis.

Infectious causes of Rhabdomyolysis

Bacterial

Gram-Positive bacteria	Gram-Negative bacteria	Mycobacteria
Streptococcus pneumoniae *Staphylococcus aureus* *Group B streptococcus* *Streptococcus pyogenes* *Listeria spp.* *Staphylococcus epidermidis* *Bacillus spp.* ***Clostridium spp.*** *Viridans streptococci* *Streptococcus suis* *β-hemolytic streptococci* *Streptococcus pyogenes*	*Legionella spp.* *Francesella tularensis* *Salmonella spp.* *Vibrio spp.* *Brucella spp.* *Escherichia coli* *Herbicola lathyri* *Klebsiella spp.* *Aeromonas* *Haemophilus influenza* *Neisseria spp.*	*Intravesical instillation of BCG* *Tuberculosis*

Fungal / Protozoal and Helminthic

Fungal	Protozoal and Helminthic
Candida spp. *Aspergillus spp.* *Mucor spp.*	*Plasmodium spp.* *Toxoplasma gondii* *Trichinosis*

Miscellaneous infections causes

Spirochetes	Rickettsial	Mycoplasma
Leptospira spp. *Borrelia burgdorferi*	*Rickettsia conorii* *Rickettsia tsutsugamushi* *Ehrlichia equi* *Ehrlichia chaffeensis* *Coxiella burnetti* *Anaplasma phagocytophilum*	*Mycoplasma pneumonia*

Poisons

Snakes	Spider and Insects
South American rattlesnake	***Hornets***
Tiger snake	*Wasps*
Majove rattlesnake	*Bees*
Russel viper	*Desert centipdede*
	Redback spider
	Taipan

215. Answer is C (Hyperthyroidism)

Hypothyroidism is a cause for Rhabdomyolysis and not hyperthyroidism

Metabolic causes of Rhabdomyolysis
Hypokalcemia
Hypophosphatemia
Hypothyroidism (Myxoedema)
Diabetic ketoacidosis
Diabetic hyperosmolar non ketotic coma
Hereditary muscle enzyme deficiencies
Carnitine deficiency

216. Answer is C (Hypercalcemia): *Primer on kidney disease 4th/310, 311*

Rhabdomyolysis is associated with hypocalcemia and not hypercalcemia

Hyperphosphatemia promotes the deposition of calcium phosphate in injured muscle thereby contributing to hypocalcemia.

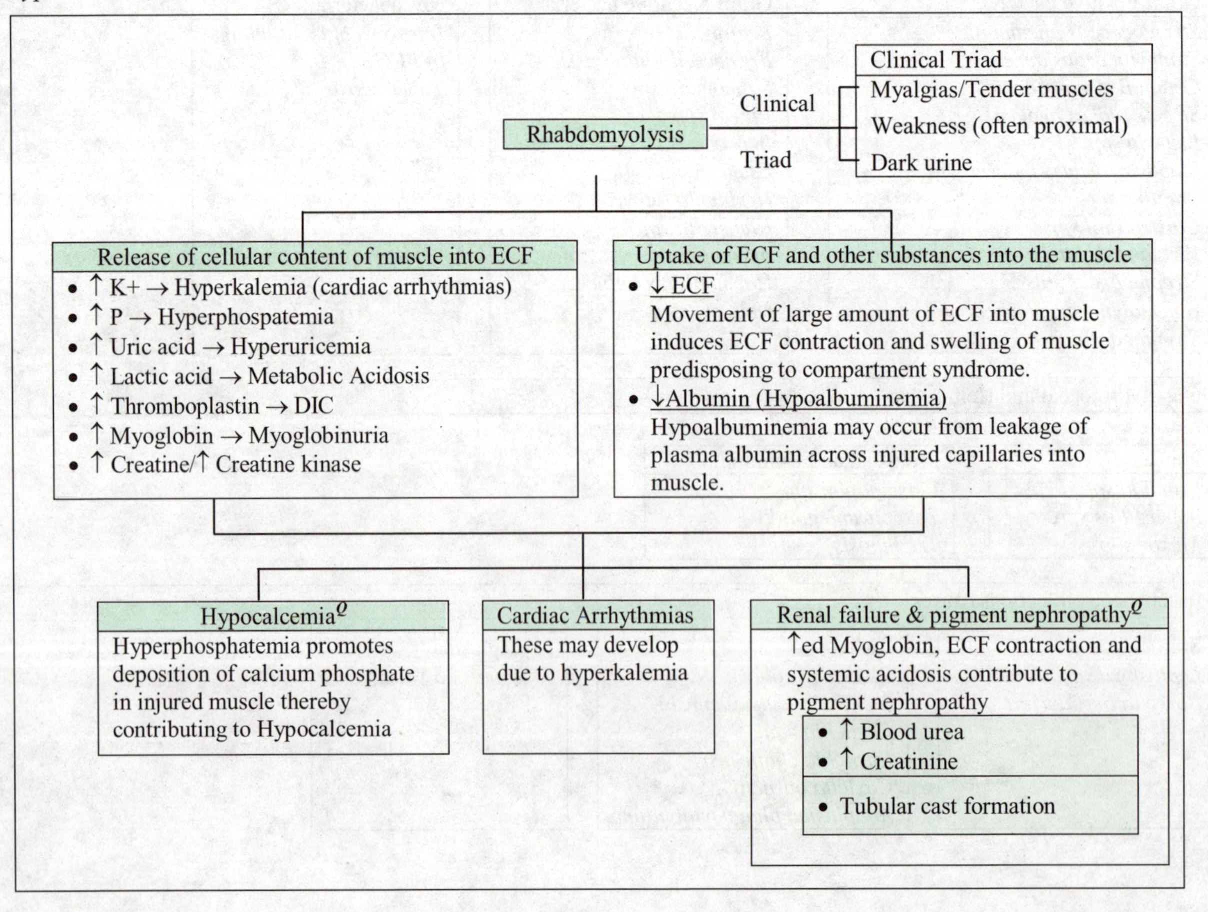

217. Answer is C (Hemoglobinuria): *Refer previous question*

Hemoglobinuria is not a feature of Rhabdomyolysis

Acute muscular weakness is seen in Rhabdomyolysis

'Pain and swelling of the involved muscles and weakness of limbs occur especially in proximal distribution'.

– Current Diagnosis and Treatment in Emergency Medicine 6th/650

'Acute proximal muscle weakness, pain, swelling, tenderness and cramping of affected muscles is the most frequent feature'. – Skeletal Muscle 1st (2002)/8

Myoglobnuria is a feature of Rhabdomyolysis

Rhabdomyolysis leads to leakage of Myoglobin from muscle into the plasma and from plasma into urine causing myoglobinuria. Rhabdomyolysis and Myoglobinuria reflect similar clinical conditions and are often grouped as Rhabdomyolysis – Myoglobinuria syndrome.

Rhabdomyolysis may present with Acute Renal failure

Acute Renal failure is the major potential complication of Rhabdomyolysis.

Miscellaneous

218. Answer is A (Carcinoma of urinary bladder) : *Bailey 23rd/1229*

***"Painless haematuria is by far the most common symptom and should be regarded as indicative of bladder carcinoma unless proven otherwise."** - Bailey*

*The patient in question is **65 years of age and a smoker**, both factors being predisposition to bladder carcinomas and presenting with the most common symptom of **painless haematuria** thus almost deliniating the diagnosis.*

Some facts about Bladder Carcinoma :

- *Most common type of bladder carcinoma : Transitional cell carcinoma*
  Most common type in areas where bilharzia is endemic - Pure Squamous cell
  Most common type arising from urachal remnant - Primary adenocarcinoma.
- Predisposing factors that have been asked :

Naphthylamine / Aniline dyes	Phenacetin exposure
Cigarette smoking	Cyclophosphamide exposure
Bilharzia industries	Tyre, Rubber, cable and Dye

- *Tumors of urothelium i.e. Pelvis, ureter and bladder are most commonly Transitional cell carcinomas.*
  But tumors of urethra are most commonly - squamous cell carcinomas.

219. Answer is C (Urine tumor markers) : *Devita 6th/1397; Harrison 16th/579*

Urine tumor markers are the single best answer of exclusion as these are neither sensitive nor specific enough to replace cystoscopy and cytology.

- *'Individuals older than 40 years of age who develop haematuria , should have a **urine specimen for cytology and undergo cystoscopy and imaging of the urinary tract with an intravenous pyelogram or CT scan.**-Devita/Harrison*

Recommended investigations in individuals greater than 40 years who develop haematuria include: *Devita/H16th*
Urinary cytology[Q] for malignant cells
Cystocopy
Imaging of the urinary tract with Intravenous Pyelogram or CT scan[Q]

- ***Other urine assay' (tumor markers)*** have been used to diagnose disease and follow up patients including flow cytometry, blood group antigens (Lewis x), cytokeratins, nuclear matrix proteins, Fibrin degradation products and telomerose. ***None is sensitive or specific enough to replace cystoscopy and urine cytology.*** *- Devita*

220. Answer is D (Urine microscopy for malignant cytology): *Bailey & Love 24th/1463; Harrison 16th/539; Devita 6th/ 1397*

Urine microscopy for malgnant cytology is the single best investigation amongst the options provided

- Painless Gross Haematuria in a 60 year old smoker requires investigation to exclude carcinoma of the bladder.

Recommended investigations in individuals greater than 40 years who develop haematuria include: *Devita/H16th*
• ***Urinary cytology***[Q] for malignant cells • ***Cystocopy*** • ***Imaging of the urinary tract with Intravenous Pyelogram or CT scan***[Q]

Amongst these recommended diagnostic procedures only 'urinary cytology for malignant cell's has been provided amongst the options and hence is the single best answer of choice.

- **USG is not a recommended investigation for eliciting bladder tumours**

USG by external, transrectal or transurethral route may define moderate size masses but it will not distinguish benign masses from solid masses. Also, it is unlikely to pick up small bladder tumours. *It has not been recommended as a first line investigation for eliciting bladder tumours.*

- **Routine Urine Microscopy and Plain X-Ray KUB will not give desired / sufficient information.**

221. Answer is B (Renal Parenchymal Disease): *Giai 7th/432; Nelson's 18th/1988; Manual of Endocrinology and Metabolism 4th/208; Hypertension Secrets (2002)/66; CPPT 19th/665*

Renal Parenchymal Disease is the most common cause of hypertension in children and should be considered in the evaluation of all asymptomatic children with hypertension

Essential hypertension *is uncommon in children and accounts for only 5-10% of cases.* A diagnosis of essential hypertension in children should be considered only after excluding other secondary causes especially renal parenchymal disease. Absence of significant history and a normal urine examination does not exclude renal parenchymal as the cause

Coarctation of Aorta *may present with hypertension in children but this is an uncommon cause* and usually presents with a charachteristic finging of blood pressure differential of > 10 mm Hg between upper and lower extremities, systolic hypertension in upper extremity along with decreased or absent femoral pulses

Polycystic kidney Disease *does not usually present with hypertension in children.* Hypertension usually becomes clinically apparent in middle age and hence the condition is also called 'Adult' polycystic kidney disease.

222. Answer is B (Pyeloplasty): *Nelson's 18th/2237; 'Ultrasound of the Urogenital system' by Baxter & Sidhu 1st/92, 93; Essentials of Pediatric Urology 2nd/83, 84, 85, 86, 87; Campbell's Urology 8th/468; Textbook of Reconstructive Urological Surgery (2008) 1st/Chapter 16*

The child in question is presenting with charachteristic feature of PUJ obstruction. He is a candidate for surgical management as differential function is only 19%. Open pyeloplasty (Anderson- Hynes dismembered pyeloplasty) is universally regarded as the gold standard operation of choice.

Ureteropelvic Junction Obstruction (UPJ Obstruction)
• UPJ obstruction is the *most common obstructive lesion in childhood*[Q] and is the *most common cause of hydronephrosis found on prenatal and early postnatal ultrasonography*[Q]. • It is most commonly caused by intrinsic stenosis of a segment of ureter which is usually localized to the region of pelviureteric junction. Other causes include ureteric folds & extrinsic obstruction by crossing lower pole vessels.
Presentation
• ***Hydronephrosis*** revealed by maternal USG ***(Dilated renal pelvis but normal ureter)*** • Palpable Renal Mass in new borns or infants • ***Abdominal flank or Back pain typically*** exacerbated by drinking large volumes of liquid • UTI / Haematuria after minimal trauma
Epidemiology
• Left side more commonly involved than right (Bilateral = 10%) • Male more commonly involved than females (M:F= 2:1)
Initial Diagnosis by Ultrasonography
• ***Hydronephrosis with dilated renal pelvis*** • Ureter if visualized is of normal caliber (not delated)

Renal Differential function

Nuclear Renography is used to determine Renal Differential function

- ***A differential function of <40% is considered significant and often an indication for surgical management***
- *Differential function of < 10% is often considered an arbitrary cut off for nephrectomy*

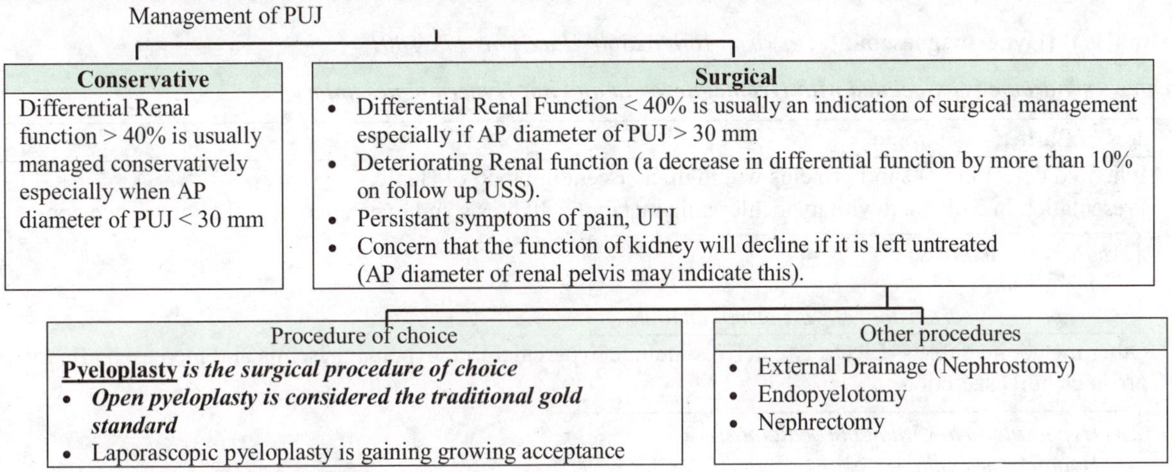

Management of PUJ

Conservative	Surgical
Differential Renal function > 40% is usually managed conservatively especially when AP diameter of PUJ < 30 mm	• Differential Renal Function < 40% is usually an indication of surgical management especially if AP diameter of PUJ > 30 mm • Deteriorating Renal function (a decrease in differential function by more than 10% on follow up USS). • Persistant symptoms of pain, UTI • Concern that the function of kidney will decline if it is left untreated (AP diameter of renal pelvis may indicate this).

Procedure of choice	Other procedures
<u>Pyeloplasty</u> ***is the surgical procedure of choice*** • ***Open pyeloplasty is considered the traditional gold standard*** • Laporascopic pyeloplasty is gaining growing acceptance	• External Drainage (Nephrostomy) • Endopyelotomy • Nephrectomy

External Drainage (Nephrostomy)

This is used to provide temporary drainage particularly when children present with pyonephrosis or ***when differential renal function is <10-15%*** to assess potential recovery of function before considering definitive surgery.

Endopyelotomy

Endopyelotomy involves incising the UPJ junction by either a retrograde or antegrade route, by a minimally invasive approach. ***The success rate is inferior to open pyeloplasty. A large hydronephrosis and differential renal function <20% are considered relative contraindications for Endopyelotomy.***

Nephrectomy

Nephrectomy may be considered when renal differential function is very low and the likelihood of functionl recovery is minimal. ***Most pediatric urologists consider an arbitrary cut off for differential function in the range of 10-15%.*** However a reconstructive procedure (pyeloplasty) should always be considered as the procedure of choice to salvage the kidney.

223. Answer is A (Diabetes mellitus): *Harrisons 15th/1590 Fundamentals of diagnostic Radiology 3rd/885*

Diabetes Mellitus is not associated with contracted (small) kidneys.

The kidneys are typically normal or increased in size in diabetic nephropathy – Harrisons

Causes of Contracted Kidneys

- *Chronic Glomerulonephritis (Bilateral)*
- *Nephrosclerosis because of systemic hypertension (Bilateral)*
- *Chronic pyelonephritis (Usually unilateral)*
- *Global renal infarction (Unilateral)*
- *Radiation nephritis (Unilateral)*
- *Renal artery stenosis (Unilateral)*
- *Post obstructive atrophy (Unilateral)*

Note that Acute Glomerulonephritis, and acute pyelonephritis are associated with enlarged kidneys but chronic cases are associated with contracted kidneys

224. Answer is C (Diabetes Mellitus): *Refer Previous questions*

The kidneys are typically normal or increased in size in diabetic nephropathy *- Harrison 14th / 1546, 15th/1590*

Most forms of chronic renal insufficiencies lead to shrinkage or decrease in size of the kidney.

<u>Notable exceptions, wherein kidney size is usually normal or increases include</u> :

1. Diabetic nephropathy Q
2. Amyloidosis Q
3. Polycystic kidney disease Q

Kidney is contracted/shrunken in the remaining three conditions
- Benign nephrosclerosis Q
- Chronic pyelonephritis Q
- Chronic glomerulonephritis Q

225. Answer is B (Hypermagnesemia): *Harrison 18th/p2360 Harrisons 17th/1801*

Bartter's syndrome is associated with Hyomagnesemia and not Hypermagnesemia.

Features of Bartter's syndrome

- Inherited defect in transport proteins within thick ascending loop of Henle.
- Presentation in childhood with hypochloremic metabolic alkalosis and hypokalemia without hypertension

*Metabolic Alkalosis*Q
*Hypokalemia*Q
*Absence of Hypertension: BP is normal or low*Q

- Other metabolic defects /Electrolyte defects include hypercalciuria, hypomagnesemia and increased urinary prostaglandiN secretion

- *Hypercalciuria with nephrocalcinosis*
- *Hypomagnesemia*
- *↑ urinary PGE2*

- Clinical presentation includes polyuria, polydypsia, salt craving and growth retardation or failure to thrive.

- *Polyurea, polydipsia, salt craving*
  (Fetal polyurea in antenatal period may cause polyhydramnios and premature labor)
- *Growth retardation or failure to thrive*
- *Fever, vomiting & diarrhea may occur due to PGE2 over production*

- Patients who survive early childhood may develop chronic renal failure

CRF is a known complication

226. Answer is D (Hepatitis) : *Critical care Medicine 3rd/236 Rudolph Pediatrics 21st/1711*

Chronic Active Hepatitis is a cause for distal type I Renal tubular acidosis which is associated with increased urinary loss of potassium

"A high urinary K+ excretion with systemic acidosis is a charachteristic feature of renal tubular acidosis. Chronic Active Hepatitis is an established cause for distal renal tubular acidosis and may hence be associated with urinary K^+ excretion.

227. Answer is C (Glomerulonephritis): *KDT 5th/717*

Nephrotoxicity due to Amphoterecin B does not manifest as Glomerulonephritis.

Renal adverse effects of Amphotericin B :

Nephrotoxicity is the most important long term toxicity of Amphotericin B - KDT

Manifestations of Nephrotoxicity of Amphotericin B are :
- ***Azotemia***
- ***Reduced G.F.R***
- ***Acidosis (RTA)***
- ***Hypokalemia***
- ***Inability to concentrate*** *urine*

Nephrotoxity reverses slowly though often incompletely after stoppage of therapy.

228. Answer is C (FK 506): *NICE Guidelines 'Immunosuppression therapy for renal transplantation in adults' (www.nice.org.uk/pdf/TA085 guidance.pdf) ; KDT 5th/790*

The most common regimens include triple therapy with cyclosporine, azathioprine and prednisolone.

Immunosuppression has customarily constituted triple therapy with : (NICE Guidelines)

1. *A calcineurin inhibitor (cyclosporin);*
2. *An antiproliferative agent (azathioprine); and*
3. *A corticosteroid (prednisolone)*

However, a small number of treatment centers use a policy of initial monotherapy with a calcineurin inhibitor, adding in other agents if necessary.

Immunosuppressive therapy for renal transplantation in adults

Induction therapy

- Is a course of intensive immunosuppressive for about 2 weeks immediately post operatively (though often started immediately pre-operatively) with the aim of 'switching off' the immune system after transplantation to reduce the likelihood of accelerated rejection and acute rejection.
- It has also been used as a means of reducing exposure to calcineurin inhibitors in the early stages after transplantation when the graft may be particularly vulnerable to their nephrotoxic effects.
- The term induction therapy has usually been linked with the use of the following agents:
  - The polyclonal antibodies antithymocyte immunoglobulin (ATG)
  - The antilymphocyte immunoglobulin (ALG), and
  - The monoclonal antibody muromonab-CD3 (OKT3)

Initial therapy

- Is the treatment given to all recipients (except where the donor is an identical twin) for 0-3 months after transplantation.
- Initial therapy is usually 'triple therapy', in which a clacineurin inhibitor (traditionally cyclosporine) is used as the 'primary agent' in combination with a corticosteroid (prednisolone) and azathioprine.
- Occasionally, dual therapy (cyclosporine plus costicositeroid) is used.

Maintenance therapy

- Is the treatment that patients receive long-term, throughout the duration of allograft survival
- Maintenance therapy is often identical to initial therapy (triple therapy) but at a reduced dosage because the transplanted kidney becomes immunologically more stable with increasing time.
- However, agents used in maintenance therapy may be altered in response to
  - Development of acute rejection, severe infections or toxicity.
  - Poor tolerability leading to non-adherence

NOTES

Gastrointestinal System

ESSENTIAL REVISION NOTES

Esophageal Conditions

Dysphagia (General / Differential Diagnosis):

Esophageal Dysphagia

Progressive	Intermittent
• *Achalasia* • *Progressive systemic sclerosis* • *Peptic stricture* • *Carcinoma*	• *Lower esophageal ring/Shatzki ring* • *Diffuse esophageal spasm* • *Zenker's diverticulum*

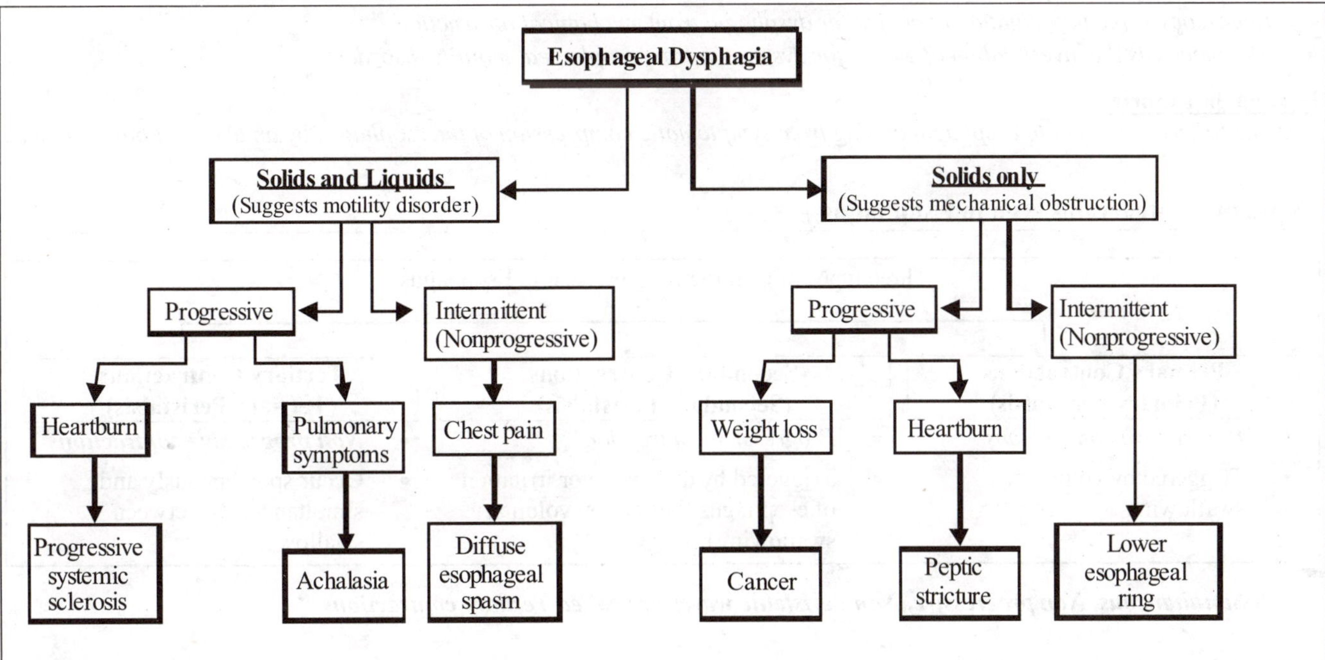

- **Achlasia Cardia** is associated with *Progressive dysphagia* to *both solids and liquids*
  Rat-tail esophagus with a dilated proximal esophagus and narrow lower end suggests a diagnosis of Achlasia cardia. (Dhingra 4th/305)
- **Esophageal carcinomas** are associated with *progressive dysphagia*. Dysphagia is *initially only for solids* at presentation (may prgress to cause dysphagia to liquids also)
  Narrow and irregular esophageal lumen suggests a diagnosis of esophageal carcinoma (Dhingra 4th/306)
- **GERD** is associated with *progressive dysphagia* to *solids alone* at presentation.
  Stricture or ulcer in the esophagus suggests a diagnosis of Gastrophageal Reflux disease (GERD)
- **Diffuse esophageal spasm** is associated with non-progressive dysphagia to both solids and liquids.
  The charachteristic barium swallow findings in diffuse esophageal spasm is the corkscrew esophagus (appearance of curling or multiple ripples in the wall, sacculations and pseudodiverticula)
- **Lower esophageal rings (Schatzki's ring**) *is associated with Non- progressive (episodic) dysphagia only for solids. The ring is apparent as a constriction in the lower esophagus on barium swallow.*

Investigations for Esophageal Dysphagia

Esophageal Dysphagia

Initial investigation should be Barium swallow[Q]

Dysphagia for both liquids & solids

Suggests esophageal motility disorder
- *Achalasia*
- *Diffuse Esophageal spasm*

↓

Investigation of choice is Manometry

Dysphagia for solids alone

Suggests mechanical obstruction
- *Carcinoma*
- *Stricture*
- *Web*

↓

Investigation of choice is endoscopy

- *Barium swallow is the recommended initial investigation for a case of Esophageal Dysphagia*
  'In evaluating a patient with dysphagia, a barium swallow should be the first test performed'-Current Otorhinology 2nd/488
- *Endoscopy is the investigation of choice for dysphagia from mechanical obstruction*
- *Manometry is the investigation of choice for dysphagia from esophageal motility disorders*

Dysphagia Lusoria

Dysphagia Lusoria refers to dysphagia arising from symptomatic compression of the esophagus by an aberrant blood vessel.

Types of Contractions seen in Esophagus

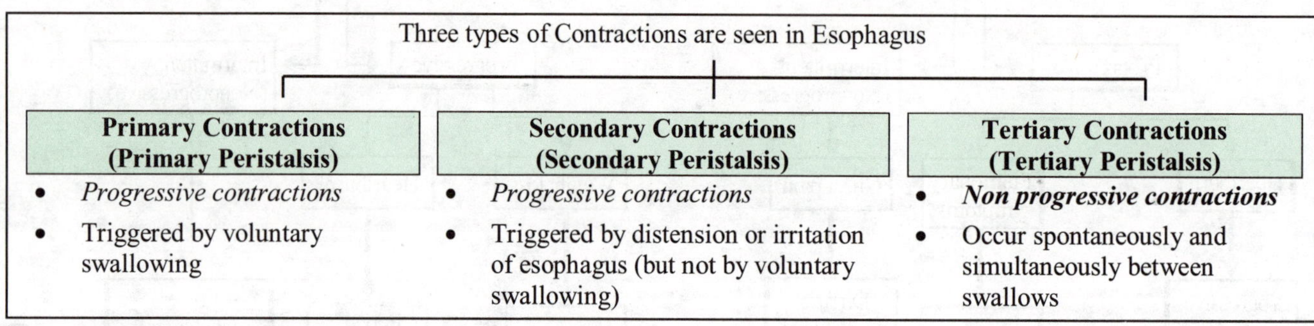

Simultaneous, Non progressive, Non Peristaltic waves are called Tertiary contractions

Achalasia Cardia

Achalasia Cardia (Primary esophageal motility disorder)

Physiological Characteristic

- Absence of esophageal peristalsis
- Increased pressure of LES
- Failure of LES to relax in response to swallowing

Pathogenesis

- True etiology unknown
- Degeneration of Myenteric plexus of Aurerbach's with loss of postganglionic inhibitory neurons is noted (These neurons contain NO and VIP which mediate LEs relaxation)
- Sparing of postganglionic cholinergic fibres (Increased Les resting pressure and insufficient relaxation)

Presentation

- Dysphagia is the most common symptom
  Dysphagia is present for both solids and liquids and is progressive
- Regurgitation is the second most common symptom
- Chest pain may also occur

Investigations

- *Esophageal Manometry is the key test in establishing the diagnosis*

Physiological /Manometric features of Achalasia
•*Elevated Resting pressure of LES (>45 mmHg)*[Q] •*Incomplete LES relaxation (in response to swallowing)* [Q] •*Absence of distal esophageal peristalsis* [Q]

- *Barium swallow should be the initial test performed*

Diagnosis suggested by:
•*Dilated sigmoid oesophagus* •*Persistant beak like narrowing of distal oesophagus*

Complications

- *Achalasia is a risk factor for Esophageal carcinomaQ*
- Achalasia predisposes to squamous cell carcinoma[Q]

Treatment

Surgical Treatment

- *Laparoscopic Heller's myotomy*[Q] *and partial fundoplication is the procedure of choice*
  Esophagectomy is not used in the treatment

Non surgical treatment includes medications that reduces LES pressure

- Intrasphinteric injection of botulinum toxin and/or
- Pneumatic dilatation

Diffuse Esophageal Spasm

Diffuse Esophageal spasm (Corkscrew esophagus)

Diffuse Esophageal spasm is a poorly understood hypermotility disorder of the oesophagus

Presentation

- The clinical presentation is typically that of *Chest pain and Dysphagia*
- ***'The most common symptom is intermittent chest pain***[Q] (>dysphagia)
- Chest pain mimics angina or pain of coronary artery disease
  - *Squeezing pressure in the chest that may radiate to the Jaw, arms or upper back*
  - *Symptoms are aggravated by emotional stress, exertion (or related to eating)*

Chest pain[Q]
Dysphagia[Q]

Diagnosis

Manometry is the key to establish the diagnosis

The diagnosis is usually made by an esophagogram (Barium swallow) and monometric study

Ambulatory pH monitoring should be performed to rule out abnormal reflux

Esophagogram (Barium Swallow)

- *Corkscrew esophagus*[Q] is *classical of Diffuse esophageal* spasm (seen in about 30% of cases)

(Radiological evidence of tertiary contractions)

Manometry

- ***Manometry is the key to establish the diagnosis (CSDT)***
  Correlation of subjective complains with evidence of spasm (induced by vagomimetic drug bethenechol) on manometric studies prvide convincing evidence- Sabiston
- *Esophageal monometry is the only test that distinguishes diffuse esophageal spasm from other primary esophageal motor disorders* - CSDT
- *An ambulatory motility record (ambulatory manometry) is preferred over standard manometry* as contractions are intermittent and normal peristalsis is seen in between. *Ambulatory manometry is the single best investigation with a sensitivity of 90% and specificity of 100%*

Ambulatory 24 hour pH monitoring

Gastro esophageal reflux disease may mimic diffuse esophageals spasm Ambulatory pH monitoring must be performed to rule out abnormal reflux which is the most common cause of non cardiac chest pain

***Diffuse esophageal spasm is synonymous with 'corkscrew esophagus' or Rosary esophagus* - Bailey**

In diffuse esophageal spasm, barium swallow shows that normal sequential peristalsis below the aortic arch is replaced by uncoordinated simultaneous contractions that produce the appearance of curling or multiple ripples in the wall, sacculations, and pseudodiverticula- the "corkscrew" esophagus.

Zenker's Diverticulum

What it is :

It is a *pulsion diverticulum*[Q], where pharyngeal *mucosa*[Q] herniates *through the Killihan's dehiscence*[Q] (a weak area *between two parts of Inferior Constrictor*[Q]). **(Zenker's Diverticulum occurs in the pharynx and not in the esophagus)**

- Zenker's diverticulum originates from the posterior wall of the pharynx through the killian's dehiscence
- Killian's dehiscence is a weak area between
  - Oblique fibres of the Thyropharyngeus (part of inferior constrictor muscle) superiorly
  - Transverse fibres of the cricopharyngeus (part of the inferior constrictor muscle) inferiorly
- Herniation *starts in the midline posteriorly*, however as the out pouching enlarges, it localizes to one side of the oesophagus most commonly on the left side.

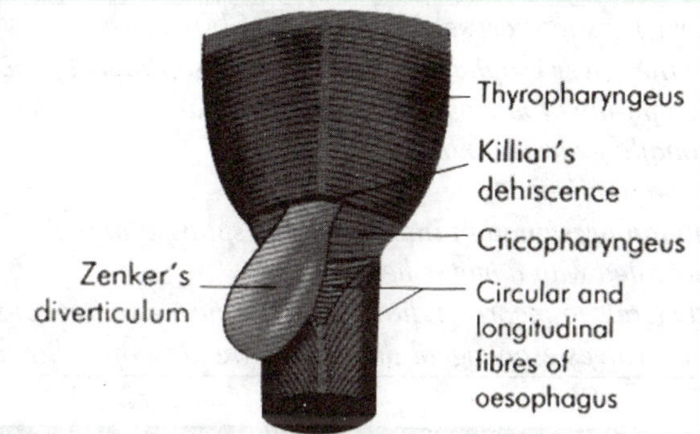

Hypopharyngeal (Zenker's) diverticulum.

Hypopharyngeal mucosa herniates through the Killian's dehiscence a weak area between two parts of inferior constrictor

- **Zenker's diverticulum is an acquired diverticulum and not a congenital diverticulum**
  These are acquired pulsion diverticulae that usually occur in people older than 60 years as their pharyngeal muscle tone and elasticity decreases.
- **Zenker's diverticulae are false diverticulae**
  Zenker's diverticulum *is a false diverticulum* because it does not contain all the anatomic layers of the esophageal wall
  Zenker's diverticulum involves protrusion of *only the mucosa (and submucosa)* through the posterior muscle layers

Age of presentation

This condition is usually seen after 60 years of age (*elderly*) [Q]

Symptomatology / presentation

- ***Dysphagia***[Q] : As mouth of the sac is wider than the opening of esophagus, food preferentially enter the sac. When the pouch gets filled with food, it presses on the esophagus & produces ***Dysphagia***. [Q]
- ***Gurgling Sound***[Q] is produced during swallowing.
- ***Halitosis*** or foul smell is frequently associated
- ***Cough & Aspiration pneumonia***[Q] : food eaten *over the last few days*[Q] may regurgitate as it collects in the pouch causing cough and aspiration pneumonia.
- ***Malnutrition***[Q] : Patient is often malnourished due to dysphagia.

The most frequent complications of Zenker diverticulum is 'aspiration' into the tracheobronchial tree which can in turn present with pneumonia and Lung Abscess.

Investigations

- Barium swallow is the diagnostic procedure of choice for Zenker's diverticulum
  Zenker's diverticulum are often identified by Lateral x-rays on Barium swallow

Treatment

- *Simple Excision of pouch*
- *Excision of pouch and cricopharyngeal myotomy* [Q]
- *Dahlman's procedure*[Q] : Done in poor-risk debilitated patients. The partition wall between esophagus and pouch is divided by diathermy.

Oesophageal Ring

Schatzki ring is a mucosal / submucosal ring at the squamo-columnar junction of distal esophagus that may present with intermittent dysphagia.

Schatzki Ring (Oesophageal Ring)

- *It is a characteristic short segment of luminal stenosis*
- ***Occurs in the lower esophageal at the gastroesophageal junction (squamo-columnar junction)***
- ***It is made up only of mucosa and submucosa and narrows the lumen only to a few millimeters.***
- *True aetiopathogenesis is not known*
- *Usually asymptomatic*
- ***Most common presentation intermittent dysphagia only for solids.***
- *Often associated with a hiatus hernia.*
- *Frequently leads to incorrect diagnosis of diffuse esophageal spasm*
- *Treatment involves esophageal dilatation or endoscopic diathermy/laser.*

Oesophageal Web (In association with Plummer Vinson Syndrome)

Plummer Vinson syndrome refers to the combination of hypopharyngeal webs and iron deficiency ***anemia in middle aged women***

Plummer Vinson Syndrome (Patterson Kelly)

- ***Upper esophageal web***
- *Iron deficiency anemia*
- *Koilonychia*
- *Glossitis and angular stomatitis*

Mallory Weiss Syndrome:

Mallory-Weiss Syndrome is associated with a tear of the gastric mucosa near the squamocolumnar mucosal junction

Mucosal Tear (Mallory-Weiss Syndrome)

- The tear usually involves the gastric mucosa near the squamocolumnar mucosal junction near cardia
- This tear is usually caused by vomiting, retching, or vigorous coughing.
- The tear is usually linear.
- Patients present with upper gastrointestinal bleeding ***(Hemetemesis)***
- Association with alcoholism and hiatus hernia
- In most patients, bleeding ceases spontaneously
  (Continued bleeding may respond to vasopressin therapy or angiographic embolization. Surgery is rarely needed)

Barret's Esophagus

Barret's Esophagus

- *Barret's esophagus is a metaplasia of the esophageal mucosa caused by replacement of squamous epithelium with columnar epithelium.*
  Specialized intestinal epithelium (intestinal metaplasia) is the most common and most important type of columnar epithelium seen in Barret's esophagus.

Barret's esophagus (columnar metaplasia)

Metaplasia of squamous epithelium into columnar epithelium

↓

Three types of Columnar Epithelium may be seen

Gastric Type	Junctional Type	Intestinal Type
Morphologically indistinguishable from normal gastric epethelia	*Morphologically indistinguishable from normal gastric epethelia*	*Morphologically distinct and readily distinguishable from gastric epethelia* • This is the most common type • Most commonly associated with dysplasia & carcinoma

- *Metaplasia characteristically affects the distal (lower) oesophagus*[Q]
- *It is consequence of severe reflex esophagitis*[Q]

Epidemiology

- *More common in men*[Q] *(Males > Females)*
- *More common in whites*[Q] *(Whites > Blacks)*
- *More common with increasing age*[Q] *(incidence increases with age)*

Complications

- *Peptic Ulcer (Barret's Ulcer: Chronic Peptic Ulceration in the columnar lined mucosa)*
- *Strictures (Can lead to high (midoesophageal) and long strictures)*
- ***Considered a premalignant condition***[Q]
  Type of cancer associated in an adenocarcinoma[Q]*(Dysplagia – cancer sequence)*
  Columnar metaplasia that carries maximum risk of adenocarcinoma is intestinal metaplasia (intestinal epithelium) [Q]

Diagnosis

- **Diagnosis can be suggested by Endoscopy**
  Endoscopy shows a 'salmon pink' epithelium above the gastroesophageal junction which replaces the whitish squamous epithelium.

- **Diagnosis is confirmed by biopsy**
  Diagnosis is confirmed by pathological examination and requires the identification of columnar (intestinal) type epithelium characterized by the presence of goblet cells.

Treatment

- *Barret's metaplasia once established does not regress with conservative management*
- *Although medical treatment does not regress the metaplastic changes, it is still advocated to prevent continued insult*

Esophageal Carcinoma

Histological Variants of Esophageal Carcinoma

- ***By far the most common esophageal cancer world wide is squamous cell carcinoma*** *(Prevalence)*
- *Most prevalent esophageal cancer world-wide (old + new cases) is squamous cell ca*
- *Most common esophageal cancer world-wide (new cases) is Adenocarcinoma*
- ***Most common esophageal cancer in India is Squamous cell Carcinoma***

Site of Esophageal Carcinoma

- ***The lower third of the esophagus is the most common site of esophageal cancer and accounts for about 50% of all esophageal cancers.***

Site of esophageal cancer (All histological types)	% of total
Upper 1/3rd	15%
Middle 1/3rd	35%
Lower 1/3rd	***50%***

- ***Most common site of Esophageal carcinoma in India is middle one third of the esophagus***
  Eighty to ninety percent of esophageal cancers in India are squamous cell carcinomas, and the most common site is middle 1/3rd of esophagus

Site of Esophageal Carcinoma based on histological type

- ***The most common site of squamous cell (histological subtype) is middle 1/3 of esophagusQ***
- ***The most common site of adenocarcinoma (histological subtype) is lower 1/3rd of esophagusQ.***
  Esophageal Adenocarcinoma invariably arises from Barret's esophagus (Barret's ulcer) which is characteristically located in the distal esophagus around the gastroesophageal junction

Epidemiology

- ***Men > Women (≈ 4 : 1) (More common in Men)***
- ***Predominantly*** *affects older age group (> 50 years)*

Predisposing factors for carcinoma esophagus :

1. ***Alcohol consumption*** Q
2. ***Smoking cigarettes*** Q
3. **Ingested Carcinogens**
   - *Nitrates* Q
   - Smoked opiates
   - Fungal toxins in pickled vegetables
4. **Mucosal damage**
   - ***Chronic Achalasia*** Q
   - Lye ingestion / Hot tea
   - Radiation induced strictures Q
5. **Host Susceptibility**
   1. *Patterson Kelley syndrome* Q *or* ***Plummer Vinson syndrome*** Q
      Esophageal web Q *+ Glossitis* Q *+ Iron deficiency* Q
   2. ***Tylosis palmaris et plantaris*** Q *: Congenital hyperkeratosis* Q *and pitting of palms and soles* Q
6. *Chronic Gastric Reflux, ie. Barrett's esophagus for Adenocarcinoma* Q

Risk factors for Esophageal Adenocarcinoma

- ***Barrets esophagus***
- *Gastroesophageal Reflux Disease (GERD)*
- ***Scleroderma***
- *Smoking*
- *Alcohol*
- *History of colon cancer*
- *Medications : Long term use (> 5 years) of Theophylline & β agonists.*

Presentation

Dysphagia is the most common symptom

Esophageal carcinomas are associated with *progressive dysphagia*. Dysphagia is *initially only for solids* at presentation (may prgress to cause dysphagia to liquids also)

Investigation

Investigation of choice is Endoscopy

Treatment

- ***Chemotherapy for esophageal cancer has improved considerably with the advent of regimens containing Cisplatin.*** *The best responses are seen in Squamous cell carcinomas*
- ***Surgical Treatment*** *involves complete Esophagectomy*
  Stomach appears to be the 'conduit' of choice *after partial or complete Esophagectomy because of ease in mobilization and its ample vascular supply*

Stomach and Duodenum

Peptic Ulcer Disease & H. Pylori Infection

Aetiological Factors in peptic ulceration:

Aetiological Factors in peptic ulceration

Primary Aetiologcial Factors (selected)	Associated Factors / Conditions (selected)
• *H. pylori infection* • *NSAID's and other drugs eg. steroids* • *Stress – Head injury / Burns* • *Bile Reflux* • *Smoking / Alcohol use* • *Genetic Factors*	• *Endocrinal Disorders* - *MEN* - ***Primary Hyperparathyroidism*** - ***Zollinger Ellison Syndrome***[Q] - *Cushing's syndrome* • ***Cirrhosis***[Q] • *Chronic Renal Failure* • *Chronic Pulmonary Disease* • *Chronic Paracreatic Disease* • *Alpha 1 Antitrypsin deficiency*

Aetiological factors in Gastric Ulcers vs Duodenal Ulcers:

Causal factor	Gastric ulcer	Duodenal ulcer
Hellicobacter pylori	Important	Very important
NSAIDs and aspirin	Important	Important
Acid	***Normal or low acid output***	***High or normal acid output***
Bile reflux	Important	Unimportant
Smoking	Important	Important
Stress	Evidence for head injuries and burns only	
Family history	Uncommon	Common

Gastric ulcers are associated with normal or decreased gastric acid output. High Acid output is a feature of Duodenal Ulcers.

H.pylori Infection

- H. Pylori is a gram negative, spiral, flagellated bacillus
- H. Pylori *infection is more prevalent in developing countries.*
  The prevalence of H. pylori is approx. 30% in U.S. and other developed countries as against > 80% in most developing countries. The chances of reinfection are also high in developing countries
- H. Pylori eradication decreases the likelihood of occurrence of complications and recurrence

Diseases associated with H. Pylori infection:

Diseases associated with H. Pylori infection
1. Duodenal ulcer
2. Gastric ulcer
3. Chronic superficial gastritis
4. Chronic atrophic gastritis
5. Gastric adenocarcinoma
6. Lymphoproliferative disease (MALT)
7. Gastroesophageal reflux disease

MALT stands for Mucosa Associated Lymphoid Tissue Lymphoma

Gastritis associated with H. Pylori Infection:

Gastritis due to H. pylori infection is predominantly antral

Antral gastritis is associated with DU formation.

Gastritis involving the corpus is also seen

This predisposes to development of gastric ulcer, gastric atrophy and ultimately gastric carcinoma.

Antral predominant gastritis	*Corpus Predominant atrophic gastritis*	*Non atrophic pangastritis (chronic superficial gastritis)*
Duodenal ulcer	Gastric ulcer Gastric adenocarcinoma	MALT Lymphoma

Diagnostic tests used for H pylori:

Invasive	Non invasive
1. Endoscopy based Biopsy Urease test	***1. Urea breath tests :***
• Here specimen from antral biopsy are tested for "Urease". • It is the most convenient endoscopy based test. • It is *quick*[Q] and *simple*[Q] however it is neither fully sensitive nor fully specific	• Here patient drinks a labelled urea solution and blows into a tube. • If H. Pylori urease is present, the urea is hydrolysed and labelled carbondioxide is detected in breath samples. • It is thus a simple, safe test and cheaper than endoscopy
2. Histology :	***2. Serological :***
Here the biopsy specimen is subjected to histological examination. It is *accurate*[Q], but time consuming	• Here specific IgG levels in serum are assessed. • Does not differentiate between active and remote infection. • Nevertheless it is particularly suited as an *epidemiological tool*
3. Culture :	***3. Stool antigen test :***
• Here the biopsy specimen is put in a culture medium. • This is accurate [Q], and permits determination of antibiotic susceptiblities, but is also time consuming.	• New test appears less accurate than urea breath test • Useful for follow up after treatment

Diagnostic Tests for Helicobacter pylori *– Harrison*

Test	Sensitivity	Comments
Serology	95	Does not differentiate between active and remote infection; **epidemiologic tool**; titer decreases slowly after eradication
Urease assay		
Breath	90-95	Simple ; may be used to monitor therapy
Biopsy	90-98	Requires endoscopy
Histology		Requires endoscopy; may be essential if antibiotic resistance emerges
Culture	70-95	Requires endoscopy'; may be essential if antibiotic resistance emerges

ELISA (An enzyme linked immuno-sorbant assay) is the most commonly used serological method.
ELISA has proved to be sensitive and specific and is ***particularly suited for Epidemiological studies***

Urease breath test (Non Invasive Test) is the test of choice for documenting eradication is.

Urease breath test detects H. pylori infection by 'bacterial urease activity' and remains positive till the bacteria have not been eradicated with treatment. ***Thus urease breath test becomes negative only after eradication of organism following treatment and not with chronic infection.***

Assessing success of Treatment / Eradicatiion of H. Pyrlori :

- Assessment should be done atleast 4 weeks after completin of anti H. Pylori therapy.
- In the assessment of treatment success non-invasive tests are normally preferred. – Harrison

Assessment of success of treatment

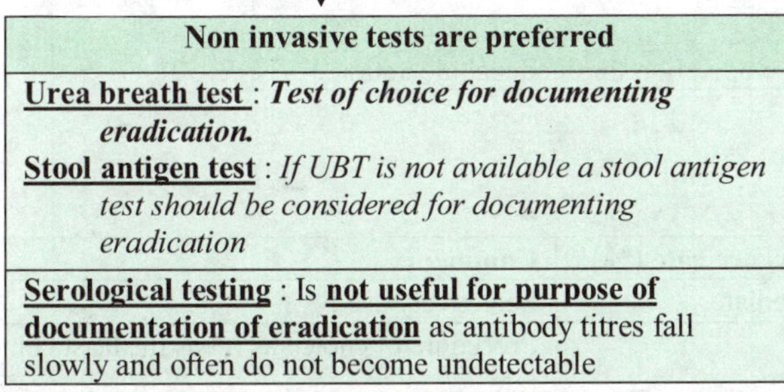

Non invasive tests are preferred

Urea breath test : ***Test of choice for documenting eradication.***

Stool antigen test : *If UBT is not available a stool antigen test should be considered for documenting eradication*

Serological testing : Is **not useful for purpose of documentation of eradication** as antibody titres fall slowly and often do not become undetectable

Inasive tests are not preferred

Biopsy based tests
(Biopsy Urease test, Histology / Culture) *are invasive tests based on Endoscopic biopsy.*

These may be used to document eradication but are not preferred for this purpose.

Treatment of H.Pylori Infection

Indications of Treatment :
H-Pylori related duodenal and gastric ulceration
Low grade B cell MALT Lymphoma

H.pylori should be eradicated.

Recommended Regimens for Eradication of H.Pylori

Recommended Regimens for Eradication of H. Pylori *(Harrison)*

TRIPLE THERAPY

1. Bismuth subsalicylate plus Metronidazole plus Tetracycline
2. Ranitidine bismuth citrate plus Tetracycline plus Clarithromycin or Metronidazole
3. PPI plus Clarithromycin plus Metronidazole or Amoxicillin

QUADRUPLE THERAPY

PPI plus Bismuth subsalicylate plus Metronidazole plus Tetracycline

*All PP1 (*Omeprazole (20mg), Lansaprazole (30mg) *Rabeprazole (20 mg), Pantaprazole (40 mg),) are given twice daily except Esmeprazole (40 mg once daily)*

The most successful are the Triple and Quadruple multi-drug regimens:

Name	Drug 1	Drug 2	Drug 3	Drug 4
OCA	Omeprazole (20 mg BD)	Clarithromycin (500 mg BD)	Amoxicillin (1g BD)	
OCM	Omeprazole (20 mg BD)	Clarithromycin (500 mg BD)	Metronidazole (500 mg BD)	
OBTM	Omeprazole (20 mg BD)	Bismuth Subsalicylate (2 tabs QID)	Tetracycline (500 mg QID)	Metronidazole

Peptic Ulcers: Gastric Ulcers and Duodenal Ulcers

- ***The most common site for peptic ulceration is the First part of duodenum***

Sites in order of decreasing frequency :
1. Duodenum, 1st portion Q *2. Stomach, usually antrum* Q *3. At the gastro-esophageal junction, in the setting of gastroesophageal reflux* Q *4. Within the margins of a gastrojejunostomy* Q *5. In the duodenum, stomoch or jejunum of patients with Zollinger- Ellison Syndrome* Q *6. Within or adjacent to a Meckels diverticulum that contains ectopic gastric mucosa* Q

- ***The most common site of gastric ulcers (benign) is on the lesser curvature straddling the incisura angularis.***
- ***The most common complication of both acute and chronic peptic ulcers is gastrointestinal haemorrhage.***
- ***The most common arterial source of a hemorrhage in duodenal ulcers is the gastroduodenal artery.***
- ***Highly selective vagotomy is the procedure of choice for the management of chronic duodenal ulcers, except in situations where ulcer recurrence rates are high.***

Highly selective vagotomy:

- In highly selective vagotomy nerves of Latarjet supplying the antrum are preserved. Q
- A drainage procedure is not required Q
- Operation mortality is lower than in any other definitive operation for duodenal ulceration. Q

- ***Vagotomy with Antrectomy is associated with lowest recurrence rates.***
  Operations for duodenal ulcers:

Operation/Procedure	Mortality	Recurrence rate (%)	Comments
Vagotomy and drainage	Intermediate	Intermediate	Selectively used
Highly selective vagotomy	Low (minimum)	***High***	Procedure of choice as it has the least complication rate
Vagotomy and antrectomy	*High*	***Low (minimum)***	Procedure with least recurrence rate. Procedure of choice when recurrence is the major problem

Operation with maximum reduction in acid production	Operation with minimum operative mortality	The most widely used procedure in India
Truncal vagotomy and antrectomy	Highly selective vagotomy	Truncal vagotomy plus a drainage procedure *Gastrojejunostomy is at present the most widely used procedure.*

Stress ulcers

- *Stress ulcers after head trauma : Cushing's Ulcers*
- *Stress ulcers after severe burns : Curling's Ulcers*

Cushings ulcers :
Are acute ulcers of the upper GI tract associated with intracranial injury or an *increase in intracranial pressure.*

These ulcers my involve the
Stomach Q *Proximal duodenum* Q *Esophagus* Q

Complication : Haemorrhage and perforation Q
Treatment: Correction of increased intracranial pressure + usual treatment of acute erosions and ulceration.

Pyloric Stenosis : Gastric Outlet Obstruction

Pyloric Stenosis

- Pyloric Stenosis refers to Gastric Outlet Obstruction, classically resulting from hypertrophy of musculature of the pylorus adjacent to the antrum.
- Gastric outlet obstruction in a patient with peptic ulcer disease usually suggests pyloric stenosis.
- Commonly the stenosis is found in the first part of the duodenum, the most common site for a peptic ulcer. (The *term pyloric stenosis may be a misnomer as the stenosis is seldom at the pylorus)*

Epidemiology

- First born male child is characteristically most commonly affected
- It is four times more common in males as in females
- The condition does not present at birth. It is most commonly seen 4 weeks after birth

Presentation

- Vomiting is the presenting symptom (child vomits milk and *no bile is present*[Q])
  The vomiting of hydrochloric acid results in hypochloremia and alkalosis i.e. hypochloremic alkalosis[Q]
  Metabolic alkalosis with paradoxical aciduria is typical
- ***Immediately after vomiting the child is hungry i.e. loss of appetite does not occur.***
- Weight loss is striking and rapidly the infant becomes emaciated and dehydrated.
  However, greater awareness of pyloric stenosis has led to earlier identification of patients and hence with ***fewer incidences of chronic malnutrition and severe dehydration*** - *Nelson 10th/1130*

Diagnosis

- The diagnosis is usually made with a test feed : In this the baby is fed with the bottle by a nurse or mother and surgeon : palpates the abdomen with a warm hand to detect the lump and observes the characteristic peristatic waves pass across the upper abdomen.
- Ultrasonography is the investigation of choice
- Pathologically musculature of pylorus adjacent to antrum is grossly hypertrophied

Treatment

- Hyperchloremic alkalosis is common and following diagnosis first concern is to correct metabolic abnormalities - child is rehydrated with dextrose saline & potassium[Q]
- Treatment *of choice : Ramsted's operation - 'Pyloromyotomy'*

Dumping Syndromes

DUMPING SYNDROMES: POST-CIBAL SYNDROMES

DUMPING SYNDROME refers to a syndrome of abdominal and vasomator symptoms which results from dumping of food stuffs with a high osmotic load, from the stomach, into the small bowel.

TYPES OF DUMPING SYNDROMES

Dumping Syndrome is actually of two types:

- **Early dumping syndrome** : *Loss of storage capacity of stomach and ablation, by pass or destruction of pylorus, results in rapid emptying of hyperosmolar chyme into duodenummm and small intestine*. Extracellular fluid then shifts into the intestinal lumen to restore isotonicity resulting in decreased intravascular volume, which gives rise to the vasomotor symptoms.
- **Late dumping syndrome:** This is *Reactive hypoglycemia*[Q]. The carbohydrate load in thesmall intestine later causes a rise in plasma glucose, which in turn causes insulin levels to rise causing a secondary hypoglycemia.

TREATMENT OF DUMPING SYNDROMES

- Both types of postcibal syndrome are treated by dietary measures including:
  - Limitation of sugar containing liquids and solids,
  - Elimination of liquids at meal time, and
  - Eating of frequent small meals.
- In severe cases, symptoms may improve, with the somatostatin-analogue *Octreotide*.

There is no role of surgery in management of post cibal syndromes.

Menetrier's disease

Menetrier's disease is characterized by hypertrophy of gastric mucosa and not by exophytic growth.

Menetrier's disease
Menetrier's disease is a relatively rare disorder of the stomach characterized by large tortuous mucosal folds
Etiology
• Etiology is unknown • Over expression of growth factors such as TGF are suggested
Pathology
Gross • Marked Hypertrophy of gastric folds/Rugae[Q] • Hypertrophy results from hyperplasia of mucus producing cells (mucosa)[Q] • Hypertrophy is most prominent in the body and fundus [Q] Histological/microscopic • Massive foveolar hyperplasia (Hyperplasia of surface and glandular mucosal cells). • Pits of gastric glands elongate and may become tortuous • Lamina propria may contain a mild chronic inflammatory infiltrate (Note: Although lamina propria may contain an inflammatory infiltrates, Menetrier's disease is not considered a form of gastritis
Clinical picture
• Protein losing enteropathy is characteristic Excessive protein is lost from the thickened mucosa into the gut which results in hypoprotenemia and edema • ***Gastric acid secretion is usually reduced or absent*** This happens because mucosal cell hyperplasia replaces most of the parietal cells. • Epigastric pain accompanied by nausea, vomiting anorexia and weight loss Overt bleeding is unusual but occult gastrointestinal bleeding may occur
Differential Diagnosis
DD includes conditions that may present with large gastric folds: ZES Malignancy Infiltrative disorders eg sarcoidosis Infectious etiology (CMV, Histoplasmosis, syphilis)
Prognosis
These is an increased risk of adenocarcinoma of stomach in adults with menetrier's disease (CSDT)

Carcinoma Stomach

Risk Factors for Carcinoma Stomoch:

Risk factors for stomach carcinoma :
1. Long term ingestion of high concentration of nitrates in dried smoke and salted foods. Q 2. Loss of gastric acidity - Atrophic gastritis Q - Partial gastrectomy (peptic ulcer surgery) Q - Pernicious anemia Q 3. Infection with H. pylori Q 4. Intestinal metaplasia Q *(metaplasia type II* and III) 5. Gatric ulcer & polyps Q (Q *No association has been found between deodonal ulcer and gastric cancer*) 6. Menetrier's disease Q: extreme hypertrophy of gastric rugal folds. 7. Blood group A Q 8. Cigarette smoking, Dust ingestion, Ingestion of spirits, Genetic factors have also been implicated.

Premalignant conditions for Gastric Adenocarcinoma:

Premalignant lesions for Gastric Adenocarcinoma
• Chronic Atrophic Gastritis (H. pylori > Pernicious Anemia) • Intestinal Metaplasia Type II and Type III *(Intestinal Metaplasia type I is not associated with increased risk)* • Gastric Dysplasia • Gastric polyps (Adenomatous polyps) *(Hyperplastic polyps are generally not considered premalignant as the rate of malignant transformation in these polyps is <1% and confined to polyps > 1cm)* • Previous Gastrectomy • Menetrier's Disease • Gastric ulcers (long standing gastric ulcers : Low risk)

Gastric adenocarcinoma may be associated with long standing gastric peptic ulcers (small risk) but not with duodenal ulcers

Gastric Polyps and Premalignant Potential:

Gastric Polyps and Premalignant Potential

Hyperplastic Polyps	Adenomatous Polyps
• Hyperplastic Polyps account for >75% of all gastric polyps • These are not considered premalignant lesions and do not appear to have any significant malignant potential (< 1%)	• Adenomatous Polyps account for < 25% of all gastric polyps • These are considered premalignant lesions They are most commonly found in the antrum of stomach and have significant malignant potential

The most common site of gastric adenocarcinoma:

- ***The most common site of gastric adenocarcinoma is antrum***
  '40% tumors are in the antrum, predominantly on the lesser curvature, 30% arise in the body and fundus, 25% at the cardia and 5% involve the whole organ'- CSDT
- **The most common site of Gastric Adenocarcinoma secondary to h.pylori Infection is Antrum**
- **The most common site of Gastric Adenocarcinoma secondary to Pernicious anemia is Fundus and Body**

Gastric cancer secondary to:	Location / Site
H. Pylori	Antrum > body > fundus
Pernicoius Anemia	Fundus and body (not antrum)

Atrophic glands with extensive intestinal metaplasia are most charachteristically confined to the fundus in patients with pernicious anaemia.Gastric cancer in case of pernicious anemia is most often located in the fundus or body of the stomach rather in the Antrum.

Classification of Gastric Carcinoma

Based on Layers of the stomach wall involved :

Early gastric cancer:	Cancer limited to the mucosa and submucosa with or without lymph node involvement.
Late gastric cancer:	Cancer involving the muscularis.

Based on Macroscopic Growth Pattern

In Ca Stomach, three macroscopic growth patterns are recognized, and may be evident in both early and advanced gastric cancer stages:

a.	Exophytic (Type I):	Protruded in early stages, Cauliflower like polypoidal growth in advanced stages.
b.	Flat or depressed (Type II) :	With no obvious tumor mass in mucosa eg. Superficial spreading type
c.	Excavated arc Ulcerated (Type III) :	Shallow or deeply erosive crater is present in the wall of stomach.

- ***Early cases of type I & type II are potentially curable*** *- Bailey 22nd / 693*
  The prognosis depends on depth of invasion and extent of nodal and distant metastasis.
- ***Superficial spreading type indicates an early stage of type II malignancy. It therefore is potentially curable.***
- ***'Linitis plastica'*** is characterized by ***extensive infiltration of malignancy*** into a broad region of gastric wall or entire stomach creating a rigid, thickened *leather-bottle like stomach.*

Guidelines for management of Gastric carcinoma:

- Surgical resection remains the mainstay of treatment of gastric cancer either for cure or for palliation
- ***The extent of gastric resection*** depends on the site of tumor in the stomach.
  Tumors in the distal third or antrum of stomach require a subtotal gastrectomy (partial gastrectomy) while tumors of the middle or proximal third of the stomach require a total gastrectomy

Distal Third /Antrum Gastric cancer	*Middle Third / Proximal Gastric cancer*
Subtotal Gastrectomy	*Total Gastrectomy*

Patients with curable cancers of the stomach should also undergo a D2 lymphadenectomy

- ***The extent of resection of adjacent*** **structures (pancreas, spleen etc)** depends on the location of primary tumor and local invasion

  Pancreatic Resection

  The distal pancreas should not be removed a part of a resection for a cancer of the distal two third of the stomach (unless there is direct invasion)

  The distal pancreas should be removed only when there is direct invasion and still a chance of a curative procedure in patients with carcinoma of the proximal stomach

  Splenic resection

  Splenectomy is not indicated unless the tumor directly invades the spleen or involves the splenic hilar lymph nodes. Resection of spleen and splenic hilar lymph nodes *may be considered* in patients with *tumors of the proximal stomach* located in the greater curvature / posterior wall of the stomach close to the splenic hilum *where the incidence of splenic hilar nodal involvement is likely to be high*

Splenic hilar lymph nodes are generally not involved in distal third / antral gastric cancers

Adjacent structure	Distal Third / Antrum Gastric cancer	Proximal Gastric cancer
Pancreas	• *Should not be removed routinely* • *Resected if there is direct invasion*	• *Should not be removed routinely* • *Resected if there is direct invasion and/or still a chance of curative procedure*
Spleen	• *Should not be removed routinely* • *Resected if there is direct invasion or involvement of splenic hilar lymph nodes (This is unlikely)*	• *May require splenectomy to include the draining lymph nodes especially if lesion is located on the greater curvature / posterior wall, close to the splenic hilum*

The most common benign neoplasms of the stomach are Leiomyomas [Q].

Malabsorption Syndrome and Disorders of Small Intestine

Steatorrhea

Steatorrhea *is typically defined as increased excretion of fat in stool (excretion of > 7.0 gm of fat in stool during 24 hours while the patient is on a diet containing no more than 100gm of fat per day).*
Steatorrhea essentially represents malabsorption of fat.

This may be caused by several conditions including**:**

- *Acute or chronic Liver disease / Biliary Disease*
- *Mucosal disease (eg. Celiac disease / Crohn's disease)*
- *Reduced absorptive surface (Small Bowel Syndrome)*
- *Reduced contact time (Laxative abuse, Carcinoid syndrome)*
- *Disturbed mesenteric blood supply (Mesenteric ischemia)*
- *Disturbed mesenteric lymphatic drainage (Tuberculosis, Malignancy)*
- ***Pancreatic exocrine deficiency (Reduced Pancreatic Lipase)***

D-xylose test

D-xylose is a carbohydrate that is absorbed almost exclusively in the proximal small bowel without the help of pancreatic enzymes. A positive D-xylose test indicates malabsorption due to intestinal mucosal disease and thus is used as a test for assessment of mucosal function.

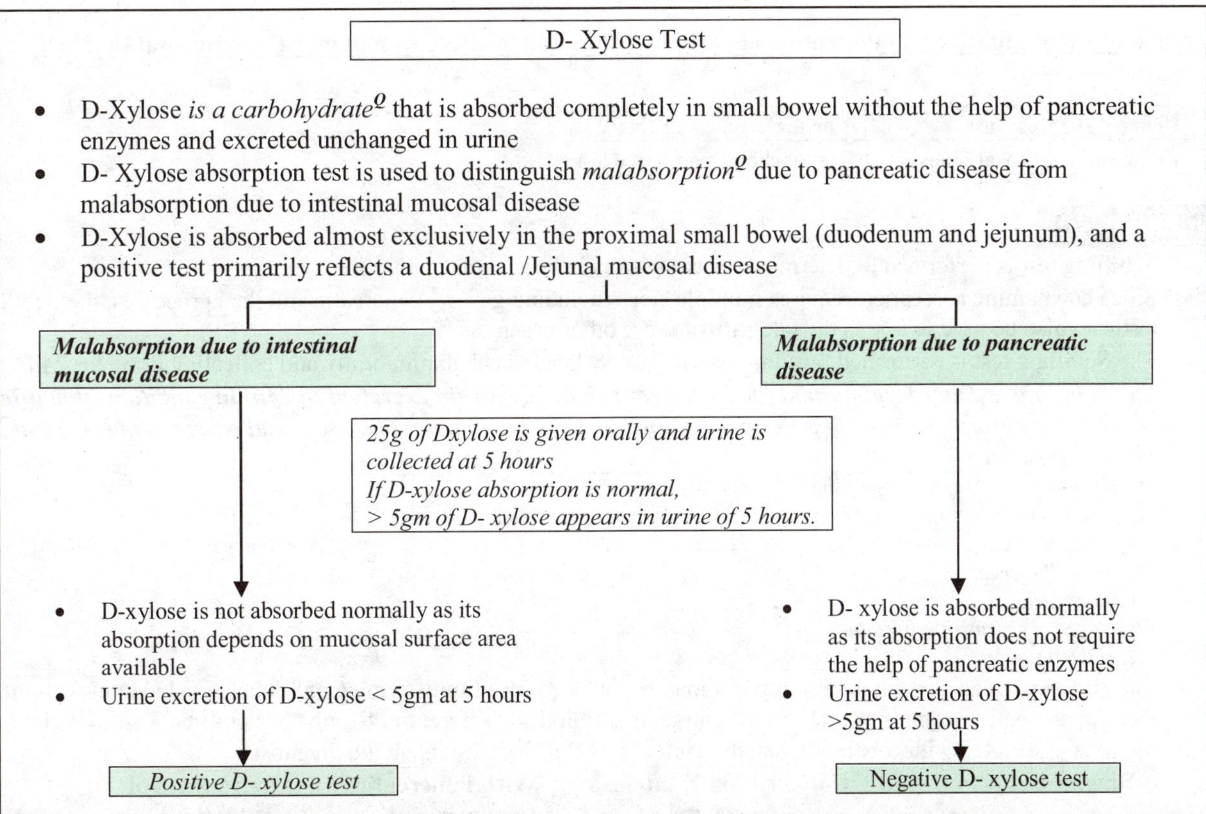

Pancreatic insufficiency is associated with a Negative D- xylose test (Normal D-xylose excretion)

D-xylose absorption test *is the most commonly employed test for carbohydrate absorption*

Causes of Positive D-Xylose Test

D-xylose Test

Positive test	False positive test
Decreased (↓) D- Xylose excretion in urine due to malabsorption from gastrointestinal mucosal disease	*Decreased D-xylose excretion in urine due to causes other than malabsorption from small bowel mucosal disease*
Causes Include	Causes Include
• ***Celiac disease*** • *Tropical sprue* • *Whipple's disease* • *Other mucosal diseases*	• ***Bacterial overgrowth*** • ***Renal insufficiency*** • *Delayed gastric emptying* • *Rapid intestinal transit* • *Vomiting* • ***Ascites /Pleural Effusion*** *(Third space collections)*

- **Blind loop syndrome** may be associated with a reduced functional intestinal mucosa and bacterial overgrowth. This condition may thus lead to both, a positive or false positive D- xylose test depending on the pathophysiology involved.
  Blind loop syndrome and *Antibiotic therapy may cause false positive D-xylose test due to* ***bacterial overgrowth***
- **Pyloric stenosis** *may cause false positive results due to delayed gastric emptying and persistant vomiting.*
- **Ascitis** *is an established cause for false positive D- xylose test due to large collection of fluid in third space*

After a positive D-xylose test is obtained, a jejunal biopsy should be performed to diagnose the mucosal abnormality

Evaluation of small intestine malabsorption of carbohydrates due to altered small intestinal mucosal function

Urinary D-xylose test	Non invasive test of choice
Endoscopic mucosal biopsy	Test of choice / preferred test

Schilling Test:

- Schilling test is performed to determine the cause of cobalamine malabsorption.
- Since cobalamine absorption requires multiple steps including gastric, pancreatic and ileal processes, the Schilling test can also be used to assess the integrity of these other organs.
- The Schilling test is performed by administering Co58-labeled cobalamin orally and collecting urine for 24h
- The ***Schilling test may be abnormal (defined as less than 10 percent excretion in 24h) in conditions that affect cobalamine absorption including Pernicious anemia, Chronic Pancreatitis, Bacterial overgrowth syndrome and Ileal dysfunction***

Conditions with Abnormal Schilling's Test (Abnormal Cobalamine Absorption)
Pernicious anemia ***Chronic Pancreatitis*** ***Achlorhydria*** ***Bacterial overgrowth syndrome*** ***Ileal dysfunction***

- The etiology for an abnormal Schilling test may be deduced by administering Co58-labeled cobalamin with intrinsic factor, pancreatic enzymes or after 5-day course of antibiotics. Differential Results of Schilling Test in various diseases associated with cobalamin malabsorption may thus help establish the diagnosis.

Diagnosis	**^{58}Co-Cbl**	**With Intrinsic Factor**	**With Pancreatic Enzymes**	**After 5 Days of Antibiotics**
Pernicious anemia	*Reduced*	*Normal*	*Reduced*	*Reduced*
Chronic pancreatitis	*Reduced*	*Reduced*	*Normal*	*Reduced*
Bacterial overgrowth	*Reduced*	*Reduced*	*Reduced*	*Normal*
Ileal disease	*Reduced*	*Reduced*	*Reduced*	*Reduced*

Differential Diagnosis of Various conditions presenting with Malabsorption using D-Xylose, Schilling's Test and Mucosal Biopsy

	D-Xylose Test	Schilling Test	Duodenal Mucosal Biopsy
Chronic pancreatitis	Normal	50% abnormal; if abnormal, normal with pancreatic enzymes	Normal
Bacterial overgrowth syndrome	Normal or only modestly abnormal	Often abnormal; if abnormal, normal after antibiotics	Usually normal
Ileal disease	Normal	Abnormal	Normal
Celiac sprue	Decreased	Normal	Abnormal: probably "flat"
Intestinal lymphangiectasia	Normal	Normal	Abnormal: "dilated lymphatics"

Malabsorption syndromes based on lesions seen on intestinal Biopsy

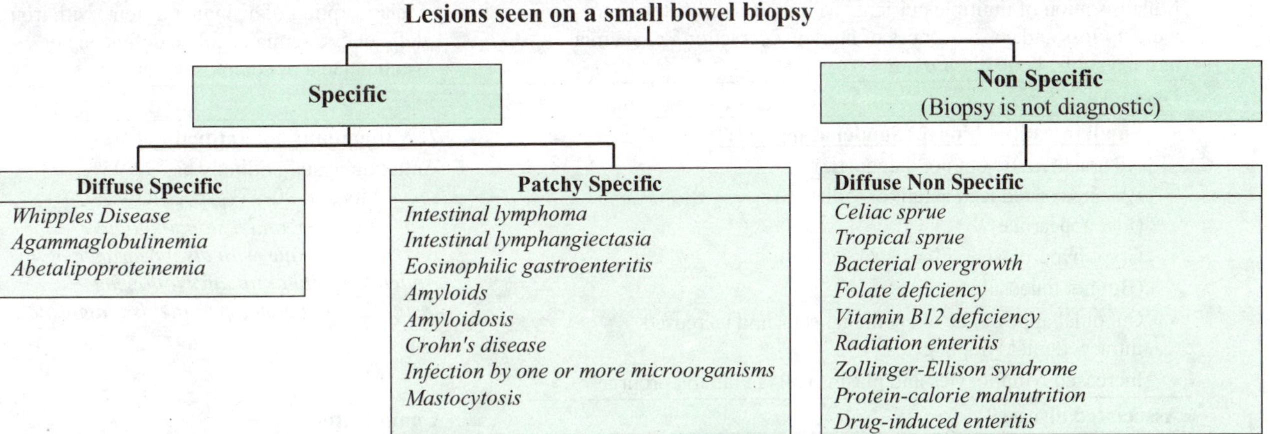

Disease that can be Diagnosed by Small-Intestinal Mucosal Biopsies

Lesions	Pathologic Findings
Diffuse, specific	
• *Whipple's disease*	Lamina propria contains macrophages containing PAS + material
• *Agammaglobulinemia*	No plasma cells; either normal or absent villi ("flat mucosa")
• Abetalipoproteinemia	Normal villi; epithelial cells vacuolated with fat postprandially
Patchy, specific	
• *Intestinal lymphoma*	Malignant cells in lamina propria and submucosa
• *Intestinal lymphangiectasia*	Dilated lymphatics; clubbed villi
• *Eosinophilic gastroenteritis*	Eosinophil infiltration of lamina propria and mucosa
• *Amyloidosis*	Amyloid deposits
• *Crohn's disease*	Noncaseating granulomas
• *Infection by one or more microorganisms*	Specific organisms
• *Mastocytosis*	Mast cell infiltration of lamina propria
Diffuse, nonspecific	
• *Celiac sprue*	Short or absent villi; mononuclear infiltrate; epithelial cell damage; hypertrophy of crypts
• *Tropical sprue*	Similar to celiac sprue
• *Bacterial overgrowth*	Patchy damage to villi; lymphocyte
• *Folate deficiency*	Short villi; decreased mitosis in crypts; megalocytosis
• *Vitamin B12 deficiency*	Similar to folate deficiency
• *Radiation enteritis*	Similar to folate deficiency
• *Zollinger – Ellison syndrome*	Mucosal ulceration and erosion from acid
• *Protein –calorie malnutrition*	Villous atrophy; secondary bacterial overgrowth
• *Drug-induced enteritis*	Variable histology

Celiac Disease

Celiac disease

Malabsorption syndrome of non-infectious etiology without systemic features.

Etiology

Environmental factors	**Immunogenic factors**	**Genetic factors**
Intolerance to ***gliadin*** a component of gluten, present in wheat, barley, rye and oats	Ig A antibodies are present - ***IgA antiendomysial*** - IgA antigliadin - IgA anti tissue tranglutaminase ***Antiendomysial antibody has 90-95% Sensitivity and 90-95% Specificity***	95% express ***HLA-OQ2 allele***[Q]

Presentation

Malabsorption of multiple nutrients with diarrhea, steatorrhea, weight / loss and consequences of nutrients depletion i.e. anemia and metabolic bone disease

or

Malabsorption of a single nutrient, with iron deficiency anemia or folate deficiency or osteomalacia or edema from protein loss.

Diagnosis

1. **Small intestinal biopsy (duodenal/jejunal)**[Q]
   (Charachteristic but not diagnostic)[Q]
   Absence or reduced height of villi
   (Flat appearnce)[Q]

- Crypt hyperplasia, villous atrophy (But not mucosal atrophy)[Q]
- Cuboidal appearance of epethelial cells and increased intraepethelial lymphocytes
- Increased lymphocytes and plasma cells in lamina propria[Q]

2. **Antiendomysial antibodies**[Q]
   Antiendomysial antibody has 90-95% sensitivity and 90-95% specificity.
   Prompt clinical and histopathological response, together with disappearance of Ig Antiendomysial antibodies following institution of a gluten free diet is diagnostic.

Associated disease[Q]

- Dermatitis Herpetoformis[Q]
- Diabetes mellitus type I[Q]
- IgA deficiency

Complications

- Increased incidence of both gastro intestinal and non gastrointestinal neoplasms as well as ***Intestinal lymphomas.***[Q]

Management

Gluten free diet + Glucocorticoids or immunosupressive agents.[Q]

Approach to diagnosis of Celiac Disease

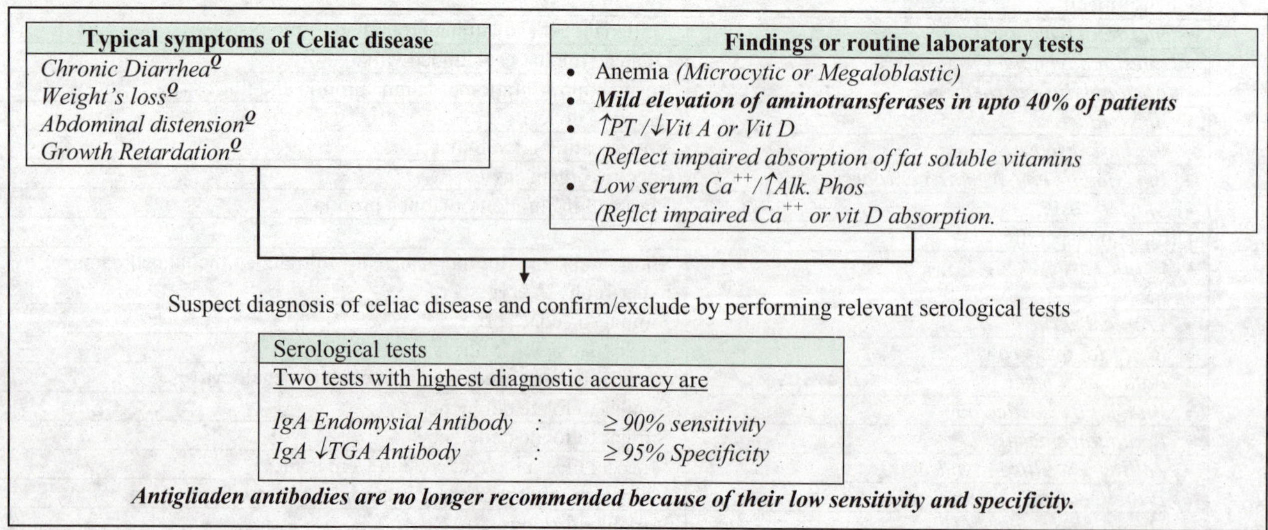

Diagnosis of Celiac Sprue

Serological tests ········▶	Endoscopic mucosal biopsy *of distal duodenum or proxi- mal jejunum* ········▶	Prompt clinical and histo-pathological response following institution of gluten free diet.
Serological tests (*CMDT*)	**Endoscopic mucosal biopsy**	**Diagnosis**
▪ ***Two serological tests with highest diagnostic accuracy are*** 1. IgA antiendomysial antibody 2. IgA anti – tTG antibody ▪ Both tests have a > 90% sensitivity and > 95% specificity.	• Findings are ***characteristic but not specific / diagnostic***. • Biopsy of distal duodenum or proximal jejunum is performed. • <u>Finding are restricted to mucosa and include</u> : – Loss or blunting of villi / flat villi – Hypertrophy of intestinal crypts – Infiltration of lamina propria will lymphocytes / plasma cells – Cuboidal appearance of epithelial cells and increased intraepithelial lymphocytes.	• **<u>Diagnosis of celiac sprue requires</u>** Presence of characteristic histopathological changes on biopsy together will prompt clinical and hispathological response following institution of gluten free diet. • IgA antiendomysial Ab or IgA anti – tTGA Ab should also disappear after a gluten free diet.
<u>IgG or IgA antigliadin antibodies</u> are present in 85% of patients with celiac sprue. However their specificity is relatively low (80 – 90%) which limits their usefulness as screening test.		
Small bowel biopsy is still recommended to confirm diagnosis.		

Antiendomysial antibody > Anti tissue transglutaminase antibody > Antireticular antibody> Antigliadin antibody			
<u>Antigliadin (IJP) Antibodies (AGN)</u>	**<u>Anti reticulin IJP Antibodies (ARA)</u>**	**<u>Antiendomysial Antibiotics (Anti EMA)</u>**	**<u>Anti tissue transglutaminase antibody (Anti-tTGA)</u>**
• First immunological assay to be tested were antigliadin antibodies. • The variability and lower accuracy make them *unsuitable for diagnostic and screening purposes* • Antigliadin assays have been replaced by more specific and sensitive tests using other antibodies	• Second antibody identified in literature was the antireticulin antibodies. • There are atleast 5 types of antireticulin antibodies but only one type is associated with celiac disease. • These antibodies are *not very sensitive and are not used in routine practice.*	• Antiendomysial antibodies have ***high sensitivity and specificity*** for the diagnosis of celiac disease. • These antibodies are directed against endomysium or 'Intermyofibril substance' of smooth muscle. • The antigen recognized by these antibodies is 'tissue transglutaminase'.	• Major breakthrough for serological diagnosis of celiac disease. • Antitissue transglutaminase antibodies (Anti-tTGA) are ***also highly sensitive and specific but performance of anti EMA is superior to Anti-tTGA***

<u>Pathologic morphology of celiac disease:</u>

The mucosa appears flat or scalloped or may be visually normal. Biopsy specimens demonstrate diffuse enteritis, with the following features.

Small Intestinal Biopsy (duodenal /jejunal) in Celiac disease (Characteristic but not diagnostic[Q])
• *Absence or reduced height of villi (Flat appearance)*[Q] • *Crypt hyperplasia, villous atrophy (but not mucosal atrophy)*[Q] • *Cuboidal appearance of epithelial cells and increased intraepithelial lymphocytes* • *Increased lymphocytes and plasma cells in lamina propria*[Q]

The villi	The surface epithelium	The crypts	The lamina propria
show marked atrophy or total loss.	shows vacuolar degeneration, loss of the microvillus brush border, and an increased number of intraepithelial lymphocytes.	exhibit increased mitotic activity and are elongated, hyperplastic and tortuous, so the overall mucosal thickness remains the same.	has an overall increase in plasma cells, lymphocytes, macrophages, eosinophils and mast cells.

*All these **structural changes are more marked in the proximal small intestine** [Q] than in the distal because it is the duodenum and proximal jejunum that are exposed to the highest concentration of the dietary gluten.*

The overall mucosal thickness remains the same in Celiac Disease
Mucosal atrophy and presence of Giardia Lambia are not seen in biopsy from celiac disease.

Associations of Celiac Disease:

Associations of Celiac Disease (CMDT & Harrisons)

- ***Dermatitis Herpetiformis***
- Other autoimmune disease including: *(CMDT)*
  - *Addison's disease*
  - *Grave's disease*
  - *Diabetes mellitus- Type I (Harrisons)*
  - *Myaesthenia Gravis*
  - *Slogren syndrome*
  - *Atrophic Gastritis*
  - *Pancreatic insufficiency*
- IgA deficiency *(Harrisons)*
- Lymphomas *(Harrisons)*

Note

Celiac disease is associated with an increased risk of cancer including Lymphomas (NHL, Intestinal T cell Lymphoma)

The possibility of Lymphoma must be considered whenever a patient with celiac sprue previously doing well on a gluten free diet is no longer responsive to gluten free diet' - Harrisons

Vitamin Deficiency in Patients with Celiac disease:

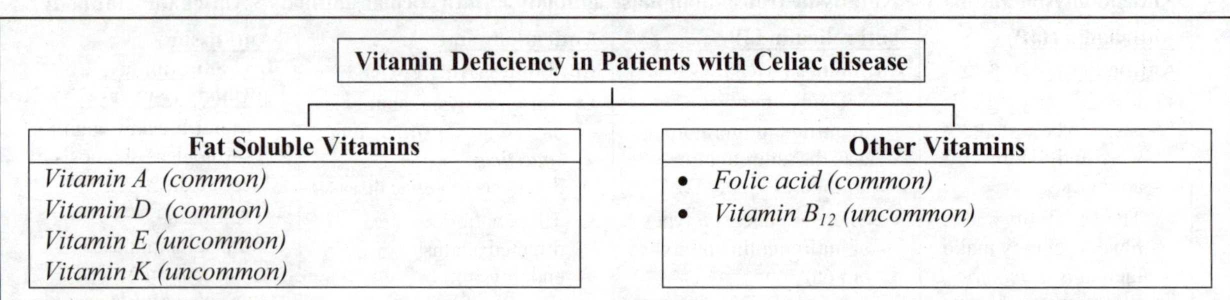

Treatment of Celiac Disease:

The mainstay of treatment for celiac sprue is administration of of a glutin free diet.
'Removal of all glutin from the diet is essential to therapy'. – CMDT

Whipple's Disease

Whipple's Disease

Malabsorption syndrome with systemic features with infectious etiology

Etiology

Gram negative actinomycete^Q Tropheryma whippelii

Biopsy/ Histopathology

Biopsy is Abnormal and specific/diagnostic

***The Hallmark of Whipple's disease is a** small intestinal mucosa laden with macrophages. **Accompanying changes include** lymphatic dilatation **suggesting lymphatic blockage. The lymphatic blockage is believed to be responsible for** lipid deposition **in the villi** – Robbins*

Histopathological findings in Whipple's disease

Characterisitc findings / Specific finding (Hallmark of disease)	Associated findings
• Small intestinal mucosa laden with ***foamy macrophages in the lamina propria***, which are characteristically, Periodic – Acid – Schiff (PAS) positive. • These PAS positive macrophages (monocytes) also *contain gram positive – acid fast bacillus T. whipleii^Q*. (The substance in macrophages that stains positive with PAS is thought to be remnants of the cell wall of phagocytosed bacilli) Note : *PAS positive macrophages are not pathognomic for Whipple's disease. They have also been isolated in other diseases eg. Mycobacterium Avium Intercellulare & Mycobacterium Tuberculosis.*	• Villi may be thickenned, widened or blunted • Small intestinal mucosal and ***submucosal lymphatic vessels are dilated*** • Lipid droplets / Lipid vacuoles / ***Lipid deposition may be seen*** • The number of lamina propria plasma cells, ***lymphocytes*** and eosinophills ***are decreased*** *(Samter's Immunologic Diseases by Austen and Samter 2nd /704)* *'The number of intraepethelial lymphocytes is not increased'* *(Sternberg's Diagnostic Surgical Pathology 4th/1481)*

Presentation

Features of malabsorption

Multisystemic involvement along with Fever, Lymphadenopathy and Arthralgias ^Q

- CNS invovement is seen in about 10% of patients. Manifestations include
  - ***Dementia*** ^Q (confusion and memory loss)
  - Seizures, Coma, Myoclonus ^Q
- Cranial N. findings include Nystagmus and Ophthalmoplegia ^Q

  Non specific symptoms like Confusion and Memory loss (Dementia) in all likelihood, should be more common a presentation than seizures.

  Ophthalmopegia is due to cranial nerve involvement and not supra-nuclear in type.

Treatment

Etiology is infectious so treatment is with Antibiotics

Trimethoprim+sufamethoxocate

Differential Diagnosis of the three major forms of Malabsorption Syndromes:

Whipple's Disease	*Tropical Sprue*	*Coeliac Disease*
Malabsorption syndrome with systemic features with infectious etiology	Malabsorption syndrome of infectious etiology without systemic features	Malabsorption syndrome of non infectious etiology without systemic features
Etiology	**Etiology**	**Etiology**
Gram negative actinomycete[Q] Tropheryma whippelii	Caused by some strains of E.coli	Caused by intolerance to 'gliadin' gluten a protein found in wheat rye, barley[Q].
Biopsy	**Biopsy**	**Biopsy**
Biopsy is Abnormal and specific/diagnostic	**Biopsy is abnormal but not specific/diagnostic**	**Biopsy is abnormal but not specific/diagnostic**
Lamina Propria is infiltrated with macrophages containing PAS positive glycoproteins and rod shaped bacilli Dilated lymphatics	Shortened, thickened villi increased crypt depth infiltration by mononuclear cells	Blunting and flattening surface with villi either absent or broad and short Crypts are elongated Dense infiltration of inflammatory cells in lamina propria
Clinical features	**Clinical features**	**Clinical features**
Features of malabsorption + Array of systemic features	Features of malabsorption	Features of malabsorption
Management	**Management**	**Management**
Etiology is infectious so treatment is with Antibiotics Trimethoprim+sufamethoxocate	Etiology is infectious so treatment is with antibiotics (Sulfonamide/ Tetracycline)	Etiology is not infectious but immune Glutin free diet (no antibiotics) + Glucocorticoids or immunosuppressive agents

Intestinal Angina

What is Intestinal Angina : Journal of Emergency Medicine : Review Article.

- Intestinal angina refers to the clinical syndrome seen in association with ***Chronic Mesenteric Ischaemia.***
- It is characterized by reduced mesenteric blood flow that interferes with physiological function but does not cause infarction.
- Mesentric angina is the result of intestinal hypoperfusion through two of the three major vessels supplying the small intestine.
  - Superior Mesentric Artery
  - Celiac artery
  - Inferior Mesentric Artery

Presentation

- Post Prandial Abdominal Pain: *Abdominal pain that starts about 30 minutes after eating and lasts for one to two hours.*
- Fear of eating and weight loss: Once the patient realizes the relationship between eating and pain.
- Diarrhea, Nausea, Vomiting

Diagnosis

*Gold standard for confirmation of mesenteric arterial occlusion (**chronic** mesenteric ischaemia) is Angiography (Note that Gold standard for diagnosis of **acute** mesenteric ischaemia is Laparotomy[Q]. Surgical exploration should not be delayed).*

Short Bowel Syndrome

Short bowel syndrome: *(Myriad of clinical problems that follow resection of warying length of small intestine)*

Causes:

1. *Mesentric vascular disease: mesenteric ischaemia*[Q]
2. *Primary mucosal and submucosal disease – Crohn's disease*[Q]
3. *Operations without preexisting small intestinal disease – jejunoilial bypass for obesity*[Q]

Manifestation resulting from resection of varying length of small intestine

Diarrhea and Steatorrhea [Q]	↑ed Renal calcium oxalate calculi	↑ed Cholesterol gall stones [Q]	Gastric hypersecretion of acid [Q]
Multiple factors contribute to diarrhea and steatorrhea such as: • Absence of intestinal mucosa required for absorption of lipid and fluid and electrolytes • Stimulation of colonic fluid and electrolyte secretion by increased bile acids that enter colon • Decreased intestinal transit and bacterial overgrowth from absence of ilio caecal valve • Reduced pH in duodenum from gastric acid hypersecretion.	• There occurs increased absorption of oxalates by large intestine in patients with a small intestinal resection with intact colon • Hyperoxaluria and renal calcium oxalate crystals form **Treatment:** • Dietry restriction of oxalate containing feed (spinach, tea) • Cholestyramine an anion binding resin and calcium	Due to a decrease in the bile acid pool size and resulting super saturation of cholesteral in gall-bladder bile.	Related to reduced hormonal inhibition of acid secretion or increased gastrin levels due to reduced small intestine catabolism of gastrin.

Short bowel syndrome is characterized by increased gastrin levels (hypergastrinemia) due to reduced small intestinal catabolism of gastrin

Vitamin Deficiencies in Short Bowel Syndrome:

Vitamin Deficiencies in Short Bowel Syndrome

Short Bowel Syndrome with Extensive Jejunal Resection

- This is associated primarily with deficiency of fat soluble vitamins (A, D, E, K)
- *The most common fat-soluble vitamins that are deficienct are vitamin A and D and to a lesser extent vitamin E followed by vitamin K.*

Vitamin A, D > Vitamin E >> Vitamin K

Deficiency of vitamin K is uncommon as vitamin K is synthesized by colonic bacteria

- 60% of vitamin K is synthesized by colonic bacteria
- 40% of vitamin K is received by dietary intake
- *Deficiency of vitamin K is therefore uncommon in patients with short bowel syndrome who have an intact colon.*
- *Deficiency of vitamin K is however common in those patients with short bowel syndrome who do not have a residual colon.*

Short Bowel Syndrome with Extensive ileal resection

- This is associated primarily with deficiency of vitamin B12 since vitamin B12 is only absorbed in the terminal ileum.
- Fat soluble vitamin deficiencies may also occur due to fat malabsorption from decrease in concentration of bile acids / salts.

  (Bile acids are absorbed only from the ileum)

Vitamin B12 > Fat solubleVitamin

The ileum has the capacity to adapt and compensate for jejunal resection. The jejunum does not have the capacity to adapt and compensate for ileal resection (as the terminal ileum has the exclusive capacity to reabsorb bile salts &vit B_{12})

Cyanocobalamine (Vitamin B12) deficiency is the most common deficiency in patients with short bowel syndrome associated with loss of ileum (ileal resection) since vitamin B12 is absorbed only in the ileum.

Inflammatory Bowel Disease

Ulcerative Colitis and Crohn's Disease

DISTINGUISHING FEATURES OF CROHN'S DISEASE AND ULCERATIVE COLITIS :

FEATURE	CROHN'S DISEASE	ULCERATIVE COLITIS
A. Macroscopic features		
1. Distribution	Segmental with ***skip areas*** [Q]	Continuous *without skip areas*[Q]
2. Location	Commonly terminal ileum and /or ascending colon	Commonly rectum sigmoid colon and extending upwards
3. Extent	Usually involves the entire thickness of the affected segment of bowel wall	Usually superficial, confined to mucosal layers
4. Ulcers	Serpiginous ulcers, that may develop into deep *Fissures* [Q]	Superficial mucosal ulcers without fissures
5. Pseudopolyps	Rarely seen	*Commonly present* [Q]
6. Fibrosis	Common	Rare
7. Shortening	Due to fibrosis	Due to contraction of muscularis
B. Microscopic features		
1. Depth of inflammation	*Typically transmural* [Q]	*Mucosal* [Q] and Submucosal
2. Type of inflammation	*Non-caseating granulomas* [Q] and infiltrate of mononuclear cells (lymphocytes, plasma cells and macrophages) (Crypt abscess may also be seen)	*Crypt abscess* and non-specific acute and chronic inflammatory cells (lymphocytes, plasma cells neutrophils, eosinophils, mast cells)
3. Mucosa	Patchy ulceration	Hemorrhagic mucosa with ulceration
4. Submucosa	Widened due to edema and lymphoid aggregates	Normal or reduced in width
5. Muscularis	Infiltrated by inflammatory cells	Usually spared, except in cases of ***Toxic Megacolon*** [Q]
6. Fibrosis	Present	Usually absent
C. Complications		
1. Fistula formation	Internal and external fistulae in 10% cases	*Extremely rare* [Q]
2. Malignant changes	Less common but present	May occur in disease of more than 10 years duration (*more common* [Q])
3. Fibrous strictures	*Common* [Q]	*Never* [Q]
4. Toxic Megacolon	--	Risk present[Q]
5. Named Features	*Hose pipe appearance*[Q] *Cobble-Stone appearance*[Q]	*Garden hose appearance* [Q] *Pseudopolyps* [Q]

Serological Markers for Inflammatory Bowel Disease

Serological markers for inflammatory bowel disease

Perinuclear Antineutrophil Cytoplasmic Antibodies (p ANCA)
- Positive in 60 - 70% of U.C. patients (and 5 - 10% of CD patients)

Antisaccharomyces Cerevisiae Antibodies (ASCA)
- Positive in 60 - 70% of CD patients (and 10 - 15% of U.C. patients)

- *p ANCA +ve with ASCA -ve* = *97% specificity for UC*
- *p ANCA +ve with ASCA +ve* = *97% specificity for CD*

Antibody	G.I. Disorder
Antiendomysial antibody[Q]	*Celiac sprue*
Antisaccharomyces cerevisiae antibody[Q]	*Crohn's disease*
Antineutrophilic cytoplasmic antibody[Q]	*Ulcerative colitis*

Extraintestinal diseases associated with inflammatory bowel disease:

Joint manifestations:	**Ocular manifestations:**	**Skin manifestations:**	**Hepatic manifestations:**
Arthralgia to acute arthritis Ankylosing spondylitis Sacroilitis	Episcleritis Recurrent iritis Uveitis	Erythema nodosum Pyoderma gangrenosum[Q] **Aphthous ulcers**	Nonspecific focal hepatitis Fatty liver Pericholangitis **Sclerosing cholangitis** Autoimmune chronic active hepatitis **Cirrhosis**

	Ulcerative Colitis	**Crohn's Disease**
Clinical		
Gross blood in stool	***Yes***	***Occasionally***
Mucus	***Yes***	***Occasionally***
Systemic symptoms	Occasionally	Frequently
Pain	Occasionally	Frequently
Abdominal mass	Rarely	Yes
Significant perineal disease	No	Frequently
Fistulas	No	Yes
Small-intestinal obstruction	No	Frequently
Colonic obstruction	Rarely	Frequently
Response to antibiotics	No	Yes
Recurrence after surgery	No	Yes
ANCA-positive	***Frequently***	***Rarely***
ASCA –positive	Rarely	Frequently
Endoscopic		
Rectal sparing	Rarely	Frequently
Continuous disease	Yes	Occasionally
Cobblestoning	No	Yes
Granuloma on biopsy	No	Occasionally
Radiographic		
Small bowel significantly abnormal	No	Yes
Abnormal terminal ileum	Occasionally	Yes
Segmental colitis	No	Yes
Asymmetric colitis	No	Yes
Stricture	Occasionally	Frequently
Epidemiology of IBD		
Age of onset	15-30 and 60-80	15-30 & 60-80
Male : Female ratio	1:1	≈1.5 : 1
Smoking	May prevent disease	May cause disease
Oral contraceptives	No increased risk	Odds ratio 1.4
Appendectomy	Protective	Not protective
Monozygotic twins	6% concordance	58% concordance
Dizygotic twins	0% concordance	4% concordance

Management Protocol for Inflammatory Bowel Disease:

The mainstay of therapy for inflammatory bowel disease remains 5- Aminosalicylic derivatives

Colonic Disorders

Irritable Bowel Syndrome (IBS)

Charachterisitc Symptoms and Diagnostic Criteria for Irritiable Bowel Syndrome (IBS)

Symptoms that cumulatively support the diagnosis of Irritable Bowel Syndrome:

- *Abnormal stool frequency*[Q] *(for research purposes, "abnormal" defined as > 3 bowel movements/week)*
- *Abnormal stool formation*[Q] *(lumpy/hard or loose/watery stool)*
- *Abnormal stool habits*[Q] *(straining, urgency, or feeling of incomplete evacuation)*
- *Passage of mucus*[Q]
- *Bloating or feeling of abdominal distention*

The diagnosis of a functional bowel disorder always presumes the absence of a structural or biochemical explanation for the symptoms.

Diagnostic criteria for Irritable Bowel Syndrome

Recurrent abdominal pain or discomfort at least 3 days per month in the last 3 months associated with two or more of the following

1. *Improvement with defecation*[Q]
2. *Onset associated with a change in frequency of stool*[Q]
3. *Onset associated with a change in form (appearance) of stool*[Q].

Criteria fulfilled for the last 3 months with symptom onset at least 6 months prior to diagnosis.

Discomfort means an uncomfortable sensation not described as pain. In pathophysiology research and clinical trails, a pain/discomfort frequency of at least 2 days a week during screening evaluation is required for subject eligibility.

Red flag" conditions in irritable bowel syndrome that suggest possibility of another disease

"Red flag" conditions in irritable bowel syndrome that suggest possibility of another disease

Presence of any of the following calls for further investigation to rule out other disease processes:

- *Fever*
- *Blood in stools*
- *Nocturnal pain*
- *Abnormal physical findings*
- *Onset in patients>50 years of age*
- *Weight loss or anorexia*
- *Anemia*
- *Abnormal blood studies*
- *Family history of inflammatory bowel disease or malignancy*

IBS may be associated with diarrhea or constipation

The most common pattern in IBS is constipation alternating with diarrhea

Young age and Female sex are epidemiological risk factors for IBS

Onset in patients>50 years of age is a red flag sign and raises the possibility of another condition

IBS may be associated with Anxiety and stress

Onset of symptoms in periods of stress supports a diagnosis of IBS.

IBS is charachteristically associated with absence of blood in stool

Presence of blood in stool is a 'Red Flag' sign that suggests possibility of another disease.- Harrison's 17th/1901

Irritable Bowel syndrome (IBS) is a benign functional bowel disorder

IBS does not predispose to malignancy in the long term

Possible Drugs for a Dominant Symptom in IBS: *(Harrison's 18th/2501)*

Diarrhea	Constipation	Abdominal Pain
• *Lopepramide* • *Cholestyramine resin* • *Alosetron*	• *Psyllium husk* • *Methylcellulose* • *Calcium polycarbophil* • *Lactulose syrup* • *70% sorbitol* • *Polyethylene glycol 3350* • *Lubiprostone (Amitiza)* • *Magnesium hydroxide*	• *Smooth-muscle relaxant* • *Tricyclic antidepressants* • *Selective serotonin reuptake inhibitors*

Colorectal Carcinomas

Hereditary gastrointestinal polyposis syndromes

Non-malignant polyps[Q] (Rare/Small Malignant potential)	
Hamartomatous polyps[Q]	***Hyperplastic polyps***[Q]
Juvenile ***polyposis***[Q] *Peutz Jeghers syndrome*[Q]	

Malignant polyps[Q]
Adenomatous Polyps[Q]
Familial adenomatous polyposis[Q] *Gardner's syndrome*[Q] *Turcot's syndrome*[Q] *Lynch syndrome*[Q]

Review of Hereditary gastrointestinal polyposis syndromes

Hereditary *autosomal dominant*[Q] gastrointestinal polyposis syndromes

↓ ↓

High Malignant Potential[Q] *(Histologically adenomas[Q])*		
Syndrome	**Distribution**	**Associated**
Familial colonic Polyposis	Large intestine	None
Gardner's syndrome	*Large intestine > small intestine*	Osteomas Lipomas Fibromas Epidermal cyst *Ampullary Ca* Desmoid
Turcot's syndrome	Large intestine	Brain Tumours

Rare (small) Malignant Potential[Q] *(Histologically hamartomas[Q])*		
Syndrome	**Distribution**	**Associated**
Peutz Jagher's syndrome	SI > LI > Stomach	**Mucocutaneous pigmentations** Tumours of ovary, Breast, pacnreas, endometrium
Juvenile polyposis syndrome	LI > SI > Stomach	Various congenital abnormalities

Clues to Diagnosis for Heriditable (Autosomal dominant) Gastrointestinal polyposis syndromes:

Neoplastic polyps:

Multiple Adenomalous polyps (Adenomas) - are a very common risk factor for colorectal malignancy. Infact if the polyposis is not treated surgically, colorectal cancer will develop in almost all patients (100%), before age 40

Clues to diagnosis:

Adenomas in large intestine with no associated lesions	**Familial Polyposis coli**
Adenomas in large intestine associated with osteomas, fibromas or lipomas	**Gardner's Syndrome**
Adenomas in large intestine associated with brain tumors	**Turcot's syndrome**

***Non-Neoplastic Polyps*:** Peutz Jegher's syndrome and Juvenile polyposis, are two autosomal dominant, heritable conditions, associated with polyps in G.I.T. These polyps are however harmatomas and do not have malignant potential.

Clues to their diagnosis:

Hamartomatous polyps throughout GIT associated with mucocutaneous pigmentation and tumors of pancreas ovary, breast, lung, uterus.	**Peutz Jeghers Syndrome** *(in small intestine[Q]>Large intestine[Q]>Stomach[Q])*
Hamartomatous polyps throughout GIT associated with various congenital anomalies.	**Juvenile Polyposis** *(in large Intestine[Q]> small intestine[Q]> stomach[Q])*

Peutz-Jegher's syndrome

Mucocutaneous pigmentation along with gastrointestinal manifestations of abdominal pain and anemia suggest the diagnosis of Peutz-Jegher's syndrome.

Peutz Jagher's Syndrome

Peutz-Jaghers syndrome is a rare autosomal dominant, inherited syndrome characterized by mucocutaneous pigmentation and gastrointestinal polyposis.

Autosomal Dominant Inheritance[Q]
Family history often positive[Q]

Mucocutaneous Pigmentation

- Mucocutancous pigmentation involving lips, buccal mucosa and skin is characteristic (Digits, nails, pains, soles genitalia or any mucosal surface may be involved)

Gastrointestinal Polyposis

- Hamartomatous polys (Harrison's) Small intestine > Large intestine > Stomach

May present with:
Intussusception or obstruction
(Abdominal pain, bleeding, Anemia)

Although hamartomas are not malignant, a small percentage of patients (13%) may develop malignancies of intestinal organs specially stomach and duodenum

Neoplasm's of Non intestinal organs

- Patients with this syndrome have increased risk of developing carcinomas of
  - Ovary
  - Breast
  - Pancreas
  - Endometrium

Syndrome[Q]	*Distribution*[Q]	*Histological type*[Q]	*Malignant potential*[Q]	*Associated*[Q]
Peutz Jegher's Syndrome	Small intestine > Large intestine > stomach	Hamartoma	Rare	• Mucocutaneous pigmentation • Tumors of non-intestinal organs - Ovary, - Breast - Pancreas - Endometrium

Although hamartomas are not malignant, a small percentage (13%) of patients develop malignancies[Q] *of intestinal organs, specially stomach and duodenum (NOT COLON).*

Prognostic Factors for Colorectal Carcinoma:

The most important prognostic factor of colorectal carcinoma is the 'stage of disease'.

The 'stage of disease' gives information related to depth of penetration into bowel wall and extent of regional lymph node spread, both of which are the two most important independent prognostic factors.

Most important prognostic factors
'Extent of Regional Lymph node spread' and 'Depth of tumor invasion' are the most important determinants of prognosis

Single most important prognostic factor

Stage of disease[Q]

Stage of disease gives information on both the depth of tumor penetration into the bowel wall and the extent of regional lymph node involvement

'Stage' of disease is a superior prognostic factor in comparison to Lymph node status alone

Single most important independent prognostic factor

Lymph node status[Q]

Single most important independent prognostic factor is the Lymph nodal status or the number of positive nodes

- Devita 7th / 1069

- Gastrointestinal Oncology (2004) / 684

Pancreatic Disorders

Pancreatitis

Ranson's criteria for prognosis in acute pancreatitis include: (Adverse factors)

At the time of Admission	During initial 48 hours
1. *Age > 55 years*[Q]	1. *Fall in haematocril > 10%*
2. *Leucocytosis > 16.000/μl* [Q]	2. *Fluid deficit > 4000 ml*
3. *Hyperglycemia > 200 mg/dl*	3. *Hypocalcemia < 8 mg/dl*[Q]
4. *Serum LDH > 400 IU/L*	4. *Hypoxemia < 5mg/dl*
5. *Serum AST > 250 IU/L*	5. *Increased BUN > 5mg/dl*
	6. *Hypoalbuminemia < 3.2 g/dl*

Serum amylase does not form any cirteria for prognosis in acute pancreatitis. (Remember this fact)
Prothrombin time is not included as an index in Ranson's criteria

The prognosis is best in patients where pancreatitis is caused by a remediable cause such as cholelithiasis.
'Eradication of gall stone disease' prevents further attacks of pancreatitis. *-Oxford text*

Diagnosis of Acute Pancreatitis:

Serum Amylase

The diagnosis of acute pancreatitis is usually established by detection of an increased level of serum amylase. Serum amylase level is the standard laboratory test carried out to confirm the diagnosis of acute pancreatitis.

Measurement during first 24 hours of onset of pain	Measeurement late after presentation
An elevation of three times the upper limit of normal clinches the diagnosis (provided overt salivary gland disease and gut perforation or infarction are excluded)	After 48-72 hrs even with continuing evidence of pancreatitis, total serum levels tend to return to normal With a late presentation thus, serum amylase levels may give a false negative result.

Serum amylase level may be increased in several other conditions

Remember: [Q]

There is no definitive correlation between the severity of pancreatitis and the degree of serum amylase elevation. An elevated serum lipase [Q] or trypsin value is more specific / diagnostic of acute pancreatitis than serum amylase – (Lipase is the single best enzyme to measure for acute pancreatitis [Q]).

Serum Lipase

Serum lipase elevation is the most specific laboratory test for establishing a diagnosis of Acute Pancreatitis
'A three fold elevated serum lipase value is usually diagnostic of acute pancreatitis' – Harrison

An elevated serum Lipase level is more specific for pancreatitis than a serum amylase level because many other pathologic conditions may present with an elevated amylase level. Serum lipase is therefore the single best answer of choice.

Purtscher's retinopathy *is a relatively unusual complication of acute pancreatitis.* It is manifested by ***sudden and severe loss of vision***. It is believed to be due to occlusion of the posterior retinal artery with aggregated granulocytes.

Peculiar Fundoscopic appearance :

Cotton wool spots and hemorrhages confined to an area limited by the optic disk and macula.[Q]

Pseudopancreatic cyst_*('pseudo' because they do not have an epithelial lining)*

- *Pseudocyst is the most common complication of acute pancreatitis usually occurring after 2-3 week*
- *Most comon cause of pancreatic pseudocyst is Pancreatitis (90%)(The second most common cause is trauma (10%))*
- *Most common site for pseudopancreatic cyst is the body and tail of pancreas*
- *The investigation of choice for Pseudopancreatic Cyst is Ultrasonography*
- *Treatment is indicated for Pseudocyst > 5cm diameter and more than 6 weeks old*[Q]

Indications for Drainage :
1. Pseudocyst > 5cm in diameter.[Q] *2. Persisting for > 6 weeks.*[Q]

**A singnificant number of pseudocysts will resovle sponteaneously more than 6 weeks after their formations*[Q]

- *Initial procedure in the management of uncomplicated persistant pancreatic pseudocysts is Percutaneous aspiration*
- *Surgical internal drainage in the form of cystojejunostomy continues to be the treatment of choice.*

Treatment of Pancreatic Psuedocyst :

If the Pseudocyst is shrinking, & in stable patients who are free of complications	***If the pseudocyst is expanding, or not responding to above treatment, or is complicated by rupture, hemorrhage or abscess formation.***
Conservative treatment is indicated.* Alternatively, a USG / CT guided single or repeated needle aspiration can be done.	Operative treatment is indicative Either external or preferably internal drainage of the cyst can be done

Percutaneous aspiration has emerged as a simple and frequently used initial procedure in the management of uncomplicated persistant pancreatic pseudocysts. However ***it cannot be termed as the treatment of choice. Surgical internal drainage in the form of cystojejunostomy continues to be the treatment of choice.***

Pseudopancreatic cyst:

Etiology :	**Site :**	**Diagnosis:**
Pancreatitis (90%)(Most common)[Q] *Trauma (10%)*[Q]	***85% are seen in body and tail*** *15% are seen in head*	*- Serum amylase level is elevated*[Q] *- Sonography is the investigation of choice*[Q] *- X-Ray : Pseudocysts may be localized, displacing some portion of git.*[Q]
Complications :	**Factors indicating possibility of hemorrhage**	
Pain due to expansion *Haemorrhage* *Rupture* Abscess	Increase in size *Localized brui over mass*[Q] *Sudden decrease in Hb or hematocrit*[Q]	
Management		
• *Pseudocyst > 5cm diameter is an indications for drainage*[Q] • Pseudocyst *less than 5 cm* in diameter and *less than 6 weeks old should be observed*[Q], as they tend to resolve spontaneously • *Initial management : US/CT guided, single or repeated needle aspirations* • Later : patients who do not respond to above modality are treated with surgical therapy preferred modality : *Internal drainage of cyst by cystojejunostomy.*[Q]		

Zollinger Ellison Syndrome

Zollinger Ellison Sydrome is characterized by unregulated secretion of gastrin leading to hypersecretion of gastric acid and the resulting manifestations.

'Gastrinomas' (non β cell tumour)[Q]
↓
Increased gastrin[Q] **secretion**
↓
Gastric acid hypersecretion[Q]
↓
Peptic ulceration[Q]
(And diarrhea)

Peptic ulceration[Q]

- ***Most common manifestation***, occuring in 90% of patient
- ***Most common site is duodenum (duodenal bulb)***
- **Clinical situations that raise special suspicion include :**
  a. *Ulcers beyond the duodenal bulb (second part of duodenum and beyond) because these are unusual locations for ulcers in Peptic ulcer diseases.*[Q]
  b. *Ulcers refractory to standard medical therapy*[Q]
  c. ***Ulcers are recurrent***[Q]
  d. *Ulcers presenting with frank complications.*[Q]

Diarrhea[Q]

- ***Is a common manifestation Q***
- ***Etiology is multifactorial, and it may have a secretory component*** *as well.*

Presenting symptom in order of frequency
• Abdominal pain (70-100%)
• Diarrhea (37-73%)
• Gastroesophageal reflux disease (GERD) (30-35 years)

Observations in patients with peptic ulcer disease that should suggest a diagnosis of ZES

Observation that should suggest the diagnosis
• *Peptic ulcer disease (PUD) with diarrhea*
• *PUD in an unusual location or with multiple lesions*
• *PUD that is refractory to treatment or persistent*
• *PUD that is associated with findings suggestive of MEN I*
• *PUD without H. pylori infection.*

Chronic unexplained diarrhea should also suggest gastrinoma

Diagnosis of Zollinger Ellison Syndrome

STEP I	Assess fasting gastrin level	Gastrin levels are increased
STEP II	Assess acid secretion : BAO estimation	BAO is increased ; BAO / MAO is increased
STEP III	Perform provocative test if required.	i.v. secretin induces substantial increase in serum gastrin.

Zollinger Elision syndrome is characterized by an increased basal gastric acid output. The ratio of BAO to MAO (maximal acid output) is increased.

Gastrin provocative tests *are used when acid secretory studies are not contributory* and include :

- *Secretin stimulation test*[Q]*: most sensitive and specific*[Q]
- Calcium infusion test
- Standard meal test

Secretin injection test is the most valuable provocative test in identifying patients with ZES

Histamine stimulation is not used and it does not bring about massive release of HCl in such patients.

Treatment of ZES

PPIs are the treatment of choice for Zollinger - Ellison Syndrome and have decreased the need for total gastrectomy.

Insulinomas

- *Insulinomas are endocrine tumors of pancreas derived from Beta cells* ectopically secrete Insulin and result in Hypoglycemia

Classic presentation of ***insulinoma*** : ***'Whipple's triad'***[Q] **:** *- Harrison 14th/589*
1. *Fasting hypoglycemia* [Q] 2 *Symptoms of hypoglycemia* [Q] 3. *Immediate relief after I.V. glucose administration* [Q]

- *They are generally small (>90% < 2 cm), usually single (90%) and usually benign (only 5-15% are malignant)*
- *The most common site of Insulinomas is the Pancreas.*

Insulinomas

Insulinomas are Endocrine tumors of the pancreas derived from Beta cells that ectopically secrete Insulin and result in Hypoglycemia

Average age of occurrence is 40-50 years

- *Generally Small* [Q] (>90% are < 2cm)
- *Usually single* [Q] (Not multiple in 90%)
- *Usually Benign* [Q] (5-15% are malignant)
- *Invariably occur in the pancreas* [Q] (Distributed equally in pancreatic Head, Body and Tail)

Symptoms due to Hypoglycemia

Most common symptoms are due to the effect of hypoglycemia on the central nervous system (Neuroglycemic Symptoms)

- Confusion
- Headache
- Disorientation
- Visual difficulties
- Irrational behavior (even coma)

Symptoms due to Excessive Catecholamine Release secondary to Hypoglycemia

- *Sweating*
- *Tremor*
- *Palpitation*

- *Insulinoma is characterised by an increase in weight (weight gain) and not by weight loss. Weight* ***gain may result from increased food ingested to combat symptoms of hypoglycemia.***

Diagnosis of Insulinomas

- *Diagnosis of Insulinoma requires demonstration of inappropriately high levels of plasma Insulin (and C-peptide) in the presence of documented hypoglycemia (Achieved by 72 hour fast test).*
- *Absolute values of Insulin or C- peptide are not reliable in establishing a diagnosis unless hypoglycemia is documented*
- ***The Gold standard test for diagnosis of Insulinoma is a supervised '72 hour fast' test***
  The '72 hour fast' test allows demonstration of hypoglycemia, together will elevated levels of Insulin and C-peptide and thus becomes the most reliable – gold standard test for establishing a diagnosis of Insulinoma

The '72 hour fast' test involves supervised fasting for upto 72 hours or until hypoglycemia can be documented *The test is considered positive if at any time when blood glucose levels drop to < 2.2mmol/l (40 mg/dl), the serum insulin levels are recorded to be greater than 6µU/ml. (and C- peptide levels > 100 pmol/l)*

Pancreatic Cholera (VIPoma; 'Verner – Morrison Syndrome' or 'WDHA Syndrome')

- *Pancreatic cholera is a Pancreatic endocrine tumor, most commonly of the Delta cells, characterized by net secretion of salt and water by gut*
- Pancreatic cholera **results from excessive secretion of VIP from endocrine tumors i.e. VIPomas**

'VIP' is an important neurotransmitter ubiquitously present in CNS and G.I. tract
Known actions of VIP explain most features of the clinical syndrome. These include :
- Stimulation of small intestinal chloride secretion
- Effects on smooth muscle contractility
- Inhibition of acid secretion
- Vasodilatory effects

- Pancreatic cholera is synonymous with 'Verner – Morrison Syndrome' or 'WDHA Syndrome'
- *Features of Pancreatic Cholera and/or WDHA Syndrome*

Features of Pancreatic cholera:
• *Severe watery diarrhea* [Q] / flushing / weight loss
• ***Hypokalemia*** [Q]
• ***Hypochlorhydria*** [Q]
• ***Hypercalcemia*** [Q] ***(not Hypocalcemia)***
• ***Hyperglycemia*** [Q]
• Inordinate fecal water and electrolyte loss

WDHA Syndrome
Watery **D**iarrhea
Hypokalemia
Achlorhydria

Various Endocrinal Tumors of Pancreas:

Pancreatic Endocrinal Tumor	***Biologically active Peptides secreted***
Zollinger Ellison Syndrome	*Gastrin*
VIPoma (Verner Morrison Syndrome, Pancreatic cholera, WDHA)	*VIP*
Glucagonoma	*Glucagon*
Insulinoma	*Insulin*
Somatostatinoma	*Somatostatin*
GRFoma	*Growth hormone releasing hormone*
ACTHoma	*ACTH*

QUESTIONS

Esophageal Conditions

Dysphagia (General / Differential Diagnosis):

1. A 30 year old female patient presents with non progressive dysphagia, for both solids and liquids. The charachteristic finding on baruim swallow that will confirm the probable diagnosis is: *(AI 2008)*
   A. Dilated esophagus with narrow lower end (Rat tail esophagus)
   B. Multiple sacculations and pseudodiverticulae (Corkscrew esophagus)
   C. Narrow and irregular esophageal lumen
   D. Stricture ulcer in the esophagus
2. A lady presented with non progressive dysphagia only for solids. Barium study showed proximal esophageal dilatation with distal constriction. The most likely diagnosis is. *(AI 2010)*
   A. Peptic Stricture
   B. Carcinoma Esophagus
   C. Achalasia Cardia
   D. Lower Esophageal Ring
3. A 40 year old female patient with dysphagia to both liquids and solids and regurgitation for 3 months. The dysphagia was non-progressive. What is the most likely diagnosis? *(AIIMS May 2006)*
   A. Carcinoma of the esophagus
   B. Lower oesophageal mucosal ring
   C. Achalasia cardia
   D. Reflux esophageal with esophageal stricture
4. Intermittent dysphagia is caused by (select two best options): *(PGI June 04)*
   A. Stricture
   B. Achalasia cardia
   C. Pharyngeal diverticulum
   D. Diffuse esophageal spasm
5. Investigation of choice for dysphagia for solids:
   A. Barium swallow *(PGI Dec 03)*
   B. Endoscopy
   C. X-ray chest
   D. C. T. scan
6. A patient present with dysphagia of 4 weeks duration. Now he is able to swallow liquid food only. Which of the following is the one investigation to be done:
   A. Barium studies are the best to be done
   B. Upper GI endoscopy is to be done
   C. CT scan is needed *(PGI June 2000)*
   D. Esophageal manometry
7. Dysphagia lusoria is due to: *(AIIMS Nov 03)*
   A. Oesophageal diverticulum
   B. Aneurysm of aorta
   C. Oesophageal web
   D. Compression by aberrant blood vessel
8. Non progressive contraction of Esophagus are:
   A. Primary *(AI 2009)*
   B. Secondary
   C. Tertiary
   D. Quaternary

Achalasia Cardia

9. True about achalasia cardia is (select two best options)
   A. Dysphagia is a presenting symptom
   B. The cause is the absence of Auerbach's plexus
   C. Esophagectomy is the treatment *(PGI June 02)*
   D. Motility-improving agents are used in treatment
   E. Barium swallow shows irregular filling defect in lower esophagus
10. In achalasia cardia, true is: *(PGI June 2000)*
    A. Pressure at distal end increased with no peristalsis
    B. Low pressure at LES with no peristalsis
    C. Pressure > 50 mmHg with peristalsis
    D. Pressure at the distal end increased with normal relaxation
11. A young patient with dysphagia more for liquids than solids. He regurgitates food often at night. Radiography shows a rat tailed appearance. Likely diagnosis is : *(AIIMS May 1996)*
    A. Achlasia cardia
    B. CA oesophagus
    C. Zenker's diverticulum
    D. Diffuse esophageal spasm
12. A young patient presents with history of dysphagia more to liquid than solids. The first investigation you will do is: *(AIIMS June 03)*
    A. Barium swallow
    B. Esophagoscopy
    C. Ultrasound of the chest
    D. C.T. scan of the chest
13. Heller's operation is done for: *(AIIMS Nov 93)*
    A. Achalasia cardia
    B. Pyloric stenosis
    C. Peptic ulcer
    D. CA Esophagus

Diffuse Esophageal Spasm

14. Diffuse esophageal spasm is best diagnosed by :
    A. Endoscopy *(AI 2008)*
    B. Manaometry
    C. Barium swallow
    D. CT
15. Corkscrew esophagus is seen in which of the following conditions? *(AI 2002)*

A. Carcinoma esophagus
B. Scleroderma
C. Achalasia cardia
D. Diffuse esophagus spasm

Zenker's Diverticulum

16. A male aged 60 years has foul breath; He regurgitates food that is eaten 3 days ago. A gurgling sound is often heard on swallowing : Likely diagnosis is: *(AI 2001)*
A. Zenkers diverticulum
B. Meckels diverticulum
C. Scleroderma
D. Achalasia cardia

17. All of the following statements about Zenker's diverticulum are true Except: *(AI 2009)*
A. Acquired diverticulum
B. Lateral X-rays on Barium swallow are often diagnostic
C. False Diverticulum
D. Out pouching of the anterior pharyngeal wall, just above the cricopharyngeus muscle.

18. A man aged 60 years presents with intermittent dysphagia & foul breath. He regurgitates food that is eaten few days ago: Likely diagnosis is:
A. Zenker's diverticulum *(AI 91)*
B. Meckel's diverticulum
C. Scleroderma
D. Achalasia cardia

19. Commonest complication of Zenker's diverticulum is: *(AIIMS Nov 96)*
A. Dysphonia
B. Gastroesophageal reflux
C. Lung abscess
D. Perforation

20. Which of the following is TURE about Zenker's diverticulum: *(AI 1995)*
A. It is asymptomatic
B. Occurs in the mid-esophagus
C. Treatment is simple excision
D. It occurs in children

Oesophageal Ring / Web

21. Schatazki's ring is: *(PGI Dec 98)*
A. Mucosal ring at squamous columnar junction
B. Muscular ring
C. Dysphagia is the presenting symptom
D. Inflammatory stricture

22. All are true regarding Plummer Vinson syndrome, ***except***: *(AIIMS Dec 97)*
A. Oesophageal web
B. Predisposes to malignancy
C. Koilonchia
D. Common in elderly males

Barret's Esophagus

23. Barret's esophagus is diagnosed by: *(AIIMS Nov 06)*
A. Squamous metaplasia
B. Intestinal metaplasia
C. Squamous dysplasia
D. Intestinal dysplasia

24. All except one are true regarding Barret's oesophagus: *(AIIMS Feb 97)*
A. More incidence of squamous cell carcinoma
B. Metaplasia
C. Columnar epithelium
D. Involves lower oesophagus

25. Barret's esophagus can lead to: *(AIIMS June 98)*
A. Stricture
B. Reflux esophagitis
C. Peptic ulcer
D. Achalasia

26. All of the following are true about Barret's esophagus, Except: *(PGI June 03)*
A. Consequence of prolonged GER
B. It is premalignant
C. Lower oesophageal mucosa is replaced by intestinal type of epithelium
D. Associated with oesophageal varices
E. Predisposes to adenocarcinoma

27. False about Barret's Esophagus is: *(PGI Dec 03)*
A. Premalignant conditions
B. Can be diagnosed by seeing under endoscope
C. Biopsy is necessary to confirm diagnosis
D. Stricture may be present in high esophagus
E. None

28. What is true regarding Barret's esophagus:
A. Seen in females *(AIIMS Nov 94)*
B. Premalignant
C. Responds to conservative management
D. Squamous metaplasia is seen

29. Barret's esophagus is commonly associated with one of the following: *(AIIMS May 06)*
A. Adenocarcinoma
B. Squamous cell carcinoma
C. Sarcoma
D. Gastrointestinal stromal tumor

Esophageal Carcinoma

30. Which of the following statements about Mallory Weiss Syndrome are true: *(PGI 2009)*
A. Presents with hemoptysis
B. Shows transmural rupture
C. Chest pain and shortness of breath
D. Shows mucosal tear

31. The most prevalent esophageal cancer world wide is:
A. Squamous cell ca *(AI 1991)*
B. Adenocarcinoma
C. Sarcoma
D. Adenoid cystic carcinoma

32. Most common site of carcinoma esophagus is: *(AIIMS Feb 97)*
A. Middle 1/3rd
B. Upper 1/3rd
C. Lower 1/3rd
D. Lower end of esophagus

33. Most common site for squamous cell carcinoma esophagus is: *(AI 01)*
A. Upper third
B. Middle third
C. Lower third
D. Gastro-esophageal junction

34. The most common site of esophageal adenocarcinoma is: *(AIIMS Nov 96, June 2000)*
A. Upper 1/3rd
B. Middle 1/3rd
C. Lower 1/3rd
D. Upper 2/3rd

35. The commonest site of carcinoma esophagus in India is: *(AIIMS Nov 03)*
A. Upper 1/3rd
B. Middle 1/3rd
C. Lower 1/3rd
D. GE Junction

36. The following are predisposing factors for Esophageal carcinoma ***except*** *(AI 1996)*
A. Plummer-Vinson syndrome
B. Tylosis palmaris
C. Chronic Achalasia
D. Benzene therapy

37. Hyperkeratosis of palm and sole is seen in: *(AIIMS Dec 97)*
A. Carcinoma colon
B. Hepatoma
C. Adenocarcinoma lung
D. Ca oesophagus

38. Esophageal adenocarcinoma is predisposed by (select two best options): *(PGI June 99)*
A. Achalasia
B. Scleroderma
C. Corrossive intake
D. Barrets esophagus

39. The adenocarcinoma of esophagus-develops in *(AI 2002)*
A. Barret's esophagus
B. Long standing achalasia
C. Corrosive structure
D. Alcohol abuse

40. Adenocarcinoma of esophagus is commonly found in *(AI 1998)*
A. Achlasia acardia
B. Barret's oesophagus
C. Plummer vinson syndrome
D. Chronic smoking

41. All of the following statements about Esophageal carcinoma are true, Except: *(PGI June 98, Dec 03)*
A. More common in Men
B. Adenocarcioma is on rise
C. Most common in elderly
D. Dysphagia is most common symptom
E. Pernicious anemia is a risk factor

42. Which neo-adjuvant chemotherapy is used in Esophageal carcinoma *(AI 1996)*
A. Cisplatin
B. Cyclophosphamide
C. Doxorubicin
D. Methotrexate

43. The commonest side effect of cisplatinum in a patient using it for esophageal carcinoma is :
A. Acute tubular necrosis
B. Thrombocytopenia *(AIIMS May 01)*
C. Hepatic failure
D. Cardiomyopathy

44. Best substitute of esophagus after esophagectomy is :
A. Stomach *(AI 1996)*
B. Jejunum
C. Left colon
D. Right colon

Stomach and Duodenum

Peptic Ulcer Disease & H. Pylori Infection

45. Peptic ulcer is associated with all except one:
A. Cirrhosis *(AIIMS Feb 1997)*
B. Zollinger Ellisons syndrome
C. Primary hyperparathyroidism
D. Pernicious anemia

46. Which one is not associated with peptic ulcer:
A. Smoking cigarette *(AIIMS Nov 95)*
B. Zollinger Ellison syndrome
C. Plummer Vinsons syndrome
D. Cirrhosis

47. All of the following are associated with Gastric Ulcer's Except: *(AI 1992)*
A. H. Pylori infection
B. High Acid output
C. Smoking
D. Bile Reflux

48. Stress ulcers seen in burns are: *(PGI Dec 2000)*
A. Curling's ulcer
B. Cushing's ulcer
C. Meleney's ulcer
D. Rodent ulcer

49. Helicobacter pylori is not associated with :
A. Gastrointestinal lymphoma *(AIIMS Nov 03)*
B. Gastric cancer
C. Gastric leiomyoma
D. Peptic ulcer

50. Endoscopic biopsy from a case of H.pylori related duodenal ulcer is most likely to reveal :
A. Antral predominant gastritis *(AIIMS Nov. 04)*

B. Multifocal atrophic gastritis
C. Acute erosive gastritis
D. Gastric atrophy

51. H. pylori is known to cause all of the following *except*: *(AI 1999)*
A. Gastric ulcer
B. Duodenal ulcer
C. Gastric lymphoma
D. Fundal atrophic gastritis

52. Diagnostic tests for H. Pylori include all of the following ***except*** : *(AI 1999)*
A. Urea-breath test
B. Rapid urease test
C. Gastric biopsy & Warthin-starry stain
D. SAFA test

53. Epidemiological studies of H. pylori are done by using: *(AI 1999)*
A. Urea-breath test
B. Serological markers
C. Culture
D. Gastric-biopsy urease test

54. Which of the following is False regarding H.Pylori infection : *(AIIMS June 2000)*
A. With chronic infection urease breath test become negative
B. H.Pylori infection remain lifelong if untreated
C. Endoscopy is diagnostic
D. Toxigenic strains usually causes ulcer

55. A patient with H. Pylori infection is treated with drugs. The best method to detect presence of residual H.Pylori infection in this person is : *(AI 2007)*
A. Rapid unrease test
B. Urea breath test
C. Endoscopy and biopsy
D. Serum anti H.Pylori titre

56. All are true regarding Helicobacter pylori ***except***:
A. Less prevalent in developing countries
B. Toxicogenic strains usually causes ulcers
C. Urea breath test is positive *(AIIMS Feb 97)*
D. Gram negative organism

57. Which of the following statements about peptic ulcer disease is true : *(AIIMS May 03)*
A. Helicobacter pylori eradication increases the likelihood of occurrence of complications.
B. The incidence of complications has remained unchanged
C. The incidence of Helicobacter pylori reinfection in India is very low.
D. Helicobacter pylori eradication does not alter the recurrence ratio.

58. Which drug is ***not*** effective against H. pylori:
A. Colloidal Bismuth *(AI 1995)*
B. Metronidazole
C. Amoxicillin
D. Erythromycin

59. All of the following drugs are commonly used in regimens against H. pylori except: *(AI 2008)*
A. Oxytetracycline
B. Amoxicillin
C. Bismuth Subcitrate
D. Omeprazole

60. All are used in treatment of Helicobactor pylori, EXCEPT: *(AIIMS Dec 97)*
A. Colloid bismuth
B. Cisapride
C. Clarithromycin
D. Metronidazole

61. Common sites for Cushing ulcers include all of the following ***except*** : *(AI 1999)*
A. Esophagus
B. Stomach
C. 1st part of duodenum
D. Distal duodenum

62. Commonest site of peptic ulcer is : *(AI 1999)*
A. Ist part of Duodenum
B. IInd part of duodenum
C. Distal 1/3 of stomach
D. Pylorus of the stomach

63. The most common site of a benign (peptic) gastric ulcer is: *(AIIMS June 04)*
A. Upper third of lesser curvature
B. Greater curvature
C. Pyloric antrum
D. Lesser curvature near incisura angularis

64. Most common complication of chronic gastric ulcer is: *(AIIMS June 93)*
A. Tea pot stomach
B. Scirrhous carcinoma (adenocarcinoma)
C. Perforation
D. Haemorrhage

65. Artery to bleed in duodenal ulcer haemorrhage:
A. Splenic artery *(PGI Dec 2000)*
B. Gastroduidenal artery
C. Left gastric artery
D. Superior mesenteric artery

66. A posteriorly perforating ulcer in the pyloric antrum of the stomach is most likely to produce initial localized peritonitis or abscess formation in the following: *(AI 2003)*
A. Omental bursa (lesser sac)
B. Greater sac
C. Right subphrenic space
D. Hepato renal space (pouch of Morison)

67. All of the following are true regarding a patient with acid peptic disease ***except*** *(AI 2001)*
A. Misoprostol is the drug of choice in patients on NSAIDS
B. DU is preventable by the use of single night time H2 blockers
C. Omeprazole may help ulcers refractory to H2 blockers
D. Misoprostol is DOC in pregnant patients

68. Surgery of choice for chronic duodenal ulcer is:
A. Vagotomy + antrectomy *(AIIMS June 93)*
B. Total gastrectomy
C. Truncal vagotomy + pyloroplasty
D. Highly selective vagotomy

69. Patient presents with recurrent duodenal ulcer of 2.5 cm size; procedure of choice *(AI 2001)*
A. Truncal vagotomy and antrectomy
B. Truncal vagotomy and gastrojejunostomy
C. Highly selective vagotomy
D. Laparoscopic vagotomy and gastrojejunostomy

70. The lowest recurrence of peptic ulcer is associated with *(AI 2002)*
A. Gastric resection
B. Vagotomy + drainage
C. Vagotomy + Antrectomy
D. Highly selective vagotomy

71. Dumping syndrome is due to: *(AI 1999)*
A. Diarrhoea
B. Presence of hypertonic content in small intestine
C. Vagotomy
D. Reduced gastric capacity

72. All are true regarding Early Post-cibal syndrome, except: *(AI 2000)*
A. Distension of abdomen
B. Managed conservatively
C. Hypermotility of intestine is common
D. Surgery is usually indicated

Gastric Outlet Obstruction

73. In gastric outlet obstruction in a peptic ulcer patient, the site of obstruction is most likely to be : *(AI 2002)*
A. Antrum
B. Duodenum
C. Pylorus
D. Pyloric canal

74. What is the most characteristic of congenital hypertrophic pyloric stenosis: *(AI 2003)*
A. Affects the first born female child
B. The pyloric tumour is best felt during feeding
C. The patient is commonly marasmic
D. Loss of appetite occurs early

75. What is true regarding congenital hypertrophic pyloric stenosis : *(AI 2001)*
A. More common in girls
B. Hypochloremic alkalosis
C. Hellers myotomy is the procedure of choice.
D. Most often manifests at birth

76. In a case of hypertrophic pyloric stenosis, the metabolic disturbance is *(AI 2002)*
A. Respiratory alkalosis
B. Metabolic acidosis
C. Metabolic alkalosis with paradoxical aciduria
D. Metabolic alkalosis with alkaline urine

77. Metabolic changes associated with excessive vomitting includes the following: *(AI 1999)*
A. Metabolic acidosis
B. Hyperchloremia
C. Hypokalemia
D. Decreases bicarbonates

78. Patient with pyloric stenosis secondary to peptic ulcer, complains of profuse vomiting and Na^+ - 125meq/L, K^+ --> 2.3 meq/L and Cl^- --> 85 meq/L, BE-8meq/L should be given. *(AIIMS June 2000)*
A. Half normal saline
B. Normal saline
C. K_+ bolus
D. Hypertonic saline

Menetrier's disease

79. All are true regarding Menetrier's disease, EXCEPT:
A. Protein loss *(AIIMS Dec 94)*
B. Exophytic growth
C. Hypertrophy of gastric mucosa
D. Premalignant condition

80. All of the following statements about Menetrier's disease are true Except:
A. It is a premalignant condition
B. Usually increased acid secretion
C. May be confused with Zollinger Ellison Syndrome
D. Associated with Protein losing enteropathy

Carcinoma Stomach

81. Risk factor for development of gastric Ca :
A. Blood group O *(AI 2002)*
B. Duodenal ulcer
C. Intestinal hyperplasia
D. Intestinal metaplasia type III

82. Premalignant conditions of stomach include all, Except:
A. Gastric ulcer
B. Pernicious anemia and achlorhydria
C. Hiatus Hernia
D. Atrophic gastritis

83. Predisposing cause for carcinoma stomach are except:
A. Chronic gastric atrophy *(PGI Dec 97)*
B. Hyperplastic polyp
C. Intestinal Metaplasia grade III
D. Pernicious anemia

84. Risk factor for carcinoma stomach include all of the following, Except: *(PGI June 2000)*
A. Blood group A
B. Atrophic Gastritis
C. Duodenal Peptic ulcer
D. Partial Gastrectomy

85. Which one of the following is the most significant risk factor for development of gastric carcinoma? *(AI 2006)*
A. Paneth cell metaplasia
B. Pyloric metaplasia
C. Intestinal metaplasia
D. Ciliated metaplasia

86. Most common site for carcinoma stomach is: *(AIIMS June 93)*
A. Antrum
B. Fundus
C. Lesser curvature
D. Greater curvature

87. When carcinoma of stomach develops secondarily to pernicious anemia, it is usually situated in the: *(AI 2006)*
A. Prepyloric region
B. Pylorus
C. Body
D. Fundus

88. Early gastric cancer generally indicates : *(AIIMS May 1996)*
A. Gastric adencarcinoma detected early
B. Gastric adenocarcinoma confined to the mucosa
C. Gastric adenocarcinoma confined to the mucosa & submucosa
D. Gastric adenocarcinoma less than 1 cm. In size

89. All the following indicates early gastric cancer ***except*** *(AI 2002)*
A. Involvement of mucosa
B. Involvement of mucosa and submucosa
C. Involvement of mucosa, submucosa and muscularis
D. Involvement of mucosa, submucosa and adjacent lymph nodes

90. The best prognosis in carcinoma stomach is with: *(AI 1995)*
A. Superficial spreading type
B. Ulcerative type
C. Linitis plastica type
D. Polypoidal fungating type

91. An adult presented with hemetemesis and upper abdominal pain. Endoscopy revealed a growth at the pyloric antrum of the stomach. CT scan showed growth involving the pyloric antrum without infiltration or invasion into surrounding structures and no evidence of distant metastasis. At Laparotomy neoplastic growth was observed to involve the posterior wall of stomach and the pancreas extending 6cm up to tail of pancreas. What will be the most appropriate surgical management: *(AI 2010)*
A. Closure of the abdomen
B. Antrectomy and vagotomy
C. Partial Gastrectomy + Distal pancreatectomy
D. Partial Gastrectomy + Distal pancreatectomy + splenectomy

92. Amongst the following, the most common site for Leiomyoma is *(AI 1994)*
A. Stomach
B. Small Intestine
C. Duodenum
D. Colon

Malabsorption Syndrome and Disorders of Small Intestine

General

93. Which of the following is not a malabsorption syndrome *(DNB June 2009)*
A. Whipple's disease
B. Coeliac disease
C. Tropical sprue
D. Tangier's disease

94. Non absorbtion of fat soluble vitamins is due to: *(DNB 2009)*
A. Steatorrhea
B. Pancreatic endocrine insufficiency
C. Both
D. None

95. Test for assessment of mucosal function of GIT: *(AI 2009)*
A. D-xylose test
B. Small bowel study
C. Biopsy
D. Schilling test

96. Positive D – xylose test indicates all of the following, Except: *(AI 1992)*
A. Pancreatic insufficiency
B. Small intestinal mucosal disease
C. Impaired carbohydrate absorption in small intestine
D. Malabsorption

97. A 41 year old patient presented with chronic diarrhoea for 3 months. A d-xylose absorption test was ordered to look for: *(AIIMS Nov 02)*
A. Carbohydrate malabsorption due to mucosal disease.
B. Carbohydrate malabsorption due to chronic pancreatitis
C. Fat malabsorption due to mucosal disease.
D. Fat malabsorption due to chronic pancreatitis.

98. Best test for Small intestine malabsorption of carbohydrates is : *(AI 1997)*
A. Lund meal test :
B. Shilling test
C. D-Xylose test
D. Follacin test

99. A d-xylose test was requested on a patient with history of long standing steatorrhea '5' hour urine sample showed <4.0 gm excretion after giving 25 gm of d-xylose. The most likely diagnosis is : *(PGI 09)*
A. Chronic Pancreatitis
B. Bacterial overgrowth syndrome
C. Ileal disease
D. Celiac sprue
E. Intestinal Lymphangiectasia

100. Cause of False positive D-xylose test include all of the following, Except *(PGI 01)*

A. Bacterial overgrowth
B. Renal failure
C. Ascitis
D. Celiac sprue
E. Blind loop syndrome

101. False positive D-xylose test may be seen in (PGI June 01)
A. Blind loop syndrome
B. Ascitis
C. Antibiotic therapy
D. Pyloric stenosis
E. All of the above

102. Which of the following statements about Schilling's test are true: (PGI 2009)
A. Abnormal in pernicious anemia
B. Normal in bacterial overgrowth syndrome
C. Abnormal in ileal disease
D. Normal in chronic pancreatitis

103. A 12 year old girl has history of recurrent bulky stolls and abdominal pain since 3 year of age. She has moderate pallor and her weight and height are below the 3rd percentile. Which of the following is the most appropriate investigation to make a specific diagnosis? (AI India/AIIMS)
A. Small intestinal biopsy
B. Barium studies
C. 24-hr- fecal fat estimation
D. Urinary d-xylose test

104. Serum amylase level is raised in all except: (PGI June 98)
A. Blocked salivary duct
B. Ruptured ectopic
C. Appendicitis
D. Pancreatitis

Celiac Disease

105. A 30 year old lady presents with features of malabsorption and iron deficiency anaemia. Duodenal biopsy shows complete villous atrophy. Which of the following antibodies is likely to be present : (AIIMS Nov. 05)
A. Antiendomysial antibodies
B. Anti-goblet cell antibodies
C. Anti-saccharomyces cerevisae antibodies
D. Antineutrophil cytoplasmic antibodies

106. 30 year male with chronic diarrhoea, anemia, raised liver enzymes. Most likely associated with: (AIIMS May 07)
A. Antimitochondrial antibody
B. Anti-endomysial antibody
C. Anti-smooth muscle antibody
D. Antinuclear antibody

107. A patient presents with chronic small bowel diarrhea, duodenal biopsy shows villous atrophy. Anti endomysial antibodies and IgA TTG antibodies are positive. What is the treatment of choice? (AI 2007)
A. Gluten free diet
B. Antibiotics
C. Loperamide
D. 5-ASA

108. Which of the following circulating antibodies has the best sensitivity and specificity for the diagnosis of celiac disease? (AIIMS May 06)
A. Anti-endomysial antibody
B. Anti-tissue transglutaminase antibody
C. Anti-gliadin antibody
D. Anti-reticulin antibody

109. The histological features of coeliac disease include all of the following, ***except*** : (AI 2002)
A. Crypt hyperplasia
B. Increase in thickness of the mucosa
C. Increase in intraepithelial lymphocytes
D. Increase in inflammatory cells in lamina propyria

110. Biopsy findings of celiac disease all of the following, except (Select two best options) : (PGI 09)
A. Crypt hyperplasia
B. Villous atrophy
C. Mucosal atrophy
D. Intraepithelial lymphocytes
E. Presence of Giardia lambia

111. Proved association of celiac sprue is with: (PGI Dec 2000)
A. Dermatitis herpetiformis
B. Scleroderma
C. Pemphigus
D. Pemphoid

112. Celiac disease associated with: (PGI Dec 06)
A. Dermatitis herpetiformis
B. Type I DM
C. Lymphoma
D. Atrophic gastritis
E. All of the above

113. Celiac sprue diagnosed by (select two options): (PGI Dec 02)
A. Intestinal biopsy
B. Unequivocal response to gluten restriction
C. Finding of organism
D. Improvement on dapsone treatment
E. H/O fat malabsorption

114. Which of the following grains can be used safely in patients with celiac sprue: (PGI Dec 01)
A. Rice
B. Wheat
C. Rye
D. Barley

115. What a patient with gluten hypersensitivity can consume (select two best options): (PGI Dec 06)
A. Rice
B. Barley
C. Oat
D. Corn
E. Rye

116. Which of the following vitamin deficiencies is uncommon in celiac disease (DNB Dec 2009)
A. Vitamin D
B. Folic Acid
C. Vitamin A
D. Vitamin B_{12}

Whipple's Disease

117. In which of the following conditions of malabsorption, an intestinal biopsy is diagnostic-: *(AIIMS May 05)*
   A. Celiac disease
   B. Tropical sprue
   C. Whipple's disease
   D. Lactose intolerance
118. Macrophages containing large quantities of undigested and partial digested bacteria in intestine are seen in *(AI 2002)*
   A. Whipple's disease
   B. Amyloidosis
   C. Immunoapproliferative small instetinal disease
   D. Vibro cholerae infection
119. Histopathological findings in Whipple's disease include all of the following Except: *(AI 2008)*
   A. Marked increase in the number of macrophages in the mucosa
   B. Marked increase in the number of intraepethelial lymphocytes
   C. Dilatation of Lymphatics in the mucosa
   D. Lipid deposition in the mucosa
120. Most common CNS manifestation of Whipple's disease is : *(AI 1999)*
   A. Cerebellar ataxia
   B. Supranuclear ophthalmoplegia
   C. Seizure
   D. Dementia
121. Which of the following parastitic infestation can lead to malabsorption syndrome? *(AI 06)*
   A. Amoebiasis
   B. Ascariasis
   C. Hookworm infestation
   D. Giardiasis

Short Bowel Syndrome

122. The short bowel syndrome is characterized by all of the following ***except*** : *(AI 2004)*
   A. Diarrhea
   B. Hypogastrinemia
   C. Weight loss
   D. Steatorrhoea
123. All are complication of ileal resection, ***except*** : *(AIIMS June 97)*
   B. Megaloblastic anaemia
   C. Iron deficiency anaemia
   D. Gastric hypersecretion
   E. Malabsorption syndrome
124. Deficiency of which of the following vitamin is most commonly seen in short bowel syndrome with ileal resection: *(AI 2012)*
   A. Vitamin B12 (Cyanocobalamine)
   B. Vitamin B1 (Thiamine)
   C. Folic Acid
   D. Vitamin K
125. Which of the following vitamin deficiencies is most commonly seen in short bowel syndrome: *(AI 2012)*
   A. Vitamin B12
   B. Biotin
   C. Vitamin B1
   D. Vitamin K

Intestinal Angina

126. "Intestinal angina" is a symptom complex of the following: *(AIIMS May 06)*
   A. Postprandial abdominal pain, weight loss, acute mesenteric vessel occlusion
   B. Postprandial abdominal pain, weight loss, chronic mesenteric vessel occlusion
   C. Pre-prandial abdominal pain, weight loss, chronic mesenteric vessel occlusion
   D. Pre-prandial abdominal pain, weight gain acute mesenteric vessel occlusion

Inflammatory Bowel Disease

Ulcerative Colitis

127. A 20 year old male presents with mucus and repeated gastrointestinal bleeding. Patient is positive for ANCA. The most likely diagnosis is:
   A. Ulcerative colitis
   B. Crohn's disease
   C. Radiation colitis
   D. Ischemic bowel disease
128. A 25 year old male presents with a history of chronic diarrhea. Pathological examination reveals cryptitis and crypt abscesses. The likely diagnosis is: *(AI 2008)*
   A. Crohn's disease
   B. Ulcerative colitis
   C. Giardiasis
   D. Microscipic colitis
129. Toxic megacolon is most commonly associated with *(AI 1996)*
   A. Ulcerative colitis
   B. Crohn's disease
   C. Whipple's disease
   D. Reiter's disease
130. Pseudopolyps are features of *(AI 1994)*
   A. Crohn's disease
   B. Ulcerative colitis
   C. Celiac sprue
   D. Whipple's disease
131. Pseudopolyps are typically seen in: *(DNB Dec 2009)*
   A. Crohn's disease
   B. Ulcerative colitis
   C. Celiac disease
   D. Tropical sprue
132. What is drug of choice for ulcerative colitis : *(AIIMS May 95) (AIIMS Feb 97)*
   A. Salazopyrine
   B. Pedinisolone
   C. Mercaptopurine
   D. 5-amino salicylic acid

133. A 41 year old male patient presented with recurrent episodes of bloody diarrhea & mucus for 5 years. Despite regular treatment with adequate doses of sulfasalazine, he has had several exacerbations of his disease and required several weeks of steroids for the control for flares. What should be the next line of treatment for him? *(AIIMS Nov 03)*
A. Methotrexate
B. Azathioprine
C. Cyclosporine
D. Cyclophosphamide

134. Drug effective in ulcerative colitis is: *(AIIMS Feb 97)*
A. 5 amino salicylic acid (5-ASA)
B. Steroids
C. Salazopyrin
D. Antibiotics

Crohn's Disease

135. Skip granulomatous lesions are seen in : *(AI 1996)*
A. Ulcerative colitis
B. Crohn's disease
C. Whipple's disease
D. Reiter's disease

136. A patient gives chronic history of Diarrhoea and blood in stool presents with multiple fistulae in the perineum and multiple stricture in small intestine. The diagnosis is: *(AIIMS June 2000)*
A. Crohn's disease
B. Radiation enteritis
C. Ulcerative Colitis
D. Ischemic bowel disease

137. The presence of anti-*Saccharomyces cerevisae* antibody is a surrogate marker of one of the following: *(AI 2006)*
A. Celiac disease
B. Crohn's disease
C. Ulcerative colitis
D. Tropical sprue

138. Crohn's disease may be caused by which one of the following infectious agents: *(AI 2008)*
A. Clostridium difficle
B. Mycobacterium paratuberculosis
C. Cytomegalo virus (CMV)
D. Mycoplasma

139. Extraintestinal manifestations of Inflammatory bowel disease include all of the following, Except: *(PGI June 05)*
A. Uveitis
B. Sclerosing cholangitis
C. Osteoarthritis
D. Skin nodules

140. A 25 yrs women presents with bloody diarrhea & is diagnosed as a case of Ulcerative colitis. Which of the following condition is not associated : *(AI 2002)*
A. Sclerosing cholengitis
B. Iritis
C. Ankylosing spondylitis
D. Pancreatitis

Colonic Disorders

Irritable Bowel Syndrome (IBS)

141. Which one of the following is *not* a feature of irritable bowel syndrome? *(AIIMS May 05)*
A. Abdominal pain
B. Constipation
C. Rectal bleeding
D. Bloating

142. Which of the following features are associated with Irritable Bowel Syndrome: *(AI 1992)*
A. Weight loss
B. Anorexia
C. Abdominal distension
D. Blood in stool

143. A young girl presents with abdominal pain and a recent change in bowel habit, with passage of mucus in stool. There is no associated blood in stool and symptoms are increased with stress. The most likely diagnosis is. *(AI 2010)*
A. Irritable bowel syndrome
B. Ulcerative Colitis
C. Crohn's disease
D. Amebiasis

144. All of the following statements about Irritable Bowel syndrome are true, except: *(PGI)*
A. Associated with anxiety
B. Stress predisposes
C. Constipation
D. Diarrhea
E. Predisposes to malignancy in long term

145. Which of the following drugs is used for Irritable Bowel Syndrome of the constipating type: *(AI 2012)*
A. Lubiprostone
B. Cholestyramine
C. Alosetron
D. Rifaximin

Diarrhea and Colitis

146. Which of the following organism does not cause invasive diarrhea *(DNB June 2009)*
A. Bacillus cereus
B. Aeromonas sp
C. Rota virus
D. Shigella

147. Secretory Diarrhea is caused by all of the following, Except: *(PGI June 07)*
A. Cholera
B. Laxatives
C. Excess phenolphthalein intake
D. Clostridium difficle

148. Features of secretory diarrhea include all of the following, Except: *(AI 2009)*

A. Stool volume > 1D /day
B. Normal osmotic anion gap
C. Reduces with fasting
D. Painless

149. Indications for use of antibiotics in acute diarrhea include (select three options): *(PGI June 07)*
A. Febrile dysentery with fever ≥ 38.5
B. Immunocompromised patient
C. Elderly patient
D. Dehydration

150. A 14-year-old girl with history of prolonged fever and abdominal discomfort is observed to have splenomegaly and leucopenia. In the course of the disease she develops acute abdominal event and died. Which of the following is the likely finding on autopsy: *(AI 2012)*
A. Transverse ulcers
B. Longitudinal ulcers
C. Pinpoint ulcers
D. Pseudopolyps

151. A patient present with lower gastrointestinal bleed. Sigmoidoscopy shows ulcers in the sigmoid. Biopsy from this area shows flask-shaped ulcers. Which of the following is the most appropriate treatment : *(AIIMS Nov. 05)*
A. Intravenous ceftriaxone
B. Intravenous mentronidazole
C. Intravenous steroids and sulphasalazine
D. Hydrocortscone enemas

152. Investigation of choice for invasive amebiasis is: *(AI 02)*
A. Indirect heamagglutination
B. ELISA
C. Counter immune electrophoresis
D. Microscopy

153. Features of Typhoid Ulcers include all of the following Except: *(DNB)*
A. Bleeding
B. Perforation
C. Stricture and obstruction
D. Longitudinal orientation

154. A patient with leukemia on chemotherapy develops acute right lower abdominal pain associated with anemia, thrombocytopenia and leukopenia. Which of following is the clinical diagnosis? *(AI 2006)*
A. Appendictis
B. Leukemic colitis
C. Perforation peritonitis
D. Neutropenic colitis

Colorectal Carcinomas

155. The most pre-cancerous condition for carcinoma colon is *(AI 1995)*
A. Familial polyposis
B. Hamartomatous polyps
C. Juvenile polyps
D. Hyperplastic polyps

156. Strong correlation with colorectal cancer is seen in:
A. Peutz-Jegher's polyp *(AI 2003)*
B. Familial polyposis coli.
C. Juvenile polyposis
D. Hyperplastic polyp.

157. Which of the following colonic polyps is not pre-malignant? *(AI 2006)*
A. Juvenile polyps
B. Hamartomatous polyps associated with Peutz-Jeghers Syndrome
C. Villous adenomas
D. Tubular adenomas

158. Which one of the following conditions commonly predisposes to Colonic carcinoma? *(AI 2005)*
A. Ulcerative colitis.
B. Crohn's disease.
C. Diverticular disease.
D. Ischaemic colitis.

159. A 25-year old male had pigmented macules over the palm, sole and oral mucosa. He also had anemia and pain in abdomen. The most probable diagnosis is:
A. Albright's syndrome *(AIIMS May 05)*
B. Cushing's syndrome
C. Peutz-Jegher's syndrome
D. Incontinentia pigmenti

160. A patient presents with malena, hyperpigmentation over lips, oral mucosa and skin; and his sister is also having similar complaints. The diagnosis is :
A. Peutz Jegher's Syndrome *(AI 2000)*
B. Familial Adenomatous Polyposis
C. Gardner's Syndrome
D. Villous Adenoma

161. In Peutz-Jeghers syndrome, polyps are seen in
A. Colon *(AI 1995)*
B. Rectum
C. Small bowel
D. Stomach

162. A girl presents with complaints of malena. On examination there are pigmented lesions involving her mouth and lips. Two of her sisters also had similar complaints. Which of the following is the most probable diagnosis: *(AIIMS Nov 2000)*
A. Kornkhite Canada syndrome
B. Puetz Jegher's syndrome
C. Gardner's syndrome
D. Turcot's syndrome

163. Most important prognostic factor for colorectal carcinoma is : *(AI 2009)*
A. Site of lesion
B. Stage of lesion

C. Age of patient
D. Lymph node status

164. After undergoing surgery, for Carcinoma of colon a patient developed single liver metastatis of 2cm. What you do next : *(AI 2002)*
A. Resection
B. Chemo radiation
C. Acetic acid injection
D. Radio frequency ablation

165. A patient was operated for colonic carcinoma and later a solitary nodule was found in the liver Treatment of choice is : *(AI 1998)*
A. Surgery
B. Radiation
C. Chemotherapy
D. Conservative treatment

166. A 50-year old male, working as a hotel cook, has four dependent family members. He has been diagnosed with an early stage squamous cell cancer of anal canal. He has more than 60% chances of cure. The best treatment option is:
A. Abdomino-perineal resection *(AI 2003)*
B. Combined surgery and radiotherapy
C. Combined chemotherapy and radiotherapy
D. Chemotherapy alone

167. All of the following genes may be involved in development of carcinoma of colon Except: *(AI 2009)*
A. APC
B. Beta – Catenin
C. K- ras
D. Mismatch Repair Genes

168. Based on Epidemiological studies, which of the following has been found to be most protective against Carcinoma Colon : *(AI 2009)*
A. High fiber diet
B. Low fat diet
C. Low selenium diet
D. Low protein diet

Pancreatic Disorders

Pancreatitis

169. All the following are causes of Acute Pancreatitis *except*: *(AI 1994)*
A. Gall stones
B. Alcohol
C. Hemochromatosis
D. Hypercalcemia

170. Increased amylase may be seen in all of the following *except* : *(AI 1997)*
A. Pancreatic pseudocyst
B. Appendicitis
C. Perforated peptic ulcer
D. Ruptured ectopic pregnancy

171. Raised serum amylase levels are used to diagnose
A. Autoimmune disease *(AIIMS May 04)*
B. Degenerative diseases
C. Acute cholecystitis
D. Acute pancreatitis

172. Ranson's critaria for prognosis in acute pancreatitis include all *except* : *(AI 1998)*
A. WBC>16,000 cells/cumm
B. Age over 55 years
C. AST > 250 U/100 ml
D. S. amylase > 350 I.U.

173. Which of the following is not a prognostic factor for Acute Pancreatitis *(AIIMS Nov. 06)*
A. Serum Amylase
B. Serum Calcium
C. Serum Glucose
D. Serum AST

174. Which one is not the bad prognostic sign for pancreatitis: *(AIIMS June 2000)*
A. TLC > 16000
B. Calcium less than 8 mmom/L
C. Glucose > 200mg%
D. Prothrombin > 2 times the control

175. Which one is not poor prognostic factor for acute pancreatitis: *(AIIMS Nov 99)*
A. Hyperglycemia
B. Hypocalcemia
C. Raised LDH level in blood
D. Hyperamylasemia

176. Monu, a 30 year old male, a chronic alcoholic presents with sudden onset of epigastric pain that radiates to the back. All are seen Except:
A. Low serum lipase *(AIIMS June 01)*
B. Increased LDH
C. Hypocalcemia
D. Increased serum amylase

177. Definitive laboratory diagnosis of acute pancreatitis is done by: *(AI 1993)*
A. Serum Amylase
B. Serum Lipase
C. Hyperglycemia
D. Hypercalcemia

178. The most specific laboratory test to establish a diagnosis of acute pancreatitis is: *(PGI 08)*
A. Serum amylase
B. Serum lipase
C. Serum Alkaline phosphatase
D. Serum Calcium
E. Serum glucose

179. Cause of acute loss of vision in a patient of alcoholic pancreatitis is: *(AI 95)*
A. Purtscher's retinopathy
B. Sudden alcohol withdrawal
C. Acute congestive glaucoma
D. CRAO

180. Cause of acute loss of vision in a patient of alcoholic pancreatitis is: *(AI 1995, 2000)*

A. Purtscher's retinopathy (*AIIMS-99*)
B. Sudden alcohol withdrawal
C. Acute congestive glaucoma
D. CRAO

181. Which of the following types of pancreatitis has the best prognosis? (*AI 2004*)
A. Alcoholic pancreatitis
B. Gall stone pancreatitis
C. Post operative pancreatitis
D. Idiopathic pancreatitis

182. Medical treatment of pancreatitis includes :
A. Cholestyramine (*AIIMS May 94*)
B. Aprotinin
C. Calcium
D. Glucagon

183. Most common complication of acute pancreatitis is:
A. Pancreatic abscess (*AIIMS May 95*)
B. Pseudocyst
C. Phlegmon
D. Pleural effusion

184. Pancreatic pseudocyst most commonly occurs after
A. Trauma (*AI 1994*)
B. Pancreatitis
C. Pancreatic surgery
D. Pancreatic malignancy

185. All are ture about pseudopancreatic cyst of pancreas *except* : (*AI 1998*)
A. Common after acute pancreatitis
B. Presents as an abdominal mass
C. Serum amylase is increased
D. Most common site is in head of pancreas

186. All of the following statements about Pseudopancreatic cysts are true *except* : (*AI 1997*)
A. Percutaneous aspiration is treatment of choice
B. Cystojejunostomy is treatment of choice
C. Serum amylase levels are increased
D. Presents as an epigastric mass

Endocrinal Tumors of Pancreas

187. Which of the following is NOT secreted in pancreatic tumour : (*AIIMS Sep 96*)
A. VIP
B. Insulin
C. Somatostatin
D. ACTH

188. Zollinger-Ellison syndrome is characterized by all of the following *except* (*AI 1994*)
A. Post bulbar ulcer
B. Recurrent duodenal ulcer
C. Severe diarrhea
D. Massive HCL in response to histamine injection

189. The triad originally described by Zollinger Ellison syndrome is characterized by: (*AI 2002*)
A. Peptic ulceration, gastric hypersecretion, non beta cell tumour
B. Peptic ulceration, gastric hypersecretion, beta cell tumour
C. Peptic ulceration, achlorhydria, non beta cell tumour
D. Peptic ulceration, achlorhydria, beta cell tumour

190. All are true regarding Zollinger Ellison syndrome, *except:* (*AIIMS Dec 97*)
A. Diarrhoea
B. Recurrence after operation
C. Hypergastrinemia
D. Decreased ratio of BAO to MAO

191. Most important investigation for diagnosis of Zollinger Ellison-syndrome is : (*AI 1999*)
A. Ca^{++} infusion test
B. Secretin injection test
C. ACTH stimulation test
D. Steroid assay

192. Drug of choice in Zollinger Ellison syndrome is
A. Ranitidine (*AIIMS May 95*)
B. Omeprazole
C. Antacids
D. B-blocker

193. Treatment of choice for ZES :
A. PPI (*AI 2007*)
B. Somatostatin analogues
C. Streptozocin
D. Sucralfate

194. Gold standard test for diagnosis of Insulinoma is :
A. '72 hour' fast test (*AI 2009*)
B. Plasma Glucose levels < 3 mmol/l
C. Plasma Insulin levels > 6μU/ml
D. C- peptide levels < 50 p mol/e

195. All of the following statements about Insulinoma are true Except: (*AI/AIIMS*)
A. Most commonly found in 'Pancreas'
B. Usually Benign
C. Usually multiple
D. Derived from Beta cells

196. Which of the following statements about Insulinoma is true: (*AIIMS*)
A. Present in Pancreas
B. Mostly malignant
C. Surgery is usually not required
D. Usually multiple

197. Weight loss may be seen in all of the following *except* : (*AI 1998*)
A. Uremia
B. Pheochromacytoma
C. Adrenal insufficiency
D. Insulinoma

198. All of the following about Gastrointestinal Carcinoid tumors are true, Except: (*AI 2010*)
A. Small intestine and appendix account for almost 60% of all gastrointestinal carcinoid.
B. Rectum is spared
C. 5 year survival for carcinoid tumors is >60%

D. Appendicial carcinoids are more commin in females than males.

199. Pancreatic cholera is characterized by ***all except:*** *(AI 1996)*
A. Hypochlorhydria
B. Hypokalemia
C. Glucose intolerance
D. Hypocalcemia

200. Which of the following statements about Pancreatic Carcinoma is not true : *(AI 2009)*
A. Mutation in P^{53} gene is associated in 75% of cases
B. Hereditary Pancreatitis significantly increases the risk
C. Median survival in locally advanced (stage III) disease is 3- 6 months
D. Five year survival after curative pancreaticoduodenectomy is 15 – 20%

Cystic Fibrosis

201. Which of the following statements about Cystic fibrosis (CF) is not true: *(AI 2009)*
A. Autosomal Recessive Disorder
B. Abnormality in CFTR which leads to defective Calcium Transport
C. Predisposition to pulmonary infection with Pseudomonas
D. Cirrhosis is an established complication of CF

202. A seven year old child with recurrent chest infections and exocrine pancreatic insufficiency is suspected of having cystic fibrosis Sweat chloride levels have been observed between 40-60 mmol/l on two separate occasions. Which of the following test should be performed next to support the diagnosis of Cystic fibrosis: *(AI 2009)*
A. Repeat Sweat chloride levels on a different day
B. Demonstrate an abnormal nasal potential difference
C. Demonstrate an abnormal F508 mutation by DNA analysis
D. Demonstrate an abnormal 72 hour fecal fat collection

Miscellaneous

203. Non invasive diarrhea is caused by: *(AI 2009)*
A. Shigella
B. B. Cereus
C. Salmonella
D. Y. enterocolitica

204. Features of secretory diarrhea include all of the following, Except: *(AI 2009)*
A. Stool volume > 1L /day
B. Normal osmotic anion gap
C. Reduces with fasting
D. Painless

205. A patient on treatment with ketoconazole for a fungal disease develops Gastroesophageal Reflux Disease (GERD). Which of the following drugs should not be prescibed to him: *(AI 2012)*
A. Cisapride
B. Itopride
C. Metoclopramide
D. Domperidone

206. Which of the following is the commonest cause of lower GI bleed: *(PGI Dec 04)*
E. Angiodysplasia
F. Enteric fever
G. Diverticulosis
H. Colonic polyps
I. Hemorrhoids

207. An elderly patient presents with a prolonged history of weakness and lethargy. On examination he is found to be anemic and stool is positive for occult blood. Which of the following is the investigation of choice: *(AI 2010)*
A. Colonoscopy
B. Barium meal
C. Barium enema
D. CT abdomen

208. Massive bleeding per rectum in a 70 yr old patient is due to : *(AI 2000)*
A. Diverticulosis
B. Carcinoma colon
C. Colitis
D. Polyps

209. A man aged 60 yrs has h/o IHD and atherosclerosis. He presents with abdominal pain and maroon stools: likely diagnosis here is: *(AI 2001)*
A. Acute intestinal obstruction
B. Acute mesenteric ischemia
C. Peritonitis
D. Appendicitis

210. Intestinal hypomotility is seen in all the following ***except:*** *(AI 1995)*
A. Diabetes
B. Parkinsonism
C. Amyloidosis
D. All of the above

211. The most common cause of seizures in children with diarrhea is: *(DNB 2009)*
A. Hypokalemia
B. Hyperkalemia
C. Hyponatremia
D. Hypernatremia

212. All of the following statements stand true for telengiectasia of colon ***except*** : *(AI 1998)*
A. May be seen in person less than 40 years of age
B. May be seen in person more than 60 years of age
C. Common site is caecum
D. 50% involve rectum

213. Hypergastrinemia with hypochlorhydria is seen in: *(AI 2002)*
   A. Zollinger Ellison Syndrome
   B. VIPoma
   C. Pernicious anemia
   D. Glucagonoma

214. Hypergastrinemia with hypochlorhydria is seen in: *(AI 2002)*
   A. Zollinger Ellison Syndrome
   B. VIPoma
   C. Pernicious anemia
   D. Glucagonoma

215. A young patient presenting with massive hematemesis was found to have splenomegaly. In this case the most likely source of bleeding is: *(AI)*
   A. Duodenal ulcer
   B. Esophageal varices
   C. Erosive mucosal disease
   D. Gastric ulcer

216. All of the following statements about Mucosa Associated Lymphoid Tissue Lymphomas (MALT) are true, Except: *(PGI June 05)*
   A. Present at extranodal sites
   B. Predisposed by H. Pylori infection
   C. Present as stromal polyps
   D. Are sensitive to chemotherapy

217. The advantage of Bladder drainage over Enteric drainage after Pancreatic Transplantation is better monitoring of : *(AI 2009)*
   A. HBA1C levels
   B. Amylase levels
   C. Glucose levels
   D. Electrolyte levels

218. Parastomal hernia is most frequently seen with: *(AI 2009)*
   A. End Colostomy
   B. Loop Colostomy
   C. End Iliostomy
   D. Loop Iliostomy

ANSWERS, REFERENCES, EXPLANATIONS AND RELEVANT HIGH YIELD FACTS

Esophageal Conditions

Dysphagia (General / Differential Diagnosis):

1. **Answer is B (Multiple sacculations and pseudodiverticulae Corkscrew esophagus):** *Current Diagnosis and Treatment in Gastroenterology 2nd/288; Harrisons 16th/1742*

The presence of non progressive dysphagia to both solids and liquids suggests the diagnosis of diffuse esophageal spasm. The charachteristic barium swallow findings in diffuse esophageal spasm is the corkscrew esophagus (appearance of curling or multiple ripples in the wall, sacculations and pseudodiverticula)

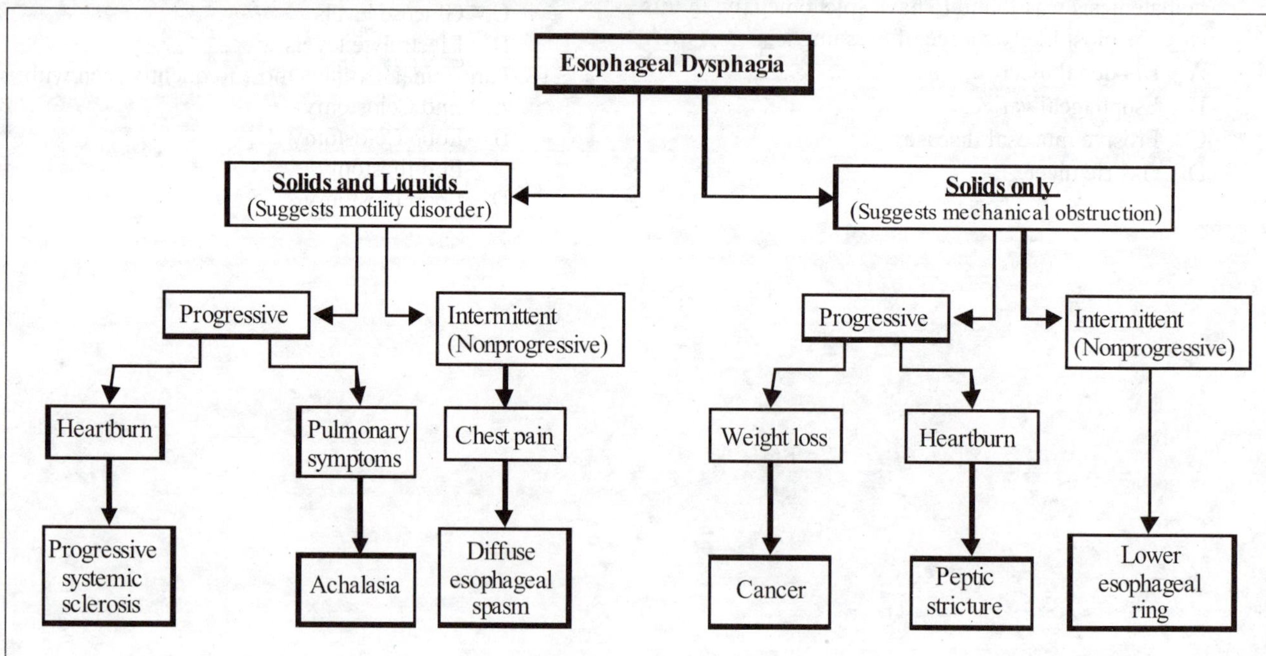

- Rat tail esophagus with a dilated proximal esophagus and narrow lower end suggests a diagnosis of Achlasia cardia. (*Dhingra 4th/305)*

  Achlasia is associated with *Progressive dysphagia* to *both solids and liquids*
- Narrow and irregular esophageal lumen suggests a diagnosis of esophageal carcinoma *(Dhingra 4th/306)*

  Esophageal carcinomas are associated with *progressive dysphagia.* Which is *initially only for solids* at presentation (may prgress to cause dysphagia to liquids also)
- Stricture or ulcer in the esophagus suggests a diagnosis of Gastrophageal Reflux disease (GERD) *(H16th/1743)* GERD is asociated with *progressive dysphagia* to *solids alone* at presentation.

2. **Answer is D (Lower esophageal ring) :** *Current Diagnosis and Treatment in Gastroenterology 2nd/288; Harrison's 17th/239, 240, 1854*

Non progressive (episodic) dysphagia only for solids is characteristic of lower esophageal rings (Schatzki's ring). The ring is apparent as a constriction in the lower esophagus on barium swallow.

Peptic stricture and carcinoma esophagus present with ***progressive*** *dysphagia for solids while Achalasia presents with* ***progressive*** *dysphagia for both solids and liquids.*

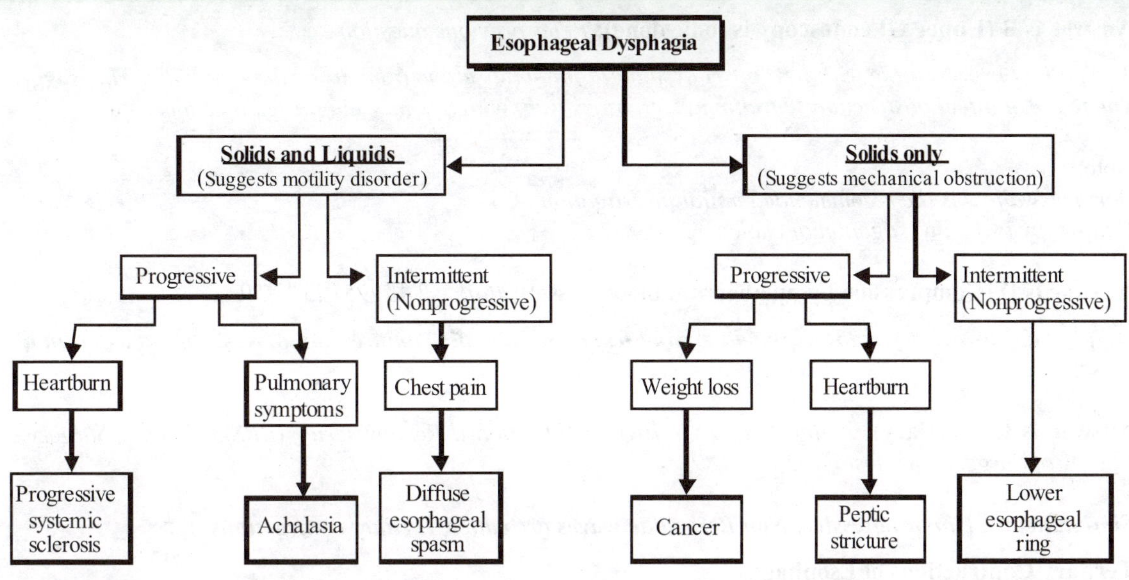

3. **Answer is C (Achalasia Cardia):** *Refer previous question*

Carcinoma Esophagus, lower esophagus ring and esophageal stricture are all associated with dysphagia for solids alone.

Presence of dysphagia for both solids and liquids suggests a diagnosis of Achalasia cardia.

Although dysphagia in Achalasia is progressive absence of progression does not exclude the diagnosis. Also amongst the options provided Achalasia is the single best answer of exclusion.

4. **Answer is C and D (Pharyngeal diverticulum) and (Diffuse esophageal spasm):** *Current Gastroenterology 2nd/288; Harrisons 16th/217; CMDT 2005/546; 09/514*

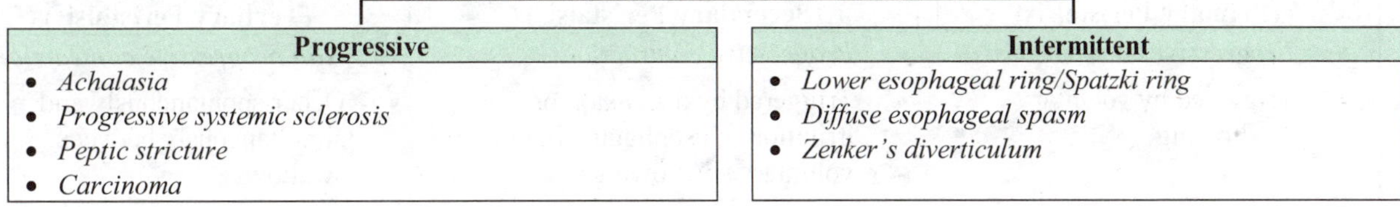

Progressive	Intermittent
• *Achalasia* • *Progressive systemic sclerosis* • *Peptic stricture* • *Carcinoma*	• *Lower esophageal ring/Spatzki ring* • *Diffuse esophageal spasm* • *Zenker's diverticulum*

5. **Answer is B (Endoscopy):** *CMDT 09/514; Refer text below*

Dysphagia for solids alone suggests a probable mechanical cause for dysphagia such as carcinoma, stricture or esophageal web. The investigation of choice for such cases is Endoscopy.

Esophageal Dysphagia

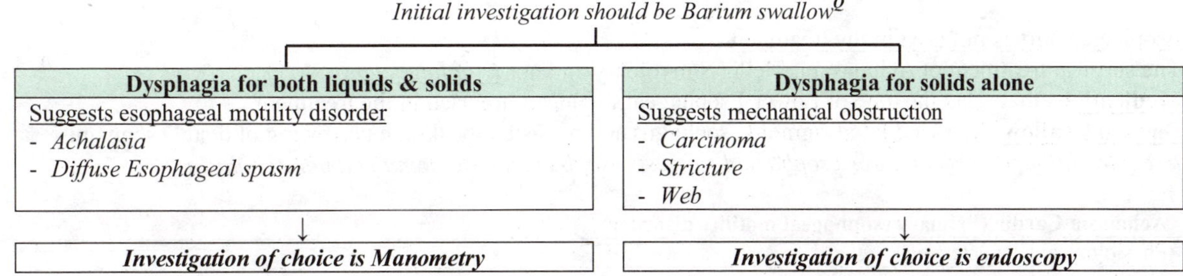

Initial investigation should be Barium swallow[Q]

Dysphagia for both liquids & solids	Dysphagia for solids alone
Suggests esophageal motility disorder - *Achalasia* - *Diffuse Esophageal spasm*	Suggests mechanical obstruction - *Carcinoma* - *Stricture* - *Web*
Investigation of choice is Manometry	***Investigation of choice is endoscopy***

6. **Answer is B (Upper GI endoscopy is to be done):** *Refer previous question*

The patient is presenting with new onset dysphagia for solids alone (able to swallow liquids). This suggests dysphagia due to mechanical obstruction (carcinoma, stricture, web) which is best diagnosed by endoscopy.

Note:
Barium swallow is the recommended initial investigation
Endoscopy is the investigation of choice.

7. **Answer is D (Compression by an aberrant blood vessel):** *Bailey 24th/995; 23rd/859*

Dysphagia Lusoria refers to dysphagia arising from symptomatic compression of the esophagus by an aberrant blood vessel.

8. **Answer is C (Tertiary):** *Bailey Love 25th/ 1010, 1011, 'Board Review series (BRS): General Surgery' (2000)/ 240, Review of Surgery' by Mostafa (2006)/189*

Simultaneous, Non progressive, Non Peristaltic waves are called Tertiary contractions.

Tertiary Contractions of Esophagus

- Tertiary contractions are simultaneous, non progressive, non peristaltic waves that can occur throughout the esophagus
- Tertiary contractions represent uncoordinated contractions of the smooth muscles that are responsible for the 'Cork Screw' appearance of esophageal spasm on Barium swallow
- Tertiary contractions do not have a physiological function and may be observed in the elderly and in patients with esophageal motility disorders.

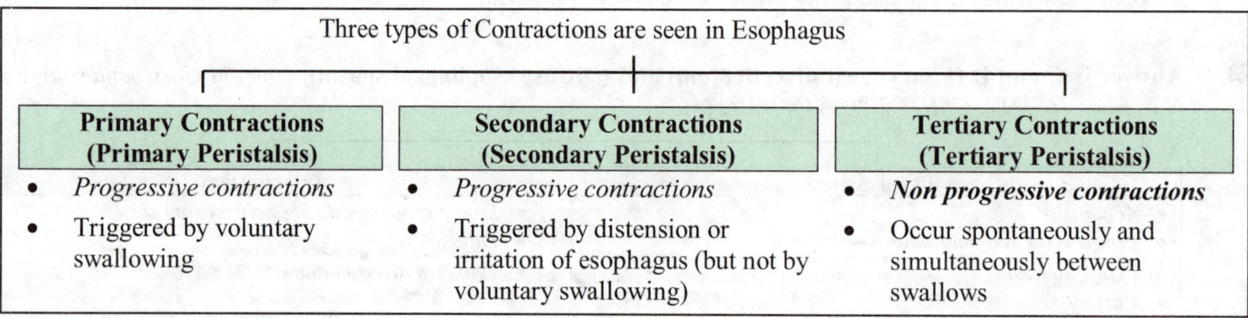

Three types of Contractions are seen in Esophagus

Primary Contractions (Primary Peristalsis)	Secondary Contractions (Secondary Peristalsis)	Tertiary Contractions (Tertiary Peristalsis)
• *Progressive contractions*	• *Progressive contractions*	• ***Non progressive contractions***
• Triggered by voluntary swallowing	• Triggered by distension or irritation of esophagus (but not by voluntary swallowing)	• Occur spontaneously and simultaneously between swallows

Achalasia Cardia

9. **Answer is A & B (Dysphagia is the presenting symptom) and (The cause is the absence of Auerbach's plexus):** *Current Diagnosis & Treatment in Otorhinolaryngology 2nd/ ; Harrison 18th/p 2430, 2431, 2432; 17th/1849, 1850*

Dysphagia is the most common presenting symptom of Achalasia which is believed to be caused by degeneration of the Myenteric plexus of Auerbach

Esophagectomy is not used in the treatment
The surgical treatment of Achalasia is Heller's myotomy and not ***Esophagectomy.***
Medications that relax the tone of Lower Esophageal Sphincter are used in the treatment.
Barium swallow shows a dilated sigmoid esophagus and persistent beak like narrowing of distal esophagus.
Irregular filling defects in lower esophageal suggests esophageal carcinoma and not Achalasia.

Achalasia Cardia (Primary esophageal motility disorder)
Physiological Characteristic
• Absence of esophageal peristalsis
• Increased pressure of LES
• Failure of LES to relax in response to swallowing

Pathogenesis
• True etiology unknown • Degeneration of Myenteric plexus of Aurerbach's with loss of postganglionic inhibitory neurons is noted (These neurons contain NO and VIP which mediate LEs relaxation) • Sparing of postganglionic cholinergic fibres (Increased Les resting pressure and insufficient relaxation)
Presentation
• Dysphagia is the most common symptom Dysphagia is present for both solids and liquids and is progressive • Regurgitation is the second most common symptom • Chest pain may also occur
Investigations
• *Esophageal Manometry is the key test in establishing the diagnosis* • *Barium swallow should be the initial test performed* <u>Diagnosis suggested by</u>: - *Dilated sigmoid oesophagus* - *Persistant beak like narrowing of distal oesophagus*
Complications
Achalasia is a risk factor for Esophageal carcinoma[Q] Achalasia predisposes to squamous cell carcinoma[Q]
Treatment
Laparoscopic Heller's myotomy[Q] and partial fundoplication is the procedure of choice Non surgical treatment includes medications that reduces LES pressure - Intrasphinteric injection of botulinum toxin and/or - Pneumatic dilatation

5

Gastrointestinal System

10. Answer is A (Pressure at distal end increased with no peristalsis): *Current Diagnosis & Treatment in Otorhinolaryngology 2nd/ ; Harrison 18th/p 2430, 2431 Harrison 17th/1849, 1850; Current Diagnosis & Treatment in Gastroenterology 2nd/287*

Achalasia is characterized by an increased pressure of LES and absence of esophageal peristalsis.

Physiological /Manometric features of Achalasia
• *Elevated Resting pressure of LES (>45 mmHg)[Q]* • *Incomplete LES relaxation (in response to swallowing)[Q]* • *Absence of distal esophageal peristalsis[Q]*

11. Answer is A (Achlasia cardia) : *Dhingra ENT 3rd/400*

Presence of dysphagia which is more for liquids than for solids along with a characteristic rat tail appearance on radiography in a young patient suggests the diagnosis of achalasia.

Malignancy (CA esophagus) usually presents with dysphagia which is more for solids than for liquids and is seen in the elderly.

Zenker's diverticulum and esophageal spasm do not show a rat tail appearance on radiography.

12. Answer is A (Barium swallow): *Current Diagnosis & Treatment in Otorhinolaryngology 2nd/488*

Presence of progressive dysphagia for both liquids and solids suggest a probable diagnosis of Achalasia Cardia. Barium swallow should be the first / initial investigation.
'In evaluating a patient with dysphagia, a barium swallow should be the first test performed'-Current Otorhinology 2nd/488

13. Answer is A (Achalasia Cardia): *Harrison 18th/p 2432 Harrison 17th/1850*
Heller's extramural myotomy of the LES is performed for Achalasia cardia and involves incising the circular muscle layer.

Diffuse Esophageal Spasm

14. Answer is B (Manometry) : *Bailey 25th/ 1039, CSDT 12th/458, Sabiston 18th/1069*

Diffuse oesophageal spasm is a type of oesophageal motility disorder. Such Motility disorders are best diagnosed by Manometry studies

'Esophageal manometry is the key test for establishing the diagnosis of diffuse esophageal spasm' – CSDT

'Esophageal manometry is the only test that distinguishes diffuse esophageal spasm from other primary esophageal motor disorders – CSDT/458

Diffuse Esophageal spasm:
Diffuse Esophageal spasm is a poorly understood hypermotility disorder of the oesophagus
Presentation

• The clinical presentation is typically that of *Chest pain and Dysphagia*
• ***'The most common symptom is intermittent chest pain*** Q (>dysphagia)
• Chest pain mimics angina or pain of coronary artery disease
  - *Squeezing pressure in the chest that may radiate to the Jaw, arms or upper back*
  - *Symptoms are aggravated by emotional stress, exertion (or related to eating)*
[Box: *Chest pain* Q / *Dysphagia* Q]

Diagnosis
Manometry is the key to establish the diagnosis *The diagnosis is usually made by an esophagogram (Barium swallow) and monometric study* *Ambulatory pH monitoring should be performed to rule out abnormal reflux*

Esophagogram (Barium Swallow)

- *Corkscrew esophagus* Q *is classical of Diffuse esophageal* spasm (seen in about 30% of cases)

(Radiological evidence of tertiary contractions)

Ambulatory 24 hour pH monitoring
Gastro esophageal reflux disease may mimic diffuse esophageals spasm Ambulatory pH monitoring must be performed to rule out abnormal reflux which is the most common cause of non cardiac chest pain

Manometry

- ***Manometry is the key to establish the diagnosis (CSDT)*** *Correlation of subjective complains with evidence of spasm (induced by vagomimetic drug bethenechol) on manometric studies prvide convincing evidence*-Sabiston
- *Esophageal monometry is the only test that distinguishes diffuse esophageal spasm from other primary esophageal motor disorders* - CSDT
- *An ambulatory motility record (ambulatory manometry) is preferred over standard manometry* as contractions are intermittent and normal peristalsis is seen in between. *Ambulatory manometry is the single best investigation with a sensitivity of 90% and specificity of 100%*

15. Answer is D (Diffuse Esophageal Spasm) : *Harrison 15th/1645; Dhingra 3rd/399; Bailey 22nd/660; 24th/1020*

***Diffuse esophageal spasm is synonymous with 'corkscrew esophagus' or Rosary esophagus* - Bailey**

In diffuse esophageal spasm, barium swallow shows that normal sequential peristalsis below the aortic arch is replaced by uncoordinated simultaneous contractions that produce the appearance of curling or multiple ripples in the wall, sacculations, and pseudodiverticula- the "corkscrew" esophagus.

Zenker's Diverticulum

16. Answer is A (Zenker's diverticulum) : *Dhingra 3rd/330*

Regurgitation of food eaten 3 days ago hints to the possibility of another sac / diverticulum which stores food. Age of the patient and gurgling sound support the diagnosis of Zenkers diverticulum.

Zenker's diverticulum

What it is :
It is a *pulsion diverticulum* Q, where pharyngeal *mucosa* Q herniates *through the Killihan's dehiscence* Q (a weak area *between two parts of Inferior Constrictor* Q).
Age of presentation
This condition is usually seen after 60 years of age (*elderly*) Q

Symptomatology / presentation
• ***Dysphagia***[Q] : As mouth of the sac is wider than the opening of esophagus, food preferentially enter the sac. When the pouch gets filled with food, it presses on the esophagus & produces ***Dysphagia.*** [Q] • ***Gurgling Sound***[Q] is produced during swallowing. • Halitosis or foul smell is frequently associated • ***Cough & Aspiration pneumonia***[Q] : food eaten *over the last few days*[Q] may regurgitate as it collects in the pouch causing cough and aspiration pneumonia. • ***Malnutrition***[Q] : Patient is often malnourished due to dysphagia.

17. Answer is D (Out pouching of the anterior pharyngeal wall, just above the cricopharyngeus muscle.) *Current Diagnosis & Treatment in Otorhinology 2nd /490, Dhingra 4th/355; Fem's Colour Atlas and Text of Clinical Medicine (2008)/560, 'Clinical scenarios in Thoracic Surgery' by Kalimi (2004) / 254*

Zenker's diverticulum is an out pouching of the posterior pharyngeal wall where pharyngeal mucosa herniates through the Killians dehiscence (a weak area between cricopharyngeus inferiorly and thyropharyngeus superiorly both being parts of the inferior constrictor).

Zenker's diverticulum originate from the posterior wall of pharynx and not from the anterior wall

- Zenker's diverticulum originates from the *posterior wall* of the pharynx through the killian's dehiscence
- Killian's dehiscence is a weak area between
  - Oblique fibres of the Thyropharyngeus (part of inferior constrictor muscle) superiorly
  - Transverse fibres of the cricopharyngeus (part of the inferior constrictor muscle) inferiorly
- Herniation *starts in the midline posteriorly*, however as the out pouching enlarges, it localizes to one side of the oesophagus most commonly on the left side.

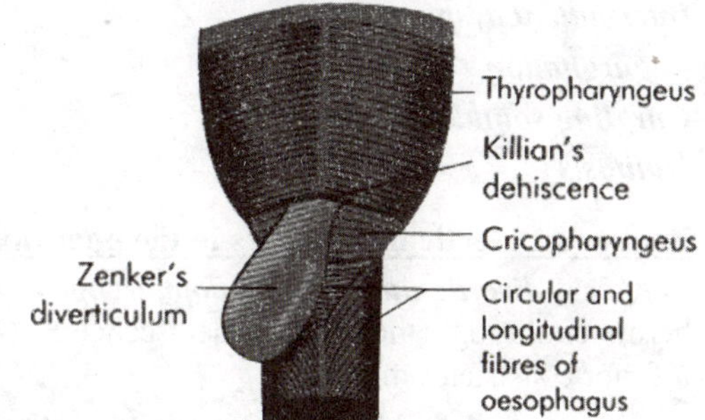

Hypopharyngeal (Zenker's) diverticulum.
Hypopharyngeal mucosa herniates through the Killian's dehiscence a weak area between two parts of inferior constrictor

Zenker's diverticulum is an acquired diverticulum and not a congenital diverticulum

Zenker's diverticulum is a *believed to be an acquired disorder* that results when mucosal and submucosal layers herniates through the killian's dehescence, a weak area between two parts of the inferior constrictor.

These are *acquired pulsion diverticulae* that usually occur in people older than 60 years as their pharyngeal muscle tone and elasticity decreases.

Zenker's diverticulae are false diverticulae

Zenker's diverticulum *is a false diverticulum* because it does not contain all the anatomic layers of the esophageal wall
Zenker's diverticulum involves protrusion of *only the mucosa (and submucosa)* through the posterior muscle layers

Zenker's diverticulum are often identified by Lateral x-rays on Barium swallow

Barium swallow is the diagnostic procedure of choice for Zenker's diverticulum

'The diagnosis is most easily made with a lateral view of cervical esophagus during barium esophagography'
- 'Gastroenterological Endoscopy' by Classes (2002) / 474

'Lateral x- Rays on barium swallow are essential because these are posterior out pouchings'
- 'Review of surgery' by Mostafa (2006) / 197

18. Answer is A (Zenker's diverticulum): *Refer previous question; Current Otolaryngology 2nd/490*

Presence of intermittent dysphagia for solids, regurgitation of food and halitosis (foul smell) suggests a diagnosis of Zenker's Diverticulum.

Essentials of Diagnosis : Zenker's Diverticulum (Current Otolaryngology)
• *Dysphagia (Intermittent)*
• *Regurgitation of undigested food (with risk of aspiration)*
• *Gurgling sounds in neck*
• *Halitosis*

19. Answer is C (Lung Abscess): *Refer text below*

The most frequent complications of Zenker diverticulum is 'aspiration' into the tracheobronchial tree which can in turn present with pneumonia and Lung Abscess.

20. Answer is C (Treatment is Simple excision) : *Dhingra 2nd / 271*

Zenker's diverticulum may be managed by simple excision of the pouch.

Zenker's diverticulum is usually symptomatic and not asymptomatic

Characteristic symptoms of Zenker's Diverticulum

Intermittent dysphagia

Regurgitation

Gurgling sound in neck

Halitosis

Zenker's Diverticulum occurs in the pharynx and not in the esophagus

Zenker's diverticulum or ***'Hypopharyngeal Diverticulum'*** is a '*Pulsion diverticulum*' where pharyngeal mucosa herniates through the Killan's dehiscence Q. (*Killan's dehiscence*Q is a weak area of pharynx between two parts of inferior constrictor muscleQ)

- Usually seen ***in elderly (after 60 years of age)***Q
- Herniation starts in midline and lies first behind the esophagus and then to its left. ***(it occurs in pharynx and not in esophagus)***. Mouth of the sac is wider than the opening of esophagus and food preferentially enters the pouch.

• ***Dysphagia is the prominent manifestation.*** It appears after a few swallows.
• When pouch gets filled with food, it presses on the esophagus.
• Gurgling sound is produced on swallowingQ
• Food may regurgitate at night when patient is recumbent causing cough and aspiration pneumonia
• Patient is malnourished due to dysphagia

Zenker's diverticulum is usually seen in elderly and not in children.

Condition is usually sen after 60 years of age (elderly)

Zenker's diverticulum may be managed by simple excision of the pouch

Treatment options for Zenker's diverticulum

- Simple Excision of pouch
- ***Excision of pouch and cricopharyngeal myotomy*** Q
- ***Dahlman's procedure***Q :Done in poor-risk debilitated patients. The partition wall between esophagus and pouch is divided by diathermy.

Oesophageal Ring / Web

21. Answer is A & C (Mucosal ring at squamo-columnar junction) & (Dysphagia is the presenting symptom): *Oxford textbook of Medicine 4th/553*

Schatzki ring is a mucosal / submucosal ring at the squamo-columnar junction of distal esophagus that may present with intermittent dysphagia.

Schatzki Ring (Oesophageal Ring)
• *It is a characteristic short segment of luminal stenosis*
• ***Occurs in the lower esophageal at the gastroesophageal junction (squamo-columnar junction)***
• ***It is made up only of mucosa and submucosa and narrows the lumen only to a few millimeters.***
• *True aetiopathogenesis is not known*
• *Usually asymptomatic*
• ***Most common presentation intermittent dysphagia only for solids.***
• *Often associated with a hiatus hernia.*
• *Frequently leads to incorrect diagnosis of diffuse esophageal spasm*
• *Treatment involves esophageal dilatation or endoscopic diathermy/laser.*

22. Answer is D (Common in elderly male): *Harrison 14th/1595; Harrison 15th/1648, 579; (Not in Harrison 16th) Kumar Clark 5th/267; Dhingra 3rd/399; Harrison 17th 1854 Harrison 18th/p 2429*

'Plummer Vinson syndrome refers to the combination of hypopharyngeal webs and iron deficiency ***anemia in middle aged women'*** *– Harrison*

Plummer Vinson Syndrome (Patterson Kelly)
- Upper esophageal web
- Iron deficiency anemia
- Koilonychia
- Glossitis and angular stomatitis

Barret's Esophagus

23. Answer is B (Intestinal Metaplasia): *Harrison 18th/p2434 Harrison 17th/1852; Current Diagnosis & Treatment in Gastroenterology/227*

Barret's esophagus is a metaplasia of the esophageal mucosa caused by replacement of squamous epithelium with columnar epithelium.
Specialized intestinal epithelium (intestinal metaplasia) is the most common and most important type of columnar epithelium seen in Barret's esophagus.

Barret's esophagus (columnar metaplasia)

Metaplasia of squamous epithelium into columnar epithelium

↓

Three types of Columnar Epithelium may be seen

Gastric Type	Junctional Type	Intestinal Type
Morphologically indistinguishable from normal gastric epethelia	*Morphologically indistinguishable from normal gastric epethelia*	*Morphologically distinct and readily distinguishable from gastric epethelia* • This is the most common type • Most commonly associated with dysplasia & carcinoma

24. Answer is A (More incidence of squamous carcinoma): *Harrison 18th/p2434 Harrison 17th/1852*

Barret's oesophagia is associated with an increased incidence of adenocarcinoma and not squamous cell carcinoma.

Barret's esophagus is associated with columnar metaplasia of distal (lower esophagus).

25. Answer is A & C (Stricture and Peptic ulcer): *Manual of Gastroenterology 4th/132*

Complications of Barret's esophageal includes peptic ulceration, strictures and adenocarcinoma.

Complications of Barret's Oesophagus

- *Peptic Ulcer (Barret's Ulcer: Chronic Peptic Ulceration in the columnar lined mucosa)*
- *Strictures*
- *Adenocarcinoma (Dysplagia – cancer sequence)*

26. Answer is a D (Associated with oesophageal varices): *Harrison 18th/p 2434 Harrison 17th/1852*

Barret's oesophagus is not associated with oesophageal varices.

Barret's oesophagus is characterized replacement of lower oesophageal mucosa by intestinal (columnar) type of epithelium. It is considered premalignant with increased risk of adenocarcinoma, and is believed to be caused by prolonged gastroesophageal reflux.

27. Answer is E (None): *Harrison 18th/p 2434 Harrison 17th/ ; Current Diagnosis and Treatment in Gastroenterology 2nd/277; Current Diagnosis and Treatment in Otorhinology 2nd/496*

All statements about Barret's Esophagus are true

- **Stricture in Barret's esophagus may present in high oesophagus**
  Barret's oesophagus can also lead to chronic peptic ulcers of the esophagus with high and long strictures
  –Harrison 17th/1852

- **Barret's esophagus is premalignant**
  Barret's esophagus can progress to adenocarcinoma

- **Diagnosis can be suggested by Endoscopy**
  Endoscopy shows a 'salmon pink' epithelium above the gastroesophageal junction which replaces the whitish squamous epithelium.

- **Diagnosis is confirmed by biopsy**
  Diagnosis is confirmed by pathological examination and requires the identification of columnar (intestinal) type epithelium characterized by the presence of goblet cells.

Barret's Esophagus

- *Metaplasia of esophageal squamous epithelium into columnar in distal oesophagus*[Q]
- *Most common type of columnar epithelium is intestinal epithelium (intestinal metaplasia)* [Q]
- *Metaplasia characteristically affects the distal (lower) oesophagus*[Q]
- *It is consequence of severe reflex esophagitis*[Q]
- *More common in men*[Q] *(Males > Females)*
- *More common in whites*[Q] *(Whites > Blacks)*
- *More common with increasing age*[Q] *(incidence increases with age)*
- *Considered a premalignant condition*[Q]
- *Type of cancer associated in an adenocarcinoma*[Q]
- *Columnar metaplasia that carries maximum risk of adenocarcinoma is intestinal metaplasia (intestinal epithelium)* [Q]
- *Can lead to chronic peptic ulceration of esophagus* [Q] *(Barret ulcer)*
- *Can lead to high (midoesophageal) and long strictures* [Q]

28. Answer is B (Premalignant condition): *Harrison 18th/p 2434 Harrison 17th/1852, 1853*

Barret's oesophagus is a premalignant condition with increased risk of adenocarcinoma.

Barret's esophagus is more common in males
More common in males (Males > Females)[Q]
More common in White (Whites > Blacks) [Q]
More common with increasing age[Q]

Barret's metaplasia once established does not respond to conservative management

'Established Metaplasia does not regress with antisecretory treatment' – Harrison

Although medical treatment does not regress the metaplastic changes, it is still advocated to prevent continued insult.

Barret's esophagus is associated with columnar metaplasia and not squamous metaplasia.

29. Answer is A (Adenocarcinoma): *Harrison 16th/1852; CMDT 2008/562; 09/516*

Barret's esophagus is a premalignant lesion and predisposes to adenocarcinoma of the lower (distal) esophagus.

Mallory Weiss Syndrome

30. Answer is D (Mucosal tear): *Harrison 18th/p 2436, 320 Harrison 17th -1854, 257*

Mallory-Weiss Syndrome is associated with a tear of the gastric mucosa near the squamocolumnar mucosal junction

Mucosal Tear (Mallory-Weiss Syndrome)
• The tear usually involves the gastric mucosa near the squamocolumnar mucosal junction near cardia • This tear is usually caused by vomiting, retching, or vigorous coughing. • The tear is usually linear. • Patients present with upper gastrointestinal bleeding ***(Hemetemesis)*** • Association with alcoholism and hiatus hernia • In most patients, bleeding ceases spontaneously (Continued bleeding may respond to vasopressin therapy or angiographic embolization. Surgery is rarely needed)

Esophageal Carcinoma

31. Answer is A (Squamous cell ca): *Current Diagnosis and Treatment in Gastroenterology/299; CSDT/469*

'By far the most common esophageal cancer world wide is squamous cell carcinoma' *– Current Gastroenterology*

'Over the past few decades there has been a progressive increase in the incidence of adenocarcinoma of the distal esophagus so that it accounts for more than 50% of all new cases of esophageal cancer. ***Squamous cell carcinoma is still the most common type world wide'*** *– CSDT/469*

Confusing inference

Most prevalent esophageal cancer world wide (old + new cases) is Squamous cell ca
Most common esophageal cancer world wide (new cases) is Adenocarcinoma

32. Answer is C (Lower 1/3rd): *Harrison 16th/524*

The lower third of the esophagus is the most common site of esophageal cancer and accounts for about 50% of all esophageal cancers.

'*About 15% of esophageal cancers occur in the upper third of esophagus (cervical esophagus), 35% in the middle third of esophagus and 50% in the lower third'* – Harrison 16th/524

Site of esophageal cancer (All histological types)	% of total
Upper 1/3rd	15%
Middle 1/3rd	35%
Lower 1/3rd	***50%***

Note:

The most common site of squamous cell (histological subtype) is middle 1/3 of esophagus^Q
The most common site of adenocarcinoma (histological subtype) is lower 1/3rd of esophagus^Q.

33. Answer is B (Middle 1/3rd): *Sabiston 17th/1119; Devita 7th/866; Robbins 7th/807*

The most common site of squamous cell carcinoma of esophagus is middle 1/3rd.

Site of squamous cell carcinoma	Percentage of total
Upper 1/3rd	20%
Middle 1/3rd	***50%***
Lower 1/3rd	30%

34. Answer is C (Lower 1/3rd): *Refer text below*

The most common site of adenocarcinoma esophagus is the lower 1/3rd of esophagus

Esophageal Adenocarcinoma invariably arises from Barret's esophagus (Barret's ulcer) which is characteristically located in the distal esophagus around the gastroesophageal junction.

35. Answer is B (Middle 1/3rd): *API 7th/1012*

Eighty to ninety percent of esophageal cancers in India are squamous cell carcinomas, and the most common site is middle 1/3rd of esophagus.

Remember

Most common site of esophageal carcinoma in India	*: Middle 1/3rd*
Most common site of esophageal carcinoma world wide	*: Lower 1/3rd*

36. Answer is D (Benzene therapy) : *Harrison 15th / 578; Harrison 16th/524; Harrison 17th/570, 571 Harrison 18th/p 764*

Benzene therapy has not been mentioned in the best of predisposing factors for carcinoma esophagus, and is the single best answer of exclusion.

Predisposing factors for carcinoma esophagus :

1. ***Alcohol consumption*** Q
2. ***Smoking cigarettes*** Q
3. **Ingested Carcinogens**
Nitrates Q Smoked opiates Fungal toxins in pickled vegetables
4. **Mucosal damage**
Chronic Achalasia Q Lye ingestion / Hot tea Radiation induced strictures Q
5. **Host Susceptibility**
1. *Patterson Kelley syndrome* Q *or* ***Plummer Vinson syndrome*** Q *Esophageal web* Q + *Glossitis* Q + *Iron deficiency* Q 2. ***Tylosis palmaris et plantaris*** Q *: Congenital hyperkeratosis* Q *and pitting of palms and soles* Q
6. *Chronic Gastric Reflux, ie. Barrett's esophagus for Adenocarcinoma* Q

37. Answer is D (Ca Esophagus) : *Harrison 15th/579; Harrison 16th/524; Harrison 17th/570, 571 Harrison 18th/p 764*

Congenital hyperkeratosis and pitting of palms and soles (i.e tylosis palmaris et plantaris) is a known etiological factor for squamous Ca of Esophagus' *– Harrison*

38. Answer is B and D (Scleroderma and Barrets esophagus): *Current Gastroenterology/300; Harrison 17th/570 Harrison 18th/p 764*

Barret's esophagus is the characteristic risk factor for adenocarcinoma esophagus.
Scleroderma also increases the risk of esophageal adenocarcinoma perhaps through the development of Barret's esophagus as the collagen deposits in the distal esophagus cause LES dysfunction.

Risk factors for esophageal adenocarcinoma *(Current Gastroenterology)*

- ***Barrets esophagus***
- *Gastroesophageal Reflux Disease (GERD)*
- ***Scleroderma***
- *Smoking*
- *Alcohol*
- *History of colon cancer*
- *Medications : Long term use (> 5 years) of Theophylline & β agonists.*

39. Answer is A (Barrett's Esophagus) : *Harrison 18th/p 764 Harrison 17th/571, 1852; Schwartz Pre-Test/Q.434*

*In **barrett's esophagus** there is a metaplastic change in the esophageal mucus membrane. The resulting columnar epithelium is susceptible to the development of the **adenocarcinoma**. The risk of developing adenocarcinoma in Barret's esophagus is 50-100 time, that of general population. If 100 patients with Barrett's esophagus are followed prospectively for one year, one adenocarcionom can be expected in that group.*
Alcohol abuse, achalasia, lye stricture and smoking are all risk factors for the development of squamous carcinoma of the esophagus.

40. Answer is B (Barret's esophagus) : *Harrison 17th/1852; Bailey Love 23rd/870*

Adenocarcinoma is seen in Barret's esophagus

Barret's esophagus is a metaplastic change in the lining mucosa of oesophagus in response to chronic gastroesophagus reflex.
In Barret's esophagus the junction between oesophageal mucosa (squammous) and gastric mucosa (columnar) moves proximally such that the lower part of esophagus now becomes lined with different types of gastric mucosa. This part of oesophagus has an increased risk for adenocarcinoma i.e.
Adenocarcinoma is seen in Barrets esophagus.

41. Answer is E (Pernicious anemia is a risk factor): *Harrison 18th/p 764 Harrison 17th/570, 571*

Pernicious anemia is a risk factor for stomach carcinoma and not for esophageal carcinoma.

Esophageal carcinoma is more common in Men and in elderly

Epidemiological feature of esophageal carcinoma

- *Men > Women (≈ 4 : 1)*
- *Predominantly affects older age group (> 50 years)*

Adenocarcinoma is on the rise
For unclear reasons the incidence of squamous cell carcinoma has decreased while the rate of adenocarcinoma has risen dramatically. – Harrison

Dysphagia is the most common symptom
The most common presentation of esophageal carcinoma is progressive dysphagia (solids then liquids)
– Current Gastroenterology/301

42. Answer is A (Cisplatin): *Harrison 18th/p 764 Harrison 17th/ 571; Bailey 23rd / 879; Bailey 24th/1015*

Chemotherapy for esophageal cancer has improved considerably with the advent of regimens containing Cisplatin.
- Bailey

The best responses are seen in Squamous cell carcinomas.

43. Answer is A (Acute tubular necrosis) : *KDT 5th/ 777*

The most important toxity of cisplatinum is renal impairment *– KDT 7th/777*
Acute tubular necrosis is a manifestation of renal impairment and hence the answer.

44. Answer is A (Stomach) : *Sabiston 16th / 744*

After a portion of esophagus is removed, or after complete esophagectomy, a conduit must be established for alimentary continuity. The stomach, colon and jejunum have all been successfully used a esophageal substitutes but the ***Stomach appears to be the 'conduit' of choice*** *because of ease in mobilization and its ample vascular supply – Sabiston*

Colon is used if the patient has undergone a partial or total gastrectomy previously, or if tumor involves the stomach to preclude a 5 cm margin.

Jejunal loops can also be used, but limited vascular supply restricts mobility.

Stomach and Duodenum

Peptic Ulcer Disease & H. Pylori Infection

45. Answer is D (Pernicious anemia): *Rubin's Pathology 5th/566; S. Das 3rd/818*

Pernicious anemia is characterized by autoimmune destruction of parietal cells leading to hypochondria (↓ acid production). It is not associated with peptic ulcer disease.

Aetiological Factors in peptic ulceration

Primary Aetiologcial Factors (selected)

- *H. pylori infection*
- *NSAID's and other drugs eg. steroids*
- *Stress – Head injury / Burns*
- *Bile Reflux*
- *Smoking / Alcohol use*
- *Genetic Factors*

Associated Factors / Conditions (selected)

- *Endocrinal Disorders*
  - *MEN*
  - ***Primary Hyperparathyroidism***
  - ***Zollinger Ellison Syndrome[Q]***
  - *Cushing's syndrome*
- ***Cirrhosis[Q]***
- *Chronic Renal Failure*
- *Chronic Pulmonary Disease*
- *Chronic Paracreatic Disease*
- *Alpha 1 Antitrypsin deficiency*

46. Answer is C (Plummer Vinson Syndrome): *Refer previous question*

Plummer Vinson Syndrome is associated with dysphagia due to esophageal web and not with peptic ulcer disease.

Zollinger Ellison syndrome, Cirrhosis and smoking are all associated with Peptic ulcer disease.

47. Answer is B (High Acid Output): *Harrison 18th/p 2441, 2442; 17th/1858; 'Textbook of Medicine' by Souhami 4th/777*

Gastric ulcers are associated with normal or decreased gastric acid output. High Acid output is a feature of Duodenal Ulcers.

'Gastric acid output (basal and stimulated) tend to be normal or decreased in Gastric Ulcer Patient's' *- Harrison*

Aetiological factors in peptic ulceration:

Causal factor	Gastric ulcer	Duodenal ulcer
Hellicobacter pylori	Important	Very important
NSAIDs and aspirin	Important	Important
Acid	***Normal or low acid output***	***High or normal acid output***
Bile reflux	Important	Unimportant
Smoking	Important	Important
Stress	Evidence for head injuries and burns only	
Family history	Uncommon	Common

48. Answer is A (Curling's Ulcer): *Harrison 18th/p 2457 Harrisons 17th/ 1869*

Stress ulcers after severe burns are called curling's ulcers

Stress ulcers after head trauma : Cushing's Ulcers
Stress ulcers after severe burns : Curling's Ulcers

49. Answer is C (Gastric leiomyoma): *Harrison 15th/961; Harrison 16th/ 1750, 887;Harrison 17th/1858, 1859 Harrison 18th/p 2442, 2443*

Gastric leiomyomas are not associated with H. pylori infections

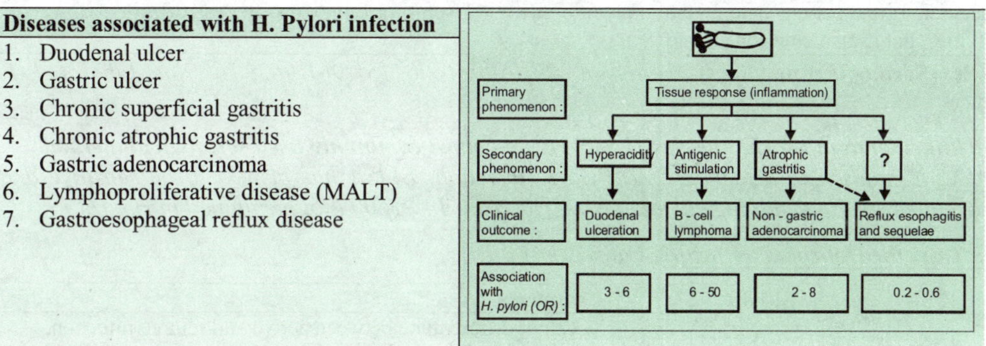

Diseases associated with H. Pylori infection
1. Duodenal ulcer
2. Gastric ulcer
3. Chronic superficial gastritis
4. Chronic atrophic gastritis
5. Gastric adenocarcinoma
6. Lymphoproliferative disease (MALT)
7. Gastroesophageal reflux disease

MALT stands for Mucosa Associated Lymphoid Tissue Lymphoma

50. Answer is A (Antral predominant gastritis) : *Harrison 16th/1750;Harrison 17th /946, 947 Harrison 18th/p 1262*

The presence of antral predominant gastritis is associated with duodenal ulcer formation.

Antral predominant gastritis	*Corpus Predominant atrophic gastritis*	*Non atrophic pangastritis (chronic superficial gastritis)*
Duodenal ulcer	Gastric ulcer Gastric adenocarcinoma	MALT Lymphoma

51. Answer is D (Fundal atrophic gastritis): *Harrison 15th/960; 16th/887,1750; 17th/946, 947; Harrison 18th/p 1262*

Chandrasoma 2nd/ 565

Gastritis due to H. pylori infection is predominantly Antral, not fundal. *Antral gastritis is associated with DU formation.*

Gastritis involving the corpus is also seen and this predisposes to development of gastric ulcer, gastric atrophy and ultimately gastric carcinoma. ***Fundal atrophic gastritis has not been mentioned.***

52. Answer is D (SAFA test) : *Harrison 14th / 942, 15th/960-61; 16th/887; 17th/947 (table-144.1) Harrison 18th/p 1263 (Table: 151.1)*
SAFA test is not used for H.pylori infection

Diagnostic tests used for H pylori include :

Invasive	Non invasive
1. Endoscopy based Biopsy Urease test	***1. Urea breath tests :***
• Here specimen from antral biopsy are tested for "Urease". • It is the most convenient endoscopy based test. • It is *quick*[Q] and *simple*[Q] however it is neither fully sensitive nor fully specific	• Here patient drinks a labelled urea solution and blows into a tube. • If H. Pylori urease is present, the urea is hydrolysed and labelled carbondioxide is detected in breath samples. • It is thus a simple, safe test and cheaper than endoscopy
2. Histology :	***2. Serological :***
Here the biopsy specimen is subjected to histological examination. It is *accurate*[Q], but time consuming	• Here specific IgG levels in serum are assessed. • Does not differentiate between active and remote infection. • Nevertheless it is particularly suited as an *epidemiological tool*
3. Culture :	***3. Stool antigen test :***
• Here the biopsy specimen is put in a culture medium. • This is accurate [Q], and permits determination of antibiotic susceptiblities, but is also time consuming.	• New test appears less accurate than urea breath test • Useful for follow up after treatment

53. Answer is B (Serological markers) : *Harrison 14th/1599, 1600, 15th/961-962; 16th/Not elaborated; 17th/947 Harrison 18th/p 1263*

An enzyme linked immuno-sorbant assay (ELISA) is the most commonly used serological method.

*'Compared with endoscopic detection of H.Pyloric infection, ELISA has proved to be sensitive and specific and is **particularly suited for Epidemiological studies'.** – Harrison 14th/1600 (not mentioned in H - 16th).*

Diagnostic Tests for Helicobacter pylori *– Harrison 14th*

Test	Sensitivity	Comments
Serology	95	Does not differentiate between active and remote infection; **epidemiologic tool**; titer decreases slowly after eradication
Urease assay		
Breath	90-95	Simple ; may be used to monitor therapy
Biopsy	90-98	Requires endoscopy
Histology		Requires endoscopy; may be essential if antibiotic resistance emerges
Culture	70-95	Requires endoscopy'; may be essential if antibiotic resistance emerges

54. Answer is A (With chronic infection urease breath test becomes negative) *Harrison 16th/887; 17th/946, 947 1858, 1859; Harrison 18th/p 1262, 1263, 2442, 2443 Microbiology by Greenwood 16th/294; Kumar&Clarke 5th/273*

*Urease breath test detects H. pylori infection by 'bacterial urease activity' and remains positive till the bacteria has not been eradicated with treatment. **Thus urease breath test becomes negative only after eradication of organism following treatment and not with chronic infection.***

- Despite a substantial humoral antibody response infection persists indefinitely (*persists life long if untreated*)
- Invasive diagnostic test are based on Endoscopic, endoscopy is a diagnostic application.
- *H. pylori produces several virulence factors that have been implicated in the damage of mucosa.*

55. Answer is B (Urea breath test) : *Harrison 16th / 1755, 887; Harrison 17th/947*

The test of choice for documenting eradication is urea breath test. – Harrison 16th / 1755

Assessing success of Treatment / Eradicatiion of H. Pyrlori :

- Assessment should be done atleast 4 weeks after completin of anti H. Pylori therapy.
- In the assessment of treatment success non invasive tests are normally preferred. – Harrison

Assessment of success of treatment

Non invasive tests are preferred	Inasive tests are not preferred
Urea breath test : *Test of choice for documenting eradication.* **Stool antigen test** : *If UBT is not available a stool antigen test should be considered for documenting eradication*	**Biopsy based tests** (Biopsy Urease test, Histology / Culture) *are invasive tests based on Endoscopic biopsy.*
Serological testing : Is **not useful for purpose of documentation of eradication** as antibody titres fall slowly and often do not become undetectable	***These may be used to document eradication but are not preferred for this purpose.***

56. Answer is A (Less prevalent in developing countries): *Harrison 18th/p 1261, 1262 Harrison 17th/ 946, 947, 1859*

H. pylori infection are more prevalent in developing countries.

- The prevalence of H. pylori is approx. 30% in U.S. and other developed countries as against > 80% in most developing countries - *Harrison*
- H. Pylori is a gram negative, spiral, flagellated bacillus - *Harrison*
- Strains producing toxins (strains possessing cag pathogenicity DNA island) are more likely to give rise to severe gastritis, peptic ulceration and gastric cancer than strains without it.
  DNA island or cag pathogenicity island is a large region of DNA which has genes that control production of toxins.

Vacuolating toxin (VaC A)
Cytotoxin (cytotoxin associated gene - Cag A)

- Urea breath test is a simple, inexpensive and consistently accurate test for H.pylori detection.

57. Answer is B (The incidence of complications has remained unchanged): *Answer of exclusion:Read text below*

- H. pylori eradication decreases the likelihood of occurrence of complications.
- The incidence of H.pylori is > 80% in most developing countries, and so the chances of reinfection are also high.
- H. pylori eradication reduced the chances of recurrence
- 'After successful eradication of H.pylori with antibiotics, ulcer recurrence rates are reduced dramatically to 5-20% at 1 year – CMDT 2003/571
- *Option 'b' **'The incidence of complications has remained unchanged'** is thus the answer of exclusion !!*

58. Answer is D (Erythromycin): *Harrison's 15th / 962, 1657; 16th/889, 1754; 17th/949, 1863 Harrison 18th/p 1265, 2449*

Erythromycin is not included in any of the successful multi drug regimens against H.pylori infection.

Indications of Treatment :
H-Pylori related duodenal and gastric ulceration
Low grade B cell MALT Lymphoma

H.pylori should be eradicated.

The most successful are the Triple and Quadruple multi-drug regimens:

Name	Drug 1	Drug 2	Drug 3	Drug 4
OCA	Omeprazole (20 mg BD)	Clarithromycin (500 mg BD)	Amoxicillin (1g BD)	
OCM	Omeprazole (20 mg BD)	Clarithromycin (500 mg BD)	Metronidazole (500 mg BD)	
OBTM	Omeprazole (20 mg BD)	Bismuth Subsalicylate (2 tabs QID)	Tetracycline (500 mg QID)	Metronidazole

59. Answer is A (Oxytetracycline): *Harrison 16th/1754; CMDT 2007/603*

Oxytetrocycline has not been mentioned as a recommended agent for eradication of H. Pylori and hence is the single best answer of choice. Tetracycline and not Oxytetracycline forms part of the regimen.
Amoxycillin, Bismuth subsalicylate and Omeprozole have all been recommended for H. Pylori eradication

Recommended Regimens for Eradication of H. Pylori *(Harrison)*

TRIPLE THERAPY

1. Bismuth subsalicylate plus Metronidazole plus Tetracycline
2. Ranitidine bismuth citrate plus Tetracycline plus Clarithromycin or Metronidazole
3. PPI plus Clarithromycin plus Metronidazole or Amoxicillin

QUADRUPLE THERAPY

PPI plus Bismuth subsalicylate plus Metronidazole plus Tetracycline

All PP1 are given twice daily except esomeprazolc (once daily)

Proton Pump inhibitors (PPI) include: Omeprazole (20mg), Lansaprazole (30mg) *Rabeprazole (20 mg), Pantaprazole (40 mg), Esmaprozole (40 mg)*

60. Answer is B (Cisapride) : *Harrison 18th/p 1264, 1265, 2449 Harrison 17th/ 948, 949, 1863; See previous question*

Cispride is not included in any of the successful multidrug regimens against H. pylori infection.

61. Answer is D (Distal Duodenum): *Harrison14th/1609, 15th/1663; (Harrison. 16th/1760; 17th 1869 – sites not elaborated) Harrison 18th/p 2457*

Distal duodenum has not been mentioned on a site for cushing ulcers

Cushings ulcers:

Are acute ulcers of the upper GI tract associated with intracranial injury or an *increase in intracranial pressure.*

These ulcers my involve the
Stomach Q
Proximal duodenum Q
Esophagus Q

Complication : Haemorrhage and perforation Q

Treatment: Correction of increased intracranial pressure + usual treatment of acute erosions and ulceration.

Memo: ***Curling's ulcers :*** *Stress ulcerations after severe burns – Robbins 7th/817*

62. Answer is A (1st part of Duodenum) : *Robbins 6th / 793; Robbins 7th/817*

First part of duodenum is the most common site for peptic ulceration.

Sites in order of decreasing frequency :
1. Duodenum, 1st portion Q
2. Stomach, usually antrum Q
3. At the gastro-esophageal junction, in the setting of gastroesophageal reflux Q
4. Within the margins of a gastrojejunostomy Q
5. In the duodenum, stomoch or jejunum of patients with Zollinger- Ellison Syndrome Q
6. Within or adjacent to a Meckels diverticulum that contains ectopic gastric mucosa Q

Peptic ulcers are usually solitary lesions less than 4 cm in diameter

63. Answer is D (Lesser Curvature near incisura angularis): *Schwartz 8th/956; Maningot's 10th/953; Textbook of Surgery by Jandra 3rd/95*

The most common site of gastric ulcers (benign) is on the lesser curvature straddling the incisura angularis.

64. Answer is D (Haemorrhage):

The most common complication of both acute and chronic peptic ulcers is gastrointestinal haemorrhage.

'Haemorrhage is the commonest complication of chronic peptic ulcers'–Morson and Dawson's Gastrointestinal Pathology 4th/146

65. Answer is B (Gastroduodenal Artery): *Bailey 24th/1026; CSDT 11th/550*

The most common arterial source of a hemorrhage in duodenal ulcers is the gastroduodenal artery.

'Bleeding ulcers in the duodenum are usually located on the posterior surface of the duodenal bulb. As the ulcer penetrates, the gastroduodenal artery is exposed and may become eroded.
Ulcers on the anterior surface of the duodenal bulb are not prone to bleed since no major blood vessels lie on the anterior surface of the duodenal bulb.' – CSDT

66. Answer is A (Omentum bursa) : *Oxford text book of surgery 2nd/1302 Love & Bailey 23rd/911; BDC 23rd /194*

"Gastric ulcers perforate into the lesser sac, which can be particularly difficult to diagnose" - Bailey
"A gastric ulcer perforates into the lesser sac, then no signs of generalised peritonitis can be seen but misleading symptoms may appear" - Schwartz

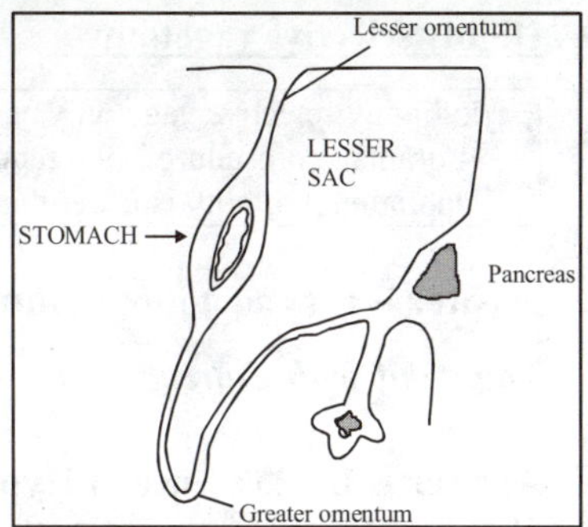

As can be seen from the figure, a posteriorly perforating ulcer of the stomach will localize in the lesser sac or omental bursa only. *(lesser sacis synonymous with omental bursa)*

67. Answer is D (Misoprostol is Drug of choice in pregnant patients) *CMDT 2009/537; 2003/575; Katzung 8th/1068*

Stimulant effect of Misoprostol on the uterus makes it contraindicated in women of child bearing age.

- **The prostaglandin analogue misoprostol** is effective in the *prevention of NSAID induced gastric and duodenal ulcer*[Q] and is the *only agent approved by the FDA for this purpose.* [Q] *CMDT-2001/609*
- Misoprostol causes a dose dependent diarrhea and its *stimulant effect on the uterus makes it contraindicated in women of child bearing age*[Q]. *Katzung 8th/1068*
- **H_2 receptor antagonist :** whereas previous recommendations were to administer these agents at least twice a day, a *single bed time dose may be just as effective and may elicit better compliance - Katzung*
  - For uncomplicated peptic ulcers, H_2 receptor antagonists may be administered twice daily or once daily at bed time, with equivalent efficacy- *CMDT 2001*
- **Proton pump inhibitors (Omeprazole) :** They are superior to H_2 receptor antagonists and to misoprostol in the healing of NSAID induced gastric ulcer.
  - Compared to H_2 Receptor antagonists, proton pump inhibitor provide faster pain relief and more rapid ulcer healing.
- **Alternate pharmacological approaches to failure of an H_2 blocker include :**
  - using a higher dose of the same H_2 blocker.
  - switching to another H_2 receptor antagonist
  - ***switching to a proton pump inhibiter*[Q] *(Omeprazole)***

68. Answer is D (Highly selective vagotomy): *Harrisons 17th/1866*

Highly selective vagotomy is the procedure of choice for the management of chronic duodenal ulcers, except in situations where ulcer recurrence rates are high.

Operations for duodenal ulcers:

Operation/Procedure	Mortality	Recurrence rate (%)	Comments
Vagotomy and drainage	Intermediate	Intermediate	Selectively used
Highly selective vagotomy	Low (minimum)	***High***	Procedure of choice as it has the least complication rate
Vagotomy and antrectomy	*High*	***Low (minimum)***	Procedure with least recurrence rate. Procedure of choice when recurrence is the major problem

69. Answer is A (Truncal vagotomy and antrectomy): *Bailey Love 23rd/908*

The question here strictly specifies recurrence as the major problem 'Recurrent duodenal ulcer'.
Hence a procedure with the minimum recurrence rate, would logically be, the best operation.
Truncal vagotomy and antrectomy are associated with minimum recurrence rate and is the answer of choice.

Note:

Operation with maximum reduction in acid production	Operation with minimum operative mortality	The most widely used procedure in India
Truncal vagotomy and antrectomy	Highly selective vagotomy	Truncal vagotomy plus a drainage procedure *Gastrojejunostomy is at present the most widely used procedure.*

Highly selective vagotomy :

- In highly selective vagotomy nerves of Latarjet supplying the antrum are preserved. [Q]
- A drainage procedure is not required [Q]
- Operation mortality is lower than in any other definitive operation for duodenal ulceration. [Q]

70. Answer is C (Vagotomy + Antrectomy) : *Repeat*

Vagotomy with Antrectomy is associated with lowest recurrence rates.

71. Answer is B (Presence of Hypertonic Contents in small intestine) : *Love & Bailey 23rd / 913; Sabiston 16th / 853; Harrison 14th / 1608, 15th/1660*

DUMPING SYNDROME refers to a syndrome of abdominal and vasomator symptoms which results from dumping of food stuffs with a high osmotic load, from the stomach, into the small bowel.
Loss of storage capacity of stomach and ablation, by pass or destruction of pylorus, results in rapid emptying of hyperosmolar chyme into duodenummm and small intestine. Extracellular fluid then shifts into the intestinal lumen to restore isotonicity resulting in decreased intravascular volume, which gives rise to the vasomotor symptoms.
Note that while reduced gastric capacity contributes, option (b) is a more accurate answer.
Dumping Syndrome is actually of two types:

- **Early dumping syndrome** (as described above)
- **Late dumping syndrome:** This is *Reactive hypoglycemia*[Q]. The carbohydrate load in thesmall intestine later causes a rise in plasma glucose, which in turn causes insulin levels to rise causing a secondary hypoglycemia.

72. Answer is D (Surgery is usually indicated) : *Harrison 14th / 1608; Harrison 15th/1660*

There is no role of surgery in management of post cibal syndromes.

Both types of postcibal syndrome are treated by dietary measures including:
- limitation of sugar containing liquids and solids,
- elimination of liquids at meal time, and
- eating of frequent small meals.

In severe cases, symptoms may improve, with the somatostatin-analogue *Octreotide*.
There is *no role of surgery* in management of post cibal syndromes.

Gastric Outlet Obstruction

73. Answer is B (Duodenum) : *Bailey 23rd / 917 ; Repeat*

Gastric outlet obstruction in a patient with peptic ulcer disease is suggestive of pyloric stenosis.
The term pyloric stenosis is normally a misnomer. The stenosis is seldom at the pylorus.
Commonly the stenosis is found in the first part of the duodenum, the most common site for a peptic ulcer.

74. Answer is B (The pyloric tumor is best felt during feeding): *Bailey Love 23rd /899*

- First born male child is characteristically most commonly affected
- It is four times more common in males as in females
- The condition does not present at birth. It is most commonly seen 4 weeks after birth

Presentation

- Vomiting is the presenting symptom (child vomits milk and *no bile is present*[Q])
- ***Immediately after vomiting the child is hungry i.e. loss of appetite does not occur.***
- Weight loss is striking and rapidly the infant becomes emaciated and dehydrated.
  However, greater awareness of pyloric stenosis has led to earlier identification of patients and hence with ***fewer incidences of chronic malnutrition and severe dehydration*** - *Nelson 10th/1130*
- The ***diagnosis is usually made with a test feed*** : In this the baby is fed with the bottle by a nurse or mother and surgeon :

  - palpates the abdomen with a warm hand to detect the lump

- observes the characteristic peristatic waves pass across the upper abdomen.

- *Pathologically musculature of pylorus adjacent to antrum is grossly hypertrophied*
- *Ultrasonography is the investigation of choice*
- *Hyperchloremic alkalosis is common and following diagnosis first concern is to correct metabolic abnormalities - child is rehydrated with dextrose saline & potassium*[Q]
- *Treatment of choice : Ramsted's operation - 'Pyloromyotomy'*

75. Answer is B (Hypochloremic alkalosis) : *Bailey Love 22nd/674, 23rd/899*

The vomiting of hydrochloric acid results in hypochloremia and alkalosis i.e. hypochloremic alkalosis[Q]

- Characteristically *first born male infant*[Q] is most commonly affected (Males > Females) [Q]
- *Onset of symptoms*, has its, peak incidence *between the third & sixth weeks of life*[Q] and *it is almost never present at birth* [Q].
- *Most common presenting symptom is vomiting*[Q] & accounts for the *hypochloremic alkalosis.* [Q]
- *The procedure of choice is a Halsted's operation*[Q] & not a Heller's myotomy.
  - *Heller myotomy is the procedure of choice for achalasia cardia.*[Q]

76. Answer is C (Metabolic alkalosis with paradoxical aciduria) : *Bailey 23rd / 917*

The vomiting of hydrochloric acid results in hypochloremia and alkalosis i.e. *hypochloremic alkalosis*[Q]
Initially the urine has a low chloride and high bicarbonate content reflecting the primary metabolic abnormality. *This bicarbonate is excreted along with sodium and so with the time the patient becomes progressively hyponatremic and more profoundly dehydrated.* ***Because of the dehydration a phase of sodium retention follows and potassium and hydrogen ions are excreted in preference. This results in urine being paradoxically acidic, and hypokalemia ensues.***

77. Answer is C (Hypokalemia) : *Harrison 14th/ 230, 15th/288-89, 279; Harrison 16th/259, 264*

Loss of gastric secretions results in Hypokalemia. *Loss of gastric contents results in volume depletion and metabolic alkalosis both of which promote kaliuresis. (Leads to hypokalemia)*

Repeated vomitings may have many deleterious effect:

Due to process of vomiting	Metabolic	Nutritional
• Pressure Rupture of esophagus [Q] : *Boerhaave's syndrome* [Q] • Linear mucosal tears in the Region of cardioesophageal junction with resultant hemetemesis- *Mallory weiss syndromes* [Q]	• Dehydration • Loss of gastric secretions (specially HCl, K^+ ions) Resulting in ***Metabolic Alkalosis and Hypokalemia*** [Q] • *HCO_3^- level will be increased* (as the person is having metabolic alkalosis) • *Hypochloremia* (due to loss of HCL)	• Malnutration • *Dental caries* [Q]

Aspiration Pneumonitis may be seen in the unconscious.

78. Answer is B (Normal saline): *Harrison 16th/254*

The patient in question has developed dehydration with mild hyponatermic dehydration with hypokalemia. ***Isotonic normal saline (.9%NaCl) is the solution of choice for intravenous replacement therapy.*** *Hypokalemia should be corrected by adding appropriate amounts of KCl to the replacement solution. – Harrison*

Management of hypovolemia with intravenous therapy :

Mild losses
Oral correction with water and sodium salts

More severe hypovolemia
↓
Intravenous therapy
↓

Patients with loss of water and electrolytes
↓

Normonatremic Mildly hyponatremic	Severe hyponatremia	Hypernatremia
Isotonic normal saline (0.9% NaCl)	Hypertonic saline (3% NaCl)	Hypotonic solutions (0.45% NaCl half N.S), (5% dextrose)

Patients with significant haemorrhage or anemia

- Blood transfusion is treatment of choice
- Colloid containing solutions are a substitute

Menetrier's disease

79. Answer is B (Exophytic growth): *Harrison 18th/p 2459 Harrison's 17th/1871, 1872; Current Surgical Diagnosis and Treatment 12th/535,536*

Menetrier's disease is characterized by hypertrophy of gastric mucosa and not by exophytic growth.

Menetrier's disease
Menetrier's disease is a relatively rare disorder of the stomach characterized by large tortuous mucosal folds
Etiology
• Etiology is unknown • Over expression of growth factors such as TGF are suggested
Pathology
Gross • Marked Hypertrophy of gastric folds/Rugae[Q] • Hypertrophy results from hyperplasia of mucus producing cells (mucosa)[Q] • Hypertrophy is most prominent in the body and fundus [Q] Histological/microscopic • Massive foveolar hyperplasia (Hyperplasia of surface and glandular mucosal cells). • Pits of gastric glands elongate and may become tortuous • Lamina propria may contain a mild chronic inflammatory infiltrate (Note: Although lamina propria may contain an inflammatory infiltrates, Menetrier's disease is not considered a form of gastritis
Clinical picture
• Protein losing enteropathy is characteristic Excessive protein is lost from the thickened mucosa into the gut which results in hypoprotenemia and edema • Gastric acid secretion is usually reduced or absent This happens because mucosal cell hyperplasia replaces most of the parietal cells. • Epigastric pain accompanied by nausea, vomiting anorexia and weight loss Overt bleeding is unusual but occult gastrointestinal bleeding may occur
Differential Diagnosis
DD includes conditions that may present with large gastric folds: ZES Malignancy Infiltrative disorders eg sarcoidosis Infectious etiology (CMV, Histoplasmosis, syphilis)
Prognosis
These is an increased risk of adenocarcinoma of stomach in adults with menetrier's disease (CSDT)

80. Answer is B (Usually increased acid secretion): *Harrison 18th/p 2459 Harrison's 17th/1872; Refer previous question*

Gastric acid secretion is usually reduced or absent (and not increased)

Gastric acid secretion is usually reduced or absent because of replacement of parictal cells' Harrison's

Menetrier's disease carries an increased risk of developing adenocarcinoma of stomach (premalignant) is associated with a protein losing enteropathy and may be confused with Zollinger Ellison Syndrome as ZES also presents with large gastric folds.

Carcinoma Stomach

81. Answer is D (Intestinal metaplasia Type III): *Harrison 15th/580; 16th/525; 17th/ 572; Harrison 18th/p765, 766 Robbins 7th/823*

Risk factors for stomach carcinoma :	
1. Long term ingestion of high concentration of nitrates in dried smoke and salted foods. Q	
2. Loss of gastric acidity	- atrophic gastritis Q - partial gastrectomy (peptic ulcer surgery) Q - pernicious anemia Q
3. Infection with H. pylori Q	
4. Intestinal metaplasia Q	
5. Gatric ulcer & polyps Q - (Q **No association has been found between deodonal ulcer and gastric cancer)**	
6. Menetrier's disease Q : extreme hypertrophy of gastric rugal folds.	
7. Blood group A Q	
8. Cigarette smoking, Dust ingestion, Ingestion of spirits, Genetic factors have also been implicated.	

82. Answer is C (Hiatus Hernia): *Gastrointestinal and Liver Diseases by Feldman, Freidman 8th/1147, 1148*

Hiatus Hernia is not considered a premalignant lesion for gastric carcinoma.

Premalignant lesions for Gastric Adenocarcinoma

- Chronic Atrophic Gastritis (H. pylori > Pernicious Anemia)
- Intestinal Metaplasia Type II and Type III
  (Intestinal Metaplasia type I is not associated with increased risk)
- Gastric Dysplasia
- Gastric polyps (Adenomatous polyps)
  (Hyperplastic polyps are generally not considered premalignant as the rate of malignant transformation in these polyps is <1% and confined to polyps > 1cm)
- Previous Gastrectomy
- Menetrier's Disease
- Gastric ulcers (long standing gastric ulcers : Low risk)

83. Answer is B (Hyperplastic Polyps): *Harrison 18th/p 766 Harrison 17th/572; Robbins 7th/823; Manual of Oncology 6th/193; Internal Medicine 5th/2046, 2047*

'Hyperplastic polyps do not appear to have malignant potential' – *Manual of Oncology 6th/193*

Gastric Polyps and Premalignant Potential

Hyperplastic Polyps	Adenomatous Polyps
• Hyperplastic Polyps account for >75% of all gastric polyps • These are not considered premalignant lesions and do not appear to have any significant malignant potential (< 1%)	• Adenomatous Polyps account for < 25% of all gastric polyps • These are considered premalignant lesions They are most commonly found in the antrum of stomach and have significant malignant potential

84. Answer is C (Duodenal Peptic ulcer): *Refer previous question*

Gastric adenocarcinoma may be associated with long standing gastric peptic ulcers (small risk) but not with duodenal ulcers

Atrophic gastritis, partial gastrectomy and blood group A have all been included in the list of risk factors for gastric adenocarcinoma.

85. Answer is C (Intestinal metaplasia): *Harrison 16th/525*

Intestinal metaplasia is the most significant risk factor for development of gastric cancer amongst the options provided.

"The risk of tumor development is greatly increased in patients in whom mucosal inflammation progresses to multifocal mucosal atrophy and intestinal metaplasia"- Robbins

'Serial endoscopic examinations of the stomach in patients with atrophic gastritis have documented replacement of the usual gastric mucosa by intestinal type cells. This process of intestinal metaplasia may lead to cellular atypia and eventual neoplasia.' - Harrison

86. Answer is A (Antrum): *CSDT 11th/557*

The most common site of gastric adenocarcinoma is antrum

'40% tumors are in the antrum, predominantly on the lesser curvature, 30% arise in the body and fundus, 25% at the cardia and 5% involve the whole organ'- CSDT

87. Answer is D > C (Fundus> Body): *Sleisenger & Fordtrans text book of Gastrointestinal disease 7th/813; An Atlas of Gastroenterology by Kapadia 1st (2002)/58; Current Gastroenterology 2nd/391*

Atrophic glands with extensive intestinal metaplasia are most charachteristically confined to the fundus in patients with pernicious anaemia.

Pernicious anemia is associated with autoimmune atrophic gastritis affecting the fundic glands.Intestinal metaplasia (premalignant for gastric carcinoma),is charachterstically seen in this area of atrophic gastritis ***.Atrophic glands with extensive intestinal metaplasia are most charachteristically confined to the fundus in patients with pernicious anaemia.Gastric cancer in case of pernicious anemia is most often located in the fundus or body of the stomach rather in the Antrum.***

Gastric cancer secondary to:	Location / Site
H. pylori	Antrum > body > fundus
Pernicoius Anemia	Fundus and body (not antrum)

88. Answer is C (Gastric adenocarcinoma confined to mucosa and submucosa): *Harrison 18th/p 765, 766 Harrison 17th/571, 572; Robbins 7th/824*

Early gastric carcinoma is defined as a lesion confined to the mucosa and submucosa regardless of the presence or absence of perigastric lymphnode metastasis *– Robbins*

89. Answer is C (Involvement of mucosa, submucosa and muscularis) : *Harrison 18th/765, 766; 17th/571, 572 Bailey 23rd / 922; Robbins 7th/824*

Early gastric cancer:	Cancer limited to the mucosa and submucosa with or without lymph node involvement.
Late gastric cancer :	Cancer involving the muscularis.

90. Answer is A (Superficial spreading type) : *Robbins 6th / 800 ; Bailey 22nd / 963; Bailey 23rd / 920, 921*

Superficial spreading type indicates an early stage of type II malignancy. It is therefore potentially curable, and thus has the best prognosis amongst the choices provided

In Ca Stomach, three macroscopic growth patterns are recognized, and may be evident in both early and advanced gastric cancer stages :

a.	Exophytic (Type I) :	Protruded in early stages, Cauliflower like polypoidal growth in advanced stages.
b.	Flat or depressed (Type II) :	With no obvious tumor mass in mucosa eg. Superficial spreading type
c.	Excavated arc Ulcerated (Type III) :	Shallow or deeply erosive crater is present in the wall of stomach.

Early cases of type I & type II are potentially curable *- Bailey 22nd / 693*

The prognosis depends on depth of invasion and extent of nodal and distant metastasis.

Superficial spreading type indicates an early stage of type II malignancy. It therefore is potentially curable, and thus has the best prognosis amongst the choices provided.

The best answer therefore is superficial spreading type which indicates an 'Early Gastric Cancer'.

'Linitis plastica' is characterized by ***extensive infiltration of malignancy*** into a broad region of gastric wall or entire stomach creating a rigid, thickened *leather-bottle like stomach.*

91. Answer is C (Partial Gastrectomy + Distal pancreatectomy): *NSSG (National Site Specific Group) Guidelines for Upper GI Cancers (NHS, UK) Official publication; 'Complications in Surgery' by Doherty (Lippincott) 2006 /398 'Diagnosis and Management of Cancer' by Mehta & Bansal (Jaypee) 1st/363; Sabiston 18th/1265*

Partial gastrectomy with distal pancreatectomy should be adequate to manage this distal gastric tumor with direct invasion into the distal pancreas.

Tumors of the distal third / antrum of stomach require a subtotal gastrectomy (Partial gastrectomy). The distal pancreas should be removed as there is direct invasion of the distal pancreas. Splenectomy is not indicated as the tumor does not directly invade the spleen, and involvement of splenic hilar lymph nodes is unlikely as the tumor is located in the distal third of the stomach (and not in the proximal stomach). This patient is best managed by subtotal gastrectomy + lymphadenectomy + distal pancreatectomy.

Guidelines for management of Gastric carcinoma

- Surgical resection remains the mainstay of treatment of gastric cancer either for cure or for palliation
- ***The extent of gastric resection*** depends on the site of tumor in the stomach.
  Tumors in the distal third or antrum of stomach require a subtotal gastrectomy (partial gastrectomy) while tumors of the middle or proximal third of the stomach require a total gastrectomy

Distal Third /Antrum Gastric cancer	*Middle Third / Proximal Gastric cancer*
Subtotal Gastrectomy	*Total Gastrectomy*

Patients with curable cancers of the stomach should also undergo a D2 lymphadenectomy

- ***The extent of resection of adjacent* structures (pancreas, spleen etc)** depends on the location of primary tumor and local invasion

Pancreatic Resection

The distal pancreas should not be removed a part of a resection for a cancer of the distal two third of the stomach (unless there is direct invasion)

The distal pancreas should be removed only when there is direct invasion and still a chance of a curative procedure in patients with carcinoma of the proximal stomach

Splenic resection

Splenectomy is not indicated unless the tumor directly invades the spleen or involves the splenic hilar lymph nodes. Resection of spleen and splenic hilar lymph nodes *may be considered* in patients with *tumors of the proximal stomach* located in the greater curvature / posterior wall of the stomach close to the splenic hilum *where the incidence of splenic hilar nodal involvement is likely to be high*

Splenic hilar lymph nodes are generally not involved in distal third / antral gastric cancers

Adjacent structure	Distal Third / Antrum Gastric cancer	Proximal Gastric cancer
Pancreas	• *Should not be removed routinely* • *Resected if there is direct invasion*	• *Should not be removed routinely* • *Resected if there is direct invasion and/or still a chance of curative procedure*
Spleen	• *Should not be removed routinely* • *Resected if there is direct invasion or involvement of splenic hilar lymph nodes (This is unlikely)*	• *May require splenectomy to include the draining lymph nodes especially if lesion is located on the greater curvature / posterior wall, close to the splenic hilum*

92. Answer is A (Stomach) : *Bailey 21st / 892; Not elaborated in later editions*

The most common benign neoplasms of the stomach are Leiomyomas º.

'Despite the fact that small bowel represents 75% of the length of Alimentary tract, *its tumors are less common than those in the stomach'.*

These statements lead us to the conclusion that within the GIT leiomyomas are more common in stomach than in other parts.

Malabsorption Syndrome and Disorders of Small Intestine

General

93. Answer is D (Tangier's Disease): *Refer text below*

Tangier's Disease is not a malabsorption syndrome.

Whipple's Disease, Celiac sprue and Tropical sprue are charachteristic / typical examples of malabsorption syndromes.

Tangier's Disease *is a genetic disorder charachterized by a severe deficiency of high density lipoprotein cholesterol (HDL-C) concentration in the plasma as well as deposition of cholesterol crystals in the tissue. Tangier's disease is synonymous with* ***Familial High Density Lipoprotein Deficiency****.*

Malabsorption Syndromes

Diffuse, specific	Patchy, specific	Diffuse, nonspecific
• *Whipple's disease* • *Agammaglobulinemia* • Abetalipoproteinemia	• *Intestinal lymphoma* • *Intestinal lymphangiectasia* • *Eosinophilic gastroenteritis* • *Amyloidosis* • *Crohn's disease* • *Infection by one or more microorganisms* • *Mastocytosis*	• *Celiac sprue* • *Tropical sprue* • *Bacterial overgrowth* • *Folate deficiency* • *Vitamin B12 deficiency* • *Radiation enteritis* • *Zollinger – Ellison syndrome* • *Protein –calorie malnutrition* • *Drug-induced enteritis*

94. Answer is A (Steatorrhea): '*Differiential Diagnosis in Medicine: From Symptom to Diagnosis (Thieme) 2007/821*

Malabsorbtion of fat soluble vitamins is typically seen in steatorrhea and pancreatic exocrine deficiency (not pancreatic endocrine deficiency).

Steatorrhea *is typically defined as increased excretion of fat in stool (excretion of > 7.0 gm of fat in stool during 24 hours while the patient is on a diet containing no more than 100gm of fat per day).*

Steatorrhea essentially represents malabsorption of fat.

This may be caused by several conditions including:

- *Acute or chronic Liver disease / Biliary Disease*
- *Mucosal disease (eg. Celiac disease / Crohn's disease)*
- *Reduced absorptive surface (Small Bowel Syndrome)*
- *Reduced contact time (Laxative abuse, Carcinoid syndrome)*
- *Disturbed mesenteric blood supply (Mesenteric ischemia)*
- *Disturbed mesenteric lymphatic drainage (Tuberculosis, Malignancy)*
- ***Pancreatic exocrine deficiency (Reduced Pancreatic Lipase)***

95. Answer is A (D-xylose test): *Harrison 18th/2467; Harrison 17th/1878*

D-xylose is a carbohydrate that is absorbed almost exclusively in the proximal small bowel without the help of pancreatic enzymes. A positive D-xylose test indicates malabsorption due to intestinal mucosal disease and thus be used as a test for assessment of mucosal function.

D- Xylose Test

- D-Xylose *is a carbohydrate*[Q] that is absorbed completely in small bowel without the help of pancreatic enzymes and excreted unchanged in urine
- D- Xylose absorption test is used to distinguish *malabsorption*[Q] due to pancreatic disease from malabsorption due to intestinal mucosal disease
- D-Xylose is absorbed almost exclusively in the proximal small bowel (duodenum and jejunum), and a positive test primarily reflects a duodenal /Jejunal mucosal disease

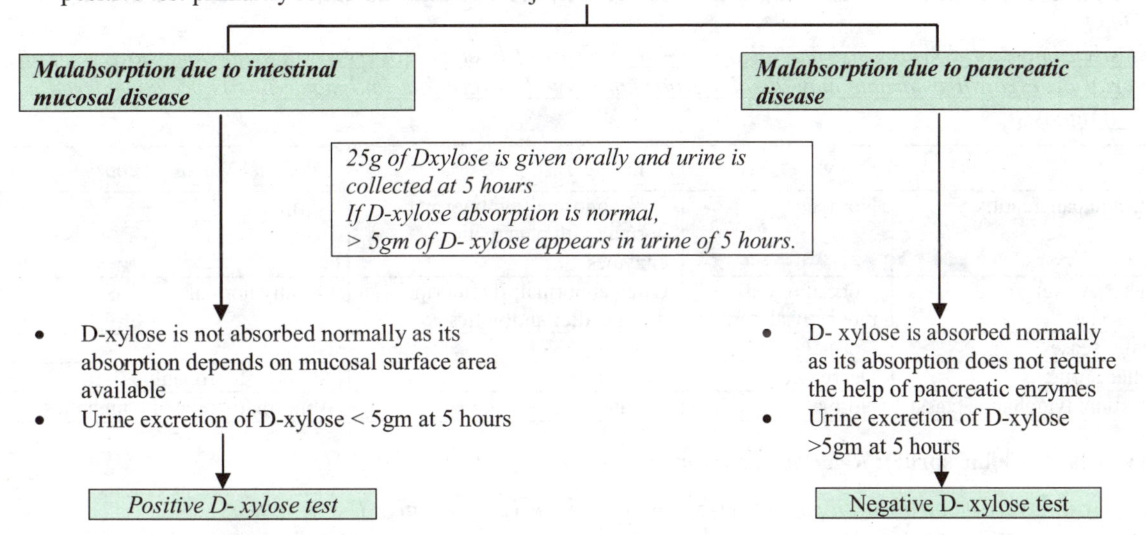

96. Answer is A (Pancreatic insufficiency): *Refer text below Harrison 18th/p 2467, 2470 Harrisons 17th / 1878, 1881, Manual of Gastroenterology 4th/ 213*

Pancreatic insufficiency is associated with a Negative D- xylose test (Normal D-xylose excretion)

97. Ans is A (Carbohydrate malabsorption due to mucosal disease): *Harrison 16th/1769; 17th/1878; 18th/p 2467*

'The urinary D-xylose test for carbohydrate absorption provides an assessment of proximal small intestine mucosal function.' *– Harrison 16th/1769*

Urinary D-xylose test:

Principle :
D-xylose is a 'pentose' that is completely absorbed almost exclusively in the proximal small intestine and excreted subsequently in the urine. The level of excreted D-xylose in urine is estimated.
Any decrease in its level in urine means abnormality in carbohydrate absorption in proximal intestine.
Procedure & interpretation
25g D-xylose is given and urine is collected for 5 hrs.
An excretion of < 4.5g primarily reflects the presence of duodenal / jejunal mucosal disease.

98. Answer is C (D-xylose test) : *Harrison 14th/1620, 15th/1672, 1634, 1674 t; 16th/1769; 17th/1878; Harrison 18th/2467*

D-xylose absorption test *is the most commonly employed test for carbohydrate absorption - Harrison*
An endoscopic mucosal biopsy is the more specific test and is now considered essential.
As endoscopic small intestinal biopsy' is not provided in the options 'D-xylose test' is the answer of the choice

Evaluation of small intestine malabsorption of carbohydrates due to altered small intestinal mucosal function

Urinary D-xylose test	Non invasive test of choice
Endoscopic mucosal biopsy	Test of choice / preferred test

'The ease of obtaining a mucosal biopsy of the small intestine by endoscopy and the false negative rate of the Dxylose test have led to its diminished use. When small intestinal disease is suspected, a small intestinal biopsy should be performed' – Harrison

99. Answer is D (Celiac sprue) : *Harrison's Gastroenterology & Hepatology 1st/165*

A Positive d-xylose test suggests a diagnosis of celiac disease
Decreased urinary excretion of d- xylose (<5.0 gm) 5 hours after administration of 25 gm D- xylose (positive test) suggests malabsorption due to intestinal mucosal disease in the proximal small bowel (duodenum and jejunum).
Celiac disease is a charachteristic cause for positive d-xylose test and the single best answer amongst the options provided
Modestly abnormal d-xylase test may also be seen in cases of bacterial overgrowth syndrome, however patients with bacterial overgrowth syndrome may also have normal d-xylose excretion, and hence this is not considered as the most likely diagnosis

	D-Xylose Test	Schilling Test	Duodenal Mucosal Biopsy
Chronic pancreatitis	Normal	50% abnormal; if abnormal, normal with pancreatic enzymes	Normal
Bacterial overgrowth syndrome	Normal or only modestly abnormal	Often abnormal; if abnormal, normal after antibiotics	Usually normal
Ileal disease	Normal	Abnormal	Normal
Celiac sprue	Decreased	Normal	Abnormal: probably "flat"
Intestinal lymphangiectasia	Normal	Normal	Abnormal: "dilated lymphatics"

100. Answer is D (Celiac sprue): *Refer text below manual of Gastroenterology 4th/ 213*

Celiac sprue is associated with a positive D- xylose and not a False positive D-xylose test.

D-xylose Test

Positive test	False positive test
Decreased (↓) D- Xylose excretion in urine due to malabsorption from gastrointestinal mucosal disease	*Decreased D-xylose excretion in urine due to causes other than malabsorption from small bowel mucosal disease*
Causes Include	Causes Include
• ***Celiac disease*** • *Tropical sprue* • *Whipple's disease* • *Other mucosal diseases*	• ***Bacterial overgrowth*** • ***Renal insufficiency*** • *Delayed gastric emptying* • *Rapid intestinal transit* • *Vomiting* • ***Ascites /Pleural Effusion*** *(Third space collections)*

After a positive D-xylose test is obtained, a jejunal biopsy should be performed to diagnose the mucosal abnormality.

Blood loop syndrome may be associated with a reduced functional intestinal mucosa and bacterial overgrowth. This condition may thus lead to both, a positive or false positive D- xylose test depending on the pathophysiology involved.

101. Answer is E (All of the above): *Refer previous question; Manual of Gastroterology 4th/213*

Blind loop syndrome and *Antibiotic therapy may cause false positive D-xylose test due to* ***bacterial overgrowth***

Pyloric stenosis may cause false positive results due to ***delayed gastric emptying and persistant vomiting.***

Ascitis is an established cause for false positive D- xylose test due to large collection of fluid in third space

102. Answer is A and C (Abnormal in pernicious anemia; Abnormal in ileal disease): *Harrison 18th/p 2467 Harrison 17th/1878*

Schilling test is abnormal in conditions that affect cobalamine absorption including Pernicious anemia, Chronic Pancreatitis, Bacterial overgrowth syndrome and Ileal dysfunction

Conditions with Abnormal Schilling's Test (Abnormal Cobalamine Absorption)
Pernicious anemia   ***Chronic Pancreatitis***   ***Achlorhydria***   ***Bacterial overgrowth syndrome***   ***Ileal dysfunction***

Schilling Test:

- Schilling test is performed to determine the cause of cobalamine malabsorption.
- Since cobalamine absorption requires multiple steps including gastric, pancreatic and ileal processes, the Schilling test can also be used to assess the integrity of these other organs.
- The Schilling test is performed by administering Co58-labeled cobalamin orally and collecting urine for 24h
- The ***Schilling test may be abnormal (defined as less than 10 percent excretion in 24h) in conditions that affect cobalamine absorption including Pernicious anemia, Chronic Pancreatitis, Bacterial overgrowth syndrome and Ileal dysfunction***
- The etiology for an abnormal Schilling test may be deduced by administering Co58-labeled cobalamin with intrinsic factor, pancreatic enzymes or after 5 day course of antibiotics.Differential Results of Schilling Test in various diseases associated with cobalamin malabsorption may thus help establish the diagnosis.

Diagnosis	**^{58}Co-Cbl**	**With Intrinsic Factor**	**With Pancreatic Enzymes**	**After 5 Days of Antibiotics**
Pernicious anemia	*Reduced*	*Normal*	*Reduced*	*Reduced*
Chronic pancreatitis	*Reduced*	*Reduced*	*Normal*	*Reduced*
Bacterialovergrowth	*Reduced*	*Reduced*	*Reduced*	*Normal*
Ileal disease	*Reduced*	*Reduced*	*Reduced*	*Reduced*

103. Answer is A (Small intestinal biopsy): *Harrisons 16th/1770, 1769; 1879, Harrison 17th/ 1879, 1880 Harrison 18th/p 2468, 2469*

'Small intestinal mucosal biopsy is essential in the evaluation of a patient with documented steatorrhea or chronic diarrhea (>3 weeks). *– Harrisons*

Failure to thrive in the background of recurrent bulky stools and abdominal pain suggests a diagnosis of chronic malabsorption. Although all options provided in the question may be used to support the diagnosis, the most appropriate investigation to make a specific diagnosis is small intestinal biopsy.

Lesions seen on a small bowel biopsy can be classified into:

Specific		**Non Specific**
Diffuse Specific	**Patchy Specific**	**Diffuse Non Specific**
Whipples Disease Agammaglobulinemia Abetalipoproteinemia	Intestinal lymphoma Intestinal lymphangiectasia Eosinophilic gastroenteritis Amyloids Amyloidosis Crohn's disease Infection by one or more microorganisms Mastocytosis	Celiac sprue Tropical sprue Bacterial overgrowth Folate deficiency Vitamin B12 deficiency Radiation enteritis Zollinger-Ellison syndrome Protein-calorie malnutrition Drug-induced enteritis

104. Answer is C (Appendicitis): *Harrison 18th/p 2632 Harrisons 17th/2004*

Appendicitis is not associated with raised amylase levels.

Pancreatitis, Ruptured ectopic and salivary gland lesions including blocked salivary duct are all associated with raised amylase levels.

Pancreatic Disease	
1. Pancreatitis A. Acute B. Chronic: ductal obstruction C. Complications of pancreatitis (i) Pancreatic pseudocyst (ii) Pancreatogenous ascites (iii) Pancreatic abscess (iv) Pancreatic necrosis	2. Pancreatic trauma 3. Pancreatic carcinoma
Non pancreatic Disorders	
1. Renal insufficiency 2. Salivary gland lesions A. Mumps B. Calculus C. Irradiation sialadenitis 3. "Tumor" hyperamylasemia A. Carcinoma of the lung B. Carcinoma of the esophagus C. Breast carcinoma, ovarian carcinoma	4. Macroamylasemia 5. Burns 6. Diabetic ketoacidosis 7. Pregnancy 8. Renal transplantation 9. Cerebral trauma 10. Drugs morphine
Other Abdominal Disorders	
1. Biliary tract disease: cholecystitis, choledocholithiasis 2. Intraabdominal disease A. Perforated or penetrating peptic ulcer B. Intestinal obstruction or infarction C. Ruptured ectopic pregnancy D. Peritonitis E. Aortic aneurysm F. Chronic liver disease G. Postoperative hyperamylasemia	

Celiac Disease

105. Answer is A (Antiendomysial antibodies): *Harrisons 16th/1770-1771; Harrison 17th/1881 Harrison 18th/p 2470, 2471*

Evidence of Malabsorption together with charachteristic histopathological changes on small intestinal biopsy in the form of complete villous atrophy suggests the diagnosis of celiac sprue / disease.

Antibody studies are frequently used to identify patients with celiac disease. *'The antiendomysial antibody has 90 to 95% sensitivity and 90 to 95% specificity' in the detection of celiac disease.* - *Harrisons 16th/1770*

Celiac disease : Review : *Harrisons 16th/1770-1772*		
Malabsorption syndrome of non infectious etiology without systemic features.		
Etiology		
Environmental factors	**Immunogenic factors**	**Genetic factors**
Intolerance to ***gliadin*** a component of gluten, present in wheat, barley, rye and oats	Ig A antibodies are present - ***IgA antiendomysial*** - IgA antigliadin - IgA anti tissue tranglutaminase ***Antiendomysial antibody has 90-95% Sensitivity and 90-95% Specificity***	95% express ***HLA-OQ2 allele***[Q]
Presentation		
Malabsorption of multiple nutrients with diarrhea, steatorrhea, weight / loss and consequences of nutrients depletion i.e. anemia and metabolic bone disease	or	Malabsorption of a single nutrient, with iron deficiency anemia or folate deficiency or osteomalacia or edema from protein loss.

Diagnosis	
1. **Small intestinal biopsy (duodenal/jejunal)**[Q] (charachteristic but not diagnostic)[Q] Absence or reduced height of villi (Flat appearnce)[Q] • Crypt hyperplasia, villous atrophy (but not mucosal atrophy)[Q] • Cuboidal appearance of epethelial cells and increased intraepethelial lymphocytes • Increased lymphocytes and plasma cells in lamina propria[Q]	2. **Antiendomysial antibodies**[Q] Antiendomysial antibody has 90-95% sensitivity and 90-95% specificity. *Prompt clinical and histopathological response, together with disappearance of Ig Antiendomysial antibodies following institution of a gluten free diet is diagnostic.*
Associated disease[Q]	**Complications**
• Dermatitis Herpetoformis[Q] • Diabetes mellitus type I[Q] • IgA deficiency	• Increased incidence of both gastro intestinal and non gastrointestinal neoplasms as well as ***Intestinal lymphomas.***[Q]
Management	
Gluten free diet + Glucocorticoids or immunosupressive agents.[Q]	

106. Answer is B (Anti-endomysial antibody): *CMDT 2008/530; 09/544; Harrison 18th/p 2470, 2471 Harrison's 17th/1881; 16th/1961, 1986*

Presence of chronic diarrhea, anemia and elevated liver enzymes is consistent with a diagnosis of Coeliac disease. ***Antiendomysial antibodies are highly sensitive and specific for diagnosis of celiac disease and the single best answer of choice amongst the options provided.***

Approach to diagnosis of Celiac Disease

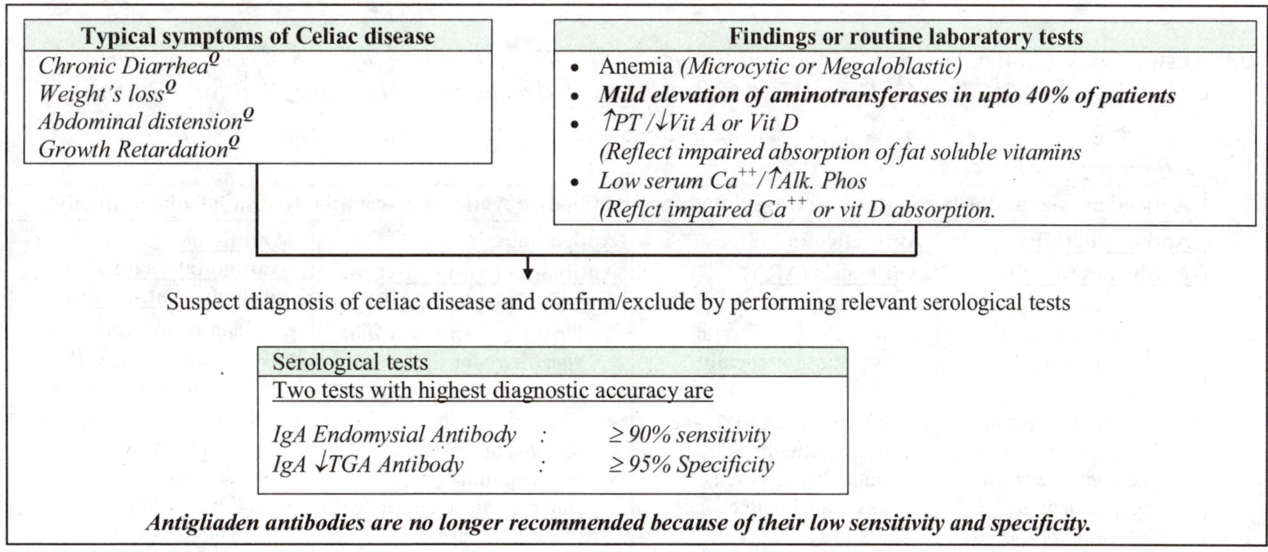

107. Answer is A (Glutin free diet) : *Harrison 16th / 1772; Harrison 17th/1880, 1881 Harrison 18th/p 2470, 2471*

Villous atrophy on duodenal biopsy together with positive serological tests for antiendomysial antibodies and IgA anti TTG antibodies suggests the diagnosis of celiac sprue.

The mainstay of treatment for celiac sprue is administration of of a glutin free diet.

'Removal of all glutin from the diet is essential to therapy'. – CMDT

'The most common cause of persistant symptoms in a patient who fulfills all the criteria of diagnosis of celiac sprue is continued intake of gluten'. – Harrison 16th

Diagnosis of Celiac Sprue

Serological tests →	**Endoscopic mucosal biopsy** *of distal duodenum or proxi- mal jejunum* →	**Prompt clinical and histo-pathological response follo-wing institution of gluten free diet.**
Serological tests (*CMDT*)	**Endoscopic mucosal biopsy**	**Diagnosis**
▪ ***Two serological tests with highest diagnostic accuracy are*** 1. IgA antiendomysial antibody 2. IgA anti – tTG antibody ▪ Both tests have a > 90% sensitivity and > 95% specificity. <u>IgG or IgA antigliadin antibodies</u> are present in 85% of patients with celiac sprue. However their specificity is relatively low (80 – 90%) which limits their usefulness as screening test. *Small bowel biopsy is still recommended to confirm diagnosis.*	• Findings are ***characteristic but not specific / diagnostic***. • Biopsy of distal duodenum or proximal jejunum is performed. • <u>Finding are restricted to mucosa and include</u> : – Loss or blunting of villi / flat villi – Hypertrophy of intestinal crypts – Infiltration of lamina propria will lymphocytes / plasma cells – Cuboidal appearance of epithelial cells and increased intraepithelial lymphocytes.	• <u>Diagnosis of celiac sprue requires</u> Presence of characteristic histopathological changes on biopsy together will prompt clinical and hispathological response following institution of gluten free diet. • IgA antiendomysial Ab or IgA anti – tTGA Ab should also disappear after a gluten free diet.

108. Answer is A (Antiendomysial antibody): *Harrison 15th / 1771; Harrison 17th/1881; Harrison 18th/p 2470, 2471 CMDT 2007/615, 616; 09/544; Diagnosis of Celiac disease 'Indian journal of Pediatrics(IJP) vol. 73 Issue 8*

Antiendomysial antibodies have a high sensitivity and specificity for diagnosis of celiac sprue and show best performance for detection of celiac sprue.

Antiendomysial antibody > Anti tissue transglutaminase antibody > Antireticular antibody> Antigliadin antibody			
<u>**Antigliadin (IJP) Antibodies (AGN)**</u>	<u>**Anti reticulin IJP Antibodies (ARA)**</u>	<u>**Antiendomysial Antibiotics (Anti EMA)**</u>	<u>**Anti tissue transglutaminase antibody (Anti-tTGA)**</u>
• First immunological assay to be tested were antigliadin antibodies. • The variability and lower accuracy make them *unsuitable for diagnostic and screening purposes* • Antigliadin assays have been replaced by more specific and sensitive tests using other antibodies	• Second antibody identified in literature was the antireticulin antibodies. • There are atleast 5 types of antireticulin antibodies but only one type is associated with celiac disease. • These antibodies are *not very sensitive and are not used in routine practice.*	• Antiendomysial antibodies have ***high sensitivity and specificity*** for the diagnosis of celiac disease. • These antibodies are directed against endomysium or 'Intermyofibril substance' of smooth muscle. • The antigen recognized by these antibodies is 'tissue transglutaminase'.	• Major breakthrough for serological diagnosis of celiac disease. • Antitissue transglutaminase antibodies (Anti-tTGA) are ***also highly sensitive and specific but performance of anti EMA is superior to Anti-tTGA***

<u>**Anti EMA and Anti-tTGA**</u>

<u>*While the performance of Anti-EMA is superior to Anti – tTGA, the discovery of Anti-tTGA is seen as a major breakthrough. Why ?*</u>

Anti-EMA	Anti – tTGA
• Anti EMA are species specific reacting only with gastrointestinal tract of primates. They are identified using indirect immunoflorescence on frozen section of monkey esophagus. • Interpretation of immunoflorescence assay is ***operator dependent and more liable to errors in less experienced hands.***	• ELISA based assays are available for detection of anti – tTGA. • Initial tests used guinea pig antigen but now human recombinant tTGA are available. • ELISA based detection is ***simpler and more accessible diagnostic test***

Recommended reading : Article on 'Diagnosis of celiac disease' by AIIMS faculty published in 'Indian Journal of Pediatric' 2006; volume 73 issue 8 (Available on internet)

A recent systemic review of the diagnostic performance of the serological tests reported in studies from 1996 to 2003 showed that in children:

Parameter	Anti-EMA	Anti-tTGA (Human Recombinant)
Specificity	100% (pooled monkey esophagus and human umbilical cord)	95 – 95% (pooled + TG guinea pig and human recombinant)
Sensitivity	96% (monkey esophagus)	96% (human recombinant)

Anti-tTGA is highly sensitive and specific but performance of anti EMA is superior to Anti-tTGA

109. Answer is B (Increase in thickness of mucosa): *Pathologic basis of Disease by Robbins 5th/797 Harrison's 16th/1770-71; 17th/1881 Harrison 18th/p 2470*

The overall mucosal thickness remains the same *- Robbins*

Pathologic morphology of celiac disease:

The mucosa appears flat or scalloped or may be visually normal. Biopsy specimens demonstrate a diffuse enteritis, with the following features.

The villi	The surface epithelium	The crypts	The lamina propria
show marked atrophy or total loss.	shows vacuolar degeneration, loss of the microvillus brush border, and an increased number of intraepithelial lymphocytes.	exhibit increased mitotic activity and are elongated, hyperplastic and tortuous, so the overall mucosal thickness remains the same.	has an overall increase in plasma cells, lymphocytes, macrophages, eosinophils and mast cells.

*All these **structural changes are more marked in the proximal small intestine** [Q] than in the distal because it is the duodenum and proximal jejunum that are exposed to the highest concentration of the dietary gluten.*

110. Answer is C and E (Mucosal atrophy & Presence of Giardia lambia): *Harrison 18th/p 2471 Harrison's 17th/1881*

Mucosal atrophy and presence of Giardia Lambia are not seen in biopsy from celiac disease.

Small Intestinal Biopsy (duodenal /jejunal) in Celiac disease (Characteristic but not diagnostic[Q])

- Absence or reduced height of villi (Flat appearance)[Q]
- Crypt hyperplasia, villous atrophy (but not mucosal atrophy)[Q]
- Cuboidal appearance of epithelial cells and increased intraepithelial lymphocytes
- Increased lymphocytes and plasma cells in lamina propria[Q]

111. Answer is A (Dermatitis Herpetiformis): *Harrisons 17th/1881 CMDT 2008/ 529, 530; 09/544*

Celiac disease is associated with Dermatitis Herpetiformis

'Dermatitis Herpetiformis is regarded as cutaneous variant of celiac disease. Almost all patients with dermatitis Herpetiformis have evidence of celiac disease on intestinal biopsy' – CMD

Associations of Celiac Disease (CMDT & Harrisons)
• ***Dermatitis Herpetiformis***
• Other autoimmune disease including: *(CMDT)*
- *Addison's disease*
- *Grave's disease*
- *Diabetes mellitus- Type I (Harrisons)*
- *Myaesthenia Gravis*
- *Slogren syndrome*
- *Atrophic Gastritis*
- *Pancreatic insufficiency*
• IgA deficiency *(Harrisons)*
• Lymphomas *(Harrisons)*

Note

Celiac disease is associated with an increased risk of cancer including Lymphomas (NHL, Intestinal T cell Lymphoma)

The possibility of Lymphoma must be considered whenever a patient with celiac sprue previously doing well on a gluten free diet is no longer responsive to gluten free diet' - Harrisons

112. Answer is E (All of the above): *Harrisons 17th/1881, 1882 CMDT 2008/530*

Celiac disease may be associated with Dermatitis Herpetiformis and other autoimmune diseases including type I D.M and Atrophic gastritis. It is also associated with increased risk of cancer including Lymphomas.

113. Answer is A and B (Intestinal biopsy and Unequivocal response to gluten restriction): *Harrison 18th/p 2470, 2471 Harrisons 17th/1881*

'The diagnosis of celiac disease requires the presence of characteristic histological changes on small intestinal biopsy together with a prompt and clinical and histological response (unequivocal response) following the institution of gluten free diet' *– Harrisons 17th/1881*

114. Answer is A (Rice): *Harrisons 16th/1772*

Rice is Gluten free and should be used in place of wheat flour in patients with Gluten sensitivity or celiac sprue

Gluten Containing Grains
• *Wheat*
• *Rye*
• *Oat*
• *Barley*
• *Spelt*

Gluten Free Grains
• *Rice*
• *Corn*
• *Millet*
• *Topioca*

115. Answer is A and D (Rice and Corn): *Refer previous question*

Rice and Corn are Gluten free grains that can be safely consumed in patients with gluten hypersensitivity

116. Answer is D (Vitamin B_{12}): *Celiac Disease for Dummies' by Blumer & Crowe (John Wiley & Sons 2010*

Vitamin B_{12} deficiency may be seen in celiac disease but the deficiency of this vitamin is uncommon in patients with celiac disease. Vitamin B_{12} is the single best Answer amongst the option provided.

'Vitamin B_{12} is absorbed from the body in the end part of small intestine (terminal ileum). Because this part of the bowel is seldom damaged - by celiac disease, Vitamin B12 deficiency is not common in this condition'- Celiac Disease for Dummies

'Vitamin D Deficiency is particularly frequent in people with celiac disease' - Celiac Disease for Dummies

'Folic acid Deficiency is fairly common in people with celiac disease' - Celiac Disease for Dummies

'Vitamin A Deficiency is common in people with celiac disease - Celiac Disease for Dummies

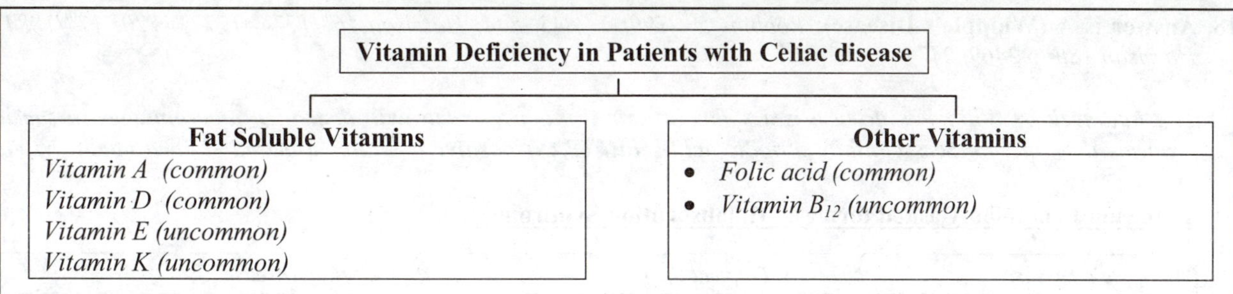

Whipple's Disease

117. Answer is C (Whipple's Disease): *Harrison 18th/2470; Harrison's 17th/1880; Harrison's 16th/1769, 1770*

An intestinal biopsy is diagnostic/specific for malabsorption due to Whipple's disease.

Three most commonly asked forms of Malabsorption Syndromes :

Whipple's Disease	***Tropical Sprue***	***Coeliac Disease***
Malabsorption syndrome with systemic features with infectious etiology	Malabsorption syndrome of infectious etiology without systemic features	Malabsorption syndrome of non infectious etiology without systemic features
Etiology	**Etiology**	**Etiology**
Gram negative actinomycete[Q] Tropheryma whippelii	Caused by some strains of E.coli	Caused by intolerance to 'gliadin' gluten a protein found in wheat rye, barley[Q].
Biopsy	**Biopsy**	**Biopsy**
Biopsy is Abnormal and specific/diagnostic	**Biopsy is abnormal but not specific/diagnostic**	**Biopsy is abnormal but not specific/diagnostic**
Lamina Propria is infiltrated with macrophages containing PAS positive glycoproteins and rod shaped bacilli Dilated lymphatics	Shortened, thickened villi increased crypt depth infiltration by mononuclear cells	Blunting and flattening surface with villi either absent or broad and short Crypts are elongated Dense infiltration of inflammatory cells in lamina propria
Clinical features	**Clinical features**	**Clinical features**
Features of malabsorption + Array of systemic features	Features of malabsorption	Features of malabsorption
Management	**Management**	**Management**
Etiology is infectious so treatment is with Antibiotics Trimethoprim+sufamethoxocate	Etiology is infectious so treatment is with antibiotics (Sulfonamide/ Tetracycline)	Etiology is not infectious but immune Glutin free diet (no antibiotics) + Glucocorticoids or immunosuppressive agents

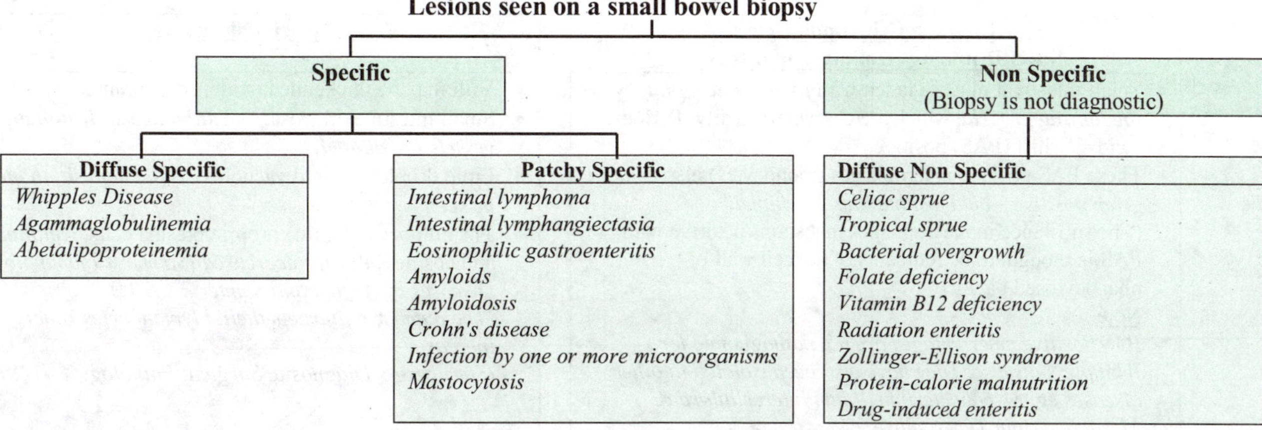

118. Answer is A (Whipple's Disease): *Robbins 5th/799; 7th/843, 844; Harrison 16th/1774, 1772, 1770; 17th/1884, 1879 Harrison 18th/p 2469, 2474*

The hallmark of Whipple's disease is a small intestinal mucosa laden with distended macrophages in the lamina propria- the macrophages contain periodic acid-schiff (PAS) positive granules and rod shaped bacilli by electron microscopy.

Three most commonly asked forms of Malabsorption Syndromes :

Whipple's Disease	*Tropical Sprue*	*Coeliac Disease*
Malabsorption syndriome with systemic features with infectious etiology	Malabsorption syndrome of infectious etiology without systemic features	Malabsorption syndrome of non infectious etiology without systemic features
Etiology	**Etiology**	**Etiology**
Gram negative actinomycete[Q] Tropheryma whippelii	Caused by some strains of E.coli	Caused by intolerance to 'gliadin' gluten a protein found in wheat rye, barley[Q].
Biopsy	**Biopsy**	**Biopsy**
Diagnostic	***Abnormal but Not Diagnostic***	***Abnormal / Characteristic but Not Diagnostic***
Lamina Propria is infiltrate with of macrophages containing PAS positive glycoproteins and rod shaped bacilli Dilated lymphatic	Shortened, thickened villi increased crypt depth infiltration by mononuclear cells	Blunting and flattening surface with villi either absent or broad and short Crypts are elongated Dense infiltration of inflammatory cells in lamina propria inflammatory
Clinical features	**Clinical features**	**Clinical features**
Features of malabsorption + Array of systemic features	Features of malabsorption	Features of malabsorption
Management	**Management**	**Management**
Etiology is infectious so treatment is with Antibiotics Trimethoprim+sufamethoxocate	Etiology is infectious so treatment is with antibiotics Antibiotic (Sulfonamide/ Tetracycline)	Etiology is not infectious but immune Glutin free diet (no antibiotics) + Glucocorticoids or immunosuppressive agents

119. Answer is B (Marked increase in the number of intraepethelial lymphocytes): *Robbins 7th/844 Samter's Immunologic Disease by Austen & Samter 2nd/ 704; Sternberg's Diagnostic Surgical Pathology 4th /1481*

The intraepethelial lymphocytes are usually, either decreased in number or normal.
Marked increase in the number of intraepethelial lymhocytes is not seen and this is the single best answer of exclusion.

The Hallmark of Whipple's disease is a small intestinal mucosa laden with macrophages**. Accompanying changes include** lymphatic dilatation **suggesting lymphatic blockage. The lymphatic blockage is believed to be responsible for** lipid deposition **in the villi** – *Robbins*

Histopathological findings in Whipple's disease

Characterisitc findings / Specific finding (Hallmark of disease)

- Small intestinal mucosa laden with ***foamy macrophages in the lamina propria***, which are characteristically, Periodic – Acid – Schiff (PAS) positive.
- These PAS positive macrophages (monocytes) also *contain gram positive – acid fast bacillus T. whipleii*[Q].
  (The substance in macrophages that stains positive with PAS is thought to be remnants of the cell wall of phagocytosed bacilli)
  Note :
  PAS positive macrophages are not pathognomic for Whipple's disease. They have also been isolated in other diseases eg. Mycobacterium Avium Intercellulare & Mycobacterium Tuberculosis.

Associated findings

- Villi may be thickenned, widened or blunted
- Small intestinal mucosal and ***submucosal lymphatic vessels are dilated***
- Lipid droplets / Lipid vacuoles / ***Lipid deposition may be seen***
- The number of lamina propria plasma cells, ***lymphocytes*** and eosinophills ***are decreased*** *(Samter's Immunologic Diseases by Austen and Samter 2nd /704)*
  'The number of intraepethelial lymphocytes is not increased'
  (Sternberg's Diagnostic Surgical Pathology 4th/1481)

Disease that can be Diagnosed by Small-Intestinal Mucosal Biopsies

Lesions	Pathologic Findings
Diffuse, specific	
• *Whipple's disease*	Lamina propria contains macrophages containing PAS + material
• *Agammaglobulinemia*	No plasma cells; either normal or absent villi ("flat mucosa")
• Abetalipoproteinemia	Normal villi; epithelial cells vacuolated with fat postprandially
Patchy, specific	
• *Intestinal lymphoma*	Malignant cells in lamina propria and submucosa
• *Intestinal lymphangiectasia*	Dilated lymphatics; clubbed villi
• *Eosinophilic gastroenteritis*	Eosinophil infiltration of lamina propria and mucosa
• *Amyloidosis*	Amyloid deposits
• *Crohn's disease*	Noncaseating granulomas
• *Infection by one or more microorganisms*	Specific organisms
• *Mastocytosis*	Mast cell infiltration of lamina propria
Diffuse, nonspecific	
• *Celiac sprue*	Short or absent villi; mononuclear infiltrate; epithelial cell damage; hypertrophy of crypts
• *Tropical sprue*	Similar to celiac sprue
• *Bacterial overgrowth*	Patchy damage to villi; lymphocyte
• *Folate deficiency*	Short villi; decreased mitosis in crypts; megalocytosis
• *Vitamin B12 deficiency*	Similar to folate deficiency
• *Radiation enteritis*	Similar to folate deficiency
• *Zollinger – Ellison syndrome*	Mucosal ulceration and erosion from acid
• *Protein –calorie malnutrition*	Villous atrophy; secondary bacterial overgrowth
• *Drug-induced enteritis*	Variable histology

120. Answer is D (Dementia) : *Harrison 14th / 1627, 15th/1667, 16th/1774; 17th/ 1884; Harrison 18th/p 2474 CMDT 2003 / 587; 09/546*

CNS manifestations in Whipples disease include dementia (presenting as confusion in memory loss) along with focal features such as Seizures. ***Non specific symptoms like Confusion and Memory loss (Dementia) in all likelihood, should be more common a presentation than seizures.***

Whipple's disease is a rare multisystemic illness caused by infection with the bacillus *'Tropheryma Whippelii'* Q

- *Essential of Diagnosis include :*
  - a. Malabsorption Q
  - b. Multisystemic involvement along with Fever, Lymphadenopathy and Arthralgias Q
  - c. Duodenal Biopsy with PAS positive macrophages Q showing characteristic bacillus (with large cytoplasmic granules)Q
- *CNS invovement is seen in about 10%* of patients. Manifestations include
  - ***Dementia*** Q (confusion and memory loss)
  - Seizures, Coma, Myoclonus Q
- *Cranial N. findings* include Nystagmus and Ophthalmoplegia Q

  Non specific symptoms like Confusion and Memory loss (Dementia) in all likelihood, should be more common a presentation than seizures.

  Ophthalmopegia is due to cranial nerve involvement and not supra-nuclear in type.

121. Answer is D (Giardiasis): *Harrison 16th/1249, CMDT 6th/1479 (Repeat)*

Giardia *should be considered in most cases of diarrhoea, especially when it is prolonged and associated with marked weight loss.* ***Syndromes*** *include, acute diarrhoea, chronic diarrhoea and* ***malabsorption.****- CMDT*
Disease manifestation of ***giardiasis*** *range from asymptomatic carriage to fulminant diarrhoea and* ***malabsorption.'***

- Harrison

Short Bowel Syndrome

122. Answer is B (Hypogastrinemia): *Harrison 15th/1676; Harrison 16th/11773; Harrison 17th/1882, 1883 Harrison 18th/p 2472, 2473*

Short bowel syndrome is characterized by increased gastrin levels (hypergastrinemia) due to reduced small intestinal catabolism of gastrin *– Harrison's*

Short bowel syndrome *(Myriad of clinical problems that follow resection of warying length of small intestine)*

Causes:

1. *Mesentric vascular disease: mesenteric ischaemia*[Q]
2. *Primary mucosal and submucosal disease – Crohn's disease*[Q]
3. *Operations without preexisting small intestinal disease – jejunoilial bypass for obesity*[Q]

Manifestation resulting from resection of varying length of small intestine

Diarrhea and Steatorrhea [Q]	↑ed Renal calcium oxalate calculi	↑ed Cholesterol gall stones [Q]	Gastric hypersecretion of acid [Q]
Multiple factors contribute to diarrhea and steatorrhea such as: • Absence of intestinal mucosa required for absorption of lipid and fluid and electrolytes • Stimulation of colonic fluid and electrolyte secretion by increased bile acids that enter colon • Decreased intestinal transit and bacterial overgrowth from absence of ilio caecal valve • Reduced pH in duodenum from gastric acid hypersecretion.	• There occurs increased absorption of oxalates by large intestine in patients with a small intestinal resection with intact colon • Hyperoxaluria and renal calcium oxalate crystals form **Treatment:** • Dietry restriction of oxalate containing feed (spinach, tea) • Cholestyramine an anion binding resin and calcium	Due to a decrease in the bile acid pool size and resulting super saturation of cholesteral in gall-bladder bile.	Related to reduced hormonal inhibition of acid secretion or increased gastrin levels due to reduced small intestine catabolism of gastrin.

123. Answer is B (Iron deficiency anaemia): *Harrison 16th/1773; Harrison 15th/1676; Harrison 17th/1882, 1883 Harrison 18th/p 2472, 2473*

Iron is primarily absorbed in duodenum therefore ileal resection will not cause iron deficiency anaemia.
All other options are true and explained in the previous question.

124. Answer is A (Vitamin B12): *'Complications in Surgery' (Lippincott Williams) 2nd (2011)/469; Sleisenger and Fordtran's Gastrointestinal Diseases 8th/2258, 2264*

Cyanocobalamine (Vitamin B12) deficiency is the most common deficiency in patients with short bowel syndrome associated with loss of ileum (ileal resection) since vitamin B12 is absorbed only in the ileum.

'Cyanocobalamine (Vitamin B12) is the most common deficiency and occurs predictably after resection of 50-60 cm of the terminal ileum'. – 'Complications in Surgery' (Lippincott Williams) 2nd (2011)/469

'Vitamin B12 and Bile acids are absorbed only in the ileum. Loss of ileum results in malabsorption of bile acids and vitamin B12 and consequent vitamin B12 deficiency' – 'Sleisenger and Fordtran's Gastrointestinal Diseases' 8th/2258, 2264

Vitamin Deficiencies in Short Bowel Syndrome

Short Bowel Syndrome with Extensive Jejunal Resection

- This is associated primarily with deficiency of fat soluble vitamins (A, D, E, K)
- *The most common fat-soluble vitamins that are deficienct are vitamin A and D and to a lesser extent vitamin E followed by vitamin K.*

Vitamin A, D > Vitamin E >> Vitamin K

Deficiency of vitamin K is uncommon as vitamin K is synthesized by colonic bacteria

- 60% of vitamin K is synthesized by colonic bacteria

Short Bowel Syndrome with Extensive ileal resection

- This is associated primarily with deficiency of vitamin B12 since vitamin B12 is only absorbed in the terminal ileum.
- Fat soluble vitamin deficiencies may also occur due to fat malabsorption from decrease in concentration of bile acids / salts.

(Bile acids are absorbed only from the ileum)

Vitamin B12 > Fat solubleVitamin

- 40% of vitamin K is received by dietary intake
- *Deficiency of vitamin K is therefore uncommon in patients with short bowel syndrome who have an intact colon.*
- *Deficiency of vitamin K is however common in those patients with short bowel syndrome who do not have a residual colon.*

The ileum has the capacity to adapt and compensate for jejunal resection. The jejunum does not have the capacity to adapt and compensate for ileal resection (as the terminal ileum has the exclusive capacity to reabsorb bile salts &vit B_{12})

125. Answer is A (Vitamin B12): *Refer previous question; 'Clinical Nutrition in Gastrointestinal Disease' by Buchman (2006)/362*

Cyanocobalamine (Vitamin B12) deficiency is the most common deficiency in patients with short bowel syndrome associated with loss of ileum (ileal resection) since vitamin B12 is absorbed only in the ileum

Short Bowel Syndrome may be associated with deficiency of fat-soluble vitamins (Vitamin A, D, E and K) and water soluble Vitamin B12 (when ileum is resected / non functional).

The most common deficiency is determined essentially by the specific segment of the small intestine (jejunum or ileum) that is resected / non functional.

Since the question does not specify the specific segment of the small intestine contributing to the short bowel syndrome, the single best answer has to be selected by a method of exclusion.

Vitamin B12 is the single best answer amongst the options provided (*since none of the commonly deficient fat soluble vitamins (A, D or E) have been provided amongst the options and deficiency of Fat soluble Vitamin K is uncommon in Short Bowel Syndrome)*

Deficiency of fat-soluble vitamin K is uncommon in short bowel syndrome*since 60% of the vitamin K is synthesized in the colon*

Deficiency of water-soluble vitamins Biotin and Thiamine is uncommon in short bowel syndrome *since thay are primarily absorbed in the duodenum and/or proximal jejunum.*

Short Bowel Syndrome is primarily associated with deficiency of fat-soluble vitamin (A, D and E) and water-soluble vitamin B12 (since this water soluble vitamin is absorbed only in the ileum)

Intestinal Angina

126. Answer is B (Postprandial Abdominal Pain, Weight loss and Chronic mesenteric vessel occlusion) : *Harrison 16th/1799; 17th/1911*

Chronic intestinal ischemia *presents with* ***intSestinal angina*** *or abdominal pain associated with need for increased blood flow to the intestine.*

Patients report abdominal pain cramping and pain following ingestion of meal (postprandial abdominal pain Weight loss and chronic diarrhea are also noted *- Harrison 16th / 1799*

What is Intestinal Angina : Journal of Emergency Medicine : Review Article.

- Intestinal angina refers to the clinical syndrome seen in association with ***Chronic Mesenteric Ischaemia.***
- It is characterized by reduced mesenteric blood flow that interferes with physiological function but does not cause infarction.
- Mesentric angina is the result of intestinal hypoperfusion through two of the three major vessels supplying the small intestine.
  - Superior Mesentric Artery
  - Celiac artery
  - Inferior Mesentric Artery

Presentation

- Post Prandial Abdominal Pain : Abdominal pain that starts about 30 minutes after eating and lasts for one to two hours.
- Fear of eating and weight loss : Once the patient realizes the relationship between eating and pain.
- Diarrhea, Nausea, Vomiting

Diagnosis

- *Gold standard for confirmation of mesenteric arterial occlusion (chronic mesenteric ischaemia) is Angiography*

- Harrison

(Note that Gold standard for diagnosis of acute mesenteric ischaemia is Laparotomy[Q]. Surgical exploration should not be delayed).

Inflammatory Bowel Disease

Ulcerative Colitis

127. Answer is A (Ulcerative Colitis): *Harrison 18th/p 2486 Harrison's 17th/1892*

Presence of mucus and blood in stool along with positive ANCA antibodies suggests a diagnosis of ulcerative colitis

Different Clinical, Endoscopic and Radiographic Features

	Ulcerative Colitis	Crohn's Disease
Clinical		
Gross blood in stool	***Yes***	***Occasionally***
Mucus	***Yes***	***Occasionally***
Systemic symptoms	Occasionally	Frequently
Pain	Occasionally	Frequently
Abdominal mass	Rarely	Yes
Significant perineal disease	No	Frequently
Fistulas	No	Yes
Small-intestinal obstruction	No	Frequently
Colonic obstruction	Rarely	Frequently
Response to antibiotics	No	Yes
Recurrence after surgery	No	Yes
ANCA-positive	***Frequently***	***Rarely***
ASCA –positive	Rarely	Frequently
Endoscopic		
Rectal sparing	Rarely	Frequently
Continuous disease	Yes	Occasionally
Cobblestoning	No	Yes
Granuloma on biopsy	No	Occasionally
Radiographic		
Small bowel significantly abnormal	No	Yes
Abnormal terminal ileum	Occasionally	Yes
Segmental colitis	No	Yes
Asymmetric colitis	No	Yes
Stricture	Occasionally	Frequently
Epidemiology of IBD		
Age of onset	15-30 and 60-80	15-30 & 60-80
Male : Female ratio	1:1	≈1.5 : 1
Smoking	May prevent disease	May cause disease
Oral contraceptives	No increased risk	Odds ratio 1.4
Appendectomy	Protective	Not protective
Monozygotic twins	6% concordance	58% concordance
Dizygotic twins	0% concordance	4% concordance

128. Answer is B > A (Ulcerative colitis > Crohn's disease): *Robbins 7th/848, 850, Harsh mohan 5th/ 582, 584*

Chronic diarrhea, crypt abscess and crypt ulcers may be seen in both forms of inflammatory bowel disease i.e, Ulcerative colitis and Crohn's disease. However ***cryptitis and crypt abscesses represent the charachteristic microscopic features in Ulcerative Colitis. Ulcerative colitis is therefore the single best answer of exclusion.***

According to Harrison

The characteristic microscopic findings in Ulcerative colitis are crypt distortion,cryptitis and crypt abscesses
(Harrisons 16th/1778, Fig 276-2)
Note
Crypt Abscesses are not specific for Ulcerative colitis and may be seen in CD or any other active inflammatory colitis.

The characteristic microscopic findings in Crohn's disease are non-casseating granulomas in all layers of the bowel wall from mucosa to serosa
However
Aphthoid ulcers and focal ***crypt abscesses*** *are also seen (early lesions) in Crohn's disease (Harrisons 16th/1779)*

Pathological examination of the bowel wall is Crohn's disease is more likely to reveal Non casseating granulomas in association with these crypt abscesses while in the case of Ulcerative colitis, crypt abscesses and cryptitis may be the only pathological finding. As the pathological examination does not mention the presence of Non casseating granulomas we may presume that these were not found during the pathological examination of specimen. ***In the absence of non casseating granulomas, the presence of cryptitis and crypt abscesses favours a diagnosis of ulcerative colitis.***

DISTINGUISHING FEATURES OF CROHN'S DISEASE AND ULCERATIVE COLITIS :

FEATURE	CROHN'S DISEASE	ULCERATIVE COLITIS
A. Macroscopic features		
1. Distribution	Segmental with ***skip areas*** [Q]	Continuous *without skip areas*[Q]
2. Location	Commonly terminal ileum and /or ascending colon	Commonly rectum sigmoid colon and extending upwards
3. Extent	Usually involves the entire thickness of the affected segment of bowel wall	Usually superficial, confined to mucosal layers
4. Ulcers	Serpiginous ulcers, that may develop into deep *Fissures* [Q]	Superficial mucosal ulcers without fissures
5. Pseudopolyps	Rarely seen	*Commonly present* [Q]
6. Fibrosis	Common	Rare
7. Shortening	Due to fibrosis	Due to contraction of muscularis
B. Microscopic features		
1. Depth of inflammation	*Typically transmural* [Q]	*Mucosal* [Q] and Submucosal
2. Type of inflammation	*Non-caseating granulomas* [Q] and infiltrate of mononuclear cells (lymphocytes, plasma cells and macrophages) (Crypt abscess may also be seen)	*Crypt abscess* and non-specific acute and chronic inflammatory cells (lymphocytes, plasma cells neutrophils, eosinophils, mast cells)
3. Mucosa	Patchy ulceration	Hemorrhagic mucosa with ulceration
4. Submucosa	Widened due to edema and lymphoid aggregates	Normal or reduced in width
5. Muscularis	Infiltrated by inflammatory cells	Usually spared, except in cases of ***Toxic Megacolon*** [Q]
6. Fibrosis	Present	Usually absent
C. Complications		
1. Fistula formation	Internal and external fistulae in 10% cases	*Extremely rare* [Q]
2. Malignant changes	Less common but present	May occur in disease of more than 10 years duration (*more common* [Q])
3. Fibrous strictures	*Common* [Q]	*Never* [Q]
4. Toxic Megacolon	--	Risk present[Q]
5. Named Features	*Hose pipe appearance*[Q] *Cobble-Stone appearance*[Q]	*Garden hose appearance* [Q] *Pseudopolyps* [Q]

129. Answer is A (Ulcerative Colitis) : *Harsh Mohan 4th / 543*

Toxic megacolon is an important complication of ulcerative colitis.

130. Answer is B (Ulcerative colitis) : *Refer previous question*

Colonic involvement with ulcerative colitis is characterised by extensive, broad based ulceration of the mucosa in the distal colon or throughout its length. ***Pseudopolyps are created by bulging upwards of isolated islands of regenerating mucosa.***

131. Answer is B (Ulcerative colitis): *Robbins 7th/848, 850; Harsh Mohan 5th/582, 584*

Pseudopolyps are typically seen in Ulcerative colitis.

DISTINGUISHING FEATURES OF CROHN'S DISEASE AND ULCERATIVE COLITIS:

FEATURE	CROHN'S DISEASE	ULCERATIVE COLITIS
Pseudopolyps	**Rarely seen**	***Commonly present*** [Q]

5

132. Answer is D (5-Aminosalicyclic acid): *Harrison 18th/2489; Harrison 17th/1815; Read text below*

'The mainstay of therapy for inflammatory bowel disease remains 5 Aminosalicyclic derrivativs. – CMDT

5 Aminosalicyclic acid:

It is used in active treatment of ulcerative colitis and Crohn's disease and during disease inactivity in order to maintain remission.

Commonly used formulations of 5 ASA are :
Sulfasalazine
Oral mesolamine agents
Azo compounds : Balsalazide, Olsalazine

133. Answer is B (Azathioprine): *Harrison 15th/ 1688; Harrison 16th/1785, 1786; Harrison 17th/1896; Harrison 18th/ 2490*

Maintenance therapy with sulfasalazine was not able to maintain the patient in remission and he required corticosteroid for the control of his exacerabations. Patient is now in remission and requines a drug which can maintain him in remission. Azathioprine reduces requirement of steroids in patients and maintains remission and this is thus the drug of choice here.

This is a case of ulcerative colitis as suggested by the recurrent episodes of bloody diarrhoea.

Clinical (1782 H/16th)	Ulcerative colitis	Crohn's disease
Cross blood stool	Yes	Occassionally
Mucus	Yes	Occassionally

Azathioprine & Mercaptopurine :

Promising drugs as maintenance therapy.

Azathioprine and 6 mercapto- purine are effective in long term management of ulcerative colitis. They reduce the requirement of steroids in patient as well as maintain the patient in remission

Cyclosporine:

It is not effective in maintenance remission without 6 MP/ Azathioprine' - *Harrison*

It's greatest value is in t/t of acute severe ulcerative colitis that does not appear to be responding adequately to glucocorticoid. However it does not reduce the rate of relapse and *is not effective as maintenance therapy.*

Methotrexate:

Methotrexate is useful in steroid dependent patient of Crohn's disease but its role in U.C. has not been mentioned.

Cyclophosphamide has no role in the management of either Crohn's disease or ulcerative colitis.

Management Protocol :

5 Aminosalicylic acid (5ASA) derivatives

(Mainstay of therapy for both U.C. & CD)

Uncontrolled ↓ *Exacerbations*

Glucocorticoids

- Effective for inducing remission in both Cd & U.C
- Glucocorticoids play no role in maintenance therapy in either UC or CD
- Once clinical remission has been achieved they should be tapered.

↓ *Maintenance*

Azathioprine and 6 Mercaptopurine

- Commonly employed in management of glucocorticoid dependent IBD
- Promising role as maintenance therapy

134. Answer is a (5-Aminosalicylic Acid): Read text below

The mainstay of therapy for inflammatory bowel disease remains 5- Aminosalicylic derivatives – CMDT

Crohn's Disease

135. Answer is B (Crohn's Disease): *Refer previous question*

Skip lesions are characteristic of Crohn's Disease

136. Answer is A (Crohn's disease): *Harrison 18th/p 2483, 2486 Harrison's 17th/1892, 1890*

Chronic diarrhea in association with significant perineal disease (multiple fistulas in perenium) and Small intestinal disease (strictures/obstruction) suggests a diagnosis of Crohn's disease.

137. Answer is B (Crohn's disease): *CMDT 2006/623; Harrison 16th/1781 - 1782*

'Antibodies to the yeast 'Saccharomyces cerevisiae' (ASCA) are found in 60 - 70% of patients with Crohn's disease and 10 - 15% of patients with ulcerative colitis.' - *CMDT 06th/623*

Serological markers for inflammatory bowel disease

Perinuclear Antineutrophil Cytoplasmic Antibodies (p ANCA)	**Antisaccharomyces Cerevisiae Antibodies (ASCA)**
• Positive in 60 - 70% of U.C. patients (and 5 - 10% of CD patients)	• Positive in 60 - 70% of CD patients (and 10 - 15% of U.C. patients)

- *p ANCA +ve with ASCA -ve* = *97% specificity for UC*
- *p ANCA +ve with ASCA +ve* = *97% specificity for CD*

Antibody	G.I. Disorder
Antiendomysial antibody[Q]	*Celiac sprue*
Antisaccharomyces cerevisiae antibody[Q]	*Crohn's disease*
Antineutrophilic cytoplasmic antibody[Q]	*Ulcerative colitis*

138. Answer is A (Clostridium Difficle): *Harrison 18th/p 2480 Harrisons 17th/ 1887, Harrisons 16th /1777.*

A possible infectious etiology includes clostridium difficle and M paratuberculosis amongst the options provided.

Clostridium difficle is the single best answer of choice when based on Harrisons 17th edition

Role of infections in Inflammatory bowel disease (Infectious etiology)

Infection with multiple pathogens may initiate inflammatory bowel disease (IBD) by triggering an inflammatory response that the mucosal & immune system may fail to control

Agents According to Harrisons 16th edition (Do not mention Clostridium difficle)

- *'Multiple pathogens (Salmonella, Shigella sp. Campylobacter sp.) may initiale IBD by triggering an inflammatory response' – H/16th*
- *Anaerobic organisms particularly Bacterioides species may be responsible for induction of inflammation - H/16th*
- **Regarding M. Paratuberculosis**

  'Three specific agents, M. paratuberculosis paramyxovirus and Helicobacter species have received greatest attention'

  However

  M paratuberculosis does not have a confirmed disease association and antimycobacterial agents are not effective in treating CD.

Agents according to Harrisons 17th edition (Include Clostridium difficle)

- *'Multiple pathogens (Salmonella, Shigella sp, Campylobacter sp,* ***Clostiridium difficle****) may initiate IBD by triggering an inflammatory response' – H/17th*
- *Anaerobic organisms particularly Bacterioides and* ***Clostridia species*** *and some aerobic species as Escherechia may be responsible for the induction of inflammation' – H/17th*

Regarding M. Paratuberculosis

Harrisons 17th edition does not mention M. Paratuberculosis amongst the list of agents implicated in causing Crohn's disease.

139. Answer is C (Osteoarthritis): *Harrison 18th/p2487, 2488 Harrisons 17th/ 1893 – 1894 Refer previous question*

Osteoarthritis is not an extraintestinal manifestation of inflammatory bowel disease
***Uveitis, Sclerosing Cholangitis, and skin nodules** (Erythema nodosum) are all recognized extraintestinal manifestations of inflammatory bowel disease.*

140. Answer is D (Pancreatitis) : *Harrison 14th / 1642; Harrison 15th/1686-7; Harrison 16th/1783, 1784;17th/1893, 1894 Harrison 18th/p 2487, 2488*

Pancreatitis is not associated with inflammatory bowel disease

Extraintestinal diseases associated with inflammatory bowel disease:

Joint manifestations:	Ocular manifestations:	Skin manifestations:	Hepatic manifestations:
Arthralgia to acute arthritis Ankylosing spondylitis Sacroilitis	Episcleritis Recurrent iritis Uveitis	Erythema nodosum Pyoderma gangrenosum[Q] **Aphthous ulcers**	Nonspecific focal hepatitis Fatty liver Pericholangitis **Sclerosing cholangitis** Autoimmune chronic active hepatitis **Cirrhosis**

Colonic Disorders

Irritable Bowel Syndrome (IBS)

141. Answer is C (Rectal Bleeding): *Harrison 18th/p2496, 2497 Harrison's 17th/1899, 1900*

Irritable Bowel syndrome is characteristically not associated with rectal bleeding.
Evidence of blood in stool should raise an alarm that a process other than IBS is operating and should prompt further investigations.
***Abdominal pain, abnormal stool formation (hard/constipation or loose/ watery stool), and Bloating** or feeling of abdominal distension are characteristic features of Irritable Bowel Syndrome.*

Symptoms that cumulatively support the diagnosis of Irritable Bowel Syndrome:

- *Abnormal stool frequency[Q] (for research purposes, "abnormal" defined as > 3 bowel movements/week)*
- *Abnormal stool formation[Q] (lumpy/hard or loose/watery stool)*
- *Abnormal stool habits[Q] (straining, urgency, or feeling of incomplete evacuation)*
- *Passage of mucus[Q]*
- *Bloating or feeling of abdominal distention*

The diagnosis of a functional bowel disorder always presumes the absence of a structural or biochemical explanation for the symptoms.

Diagnostic criteria for Irritable Bowel Syndrome

Recurrent abdominal pain or discomfort at least 3 days per month in the last 3 months associated with two or more of the following
1. *Improvement with defecation[Q]*
2. *Onset associated with a change in frequency of stool[Q]*
3. *Onset associated with a change in form (appearance) of stool[Q].*

Criteria fulfilled for the last 3 months with symptom onset at least 6 months prior to diagnosis.
Discomfort means an uncomfortable sensation not described as pain. In pathophysiology research and clinical trails, a pain/discomfort frequency of at least 2 days a week during screening evaluation is required for subject eligibility.

142. Answer is C (Abdominal distension): *Harrison 18th/p 2496, 2497 Harrison's 17th/1900; Refer previous question*

Bloating or feeling of abdominal distension is a characteristic feature of Irritable bowel syndrome

Presences of blood in stool, weight loss or anorexia are 'Red Flag' conditions in irritable bowel syndrome. Their presence should raise on alarm that a process other than IBS is operating and should prompt further investigations to rule out other disease process.

"Red flag" conditions in irritable bowel syndrome that suggest possibility of another disease

Presence of any of the following calls for further investigation to rule out other disease processes:

- *Fever*
- *Blood in stools*
- *Nocturnal pain*
- *Abnormal physical findings*
- *Onset in patients>50 years of age*
- *Weight loss or anorexia*
- *Anemia*
- *Abnormal blood studies*
- *Family history of inflammatory bowel disease or malignancy*

143. Answer is A (Irritable bowel syndrome): *Harrison 18th/p 2496, 2497, 2498 Harrison's 17th/- 1899, 1900, 1901; 'Sleisenger's and Fordtran's 'Gastrointestinal & Liver Disease' 8th/ed 2634*

Stress related increase in abdominal pain with change in bowel habit and passage of mucus in stool, together with absence of 'red flag' signs such as blood in stool in a 'young female' suggest a diagnosis of Irritable bowel syndrome.

Young age and Female sex are epidemiological risk factors for IBS

"Younger people have a higher prevalence of IBS in the community"

Although IBS may affect all ages most patients have their onset of symptoms before age of 45. Older people have a lower rate reporting frequency and onset in patients > 50 years of age is a 'Red Flag' sign that may suggest the possibility of another disease

'Women are diagnosed two or three times as often as men and make up 80% of the population with severe IBS'

– Harrison 17th/1899

Onset of symptoms in periods of stress support a diagnosis of IBS.

Onset of symptoms in periods of stress or emotional upset are suggestive of IBS' - Harrison 17th/ed 1901

IBS is charachteristically associated with absence of blood in stool

Presence of blood in stool is a 'Red Flag' sign that suggests possibility of another disease.- Harrison's 17th/1901

"Red flag" conditions in irritable bowel syndrome that suggest possibility of another disease

Presence of any of the following calls for further investigation to rule out other disease processes:

- *Fever*
- *Blood in stools*
- *Nocturnal pain*
- *Abnormal physical findings*
- *Onset in patients>50 years of age*
- *Weight loss or anorexia*
- *Anemia*
- *Abnormal blood studies*
- *Family history of inflammatory bowel disease or malignancy*

Abdominal pain with change in bowel habit together with passage of mucus in stool (in the absence of 'Red Flag' signs) supports a diagnosis of IBS.

Symptoms that cumulatively support the diagnosis of Irritable Bowel Syndrome:

- *Abnormal stool frequency*[Q] *(for research purposes, "abnormal" defined as > 3 bowel movements/week)*
- *Abnormal stool formation*[Q] *(lumpy/hard or loose/watery stool)*
- *Abnormal stool habits*[Q] *(straining, urgency, or feeling of incomplete evacuation)*
- ***Passage of mucus***[Q]
- *Bloating or feeling of abdominal distention*

144. Answer is E (Predisposes to malignancy in long term): *Harrison 18th/p 2496, 2497 Harrisons 17th / 1899, 1990*

Irritable Bowel syndrome (IBS) is a benign functional bowel disorder.
IBS does not predispose to malignancy in the long term

IBS may be associated with diarrhea or constipation

'The most common pattern in IBS is constipation alternating with diarrhea' - Harrison

IBS may be associated with Anxiety and stress

Abnormal Psychiatric manifestation are recorded in 80% of IBS patients.
Emotional disorder and stress are associated with exacerbation of symptoms in IBS

145. Answer is A (Lubiprostone): *Harrison's 18th/2500, 2501*

Lubiprostone is an effective agent for treatment of patient with constipation predominant Irritable Bowel Syndrome. Lubiprostone *is a novel chloride channel activator that stimulates chloride channels in the apical membrane of intestinal epethelial cells. Chloride secretion induces passive movement of sodium and water into the bowel lumen and improves constipation predominant IBS.*

Cholestyramine and Alosetron *are used for the management of patients with Diarrhea predominant Irritable Bowel Syndrome.*

Rifaximin is a non-absorbed oral antibiotic being evaluated for global Irritable Bowel Syndrome Symptoms. *It is not specific for constipation predominant IBS* and currently there is still insufficienct data to recommend routine use of this antibiotic in the treatment of IBS.

Possible Drugs for a Dominant Symptom in IBS: *(Harrison's 18th/2501)*

Diarrhea	Constipation	Abdominal Pain
• *Lopepramide* • *Cholestyramine resin* • *Alosetron*	• *Psyllium husk* • *Methylcellulose* • *Calcium polycarbophil* • *Lactulose syrup* • *70% sorbitol* • *Polyethylene glycol 3350* • *Lubiprostone (Amitiza)* • *Magnesium hydroxide*	• *Smooth-muscle relaxant* • *Tricyclic antidepressants* • *Selective serotonin reuptake inhibitors*

Diarrhea and Colitis

146. Answer is A (Bacillus cereus): *Harrison 17th /248; Harrison's 18th/311*

Bacillus cereus causes non invasive diarrhea secondary to small bowel hypersecretion, as a result of preformed bacterial toxins.
Rotavirus, Aeromonas sp and Shigella are all invasive organism known to cause invasive diarrhea.

Association between Pathobiology of Causative Agents and Clinical Features in Acute Infectious Diarrhea:

Toxin Producers (Diarrhea from Hypersecretion)

Pathobiology/Agents
Preformed toxin
• *Bacillus cereus* • *Staphylococcus aureus* • *Clostridium perfringens*
Enterotoxin
• *Vibrio cholera* • *Enterotoxigenic Escherichia coli* • *Klebsiella pneumonia* • *Aeromonas* species
Enteroadherent
• Enteropathogenic and Enteroadherent *E. coli* • *Giardia* organisms • Cryptosporidiosis • Helminths
Cytotoxin producers
• *C. difficile* • Hemorrhagic *E. coli*

Invasive Organisms (Invasive Diarrhea)

Minimal inflammation
• Rotavirus and norovirus
Variable inflammation
• *Salmonella* • *Campylobacter* • *Aeromonas* species • *Vibrio parahaemolyticus* • *Yersinia*
Severe inflammation
• *Shigella* species • Enteroinvasive *E. coli* • *Entamoeba histolytica*

Association between Pathobiology of Causative Agents and Clinical Features in Acute Infectious Diarrhea:

Toxin Producers (Diarrhea from Hypersecretion)

Pathobiology/Agents	Incubation Period	Vomiting	Abdominal Pain	Fever	Diarrhea
Preformed toxin					
Bacillus cereus, Staphylococcus aureus, Clostridium perfringens	1–8 h 8–24 h	3–4+	1–2+	0–1+	3–4+, watery
Enterotoxin					
Vibrio cholerae, Enterotoxigenic Escherichia coli, Klebsiella pneumoniae, Aeromonas species	8–72 h	2–4+	1–2+	0–1+	3–4+, watery
Enteroadherent					
Enteropathogenic and Enteroadherent *E. coli, Giardia* organisms, cryptosporidiosis, helminths	1–8 d	0–1+	1–3+	0–2+	1–2+, watery, mushy
Cytotoxin producers					
C. difficile	1–3 d	0–1+	3–4+	1–2+	1–3+, usually watery, occasionally bloody
Hemorrhagic *E. coli*	12–72 h	0–1+	3–4+	1–2+	1–3+, initially watery, quickly bloody

Invasive Organisms (Invasive Diarrhea)

Minimal inflammation					
Rotavirus and norovirus	1–3 d	1–3+	2–3+	3–4+	1–3+, watery
Variable inflammation					
Salmonella, Campylobacter, and *Aeromonas* species, *Vibrio parahaemolyticus, Yersinia*	12 h–11 d	0–3+	2–4+	3–4+	1–4+, watery or bloody
Severe inflammation					
Shigella species, Enteroinvasive *E. coli, Entamoeba histolytica*	12 h–8 d	0–1+	3–4+	3–4+	1–2+, bloody

147. Answer is D (Clostridium Difficle): *Manual of Gastroentrology 4th 4th/184 - Harrison 18th/p311 Harrisons 17th/249*

Clostridium difficle is typically associated with Inflammatory' diarrhea and not 'secretory' diarrhea.

Clostridium Difficle may rarely cause a secretory type of diarrhea, but it remains the single best answer of exclusion.

Causes of Secretory Diarrhea

Enterotoxins Produced by infectious organisms
- ***Vibrio cholerae***
- Enterotoxigenic E coli (ETEC)
- Staphylococcus Aureus
- Bacillus cereus
- Rota virus

Laxatives

Exogenous Laxatives
- Castor oil
- ***Phenolpthalein***
- Bisacodyl
- Senna
- Dioctyl sodium sulphosuccinate

Endogenous Laxatives
- Bile salts (Bile duct obstruction)
- Fatty acids (Pancreatic insufficiency small Intestinal mucosal disease)

Harmone Producing Tumors
- Carcinoids (serotonin)
- VIP omas
- Medullary cancer Thyroid (calcitonin)
- Gastrinoma (ZES)
- Mastocytosis (Histamine)
- Colorectal villous adenoma

Others
- Chronic Ethanol ingestion
- Bowel Rescetion, disease or fistula (↓ absorption)
- Partial bowel obstruction or fecal impaction
- Addison's disease
- Congenital electrolyte absorption defects

148. Answer is C (Reduces with fasting): *CMDT 2009/499; Manual of Gastroenterology 4th/184 – Harrison 18th/p 312 Harrisons 17th/249*

Secretory diarrhea does not reduce with fasting.

In secretory diarrhea an abnormal ion transport occurs accross intestinal epethelial cells. This diarrhea is not related to the intestinal content and hence it typically does not cease with fasting

Typical Features of Secretory Diarrhea

- ***Large volume (typically > 1L/ day)***
- ***Little change with fasting*** *(Diarrhea typically does not cease while patient fasts)*
- ***Normal stool osmotic gap*** *(osmoality of stool is close to osmolality of plasma)*
- *No anion gap*
- *Stools are watery in consistency and do not contain pus or blood*
- ***Painless***

149. Answer is A, B, and C (Febrile dysentery with fever ≥ 38.5; Immunocompromised patient; Elderly patient): *Harrisons 17th/248, 249*

Antibiotic coverage is indicated whether or not a causative organism is discovered in patients who are ***immuncompromized****, have mechanical heart valves or recent vascular grafts or* ***are elderly****. Emperical antibiotic treatment should also be started in* ***moderately to severely ill patients with febrile dysentery*** *specially when fever ≥ 38.5°C*

Indications for Antibiotic coverage

- Patients who are immuno *compromised*[Q]
- Patients with *mechanical heart valves*[Q]
- Patients with *recent vascular grafts*[Q]
- Patients who *are elderly*[Q]
- Moderately to severely ill patients with *fibrile dysentry*[Q] (Grossly bloody stools and fever ≥ 38.5°C)
- Increased fecal WBCS

150. Answer is B (Longitudinal ulcers): *Harrison 18th/1276; Current Diagnosius & Treatment in Infectious Diseases (International Edition)/561; Robin's Pathology 6th/359; Differential Diagnosis in INternal Medicine: From Symptom to Diagnosis (Thieme) 2007/148; 'Fundamentals of Surgical Pathology' by Shariff (Jaypee)/179*

Typhoid ulcers (Salmonella/Enteric Fever) occur due to ulceration of Peyer's patches. Since Peyer's patches (aggregation of lymphoid follicles in the wall of gut) are oval in shape and placed longitudinally/vertically along the antimesenteric border, the axis of typhoid ulcers is longitudinal.

History of prolonged fever and abdominal discomfort together with typical features of splenomegaly and leucopenia suggest a diagnosis of salmonelosis or 'Enteric Fever'. Enteric fever is a potentially fatal systemic illness and death may occur from life threatening complications of gastrointestinal bleeding and intestinal perforation. This most commonly occurs in the third or fourth week of illness and results from hyperplasia ulceration (longitudinal) and necrosis of the ileocecal Payer's patches at the initial site of salmonella infiltration.

Typhoid Ulcers (Enteric Fever)	Tubercular Ulcers
• Longitudinal Ulcers (as they occur over lymphoid follicles/Peyer's patches at the antimesenteric border)	• Transverse ulcers (due todirection of lymphatics)
• When they heal, they cause no features of obstruction	• When they heal they cause stenosis and obstruction due to fibrosis (since they are circular surroundings the lumen of intestine)

Enteric Fever

Enteric Fever is a potentially life threatening systemic disease characterized by fever and abdominal pain caused by dissemination of Salmonella Typhi or Salmonella Parotyphi.

Typical Hallmark Features	Non specific symptoms	Typical Findings (Signs typical, but not always present)
• ***Fever*** • ***Abdominal Discomfort*** (Pain, Anorerxia, Diarrhea or Constipation, Anorexia, Nausea, Vomiting)	• Headache • Chills/Shivering • Cough • Sweating • Myalgia • Arthralgia • Fatigue	• Rose spots • ***Splenomegaly*** • ***Leucopenia*** with a distinct left shift The lipopolysacharide endotoxin of bacteria is responsible for Leucopenia and splenomegaly • Relative Bradycardia dispite high fever • Mental state changes (Typhoid Psychosis) (Muttering Delerium/Coma vigil)

Life threatening complications primarily include ***Gastrointestinal Bleeding and/or Gastrointestinal Perforation*** which most frequently occur in the third or fourth week of illness from hyperplasia, ulceration and necrosis of the ileocoecal Payer's patches at the initial site of Salmonella infection

151. Answer is B (Intravenous Metronidazole): *Harrisons 16th/1214, 1216-1217; Harrison 17th/1278; 18th/p 1686*

Presence of the classic flask shaped ulcers' in a patient presenting with lower gastrointestinal bleeding suggests a diagnosis of 'Intestinal amebic colitits'.

'Patients with amebic colitis should be treated with intravenous or oral Metronidazole.' *- Harrisons 16/e, p 1217*

Intestinal Amebiasis (Amebic colitis)

Pathology (H 16/e, 1214)	Clinical features (H 16/e, 1215)	Treatment (H 16/e, p 1217)
• Microulcerations of the mucosa of cecum, sigmoid colon and rectum ↓ • Small ulcers will heaped up margins and normal intervening mucosa ↓ • ***Classic ' Flask-shaped' ulcers***Q Produced by submucosal extension of ulceration under viable appearing surface mucosa	• Lower abdominal pain • Diarrhea • Dysentry : stools contain little fecal matter and consist ***mainly of blood and mucus*** • Systemic features such as malaise weight loss, fever • ±Toxic megacolon • ±Tender abdominal mass (Ameboma)	***Metranidazole (Intravenous or oral)*** + Luminal agents • Iodoquinol 'Paramomycin'

152. Answer is B (ELISA) : *Ghai 5th/221*

In Extra-intestinal amebiasis, antibody detection by ELISA is the most sensitive test *- Ghai 5th/221.*
ELISA : This test is positive in more than 90% of patients and it usually reverts to normal with in 6-12 months.
IHA : May also be done in invasive Amoebiasis or liver abscess.
The interpretation of the IHA is however more difficult because titres may remain positive for as long as 10 years.

153. Answer is C (Stricture and obstruction); *Gastrointestinal Pathology by Chandrasoma(1998)/199; 'Typhoid Fever' by Khosla 1st/149*

Strictures and obstruction do not occur in typhoid ulcers.

'Typhoid Ulcers heal without significant scarring in patients that recover and hance do not produce strictures or intestinal obstruction' – Gastrointestinal Pathology

Characteristic Features of Typhoid Ulcers

- Most common site is mucosa of small intestine (Ileum) in region of lymphoid patches (Payer's patches)
- Ulcers are *oval*
- Ulcers are arranged *longitudinally (Longitudinal ulcers)*Q
- Lie in the long axis of the intestine along the *antimesenteric border*Q
- Ulcers may be single or multiple
- Ulcers may erode and cause complications *(Bleeding/perforation)*Q
  - Bleeding
  - Perforation
- ***Ulcers heal without significant scarring or fibrosis in patients who recover***
  - Strictures and intestinal obstruction almost never occurs.

154. Answer is D (Neutropenic Colitis) : *Harrisons 16th/492*

Acute Right sided lower quadrant pain following chemotherapy in an immunocompromised host in characteristic of Neutropenic colitis.

Typhilitis : Syn : Neutropenic colitis, Necrotizing colitis, Necrotizing enteropathy, ileocoecal syndrome or cecitis.

- This syndrome is classically seen in neutropenic patients after chemotherapy with cytotoxic drugs
- More common in children than adults
- More common in patients with AML/ALL than among those with other types of cancer.

- Clinically characterized by
  - Fever
  - ***Right lower quadrant pain and tenderness (Most characteristic)***
  - Associated bloody diarrhea (±)
  - Immunocompromised blood picture
- Confirmed on CT/USG Finding a thickened coecal wall.

Colorectal Carcinomas

155. Answer is A (Familial polyposis) : *Harrison 15th / 582; Harrisons 16th/528, 529; Harrison 17th/574, 575 Harrison 18th/p 768, 769, 770*

'Familial polyposis of colon' is characterized by the appearance of thousands of adenomatous polyps throughout the large bowel. If polyposis is not treated surgically, colorectal cancer will develop in almost all patients before the age of 40. *Once the multiple polyps that constitute 'Polyposis' are detected patients should undergo total colectomy*

Remember :

Non-malignant polyps^{Q} (Rare/Small Malignant potential)	
Hamartomatous polyps^{Q}	***Hyperplastic polyps^{Q}***
Juvenile ***polyposis^{Q}*** *Peutz Jeghers syndrome^{Q}*	

Malignant polyps^{Q}
Adenomatous Polyps^{Q}
Familial adenomatous polyposis^{Q} *Gardner's syndrome^{Q}* *Turcot's syndrome^{Q}* *Lynch syndrome^{Q}*

156. Answer is B (Familial Polyposis coli) : *Harrison's 15th/582; Harrison 16th/528; Harrison 17th/574, 575 Harrison 18th/p 768, 769, 770*

Familial polyposis coli if not treated surgically, colorectal cancer will develop in almost all patients before age 40. - *Harrison*

<u>Familial polyposis coli</u> *is a rare condition characterised by appearance of thousands of adenomatous polyps throughout the large bowel. Colonic polyps are rarely present before puberty but are generally evident in affected individuals by 25 years of age. If polyposis coli is not treated surgically, colorectal cancer will develop in almost all patients before age 40. – Harrison*

<u>Review of Hereditary gastrointestinal polyposis syndromes</u>

Hereditary *autosomal dominant^{Q}* gastrointestinal polyposis syndromes

High Malignant Potential^{Q} (*histologically adenomas^{Q}*)		
Syndrome	**Distribution**	**Associated**
Familial colonic Polyposis	Large intestine	None
Gardner's syndrome	*Large intestine > small intestine*	Osteomas Lipomas Fibromas Epidermal cyst *Ampullary Ca* Desmoid
Turcot's syndrome	Large intestine	Brain Tumours

Rare (small) Malignant Potential^{Q} (*histologically hamartomas^{Q}*)		
Syndrome	**Distribution**	**Associated**
Peutz Jagher's syndrome	SI > LI > Stomach	**Mucocutaneous pigmentations** Tumours of ovary, Breast, pacnreas, endometrium
Juvenile polyposis syndrome	LI > SI > Stomach	Various congenital abnormalities

157. Answer is A (Juvenile Polyps): *Sabiston 17th / 1451 – 1454*

Juvenile Polyps is the single best answer of choice.

Juvenile polyps (sporadic), in general occur singly and being hamartomatous lesions have no malignant potential-Robbins
***Juvenile polyps are benign polyps** - Sabiston*

Pathologically hamartomas are considered benign and devoid of malignant potential. However hamartomatous polyps associated with Autosomal dominant hereditary syndromes have now been established to carry a small malignant potential *(Rare)*

- ***Juvenile Polyps are benign but Juvenile Polyps in association with Juvenile Polyposis syndrome carry small malignant potential.***
  The juvenile polyps in Juvenile polyposis syndrome are usually hamartomas but they may contain adenomatous elements and may progress to adenomas. This syndrome is associated with increased risk of (9 – 25%) of colorectal cancer. Mutation in Tumor supressor gene SMAD4 are believed to cause 50 % of Reported cases.
- ***Sporadic Hamartomatous polyps are benign but Hamartomas in association with Peutz Jaghers Syndrome may carry a small malignant potential.***
  Peutz Jaghers Syndrome is associated with increased risk (2-10%) of cancer in the intestinal tract. (Sabiston)
  The malignant potential of polyps associated with Peutz Jaghers Syndrome is small – CSDT.

Review of Hereditary gastrointestinal polyposis syndromes

Hereditary *autosomal dominant*[Q] gastrointestinal polyposis syndromes

↓ ↓

High Malignant Potential[Q] *(histologically adenomas[Q])*		
Syndrome	**Distribution**	**Associated**
Familial colonic Polyposis	Large intestine	None
Gardner's syndrome	*Large intestine > small intestine*	Osteomas Lipomas Fibromas Epidermal cyst *Ampullary Ca* Desmoid
Turcot's syndrome	Large intestine	Brain Tumours

Rare (small) Malignant Potential[Q] *(histologically hamartomas[Q])*		
Syndrome	**Distribution**	**Associated**
Peutz Jagher's syndrome	SI > LI > Stomach	**Mucocutaneous pigmentations** Tumours of ovary, Breast, pacnreas, endometrium
Juvenile polyposis syndrome	LI > SI > Stomach	Various congenital abnormalities

158. Answer is A (Ulcerative colitis): *Robbins 7th/ 849*

Malignant potential is seen in both ulcerative colitis and Crohn's disease, but ulcerative colitis is a more important risk factor than Crohn's and hence the answer of choice here. Diverticular disease and ischaemic colitis do not predispose to cancer.

***The risk of cancer in CD is considerably less than in patients with chronic U.C.'** – Robbins.*

> Confusing fact:
>
> - The cancer risk in CD and UC are probably equivalent for similar extent and duration of disease – *Harrison 16th/ 1788*
> - Patients with Crohn's pancolitis have similar risk – *Schwartz 8th/ 1085*
>
> *Thus while certain texts are now suggesting that the cancer risk for both CD & UC are probably equivalent, these are other texts which identify U.C. as a significantly more important cause. As we have to pick one single best answer, the option of choice remains U.C.*

159. Answer is C (Peutz-Jegher's Syndrome): *Harrison's 17th/326; Harrison's 16th/302; Robbins 7th/859, 1189; Sternberg's diagnostic surgical pathology 4th/1548*

Mucocutaneous pigmentation along with gastrointestinal manifestations of abdominal pain and anemia suggest the diagnosis of Peutz-Jegher's syndrome.

Peutz Jagher's Syndrome

Peutz-Jaghers syndrome is a rare autosomal dominant, inherited syndrome characterized by mucocutaneous pigmentation and gastrointestinal polyposis.

Autosomal Dominant Inheritance[Q]
Family history often positive[Q]

Mucocutaneous Pigmentation	Gastrointestinal Polyposis	Neoplasm's of Non intestinal organs
• Mucocutancous pigmentation involving lips, buccal mucosa and skin is characteristic (Digits, nails, pains, soles genitalia or any mucosal surface may be involved)	• Hamartomatous polys (Harrison's) Small intestine > Large intestine > Stomach May present with: Intussusception or obstruction (Abdominal pain, bleeding, Anemia) *Although hamartomas are not malignant, a small percentage of patients (13%) may develop malignancies of intestinal organs specially stomach and duodenum*	• Patients with this syndrome have increased risk of developing carcinomas of - Ovary - Breast - Pancreas - Endometrium

160. Answer is A (Peutz Jegher's Syndrome) : *Roxburgh 16th/296*

Peutz Jegher's Syndrome is a rare autosomal dominant disorder in which ***perioral and labial pigmented macules,*** *occur in association with jejunal polyps. Presence of* ***malena may reflect polyps in jejunum****.*
Similar complains in sister indicate the ***hereditary nature*** *of this disorder.* ***Together these features confirm the diagnosis.***
'Pigmentation' *is not a feature with Gardener's and FAP, nor with villous adenoma.*

Heriditable (Autosomal dominant) Gastrointestinal polyposis syndromes :

Neoplastic polyps:

Multiple Adenomalous polyps (Adenomas) - are a very common risk factor for colorectal malignancy. Infact if the polyposis is not treated surgically, colorectal cancer will develop in almost all patients (100%), before age 40

Clues to diagnosis:

Adenomas in large intestine with no associated lesions	**Familial Polyposis coli**
Adenomas in large intestine associated with osteomas, fibromas or lipomas	**Gardner's Syndrome**
Adenomas in large intestine associated with brain tumors	**Turcot's syndrome**

Non-Neoplastic Polyps: Peutz Jegher's syndrome and Juvenile polyposis, are two autosomal dominant, heritable conditions, associated with polyps in G.I.T. These polyps are however harmatomas and do not have malignant potential.

Clues to their diagnosis:

Hamartomatous polyps throughout GIT associated with mucocutaneous pigmentation and tumors of pancreas ovary, breast, lung, uterus.	**Peutz Jeghers Syndrome** *(in small intestine*[Q]*>Large intestine*[Q]*>Stomach* [Q]*)*
Hamartomatous polyps throughout GIT associated with various congenital anomalies.	**Juvenile Polyposis** *(in large Intestine*[Q]*> small intestine*[Q]*> stomach* [Q]*)*

161. Answer is C (Small bowel) : *Harrison's 15th / 582 ; CMDT 2009 /576; Harrison 16th/528, 529; Harrison 17th/574, 575 Harrison 18th/p 768, 769, 770*

Polyps may be seen throughout the gastro intestinal tract but most commonly in the small intestine.

Peutz Jegher's syndrome:

It is an autosomal dominant condition characterized by:

- ***Hamartomatous polyps throughout the gastrointestinal tract, most notably in small intestine***[Q]

- *Mucocutaneous pigmented macules on the lips, buccal mucosa and skin*[Q]

Syndrome[Q]	*Distribution*[Q]	*Histological type*[Q]	*Malignant potential*[Q]	*Associated*[Q]
Peutz Jegher's Syndrome	Small intestine > Large intestine > stomach	Hamartoma	Rare	• Mucocutaneous pigmentation • Tumors of non-intestinal organs - Ovary, - Breast - Pancreas - Endometrium

Although hamartomas are not malignant, a small percentage (13%) of patients develop malignancies[Q] *of intestinal organs, specially stomach and duodenum (NOT COLON).*

162. Answer is B (Peutz Jagher's syndrome): *Refer previous question*

Mucocutaneous pigmentation and gastrointestinal manifestations in the form of bleeding (malena) along with a positive family history suggests a diagnosis of Peutz Jagher's syndrome.

163. Answer is B (Stage of lesion) : *Robbins 7*[th] */ 866; Harrison's 17*[th] */ 56; Devita's 7*[th] */ 1069; Gastrointestinal and Liver diseases by Feldman 8*[th] */ 2782*

The most important prognostic factor of colorectal carcinoma is the 'stage of disease'.

The 'stage of disease' gives information related to depth of penetration into bowel wall and extent of regional lymph node spread, both of which are the two most important independent prognostic factors.

Most important prognostic factors
'Extent of Regional Lymph node spread' and 'Depth of tumor invasion' are the most important determinants of prognosis

Single most important prognostic	**Single most important <u>independent</u> prognostic factor**
Stage of disease[Q]	*Lymph node status*[Q]

Stage of disease gives information on both the depth of tumor penetration into the bowel wall and the extent of regional lymph node involvement

'Stage' of disease is a superior prognostic factor in comparison to Lymph node status alone

Single most important independent prognostic factor is the Lymph nodal status or the number of positive nodes

- Devita 7th */ 1069*

- Gastrointestinal Oncology (2004) / 684

Pathologic, Molecular and Clinical Features that May Affect Prognosis in Patients with Colorectal Cancer:

Feature of Marker	***Effect of prognosis***
Pathologic	
• Surgical-pathologic stage	
Depth of bowel wall penetration	Increased penetration diminishes prognosis
Number of regional nodes involved by tumor	1-4 nodes is better than > 4 nodes
• Tumor morphology histology	
Degree of differentiation	Well-differentiated is better than poorly differentiated
Mucinous (colloid) or signet ring cell histology	Diminishes prognosis
Scirrhous histology	Diminishes prognosis
• Venous invasion	Diminishes prognosis
• Lymphatic invasion	Diminishes prognosis
• Perineural invasion	Diminishes prognosis
• Local inflammation and immunologic reaction	Improved prognosis
• Tumor morphology	Polypoid/exophytic is better than ulcerating/infiltrating
• Tumor DNA content	Increased DNA content (aneuploidy) diminishes prognosis
• Tumor size	No effect in most studies
Molecular	
• Loss of heterozygosity at chromosome 18q (DCC, DPC4)	Diminishes prognosis
• Loss of heterozygosity at chromosome 17q (p53)	Diminishes prognosis
• Loss of heterozygosity at chromosome 8p	Diminishes prognosis

• Increased labeling index for p21WAF/CIP1 protein	Improved prognosis
• Microsatellite instability	Improved prognosis
• Mutation in BAX gene	Diminishes prognosis
Clinical	
• Diagnosis in asymptomatic patients	Possibly improved prognosis
• Duration of symptoms	No demonstrated effect
• Rectal bleeding as a presenting symptom	Improved prognosis
• Bowel obstruction	Diminishes prognosis
• Bowel perforation	Diminishes prognosis
• Tumor location	May be better for colon than for rectum May be better for left colon than for right colon tumors
• Age < 30 yr	Diminished prognosis
• Preoperative CEA	Diminished prognosis with a high CEA level
• Distant metastases	Markedly diminished prognosis

164. Answer is A (Resection) : *Harrison 14 th/576; Harrison 17th/578; Harrison 18th/p 774 CMDT 2002 / 665; CMDT 2003/620*

Patients of colon cancer, with solitary hepatic metastasis without clinical or radiographic evidence of additional tumor involvement should be considered for partial liver resection, because such procedures are associated with 5-year survival rates of 25-30% when performed on selected individuals by experienced surgeons.
Resection of isolated (One to three) liver or lung metastasis result in long term survival (over 5 years in 20% - 40% of cases) - *CMDT 2002/665*

165. Answer is A (Surgery) : *Harrison 18th/p 773, 774 Harrison 17th/578; CMDT 2009/1450-51; Sabiston 16 th/964; CMDT 2003/618-619*

The presence of metastatic disease to the liver does not preclude the surgical excision of the primary tumor and even the liver metastasis.
Treatment of metastatic disease: ***presence of isolated metastasis to lung or liver, 1 to 3 in number is not a contraindication to surgery. Treatment here involves resection or cryosurgical ablation of secondries, alongwith the management of the primary.***
The reason for proceeding with surgery for colorectal CA (CRC) in presence of liver metastasis are :

1. First, if the colonic tumor is left untreated, death is imminent, and its cause will not be cancer but colonic obstruction or bleeding.
2. Second, there is a significant cure rate for patients undergoing surgery for CRC metastatic to the liver.

166. Answer is C (Combined chemotherapy and Radiotherapy) : *Bailey Love 23rd/1141*

A combination of chemotherapy and radiotherapy called as 'chemoradiation' is the preferred initial therapy for all anal canal tumors *– Bailey*

167. Answer is None (All above genes may be involved) : *'Gastrointestinal and Liver diseases' by Feldman 8th/2768 'Neoplasms of the Colon, Rectum and Anus' 2nd/ 58*

APC, K-ras and mismatch repair genes are characteristically involved in generation of cancer of colon.

β Catenin mutations *are uncommon / infrequent mutations seen in a subset of patients who have normal APC. Tumors lacking APC mutations may have activating mutations in β catenin which is the main downstream target of APC action.*

Genes involved in Development of Colorectal Cancer

Oncogenes / Protooncogenes	Tumor suppressor Genes	Mismatch Repair Genes
K – ras	• ***APC***	• *h MLH – 1*
	• DCC (Deleted in Ca Colon)	• *h MSH – 2*
	• P^{53}	• *h MSH – 3*
	• SMAD4 (DPC, MADH)	• *h MSH – 6*
	• MCC	• *h PMS – 1*
	• ***TGF – β – RII***	• *h PMS - 2*

β Catenin Gene Mutations may be seen in a subset of patient who have no mutation in APC.

- β Catenin is the main downstream target of APC action.
- APC functions to modulate extracellular signals that are transmitted to the nucleus through a cytoskeletal protein 'β catenin' which then regulates transcription and other target genes.
- APC is a tumor suppressor gene that binds to β-catenin and causes its degradation unopposed stimulation of various pathways that lead to tumor genesis.
- ***Besides inactivating mutations of APC gene, tumor genesis can also occur directly through dominant stimulatory mutations of the β-catenin gene. Such mutations are found in 15-20% of Microsattelite Instability colon cancers.***

Genes altered in sporadic Colorectal Cancer *(Gastrointestinal and Liver Diseases by Feldman 8th/2768)*

Gene	Chromosome	Percentage of tumors with Gene Alterations	Gene Class	Gene function
K-ras	12	50	Proto-oncogene	Encodes guanine nucleotide-binding protein that regulates intracellular signaling
APC	5	70	Tumor suppressor	***Regulation of β-catenin that is involved in activation of WnT/TcF signaling*** (activates c-myc, cyclin D_1)*; regulation of proliferation and apoptosis; interaction with E-cadherin (cell adhesion?)
DCC	18	70	Tumor suppressor	Netrin-1 receptor; capase substrate in apoptosis; cell adhesion
SMAD4 (DPC4, MADH4)	18	?	Tumor suppressor	Nuclear transcriptase factor in transforming growth factor (TGF-β1) signaling; regulation of angiogenesis; regulator of WAF1 promoter; downstream mediator of SMAD2
P53	17	75	Tumor suppressor	Transcription factor; regulator of cell cycle progression after cellular stress, of apoptosis, of gene expression, and of DNA repair
hMSH2	2	#	***DNA mismatch repair***	Maintains fidelity of DNA replication
hMLH1	3	#	***DNA mismatch repair***	Maintains fidelity of DNA replication
hMSH6	2	#	***DNA mismatch repair***	Maintains fidelity of DNA replication
TGF-β1 RII	3	⊕	Tumor suppressor	Receptor for signaling in the TGF-β1 pathway; inhibitor of colonic epithelial proliferation, often mutated in tumors with MSI

*β-Catenin mutations (downstream of APC) are found in 16-25% of MSI colon cancers but not in microsatellite stable (MSS) cancers
#Approximately 15% of sporadic colorectal cancers demonstrate MSI associated with alterations in mismatch repair genes (principally hMSH2 and hMLH1 but also hMSH3, hMSH6, hPMS1, and hPMS2)
⊕ Mutated in 73-90% of MSI colon cancers. Upto 55% MSS colon cancer cell lines may demonstrate a TGF-β signaling blockage distal to TGF-β1 RII.
MSI, nicrosatellite instability; TGF-β, transforming growth factor-β

168. Answer is A (High fiber diet): *Gastrointestinal and Liver Diseases by Feldman 8th/2762, Advanced Surgical Practice' by Majid & Kingsnorth (2002)/ 271 , Lange Outline Review' for USMLE STEP 3' by Goldberg 5th / 108*

Epidemiologic, case control and animal studies suggest that dietary fibers are protective against the development of colon cancer

Fat *is primarily related as a 'promoting' agent* such that high fat in diet is believed to promote carcinogenesis. *Low Fat has not been shown to have a 'protective' role in carcinogenesis* although it may reduce the incidence of colonic carcinoma indirectly by reducing a 'promoting effect'.

Low selenium *is 'possibly related' as a promoting agent*
Low Protein has *not been mentioned in relation to carcinogenesis in the colon.*

Environmental /Dietary Factors that influence Carcinogenesis is Colon (Based on Epidemiological Studies)

Promoting Factors	Inhibiting / Protective Factors
Probably Related	**Probably Protective**
• ***High Dietary Fat consumption***	• ***High fiber consumption***
• ***Low Dietary Fiber consumption***	• *Dietary Calcium*
• ***Red Meat Consumption***	• *Aspirin and NSAID's*
Possibly related (Based on Limited Data)	• *Physical Activity*
• *Bear and Ale consumption*	• *Low Body Mass*
• ***Low dietary Selenium***	• *Hormone Replacement Therapy (estrogen)*
• *Environmental carcinogens and mutagens*	**Possibly protective (Based on Limited Data)**
- *Heterocyclic amines (from charbroiled & fried meat & fish)*	• *Yellow green cruciferous vegetables*
- *Products of Bacterial Metabolism*	• *Foods rich in carotene (Vitamin A)*
	• *Vitamin C and E*
	• ***High selenium***
	• *Vitamin D*
	• *Other Cox-2 inhibitors*

Pancreatic Disorders

Pancreatitis

169. Answer is C (Hemochromatosis) : *Harrison 15th / 1793; Harrison 16th/1896;Harrison 17th/2007 Harrison 18th/p 2635*

Gall stones [Q] ***, Alcohol ingestion*** [Q] ***and Hypercalcemia*** [Q] ***(e.g. Hypoparathyroidism) have all been mentioned as causes of Acute Pancreatitis.***

Hemochromatosis has not been included [Q] as a cause in this exhaustive list.

Causes of Acute Pancreatitis:

Common Causes	Uncommon causes
Gallstones (including microlithiasis) Alcohol (acute and chronic alcoholism) Hypertrigleceridemia Endoscopic retrograde cholangiopancreatography (ERCP), Truama (especially blunt abdominal trauma) Postoperative (abdominal and nonabdominal operations) Drugs (azathioprine, 6-mercaptourine, sulfonamides, estrogens, tetracycline, valproic acid, anti-HIV medications) Sphincter of Oddi dysfunction	Vascular causes and vasculitis Connective tissue disorders Thrombotic thrombocytopenic purpura (TTP) Cancer of the pancreas Hypercalcemia Periampullary diverticulum Pancreas divisum Hereditary pancreatitis Cystic fibrosis Renal failure
Rare causes	**Causes to consider in patients with recurrent bouts of acute pancreatitis without an obvious etilogy**
Infections (mumps, coxasackievirus, cytomegalovirus, echopvirus, parasites) Autoimmune (e.g., Sjogren's syndrome)	Occult disease of the biliary tree or pancreatic ducts Drugs Hypertriglyceridemia Pancreas divisum Pancreatic cancer Sphincter of Oddi dysfunction Cystic fibrosis Idiopathic

170. Answer is B (Appendicitis) : *Harrison 14th/ 1739, 15th/1788, 1795; Harrison 16th/1893; Harrison 17th/2004 (306.2) Harrison 18th/p 2632, (Table: 312.2)*

Appendicitis alone does not cause increased amylase.

Perforated appendix, may be associated with *increased amylase*.

Causes of Hyperamylasemia and Hyperamylasuria:

Pancreatiti Disease	Non Pancreatic Disorders	Other Abdominal Disorders
I. Pancreatitis A. Acute B. Chronic : ductal obstruction C. Complications of pancreatitis 1. Pancreatic pseudocyst 2. Pancreatogenous ascites 3. Pancreatic abscess 4. Pancreatic necrosis II. Pancreatic trauma III. Pancreatic carcinoma	I. Renal insufficiency II. Salivary gland lesions A. Mumps B. Calculus C. Irradiation sialadenitis D. Maxillofacial surgery III. Tumor hypermamylasemia A. Carcinoma of the lung B. Carcinoma of the esophagus C. Breast carcinoma, ovarian carcinoma IV. Macroamylasemia V. Burns VI. Diabetic ketoacidosis VII. Pregnancy VIII. Renal transplantation IX. Cerebral trauma X. Drugs : morphine	I. Biliary tract disease : cholecystitis, choledocholithiasis II. Intraabdominal disease A. Perforated or penetrating peptic ulcer B. Interstitial obstruction or infarction C. Ruptured ectopic pregnancy D. Peritonitis E. Aortic aneurysm F. Chronic liver disease G. Postoperative hyperamylasemia

171. Answer is 'D' (Acute pancreatitis): *Harrison 16th/1897; Harrison 17th/2002, 2008; Harrison 18th/p 2636 Kumar & Clarke 5th/398*

'The diagnosis of acute pancreatitis is usually established by detection of an increased level of serum amylase' *Harrison 16th*

'Serum amylase level is the standard laboratory test carried out to confirm the diagnosis of acute pancreatitis'

Kumar & Clarke 5th

Measurement during first 24 hours of onset of pain	Measeurement late after presentation
An elevation of three times the upper limit of normal clinches the diagnosis (provided overt salivary gland disease and gut perforation or infarction are excluded)	After 48-72 hrs even with continuing evidence of pancreatitis, total serum levels tend to return to normal With a late presentation thus, serum amylase levels may give a false negative result.

Serum amylase level may be increased in acute cholecystitis, but it does not form a criteria for its diagnosis.

Remember: [Q]

There is no definitive correlation between the severity of pancreatitis and the degree of serum amylase elevation. An elevated serum lipase [Q] or trypsin value is more specific / diagnostic of acute pancreatitis than serum amylase – (Lipase is the single best enzyme to measure for acute pancreatitis [Q]).

172. Answer is D (Serum amylase > 350 IU) : *Harrison 14th/1743; Harrison 16th/not elaborated; Harrison 17th/2008 Harrison 18th/p 2636*

Serum amylase does not form any cirteria for prognosis in acute pancreatitis. (Remember this fact)

Therefore, if amylase is present as any of the options, you can easily and safely exclude it.!!

Ranson's criteria for prognosis in acute pancreatitis include : (Adverse factors)

At the time of Admission	During initial 48 hours
1. Age > 55 years [Q] *2. Leucocytosis > 16.000/μl* [Q] *3. Hyperglycemia > 200 mg/dl* *4. Serum LDH > 400 IU/L* *5. Serum AST > 250 IU/L*	*1. Fall in haematocril > 10%* *2. Fluid deficit > 4000 ml* *3. Hypocalcemia < 8 mg/dl* [Q] *4. Hypoxemia < 5mg/dl* *5. Increased BUN > 5mg/dl* *6. Hypoalbuminemia < 3.2 g/dl*

173. Answer is A (Serum Amylase) : *Harrison 16th / 1897; 14th / 1743; Harrison 17th/2008; Harrison 18th/2636, 2637*

Serum Amylase does not form any criteria for prognosis in Acute Pancreatitis.

Although elevated serum amylase level is important for establishing diagnosis of acute pancreatitis, it plays no role in predicting prognosis or severity.

"There appears to be no definite correlation between severity of pancreatitis and the degree of serum amylase elevation. After 48 to 72 hours, even with continuing evidence of pancreatitis, total serum amylase levels tend to return to normal." - Harrison

Hyperglycemia (Glucose), Hypocalcemia (Calcium) and elevated serum AST are all poor prognostic factors in accordance with Ranson's criteria as elaborated in the previous question.

174. Answer is D (Prothrombin Time > 2 sec): *Harrison 14th/1743*

Prothrombin time is not included as an index in Ranson's criteria.
It is the single best answer of choice.

TLC > 16,000, Calcium < 8 mmol/l, Hyperglycemia > 200 ***mg/dl*** *are all poor prognostic signs for acute pancreatitis in accordance with Ranson's criteria.*

175. Answer is D (Hyperamylasemia): *Refer previous question*

Serum amylase levels do not form any criteria for prognosis in acute pancreatitis.

Hyperglycemia, Hypocalcemia and raised LDH levels are poor prognostic factors according to Ranson's criteria.

176. Answer is A (Low serum Lipase): *Harrison 18th/p 2636, 2637 Harrison 17th/2008*

The presence of sudden onset epigastric pain that radiates to the back in an alcoholic patient suggests the diagnosis of Acute Pancreatitis.

Acute pancreatitis is characterized by an elevated serum lipase leve and not a low serum lipase

'An elevated serum lipase is more specific for pancreatitis than a serum amylase level'- Harrison

177. Answer is B (Serum Lipase): *Harrison 18th/p 2636, 2637 Harrisons 17th/2008*

Serum lipase elevation is the most specific laboratory test for establishing a diagnosis of Acute Pancreatitis
'A three fold elevated serum lipase value is usually diagnostic of acute pancreatitis' *– Harrison*

Serum Lipase levels and serum amylase levels are both used to establish the diagnosis of acute pancreatitis

An elevated serum Lipase level is more specific for pancreatitis than a serum amylase level because many other pathologic conditions may present with an elevated amylase level. Serum lipase is therefore the single best answer of choice.

178. Answer is B (Serum lipase) : *Harrison 18th/p 2636, 2637 Harrison's 17th/2008*

Serum lipase elevation is the most specific laboratory test for establishing a diagnosis of Acute Pancreatitis
'A three fold elevated serum lipase value is usually diagnostic of acute pancreatitis' *– Harrison*

Serum Lipase levels and serum amylase levels are both used to establish the diagnosis of acute pancreatitis

An elevated serum Lipase level is more specific for pancreatitis than a serum amylase level because many other pathologic conditions may present with an elevated amylase level. Serum lipase is therefore the single best answer of choice.

179. Answer is A (Purtscher's retinopathy) : *Harrison 18th/p 2642 Harrison's 16th/1898; 15th / 1796*

Purtscher's retinopathy is a relatively unusual complication of acute pancreatitis. It is manifested by ***sudden and severe loss of vision***. It is believed to be due to occlusion of the posterior retinal artery with aggregated granulocytes.

Peculiar Fundoscopic appearance :

Cotton wool spots and hemorrhages confined to an area limited by the optic disk and macula.[Q]

180. Answer is A (Purtscher's retinopathy) : *Harrison's 15th / 1796; Harrison 16th/1898/ Harrison 17th/2009*

Purtscher's retinopathy *is a relatively unusual complication of acute pancreatitis.* It is manifested by ***sudden and severe loss of vision***. It is believed to be due to occlusion of the posterior retinal artery with aggregated granulocytes.

Peculiar Fundoscopic appearance :[Q]

Cotton wool spots and hemorrhages confined to an area limited by the optic disk and macula.

181. Answer is B (Gall stone pancreatitis): *Oxford textbooks of surgery 2nd/1766*

The prognosis is best in patient where pancreatitis is caused by a remediable cause such as cholelithiasis. 'Eradication of gall stone disease' prevents further attacks of pancreatitis. *-Oxford text.*

The etiological mechanism probably involves the transient obstruction of pancreatic duct by a gall stone in the common bile duct at the Ampulla of Vater.
Good prognosis is also evidenced by the fact that gall stones are recoverable in the faeces of over 90% of patients within 10 days of an attack, suggesting that the obstruction is brief and that most such stones pass into the duodenum.

182. Answer is C (Calcium) : *Harrison 16th/1899; 17th/2009, 2010; Harrison 18th/p 2640, 2641 C.M.D.T. 2009/626; Kumar & Clark 5th/399*

'Calcium gluconate must be given intravenously if there is evidence of hypocalcemia with tetany'*- CMDT 2009/626*

Drugs evaluated by prospective controlled trials but found ineffective – *H/16th/ 1899*	**Drugs with some beneficial role**
Glucagon H2 blockers Protease inhibitors like Aprotinin Glucocorticoids Calcitonin NSAIDS Lexiplafant (platelet activating factor inhibitor)	Analgesic for pain (Harrison) Prophylactic anititbiotics (Harrison) Calcium gluconate (hypocalcemia or tetany) CMDT Octreotide (Harrison) : Reduced mortality but no change in complication Gabexale (Harrison) : No affect on mortality but reduced pancreatic damage.

Treatment of acute pancreatitis
• Analgesia for pain (Mepridine) • IV fluid and colloids : to maintain normal intravascular volume • No oral alimentation • Nasogastric suction: to decrease gastrin release from stomach and prevent gastric contents from entering duodenum. • Prophylactic antibiotics • Feeding : Entral nutrition by nasojejunal tube

183. Answer is B (Pseudocyst) : *Harrison 18th/p 2642 Harrison 17th/2011; Schwartz 7th/704*

*"**Pseudocyst** is the most common complication, usually occurring after 2-3 weeks" - Schwartz Handook, 7th/704*

184. Answer is B (Pancreatitis) : *Harrison 15th / 1798 ; Harrison 16th/1901; Harrison 17th/2008, 2009, 2011 Harrison 18th/p 2642, 2643*

Most common cause of pancreatic pseudocyst is Pancreatitis (90%).
The second most common cause is trauma (10%).

185. Answer is D (Mostly present in head of pancreas): *CSDT 11th/635, 638, Schwartz 7th/1256, 1257; Harrison 14th/1747; 15th/1795; 16th/1901*

Short bowel syndrome (massive small bowel resection) is associated with Hypergastrinemia.

Most common site for pseudopancreatic cyst is the body and tail of pancreas *- Harrison*

Pseudopancreatic cyst (called 'pseudo' because they do not have an epithelial lining)

Etiology :	**Site :**	**Diagnosis:**
Pancreatitis (90%) (most common)[Q] *Trauma (10%)* [Q]	***85% are seen in body and tail*** *15% are seen in head*	- *Serum amylase level is elevated* [Q] - *Sonography is the investigation of choice* [Q] - *X-Ray : Pseudocysts may be localized, displacing some portion of git.* [Q]
Complications :	**Factors indicating possibility of hemorrhage**	
Pain due to expansion *Haemorrhage* *Rupture* Abscess	Increase in size *Localized brui over mass* [Q] *Sudden decrease in Hb or hematocrit* [Q]	

Management
• *Pseudocyst > 5cm diameter is an indications for drainage* [Q] • Pseudocyst *less than 5 cm* in diameter and *less than 6 weeks **old should be observed***[Q], as they tend to resolve spontaneously • *Initial management : US/CT guided, single or repeated needle aspirations* • Later : patients who do not respond to above modality are treated with surgical therapy preferred modality : *Internal drainage of cyst by cystojejunostomy.* [Q]

186. Answer is A (Percutaneous aspiration is treatment of choice): *Harrison 14th/1747,15th/1795;16th/1901, 1902; 17th/2011, 2348; Harrison 18th/p 2642 CSDT 11th/ 635, 638, Schwartz 1256, 1257*

Percutaneous aspiration has emerged as a simple and frequently used initial procedure in the management of uncomplicated persistant pancreatic pseudocysts. However ***it cannot be termed as the treatment of choice. Surgical internal drainage in the form of cystojejunostomy continues to be the treatment of choice.***

Treatment of Pancreatic Psuedocyst :

If the Pseudocyst is shrinking, & in stable patients who are free of complications	***If the pseudocyst is expanding, or not responding to above treatment, or is complicated by rupture, hemorrhage or abscess formation.***
Conservative treatment is indicated.* Alternatively, a USG / CT guided single or repeated needle aspiration can be done.	Operative treatment is indicative Either external or preferably internal drainage of the cyst can be done

****A singnificant number of pseudocyst will resolve sponteaneously more than 6 weeks after their formations*** [Q]

Indications for Drainage :
1. Pseudocyst > 5cm in diameter.[Q] *2. Persisting for > 6 weeks.* [Q]

Endocrinal Tumors of Pancreas

187. Answer is none or D (None or ACTH): *Harrison 18th/p 3057 Harrison's 17th/2348*

VIP, Insulin Somatostatin and ACTH may all be secreted from pancreatic endocrine tumors. Amongst the options provided ACTH is the most rare peptide associated with Pancreatic Endocrine Tumors, and hence may be selected as the single best answer of exclusion.

Insulin > VIP > Somatostatin (Rare) > ACTH (Rare)

Name	Biologically active Peptides secreted	(New Cases/10^6 Population/ Year)	Tumour location
Zollinger Ellison Syndrome	Gastrin	0.5-1.5	Duodenum (70%) Pancreas (25%)
VIPoma (Verner Morrison Syndrome, Pancreatic cholera, WDHA)	VIP	0.05 – 0.2	Pancreas (90% in adult)
Glucagonoma	Glucagon	0.01 – 0.1	Pancreas (100%)
Insulinoma	Insulin	1 – 2	Pancreas (> 99%)
Somatostatinoma	Somatostatin	Rare	Pancreas (55%) Duodenum-Jejunum (44%)
GRFoma	Growth hormone releasing hormone	Unknown	Pancreas (30%) Lung (54%)
ACTHoma	ACTH	Rare	Pancreas

188. Answer is D (Massive HCl in response to histamine injection) : *Harrison 15th/1661, Harrison 16th/1894; 17th/1868 Harrison 18th/p 2455*

Massive secretion of HCl is seen in response to stimulation with Secretin (not with Histamine).

Zollinger Ellison Syndrome (as mentioned in the previous question) is characterized by unregulated secretion of gastrin leading to hypersecretion of gastric acid and the resulting manifestations. The most common presentation is with :

Peptic ulceration Q :	• ***Most common manifestation***, occuring in 90% of patient • ***Most common site is duodenum (duodenal bulb)*** • **Clinical situations that raise special suspicion include** : a. *Ulcers beyond the duodenal bulb (second part of duodenum and beyond) because these are unusual locations for ulcers in Peptic ulcer diseases.* Q b. *Ulcers refractory to standard medical therapy* Q c. ***Ulcers are recurrent*** Q d. *Ulcers presenting with frank complications.* Q
Diarrhea Q **:**	***Is the most common manifestation*** Q Etiology is multifactorial, and it may have a secretory component as well.

Gastrin provocative tests *are used when acid secretory studies are not contributory* and include :

1. *Secretin stimulation test* Q *: most sensitive and specific* Q
2. Calcium infusion test
3. Standard meal test

Histamine stimulation is not used and it does not bring about massive release of HCl in such patients.

189. Answer is A (Peptic Ulceration, Gastric Hypersecretion, Non β Cell Tumour) : *Harrison 16th/ 2227; 17th/1868 Harrison 18th/p 2455*

Zollinger Ellison Syndrome is characterised by peptic ulceration due to gastrin hyper secretion by a non beta cell tumor.

Zollinger Ellison Syndrome

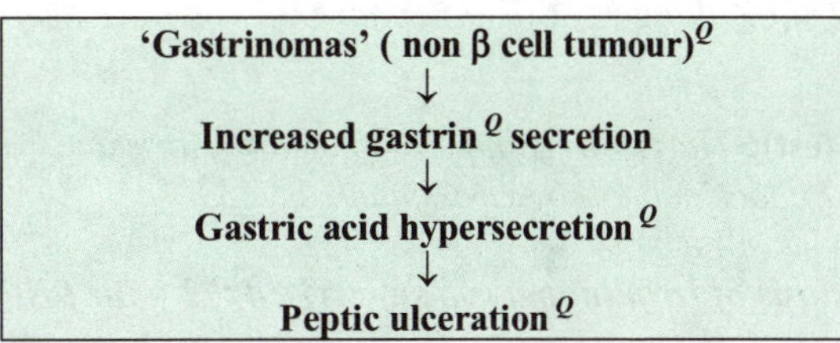

190. Answer is D (Decreased ratio of BAO to MAO): *Harrison 15th/1661; 16th/2227; 17th/1868; 18th/p 2455, 2456*

Zollinger Elision syndrome is characterized by an increased basal gastric acid output. The ratio of BAO to MAO (maximal acid output) is increased.

Presenting symptom in order of frequency
• Abdominal pain (70-100%) • Diarrhea (37-73%) • Gastroesophageal reflux disease (GERD) (30-35 years)

10-20% of patients present with diarrhea only.

Observation that should suggest the diagnosis
• Peptic ulcer disease (PUD) with diarrhea • PUD in an unusual location or with multiple lesions • PUD that is refractory to treatment or persistent • PUD that is associated with findings suggestive of MEN I • PUD without H. pylori infection.

Chronic unexplained diarrhea should also suggest gastrinoma.

<u>Diagnosis of Zollinger Ellison Syndrome</u>

STEP I	Assess fasting gastrin level	Gastrin levels are increased
STEP II	Assess acid secretion : BAO estimation	BAO is increased ; BAO / MAO is increased
STEP III	Perform provocative test if required.	i.v. secretin induces substantial increase in serum gastrin.

191. Answer is B (Secretin injection test) : *Harrison 14th/1614, 15th/1662; 16th/2227, 1891, 1894; 17th/1868 Harrison 18th/p 2455, 2456*

Secretin injection test is the most valuable provocative test in identifying patients with ZES.

<u>Secretin injection test :</u>

- In normal individuals, and patients with common Duodenal ulcer, secretin produces either no change or a small reduction or increase in serum gastrin levels. However, in ZES patients i.v. secretin induces substantial increase in serum gastrin.
- Otherwise however remember that the diagnosis of 'Gastrinoma' in a patient with clinical features consistant with ZES depends on demonstration of increased serum gastrin levels.

<u>Ca^{++} infusion test & 'Standard Test Meal' tests</u> are the other 2 provocative tests. They are not as valuable as sercretin test.

<u>ACTH stimulation test</u> is used for diagnosis of Addison's disease for which it is the only reliable test.

192. Answer is B (Omeprazole): *Harrison 15/1662; 16th/2227; 17th/1869 Harrison 18th/p 2456*

The gastric acid hypersecretion in patients with gastrinomas can be controlled in almost every case by oral gastric antisecretory drugs. ***Because of their long duration of action potency, allowing once or twice a day dosing, the proton pump inhibitors are the drug of choice*** *- Harrison*

193. Answer is A (PPI): *Harrison 16th / 1759; 17th/1869 Harrison 18th/p 2456*

PPIs are the treatment of choice for Zollinger - Ellison Syndrome and have decreased the need for total gastrectomy.
- Harrison 16th / 1759

194. Answer is A ('72 hour' fast test): *Harrison 18th/p 3066, 3067 Harrison's 17th/2354, 2355, Oxford Textbook of Medicine 4th/365, 366, 'Clinical Endocrinology' by Grossmann 2nd/534*

The Gold standard test for diagnosis of Insulinoma is a supervised '72 hour fast' test

Diagnosis of Insulinoma requires demonstration of inappropriately high levels of plasma Insulin (and C- peptide) in the presence of documented hypoglycemia (Achieved by 72 hour fast test).

Absolute values of Insulin or C- peptide are not reliable in establishing a diagnosis unless hypoglycemia is documented

The '72 hour fast test' allows demonstration of hypoglycemia, together will elevated levels of Insulin and C-peptide and thus becomes the most reliable – gold standard test for establishing a diagnosis of Insulinoma

Diagnosis of Insulinoma: '72 hour fast' test

- The diagnosis of Insulinoma requires the demonstration of an inappropriately elevated plasma insulin (and C-peptide) at the time of hypoglycemia
- The '72 hour fast' test involves supervised fasting for upto 72 hours or until hypoglycemia can be documented (<2.2 mmol/L or < 40 mg/dl)
- The test is considered positive if at any time when blood glucose levels drop to < 2.2mmol/l (40 mg/dl), the serum insulin levels are recorded to be greater than 6μU/ml. (and C- peptide levels > 100 pmol/l)
- *Studies indicate that 100% of patient with insulinoma will be detected after a supervised 72 hour fast and hence this test is considered the gold standard test*

First 24 hours :	*70-80% of patients with insulinoma can be detected*
Upto 48 hours :	*98% of patients with insulinoma can be detected*
By 72 hours:	*100% of patients with insulinoma can be detected*

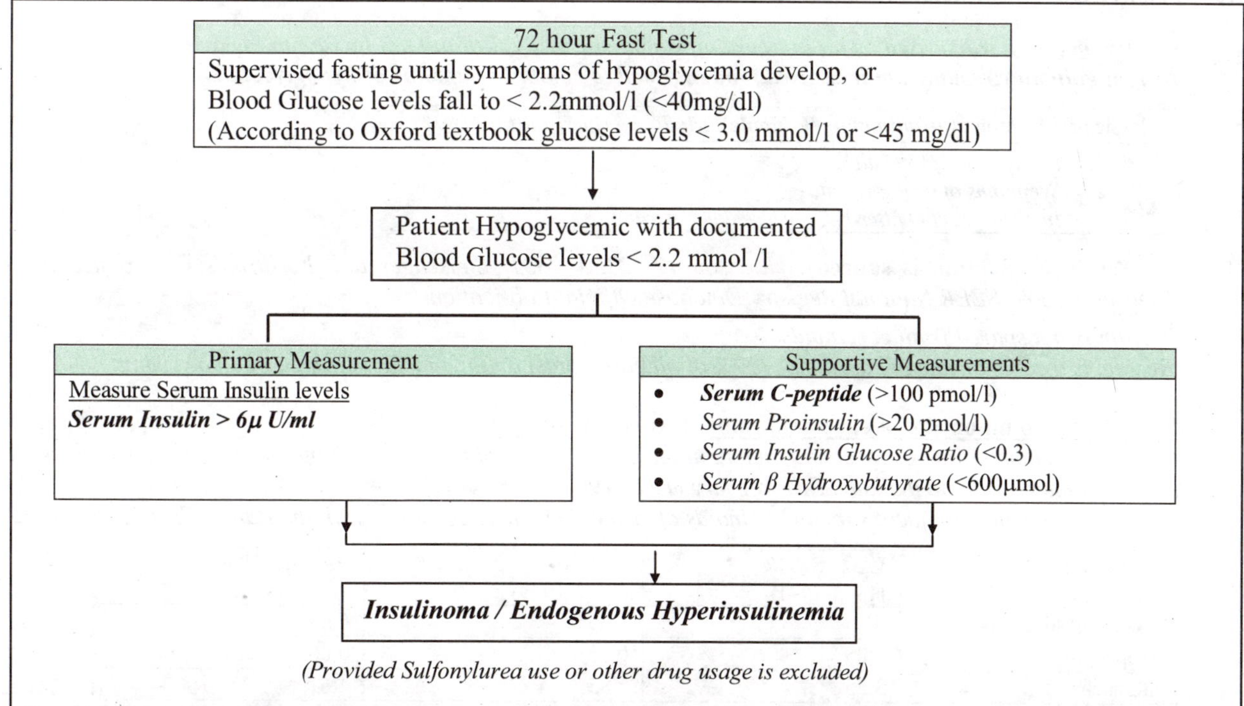

195. Answer is C (Usually multiple): *Harrison 18th/p 3066 Harrison's 17th/2354*

Insulinomas are usually single and not multiple (>90%) *– Harrison's*

Insulinomas are endocrine tumors of pancreas derived from Beta cells.
They are generally small (>90% < 2 cm), usually not multiple (90%) and only 5-15% are malignant (usually benign).

– Harrison's

Insulinomas

Insulinomas are Endocrine tumors of the pancreas derived from Beta cells that ectopically secrete Insulin and result in Hypoglycemia

Average age of occurrence is 40-50 years

- *Generally Small*[Q] (>90% are < 2cm)
- *Usually single*[Q] (Not multiple in 90%)
- *Usually Benign*[Q] (5-15% are malignant)
- *Invariably occur in the pancreas*[Q] (Distributed equally in pancreatic Head, Body and Tail)

Symptoms due to Hypoglycemia

Most common symptoms are due to the effect of hypoglycemia on the central nervous system (Neuroglycemic Symptoms)

- Confusion
- Headache
- Disorientation
- Visual difficulties
- Irrational behavior (even coma)

Symptoms due to Excessive Catecholamine Release secondary to Hypoglycemia

- *Sweating*
- *Tremor*
- *Palpitation*

196. Answer is A (Present in Pancreas): *Harrison 18th/p 3066 Harrison's 17th/2534*

The most common site of Insulinomas is the Pancreas.

197. Answer is D (Insulinoma) : *Harrison 14th/ 245; Harrison 15th/ 251; 16th/ 2227; 17th/2354 Harrison 18th/p 3066*

Insulinoma is characterised by an increase in weight (weight gain) and not by weight loss.
Weight gain may result from increased food ingested to combat symptoms of hypoglycemia.

Classic presentation of ***insulinoma*** : ***'Whipple's triad'***[Q] ***: - Harrison 14th/589***

1. *Fasting hypoglycemia*[Q]
2. *Symptoms of hypoglycemia*[Q]
3. *Immediate relief after I.V. glucose administration*[Q]

198. Answer is B (Rectum is sapred): *Harrison 17th/2350, 2351; Sleisenger and Fordtran's Gastrointestinal & Liver diseases 8th/609; SEER National Registry Database Official Publication.*

Rectum is not spared from carcinoids.
'Rectum is a common site of carcinoids (19% of all carcinoids) and the incidence appears to be rising'
– Sleisenger and Fordtran's 8th/609

Rectum is a common site of carcinoid tumors (It is not spared)
Rectum is a common site of carcinoid tumors in the gastrointestinal tract accounting for almost 19% of all carcinoid tumors of the GI tract in the late SEER registry (1992-1999).
It is the second most frequent site of Carcinoids after the ileum in accordance with the Pan SEER registry (1973-1999).

Carcinoid site	Early SEER (1973-1991)	Late SEER (1992-1999)	Pan SEER (1973-1999)
Gastrointestinal tract	61.57	67.55	64.31
Esophagus	0.05	0.06	0.06
Stomach	3.55	5.85	4.61
Small intestine	28.82	28.22	28.54
Duodenum	1.94	3.83	2.80
Jejunum	2.11	1.48	1.81
Ileum	16.23	13.35	14.92
Not specified	7.86	8.74	8.26
Colon	9.48	7.62	8.62
Appendix	6.76	2.43	4.77
Rectum	9.44	18.54	13.61

<u>**Small intestine and appendix account for almost 60% of gastrointestinal carcinoids**</u>

Small intestine and appendix together account for about 58% (≈60%) of gastrointestinal carcinoids according to the data from early SEER (1973-1991) and for about 51% of gastrointestinal carcinoids from the Pan SEER data (1973-1999)

Although the statement (option A) is not entirely correct in view of the late SEER registry and/or the Pan SEER data, this <u>may be accepted as a 'true statement' for the purpose of the question</u>.

> <u>**Site Specific incidence rate of Carcinoid Tumors**</u>
>
> *The reported anatomic distribution of carcinoid tumors varies widely amongst different textbooks depending on the source of data quoted.*
> *<u>Several textbooks including Schwartz and Sabiston, continue to mention Appendix as the most common site of gastrointestinal carcinoids</u> however these incidence rates are based on old data before the 1970's and most studies thereafter report other locations as being more frequent. <u>Results from Surveillance, Epidemiology and End Results (SEER) natural registry are now accepted as standard (Harrison.)</u>*

Five year survival is > 60%.

The five survival for all gstrointestinal carcinoids is getaer than 60 percent

5 Year Survival	Early SEER	Late SEER	Pan SEER
All Gastrointestinol Carcinoids	≈57%	≈68%	≈62.5%

Appendecial carcinoids are more common in females

'Appendecial carcinoids are more coomon in females. Two of Three cases of appendecial carcinoids are females.' - Sleisenger & Fordtradn 8th/609

The evaluation of carcinoid tumors by Pan-SEER (1973-1999) reveals a slight overall female predominance in all type of carcinoid tumors (55%).

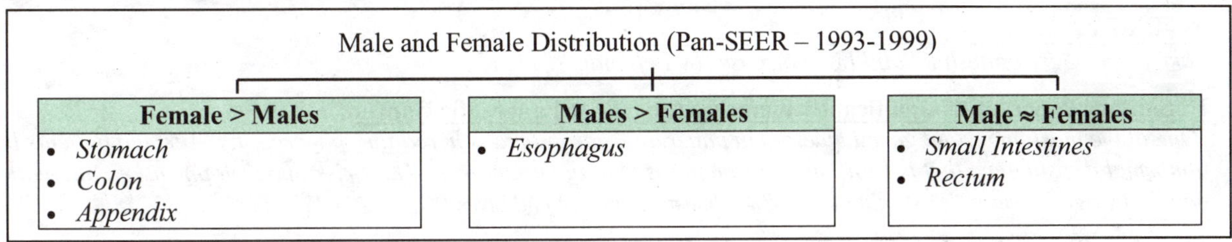

199. Answer is D (Hypocalcemia) : *Harrison 14th / 1752 ; 15th / 1803; 16th/2228, 2229; 17th/2355, 2356 Harrison 18th/p 3061, 3062*

Pancreatic cholera is a Pancreatic endocrine tumor, most commonly of the Delta cells, characterized by net secretion of salt and water by gut :

Features of Pancreatic cholera :
- *Severe watery diarrhea* Q / flushing / weight loss
- ***Hypokalemia*** Q
- ***Hypochlorhydria*** Q
- ***Hypercalcemia*** Q ***(not Hypocalcemia)***
- ***Hyperglycemia*** Q
- Inordinate fecal water and electrolyte loss

Pancreatic cholera is synonymous with 'Verner – Morrison Syndrome' or 'WDHA Syndrome'

WDHA Syndrome
Watery diarrhea
Hypokalemia
Achlorhydria

Pancreatic cholera results from excessive secretion of VIP from endocrine tumors i.e. VIPomas
'VIP' is an important neurotransmitter ubiquitously present in CNS and G.I. tract
Known actions of VIP explain most features of the clinical syndrome. These include :

- stimulation of small intestinal chloride secretion
- effects on smooth muscle contractility
- inhibition of acid secretion
- vasodilatory effects

200. Answer is C (Median Survival in locally advanced (stage III) disease is 3- 6 months) : *Integrated Medical and Surgical Gastroenterology (2004) / 206; Internal Medicine: Just the facts (MCG raw Hill) (2008) / 474; other References along with text*

Median survival of locally advanced (Stage III) disease is 6-10 months and not 3-6 months. Median survival of 3-6 months is a feature of Metastatic Stage IV disease.

Median survival in locally advanced disease (stage III) is 6 – 10 months
Metastatic disease (stage IV) is associated with a median survival of 3 – 6 months.
Stage III locally advanced disease is associated with a median survival of 6 – 10 months

Clinical / Radiological Criteria	Median Survival
• Resectable Disease (Stage I and Stage II)	15 – 20 months
• Locally Advanced Disease (Stage III)	6 – 10 months
• Metastatic Disease (Stage IV)	3 – 6 months

p^{53} mutation is seen in 75% of cases of Pancreatic cancer

Gene	Pancreatic Cancer%	Colorectal Cancer (%)
• P16	95	0
• K – ras	90	50
• ***P53***	***75***	***60***
• DPC4	55	15
• BRCA 2	7	?

Taken from Gastrointestinal and Liver disease' by Feldman 8th /1312

Hereditary Pancreatitis significantly increases the risk of Pancreatic Cancer
'One of the most important genetic factors in pancreatic carcinoma is hereditary pancreatitis. Affected patients have an abnormal trypsin gene that is transmitted as an autosomal dominant trait. Their risk of development of pancreatic cancer by age 70 years is estimated at 40%' - 'Gastrointestinal and Liver Diseases' by Feldman 8th / 1309

Five Year Survival after curative Pancreaticoduodenectomy approaches 15 -20%.

- *Overall 5-year survival rate with pancreatic cancer is 5%*
- *5 – year survival rate for patients undergoing curative tumor resection (pancreaticoduodenectomy) is 15% - 20%*

Note
Only 10% of pancreatic cancers are diagnosed at on early stage when radical resection with curative intent can be performed. - 'Pathophysiology of Disease (Lange) 5th /454'

Cystic Fibrosis

201. Answer is B (Abnormality in CFTR leads to defective Calcium Transport): *Harrison 18th/p 2147 Harrison's 17th/1632; Robbins 7th/494; Nelson's 18th ;Board Review Series 'Paediatrics' 2nd/272*

The genetic defect in cystic fibrosis produces an abnormal Cystic fibrosis Transmembrane Regulator protein (CFTR protein). This abnormal CFTR protein is associated with defective Na^+ and Cl^- transport and not defective calcium transport

Cystic fibrosis is an autosomal recessive disorder with an abnormal CFTR protein that leads to defective transport of Na^+ and Cl^-

- Cystic fibrosis is a monogenic disorder with *autosomal recessive (AR) inheritance*
- CF results from a mutation in the gene that encodes *for CF transmembrane receptor protein (CFTR)*
- The genetic mutation is located on *chromosome 7[Q]*
- The defective CFTR protein causes *dysfunction in transport of sodium and chloride (Na+ & cl-) in epithelial cells*

Cystic fibrosis predisposes to pulmonary infection with Pseudomonas

- *Cystic fibrosis airways are predisposed to chronic infections with staphylococcus and pseudomonas due to failure to clear thick viscid mucus*

Charachteristic sputum microbiology in CF patients
First organisms to be recovered are Hemophillus influenzae & staphylococcus aureces.
Thereafter Pseudomonas Aeruginosa is cultured from lower respiratory tract
Burkholderia (formerly Pseudomonas cepacia) is also recovered from CF sputum and is considered pathognomic

Cystic fibrosis may lead to cirrhosis

- *Significant liver disease occurs late in the natural history of CF*
- *Biliary Cirrhosis and multilobular cirrhosis are established complications*

Clinical Features and Diagnostic Criteria for Cystic Fibrosis:Review

Chronic Sinopulmonary disease manifested by
1. Persistent colonization/infection with typical cystic fibrosis pathogens, including Staphylococcus aureus, nontypeable, Hemophilus influenzae, ***mucoid and nonmucoid Pseudomonas aeruginosa***, Burkholderia cepase 2. Chronic cough and sputum production 3. Persistent chest radiograph abnormalities (eg. Bronchiectasis, atelectasis, infiltrates, hyperinflation) 4. Airway obstruction manifested by wheezing and air trapping 5. Nasal polyps; radiographic or computed tomographic abnormalities of paranasal sinuses 6. Digital clubbing
Gastrointestinal and nutritional abnormalities, including
1. Intestinal: meconium ileus, distal intestinal obstruction syndrome, rectal prolapse 2. Pancreatic: pancreatic insufficiency; recurrent pancreatitis 3. Hepatic: chronic hepatic disease manifested by clinical or histologic evidence of focal biliary ***cirrhosis***, or multilobular ***cirrhosis*** 4. Nutritional: failure to thrive (protein-calorie malnutrition), hypoproteinemia, edema, complications secondary to fat-soluble vitamin deficiency
Metabolic Abnormalities
1. Salt depletion syndrome 2. Hyponatremia 3. Hypochloremia 4. Hypokalemic metabolic Alkalosis
Male urogenital abnormalities resulting in obstructive azoospermia (congenital bilateral absence of vas deferens)

202. Answer is B (Demonstrate an abnormal nasal potential difference): *Nelson's 18th/1808; Harrison 18th/p 2149 Harrison's 17th/1634; Rudolph's Pediatrics 21st/1972*

Nasal Potential Difference is a sensitive test of electrolyte transport (CFTR function) that can be used to support or refute a diagnosis of cystic fibrosis when sweat chloride levels are normal or border line and two CF mutations cannot be demonstrated by DNA testing.

Diagnostic criteria for cystic fibrosis

Risk Factor For CF	PLUS	**Laboratory Evidence of CFTR Dysfunction**
• *Presence of one or more typical clinical feature (≥ 1 phenotypic symptom)*	Plus	• *Positive sweat chloride test (>60 mcq/l on two occasions)*
or		*or*
• *History of CF in sibling*	Plus	• *Identification of 2 CF mutations*
or		*or*
• *Positive Neonatal screening test*	Plus	• *Abnormal Nasal Potential Difference*

The patient in question has typical clinical features of cystic fibrosis; however the sweat chloride levels are border line (between 40-60meq/l) on two separate occasions. To establish the diagnosis of cystic fibrosis, another laboratory evidence demonstrating CFTR dysfunction is therefore required.

This can be achieved by demonstration of abnormal CF mutation by DNA analysis or by demonstrating an abnormal nasal potential difference.

The diagnostic criteria for cystic fibrosis requires demonstration of at least two CF mutations and hence ***demonstration of an abnormal F508 mutation alone is not sufficient to establish the diagnosis of CF***

An abnormal CFTR nasal potential difference is an established laboratory evidence of CFTR dysfunction and is accepted as a diagnostic criterion to establish the diagnosis of cystic fibrosis

Clinical History/Features

- Presence of one or more charachteristic clinical features
  - Respiratory (chronic obstructive pulmonary disease etc)
  - Gastrointestinal (Exacrine pancreatic insufficiency)
  - Genitourinary (Male infertility)
  - Salt loss syndrome

  Or
- History of Cystic fibrosis in sibling

  Or
- History of positive new born screening

PLUS PLUS

Laboratory evidence of CFTR Dysfunction

Positive sweat chloride test	Identification of two CF mutations	Abnormal Nasal Potential Difference (PD)
• Sweat chloride concentration >60 meq/l on two occasions • *Elevated sweat chloride levels are nearly pathognomic of cystic fibrosis*	• Commercial laboratory DNA tests, test for 30-80 most common CFTR mutations • This testing identifies individuals who carry *two CFTR mutations*	• Nasal PD measures the bioelectric voltage difference across nasal epithelium and is a sensitive test of electrolyte transport (CFTR dysfunction) • ***Nasal PD can be used to document CFTR dysfunction when sweat chloride levels are normal or borderline and two CF mutations are not identified on DNA testing.***

Miscellaneous

203. Answer is B (B. cereus) : *Harrison 18th/p 312 CMDT 2008 / 482*

Bacillus cereus causes non invasive diarrhea due to preformed enterotoxins

Shigella, Salmonella and Y. enterocolitica are causes of invasive diarrhea.

Bacterial Diarrhea

Non Invasive	Invasive
• Non invasive diarrhea is caused by the release of toxins from bacteria that disrupt the secretory process • This diarrhea is charachterized by the presence of watery stools Blood and fecal leucocytes are charachteristically bsent **Bacteria associated with Non Invasive Diarrhea** • *Staphylococcus Aureus (Preformed toxin)* • *Bacillus cereus (Preformed toxin)* • *Clostridium perfringes (preformed toxin)* • *ETEC (Enterotoxigenic E.coli)* • *Vibrio cholerae*	• Invasive diarrhea is caused by damage to gastrointestinal tissue (colonic tissue) due to direct invasion by bacteria • This diarrhea is charachterized clinically by the presence of - Fever - Bloody stools (Dysentry) - Fecal leucocytes. **Bacteria associated with Invasive diarrhea** • ***Shigella*** • ***Salmonella*** • ***Yersenia Enterocolitica*** • *Entero invasive E.coli (ETEC)* • *Aeromonas* • *Plesiomonas* • *Listeria monocytogenes*

204. Answer is C (Reduces with fasting): *CMDT 2009/499; Manual of Gastroenterology 4th/184 – Harrison 18th/p 321 Harrisons 17th/249*

Secretory diarrhea does not reduce with fasting.

In secretory diarrhea an abnormal ion transport occurs across intestinal epethelial cells. This diarrhea is not related to the intestinal content and hence it typically does not cease with fasting

Typical Features of Secretory Diarrhea

- ***Large volume (typically > 1L/ day)***
- ***Little change with fasting*** *(Diarrhea typically does not cease while patient fasts)*
- ***Normal stool osmotic gap*** *(osmolality of stool is close to osmolality of plasma)*
- *No anion gap*
- *Stools are watery in consistency and do not contain pus or blood*
- ***Painless***

205. Answer is A (Cisapride): *Harrison 18th/46; Drug Induced Long QT syndrome (2002)/45; 'The Chemotherapy Source Book (Lippincott) 4th/605*

Co-administration of ketoconazole with cisapride is contraindicated secondary to an increased risk of cardiovascular adverse effects such as 'torsades-de-pointes', ventricular tachycardia or ventricular fibrillation'.
(Taken from 'The Chemotherapy Source Book (Lippincott) 4th/605)

Ketoconazole and Prolonged QT interval

- Ketoconazole has been reported to be pro-dysrhythmic (prolonged QT interval) even without the concomitant use of other drugs that cause prolongation of the QT interval.

Ketoconazole alone can prolong the QT interval and induce Torsades-de-pointes by blocking the rapid component of delayed rectifier potassium channels (IKr)4.

- Ketoconazole also *inhibits the cytochrome P450 CYP3A4 isoenzyme.*
- Ketoconazole ***should not be co-administered with another QT prolonging drug that is metabolized by the cytochrome P450 CYP3A4 isoenzyme such as Cisapride****, Terfenadine, Astemizole, or Amitryptyline as this will result in increased concentration of the latter leading to marked prolongation of QT interval and increase the risk of Torsades-de-pointes and life threatening ventricular arrythmias.*

Important QT prolonging drugs metabolized by CYP3A4
Contraindicated for co-administration with Ketoconazole, Itraconazole, Erythromycin, Clarithromycin

- *Cisapride*
- *Terfenadine*
- *Astemizole*
- *Mizolastin*
- *TCA (Amitryptaline)*

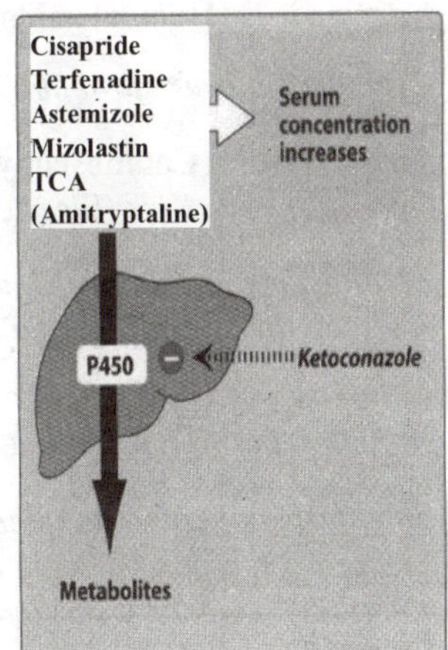

Drugs with High Risk of Generating Pharmakokinetic Interactions *(Harrison's 18th/ 46)*

Drug	Mechanism	Examples
Antacids Bile acid sequestrants	Reduced absorption	Antacids/tetracyclines Cholestyramine/digoxin
Proton pump inhibitors H_2–receptor blockers	Altered gastric pH	Ketoconazole absorption decreased
Rifampin Carbamazepine Barbiturates Phenytoin St. John's wort Glutethimide	Induction of Hepatic Metabolism	Decreased concentration and effects of : Warfarin Quinidine Cyclosporine Losartan Oral contraceptives Methadone

Tricyclic antidepressants Fluoxetine Quinidine	Inhibitors of CYP2D6	Increased effect of many β blockers Decreased codeine effect
Cimetidine	Inhibitor of multiple CYPs	Increased concentration and effects of Warfarin Theophylline Phenytoin
Ketoconazole, Itraconazole Erythromycin, Clarithromycin Calcium channel blockers Ritonavir	Inhibitor of CYP3A	Increased concentration and toxicity of some HMG-CoA reductase inhibitors, *cyclosporine*, ***cisapride***, *terfenadine (now withdrawn)* Increased concentration and effects of indinavir (With ritonavir) Decreased clearance and dose requirement for cyclosporine (with calcium channel blockers)
Allopurinol	Xanthine oxidase inhibitor	Azathioprine and 6-mercaptopurine toxicity
Amiodarone	Inhibitor of many CYPs and of P-glycoprotein	Decreased clearance (risk of toxicity) for Warfarin Digoxin Quinidine
Gemfibrazole (and other fibrates)	CYP3A inhibition	Rhabdomyolysis when co-prescribed with some HMG-CoA reductase Inhibitors
Quinidine Amiodarone Verapamil Cyclosporine Itraconazole Erythromycin	P-glycoprotein inhibition	Risk of digoxin toxicity
Phenylbutazone Probenecid Salicylates	Inhibition of renal tubular transport	Increased risk of methotrexate toxicity with salicylate

206. Answer is E (Hemorrhoids): *Harrison 17th/259*

'Hemorrhoids are probably the most common cause of Lower GIBleed (LGIB)' *– Harrisons*

207. Answer is A (Colonoscopy): *'Primary Care Medicine' by Goroll & Mulley (Lippincott) 6th/522; 'General Surgical Operations' by Kirk (Elsevier) 2006/228*

Colonoscopy is the investigation of choice in elderly patients presenting with occult fecal blood and anemia to evaluate the possibility of a colorectal cancer.

'Colonoscopy is the test of choice in a case with occult fecal blood, rectal bleeding, anemia, or weight loss in an older patient, all of which suggest the possibility of colorectal cancer' - 'Primary Care Medicine' (Lippincott)6th/522

'In elderly patients who often tolerate barium enema badly, colonoscopy should be the first-line investigation for unexplained rectal bleeding or anemia ***and is the investigation of choice for all patients with a positive fecal occult blood test'*** *- General surgical operations by Kirk (Elsevier) 2006/228.*

208. Answer is A (Diverticulosis) : *Harrison 14th/247; Harrison 15th/253; (Not elaborated in Harrison 16th)*

Although anorectal disease is the most commonm cause of bleeding per rectum in the elderly, these lesions usually cause small amount of 'bright red' blood on the surface of stool and toilet tissue (small bleeds).
Diverticulosis may give rise to massive colonic bleed. The usual presentation of diverticular hemorrhage is that of brisk painless passage of a maroon coloured stool. It is the most common cause of massive bleeding per rectum in those above 55 years of age and hence the answer here.

Common causes of Acute Lower G.I. bleeding (in descending order) over 55 years of age are :
1. Anorectal disease : Haemorrhoids and fissures
2. Diverticulosis
3. Angiodysplasia
4. Polyps and Cancer
5. Enterocolitis

209. Answer is B (Acute mesentric ischaemia) : *Harrison 14th/1652, 15th/1699, 16th/1798; Bailey Love 23rd/1074*

The onset of abdominal pain and maroon stools in an elderly patient with the background of ischaemic heart disease and atherosclerosis suggests the diagnosis of acute mesenteric ischemia.

'The most important clue to an early diagnosis of acute mesentric ischaemia is the sudden onset of severe abdominal pain in a patient with atrial fibrillation or atherosclerosis' - *Harrison*

The patient in question : is an ***old man of 60 yrs***, who has a ***history of I.H.D. & atherosclerosis*** & ***presents with abdominal pain*** thus leading us towards this diagnosis

Major clinical features of acute mesentric ishcaemia are :

1. ***Severe abdominal pain***, often colicky & periumbilical at onset, later becoming diffuse
2. Vomiting, anorexia
3. Diarrhoea and / or constipation

Examination of the abdomen reveals: Tenderness & distension.

Two features are important to be observed

- ***Bowel sounds are often normal even in face of severe infarction.*** Q
- ***Gross haemorrhage is unusual*** Q (except in ischaemic colitis) Q

Gastrointestinal bleeding therefore is mild and accounts for the maroon stools in our patient.

210. Answer is D (All of the above) : *Harrison 15th / 1697*

Intestinal hypomotility may be seen in all conditions mentioned in the questions.

Parkinsonism	• Achalasia / Pseudo-obstruction / Megacolon • Lewy bodies in myenteric plexus of esophagus and colon
Diabetes Mellitus	• Gastroparesis and intestinal & colonic dysmotility • Myenteric plexus morphologically intact
Amyloidosis	• Achalasia / Gastroparesis / Pseudo-obstruction • Amyloid deposit in both smooth muscle and myenteric plexus

211. Answer is C (Hyponatremia): *A practical Guide to Pediatric Emergency Medicine (Cambridg Univ. Press) 2011/chap. 54; Pediatric Medical student USMLE Board part II & III & IV (John Barlett 1999/46, 47.*

The most common cause of seizures in children with diarrhea is hypovolemic hyponatremia.

Diarrhea may be associated with hypovolemic hyponatremia or hypernatremia from hypotonic fluid loss. Both hyponatremia and hypernatremia may manifest with seizures. However Hyponatremia remains the most common electrolyte abnormality in diarrhea encountered in clinical practice and is hence the single best ***Answer*** *of choice amongst the options provided.*

212. Answer is D (50% involve rectum) : *Surgical Pathology by Noel Weidner /230*

'2/3 of lesions are located in the caecum and ascending colon and one quarter in the left colon'.

Thus involvement of left side of colon (or rectum) is uncommon and certainly less than 50% of cases involve rectum.

Telengiectasias consist of dilated capillaries that appear clinically as erythematous to violaceous vessels.

Telengiectaseas in colon may most commonly be due to :

1. Vascular ectasia / Angiodysplasia
   - **Angiodysplasia is a telengiectasia** of thin walled capillaries and venules in the mucosa and submucosa of colon
   - **Mean age at diagnosis is approx. 65 years** but cases **have occured in the young.**
   - **2/3 of lesions are located in coecum and ascending colon** and **one quarter in the left colon**.
2. Radiation : Telengiectaseas are the most common long term effect of radiation.
3. Hereditary hemorrhagic telengiectaseas - affect **younger patients** with a positive family history.

213. Answer is C (Pernicious anemia) : *Harrison's 16th/604*

Pernicious anemia is associated with Hypergastrinemia and Hypochlorhydria.

<u>**Pernicious anemia**</u>

- It is the most common cause of vitamin B12 deficiency in temperate climate[Q]
- It is characterised by gastric atrophy [Q] affecting the acid and pepsin secreting portion of stomach i.e. fundus and body. Antrum is spared.
  - intrinsic factor required for absorbtion of vit B12 is secreted by perietal cells, present in body and fundus of stomach and therefore ***intrinsic factor is depleted.***
  - acid secreting cells are situated in body and fundus of stomach and therefore **acid is depleted - Achlorhydria**
  - gastrin producing G cells are situated in the antrum of stomach and so spared and therefore **depletion of gastric acid results in hypertrophy of G-cells and hypergastrinemia - Hypergastrinemia**

214. Answer is C (Pernicious anemia) : *Harrison's 15th/677; Harrison 14th/655, 656; Harrison 16th/604*

Depletion of gastric acid (Hypochlorhydria) results in hypertrophy of G-cells and hypergastrinemia

<u>**Perenicious anemia**</u>

- It is the most common cause of vitamin B_{12} deficiency in temprate climate[Q]
- It is characterised by gastric atrophy[Q] affecting the acid and pepsin secreating portion of stomach i.e. fundus and body. Antrum is spared.
  - intrinsic factor required for absorbtion of vit B12 is secreted by perietal cells, present in body and fundus of stomach and therefore ***intrinsic factor is depleted.***
  - acid secreting cells are situated in body and fundus of stomach and therefore **acid is depleted achlorhydria**
  - gastrin producing G cells are situated in the antrum of stomach and so spared and therefore **depletion of gastric acid results in hypertrophy of G-cells and hypergastrinemia**

215. Answer is B (Esophagus varices) *Harrison 16th /e p. 1863, 235 ; Harrison 17th 1976-1977 Harrison 18th/p 2597, 2598*

'Massive haematemesis in the background of splenomegaly suggests variceal bleed due to portal hypertension.'

216. Answer is C (Present as stromal polyps): *Harrison 18th/p 928 Harrisons 17th / 694; Current Diagnosis & Treatment in Gastroenterology 2nd/389; Oxford Text book of Medicine 4th/589*

Stromal polyps are infrequent primary gastric malignancies classified as Gastrointestinal Stromal Cell Tumors (GSIT). These are not associated with MALT Lymphomas

- <u>**MALT Lymphomas presents at extranodal sites**</u> (Harrisons)
  MALT Lymphomas are also called 'Extranodal Margmal zone B cell Lymphomas of MALT type' and typically occur at extranodal sites as suggested by the terminology
- <u>**MALT Lymphomas are predisposed by H.Pylori**</u> (Harrison)
  Gastric presentation of MALT Lymphoma is associated with H. Pylori infection – Harrisons
- <u>**MALT Lymphomas are sensitive to chemotherapy**</u>
  Extensive MALT Lymphomas are most often treated with single agent chemotherapy such as chlorambucil- Harrison

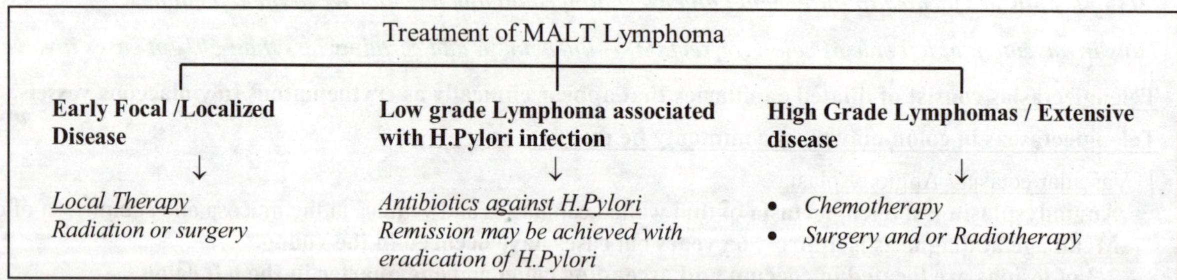

217. Answer is B (Amylase levels): *Washington Manual of surgery 5th / 413, Bailey 25th / 1425*

The major advantage of Bladder drainage is the ability to measure urinary amylase which can facilitate early diagnosis of rejection

'Urinary drainage of the pancreas has the advantage that urinary amylase levels can be used to monitor graft rejection' - Bailey 25th / 1425

Exocrine Drainage after Pancreatic Transplantation

Enteric Drainage	Bladder Drainage
The whole pancreas along with a segment of donor duodenum is transplanted into the recipient small bowel All exocrine secretions / enzymes are drained into the bowel and excreted with the stool	The whole pancreas along with a segment of donor duodenum is transplanted into the recipient bladder All exocrine secretions / enzymes are drained into the bladder and excreted via urine
Major Advantage of Enteric Drainage (Disadvantage of Bladder Drainage) • Fewer Urinary tract infections /Urological complications (Urological complications are more common with bladder drainage) • Fewer Metabolic complications (eg Acidosis) (Metabolic complications such as metabolic acidosis are more common with bladder drainage) • Lesser incidence of Reflux Pancreatitis (Reflux Pancreatitis is more common with bladder drainage)	**Major Advantages of Bladder Drainage (Disadvantage of Enteric drainage)** • *Ability to measure urinary amylase which can facilitate early diagnosis of rejection* (A fall in urinary amylase usually precedes a rise in systemic blood glucose during rejection such that anti-rejection treatment can be commenced sooner) • Lower rate of Technical failure (Procedure related complications)

218. Answer is A (End colostomy) : *PreTest Surgery 11th/299; Schwartz 8th/1074; 'Intestinal Failure' by Nightingale (2001)/62*

Parastomal hernia is the most frequent complication of End Colostomies.

Parastomal hernia is common around an end colostomy particularly if the stoma brought out is lateral to the rectus sheath and if the abdominal musculature is very weak as often occurs in the elderly.

Facts to Remember

- *Parastomal hernias are more common after a colostomy than after on Iliostomy*
- *Parastomal hernias are most frequently seen in association with end colostomies that are brought out lateral to the rectus muscle*
- *'Prolapse' are more common after a colostomy than after an Iliostomy*
- *'Prolapse' is most commonly seen after 'loop colostomies' particularly loop transverse colostomies.*

NOTES

Liver and Biliary Tract

ESSENTIAL REVISION NOTES

Jaundice

Catabolism of 'Haem' and Generation of Bilirubin

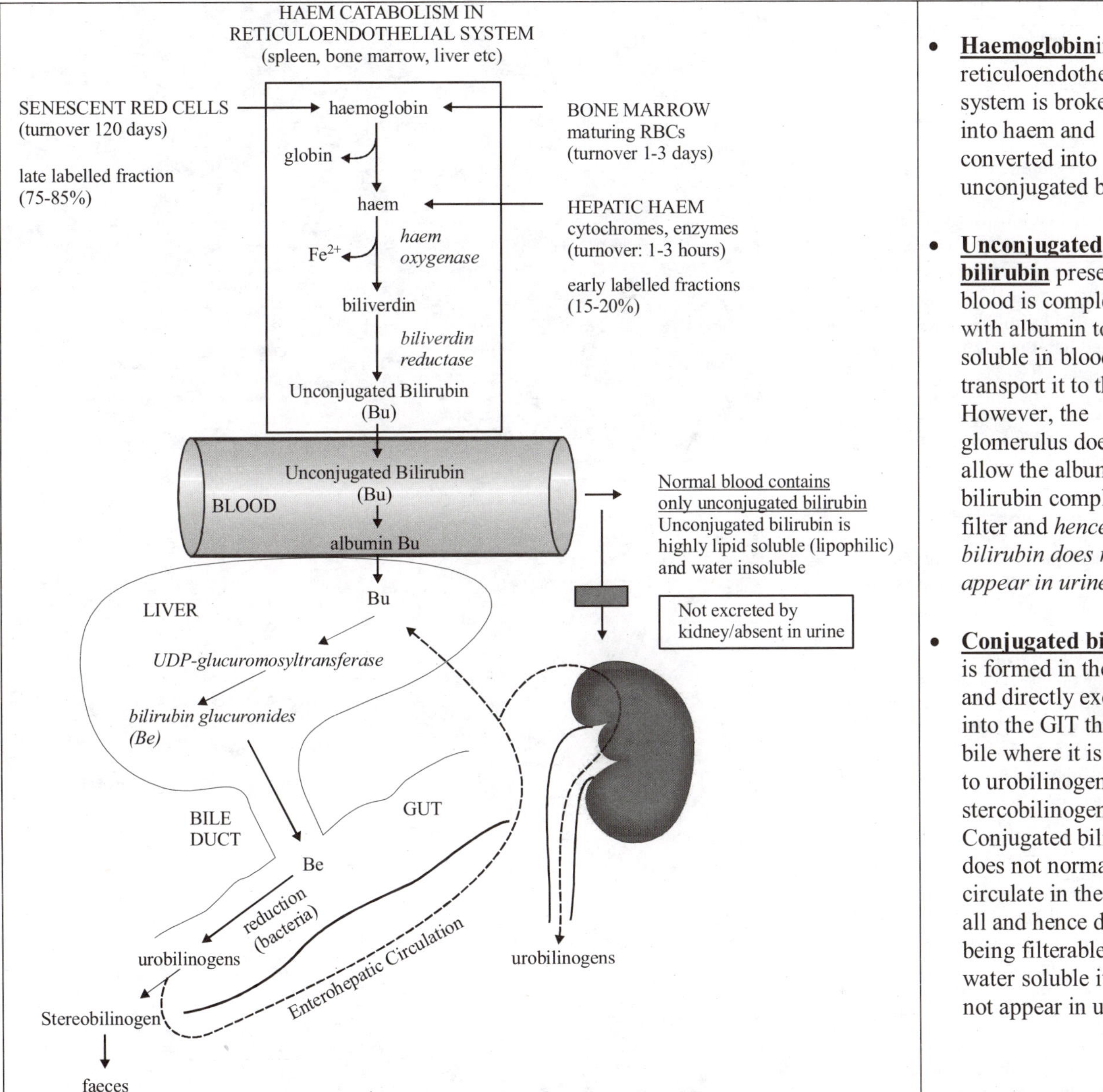

- **Haemoglobin** in the reticuloendothelial system is broken down into haem and converted into unconjugated bilirubin
- **Unconjugated bilirubin** present in blood is complexed with albumin to make it soluble in blood and transport it to the liver. However, the glomerulus does not allow the albumin bilirubin complex to filter and *hence bilirubin does not appear in urine.*
- **Conjugated bilirubin** is formed in the liver and directly excreted into the GIT through bile where it is reduced to urobilinogen and stercobilinogen. Conjugated bilirubin does not normally circulate in the blood at all and hence despite being filterable and water soluble it does not appear in urine.

Pathophysiology of different types of jaundice

Pathophysiology of different types of jaundice

- Normal blood contains unconjugated bilirubin only (no conjugated bilirubin)

> *Unconjugated bilirubin is water insoluble (lipophilic, lipid soluble) and not filterable by the kidney.*

- Unconjugated bilirubin is taken up from the systemic circulation by hepatocytes (1)
- Unconjugated bilirubin is then conjugated to bilirubin glucoronide by glucoronyl transferase within the hepatocytes (2)
- Conjugated bilirubin is then excreted into the bile from where it reaches the GIT (3)
  This is the rate-limiting step.

> *Conjugated bilirubin is water soluble and filterable by the kidney*
> **Normally**, there is no conjugated bilirubin in the systemic circulation and hence no bilirubin is filtered in the kidney or present in the urine.
> ***Abnormally***
> When there is hepatocellular dysfunction or bile flow is totally obstructed, conjugated bilirubin "leaks" into the systemic circulation
> This conjugated bilirubin may now be excreted by the kidney and be detected in urine.
> **Bilirubin in urine (bilirubinuria)**
> *Presence of bilirubin in urine suggests a diagnosis of conjugated hyperbilirubinemia either due to hepatocellular jaundice or obstructive jaundice.*

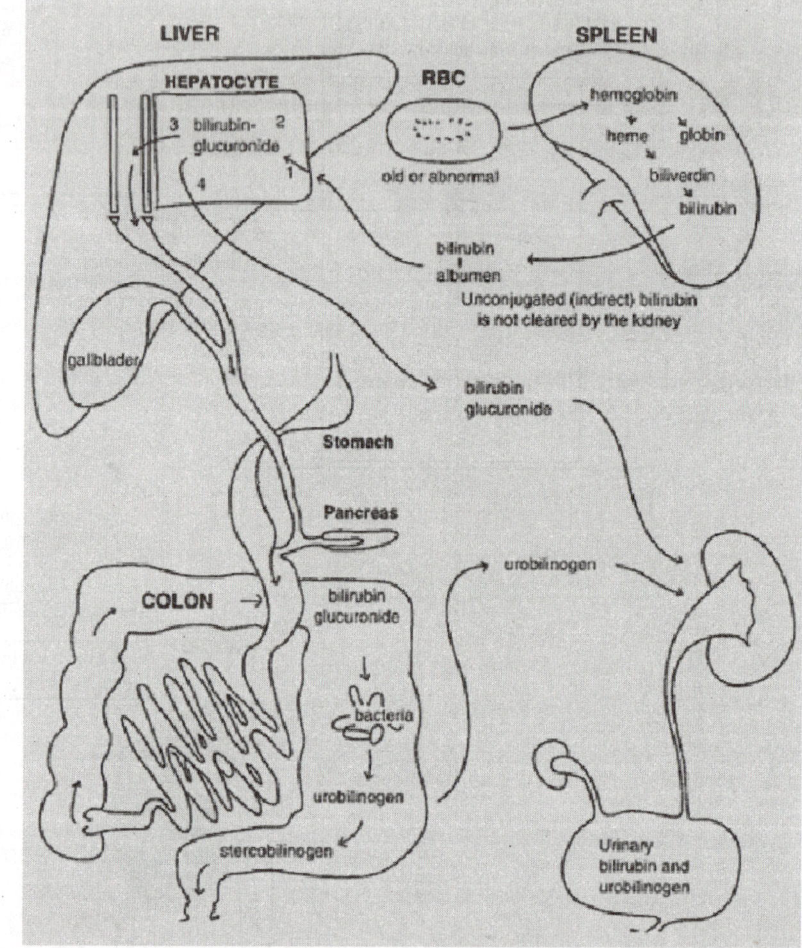

- Within the GIT conjugated bilirubin is degraded/reduced to urobilinogen and then to stercobilinogen

> Urobilinogen is water soluble and filterable by the kidney
> **Normally**, a small portion of the urobilinogen is reabsorbed from the gut and excreted by the kidney (<4 mg/day)
> **In Non-Obstructive Hyperbilirubinemia (hemolytic, hepatocellular)** the amount of urobilinogenexreated by the kidney is increased as more urobilinogen is formed and reabsorbed.
> ***Elevated levels of urobilinogen suggest primarily an non obstructive hyperbilirubinemia***
> **In Obstructive Hyperbilirubinemia**, conjugated bilirubin does not reach the GIT and hence no urobilinogen is formed
> ***Absent levels of urobilinogen suggest a diangnosis of obstructive hyperbilirubinemia***

Causes and Classification of Hyperbilirubinemia

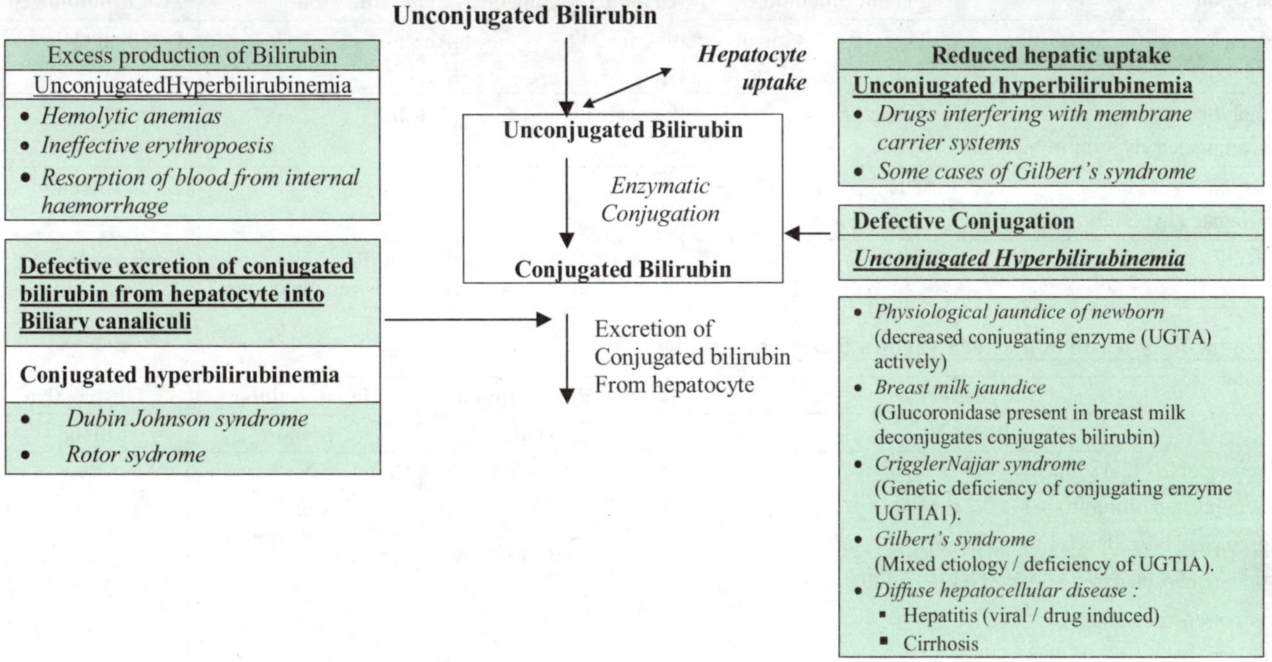

Unconjugated Bilirubin

Hepatocyte uptake

Unconjugated Bilirubin

Enzymatic Conjugation

Conjugated Bilirubin

Excretion of Conjugated bilirubin From hepatocyte

Excess production of Bilirubin
UnconjugatedHyperbilirubinemia
• *Hemolytic anemias* • *Ineffective erythropoesis* • *Resorption of blood from internal haemorrhage*

Reduced hepatic uptake
Unconjugated hyperbilirubinemia
• *Drugs interfering with membrane carrier systems* • *Some cases of Gilbert's syndrome*

Defective Conjugation
Unconjugated Hyperbilirubinemia

• *Physiological jaundice of newborn* (decreased conjugating enzyme (UGTA) actively)
• *Breast milk jaundice* (Glucoronidase present in breast milk deconjugates conjugates bilirubin)
• *CrigglerNajjar syndrome* (Genetic deficiency of conjugating enzyme UGTIA1).
• *Gilbert's syndrome* (Mixed etiology / deficiency of UGTIA).
• *Diffuse hepatocellular disease :*
  ▪ Hepatitis (viral / drug induced)
  ▪ Cirrhosis

Defective excretion of conjugated bilirubin from hepatocyte into Biliary canaliculi
Conjugated hyperbilirubinemia
• *Dubin Johnson syndrome* • *Rotor sydrome*

Indirect hyperbilirubinemia
Hemolytic disorders
Inherited • *Spherocyteosis,* • *Elliptocytosis* • *Glucose-6-phosphate dehydrogenase* • *Pyruvate kinase deficiencies* • *Sickle cell anemia* Acquired • *Microangiopathic hemolytic anemias* • *Paraoxysmal nocturnal hemoglobinuria* • *Immune* hemolysis
Ineffective erythropoiesis
• *Cobalamin and folate deficiency* • *Severe iron deficiency* • *Thalassemia*
Drugs
• *Rifampicin,* • *Probenecid,* • *Ribavirin*
Inherited conditions
• *Crigler-Najjar types I and II* • *Glibert's* syndrome

Direct hyperbilirubinemia
Inherited conditions
• *Dubin-Johnson syndrome* • *Rotor's* syndrome

Biochemical markers in various types of Jaundice

Condition	Serum Bilirubin	Urine Urobilinogen	Urine Bilirubin	Fecal urobilinogen
Normal	Direct 0.1-0.4 mg/dl Indirect 0.2-0.7 mg/dl	0-4 mg/24 h	Absent	40-280 mg/24h
Hemolytic anemia (Unconjugated Hyperbilirubinemia)	↑ Indirect	Increased	Absent	Increased
Obstructive jaundice (Conjugated hyperbilirubinemia)	↑ Direct	Absent	Present	Trace to absent
Hepatitis	↑ Direct and indirect	Decreased if micro-obstruction is present	Present if microobstruction occurs	Decreased

Distinguishing features between various forms of Jaundice:

Parameter	Hemolytic	Hepatocellular	Obstructive
Blood	**Blood**	**Blood**	**Blood**
Haemoglobin (12-18 g/dl)	Decreased	N.	N.
Unconjugated bilirubin (0.2 to 0.7 mg/dl)	↑↑	N or ↑	N
Conjugated bilirubin (0.1 to 0.3 mg/dl)	N	↑	↑
Alkaline phosphatase (3-13 KAU) (30 to 120 IU/L)	N	N or ↑	↑↑
Aminotransferases	N	↑↑	N
Cholesterol	N	N	↑
Stool	**Stool**	**Stool**	**Stool**
Colour of stool	N	N	Pale
Urine	**Urine**	**Urine**	**Urine**
Bilirubin	0	↑	↑
Urobilinogen	↑	↑	↓

Approach to a patient presenting with bilirubinemia

Hyperbilirubinemia

Unconjugated Hyperbilirubinemia	Conjugated Hyperbilinubinemia
Direct bilirubin < 15% Indirect bilirubin > 85%	Direct bilirubin > 15% Indirect bilirubin < 85%

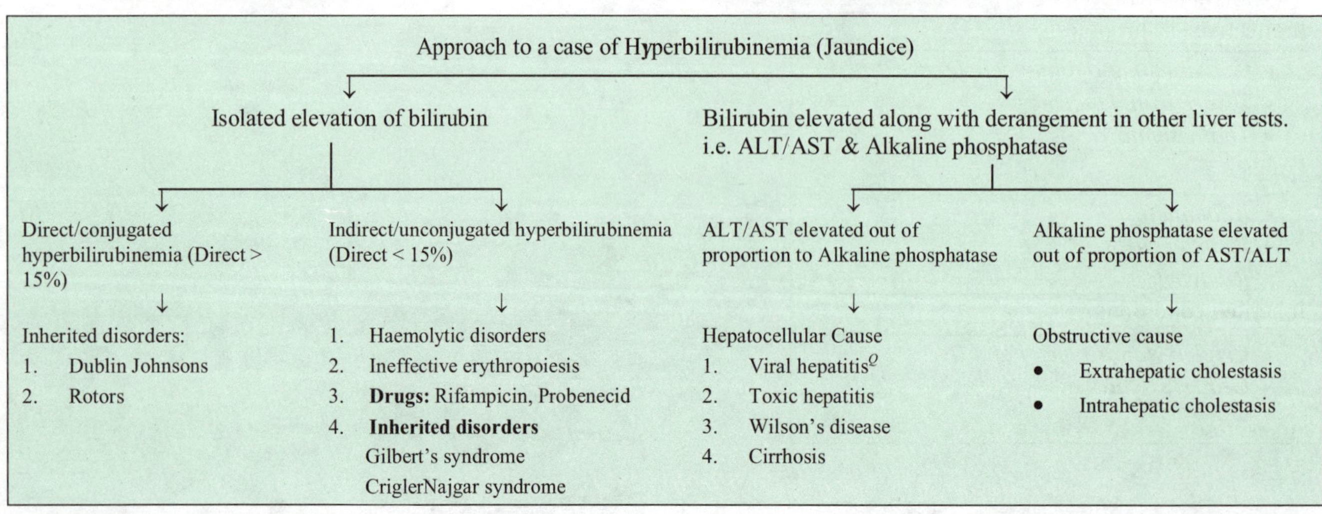

Further Approach to a patient with direct hyperbilirubinemia

If direct conjugated bilirubin is greater than 15% of the total bilirubin, it is termed as direct bilirubinemia

Bilirubin	Associated parameter	Inference
Direct bilirubinemia	Alkaline phosphatase raised out of proportion to transferases (ALT/AST)	Cholestatic obstructive jaundice
Direct bilirubinemia	Transferases (ALT/AST) Raised out of proportion to alkaline phosphatase	Hepatocellular jaundice

Further Protocol for investigating a patient with cholestatic serum profile.

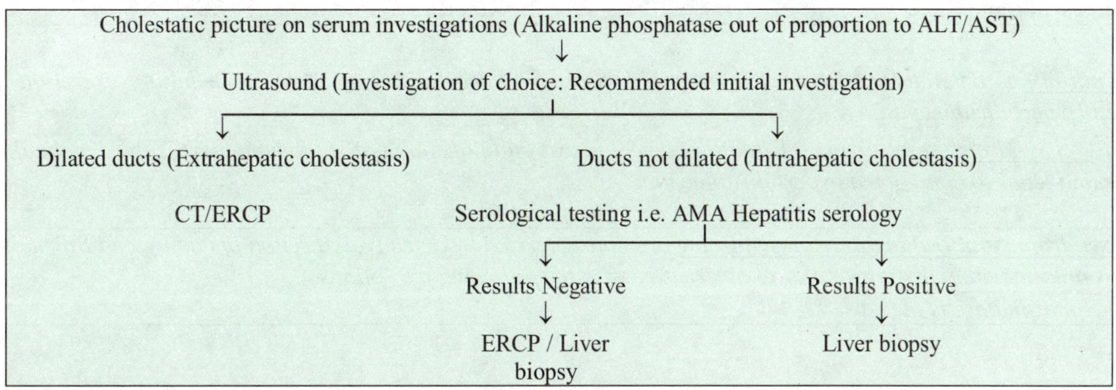

Initial investigation of choice in a case of obstructive jaundice is: ULTRASONOGRAPHY

Hepatic Enzymes and their role in determining cause of Hyperbilirubinemia

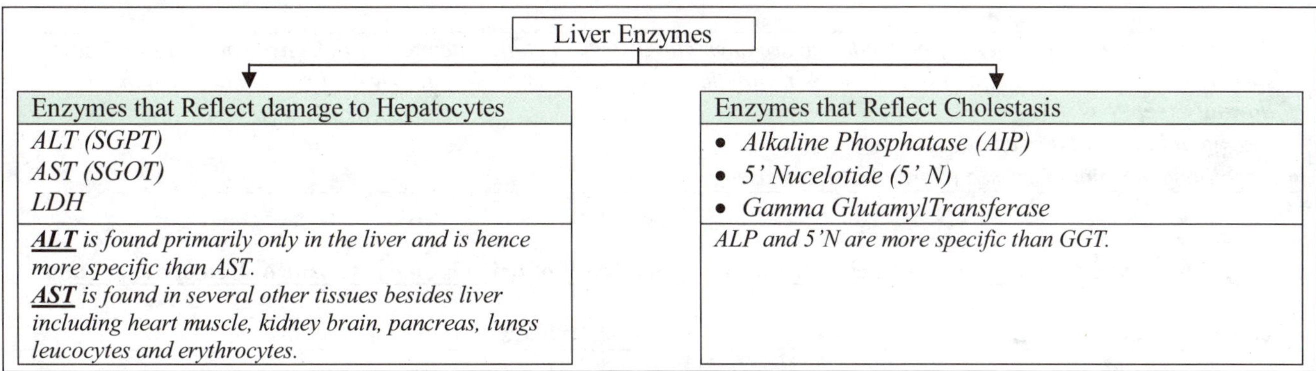

Note that true assessment of hepatic excretory function requires measurement of serum concentration of substances metabolized and transported by the liver or by determination of rate of clearance of exogenously administered dyes or drugs such as indocyanine green, caffeine, lidocaine and PABA.

Liver enzymes including those reflecting cholestasis are not true measures for detecting excretory function of hepatocytes.

Hereditary Hyperbilirubinemias

Hereditary Hyperbilirubinemias Q

Unconjugated	**Conjugated**
(Defect conjugating enzyme bilirubin glucoronyltransferase)	(Defect in biliary excretion of conjugated bilirubin)
1. CirglerNajjar Syndrome type I & type II Q 2. Gilberts syndrome Q	1. Dubin Johnson syndrome Q 2. Rotor's syndrome Q

Rotor's syndrome is an Autosomal recessive inherited disorder characterized by a defect in biliary excretion leading to Conjugated Hyperbilirubinemia.

Dubin Johnson Syndrome results from a hereditary defect in excretion of conjugated bilirubin across the canalicular membrane and leads to conjugated hyperbilirubinemia.

Rotor's syndrome and Dubin Johnson syndrome *are characterized by defective excretion of conjugated Bilirubin. They thus present with a picture similar to obstructive with the following exceptions:*

- *Alkaline phosphatase is not raised.*

Gilberts syndrome and CriglerNajjarsyndromepresent with unconjugated hyperbilirubinemia due to defect in the conjugating enzyme bilirubin glucoronyltransferase

Urinary Urobilinogens are however not elevated in these conditions. *Urobilinogen may never the less be present in urine (N or ↓) in these conditions*

Gilberts syndrome and CriglerNajjar syndrome are enymatic disorders charachterized by defective conjugation. These disorders may present with a picture similar to hemolytic jaundice with unconjugated hyerbilirubinamia, with the following exceptions.

- *Haemoglobin is not decreased*
- *Urobilinogen is not increased (Normal or Decreased)*

Unconjugated Hyperbilirubinemia with elevated urobilinogen levels of urine is characteristic of Hemolytic anemia

Condition / syndrome	Hyperbilirubinemia	Urinary Urobilinogen*(N=0-4 mg/24 hrs)*
Hemolytic Anemia	*Unconjugated (Indirect)*	*Increased*
Gilbert's syndrome	*Unconjugated (Indirect)*	*Normal or Decreased*
CriglerNajjar	*Unconjugted (Indirect)*	*Normal or Decreased*

Dubin Johnson Syndrome : Review

During Johnson syndrome is an ***autosomal recessive***[Q] hereditary disorder presenting with ***conjugated hyperbilirubinemia***[Q] due to ***defect in hepatic excretory function across the canalicular membrane of hepatocyte.***[Q]

Clinical presentation

- Most patient are asymptomatic (subclinical chemical hyperbilirubinemia)
- ***Unexplained low grade jaundice during teenage years <u>Often exacerbated by</u> :***
  - ***Oral contraceptive use***
  - Pregnancy
  - Intercurrent illness
- Physical examination is usually normal (occasional patient may have hepatosplenomegaly)

Laboratory studies

- ***<u>Conjugated Hyperbilirubinemia</u>*** : Total bilirubin is ***typically between 2 – 5 mg/dl*** *(34 – 85 µmol/L)*

May occasionally be Normal or as high as 20-25 mg/dl(340-430 µmol/L)

- **<u>Bilirubinuria</u>** : Typically present as hyperbilirubinemia is conjugated
- ***<u>Other Routine Liver Function Tests</u> including Serum Transaminases and Alkaline Phosphatase are essentially Normal***

Diagnosis

<u>Bromsulphaleintest</u>:*Elaborated above*

<u>Corporphyrin test</u>
<u>(Preferential urinary excretion of corporphyrin-I)</u>

Corporphrins are byproducts of hemebiosnthesis
There are two naturally occurring corporphyrins – I & III
Normally approx. 75 % of corporpyrin in urine is isomer III
In urine of patients with D-J Syndrome total corporphyrin content in urine is norma but > 80 % is Isomer I

<u>Histology :</u>

Deposition of melanin like pigment occurs in the liver causing ***liver to appear dark or completely black.***

Pigment is thought to be derived from epinephrine metabolites that are not excreted normally

CriggerNajjar syndrome

CriggerNajjar syndrome is primarily an autosomal recessive hereditary disorder charchterized by unconjugated hyperbilirubinemiadue to defect in the conjugating enzyme bilirubin glucoronyltransferase

Principal Characteristics Criggler-Najjar Syndromes

Feature	Crigler-Najjar Syndrome	
	Type1	**Type II**
Total serum bilirubin, µmol/L (mg/dl)	310-755 (usually > 345) [18-45 (usually >20)]	100-430 (usually <345) [6-25(usually <20)]
Routine liver tests	Normal	Normal
Response to Phenobarbital	None	Decreases bilirubin by>25%
Kernicterus	Usual	Rare
Hepatic histology	Normal	Normal
Bile characteristics		
Color	Pale or colorless	Pigmented
Bilirubin fractions monoconjugates	>90% unconjugated	Largest fraction (mean: 57%)
Bilirubin UDP-glucuronosyl-transferase	Typically absent; traces in some patients	Markedly reduced:0-10% of normal
Inheritance (all autosomal)	Recessive	Predominantly recessive

<u>Kernincterus</u> *is characteristic features of type I CrigglerNajjar syndrome; Kernincterus is extremely rare in Type II CrigglerNajjar syndrome.*
<u>Phenobarbital</u> *is extremely effective and useful in type II CrigglerNajjar syndrome and reduces bilirubin levels by > 25%.*

Viral Hepatitis

Diagnosis of Acute viral Hepatitis:

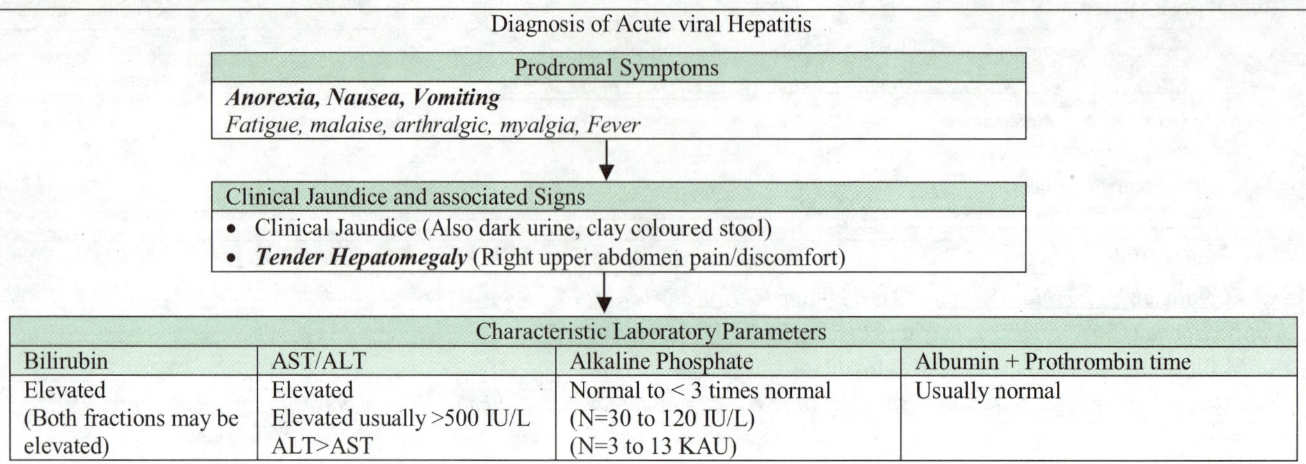

Bilirubin	AST/ALT	Alkaline Phosphate	Albumin + Prothrombin time
Elevated (Both fractions may be elevated)	Elevated Elevated usually >500 IU/L ALT>AST	Normal to < 3 times normal (N=30 to 120 IU/L) (N=3 to 13 KAU)	Usually normal

Note:
ALT is synonymous with SGPT[Q]
AST is synonymous with SGOT[Q]

Pathology of Acute Viral Hepatitis:

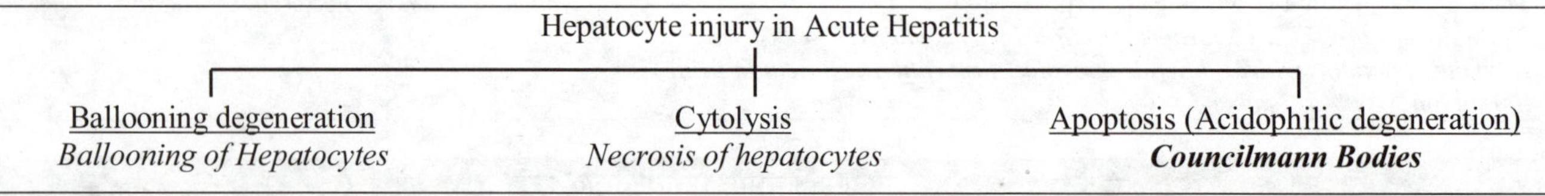

Councilman bodies are acidophilic /eosinophilic apoptotic bodies seen in Acute Viral hepatitis and represent irreversible hepatocyte damage.

Pathology of Chronic Viral Hepatitis:

Histopathological Classification of Chronic Hepatitis

Chronic Active Hepatitis (Periportal or Interface Hepatitis)

Chronic Hepatitis with histopathological features suggesting a progressive course

Biopsy Features

- *Hepatic architecture is distorted*
- *Inflammation extends beyond the portal tract (Portal tract infiltration is common with early portal tract fibrosis)*
- *Lamina Limitans is breached and hepatic lobules are invaded*
- *Piecemeal necrosis & bridging necrosis is typically seen in Lobules*

Chronic Persistant Hepatitis (Portal Hepatitis)

Chronic Hepatitis with histopathological features suggesting a beingn and self limiting course

Biopsy Features

- *Hepatic architecture is maintained*
- *Inflammation is limited to portal tracts (Portal tract infiltration is typical but portal tract fibrosis is minimal)*
- *Minimal/No breach of Lamina Limitans*
- *Minimal /No Piecemeal necrosis or Bridging necrosis in Lobules*

Clinical and epidemiologic features of viral hepatitis:

Features	HAV	HBV	HCV	HDV	HEV
Incubation (days)	15-45	30-180	15-160	30-180	14-60
Age	Children, young Adults	Young adults	Any age but more in adult	Any age	Young adults
Transmission					
Fecal-oral	+++	---	---	---	+++
Percutaneous	Unusual	+++	+++	+++	---
Perinatal	---	+++	+	+	---
Sexual	+	++	+	++	---
Clinical					
Severity	Mild	Occasionally Severe	Moderate	Occasionally Severe	Mild
Fulminant	.1%	.1%-1%	.1%	5-20%	1-2%
Progression to chronicity	None	Occasional (1-10%)	Common (50-70%)	Common	None
Carrier	None [Q]	01%-30%	1.5 to 3.2%	Variable	None [Q]
Cancer	None [Q]	+nt	+nt	Variable	None [Q]
Prognosis	Excellent	Worse with age	Moderate	Acute: good Chronic: poor	Good
Prophylaxis	IgG Vaccine	HBIG Recombinant vaccine	None	-	Unknown

[Q] *HCV is the most common Virus associated with transfusion-associated hepatitis*
[Q] *No vaccine / prophylaxis is available for HCV*
[Q] *Malignant potential is present with HCV (also with HBV)*
[Q]*Progression to chronicity is seen with hepatitis B and Hepatitis C*
[Q]*Perinatal transmission is most significant with hepatitis B*
[Q]*Hepatitis B, C and D are essentially spread by parenteral routes.*
[Q]*HepatitisA& E are non-parenteral hepatitis.*
[Q]*Hepatitis B is not transmitted through fecal-oral route (stool).*
[Q]*Most common hepatitis to progress to chronicity is hepatitis C*
[Q] *Most common cause of fulminant Hepatitis in pregnant women is Hepatitis E*
[Q] *Most common cause of epidemic hepatitis is Hepatitis E*
[Q] *Most common cause of sporadic hepatitis in adults is Hepatitis E*
[Q] *Most common cause of sporadic Hepatitis in children is Hepatitis A*

Anti-Liver Kidney Microsomal Antibodies (anti-LKM antibodies)

*Anti-Liver **K**idney **M**icrosomal (LKM) antibodies* are detected in the sera of patients with different types of acute or chronic liver disease.

These antibodies are target against *Cytochrome P-450 components (antigens)*

Three types of LKM antibodies have been most extensively studied

Microsomal Antibodies	Antigen	Disease
Anti-LKM1	Cytochrome P450 2D6	• ***Autoimmune Hepatitis type II*** • ***Chronic Hepatitis C (10%)***
Anti-LKM2	Cytochrome P450 2C9	• ***Drug induced Hepatitis*** (Tienilic acid induced Hepatitis)
Anti-LKM3	Cytochrome P450 1A2	• ***Chronic Hepatitis D***

Hepatitis B

Genomic structure of Hepatitis B:

'S' Gene	'C' Gene	'P' Gene	'X' Gene
Codes for the envelope protein, Hbs Ag.	Codes for two nucleocapsid protein. a. Hbc Ag: The intracellular core protein. b. Hbe Ag: A soluble non particulatenucleocapsid protein.	Codes for DNA polymerase This DNA polymerase has two acitivities: a. DNA dependent DNA Polymerase b. ***RNA dependent Reverse Transcriptase.***	Codes for Hbx Ag. It is a small non particulate protein, that can transactivate the transcription of cellular and viral gene.

The reverse transcriptase activity is a property of DNA polymerase which is coded by 'P' gene

Serology of Hepatitis B

Hbs Ag	Anti Hbs Ag
Indicates that the person is infected with the virus. The infection may manifest as 'disease' either acute or chronic, or be just present as in carrier state Hbs Ag thus indicated as possible: - Acute disease - Chronic disease - Carrier state	With the development of antibody to Hbs Ag i.e. Anti Hbs Ag, the Hbs Ag antigen disappears from the serum - Patient is immune (with immunization Antibody develops and Hbs Ag disappears) - Patient is protected Anti Hbs Ag indicates good immunity [Q] Anti Hbs Ag indicates protection against Hepatitis B [Q]
Hbc Ag	**Anti Hbc Ag**
It is a hidden component of the viral core and is not detectable at all	Antibodies to Hbc Ag develop early in the course of disease Anti Hbc Ag is the first antibody to appear after an acute infection and persists in serum even during the recovery phase - When acute antibody is of IgM type - When chronic antibody is of IgG type
Hbe Ag	**Anti Hbe Ag**
Denotes high infectivity [Q] and active disease	Denotes low infectivity

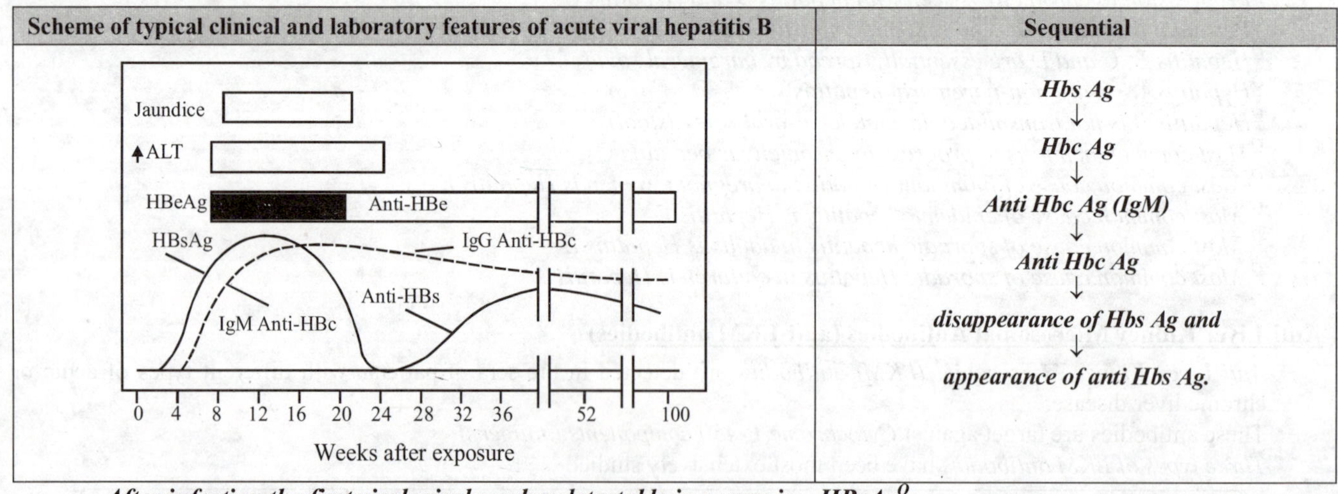

Scheme of typical clinical and laboratory features of acute viral hepatitis B	Sequential
	Hbs Ag ↓ ***Hbc Ag*** ↓ ***Anti Hbc Ag (IgM)*** ↓ ***Anti Hbc Ag*** ↓ ***disappearance of Hbs Ag and*** ↓ ***appearance of anti Hbs Ag.***

- ***After infection the first virological marker detectable in serum is – HBsAg*** [Q]

Commonly Encountered Serologic Patterns of Hepatitis B Infection:

HBsAg	Anti-HBs	Anti-HBc	HBeAg	Anti-HBe	Interpretation
+	–	IgM	+	–	Acute hepatitis B, high infectivity
+	–	IgG	+	–	Chronic hepatitis B, high infectivity
+	–	IgG	–	+	Late acute or chronic hepatitis B, Low infectivityHBeAg–negative ("precore–mutant") hepatitis B (chronic or, rarely, acute)
+	+	+	+/–	+/–	1. HBsAg of one subtype and heterotypic anti–HBs (common) 2. Process of seroconversion from HBsAg to anti– HBs (rare)
–	–	IgM	+/–	+/–	1. Acute hepatitis B *2. Anti–HBc "window"*
–	–	IgG	–	+/–	1. Low–level hepatitis B carrier 2. Hepatitis B in remote past
–	+	IgG	–	+/–	Recovery from hepatitis B
–	+	–	–	–	1. Immunization with HBsAg (after vaccination) 2. Hepatitis B in the remote past (?) 3. False–positive

- **Only marker detected in window period of Hepatitis B is IgM type Anti HBc**

  Presence of IgM Anti-HBc without HBs Ag may suggest acute hepatitis B in the window period.

HbsAg	Anti-HBs	Anti-HBc	HBeAg	Anti-HBe	Interpretation
+	-	***IgM***	+	-	Acute Hepatitis B, high infectivity
-	-	***IgM***	+/-	+/-	1. Acute Hepatitis B 2. Anti—HBc "window"

Occasionally a gap of several weeks or longer may separate the disappearance of HBsAg and the appearance of Anti-HBs after an acute infection with Hepatitis B virus. During this 'gap' or 'window' period, presence of Anti-HBc may represent the only serological evidence of current or recent HBV infection

- **The most reliable marker of acute HBV infection is IgM Anti HBc Antibody**

  Hbs Ag is present in recent hepatitis B infection but it ***is not specific to acute infection***
  IgM anti- HBc is specific for acute or recent hepatitis, and hence is the marker of choice for acute hepatitis B.

  Although Hbs Ag is the earliest virological marker in serum of patients with acute viral hepatitis B; it does not help in establishing the diagnosis of acute Hepatitis B infection.This is so because presence of Hbs Ag only denotes the fact that the patient is a carrier of the above infection and such a patient may well be a case of chronic hepatitis B.
  It is the presence of IgM anti HBc that confirms an acute hepatitis B infection.
  Acute Hepatitis B is characteristically diagnosed by the presence of IgM anti HBc with HBs Ag.
  Presence of IgM anti HBc without HBs Ag may suggest acute hepatitis in the window period.

- **Vaccination or immunization against HBs Ag is suggested by Isolated Anti-HBs Ag in serum**

  Isolated Anti-HBs Ag in serum is seen in immunization with HBs Ag.
  The marker for determining efficacy of hepatitis B vaccination is Anti – HBs Ag

- **High Infectivity or active disease is indicated by HBeAg**
  The principal clinical usefulness ofHBe Ag is as an indicator of relative infectivity

Markers for Active Hepatitis B (Persistent Replication; High Infectivity: Active Disease)

Markers for Active Hepatitis B
(*Persistent Replication; High Infectivity: Active Disease)*

- *HBV DNA*
- *HBV DNA polymerase*
- *HBe Ag*

HBV DNA is the most sensitive marker of active Hepatitis B virus replication

HBV DNA[Q]> HBV DNA polymerase[Q]>HBeAg[Q]

AST & ALT levels are not considered markers for active viral replication

Markers for Hepatitis B Virus Replication

HBV DNA

- ***HBV DNA is the most sensitive and specific marker of virus replication***
- HBV DNA may provide both, a qualitative and quantitative estimate of virus replication
- *HBV DNA estimation as a measure of virus replication has largely replaced the determination of DNA polymerase*
- ***The Gold standard for confirmation of viral replication is HBV DNA detection***

HBV DNA Polymerase

- ***HBV DNA polymerase is considered the traditional marker active viral replication***
- HBV DNA polymerase activity usually parallel's serum HBV DNA levels
- Both HBV DNA and HBV DNA polymerase are markers for the complete virion.

HBe Ag levels

- ***HBeAg is considered a convenient and readily detectable qualitative marker of HBV replication and relative infectivity***

The HBe Ag if detectable is considered a marker for active viral replication, but the lack of HBe Ag does not exclude viral replication

Markers for HBV Replication

Quantitative Markers

***HBe Ag** is a qualitative marker for HBV replication*

Quantitative Markers

- ***HBV DNA** is a quantitative definitive marker for HBV replication*
- ***DNA polymerase** is a definitive marker for HBV replication*

Various Chronic Hepatitis B Categories

Chronic Hepatitis B (*HBs Ag + ve with IgG Anti HBc)*

Chronic Hepatitis B can be divided into two categories
Based on activity of the virus and evidence of liver damage

Inactive HBs Ag Carrier state

- Patients with negligible virus replication (HBV DNA levels ≤ 10^3virions/ml) and /or no clinical signs and symptoms of liver damage and normal liver enzyme levels are characterized as inactive HBV carriers
  Inactive HBV carriers harbor Hepatitis B virus antigen (HBs Ag), but are clinically asymptomatic, have a normal physical examination with normal liver enzymes (AST & ALT). HBe Ag is typically negative and levels of HBV DNA are less than 10^3-10^4virions/ml
- Such patients have minimal (if any) liver inflammation or damage, and usually live a normal life. However compared to the general population these patients remain at risk for hepatocellular carcinoma
- Treatment is currently not recommended for Inactive HBV carrier. However *regular observation is advised* as there is a risk for reactivation of virus.

Chronic Hepatitis B (Active)

- Patients with active virus replication (HBV DNA levels > 10^3 -10^4virions/ml) and /or clinical signs and symptoms of liver damage or elevated liver enzyme levels are characterized as chronic hepatitis B patients.
- Depending on the presence or absence of HBe Ag two type of chronic (active) hepatitis B may be identified.

HBe Ag positive chronic hepatitis B

These HBs Ag positive, individuals are also positive for HBe Ag and show detectable HBV DNA levels. Such patients are in the replicative phase of chronic hepatitis B infection, have persistently or intermittently elevated liver enzymes and liver biopsy results typically reveals inflammation and damage

Patients with chronic (active) hepatitis B may become inactive (relatively non replicative) over time (rate of ~10 % per year) by becoming negative for HBe Ag and HBV DNA (HBV DNA < 10^3 - 10^4) virions/ml) Liver injury tend to subside in such patients and these may then be characterized as 'inactive carriers'

HBe Ag negative chronic hepatitis B (Precore mutant)

Such HBs Ag positive individuals are negative for HBe Ag but show detectable HBV DNA levels. Such patients are also in the replicative phase of chronic hepatitis B (despite negative HBe Ag) and have persistently or intermittently elevated liver enzymes and liver biopsy results typically reveal severe inflammation and damage

Negative HBe Ag Status *results from a mutant strain of hepatitis B that is characterized by the failure of the virus to make the hepatitis B 'e' antigen (HBe Ag)*. This mutation is called the ***'precore' mutation*** as it prevents the translation of a precore protein to prevent HBe antigen production.
This mutation does not however affect the ability of the virus to replicate

Evidence of chronic active hepatitis B (suggested by elevated liver enzymes) in patients with detectable HBV DNA but negative HBe Ag suggests a diagnosis of precore mutant chronic hepatitis B

Precore mutant form of chronic hepatitis B

- Represents an infection with a molecular variant of the hepatitis B virus that results in an *unusual serologic – clinical profile*.
- ***Such patients have severe chronic hepatitis B infection with detectable HBV DNA levels, but HBe Ag antigen is typically negative***
- This *results from an infection with an HBV mutant that contains an alteration in the precore regions rendering the virus incapable of encoding HBe Ag*
- Patients with such mutations in the precore region are unable to secrete HBe Ag, have a negative HBe Ag phenotype but *tend to have severe liver disease that progresses more rapidly to cirrhosis*
- *Characteristic of such HBe Ag negative (precore mutant) chronic hepatitis B are lower levels of HBV DNA (≤ 10^5 copies /ml) and one of several patterns of aminotransferase activity – persistent elevation, periodic fluctuation above the normal range and periodic fluctuations between the normal and elevated range*
- *HBe Ag negative chronic hepatitis B with mutation in the pre-core region is now the most frequently encountered form of hepatitis B in the Mediterranean countries and in Europe.*

Assessment of need for Antiviral therapy in Chronic Hepatitis B

Antiviral therapy is indicated for patients with active HBV replication
Active HBV replication is best assessed by measuring serum HBe Ag levels and HBV DNA levels

Markers for Active HBV Replication
HBeAg[Q]
HBV – DNA[Q]

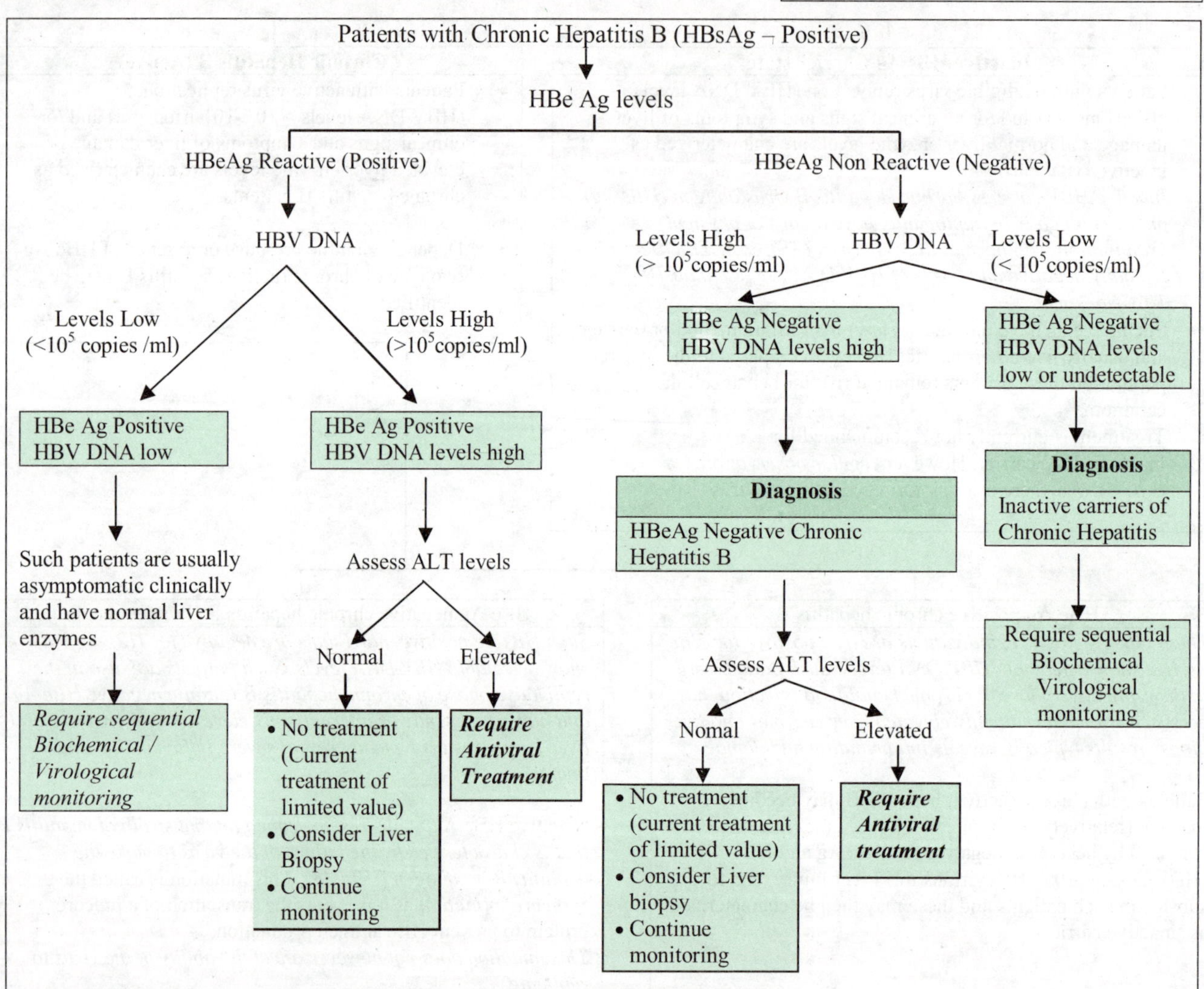

Seven drugs have been approved for treatment of chronic Hepatitis B (Harrisons)

1. *Interferon α(and Pegylated Interferon)*
2. *Lamuvudine (oral)*
3. *Adefovir (oral)*
4. *Entecavir (oral)*
5. *Dipivoxil (oral)*
6. *Telbivudine*
7. *Tenofavir*

Recommendations for Treatment of Chronic Hepatitis B

Based on practice guidelines of the American Association for the Study of Liver Diseases (AASLD).

HBeAg status	Clinical	HBV DNA (IU/ml)	ALT	Recommendation
HBeAg-reactive	Mild or Inactive Liver disease	>2 x10^4	≤2 x ULN	No treatment; monitor. In patients >40, with family history of hepatocellular carcinoma, and/or ALT persistently at the high end of the twofold range, liver biopsy may help in decision to treat
	Chronic hepatitis	>2 x 10^4	>2 x ULN	Treat[e]
	Cirrhosis compensated	>2 x 10^3	<or> ULN	Treat[e] with oral agents, not PEG IFN
		<2 x 10^3	>ULN	Consider treatment
	Cirrhosis decompensated	Detectable	<or> ULN	Treat[e] with oral agents[g], not PEG IFN; refer for liver transplantation
		Undetectable	<or> ULN	Observe; refer for liver transplantation
HBeAg-negative	Mild or Inactive Liver disease	≤2 x 10^3	≤ULN	Inactive carrier; treatment not necessary
	Chronic hepatitis	>10^3	1->2 x ULN	Consider liver biopsy; treat[h] if biopsy shows moderate to severe inflammation or fibrosis
	Chronic hepatitis	>10^4	>2 x ULN	Treat[h,i]
	Cirrhosis compensated	>2 x 10^3	<or> ULN	Treat[e] with oral agents, not PEG IFN
		<2 x 10^3	>ULN	Consider treatment
	Cirrhosis decompensated	Detectable	<or> ULN	Treat[h] with oral agents[g], not PEG IFN; refer for liver transplantation
		Undetectable	<or> ULN	Observe; refer for liver transplantation

[e] One of the potent oral drugs with a high barrier to resistance (entecavir or tenofovir) or PEG IFN can be used as first-line therapy. These oral agents, but not PEG IFN, should be used for interferon-refractory/intolerant and immunocompromised patients. PEG IFN is administered weekly by subcutaneous injection for a year; the oral agents are administered daily for at least a year and continued indefinitely or until at least 6 months after HBeAgseroconversion.

[g] Because the emergence of resistance can lead to loss of antiviral benefit and further deterioration in decompensated cirrhosis, a low-resistance regimen is recommended-entecavir or tenofovirmonotherapy or combination therapy with the more resistance-prone lamivudine (or telbivudine) plus adefovir. Therapy should be instituted urgently.

[h] Because HBeAgseroconversion is not an option, the goal of therapy is to suppress HBV DNA and maintain a normal ALT. PEG IFN is administered by subcutaneous injection weekly for a year; caution is warranted in relying on a 6-month posttreatment interval to define a sustained response, because the majority of such responses are lost thereafter. Oral agents, entecavir or tenofovir, are administered daily, usually indefinitely or, until as very rarely occurs, virologic and biochemical responses are accompanied by HBsAgseroconversion.

[i] For older patients and those with advanced fibrosis, consider lowering the HBV DNA threshold to >2 x 10^3 IU/ml.

Abbreviations: ULN, upper limits of normal;PEG IFN, pegylated interferon.

Prognosis in HBV Infection

Prognosis in HBV Infection
Acute HBV infection ≤ simultaneous HBV – HDV confection << HDV super-infection on HBV infection
(Best prognosis) *(Worst prognosis)*

[Q]HDV superinfection of a person with chronic Hepatitis B (HBV) has the worst prognosis with high likelihood of fulminant hepatitis and death

Glomerulonephritis associated with Hepatitis B

Glomerulonephritis during chronic Hepatitis B infection
Membranous Glomerulonephritis (MGN) *Membranoproliferative Glomerulonephritis (MPGN)* *Mesanglocapillary glomerulonephritis*

Note

MGN is most commonly seen ***in children***[Q]
MPGN is most commonly seen ***in adults***[Q]

Hepatitis C

Essential Features of Hepatitis C

- *HCV is the most common Virus associated with transfusion-associated hepatitis* [Q]
- *Themost common/prominent mode of transmission is through percutaneous route*
- *Hepatitis C does not spread through feco-oral route*
- *No vaccine / prophylaxis is available for HCV* [Q]
- *Malignant potential is present with HCV (also with HBV)* [Q]
- ***Hepatitis C is associated with Anti-LKM antibodies.***

LKM antibodies stand for antibodies against Liver-Kidney microsomes.

LKM antibodies may be seen in

- *Type II autoimmune hepatitis (anti LKM-I)*
- *Drug induced hepatitis (anti LKM-II)*
- *Chronic hepatitis C (Usually anti-LKM-1)*
- *Chronic hepatitis D (anti LKM-III)*

Extrahepatic Manifestations of Hepatitis C

Extrahepatic manifestations in viral hepatitis C: *'Hepatology' by Kuntz*

- *Agranulocytosis*
- *Aplastic anaemia*
- *Corneal ulceration*
- *Cryoglobulinaemia*
- *Diabetes mellitus (type I)*
- *Erythema exsudativummultiforme*
- *Glomerulonephritis*
- *Guillain-Barre syndrome*
- *Hyperlipasaemia*
- *Lichen planus*
- *Non-Hodgkin lymphoma*
- *Polyarteritisnodosa*
- *Polyarthritis*
- *Polyneuritis*
- *Porphyria cutaneatarda*
- *Sialadenitis*
- *Sjogren's syndrome /Sicca syndrome*
- *Thrombocytopenia*
- *Thyroiditis*

Hepatitis C is also associated with ***essential mixed cryoglobulinemia (EMC)*** *- Harrison 14th/1683*

Essential mixed cryoglobulinemia is an extrahepatic manifestation of viral hepatitis. It was reported initially to be associated with hepatitis B. Recent reevaluation of patients with EMC suggests that association is with chronic HCV infection rather than HBV infection.

Diagnosis and Management of Chronic Hepatitis C

Antibodies against HCV in the blood indicate infection with Hepatitis C virus.If the infection persists for more than 6 months and HCV RNA levels confirm viral replication, then the person can be confirmed as having chronic hepatitis C.

HCV RNA levels in the setting of elevated antibodies to HCV for 6 months determine serological diagnosis of chronic hepatitis.

Antibodies against HCV for 6 months
↓
Determine HCV RNA levels

- Detectable HCV RNA Levels in serum → Patient has Chronic Hepatitis C
- No detectable HCV RNA Levels in serum → Patient is unlikely to have Chronic hepatitis C

Antibodies against HCV (anti- HCV) in the blood indicate infection with the HCV. Persistance of antibodies for 6 months suggests a diagnosis of chronic hepatitis C. Patients with chronic hepatitis C, even with normal ALT levels are candidates for Liver biopsy to establish a histo-pathological diagnosis of chronic hepatitis. ***Patients with at least moderate grade and stage are candidates for antiviral therapy with PEG IFN and ribararin regardless of the ALT levels***

'Although patients with persistantly normal ALT levels tend not to progress histologically, they respond to antiviral therapy just as well as do patients with elevated ALT levels. Such patients are potential candidates for antiviral therapy'

- Harrisons 17th/ 1965

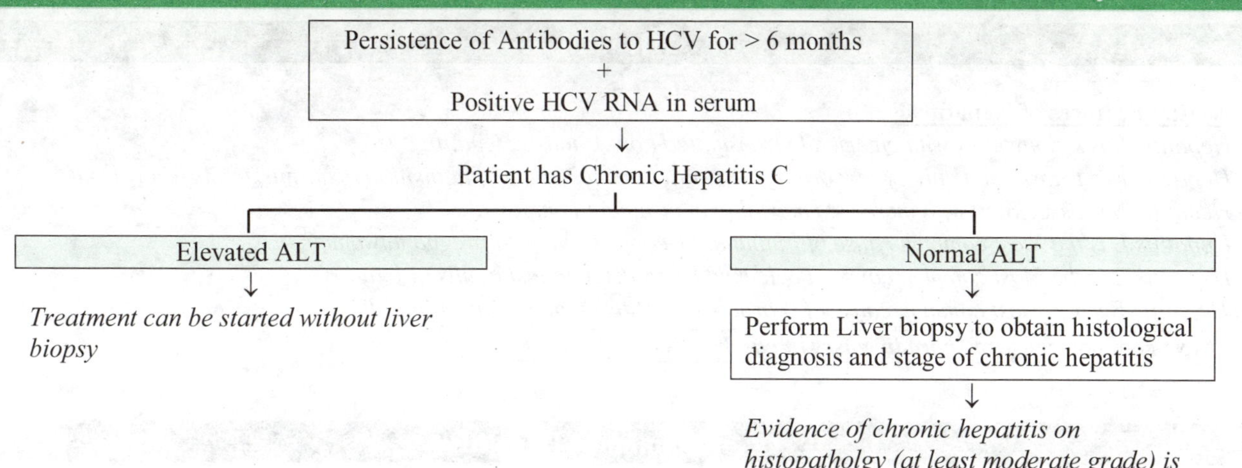

Treatment of Choice for Chronic Hepatitis C

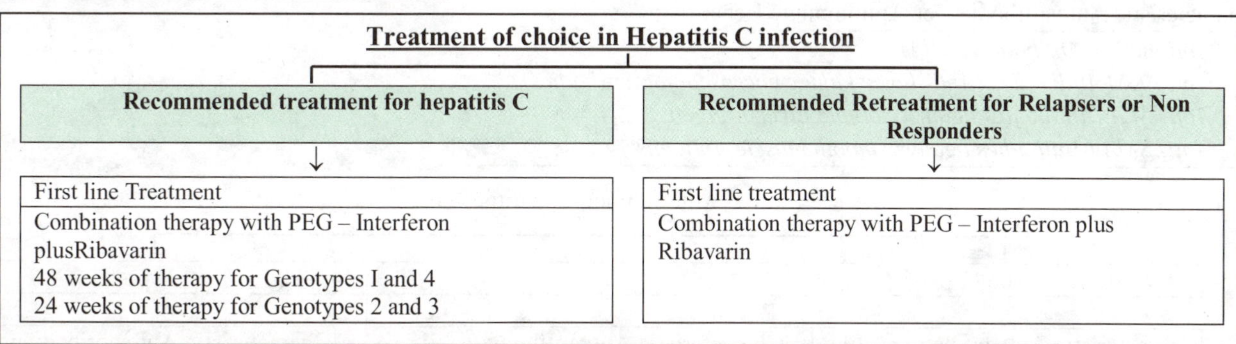

Chronic hepatitis C: 'Evidence Based medicine Guidelines' 1st (2005) / 330

- Increased serum ALT 6 months after the onset of symptoms: (normal ALT does not, however, rule out chronic hepatitis).
- A patient with a positive HCV-PCR-test and permanently elevated ALT most probably has a mild chronic hepatitis and treatment decisions can be made without liver biopsy in genotypes 2 and 3.
- Liver biopsy is indicated in a patient with positive HCV-PCR- test and normal ALT, and with genotypes 1 and 4 before considering therapy. Signs of chronic hepatitis in the biopsy are an indication for treatment.
- Information on the genotype of the virus is important to guide treatment decisions. Treatment is more effective for genotypes 2 or 3 than for genotypes 1 and 4.
- Treatment with a combination of interferon alpha or pegylated interferon alpha and ribavirin is used for 48 weeks for genotypes 1 and 4 and for 24 weeks for genotypes 2 and 3.
- When treating genotypes 1 or 4. If there is no response at 12 weeks (HCV-PCR still positive), the treatment is discontinued.
- Liver transplantation is indicated if the expected survival is about 6 months

Prognostic Markers for response to antiviral therapy in the treamtment of chronic hepatitis C

Reduced Responsiveness

- ***Genotype 1***
- High levels of HCV RNA
- ***Adranced fibrosis (ciorrhosis, bridging fibrosis)***
- Long duration disease
- ***Age > 40 years***
- Immunosupression
- African American
- Obesity
- Hepatic steatosis
- Reduced adherence
- Male sex (*Handbook of Gastroenterology*)

Sustained Responsiveness

- Genotype 2 and 3
- Low levels of HCV RNA
- Minimal fibrosis
- Short duration disease
- Age < 40 years
- Immunocompetance

Others

- Absence of obesity
- Absence of Hepatic steatosis
- Increased Adherence
- Female sex (*Handbook of Gastroenterology*)

Hepatitis E

Essential Features of Hepatitis E

- *Hepatitis E is synonymous with enterically transmitted non-A non-B Hepatitis*
- *Hepatitis E is transmitted only by fecooral route (Most common route of aquisition /transmission is fecoralroute[Q])*
- *Hepatitis E is associated with increased mortality in pregnant females*
- *Hepatitis E is the Most common cause of Fulminant Hepatitis amongst pregnanatwomen[Q]*
- *Hepatitis E is the Most common cause of epidemic Hepatitis amongst adults in India[Q]*
- *Hepatitis E is the Most common cause of sporadic Hepatitis amongst adults in India[Q]*

Most common cause of ***sporadic cases in children is - Hepatitis A***. [Q]

Autoimmune Hepatitis

Charachterisitic Features of Autoimmune Hepatitis

Characteristic Autoantibodies for Autoimmune Hepatitis

- *Antinuclear Antibodies (ANA)*
- *Anti LKM Antibodies (Anti- Liver-kidney microscomal antibodies)*
- *Anti- SLA (Antibodies against Soluble Liver Antigens)*
- *Anti- SMA (Antibodies against smooth muscle Antigens*

Autoimmune Hepatitis

Type I	Type II	Type III
Characteristic Autoantibody profile	Characteristic Autoantibody Profile	Characteristic Auto antibody profile
ANA ++ *SMA ++*	***Anti LKM1 ++***	***Anti – SLA ++*** ***ANA +/- ; SMA +/-***
Associated Antibody Profile	Associated Antibody Profile	Associated Antibody profile
P ANCA *Anti – Actin* *Anti – ASGPR*	*Anti- LC1* *Anti – ASGPR*	*Anti – ASGPR*

ANA (Antinuclear Antibodies); anti- ASGPR (antibody to asialoglycoprotein receptor); anti LC1 (antibody to Liver cytosol type I); anti- LKM1 (antibody to soluble liver kidney microsome Type I); anti, SLA (antibody to soluble liver antigen). 'Autoimmune hepatitis has been recognized to recur in upto 40% of transplanted livers as immunosupression is reduced.' - CMDT' 2006 / 663

Autoimmune Hepatitis has a high incidence of recurrence after Liver Transplantation

Recurrance of primary disease following liver transplantation

Auto immune Hepatitis	Primary billary Cirrhosis	Wilson's disease Alpha$_1$ –Antitrypsin deficiency
Disease has been recognized to recur in upto 40% of transplanted livers as immunosupression is reduced *(CMDT)*	Disease recurs in the graft in 20% by 3 years' – *CMDT*	'Hereditary disorders such as Wilson's disease and α_1 antitrypsin deficiency have not recurred after liver transplantation' – *Harrisons 16/e, p 1878*

Alcoholic Hepatitis

Feature of Alcoholic Hepatitis

Feature of Alcoholic Hepatitis

Features suggesting Hepatocyte injury (Enzyme studies)	Features suggesting dearrangementinHepatocyte function
AST/ALT	**Bilirubin**
• Levels are increased • Increased is less than 8 fold (< 400u/L) • AST is elevated greater than ALT • AST: ALT Ratio >1 AST: ALT>2 is suggestive AST: ALT>3 is highly suggestive	• May be markedly elevated • Both fractions (direct/indirect) may be elevated **Albumin** • Often decreased (Hypoalbuminemia) • Albumin <2.5 mg/dlsuggests severe alcoholic hepatitis
Alkaline Phosphatase	
• Levels are increased (may be normal) • Increase is moderate (<3 times normal) Normal to < 3 times normal elevation	**Prothrombintime** • Often prolonged • Fails to correct with parentralvitK(Coagulopathy)
Gamma GlutamylTranspeptidase (GGT)	Others
• Levels are increased • Note that GGT elevation is not specific to alcohol GGT is easily inducible and may be elevated in all forms of fatty liver	• *Polymorphonuclear cells (Neutrophils)* are often increased and if > 5500/μl predict severe alcoholic hepatitis. • *Hypertriglyceredemia* and *Hypercholesterolemia* may be associated with alcoholic fatty liver.

Pattern of aminotranferases and etiology of hepatitis

Alcoholic Hepatitis	Non Alcoholic Hepatitis (Viral/toxin induced)
• AST/ALT Ratio > 1 (>2 or >3 may be seen) • AST/ALT elevation is moderate and rarely >400 u/L (Less than 8 fold increase) • AST is elevated more than ALT	• AST/ALT ratio <1 • AST/ALT elevation is usually more marked and often >500 u/L (More than 8 fold increase) • ALT is elevated more than AST

The low level of ALT in alcoholic liver disease is due to an alcohol-induced deficiency of pyridoxal Phosphate.

In alcoholic liver disease the AST rises out of proportion to ALT such that the ratio of AST and ALT may become greater than 2.

AST (SGOT) out of proportion to ALT (SGPT) seen in [Q]
1. Alcoholic hepatitis [Q]
2. Fatty liver in pregnancy [Q]

Stigmata of Alcoholic hepatitis / cirrhosis that aid in diagnosis:

1. *Bilateral enlarged parotids* [Q]
2. *Gynaecomastia*[Q]
3. *Testicular atrophy with loss of body hair* [Q]
4. *Wasting of muscle mass* [Q]
5. *Duputyrens contracture* [Q]

[Q]***Pentoxyfylline has shown to reduce mortality from renal failure in alcoholic hepatitis.***

Non-Alcoholic Fatty Liver Disease (NAFLD/NASH)

Causes of Non- Alcoholic Fatty Liver Disease (NAFLD) or Non-Alcoholic Steato-Hepatitis (NASH)

Causes of Non-Alcoholic Fatty Liver Disease (NAFLD) or Non-Alcoholic Steato-Hepatitis (NASH)

- *Obesity (present in > 40% cases)*
- *Diabetes mellitus (present in > 20% cases)*
- *Hypertriglyceredemia (>20%)*
- *Endocrinopathies (Cushing's and Hypopituitarism, PCOS)*
- *Metabolic disorders (Hyperbetalipoproteinemia)*
- *Obstructive sleep apnea*
- *Starvation and Refeeding syndrome*
- *Total parentral Nutrition*
- *Medications and poisons*
  -Corticosteroids - diltiazem - irinotecan
  - Antiretroviral therapy, -Amiodarone- tamoxifen
  -Oxaliplatin - CCl_4& Yellow phosphorus

Commonest **Associations of NAFLD / NASH** *(Robbins)*

- *Obesity*
- *Dyslipidemia*
- *Hyperinsulinemia (Insulin resistance is a charachteristicfeature[Q])*
- *Diabetes*

- *NAFL is now considered the most common cause of 'cryptogenic cirrhosis' – Robbins 7th/908*
- *Most patients with NAFLD come to medical attention as a result of incidentally elevated liver enzymes*
  - *ALT > AST*
  - *Aminotransferases are usually only mildly elevated 2 times normal*

Treatment of NAFLD or NASH

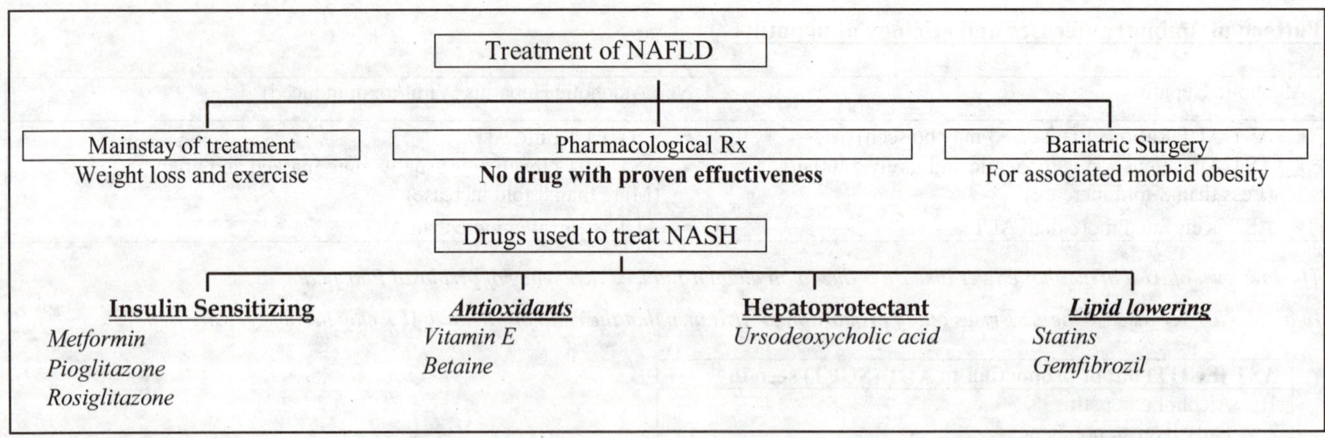

Cirrhosis and its Complications

Morphological Classification of Cirrhosis

Morphological ClassificationofCirrhosis

Macronodular Cirrhosis (Parenchymal nodules > 3mm)

Aetiology	Frequency
• *Chronic viral hepatitis*	*10-20%*
• *Wilson's disease*	*Rare*
• *α-Antitrypain deficiency*	*Rare*
• *Various drugs and toxins*	*Rare*
• *Hereditary haemorrhagic telangiectasis*	*Rare*
• *Cryptogenic cirrhosis*	*Common*

Micronodular Cirrhosis (Parenchymal nodules < 3mm)

Aetiology	Frequency
• *Alcohol*	*60-70%*
• *'Primary' biliary cirrhosis*	*5%*
• *Large bile duct obstruction*	*<5%*
• *Haemochromatosis*	*5%*
• *Intestinal bypass*	*Rare*
• *Cystic fibrosis*	*Rare*
• *Indian childhood cirrhosis*	*Rare*

[Q]***Postnecrotic cirrhosis is charachterized by a shrunken liver with reduced liver span.***

[Q]**In advanced stages of cirrhosis major blood supply to Liver is from hepatic artery**

Normally 80% of blood flow toliver comes from the portal vein and 20% of the blood supply is contributed by the hepatic artery

In cirrhosis the blood flow to liver from the portal vein is reduced due to increased pressure and a compensatory increase in the blood to liver through the hepatic artery occurs

Stigmata of Chronic Liver Disease / Cirrhosis

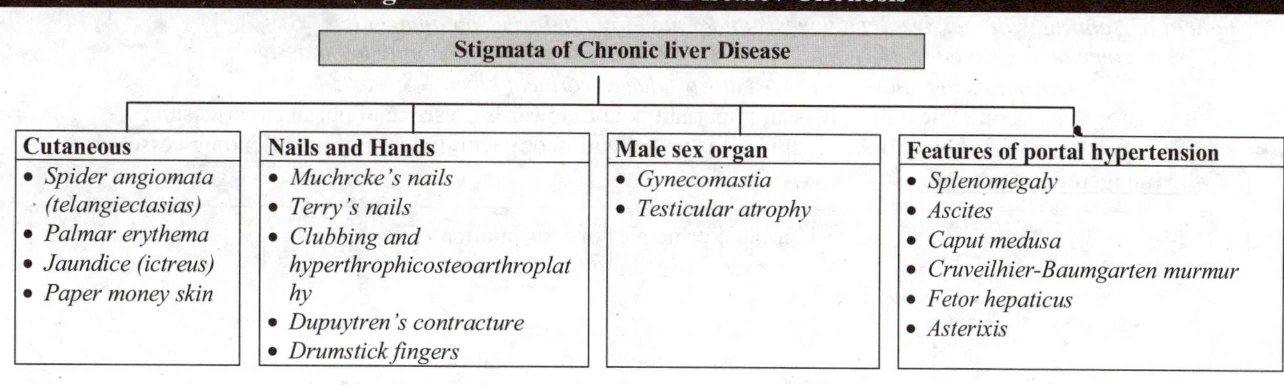

Portal Hypertension

- **Portal hypertension**refers to increased pressure in the portal vein and most commonly results from increased resistance to portal blood flow.

Normal Pressure in the Portal Vein	
cm (Saline)	*10 – 15 cm saline*
mm (Hg)	*5 – 10 mmHg*

- ***Portal hypertension in patients with cirrhosis most commonly results from increased resistance at the level of sinusoids***

Increased resistance can occur at three levels:

Presinusoidal	Sinusoidal	Post sinusoidal
• Anatomically outside the liver eg. Portal vein thrombosis • Within the liver but proximal to sinusoids eg. Schistosomiasis	***Cirrhosis*** *When cirrhosis is complicated by portal hypertension, the increased resistance is usually sinusoidal*	• Outside liver, at level of hepatic veins - ***Budd chiarri syndrome*** • In the inferior vena cava - Thrombosis • In the liver but distal to sinusoid - Venoocclusive disease

- Cirrhosis is the most common cause of portal hypertension in the United States.[Q]
  Portal vein obstruction is the second most common cause. [Q]
- *The most charachteristic features of Portal Hypertension are hematemesis from esophageal varices and splenomegaly*

The most constant finding in patients with portal hypertension is splenomegaly (present in 80% of patients).-CSDT

- ***Presence of massive haematemesis in the background of moderate splenomegaly suggests a diagnosis of esophageal varices secondary to portal hypertension.***

Esophageal Varices

Oesophagealvariceal bleeding secondary to portal hypertension should always be the initial diagnosis in a young patient presenting with massive hematemesis and a moderate to large splenomegaly'

- *Most common presentation of esophageal varices is* ***Hematemesis which may be 'massive'***
  Massive hematemesis in children is almost always due to variceal bleed – Shwartz
- Presence of moderate splenomegaly is an important pointer towards presence of portal hypertension.
- The management of choice for variceal bleed is urgent endoscopy with ligation of the offending vessel

Management protocol :

Cardinal principles of resuscitation
(**A**irway / **B**reathing / **C**irculation)
↓
Urgent endoscopy
(diagnostic + therapeutic modality)
Ligation is the endoscopic therapy of choice for variceal bleeding
Endoscopic Sclerotherapy is another option
Acute treatment with octreotide (preferred over vasopressin) is the medical management of choice

Principles :

- Once the patient is hemodynamically stable urgent endoscopy should be performed
- Ligation is the endoscopic therapy of choice for esophageal varices because it has requires fewer treatment sessions.
- Endoscopic Sclerotherapy is another option
- Acute treatment with octreotide (preferred over vasopressin) is the medical management of choice
- In patients who have persistent or recurrent bleeding despite endoscopic and medical therapy, TIP is recommsended (TIPS is Transjugular intrahepatic portosystemic shunt)

Ascitis

Causes of Chylous and Mucinous Ascitis

ChylousAscitis refers to a turbid milky or crcamy peritoneal fluid due to the presence of thoracic or intestinal lymph. It is most often a result of lymphatic obstruction from the cause mentioned below.

Causes of ChylousAscitis
• Trauma • Tumor • Tuberculosis • Filariasis • Congenital anomalies • Nephrotic syndrome

Causes of Mucinous Ascitis
• Pseudomyxomaperitonei • Colloid carcinoma stomach with peritoneal implants • Colloid carcinoma colon with peritoneal implants ***Colloid carcinoma of stomach causes mucinous ascities*** *– Harrisons*

Treatment of Ascitis:

Treatment of Ascitis: Oxford Textbook of Medicine: Recommendations

- ***Bed Rest*** *is of little value*
- ***Dietry sodium Restriction*** *is the first line management*
- ***Diuretic therapy*** *is the mainstay of treatment of Ascitis (Spironolactone should be employed as the* ***first line drug)***
- ***Large volume paracentesis****should initially be carried out on patients with moderate or marked ascitis*

Large volume Therapeutic Paracentesis is not recommended for SBP
Diagnostic paracentesis is indicated in SBP for establishing the diagnosis but large volume paracentesis should be avoided - Schiff's Diseases of the Liver

- ***Shunts (TIPS)*** *may be used in cases of Refractory Ascitis in whom recurrent paracentesis is too frequent or poorly tolerated, or in those with a hepatic hydrothorax*

[Q]**Abdominal ultrasound may detect as little as 100 ml of ascitic fluid**
Ultrasound is thus a useful investigation for the diagnosis of minimal ascitis – CCDT

[Q]**HemorrhagicAscitis is diagnosed when RBC count >10, 000 / mm^3**
An RBC count of 10,000 / mm^3 is the threshold for pink appearance and hemorrhagic ascitis is thus diagnosed when ascitic RBC count is > 10,000 / mm^3 - Schiff's diseases of the Liver

[Q]**Spontaneous Bacterial peritonitis (SBP) is diagnosed when Neutrophil count > 250/mm^3**
The diagnosis of SBP is made when the absolute neutrophil count > 250 / mm3 – Harrisons

Primary Biliary Cirrhosis

Primary biliary cirrhosis is a disease characterized by chronic inflammation and fibrous obliteration of intrahepatic bile ductules due to an unknown (primary) stimulus.

Etiology / pathogenesis :

PBC is believed to be due to an autoimmune [Q] etiology as it is often associated with other autoimmune disorders [Q] such as

1. CREST [Q] :**C**alcinosis, **R**aynaud's, **E**sophageal dysmotility, **S**clorodactyly**T**alenglectasia
2. SICCA SYNDROME [Q]
3. Autoimmune thyroiditis [Q]
4. Renal tubular acidosis

- Antimitochondrial Antibody (IgG) is positive

Clinical feature :

- Most patients are asymptomatic [Q]
- Pruritis is commonest / earliest symptom [Q]

> ***'The earliest symptom is 'pruiritis' which may be either generalized or limited initially to the plams and soles.'***- Harrison

- Jaundice [Q]
- Melanosis: gradual darkening of exposed areas of skin [Q]
- Deficiency of fat soluble vitamins due to malabsorption[Q]
  - Vit D deficiency : bone pain - osteomalacia[Q]
  - Vit K deficiency : bleeding – bruising [Q]
  - Vit A deficiency : Night blindness [Q]
- *Xanthelismanxanthomas*[Q] due to protracted elcvaliar of serum lipids.

Lab Findings :

- ↑↑ Serum alkaline phosphatase [Q] (2-5 fold)
- ***Positive antimitochondrialantibody***: [Q]Sensitive and specific
  Antimitochondrial' Antibodies (AMA) are present in about 90% of patients with PBC' – Harrison
- ***Hyperlipidemia (Abnormal Lipoprotein)***
  'The serum levels of cholesterol increase strikingly in PBC and an abnormal lipoprotein (Lipoprotein- x) appears which is found in many forms of chronic cholestasis' – Rubin's pathology

Primary Sclerosing Cholangitis

Primary SclerosingCholongitis

Progressive Idiopathic obliteration of intrahepatic or extrahepatic bile ducts

Note

Smoking is associated with a decreased risk of PSC

Conditions with decreased risk from smoking
• *Ulcerative Colitis* • *Primary biliary sclerosis*

- *Most common in Men aged 20- 50 years (M > F)* [Q]
- *Characteristically associated with ulcerative colitis (IBD)* [Q] *(and less commonly with crohn's disease)*
- *Characteristic increased risk of cholangiocarcinoma (10%)*

Presentation	Characteristic LaboratoryFeature	Diagnostic study of choice
• **Progressive obstructive jaundice.** Patient presents with progressive jaundice, pruiritis and other features of cholestasis	• **GGT is typically elevated** ***Asymptomatic elevation of GGT is the earliest finding*** • **ALP & bile acids are ↑ed**	*ERCP or MRCP is the diagnostic study of choice demonstrating irregularities of the biliary tree*

'The ultimate treatment of PSC is Liver transplantation' – Harrison

Non-Cirrhotic Portal Hypertension (NCPF and EHPVO)

- ***Non-Cirrhotic Portal Hypertension is charachterized by features of portal hypertension along with a moderate/large splenomegaly with conspicuous absence of features of liver cell failure***
- **Non-cirrhotic portal hypertension** encompasses two distinct pathological condition that present with similar clinical features.

Non cirrhotic portal fibrosis Extrahepatic portal obstruction

- *Signs of Liver failure such as Jaundice and Ascitis are uncommon in EHPVO and NCPF. Their presence favors a diagnosis of cirrhosis and their absence makes cirrhosis unlikely*

Non Cirrhotic Portal Hypertension is suspected in a patient presenting with symptoms of portal hypertension with:
• Moderate/Large Splenomegaly • ***NO*** FEATURES SUGGESTIVE OF LIVER CELL FAILURE - No Jaundice (uncommon) - No Ascitis (uncommon) - No Hepatomegaly (uncommon) - No Stigmata of liver cell failure (uncommon)

- *Distinction between the two conditions should ideally be made by further investigations as the similarly in presentation makes clinical criteria unreliable.*
  Neverthless if we do have to choose one single best option the following clues may be helpful.

Features	EHPVO	NCPF
• Defination	***Extra-hepatic portal vein obstruction*** *refers to features of portal hypertension resulting from an extrahepatic block to the portsl venous system either from congenital malformations or acquired causes like thrombosis*	***Non-cirrhotic portal fibrosis*** *is a condition of liver characterized by widespread fibrosis of the liver (mainly portal, subcapsular and rarely perisinusuoidal) causing wide variation in the normal architecture but there is no true cirrhosis.*
• ***Age***	***Children (1st & 2nd decade)*** *EHPVO may present in two age groups* *Children(1st & 2nd decade) (Congenital malformations)* *Adults (4th & 5th decade) (Thrombotic event)*	*Adults (3rd & 4th decade)* *NCPF presents in young adults most commonly during the third and fourth decade*
• ***Gender***	***M > F***	*F > M* *NCPF is more common in females*
• Onset	*The onset of symptoms is gradual*	*The onset is gradual in children where the cause is congenital malformation* *The onset is acute in adults where the cause is usually a thrombotic even*
• ***Splenomegaly (Mass in Left upper quadrant)***	***Mild /Moderate*** *Mass in left upper quadrant (splenomegaly) is four times less common in patients with EHPH*	***Moderate / Large*** *Mass in left upper quadrant (splenomegaly) is about 4 times more common in NCPF than EHPH*
• Variceal bleed (Hemetemesis / Malena)	+ +	+ +
• Jaundice / Ascitis Encephalopathy	*± (Absent / Transient)*	*± (Absent / Transient)*
• LFT	*Normal*	*Normal*
• Site of block along portal venous system	*Large branches are thrombosed (Main trunk; 1st order branches)*	*Small branches are involved (3rd order and 4th order branches)*
• USG	*Portal / Splenic vein block 'Portal covernoma'*	*Normal splenoportal axis*

Most common cause of Portal Hypertension in India

Portal Hypertension in Indian Children	Portal Hypertension in Indian Young Adults
The most common cause of Portal Hypertension in Indian Children is EHPVO	*The most common cause of Portal Hypertension in Indian Adults is NCPF*
NCPF is the most important causes of intrahepatic non-cirrhotic portal hypertension in India. [Q]	

'More than three quarters of Indian Children with portal hypertension were found to have extra hepatic portal vein obstruction (EHPVO) and Indian studies have shownextra hepatic portal vein obstruction (EHPVO) to be the commonest non cirrhotic cause for portal hypertension in children'

- 'Diseases of the Liver and Biliary System in Children' by Kelly 3rd /559

Clinical Differentiation of NCPF, EHPVO and Cirrhosis in patients with features of Portal Hypertension

Parameter	EHPVO	NCPF	Cirrhosis
Mean age (years)	10	28	40
Ascites	Absent/transient after bleed	Absent/transient after bleed	+ to +++
Encephalopathy	-	-	+
Jaundice signs of liver failure	-	-	+
Liver function tests	Normal*	Normal	Deranged
Liver Gross Microscopic	 Normal/small Normal	 Normal, rarely irregular Normal portal/fibrosis	 Shrunken, nodular Necrosis, regeneration
Splenoportovenography/US	Portal/splenic vein block	Normal splenoportal axis, 'withered tree' appearance, periportal fibrosis	Dilated, patent portal and splenic vein

*Occasional impairment may be observed
NCPF, non-cirrhotic portal fibrosis; EHPVO, extrahepatic portal vein obstruction; US, ultrasound

Etiology of NCPF

- The precise etiology of NCPF remains an enigma.
- Infection, Chemicals and Immune mechanisms have all been implicated

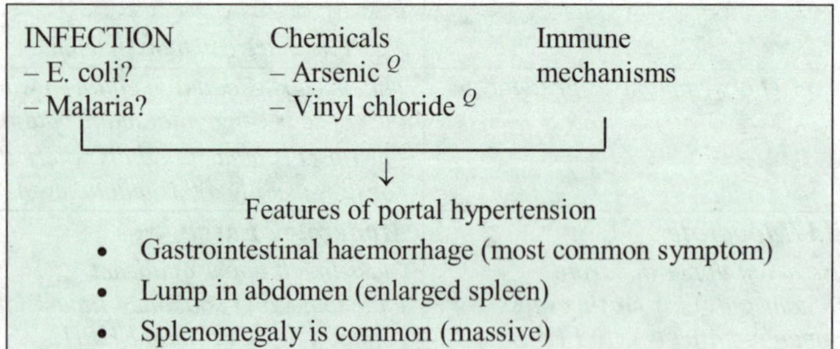

The implicated chemical agents include:
- ***Arsenic***
- Copper
- Vinyl chloride

"Chronic ingestion of Arsenic has been incriminated in causation of NCPF. High Hepatic arsenic levels in patients with NCPF have been reported" *– API 7th/ 621*

Arsenic in also associated with the following cancers [Q]
1. Skin cancer [Q] (Chandrasoma Taylor 3rd/ 285)
2. Lung cancer [Q] (Chandrasoma Taylor 3rd/ 285)
3. Hepatic angiosarcoma[Q] (Chandrasoma Taylor 3rd/ 185)

Hepatic Encephalopathy / Hepatic failure

Common precipitants of Hepatic Encephalopathy

Increased nitrogen load as in	Electrolyte and Metabolic imbalance such as in
1. *GI bleeding* [Q]	1. *Hypokalemia* [Q]
2. *Excessive dietary protein intake* [Q]	2. *Alkalosis* [Q]
3. *Azotemia* [Q]	3. *Hypoxia* [Q]
4. *Constipation* [Q]	4. *Hyponatremia*[Q]
Drugs	**Miscellaneous conditions like**
CNS depressant agents like narcotics, tranquillizers, sedatives [Q]	Infection [Q], surgery [Q], superimposed acute liver disease. [Q]

Anaemia may lead to cellular hypoxia at the level of liver cells and thus precipitates encephalopathy [Q]
Hypothyroidism, though not mentioned as a direct precipitating factor, may contribute towards precipitating encephalopathy by causing *'constipation'* or slowing down the intellectual and motor activity.

Initial Laboratory abnormalities and Prognostic Factors in Hepatocellular Failure

- ***Patients with early hepatocellular failure may present with isolated prolongation of Prothrombin Time (PT)***

  An increased prothrombin time is the most frequently observed first laboratory test suggesting the possibility of hepatocellular failure. Early liver failure may be suspected based on isolated prolongation of the Prothrombin Time (PT).

- ***Prolonged Prothrombin Time and Factor V levels are important prognostic Factors***

Coagulation factors as Laboratory Prognostic markers in patients with acute liver failure include the following:
1. ***Prothrombin time (King's criteria)***
2. ***Factor V levels (Clinchy's criteria)***
3. INR (CMDT)

'The standard liver blood tests (AST, ALT, ALP, Bilirubin, Ammonia) have no discriminatory value affecting survival The extent to which plasma levels of liver derived coagulation factors are depressed correlates with the severity of the hepatic lesion.'

Diagnostic Criteria for Hepatic Encephalopathy

The diagnosis of hepatic encephalopathy should be considered when four major factors are present
1. Acute or chronic hepatocellular disease and/or extensive portal systemic collateral shunts
2. Disturbance of awareness and mentation, which may progress from forgetfulness and confusion to stupor and finally coma.
3. Shifting combinations of neurological signs including asterixis, rigidity, hyperreflexia, extensor plantar signs and rarely seizures.
4. A characteristic but (nonspecific), symmetric, high voltage, triphasic slow wave (2 or 5/second) pattern on electroencephalogram.

Typical Causes of Flapping Tremors

Asterexis (Flapping tremor) is most commonly seen in metabolic encephalopathies due to hepatic, renal (uremia) and respiratory failure (CO_2Nercosis).

Typical Metabolic Encephalopathies	
• ***Hepatic Encephalopathy*** • ***Uremic Encephalopathy*** • ***Respiratory failure with CO_2 Retention (CO_2 Narcosis)***	*Typically Metabolic Encephalopathies due to hepatic, renal and respiratory failure are the most common causes.*

'Thyrotoxicosis (Hyperthyroidism) is associated with rapid fine tremors and not flapping tremors (irregular coarse tremor) also called Asterixis.

Hepatorenal syndrome

- Hepatorenal syndrome is defined as a state of functional renal failure (Reduced GFR) in patients with severe liver disease
- ***Structurally /Histologically the kidneys are normal and recover function after successful liver transplantation.***
- The pathogenetic hallmark of hepatorenal syndrome is intense renal vasoconstriction with coexistent systemic vasodilatation
- The diagnosis of hepatorenal syndrome is considered in accordance with the following diagnostic criteria.

Diagnostic of Hepatorenal Syndrome
Major criteria
• *Low glomerular filtration rate, as indicated by serum creatinine> 1.5 mg/dL or 24-hr creatinine clearance < 40 mL/min* • *Absence of shock, ongoing bacterial infection, fluid losses, and current treatment with nephrotoxic drugs* • *No sustained improvement in renal function (decrease in serum creatinine to 1.5 mg/dL or increase in creatinine clearance to 40 mL/min) after diuretic withdrawal and expansion of plasma volume with 1.5L of a plasma expander* • *Proteinuria <500 mg/dL and no ultrasonographic evidence of obstructive uropathy or parenchymal renal disease*
Additional criteria
• *Urine volume < 500 mL/d* • *Urine sodium < 10 meq/L* • *Urine osmolality greater than plasma osmolality* • *Urine red blood cells <50/high- power field* • *Serum sodium concentration < 130 mEqL*
Note: All major criteria must be present for the diagnosis of hepatorenal syndrome. Additional criteria are not necessary for the diagnosis but provide supportive evidence.

Hepatocellular Carcinoma

Risk factors for hepatocellular carcinoma:

Major etiological factors - *Robbins*	**Other etiological factors** – *Harrison*
• Viral infection *Hepatitis C infection* *Hepatitis B infection* • Chronic alcoholism • Food contaminants: Alfatoxins	• Alphal antitrypsin deficiency • Hemochromatosis • Tyrosinemia • Primary biliary cirrhosis • Exposure to thoriumdioxide or vinyl chloride • Long term androgenic steroid administration • Exposure to estrogen

Hepatocellular Carcinoma: Epidemiological Characterisitcs and Clinical Features

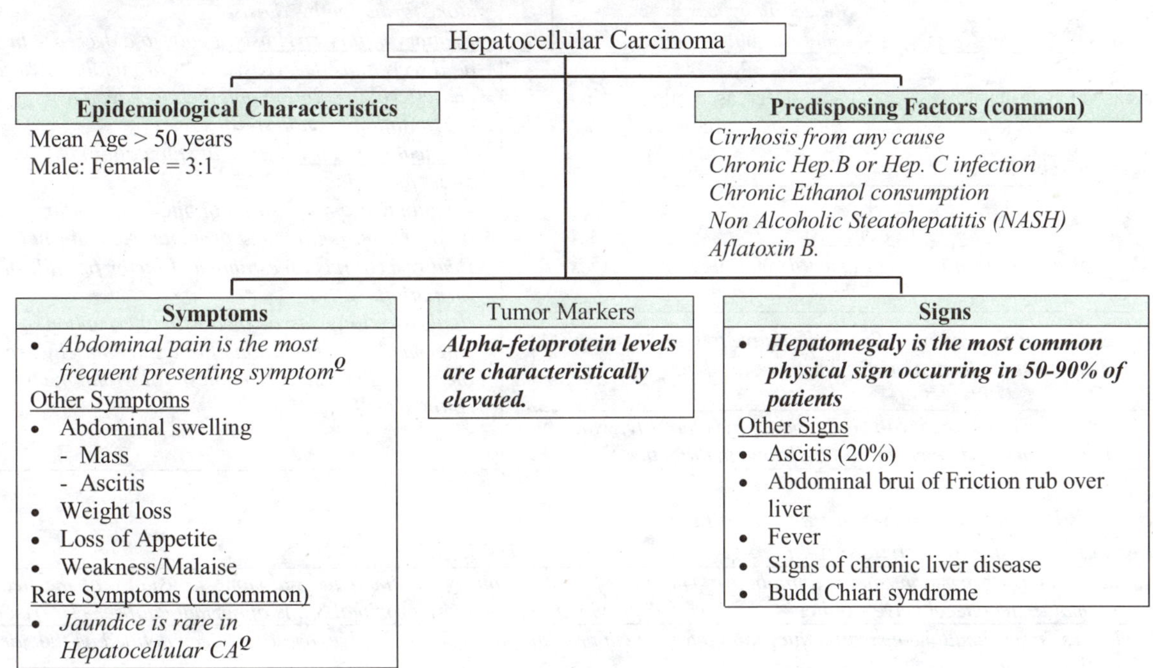

Most common clinical manifestations of hepatocellular carcinoma:
• Abdominal pain and Abdominal Liver mass The most common presenting features are abdominal pain with detection of an abdominal mass in the right upper quadrant
Uncommon / inconstant features
• Jaundice: Jaundice is ***rare***, unless significant deterioration of liver function or mechanical obstruction of bile duct occurs • Esophageal variceal bleeding: Gastrointestinal or esophageal variceal bleeding are ***inconstant*** findings

Characteristic features of fibrolamellar carcinoma

Characteristic features of fibrolamellar carcinoma
• Distinctive variant of Hepatocellular carcinoma • Occurs in young adults (20 to 40 years of age) • *Equal sex incidence (Robbins); More common in females -Chandrasoma Taylor* • No association with HBV or cirrhosis • Well circumscribed mass (localized) *Non encapsulated but well circumscribed – Harrison* *Grossly encapsulated – Chandrasoma Taylor* • ***No AFP elevation*** *-Chandrasoma Taylor* • Better prognosis: Slow growth and longer survival.

Hepatoblastoma is a malignant liver tumor of infancy i.e. typically associated with very high serum AFP levels. *The lesions are usually solitary, may be resectable and have a better five year survival than that of HCC.*

Disorders of Biliary Tract

Factors favouring the formation of Bile stones

Bile salts and phospholipids in bile keep cholesterol in solution by the formation of micelles.
An ***excess of cholesterol relative to bite salts* and phospholipids** allows cholesterol to form crystals and such bile is called ***Lithogenic or Super-saturated bile***.

Factors favouring the formation of Bile stones

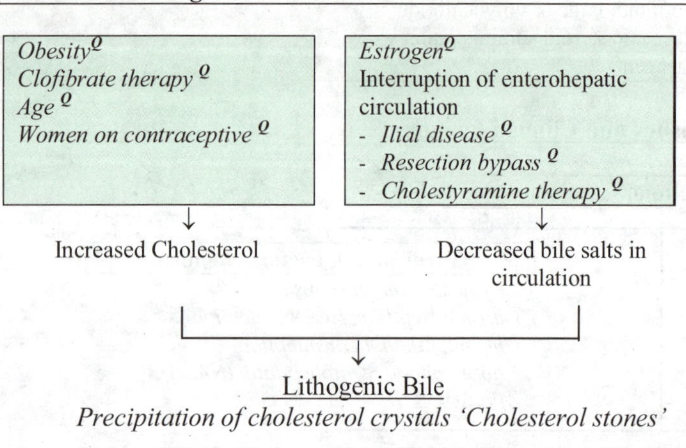

It is increased concentration of cholesterol relative to bile salts in bile that promotes gall stone formation. Serum cholesterol may well be normal.

- ***Diabetes mellitus** is associated with Gall bladder hypomotility, which may contribute to increased incidence of gallstone in diabetics.*

- ***Clofibrate therapy**: This drug is used to excrete cholesterol in hyperlipoprotenemialt therefore increases the concentration of cholesterol in bile.*
- ***Hyperalimentation:** Parental supplementation leads to hypofunction of Gall bladder, thus contibuting to gall stone formation by 'Stasis'.*
- ***Primary biliary cirrhosis:** Leads to a decrease in bile acid secretions. Decreased salts are unable to keep cholesterol in solution and therefore lead to precipitation of cholesterol stones*
- ***Truncal vagotomy**(not vagal stimulation) enhances Stone formation*
  Vagotomy promotes stasis of bile by inhibiting gall bladder contractility and promotes stone formation.
- ***Ileal resection is an established factor for gall stone formation.***
  Ileal resection is associated with interruption of enterohepatic circulation of bile salts thereby decreasing the ratio of bile salts to cholesterol within the bile (Lithogenic bile)

- ***Cholelithiasis is more common in women than men***
- ***The most common site of obstruction due to gallstone is the terminal ileum.***

'Classically there is obstruction / impaction about 60 cm proximal to ileocaecal valve'- Bailey	'The site of obstruction by the impacted gallstone is usually at the ileocaecal valve" provided that the more proximal S.I. is of normal calibre. - Harrisons
If both choices come simultaneously in a question go for 60 cm proximal to ileacoecal valve, as, it has been defined as the narrowest part of small intestine.	

- ***The most common site of Biliary – enteric fistulas is the duodenum (Cholecystoduodenal fistula)***

Type of fistula	Percent	Comment
Cholecystoduodenal	*≈ 75%*	*Most common type (duodenum)*
Cholecysto colic	*≈ 16%*	*Second most common (colon)*

- ***Medical therapy for gall bladder stone is amenable for stones < 15 mm (preferably <10 mm)***

Prerequisitesfor medical therapy:

1. *Gall bladder should be functioning [Q]*
2. *Stones should be radioluscent[Q]*
3. *Size should be small preferably <10-15 mm [Q](<10mm-Harrison)*
4. *Stones should be 'cholesterol stones' only (obvious by thier mechanism of action) [Q]*

Medical therapy for Gall stone dissolution	Mechanism of action:
UDCA (Ursodeoxycholic acid) [Q] *CDCA (Choledeoxycholic acid) [Q]*	*Inhibit HmG CoA reductase activity [Q], which in turn results in decreased hepatic cholesterol synthesis.Allows dispersion of 'cholesterol' from stones by physicochemical means.*

- ***Prophylactic cholecystectomy is not warranted in an asymptomatic patient.***

Saint's Triad and Charcot's Triad

Saint's triad (Association of)
Diverticular disease
Gall stone/Cholelithiasis
Hiatus Hernia

Charcot's triad
Abdominal pain
High fever with rigors
Jaundice

Predisposing factors of cholangiocarcinoma

The predisposing factors of cholangiocarcinomainclude :

1. Chronic hepato-biliary parasite infection Q
   (Clonorchiasis or Asiatic cholangio-hepatitis) Q
2. Congenital Anomaly with ectatic ducts (Choledochal cyst). Q
3. Sclerosing cholangitis Q
4. Ulcerative colitis Q
5. Occupational exposure to carcinogens Q
   (Rubber + Automotive plants)

- *Cholelithiasis is not clearly a predisposing factor for Cholangiocarcinoma– Harrison*
- *Chronic pancreatitis does not predispose to cholangiocarcinoma*

Nodular lesions that arise at the bifurcation of hepatic ducts are called ***Klastskin tumors***. Q

Factors, which indicate possibility of malignancy in Gall bladder Polyps

Factors which indicate possibility of malignancy in Gall bladder Polyps	
• *Age > 50 years*Q	• *Presence of a single polyp*Q
• *Sessile Polyps*Q	• *Polyp > 1.0 cm in size*Q
• *Rapid change in size of polyp*Q	• *Associated Gall stones*Q

Management Protocol for Asymptomatic Gall Bladder Polyps

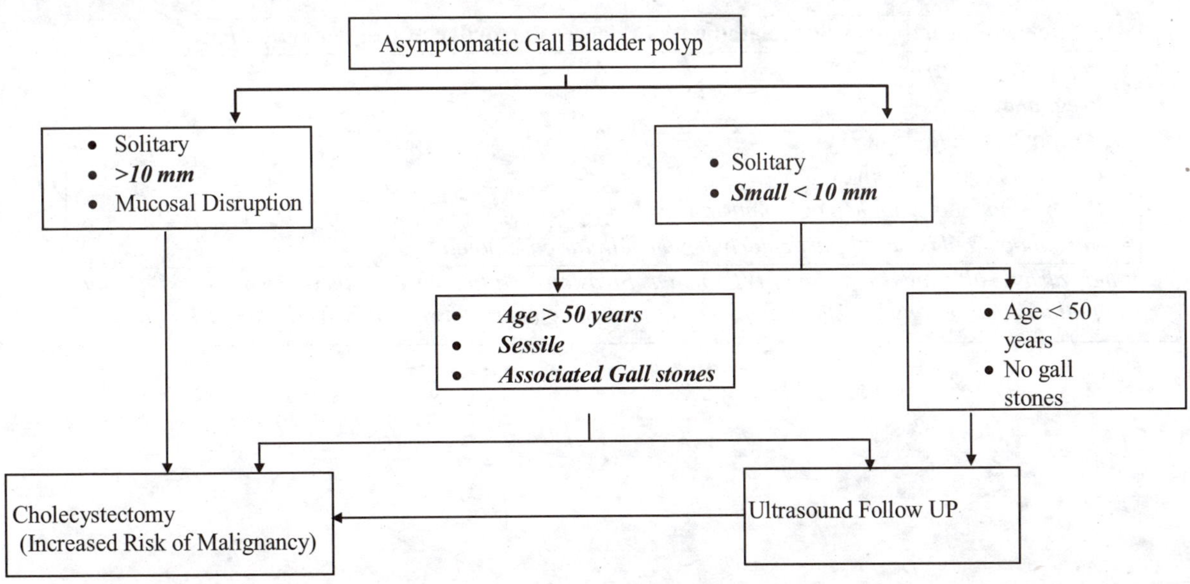

Causes of air in biliary tract

Air coming from GI tract through fistulas caused by	Air Produced with in Biliary tract	Air coming from GI tract d/t failure of closure of sphincter of oddi/t reflux of duodenal gas
• Trauma • Surgery • ***Malignancy***[Q] • Duodenal Ulcer • ***Gall stone ileus***[Q]	• *Emphysematous cholecystitis*[Q]	• Passage of Stone • Passage of Ascaris (Biliary ascariasis) • Surgery (endoscopic sphincterotomy, sphincteroplasty, ***papillotomy***)

[Q]***Sclerosing cholangitis is not associated with air in the biliary tract***

Budd Chiari Syndrome:

- ***Budd chiari syndrome by definition is 'occlusion of hepatic vein'***
  Budd chiari syndrome is characterized by post sinusoidal obstruction outside the liver at the level of hepatic veins
- It is a clinical complex characterized by -
  - *Liver enlargement (hepatomegaly)*
  - *Ascitis*
  - *Abdominal pain*
- It is produced as a result of obstruction of two or more major hepatic veins and results from increased intrahepatic blood pressure and an inability of the massive hepatic blood from to shunt around the blocked outflow tract
  - *Obstruction of two or more major hepatic veins produces Budd chiari syndrome*
  - *Obstruction of a single main hepatic vein by thrombosis is clinically silent*
- The most common cause of Hepatic vein obstruction producing Budd chiari syndrome is Hepatic Vein Thrombosis.
  The most common cause of Hepatic Vein Thrombosis causing Budd Chairi Syndrome is Polycythemia Vera

Hepatic vein thrombosis is associated with in decreasing order of frequency:*Robbins*
- *Polycythemia vera*[Q]
- *Pregnancy*
- *Postpartum state*
- *Use of oral contraceptives*
- *Paroxysmal nocturnal hemoglobinuria (PNH)* [Q]
- *Intraabdominal cancers, particularly hepatocellular carcinoma.*

It may also result from occlusion of IVC such as invasion by a tumour but this is certainly less common.
Idiopathic membranous obstruction of IVC is the most common cause of this syndrome in Japan

Wilson's Disease

The basic defect in Wilson's disease is reduced biliary excretion of copper due to a mutation of gene on chromosome 13, which promotes copper excretion. This leads to accumulation of copper initially in the liver and subsequently in plasma and other systems once liver is saturated. *Serum ceruloplasmin is the main copper binding protein in the blood and once excess copper spills into the blood,* ***levels of free ceruloplasmin are decreased.*** *Also excess copper is eventually excreted in urine and hence* ***urinary copper levels are increased or high.***

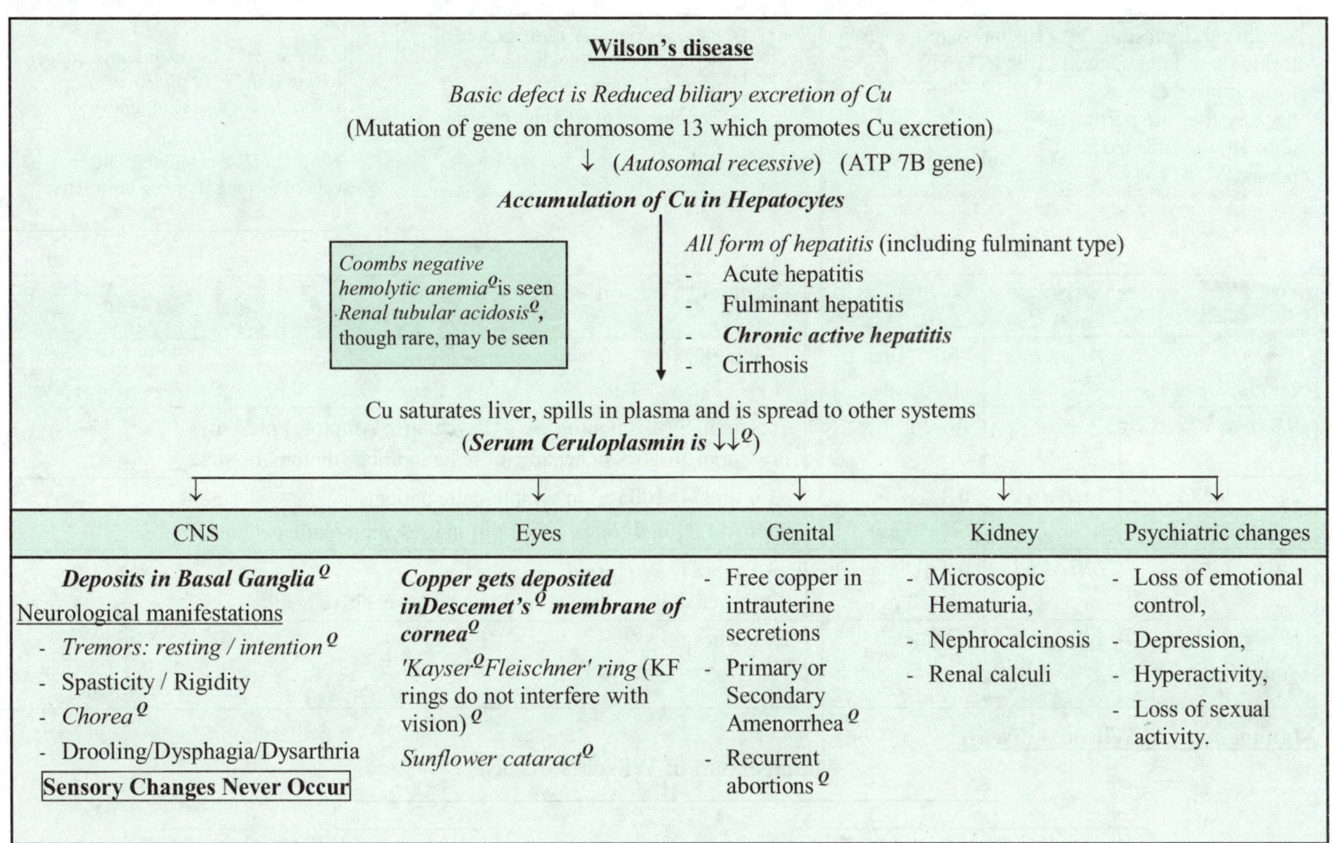

Kayser – Fleischer Rings (KF Rings) and Wilson's disease

Kayser – Fleischer Rings (KF Rings)

- *Brownish yellow discolourations[Q] seen in limbic zone of cornea*
- *Result from deposition of copper in Descemet'smembrane[Q] of the cornea*
- *Do not interfere with vision[Q]*
- *Charachteristically seen in Wilson's disease[Q] but are not pathognomic[Q] of Wilson's disease* and may be seen in other conditions

Conditions that may present with KF rings
• ***Wilson's disease (characteristic[Q])***
• *Chronic Active Hepatitis / Autoimmune Hepatitis*
• *Primary Biliary Cirrhosis*
• *Intrahepatic cholestatic syndromes*

- *Present in almost all patients of Wilsons disease with Neurological /Psychiatric symptoms (99% of patients)[Q]*
- *Present in only 30-50% of patients of Wilson's disease with only hepatic manifestations*
- *Absence of KF rings does not exclude the diagnosis of Wilson's disease[Q]*
- *May* occasionally be visible to the naked eye without magnification but *definite diagnosis can only be made by an ophthalmologist using a slit lamp[Q]*

Recommended Tests for Wilson's disease:

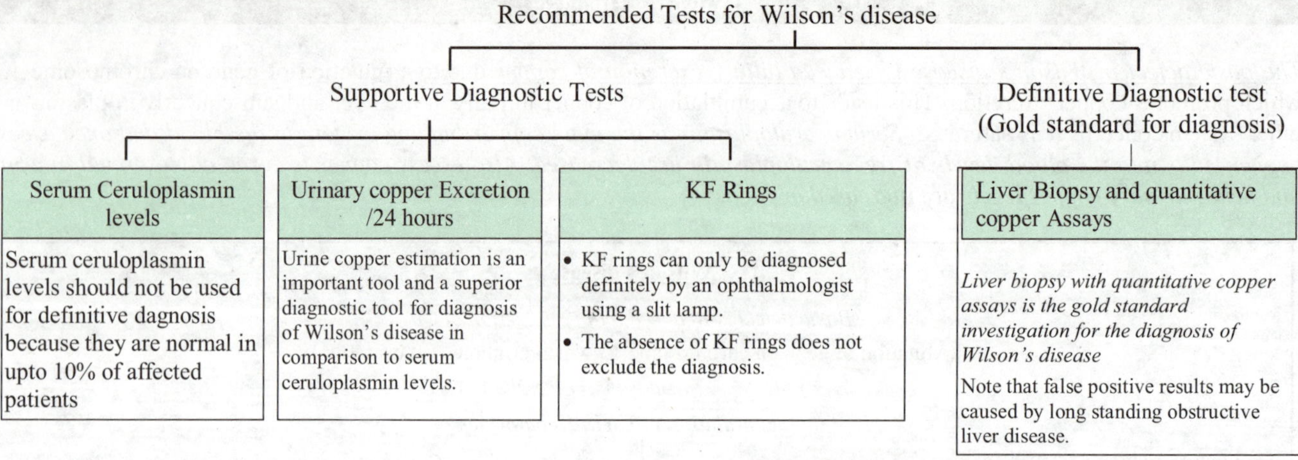

Test	Wilson's Disease	Normal Value	Comment (Wilson's Disease)	Usefulness
Serum Ceruloplasmin	***Decreased***	180-350mg/L (18-35 mg/dL)	Low in 90%	+
KF rings	*Present*	Absent	Present in 99% if neurologic or psychiatric symptoms present Present in 30-50% in hepatic presentation/presymptomatic state	++
24-h urine Cu	***Increased***	0.3-0.8 μmol (20-50 μg)	>1.6 μmol (>100 μg) in symptomatic patients 0.9 to >1.6 μmol (60 to > 100 μg) in presymptomatic patients	+++
Liver Cu	*Increased*	0.3–0.8 μmol/g (20-50 μg)	>3.1 μmol (>200 μg) (Obstructive liver disease can cause false-positive results)	++++
Haplotype Analysis	*2 Matches*	0 Matches	2 Matches	++++ (Siblings only)

Management of Wilson's disease:

Management of Wilson's disease

- Wilson's disease with initial Hepatic manifestations (Hepatitis/cirrhosis)
  - Without evidence of Hepatic decompensation
    - *Zinc is the therapy of choice*
  - With evidence of hepatic decompensation
    - Chelater (Trientene preferred) Along with zinc is the therapy Of choice
- Wilson's disease with initial Neorological/Psychiatric Presentation
  - *Tetrathromolybdate is the drug of choice*

Zinc is the therapy of choice for patients with hepatitis or cirrhosis without evidence of hepatic decompensation or neuropsychiatric symptoms.Zinc is also the treatment of choice for maintainance therapy in Wilson's disease

Zinc is the treatment of choice in Wilson's disease for

- *Initial therapy in patients with hepatitis without decompensation*[Q]
- *Maintainance therapy*
- *Presymptomatic patient*
- *Pediatric patients*
- *Pregnant patients*

Hematochromatosis

Hematochromatosis (Disorder of iron storage)

Inappropriate increase in intestinal absorption results in deposition of excessive amounts of iron in parenchymal cells with eventual tissue damage and impaired function of organs

Serum iron ↑ed
% Transferrin saturation ↑ed
Serum ferritin ↑ed
Elevation in percent Transferrin saturation is the earliest phenotypic marker of herditaryhemochromatosis[Q]

Liver	Skin	Pancreas	Joints	Heart	Hypogonadism
• Usually *first organ to be affected* • Hepatomegaly is seen in 95% of symptomatic patients • Cirrhosis may occur (Micronodular) • Hepatocellular carcinoma (30% of patients with cirrhosis). • It is the *most common cause of death in treated patients.*	• ***Excessive skin (Bronzing of skin) pigmentation*** is present in 90% of symptomatic patients • Usually diffuse and generalized. May be more pronounced on Face, Neck, Extensor aspect of forearm, dorsa of hands, lower legs and genitalia and ears • Usually results from increased melanin and iron in dermis	Involvement of pancreas *results in Diabetes mellitus* which is seen in 65% of symptomatic patients	• ***Arthropathy*** develops in 25-50% of patients • *The joints of hands especially the 2nd and 3rd MCP joints are the first to be involved* • Progressive polyarthritis involving wrist, knees, hips and ankles may also be seen	• Heart is involved in 15% of symptomatic patients • The most common manifestation is congestive heart failure • Cardiomyopathy and cardiac arrhythmias may be seen	• Results from impairment of Hypothalmopituitary function by iron deposition which leads to decreased production of gonadotrophins.

The charachteristic clinical features of Haemochromatosis in order of frequency are[Q]***:***

- *Hepatomegaly (95%)*
- *Skin pigmentation (90%)*
- *Diabetes mellitus (65%)*
- *Arthropathy (25-50%)*
- *Cardiac disease (15%)*
- *Hypogonadism*

<u>Bronze Diabetes</u>
The combination of skin hyperpigmentation and insulin deficiency (diabetes) is called Bronze diabetes.

<u>Tests Recommended for screening for Hereditary Hematochromatosis</u>

Tests Recommended for screening for HereditaryHematochromatosis

Transferrin Saturation

- *A transferrin saturation of more than 45% is the earliest phenotypic abnormality in hereditary hematochromatosis*
- *Transferrin saturation is considered the best initial screening test for hereditary hematochromotosis*
- Transferrin saturation has a high sensitivity of >90% in diagnosing hereditary hematochromatosis

Iron binding capacity (Unbound /Unsaturated)

- *Unbound Iron binding capacity is an alternative screening test.*
- *Unbound Iron binding capacity UIBC=TIBC-Serum Iron*
- *Unbound iron binding capacity is decreased in hematochromatosis*

Treatment of Haematochromatosis

Therapy of Haematochromatosis involves removal of excessive body iron and supportive treatment of damaged organs

Removal of Excessive Body iron
• ***<u>Phlebotomy is the treatment of choice</u>*** Iron removal is best accomplished by once or twice weekly phlebotomy of 500ml, - These should be continued until the serum ferritin level is < 50μg/L (May be required for 1-2 years) - Thereafter phlebotomies are performed at appropriate intervals to maintain ferritin levels between 50-100μg/L (usually one phlebotomy every 3 months)
• **<u>Chelating agents</u>***(such as Desferoxamine) are alternative agents and indicated when anemia and hypoproteinemia are severe enough to preclude phlebotomy*

Alcohol consumption should be eleminated[Q] as it increases the risk of cirrhosis in hematochromatosis nearly ten fold.

<u>Algorithm for diagnosis and management of a patient with suspected Hmatochromatosis:</u>

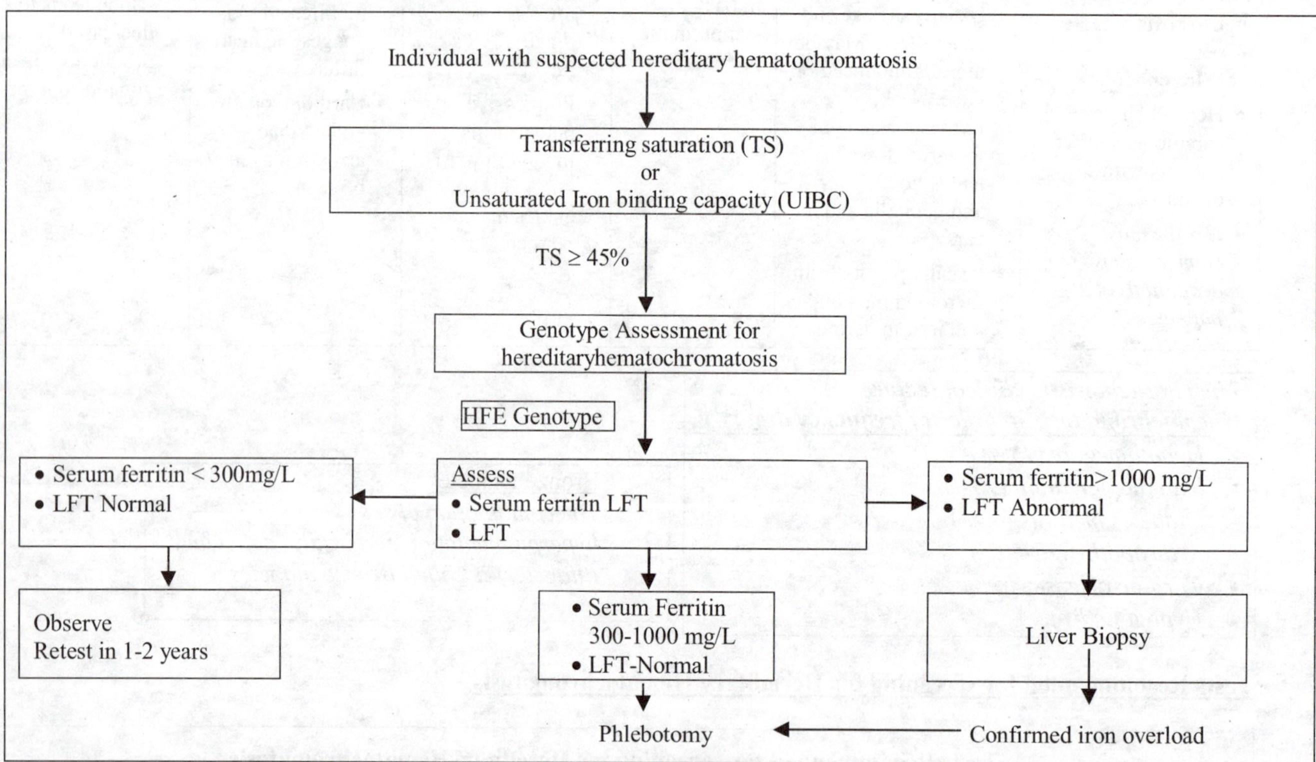

Note

Serum ferritin levels are a good index of body iron stores and are raised early during the cause of disease. Yet serum ferritin levels should not be used as initial screening test to detect hereditary hematochromatosis.

This is because serum ferritin also acts as an acute phase reactant and its levels are increased in variable infections and inflammatory conditions without iron overload. Also the serum concentration of ferritin may be increased in patients with hepatocellular injury as in viral hepatitis, alcoholic fatty liver disease or alcoholic liver diseases due to increased release from tissue cell.

QUESTIONS

Jaundice

1. Following are causes of unconjugated hyperbilirubinemia, ***except***: *(AIIMS Dec 94)*
   A. Hemolytic anemia
   B. Large hematoma
   C. Rotor syndrome
   D. Megaloblastic anemia
2. Conjugated hyperbilirubinemia is seen in: *(AIIMS May' 2006)*
   A. Gilbert's syndrome
   B. Criggler Najjar syndrome
   C. Breast milk jaundice
   D. Dubin Johnson syndrome
3. Bilirubin is absent in urine because it is- *(AIIMS Nov 99)*
   A. Distributed in the body fat
   B. Conjugated with glucoron
   C. Not filtered
   D. Lipophilic
4. A young male presents with elevated bilirubin levels. Examination of urine shows presence of bilirubin while urobilonogen is absent. Likely diagnosis is: *(AI 1991)*
   A. Hepatitis
   B. Hemolytic jaundice
   C. Obstructive jaundice
   D. Gilbert's syndrome
5. A patient presents with unconjugated hyperbilirubinemia and presence of urobilinogen in urine. Which amongst the following is the least likely diagnosis: *(AI 2010)*
   A. Hemolytic jaundice
   B. Crigler Najjar syndrome
   C. Gilbert's syndrome
   D. Dubin Johnson syndrome
6. A patient presents with unconjugated hyperbilirubinemia and elevated urobilinogen levels in urine. The most likely diagnosis is: *(AI 2010)*
   A. Hemolytic Jaundice
   B. Crigler Najjar syndrome
   C. Gilbert's syndrome
   D. Dubin Johnson syndrome
7. A 8 year old child presents with Total bilirubin levels of 2.4 mg/dl Urinary Urobilinogen levels are increased and Bilirubin is absent in urine. The most likely diagnosis is
   A. Hepatitis
   B. Hemolytic jaundice
   C. Obstructive jaundice
   D. Dubin Johnson's syndrome
8. A young male with gallbladder stones shows the following test results; serum bilirubin 2.5, Hb 6; urine test positive for urobilinogen; diagnosis is: *(AI 2001)*
   A. Hemolytic jaundice
   B. Obstructive jaundice
   C. Hepatocellular jaundice
   D. Protoporphyria
9. A 30 year-old male has jaundice. Blood examination shows total serum bilirubin 28 mg%, direct bilirubin 16 mg % and alkaline phosphatase 184 KA units. The Diagnosis is : *(AIIMS June 99)*
   A. Haemolytic jaundice
   B. Viral hepatitis
   C. Chronic active hepatitis
   D. Obstructive jaundice
10. A young pt presents with jaundice. Total bilirubin is 21, direct is 9.6, alkphosis 84 KA units. Diagnosis is: *(AI 2001)*
    A. Hemolytic jaundice
    B. Viral hepatitis
    C. Chronic active hepatitis
    D. Obstructive jaundice
11. True statement about unconjugated hyperbilirubinemia (select three options) *(PGI Dec 05)*
    A. 85% of the total should be indirect
    B. Seen in hemolytic anemia
    C. Seen in ↑ hemoglobin destruction (↑ bilirubin production)
    D. 50% of the total should be indirect
    E. It is seen in Biliary atresia and neonatal hepatitis
12. 5'-Nucleotidase activity is increased in: *(AI 2005)*
    A. Bone diseases.
    B. Prostate cancer.
    C. Chronic renal failure.
    D. Cholestatic disorders.
13. Abnormal excretory function of hepatocytes may be assessed by: *(PGI June 07)*
    A. Increased PT
    B. Increased ALT
    C. Increased Alkaline Phosphatase
    D. Increased gamma GT
14. Increased B_{12} level is seen in all, ***except***: *(AI 2000)*
    A. Cirrhosis
    B. Primary hepatocellular Ca
    C. Hepatitis
    D. Cholestatic jaundice
15. A 56 year old man presents to his internist with jaundice. The patient is receiving no medication and his only symptomatic complaints is mild fatigue over the past 2 months. Physical examination is remarkable only for the presence of scleral icterus. The patient has no significant past medical history. Analysis of serum chemistry reveals the following: *(AIIMS Nov 99)*
    SGOT : 0.58 microkat/L (35U/L)
    SGPT : 0.58 microkat/L (35U/L)
    Total bilirubin : 91.7 micron mol/L (7 mg/dL)
    Direct Bilirubin : 85.5 micron mol/L (5mg/dL)
    Alkaline phosphatase:12 micron kat/L (720U/L)
    Which of the following is the next appropriate diagnostic step?
    A. Ultrasound

B. Liver biopsy
C. Review of peripheral blood smear
D. Endoscopicretrograde cholangiopancreatography (ERCP)

16. The test used to diagnose Dubin Johnson syndrome is *(AI 2007)*
A. Serum transminases
B. BSP test
C. Hippurate test
D. Gamma glutamyl transferase level

17. True about Crigler Najjar type II syndrome is: *(PGI Dec 97)*
A. Diglucuronide deficiency
B. Recessive trait
C. Kernicterus is seen
D. Phenobarbitone is not useful

Viral Hepatitis

General

18. A 50 year old lady presented with history of pain upper abdomen, nausea, and decreased appetite for 5 days. She had undergone cholecystectomy 2 years back. Her bilirubin was 10 mg/dl, SGPT 900 IU/L SGOT 700 IU/L and serum alkaline phosphatase was 280 IU/L. What is the most likely diagnosis - *(AIIMS Nov 05)*
A. Acute pancreatitis
B. Acute cholangitis
C. Acute viral hepatitis
D. Posterior penetration of peptic ulcer

19. Councilman Bodies are seen in: *(AIIMS Nov 07)*
A. Wilson disease
B. Alcoholic hepatitis
C. Acute viral hepatitis
D. Auto immune hepatitis

20. The commonest hepatotropic virus progressing to chronicityis : *(AIIMS May 01)*
A. HEV
B. HAV
C. HBV
D. HCV

21. Chronic hepatitis is caused by (select two options): *(PGI June 03)*
A. Hepatitis A
B. Hepatitis B
C. Hepatitis C
D. Hepatitis E
E. Hepatitis G

22. Which of the following hepatitis viruses have significant perinatal transmission : *(AI 2003)*
A. Hepatitis E virus
B. Hepatitis C virus
C. Hepatitis B virus
D. Hepatitis A virus

23. Non-parenteral hepatitis is : *(AI 2000)*
A. Hepatitis E
B. Hep B
C. Hep C
D. Hep D

24. All of the following are correctly matched, Except *(AIIMS Nov 2010)*
A. LKM1 - Autoimmune Hepatitis
B. LKM2 - Drug Induced Hepatitis
C. LKM1 - Chronic Hepatitis C
D. LKM2 - Chronic Hepatitis D

25. Which of the following Hepatitis has worst prognosis *(DNB Dec 2010)*
A. HBV Infection
B. HDV Infection
C. HBV – HDV Coinfection
D. HDV super- infection on HBV

Hepatitis B

26. Acute infection of hepatitis B virus is diagnosed by: *(AIIMS Feb 97)*
A. IgM antibody of Hb_s Ag
B. IgM antibody of Hb_c Ag
C. IgM antibody of Hb_e Ag
D. IgG antibody of Hb_c Ag

27. Chronic Active Hepatitis can be best differentiated from Chronic Persistant Hepatitis by: *(DNB 2011)*
A. HBs Ag
B. Antibody to HBs Ag
C. Histopathology
D. None of the above

28. Hepatitis B can be transmitted through all of the following, except *(DNB 2011)*
A. Semen
B. Blood
C. Breast milk
D. Fecal-oral (stool)

29. Chances of vertical transmission of Hepatitis B may be high as *(DNB 2011)*
A. 25%
B. 40%
C. 60%
D. 90%

30. The first virological marker following acute infection with HBV is : *(AI 1999)*
A. HBs Ag
B. Anti HBs Ag
C. IgM anti HBc Ag
D. Anti HBe Ag

31. Early diagnosis of acute hepatitis-B infection is made by *(AIIMS Nov 03)*
A. Presence of Hbe Ag in serum
B. Presence of IgM anti-HBc in serum
C. Presence of Hbs Ag in serum
D. Presence of IgG anti-HBc in serum

32. Early diagnosis of active hepatitis B infection is done by : *(AIIMS June 2000)*
A. IgM HBcAg antibody
B. HBsAg
C. HBcAg
D. IgE HBsAg antibody

33. Which of the following markers in the blood is the most reliable indicator of recent hepatitis B-infection? *(AIIMS May 03)*

A. HBsAg
B. IgG anti – HBs
C. IgM anti – HBc
D. IgM anti – Hbe

34. Which of the following is a marker for Active Hepatitis B *(DNB 2012)*
A. HBe Ag
B. IgM Anti HBs Ag
C. HBs Ag
D. Ig G Anti HB1 Ag

35. All of the following are markers of active replicative of chronic hepatitis B, except: *(AIIMS Nov 08)*
A. HBV DNA
B. HBV DNA Polymerase
C. HBeAg
D. AST & ALT

36. Which of the following is the most sensitive marker of active Hepatitis B virus replication : *(PGI 08)*
A. HBV DNA
B. HBV DNA polymerase
C. HBeAg
D. Transaminases

37. Acute hepatitis B is diagnosed by: *(PGI Dec 04)*
A. HBsAg
B. Hbe AG
C. Anti- HBs AG
D. IgM anti – HBc
E. HBV DNA

38. A 35-year-old male patient presented with history of jaundice for 15 days. The onset was preceded by a prodromal illness. His serum tested positive for HBsAg. A clinical diagnosis of acute Hepatitis B was made. What should be the next best confirmatory investigation *(AIIMS May 04)*
A. Anti-HBeAg antibody
B. HBe antigen
C. Anti-HBe IgM antibody
D. HBV DNA by PCR

39. A thirty-year man presented with nausea, fever and jaundice of 5 days duration. The biochemical tests revealed a bilirubin of 6.7 mg/dl (conjugated 5.0 mg/dl) with SGOT/ SGPT (AST/ALT) of 1230/900 IU/ml. The serological tests showed presence of HBs Ag. IgM anti-HBc and Hbe Ag. The most likely diagnosis is: *(AIIMS Nov 02)*
A. Chronic hepatitis B infection with high infectivity.
B. Acute hepatitis B infection with high infectivity.
C. Chronic hepatitis infection with low infectivity.
D. Acute hepatitis B infection with low infectivity.

40. A male patient is observed to be HBs Ag antigen positive HBe Ag antigen negative and anti-HBe antibody positive. HBV DNA copies are observed to be 100,000/ml while SGOT and SGPT are elevated to 6 times the upper limit of normal value. What is the likely diagnosis: *(AI 2010)*
A. HBV surface mutant
B. HBV precore mutant
C. Wild HBs Ag
D. Inactive HBV carrier

41. A patient is found to be positive for HBs Ag on routine laboratory evaluation. Other serological tests for hepatitis are unremarkable. He is clinically asymptomatic and liver enzymes are within the normal range. Which of the following best describes his diagnosis: *(AI 2010)*
A. Inactive HBV carrier
B. Acute Hepatitis B
C. Chronic Hepatitis B
D. Active HBV carrier

42. The following is a marker of acute hepatitis B infection: *(AIIMS Nov 07)*
A. DNA polymerase
B. Hepatitis core antigen
C. Anti HBs
D. IgG to core antigen

43. All of the following are seen in active chronic hepatitis B except: *(AIIMS Nov 07)*
A. IgM against core antigen
B. Total core antibody
C. HbeAg
D. HbsAg

44. In a patient only Anti HBsAg is positive in serum, all other viral markers are negative. This indicates : *(AIIMS June 2000)*
A. Acute hepatitis
B. Chronic active hepatitis
C. Persistent carrier
D. Immunized person with hepatitis B vaccine

45. A patient is found to be positive only for Anti HBsAg. All other viral markers are negative.The likely diagnosis is : *(PGI 2009)*
A. Vaccination
B. Chronic hepatitis B
C. Acute hepatitis B
D. Fulminant hepatitis B

46. The marker for determining efficacy of hepatitis B vaccination is: *(DNB 2010)*
A. HBs Ag
B. IgM Anti HBc
C. IgG Anti HBc
D. Anti – HBs Ag

47. The only serological marker present in the 'window period' of Hepatitis B is *(DNB 2011)*
A. Anti HBc
B. HBs Ag
C. Anti HBS Ag
D. HBe Ag

48. All of the following should be included during preliminary evaluation of a case of suspected Acute viral hepatitis except: *(AIIMS June 2000)*
A. Hbs Ag
B. IgM anti HBc

C. Anti-HCV
D. IgM anti HBe.

49. A 30-year-old patient presented with history of jaundice for 30 days. His liver function tests showed bilirubin of 100mg/dl, SGOT/SGPT-1100/1450, serum alkaline phosphatase-240 IU. He was positive for Hbs Ag. What should be the confirmatory test to establish Acute hepatitis B infection?
A. IgM Anti-HBc antibody (AIIMS May 06)
B. HbeAg
C. HBV DNA by PCR
D. Anti-HBc antibody

50. Hepatitis B infectivity is indicated by: (AI 1994)
A. Anti-HBsAg
B. HBsAg + HBeAg
C. Anti-HBsAg – Anti-HBc
D. Anti-HBeAg + Anti-Hbs Ag

51. HBV Replication is indicated by all of the following, Except: (PGI Dec 06)
A. HBV DNA
B. DNA polymerase
C. HBe Ag
D. HBs Ag

52. Hera lal 35 years old man was found +ve for HBsAg & HBeAg, accidentally during screening of blood donation. On Lab examination SGOT & SGPT are Normal. What should you do next : (AI 2002)
A. Liver biopsy
B. Interferon therapy
C. Observation
D. HBV-DNA estimation

53. A person is screened for blood Donation. Which of the following serology is safe for Blood donation.
A. Anti HBsAg positive (PGI June 03)
B. HBsAg positive
C. Anti HBC positive (IgM)
D. HBcAg positive

54. A blood donor is not considered for safe transfusion, if he has : (AI 2000)
A. Anti HBs Ag +ve
B. Anti HBs Ag and HBc Ag +ve
C. Hbs Ag +ve, & IgM anti HBc +ve
D. Anti HBe +ve

55. Reserve transcriptase of hepatitis B virus is coded on the following gene : (AI 2000)
A. C gene
B. S gene
C. P gene
D. X gene

56. A young male was found to be HBsAg positivity and HBe Ag negative. His liver enzymes were normal. The next step in management of this young male should be: (AI 2008)
A. Lamivudine therapy
B. Lamivudine plus IFN therapy
C. Start IFN therapy
D. Serial monitoring

57. A 26 year old man was observed to be positive for HBs Ag but negative for HBe Ag. The AST / ALT levls were observed to be within normal limits. The next step in management of this patient should be
A. Serial monitoring (DNB 2011)
B. Antiviral treatment with Lamivudine monotherapy
C. Antiviral treatment with Lamivudine and pulsed IFN
D. Antiviral treatment with IFN Alfa alone

58. Lamivudine is recommended for treatment of chronic hepatitis B when: (DNB 2012)
A. HBe Ag positive
B. HBe Ag Negative
C. ALT > 2 xULN
D. Viral DNA > 102 copies

59. Which one of the following pairs regarding Hepatitis B is not correctly matched (AIIMS Nov 2010)
A. Acute Viral Hepatitis B - Supportive care
B. Acute Viral Hepatitis B - Antiviral therapy
C. Chronic Viral Hepatitis B - Supportive care
D. Chronic Viral Hepatitis B - Antiviral therapy

60. All of the following statements about Hepatitis B are true, Except (AIIMS Nov 2010)
A. Vertical Transmission is more common than horizontal transmission in non-endemic areas
B. Age of onset determines prognosis
C. Period of communicability lasts several months
D. Virus can be detected in blood one month before jaundice

61. Extrahepatic Manifestations of Hepatitis B include all of the following Except (PGI June 01)
A. Aplastic Anemia
B. Gullian Barre syndrome
C. Pancreatitis
D. Gall stone disease
E. Cryoglobulinemia

62. HBs Ag positive person may have all of the following associated Renal lesions, Except: (PGI Dec 06)
A. Membranous Glomerulonephritis (MGN)
B. Membrano proliferative Glomerulnephritis (MPGN)
C. Mesangiocapillary Glomerulonephritis
D. Focal Segmental Glomerulosclerosis (FSGS)

63. Interferon treatment is recommended in chronic hepatitis B in patients with: (PGI June 07)
A. ↑ HBV DNA and Normal ALT
B. ↑ HBV DNA and ↑ ALT
C. ↑ HBV DNA and compensated cirrhosis
D. ↑ HBV DNA and decompensated cirrhosis

64. Agents Recommended for treatment of chronic

Hepatitis B include all of the following, Except.
A. Interferon (PGI June 05)
B. Lamuvudine
C. Adefovir
D. Entecevir
E. Famcyclovir

Hepatitis C

65. Chronic liver disease is most commonly caused by : (AI 2000)
A. Hepatitis B
B. Hepatitis A
C. Hepatitis C
D. Hepatitis E

66. Hepatitis C virus is associated with : (AI 2000)
A. Anti LKM antibody
B. Scleroderma
C. Cryoglobulinemia
D. Polyarteritis nodosa

67. Extrahepatic Manifestations of Hepatitis C include all of the following Except: (PGI June 04)
A. Lichen Planus
B. Celiac Disease
C. Glomerulonephritis
D. Cryoglobulinemia
E. Polyarthritis

68. Hepatic C is associated with all except: (PGI June 08)
A. PAN
B. Dermatomyositis like syndrome
C. Lichen Planus
D. Psoriasis

69. A 30 year old patient with H/O antibodies to HCV for 6 months duration and his AST/ALT is normal. There is no symptom or stigmata of liver disease. The most appropriate approach: (PGI June 04)
A. Reassure the patient
B. Repeat titre every three years
C. Repeat enzymes every year
D. Do liver biopsy & start antiviral drugs accordingly.

70. A 30 year old patient with H/O persistant antibodies to HCV for 6 months duration and his AST/ALT is normal. There is no symptom or stigmata of liver disease. The most appropriate approach:
A. Reassure the patient (PGI June 04)
B. Repeat titre every three years
C. Repeat enzymes every year
D. Do liver biopsy & start antiviral drugs accordingly.
E. Determine HCV RNA levels

71. A 55 year old male patient was diagnosed to have chronic hepatitis C. He responded to treatment with interferon. However, after one year of follow up he showed a relapse of disease. Which of the following would be the next most appropriate choice?
A. Ribavarin and interferon (AIIMS Nov 03)
B. Lamivudine and interferon
C. Nevirapine and lamivudine
D. Indinavir and ribavarin.

72. A 55 year old male patient was diagnosed to have chronic hepatitis C. He responded to treatment with interferon. However, after one year of follow up he showed a relapse of disease. Which of the following would be the next most appropriate choice?
A. Ribavarin and interferon (AIIMS Nov 03)
B. Lamivudine and interferon
C. Nevirapine and lamivudine
D. Indinavir and ribavarin.

73. Sustained Response to antiviral therapy (IFN + Ribavarin) in hepatitis C is indicated by
A. High HCV-RNA (PGI Dec 04)
B. Cirrhosis
C. Age > 40 years
D. Genotype I
E. Female sex

Hepatitis E

74. True regarding hepatitis E virus is: (AIIMS Dec 98)
A. Seen in Post transfusion cases
B. Associated with increased mortality in pregnant female
C. Associated with hepatitis B virus
D. Acquired by feco-oral route

75. The most common route of spread in hepatitis E is:
A. Blood transfusion (AI 1995)
B. Feco-oral
C. Intercourse
D. IV injection

76. During an epidemic of hepatitis E, Fatality is maximum in : (AI 2000)
A. Pregnant women
B. Infants
C. Malnourished male
D. Adolescents

77. Fulminant Hepatitis E is typically seen in: (DNB)
A. Pregnant women
B. Infants
C. Adolescents
D. Malnourished males

78. Which hepatitis is most dangerous in pregnancy:
A. Hepatitis A (AIIMS May 95)
B. Hepatitis B
C. Hepatitis C
D. Hepatitis E

79. Which hepatitis virus has worst prognosis in pregnancy : (AIIMS Feb 97)
A. HBV
B. HCV
C. HEV
D. HAV

80. Most common type of hepatitis responsible for epidemics in India is : *(AI 1997)*
   A. Hepatitis A
   B. Hepatitis B
   C. Hepatitis C
   D. Hepatitis E
81. Most common cause of acute sporadic hepatitis in India is *(DNB 2012)*
   A. Hepatitis E
   B. Hepatitis B
   C. Hepatitis C
   D. Hepatitis D

Autoimmune and Granulomatous Hepatitis

82. Characteristic Auto antibodies of Autoimmune Hepatitis include all of the following, Except:
   A. Antinuclear Antibodies (ANA) *(PGI Dec 06)*
   B. Anti SLA
   C. Anti LKM1
   D. ANCA
83. Granulomatous hepatitis may be seen with :
   A. Carbamazepine *(AI 1996)*
   B. Allopurinol
   C. Phenylbutazone
   D. All of the above

Alcoholic Hepatitis

84. Features of Alcoholic hepatitis include all of the following except: *(AI 1991)*
   A. Elevated bilirubin
   B. Prolonged prothrombin time
   C. Elevated serum albumin
   D. Anemia
85. Ratio of AST/ALT > 1 is present in *(AIIMS May 07)*
   A. Non alcoholic steatohepatitis
   B. Alcoholic hepatitis
   C. Wilson's disease
   D. All of the above
86. Which is **not** true about alcoholic hepatitis :
   A. Gamma glutamyl transferase is raised
   B. SGPT is raised > SGOT *(AIIMS May 95)*
   C. SGOT is raised > SGPT
   D. Alkaline phosphatase is raised
87. Which of the following enzyme assay is useful to diagnose alcoholism *(AIIMS Dec 94)*
   A. SGOT
   B. SGPT
   C. Alkaline phosphatase
   D. Glutamyl aminotransferase
88. Which is useful to decrease mortality and renal failure in acute liver disease due to alcoholism:
   A. Pentoxyfylline *(AIIMS May 07)*
   B. Orlistat
   C. S-Adenosyl methionine
   D. Syrlamysin

Non Alcoholic Fatty Liver Disease (NAFLD/NASH)

89. Non Alcoholic steatohepatitis is seen in all, except:
   A. Diabetes *(PGI June 05)*
   B. Obesity
   C. Hypertriglyceridemia
   D. Total Parentral Nutrition
   E. Gall stone disease
90. All of the following statements about Non Alcoholic Fatty Liver disease are true, except: *(PGI June 01)*
   A. Common in Diabetics
   B. Clofibrate provides effective treatment
   C. Commonest cause of cryptogenic cirihosis
   D. Associated with elevated transminases

Ascitis

91. Chylous ascities is caused by all of the following ***except***: *(AIIMS Nov 02)*
   A. Colloid carcinoma of stomach.
   B. Tuberculosis.
   C. Trauma.
   D. Nephrotic syndrome.
92. Which of the following statement about ascitis is true: *(PGI June 05)*
   A. Hemorrhagic ascitis is diagnosed when RBC count > 1,000/mm^3
   B. SBP is diagnosed when Neutrophil count > 500/mm^3
   C. Large volume paracentesis is indicated in SBP
   D. USG can detect as little as 100 ml of peritoneal fluid
   E. Norfloxacin is the drug of choice in SBP
93. First line of treatment in Ascitis is: *(PGI June 96)*
   A. Salt Restriction
   B. Diuretics
   C. Paracentesis
   D. Shunt

Cirrhosis and its Complications

Cirrhosis: General

94. Micronodular cirrhosis is commonly seen in all except: *(AIIMS Nov 07)*
   A. Chronic hepatitis B
   B. Alcoholic liver disease
   C. Hemochromatosis
   D. Chronic extrahepatic biliary obstruction
95. In hepatic cirrhosis, which of the following is increased: *(PGI June 97)*
   A. Alpha 1 globulin
   B. Alpha 2 globulin

C. Gamma globulin
D. All of the above

96. A patient presents with esophageal varices and a liver span of 10cm. All of the following are likely causes, except: *(PGI Dec 04)*
A. Haemochromatosis
B. Alcoholic liver disease
C. Veno-occlusive disease
D. Post necrotic cirrhosis
E. Budd-chiary syndrome

97. Enlarged liver with Hepatocellular dysfunction may be seen in all of the following, except: *(PGI June 05)*
A. Wilson's disease
B. Budd Chirai syndrome
C. Alcoholic hepatitis
D. NASH
E. Post necrotic syndrome

Primary Biliary Cirrhosis & Sclerosing Cholangitis

98. Most common symptom of primary biliary cirrhosis is *(AI 1996)*
A. Pruritis
B. Abdominal pain
C. Jaundice
D. Bleeding

99. All of the following statements about primary sclerosing cholangitis are true, Except: *(AI 1992)*
A. Increased risk associated with smoking
B. Associated with Ulcerative colitis
C. GGT elevation occurs early
D. Pruritis is a common presenting symptom

100. All of the following statements about primary sclerosing cholangitis are true, Except: *(PGI Dec 03)*
A. Increased incidence in females
B. Associated with Inflammatory bowel disease
C. May involve both intra and extra hepatic ducts
D. ERCP is a sensitive investigation

101. All of the following statements are correct, Except:
A. Antimitochondrial antibodies are positive in primary biliary cirrhosis
B. In late stage of PSC treatment is liver transplantation
C. In advanced stages of cirrhosis major blood supply to liver comes from Hepatic vein
D. Elevated lipoprotein-X in PBC

Non Cirrhotic Portal Fibrosis

102. A child presents with massive hemetemesis and systemic hypotension. He has no fever or other significant history. Examination reveal massive splenomegaly but no hepatomegaly. Likely diagnosis is *(AIIMS Nov 01)*
A. Hepatocellular carcinoma
B. Bleeding duodenal ulcer
C. Oesophageal varices
D. Non-cirrhotic portal fibrosis

103. A 12 year old boy presents with hemetemesis, malena and mild splenomegaly. There is no obvious jaundice or ascitis. The most likely diagnosis is
A. EHPVO
B. NCPF
C. Cirrhosis
D. Malaria with DIC

104. A 23 year old male has presented with repeated episodes of hematemesis. There is no history of jaudice or liver decompensation. On examination ther significant findings include splenomegaly (8 cms below costal margin), and presence of esophageal varices. There is no ascites or peptic ulceration. The liver function tests are normal. The most likely diagnosis is :
A. Extahepatic portal venous obstruction
B. Non cirrhotic portal fibrosis
C. Cirrhosis
D. Hepatic venous outflow tract obstruction

105. Ingestion of arsenic causes : *(AIIMS May 01)*
A. Hepatic carcinoma
B. Hepatic adenoma
C. Non cirrhotic portal fibrosis
D. Hepatic cirrhosis

106. Which of the following is the most common presenting symptom of non-cirrhotic portal hypertension? *(AI 2006)*
A. Chronic liver failure
B. Ascites
C. Upper gastrointestinal bleeding
D. Encephalopathy

Portal Hypertension

107. In patients with cirrhosis of the liver the site of obstruction in the portal system is in the : *(AI 2004)*
A. Hepatic vein
B. Post sinusoidal
C. Extra hepatic portal vein
D. Sinusoids

108. Normal portal venous pressure is: *(AI 1994)*
A. 3-5 cm saline
B. 5-10 cm saline
C. 10-15 cm saline
D. 15-20 cm saline

109. An 18 yr old male presents with massive hematemesis; he has history of fever for the past 14 days for which he was managed with drugs; moderate splenomegaly is present; diagnosis is: *(AI 2001)*
A. NSAID induced duodenal ulcer
B. Drug induced gastritis
C. Esophageal varices
D. None of the above.

110. A young boy, Rahul presents with massive hemetemesis. He had fever for 15 days few days back

which was treated with few drugs. Clinical examination reveal moderate splenomegaly). No other history is positive) Probable diagnosis is:
A. Drug induced gastritis (AIIMS Nov 01)
B. Oesophageal tear
C. Bleeding duodenal ulcer
D. Oesophageal varices

111. A young patient presenting with massive hematemesis was found to have splenomegaly. In this case the most likely source of bleeding is :
A. Duodenal ulcer
B. Esophageal varices
C. Erosive mucosal disease
D. Gastric ulcer

112. A man presents with history of hemetemesis of about 500 ml of blood. On examination, spleen is palpable 5 cms below the left costal margin. The most likely diagnosis is: (AI 2012)
A. Portal Hypertension
B. Gastric ulcer
C. Drug induced
D. Mallory Weiss Tear

113. All can be used as endoscopic sclerosants in the treatment of variceal bleeding, ***except***:
A. Polydochyl (AIIMS Nov 01)
B. Cynoacrylate
C. Alcohol
D. Acetic acid

114. A 40 year old patient, a known case of cirrhosis develops acute episode of GI bleed. Initial therapy given for 6 hours. Which of the following procedure is useful : (AIIMS June 99)
A. Nasogastric aspiration
B. Urgent endoscopy
C. Sedation
D. Ultrasound

115. A 45 - year old cirrhotic patient presented with severe haematemesis. The management of choice is :
A. Whole blood transfusion is the best
B. Colloids are preferred over crystalloids
C. Normal saline infusion (AIIMS June 99)
D. IV fluid with diuretics

Hepatic Encephalopathy / Hepatic failure

116. Hepatic-encephalopathy may be precipitated by all of the following ***except*** : (AI 1999)
A. Anemia
B. Barbiturates
C. Hyperkalemia
D. Hypothyroidism

117. Stigmata of chronic Liver disease include all of the following, except (DNB 2010)
A. Parmar Erythema
B. Spinder naevi
C. Testicular Atrophy
D. Subcutaneous nodules

118. Skin stigmata of Liver disease include all of the following, Except (DNB 2011)
A. Parmar Erythema
B. Paper money skin
C. Drumstick fingers
D. Subcutaneous nodules

119. Which of the following is *not* a precipitating factor for hepatic encephalopathy in patients with chronic liver disease? (AIIMS May 05)
A. Hypokalemia
B. Hyponatremia
C. Hypoxia
D. Metabolic acidosis

120. Hepatic Encephalopathy is predisposed by all, Except: (PGI June 03)
A. Hyperkalemia
B. Dehydration
C. Constipation
D. GI Bleeding
E. SBP

121. Features of Acute Fulminant Hepatic failure include all of the following Except: (PGI June 01)
A. Hyperglycemia
B. Hypomagnesemia
C. Hepatorenal syndrome
D. Intracranial hemorrhage
E. Coagulopathy

122. In child with acute liver failure, the most important prognostic factor for death is- (AIIMS 06)
A. Increasing transaminase
B. Increasing bilirubin
C. Increasing prothrombin time
D. Gram negative sepsis

123. In patients with acute liver failure, the best prognostic indicator is: (AIIMS May 01)
A. Serum albumin
B. Serum alpha feto protein
C. Serum bilirubin
D. Factor V estimation

124. The first laboratory test that becomes abnormal in acute hepatocellular failure is: (DNB)
A. Prothrombin time (PT)
B. APTT
C. Decreased Albumin
D. Increased Arterial Ammonia

125. A symmetric high-voltage, triphasic slow wave pattern is seen on EEG in the following
A. Hepatic encephalopathy (AIIMS May 06)
B. Uremic encephalopathy
C. Hypoxic encephalopathy
D. Hypercarbic encephalopathy

126. Flapping Tremors may be associated with all of the following, Except (DNB 2010)
A. Hepatic encephalopathy
B. Uremia
C. CO_2 Narcosis
D. Thyrotoxicosis

127. Following liver transplantation, recurrence of primary disease in the liver most likely occures in: *(AIIMS Nov. 05)*
   A. Wilson disease
   B. Autoimmune hepatitis
   C. Alpha - 1 antitrypsin deficiency
   D. Primary biliary cirrhosis

Hepatorenal Syndrome

128. Features of Hepatorenal syndrome are (select two options): *(PGI June 06)*
   A. Urine sodium < 10 meq/l
   B. Normal renal histology
   C. Renal function abnormal even after liver become normal
   D. Proteinuria < 500 mg/day

129. Which of the following statements is incorrect with regard to Hepatorenal syndrome in a patient with cirrhosis *(AI 2003)*
   A. Createnine clearance < 40 ml/min
   B. Urinary sodium < 10mq/L
   C. Urine osmolality lower than plasma osmolality
   D. No sustained improvement in renal function after volume expansion.

130. Which of the following statements is incorrect with regard to heptorenal syndrome in a patient with cirrhosis
   A. The creatinine clearance is > 40 ml/min
   B. The urinary sodium is less than 10 mmol/L
   C. The urine osmolality is lower than the plasma osmolality *(AIIMS Nov 2004)*
   D. There is poor response to volume expansion

Hepatocellular Carcinoma

131. All of the following are risk factors for Hepatocellular carcinoma ***except***: *(All India)*
   A. Hepatitis C infection
   B. Alcoholism
   C. Alfatoxins
   D. Animal fat in diet

132. Lalloo, 60 years of age, a known case of cirrhosis liver, presents with increased levels of Alpha feto protein, hepatomegaly 3 cm below costal margin.USG showed lesions involving the right lobe of the liver. What is the most probable diagnosis : *(All India)*
   A. Focal nodular hyper-plasia
   B. Hepatocellular carinoma
   C. Hepatic adenoma
   D. Metastasis

133. All of the following are important clinical manifestations of hepatocellular carcinoma ***except***: *(All India)*
   A. Jaundice
   B. Abdominal pain
   C. Abdominal mass
   D. Ascitis

134. 38 year old man Babbu, a chronic alcoholic, presents with pain in abdomen. On examination his liver is enlarged and serum α fetoprotein is elevated. The most likely diagnosis is: *(AI 2000)*
   A. Hepatocellular carcinoma
   B. Liver cell hyperplasia
   C. Hepatic adenoma
   D. Hepatitis

135. Increase in alpha-fetoprotein is seen in : *(AIIMS June 2000)*
   A. Hepatoblastoma
   B. Neuroblastoma
   C. Thymoma
   D. Angiosarcoma

136. Which of the following statements is not true regarding α-fetoprotein : *(AI 1999)*
   A. High levels are seen in fibrolamellar hepatic carcinoma
   B. Pre-operative high level indicates worse prognosis
   C. High level are seen in stomach carcinoma
   D. Levels may be increased in hepatitis

137. All are features of hepatocellular carcinoma, ***except***: *(AIIMS Sept 96)*
   A. Not common in Asian
   B. Liver biopsy is diagnostic
   C. Raised titre of HBV and HCV antibodies
   D. Fibrolameller type is having good prognosis

138. About fibrolamellar carcinoma, TRUE is : *(AIIMS May 94)*
   A. Diffuse in nature
   B. Occurs after 60 years of age
   C. Cirrhosis is the most common presenting feature
   D. Has better prognosis

139. All of the following are true about fibrolamellar carcinoma of the liver ***except*** : *(AI 2001)*
   A. More common in females
   B. Better prognosis than HCC
   C. AFP levels always greater than 1000
   D. Occur in younger individuals

Budd Chiari Syndrome

140. Budd-chiari syndrome is most commonly due to: *(AI 1999)*
   A. Hepatic vein obstruction
   B. Acute portal hypertension
   C. Congenital portal hypertension
   D. IVC- obstruction

141. What is the most common cause for Budd chiari syndrome : *(AIIMS Nov 2000)*
   A. Right ventricular failure
   B. PNH
   C. Valve in hepatic veins
   D. Polycythemia vera

142. Commonest cause of Budd Chiary syndrome is: *(AI 1997)*
   A. Valve in the IVC
   B. Hepatocellular carcinoma
   C. Paroxysmal nocturnal hemoglobinuria
   D. Renal cell carcinoma

143. Most common cause of Budd Chiari syndrome is:

A. Idiopathic (AIIMS May 97)
B. Valves in hepatic veins
C. Hepatocellular carcinoma
D. Thrombosis of hepatic veins

144. In Budd Chiari syndrome, the site of venous thrombosis is : (AI 2004)
A. Infrahepatic inferior vena cava
B. Infrarenal inferior vena cava
C. Hepatic veins
D. Portal veins

Disorders of Biliary Tract

145. 5'-Nucleotidase activity is increased in: (AI 2005)
A. Bone diseases
B. Prostate cancer.
C. Chronic renal failure.
D. Cholestatic disorders.

146. Lithogenic bile has the following properties : (AI 1996)
A. ↓ Bile and ↑ Cholesterol ratio
B. ↑ Bile and ↓ cholesterol ratio
C. Equal bile and cholesterol
D. Cholesterol only

147. Gall bladder stone formation in influenced by all ***except:*** (AI 1998)
A. Clofibrate therapy
B. Hyperalimentation
C. Primary biliary cirrhosis
D. Hypercholesterolemia

148. Stone formation in Gall bladder is enhanced by all ***except*** : (AI 1996)
A. Clofibrate therapy
B. Ilial resection
C. Cholestyramine therapy
D. Vagal stimulation

149. Incidence of gall stone is high in: (AIIMS Nov 93)
A. Partial hepatectomy
B. Ileal resection
C. Jejunal resection
D. Subtotal gastrectomy

150. True statement about gall stones are All/Except:
A. Lithogenic bile is required for stone formation
B. May be associated with carcinoma gall bladder
C. Associated with diabetes mellitus (AIIMS Nov 99)
D. More common in males between 30-40 years of age

151. Most common site for impaction of gell stones in gall stone lieus is : (AI 1999)
A. Ist part of duodenum
B. IInd part of duodenum
C. Terminal ileum
D. Colon

152. The most common site of intestinal obstruction in gallstone ileus is: (AIIMS May 05, AI 04)
A. Duodenum
B. Jejunum
C. Ileum
D. Sigmoid colon

153. Internal fistula is most common between gall bladder and: (AIIMS June 93)
A. Colon
B. Duodenum Ist part
C. Jejunum
D. Transverse colon

154. The treatment of choice for silent stones in Gall bladder is : (AI 1997)
A. Observation
B. Chenodeoxycholic acid
C. Cholecystectomy
D. Lithotripsy

155. Which of the following is not an indication for cholecystectomy: (AIIMS May 05)
A. A. 70 year old male with symptomatic gall stone
B. B. 20 years old male with sickle cell anemia and symptomatic gallstones
C. C. 65 year old female with a large gallbladder polyp
D. D. 55 year old with an asymptomatic gallstone

156. A 69 year old male patient having coronary artery disease was found to have gall bladder stones while undergoing a routine ultrasound of the abdomen. There was no history of biliary colic or jaundice at any time. What is the best treatment advice for such a patient for his gallbladder stones:
A. Open cholecystectomy (AIIMS Nov 03, AI 03)
B. Laparoscopic cholecystectomy
C. No surgery for gallbladder stones
D. ERCP and removal of gallbladder stones

157. Medical treatment for gall bladder stone is amenable for : (AI 1998)
A. Stones less than 15 mm in size
B. Radioopaque stone
C. Calcium bilirubinate oxalate stone
D. Nonfunctioning stones associated with gall bladder

158. All of the following are required for visualization of gall bladder in an oral cholecystogram ***except***:
A. Motor mechanism of gall bladder (AI 1997)
B. Patency of cystic duct
C. Ability to absorb water
D. Functioning hepatocytes

159. All are component of saint's triad except:
A. Renal stones (AIIMS Nov 95)
B. Hiatus hernia
C. Diverticulosis coli
D. Gall stones

160. Charcot's triad includes all of the following ***except*** (AI 1996)
A. Pain
B. Fever
C. Jaundice

D. Vomiting

161. All of the following are known predesposing factors for cholangiocarcinoma ***except*** : (AI 1997)
   A. CBD stones
   B. Clonorchis sinensis
   C. Ulcerative colitis
   D. Primary sclerosing cholangitis

162. Which of the following does not predispose to Cholangiocarcinoma (AI 1996)
   A. Ulcerative colitis
   B. Clonorchis sinensis
   C. Choledochal cyst
   D. Chronic pancreatitis

163. Risk factors for malignant change in an asymptomatic patient with a gall bladder polyp on ultrasound include all of the following, Except: (AI 2009)
   A. Age > 60 years
   B. Rapid increase in size of polyp
   C. Size of polyp > 5 mm
   D. Associated Gall stones

Wilson's Disease

164. All the following are features of Wilson's disease ***except***: (AI 1996)
   A. Increased copper content in liver
   B. Increased ceruloplasmin
   C. Mental changes
   D. Features of chronic active hepatitis

165. Which of the following statements about Wilson's disease is true: (AI 2010)
   A. Low serum ceruloplasmin and low urinary copper
   B. Low serum ceruloplasmin and high urinary copper
   C. High serum ceruloplasmin and low urinary copper
   D. High serum ceruloplasmin and high urinary copper

166. A 12 years old girl with tremors and emotional liability has golden brown discolouration in liability has golden brown discolouration in liability has golden brown discolouration in Descement's membrane. The most likely diagnosis is- (AI 04)
   A. Fabry's disease
   B. Wilson's disease
   C. Glycogen storage disease
   D. Acute Rheumatic fever

167. All of the following are features of wilson's disease, except- (AIIMS Dec 97)
   A. Hemolytic anemia
   B. Testicular atrophy
   C. Chorea
   D. Chronic active hepatitis

168. Kayser- Fleischer rings (KF rings) are seen in: (AI 2010)
   A. Pterygium
   B. Hematochromatosis
   C. Wilson's disease
   D. Menke's kinked hair syndrome

169. All of the following statements about. Wilson's disease are true, EXCEPT- (AIIMS May 04)
   A. It is an autosomal recessive disorder
   B. Serum ceruloplasmin level is < 20 mg/dl
   C. Urinary copper excretion is <100 μg/dl
   D. Zinc acetate is effective as maintenance therapy

170. A 14 year old boy presents wit recurrent episodes of hepatitis Opthalmoscopic evalution reveals KF rings and serum ceruloplasmin levels are < 20 mg/dl. The treatment of choice for initial therapy is
   A. Zinc
   B. Pencillamine
   C. Tetrathromolybdate
   D. Hepatic transplantation

Hemochromatosis

171. A patient presents with Arthritis, hyperpigmentation of skin andhypogonadism, likely diagnosis is- (AI 2001)
   A. Hemochromatosis
   B. Ectopic ACTH secreting tumour of the lung
   C. Wilson's disease
   D. Rheumatoid arthritis

172. Earliest phenotypic manifestation of Idiopathic hereditary hemochromatosis is- (AIIMS May 07)
   A. Post prandial increase in serum iron concentration
   B. Elevated serum ferritin level
   C. Slate grey pigmentation of skin
   D. Increased transferrin saturation

173. Lallo, aged 54 years, who is a known diabetic patient develops cirrhosis. There is associated skin hyperpigmentation and restrictive cardiomyopathy which of the following is the best initial test to diagnose this case. (AIIMS Nov 2000)
   A. Iron binding capacity
   B. Serum ferritin
   C. Serum copper
   D. Serum ceruloplasmin

174. All are seen in hemochromatosis except-
   A. Hypogonadism
   B. Arthropathy
   C. Bronze diabetes
   D. Desferrioxamine is the treatment of choice.

Miscellaneous

175. Which of the following statements regarding liver enzymes is true (DNB Dec 2012)
   A. ALT is less specific indicator of liver injury than AST

B. Absolute levels of aminotransferase correlate with outcome
C. Glutathione-S- Transferase is used as a hepatic prognostic marker after surgery
D. None of the above

176. Increased LDH is an important marker for: *(DNB 2011)*
A. Bulky Disease
B. Lymphoma
C. Liver metastasis
D. Lung metastasis

177. Significant weight loss is defined as: *(DNB)*
A. 5% weight loss in 1-2 months
B. 5% weight loss in 2-3 months
C. 10% weight loss in 1-2 months
D. 10% weight loss in 2-3 months

178. Indications for Liver Transplantation include: *(PGI 09)*
A. Hemochromatosis
B. Primary Biliary Cirrhosis
C. Sclerosing cholangitis with ulcerative colitis
D. Sclerosing cholangitis without ulcerative colitis
E. Biliary

179. Quantitative assessment of liver function can be done by: *(PGI Dec 05)*
A. Degree of ↑ Transaminases
B. Degree of ↑ Alkaline phosphatase
C. Degree of ↑ GGT
D. Estimation of Galactose Elimination capacity

180. Hepatomegaly is a feature of all of the following, Except : *(AI 2009)*
A. Von Girke's Disease
B. Hurler's Disease
C. Nieman Pick Disease
D. Hepatic porphyrias

181. Which one of the following serum levels would help in distinguishing an acute liver disease from chronic liver disease? *(AI 2005)*
A. Aminotransaminase.
B. Alkaline phosphatase.
C. Bilirubin.
D. Albumin.

182. Air in biliary tract is seen in all except: *(AIIMS 1995)*
A. Gall stone ileus
B. Sclerosing cholangitis
C. Carcinoma gall bladder
D. Endoscopic papillotomy

183. Treatment of choice for Echinococcus granulosus is. *(DNB 2010)*
A. Albendazole
B. Mebendazole
C. Thiobendazole
D. Praziquantel

184. Bland cholestasis is caused by all of the following drugs, except *(PGI Dec-04)*
A. Androgen
B. OCP
C. Cyclosporine
D. Estrogen
E. Chlorpromazine

ANSWERS, REFERENCES, EXPLANATIONS AND RELEVANT HIGH YIELD FACTS

Jaundice

1. **Answer is C (Rotor syndrome):** *Harrisons 15th/257, 16th/240; 17th/ 263 (t-43.1); 18th/p 326 (t:42.1); Robbins 7th/888;*

Rotor's syndrome is an Autosomal recessive inherited disorder characterized by a defect in biliary excretion leading to conjugated hyperbilirubinemia.

Hereditary Hyperbilirubinemias Q

Unconjugated (defect conjugating enzyme bilirubin glucoronyl transferase)	Conjugated (defect in biliary excretion of conjugated bilirubin)
1. Cirgler Najjar Syndrome type I & type II Q 2. Gilberts syndrome Q	1. Dubin Johnson syndrome Q 2. Rotor's syndrome Q

Causes of Isolated Hyperbilirubinemia

Indirect hyperbilirubinemia	Direct hyperbilirubinemia
A. Hemolytic disorders 1. Inherited a. Sperocyteosis, elliptocytosis Glucose-6-phosphate dehydrogenase and pyruvate kinase deficiencies b. Sickle cell anemia 2. Acquired a. Microangiopathic hemolytic anemias b. Paraoxysmal nocturnal hemoglobinuria c. Immune hemolysis B. Ineffective erythropoesis 1. Cobalamin, folate, thalassemia, and severe iron deficiencies C. Drugs 1. Rifampicin, probenbecid, ribavirin D. Inherited conditions 1. Crigler-Najjar types I and II 2. Glibert's syndrome	A. Inherited conditions 1. Dubin-Johnson syndrome 2. Rotor's syndrome

2. **Answer is D (Dubin Johnson syndrome):** *Robbin's 7th / 888; Harrison 17th/ 263 Harrison 18th/p 326*

Dubin Johnson Syndrome results from a hereditary defect in excretion of conjugated bilirubin across the canalicular membrane and leads to conjugated hyperbilirubinemia.

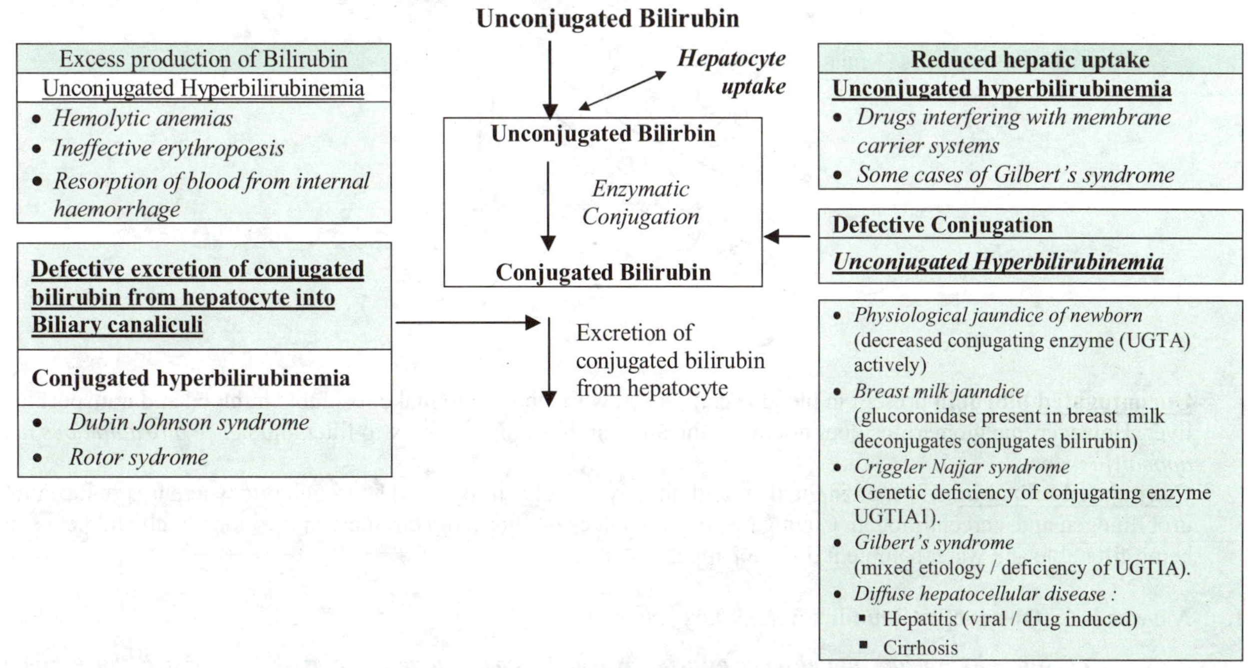

3. **Answer is C and D (Not filtered and lipophilic)**: *Harrison's 16th/240, 241, 242; 17th/262,263,264; 18th/325, 326, 327*

Normal urine does not contain bilirubin because normal blood contains bilirubin in the uncongugated form. Unconjugated bilirubin is lipid soluble or lipophilic (water insoluble) because it is transported in the blood as a complex with albumin (albumin-bilirubin complex) which is not allowed to filter through the glomerulus.

Although conjugated bilirubin is water soluble and filterable at the glomurulus, conjugated bilirubin is not present in the blood normally and hence does not filter to appear in the urine.

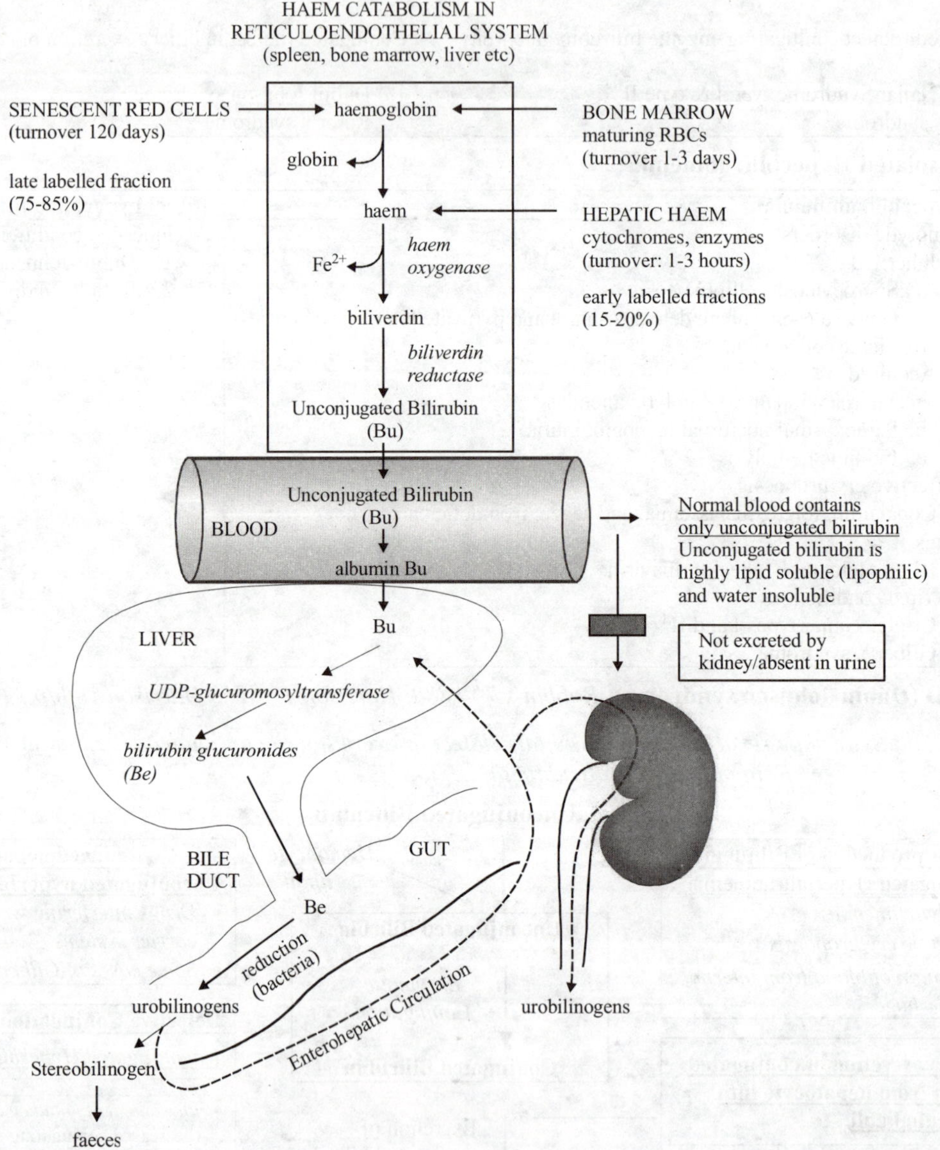

Unconjugated bilirubin present in blood is complexed with albumin to make it soluble in blood and transport it to the liver. However, the glomerulus does not allow the albumin bilirubin complex to filter and *hence bilirubin does not appear in urine*.
Conjugated bilirubin is formed in the liver and directly excreted into the GIT through bile where it is reduced to urobilinogen and stercobilinogen. Conjugated bilirubin does not normally circulate in the blood at all and hence despite being filterable and water soluble it does not appear in urine.

4. **Answer is C (Obstructive Jaundice):** *Refer text below*

Presence of Bilirubin in urine and absence of urinary urobilonogen suggests a diagnosis of obstructive jaundice.

Pathophysiology of different types of jaundice

- Normal blood contains unconjugated bilirubin only (no conjugated bilirubin)

  Unconjugated bilirubin is water insoluble (lipophilic, lipid soluble) and not filterable by the kidney.

- Unconjugated bilirubin is taken up from the systemic circulation by hepatocytes (1)
- Unconjugated bilirubin is then conjugated to bilirubin glucoronide by glucoronyl transferase within the hepatocytes(2)
- Conjugated bilirubin is then excreted into the bile from where it reaches the GIT (3)
  This is the rate limiting step.

  Conjugated bilirubin is water soluble and filterable by the kidney

  Normally, there is no conjugated bilirubin in the systemic circulation and hence no bilirubin is filtered in the kidney or present in the urine.

  Abnormally

  When there is hepatocellular dysfunction or bile flow is totally obstructed, conjugated bilirubin "leaks" into the systemic circulation This conjugated bilirubin may now be excreted by the kidney and be detected in urine.

  Bilirubin in urine (bilirubinuria)

  Presence of bilirubin in urine suggests a diagnosis of conjugated hyperbilirubinemia either due to hepatocellular jaundice or obstructive jaundice.

- Within the GIT conjugated bilirubin is degraded/reduced to urobilinogen and then to stercobilinogen

  Urobilinogen is water soluble and filterable by the kidney

  Normally, a small portion of the urobilinogen is reabsorbed from the gut and excreted by the kidney (<4 mg/day)

  In non obstructive hyperbilirubinemia (hemolytic, hepatocellular) the amount of urobilinogen exreated by the kidney is increased as more urobilinogen is formed and reabsorbed.

  Elevated levels of urobilinogen suggest primarily an non obstructive hyperbilirubinemia

  In obstructive hyperbilirubinemia, conjugated bilirubin does not reach the GIT and hence no urobilinogen is formed

  Absent levels of urobilinogen suggest a diangnosis of obstructive hyperbilirubinemia

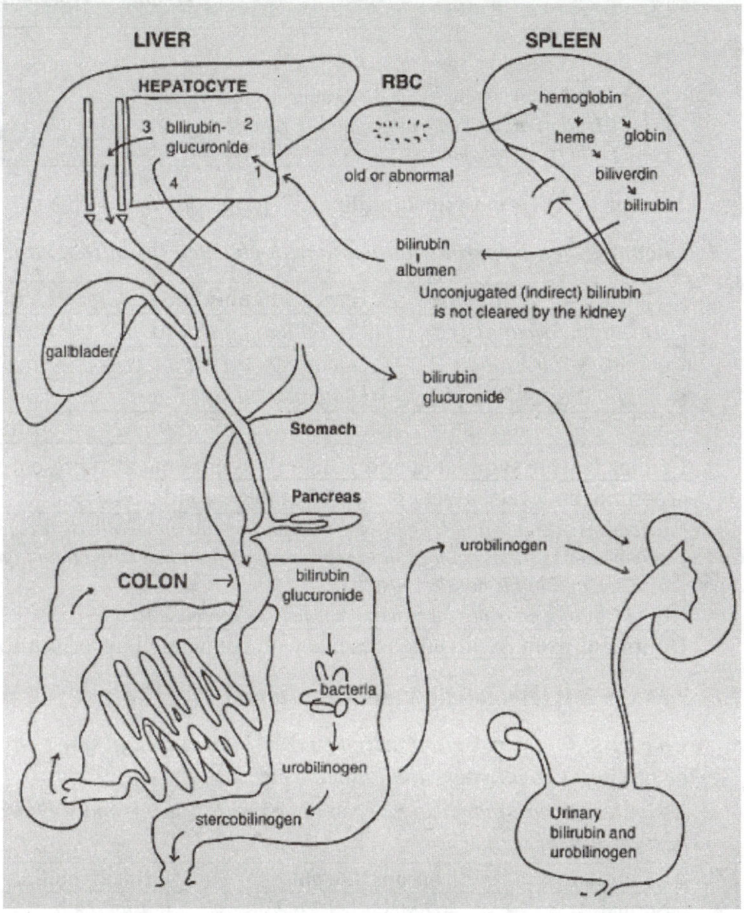

Condition	Serum Bilirubin	Urine Urobilinogen	Urine Bilirubin	Fecal urobilinogen
Normal	Direct 0.1-0.4 mg/dl Indirect 0.2-0.7 mg/dl	0-4 mg/24 h	Absent	40-280 mg/24h
Hemolytic anemia	↑ Indirect	Increased	Absent	Increased
Hepatitis	↑ Direct and indirect	Decreased if micro-obstruction is present	Present if microobstruction occurs	Decreased
Obstructive jaundice	↑ Direct	Absent	Present	Trace to absent

5. Answer is D (Dubin Johnson Syndrome): *Harrison 18th/p 325, 326 Harrison's 17th/263, 264, 262*

Dubin Johnson syndrome is associated with conjugated hyperbilirubinemia & not unconjugated hyperbilirubinemia. *Dubin Johnson Syndrome results from a hereditary defect in excretion of conjugated bilirubin across the canalicular membrane and leads to conjugated hyperbilirubinemia.*

Dubin Johnson syndrome is an inherited disorder charachterized by defective excretion of conjugated bilirubin from hepatocytes into biliary canaliculi. It thus presents with a clinical picture similar to obstructive jaundice with conjugated hyperbilirubinemia and absence of urobilinogen in urine.

Hemolytic Anemia typically presents with unconjugated hyperbilirubinemia and elevated urinary urobilinogens. **Gilberts syndrome and Crigler Najjar syndrome** also present with unconjugated hyperbilirubinemia. Urinary Urobilinogens are however not elevated in these conditions. *Urobilinogen may never the less be present in urine (N or ↓) in these conditions*

Hereditary Hyperbilirubinemias Q

Unconjugated (defect in conjugating enzyme bilirubin glucoronyl transferase)	Conjugated (defect in biliary excretion of conjugated bilirubin)
3. ***Cirgler Najjar Syndrome type I & type II*** Q	***Dubin Johnson syndrome*** Q
4. ***Gilberts syndrome*** Q	Rotor's syndrome Q

6. **Answer is A (Hemolytic Jaundice):** *Refer text below*

Unconjugated Hyperbilirubinemia with elevated urobilinogen levels of urine is characteristic of Hemolytic anemia

Condition / syndrome	Hyperbilirubinemia	Urinary Urobilinogen *(N=0-4 mg/24 hrs)*
Hemolytic Anemia	*Unconjugated (Indirect)*	*Increased*
Gilbert's syndrome	*Unconjugated (Indirect)*	*Normal or Decreased*
Crigler Najjar	*Unconjugted (Indirect)*	*Normal or Decreased*
Dubin Johnson's	*Conjugated (Direct)*	*Absent*

Crigler Najjar syndrome and Gilbert's syndrome also present with unconjugated hyperbilirubinemia, however urobilinogen levels are not increased in these conditions.

Gilberts syndrome and Crigler Najjar syndrome are enymatic disorders charachterized by defective conjugation. These disorders may present with a picture similar to hemolytic jaundice with unconjugated hyer bilirubinamia, with the following exceptions.
a. Haemoglobin is not decreased
b. *Urobilinogen is not increased (Normal or Decreased)*

Dubin Johnson Syndrome presents with conjugated hyperbilirubinemia and absent urobilinogen in urine

7. **Answer is B (Hemolytic Jaundice):** *Harper 27th/292*

Combination of increased urinary urobilinogen and absence of bilirubin in urine is suggestive of hemolytic jaundice or unconjugated hyperbilirubinemia.

A similar picture may also be seen in hepatitis but it is more charachteristic of hemolytic jaundice which is the single best answer of choice

Condition	Serum Bilirubin	Urine Urobilinogen	Urine Bilirubin	Fecal urobilinogen
Normal	Direct 0.1-0.4 mg/dl Indirect 0.2-0.7 mg/dl	0-4 mg/24 h	Absent	40-280 mg/24h
Hemolytic anemia	↑ Indirect	Increased	Absent	Increased
Hepatitis	↑ Direct and indirect	Decreased if micro-obstruction is present	Present if microobstruction occurs	Decreased
Obstructive jaundice	↑ Direct	Absent	Present	Trace to absent

8. **Answer is A (Haemolytic jaundice):** *Harrisons 15th/256, Harrison 16th/238 Read text below; Harrison 17th/ 262, 263, 264*

All findings in the question corroborate with a haemolytic picture.

- *Presence of Urobilinogen in urine rules out an obstructive cause for jaundice.*
- *Decrease in haemoglobin and elevated bilirubin levels are consistent with a haemolytic cause.*
- *Gall stones can be explained by precipitation of bilirubin (Bilirubinate crystals)*

Distinguishing features between various forms of Jaundice :

Parameter	Hemolytic	Hepatocellular	Obstructive
Blood	**Blood**	**Blood**	**Blood**
Haemoglobin (12-18 g/dl)	Decreased	N.	N.
Unconjugated bilirubin (0.2 to 0.7 mg/dl)	↑↑	N or ↑	N
Conjugated bilirubin (0.1 to 0.3 mg/dl)	N	↑	↑
Alkaline phosphatase (3-13 KAU) (30 to 120 IU/L)	N	N or ↑	↑↑
Aminotransferases	N	↑↑	N
Cholesterol	N	N	↑
Stool	**Stool**	**Stool**	**Stool**
Colour of stool	N	N	Pale
Urine	**Urine**	**Urine**	**Urine**
Bilirubin	0	↑	↑
Urobilinogen	↑	↑	↓

Note :

- **Gilberts Syndrome and Criggler Najjar syndrome:** are enzyme disorders characterized by defective conjugation.
  They thus present with a picture similar to Hemolytic with the following exceptions:
  a. Hb is not decreased
  b. Urobilinogen is not increased (N or ↓)
- **Rotor's syndrome and Dubin Johnson syndrome** are characterized by defective excretion.
  They thus present with a picture similar to obstructive with the following exceptions: Alkaline phosphatase is not raised.

9. Answer is D (Obstructive jaundice): *Harrison 15th/256; 16th/240; See previous question; Harrison 17th/ 262, 263*

The patient in question has high conjugated bilirubin levels (direct bilirubin > 50% of total bilirubin), along with alkaline phosphatase levels more than 6 times normal. The answer of choice therefore is obstructive jaundice.

Approach:

If direct conjugated bilirubin is greater than 15% of the total bilirubin, it is termed as direct bilirubinemia.

A patient presenting with direct bilirubinemia is further approached as follows:

Bilirubin	Associated parameter	Inference
Direct bilirubinemia	Alkaline phosphatase raised out of proportion to transferases (ALT/AST)	Cholestatic obstructive jaundice
Direct bilirubinemia	Transferases (ALT/AST) Raised out of proportion to alkaline phosphatase	Hepatocellular jaundice

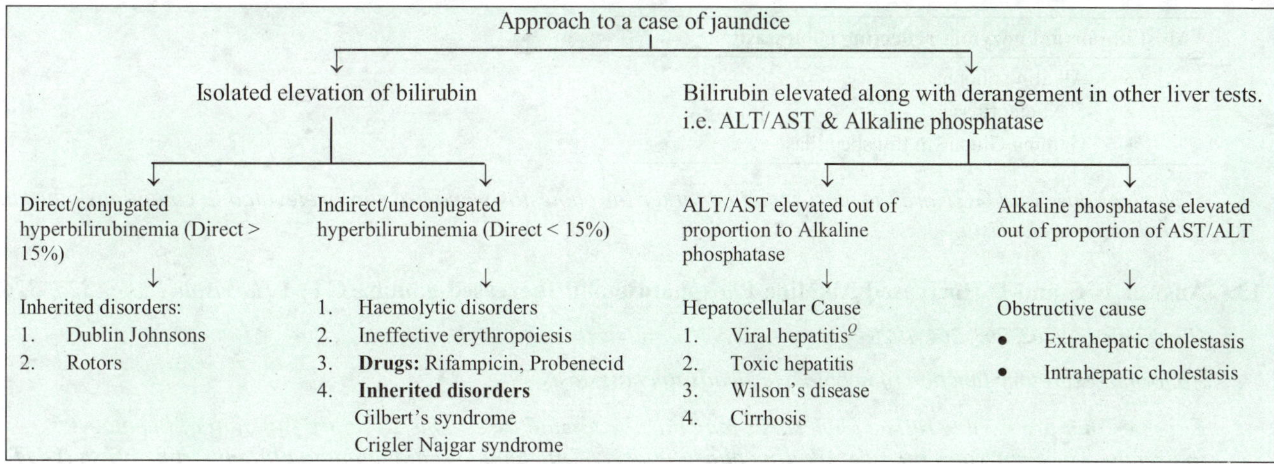

10. Answer is D (Obstructive jaundice): *Read text below; Harrisons 14th/254, 1664; 15th/256; 16th/240; 17th/ 262, 263; 18th/p 325*

Direct bilirubinemia (conjugated birirubin > 15% of total bilirubin) along with high serum alkaline phosphatase (6-7 times normal) suggests the diagnosis of obstructive jaundice.

	Normal	Patient	Inference
Total bilirubin (mg/dl)	0.3 to 1.0	21.0	Direct bilirubin is 45% of total bilirubin
Conjugated bilirubin (mg/dl)	0.1 to 0.3	9.6	**Direct bilirubinemia**
Alkaline phosphatase	3-13 KAV	84 KA	Alkaline phosphatase is raised by atleast six times:**Significant rise**

Rise in conjugated bilirubin level *may be seen with both, hepatocellular disease (Viral/ infective Hepatitis) and Obstructive jaundice but association with significantly elevated ALP limits our diagnosis to obstructive damage.*

Rise in alkaline phosphatase levels

Patient with **parenchymal disease of liver** i.e. hepatocellular disorders : *may show increase in alkaline phosphatase levels but the increase is only slight to moderate and usually not more than two times normal*

Obstructive lesion: *Striking increase in alkaline phosphatase* is more suggestive of an obstructive lesion

In the given question rise in alkaline phosphatase is about 6 to 7 times normal and thus is more in favour of an obstructive cause.

11. Answer is A, B, C (85% of the total should be indirect, Hemolytic anemia, Seen in ↑ hemoglobin destruction (↑ bilirubin production): *Harrison's 17th/262*

Unconjugated Hyperbilirubinemia is associated with > 85% indirect bilrubin or less than 15% of direct bilirubin.

Hemolytic disorders and increased hemoglobin destruction cause unconjugated or indirect hyperbilirubinemia.

Biliary atresia and neonatal hepatitis lead to conjugated hyperbilirubinemia.

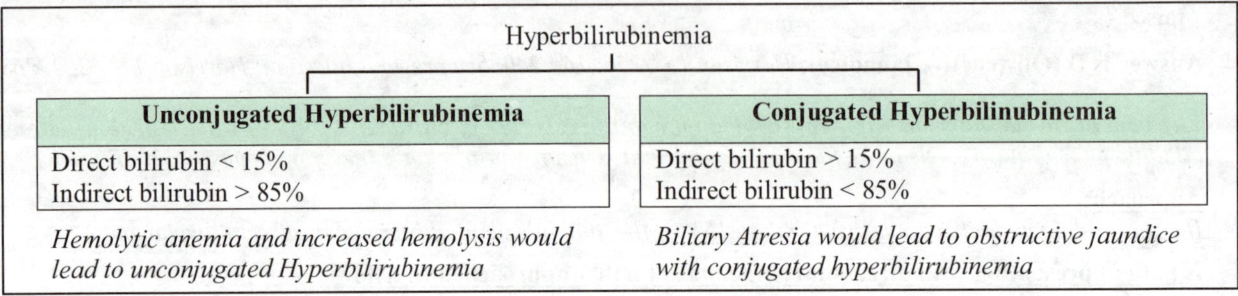

12. Answer is D (Cholestatic disorders) : *Harrison 16th/1815*

5' Nucleotidase reflects cholestasis and is rarely elevated in conditions other than liver disease.

Most important enzymes reflecting cholestasis
• Alkaline phophatase • 5' Nucleotidase • Gamma Glutanym transpeptidase

5' Nucleotidase and GGT are the most specific marker for cholestasis and are rarely elevated in conditions other than liver disease – Harrison

13. Answer is C and D (Increased Alkaline Phosphatase and Increased gamma GT) : *Harrison 18th/p 325, 326, 327 Harrison's 17th/262, 263, 264, 1925*

Abnormal excretory function of hepatocytes leads to cholestasis.

Enzymes that are used to reflect cholestasis may thus be used to assess the excretory function of hepatocytes indirectly. These enzymes include Alkaline phosphatase, 5' nucleotidase and gamma glutamy transferase (GGT)

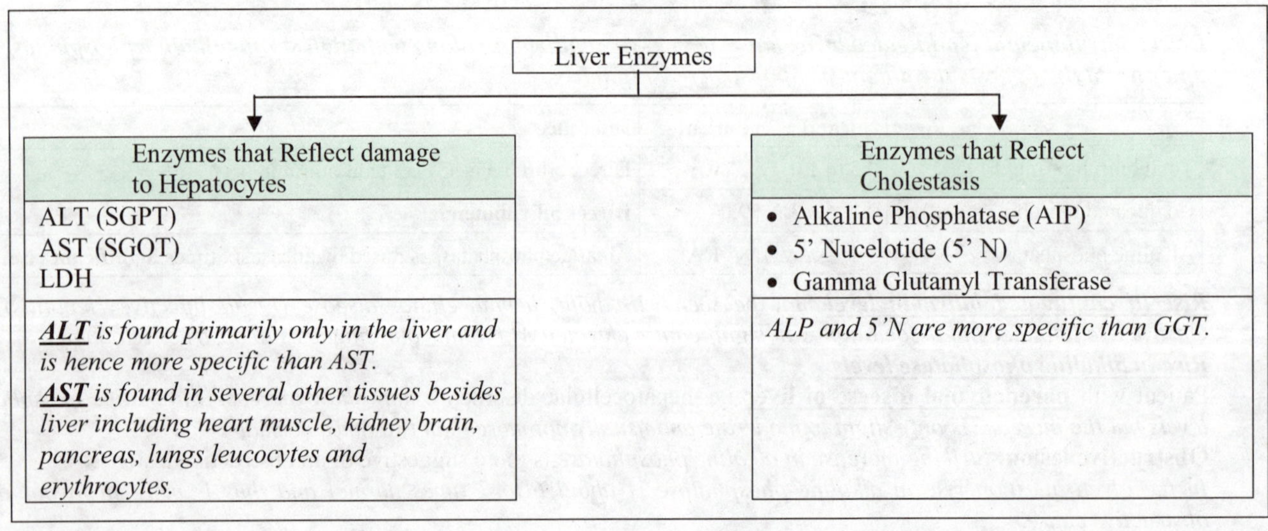

Note that true assessment of hepatic excretory function requires measurement of serum concentration of substances metabolized and transported by the liver or by determination of rate of clearance of exogenously administered dyes or drugs such as indocyanine green, caffeine, lidocaine and PABA.
Liver enzymes including those reflecting cholestasis are not true measures for detecting excretory function of hepatocytes. However, amongst the options provided these are the best answers of exclusion as they may provide an indirect assessment of excretory function of hepatocytes.

14. Answer is D (Cholestatic jaundice)

15. Answer is A (Ultrasound): *Harrisons 16th/240 (fig 38-1); see below; Harrison 17th/ 263, 264 Harrison 18th/p 325*

Initial investigation of choice in a case of obstructive jaundice is: ULTRASONOGRAPHY
The patient in question has an obstructive form of jaundice, as is indicated by marked elevation of conjugated bilirubin together with a significant rise is Alkaline phosphatase. Patient: should therefore be next subjected to ultrasonography to confirm the diagnosis and if possible locate the site of block.

Protocol for investigating a patient with cholestatic serum profile.

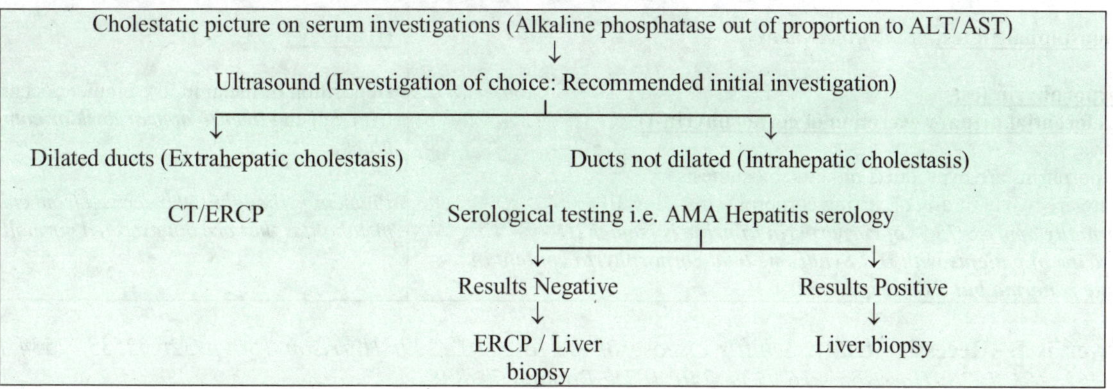

16. Answer is B (Bromsulphalein / Sulfobromophthalein) :*Harrison 16th / 1821; 17th/ 1930 Harrison 18th/p 2535, 2536*

The appearance of late rise in plasma level of Bromsulphalein, BSF / Sulfobromophthalein in the clearance of this dye has been considered as a pathognomic sign of Dubin Johnson syndrome
– Metabolism of Bromsulphalein in D-J syndrome; Digestive diseases and Sciences Vol/17 numbers 6.

Patients with D - J syndrome exhibit a characteristic rise in plasma concentration of Bromsulphalein at 90 minutes after injection due to reflux of conjugated BSP into circulation from Hepatocyte. *– Harrison*

Bromsulphalein test for Dubin Johnson syndrome : *Harrison 16th / 1821*
• *Dubin Johnson syndrome is characterized by a Familial / Autosomal Recessive defect in Hepatic excretory function (from hepatocyte to biliary canaliculi)*   • *Biliary excretion of a number of anionic compounds is compromised including that of sulfobromphthalein (Bromsulphalein, BSP), a synthetic dye (cholecystographic agent).*   • *To test for D – J syndrome, the role of disappearance of BSP from plasma is determined after its bolus intravenous administration.*   • *Patients with D - J syndrome exhibit a characteristic rise in its plasma concentration at 90 minutes after injection due to reflux of conjugated BSP into circulation from Hepatocyte. – Harrison*

Dubin Johnson Syndrome : Review

During Johnson syndrome is an ***autosomal recessive***[Q] hereditary disorder presenting with ***conjugated hyperbilirubinemia***[Q] due to ***defect in hepatic excretory function across the canalicular membrane of hepatocyte.***[Q]

Clinical presentation

- Most patient are asymptomatic (subclinical chemical hyperbilirubinemia)
- ***Unexplained low grade jaundice during teenage years Often exacerbated by :***
  - ***Oral contraceptive use***
  - Pregnancy
  - Intercurrent illness
- Physical examination is usually normal (occasional patient may have hepatosplenomegaly)

Laboratory studies

- ***Conjugated Hyperbilirubinemia*** : Total bilirubin is ***typically between 2 – 5 mg/dl*** *(34 – 85 μmol/L)*
  May occasionally be Normal or as high as 20-25 mg/dl(340-430 μmol/L)
- **Bilirubinuria** : Typically present as hyperbilirubinemia is conjugated
- ***Other Routine Liver Function Tests including Serum Transaminases and Alkaline Phosphatase are essentially Normal***

Diagnosis

Bromsulphalein test : *Elaborated above* **Corporphyrin test** **(Preferential urinary excretion of corporphyrin-I)** Corporphrins are byproducts of heme biosnthesis There are two naturally occurring corporphyrins – I & III ***Normally approx. 75 % of corporpyrin in urine is isomer III*** ***In urine of patients with D-J Syndrome total corporphyrin content in urine is norma but > 80 % is Isomer I***	**Histology :** Deposition of melanin like pigment occurs in the liver causing ***liver to appear dark or completely black***. *Pigment is thought to be derived from epinephrine metabolites that are not excreted normally*

17. Answer is B (Recessive trait): *Schiff's disease of the liver 10th/229; Harrison 18th/p 326, 2533, 2534 Harrison's 17th/262, 263, 1928; Harrison's 16th/239, 240, 1818; Robbins 7th/888*

Crigger Najjar syndrome is inherited as an autosomal recessive trait.
Crigger Najjar Syndrome (Type II) is associated with a deficient activity of Bilirubin UDP - Glucoronyl Transferase activity (UGITAL) and not with ***diglucornide deficiency****.*

Kernincterus *is a characteristic features of type I Criggler Najjar syndrome and Kernincterus is extremely rare in type II Criggler Najjar syndrome.*

Phenobarbital *is extremely effective and useful in type II Criggler Najjar syndrome and reduces bilirubin levels by > 25%.*

Principal Characteristics Criggler-Najjar Syndromes

Feature	Crigler-Najjar Syndrome	
	Type1	**Type II**
Total serum bilirubin, μmol/L (mg/dl)	310-755 (usually > 345) [18-45 (usually < 20)]	100-430 (usually <345) [6-25(usually <20)]
Routine liver tests	Normal	Normal
Response to Phenobarbital	None	Decreases bilirubin by>25%
Kernicterus	Usual	Rare
Hepatic histology	Normal	Normal
Bile characteristics		
Color	Pale or colorless	Pigmented
Bilirubin fractions monoconjugates	>90% unconjugated	Largest fraction (mean: 57%)
Bilirubin UDP-glucuronosyl-transferase	Typically absent; traces in some patients	Markedly reduced:0-10% of normal
Inheritance (all autosomal)	Recessive	Predominantly recessive

Viral Hepatitis

General

18. Answer is C (Acute viral Hepatitis): *Harrison 18th/p 2549, 2550, 2530 Harrison's 17th/1926, 1941, 1942*

Prodromal symptoms of nausea and anorexia, presence of pain in upper abdomen together with characteristic laboratory features (elevated bilirubin, elevated SGOT and SGPT>500 with SGPT > SGOT, and elevated alkaline phosphates to < 3 times normal) suggest the diagnosis of viral hepatitis.

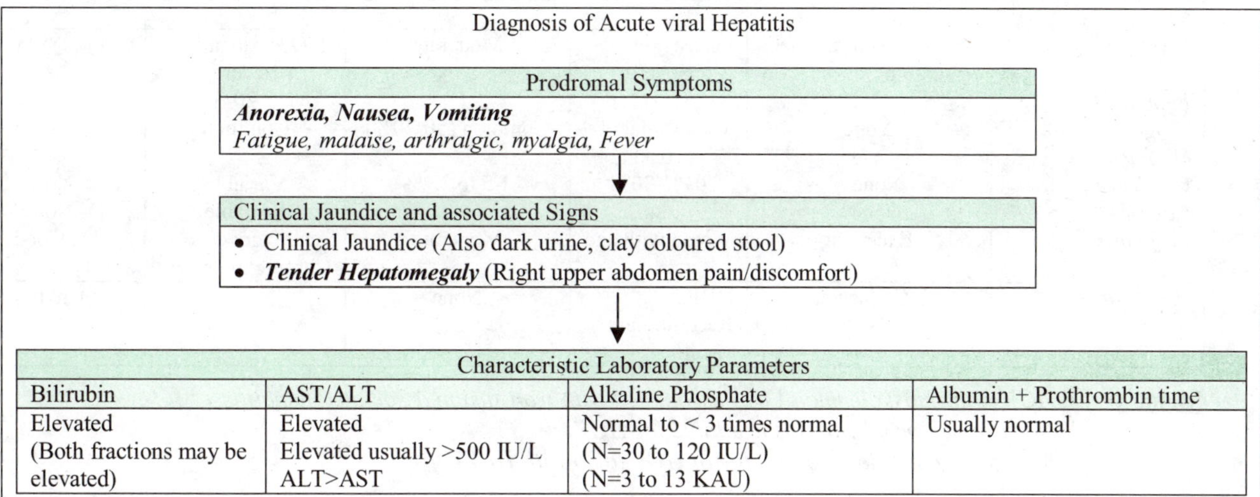

Characteristic Laboratory Parameters			
Bilirubin	AST/ALT	Alkaline Phosphate	Albumin + Prothrombin time
Elevated (Both fractions may be elevated)	Elevated Elevated usually >500 IU/L ALT>AST	Normal to < 3 times normal (N=30 to 120 IU/L) (N=3 to 13 KAU)	Usually normal

Note:

ALT is synonymous with SGPT[Q]

AST is synonymous with SGOT[Q]

19. Answer is C (Acute viral Hepatitis): *Robbins 7th/899; 'Pathology' by wolf (1998)/572*

Councilman bodies are acidophilic /eosinophilic apoptotic bodies seen in Acute Viral hepatitis and represent irreversible hepatocyte damage.

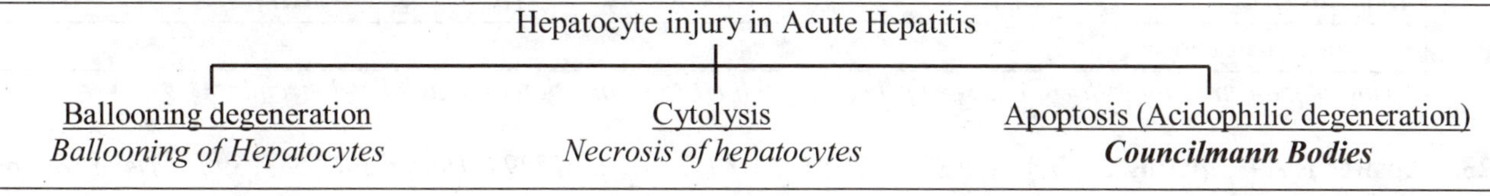

20. Answer is D (HCV): *Harrison 15th/1728; Harrisons 16th/ 1849, 1829; 17th/ 1945, 1939 Harrison 18th/p 2553, 2546*

Most common hepatitis to progress to chronicity is Hepatitis C.

'Chronic hepatitis follows acute hepatitis in 50-70% of cases. Even in hose with a return to normal in AST/ALT levels after acute hepatitis C, chronic infection is common adding upto 85-90% likelihood of chronic HCV infection after acute hepatitis C.' – Harrison 16th/ 1849

Parameter	HAV	HBV	HCV	HDV	HEV
Progression to chronicity	None	Occasional (1-10%)	Common (50-70%)	*Common	None

** In acute HBV/HDV co infection, the frequency of chronicity is the same as that for HBV. In HDV superinfection chronicity is variable*

Clinical and epidemiologic features of viral hepatitis:

Features	HAV	HBV	HCV	HDV	HEV
Incubation (days)	15-45	30-180	15-160	30-180	14-60
Age	Children, young Adults	Young adults	Any age but more in adult	Any age	Young adults
Transmission					
Fecal-oral	+++	---	---	---	+++
Percutaneous	Unusual	+++	+++	+++	---
Perinatal	---	+++	+	+	---
Sexual	+	++	+	++	---
Clinical					
Severity	Mild	Occasionally Severe	Moderate	Occasionally Severe	Mild
Fulminant	.1%	.1%-1%	.1%	5-20%	1-2%
Progression to chronicity	None	Occasional (1-10%)	Common (50-70%)	Common	None
Carrier	None [Q]	01%-30%	1.5 to 3.2%	Variable	None [Q]
Cancer	None [Q]	+nt	+nt	Variable	None [Q]
Prognosis	Excellent	Worse with age	Moderate	Acute: good Chronic: poor	Good
Prophylaxis	IgG Vaccine	HBIG Recombinant vaccine	None	-	Unknown

Memo : [Q] *HCV is the most common Virus associated with transfusion associated hepatitis*
[Q] *No vaccine / prophylaxis is available for HCV*
[Q] *Malignant potential is present with HCV (also with HBV)*

21. **Answer is B and C (Hepatitis B and Hepatitis C) :** *Repeat*

Progression to chronicity is seen with hepatitis B and Hepatitis C

22. **Answer is C (Hepatitis B):** *Harrison's 15th/ 1748; Harrisons 16th/1829 t; Harrison 17th/ 1939 Harrison 18th/p 2546*

Perinatal transmission is most significant with hepatitis B

Perinatal transmission of various Hepatitis viruses as described in Harrison's Text:

Hepatitis virus	HAV	HBV	HCV	HDV	HEV
Perinatal transmission	-	+++	-	+	-

Perinatal transmission with HCV is seen primarily with HIV co-infection and high level viremia

23. **Answer is A (Hepatitis E):** *Harrison's 14th/ 1684; 15th/ 1728 t; 16th/1829 t; Harrison 17th/ 1939 Harrison 18th/p 2546*

Hepatitis B, C and D are essentially spread by parenteral routes.
Hepatitis A & E are non parenteral hepatitis.

24. **Answer is D (LKM2 – Chronic Hepatitis D):** *Harrison's 17th/1968; 'Hepatobiliary Tract & Pancreas' by Reddy (Mosby) 1st (2004)/145; 'Self Assessment Colour Review of Hepatobiliary Medicine' 1st/150 (Q144)*

Hepatitis D is associated with Anti LKM3 Antibodies and not Anti LKM2 antibodies

Anti-Liver Kidney Microsomal Antibodies (anti-LKM antibodies)

*Anti-**L**iver **K**idney **M**icrosomal (LKM) antibodies* are detected in the sera of patients with different types of acute or chronic liver disease.

These antibodies are target against *Cytochrome P-450 components (antigens)*

Three types of LKM antibodies have been most extensively studied

Microsomal Antibodies	Antigen	Disease
Anti-LKM1	Cytochrome P450 2D6	• ***Autoimmune Hepatitis type II*** • ***Chronic Hepatitis C (10%)***
Anti-LKM2	Cytochrome P450 2C9	• ***Drug induced Hepatitis*** (Tienilic acid induced Hepatitis)
Anti-LKM3	Cytochrome P450 1A2	• ***Chronic Hepatitis D***

25. Answer is D (HDV super-infection on HBV): *Harrison's 18th/2552*

HDV superinfection of a person with chronic Hepatitis B (HBV) has the worst prognosis with high likelihood of fulminant hepatitis and death.

'Among patients ill enough to be hospitalized for acute hepatitis B infection the case fatality rate is 1%. Patients with simultaneous acute hepatitis B and hepatitis D do not necessarily experience a higher mortality rate than do patients with acute hepatis B alone, however in several recent outbreaks of acute simultaneous HBV and HDV infection amongst injection drug users the case fatality rate has been ~ 5%. ***In the case of HDV super infection of a person with chronic hepatitis B, the likelihood of fulminant hepatitis and death is increased substantially. In out breaks of severe HDV super infection in isolated populations with a high hepatitis B carrier state the mortality has been recorded in excess of 20%*** *- Harrison's 18th/2552*

Prognosis in HBV Infection
Acute HBV infection ≤ simultaneous HBV – HDV confection << HDV super-infection on HBV infection *(Best prognosis)* *(worst prognosis)*

Hepatitis B

26. Answer is B (IgM antibody to Hb_c Ag): *Read text below; Various texts; Harrison 18th/p 2550, 2551, 2539, 2540; Harrison 17th/ 1933, 1934, 1943, 1944*

Acute infection is best indicated by an IgM anti Hb_c Ag.

Serology of Hepatitis B

	HBSAg	Anti HBsAg	HBe Ag	Anti HBeAg	Anti HBcAg
Acute HBV (with high infectivity)	+	-	+		IgM
Acute HBV (with low infectivity)	+	-		+	IgM
Chronic HBV (High infectivity)	+	-	+		IgG
Chronic HBV (low infectivity)	+	-		+	IgG

Hbs Ag would be positive even in chronic infection and hence cannot be used to establish a diagnosis of acute Hepatitis B infection.

Hbs Ag	Anti Hbs Ag
Indicates that the person is infected with the virus. The infection may manifest as 'disease' either acute or chronic, or be just present as in carrier state Hbs Ag thus indicated as possible: - Acute disease - Chronic disease - Carrier state	With the development of antibody to Hbs Ag i.e. Anti Hbs Ag, the Hbs Ag antigen disappears from the serum - Patient is immune (with immunization Antibody develops and Hbs Ag disappears) - Patient is protected Anti Hbs Ag indicates good immunity [Q] Anti Hbs Ag indicates protection against Hepatitis B [Q]
Hbc Ag	**Anti Hbc Ag**
It is a hidden component of the viral core and is not detectable at all	Antibodies to Hbc Ag develop early in the course of disease Anti Hbc Ag is the first antibody to appear after an acute infection and persists in serum even during the recovery phase - When acute antibody is of IgM type - When chronic antibody is of IgG type
Hbe Ag	**Anti Hbe Ag**
Denotes high infectivity [Q] and active disease	Denotes low infectivity

Window period is a period during recovery phase when both of these are negative and the diagnosis may be missed if test includes only Hbs Ag and Anti Hbs Ag.

27. Answer is C (Histopathology): *Textbook of pathology by Dutta (Jaypee) 2nd/755; 'Biopsy Interprelation of Liver' by Geller & Petrovic (Lippincott Williams) 2nd/108*

Chronic Active Hepatitis and Chronic Persistant Hepatitis (CPH) are histopathological classification systems for various forms of chronic hepatitis based on findings on biopsy specimens. *This classification system is however obsolete now and should not be used.*

Histopathological Classification of Chronic Hepatitis

Chronic Active Hepatitis (Periportal or Interface Hepatitis)	Chronic Persistant Hepatitis (Portal Hepatitis)
Chronic Hepatitis with histopathological features suggesting a progressive course **Biopsy Features** • *Hepatic architecture is distorted* • *Inflammation extends beyond the portal tract (Portal tract infiltration is common with early portal tract fibrosis)* • *Lamina Limitans is breached and hepatic lobules are invaded* • *Piecemeal necrosis & bridging necrosis is typically seen in Lobules*	Chronic Hepatitis with histopathological features suggesting a beingn and self limiting course **Biopsy Features** • *Hepatic architecture is maintained* • *Inflammation is limited to portal tracts (Portal tract infiltration is typical but portal tract fibrosis is minimal)* • *Minimal/No breach of Lamina Limitans* • *Minimal /No Piecemeal necrosis or Bridging necrosis in Lobules*

28. Answer is D (Fecal-oral route): *Harrison's 18th/2546*

Hepatitis B is not transmitted through fecal-oral route (stool).

Transmission of Viral Hepatitis:

Feature	HAV	HBV	HCV	HDV	HEV
Transmission					
Fecal-oral	+++	–	–	–	+++
Percutaneous	Unusual	+++	+++	+++	–
Perinatal	–	+++	±	+	–
Sexual	±	++	±	++	–

29. Answer is D (90%): *Harrison's 18th/2547*

The rate of perinatal transmission of hepatitis B (HBV) essentially depends on the presence or absence of HBe Ag and viral replication. The rate of perinatal transmission of HBV may be as high as 90% in neonates born to mothers who are positive for HBe AG.

'The likelihood of perinatal transmission of HBV correlates with the presence of HBe Ag and high level viral replication. ***90% of HBe Ag positive mothers*** *but only 10-15% of Anti-HBe Ag negative mothers transmit HBV to their offspring' - Harrison's 18th/2547*

'Transmission of infection from an HBV carrier mother to her neonate accounts for the majority of new infections in the world today. Sixty to 90% of Hepatitis B surface antigen (HBs Ag) positive mothers who are Hepatitis B 'e' antigen (HBe Ag) positive transmit the disease to their offspring, whereas mothers who are positive for antibody to HBe Ag (Anti - HBe) do so less frequently (15-20%). - Sleisenger & Fordtran's Gastrointestinal & Liver Disease 8th/1647

30. Answer is A (HBs Ag): *Harrison 14th/ 1679, Harrison 15th/ 1721; Harrison 16th/1825; Harrison 17th/ 1933, 1934, 1943 Harrison 18th/p 2539, 2550, 2551*

The earliest marker appearing in serum in acute Hepatitis B infection is HBs Ag.

- ***After infection the first virological marker detectable in serum is – HBsAg ^{Q} – Harrisons 16th***
  - it precedes elevation of serum aminotransferases as well as clinical symptoms. ^{Q}
  - it remains elevated during the entire icteric or symptomatic phase of acute hepatitis B & beyond. ^{Q}

  Anti Hbs Ag appears only after Hbs Ag has disappeared (occasionally after a gap of several weeks).
- **IgM Anti HBcAg** is demonstrable in serum *beginning within 1-2 weeks after the appearance of HBsAg.* ^{Q} HBcAg is sequestrated and not detectable routinely in the serum. ^{Q}
- **Anti HBe Ag** appears shortly before disappearance of Hbs Ag. HBeAg appear concurrently or shortly after HBsAg ^{Q}. This too is detectable during the acute phase.

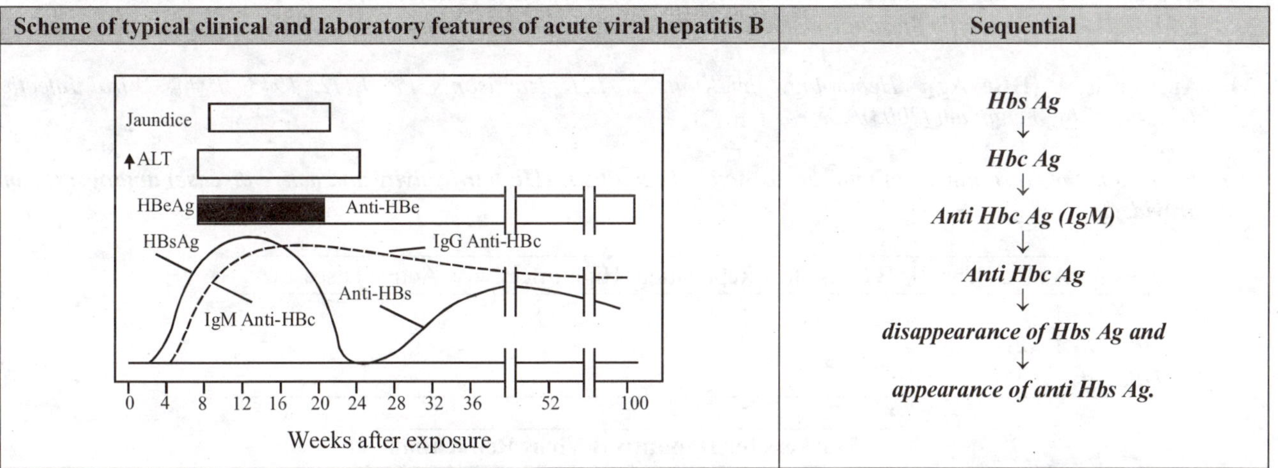

31. Answer is B (Presence of IgM anti-HBc in serum): *Harrison 16th/ 1833; 17th/ 1933, 1934 Harrison 18th/p 2539, 2540*

Although Hbs Ag is the earliest virological marker in serum of patients with acute viral hepatitis B, it does not help in establishing the diagnosis of acute Hepatitis B infection. *This is so because presence of Hbs Ag only denotes the fact that the patient is a carrier of the above infection and such a patient may well be a case of chronic hepatitis B.*

It is the presence of IgM anti HBc that confirms an acute hepatitis B infection.

Diagnostic interpretation	HBs Ag	IgM Anti HBc
Acute hepatitis B infection	+	+
Chronic Hepatitis B infection	+	-
Acute Hepatitis B infection (Below Hbs Ag detection threshold)	-	+

As is evident from the above chart, ***the basis of diagnosis of acute Hepatitis B infection is either presence of both Hbs Ag & anti HBc IgM or only IgM anti HBc. Presence of HBs Ag alone cannot be used in establishing the diagnosis of acute hepatitis B infection.***

32. Answer is A (IgM Anti HBc Antibody): *Harrison 18th/2539, 2540, 2544 Harrison's 17th/1938, 1934, 1943; Harrison's 16th/1823, 1824, 1833; Hepatology Principles and Practice by Kuntz 2nd /117*

IgM Anti HBc Antibody is the most reliable marker of acute HBV infection

IgM Anti HBc Antibody is known to be the most reliable marker of an acute HBV infection since it is detectable even during the so called serological gap and is charachteristically absent in chronic infections (IgG HBc Antibody is present in chronic infections)-Hepatology: Principles and Practice' 2nd/117

	HBsAg	HBeAg	IgM anti-HBc	IgG anti-HBc	Anti-HBs	Anti-HBe	HBVDNA	Interpretation
Acute HBV	+	+	+		-		+++	Early phase
Infection	-	-	+		-	+	+	Window phase
	-	-	-	+	+	+	±	Recovery phase
Chronic HBV	+	-	-	+	-	+	±	Inactive carrier state
Infection	+	-	-	+	-	+	++	HBeAg-chronic hepatitis
	+	+	-	+	-	-	+++	HBeAg+chronic hepatitis

HbsAg, hepatitis B surface antigen;**HBeAg**, hepatitis B e antigen;**IgM**, immunoglobulin M;**anti-HBc**, hepatitis B core Antibody; **IgG**, immunoglobulin G; **anti-HBs**, hepatitis B surface antibody; **anti-HBe**, hepatitis B e antibody

33. Answer is C (IgM anti-HBc): *Harrison 16th/1832, 1833; 17th/ 1932, 1933, 1935; 18th/2538, 2539, 2540, 2541*

Hbs Ag is present in recent hepatitis B infection but it ***is not specific to acute infection*** (*it may also be seen in carriers*). ***IgM anti- HBc is specific for acute or recent hepatitis, and hence is the answer of choice.***

34. Answer is A (HBe Ag): *'Hepatology' by Kuntz 3rd/121; Harrison's 17th/1942, 1943, 1944; 'Viral Infections & Treatment' by Weigmann (2003)/225*

HBe Ag is the most important marker for Active Hepatitis B (High infectivity and active disease) amongst the options provided.

Markers for Active Hepatitis B (Persistent Replication; High Infectivity: Active Disease)
• *HBV DNA* • *HBV DNA polymerase* • *HBe Ag*

Markers for Hepatitis B Virus Replication

HBV DNA	HBV DNA Polymerase	HBe Ag levels
• ***HBV DNA is the most sensitive and specific marker of virus replication*** • HBV DNA may provide both, a qualitative and quantitative estimate of virus replication • *HBV DNA estimation as a measure of virus replication has largely replaced the determination of DNA polymerase* • ***The Gold standard for confirmation of viral replication is HBV DNA detection***	• ***HBV DNA polymerase is considered the traditional marker active viral replication*** • HBV DNA polymerase activity usually parallel's serum HBV DNA levels • Both HBV DNA and HBV DNA polymerase are markers for the complete virion.	• ***HBeAg is considered a convenient and readily detectable qualitative marker of HBV replication and relative infectivity*** *The HBe Ag if detectable is considered a marker for active viral replication, but the lack of HBe Ag does not exclude viral replication*

35. Answer is D (AST & ALT) : *'Hepatology' by Kuntz 3rd/121; Harrison's 17th/1942, 1943, 1944; Harrison 18th/p 2549, 2550, 2551, 2552 'Viral Infections & Treatment' by Weigmann (2003)/225*

AST & ALT levels are not considered markers for active viral replication

HBV DNA, HBV DNA polymerase and HBeAg levels are all considered markers for active viral replication, with HBV DNA being the most sensitive marker (gold standard)

Markers for Hepatitis B Virus Replication

HBV DNA	HBV DNA Polymerase	HBe Ag levels
• ***HBV DNA is the most sensitive and specific marker of virus replication*** • HBV DNA may provide both, a qualitative and quantitative estimate of virus replication • *HBV DNA estimation as a measure of virus replication has largely replaced the determination of DNA polymerase* • ***The Gold standard for confirmation of viral replication is HBV DNA detection***	• ***HBV DNA polymerase is considered the traditional marker active viral replication*** • HBV DNA polymerase activity usually parallel's serum HBV DNA levels • Both HBV DNA and HBV DNA polymerase are markers for the complete virion.	• ***HBeAg is considered a convenient and readily detectable qualitative marker of HBV replication and relative infectivity*** *The HBe Ag if detectable is considered a marker for active viral replication, but the lack of HBe Ag does not exclude viral replication*

36. Answer is A (HBV DNA): *Refer previous question*

HBV DNA is the most sensitive marker of active Hepatitis B virus replication

'HBV DNA is the most sensitive marker of virus replication. The detection of HBV DNA as the most sensitive marker of virus replication end as such proof of infectivity has replaced the determination of DNA polymerase'

– 'Hepatology' by Kuntz 3rd/121

'The gold standard for confirmation of viral replication is qualitative HBV DNA detection'

– 'Viral Infections & Treatment' by Weigmann (2003)/225

Markers for HBV Replication
HBV DNA^Q > HBV DNA polymerase^Q > HBe Ag^Q

37. Answer is A and D (HBsAg and IgM anti – HBc) : *Harrison 18th/p 2550 Harrisons 17th/1943*

Acute Hepatitis B is characteristically diagnosed by the presence of IgM anti HBc with HBs Ag. Presence of IgM anti HBc without HBs Ag may suggest acute hepatitis in the window period.

HbsAg	Anti-HBs	Anti-HBc	HBeAg	Anti-HBe	Interpretation
+	-	***IgM***	+	-	Acute Hepatitis B, high infectivity
-	-	***IgM***	+/-	+/-	1. Acute Hepatitis B 2. Anti—HBc "window"

38. Answer is None: *Harrison 18th/p 2550, 2551 Harrison's 17th/1944, 1943; Harrison's 16th/1823, 1824*

The next best investigation to confirm the diagnosis of acute hepatitis B infection should be serological measurement of IgM anti, HBc antibody, which is not provided amongst the options (probably HBc Ag has been misprinted as HBeAg) ***Neither of the options provided (HBeAg, Anti HbeAg, antiHBeAg (Igm) or HBV DNA) can confirm a diagnosis of Acute Hepatitis.***

39. Answer is B (Acute hepatitis B infection with high infectivity): *Harrisons 16th/1832, 1833; Harrison 17th/ 1935, 1942, 1943, 1944 Harrison 18th/p 2540, 2550, 2551*

Presence of Anti HB IgM and Hbs Ag indicates acute infection. Presence of Hbe Ag indicates high infectivity

40. Answer is B (HBV pre-core mutant): *Harrison 18th/p 2541, 2542 Harrison's 17th/1935, 1936; 'Blueprints Pocket Gastroenterology' by Grover (Lippincott-Williams) 1st (2007)/115*

Evidence of chronic active hepatitis B (suggested by elevated liver enzymes) in a patients with detectable HBV DNA but negative HBe Ag suggests a diagnosis of precore mutant chronic hepatitis B

6

Liver and Biliary Tract

Precore mutant chronic hepatitis B

- Precore mutant form of chronic hepatitis B represents an infection with a molecular variant of the hepatitis B virus that results in an *unusual serologic – clinical profile*.
- ***Such patients have severe chronic hepatitis B infection with detectable HBV DNA levels, but HBe Ag antigen is typically negative***
- This *results from an infection with an HBV mutant that contains an alteration in the precore regions rendering the virus incapable of encoding HBe Ag*
- Patients with such mutations in the precore region are unable to secrete HBe Ag, have a negative HBe Ag phenotype but *tend to have severe liver disease that progresses more rapidly to cirrhosis*
- *Characteristic of such HBe Ag negative (precore mutant) chronic hepatitis B are lower levels of HBV DNA ($\leq 10^5$ copies /ml) and one of several patterns of aminotransferase activity – persistent elevation, periodic fluctuation above the normal range and periodic fluctuations between the normal and elevated range*
- *HBe Ag negative chronic hepatitis B with mutation in the pre-core region is now the most frequently encountered form of hepatitis B in the Mediterranean countries and in Europe.*

	HBs Ag	Anti HBs Antibody	Anti HBc Antibody	HBe Ag	Anti HBe Antibody	HBV DNA
Acute Hepatitis B (early)	+	-	-	+	-	+
Acute Hepatitis B (window period)	+	-	IgM	+	-	+/-
Acute Hepatitis B (recovery)	+	+	IgG	-	+	-
Chronic Hepatitis B, high replication	+	-	IgG	+	-	+
Chronic Hepatitis B, low/non-replicative phase	+	-	IgG	-	+	-
Chronic Hepatitis B Precore Mutant	+	-	IgG	-	+	+
Chronic Hepatitis B inactive carrier	+	-	IgG	-	+/-	Low-level +
Chronic hepatitis B reactivation	+	-	IgM	+	-	+
Hepatitis B vaccine	-	+	-	-	-	-

41. Answer is A (Inactive HBV carrier): *Harrison 18th/p 2550, 2551 Harrison's 17th/1943; 'Blue Prints Pocket Gastroenterology' by Grover (Lippincott) 1st (2007) /114; Hepatitis B Research Advances' by Willis (2007) /12*

Absence of clinical signs and symptoms of liver damage and normal liver enzymes in an HBs Ag positive individual with otherwise unremarkable serological tests suggests a diagnosis of Inactive HBV carrier state.

'An inactive hepatitis B carrier is defined as one with HBs Ag in serum but without HBe Ag with normal liver function tests and with low/ undetectable levels of HBV DNA ($< 10^3$-10^4 virions/ml) - 'Blue Prints Pocket Gastroenterology' by Grover (Lippincott Williams) 1st (2007) /114

Chronic Hepatitis B carriers (*HBs Ag + ve with IgG Anti HBc*)

Chronic Hepatitis B virus carriers can be divided into two categories based on activity of the virus and evidence of liver damage

Inactive HBs Ag Carrier state

- Patients with negligible virus replication (HBV DNA levels $\leq 10^3$ virions/ml) and /or no clinical signs and symptoms of liver damage and normal liver enzyme levels are characterized as inactive HBV carriers *Inactive HBV carriers harbor Hepatitis B virus antigen (HBs Ag), but are clinically asymptomatic, have a normal physical examination with normal liver enzymes (AST & ALT). HBe Ag is typically negative and levels of HBV DNA are less than 10^3-10^4 virions/ml*
- Such patients have minimal (if any) liver inflammation or damage, and usually live a normal life. However compared to the general population these patients remain at risk for hepatocellular carcinoma
- Treatment is currently not recommended for Inactive HBV carrier. However *regular observation is advised* as there is a risk for reactivation of virus.

Chronic Hepatitis B (Active)

- Patients with active virus replication (HBV DNA levels > 10^3 -10^4 virions/ml) and /or clinical signs and symptoms of liver damage or elevated liver enzyme levels are characterized as chronic hepatitis B patients.
- Depending on the presence or absence of HBe Ag two type of chronic (active) hepatitis B may be identified.

HBe Ag positive chronic hepatitis B

These HBs Ag positive, individuals are also positive for HBe Ag and show detectable HBV DNA levels. Such patients are in the replicative phase of chronic hepatitis B infection, have persistently or intermittently elevated liver enzymes and liver biopsy results typically reveals inflammation and damage

Patients with chronic (active) hepatitis B may become inactive (relatively non replicative) over time (rate of ~10 % per year) by becoming negative for HBe Ag and HBV DNA (HBV DNA < 10^3 - 10^4) virions/ml) Liver injury tend to subside in such patients and these may then be characterized as 'inactive carriers'

HBe Ag negative chronic hepatitis B (Precore mutant)

Such HBs Ag positive individuals are negative for HBe Ag but show detectable HBV DNA levels. Such patients are also in the replicative phase of chronic hepatitis B (despite negative HBe Ag) and have persistently or intermittently elevated liver enzymes and liver biopsy results typically reveal severe inflammation and damage

Negative HBe Ag Status *results from a mutant strain of hepatitis B that is characterized by the failure of the virus to make the hepatitis B 'e' antigen (HBe Ag)*. This mutation is called the ***'precore' mutation*** as it prevents the translation of a precore protein to prevent HBe antigen production.
This mutation does not however affect the ability of the virus to replicate

42. **Answer is A (DNA polymerase):** *Current Diagnosis and Treatment in Infectious Diseases 1st/437*

DNA polymerase is a marker for active viral replication.
DNA polymerase are usually associated with Acute viral hepatitis B when there is active viral replication and hence DNA polymerase is the single best answer amongst the options provided

Note that although DNA polymerase is often present in acute Hepatitis B infection, its presence suggests active virus replication (like HbeAg, HBV DNA) and it should not be used as a laboratory marker for acute hepatitis B infection.

'During the acute episode of disease when there is active viral replication large amounts of HBsAg and Hepatic B virus DNA can be detected in the serum as can fully developed virions and high levels of DNA polymerase and HBeAg'-*Current Diagnosis and Treatment in Infections Disease/437*

43. Answer is A (IgM against core antigen): *Harrison's 16th/1832; Pathology by Wolf (1998)/582*

IgM antibody against core antigen is a diagnostic of an acute infection with hepatitis B virus. IgM antibodies against core antigen are characteristically absent in patients with chronic hepatitis B.
(Absent in both forms of chronic hepatitis, namely, chronic active hepatitis and chronic persistent hepatitis)

Chronic Hepatitis

Chronic Persistent Hepatitis
(Low infectivity; HBeAg-ve chronic Hepatitis)

HBsAg	+ve
HBeAg	-ve
IgM HBc	-ve
HBV DNA	+ve

Chronic Active Hepatitis
High infectivity; HBeAg+ve chronic Hepatits

HBsAg	+ve
HBeAg	+ve
IgM Anti HBc	-ve
IgG Anti HBc	+ve
HBV DNA	+ve

44. Answer is D (Immunized person with hepatitis B vaccine): *Harrison, 15th/1731; 16th/1832 See previous question; Harrison 17th/ 1943 Harrison 18th/p 2550*

Isolated Anti-HBs Ag is seen in immunization with HBs Ag.

Commonly Encountered Serologic Patterns of Hepatitis B Infection:

HBsAg	Anti-HBs	Anti-HBc	HBeAg	Anti-HBe	Interpretation
+	–	IgM	+	–	Acute hepatitis B, high infectivity
+	–	IgG	+	–	Chronic hepatitis B, high infectivity
+	–	IgG	–	+	Late acute or chronic hepatitis B, low infectivityHBeAg–negative ("precore–mutant") hepatitis B (chronic or, rarely, acute)
+	+	+	+/–	+/–	1. HBsAg of one subtype and heterotypic anti–HBs (common) 2. Process of seroconversion from HBsAg to anti– HBs (rare)
–	–	IgM	+/–	+/–	1. Acute hepatitis B 2. Anti–HBc "window"
–	–	IgG	–	+/–	1. Low–level hepatitis B carrier 2. Hepatitis B in remote past
–	+	IgG	–	+/–	Recovery from hepatitis B
–	+	–	–	–	1. Immunization with HBsAg (after vaccination) 2. Hepatitis B in the remote past (?) 3. False–positive

45. Answer is A (Vaccination): *Harrison 18th/p 2550 Harrison 17th/1943*

Isolated Anti-HBs Ag in serum is seen in immunization with HBs Ag.

Possible Causes of Isolated Anti-HBsAg Positivity in serum (Other markers negative)
• Immunization with HBsAg (after vaccination) • Hepatitis B in the remote past (?) • False-positive

46. Answer is D (Anti-HBs Ag): *Harrison 17th /1943; Harrison's 18th/2550*

Anti-HBsAg is the only serological marker to appear after immunization with hepatitis vaccine.

Diagnostic interpretation	Hbs Ag	Anti Hbs	Anti HBc	Hbc Ag	Anti Hbe
Immunization with Hbs Ag (? Hepatitis B is remote past) (? False positive)	-	+	-	-	-

Isolated Anti-HBs Ag in serum is seen in immunization with HBs Ag.

Possible Causes of Isolated Anti-HBsAg Positivity in serum (Other markers negative)
• *Immunization with HBsAg (after vaccination)* • *Hepatitis B in the remote past (?)* • *False-positive*

47. Answer is A (Anti-HBc): *Harrison's 18th/2550*

IgM type Anti HBc may be the only serological marker during window period of Hepatitis B.

Presence of IgM Anti-HBc without HBs Ag may suggest acute hepatitis B in the window period.

HbsAg	Anti-HBs	Anti-HBc	HBeAg	Anti-HBe	Interpretation
+	-	***IgM***	+	-	Acute Hepatitis B, high infectivity
-	-	***IgM***	+/-	+/-	1. Acute Hepatitis B 2. Anti—HBc "window"

Occasionally a gap of several weeks or longer may separate the disappearance of HBsAg and the appearance of Anti-HBs after an acute infection with Hepatitis B virus. During this 'gap' or 'window' period, presence of Anti-HBc may represent the only serological evidence of current or recent HBV infection

48. Answer is D (IgM anti HBe): *Harrisons 16th/ 1833; 17th/1934, 1935, 1942, 1943, 1944; 18th/2539, 2540, 2550, 2551*

If a clinical diagnosis of acute viral hepatitis (of any type) is suspected, the patient should undergo the following four serological tests.

1. **HBsAg** – *To detect hepatitis B infection*
2. **IgM Anti HBc** – *To detect whether the hepatitis B infection is acute or chronic.*
3. **IgM Anti HAV** – *To establish the presence of acute hepatitis A infection.*
4. **Anti HCV** - *To establish the presence of acute hepatitis C infection.*

Simplified Diagnostic Approach in Patients Presenting with Acute Hepatitis - *Harrison*

HbsAg	IgM Anti-HAV	IgM Anti-HBc	Anti-HCV	Diagnostic Interpretation
+	-	+	-	Acute hepatitis B
+	-	-	-	Chronic hepatitis B
+	+	-	-	Acute hepatitis A superimposed on chronic hepatitis B
+	+	+	-	Acute hepatitis A and B
-	+	+	-	Acute hepatitis A and B (HBs Ag below detection threshold)
-	-	+	-	Acute hepatitis B (HbsAg below detection threshold)
-	-	-	+	Acute hepatitis C

49. Answer is A (IgM - Anti - HBc antibody) : *Harrison 16th / 1833, 1832; Harrison 17th/ 1943 Harrison 18th/p 2550*

If IgM - Anti - HBc is present the Hepatitis B infection is considered acute - *Harrison 16th / 183*

The presence of Hepatitis B virus infection is represented by the presence of HBs Ag and IgM Anti - HBc antibody.

- If IgM Anti HBc is present the HBV infection is considered acute.
- If IgM Anti HBc is absent the HBV infection is considered chronic.

HBs Ag	IgM Anti - HBc	Diagnostic interpretation
+	+	Acute Hepatitis B
+	-	Chronic Hepatitis B
-	+	Acute Hepatitis B (HBs Ag below detection threshhold)

- The presence of **HBeAg** only denotes High infectivity and active disease.
  HBeAg may be present in both Acute and Chronic Hepatitis B infection.

- **HBV DNA** like HBe Ag is an indicator of HBV replication - *Harrison 16th*
  The presence of HBV DNA therefore also represents an indicator for infectivity and active disease and may be seen both in acute and chronic Hepatitis B infection.
  HBV DNA detection has high sensitivity and may be detected when HBe Ag is still undetectable.

50. Answer is B (HBs Ag + HBe Ag): *Harrison 15th/1731; 16th/1832; 17th/1934 Harrison 18th/p 2550*

HBe Ag: Its principal clinical usefulness is an indicator of relative infectivity – Harrison
HBs Ag: *Its presence in serum indicates infection / pervious vaccination with hepatitis B virus.*

	HBs Ag	Anti- HBsAg	Anti Hbe	HBe Ag	Anti-Hbe
Acute HBV infection High infectivity	+	-	IgM	+	-
Chronic HBV infection High infectivity	+	-	IgG	+	-

Thus, the presence of the above two markers indicate an infection with hepatitis B virus and high infectivity. Q
Whether the infection is acute or chronic can, however, only be commented if status of anti-HBe marker is clear.

51. Answer is D (HBs Ag) : *Harrison 18th/p 2540, 2541 Harrison 17th/1933, 1935; CPDT 16th/662*

HBsAg is not a marker for active HBV Replication. Serological markers for active viral replication include HBe Ag, presence of DNA polymerase and circulating HBV DNA

Markers for HBV Replication

Quantitative Markers	Quantitative Markers
HBe Ag *is a qualitative marker for HBV replication*	• ***HBV DNA*** *is a quantitative definitive marker for HBV replication* • ***DNA polymerase*** *is a definitive marker for HBV replication*

Serological markers for Active viral Replication
1.HBV DNA (Definitive)
2.HBV DNA polymerase (Definitive)
3.HBeAg (Qualitative)

52. Answer is D (HBV-DNA estimation): *Harrison 16th/1832; 17th/ 1933-34, 1943-44; 18th/2540, 2541, 2550, 2551*

Like Hbe Ag, serum ***HBV DNA*** *is an indicator of HBV replication,* ***but tests for HBV DNA are more sensitive and quantitative****- Harrison 16th/1832*
The marker HBV DNA is useful in following the course of HBV replication and thus deciding need for antiviral chemotherapy.

Interferon therapy would be started after adjudging its need as indicated by HBV DNA testing.

Liver biopsy would be too radical at this stage.

53. Answer is A (Anti HBsAg positive): *Harrisons 17th/1943 Harrison 18th/p 2550*

Presence of Anti HBsAg positive status indicates either immunization with HBs Ag or Hepatitis B in the remote past with complete recovery such patients are considered safe for blood transfusion.

HbsAg	Anti-HBs	Anti-HBc	HBeAg	Anti-HBe	Interpretation
-	+	IgG	-	+/-	Recovery from hepatitis B
-	+	-	-	-	1. Immunization with HbsAg (after vacciniation) 2. Hepatitis B in the remote past (?) 3. False-positive

54. Answer is C (Hbs Ag+ and IgM anti-HBc+): *Harrison 14th/ 1688; Harrison 15th/ 1731; Harrison 16th/1832; Harrison 17th/ 1933, 1934, 1943 Harrison 18th/p 2540, 2541, 2550*

Presence of 'HBsAg +ve' status along with an IgM type of anti HBc is indicative of acute viral hepatitis B. Such a patient is certainly not considered safe for transfusion.

- ***Anti HbsAg +ve alone*** **:** Indicate either
  1. Immunization with HBsAg
  2. Remote past infection
  3. False positive

  Such a patient is considered safe.
- ***Hbc'Ag' is never detectable in the serum***, and this is a false proposition altogether.
- **Anti Hbe +ve** alone is insufficient data to comment up on. However presence of anti Hbe Ag. indicates HBV infection with low infectivity. *Although transfusion is not advisable in this case, this person is safer than option (c).*

55. Answer is C ('P' gene): *Harrison's 14th/ 1679; 15th/1722; 16th/1823; 17th/ 1933 Harrison 18th/p 2538, 2539, 2540*

The reverse transcriptase activity is a property of DNA polymerase which is coded by 'P' gene.

Genomic structure of Hepatitis B:

'S' Gene	'C' Gene	'P' Gene	'X' Gene
Codes for the envelope protein, Hbs Ag.	Codes for two nucleocapsid protein. a. Hbc Ag: The intracellular core protein. b. Hbe Ag: A soluble non particulate nucleocapsid protein.	Codes for DNA polymerase This DNA polymerase has two acitivities: a. DNA dependent DNA Polymerase b. ***RNA dependent Reverse Transcriptase.***	Codes for Hbx Ag. It is a small non particulate protein, that can transactivate the transcription of cellular and viral gene.

56. Answer is D (Serial Monitoring) : *Harrison 18th/p 2569-2577 Harrisons 17th/1957- 1962*

Antiviral therapy (IFN, Lamuvidene, Adefovir, Entecovir) for chronic hepatitis B is indicated for patients with active HBV replication. Negative HBe Ag and Normal levels of liver enzymes suggest that the patient is either in a ***non replicative phase of chronic hepatitis****, or, is an inactive carrier of chronic Hepatitis.*

Such patients are best managed by sequential monitoring (biochemical and virological) over many months and are not considered candidates for antiviral therapy

Assessment of need for Antiviral therapy in Chronic Hepatitis B

Antiviral therapy is indicated for patients with active HBV replication
Active HBV replication is best assessed by measuring serum HBe Ag levels and HBV DNA levels

Markers for Active HBV Replication
HBe Ag[Q]
HBV – DNA[Q]

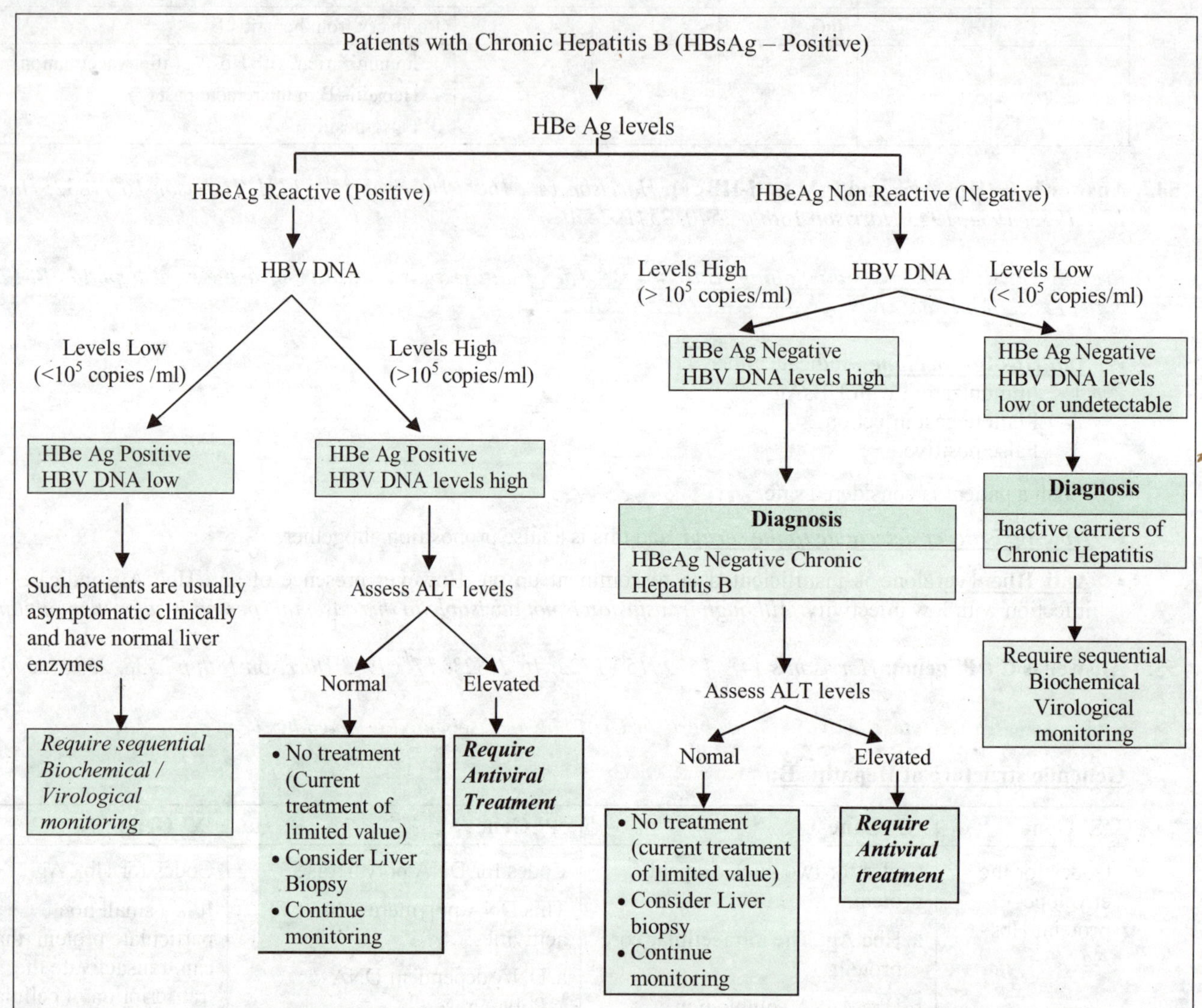

The patient in question is negative for HbeAg and has normal ALT levels. He is thus not a candidate for antiretroviral therapy. Such patients are best managed by sequential monitoring (biochemical and virological) over many months.

57. Answer is A (Serial monitoring): *Harrison's 18th/2576*

HBe Ag Negative individuals with ALT ≤ upper limit of normal do not require anti-viral treatment. Such individuals may be monitored sequentially with biochemical or virological markers.

The patient in question is negative for HbeAg and has normal ALT levels. He is thus not a candidate for antiretroviral therapy. Such patients are best managed by sequential monitoring (biochemical and virological) over many months.

Seven drugs have been approved for treatment of chronic Hepatitis B (Harrisons)

1. *Interferon α (and Pegylated Interferon)*
2. *Lamuvudine (oral)*
3. *Adefovir (oral)*
4. *Entecavir (oral)*
5. *Dipivoxil (oral)*
6. *Telbivudine*
7. *Tenofavir*

Recommendations for Treatment of Chronic Hepatitis B

Based on practice guidelines of the American Association for the Study of Liver Diseases (AASLD).

HBeAg status	Clinical	HBV DNA (IU/ml)	ALT	Recommendation
HBeAg-reactive	Mild or Inactive Liver disease	$>2 \times 10^4$	≤ 2 x ULN	No treatment; monitor. In patients >40, with family history of hepatocellular carcinoma, and/or ALT persistently at the high end of the twofold range, liver biopsy may help in decision to treat
	Chronic hepatitis	$>2 \times 10^4$	>2 x ULN	Treat[e]
	Cirrhosis compensated	$>2 \times 10^3$	< or > ULN	Treat[e] with oral agents, not PEG IFN
		$<2 \times 10^3$	>ULN	Consider treatment
	Cirrhosis decompensated	Detectable	< or > ULN	Treat[e] with oral agents[g], not PEG IFN; refer for liver transplantation
		Undetectable	< or > ULN	Observe; refer for liver transplantation
HBeAg-negative	Mild or Inactive Liver disease	$\leq 2 \times 10^3$	$\leq$ULN	Inactive carrier; treatment not necessary
	Chronic hepatitis	$>10^3$	1->2 x ULN	Consider liver biopsy; treat[h] if biopsy shows moderate to severe inflammation or fibrosis
	Chronic hepatitis	$>10^4$	>2 x ULN	Treat[h,i]
	Cirrhosis compensated	$>2 \times 10^3$	< or > ULN	Treat[e] with oral agents, not PEG IFN
		$<2 \times 10^3$	>ULN	Consider treatment
	Cirrhosis decompensated	Detectable	< or > ULN	Treat[h] with oral agents[g], not PEG IFN; refer for liver transplantation
		Undetectable	< or > ULN	Observe; refer for liver transplantation

[e] One of the potent oral drugs with a high barrier to resistance (entecavir or tenofovir) or PEG IFN can be used as first-line therapy. These oral agents, but not PEG IFN, should be used for interferon-refractory/intolerant and immunocompromised patients. PEG IFN is administered weekly by subcutaneous injection for a year; the oral agents are administered daily for at least a year and continued indefinitely or until at least 6 months after HBeAg seroconversion.

[g] Because the emergence of resistance can lead to loss of antiviral benefit and further deterioration in decompensated cirrhosis, a low-resistance regimen is recommended-entecavir or tenofovir monotherapy or combination therapy with the more resistance-prone lamivudine (or telbivudine) plus adefovir. Therapy should be instituted urgently.

[h] Because HBeAg seroconversion is not an option, the goal of therapy is to suppress HBV DNA and maintain a normal ALT. PEG IFN is administered by subcutaneous injection weekly for a year; caution is warranted in relying on a 6-month posttreatment interval to define a sustained response, because the majority of such responses are lost thereafter. Oral agents, entecavir or tenofovir, are administered daily, usually indefinitely or, until as very rarely occurs, virologic and biochemical responses are accompanied by HBsAg seroconversion.

[i] For older patients and those with advanced fibrosis, consider lowering the HBV DNA threshold to $>2 \times 10^3$ IU/ml.

Abbreviations: ULN, upper limits of normal; PEG IFN, pegylated interferon.

58. Answer is C (ALT > 2x ULN): *Harrison's 18th/2576*

The primary indication of antiviral treatment in chronic hepatitis B is elevation of ALT levels to more than 2 times the upper limit of normal.

Antiviral treatment is recommended for treatment of chronic hepatic B in both HBe Ag positive and HBe Ag negative individuals when HBV DNA > 2×10^4 U/ml and ALT > 2 times ULN.

Lamivudine is the first of the nucleoside analogues to be approved and may be used for Antiviral treatment in such cases although newer, more potent agents are now generally preferred.

59. Answer is B (Acute Viral Hepatitis B - Antiviral therapy): *Harrison 18th/p 2554 Harrison's 17th/1946, 1956: 'Clinical Hepatology: Principles & Practice of Hepatobiliary Disease' (Springer, 2010) /761*

Acute Viral Hepatitis B is not an indication of Antiviral therapy. Antiviral therapy is not indicated for Acute Hepatitis B.

Acute Hepatitis B is not an approved indication for Antiviral Therapy

In the vast majority of patients Acute Hepatitis B is a self limiting disease that results in viral elimination and complete healing.

'In Hepatitis B among previously healthy adults who present with clinically apparent hepatitis, recovery occurs in ~ 99%; therefore antiviral therapy is not likely to improve the rate of recovery and is not required'- Harrison's 17th/1946

'The administration of Antiviral therapy (lamivudine) to patients with acute hepatitis B may slow the development of protective Anti- HBs titres. Therefore antiviral treatment is not recommended in patients with uncomplicated acute viral hepatitis B' - Clinical Hepatology (Springer, 2010) /761

Note *(Harrison's 17th/1946; Clinical Hepatology (2010)/761)*

Antiviral therapy with nucleos(t)ide analogs might be considered for fewer than 1% of patients with acute viral hepatitis B who present with a fulminant clinical course. Although ***at present severe/fulminant acute hepatitis B is not an approved indication of antiviral therapy*** *and there is no data to support such an approach most authorities would recommended institution of antiviral therapy for severe acute Hepatitis B*

60. Answer is A (Vertical Transmission is more common than horizontal transmission in non-endemic areas): *Harrison 18th/p 2547 Harrison's 17th/Park 20th/186, 187*

Vertical transmission is more common that horizontal transmission in endemic Areas (not in non-endemic areas)

Age of onset determines prognosis

'The outcome of HBV infection is age dependent. The development of chronic hepatitis B is inversely related to age and occurs in approximately 95% of persons infected perinatally, in 80% of persons infected in early childhood and in 5-10% infected after 5 years of age' – Park 20th/188

Period of communicability lasts several months

'The period of communicability is usually several months. The virus is present in the blood during the incubation period (for a month before jaundice) and acute phase of disease' – Park 20th/187

Virus can be detected in blood one month before jaundice

'Circulating HBsAg precedes elevation of aminotransferases and clinical symptoms (jaundice) by 2-6 weeks and remains detectable during the entire icteric or symptomatic phase of acute 'Hepatitis B' and beyond'
– Harrison's 17th/1933

Vertical transmission is more common in Endemic areas

'Perinatal transmission (vertical) is uncommon in North America and Europe (Non-Endemic areas) but occurs with great frequency and is the most common mode of HBV perpetuation in the Far East and developing countries (Endemic areas)' – Harrison's 17th/1940,1947

61. Answer is D (Gall stone disease): *Harrison 18th/p 2547 Hepatology: Principles and Practice 2nd/431 Liver Immunology: Principles and Practice (2007) / 210*

Gallstone disease has not been mentioned in the list for extrahepatic manifestations of Hepatitis B

Extrahepatic manifestations in viral hepatitis B:

- *Aplastic Anemia*
- *Cryoglobulinaemia*
- *Diabetes mellitus*
- *Dermatomyositis-like syndrome*
- *Gianotti- Crosti syndrome*
- *Glomerulonephritis*

- *Guillain- Barre syndrome*
- *Myasthenia gravis*
- *Pericarditis and myocarditis*
- *Pancreatitis*
- *Peripheral Neuropathy*
- *Polyarleritis Nodosa*
- *Polyarthritis*
- *Polymyalgia rheumatica*
- *Polymyositis*
- *Porphyria cutanea tarda*
- *Psychosis*
- *Raynaud's syndrome*
- *Serum sickness like illness*
- *Splenomegaly and lymph node enlargement*
- *Skin alterations*
- *Thrombopenic purpura*
- *Thyroiditis*
- *Urticaria*

62. Answer is D (Focal Segmental Glomerulosclerosis) : *Harrisons 17th/ 1796 ; Liver Immunology; Principles & Practice (2007) / 211 'Viral Hepatitis' be vilson (1997) / 332*

Focal Segmental Glomerulosclerosis (FSGS) has not been mentioned in association with hepatitis B associated Glomerulonephritis

Glomerulonephritis associated with Hepatisis B include, MGN, MPGN and Mesangiocapillary GN

Glomerulonephritis during chronic Hepatitis B infection
Membranous Glomerulonephritis (MGN)
Membranoproliferative Glomerulonephritis (MPGN)
Mesanglocapillary glomerulonephritis

Note

MGN is most commonly seen ***in children***[Q]
MPGN is most commonly seen ***in adults***[Q]

63. Answer is B (↑ HBV DNA and ↑ ALT) : *Harrison 18th/p 2583 Harrison 17th/ 1961*

Antiviral therapy with interferon is indicated in patients with active viral replication (↑ HBV DNA) and elevated ALT levels

Patient with active DNA replication (↑ HBV DNA) and cirrhosis (compensated or decompensated) should not be treated with Interferon therapy These patients should be treated with other oral agents and IFN

Indications for Interferon Therapy
Chronic Hepatitis with ↑ HBV DNA and Elevated LFT

64. Answer is E (Famcyclovir): *Harrison 18th/p 2569 Harrisons 17th/ 1957*

Famcyclovir is not an approved drug for treatment of chronic hepatitis B

Seven drugs have been approved for treatment of chronic Hepatitis B (Harrisons)
1. Interferon alpha and Pegylated Interferon (PEG)
2. Lamuvudine (oral)
3. Adefovir (oral)
4. Entecavir (oral)
5. Dipivoxil (oral)
6. Telbivudine
7. Tenofovir

Hepatitis C

65. Answer is C (Hepatitis C): *Harrison 18th/p 2546 Harrison's 17th/1939; Harrison's 16th/1829; Refer previous question*

Most common hepatitis to progress to chronicity is hepatitis C

Parameter	HAV	HBV	HCV	HDV	HEV
Progression to chronicity	None	Occasional (1-10%)	Common (50-70%)	*Common	None

** In acute HBV/HDV co infection, the frequency of chronicity is the same as that for HBV. In HDV superinfection chronicity is variable*

Clinical and epidemiologic features of viral hepatitis:

Features	HAV	HBV	HCV	HDV	HEV
Incubation (days)	15-45	30-180	15-160	30-180	14-60
Age	Children, young Adults	Young adults	Any age but more in adult	Any age	Young adults
Transmission					
Fecal-oral	+++	---	---	---	+++
Percutaneous	Unusual	+++	+++	+++	---
Perinatal	---	+++	+	+	---
Sexual	+	++	+	++	---
Clinical					
Severity	Mild	Occasionally Severe	Moderate	Occasionally Severe	Mild
Fulminant	.1%	.1%-1%	.1%	5-20%	1-2%
Progression to chronicity	None	Occasional (1-10%)	Common (50-70%)	Common	None
Carrier	None Q	01%-30%	1.5 to 3.2%	Variable	None Q
Cancer	None Q	+nt	+nt	Variable	None Q
Prognosis	Excellent	Worse with age	Moderate	Acute: good Chronic: poor	Good
Prophylaxis	IgG Vaccine	HBIG Recombinant vaccine	None	-	Unknown

Memo : Q *HCV is the most common Virus associated with transfusion associated hepatitis*
Q *No vaccine / prophylaxis is available for HCV*
Q *Malignant potential is present with HCV (also with HBV)*

66. Answer is A (Anti-LKM antibody): *Harrison 14th/1687, 1703; 15th/1751, 1747; 16th/1828; 17th/1942; 18th/2550*

Hepatitis C is associated with Anti-LKM antibodies. *Hepatitis C may possibly also be associated with cryoglobulinemia but in view of its definite association with anti-LKM antibodies, this is the single best answer.*

LKM antibodies stand for antibodies against Liver-Kidney microsomes.

LKM antibodies may be seen in
- Type II autoimmune hepatitis (anti LKM-I)
- Drug induced hepatitis (anti LKM-II)
- Chronic hepatitis C
- Chronic hepatitis D (anti LKM-III)

Note that species of LKM antibodies in hepatitis C and hepatitis D are different from each other as well as from LKM antibodies in autoimmune hepatitis type II.

- *Hepatitis C is also associated with* ***essential mixed cryoglobulinemia (EMC)*** *- Harrison 14th/1683*
  Essential mixed cryoglobulinemia is an extrahepatic manifestation of viral hepatitis. It was reported initially to be associated with hepatitis B. Recent reevaluation of patients with EMC suggests that association is with chronic HCV infection rather than HBV infection.
- ***PAN*** *is associated with hepatitis B virus and not with hepatitis C.*
- ***Scleroderma*** *is not associated with Hepatitis C.*

67. Answer is B (Celiac disease): *'Hepatology: Principles and Practice' by Kuntz 2nd/443*

Celiac disease has not been mentioned in list of extrahepatic manifestations of hepatitis C

Extrahepatic manifestations in viral hepatitis C: *'Hepatology' by Kuntz*

- *Agranulocytosis*
- *Aplastic anaemia*
- *Corneal ulceration*
- *Cryoglobulinaemia*
- *Diabetes mellitus (type I)*
- *Erythema exsudativum multiforme*
- *Glomerulonephritis*
- *Guillain-Barre syndrome*
- *Hyperlipasaemia*
- *Lichen planus*
- *Non-Hodgkin lymphoma*
- *Polyarteritis nodosa*
- *Polyarthritis*
- *Polyneuritis*
- *Porphyria cutanea tarda*
- *Sialadenitis*
- *Sjogren's syndrome /Sicca syndrome*
- *Thrombocytopenia*
- *Thyroiditis*

68. Answer is B and D (Dermatomyositis like syndrome> Psoriasis): *'Dermatology byBurg dorf (Thieme Clinical companion Series) 2006/66*

Dermatamyositis like syndrome has not been mentioned in association with Hepatitis C infection.

Psoriasis has also not been linked to Hepatitis C virus directly although it may be seen in patients treated with Interferon α

Lichen planus and PAN are established associations of both, hepatitis B and hepatitis C.

Dermatoses associated with Hepatitis B	Dermatoses associated with Hepatitis C
• Gianotti-Crosti syndrome • Lichen planus • Mixed cryoglobulinemia • Erythema nodosum • Pyoderma gangrenosum • Polyarteritis nodosa • Urticaria • Leukocytoclastic vasculitis • Serum sickness-like prodrometeinuria, or hematuria • Dermatomyositis-like syndrome	• B-cell lymphoma (lymphoplasmacytic lymphoma, Waldenstrom macroglobulinemia) associated with mixed cryoglobulinemia. • Leukocytoclastic vasculitis • Polyarteritis nodosa • Porphyria cutanea tarda • Lichen planus • Urticaria

*Many dermatoses formerly associated with HBV infection have turned out to be more often or exclusively associated with HCV. Thus, both of these lists should be viewed as working formulations.

69. Answer is D (Do liver biopsy and start antiviral treatment accordingly): *Harrison 18th/p 2582 Harrisons 17th/ 1965*

Antibodies against HCV (anti- HCV) in the blood indicate infection with the HCV. Persistance of antibodies for 6 months suggests a diagnosis of chronic hepatitis C. Patients with chronic hepatitis C, even with normal ALT levels are candidates for Liver biopsy to establish a histo-pathological diagnosis of chronic hepatitis. ***Patients with at least moderate grade and stage are candidates for antiviral therapy with PEG IFN and ribararin regardless of the ALT levels***

'Although patients with persistantly normal ALT levels tend not to progress histologically, they respond to antiviral therapy just as well as do patients with elevated ALT levels. Such patients are potential candidates for antiviral therapy'
- Harrisons 17th/ 1965

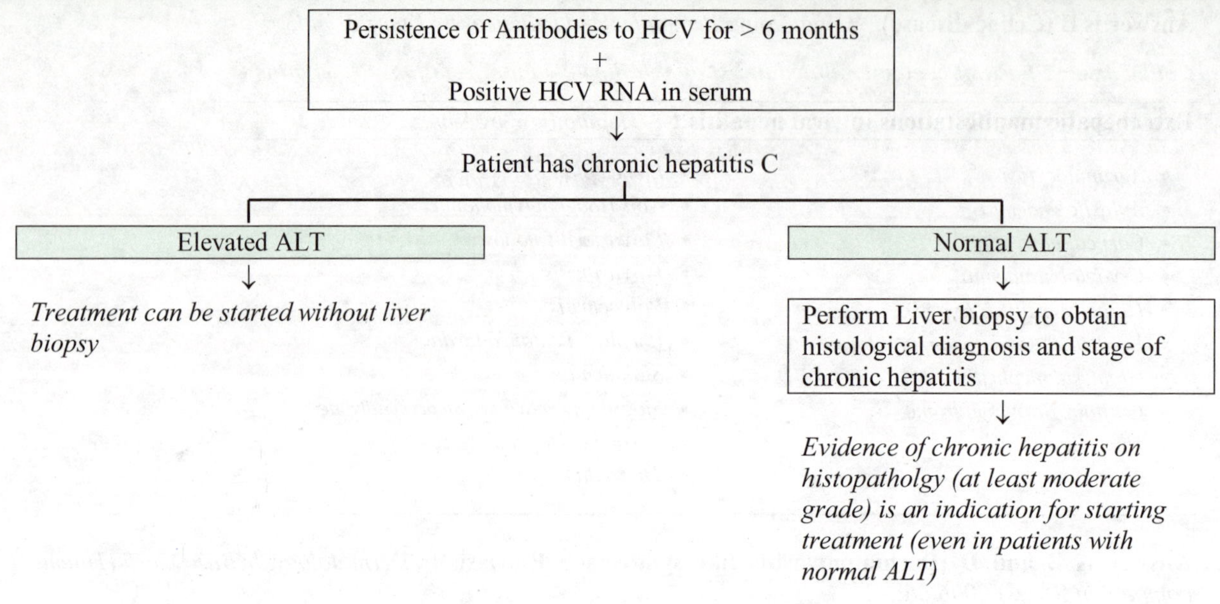

Chronic hepatitis : 'Evidence Based medicine Guidelines' 1st (2005) / 330

- Increased serum ALT 6 months after the onset of symptoms: (normal ALT does not, however, rule out chronic hepatitis).
- A patient with a positive HCV-PCR-test and permanently elevated ALT most probably has a mild chronic hepatitis and treatment decisions can be made without liver biopsy in genotypes 2 and 3.
- Liver biopsy is indicated in a patient with positive HCV-PCR- test and normal ALT, and with genotypes 1 and 4 before considering therapy. Signs of chronic hepatitis in the biopsy are an indication for treatment.
- Information on the genotype of the virus is important to guide treatment decisions. Treatment is more effective for genotypes 2 or 3 than for genotypes 1 and 4.
- Treatment with a combination of interferon alpha or pegylated interferon alpha and ribavirin is used for 48 weeks for genotypes 1 and 4 and for 24 weeks for genotypes 2 and 3.
- When treating genotypes 1 or 4. If there is no response at 12 weeks (HCV-PCR still positive), the treatment is discontinued.
- Liver transplantation is indicated if the expected survival is about 6 months

70. Answer is E (Determine HCV RNA levels)

Antibodies against HCV in the blood indicate infection with Hepatitis C virus. If the infection persists for more than 6 months and viral replication is confirmed by HCV RNA levels, then the person can be confirmed as having chronic hepatitis C.

The next step in the management of the patient in question would be to establish a serological diagnosis of chronic hepatitis (which can be determined by HCV RNA levels in the setting of elevated antibodies to HCV for 6 months).

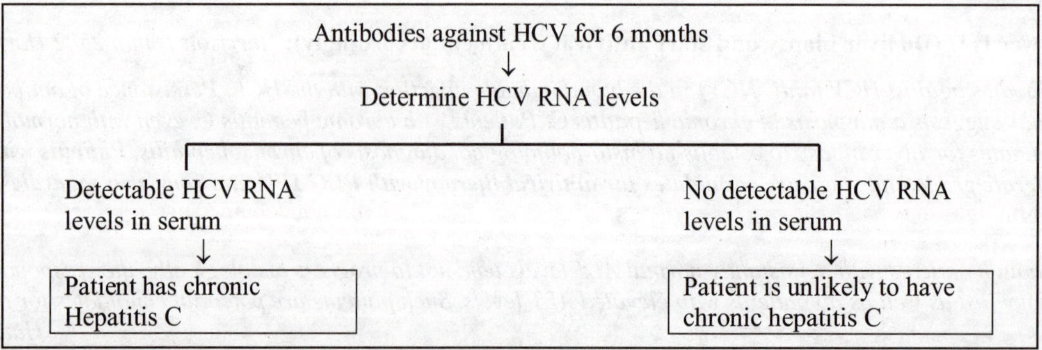

Once a diagnosis of chronic hepatitis C is suggested by the presence of HCV RNA, levels of ALT should be determined to plan appropriate treatment as indicated in the previous question.

71. Answer is A (Ribavarin and interferon): *Harrison 18th/p 2583 Harrison's 17th/1965; Harrison's 16th/1852*

The patient in question is a relapser after previous standard interferon monotherapy.
The recommended treatment of choice for such patients is a course of Interferon plus Ribavarin.

'A course of Interferon plus Ribavarin is the recommended treatment of choice for Relapsers after a previous course of standard monotherapy with interferon or combination interferon/ribavarin therapy'- Harrison's

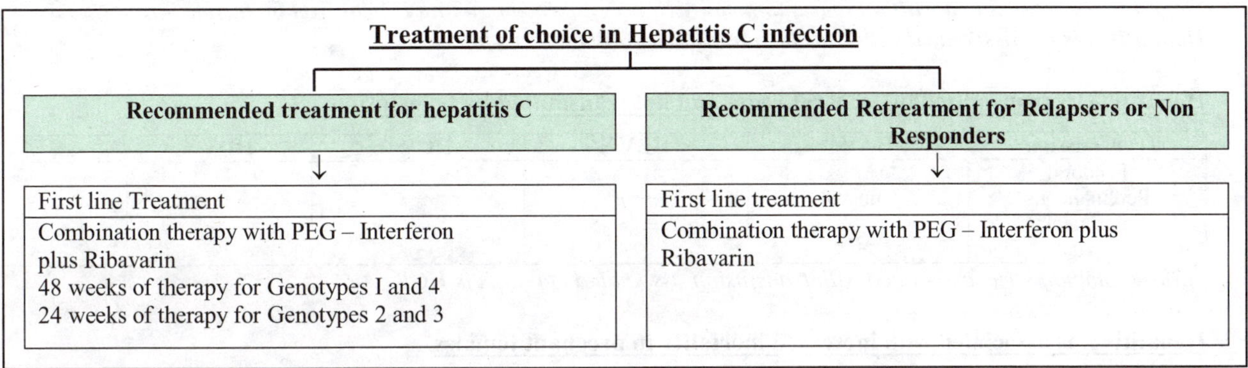

72. Answer is A (Ribavarin and interferon): *Harrison 15th/ 1749, Table 297-6; Harrison 16th/ 1852, 1851; Harrison 17th/ 1965 Harrison 18th/p 2582, 2583*

'Patients who have relapsed after a course of interferon monotherapy are candidates for retreatment with combination regulated interferon plus ribavarin therapy.' *– Harrison 16th/ 1852*

Indication Of Therapy:

1. Elevated ALT
2. Portal bridging fibrosis or moderate to severe hepatitis on liver biopsy
3. Detectable HCV RNA

Treatment options / Regimens:

First line treatment (treatment of choice)	Alternate regimen (if ribavarin is C/I)
Combination pegylated IFN plus ribavarin	*Pegylated interferon monotherapy*

Pegylated IFN are long acting IFN's bound to polyethylene glycol. Such pegylated IFN have a substantially longer half life, achieve prolonged concentration, permitting administration once a week.

73. Answer is E (Female sex): *Harrison 18th/p 2583 Harrisons 17th/1965 Hand book of Gastroenterology 1st / 129*

Female sex is a favourable feature, associated with sustained responsiveness to antiviral therapy Male sex is associated with reduced responsiveness.

Reduced Responsiveness

- ***Genotype 1***
- High levels of HCV RNA
- ***Adranced fibrosis (ciorrhosis, bridging fibrosis)***
- Long duration disease
- ***Age > 40 years***
- Immunosupression
- African American
- Obesity
- Hepatic steatosis
- Reduced adherence
- Male sex (*Handbook of Gastroenterology*)

Sustained Responsiveness

- Genotype 2 and 3
- Low levels of HCV RNA
- Minimal fibrosis
- Short duration disease
- Age < 40 years
- Immunocompetance

Others

- Absence of obesity
- Absence of Hepatic steatosis
- Increased Adherence
- Female sex (*Handbook of Gastroenterology*)

Hepatitis E

74. Answer is B and D (Associated with increased mortality in pregnant women and Acquired by Fecooral route): *Ananthnarayanan 6th/519; Park 18th/174l; Harrison's 17th/1934, 41, 44; Harrison's 18th/1829, 1831, 1834 Harrison 18th/p 2538, 2548, 2552*

Hepatitis E is associated with increased mortality in pregnant women and is acquired by fecooral route.
Hepatitis E is not associated with transfusion with Hepatitis B virus infection.

Hepatitis E is transmitted by fecooral route and not transmitted by transfusion

Transmission[Q]	HAV [Q]	HBV [Q]	HCV [Q]	HDV [Q]	HEV [Q]
Fecooral	+++	-	-	-	+++
Percutaneous	Unusual	+++	+++	+++	-
Perinatal	-	+++	±	+	-
Sexual	±	++	±	++	-

[Q] *Most common virus associated with transfusion associated hepatitis is HCV.*

Hepatitis E is associated with increased mortality in pregnant females

A unique feature of Hepatitis E virus is the clinical severity and high case fatality rate of 20-40% in pregnant women, especially in the last trimester of pregnancy.

Hepatitis D is associated with Hepatitis B infection and not Hepatitis E

75. Answer is B (Feco-oral): *Park 17th/ 165; Harrison 16th / 1829±, 1831; 17th/ 1939, 1941 Harrison 18th/p 2538, 2548*

Hepatitis E is synonymous with Enterically transmitted non-A non-B Hepatitis.
The infection caused by hepatitis E is essentially a water borne disease- Water or Food supplies, contaminated with feces in which the virus is excreted, have been implicated in major outbreaks reported in all parts of the world.

Transmission[Q]	HAV [Q]	HBV [Q]	HCV [Q]	HDV [Q]	HEV [Q]
Fecooral	+++	-	-	-	+++
Percutaneous	Unusual	+++	+++	+++	-
Perinatal	-	+++	±	+	-
Sexual	±	++	±	++	-

[Q] *Most common virus associated with transfusion associated hepatitis is HCV.*

76. Answer is A (Pregnant women): *Ananth Narayan 6th/ 519; Park 18th /174; 17th/ 1944-45 Harrison 18th/p 2552, 2553*

A unique feature of Hepatitis E virus is the clinical severity and high case fatality rate of 20-40% in pregnant women, especially in the last trimester of pregnancy.

77. Answer is A (Pregnant women): *Harrison 17th /1939, 1941; Harrison's 18th/174; Robbins 7th/891;De swiet's Medical Disorders in Obstetric Practice (John Wiley & Sons) 2010/230*

Fulminant Hepatitis E is typically seen in pregnant women especially in the last trimester.

'A unique feature of Hepatitis E virus is the clinical severity and high case fatality rate (20-40%) in pregnant women, especially in the last trimester of pregnancy'. - Park

'Hepatitis E can lead to fulminant hepatitis which happens most frequently amongst pregnant women than any other subgroup' – De Swiet's Medical Disorder in Obstetric Practice.

78. Answer is D (Hepatitis E): *See previous question; Harrison 18th/p 2552, 2553 Harrison 17th/ 1944-45*

79. Answer is C (HEV): *See previous question; Harrison 18th/p 2552, 2553 Harrison 17th/ 1944-45*

80. Answer is D (Hepatitis E): *Park 18th/174; Harrison 18th/2538, 2548; 17th/1939, 1941, Park 17th/165, Ananth Narayan 7th/559*

Epidemics are almost exclusively caused by enterically transmitted NON A NON B Hepatitis virus - i.e. Hepatitis E.[Q]
- Park

Sporadic cases :
Most common cause of ***sporadic cases in adults is - Hepatitis E*** [Q]
Most common cause of ***sporadic cases in children is - Hepatitis A.*** [Q]

81. Answer is A (Hepatitis E) : *Zokin & Boyer's Hepatology: A textbook of Liver Diseases (Elsvier)2011/612; Schiff's Diseases of the Liver (John Willey & Sons)2011/chapter 23*

The most common cause of acute sporadic hepatitis amongst adults in India is Hepatitis E.

'In India HEV infection is the most common cause of acute sporadic hepatitis and account s for upto 70% of such cases amongst adults' - Zokin & Boyer's Hepatology

'Hepatitis E is the second leading cause of acute clinical hepatitis in adults in North African and the middle east (after Hepatitis B) and is the most common cause in Nepal, India and throughout central & south east Asia.
- Schiff - Diseases of the Liver

'Hepatitis E is the most common cause of a sporadic and epidemic Hepatitis amongst adults in Asia (India) and the second most common cause amongst adults (after HBV) in the middle east and north Africa'
- De Sweet's Medical Disorder in Obstetric Practice

Hepatitis E (HEV)

- *Most common cause of sporadic Hepatitis amongst adults in India*[Q]
- *Most common cause of epidemic Hepatitis amongst adults in India*[Q]
- *Most common cause of Fulminant Hepatitis amongst pregnanat women*[Q]
- *Most common route of aquisition /transmission is fecoral route*[Q]

Autoimmune and Granulomatous Hepatitis

82. Answer is D (ANCA): *Harrison 18th/2586; Harrisons 17th/1967 Oxford Textbook of Medicine 4th/ 722*

The characteristic autoantibodies in autoimmune hepatitis include ANA, Anti SLA and, Anti LKM antibodies and anti SMA antibodies

Although p ANCA may be seen in patients with type I autoimmune hepatitis, these antibodies are not considered characteristic for any type of autoimmune hepatitis.

Characteristic Autoantibodies for Auto immune Hepatitis

- *Antinuclear Antibodies (ANA)*
- *Anti LKM Antibodies (Anti- Liver-kidney microscomal antibodies)*
- *Anti- SLA (Antibodies against Soluble Liver Antigens)*
- *Anti- SMA (Antibodies against smooth muscle Antigens*

Autoimmune Hepatitis

Type I	Type II	Type III
Characteristic Autoantibody profile	**Characteristic Autoantibody Profile**	**Characteristic Auto antibody profile**
ANA ++ *SMA ++*	***Anti LKM1 ++***	***Anti – SLA ++*** ***ANA +/- ; SMA +/-***
Associated Antibody Profile	**Associated Antibody Profile**	**Associated Antibody profile**
P ANCA *Anti – Actin* *Anti – ASGPR*	*Anti- LC1* *Anti – ASGPR*	*Anti – ASGPR*

ANA (Antinuclear Antibodies); anti- ASGPR (antibody to asialoglycoprotein receptor); anti LC1 (antibody to Liver cytosol type I); anti- LKM1 (antibody to soluble liver kidney microsome Type I); anti, SLA (antibody to soluble liver antigen).

83. Answer is D (All of the above): *Harrison 15th/e 1739, 1759; 16th/ 1840, 1872; Harrison 17th 1739, 1759 (17th/ not elaborated)*

Granulomatous Hepatitis has been implicated with the following drugs:
1. ***Phenylbutazone*** ^Q^
2. *Sulfonamides* ^Q^
3. *INH* ^Q^
4. ***Allopurinol*** ^Q^
5. *Quinidine* ^Q^
6. ***Carbamazepine*** ^Q^

Alcoholic Hepatitis

84. Answer is C (Elevated serum Albumin): *Harrison 18th/p 2590, 2530 Harrison's 17th/1970, 1971, 1926,264*

Alcoholic hepatitis is associated with hypoalbuminemia or decreased serum albumin levels (and not elevated serum albumin).

'Severe alcoholic hepatitis is heralded by coagulopathy (prothrombin time>5 sec), hypoalbuminemia (albumin<25g/L or 2.5 g/dl) elevated bilirubin levels (>137µmol/l or > 8mg/dl), anemia, renal failure and ascitis.- Harrison's

Feature of Alcoholic Hepatitis

Features suggesting Hepatocyte injury (Enzyme studies)	Features suggesting dearrangement in Hepatocyte function
AST/ALT : Levels are increased : Increased is less than 8 fold (< 400u/L) : AST is elevated greater than ALT : AST: ALT Ratio >1 AST: ALT>2 is suggestive AST: ALT>3 is highly suggestive	**Bilirubin** : May be markedly elevated Both fractions (direct/indirect) may be elevated
	Albumin : Often decreased (Hypoalbuminemia) (Albumin <2.5 mg/dl) suggests severe alcoholic hepatitis
Alkaline Phosphatase: Levels are increased (may be normal) Increase is moderate (<3 times normal) Normal to < 3 times normal elevation	**Prothrombin time** : Often prolonged Fails to correct with parentral vit K (Coagulopathy)
Gamma Glutamyl Transpeptidase (GGT) : Levels are increased : Note that GGT elevation is not specific to alcohol GGT is easily inducible and may be elevated in all forms of fatty liver	Others : *Polymorphonuclear cells (Neutrophils)* are often increased and if > 5500/µl predict severe alcoholic hepatitis. *Hypertriglyceredemia* and *Hypercholesterolemia* may be associated with alcoholic fatty liver.

85. Answer is B (Alcoholic Hepatitis): *Harrison 18th/2529, 2590; 17th/1925,1970,1971; Harrison's 16th/1815, 1855, 1856*

An AST/ALT ratio of greater than 1 suggests a diagnosis of alcoholic hepatitis

Pattern of aminotranferases and etiology of hepatitis

Alcoholic Hepatitis	Non Alcoholic Hepatitis (Viral/toxin induced)
• AST/ALT Ratio > 1 AST: ALT>2:1 is suggestive AST: ALT>3:1 is highly suggestive	• AST/ALT ratio <1
• AST/ALT elevation is moderate and rarely >400 u/L	• AST/ALT elevation is usually more marked and often >500 u/L
• AST is elevated more than ALT	• ALT is elevated more than AST
The low level of ALT in alcoholic liver disease is due to an alcohol induced deficiency of pyridoxal Phosphate.	

86. Answer is B (SGPT > SGOT): *Harrison 15th/ 1713; 1753; 16th/ 1856, 1857, 1815; 17th/ 1925 Harrison 18th/p 2529*

AST is synonymous with SGOT & ALT is synonymous with SGPT
In general AST and ALT levels rise parallel to each other. ***In alcoholic liver disease the AST rises out of proportion to ALT such that the ratio of AST and ALT may become greater than 2.***

Stigmata of Alcoholic hepatitis / cirrhosis that aid in diagnosis :

1. Bilateral enlarged parotids Q
2. Gynaecomastia Q
3. Testicular atrophy with loss of body hair Q
4. Wasting of muscle mass Q
5. Duputyrens contracture Q

AST (SGOT) out of proportion to ALT (SGPT) seen in Q
1. Alcoholic hepatitis Q
2. Fatty liver in pregnancy Q

Gamma Glutamyl transferase levels correlate with levels of Alkaline phosphatase and are a sensitive indicater of biliary tract disease – obstructive jaundice. *It is not an indicator of alcoholic liver disease.*
Remember : GGT is the most sensitive indicator of biliary tract disease

87. Answer is A (SGOT): *Harrison 15th/e 1753; 16th/ 1857, 1515, 1815; 17th/ 1925, 1970, 1971; 18th/p 2529, 2590*

All the enzymes given in the options are elevated in Alcoholic hepatitis. Although none of the options appear to be appropriate, the best options amongst these should be AST or SGOT.
In alcoholic hepatitis, in contrast to other causes of fatty liver, the AST and ALT are usually elevated two to seven fold. *In general AST and ALT levels rise parallel to each other. In alcoholic liver disease the AST rises out of proportion to ALT such that the ratio of AST and ALT may become greater than 2. AST (SGOT) is therefore the single best answer.*

AST/ALT > 2:1 is ***suggestive*** of alcoholic liver disease.
AST/ALT > 3 : 1 is ***highly suggestive*** of alcoholic liver disease.

Laboratory diagnosis of alcoholic fatty liver and alcoholic hepatitis.

Test	Comments
AST	• Increase two to seven fold, less than 400U/L, greater than ALT
ALT	• Increased two to seven fold, less than 400 U/L
AST/ALT	• Usually less than 1
GGTP	• Not specific to alcohol, easily inducible, elevated in all forms of fatty liver.
Bilirubin	• May be markedly increased in alcoholic hepatitis despite modest elevation in alkaline phosphatase
PMN	• If > 5500/mL, predicts severe alcoholic hepatitis when discriminant function > 32

Alkaline phosphatase levels may increase but it is not specific to alcohol liver disease

Macrocytosis may be seen. (Raised MCV)

Alcoholism is also associated with:

- Hypertriglyceremia
- Hypercholesterolemia
- Hyperbilirubinemia
- Increase in circulating polymorphonuclear leucocytes > 5500/μl.

88. Answer is A (Pentoxyfylline): *Davidson's 20th/971*

Pentoxy fylline has shown to reduce mortality from renal failure in alcoholic hepatitis.

'In severe alcoholic hepatitis oral pentoxyfylline reduces inpatient mortality, particularly from hepatorenal failure'
- Davidson

Non Alcoholic Fatty Liver Disease (NAFLD/NASH)

89. Answer is E (Gall stone disease): *CMDT 2007 / 683; 09/600; Robbins 7th / 907, 908*

Gall stone disease has not been mentioned as a cause / association of NASH

Causes of Non Alcoholic Fatty Liver Disease (NAFLD) or Non Alcoholic Steato hepatitis (NASH)

- *Obesity (present in > 40% cases)*
- *Diabetes mellitus (present in > 20% cases)*
- *Hypertriglyceredemia (>20%)*
- *Endocrinopathies (Cushing's and hypopituitarism, PCOS)*
- *Metabolic disorders (Hyperbetalipoproteinemia)*
- *Obstructive sleep apnea*
- *Starvation and Refeeding syndrome*
- *Total parentral Nutrition*
- *Medications and poisons*
  - *Corticosteroids* - *diltiazem* - *irinotecan* - *Antiretroviral therapy*
  - *Amiodarone* - *tamoxifen* - *oxaliplatin* - *CCl_4 & Yellow phosphorus*

6

90. Answer is B (Clofibrate provides effective treatment): *Harrison 18th/2604, 2605; 17th/ 1982 ; Robbins 7th/ 907, 908*

Clofibrate is a lipid lowering drug that decreases hepatic triglyceride content. Based on this, usefulness of clofibrate has been evaluated in the treatment of NASH, however clofibrate has not been found to be effective in the treatment of NASH.

Non Alcoholic fatty Liver Disease (NAFLD) is common in Diabetics

Commonest **Associations of NAFLD / NASH** *(Robbins)*

- *Obesity*
- *Dyslipidemia*
- *Hyperinsulinemia (Insulin resistance is a charachteristic feature[Q])*
- *Diabetes*

NAFLD is believed to be the commonest cause of cryptogenic cirrhosis

NAFL is now considered the most common cause of 'cryptogenic cirrhosis' – Robbins 7th/908

Spectrum of NAFLD

- *Simple steatosis (Early)*
- *Steatohepatitis (NASH) : Non Alcoholic Steatohepatitis) (Intermediate)*
- *Fibrosis and cirrhosis (Advanced)*

NAFLD is associated with elevated transminases (transaminitis)

'Most patients with NAFLD come to medical attention as a result of incidentally elevated liver enzymes' – Harrison

- ALT > AST
- Aminotransferases are usually only mildly elevated 2 times normal

Clofibrate has not been found to be effective in the treatment of NAFLD: *'Fatty Liver Disease:NASH & related disorders' (2005)/ 202*

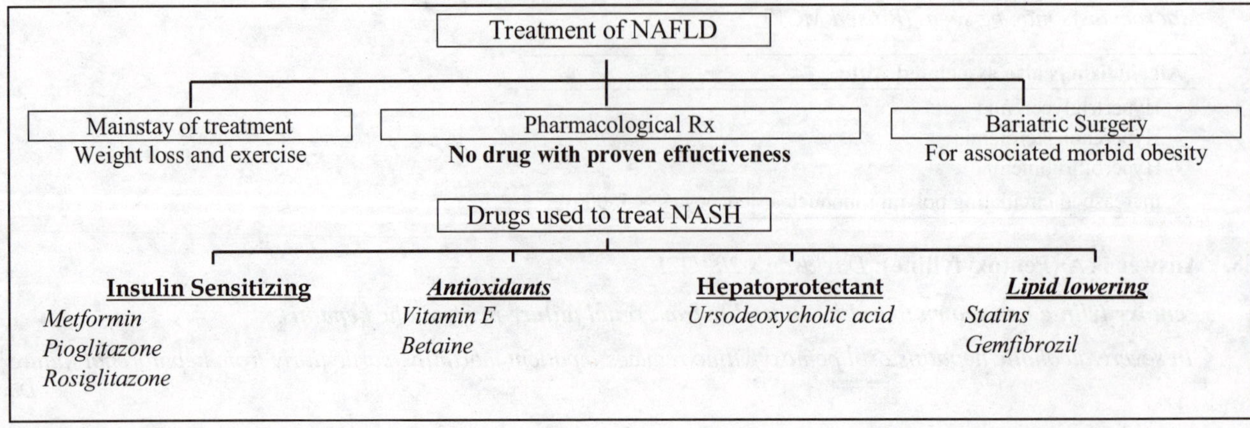

Ascitis

91. Answer is A (Colloid carcinoma of stomach): *Harrison 15th/ 261; 16th/245; Harrison 17th/268 Harrison 18th/p 332*

Colloid carcinoma of stomach causes mucinous ascities – *Harrisons 16th/ 245*
Chylous Ascitis refers to a turbid milley or crcamy peritoneal fluid due to the presence of thoracic or intestinal lymph. It is most often a result of lymphatic obstruction from the cause mentioned below.

Causes of Chylous Ascitis	Causes of Mucinous Ascitis
Trauma	Pseudomyxoma peritonei
Tumor	Colloid carcinoma stomach with peritoneal implants
Tuberculosis	Colloid carcinoma colon with peritoneal implants
Filariasis	
Congenital anomalies	
Nephrotic syndrome	

92. Answer is D (USG can detect as little as 100 ml of peritoneal fluid): *Current Critical Care Diagnosis & Treatment 3rd/717; Harrisons 17th/267, 268, 1979; Harrison 18th/p 2601, 333 Refer text below*

Abdominal ultrasound may detect as little as 100 ml of ascitic fluid ultrasound is thus a useful investigation for the diagnosis of minimal ascitis – *CCDT 3rd/717*

Hemorrhagic Ascitis is diagnosed when RBC count >10, 000 / mm^3 (Not >1000/mm^3)
An RBC count of 10,000 / mm^3 is the threshold for pink appearance and hemorrhagic ascitis is thus diagnosed when ascitic RBC count is > 10,000 / mm^3 - Schiff's diseases of the Liver 10th/ 996

Spontaneous Bacterial peritonitis (SBP) is diagnosed when Neutrophil count > 250/mm^3
The diagnosis of SBP is made when the absolute neutrophil count > 250 / mm3 – Harrisons 17th/1979

The drug of choice for treatment of SBP are cephalosporins & not Norfloxacin
Cefotaxime is considered the drug of choice for emperic therapy of SBP

Large volume Therapeutic Paracentesis is not recommended for SBP
Diagnostic paracentesis is indicated in SBP for establishing the diagnosis but large volume paracentesis should be avoided - Schiff's Diseases of the Liver 10th/ 561

93. Answer is A (Salt Restriction): *Harrison 18th/p 2600 Harrisons 17th/ 1978; Oxford Textbook of Medicine 4th/736*

The first line treatment of Ascitis is dietary salt restriction.

Treatment of Ascitis: Oxford Textbook of Medicine : Recommendations

- ***Bed Rest*** *is of little value*
- ***Dietry sodium Restriction*** *is the first line management*
- ***Diuretic therapy*** *is the mainstay of treatment of Ascitis (Spironolactone should be employed as the* ***first line drug)***
- ***Large volume paracentesis*** *should initially be carried out on patients with moderate or marked ascitis*
- ***Shunts (TIPS)*** *may be used in cases of Refractory Ascitis in whom recurrent paracentesis is too frequent or poorly tolerated, or in those with a hepatic hydrothorax*

Cirrhosis and its Complications

Cirrhosis: General

94. Answer is A (chronic Hepatitis B): *'Pathology: Basic and systemic' by Woolfe (1998)/587,597*

Chronic viral hepatitis including Chronic Hepatitis B is associated with macronodular Cirrhosis and not micronodular cirrhosis.

Alcohol, hematochromatosis and large bile duct obstruction are all associated with micronodular cirrhosis.

Morphological Classification of Cirrhosis

Macronodular Cirrhosis (Parenchymal nodules > 3mm)		**Micronodular Cirrhosis (Parenchymal nodules < 3mm)**	
Aetiology	**Frequency**	**Aetiology**	**Frequency**
• *Chronic viral hepatitis*	*10-20%*	• *Alcohol*	*60-70%*
• *Wilson's disease*	*Rare*	• *'Primary' biliary cirrhosis*	*5%*
• *α-Antitrypain deficiency*	*Rare*	• *Large bile duct obstruction*	*<5%*
• *Various drugs and toxins*	*Rare*	• *Haemochromatosis*	*5%*
• *Hereditary haemorrhagic telangiectasis*	*Rare*	• *Intestinal bypass*	*Rare*
		• *Cystic fibrosis*	*Rare*
• *Cryptogenic cirrhosis*	*Common*	• *Indian childhood cirrhosis*	*Rare*

95. Answer is C (Gamma Globulins): *Harrison 18th/p 2530 Harrisons 17th / 1925*

Gamma Globulins are increased in chronic liver disease such as chronic Hepatitis and cirrhosis - Harrison

Gamma Globulins are produced by B Lymphocytes and not in hepatocytes

Gamma globulins are increased in chronic liver diseases such as chronic hepatitis and cirrhosis

In cirrhosis the increased serum gamma globulin concentration is due to the increased synthesis of antibodies, some of which are directed against intestinal bacteria, This occurs because the cirrhotic liver fails to clear bacterial antigens that normally reach the liver through the hepatic circulation

Alpha Globulins (α_1 and α_2) and Beta Globulins are produced primarily by hepatocytes

Their concentrations are thus likely to fall with impaired function of hepatocytes in chronic liver diseases like cirrhosis

96. Answer is D (Post necrotic cirrhosis): *Harrisons 16th/ 858, 1859; Robbins 7th / 919*

Post necrotic cirrhosis is charachterized by a shrunken liver with reduced liver span.

The normal liver span measures about 12- 15 cm and a lover span of 19cm suggests and chlorged liver. Presence of esophageal varices suggests portal hypertension due to advanced liver disease / cirrhosis or occlusion of portal vein.

Venoocclusive disease, Budd chiari syndrome, Hematochromatosis and Alcohol liver disease may all present with an enlarged liver and portal hypertension (esophageal varices).

97. Answer is E (Post necrotic cirrhosis): *Robbins 7th/ 905, 967, 909, 911, 919, Harrisons 16th/ 858, 1859*

Liver is typically shrunken in size and not enlarged in post necrotic cirrhosis.

Alcoholic hepatitis, NASH, Wilson's disease and Budd chiari syndrome may all present with enlarged liver and hepatocellular dysfunction.

Primary Biliary Cirrhosis & Sclerosing Cholangitis

98. Answer is A (Pruritis): *Harrison 15th/ 1757; Harrisons 16th/ 1860; Harrison 17th/ 1974 Harrison 18th/p 2595*

'The earliest symptom is 'pruiritis' which may be either generalized or limited initially to the plams and soles.'
– Harrison

Primary Biliary Cirrhosis

Primary biliary cirrhosis is a disease characterized by chronic inflammation and fibrous obliteration of intrahepatic bile ductules due to an unknown (primary) stimulus.

Etiology / pathogenesis :

PBC is believed to be due to an autoimmune Q etiology as it is often associated with other autoimmune disorders Q such as

1. CREST Q : **C**alcinosis, **R**aynaud's, **E**sophageal dysmotility, **S**clorodactyly **T**alenglectasia
2. SICCA SYNDROME Q
3. Autoimmune thyroiditis Q
4. Renal tubular acidosis

- Antimitochondrial Antibody (IgG) is positive

Clinical feature :

- Most patients are asymptomatic Q
- Pruritis is commonest / earliest symptom Q
- Jaundice Q
- Melanosis: gradual darkening of exposed areas of skin Q
- Deficiency of fat soluble vitamins due to malabsorption Q
  - Vit D deficiency : bone pain - osteomalacia Q
  - Vit K deficiency : bleeding – bruising Q
  - Vit A deficiency : Night blindness Q
- *Xanthelisman & xanthomas* Q due to protracted elcvaliar of serum lipids.

Lab Findings :

- ↑↑ Serum alkaline phosphatase Q (2-5 fold)
- **Positive antimitochondrial antibody** :Q Sensitive and specific
- Hyperlipidemia Q

99. Answer is A (Increased risk associated with smoking) *CPDT 16th/ 675 CMDT 2008/707;09/622; Harrisons 17th/2001, 1975 Harrison 18th/p 2627, 2596*

Smoking is associated with a decreased risk of developing primary sclerosing cholangitis (and not an increased risk)
'As in ulcerative colitis, smoking is associated with a decreased risk of primary sclerosing cholangitis' – CMDT

Two important conditions with decreased risk from smoking

- *Ulcerative colitis (UC)*Q
- *Primary sclerosing cholangitis (PSC)* Q

Primary Sclerosing Cholongitis

Progressive Idiopathic obliteration of intrahepatic or extrahepatic bile ducts

Note
*Smoking is associated with a decreased risk of PSC (and UC)*Q

- *Most common in Men aged 20- 50 years (M > F)*
- *Characteristically associated with ulcerative colitis (IBD) (and less commonly with crohn's disease)*
- *Characteristic increased risk of cholangiocarcinoma (10%)*

Presentation	Characteristic Laboratory Feature	Diagnostic study of choice
• **Progressive obstructive jaundice.** Patient presents with progressive jaundice, pruritis and other features of cholestasis	• **GGT is typically elevated** ***Asymptomatic elevation of GGT is the earliest finding*** • **ALP & bile acids are ↑ed**	*ERCP or MRCP is the diagnostic study of choice demonstrating irregularities of the biliary tree*

100. Answer is A (Increased incidence in Females): *CMDT 2008/603;09/622; CPDT 16th/675; Harrison 18th/p 2596 Harrisons 17th/2001, 1975 Refer previous question*

Primary sclerosing cholangitis is characteristically more common in men than women

'PSC is most common in men aged 20 to 50 years' – CMDT

101. Answer is C (In advanced stages of cirrhosis major blood supply to liver comes from Hepatic vein) *Harrison 18th/p 2595, 2596 Harrisons 17th/ 1974*

In advanced stages of cirrhosis major blood supply to Liver comes from Hepatic artery and not from hepatic vein

Antimitochondrial Antibodies are positive in PBC *(Harrisons 17th/ 1974)*
'Antimitochondrial' Antibodies (AMA) are present in about 90% of patients with PBC' – Harrison

Elevated Lipoprotein Y is seen in PBC: *Rubin's Pathology 5th/ 328*
' The serum levels of cholesterol increase strikingly in PBC and an abnormal lipoprotein (Lipoprotein- x) appears which is found in many forms of chronic cholestasis' – Rubin's pathology

In Late stages of PSC treatment is Liver Transplantation *(Harrisons 17th/1975)*
'The ultimate treatment of PSC is Liver transplantation' – Harrison

In advanced stages of cirrhosis major blood supply to Liver is from hepatic artery
Normally 80% of blood flow to liver comes from the portal vein and 20% of the blood supply is contributed by the hepatic artery

In cirrhosis the blood flow to liver from the portal vein is reduced due to increased pressure and a compensatory increase in the blood to liver through the hepatic artery occurs

Hepatic veins drain blood away from the liver and do not contribute in the blood supply to the liver

Non Cirrhotic Portal Fibrosis

102. Answer is D (Non cirrhotic portal fibrosis): *API 6th 591; API 7th/ 621; Harrison 17th 621*

Young patients presenting with features of portal hypertension along with a moderate/large splenomegaly with conspicuous absence of features of liver cell failure suggests a diagnosis of NCPF.

NCPF is suspected in a patient presenting with symptoms of portal hypertension with:
• YOUNG AGE • Moderate/Large Splenomegaly • ***NO*** FEATURES SUGGESTIVE OF LIVER CELL FAILURE - No Jaundice (uncommon) - No Ascitis (uncommon) - No Hepatomegaly (uncommon) - No Stigmata of liver cell failure (uncommon)

Non cirrhotic portal fibrosis is a condition of liver characterized by widespread fibrosis of the liver (mainly portal, subcapsular and rarely perisinusuoidal) causing wide variation in the normal architecture but there is no true cirrhosis.

NCPF is the most important causes of intrahepatic non cirrhotic portal hypertension in India. [Q]

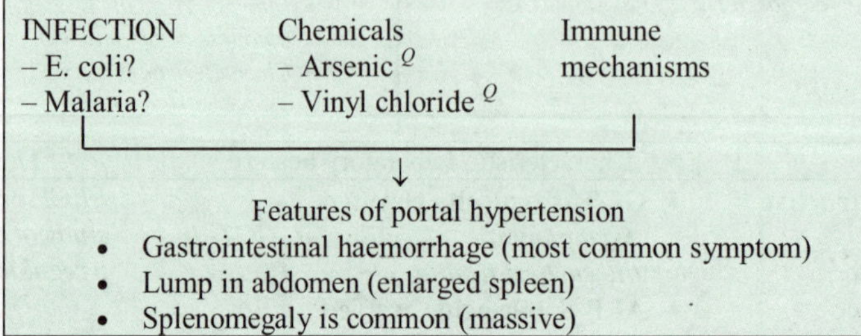

103. Answer is A (EHPVO) : *'Tropical Hepato – Gastroenterology' by Tandon (Elsevier, India) 2007 /396, 397 'Non cirrhotic Portal Fibrosis: Current concepts and Management': Journal of Gastroenterology and Hepatology (2002) 17, 526- 534: 'Portal Hypertension : Pathogenesis & Management' by Helmy (2006) /354, 355; 'Comprehensive Clinical Hepatology' by Bacon, O,Gardy (2006) /553; 'Diseases of the Liver and Biliary System in Children' by Velly 3rd /559; 'Current Diagnosis & Treatment Surgery' by Doherty /537*

Presence of hemetemesis, malena and splenomegaly suggests a diagnosis of portal hypertension. The most common cause of portal hypertension in a male child (12 year old boy) is Extra Hepatic Portal Vein Obstruction (EHPVO). EHPVO is therefore the single best answer by exclusion

Non Cirrhotic Portal Fibrosis *presents in a similar fashion clinically, however it is more common in females and in an adult population (third or fourth decade). NCPF is usually associated with a moderate/large (massive) splenomegaly*

Cirrhosis *is an uncommon cause of portal hypertension in children and the absence of jaundice and ascitis makes this diagnosis more unlikely.*

'An infant or child presenting with hemetemesis and mild/moderate splenomegaly in the absence of features of chronic liver disease is likely to be suffering from EHPVO. In adults, one needs to exclude diseases such as NCPF and compensated cirrhosis - 'Portal Hypertension': by Roberto De Franchis (Wiley - Blackwell) 2006 /314

Age of presentation favors a diagnosis of EHPVO over NCPF

Age at presentation is an important factor in distinguishing EHPVO from NCPF

- Indian Journal of Gastroenterology; 1984; Vol 3; No 4; 201-202

Features	EHPVO	NCPF
• Age	***Children (1st & 2nd decade)***	*Adults (3rd & 4th decade)*
• Gender	***M > F***	*F > M*
• Variceal bleed (Hemetemesis / Malena)	+ +	+ +
• ***Splenomegaly***	***Mild /Moderate***	***Moderate / Large***
• Jaundice / Ascitis Encephalopathy	*± (Absent / Transient)*	*± (Absent / Transient)*
• LFT	*Normal*	*Normal*
• Site of block along portal venous system	*Large branches are thrombosed (Main trunk; 1st order branches)*	*Small branches are involved (3rd order and 4th order branches)*
• USG	*Portal / Splenic vein block 'Portal covernoma'*	*Normal splenoportal axis*

'More than three quarters of Indian Children with portal hypertension were found to have extra hepatic portal vein obstruction (EHPVO) and Indian studies have shown extra hepatic portal vein obstruction (EHPVO) to be the commonest non cirrhotic cause for portal hypertension'

- 'Diseases of the Liver and Biliary System in Children' by Kelly 3rd /559

'In a prospective study 'Yaccha et.al' provided support for the hypothesis that the etiology of upper gastro intestinal bleeding in children may differ between developed and developing countries. They showed that 95% of children had upper gastrointestinal variceal bleeding, 92% of whom had bleeding due to EHPVO, a figure significantly higher than that seen in the west' - Disease of the Liver & Biliary system in Children by Kelly 3rd /560

Portal Hypertension in Indian Children	Portal Hypertension in Indian Young Adults
The most common cause of Portal Hypertension in Indian Children is EHPVO	*The most common cause of Portal Hypertension in Indian Adults is NCPF*

Absence of Jaundice and Ascitis makes a diagnosis of cirrhosis unlikely

Signs of Liver failure such as Jaundice and Ascitis are uncommon in EHPVO and NCPF. Their presence favors a diagnosis of cirrhosis and their absence makes cirrhosis unlikely

Differentiating features between extrahepatic portal vein obstruction, non-cirrhotic portal fibrosis and cirrhosis of liver:

Parameter	EHPVO	NCPF	Cirrhosis
Mean age (years)	10	28	40
Ascites	Absent/transient after bleed	Absent/transient after bleed	+ to +++
Encephalopathy	-	-	+
Jaundice signs of liver failure	-	-	+
Liver function tests	Normal*	Normal	Deranged
Liver			
Gross	Normal/small	Normal, rarely irregular	Shrunken, nodular
Microscopic	Normal	Normal portal/fibrosis	Necrosis, regeneration
Splenoportovenography/US	Portal/splenic vein blovk	Normal splenoportal axis, 'withered tree' appearance, periportal fibrosis	Dilated, patent portal and splenic vein

*Occasional impairment may be observed

NCPF, non-cirrhotic portal fibrosis; EHPVO, extrahepatic portal vein obstruction; US, ultrasound

104. Answer is B (Non cirrhotic portal fibrosis) : *API 7th/621, 622; Various other texts;other texts*

Features of portal hypertension in an adult with a large splenomegaly (8cm below coastal margin) with no history of jaundice or liver decompensation suggests a diagnosis of Non-cirrhotic portal hypertension.

Non cirrhotic portal hypertension encompasses two distinct pathological condition that present with similar clinical features.

Non cirrhotic portal fibrosis Extrahepatic portal obstruction

Distinction between the two conditions should ideally be made by further investigations as the similarly in presentation makes clinical criteria unreliable.

Neverthless if we do have to choose one single best option the following clues may be helpful.

NCPF	Extrahepatic portal hypertension
NCPF presents in young adults most commonly during the third and fourth decade	EHPH may present in two age groups children (1st & 2nd decade) (congenital malformations) Adults (4th & 5th decade) (thrombotic event)
Mode of presentation	
The onset of symptoms is gradual	The onset is gradual in children where the cause is congenital malformation The onset is acute in adults where the cause is usually a thrombotic even
Mass in left upper quadrant (splenomegaly) is about 4 times more common in NCPF than EHPH	Mass in left upper quadrant (splenomegaly) is four times less common in patients with EHPH

Thus a young adult presenting with a gradually progressive cause and a moderate to massive splenomegaly suggests the diagnosis of Non cirrhotic portal fibrosis.

105. Answer is C (Non cirrhotic portal fibrosis): *API 6th/ 591; API 7th/ 621*

***"Chronic ingestion of Arsenic has been incriminated in causation of NCPF. High Hepatic arsenic levels in patients with NCPF have been reported"** – API 7th/ 621*

The precise etiology of NCPF remains an enigma.

The implicated chemical agents include:

1. Arsenic
2. Copper
3. Vinyl chloride

Arsenic in also associated with the following cancers Q
1. Skin cancer Q (Chandrasoma Taylor 3rd/ 285)
2. Lung cancer Q (Chandrasoma Taylor 3rd/ 285)
3. Hepatic angiosarcoma Q (Chandrasoma Taylor 3rd/ 185)

106. Answer is C (Upper gastrointestinal bleeding): *Schwartz 7th/1420, 1421; www.emedicine.com/ RADIO/topic570.htm*

Most common presenting symptom of extrahepatic portal hypertension is acute gastrointestinal bleeding.

Acute gastrointestinal bleeding is the single best answer as explained below.

- *'**Hematemesis** resulting from bleeding esophageal varices is the most common presentation in patients with portal hypertension'- emedicine*
- ***Ascites** is not a usual accompaniment of extrahepatic portal venous obstruction, but has been noted occasionally.- Schwartz*
- ***Encephalopathy** rarely occurs in patients with obstruction of the extrahepatic portal venous system without hepatocellular dysfunction- Schwartz*
- ***Chronic liver failure** in the setting of portal hypertension suggests cirrhosis as the underlying cause. It is less likely with non-cirrhotic portal hypertension.*

Note:
The most constant finding in patients with portal hypertension is splenomegaly (present in 80% of patients).
-CSDT 11th/580.

(Splenomegaly has not been provided amongst the options and hence upper gastrointestinal bleeding is the single best answer beyond any doubt.)

Portal Hypertension

107. Answer is D (Sinusoids): *Harrison 15th/e 1759; Harrison 16th/ 1863; Harrison 17th/ 1976 Harrison 18th/p 2597, 2598*

'When cirrhosis is complicated by portal hypertension the increased resistance is usually sinusoidal'-*Harrison's 15th/1759*
Portal hypertension (> 10 mm Hg: Normal portal pressure = 5 to 10 mmHg) most commonly results from increased resistance to portal blood flow.

Increased resistance can occur at three levels:

Presinusoidal	Sinusoidal	Post sinusoidal
• Anatomically outside the liver eg. Portal vein thrombosis • Within the liver but proximal to sinusoids eg. Schistosomiasis	***Cirrhosis*** *When cirrhosis is complicated by portal hypertension, the increased resistance is usually sinusoidal*	• Outside liver, at level of hepatic veins - ***Budd chiarri syndrome*** • In the inferior vena cava - Thrombosis • In the liver but distal to sinusoid - Venoocclusive disease

Remember :
1. Cirrhosis is the most common cause of portal hypertension in the United States.[Q]
2. Portal vein obstruction is the second most common cause. [Q]

108. Answer is C (10-15 cm Saline): *Harrison 14th/ 1710; Harrison 15th/ 1759; Harrison 16th/ 1863; Harrison 17th/ 1976 Harrison 18th/p 2597*

Normal pressure in portal vein is low '10 – 15 cm saline' *– Harrison 14th/ 1710.*
Normal pressure in portal vein is low '5 – 10 mm Hg' *– Harrison 16th/e 1863*

Normal pressure in portal vein :

cm (Saline)	mm (Hg)
10 – 15 cm saline	5 – 10 mmHg

109. Answer is C (Esophageal varices) : *Nelson 16th/e 1226*

Presence of massive haematemesis in the background of moderate splenomegaly suggests a diagnosis of esophageal varices secondary to portal hypertension.

Esophageal varices :
- *Most common presentation of esophageal varices is **Hematemesis.***
- *'**Splenomegaly**, sometimes with hypersplenism, is the next most common presenting feature in the portal vein obstruction.'*

110. Answer is D (Oesophageal varices) : *Read text below; Harrison 18th/p 2598 Harrison 17th 1976, Pretest Sugery 8th/ 8320*

'Oesophageal variceal bleeding secondary to portal hypertension should always be the initial diagnosis in a young patient presenting with massive hematemesis and a moderate to large splenomegaly'

Features in favour of oesophageal varices:

- Most common presentation of oesophageal varices is G.I. bleed, which may be 'massive'.
  - Massive hematemesis in children is almost always due to variceal bleed – Shwartz
  - Gastrointestinal bleed in peptic ulcer disease usually occurs in persons who are > 60 years old i.e. (it certainly is an uncommon presentation in a young boy) – Harrison
  - Erosive drug induced gastritis is usually superficial therefore hemodynamically significant 'massive' bleeding is rare
- Patients presents with moderate splenomegaly which is an important pointer towards presence of portal hypertension.
- Absence of any significant history of altered liver function in the presence of portal hypertension could well be attributed to an extrahepatic causes of portal hypertension.

111. Answer is B (Esophagus varices) *Harrison 16th /e p. 1863, 235, ; Harrison 18th/p 2598 Harrison 17th 1976-1977*

'Massive haematemesis in the background of splenomegaly suggests variceal bleed due to portal hypertension.'

112. Answer is A (Portal Hypertension): *Harrison 18th/320, 2598*

Hemetemesis in a patient with palpable splenomegaly suggests a diagnosis of variceal blood secondary to portal hypertension.
Hemetemesis from Gastric ulcer, Mallory Weiss tear and/or drug induced gastritis is not associated with splenomegaly.

113. Answer is D (Acetic Acid): *KDT 5th/ 560; API 7th/ 615; KDT 5th/560*

Acetic acid has not been mentioned as a sclerosing agent.

Sclerosing agents are irritants which cause inflammation, coagulation and ultimately fibrosis when injected into hemorrhoids or varicose vein mass. They are used only for local injection.
Endoscopic sclerotherapy involves local injection of sclerosants into variceal columns especially in lower 5 cm of oesophagus.

These Sclerosing agents include:
1. Polidocanal (Polydochyl)
2. N butyl – cyanoacrylate (glue injection)
3. Absolute alcohol & Phenol
4. Ethalonalamine maleate / Oleate
5. Sodium tetradecyl sulphate

114. Answer is B (Urgent endoscopy): *Harrisons 16th/ 236; Harrisons 14th/ 248. ; Harrison 18th/p 2598, 2599, 320, 321 Harrison 17th 258, 1977*

Acute episode of GI bleeding in a known patient of cirrhosis suggests a clear cut diagnosis of variceal bleed. ***Urgent endoscopy is the modality of choice following haemodynamic stabilization as it is both a diagnostic and therapeutic modality.***

Management protocol :

Cardinal principles of resuscitation (**A**irway / **B**reathing / **C**irculation) ↓ **Urgent endoscopy** (diagnostic + therapeutic modality) Ligation is the endoscopic therapy of choice for variceal bleeding (Harrison 16th/236)
Other options : Endoscopic sclerotherapy Q / IV oetreotide Q (Medical management)

Principles :

- Once the patient is hemodynamically stable urgent endoscopy should be performed
- Ligation is the endoscopic therapy of choice for esophageal varices because it has requires fewer treatment sessions.
  - Less rebleeding
  - Fewer mortality rate
  - Fewer local complication
- Acute treatment with octreotide (preferred over vasopressin) is the medical management of choice
- In patients who have persistent or recurrent bleeding despite endoscopic and medical therapy, TIP is recommsended (TIPS is Transjugular intrahepatic portosystemic shunt)

115. Answer is A (Whole Blood transfusion is the best): *Kumar & Clarke 5th/ 677; Harrison 16th/ 254; 15th/ 274; Harrison 17th/ 259 Harrison 18th/p 321, 322*

'The overriding principle aim is to replace what is missing. Haemorrhage involves loss of whole blood, and the rationale treatment of acute haemorrhage therefore is the infusion of whole blood or a combination of red cells and a plasma substitute' – *Kumar Clarke 5th/ 677*

Management of hypovolemia : *Harrisons 16th/ 254; Kumar Clarke 5th/ 678.*

The therapeutic goals are to restore normovolemia with fluid similar in composition to that lost and to replace ongoing losses.

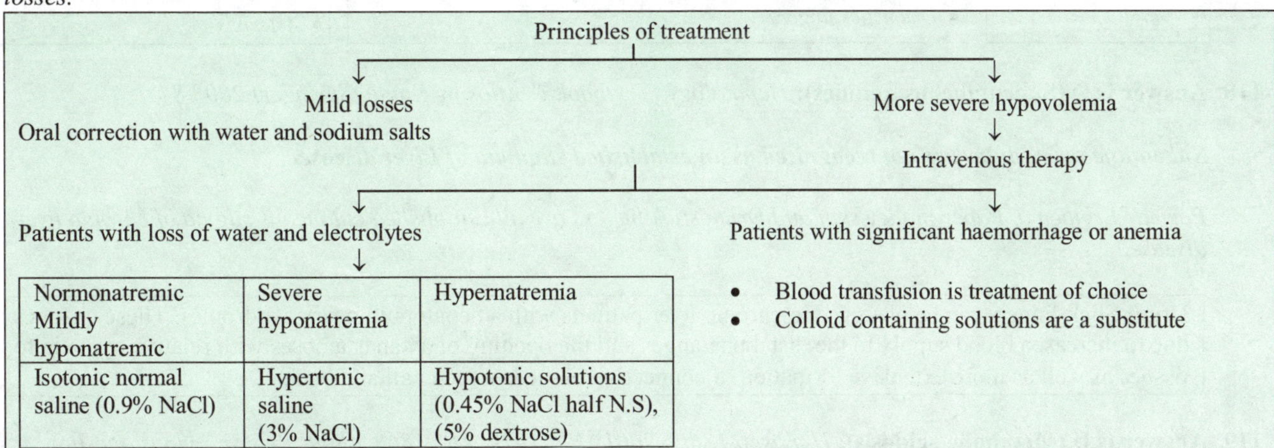

Hepatic Encephalopathy / Hepatic failure

116. Answer is C (Hyperkalemia): *Harrison 14th/ 1715, 1716; 15th/ 1765 t; 16th/ 1868. ; Harrison 17th/1979 Harrison 18th/p 2601*

It is Hypokalemia and not hyperkalemia that precipitates encephalopathy.

Hypokalemia *may contribute to systemic alkalosis and thereby cause an increase in the amount of non-ionic ammonia (NH_3), which readily crosses the BBB and accumulates in CNS worsening or precipitating encephalopathy.*

Common precipitants of Hepatic Encephalopathy include :

- Anaemia may lead to cellular hypoxia at the level of liver cells and thus ppt. encephalopathy [Q]
- Barbiturates are CNS depressant drugs and their injudicious use, therefore may precipitate hepatic [Q] encephalopathy.
- Hypothyroidism, though not mentioned as a direct precipitating. factor, may contribute towards precipitating encephalopathy by causing 'constipation' or slowing down the intellectual and motor activity.

Increased nitrogen load as in	Electrolyte and Metabolic imbalance such as in
1. *GI bleeding* [Q] 2. *Excessive dietary protein intake* [Q] 3. *Azotemia* [Q] 4. *Constipation* [Q]	1. *Hypokalemia* [Q] 2. *Alkalosis* [Q] 3. *Hypoxia* [Q] 4. *Hyponatremia* [Q]
Drugs	**Miscellaneous conditions like**
CNS depressant agents like narcotics, tranquillizers, sedatives [Q]	Infection [Q], surgery [Q], superimposed acute liver disease. [Q]

117. Answer is D (Subcutaneous nodules): *Chamberlain's Symptoms and Signs of Clinical Medicine 13th/382; Hepatology. Textbook & Atlas by Kuntz (Springer) 2008/84; Principles & Practice of Palliative Care & Supportive Oncology (Lippincott Williams) 2007/328*

Subcutaneous nodules are generally not seen as a stigmata of chronic liver disease.

Chronic Liver Disease manifests with loss of subcutaneous fatty tissue resulting in paper thin skin with marked folds (paper-money skin).

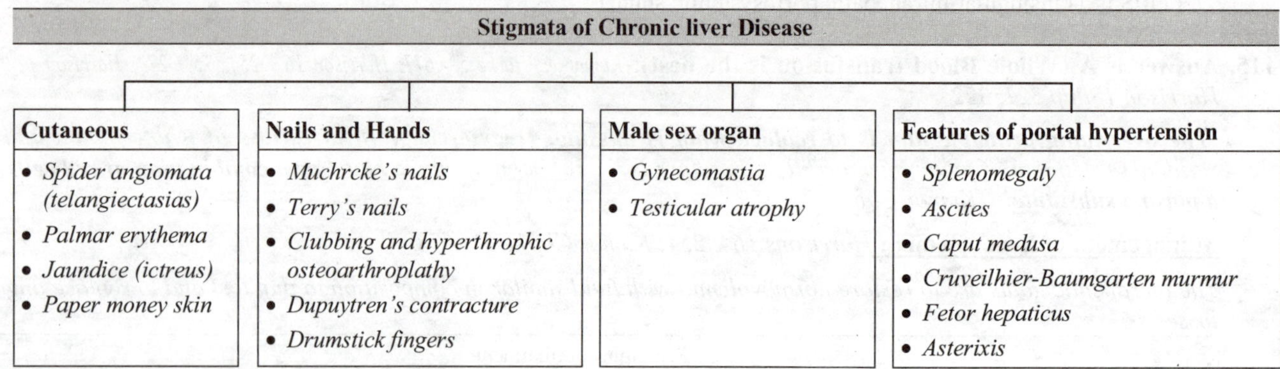

6 Liver and Biliary Tract

118. Answer is D (Subcutaneous nodules): *Hepatology: Textbook & Atlas by Kunte (Springer) 2008/84*

Subcutaneous nodules are not recognized as an established stigmata of Liver disease.

Parmar Erythema, Paper-money skin and Drum stick fingers are all established cutaneous stigma of chronic liver disease.

Drum-Stick fingers can be observed in chronic liver patients with a hepatopulmonary syndromes. These changes are due to increased blood supply to the distal phalanges and the opening of av anastamoses with relative hypoxia to tissues as well as more extensive formation of connective tissue between nail and bone.

119. Answer is D (Metabolic acidosis): *Harrison 18th/p 2601; 17th/1979; 16th/1868, 1869; Refer previous question*

Hepatic encephalopathy is precipitated by metabolic alkalosis and not by metabolic acidosis.

Electrolyte and Metabolic imbalances that precipitate Hepatic Encephalopathy

Hypokalemia
Alkaosis (Metabolic Alkalosis)
Hypoxia
Hyponatremia

120. Answer is A (Hyperkalemia): *Harrison 18th/p 2601 Harrisons 17th /1979*

Hepatic Encephalopathy is predisposed by Hypokalemia and not by Hyperkalemia

121. Answer is A (Hyperglycemia) : *Refer text below; Current Gastroenterology Diagnosis & Treatment*

Fulminant hepatic failure is associated with hypoglycemia and not with hyperglycemia

Hypoglycemia is a common complication of severe fulminant hepatic failure. The pathophysiology of hypoglycemia is multifactorial including impaired hepatic glucose release, impaired hepatic gluconeogenesis and elevated serum insulin levels. All patients with fulminant hepatic failure are recommended to recieve a continuous intravenous infusion of 10% dextrose to counteract hypoglycemia.

COMPLICATIONS IN ACUTE HEPATIC FAILURE	
Metabolic	**Neurologic**
Hypoglycemia	*Encephalopathy*
Hypophosphatemia	*Cerebral edema*
Hypokalemia	*Seizures*
Hyponatremia	*Intracranial hemorrhage*
Hypomagnesemia	**Multiorgan dysfunction**
Acid-base disturbance	*Pancreatitis*
Respiratory alkalosis	*Pulmonary edema / hemorrhage*
Metabolic acidosis	*Shock*
Hematologic	*Acute tubular necrosis*
Aplastic anemia	*Hepatorenal syndrome*
Coagulopathy	*Respiration failure*
Disseminated intravascular coagulopathy	*Sepsis*
Ascitis	

122. Answer is C (Increasing prothrombin time): *Pediatric Hepatology (1990)/353; Harrison 18th/p 2530 Harrison's 17th/1926; Harrison's 16th /1816*

It is difficult to choose one best prognostic factor as most criteria use a combination of various markers to assess the results.

Amongst the options provided the most important prognostic factors predicting survival is prothrombin time.

This is so because, coagulation factors have short serum half lives and their levels thus best determines the current status of liver function. The severity of hepatic lesion and mortality correlates best with the extent to which plasma levels of liver derived coagulation factors are depressed. ***Prothrombin time*** *collectively measures factors II, VII, IX and X and gives a choice approximation of the extent to which these factor are depressed Marked prolongation of prothrombin time to > 5 seconds above control and not corrected by parentral vitamin K is a poor prognostic sign reflecting higher mortality and poor survival.*

Pediatric Hepatology (1990)/353

'The standard liver blood tests (AST, ALT, ALP, Bilirubin, Ammonia) have no discriminatory value affecting survival The extent to which plasma levels of liver derived coagulation factors are depressed correlates with the severity of the hepatic lesion.'

123. Answer is D (Factor V estimation): *API 7th/ 602; CMDT 2003/ 637; 09/592*

It is difficult to choose one best prognostic factor as most criteria use a combination of various markers to assess the results. ***However amongst the options provided 'factor V' estimation should be the choice to pick.***
This is so because, coagulation factors have short serum half lives and their levels thus best determines the current status of liver function. The severity of hepatic lesion and mortality correlates best with the extent to which plasma levels of liver derived coagulation factors are depressed.
Prothrombin time which collectively measures factors II, VII, IX and X has not beenprovided amongst the options.
Levels of coagulation Factor V have also been shown to predict prognosis in patients with acute liver failure.
Accordingly perhaps 'Clinchy (France)' has use 'factor V levels' as an isolated prognostic marker in his criteria i.e. 'Clinchy criteria'

Clinchy Criteria (France)

Factor V levels < 20% of normal in patients < 30 years of age Factor V levels < 30% of normal in patients < 30 years of age
NB: The above factors indicate poor prognosis.

Coagulation factors as Laboratory Prognostic markers in patients with acute liver failure include the following:
1. Prothrombin time (King's criteria) 2. Factor V levels (Clinchy's criteria) 3. INR (CMDT)

124. Answer is A (Prothrombin time (PT)): *Schiff's diseases of the liver (Lippincott Williams, 2007)10th*

An increased prothrombin time is the most frequently observed first laboratory test suggesting the possibility of hepatocellular failure. Early liver failure may be suspected based on isolated prolongation of the Prothrombin Time (PT).

- **Prolonged PT** *is an early sensitive indicator of hepatic synthetic dysfunction due to the short half life of factor VII (2-6 hours) which the failing liver cannot maintain.*
- **APTT** *is prolonged after PT in Liver Disease.*
- **Albumin** has a long half life of about 20 days and hence reduced albumin will manifest only after 20 days of onset of Reduced synthetic function of Liver.
- **Increased arterial ammonia** is also a sign of acute liver failure, however increased arterial ammonia is primarily vieved as an important factor in the development of hepatic encephalopathy.

Patients with early hepatocellular failure may present with isolated prolongation of PT

'Patient with liver disease may have only a prolonged PT (normal APTT and thrombin time) reflecting a decrease in factor VII which is the first to be reduced in liver disorders because of its short half life of 2-6 hours'

'Factor VIIa is an essential enzyme in the extrinsic pathway of coagulation. The pathway is evaluated by PT. Because factor VII has the shortest half life of the procoagulant proteins, patient with early liver disease may present with an isolated prolonged PT' - *Hematology / Oncology Secrets / 82*

'Increased Prothrombin Time has a high prognostic value, particularly for patients with acute hepatocellular failure. An abnormal prothrombin time with confirmed prolongation of more than 5-6 seconds above control is the single laboratory test that draws attention to the possibility of the development of flummant hepatic necrosis (acute hepato cellular failure) in the course of acute viral hepatitis. Such a prolonged prothrombin time often precedes by days the manifestations of liver failure' - *Schiff's Disease of the Liver 10th/52*

'Most coagulation factors are produced in the liver (except VWF) and development of liver disease may result in prolongation of both PT and APTT. However because factor VII (Extrinsic pathway; measured by PT) has the shortest half life amongst all vitamin K dependent factor, PT will be the first to be prolonged. Development of Liver disease will lead to deficiency of factor VII first and initial prolongation of only the Prothrombin Time. With further deterioration of liver function both the PT and APTT will be prolonged' - *'Clinical Anesthesia' by stoelting (Lippincott Williams) 2009/396*

125. Answer is A (Hepatic encephalopathy): *Harrison 16th/1868*

Symmetric, high voltage, triphasic slow wave (2-5/second) pattern on Electroencephalogram (EEG) is characteristic (but non specific) of hepatic encephalopathy- *Harrison 16th/1868*

The diagnosis of hepatic encephalopathy should be considered when four major factors are present
1. Acute or chronic hepatocellular disease and/or extensive portal systemic collateral shunts
2. Disturbance of awareness and mentation which may progress from forgetfulness and confusion to stupor and finally coma.
3. Shifting combinations of neurological signs including asterixis, rigidity, hyperreflexia, extensor plantar signs and rarely seizures.
4. A characteristic but (nonspecific), symmetric, high voltage, triphasic slow wave (2 or 5/second) pattern on electroencephalogram.

126. Answer is D (Thyrotoxicosis): *Marsden's Book of movement Disorders (Oxford Press) 2012/1008; Sapira's Art and Science of Bediside Diagnosis 4th/549*

'Thyrotoxicosis (Hyperthyroidism) is associated with rapid fine tremors and not flapping tremors (irregular coarse tremor) also called Asterixis.

Asterexis (Flapping tremor) is most commonly seen in metabolic encephalopathies due to hepatic, renal (uremia) and respiratory failure (CO_2 Nercosis).

Causes of Asterixis /Flapping Tremor (Coarse irregular tremor)	
Typical Metabolic Encephalopathies	
• ***Hepatic Encephalopathy*** • ***Uremic Encephalopathy*** • ***Respiratory failure with CO_2 Retention (CO_2 Narcosis)***	*Typically Metabolic Encephalopathies due to hepatic, renal and respiratory failure are the most common causes.*
Other Metabolic Encephalopathies	
• *Hyperglycemia / Hypoglycemia* • *Electrolyte Disturbances (Hypokalemia, Hypomagnesemia etc)*	
Medication side Effects / Intrications	
• *Bromide intoxication* • *Phenytoin intoxication* • *Chloral Hydrate intoxication* • *Glutathemide intoxication* • *Intravenous ammonium chloride*	• *Gabapentin / Pregabalin* • *Valproate /Carbamazapine / Clozapine* • *Lithium / Levodopa* • *Metrizamide / Ifosfamide*
Gastrointestinal Disease	
• *Whipple's Disease* • *Malbsorption syndrome / Idiopathic Steatorrhea* • *Toxic Megacolon of Ulcerative Calitis*	
Structural lesions	
• *Vascular Infarction / Haemorrhage (brainstem / intraventruculer)* • *Subdural Empyema / hematoma* • *Encephalitis* • *Post-anoxic action myoclonus* • *Brain tumors* • *Post –surgical scars*	
Miscellaneous	
• *Congestive Cardiac Failure* • *Chronic Dialysis* • *Septisemia*	

127. Answer is B (Autoimmune hepatitis): *CMDT 2006/663,675; 09/597; Harrison 18th/p 2611, 2612 Harrison 17th/ 1987,1988; 16th/1877-1878*

Amongst the options provided, recurrence of primary disease in the liver following liver transplantation is most common with auto immune hepatitis.

'Autoimmune hepatitis has been recognized to recur in upto 40% of transplanted livers as immuno supression is reduced.' - CMDT' 2006 / 663

Recurrance of primary disease following liver transplantation		
Auto immune Hepatitis	**Primary billary Cirrhosis**	**Wilson's disease Alpha$_1$ –Antitrypsin deficiency**
Disease has been recognized to recur in upto 40% of transplanted livers as immunosupression is reduced *(CMDT)*	Disease recurs in the graft in 20% by 3 years' – *CMDT*	'Hereditary disorders such as Wilson's disease and α_1 antitrypsin deficiency have not recurred after liver transplantation' – *Harrisons 16/e, p 1878*

Hepatorenal Syndrome

128. Answer is A & B (urine Na < 10 meq/l and Normal Renal Histology): *Walker's Pediatric Gastrointestinal Disease 5th/1140; Washington Manual of Medical Therapeutics 32nd/506*

Hepatorenal syndrome is associated with normal renal histology and supported by a urine sodium excretion < 10meq/L

Hepatorenal syndrome

- Hepatorenal syndrome is defined as a state of functional renal failure (Reduced GFR) in patients with severe liver disease
- ***Structurally /Histologically the kidneys are normal and recover function after successful liver transplantation.***
- The pathogenetic hallmark of hepatorenal syndrome is intense renal vasoconstriction with coexistent systemic vasodilatation
- The diagnosis of hepatorenal syndrome is considered in accordance with the following diagnostic criteria.

Diagnostic of Hepatorenal Syndrome
Major criteria
• *Low glomerular filtration rate, as indicated by serum creatinine > 1.5 mg/dL or 24-hr creatinine clearance < 40 mL/min*
• *Absence of shock, ongoing bacterial infection, fluid losses, and current treatment with nephrotoxic drugs*
• *No sustained improvement in renal function (decrease in serum creatinine to 1.5 mg/dL or increase in creatinine clearance to 40 mL/min) after diuretic withdrawal and expansion of plasma volume with 1.5L of a plasma expander*
• *Proteinuria <500 mg/dL and no ultrasonographic evidence of obstructive uropathy or parenchymal renal disease*
Additional criteria
• *Urine volume < 500 mL/d*
• *Urine sodium < 10 meq/L*
• *Urine osmolality greater than plasma osmolality*
• *Urine red blood cells <50/high- power field*
• *Serum sodium concentration < 130 mEqL*
Note: All major criteria must be present for the diagnosis of hepatorenal syndrome. Additional criteria are not necessary for the diagnosis but provide supportive evidence.

129. Answer is C (Urine osmolality is lower than plasma osmolality): *Refer previous question*

Hepatorenal syndrome is associated with urine osmolality greater than plasma osmolality (and not lower than plasma osmolality).

Creatinine clearance < 40 ml/minute and poor response to volume expansion are major diagnostic features of hepatorenal syndrome while urinary sodium of less than 10 mmol/L is an additional criteria that provides supportive evidence.

130. Answer is A > C (The creatinine clearance is > 40 ml/min) : *Refer previous question.*

Hepatorenal syndrome is associated with creatinine clearance < 40 ml/min which is a major criteria in the diagnsis of hepatorenal syndrome and the single best answer of choice
Hepatorenal syndrome is also associated with a urine osmolaity that is higher (and not lower) than plasma osmolality. However this is an additional or supportive criteria that is not necessary for diagnosis and hence this is not the answer of choice.

Hepatocellular Carcinoma

131. Answer is D (Animal fat in diet): *Harrison 16th/534, 527; Robbins 7th/924; Harrison 17th/ 580 Harrison 18th/p 777*

Animal fat in diet is a known risk factor for development of colorectal cancer. It has not been mentioned as a risk for hepatocellular carcinoma

Risk factors for hepatocellular carcinoma:

Major etiological factors - *Robbins*	**Other etiological factors** – *Harrison*
1. Viral infection	Alphal antitrypsin deficiency
Hepatitis C infection	Hemochromatosis
Hepatitis B infection	Tyrosinemia
2. Chronic alcoholism	Primary biliary cirrhosis
3. Food contaminants: Alfatoxins	Exposure to thoriumdioxide or vinyl chloride
	Long term androgenic steroid administration
	Exposure to estrogen

132. Answer is B (Hepatocellular Carcinoma): *Harrison 18th/p 777, 778, 779 Harrison's 17th/580,581,582*

Presence of elevated Alphafetoprotein levels (tumor marker) and hepatomegaly (most common clinical sign) in a sixty year old patient with cirrhosis (predisposing factor) suggests the diagnosis of hepatocellular carcinoma.

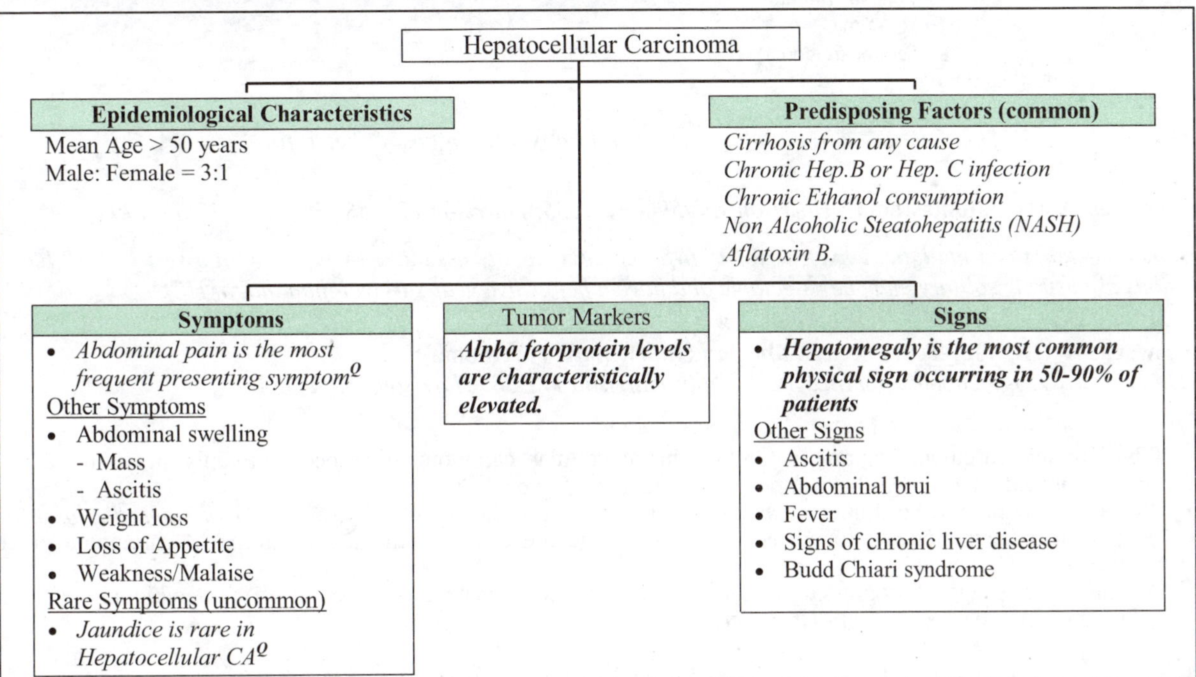

133. Answer is A (Jaundice): *Harrison 16th/534; Robbins 581*

Jaundice is rare in hepatocellular carcinoma- *Harrison*

Clinical manifestations of hepatocellular carcinoma:
• Abdominal pain and Abdominal mass - The most common presenting features are abdominal pain with detection of an abdominal mass I the right upper quadrant- *Harrison 16th/534* • Ascites - Blood tinged ascites occur in about 20% of cases – *Harrison 16th/534* • Friction rub or brui: - A friction rub or brui may be over the liver • Malaise, fatigue, weight loss
Uncommon / inconstant features
• Jaundice - Jaundice is ***rare***, unless significant deterioration of liver function or mechanical obstruction of bile duct occurs-*Harrison 16th/534* • Esophageal variceal bleeding - Gastrointestinal or esophageal variceal bleeding are ***inconstant*** findings – *Robbins*

134. Answer is A (Hepatocellular carcinoma) : *Robbins 7th/926; Harrison 18th/p 779 Harrison 17th/ 582*

Presence of elevated serum α fetopotein in the background of chronic history of alcohol consumption (risk factor for HCC) leads us to the diagnosis pf hepatocellular carcinoma.

AFP is the most specific and an ideal tumor marker for primary Ca of the liver i.e, Hepatocellular Carcinoma

The presence and persistence of high levels of serum AFP (Over 500 to 1000mg/L) in an adult with liver disease, and without an obvious gastrointestinal tumor strongly suggests Hepatocellular C_A.

AFP levels as tumor marker
1. Liver cell carcinoma: Hepatocellular carcinoma Hepatoblastoma
2. Non seminomatous germ cell tumors of testes and ovary: Choriocarcinoma Embryonal carcinoma Yolk sac tumors Teratoma Teratocarcinoma
3. Gastrointestinal tumors

AFP levels may also be increased in non neoplastic conditions like cirrhosi & hepatitis.

135. Answer is A (Hepatoblastoma): *Harrison 15th/590; 16th/535; Harrison 17th/ 582 Harrison 18th/p 779*

Hepatoblastoma is a malignant liver tumor of infancy i.e. typically associated with very high serum AFP levels. *The lesions are usually solitary, may be resectable and have a better five year survival than that of HCC.*

136. Answer is A (High levels are seen in fibrolamellar hepatic carcinoma):
- Harrison 16th/534; Chandrasoma Taylor 3rd/660; Harrison 17th 585 Harrison 18th/p 784

Fibrolamellar variant has no AFP elevation.

- Fibrolamellar carcinoma is rare variant of hepatocellular carcinoma that occurs mainly in young adults and characteristically has no AFP elevation – *Chandrasoma Taylor 3rd/660*
- Alpha fetoprotein may be slightly elevated in some cases of hepatitis and cirrhosis – *Chandrasoma Taylor 3rd/660*
- Alpha feto protein may be found as a result of large metastasis from gastric (stomach) carcinoma or colonic carcinomas – *Harrisons*
- A rising level suggests progression of tumor or recurrence after hepatic resection or therapeutic approach such as ablation or chemoembolization.- *Harrison*

137. Answer is A (Not common in Asians): *Harrison, 15th/ 588; 16th/534; Harrison 17th/ 580 Harrison 18th/p 777*

Primary hepatocellular carcinoma is specially prevalent in regions of Asia and Sub-Saharan Africa.

- Primary hepatocellular carcinoma is specially prevalent in regions of Asia and Sub-Saharan Africa.
- The principal reason for high incidence of HCC in parts of Asia and Africa is the frequency of chronic infection with hepatitis B virus and hepatitis C virus. *Raised titres of HBV and HBC markers are thus important etiological predictors.*
- *Percutaneous liver biopsy is diagnostic* provided the sample is taken from an area localized by ultrasound or CT – *Harrison*
- *Fibromellar variant grows slowly and is associated with a longer survival if treated - Harrison*
(It has thus a better prognosis)

138. Answer is D (Has better prognosis): *Harrison 15th 590; Chandrasoma Taylor 3rd/660, Robbins 7th/925; Harrison 17th/ 585 Harrison 18th/p 784*

Fibrolamellar carcinoma grows slowly and is associated with a longer survival if treated. It has a distinctly better prognosis.

Characteristic features of fibrolamellar carcinoma
• Distinctive variant of Hepatocellular carcinoma
• Occurs in young adults (20 to 40 years of age)
• *Equal sex incidence (Robbins); More common in females -Chandrasoma Taylor*
• No association with HBV or cirrhosis
• Well circumscribed mass (localized) *Non encapsulated but well circumscribed – Harrison* *Grossly encapsulated – Chandrasoma Taylor*
• No AFP elevation -*Chandrasoma Taylor*
• Better prognosis: Slow growth and longer survival.

139. Answer is C (AFP levels always greater than 1000) : *Harrison 14th/580, 15th//590, 16th / 535; Chandrasoma Taylor 3rd / 660; Harrison 17th/ 585 Harrison 18th/p 784*

Fibrolamellar variant has no AFP elevation - Chandrasoma Taylor
Equal sex incidence - Robbins
More common in females -Chandrasoma Taylor
Although Robbins and Chandrasoma Taylor are contradicting each other as far as distribution of the tumor in the two sexes is concerned, elevation of AFP appears certainly not to be so significant as to rise to levels greater than 1000. The single best answer is undoubtedly option 'C'.

Budd Chiari Syndrome

140. Answer is A (Hepatic vein obstruction): *Harrison 14th/ 1709; 15th/ 1759; 16th/ 1862; Robbins 7th/ 919; 6th/ 883; Harrison 17th/ 733*

Budd chiari syndrome by definition is 'occlusion of hepatic vein'
Obstruction of two or more major hepatic veins produces Budd chiari syndrome
Obstruction of a single main hepatic vein by thrombosis is clinically silent

Budd Chiari Syndrome:

- It is a clinical complex characterized by -
  - Liver enlargement (hepatomegaly)
  - Ascitis
  - Abdominal pain
- It is produced as a result of obstruction of two or more major hepatic veins and results from increased intrahepatic blood pressure and an inability of the massive hepatic blood from to shunt around the blocked outflow tract
- The most common cause of hepatic vein obstruction producing Budd chiari syndrome is hepatic vein thrombosis.

It may also result from occlusion of IVC such as invasion by a tumour but this is certainly less common.
Idiopathic membranous obstruction of IVC is the most common cause of this syndrome in Japan.

141. Answer is D (Polycythemia vera): *Robbins 6th/ 883; 7th/919; (Not elaborated in sequential order in Robbins 7th)*

Amongst the options provided Polycythemia vera is the commonest cause of Budd chiary syndrome.
Budd chiari syndrome includes acute, subacute or chronic occlusion of hepatic vein most commonly caused by hepatic vein thrombosis.

Hepatic vein thrombosis is associated with in decreasing order of frequency: *Robbins 6th/ 883*
- Polycythemia vera [Q]
- Pregnancy
- Postpartum state
- Use of oral contraceptives
- Paroxysmal nocturnal hemoglobinuria (PNH) [Q]
- Intraabdominal cancers, particularly hepatocellular carcinoma.

142. Answer is C (Paroxysmal nocturnal hemoglobinuria): *Robbins 6th/ 1883: Previous question.*

The most common cause of hepatic vein thrombosis from the list mentioned in the previous question amongs the above is Paroxysmal nocturnal hemoglobinuria, and hence is the answer of choice here.

143. Answer is D (Thrombosis of hepatic veins): *Refer previous question.*

Most common cause of Budd Chiari Syndrome is hepatic vein obstruction
Most common cause of hepatic vein obstruction causing Budd Chiari Syndrome is 'thrombosis of hepatic veins'.

144. Answer is C (Hepatic vein): *Refer previous question*

Budd chiari syndrome is characterized by post sinusoidal obstruction outside the liver at the level of hepatic veins
– Harrison

Disorders of Biliary Tract

145. Answer is D (Cholestatic diseases) : *Harrison 16th/1815; Harrison 17th/ 1925 Harrison 18th/p 2529*

5' Nucleotidase reflects cholestasis and is rarely elevated in conditions other than liver disease.

Most important enzymes reflecting cholestasis
• Alkaline phophatase
• 5' Nucleotidase
• Gamma Glutanym transpeptidase

5' Nucleotidase and GGT are the most specific marker for cholestasis and are rarely elevated in conditions other than liver disease - Harrison

146. Answer is A (Decreased Bile and Increased cholesterol ratio): *Harrison 16th/1881, 1882; Harrison 17th/ 1991, 1992*

Bile salts and phospholipids in bile keep cholesterol in solution by the formation of micelles.
An ***excess of cholesterol relative to bite salts and phospholipids*** allows cholesterol to form crystals and such bile is called ***Lithogenic or Super-saturated bile***.

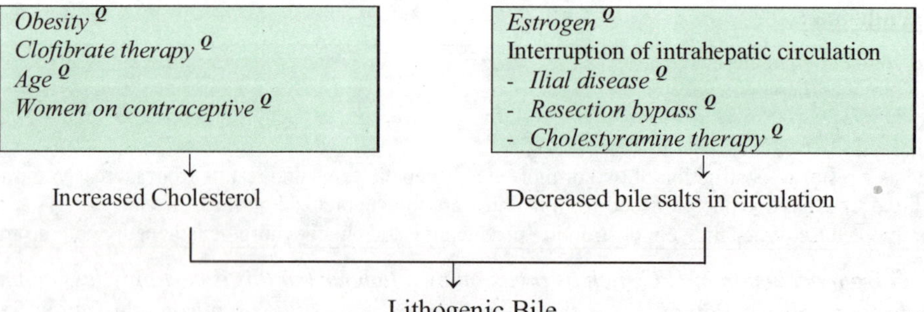

Precipitation of cholesterol crystals 'Cholesterol stones'

147. Answer is D (Hypercholesterolemia): *Harrison 14th/1728; 15th/1781; 16th/1881, 1882; 17th/ 1992, 1993 Harrison 18th/p 2617, 2618*

It is increased concentration of cholesterol relative to bile salts ***in bile*** *that promotes gall stone formation. Serum cholesterol may well be normal.*

All other options are known local factors that promote gall stone formation and hence Hypercholesterolemia is the single best answer of exclusion.

Formation of Gall stones is promoted by following factors :

1. ***Increased concentration of cholesterol*** relative to bile salts **in bile**. (***With or without hypercholesterolemia***)
2. Stasis
3. Infection

Clofibrate therapy :
This drug is used to excrete cholesterol in hyperlipoprotenemia
It therefore increases the concentration of cholesterol in bile.
Hyperalimentation :
Parental supplementation leads to hypofunction of Gall bladder, thus contibuting to gall stone formation by 'Stasis'.
Primary biliary cirrhosis :
Leads to a decrease in bile acid secretions. Decreased salts are unable to keep cholesterol in solution and therefore lead to precipitation of cholesterol stones

148. Answer is D (Vagal stimulation): *Bailey 23rd/975; Repeat*

Stone formation is enhanced by Truncal vagotomy (not by vagal stimulation).
Vagotomy promotes stasis of bile by inhibiting gall bladder contractility and promotes stone formation.
All other options have been explained in the previous questions.

149. Answer is B (Ileal resection): *Refer previous question*

Ileal resection is an established factor for gall stone formation.

Ileal resection is associated with interruption of enterohepatic circulation of bile salts thereby decreasing the ratio of bile salts to cholesterol within the bile (Lithogenic bile)

150. Answer is D (More common in males between 30-40 years of age): *Bailey and Love 24th/1103; 23rd/974*

Cholelithiasis is more common in women than men

Lithogenic bile is required for gall stone formation and gall stones.
May be associated with increased risk of carcinoma gall bladder.

Diabetes mellitus *is associated with Gall bladder hypomotility which may contribute to increased incidence of gall stone in diabetics.*

151. Answer is C (Terminal ileum): *Love &Bailey 23rd/1066; Harrison 14th/1732,15th/1783, 16th/1886; Sabiston 16th/1095;*

'Classically there is obstruction / impaction about 60 cm proximal to ileocaecal valve'- Bailey
'The site of obstruction by the impacted gall stone is usually at the ileocaecal valve" provided that the more proximal S.I. is of normal calibre. *- Harrisons*
If both choices come simultaneously in a question go for 60 cm proximal to ileacoecal valve, as, it has been defined as the narrowest part of small intestine.

152. Answer is C (Ileum): *Refer previous question*

Thye most common site of obstruction due to gall stone is the terminal ileum.

153. Answer is B (Duodenum 1st part): *Hamilton Bailey 10th/432; Diseases of Gall bladder and Bile duct 1st/188*

The most common site of Biliary – enteric fistulas is the duodenum (Cholecystoduodenal fistula)

Type of fistula	Percent	Comment
Cholecystoduodenal	≈ 75%	Most common type (duodenum)
Cholecysto colic	≈ 16%	Second most common (colon)

154. Answer is A (Observation) : *Bailey 23rd/974; Harrison 14th/1729, 15th/1780; 16th / 1884*

Prophylactic cholecystectomy is <u>not</u> warranted in an asymptomatic patient. *As the question does not provide us with any details to decide upon the possibility of medical therapy observation remains the management of choice.*
Gallstone disease in an asymptomatic patient or in a patient whose symptoms are not referable to cholelithiasis is called ***<u>'Silent' or Asymptomtic Gallstones</u>***, & is a common clinical problem.
Prophylactic cholecystectomy is <u>not</u> warranted.
This also applies to Diabetes with silent Gallstones.

155. Answer is D (55 year old with an asymptomatic gallstone): *Refer previous question*

Prophylactic cholecystectomy is not warranted in an asymptomatic patient.

156. Answer is C (No surgery for gallbladder stones): *Refer previous question*

Prophylactic cholecystectomy is not warranted in an asymptomatic patient.

157. Answer is A (Size of stone less than 15mm) : *Harrison 14th/1730; Harrison 15th/1781; 16th / 1884; Harrison 17th/ 1995*

Harrison 18th/p 2621

Medical therapy for gall bladder stone is amenable for stones < 15 mm (preferably <10 mm)

Prerequisites for medical therapy :
1. Gall bladder should be functioning Q
2. Stones should be radioluscent Q
3. Size should be small preferably < 15 mm Q *- Harrison 14th (<10mm-Harrison 16th)*
4. Stones should be 'cholesterol stones' only (obvious by thier mechanism of action) Q

(*Newer edition of Harrison has mentioned the size of stone to be preferably < 10 mm rather than < 15 mm but we will go with same answer because the question was framed in older times*).

Medical therapy for Gall stone dissolution consists of administration of :
UDCA (Ursodeoxycholic acid) Q
CDCA (Choledeoxycholic acid) Q

Mechanism of action:
Inhibit HmG CoA reductase activity Q, which in turn results in decreased hepatic cholesterol synthesis.
Allows dispersion of 'cholesterol' from stones by physicochemical means.

158. Answer is A (Motor mechanisms of Gall bladder): *Bailey 23rd / 967*

Functioning motor mechanism of the gall bladder is not a prerequisite* Q*, & even in its absence, the contrast can be concentrated in the Gall bladder & be visible radiographically.

Oral Cholecystogram (also called *Graham Cole test*)Q

- *Ipanoid Acid tablets* Q (contrast) is taken the right before the test.
- The contrast is absorbed, secreted into the bile by the liver (i.e. *functioning hepatocytes required*) Q passes through the cystic duct into the gal bladder (i.e. *patent cystic duct is required*). But is then concentrated in the Gall Bladder (ability to absorb water is required)
- *Functioning motor mechanism of the gall bladder is not a prerequisite* Q, & even in its absence, the contrast can be concentrated in the Gall bladder & be visible radiographically.
- Since *a negative test can result from so many causes, it is NOT diagnostic of Gall stone Disease.* Q

159. Answer is A (Renal stones): *Bailey 23rd/975*

Renal stones are not a feature of Saint's triad

Saint's triad (Association of)
Diverticular disease
Gall stone/Cholelithiasis
Hiatus Hernia

160. Answer is D (Vomiting): *Clinical Surgery by Thompson/289*

Charcot's triad constitute the classical presentation of acute cholangitis and includes:

Charcot's triad
Abdominal pain
High fever with rigors
Jaundice

161. Answer is A (CBD stone) : *Harrisons 14th/580, 15th/590; 16th/536; Harrison 17th/ 585 Harrison 18th/p 784*

Cholelithiasis is not clearly a predisposing factor for Cholangiocarcinoma - Harrison

The predisposing factors of cholangiocarcinoma include :
1. Chronic hepato-biliary parasite infection Q (Clonorchiasis or Asiatic cholangio-hepatitis) Q
2. Congenital Anomaly with ectatic ducts (Choledochal cyst). Q
3. Sclerosing cholangitis Q
4. Ulcerative colitis Q
5. Occupational exposure to carcinogens Q (Rubber + Automotive plants)

Note: *Nodular lesions that arise at the bifurcation of hepatic ducts are called* ***Klastskin tumors***. Q

162. Answer is D (Chronic pancreatitis) : *Refer previous question; Harrison 17th/ 585 Harrison 18th/p 784*

Chronic pancreatitis does not predispose to cholangiocarcinoma

163. Answer is C (Size of polyp > 5mm) *Schwartz 8th / 1214, Manual of Gastroenterology 4th/ 457; 'Mastery of surgery' by Fischer 5th/ 1025, Basis and New Aspects of Gastrointestinal Ultrasonography' (2005)/117*

Risk factor for malignant change in an Adenomatous Gall bladder polyp is a size greater than 1.0 cm (10mm). Polyps smaller than 1.0 cm seldom undergo malignant transformation.

'Malignancy should be considered when polyp exceeds 1 cm in diameter or when rapid growth of polyp is seen on sonographic follow-up' - 'Diagnostic Ultrasound' by Goldberg – 2nd/ 454

Factors which indicate possibility of malignancy in Gall bladder polyps
• *Age > 50 years*[Q]
• *Presence of a single polyp*[Q]
• *Sessile Polyps*[Q]
• *Polyp > 1.0 cm in size*[Q]
• *Rapid change in size of polyp*[Q]
• *Associated Gall stones*[Q]

(*Taken from 'Basic and New Aspects of Gastrointestinal Ultrasonography* (2005 / 117))

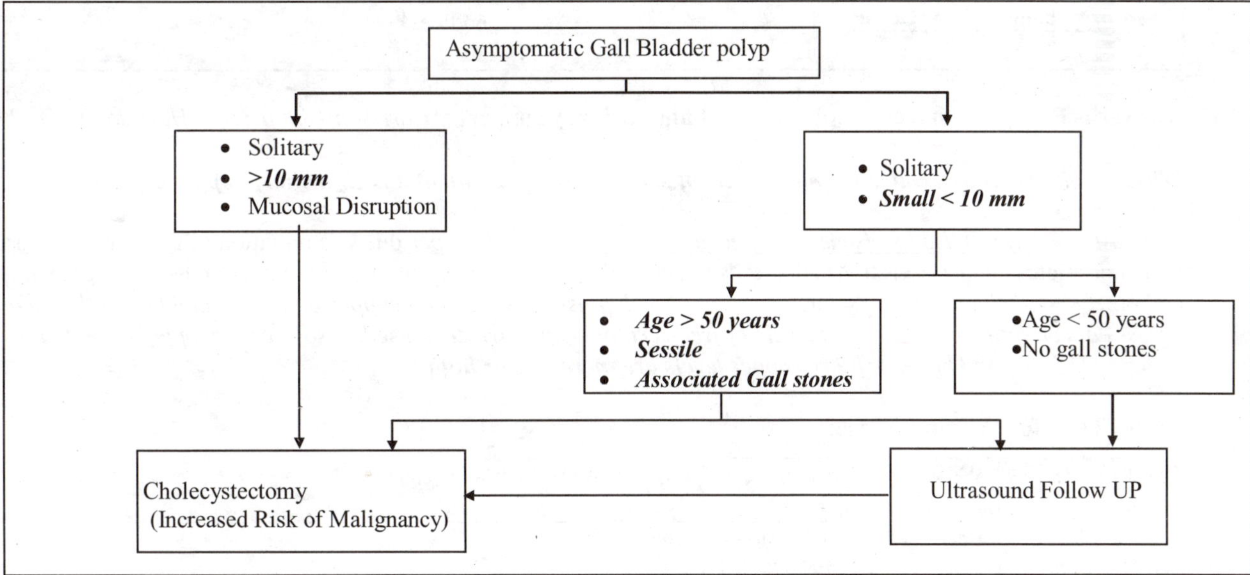

Wilson's Disease and Hemochromatosis

164. Answer is B (Increased Ceruloplasmin) : *Harrison 15th / 2274; 16th/2314; 17th/ 1981, 1982 Harrison 18th/p 2604*

In Wilson's disease, Ceruloplasmin levels are decreased (not increased).

In Wilson's disease excess Cu saturates liver and spills in the plasma thereby decreasing ceruloplasmin levels. (Serum Ceruloplasmin is ↓↓ Q)

Serum Ceruloplasmin levels	
Normal	180-350mg/L (18-35 mg/dl)
Wilson's Disease	Low in 90%

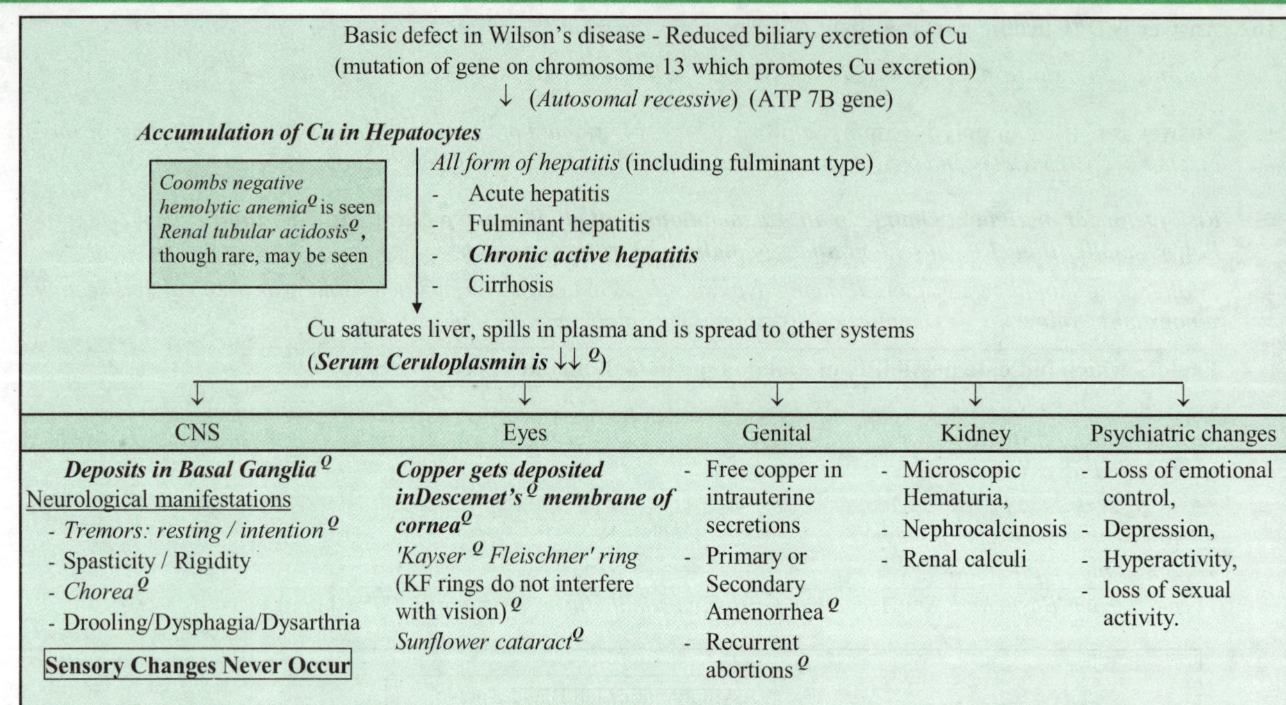

165. Answer is B (Low serum ceruloplasmin and high urinary copper) : *Harrison 18th/p 3189 Harrison's 17th/2450*

Wilson's disease is associated with low levels of serum ceruloplasmin and high urinary copper excretion

The basic defect in Wilson's disease is reduced biliary excretion of copper due to a mutation of gene on chromosome 13 which promotes copper excretion. This leads to accumulation of copper initially in the liver and subsequently in plasma and other systems once liver is saturated. *Serum ceruloplasmin is the main copper binding protein in the blood and once excess copper spills into the blood, **levels of free ceruloplasmin are decreased.** Also excess copper is eventually excreted in urine and hence **urinary copper levels are increased or high.***

Useful Tests for Wilson Disease:

Test	Wilson's Disease	Normal Value	Comment (Wilson's Disease)	Usefulness
Serum ceruloplasmin	***Decreased***	180-350mg/L (18-35 mg/dL)	Low in 90%	+
KF rings	*Present*	Absent	Present in 99% if neurologic or psychiatric symptoms present Present in 30-50% in hepatic presentation/presymptomatic state	++
24-h urine Cu	***Increased***	0.3-0.8 μmol (20-50 μg)	>1.6 μmol (>100 μg) in symptomatic patients 0.9 to >1.6 μmol (60 to > 100 μg) in presymptomatic patients	+++
Liver Cu	*Increased*	0.3–0.8 μmol/g (20-50 μg)	>3.1 μmol (>200 μg) (obstructive liver disease can cause false-positive results)	++++
Haplotype analysis	*2 Matches*	0 Matches	2 Matches	++++ (Siblings only)

166. Answer is B (Wilson's Disease): *Harrison 18th/p 3188 Harrisons 17th/2449, 2450; Harrisons 16th/2313,2314; Refer previous question*

Psychiatric manifestations in the form of emotional lability along with neurological manifestations in the form of tremors and the characteristic 'Kayser Fleisher Rings' (golden brown discolouration of descemet's membrane) are diagnostic of Wilsons disease.

167. Answer is B (Testicular Atrophy): *Harrison 18th/p 3187, 3188 Harrisons 17th/2449, 2450, 2451; Harrisons 16th/2313,2314*

Testicular Atrophy is not documented as a feature of Wilson's disease.
Hemolytic Anemia, Chorea and Chronic active hepatitis are documented manifestations of Wilson's disease.

Hemolytic Anemia is a feature of Wilson disease
Hemolytic Anemia may occur in severe hepatic failure because large amounts of copper derived from Hepatocellular damage are released into the blood stream.
'The association of hemolysis and liver disease makes Wilson's a likely diagnosis'- Harrison

Chorea is a feature of Wilson's disease
Chorea is an established Neurological manifestation of wilson's disease

Chronic Active hepatitis is a feature of Wilson's disease
Wilson's disease may present as fatty change, acute hepatitis, chronic active hepatitis, cirrhosis or massive hepatic necrosis.

168. Answer is C (Wilson's disease): *Harrison 18th/p 3188 Harrisons 17th/ 2450; Greenberg's Text Atlas of Emergency Medicine (2005)/114*

KF rings are a charachteristic feature of Wilson's disease.

Kayser – Fleischer Rings (KF Rings)

- *Brownish yellow discolourations*[Q] *seen in limbic zone of cornea*
- *Result from deposition of copper in Descemet's membrane*[Q] *of the cornea*
- *Do not interfere with vision*[Q]
- *Charachteristically seen in Wilson's disease*[Q] *but are not pathognomic*[Q] *of Wilson's disease* and may be seen in other conditions

Conditions that may present with KF rings
• ***Wilson's disease (characteristic*[Q]*)***
• *Chronic Active Hepatitis / Autoimmune Hepatitis*
• *Primary Biliary Cirrhosis*
• *Intrahepatic cholestatic syndromes*

- *Present in almost all patients of Wilsons disease with Neurological /Psychiatric symptoms* (99% of patients)[Q]
- Present in only 30-50% of patients of Wilson's disease with only hepatic manifestations
- Absence of KF rings does not exclude the diagnosis of Wilson's disease[Q]
- May occasionally be visible to the naked eye without magnification but *definite diagnosis can only be made by an ophthalmologist using a slit lamp*[Q]

169. Answer is C (Urinary copper excretion is <100μg/day): *Harrison 18th/p 3188, 3189 Harrisons 17th/2450; Harrisons 16th/2313,2314*

Urine copper is an important diagnostic too. Symptomatic patients invariably have urine copper levels > 100 μ (>1.6 umol) per 24 hours.

Wilson's disease is an autosomal recessive disorder

It is caused by a mutation of a gene on chromosome 13[Q] *which promotes Cu excretion (ATP 7B gene)*

Symptomatic patients with Wilson's disease invariably have urinary copper excretion of >100 μg per 24 hours (>1.6 μmol /24 hr)

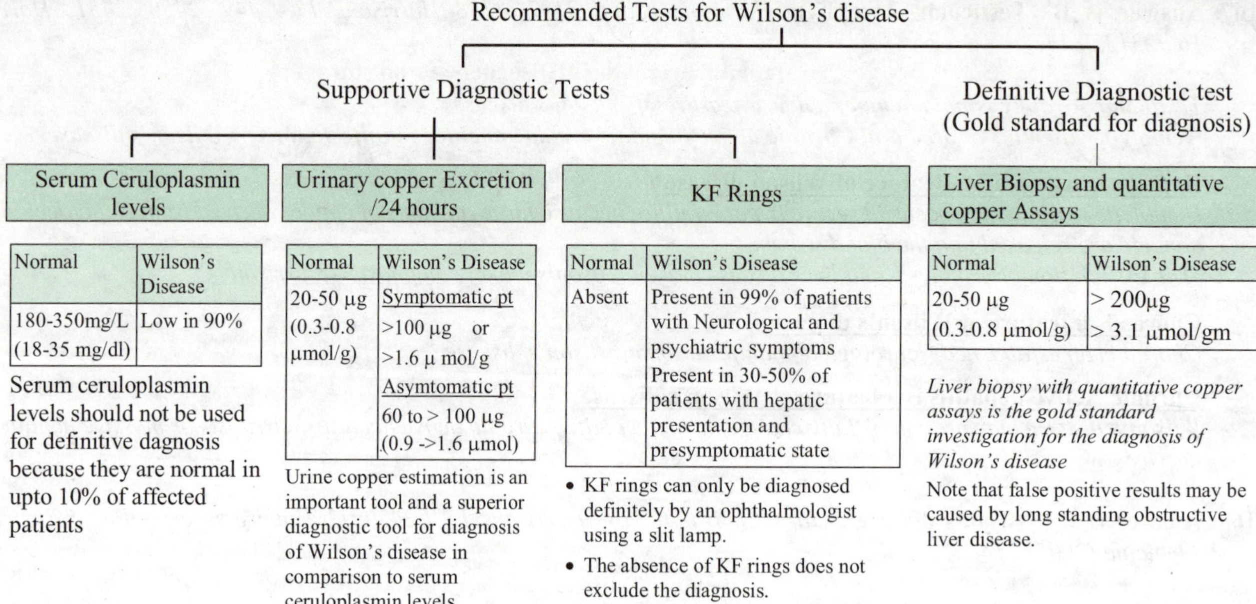

Serum Ceruloplasmin levels

Normal	Wilson's Disease
180-350mg/L (18-35 mg/dl)	Low in 90%

Serum ceruloplasmin levels should not be used for definitive dagnosis because they are normal in upto 10% of affected patients

Urinary copper Excretion /24 hours

Normal	Wilson's Disease
20-50 μg (0.3-0.8 μmol/g)	Symptomatic pt >100 μg or >1.6 μ mol/g Asymtomatic pt 60 to > 100 μg (0.9 ->1.6 μmol)

Urine copper estimation is an important tool and a superior diagnostic tool for diagnosis of Wilson's disease in comparison to serum ceruloplasmin levels.

KF Rings

Normal	Wilson's Disease
Absent	Present in 99% of patients with Neurological and psychiatric symptoms Present in 30-50% of patients with hepatic presentation and presymptomatic state

- KF rings can only be diagnosed definitely by an ophthalmologist using a slit lamp.
- The absence of KF rings does not exclude the diagnosis.

Liver Biopsy and quantitative copper Assays

Normal	Wilson's Disease
20-50 μg (0.3-0.8 μmol/g)	> 200μg > 3.1 μmol/gm

Liver biopsy with quantitative copper assays is the gold standard investigation for the diagnosis of Wilson's disease

Note that false positive results may be caused by long standing obstructive liver disease.

Zinc is the treatment of choice for maintainance therapy in Wilson's disease

Zinc is the treatment of choice in Wilson's disease for

- *Initial therapy in patients with hepatitis without decompensation*[Q]
- *Maintainance therapy*
- *Presymptomatic patient*
- *Pediatric patients*
- *Pregnant patients*

170. Answer is A (Zinc): *Harrison 18th/p 3188 Harrisons 17th/2451: Harrisons 16th/2313,2314*

Presence of KF rings and decreased ceruloplasmin levels suggest the diagnosis of Wilson's disease.
The patient in question is presenting with intial hepatic disease without any evidence of hepatic decompensation.
Zinc is the therapy of choice for patients with hepatitis or cirrhosis without evidence of hepatic decompensation or neuropsychiatric symptoms.

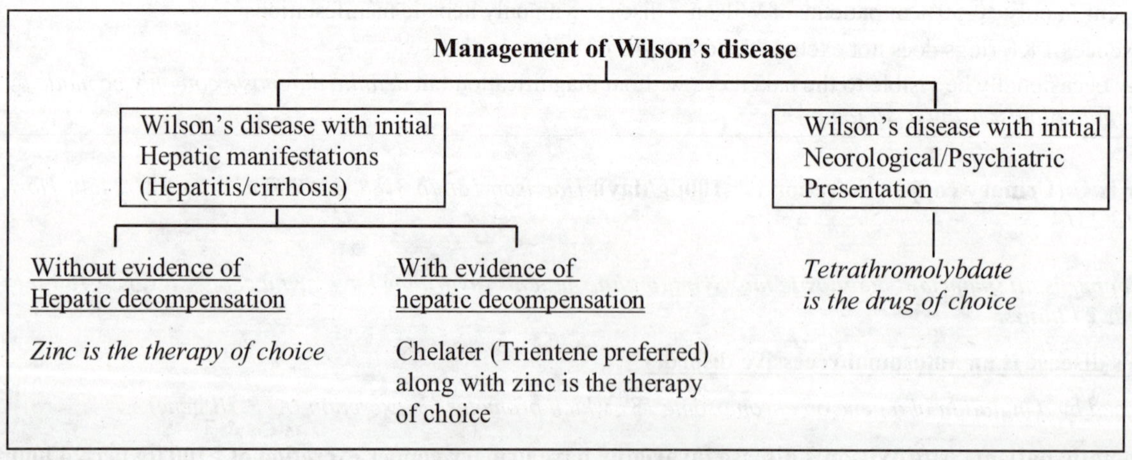

Hematochromatosis

171. Answer is A (Hemochromatosis): *Harrisons 16th/2288-2303; Harrisons 17th/2433 Harrison 18th/p 3164, 3165*

The association of Arthritis, hyperpigmentation of skin and hypogonadism suggests the diagnosis of hematochromatosis.

Hematochromatosis (Disorder of iron storage)

Inappropriate increase in intestinal absorption results in deposition of excessive amounts of iron in parenchymal cells with eventual tissue damage and impaired function of organs

Serum iron ↑ed
% Transferrin saturation ↑ed
Serum ferritin ↑ed
Elevation in percent Transferrin saturation is the earliest phenotypic marker of herditary hemochromatosis[Q]

Liver	**Skin**	Pancreas	**Joints**	Heart	***Hypogonadism***
• Usually *first organ to be affected* • Hepatomegaly is seen in 95% of symptomatic patients • Cirrhosis may occur (Micronodular) • Hepatocellular carcinoma (30% of patients with cirrhosis). • It is the *most common cause of death in treated patients.*	• ***Excessive skin (Bronzing of skin) pigmentation*** is present in 90% of symptomatic patients • Usually diffuse and generalized. May be more pronounced on Face, Neck, Extensor aspect of forearm, dorsa of hands, lower legs and genitalia and ears • Usually results from increased melanin and iron in dermis	Involvement of pancreas *results in Diabetes mellitus* which is seen in 65% of symptomatic patients	• ***Arthropathy*** develops in 25-50% of patients • *The joints of hands especially the 2nd and 3rd MCP joints are the first to be involved* • Progressive polyarthritis involving wrist, knees, hips and ankles may also be seen	• Heart is involved in 15% of symptomatic patients • The most common manifestation is congestive heart failure • Cardiomyopathy and cardiac arrhythmias may be seen	• Results from impairment of Hypothalmo pituitary function by iron deposition which leads to decreased production of gonadotrophins.

Treatment of Haematochromatosis

Therapy of Haematochromatosis involves removal of excessive body iron and supportive treatment of damaged organs

Removal of Excessive Body iron

- ***Phlebotomy is the treatment of choice***
  Iron removal is best accomplished by once or twice weekly phlebotomy of 500ml,
  - These should be continued until the serum ferritin level is < 50μg/L (May be required for 1-2 years)
  - Thereafter phlebotomies are performed at appropriate intervals to maintain ferritin levels between 50-100 μg/L (usually one phlebotomy every 3 months)
- **Chelating agents** *(such as Desferoxamine) are alternative agents and indicated when anemia and hypoproteinemia are severe enough to preclude phlebotomy*

Alcohol consumption should be eleminated[Q] *as it increases the risk of cirrhosis in hematochromatosis nearly ten fold.*

The charachteristic clinical features of Haemochromatosis in order of frequency are[Q] ***:***

- *Hepatomegaly (95%)*
- *Skin pigmentation (90%)*
- *Diabetes mellitus (65%)*
- *Arthropathy (25-50%)*
- *Cardiac disease (15%)*
- *Hypogonadism*

172. Answer is D (Increased Transferrin Saturation): *Harrison 18th/p 3165, 3166 Harrisons 17th/2431,2432Mayo clinic Gastroenterology and Hepatology Board Review by Hauser 2nd/323; Clinical Laboratory medicine by Mc Clatchey 2nd/839*

'A transferrin saturation of more than 45% is the earliest phenotypic abnormality in hereditary hematochromatosis'
- Hauser 2nd/3232

Transferrin saturation and measurement of unbound iron bindeng capacity are recommended for initial scrceening of individuals

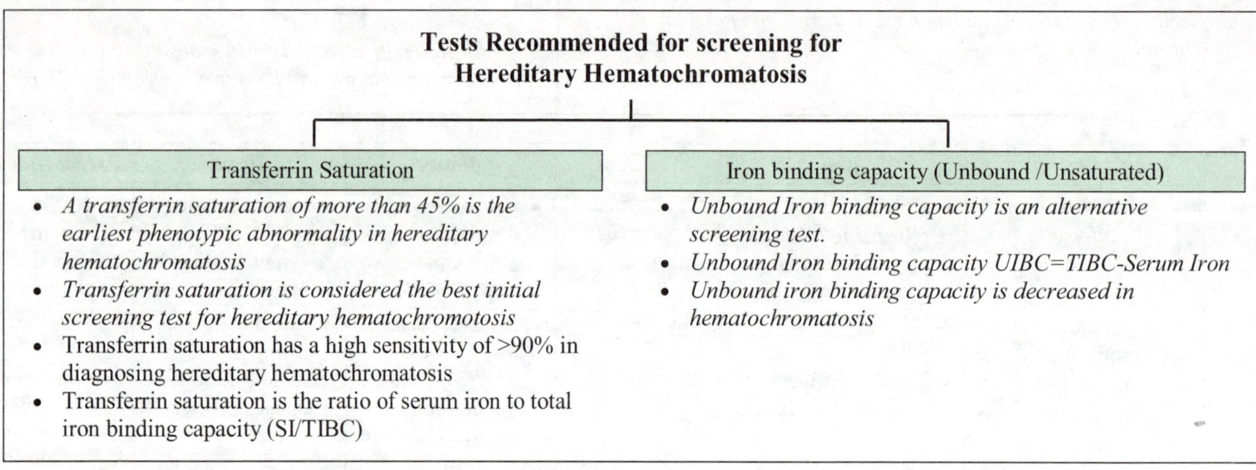

173. Answer is A (Iron binding capacity): *Harrison 18th/p 3165, 3166 Harrisons 17th/2433*

The presence of hyperpigmentation and diabetes (bronze diabetes) together with restrictive cardiomyopathy and cirrhosis suggests a diagnosis of hereditary hematochromatosis.

The best initial test to diagnose hereditary hematochromatosis are Transferrin saturation and unsaturated Iron binding capacity

As transferrin saturation is not provided amongst the options, Iron binding capacity is the single best answer of choice.

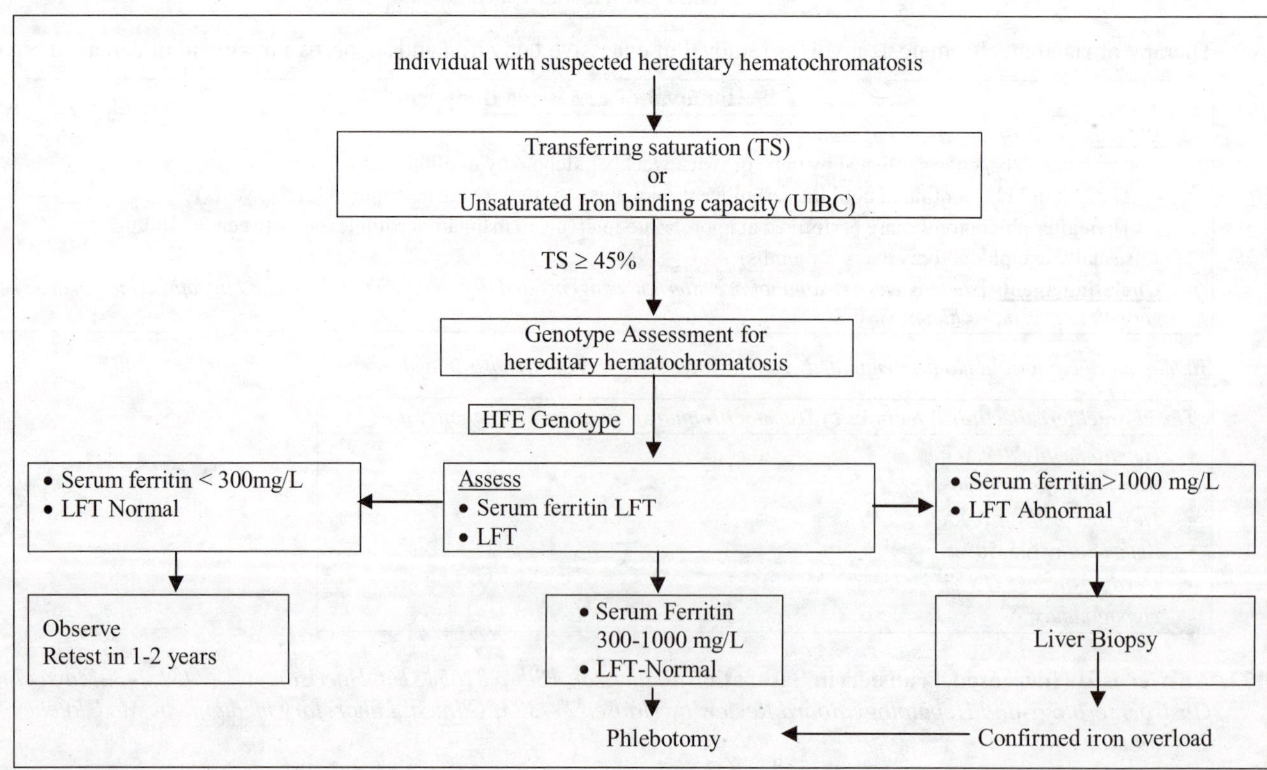

Note

Serum ferritin levels are a good index of body iron stores and are raised early during the cause of disease. Yet serum ferritin levels should not be used as initial screening test to detect hereditary hematochromatosis.
This is because serum ferritin also acts as an acute phase reactant and its levels are increased in variable infections and inflammatory conditions without iron overload. Also the serum concentration of ferritin may be increased in patients with hepatocellular injury as in viral hepatitis, alcoholic fatty liver disease or alcoholic liver diseases due to increased release from tissue cells.

174. Answer is D (Desferrioxamine is the treatment of choice): *Harrison 18th/3166; 17th/2433; Harrisons 16th/2288,2203*

The treatment of choice for Hematochromatosis is removed of excess body iron by Phlebotomy and not with the use of chelating agents like desfernoxamine.

Phlebotomy is the treatment of choice in Hematochromatosis

Treatment of Haematochromatosis

Therapy of Haematochromatosis involves removal of excessive body iron and supportive treatment of damaged organs

Removal of Excessive Body iron
• ***Phlebotomy is the treatment of choice*** Iron removal is best accomplished by once or twice weekly phlebotomy of 500ml, - These should be continued until the serum ferritin level is < 50µg/L (May be required for 1-2 years) - Thereafter phlebotomies are performed at appropriate intervals to maintain ferritin levels between 50-100 µg/L (usually one phlebotomy every 3 months) • **Chelating agents** *(such as Desferoxamine) are alternative agents and indicated when anemia and hypoproteinemia are severe enough to preclude phlebotomy*

Alcohol consumption should be eleminated[Q] as it increases the risk of cirrhosis in hematochromatosis nearly ten fold

Arthropathy, Hypogonadism, Diabetes and Bronzing (pigmentation) of skin are all characteristic manifestation of hematochromatosis

The charachteristic clinical features of Haemochromatosis in order of frequency are[Q] :
• *Hepatomegaly (95%)* • *Skin pigmentation (90%)* • *Diabetes mellitus (65%)* • *Arthropathy (25-50%)* • *Cardiac disease (15%)* • *Hypogonadism*

Note: The combination of skin hyperpigmentation and insulin deficiency (diabetes) is called Bronze diabetes.

Miscellaneous

175. Answer is C (Glutathione-S- Transferase is used as a hepatic prognostic marker after surgery): *Harrison's 18th/2528; Schiff Diseases of the Liver 11th/chapter 2; Biomarkers of Disease. An Evidence Based Approach (Cambridge University Press) 2006/169*

Glutathione – S – Transferase is an emerging enzyme marker for post-transplant monitoring (surgery) as an aid to the diagnosis of acute allagraft rejection
ALT is a more specific indicator of liver injury than AST and absolute levels of aminotransferase do not correlate with outcome.

ALT is a more specific indicator of Liver injury than AST

'AST (Aspartate Aminotransferase) is found in the liver, cardiac muscle, skeletal muscle, kidneys, brain, pancreas, lung, leukocytes and erythrocytes in decreasing order of concentration.
ALT is found primarily in the liver and is therefore a more specific indicator of Liver injury *- Harrison's 18th/2528*

Absolute level of Aminotransferase elevation do not correlate with outcome

'There is poor correlatation between extent of Liver cell Necrosis and the elevation of serum aminotransferase levels in chronic liver diseases. Similarly, absolute elevation of aminotransferase levels is of little value in predicting the outcome of acute hepatocellular disorders' - Schiff's Deseases of the Liver

Serum Glutathione – S- Transferase may be used as a prognostic marker after transplant surgery

'Serum Alpha – Glutathione – S – Transferase is an emerging static test indicating hepatocellular damage. As in vivo plasma half life of this enzyme is less than 60-90 minutes, this enzyme offer advantages in post-transplant monitoring as an aid to the diagnosis of acute allagraft rejection. Recent investigations have indicated that monitoring of GST reduced both mortality and morbidity in liver transplant recipients. GST showed a distinct higher sensitivity (81%) for acute rejection than conventional liver function tests (the specificity however was relatively low (45%).

- Biomarkers of Disease: Evidence Based Approach

Glutathione – S-Transferase (GST) - *Miller's Anesthesia (Elsevier) 2010/426*
Glutathione-S-Transferase is a sensitive and specific test for some patterns of Liver injury. The enzyme has a brief plasma half life (90 minutes) and is released rapidly into circulation following hpatocellular injury. Thus serial GST measurements can reveal time course of hepatic injury from its onset to its resolution. In contrast to AST and ALT which reside in Acinar Zone I, GST localizes in Acinar Zone III (centrilobular region). This zone contains the hepatacyte population with highest susceptibility to injury from hypoxia or reactive drug metabolites. Accordingly GST would be more sensitive than AST or ALT as a marker of contrilobular necrosis in its incipient stage.

176. Answer is A (Bulky Disease): *Essentials of Clinical Oncology (Jaypee)2005/324; Principles & Practice of Surgical Oncology (Lippincott Williams) 2009/964*

The most important role of serum LDH is to estimate the tumor bulk (volume of tumor).

'LDH levels are elevated in large volume bulky tumors of any histology. LDH levels when elevated correlate well with the volume of tumor' – The Essential of clinical oncology.

'LDH elevation provides a useful guide to bulk of disease; Bulky Disease (In Hodgkin's Lymphoma) is a node mass more than 10 cm in diameter' - 'Essential Revision notes for MRCP' by Katra (PasTest)2004/288

Serum LDH is a non specific marker elevated in a variety of tumors.

177. Answer is A (5% weight loss in 1-2 months): *Medical Nutrition & Disease:A case based approach (John Wiley & Sons)2009/10*

Significant weight loss is defined as 5% weight loss in 1 month.

Percent weight change over a period of time is calculated using the person's current body weight and person's usual body weight.

$$\text{Percent weight change} = \frac{\text{Usual weight} - \text{Current weight}}{\text{Usual weight}}$$

Severity of weight loss is thereby defined by percent change in a defined period of time

Time	Significant weight	Severe weight loss
1 week	*1-2%*	*>2%*
1 month	*5%*	*>5%*
3 months	*7.5%*	*7.5%*
6 months	*10%*	*10%*
1 year	*20%*	*20%*

178. Answer is All (All of the above) : *Current Diagnosis and Treatment in Gastroenterology, Hepatology and Endoscopy (2009)/518, Harrison's 17th/1984*

Biliary atresia is an indication for Liver transplantation in children while primary Biliary Cirrhosis, Sclerosing cholangitis and Hematochromatosis an established indications for Liver transplantation in adults

Indication for Liver Transplantation:

Children	Aduts
Biliary atresia	Primary biliary cirrhosis
Neonatal hepatitis	Secondary biliary cirrhosis
Congenital hepatic fibrosis	Primary sclerosing cholangitis
Alagille's disease[a]	Autoimmune hepatitis
Byler's disease[b]	Caroli's disease[c]
α1-Antitrypsin deficiency	Cryptogenic cirrhosis
Inherited disorders of metabolism	Chronic hepatitis with cirrhosis
Wilson's disease	Hepatic vein thrombosis
Tyrosinemia	Fulminant hepatitis
Glycogen storage diseases	Alcoholic cirrhosis
Lysosomal storage diseases	Chronic viral hepatitis
Protoporphyria	Primary hepatocellular malignancies
Crigler-Najjar disease type 1	Hepatic adenomas
Familial hypercholesterolemia	Nonalcoholic steatohepatitis
Primary hyperoxaluria type 1	Familial amyloid polyneuropathy
Hemophilia	

[a]Arteriohepatic dysplasia, with paucity of bile ducts, and congenital malformations, including pulmonary stenosis.
[b]Intrahepatic cholestasis, progressive liver failure, mental and growth retardation
[c]Multiple cystic dilatations of the intrahepatic biliary tree.

Hematochromatosis is also an indication for Liver Transplantation

'Among genetic and metabolic conditions, Hematachroatosis is the most common reason for Liver Transplantation' - *Current Gastroenterology & Hepatology (LANGE) 2009/518*

179. Answer is D (Estimation of Galactose Elimination capacity): *'Textbook of Hepatology' by Rodes 3rd / 475*

Estimation of Galactose Elimination capacity (GEC) is an example of quantitative liver tests

Liver Function tests

Non quantitative Tests for Liver Function	Quantitative tests for Liver Function
Although generally termed as Liver function tests, these are either not related to function or only reflect given aspects of liver function and are not over all parameters of latter	Quantitative tests for Liver function measure the true functional reserve of the liver
These Include	These Include
• *Serum Bilirubin* • *Serum Alkaline phosphatase* • *Serum Transminases* • *Serum Bile Acids* • *Serum Albumin* • *Serum prothrombin time, etc*	• ***Galactose Elimination capacity*** • *Urea synthesis capacity* • *Inducyanine clearance* • *Sorbitol clearance* • *Caffeine clearance* • *Aminopyrine Breath test* • *Ketoisocaproic acid breath test*

180. Answer is D (Hepatic Porphyrias): *Harrison's 16th/2316,2320; Oxford Textbook of Medicine 4th/69, Gastrointestinal and Liver Disease by Feldman 8th/1623*

Frank Hepatomegaly is rare in hepatic porphyrias

Although hepatomegaly may occasionally be seen in hepatic porphyrias, frank hepatomegaly is rare and not a prominent manifestation of hepatic porphyria .Hepatic porphyria is therefore the single best answer by exclusion

Frank signs of hepatomegaly are rare in Hepatic Porphyrias but have been noted.

Hepatic involvement in porphyria is variable

Patients with *acute hepatic porphyria* generally have elevation of serum aminotransferases and bile acid levels.

Patients with *chronic hepatic porphyrias* (porphyria cutanea tarda) may show liver enlargement with fatty infiltration ***but frank signs of hepatomegaly and iron overload are rare***

Hepatomegaly is a prominent manifestation of Hurler's syndrome, Nieman Pick disease and Von Girke's Disease

(Harrison's 16th/2316,2320)

Condition		***Hepatomegaly***
Hurler's syndrome	(Mucopolysacharidosis)	Prominent
Nieman Pick Disease	(Glycosphingolipidosis)	Prominent
Von Girke's Disease	(Hepatic Glycogen Storage Disease)	Prominent

181. Answer is D (Albumin): *Harrisons 16th/ 1815*

Only minimal changes in serum albumin are seen in acute liver conditions. Hypoalbuminemia is common in chronic liver disorders such as cirrhosis. In hepatitis serum albumin levels of less than 3g/dl (hypoalbuminemia) should raise the possibility of chronic liver disease' *– Harrisons 16th/ 1815*

Albumin as marker for liver dysfunction
• Serum albumin is synthesized exclusively by hepatocytes • Serum albumin has a long half life and is degraded very slowly (approx 4% is degraded per day.) Because of this slow turnover, the serum albumin is not a good indicator of acute hepatic dysfunction. • Acute liver conditions are associated with only minimal changes in serum albumin (Albumin levels may be normal or minimally altered in viral hepatitis drug related hepato-toxity and obstructive jaundice) • Chronic liver conditions are associated with hypoalbuminemia reflecting decreased albumin synthesis from severe and prolonged liver dysfunction.

Remember: Hypoalbuminemia is not specific for liver disease and may occur in protein malnutrition of any cause, protein losing enteropathies nephritic syndrome and chronic infections.

- **Aminotransferases** are used as indicators of extent of hepatocellular injury. They may be elevated in both acute and chronic hepatocellular disorders.
- **Alkaline phosphatase** is an enzyme used as markers of cholestasis and again may be elevated in both acute and chronic cholestatic disorders.
- **Bilirubin** levels also may be elevated in both acute and chronic liver disease.

182. Answer is B (Sclerosing Cholangitis): *Sutton 7/e P-714; Grainger 4/e P-984; CSDT 2003-600*

Sclerosing cholangitis is not associated with air in the biliary tract.

Causes of air in biliary tract

Air coming from GI tract through fistulas caused by	**Air Produced with in Biliary tract**	**Air coming from GI tract d/t failure of closure of sphincter of oddi** l/t reflux of duodenal gas
• Trauma • Surgery • ***Malignancy***[Q] • Duodenal Ulcer • ***Gall stone ileus***[Q]	• *Emphysematous cholecystitis*[Q]	• Passage of Stone • Passage of Ascaris (Biliary ascariasis) • Surgery (endoscopic sphincterotomy, sphincteroplasty, ***papillotomy***)

183. Answer is A (Albendazole): *Harrison 18th /1763; Goodman Gillman 11th/710*

The drug of choice for treatment of Echinococcus granulosus infection (Hydatid cyst) is ***Albendazole***.

184. Answer is E (Chlorpromazine): *CMDT 2008 / 582; Harrisons 17th*

Chlorpromazine is associated with inflammatory cholestasis and not with Bland (non inflammatory) cholestasis.

Cholestatic Reactions

Non Inflammatory (Bland)	**Inflammatory**
Bland cholestasis is characterized by cholestasis in the absence of inflammation (hepatitis). *This is believed to result from inhibition of various hepatobiliary transport systems.* Important Drugs causes Bland cholestasis • *Estrogen and OCP* • *Anabolic steroids and / or 17 α substituted androgens* • *Indinavir* • *Mercaptopurine* • *Methyl testesterone* • *Cyclosporine*	*Inflammatory cholestasis is charachterized by inflammation of portal tracts with bile duct injury often associated with allergic features like eosinophilia* Important drugs causing inflammatory cholestasis • *Amoxiciline – Clavulanic acid* • *Azathioprine* • *Azithromycin* • *Captopril* • *Cephalosporins* • *Chlorthiazide* • *Chlorpromazine* • *Chlorpropamide* • *Erythromycin* • *Pencillamine* • *Prochlorperazine* • *Semisynthetic pencillins* • *Sulphadiazine*

Connective Tissue Disorders

ESSENTIAL REVISION NOTES

ILLUSTRATION - 1

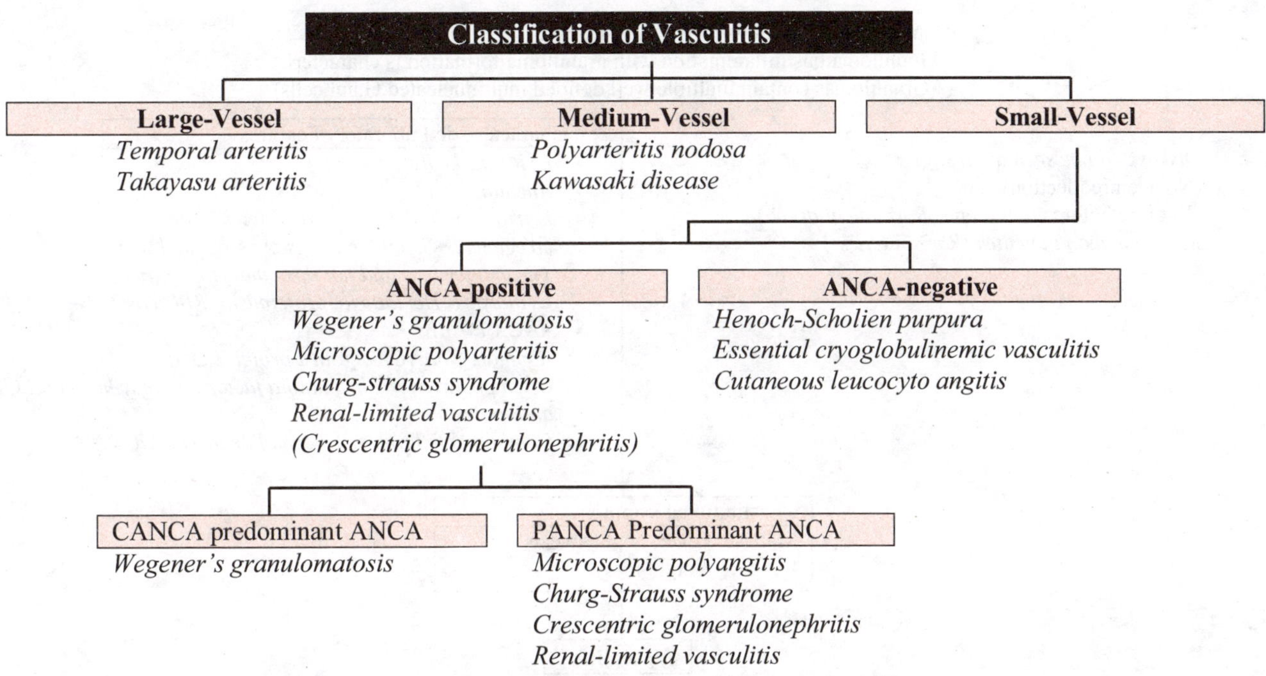

Classification of Vasculitis into Granulomatous & Non-Granulomatous

Granulomatous Vasculitis	Non Granulomatous Vasculitis
• *Giant Cell (Temporal) Arteritis*[Q]	• *Polyarteritis Nodusa (classic PAN)*[Q]
• *Takayasu Arteritis*[Q]	• *Kawasaki Disease*[Q]
• *Wegener's Granulomatosis*[Q]	• *Microscopic Polyangitis*[Q]
• *Churg- strauss syndrome*[Q]	• *Henoch – Sehonlein Purpura*[Q]
	• *Essential Cryoglobulinemic vasculitis*
	• *Cutaneous Leucocytoclastic Angiitis*[Q]

ILLUSTRATION - 2

Wegener's Granulomatosis

- Small vessel vasculitis (cANCA – positive)
- Granulomatous inflammation with granuloma formation is characteristic (Granulomas contain multiple well defined multinucleated Giant cells)

- *Disease can be seen at any age* (No age predilection) (But rare before adolescence *Rare in children*Q)
- *More common in whites (Rare in blacks)*

Characteristic Laboratory Features

- *ESR (markedly elevated)*
- *Anemia*
- *Leukocytosis and Elevated platelet count (Wegener's Granulomatosis is associated with Thrombocytosis and not thrombocytopenia)*
- *Urinalysis: Hematuria, proteinuria, RBC cast*
- *ANCA Positive (Primarily cANCA-Against proteinase 3)*
- *Often positive for Rheumatoid factor and may have anti GBM antibodies*
- *Compliments levels are normal or increased*

Constitutional symptoms

Malaise, Fever, Night sweats
Fatigue, Weight loss

Vasculitis

Charachteristic Triad

Vasculitis of upper Respiratory Tract (Ear Nose Throat- ENT) — (Most common – 95%)

Nose
- Nasal involvement with *septal perforation*Q and collapse of nasal bridge (saddle nose deformity)

Ear
- *Otitis media* (conductive deafness) (sensorineural deafness may also occur late in disease)

Throat and mouth
- *Strawberry gum and gum ulcers*Q
- *Mucosal ulceration of Nasopharynx*Q
- *Subglottic stenosis*Q Results from inflammation and scarring of trachea below the vocal cords and is largely specific to WG.

Vasculitis of Lower Respiratory Tract (Lungs) — 2nd most common ≈85-90%

- Cough, Haemoptysis and Dyspnea
- Multiple bilateral *cavitatory nodular infiltrates*Q on X-ray *(Wegener's causes cavitatory lesions in the lung*Q*)*

Vasculitis of Kidney (Renal) — Develop in 80% of patients

- Present with Rapidly progressive Glomerulonephritis *(Crescentric GN)*Q
- Present with *hematuria proteinuria and RBC cast in urine*Q

Other Vasculitis (less common)

Skin (46%)

*Palpable purpura*Q, subcutaneous nodules, ulcers, vesicobullous lesions, splinter haemorrhages, *digital ischaemias and gangrene may occur*Q

Joints

Arthralgia, Migratory arthritis (Arthritis is not destructive)

Eyes (52%)

- Orbital pseudo tumors behind the eye may lead to proptosis and visual loss
- Scleritis/Episcleritis
- Keratitis
- Conjunctivitis
- Uveitis

Peripheral Nerve

Mononeuritis multiplex may occur

Gastrointestinal (uncommon)

Mesenteric vasculitis may occur but is uncommon

ILLUSTRATION - 3

Polyarteritis Nodosa (Classical PAN)

Classic PAN is a disorder characterized by Necrotizing inflammation of small or medium arteries (ANCA Negative) (spares arterioles or capillaries)
Classic PAN spares the smallest blood vessels (arterioles or capillaries) and is classified as a Medium vessel vasculitis.

Distinguishing Features
• Does not involve lung[Q] • Involves kidneys but does not cause glomerulonephritis *(RBC casts are not seen in PAN)* • *Disease is confined to arterial rather than venous circulation*[Q] • *Does not cause granulomatous inflammation*[Q] • *ANCA Negative*[Q]
• RBC cast Negative (Absent)

- *PAN can involve virtually any organ with the exception of lung*[Q]
- *Renal involvement is common and is characterized by arteritis without glomerulonephritis*[Q]

Renal involvement Present	Hematuria and protenuria may be seen Serum creatinine may be elevated
No Glomerulonephritis	RBC cast are absent

Constitutional symptoms: Common
Fever Malaise, Weight loss and Myalgia

Vasculitis of Skin
- Livido Reticular is Diffuse distribution over extremities and buttocks
- Nodules, papules and ulcers
  Frequently involve the lower extremities
  Heal with scarring
- Digital Ischaemia leading to gangrene
  This is often accompanied by splinter haemorrhage and leads to tissue loss
- Palpable purpura
  Concentrated over buttocks and lower extremity

Vasculitis of Peripheral Nerves

Mononeuritis Multiplex is common

Common manifestation seen in upto 60% of cases
Usually asymmetrical (May be symmetric)
May present as wrist drop or foot drop.

Vasculitis of Gastrointesinal tract (Mesentric vessels)
- Abdominal pain
  Post parandial abdominal pain or intestinal angina is common
- Gastrointestinal bleeding
  Malena may be a presenting symptom

- *Hepatitis B is an established etiological agent and has a strong association for PAN, Hepatitis B serology should be done in cases of PAN)*

Vasculitis of Kidney (Renal vasculitis)

Involves renal artery and smaller medium sized muscular arteries

Presents as Renovascular Hypertension

Glomercular vessels are not involved
No Glomerulonephritis
(No RBC cast in urine)

Other Features of vasculities

Joints
Arthralgias of large joints (Knees, ankles, elbow) are common and seen in upto 50% of patients
Cardiac
Congestive heart failure, MI and pericarditis may be seen
CNS
CVA, Seizures and altered mental status may occur
Genitourinary
Testicular, ovarian or epidiymal pain

ILLUSTRATION - 4

Giant cell Arteritis (Temporal Arteritis)

- Large vessel vasculitis that preferentially affects the extracranial branches of the external carotid artery (Most commonly the temporal artery)
- Typically causes granulomatous inflammation.

Characteristic patient (Risk Patient)

Elderly (>55 years of age)[Q]
Age is the most important Risk factor
Disease is almost exclusively seen in patients > 55 years old age
More common in women (Women > Men)
More common in whites (White >Black)

Characteristic Laboratory Features

- *Anemia*
- *Raised ESR (Elevated ESR)*[Q] *(>50 mm/hr in 90% of cases)*[Q]

Constitutional Symptoms due to Systemic nature of vasculitis (Seen in almost all patients)

Malaise, Fatigue, Loss of Appetite, Weight loss
Fever develops in about 40 % of patients.

Typical Presentation

Symptoms due to vasculitis

Vasculitis of Temporal Artery

Head ache
- *Most common symptom*[Q]
- Most commonly localized over the temporal region
- Typically described as dull aching pain
- Often associated with scalp tenderness
  Patients present with typical pain in scalp when they comb or brush their hair some patients may localized tenderness to temporal artery which may be thickened and nodular.

Jaw Claudication
Most specific symptom[Q]
Typically present with pain in the masseter muscle on prolonged chewing

Vasculitis of ophthalmic Artery

Visual loss/Blindness
- *Most feared complication (symptom)*[Q] of G.C.A because it is usually irreversible
- Visual loss is usually caused by occlusion of posterior ciliary branch of ophthalmic Artery (Anterior ischaemic optic neuropathy)
- Risk of blindness correlates with high levels of interleukin 6 and other markers of strong inflammatory response.
- Visual loss may be transient or permanent and monocular or binocular

Diplopia
Diplopia is the other most common visual symptom

Symptoms of Polymyalgia Rheumatics

Nearly 40% of patient of GCA also present with symptoms of plymyalgia Rheumatics

Typically present with pain and stiffness in the neck, shoulder and hip girdle that are much worse in the morning

Patient complains of difficulty getting out of bed, arising from the toilet or brushing their teeth (shoulder is most commonly involved >hip)

Important Criteria to diagnosis PMR
- Age>50years
- Aching and stiffness for at least 1 month affecting at least 2 out of 3 areas (Shoulder/Neck/Pelvic girdle)
- Morning Stiffness lasting atleast one hour
- ESR>40 mm/hr
- Rapid response to Prednisolone

ILLUSTRATION - 5

KAWASAKI DISEASE

Medium vessel vasculitis associated with mucocutaneous lymph node syndrome
(Non Granulomatous inflammation)
(Immune mediated injury to vessel endothelium with ***infiltration of mononuclear cells***[Q])

Primarily affects children[Q]
(80% cases occur < 5 years of age)

There is no diagnostic test for Kawasaki disease
2D Echocardiography or Angiography should be performed in suspected cases to exclude serious coronary complications

- *Thrombocytosis*[Q] *(Platelet count)*
- *↑ESR*[Q] */ ↑CRP*[Q]
- *Leucocytosis*[Q]

Constitutional symptoms

Fever *is the most important constitutional symptom*

Mucocutaneous Lymph node Features

Mucocutaneous Features

Changes in Extremities

Erythema of palms and soles[Q]
Edema of hands and feet[Q]
Periungual peeling of fingers[Q]

Changes in Lips and oral cavity

Erythema[Q]
Lip cracking[Q]
Strawberry tongue[Q]
Injection of oral and pharyngeal mucosa[Q]

Rash

Polymorphous Exanthem[Q]

Conjunctival changes

Bilateral bulbar conjunctival congestion without exudates[Q]
(Non purulent conjunctivitis)[Q]

Lymph node features

Cervical Lymphadenopathy

- Usually Unilateral[Q]
- Non suppurative[Q]
- Usually >1.5 cm

Vasculitis

Vasculitis of the coronary artery

- Vasculitis of the coronary arteries is the *most dreaded complication*[Q]
- It is associated with coronary artery aneurysm *(seen in 25% of untreated patients*[Q]*)*
- Although generally benign and self limiting it *may be associated with fatal complications* (upto 3% of cash)

Other manifestation include

Pericarditis
Myocarditis
MI (Ischaemia and Infarction)
Cardiomegaly

Strong association has been reported between a novel form of S. aureus that releases TSS toxin-1 and Kawasaki disease[Q]*. However the disease is unresponsive to antibiotics.*

ILLUSTRATION - 6

H. S. Purpura / Anaphylactoid Purpura

- **Small vessel vasculitis**[Q] (ANCA – Negative[Q])
- Pathogenic mechanism of vasculitis is **immune complex deposition**[Q]
- The most common class of Antibodies deposited in immune complexes is **IgA**[Q]

- *Usually seen in children*[Q]
  (Peak incidence in age of 4-7 years)
- May be seen in infants and adults[Q]
  (Most common vasculitis in children[Q]*)*

Characteristic Laboratory Features

- *ANCA Negative*[Q]
- *Elevated serum IgA*[Q]
- *Elevated ESR*[Q]
- *Mild Leukocytosis and Normal Platelet count*[Q]
- *No Thrombocytopenia* [Q]
  Purpura in H.S. Purpura is due to vasculitis and not due to thrombocytopenia
- Hematuria (RBC), Proteinuria and RBC cast (Glomerulonephritis) on Urinalysis
- Despite immune complex mechanism involved *serum complement levels are usually normal*[Q]

Constitutional symptoms
Malaise, Fever, Night sweats, Weight loss and Fatigue

Vasculitis

Vasculitis of Skin (cutaneous)	Vasculitis of Toints (Arthralgias)	Vasculitis of Gastrointesinal tract	Vasculitis of kidney
Palpable purpura[Q] Most commonly distributed over the buttocks and lower extremity	• ***Polyarthralgias***[Q] in absence of frank arthritis (Non deforming in nature) • Mainly involves large joints of the lower extremity • Joint involvement is often migratory	***Colicky Abdominal pain***[Q] is the most charachteristic manifestation . *Other manifestations:* • Passage of blood & mucus per rectum • Nausea/vomiting • Diarrhea / constipation	***Mild glomerulonephritis***[Q] leading to proteinuria, ***microscopic haematuria***[Q] and RBC cast in urine are the charachteristic renal manifestation

ILLUSTRATION - 7

Behcet's syndrome

Behcet's syndrome is a chronic multisystem relapsing vascular inflammatory disease (vasculitis) of unknown origin
Behcet's disease is primarily a small vessel vasculitis but it can also involve large vessels both arteries and veins.
Behcet's disease is associated with HLA-B5 rather than HLA B27

- *Disease pf young people (20 par)* [Q]
- *Male's affected equally as females*[Q]

HLA B5 positive[Q]

Diagnostic criteria
Essential criteria plus two of the non essential criteria are required for diagnosis

Essential criteria

Recurrent oral Ulceration
- *Oral ulceration is the hallmark of disease*[Q]
- *These are sin qua non for the diagnosis*
- Types of Ulcers include
  - Minor Aphthous
  - Major Aphthous
  - Herpetiform ulcers
- Features of oral ulcers
  - *Painful*[Q]
  - Shallow with a central yellowish necrotic base
  - Appear singly or in crops
  - Subside without leaving scars[Q] (persist for 1-2 weeks)

Non-Essential criteria

Recurrent Genital Ulcers
- Less common but more specific
- Do not affect glans or urethra
- Produce scars (scrotal scars)

Eye lesions : Uveitis
- Anterior Uveitis (Recurrent Hypopyon)
- Posterior uveitis
- Retinal vasculitis

Skin lesions
- Erythema nodosum
- Pseudofolliculitis
- Pseudopustular lesions
- Acneform nodules

Positive Pathergy Test
- Pathergy refers to hyperreactivity of skin to any intracutaneous injection or needle stick
- Pathergy is characteristic feature of Behcet's although the mechanism is unknown
- Pathergy test is said to be positive if a papule or pustule >2mm develops 24-48 hrs after needle prick to a depth of 5 mm.

Other Clinical Features

Arthritis
Non deforming Arthritis commonly affects knees and ankles

Thrombophlebitis : Vascular lesions
- Superficial or deep peripheral vein thrombosis (25% of patients)
- Arterial thrombosis may be seen

Neurological involvement (5-10%)
Dural vein thrombosis nay be seen

Pulmonary symptoms
Pulmonary artery vasculitis may occur and present with dyspnea, cough, chest pain, hemoptysis

Gastro intestinal involvement
Consists of mucosal ulceration of Gut similar to Crohn's disease

ILLUSTRATION - 8

Reiter's syndrome/Reactive Arthritis

Reiter's syndrome and Reactive arthritis are regarded as spectrum of same disease

- *Usually develops in young adults*
- *HLA B27 positive*
- *Features of seronegative spondyloarthropathy*

Usually follows gastroenteritis or genitourinary tract infection
Gastroenteritis (Shigella, Salmonella, Campylobacter or Yersenia)
(History of travel to endemic region may be positive)
Genitourinary infection with Chlamydia trachomatis

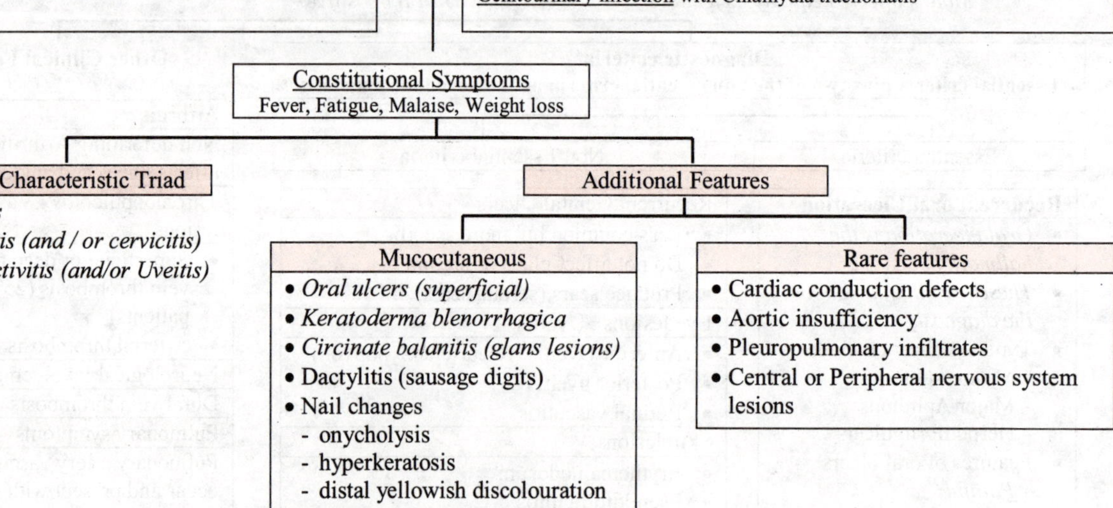

Mucocutaneous Manifestations of Reactive Arthritis/Reiter's syndrome

Oral Ulcers
- Superficial
- Transient
- Painless/Asymptomatic

Keratoderma Blenorrhagica
- ***Characteristic skin lesion of Reactive Arthritis***
- Consists of vesicles that become hyperkeratotic and form crust before disappearing
- Most common on palms & soles

Circinate Balanitis
- These are common lesions seen on glans penis
- Consists of vesicles that rupture to form painless superficial erosions
- May form crusts

ILLUSTRATION - 9

Churg Strauss Syndrome

- Small (medium) vessel necrotizing vasculitis vessel (ANCA positive)
- Granulomatous inflammation / reactions is a charachterictic histopathological feature that may be present in the tissues or walls of the vessels themselves (infiltration of tissues with eosinophils[Q])

- Mean age = 48 years (Disease can be seen at any age with possible exception of infants)
- Female to male ratio is 1.2:1 *(More common in females)*

Characteristic Laboratory Features
- Striking eosinophilia (>1000 cells /μl) (seen in > 80% of patients)
- Evidence of Inflammation (↑ESR: ↑fibrinogen; ↑alpha2 - globulin)
- ANCA positive
- ANCA is usually anti-myeloperoxidase

Constitutional Symptoms
Fever, malaise
Anorexia, Weight loss

Asthma
- Severe asthmatic attacks and presence of pulmonary infiltrates dominates the clinical picture

Allergic Rhinitis and sinusitis may be seen in about 61% of patients

Eosinophilia

Marked Peripheral and Tissue eosinophilia

Extravascular Granuloma formation

Extravascular Granuloma formation is a typical feature of Churg Strauss syndrome

Intravascular granuloma may also be seen

Vasculitis of multiple organ systems
- Any organ may be involved
- Mononeuritis multiplex is second most common manifestation (~72%)
- Skin lesions such as purpura & skin nodules are common (~51%)
- Heart disease ~ 14%
- Kidney involvement is less common and renal failure is rare

ILLUSTRATION - 10

Comparison of the Features of MPA, WG, and PAN

	MPA	WG	PAN
Vessel size	*Small to medium*	*Small to medium*	*Medium*
Vessel type	*Capillaries, venules and arterioles; sometimes arteries and veins*	*Capillaries, venules, and arterioles; sometimes arteries and veins*	*Muscular arteries*
Granulomatous inflammation	*No*	*Yes*	*No*
Lung involvement	*Yes (pulmonary capillaries)*	*Yes (pulmonary nodules, often cavitary)*	*No*
Glomerulonephritis	*Yes*	*Yes*	*No*
Renin-mediated hypertension	*No*	*No*	*Yes*
ANCA-positive	*75%*	*60-90%*	*No*
Hepatitis B association	*No*	*No*	*Yes (<10% od cases now)*
Microaneurysm	*Rarely*	*Rarely*	*Typically*
Likelihood of disease recurrence	*33%*	*>50%*	*≤ 10%*

MPA, microscopic polyangitis; **WG**, Wegener granulomatosis; **PAN**, Polyarteritis nodosa; ANCA, Antineutrophil cytoplasmic antibody

Organs Systems involved in Small Vessel Vasculitis

Organ involvement throughout disease course	Wegner's granulomatosis	Microscopic polyangitis	Churg-Strauss syndrome
Upper respiratory tract	*80%*	*Uncommon*	*55%*
Lower respiratory tract	***70%***	***30%***	***100%***
Eye	*46%*	*10%*	*6%*
Kidney	*80%*	*90%*	*33%*
Peripheral nervous system	35%	20%	67%
Gastrointestinal system	5%	5%	17%
Heart	Uncommon	Uncommon	28%
Skin	50%	25%	44%
Constitutional symptoms	95%	90%	94%

ILLUSTRATION - 11

Cryoglobulinemia

- Cryoglobulins are immunoglobulins that precipitate as serum is cooled below core body temperature (below 37° C) and re-dissolve on re-warming.
- Cryoglobulinemia is characterized by the presence of cryoglobulins in the serum.
- Cryoglobulinemia is most commonly classified into three types in accordance with the Brouet Classification based on the components of the cryoprecipitate.

Type I (Simple Cryoglobulinemia) and Type II, Type III (Mixed cryoglobulinemia)

Feature	Type I (Simple Cryoglobulinemia)	Type II (Mixed Cryoglobulinemia)	Type III (Mixed Cryoglobulinemia)
Cryoglobulin	Single Monoclonal	Mixed Monoclonal`	Mixed Polyclonal
Molecular composition	Monoclonal IgM or Monoclonal IgG Composed entirely of Monoclonal Immunoglobulins, usually IgM or IgG	Monoclonal IgM* (>IgG*) Polyclonal IgG Composed of Monoclonal Immunoglobulins usually IgM along with Polyclonal Immunoglobulin usually IgG	Polyclonal IgM and Polyclonal IgG Composed of polyclonal immunoglobulin of more than once isotype such as polyclonal IgM and polyclonal IgG
Rheumatoid Factor Activity	Rheumatoid factor activity is absent (rarely present) Monoclonal IgM in Type I Syndrome does not have Rheumatoid Factor Activity	Rheumatoid Factor activity is strongly positive Monoclonal IgM in Type II Syndrome has Rheumatoid Factor activity against IgG	Rheumatoid factor activity is positive Polyclonal IgM has Rheumatoid factor activity
Complement Activation in Vitro	Do not activate the complement cascade Complement levels normal	Activate the complement cascade Complement levels reduced	Activate the complement cascade Complement levels reduced.
Predominant clinical manifestation	Primarily related to Hyperviscosity and consequent thrombosis • Acrocyanosis • Retinal Hemorrhages • Raynaud's phenomenon with digital ulceration • Livido reticularis • Arterial reticularis • Arterial Thrombosis	Primarily related to vasculitis due to immune complex formation and activation of complement • Cutaneous vasculitis • Renal Glomerulonephritis • Neuropathy (Vasculitis) • Abdominal pain (mesenteric vasculitis) • Arthralgia & myalgia Mitzer's Triad: Purpura + Arthralgia + Weakness	
Associations	Lymphoproliferative Diseases • Multiple Myeloma • 'Waldenstroms Macroglobulinemia' • Monoclonal Gammopathy	• Chronic hepatitis C • Autoimmune disease • Sjogren's syndrome • CLL • NHL	Autoimmune Diseases • Systemic Lupus Erythematous • Rheumatoid Arthritis • Inflammatory Bowel Disease • Biliary Cirrhosis Chronic Infections • Viral (EBV, CMV, HIV, Hep.E) • Bacterial *(Leprosy, Spirochetal etc)* • Fungal and/or Parasitic

ILLUSTRATION - 12

Hypersensitivity Vasculitis

- *Hypersensitivity vasculitis refers to small vessel vasculitis that is restricted to the skin and not associated with any other form of primary or secondary vasculitis.*

Implicit in the definition is that this condition is not associated with medium or large vessel disease at other sites, nor with small vessel disease in other organs (only skin)
Microscopic polyangitis affects the skin and also internal organs and hence is not considered part of hypersensitivity vasculitis

- *The typical histopathological feature of cutaneous vasculitis is the presence of leukocytoclastic vasculitis of small vessels.*

Vasculitis is charachterized by Leukocytoclasis – Harrison's
Synonyms for Hypersensitivity vasculitis include: cutaneous small vessels vasculitis, leucocytoclastic vasculitis, cutaneous leucocytoclastic angitis etc.

- *'Post-capillary venules are the most commonly involved vessels. Capillaries and arterioles may be involved less frequently' – Harrison*

American College of Rheumatology 1990 Criteria for the Classification of Hypersensitivity Vasculitis

- Age at disease onset > 16 years
- Medication at disease onset
- Palpable purpura
- Maculopapular rash
- Biopsy including arteriole and venule, showing granulocytes in a perivascular or extravascular location

For purposes of classification, hypersensitivity vasculitis may be diagnosed if the patient meets at least three of these five criteria.
Sensitivity = 71%; specificity = 83.9%.

Laboratory and Radiographic Work-up of Patients with Possible Hypersensitivity Vasculitis

Test	Result
Complete blood cell count	Normal
Electrolytes	Normal
Liver function test	Normal
Urinalysis with microscopy	Normal
Erythrocyte sedimentation rate/CRP	Mild to moderate elevation in <50% of patients
Antinuclear antibody (ANA)	Negative
Rheumatoid factor	Negative
C3, C4	Normal
Antineutrophil cytoplasmic antibody (ANCA)	Negative
Antihepatitis B and C assays	Negative
Cryoglobulins	Negative
Chest radiography	Normal

ILLUSTRATION - 13

Serological markers for inflammatory bowel disease

Serological markers for inflammatory bowel disease

Perinuclear Antineutrophil Cytoplasmic Antibodies (p-ANCA)	Antisaccharomyces Cerevisiae Antibodies (ASCA)
• Positive in 60 - 70% of U.C. patients (And 5 - 10% of CD patients)	• Positive in 60 - 70% of CD patients (And 10 - 15% of U.C. patients)

- p ANCA +ve with ASCA -ve = 97% specificity for UC
- p ANCA +ve with ASCA +ve = 97% specificity for CD

Antibody	G.I. Disorder
Antiendomysial antibody[Q]	Celiac sprue
Antisaccharomyces cerevisiae antibody[Q]	Crohn's disease
Antineutrophilic cytoplasmic antibody[Q]	Ulcerative colitis

Antinuclear antibodies in Autoimmune diseases :

1. Anti double stranded DNA (anti dsDNA)	*SLE*
2. Anti histone antibodies	*Drug induced lupus erythematosis*
3. Anti Sm antibody[Q] (antibody to core[Q] protein of small nuclear ribonucleoprotein particles/smith antigen[Q])	*SLE*
4. SSA (Ro) / **5. SSB (La)** — **antibodies to ribonucleoproteins antigens[Q]**	*Sjogren syndrome*
6. Antibodies of ribonucleoprotein antigen[Q] containing ULRNP	*Mixed connective tissue disease*
7. Anti DNA topoisomerase antibody (Scl 70)[Q]	*Systemic sclerosis (diffuse)*
8. Anti centromeric antibody[Q]	*Limited Scleroderma (crest)*
9. Histidyl-tRNA synthetase	*Inflammatory myopathy*
10. Anti mitochondrial antibody[Q]	*Primary biliary cirrhosis*

Best Markers for SLE

Most sensitive stest for SLE	Anti nuclear antibodies
Most specific test for SLE	Anti Sm Antibody and Anti Ds DNA (Anti Sm Antibody > Anti Ds DNA)

Anti Smith Antibodies (Anti Sm) is found in 25 to 30% of SLE patients and is the most specific diagnostic test for SLE. – *Interpretation of diagnostic tests 8th/1034*

Anti Ds DNA is almost as specific as anti Sm antibodies but only when present in high titres

Anti Sm antibodies have high specificity for SLE but low sensitivity being found in < 30% of patients with SLE

Anti Ds DNA is more sensitive than Anti Sm Antibodies being found in upto 70% of patients with SLE but it is almost equally specific than Anti Sm Antibodies when present in high titres. Low titres of Anti Ds DNA are less specific for SLE than low titres of Anti Sm Antibodies.

Antibody	Prevalence %	Clinical Utility
Anti-dsDNA	70	***High titres are SLE specific*** In some patients correlate with disease activity, nephritis, vasculitis
Anti-Sm	25	***Specific for SLE*** No definite clinical correlations

The best marker for Drug Induced Lupus

The best marker for Drug Induced Lupus is Antihistone Antibodies. *Antihistone Antibodies are positive in >95% of patients with drug induced lupus.*

Drug induced Lupus is rarely associated with anti ds DNA and is commonly associated with antibodies to histone (antihistone antibodies)

The best marker for Limited Cutaneous Scleroderma (CREST Syndrome)

Anticentromere antibodies are characteristic of CREST syndrome.

Anticentromere antibodies are present in 40 - 80% of patients with limited cutaneous scleroderma or crest syndrome.

Anticentromere antibodies are found in only about 2% to 5% of patients with diffuse cutaneous scleroderma, and rarely in other connective tissue disease.- Harrison

Systemic sclerosis subsets[Q]

Diffuse cutaneous	Limited cutatneous
Anti-topoisomerase - I antibody	Anticentromere antibody

The best marker for Diffuse Scleroderma or Systemic Sclerosis

Anti DNA topoisomerase antibody (Scl 70) are characteristic of Diffuse Sceroderma or Systemic Sclerosis

Systemic Lupus Erythrmatosis (SLE)

Diagnostic criteria for Systemic Lupus Erythematosus:

1. Malar rash	Fixed erythema, flat or raised, over the malar eminences
2. Discoid rash	Erythematous circular raised patches with adherent keratotic scaling and follicular plugging; atrophic scarring may occur
3. Photosensitivity	Exposure to ultraviolet light causes rash
4. Oral ulcers	Includes oral and nasopharyngeal ulcers, observed by physician
5. Arthritis	*Nonerosive arthritis* of two or more peripheral joints, with tenderness, swelling, or effusion
6. Serositis	Pleuritis or pericarditis documented by ECG or rub or evidence of effusion
7. Renal disorder	***Proteinuria >0.5 g/d*** or ≥3+, or cellular casts
8. Neurologic disorder	Seizures or psychosis without other causes
9. Hematologic disorder	Hemolytic anemia or ***Leukopenia (<4000/μL) or*** ***Lymphopenia (<1500μL) or*** ***Thrombocytopenia (<100,000μL)*** in the absence of offending drugs
10. Immunologic disorder	***Anti-dsDNA***, anti-Sm, and/or anti-phospholipid
11. Antinuclear antibodies	***An abnormal titer of ANA*** by immunofluorescence or an equivalent assay at any point in time in the absence of drugs known to induce ANAs

Note: ANA, antinuclear antibodies; dsDNA, double-strand DNA; ECG, electrocardiography.

If ≥4 of these criteria, well documented, are present at any time in a patient's history, the diagnosis is likely to be SLE. Specificity is ~95%; sensitivity is ~75%.

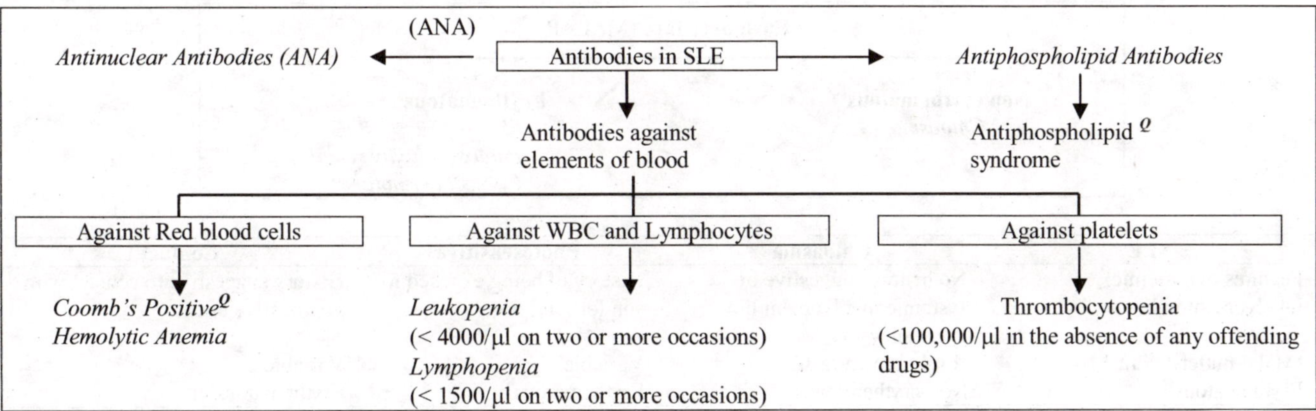

Note

- *SLE is characterised typically by a non-erosive Arthritis* (erosions are rare).

Diagnostic criteria for arthritis in SLE includes
Non erosive arthritis involving two or more peripheral joints characterised by tenderness, swelling or effusion

- *Shrinking lung syndrome is a pulmonary manifestation of SLE.*

Shrinking Lung Syndrome

- Shrinking lung syndrome is a rare manifestation / complication of SLE and is characterized by diaphragmatic weakness or dysfunction.
- Shrinking lung syndrome is associated with restrictive physiology and abnormalities of ventilation and the absence of overt parenchymal or vascular disease.
- The restriction is due to selective weakness of muscles of respiration including the diaphragm

- ***Wire loop lesions are characteristic of SLE Nephritis or Lupus Nephritis***

Wire loop lesions:

- Wire loop lesions represent local PAS – Positive thickening of glomerular capillary walls and are characteristically seen in Lupus Nephritis (SLE)
- These lesions result from subendothelial deposits between endothelium and basement membrane. When extensive and confluent, these subendothelial deposits create a homogenous thickening of the capillary wall which can be seen in light microscopy as 'Wire loop lesion'
- Wire loop lesions are most characteristic of Lupus Nephritis Class IV or Diffuse Lupus Nephritis
  These may however also be seen in Class III (Focal Lupus Nephritis) and Class V (membranous) Lupus Nephritis.

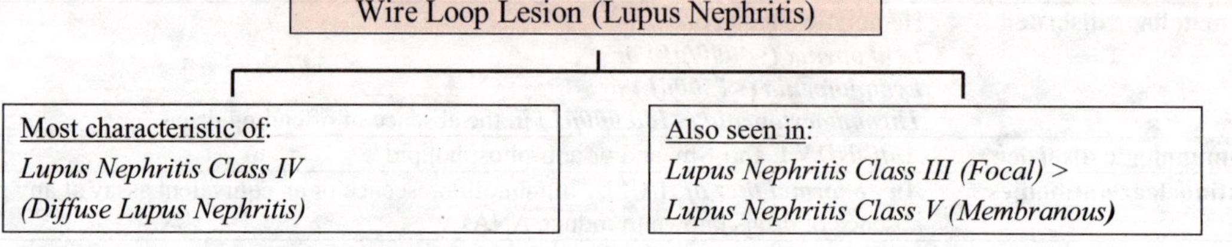

- ***Malar Rash in SLE is typically Fixed erythematous, flat or raised, over the malar eminences***
  Non-erythematous malar rash in a woman of childbearing age suggests diagnosis of chloasma.

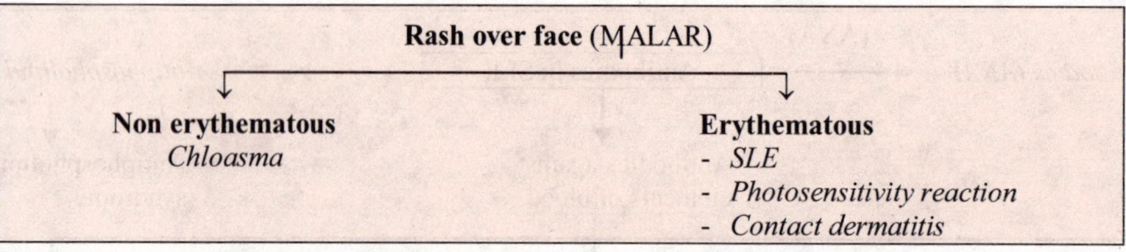

SLE	Chloasma	Photosensitive	Contact
Features of systemic[Q] involvement in history	No history suggestive of systemic involvement h/o Pregnancy	History of being exposed to sun for long time	History suggestive to contact with provocative agent
'Malar butterfly[Q] rash'	'Light brown rash'	Variable	Variable
Erythematous[Q]	Non-erythematous	Erythematous	Erythematous

- ***Bilateral parotid enlargement is not a feature of SLE.***

Causes of Bilateral parotid enlargement			
Viral infections	Metabolic causes	Endocrinal	Miscellaneous
• *Mumps*[Q] • *Influenza*[Q] • *Epstein barr virus* • *Coxackie virus A* • *CMV* • *HIV*	• *Diabetes mellitus*[Q] • *Hyper lipoproteinemia* • *Chronic pancreatitis*[Q] • *Cirrhosis*	• Acromegaly • Gonadal hypofunction	• Sarcoidosis • Amyloidosis • Sjogren syndrome

- ***Indications for use of Corticosteroids in SLE***

Indications for corticosteroids in SLE: *CMDT*		
1. *Thrombocytopenic purpura*[Q]	2. *Hemolytic anemia*[Q]	3. *Myocarditis*[Q]
4. *Pericarditis*[Q]	5. *Convulsions*[Q]	6. *Nephritis*[Q]

Drug induced lupus

Drug Induced Lupus is defined as a syndrome of SLE like symptoms and positive ANA, that appears during therapy with certain medications and biological agent.

Drug induced Lupus

- *Syndrome of Positive ANA with symptoms such as fever, malaise, arthritis, intense arthralgia/myalgia,* ***serositis*** *and or rash (ANA usually appears before symptoms)*
- *Predominant in Caucasians*
- *Less female predilection than SLE*
- *Commonly associated with Anti-Histone*
- *Rarely associated with Anti- ds DNA*
- *Rarely involves kidney or brain*

Renal involvement is rare in Drug Induced Lupus

- *Syndrome usually appears during therapy with certain medications and biologic agents*
- *Syndrome usually resolves over several weeks after discontinuation of the offending medication.*

Differences from classical SLE

- *Less predilection for females than SLE*
- *Rarely involves kidneys and brain (CNS involvement is rare[Q])*
- *Rarely associated with Anti-ds-DNA antibodies (Most common ANA are Antihistone Antibodies)*
- *Usually resolves (remits) after discontinuation of offending medication.*

Persons with HLA-D and 4 allele are of a greater risk of developing Lupus Erythematosus after administration of Hydalazine.

Offending agents

Agent	Risk	Agent	Risk
Antiarrhythmics		**Anticonvulsants**	
Procainamide (Pronestyl)	High	Carbamazepine (Tegretol)	Low
Quinidine (Quinaglute)	Moderate	Phenytoin (Dilantin)	Very low
Disopyramide (Norpace)	Very low	Trimethadone (Tridone)	Very low
Propafenone (Rythmol)	Very low	Primidone (Mysoline)	Very low
Amiodarone (Cordarone)	Very low	Ethosuxamide (Zarontin)	Very low
Antihypertensives		**Antithyroidals**	
Hydralazine (Apresoline)	High	Propylthiouracil (Propylthyracil)	Low
Methyldopa (Aldomet)	Low	**Anti-inflammatories**	
Captopril (Capoten)	Low	D-Penicillamine (Cuprimine)	Low
Acebutolol (Sectral)	Low	Sulfasalazine (Arunfidine)	Low
Enalapril (Vasotec)	Very low	Phenylbutazone (Butazolidin)	Very low
Clonidine (Catapres)	Very low	TNF-α inhibitors (Remicade)	Very low
Atenolol (Tenormin)	Very low	Mesalamine (Asacol)	Very low
Labetalol (Normodyne)	Very low	Zafirlukast (Accolate)	Very low
Pindolol (Visken)	Very low	**Diuretics**	
Minoxidil (Loniten)	Very low	Chlorthalidone (Hygroton)	Very low
Prazosin (Minipress)	Very low	Hydrochlorothiazide (DiuchlorH)	Very low
Lisinopril	Very low	**Antihyperlipidemics**	
Antipsychotics		Lovastatin (Mevacor)	Very low
Chlorpromazine (Thorazine)	Low	Simvastatin (Zocar)	Very low
Phenelzine (Nardil)	Very low	Atorvastatin (Lipitor)	Very low
Chlorprothixene (Taractan)	Very low	**Miscellaneous**	
Lithium carbonate (Eskalith)	Very low	Aminoglutethimide (Cytadren)	Very low
Perphanazine (Trilafon)	Very low	Interferon –a (Wellferon) - β - γ	Very low
Antibiotics		Timolol eye drops (Timoptic)	Very low
Isoniazid (INH)	Low	Ticlopidine (Ticlid)	Very low
Minocycline (Minocin)	Low		
Nitroturantoin (Macrodantin)	Very low		

Rheumatoid arthritis:

It is a chronic systemic inflammatory disease of unknown cause characterized by persistent involvement of synovial membrane of multiple joints and variety of systemic manifestations.

Diagnostic criteria :	
Morning stiffness: [Q]	Stiffness in and around joints lasting 1 hour before maximal improvement. *Constitutional features indicative of the inflammatory nature of disease such as Morning stiffness* ***"support the diagnosis"*** *– Harrison*
Arthritis: [Q]	• *Symmetrical*[Q], involving same joint areas on both sides of body simultaneously • *Multiple*[Q]: It commonly involves three or more joint areas, predominantly of the joint areas in hand (peripheral) [The 14 possible joint areas involved include bilateral PIP, MCP, Wrist, elbow, knee, ankle and MTP (*DIP are not involved*)] *The Typical picture of bilateral symmetrical inflammatory polyarthritis involving small and large joints in both upper and lower extremity with sparing of axial skeleton except the cervical spine "<u>suggest the diagnosis of Rheumatoid Arthritis</u>" – Harrison*
Rheumatoid nodules[Q]*:*	*Demonstration of subcutaneous nodules is* ***"Helpful diagnostic feature"*** *– Harrison*
Serum Rheumatoid factor[Q]***:***	***An IgM antibody directed against the Fc fragment of IgG is present in sera of more than 75% of patients.***
Radiographic changes[Q]***:***	***Juxta articular osteoporosis***[Q]***,*** Joint erosion with Narrowing of joint spaces.

Presence of Rheumatoid factor, inflammatory synovial fluid and Radiographic findings ***Substantiate the diagnosis*** *– Harrison*

<u>Women are affected 3 times more commonly than men</u>

'Women are affected approximately three time more often than men' Harrison's 17th / 2083.

<u>Pathology is not limited to articular cartilage alone and arthritis is typically 'erosive'</u>

The potential of the synovial inflammation to cause cartilage damage and bone erosions and subsequent changes in joint integrity is the hallmark of the disease.

Rheumatoid Arthritis is charachterized by erosive arthritis

<u>DIP joints are usually/typically spared</u>

'RA most often causes symmetric arthritis with characteristic involvement of certain specific joints such as the proximal interphalangeal and metacarpophalangeal joints. The distal interphalangeal joints are rarely involved'.- Harrisons

<u>Axial skeleton involvement is usually limited to Upper Cervical Spine</u>

Rheumatoid arthritis commonly involves the joints of hands, wrist, elbow, knees, ankle, and feet in a symmetrical manner. ***Axial skeleton involvement is usually limited to Upper Cervical Spine*** *–Harrison*

<u>Extra articular manifestations are seen in upto 40 percent of patients</u>

'It is estimated that as many as 40% of patients may have extraarticular manifestations, and in ~15% these are severe'

-Harrison's

<u>Rheumatoid nodules are seen in approximately 20% of patients</u>

'Rheumotoid nodulels may develop in 20-30% of persons with RA' – Harrison's

<u>Typically the pleural fluid contains very low levels of glucose</u>[Q]

'Pleuropulmonary manifestations include ***'Pleuro-Pulmonary nodules'***[Q]*, Pleural disease, Interstitial fibrosis, Pneumonitis, Arteritis. Typically the pleural fluid contains very low levels of glucose*[Q] *– Harrison*

<u>Rheumatoid arthritis is associated with Normocytic Normochromic Anemia of Chronic Disease</u>

'Normochromic, normocytic anaemia is frequently present in Rheumatoid arthritis. It is thought to reflect ineffective erythropoesis, large stores of iron are found in the bone marrow' – Harrisons 17th/2088

Rheumatoid arthritis is most strongly associated with the **Class II**[Q] MHC allele **HLA DR4**[Q] and related alleles

Rheumatoid arthritis is associated with multiple HLA-DR subtypes, but the strongest association has been reported with HLA DR4

'The class II MHC allele HLA DR4 and related alleles are knkwn to be major genetic risk factors for RA' – Harrison

HLA-B27 antigen is associated with seronegative spondyloarthropathies and not Rheumatoid Arthritis

Rheumatoid Arthritis is best diagnosed by Anti-CCP Antibodies

'Anti CCP antibodies are the most specific blood test for rheumatoid arthritis (specificity ~95%)' - CMDT

Felty's syndrome is seen in association with Rheumatoid Arthritis

Felty's syndrome consists of
- *Chronic rheumatoid arthritis*[Q] - *Splenomegaly*[Q] - *Neutropenia*[Q]

Anaemia or *thrombocytopenia* may be associated with Felty's syndrome.

Rheumatoid Factor and Rheumatoid Arthritis

- A ***Rheumatoid Factors is an antibody*** (auto-antibody) *of any immunoglobulin class* (directed against Fc fragment of human IgG)
- *Rheumatoid factor in Rheumatoid Arthritis belongs to the IgM class* [Q] *(directed against Fc fragment of IgG)* [Q]
- IgM Rheumatoid factor is positive in about 75% to 80% of patients with Rheumatoid arthritis
- The presence of RA factor is not specific for R.A.
- The presence of Rheumatoid factor does not establish the diagnosis of RA

Causes of False Positive Rheumatoid factor	
• ***SLE (Associated with a positive Coomb's test)***	• Tuberculosis
• Sjogren syndrome	• Leprosy
• Chronic Liver disease	• ***Syphilis (Associated with a positive VDRL)***
• Sarcoidosis	• Subacute bacterial endocarditis
• Interstitial Pulmonary Fibrosis	• Visceral leishmaniasis
• Infectious mononucleosis	• Schistosomiasis
• ***Hepatitis B (Associated with HbsAg)***	• Malaria

- Rheumatoid factor is only of prognostic significance because patients with high titres tend to have more severe and progressive disease with extraarticular manifestations

DMARDs *(Disease Modifying Anti-Rheumatoid Drugs)*

DMARD's include agents that appear to have the capacity to alter the course of Rheumatoid Arthritis.

DMARDs
1. Methotrexate[Q] 2. *Gold* compounds[Q] 3. *D-Penicillamine* 4. Anti-malarials eg. *Chloroquines*[Q] 5. Sulfasalazine
Methotrexate is the DMARD of choice.

Scleroderma / Systemic Sclerosis

Scleroderma (Systemic sclerosis) is a multisystemic disorder of unknown cause. It is characterized by fibrosis of the skin, blood vessels and visceral organs.

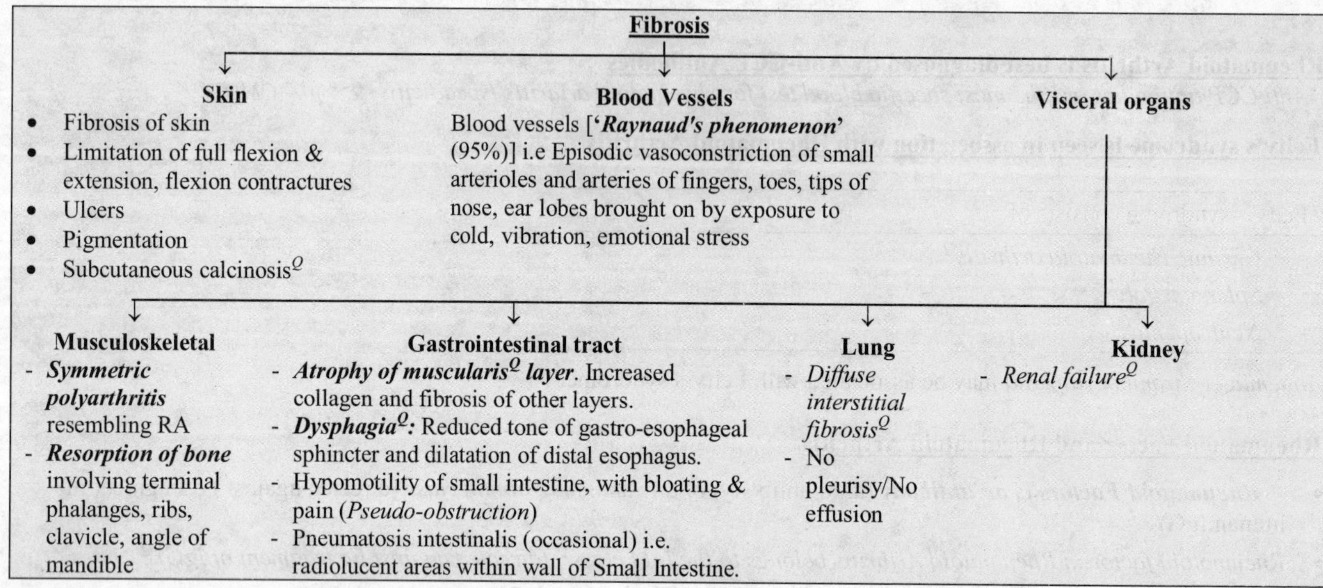

Subsets of systemic sclerosis (SSC): Limited cutaneous SSC versus Diffuse Cutaneous SSC

Features	Limited cutaneous SSc	Diffuse cutaneous SSc
Skin involvement	Limited to fingers, distal to elbows, face; Slow progression	Diffuse: finger, extremities, face, trunk; Rapid progression
Raynaud's phenomenon	Preceds skin involvement; associated with critical ischemia	Onset contemporaneous with skin involvement
Pulmonary Involvement		
Pulmonary fibrosis	May occur, moderate	Frequent, early and severe
Pulmonary arterial hypertension	Frequent, late, may be isolated	May occur, associated with pulmonary fibrosis
Renal Involvement		
Scleroderma renal crisis	Very rare	Occurs in 15%; early
Calcinosis cutis	Frequent, prominent	May occur, mild
Characteristic autoantibodies	Anticentromere	Antitopoisomerase (Scl - 70)
Systemic symptoms	Infrequent systemic symptoms such as Arthralgias, weight loss and pulmonary symptoms	Significant systemic symptoms such as Arthralgias, weight loss and tendon friction rubs

Features of 'CREST' syndrome in association with antinuclear antibodies is sufficient to establish diagnosis of limited form of Limited 'systemic sclerosis'

CREST syndrome	
C	*Calcinosis*
R	*Raynauld's*
E	*Esophageal dysmotility*
S	*Sclerodactyly*
T	*Telengactasia*

The skin of extremities and trunk may be darkly pigmented. Diffuse tanning in the absence of sun exposure may be a very early manifestation of skin involvement – Harrisons

<u>**Systemic sclerosis is not a disease of young individuals**</u>

The mean age of presentation of systemic sclerosis is 50 years – Current Diagnosis & Treatment in Rheumatology 2nd/228
The peak incidence of systemic sclerosis is 50-60 years – Robbins 7th/239
The most common age of onset in the range of 30-50 years – Harrison 17th/2097

<u>**Systemic sclerosis is more common in women**</u>

Like other connective tissue disorders systemic sclerosis shows a female predominance- Harrison 17th/2097
Systemic sclerosis is primarily a disease of women (female to male ratio is 3:1) – Robbin's 7th/239

Reynaud's Phenomenon and Scleroderma

- Reynaud's phenomenon (RP) is the clinical syndrome of episodic color change of the digits in response to cold and in some patients, emotional stress. ***The typical sequence*** *is pallor (arterial constriction) followed by cyanosis (vasospasm and desaturation) of hemoglobin.*
- Reynaud's Phenomenon *may be associated with a variety of connective tissue disorders including SLE, Rheumatoid arthritis, scleroderma and dermatomyositis* (all options provided in question), ***however its association with scleroderma is exceptionally strong.***

- Reynaud's Phenomenon is associated with virtually every patient of scleroderma (or Systemic Sclerosis) (98-99%)

Feature	*Limited Scleroderma (59%)*	*Diffuse Scleroderma*
Reynaud's Phenomenon	*99%*	*98%*

- Reynaud's phenomenon is the ***presenting initial complaint in 70% of patient's with scleroderma***
- Reynaud's phenomenon precedes other symptoms of scleroderma briefly (< 2 years) in diffuse scleroderma while it precedes other symptoms by several years (>2 years) in the limited form (limited scleroderma)

Sjogren Syndrome

<u>**Sjogren syndrome:**</u>

Sjogren's syndrome is a clinicopathologic entity characterized by *dry eyes* (keratoconjunctivitis sicca) and *dry mouth* (xerostomia) resulting from *immunologically mediated destruction of the lacrimal and salivary glands.*

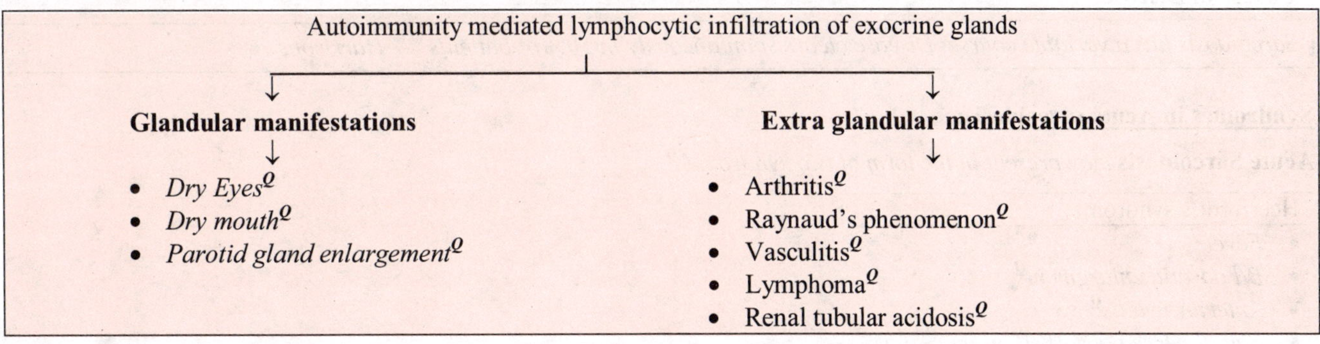

Being an autoimmune disorder this disorder is associated with a number of other disorders of autoimmune origin.

Sarcoidosis

What is Sarcoidosis

Sarcoidosis is a chronic multisystem disorder of unknown cause characterized by accumulation of T lymphocytes and mononuclear phagocytes in various tissues of body

Pathology and Clinical Manifestations

Sarcoid granulomas: The inflammatory process in sarcoidosis is characterized by formation of sarcoid granulomas in various organs

Giant Cells within granulomas can be of Langerhan's or Foreign-body variety and often contain inclusions bodies:

Inclusions seen in giant cells in sarcoidosis. (Remember as **SAR**coidosis)
***S**chaumann bodies*[Q]
***A**steroid bodies*[Q]
***R**esidual bodies*[Q]

Non caseating **SAR**coid granulomas in affected organs

Lung (90%)

- ***Interstitial lung disease***[Q] Fibrosis of lung parenchyma
- Pleura is involved in 1-5% of cases o/e ***pleural effusion***[Q]
- *Cavitation **is rare***[Q]

Lymph nodes (75-90%)

- *B/l hilar lymphadenopathy is the hallmark of sarcoidosis*
- Parotid enlargement B/l involvement is the rule

Skin

- ***Erythema nodosum***[Q]
- ***Lupus perenium***[Q] (purple blue shiny swollen lesions on nose, cheeks, lips, ears).

Others

Eye	Uveitis
Kidney (rare)	Renal hypercalcemia with or without hypercalcuria
Skeletal	Arthritis
Nervous system	Peripheral neuropathy.
Heart	Cor pulmonle

Neurological findings are observed in about 5% of patients with sarcoidosis. "Seventh nerve involvement with unilateral facial paralysis is most common. It occurs suddenly and is usually transient."

Course of Disease

Sarcoidosis has a variable course. Disease clears spontaneously in 50% of patients[Q] *– Harrisons*

Syndromes in Acute sarcoidosis:

Acute Sarcoidosis *may present in the form of two syndromes*[Q]

Heerfordt's syndrome[Q]

- *Fever*[Q]
- *B/l parotid enlargment*[Q]
- *Anterior uveitis*[Q]
- *Facial nerve palsy (VIIth nerve)*[Q]

Löfgren's syndrome

- Joint symptoms
- Erythema nodosum
- X-ray finding of bilateral hilar adenopathy

Uveoparotid fever (Heerfordt syndrome) is seen in Sarcoidosis[Q]
Lofgren's syndrome is seen in Sarcoidosis[Q]

Investigations in a Suspected case of Sarcoidosis

Ancilliary	Confirmatory
• Blood: *ACE*[Q] • *X ray chest*[Q] • *Skin test for anergy*[Q] • *Gallium 67*[Q]	• ***BIOPSY***

***X-Ray chest*:**

- *Bilateral hilar lymphadenopathy is the hallmark of disease*
- Parenchymal involvement may or may not be present ***(clear lung fields)***[Q]
- ***Egg shell calcification of hilar nodes may be seen***[Q]

> Sarcoidosis of the lung is primarily an interstitial lung disease in which the inflammatory process involves the alveoli, small bronchi and small blood vessels.
> Of individuals with **sarcoidosis** 90% have abnormal findings on Chest X-Ray
> ***Cavitation is Rare in sarcoidosis***[Q] ***(Cavitation is* seen in <5% patients with sarcoidosis)**

***Kveim siltzbach test*[Q]*: Skin test*[Q]:**

- Intradermal injection of a heat-treated suspension of a sarcoidosis spleen extract
- Tuberculin test may be negative due to the presence of skin anergy

***Angiotensin converting enzyme (ACE) in blood*[Q]**

- *ACE is elevated in 2/3 of patients with sarcoidosis Q (60%)*[Q]
- *ACE levels indicate activity of disease*[Q]
- *ACE* levels provide an important method of monitoring the course of disease.[Q]

(The cells in granuloma release angiotensin converting enzyme into the serum)

Gallium 67 scan

- Gallium 67 lung scan is usually abnormal showing a pattern of diffuse uptake

Bronchoalveolar lavage: Lavage fluid is typically characterized by

- *Increase in Lymphocytes*[Q]
- *High CD4 / CD8 cell ratio*[Q]

CD4/CD8 counts in the blood may be normal

'While there is marked enhancement of number of T-Helper cells at the sites of disease the number of T-Helper cells in the blood are normal' – *Harrison*

Lung function abnormalities

- *Typical for interstitial lung disease.*

***Biopsy*:**

- Biopsy is mandatory to make a definitive diagnosis of sarcoidosis
- Characteristic finding is a typical non casseating granuloma[Q]

Seronegative Spondyloarthropathies

Seonegative Spondyloarthropathies: Conditions associated with HLA-B27

Seronegative spondyloarthropathies

- *Ankylosing spondylitis*
- *Reactive Arthritis (and Reiter's syndrome)*
- *Psoriatic Arthritis and spondylitis*
- *Enteropathic Arthritis (Arthropathy of Inflammatory Bowel Disease)*
- *Undifferentiated spondylorathropathy*

HLA B27 is typically associated with seronegative spondyloarthropathies like Ankylosing Spondylitis

Charachterisitic Features of Seronegative Spondyloarthropathies

The seronegative spondyloarthritis have the following in common:

- ***Negative RF*** *(Absence of Auto-antibodies in serum: Seronegative)*
- ***Strong association with HLA-B27 antigen***
- ***Oligoarthritis (asymmetrical)***
- ***Enthesitis*** *(inflammation at sites of insertion of fascia, ligament or tendon to bone)*
- *Inflammatory arthritis of spine or large peripheral joints or both (axial and sacroiliac joints)*
- ***Extra-articular features (eyes-uveitis, skin, genitourinary tract)***
- *Familial predisposition and onset usually before the age of 40*

Seronegative Spondyloarthropathies are typically associated with HLA-B27

HLA-B27	• ***Seronegative Spondyloarthropathies*** • ***Anterior Uveitis***

Important conditions associated with certain other HLA Types	
HLA-B5	• *Behcet's Syndrome* ***Behcet's Syndrome is not associated with HLA-B27***[Q]
HLA-B8	• *Myesthenia Gravis (Also with HLA-DR3)* • *Hyperthyroidism (Grave's Disease)*
HLA-DW4/DR4	• *Rheumatoid Arthritis*
HLA-DR3	• *Gluten Sensitive Enteropathy* • *Diabetes Mellitus Type-I (this also has DR2 and DR4)* • *Myesthenia Gravis (along with HLA-B8)*
HLA-DR2	• *Narcolepsy* *Narcolepsy is associated with HLA DR2 and has exceptionally high relative risk of more than 100%*

Treatment for Seronegative Spondyloarthropathies

Non steroidal anti-inflammatory drugs are the medications of choice in seronegative spondyloarthropathies. Indomethacin is the preferred NSAID for most of the seronegative spondyloarthropathies.

Charachteristic Pattern of Small Joint Involvement in Osteoarthritis

Sparing of wrist and metacarpophalangeal joint with involvement of base of thumb (i.e. carpometacarpal joint) is very characteristic of 'osteoarthritis'.

- ***DIP*** *is the most common form of idiopathic O.A.* [Q] *(PIP involvement is also common)*

Herbeden's nodes or bony enlargement of distal interphalangeal joints are the most common form of idiopathic osteoarthritis

Bouchard's nodes	Herbeden's nodes
Bony enlargement of PIP joint in osteoarthritis	Bony enlargement of DIP joint in osteoarthritis

- *Base of thumb (Ist carpometacarpal joint) is the 2nd most common site of involvement in idiopathic osteoarthritis* [Q]
- ***Wrists and Metacarpophalangeal joints are generally not involved in Osteoarthritis*** *– Harrison 16th/2040*

Sparing of wrist and metacarpophalangeal joint with involvement of base of thumb (i.e. carpometacarpal joint) is very characteristic of 'osteoarthritis'.

Charachteristic Pattern of Small Joint Involvement in Psoriatic Arthritis

Psoriatic arthritis involves PIP, DIP and metacarpophalangeal joints, and may or may not involve the wrist.

Charachteristic Pattern of Small Joint Involvement in Rheumatoid Arthritis

DIP joints are usually/typically spared

'RA most often causes symmetric arthritis with characteristic involvement of certain specific joints such as the proximal interphalangeal and metacarpophalangeal joints. The distal interphalangeal joints are rarely involved'.- Harrisons

Review of Small Joint Involvement in OA, RA and Psoriatic Arthritis

Osteoarthritis	Rheumatoid arthritis	Psoriatic arthritis
• Involvement of PIP, DIP and Ist carpometacarpal joint (base of thumb) • ***Sparing of MCP and wrist***	• Involvement of any small joints of the hand i.e. PIP, MCP, wrist. • ***Sparing of DIP***	• Involvement of PIP, DIP, MCP and wrist • Sparing of any joint may or may not be present.

- ***Involvement of DIP makes rheumatoid arthritis unlikely.*** *DIP is spared in rheumatoid arthritis.*
- ***Involvement of metacarpophalangeal joints makes osteoarthritis unlikely.*** *Metacarpophalangeal joints and carpometacarpal joint with the exception of base of thumb are spared in osteoarthritis.*

Gout

What is Gout
• *Gout is primarily a disorder of purine metabolism resulting from overproduction of uric acid*
Etiology
• *Uric acid is the final breakdown product of purine degradation in humans.* • *Primary Gout may results from either increased production or impaired excretion of metabolic end products of purine metabolism (Uric Acid)* ***The most common mechanism of hyperuricemia in gout is a defect in the renal handing of uric acid (and not uric acid over production)*** *'Over 90% of individuals with sustained hyper uricemia have a defect in the renal handling of uric acid' – Harrisons* *'Fewer than 5% of patients with gout are hyper uricemic because of urate overproduction' – Current Rheumatology*
Epidemiology
• Commoner in Caucasians • ***More wide spread in men than in women***[Q] (20: 1) Women are seldom affected *until after menopause.* Often there is a family history. • ***Usually men over the age of 30 years***[Q]; • Sterotype patient is *obese, rubicund, hypertensive and fond of alcohol* and may be ***nudged into an attack by uncontrolled administration of diuretics or aspirin***[Q]
Pathology
• *Gout is caused whenever synovial fluid is supersaturated with uric acid resulting in the formation and deposition of crystals of* ***mono – sodium-urate- monohydrate in joints and peri-articular tissues***[Q] and recurrent attacks of acute synovitis • Tophi are nodular deposits of *monosodium urate monohydrate crystals*, with an associated *foreign body reaction. These form in extra articular and articular structures and cause deformity and destruction of hard and soft tissue* . Tophi suggest chronic gout and sites of deposition in minute clumps in connective tissue include***articular cartilage***[Q] , ***tendon (not muscle)***[Q], ***bursae***[Q]., periarticular tissue, ***synovium & joints***, pinnae (cartilage) of ear , ligaments, articular ends of bone , ***subcutaneous tissue***[Q], kidney etc. Tophi may ulcerate through skin or destroy cartilage & periarticular bone
Presentation
• Acute attack is typically charachterized by sudden onset of severe joint pain • ***The skin is red, shiny, swollen, hot and extremely tender suggesting a cellulitis or septic arthritis***[Q] • The ***commonest sites are metatarsophalangeal joint of big toe***[Q] > ankle & finger joints and olecranon bursae. • Usually comes out of blue buy history of a precipitating factor such as minor trauma, illness, unaccustomed exercise, alcohol, ACTCH, steroid withdrawl or drugs including hypouricemic therapy can often be elicited
Investigations
• **Definitive diagnosis of gout requires aspiration of the involved joint and demonstration of intracellular monosodium urate crystals in synovial fluid.** *Under polarized light these are demonstrated as 'strongly negative birefringent needle shaped crystals'* • **Serum uric acid levels may be normal in Acute Gout** *Gout is caused whenever; synovial fluid is supersaturated with uric acid, irrespective of serum concentration of uric acid.* ***The serum levels of uric acid can be normal or even low at the time of an attack*** *and hence its determination is not diagnostic.* • X- rays show only soft tissue swelling. Chronic gout may result in joint space narrowing & secondary OA • Tophi appear as characteristic ***punched out cysts or deep erosions with over hanging bony edges***[Q] **(Martel's or G' sign)**. These well-defined erosions are larger & slightly further from joint margin than typical RA erosions.

Management

Acute Gout	Chronic Tophaceous Gout
Antiinflammatory drugs such as NSAIDs are the drugs of choice *Uricocurics such as Allopurinol should not be started in acute attacks as they may actually precipitate an acute attack* ***Allopurinol should never be started in acute gout as it may actually precipitate an acute attack***	Hypouricemic agents such as Allopurinol are the agents of choice in patients who already have tophi or chronic gouty arthritis Hypourecemic agents **Xanthene oxidase inhibitors** • Allopurinol **Uricosuric agents** • Probenecid • Benzbromarone

Hyperuricemia and Gout

- ***Gout is common in Hypercurecemic patients***
- The rate of urate deposition in joint and articular destruction correlate with the duration and severity of hyperuricemia.
- The complications of gout correlate with both duration & severity of hyperuriacemia
- ***Although the risk of developing clinical features of gout increases with increasing levels of serum uric acid, only a fraction of those with hyperuricaemia develop symptoms***[Q]
- ***Any factor that causes either an abrupt increase or decrease in the serum urate levels may provoke an acute attack, the best correlations being factors that cause an abrupt fall***[Q].
- ***Serum uric acid levels can be normal or low at the time of acute attack***[Q]
- ***Despite these limitations, serum uric acid is almost always elevated at some time***[Q] and can be used to follow the cource of hypouricemic therapy.

There is no indication of treating asymptomatic Hyperuricemia
The vast majority of hyperuricemic patients are asymptomatic and are at no clinical risk because of it.
Asymptomatic hyperuricemia does not mean Gout and requires no treatment

Renal Disease In Gout

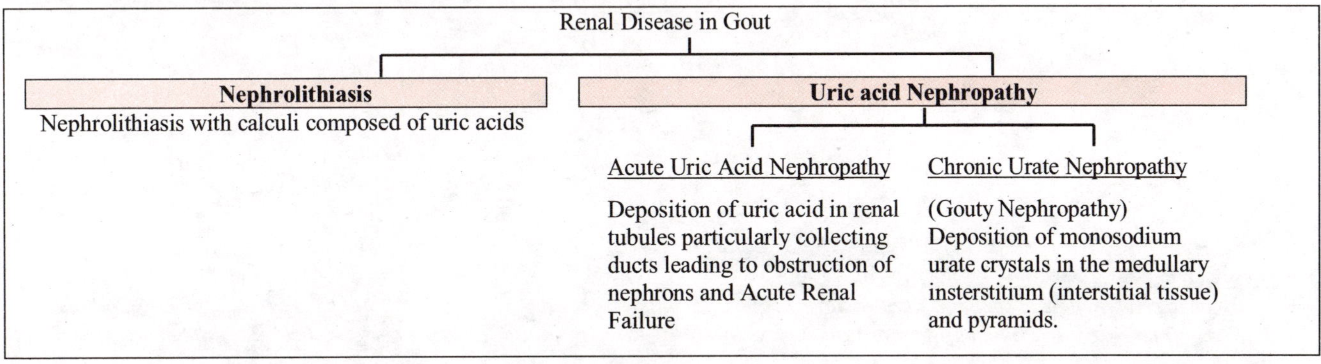

Charcot's Joint

Neuropathic joint Disease/Charcot's joint

- It is progressive destructive arthritis arising from loss of pain sensation and proprioception (position sense).
- *Destructive arthritis and swollen joints in the absence of pain suggest a diagnosis of neuropathic joint disease (Charcot joint).*

Clinical Presentation

- Begins in a single joint and then progresses to involve other joints
- The involved joint becomes progressively enlarged from bony overgrowth and Synovial effusion (swelling).
- The markedly swollen joint is neither tender nor warm.
- ***Loose bodies may be palpated*** in the joint cavity.
- ***The amount of pain experienced by the patient is less than would be anticipated*** based on the degree of joint involvement (sudden pain may be experienced from intraarticular fractures of osteophytes or condyles).

> The paradox is diagnostic i.e. the amount of pain experienced is less than would be anticipated based on degree of joint involvement.

- Joint instability, Subluxation, crepitus occur as the disease progresses
- Patients complains of weakness, swelling, instability, laxity & progressive deformity involving the joint , but minimal pain
- Features of underlying disease

Radiological Features

- Similar to Osteoarthritis with joint space narrowing, subchondrial bone sclerosis, osteophytes and loose bodies However Charcot's joint show more marked destructive and hypertrophic changes.
  The process is usually more rapid.
- Joint swelling and appearance of intraarticular calcification are further clues.

Disorders associated with Charcot's Joints (Neuropathic joints)

Disorders associated with Neuropathic joint disease (Charcot's joint)	
Diabetes mellitus	*Amyloidosis*
Tabes dorsalis	*Leprosy*
Meningomyelocele	*Congenital indifference to pain*
Syringomyelia	*Peroneal muscular atrophy*

Charachteristic Joints involved based on underlying disorder

Tabes dorsalis[Q]	Syringomyelia[Q]	Diabetes[Q]
Knee, hips, ankles	Glenohumeral joint, elbow & wrist.	Tarsal and metatarsal joints

Marfan's Syndrome

Marfan Syndrome : Review

Marfan's syndrome is a genetic disorder of the connective tissue of the body manifested principally by changes in the skeleton, eye and cardiovascular system

Mutation in the fibrillary gene[Q] (15 q 21.1)[Q]

↓

Loss of fibrillary fibre base for deposition of elastin

↓

Alteration in connective tissue in various parts of the body particularly in

Skeletal changes of marfans syndrome	Cardiovascular changes[Q]	Ocular changes[Q]
- *Patients are usually* ***tall***[Q] - *Have long limbs*[Q] - *The ratio of upper segment to lower segment is usually 2 SDs below the mean for age, race & sex* - ***Arachnodactyly*** *(fingers are long and slender, spider like in appearance)*[Q] - *Pectus Excavatum, Pectum Carinatum*[Q] - *Scoliosis, Kyphosis*[Q]	- *Mitral valve prolapse &*[Q] - *Mitral valve progresses to Mitral valve Regurgitation* - *Aortic aneurysm occurs it can leads to Aortic Regurgitation* • Associated changes - *Spontaneous pneumothorax*[Q] - *Inguinal & incisional hernias* - *Striae may occur over the shoulders & buttocks.*	- ***Dislocation of the lens (ectopia lentis)***[Q] - *Elongation of globe (Myopia)*[Q] - *Retinal detachment.*[Q]

Marfan's syndrome most commonly involves the ascending aorta.

'Dilation of the ascending aorta at the level of aortic sinuses is the most common and charachteristic cardiovascular manifestation of Marfan's syndrome'.

Most common cardiovascular Manifestations of Marfan's syndrome

The most common cardiovascular manifestations of Marfan's Syndrome are *Mitral valve prolapse* and *Dilation of Ascending Aorta*

Annula-Aortic Ectasia (Dilation of Ascending Aorta at level of aortic sinuses)	***Mitral Valve Prolapse***[Q]
• Annule aortic ectasia is a specific subgroup of aortic aneurysms affecting the root of aorta and the aortic annulus. This entity is charachteristic/typical of Marfan's syndrome *(Cystic Medial Necrosis*[Q]*)* • Annuloaortic ectasia results in ***dilation of ascending aorta*** initially at level of aortic sinuses • May lead to Aortic Regurgitation, Ruptured Aneurysm and/or Aortic Dissection	• Mitral valve prolapse is usually progressive and leads to *Mitral Regurgitation*[Q]

Major Cardiovascular Criteria for Marfan's	Minor Cardiovascular Criteria for Marfan's
• *Dilation of ascending aorta with or without aortic regurgitation and atleast involving the sinus of valsava* • *Dissection of Ascending Aorta*	• *Mitral valve prolapse with or without mitral regurgitation*

QUESTIONS

Vasculitis

General

1. All of the following are small vessel vasculitis, Except: *(AI 1991)*
   A. Wegner's granulomatosis
   B. Microscopic polyangitis
   C. Polyarteritis Nodosa
   D. Henoch-Schonelin purpura
2. Which of the following is a 'Small Vessel Vasculitis': *(AI 2012)*
   A. Polyarteritis Nodosa (PAN)
   B. Microscopic polyangitis
   C. Giant cell vasculitis
   D. Takayasu's Disease
3. All of the following are small vessels vasculitis, Except: *(PGI Dec 2000)*
   A. Classical PAN
   B. Wegner's granulomatosis
   C. HSP
   D. Churg Strauss Syndrome
   E. Microscopic Polyangitis
4. Which of the following are Small Vessel Vacuitides (Select two best options): *(PGI 2009)*
   A. HUS
   B. HSP
   C. Kawasaki disease
   D. Churg-Strauss Syndrome
5. ANCA is found in all of the following Except:
   A. A. Wegner's granulomatosis *(PGI June 02)*
   B. Churg-Strauss disease
   C. Microscopic polyangitis
   D. Takayasu arteritis
   E. SLE
6. ANCA positive vasculitis include all of the following Except: *(PGI Dec 06)*
   A. Wegner's granulomatosis
   B. Churg strauss syndrome
   C. Microscopic PAN
   D. Good pasture's syndrome
7. ANCA is NOT associated with which of the following diseases : *(AIIMS Nov. 2000)*
   A. Wegener's granulomatosis
   B. Henoch schonlein purpura
   C. Microscopic PAN
   D. Churg Strauss syndrome
8. ACNA is sensitive and specific for: *(AIIMS Dec 98)*
   A. Post streptococcal glomerulonephritis
   B. Idiopathic cresentic glomerulonephritis.
   C. Diffuse glomerulosclerosis
   D. Henoch's schonlein purpura
9. CANCA Positivity is specific for:
   A. Polyarteritis Nodosa
   B. Wegener's granulomatosis
   C. Henoch shontein purpura
   D. Churg strouss syndrome
10. c-ANCA is characteristic for : *(AIIMS Dec 98)*
    A. Polyarteritis Nodosa
    B. R.P.G.N.
    C. Henoch's Schonlein Purpura
    D. Wegeners granulomatosis
11. C-ANCA is associated with: *(PGI- June 08)*
    A. Wegener's Granulomatosis
    B. Microscopic Polyangitis
    C. Churg- Strauss Syndrome
    D. Polyarteritis Nodosa (PAN)
12. c-ANCA positivity indicates, antibody formed against: *(AI 07)*
    A. Proteinase 3
    B. Myeloperoxidase
    C. Cytoplasmic antinuclear antibody
    D. Anti centromere antibody
13. p-ANCA is characteristic for: *(AIIMS Dec 92)*
    A. PAN
    B. Microscopic polyangitis
    C. Wegener's granulomatosis
    D. Henoch-Schonlein purpura
14. The presence of anti-saccharomyces cerevisae antibody is a surrogate marker of one of the following: *(AI 06)*
    A. Coeliac disease
    B. Crohn's disease
    C. Ulcerative colitis
    D. Tropical sprue
15. Antiendomysial Antibody is typically seen in:
    A. Celiac Disease *(DNB)*
    B. SLE
    C. Tropical sprue
    D. Collagenous Colitis
16. All of the following condition are associated with granulomatous pathology, except: *(AI 2010)*
    A. Wegner's Granulomatosis (WG)
    B. Takayasu Arteritis (TA)
    C. Polyarteritis Nodosa (Classic PAN)
    D. Giant Cell Arteritis (GCA)

Wegener's Granulomatosis

17. A person with involvement of upper respiratory tract, lungs and kidney shows evidence of granulomas on histo pathology. The most likely diaglosis is: *(DNB)*
    A. Wegener's Granulomatosis
    B. Goodpasture Syndrome
    C. Tuberculosis
    D. Sarcoidosis
18. A 20 year old woman presents with bilateral conductive deafness, palpable purpura on the legs and hemoptysis. Radiograph of the chest shows a thin-walled cavity in left lower zone. Investigations reveal total leukocyte count 12000/mm^3, red cell casts in the urine and serum creatinine 3mg/dL. What is the most probable diagnosis?

A. Henoch-Schonlein purpura (AI 2004)
B. Polyarteritis nodosa
C. Wegener's granulomatosis
D. Disseminated tuberculosis

19. A 25 years old female develops serous otitis media of left ear with cough and occasional hemoptysis and hematuria and epistaxis for one and half months her. Hemoglobin is 7 gm. B.P. > 170/100, ptoreinuria +++, RA positive (+ve) and ANCA positive (+ve), the likely cause is- (AIIMS June 99)
A. Wegener's granulo matosis
B. Rheumiatoid arthritis
C. Rapidly proliferative glomerulonephritis
D. Good pasteur's syndrome

20. A 25 years old female develops serous otitis media of left ear with cough and occasional hemoptysis and hematuria and epistaxis for one and half months her hemoglobin is 7 gm. B.P is > 170/100, proteinuria +++, RA – ve and ANCA – ve, the likely cause is-
A. Wegener's granulomatosis
B. Rheumiatoid arthritis (AIIMS June 99)
C. Rapidly proliferative glomerulonephritis
D. Goodpasteur's syndrome

21. Wegener's granulomatosis does not affect:
A. Kidney (DNB Jun 2010)
B. Lungs
C. Eye
D. Liver

22. Cavitating lesion in lung is seen in: (PGI Dec 99)
A. PAN
B. SLE
C. Wegner's granulomatosis
D. Sjognern's syndrome

Polyarteritis Nodosa

23. In polyarteritis nodosa, aneurysms are seen in all, *except*: (AIIMS Dec 95)
A. Kidney
B. Lung
C. Liver
D. Pancreas

24. A 30 years old male patient presents with complaints of weakness in right upper and both lower limbs of last 4 months. He developed digital infarcts involving 2nd and 3rd fingers on right side and 5th finger on left side. On examination, BP was 160/140 mm Hg, all peripheral pulses were palpable and there was asymmetrical neuropathy. Investigations showed a Hb 12 gm, TLC-12000 Cu mm, Platelets 4,30,000, ESR-49 mm. Urine examination showed proteinuria and RBC – 10-15/hpf with no casts. Which of the following is the most likely diagnosis? (AI 05)
A. Polyarteritis nodosa
B. Systemic lupus erythematosus
C. Wegener's granulomatosis
D. Microscopic polyangitis

25. An 18 year old boy presents with digital gangrene in 3rd & 4th fingers for last 2 weeks. On examination the BP is 170/110 mm of Hg and all peripheral pulses were palpable. Blood & Urine examination were unremarkable. Antinuclear antibody, Antibody to ds DNA & DNA & ANCA were negative. Most likely diagnosis is: (AI 2004)
A. Henoch-Schonlein purpura
B. Polyarteritis nodosa
C. Wegener's granulomatosis
D. Disseminated tuberculosis

26. A 30 year old male presents with numbness of both lower limbs and right upper limb.
Examination reveals pulse 88/minutes and BPI 160/110 mm of Hg. He also has digital gangrene involving right 2nd and 3rd finger, urine routine examination is unremarkable. Microscopic examination shows RBC's. Hemogram and serum biochemistry is within normal limits. What is the most probable diagnosis?
A. Systemic lupus erythematosus
B. Polyarteritis nodosa (AIIMS May. 2006)
C. Malignant hypertension
D. Chugh-Strauss syndrome

27. A patient presents with melaena normal renal function, hypertension and mononeuritis multiplex. The most probable diagnosis is: (AIIMS Nov 04)
A. Classical polyarteritis nodosa
B. Microscopic polyangiitis
C. Henoch-Schonlein purpura
D. Buerger's disease

28. Biopsy in PAN shows: (PGI June 98)
A. Necrotizing arteritis
B. Atrophy
C. Granulomatous lesion
D. Ring lesion

Microscopic Polyangitis (MPA)

29. Which of the following is not true about Churg Strauss Syndrome (DNB June 2009)
A. Asthma
B. Peripheral eosinophilia
C. Vasculitis of multiple organ systems
D. Intravascular Granulomas

30. All of the following statements about Churg Strauss Syndrome are true, except:
A. Marked Eosinophilia
B. Mononeuritis multiplex is common
C. Renal failure is common
D. Often associated with Allergic Rhinitis

31. Which of the following is more frequently seen in Churg Strauss Syndrome in comparison to Wegener's Granulomatosis
A. Renal involvement
B. Lower Respiratory Tract involvement
C. Eye involvement
D. Upper Respiratory Tract involvement

32. Feature of microscopic polyangitis is: *(PGI Dec 99)*
    A. IgG deposits in kidney
    B. Bronchospasm
    C. Renal involvement in 80% of cases
    D. All of the above

33. All of the following features may be used to distinguish PAN from microscopic Polyangitis, Except: *(PGI June 1996)*
    A. ANCA positivity
    B. RBC cast in urine
    C. Necritizing vasculitis
    D. HBV infection

Giant Cell Arthritis

34. All of the following are true about Temporal Arteritis *except*: *(AI 1996)*
    A. Polymyalgia Rheumatica *(AIIMS-May 95)*
    B. Anemia
    C. Low ESR
    D. Sudden blindness

35. An elderly female presents to the emergency department with history of fever, headache and double vision. Biopsy of temporal artery revealed panarteritis. The most likely diagnosis is
    A. Nonspecific Arteritis *(AIIMS Nov 09)*
    B. Polyarteritis Nodosa
    C. Wegener's Granulomatosis
    D. Temporal Arteritis

36. Which of the following is the most frequent presenting symptoms in patients with giant cell arteritis
    A. Headache *(AI 1991, 1999)*
    B. Jaw claudication
    C. Polymyalgin Rheumatica
    D. Blindness

37. All of the following statements about temporal arteritis are true, Except: *(AI 2009)*
    A. More common in females
    B. Worsens on exposure to heat
    C. Seen in elderly women
    D. Can lead to sudden bilateral blindness

38. The investigation of choice for diagnosis of Giant cell Arteritis is *(AI-1990)*
    A. Temporal Artery biopsy
    B. Colour Doppler of Temporal Artery
    C. CT Angiography
    D. MRI

Kawasaki Disease

39. All of the following are clinical manifestation of Kawasaki disease, Except:
    A. Pedal Edema *(AIIMS Feb 97)*
    B. Cervical Lymphadenopathy
    C. Strawberry tongue
    D. Exudative conjunctivitis

40. Kawasaki disease is associated with all of the following features *except*: *(AI 1996)*
    A. Erythema
    B. Posterior cervical Lymphadenopathy
    C. Thrombocytopenia
    D. Conjunctivitis

41. Kawasaki disease is associated with all of the following clinical features *except*:
    A. Truncal rash *(AIIMS Dec 98)*
    B. Posterior cervical lymphadenopathy
    C. Thrombocytopenia
    D. Pericarditis

42. All of the following statements about Kawasaki disease are true, Except: *(AI 1992)*
    A. Immunoglobulin are the treatment of choice
    B. Prognosis is good
    C. Thrombocytopenia
    D. Elevated ESR

43. Which of the following statements regarding Kawasaki disease is True: *(AI 2008)*
    A. Associated with coronary artery aneurysm in up to 25% of untreated cases
    B. It is the most common cause of vasculitis in children
    C. IV immunoglobulins are recommended only if coronary artery is involved
    D. Lymph node biopsy is used for diagnosis

44. All are features of Kawasaki disease, *except*
    A. Peak incidence at age > 5 years
    B. Aneurysm of coronary artery
    C. Enlarged lymphnodes *(AIIMS Feb 97)*
    D. Fever

45. The treatment of choice for Kawasaki disease is:
    A. Cyclosporine *(AIIMS May 2005)*
    B. Prednisolone
    C. Immunoglobulins
    D. Methotrexate

46. Treatment of choice for Kawasaki Disease is:
    A. IV Immunoglobulins *(AIIMS Nov 2011)*
    B. Steroids
    C. Dapsone
    D. Methotrexate

47. Treatment of choice for Kawasaki Disease
    A. Immunoglobulins *(AIIMS May 09)*
    B. Corticosteroids
    C. Azathioprine
    D. Methotrexate

Henoch Schonlein Purpura

48. A 24 year old male presents with abdominal pain, rashes, palpable purpura and, arthritis. The most probable diagnosis is. *(AI 08)*
    A. Henoch Schonlein Purpura (HSP)
    B. Sweet syndrome
    C. Meningococcemia
    D. Hemochromatosis

49. A 5-year-old child presents with non-blanching purpura over the buttocks and lower limbs along with colicky abdominal pain. Further evaluation revealed deposition of IgA immune complexes. The most likely diagnosis is: *(AIIMS 2011)*
   A. Henoch Shonlein Purpura
   B. Kawasaki Disease
   C. Wegner's Granulomatosis
   D. Takayasu Disease

50. Henoch Schönlein purpura is characterized by all ***except*** *(AI 1994)*
   A. Thrombocytopenia
   B. Glomerulonephritis
   C. Arthralgia
   D. Abdominal pain

51. All of the following are true about HSP, Except: *(PGI Dec 2000)*
   A. A. Palpable Purpura
   B. Kidney's commonly affected
   C. ANCA Negative
   D. Thrombocytopenia

52. A 20 year old girl presents with abdominal pain, arthralgia and a palpable purpuric rash all over the body. The most likely diagnosis is: *(DNB)*
   A. Henoch Schonlein Purpura (HSP)
   B. Kowasaki Disease
   C. Hemolytic Uremic Syndrome (HUS)
   D. Idiopathic Thrombocytopenic Purpura (ITP)

53. All are true of Henoch Scholein' s purpura, ***except*** : *(AI 2000)*
   A. Thrombocytopenia
   B. Abdominal pain
   C. Arthritis
   D. GI bleed

54. True about Henoch Scholien purpura: *(PGI June 07)*
   A. Abdominal pain
   B. Can lead to end stage renal disease
   C. Palpable purpura
   D. Intussusception
   E. All of the above

55. One of the following is a characteristic of Henoch - Schonlein Purpura: *(AI 2002)*
   A. Blood in stool
   B. Thrombocytopenia
   C. Intracranial hemorrhage
   D. Susceptibility to infection

56. A 8 year old male had non blanching rashes over the shin and swelling of knee joint with haematuria +++ and protein +. Microscopic analysis of his renal biopsy specimen is most likely to show- *(AIIMS Nov 07)*
   A. Tubular necrosis
   B. Visceral podocyte fusion
   C. Mesangial deposits of IgA
   D. Basement membrane thickening

57. Henoch - Schonlein purpura is characterized by the deposition of the following immunoglobulin around the vessels : *(AIIMS Nov. 05)*
   A. IgM
   B. IgG
   C. IgA
   D. IgE

58. Henoch Schonlein Purpura presents with deposition of *(DNB)*
   A. IgG
   B. IgM
   C. IgA
   D. IgE

Behcet's Syndrome

59. All the following are features of Behçet's syndrome ***except*** : *(AI 1994)*
   A. Recurrent aphthous stomatitis
   B. Multi-system involvement
   C. Seen only in the tropics
   D. Common in youngsters

60. Behcet's syndromes is characterized by all, Except: *(PGI Dec 2000)*
   A. Myocarditis
   B. Erythema Nodosum
   C. Oral and Genital ulcers
   D. Thrombophlebitis

61. Recurrent Bilateral Hypopyon formation associated with thrombophlebitis is most consistent with which of the following: *(AI 2009)*
   A. HLA B 27 associated uveitis
   B. Behcet's syndrome
   C. Syphilis
   D. Herpes Zoster

Cryoglobulinemia

62. Type I Cryoglobulinemia is associated with all of the following, except: *(AI 2012)*
   A. Hyperviscosity
   B. Monoclonal IgM paraprotein
   C. Normal complement levels
   D. Strongly Positive Rheumatoid factor

Hypersensitivity Vasculitis

63. Which of the following is most commonly involved in Hypersensitivity vasculitis: *(AIIMS May 09)*
   A. Capillaries
   B. Arterioles
   C. Post-capillary venules
   D. Medium sized arteries

Connective Tissue Disorders & Joint Disorders

64. Anti-double stranded DNA is highly specific for : (AIIMS June 97)
    A. Systemic sclerosis
    B. S.L.E.
    C. Polymyositis
    D. Rheumatic sclerosis
65. Anti ds DNA is most specific for: (PGI Dec 03)
    A. SLE
    B. Rheumatoid arthritis
    C. Scleroderma
    D. Polymyositis
    E. Sjogren's syndrome
66. Most specific Antibodies for SLE are: (PGI Dec 2000)
    A. Anti-Ro
    B. Anti-Jo
    C. Anti-Sm
    D. Anti-ds DNA
    E. Anti-La
67. Best marker for drug induced lupus is : (AI 2007)
    A. Antihistone antibodies
    B. Anti ds DNA
    C. ANA
    D. Anti smith Ab
68. Drug induced lupus can be identified by: (AI 06)
    A. Anti-histone antibodies
    B. Double stranded DNA antibodies
    C. Antinuclear antibodies
    D. Anti-SM antibodies
69. Anticentromere antibodies are most commonly associated with : (AI 06)
    A. Diffuse cutaneous systemic sclerosis
    B. Mixed connective tissue disease
    C. CREST syndrome
    D. Polymyositis

Systemic Lupus Erythrmatosis (SLE)

70. Which of the following parameters are included in the Revised (ACR) Criteria for SLE: (PGI 2009)
    A. ANA
    B. Anti DS-DNA Antibody
    C. Lymphopenia <10000/microL
    D. Proteinuria >7500mg/d
    E. Leucocytopenia<1000/microL
71. Characteristic feature of SLE is: (PGI Dec 99)
    A. Uveitis
    B. Joint deformity
    C. Polyserositis
    D. Cavitating lesion in lung
72. A 23-year old woman has experienced episodes of myalgias, pleural effusion, pericarditis and arthralgias without joint deformity over course of several years. The best laboratory screening test to diagnose her disease would be: (AI 2003)
    A. CD4 lymphocyte count
    B. Erythrocyte sedimentation rate
    C. Antinuclear antibody
    D. Assay for thyroid hormones
73. Erosive arthritis is seen in all, except: (AI 2000)
    A. SLE
    B. Gout
    C. Osteoarthritis
    D. Old age
74. Joint erosions are not a feature of : (AI 06)
    A. Rheumatoid arthritis
    B. Psoriasis
    C. Multicentric reticulohistiocytosis
    D. Systemic lupus erythematosus
75. In which of the following arthritis erosions are *not* seen: (AIIMS May 05)
    A. Rheumatoid arthritis
    B. Systemic lupus erthematosus (SLE)
    C. Psoriasis
    D. Gout
76. All of the following are true about SLE except: (PGI Dec 06)
    A. Autoimmune Hematolytic Anemia
    B. ↑ed ANA
    C. Anti-ds DNA
    D. Raynaud's phenomenon
    E. Joint deformity
77. Shrinking lung is a feature of: (PGI June 99)
    A. SLE
    B. Rheumatoid arthritis
    C. Scleroderma
    D. Sarcoidosis
78. Deposition of Anti ds DNA Ab in kidney, skin, choroid plexus and joints is seen in: (AI 2007)
    A. SLE
    B. Good pasture
    C. Scleroderma
    D. Raynauds disease
79. Autoimmune destruction of platelet is seen in : (AIIMS May 95)
    A. SLE
    B. Rheumatoid arthritis
    C. Reiter disease
    D. Polyarteritis nodosa
80. All of the following are known to cause Lupus like syndrome, except (AIIMS Nov 2010)
    A. INH
    B. Penicillin
    C. Hydralazine
    D. Sulphonamide
81. All of the following are true about Drug induced Lupus; Except: (PGI June 07)
    A. Anti histone antibody
    B. Rare anti ds DNA
    C. Renal involvement
    D. Serositis

82. In SLE, characteristic kidney lesion is: *(PGI Dec 98)*
A. Mesangial proliferation
B. Tubular fibrin deposits
C. Wire loop lesions
D. IgG deposits

83. Wire loop lesions are often characteristic for the following class of lupus nephritis: *(AIIMS May 04)*
A. Mesangial proliferative glomerulonephritis(WHO class II)
B. Focal proliferative glomerulonephritis (WHO class III)
C. Diffuse proliferative glomerulonephritis (WHO class IV)
D. Membranous glomerulonephritis (WHO class V)

84. All of the following factors are associated with adverse prognosis and high risk of Renal progression in Lupus Nephritis, Except: *(PGI Dec 03)*
A. High levels of Anti-ds DNA
B. Persistant proteinuria (Nephrotic range> 3gm/day)
C. Hypocomplementenemia
D. Anti LA (SSB)

85. 30-year old Basanti presents with light brown lesions involving both her cheeks. The lesions had never been erythematous. Which of the following is the most probable diagnosis: *(AIIMS Nov. 2000)*
A. SLE
B. Chloasma
C. Air borne contact dermatitis
D. Photo sensitive reaction

86. A female developed brown macule on the cheek, forehead and nose after exposure to light following delivery of a baby, the diagnosis is
A. SLE *(AIIMS June 2000)*
B. Chloasma
C. Photodermatitis
D. Acne rosacea

87. Features of SLE include all of the following except:
A. Recurrent abortion *(AI 1998)*
B. Sterility
C. Coomb's positive hemolytic anemia
D. Psychosis

88. Antiphospholipid Antibody (APLA) syndrome is associated with all of the following except: *(AI 2010)*
A. Bleeding disorders
B. Thrombotic disorders
C. Coagulation disorders
D. Recurrent fetal loss

89. All of the following statements about Antiphospholipid Antibody Syndrome (APLAb) are true, Except : *(AI 2010)*
A. Single titre of Anticardiolipin is diagnostic
B. Commonly presents with recurrent fetal loss
C. May cause pulmonary hypertension
D. Warfarin is given as treatment

90. Anti Phospholipid Syndrome (APS) is associated with all of the following Except: *(AI 2008)*
A. Pancytopenia
B. Recurrent abortions
C. Venous thrombosis
D. Pulmonary hypertension

91. Lupus anticoagulants may cause all of the following except: *(AI 1998)*
A. Recurrent abortion
B. False +ve VDRL results
C. Increase prothrombin time
D. Arterial thrombosis

92. The following condition is not associated with an Anti-phopholipid syndrome : *(AI 2002)*
A. Venous thrombosis
B. Recurrent foetal loss
C. Thrombocytosis
D. Neurological manifestations

93. Which of the following is recommended in a woman with Antiphospholipid Antibodies and history of prior abortions / still birth. *(AI 2010)*
A. Aspirin only
B. Aspirin + Low molecular weight Heparin
C. Aspirin + Low molecular weight Heparin + Prednisolone.
D. No Treatment

94. Bilateral parotid enlargement occurs in all, Except:
A. Sjogren's syndrome *(AIIMS June 97)*
B. SLE
C. HIV
D. Chronic pancreatitis

95. Bilateral parotid gland enlargement is seen in all of the following except: *(AI 1998)*
A. Sarcoidosis
B. SLE
C. Chronic pancreatitis
D. Sjogern's syndrome

96. Indications of steroids in SLE are all except:
A. Myocarditis *(AI 1998)*
B. Endocarditis
C. Thrombocytopenia
D. Neuropsychiatric symptoms

97. Low doses of aspirin therapy is essentially advised for all of the following conditions except: *(AI 1997)*
A. SLE
B. IUGR
C. Post myocardinal infarction
D. Pre ecclampsia

Rheumatoid Arthritis and Other Joint Arthritis

98. All of the following are seen in inflammatory polyarthritis, except *(AIIMS May 94)*
A. New bone formation
B. Erythema
C. Increased ESR
D. Morning stiffness more than one hour

99. All the following are true about Rheumatoid arthritis except: *(AI 1994)*
 A. Positive for Anti-IgG antibody
 B. Juxta-articular osteoporosis
 C. Morning stiffness
 D. C Reactive protein indicates better prognosis

100. Which of the following is *true* regarding Rheumatoid arthritis: *(AI 1994)*
 A. Typically involves small and large joints symmetrically but spares the cervical spine
 B. Causes pleural effusion with low sugar
 C. Pulmonary nodules are absent
 D. Enthesopathy prominent

101. All of the following are true about Rheumatoid Arthritis, Except (Select three options): *(PGI 2009)*
 A. PIP and DIP Joints involved equally
 B. Pathology limited to articular cartilage
 C. Women are affected 3 times more commonly than men
 D. Rheumatoid nodules are seen in 20% of patents
 E. 20 percent of patients have extra articular manifestations

102. A middle aged female presents with polyarthritis, elevated Rheumatoid factor and ANA levels. Which of the following features will help in differentiating Rheumatoid arthritis from SLE *(AIIMS Nov 08)*
 A. Soft tissue swelling in PIP Joint
 B. Juxta-articular osteoporosis on X ray
 C. Articular erosions on X Ray
 D. Elevated ESR

103. True regarding felty's syndrome is all, EXCEPT:
 A. Splenomegaly *(AIIMS Dec 97)*
 B. Rheumatoid arthritis
 C. Neutropenia
 D. Nephropathy

104. Which part of the spine is most commonly affected in Rheumatoid arthritis:
 A. Cervical *(AI 1994) (AIIMS Feb 97)*
 B. Lumbar
 C. Thoracic
 D. Sacral

105. Which radiological feature would help differentiate rheumatoid arthritis with SLE? *(AIIMS Nov 2008)*
 A. Erosion
 B. Juxta-articular osteoporosis
 C. Subluxation of MCP joint
 D. Swelling of PIP joint

106. Rh factor is a: *(AI 2008)*
 A. Antibody
 B. Mucopolysaccharide
 C. Lipoprotein
 D. Glycoprotien

107. Rheumatoid factor is: *(PGI Dec 01)*
 A. IgG
 B. IgM
 C. IgD
 D. IgE
 E. IgM

108. Rheumatoid factor in Rheumatoid arthritis is:
 A. IgG *(PGI Dec 03)*
 B. IgM
 C. IgA
 D. IgD
 E. IgE

109. Rheumatoid factor in rheumatoid arthritis is important because: *(AI 2002)*
 A. RA factor is associated with bad prognosis
 B. Absent RA factor rules out the diagnosis of Rheumatoid arthritis
 C. It is very common in childhood Rheumatoid arthritis
 D. It correlates with disease activity

110. False positive rheumatoid factor can be associated with all except: *(AI 2009)*
 A. Inflammatory bowel disease
 B. HbsAg
 C. VDRL
 D. Coombs test

111. Which of the following is the most specific test for Rheumatoid Arthritis *(AIIMS Nov. 06)*
 A. Anti- ccp antibody
 B. Anti IgM antibody
 C. Anti IgA antibody
 D. Anti IgG antibody

112. Rheumatoid Arthritis is best diagnosed by:
 A. Anti-CCP Antibodies *(AIIMS Nov 2011)*
 B. IgA Rheumatoid Factor
 C. IgG Rheumatoid Factor
 D. IgM Rheumatoid Factor

113. Type of anemia seen in Rheumatoid arthritis is: *(AIIMS Dec 97)*
 A. Microcytic hypochromic anaemia
 B. Macrocytic hypochromic anaemia
 C. Normocytic hypochromic anaemia
 D. Normocytic normochromic anaemia

114. Causative agent for rheumatoid arthritis is: *(AI 2008)*
 A. Mycoplasma
 B. Mycobacaterium avium
 C. Yersinia
 D. Herpes virus

115. Which of the following HLA subtype is most characteristically associated with Rheumatoid arthritis: *(PGI June 01)*
 A. HLADR1
 B. HLADR2
 C. HLADR3
 D. HLADR4
 E. HLADR5

116. All of the following are true about Rheumatoid Arthritis, Except: *(PGI Dec 01)*

A. HLA-DR determine genetic susceptibility
B. HLA-B27 determine genetic susceptibility
C. Anemia
D. Subcutaneous nodules
E. Joint deformity

117. The following are rheumatoid disease modifying drugs except: *(AI 1995)*
A. Chloroquine
B. Gold
C. Penicillamine
D. BAL

118. Gold salts can be used in: *(AI 1994)*
A. Ankylosing spondylitis
B. Rheumatoid arthritis
C. Osteoarthritis
D. Behçet's syndrome

119. Indication of systemic steroids in rheumatoid arthritis is: *(AI 1997)*
A. Mononeuritis multiplex
B. Carpul tunnel syndrome
C. Presence of deformities
D. Articular cartilage involvement

120. Hemophilia with Rheumatoid arthritis, analgesic of choice is: *(PGI Dec 98)*
A. Ibuprofen
B. Asprin
C. Acetaminophen
D. Phenylbutazone

121. Which of the following is not true about JRA? *(AI 2009)*
A. Fever
B. Rheumatoid nodules
C. Uveitis
D. Raynaud's phenomenon

Scleroderma / Systemic Sclerosis

122. All the following are features of Scleroderma ***except*** : *(AI 1995)*
A. Dysphagia
B. Raynaud's phenomenon
C. Skin contracture
D. Calcification in all the long bones

123. A 35 year old lady complains dysphagia, Raynaud's phenomenon, sclerodactyly. Investigations show antinuclear antibody. The likely diagnosis is : *(AIIMS June 99)*
A. Systemic lupus erythematosis
B. Systemic sclerosis
C. Mixed connective tissue disorder
D. Rheumatoid arthritis

124. All of the following features about generalized (diffuse) systemic sclerosis are true, Except: *(PGI June 07)*
A. Raynaud's phenomenon seen years before skin changes
B. Trunk involvement
C. Anti centromere antibodies are characteristic
D. Frequent systemic symptoms
E. All statements are true

125. Vasanti, 28-year-old, presents with complaints of tightness of fingers. There is also history of dysphagia. Which of the following is the probable diagnosis: *(AIIMS Nov. 2000)*
A. Dermatomyositis
B. Scleroderma
C. Rheumatoid arthritis
D. Polyarteritis nodosa

126. Features of systemic sclerosis include all of the following, Except: *(PGI June 03)*
A. Calcinosis
B. Sclerodactyly
C. Hyperpigmentation (Melanin deposition)
D. More common in women
E. More common in young patients

127. A 14 year old girl on exposure to cold has pallor of extremities followed by pain and cyanosis. In later stages of life she is most prone to develop: *(AIIMS Nov 08)*
A. SLE
B. Scleroderma
C. Rheumatoid Arthritis
D. Dermatomyositis

Sjogren Syndrome

128. All of the following may be associated with Sjogron syndrome, ***except*** : *(AIIMS Dec 95)*
A. Dry eyes
B. Dry mouth
C. Parotid gland enlargement
D. Systemic manifestations

129. Sicca syndrome is associated with all, Except : *(AIIMS Feb 97)*
A. Midline granuloma
B. Chronic active hepatitis
C. Rheumatoid arthritis
D. Scleroderma

Sarcoidosis

130. B/L hilar lymphadenopathy, along with non caseating granulomas is a characteristic feature of: *(AI 1997)*
A. Sarcoidosis
B. Scleroderma
C. SLE
D. Stein-leventhal syndrome

131. Following cranial nerve is most commonly involved in patients with sarcoidosis: *(AIIMS Nov 02)*
A. II Cranial nerve.
B. III Cranial nerve.
C. VII Cranial nerve.
D. IX Cranial nerve.

132. All are correct regarding sarcoidosis ***except*** : *(AIIMS Dec 98)*
A. Often cavitate
B. Spontancous remission is usual
C. Tuberculine test is negative
D. B/L hilar lymphadenopathy.

133. A woman is admitted with complains of low-grade fever of 6 weeks duration. Chest radiograph reveals bihilar adenopathy with clear lung fields. All of the following investigations will be useful in differential diagnosis *except*: *(AI 2004)*
A. CD4/CD8 counts in the blood
B. Serum ACE levels
C. CECT of chest
D. Gallium scan

134. Uveoparotid fever is seen in: *(PGI June 98)*
A. SLE
B. Sjogren's syndrome
C. Rheumatoid Arthritis
D. Sarcoidosis

Seronegative Spondyloarthropathies

135. All are seronegative (spondyloepiphyseal) arthritis with ocular manifestations, EXCEPT: *(AIIMS Nov 01)*
A. Ankylospondilitis
B. Ritter's disease
C. Rheumatoid arthritis
D. Psoriatic arthritis

136. HLA-B27 is typically associated with:
A. Rheumatoid Arthritis *(AIIMS Nov 09)*
B. Ankylosing spondylitis
C. Sjogren's syndrome
D. Scleroderma

137. Features of seronegative spondyloarthropathy include all of the following, Except: *(PGI June 01)*
A. Strong association with HLA B27
B. Negative Rheumatoid Factor
C. Symmetrical Polyarthritis
D. Enthesitis
E. Extraarticular feature including uveitis

138. All are seronegative (spondyloepiphyseal) arthritis with ocular manifestations, except-
A. Ankylospondilitis *(AIIMS Nov 01)*
B. Ritter's disease
C. Rheumatoid arthritis
D. Psoriatic arthritis

139. Ankylosing spondylitis in associated with:
A. HLA-B27 *(AI 1999)*
B. HLA-B-8
C. HLA-DW4/DR4
D. HLA-DR3

140. All the following diseases are associated with HILA B-27 & Uveitis, except: *(AI 2000)*
A. Bechcet's syndrome
B. Psoriasis
C. Ankylosing Spondylitis
D. Reiter's syndrome

141. HLA B 27 is associated with all Except (choose two options): *(PGI Dec 98)*
A. Ankylosing spondylitis
B. Pernicious anemia
C. Behcet's syndrome
D. Reiter's syndrome

142. Treatment of choice in seronegative spondy-larthritis is: *(AIIMS Nov 93)*
A. Phenylbutazone
B. Aspirin
C. Indomethacin
D. Corticosteroid

143. A 35 - year old male develops involvements of PIP, DIP and metacarpophalangeal joints with sparing of wrist and carpometacarpal joints. The probable diagnosis is:
A. Psoriatic arthopathy *(AIIMS June 99)*
B. Osteo arthritis
C. Rheumatoid arthritis
D. Pseudo gout

144. A patient presents with foreign body sensation in eye and swollen knee joint after a leisure trip. The most probable diagnosis is: *(AI 2009)*
A. Sarcoidosis
B. Reiter's disease
C. Behcet's disease
D. SLE

145. What is not seen in Reiters syndrome: *(AIIMS Nov 08)*
A. Subcutaneous nodules
B. Keratoderma blennorrhagicum
C. Circinate balanitis
D. Oral ulcers

146. Which of the organisms most commonly causes reactive arthritis? *(AIIMS Nov 08)*
A. Ureaplasma urealyticum
B. Group A beta hemolytic streptococci
C. Borrelia burggorferi
D. Chlamydia

147. Keratoderma Blenorrhagica is typically seen in
A. Rheumatoid Arthritis *(DNB June 2010)*
B. Psoriatic Arthritis
C. Reactive Arthritis
D. Ankylosing spondylitis

Osteoarthritis

148. Proximal interphalangeal, distal interphalangeal & Ist carpometacarpal joint involvement and sparing of wrist is a feature of: *(AIIMS Dec 95)*
A. Rheumatoid arthritis
B. Pseudogout
C. Psoriatic arthropathy
D. Osteoarthritis

149. Least common site to be involved in osteoarthritis amongst the following is:
A. Hip joint *(AI 1997)*
B. Knee joint
C. Carpometacarpal joint of thumb
D. Metacarpophalangeal joint

150. A 35 year old male patient develops involvement of proximal and distal interphalangeal joints and Ist canpo-metacarpal joints with sparing of wrist and metacarophalangeal joint. The Diagnosis is: *(AI 2000)*
A. Osteoarthritis
B. Psoriatic arthropathy
C. Rheumatoid arthritis
D. Pseudogout

151. Herbeden's arthropathy affects *(AI 2005)*
A. Lumbar spine
B. Symmetrically large joints
C. Sacroiliac joints
D. Distal interphalangeal joints

Gout

152. Gout is a disorder of: *(AI 2010)*
A. Purine Metabolism
B. Pyrimidine Metabolism
C. Ketone Metabolism
D. Protein metabolism

153. Clinical features of Gout include: *(PGI)*
A. Severe joint pain
B. Involvement of small joints
C. Deposition of monosodium urate crystals in syynovium
D. Chondrocalcinosis
E. All of the above

154. All of the following statements about primary Gouty Arthritis are true, Except: *(AI 2010)*
A. 90% of cases are caused by over production of uric acid
B. Uric acid levels may be normal at the time of an acute attack
C. Men are more commonly affected than women (Male > Females)
D. Definitive diagnosis requires aspiration of synovial fluid

155. All of the following are true about Gout, except:
A. Occurs due to accumulation of urate crystals in joint *(PGI June 02)*
B. Can be pptd by pyrazinamide
C. Birefringement crystals are present in joint
D. Occurs more in females
E. Due to decreased excretion of uric acid

156. All of the following statements about an attack of gouty arthritis are true, except: *(DNB June 2009)*
A. Joint aspirate reveals negative birefringent crystals
B. Allopurinol should be started immediately
C. Colchicine is known to provide relief
D. Serum uric acid levels may be normal

157. All of the following conditions are observed in Gout except: *(AIIMS May 05)*
A. Uric acid nephrolithiasis
B. Deficiency of enzyme Xanthine oxidase
C. Increase in serum urate concentration
D. Renal disease involving interstitial tissues

158. What is not true about gout: *(AIIMS May 95)*
A. Abrupt increase in serum urate levels is more common a cause for acute gout than an abrupt fall in urate levels.
B. Patient may be asymptomatic with high serum uric acid for years
C. Development of arthritis correlates with level of serum uric acid
D. Uric acid crystals are best seen by polarising light microscope

159. False regarding gouty arthritis is: *(AIIMS Nov 93)*
A. Synovial fluid analysis is diagnostic
B. Alloputinol is the treatment of choice in acute gout
C. Arthritis occurs after long attack of hyperuricemia
D. Levels of uric acid in blood and severity of gout has good correlation

160. Specific test for gout is: *(AIIMS Sept 96)*
A. Raised serum uric acid level
B. Raised uric acid in synovial fluid of joint
C. Raised urea level
D. Raised urease enzyme level

161. All are used in treatment of acute gout, EXCEPT: *(AIIMS May 93)*
A. Aspirin
B. Naproxen
C. Allopurinol
D. Colchinine

Charcot's Joint

162. A 60-year old man with diabetes mellitus presents with painless, swollen right ankle joint. Radiographs of the ankle show destroyed joint with large number of loose bodies. The most probable diagnosis is: *(AI 2003)*
A. Charcot's joint
B. Clutton's joint
C. Osteoarthritis
D. Rheumatoid arthritis

163. A 60-year old man with diabetes mellitus presents with painless, swollen right ankle joint. Radiographs of the ankle show destroyed joint with large number of loose bodies. The most probable diagnosis is: *(AI 2003)*
A. Charcot's joint
B. Clutton's joint
C. Osteoarthritis
D. Rheumatoid arthritis

164. Charcot's joint includes all of the following Except: *(AIIMS Nov 06)*
A. Syrimgomyelia
B. Leprosy
C. Diabetes
D. Arthrogryposis multiple congenital

Polymyositis / Deratomyosistis

165. Primary idiopathic polymyositis does not involve:
   A. Pelvic girdle muscles *(AIIMS-97)*
   B. Neck muscles
   C. Ocular muscles
   D. Pharyngeal muscle
166. Which is NOT a feature of polymyositis?
   A. Pharyngeal muscle involvement
   B. Gottron's rash *(AIIMS-97)*
   C. Proximal muscle involvement
   D. Pain in limbs

Fibromyalgia

167. Which of the following statements about Fibromyalgia is true: *(AI 2012)*
   A. More common in Males
   B. Sleep EEG studies have shown disruption in REM sleep
   C. Increased Cortisol response to stress
   D. SPECT studies have reduced blood flow to the thalamus

Marfan's Syndrome

168. A young, tall, thin, male with archnodactyly has ectopia lentis in both eyes. The most likely diagnosis is : *(AIIMS Nov. 05)*
   A. Marfan's syndrome
   B. Marchesani's syndrome
   C. Homocystinuria
   D. Ehler's danlos syndrome
169. Marfan's syndrome most commonly involves
   A. Ascending Aorta
   B. Descending Aorta
   C. Arch of Aorta
   D. Aortic valves

Wilson's Disease

170. A 12 years old girl with tremors and emotional liability has golden brown discolouration in liability has golden brown discolouration in liability has golden brown discolouration in Descement's membrane. The most likely diagnosis is- *(AI 04)*
   A. Fabry's disease
   B. Wilson's disease
   C. Glycogen storage disease
   D. Acute Rheumatic fever
171. All of the following are features of wilson's disease, except- *(AIIMS Dec 97)*
   A. Hemolytic anemia
   B. Testicular atrophy
   C. Chorea
   D. Chronic active hepatitis
172. All of the following statements about. Wilson's disease are true, EXCEPT- *(AIIMS May 04)*
   A. It is an autosomal recessive disorder
   B. Serum ceruloplasmin level is < 20 mg/dl
   C. Urinary copper excretion is <100 μg/dl
   D. Zinc acetate is effective as maintenance therapy
173. Which of the following statements about Wilson's disease is true: *(AI 2010)*
   A. Low serum ceruloplasmin and low urinary copper
   B. Low serum ceruloplasmin and high urinary copper
   C. High serum ceruloplasmin and low urinary copper
   D. High serum ceruloplasmin and high urinary copper
174. Wilson's disease is best diagnosed by
   A. Increased serum ceruloplasmin
   B. Increased urinary copper excretion
   C. Decreased Liver copper *(DNB June 11, 10)*
   D. Absence of KF rings
175. A 14 year old boy presents wit recurrent episodes of hepatitis Opthalmoscopic evalution reveals KF rings and serum ceruloplasmin levels are < 20 mg/dl. The treatment of choice for initial therapy is
   A. Zinc
   B. Pencillamine
   C. Tetrathromolybdate
   D. Hepatic transplantation

Hematochromatosis

176. A patient presents with Arthritis, hyperpigmentation of skin andhypogonadism, likely diagnosis is-
   A. Hemochromatosis *(AI 2001)*
   B. Ectopic ACTH secreting tumour of the lung
   C. Wilson's disease
   D. Rheumatoid arthritis
177. Which of the following statements about Hematochromatosis is not true *(DNB June 2011)*
   A. Hypogonadism may be seen
   B. Arthropathy may occur
   C. Diabetes Mellitus may develop
   D. Desferrioxamine is treatment of choice
178. Earliest phenotypic manifestation of Idiopathic hereditary hemochromatosis is- *(AIIMS May 07)*
   A. Post prandial increase in serum iron concentration
   B. Elevated serum ferritin level
   C. Slate grey pigmentation of skin
   D. Increased transferrin saturation
179. Lallo, aged 54 years, who is a known diabetic patient develops cirrhosis. There is associated skin hyperpigmentation and restrictive cardiomyopathy which of the following is the best initial test to diagnose this case. *(AIIMS Nov 2000)*

A. Iron binding capacity
B. Serum ferritin
C. Serum copper
D. Serum ceruloplasmin

180. All of the following statements about hereditary hemochromatosis are true Except *(AI 2008)*
A. Arthropathy involving small joints of hands may be seen
B. Skin pigmentation is a frequent presentation
C. Desferroxamine is the treatment of choice
D. Hypogonadism may be seen

181. All are seen in hemochromatosis except- *(AI 2008)*
A. Hypogonadism
B. Arthropathy
C. Bronze diabetes
D. Desferrioxamine is the treatment of choice.

182. Which of the following statements about Hemochromatosis is true: *(AI 2009)*
A. Shows complete penetrance
B. Inherited as an autosomal recessive disorder
C. Phlebotomy is curative
D. More common in Females

Miscellaneous

183. Most common cause of death in Primary Amyloidosis is *(DNB)*
A. Respiratory failure
B. Renal Failure
C. Cardiac Failure
D. Septicemia

184. True about Raynaud's disease are all except: *(AI 2007)*
A. More common in females
B. Good prognosis
C. Positive antinuclear phenomenon
D. Most common cause of Raynoud's phenomenon

185. A Ten year old boy presents to the pediatric emergency unit with seizures. Blood pressure in the upper extremity measured as 200/140 mm Hg. Femoral pulses were not palpable. The most likely diagnosis amongst the following is: *(AI 2010)*
A. Takayasu Aortoarteritis
B. Renal parenchymal disease
C. Grandmal seiures
D. Coarctation of Aorta

186. Renal artery stenosis may occur in all of the following, except : *(AI 06)*
A. Atherosclerosis
B. Fibromuscular dysplasia
C. Takayasu's arteritis
D. Polyarteritis nodosa

187. What is the best method for confirming amyloidosis : *(AI 2007)*
A. Colonoscopy
B. Sigmoidoscopy
C. Rectal biopsy
D. Tongue biopsy

188. Select two medications for IV immunoglobulin infusions: *(PGI June 02)*
A. Myesthenia gravis
B. Idiopathic thrombocytopenic purpura
C. Takayasu arteritis
D. Hemolytic uremic syndrome
E. Multiple myeloma

189. Which of the following disease is/are mediated through complement activation: *(PGI Dec 03)*
A. Atopic dermatitis
B. Graft versus host disease
C. Photoallergy
D. Necrotizing vasculitis
E. Urticaria

190. Intravenous immunoglobulin is given in: (select three options) *(PGI June 04)*
A. Kawasaki disease
B. GB syndrome
C. Heart block
D. Atrial fibrillation
E. Myasthenia gravis

191. Immunoglobulins used in Rx of: (select three optinos) *(PGI Dec 06)*
A. Myathenia
B. I.T.P.
C. PAN
D. Wegener's granulomatosis
E. Guillian Barre syndrome

192. Immunoglobulins infusion is indicated in all Except: *(PGI June 07)*
A. Wiskott Aldrich syndrome
B. X-linked Aggamaglobulinemia
C. Kawasaki disease
D. PAN

193. IV Immunoglobulins are indicated in all Except: *(PGI June 03)*
A. Kawasaki Disease
B. PAN
C. GBS
D. Bruton's Hypogammaglobulinemia

194. Plasmapharesis is used in all of the following except: *(AI 2010)*
A. Myaesthenic crisis
B. Cholinergic crisis
C. Gullian Barre syndrome
D. Polymyositis

ANSWERS, REFERENCES, EXPLANATIONS AND RELEVNT HIGH YIELD FACTS

Vasculitis

1. **Answer is C (Polyorteritis Nodosa):** *Current Diagnosis and Treatment in Rheumatology 2nd/260 Rudolph Pediatrics 21st/1560*

Classic Polyarteritis nodosa does not involve capillaries and venules and is classified as a medium vessel vasculitis.

Micorscopic polyangitis (Microscopic PAN), Wegener's granulomatosis and Henoch Scholein purpura are all classified as small vessel vasculitis.

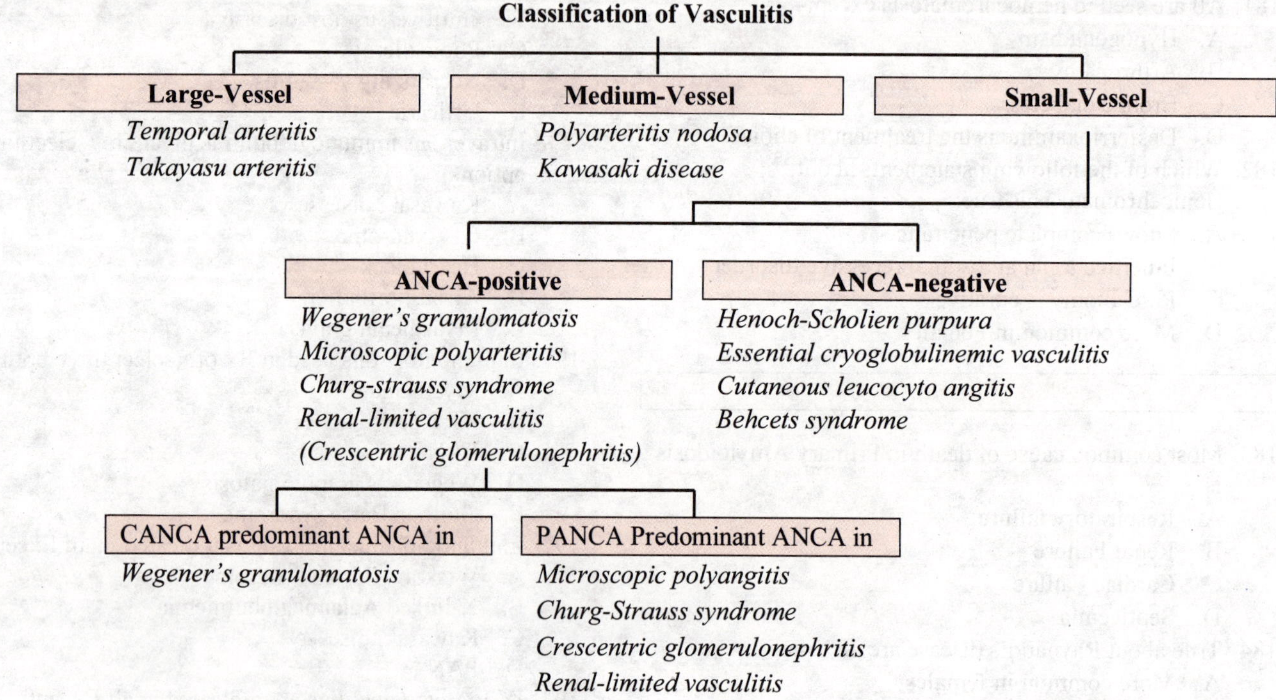

2. **Answer is B (Microscopic polyangitis):** *Harrison 18th/2742*

Miscroscopic Polyangitis (Microscopic Polyarteritis) is classified as 'Small Vessel Vasulitis'

Polyarteritis Nodosa (PAN) is classified as 'Medium Vessel' vasculitis, while, Giant cell vasculitis(Temporal) and Takayasu disease are both classified as 'Large Vessel' vasculitides.

3. **Answer is A (Classical PAN):** *Refer text below*

Classical PAN is a predominantly medium vessel vasculitis and not a small vessel vasculitis.

4. **Answer is B and D (HSP; Churg-Strauss Syndrome):** *Harrison 17th/2120; Repeat; Harrison 18th/p2786*

Henoch Schonlein Purpura (HSP) and Churg-Strauss Syndrome (CSS) are typical examples of small vessel vasculitides

Kawasaki disease is a medium vessel vasculitis while HUS is classified as a thrombotic microangiopathy and not as a vasculitis.

5. **Answer is D (Takayasu Arteritis):** *Harrison 17th/2120; Rheumatology Secret's 2nd/60, 61; 'Heptinstall's Pathology of the Kidney' 6th/647; Davidson 20th/83; Harrison 18th/p2786, 2787*

Takayasu Arteritis is not associated with ANCA

Wegner's granulomatosis *is characteristically associated with c-ANCA while* ***Churg-Strauss syndrome*** *and* ***Microscopic polyagnitis*** *is characteristically asscoaited with p-ANCA against Myeloperoxidase (MPO positive p-ANCA)*

SLE *may be associated with atypical p-ANCA not against myeloperoxidase (MPO negative p-ANCA)*

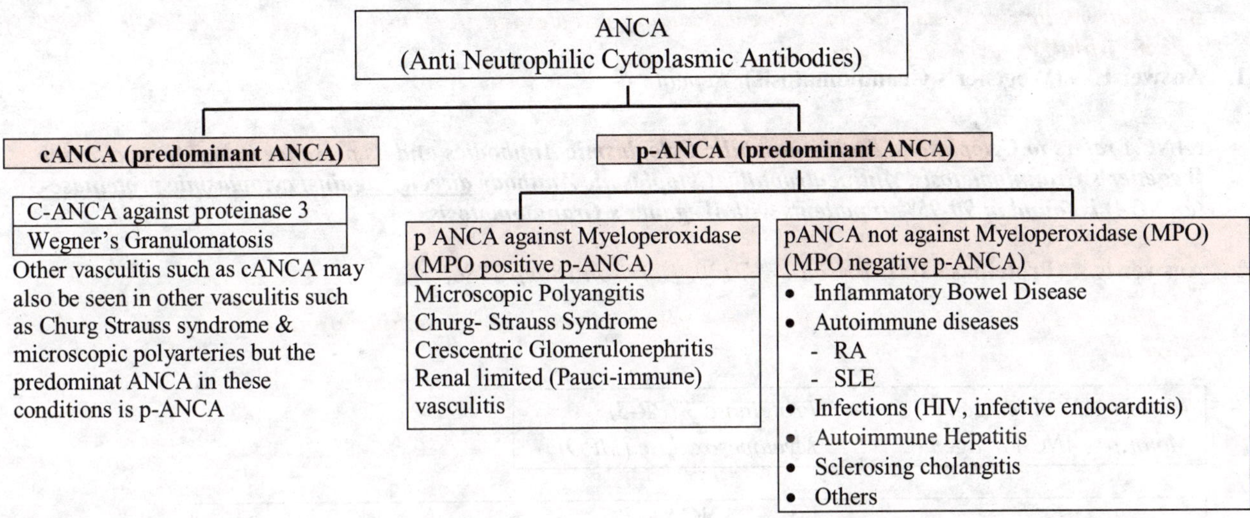

Note:
If p-ANCA is not against Myeloperoxidase (or CANCA is not against Proteinase-3), look for causes other than Vasculitis for the positive ANCA.

6. **Answer is D (Good pasture's syndrome):** *Refer text below*

   Goodpasture's syndrome is not classified as an ANCA positive vasculitis.

7. **Answer is B (H.S. Purpura) :** *Harrison 15th/1957; Harrison 16th/2002; Harrison 17th/2120; Harrison 18th/p2786*

   H.S. purpura is not associated with any antinuclear cytoplasmic antibody (ANCA). It is an example of ANCA negative vasculitis.

   ANCA (Antineutrophic cytoplasmic antibodies):

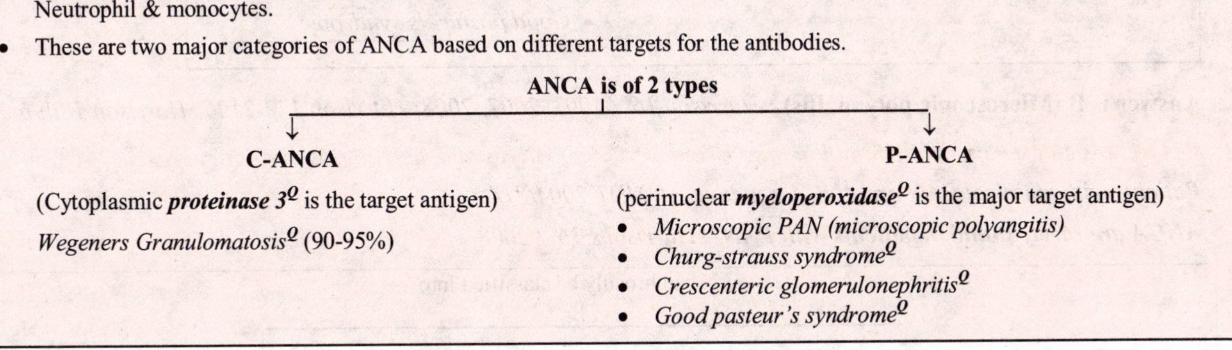

8. **Answer is B (Idiopathic crecentric glomerulonephritis)** *[Ref: Answer One] ; Harrison 17th/2120; Harrison 18th/p2786*

   Crescentric glomerulonephritis is associated with antimyeloperoxidase antibodies.

   The major target for perinuclear ANCA (p-ANCA) is the enzyme myeloperoxidase.

9. **Answer is B (Wegener's granulomatosis):** *Harrisons 17th/2123*

CANCA refers to Cytoplasmic Antineutrophilic cytoplasmic antibodies and its presence is highly specific for Wegener's granulomatosis

10. **Answer is D (Wegener's granulomatosis) :** *Harrison 16th/2002; Harrison 17th/2120; Harrison 18th/p 2786*

Antineutrophilic cytoplasmic antibody directed against cytoplasmic proteinase-3 (cANCA) is found in 90-95% if patients with Wegener's granulomatosis.

11. **Answer is A (Wegener's Granulomatosis):** *Repeat*

cANCA refers to Cytoplasmic Antineutrophilic Cytoplasmic Antibodies and its presence is highly specific for Wegener's Granulomatosis. Antineutrophilic Cytoplasmic Antibody directed against cytoplasmic proteinase-3 (cANCA) is found in 90-95% if patients with Wegener's Granulomatosis.

12. **Answer is A (Proteinase 3):** *Harrison 17th/2120; Harrison 18th/p 2786;*

Proteinase – 3 (a 29 – kDA serine proteinase) present in neutrophil azurophilic granules is the major c-ANCA antigen.

Major c-ANCA antigen	:	*Proteinase 3 (PR-3)*
Major p – ANCA antigen	:	*Myeloperoxidase (MPO)*

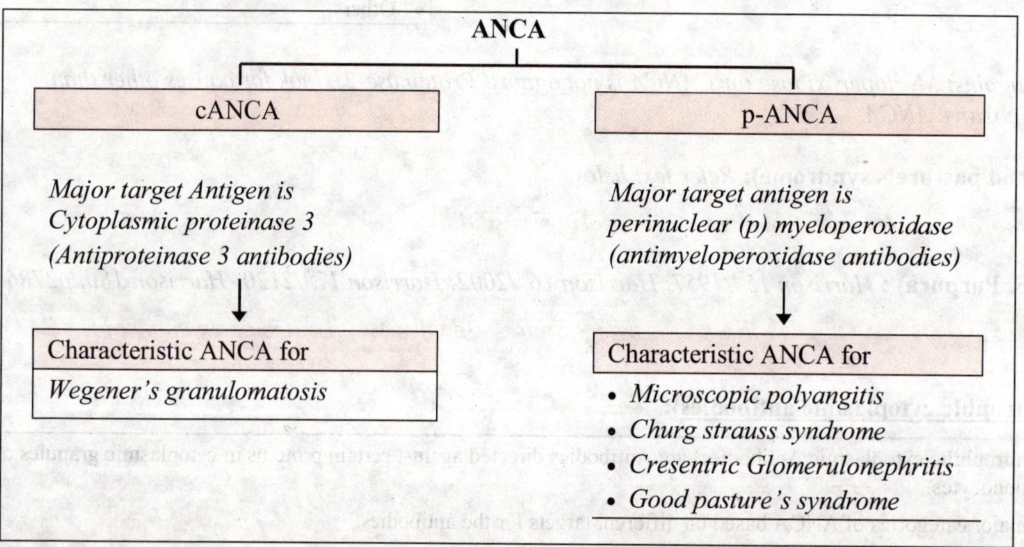

13. **Answer is B (Microscopic polyangitis) :** *Harrison 16th/ 2003, 2007, 2008; Harrison 17th/2126; Harrison 18th/p 2743*

P-ANCA is characteristically found in microscopic PAN i.e. microscope polyangitis & not in classical PAN.

***Patients with classical PAN are ANCA negative** – CMDT 2004/814*

***ANCA are rarely found in patients with PAN** – Harrisons 16th/ 2008*

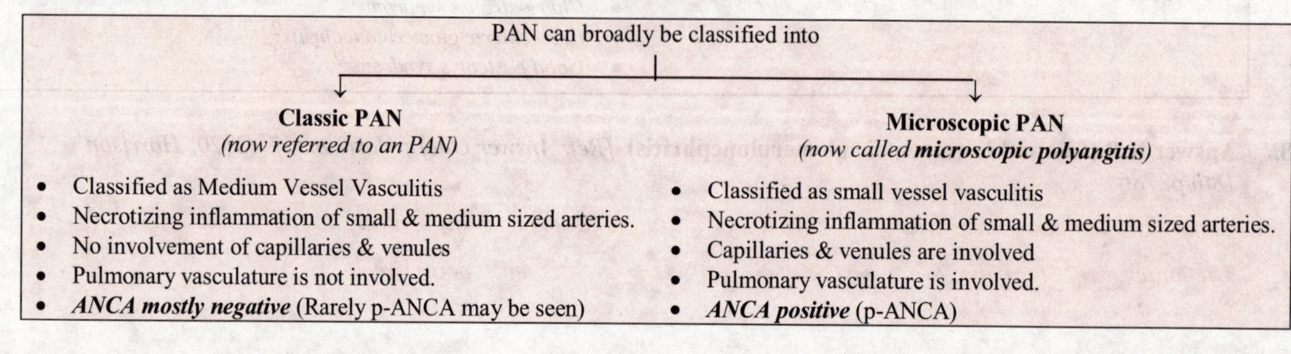

14. Answer is B (Crohn's disease): *CMDT 6th/623; Harrison 16th/1781 - 1782; Harrison 17th/1891*

'Antibodies to the yeast 'Saccharomyces cerevisiae' (ASCA) are found in 60 - 70% of patients with Crohn's disease and 10 - 15% of patients with ulcerative colitis.' - *CMDT 6th/ 623*

Serological markers for inflammatory bowel disease	
Perinuclear Antineutrophil Cytoplasmic Antibodies (p ANCA)	**Antisaccharomyces Cerevisiae Antibodies (ASCA)**
• Positive in 60 - 70% of U.C. patients (and 5 - 10% of CD patients)	• Positive in 60 - 70% of CD patients (and 10 - 15% of U.C. patients)
• p ANCA +ve with ASCA -ve =	97% specificity for UC
• p ANCA +ve with ASCA +ve =	97% specificity for CD

Antibody	G.I. Disorder
Antiendomysial antibody[Q]	Celiac sprue
Antisaccharomyces cerevisiae antibody[Q]	Crohn's disease
Antineutrophilic cytoplasmic antibody[Q]	Ulcerative colitis

15. Answer is A (Celiac Disease): *Harrison 17th /1880, 1881*

Antiendomysial antibodies are trypically seen in celiac disease.

Diagnosis of Celiac Sprue

Serological tests →	**Endoscopic mucosal biopsy** *of distal duodenum or proximal jejunum* →	**Prompt clinical and histopathological response following institution of gluten free diet.**
Serological tests (*CMDT*)	**Endoscopic mucosal biopsy**	**Diagnosis**
▪ ***Two serological tests with highest diagnostic accuracy are*** 1. IgA antiendomysial antibody 2. IgA anti – tTG antibody ▪ Both tests have a > 90% sensitivity and > 95% specificity. IgG or IgA antigliadin antibodies are present in 85% of patients with celiac sprue. However their specificity is relatively low (80 – 90%) which limits their usefulness as screening test. *Small bowel biopsy is still recommended to confirm diagnosis.*	• Findings are ***characteristic but not specific / diagnostic***. • Biopsy of distal duodenum or proximal jejunum is performed. • Finding are restricted to mucosa and include : – Loss or blunting of villi / flat villi – Hypertrophy of intestinal crypts – Infiltration of lamina propria will lymphocytes / plasma cells – Cuboidal appearance of epithelial cells and increased intraepithelial lymphocytes.	• **Diagnosis of celiac sprue requires** Presence of characteristic histopathological changes on biopsy together will prompt clinical and hispathological response following institution of gluten free diet. • IgA antiendomysial Ab or IgA anti – tTGA Ab should also disappear after a gluten free diet.

16. Answer is C (Polyarteritis Nodosa (Classic PAN)): *Harrison's 17th/2125; Current Rheumatology 2nd/297; Robbins 8th/ed; 'Vasculitis' by Ball & Bridges 2nd/286; Harrison 18th/p 2792*

Polyarteritis Nodosa or Classic PAN is not associated with a granulomatous pathology

'Granulomas are charachteristically not found in PAN'- Harrison
'Absence of granulomatous inflammation is charachteristic feature of PAN' – Current Rheumatology

Wegener's Granulomatosis, Takayasu Arteritis and Giant cell arteritis are all granulomatous vasculitis

Classification of Vasculitis into Granulomatous & Non-Granulomatous

Granulomatous Vasculitis	Non Granulomatous Vasculitis
• *Giant Cell (Temporal) Arteritis*[Q]	• *Polyarteritis Nodusa (classic PAN)*[Q]
• *Takayasu Arteritis*[Q]	• *Kawasaki Disease*[Q]
• *Wegener's Granulomatosis*[Q]	• *Microscopic Polyangitis*[Q]
• *Churg- strauss syndrome*[Q]	• *Henoch – Sehonlein Purpura*[Q]
	• *Essential Cryoglobulinemic vasculitis*
	• *Cutaneous Leucocytoclastic Angiitis*[Q]

Wegener's Granulomatosis *(Refer Illustration 2 in Review Notes)*

17. Answer is A (Wegener's Granulomatosis)

The charachteristic triad of vasculitis involving the upper respiratory tract, the lower respiratory tract (Lungs) and kidney along with granuloma formation on histopatholgy suggests a diagnosis of Wegener's granulomatosis.

18. Answer is C (Wegener's granulomatosis) : *Harrison 15th / 1961, 1962; 16th / 2004; CMDT 2009 / 747; Harrison 17th/2121-2123; Harrison 18th/p 2789, 2791*

The patient in question has been depicted to have one manifestation each of the classical triad as mentioned below along with skin lesion in the form of palpable purpura and hence the answer is clearly Wegener's granulomatosis.

Wegener's granulomatosis in its classical form presents as characteristic triad of –

- Upper respiratory infection (ENT manifestations): includes otitis media (conductive deafness)
- Lower respiratory tract infection (Lung): includes haemoptysis and radiological cavity.
- Renal involvement: includes red cell casts and raised serum creatinine.

Skin lesions are seen in 46% of patients and may take the form of palpable purpura.

Wegener's granulomatosis: Review

Wegener's granulomatosis is a distinct clinicopathological entity characterized -		
Clinically		
• **Triad of**		
Upper respiratory tract manifestation (ENT)	Lower respiratory tract[Q] manifestations (Lung)	Renal manifestations[Q]
- Otitis media (conductive deafness) - Paranasal sinus pain & drainage - Septal perforation[Q] - Other manifestations	- Cough, haemoptysis, dyspnea[Q] - Multiple bilateral cavitatory nodular infiltrates	- Rapidly progressive renal failure[Q] - Crescentric glomerulonephritis[Q]
• Fever[Q], ***skin manifestation***[Q] in the form of papules, vesicles, palpable purpura etc eye manifestations[Q], joint manifestations[Q] cardiac manifestations[Q] and nervous system manifestations[Q].		

Pathologically by
• Necrotizing vasculitis[Q] of small[Q] arteries and veins • Intravascular and extravascular granuloma formation [Q] Granulomas contain multiple well defined multinucleated giant cells [Q] Bronchoalveolar lavage fluid contains high percentage of neutrophils compared to other granulomatous diseases which contain increased number of Lymphocytes [Q] c-ANCA is the predominant ANCA in the disease
Characteristic laboratory findings include:
1. Positive c-ANCA[Q] 2. Elevated ESR (mild elevation) 3. RF[Q] (often elevated) 4. Hypergammaglobunemia (particularly IgA class)[Q] • Hypocomplementemia is not seen despite presence of circulating immune complexes[Q]

Treatment of choice is: cyclophosphamide[Q]

19. Answer is A (Wegener's granulomatosis): *Current Rheumatology Diagnosis and treatment 2nd/281; Harrisons 17th/2123; Harrison 18th/p 2790, 2791*

The patient in question is presenting with the charachteristic triad of Wegener's granutomatosis namely, vasculitis of the upper respiratory tract (serious otitis media and epistaxis), vasculitis of the lower respiratory tract (hemoptysis) and vasculitis of the kidney (proteinuria)

Presence of ANCA and Rheumatoid factor further support the diagnosis of Wegener's granulomatosis which is the single best answer of choice.

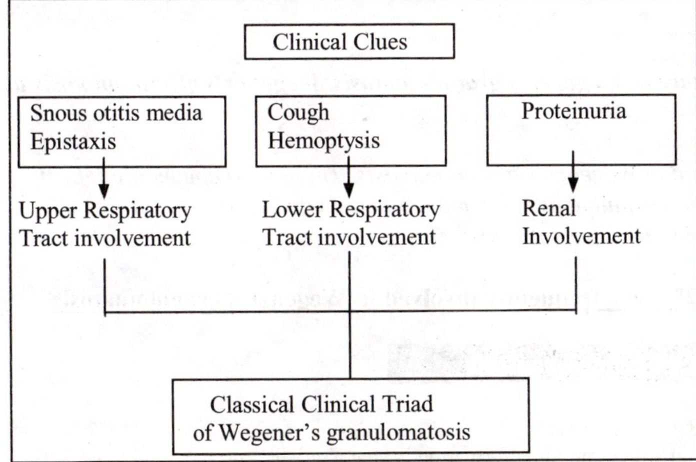

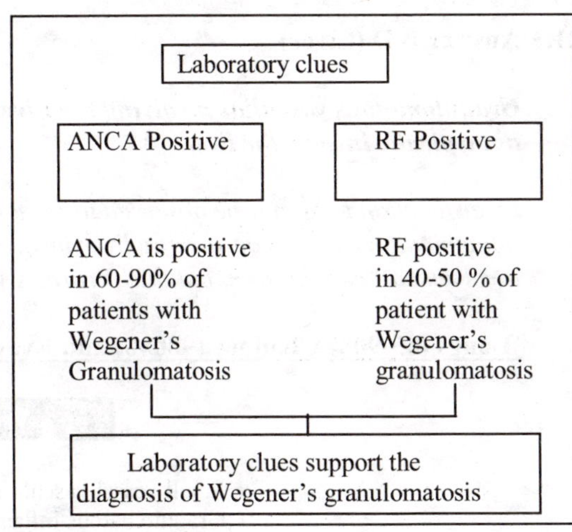

20. Answer is A>D (Wegener's granulumatosis > Goodpasture's Syndrome); *Current Diagnosis and Treatment in Rheumatology 2nd/281, Current Critical Care Diagnosis and Treatment; Harrisons 17th/2122,2123,1788; Harrison 18th/p 2342, 2790, 2791*

The patient in question is presenting with characteristic clinical triad of Wegener's granulomatosis, namely, Vasculitis of upper respiratory tract (serous otitis media, epistaxis), Vasculitis of lower respiratory tract (cough and hemoptysis) and vasculitis of the kidney (proteinuria)

Although positive ANCA assays are often instrumental in suggesting the diagnosis of WG, Negative ANCA assays do not preclude the diagnosis, 10% of patients with disseminated WG and upto 30% of patients with limited WG may be negative for ANCA

The clinical picture is classical of Wegner's Granulomatosis. However, the absence of ANCA confuses the diagnosis. Nevertheless the presence or absence of ANCA should be adjunctive and in the presence of a classical clinical picture of WG, tissue diagnosis (biopsy) should be performed to confirm the diagnosis.

Definitive diagnosis of WG is established by tissue biopsy and not by presence or absence of ANCA

Pulmonary + Renal Syndrome

Pulmonary (Hemoptysis) + Renal (Proteinuria) manifestations

Wegener's granulomatosis	Goodpasture's syndrome
Classical Clinical presentation is one of a young Male/Female (male: female=1:1) presenting with upper respiratory tract features (Otitis media, Epistaxis) along with hemoptysis and acute glomerulonephritis+	*Classical clinical presentation is one of a young male smoker (male : female=3-4:1) presenting with hemoptysis and signs of acute glomerulonephritis* Although disease may be preceeded by an upper respiratory tract infection, upper respiratory tract involvement features like otitis media and epistaxis are not characterstic of good pasture's syndrome
ANCA is usually positive and suggests the diagnosis ***Negative ANCA does not preclude the diagnosis. In the presence of classical clinical picture a provisional diagnosis of WG should be made on clinical ground and confirmed/ excluded by tissue biopsy*** *The patient in question is presenting with classical clinical triad of Wegener's granulomatosis. Although ANCA is negative a negative ANCA does not preclude the diagnosis of WG. Based on the strong clinical suspicion, WG should the single best initial provisional diagnosis and tissue biopsy should be performed.*	*ANCA is usually negative* *Diagnosis is made by detecting serum levels of Anti GBM antibodies* ↓ *The patient in question is not presenting with classical clinical features of good pasture's syndrome and serum levels of Anti GBM antibodies have not been provided in the question. These make a diagnosis of Good pasture's syndrome less likely.*

21. Answer is D (Liver)

Granulomatous vasculitis involving the Liver is rare in Wegener's granulomatosis. Wegener's granulomotosis does not typically involve the liver.

Liver function tests may be observed to be abnormal in Wegener's granulomatosis. These most commonly reflect inflammation rather than specific liver involvement. Granulomata and hepatic blood vessel involvement (Liver involvement) may be seen, but this is rare.' - Vasculitis in Clinical Practice

'Lungs (85-90%), Kidney (~80%) and Eyes (~52%) are frequently involved in Wegener's granulomatosis

Wegener's Granulomatosis

- Small vessel vasculitis (cANCA – positive)
- Granulomatous inflammation with granuloma formation is characteristic (Granulomas contain multiple well defined multinucleated Giant cells)

- *Disease can be seen at any age*
  (No age predilection)
  (But rare before adolescence *Rare in children*[Q])
- *More common in whites (Rare in blacks)*

Characteristic Laboratory Features

- *ESR (markedly elevated)*
- *Anemia*
- *Leukocytosis and Elevated platelet count (Wegener's Granulomatosis is associated with Thrombocytosis and not thrombocytopenia)*
- *Urinalysis: Hematuria, proteinuria, RBC cast*
- *ANCA Positive (Primarily cANCA-Against proteinase 3)*
- *Often positive for Rheumatoid factor and may have anti GBM antibodies*
- *Compliments levels are normal or increased*

Constitutional symptoms

Malaise, Fever, Night sweats
Fatigue, Weight loss

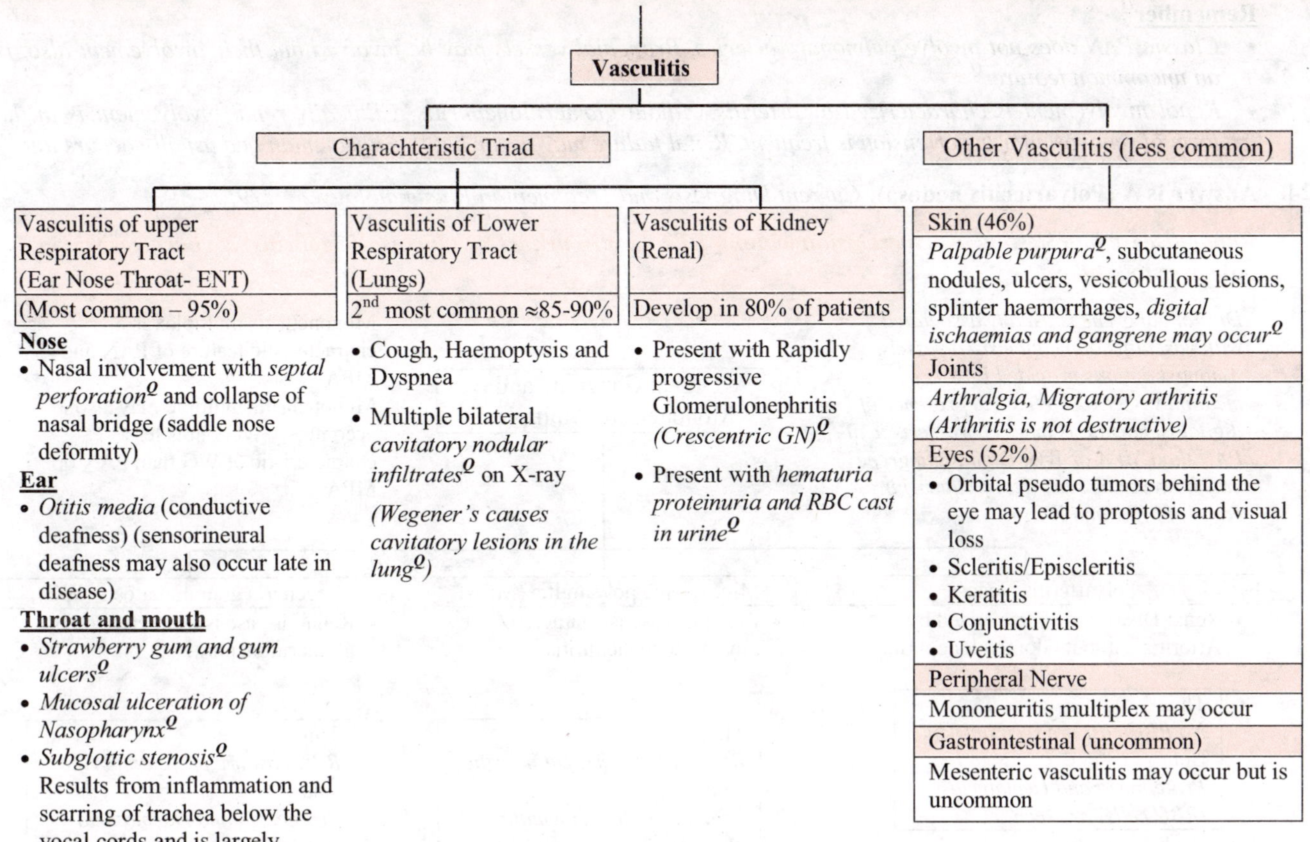

22. Answer is C (Wegener's granulomatosis): *Harrison 17th/1960, 2122, 2123: Repeat: Refer Coloured Plate; Harrison 18th/p 2790, 2791*

Cavitatory lesions of lungs are characteristic of Wegener's granulomatosis.

Polyarteritis Nodosa *(Refer Illustration – 3 in Review Notes)*

23. Answer is B (Lung): *Harrison 15th/1958; Harrison 16th/2007, 2008; Harrison 17th/2124; Harrison 18th/p 2125, 2794*

'PAN (classic PAN) does not involve pulmonary arteries although bronchial vessels may be involved. Aneurysmal dilatation upto 1 cm in size along the involved arteries is characteristic of PAN.' *-Harrison 16th/2007.*

Classical PAN: Review

Classical PAN is a multisystem necrotizing vasculitis of small & medium sized muscular arteries in which involvement of renal & visceral arteries is characteristic

Clinical Manifestations Related to Organ System Involvement in Classic Polyarteritis Nodosa

Renal	Hypertension, Renal failure
Musculoskeletal	Arthritis, arthralgia, myalgia
Peripheral nervous system	Peripheral neuropathy, mononeuritis multiplex
Gastrointestinal tract	Abdominal pain, nausea and vomiting, bleeding, bowel infarction and perforation, cholecystitis, hepatic infarction, pancreatic infarction
Skin	Rash, purpura, nodules, cutaneous infarcts, livedo reticularis, Raynaud phenomenon
Cardiac	Congestive heart failure, myocardial infarction, pericarditis
Genitourinary	Testicular, ovarian, or epididymal pain
Central nervous system	Cerebral vascular accident, altered mental status, seizure

Remember[Q]

- *Classic PAN does not involve pulmonary arteries. Bronchial vessels may be involved but their involvement also, is an uncommon feature.* [Q]
- *Renal involvement is characterized by arteritis without glomerulonephritis. Clinically renal involvement is in the form of renovascular hypertension is frequent. Renal failure may occur but it is uncommon and usually occurs late.*[Q]

24. Answer is A (Polyarteritis nodosa): *Current Diagnosis and Treatment in Rheumatology 2nd/279;*

Renal disease manifesting as hypertension without RBC cast in urine (No glomerulonephritis) is characteristic of polyarteritis Nodosa

Digital gangrene is usually associated with vasculitis of medium sized vessels. Amongst options provided PAN is a medium vessel vasculitis and presence of digital ischaemia is more characteristic of PAN than MPA or WG. Digital gangrene may however be seen (less frequent) in cases of MPA and WG.

Digital Gangrene and Mononeuritis Multiplex

Mononeuritis multiplex is a characteristic feature of PAN and MPA
Mononeuritis multiple may also accompany WG but is less characteristic of WG than PAN or MPA

Polyarteritis Nodosa	Microscopic polyangitis (MPA)	Wegener's granulomatosis (WG)
• Renal Disease is characterized by Arteritis without Glomerulonephritis	• Renal disease is characterized by glomeruloneonephritis	• Renal disease is characterized by glomerulonephritis
Thus *No RBC cast are seen in Urine* But *Proteinuria and Hematuria (RBC cells) are seen*	Thus *RBC cast are present in urine* And *Proteinuria and Haematuria are seen*	Thus *RBC cast are present in urine* And *Protenuria and Haematuria are seen*
• Renal disease is characterized by intraperenchymal inflammation with involved of medium sized muscular arteries within the kidney.	• Renal disease is not associated with involvement of medium sized muscular arterus	• Renal disease is not associated with involvement of medium sized arteries
This presents as Renin mediated Hypertension which is a prominent features.	*Renin mediated hypertension is not associated*	*Renin mediated Hypertension is not associated*

25. Answer is B (Polyarteritis Nodosa) : *Harrison 15th /1959; Harrison 16th/2007, 2008; Harrison 17th/2124; Harrison 18th/p 2794*

The clinical presentation of the patient in question is consistent with a diagnosis of Polyarteritis Nodosa.

The clinical presentation of patient in question gives us the following 'leads' in approaching the diagnosis.

- Digital gangrene in the setting of normal peripheral pulses.
- Presence of hypertension
- Negative antinuclear antibodies
- Negative anti dsDNA
- Negative ANCA

Polyarteritis Nodosa: PAN

- Classic Polyarteritis nodosa is characterized by necrotizing inflammation of medium sized muscular arteries.
- In classic Polyarteritis Nodosa, skin findings include livido reticularis, subcutaneous nodules and skin ulcers. **Digital gangrene**[Q] is not an unusual occurance – *CMDT/ 2004/813*
- Involvement of renal arteries leads to renin mediated ***hypertension***[Q].
- Patients with classic PAN are **ANCA negative** – *CMDT 2004/814*
- Positive ANCA (pANCA) are found in low percentage (< 20%) of patients with classical PAN- *Harrison* [ANCAs that produce a p-ANCA pattern on immunofluorescence testing are frequently associated with microscopic polyangitis and not classical PAN.
- Polyarteritis nodosa is a term given to necrotizing arteritis of medium sized vessels. – *CMDT 2004*
- Microscopic polyangitis may involve medium sized as well as small blood vessels and its spectrum overlaps that of PAN.
- The clinical presentation of patient in question is consistent with a diagnosis of PAN.

Takayasu's disease is also known as 'pulseless disease' and absence of peripheral pulses is a clinical hallmark of disease. *The presence of all peripheral pulses makes this diagnosis unlikely.*
SLE: *Absence of ANA and Anti ds DNA almost rules out the possibility of SLE as a probable diagnosis.*

Wegener's granulomatosis is a necrotizing granulomatous vasculitis of small arteries and skin manifestations does not include digital gangrene.
Antineutrophil cytoplasmic antibodies (ANCA) occur is about 90% of patients with active Wegner's granulomatosis. *Absence of ANCA in blood strongly points against a diagnosis of Wegener's granulomatosis*

26. Ans. is B i.e. (Polyarteritis nodosa) *Repeat : Harrison 16th / 2007-2008; CMDT 2009 / 744; Refer previous question; Harrison 17th/2124; Harrison 18th/p 2794*

Polyarteritis nodosa is the single best answer amongst the options provided.

- ***Numbness of multiple limbs indicates*** peripheral neuropathy / mononeuritis multiplex.

  'PAN is amongst the forms of vasculitis most commonly associated with vasculitic neuropathy'- CMDT.

- ***Digital gangrene*** forms part of the typical skin findings in PAN.

  'Typical skin findings in PAN include Livido Reticularis, subcutaneous nodules and skin ulcers. ***Digital gangrene is not uncommon'*** *- Harrison*

- ***Hypertension (BP = 160/110mmHg) is a common manifestation of renal involvement in PAN.***

  'Involvement of renal arteries leads to a renin mediated hypertension (much less characteristic of vasculitides involving smaller vessels).

- ***Renal function*** may be normal unless renal failure supervenes which is often late in the course of classic PAN.

  Also ***microscopic haematuria*** though uncommon with renal involvement in PAN may well be seen from haemorrhage due to microaneurysms. *Harrison 16th / 2007*

  (Remember that pathology in the kidney in classic PAN is that of Arteritis without Glomerulonephritis).

  PAN is the answer of choice as if satisfies most diagnostic hint provided in the question.

27. Answer is A (Classic PAN) : *Harrision 16th/2007; API 7th/1183; Harrison 17th/2124, 2125, 2656; Harrison 18th/p 2794*

Amongst the options provided, mononeuritis multiplex is a feature of classical PAN and microscopic polyangitis. Presence of hypertension (infrequent in microscopic polyangitis) and normal renal function (infrequent in microscopic polyangitis) leads us to a diagnosis of classical polyarteritis nodosa.

Renal involvement in classic PAN	Renal involvement in microscopic polyangitis
Pathology in kidney is that of arteritis without glomerulonephritis (involves small & medium sized muscular arteries)	Pathology in kidney is that of glomerulonephritis
Renal impairment is uncommon – API 7th/1183	*Rapid renal impairment is characteristic – API 7th/1183*
Hypertension is frequent	*Hypertension is infrequent- API 7th/1183*
Renal involvement is mainly in the form of Renovascular hypertension – *API 7th/1183*	

Causes of mononeuritis multiplex : *Harrison 14th/2467 (not elaborated in Harrison 16th)*

Common causes	Uncommon causes
Classic polarteritis nodosa	Mixed cryoglobulinemia
Microscopic polyangitis	Sjogren syndrome
RA	Wegner's granulomatosis
SLE	Progressive systemic sclerosis
Mixed connective tissue disease	Churg-strauss allergic granulomatosis
	Hypersensitivity angitis
	Leprosy
	Amyloidosis
	Diabetes

28. Answer is A (Necrotizing arteritis): *Harrison 17th/2124; Harrison 18th/p 2794*

PAN is characterized by necrotizing vasculitis of small and medium sized muscular arteries. The vascular lesion in PAN is necrotizing inflammation of small and medium sized muscular arteries.

Microscopic Polyangitis (MPA) and Churg Strauss Syndrome

29. Answer is D (Intravascular Granulomas): *Harrison's 18th/2793*

Churg Strauss Syndrome is typically charachterized by extravascular granulomas.

'Churg Strauss Syndrome also referred to allergic angitis and granulomatosis is charachterized by asthma, peripheral and tissue eosinophilia, extravascular granuloma formation and vasculitis of multiple organ systems' - Harrison's 18th

'Churg Strauss Syndrome is typically associated with Cutaneous Extravascular Necrotizing Granulomas (CENG)'.
- Practical Immunodermatology

Note that intravascular granulomas present within the walls of the vessels themselves may also be seen in Churg Strauss Syndrome. This is however not a charachteristic feature.

Churg Strauss Syndrome

- Small (medium) vessel necrotizing vasculitis vessel (ANCA positive)
- Granulomatous inflammation / reactions is a charachterictic histopathological feature that may be present in the tissues or walls of the vessels themselves (infiltration of tissues with eosinophils[Q])

- Mean age = 48 years (Disease can be seen at any age with possible exception of infants)
- Female to male ratio is 1.2:1 *(More common in females)*

Characteristic Laboratory Features

- Striking eosinophilia (>1000 cells /μl) (seen in > 80% of patients)
- Evidence of Inflammation (↑ESR: ↑fibrinogen; ↑alpha2 - globulin)
- ANCA positive
- ANCA is usually anti-myeloperoxidase

Constitutional Symptoms
Fever, malaise
Anorexia, Weight loss

Asthma

- Severe asthmatic attacks and presence of pulmonary infiltrates dominates the clinical picture

Allergic Rhinitis and sinusitis may be seen in about 61% of patients

Eosinophilia

Marked Peripheral and Tissue eosinophilia

Extravascular Granuloma formation

Extravascular Granuloma formation is a typical feature of Churg Strauss syndrome

Intravascular granuloma may also be seen

Vasculitis of multiple organ systems

- Any organ may be involved
- Mononeuritis multiplex is second most common manifestation (~72%)
- Skin lesions such as purpura & skin nodules are common (~51%)
- Heart disease ~ 14%
- Kidney involvement is less common and renal failure is rare

30. Answer is C (Renal failure is common): *Harrison's 18th/2793*

The Renal involvement in Churg Strauss Syndrome is not prominent and renal failure is rare.

*'The Renal disease in Churg Strauss Syndrome is less common and **generally** less severe than with granulomatosis with polyangitis (Wegener's) and microscopic polyangitis'- Harrison's 18th/2793*

'Renal failure is rare in Churg Strauss syndrome - Pulmonary Involvement in Systemic Autoimmune Disease

31. Answer is B (Lower Respiratory Tract involvement): *Oxford Desk Reference: Nephrology (Oxford University Press) 2009/169*

Lower Respiratory Tract involvement is typically more common in Churg Strauss Syndrome in comparison to Wegener's Granulomatosis.

Organs involved in small vessels vasculitis:

Organ involvement throughout disease course	**Wegner's granulomatosis**	**Microscopic polyangitis**	**Churg-Strauss syndrome**
Upper respiratory tract	*80%*	*Uncommon*	*55%*
Lower respiratory tract	***70%***	***30%***	***100%***
Eye	*46%*	*10%*	*6%*
Kidney	*80%*	*90%*	*33%*
Peripheral nervous system	35%	20%	67%
Gastrointestinal system	5%	5%	17%
Heart	Uncommon	Uncommon	28%
Skin	50%	25%	44%
Constitutional symptoms	95%	90%	94%

32. Answer is C (Renal involvement in 80% of cases): *Current Rheumatology Diagnosis & Treatment (CRDT) 2nd/287; Harrison 17th/2125, 2126; Harrison 18th/p 2793, 2794*

Renal involvement is seen in at least 80% ofpatients with MPA.

<u>Renal involvement is seen in at least 80% of patients with MPA</u>
Renal involvement is seen in at least 80% of patients with MPA - CRDT
Glomerulonephritis occurs in atleast 79% of patients – Harrison

<u>Microscopic polyangitis is not associated with IgG Deposits in kidney</u>
Microscopic Polyangitis is a pauci-immune glomerulonephritis.
Immunofluorescence and electron microscopy show no immune deposits

<u>Microscopic Polyangitis is not associated with bronchospasm</u>
Asthma (bronchospasm) and Eosinophilia are features of Churg-Strauss Syndrome and are typically absent in microscopic polyangitis.

Features	H.S. purpura	Microscopic Polyangitis	Wegner's Granulomatosis	Churg-Strauss syndrome
Deposits in kidney	+ nt (IgA deposits)	-	-	-
Bronchospasm (Asthma)	-	-	-	+
Eosinophilia	-	-	-	+
Predominant ANCA	-	p-ANCA	c-ANCA	p-ANCA

33. Answer is C (Necrotizing vasulitis): *Refer text below*

Both polyarteritis nodosa and microscopic polyangitis are characterized by histologicaly by necrotizing vasculitis.

Clinical Features	PAN	MPA
Kidney Involvement		
• *Renal vasculitis with infarcts and microaneurysms*	Yes	No
• *Rapidly progressive glomerulonephritis with crescents*	No	Yes
Lung involvement		
• *Alveolar hemorrhage*	No	Yes
Laboratory data		
• *HBV-infection*	Yes (10%)	No
• *ANCA*	Negative	Positive (p-ANCA)
Abnormal angiogram with microaneurysms	Yes	No
• *Histology*	Necrotizing vasculitis	Necrotizing vasculitis (no granulomas)
• *Relapses*	Rare	Common

Giant Cell Arthritis *(Refer Illustration - 4 in Review Notes)*

34. Answer is C (Low ESR): *Harrison 15th/1963; Harrison 16th/2009; Harrison 17th/2126; Harrison 18th/p 2795*

Temporal arteritis is characterised by an increased ESR.

TEMPORAL ARTERITIS / GIANT CELL ARTERITIS / CRANIAL ARTERITIS :

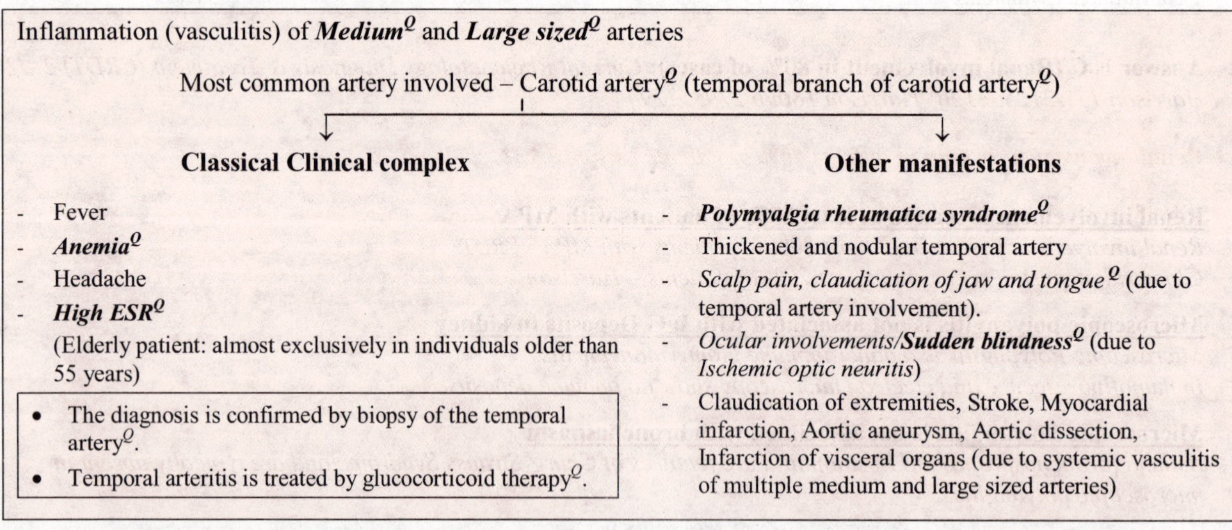

35. Answer is D i.e. (Temporal Arteritis): *Harrison's 17th/2126, 2127; Current Rheumatology 2nd/264,265; Robbins 8th/512; Textbook of Medicine by Mouxham 4th/1184; Harrison 18th/p 2795, 2796*

The clinical complex of fever, headache and diplopia together with panarteritis on biopsy of temporal artery suggests the diagnosis of temporal arteritis.

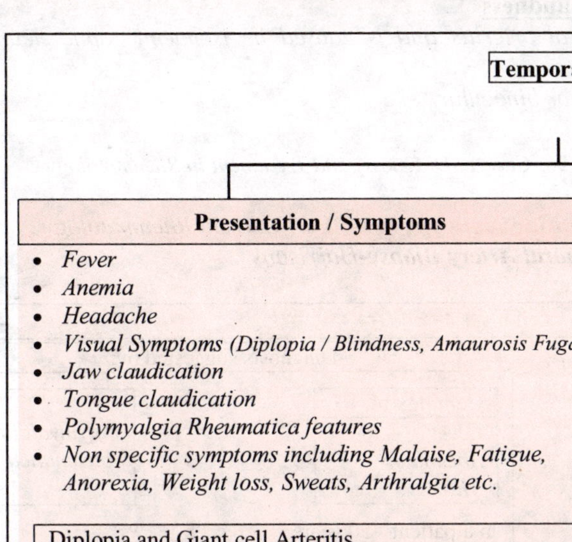

Temporal Arteritis

Age > 50y

Sex: F > M

Presentation / Symptoms	Biopsy of Temporal Artery
• *Fever* • *Anemia* • *Headache* • *Visual Symptoms (Diplopia / Blindness, Amaurosis Fugax)* • *Jaw claudication* • *Tongue claudication* • *Polymyalgia Rheumatica features* • *Non specific symptoms including Malaise, Fatigue, Anorexia, Weight loss, Sweats, Arthralgia etc.*	• **Panarteritis** *Temporal Arteritis is characterized histologically by* ***'Panarteritis'*** *with inflammatory mononuclear cell infiltrates and Giant cell formation* - *Nodular intimal thickening* - *Granulomatous inflammation with Multinucleated Giant cells* - *Elastic Lamina fragmentation* • **Patchy with ship lesions** *Inflammatory changes may not affect the entire length of the artery and 'skip lesions' are common.*

Diplopia and Giant cell Arteritis
About one third of patients present with visual symptoms, ***chiefly diplopia*** *or visual loss.* *- Current Rheumatology 2nd/265*

36. Answer is A (Headache): *Current and Diagnosis and Treatment in Rheumatology 2nd/264; Harrisons 17th/2126; Harrison 18th/p 2795*

The most common presenting symptom in giant cell Arteritis is Headache

Headache is the predominant symptom-Harrison 17th/2126
Headache is the most common Symptom- Current Rheumatology 2nd/264

Classic Presenting Manifestation of Giant Cell Arteritis (Current Rheumatology)	
Headache	70% (most common symptoms)
Jaw Claudication	50%
Polymyalgia Rheumatica	40%
Blindness	20%

Facts to Remember

Characteristic Clinical manifestation of Temporal Arteritis include a complex of:
Fever and or constitutional symptoms
Anemia (80%)
ESR (90%)
Headache (70%)

37. Answer is B (Worsens on exposure to heat): *Harrison 17th/2126; Harrison 18th/p 2795*

Worsening of symptoms on exposure to heat is not a feature of temporal arteritis.

Temporal Arteritis is more common in women *(Harrison 17th/2126)*

Epidemiological features of Temporal Arteritis

More common in women than Men (Women > Men)
More common in whites than blacks (Whites > blacks)

Temporal arteritis is primarily a disease of the elderly

Giant cell arteritis (Temporal arteritis) occurs almost exclusively in individuals > 50 years – Harrison

Temporal Arteritis can lead to sudden onset bilateral blindness

Blindness is the most dreaded complication of Temporal arteritis and is caused by ischaemic optic neuropathy, particularly in untreated patients.

Visual loss may be transient or permanent and monocular or binocular.

38. Answer is A (Temporal Artery Biopsy): *Harrisons 17th/2126; Current Diagnosis and Treatment in Rheumatology 2nd/2126; Harrison 18th/p 2795, 2796*

Temporal artery biopsy is the gold standard test for diagnosing giant cell Arteritis – *Current Rheumatology*

The diagnosis of giant cell Arteritis is confirmed by Temporal Artery Biopsy-*Harrisons*

Diagnosis of Giant cell Arteritis (GCA)

- *Diagnosis of GCA is suggested clinically by demonstration of complex of fever, anemia and high ESR with or without polymyalgia Rheumatica in a patient > 50 years.*
- *Diagnosis is confirmed by biopsy of temporal artery (Gold standard).*
- *Colour duplex ultrasonography of affected temporal artery can show a characteristic halo of edema and stenosis but this investigation is no more sensitive for the diagnosis of GCA than careful physical examination (Current Rheumatology).*
- *CT Angiography and MRI may be useful for assessment of Temporal Artery but are not the investigations of choice.*

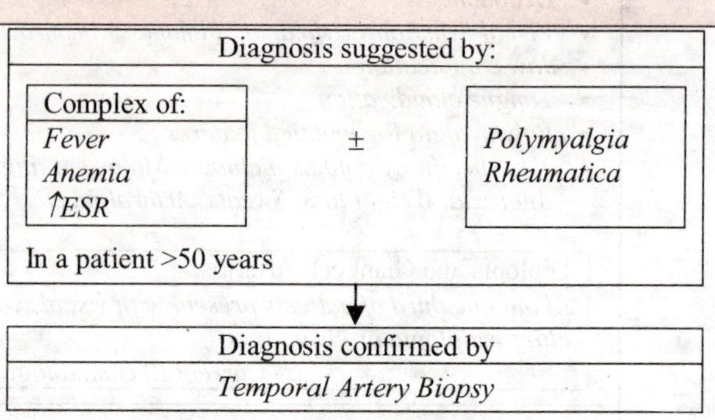

Kawasaki Disease *(Refer Illustration-5 in Review Notes)*

39. Answer is D (Exudative conjunctivitis): *Nelsons 18th/1038*

Kawasaki disease is associated with non exudative conjunctivitis

Diagnostic criteria for Kawasaki disease include bilateral bulbar conjunctival injection ***without exudate*** *as one of their diagnostic criteria.*

Classic Clinical criteria for Kawasaki Disease (Diagnosis is based on clinical signs)
Fever persisting at least 5 days Presence of at least 4 principal features • Changes in extremities - *Erythema of palms soles* - ***Edema of hands, feet*** - *Periungual peeling of fingers,toes in weeks 2 and 3* • Polymorphous exanthem • ***Bilateral bulbar conjunctival injection without exudate*** • Changes in lips and oral cavity - *Erythema, lips cracking,* ***strawberry tongue****, diffuse injection of oral and pharyngeal mucosa* • Cervical lymphadenopathy (>1.5cm diameter usually unilateral) Exclusion of other diseases with similar findings Patients with fever at least 5 days and < 4 principal criteria can be diagnosed with Kawasaki disease when coronary artery abnormalities are detected with 2DE or angiography.

Characteristic Laboratory Findings (There is no diagnostic test for KD)
• *Leukocytosis with neutrophilia and immature forms* • *Elevated erythrocyte sedimentation rate (ESR)* • *Elevated C- reactive protein (CRP)* • *Anemia* • *Abnormal plasma lipids* • *Hypoalbuminemia* • *Hypernatrenia* • *Thrombocytosis after week 1* • *Sterile pyuria* • *Elevated serum transaminases* • *Elevated serum gamma glutamyl transpeptidase* • *Pleocytosis of cerebrospinal fluid* • *Leukocytosis in synovial fluid*

40. Answer is C (Thrombocytopenia): *Harrison 15th / 1966, 1968; Harrisons 16th/2012; Harrison 17th/2130; Harrison 18th/p 2800*

Kawasaki disease is associated with thrombocytosis (not thrombocytopenia).

Kawasaki disease (mucocutaneous[q] lymph node[q] syndrome):

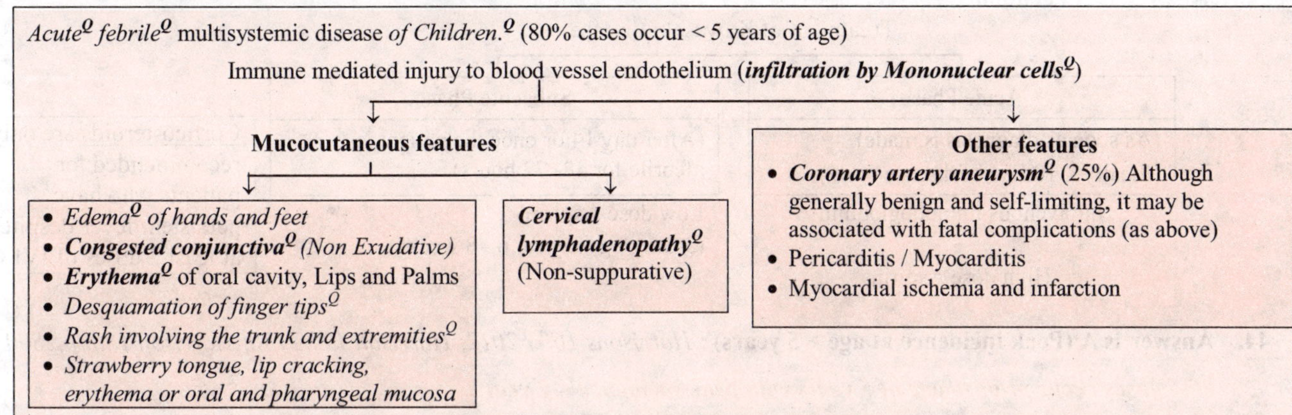

Strong association has been reported between a novel form of S. aureus that release TSS toxin-1 & Kawasaki disease.[Q] *However, the disease is unresponsive to antibiotics.*[Q]

41. Answer is C (Thrombocytopenia) : *Harrisons 16th / 2012; Refer previous question; Harrison 17th/2130; Harrison 18th/p 2800*

Kawasaki disease is associated with thrombocytosis and not thrombocytopenia.

Characteristic laboratory findings include	Treatment of Choice	Prognosis
Increased ESR[Q] ***Thrombocytosis***[Q]	*High dose intravenous immunoglobulins*[Q]	***Prognosis for uneventful recovery is excellent.***[Q]

42. Answer is C (Thrombocytopenia) : *Harrisons 17th/2130; Nelsons 18th/1038; Harrison 18th/p 2800*

Kawasaki disease is associated with thrombocytosis and not thrombocytopenia.

Characteristic laboratory findings include	Treatment of Choice	Prognosis
Increased ESR[Q] ***Thrombocytosis***[Q]	*High dose intravenous immunoglobulins*[Q]	***Prognosis for uneventful recovery is excellent.***[Q]

43. Answer is A (Associated with coronary artery aneurysms in up to in 25% of untreated cases)

'Coronary artery aneurysm develops in up to 25% of untreated patients' *– Nelson 18th/ 1038*

The most common cause of vasculitis in children is Henoch Schonlein Purpura (HSP)

Although Ghai's textbook mentions Kawasaki disease as the most common vasculitis in children, most other standard textbooks (Rudolph Pediatrics, Current Rheumatology Diagnosis and Treatment, CPDT etc) mention HSP as the most common vasculitis in children.

'HSP is the most common form of vasculitis in children' - Current Rheumatology Diagnosis & Treatment (CRDT) / 286

'HSP is the most common vasculitis of childhood with an annual incidence of 15/100,000 children'

- Rudolph's Fundamentals of Pediatrics 3rd /284

Coronary artery aneurysms develop in up to 25% of untreated patients

(25% according to Nelson, 15-25% according to CPDT and 15-30% according to Ghai)

Coronary artery aneurysms *are the* most serious complication[Q] seen in cases of Kawasaki disease

These are usually seen in the 2nd or 3rd week of illness (Rarely before day ten[Q] *(CPDT))*

These are best detected by two dimensional echocardiography[Q] *(Nelson)*

Lymph node biopsy does not aid the diagnosis of Kawasaki disease (Not used)

The diagnosis of Kawasaki disease is based on presence of specific clinical signs (clinical criteria). There is no specific laboratory test

Treatment with Intravenous Immunoglobulins (IVIG) should be started as soon as possible after diagnosis and not only if coronary artery is involved.

Treatment of Kawasaki disease

Acute Phase	Subacute Phase
(As soon as diagnosis is made) (Ideally < 10days of disease onset)	(After day 14 or once the patient is afebrile for 48- 72 hours)
Intravenous immunoglobulin + High dose Aspirin	Low dose Aspirin (3-5mg/hg /day for 6 –8 weeks)

Corticosteroids are only recommended for patients who have persistent fever despite at least 2 doses of IVI G

44. Answer is A (Peak incidence at age > 5 years) : *Harrisons 16th / 2012; Harrison 17th/2130; Harrison 18th/p 2800*

80% cases occur prior to age of 5 years with peak incidence < 2 years.

- Kawasaki disease is an Acute ***febrile***[Q] multisystem ***disease of children***[Q]
- Prolonged fever over 5 days that is unresponsive to antibiotics is seen.
- Although the disease is generally benign & self limiting it is associated c coronary artery aneurysm in 25% of cases
- Non suppurative cervical lymphadenopathy is characteristic

45. Answer is C (Immunoglobulins): *Nelsons 18th/1038; Harrisons 17th/2130;*

The treatment of choice in Kawasaki disease is intravenous immunglobulins

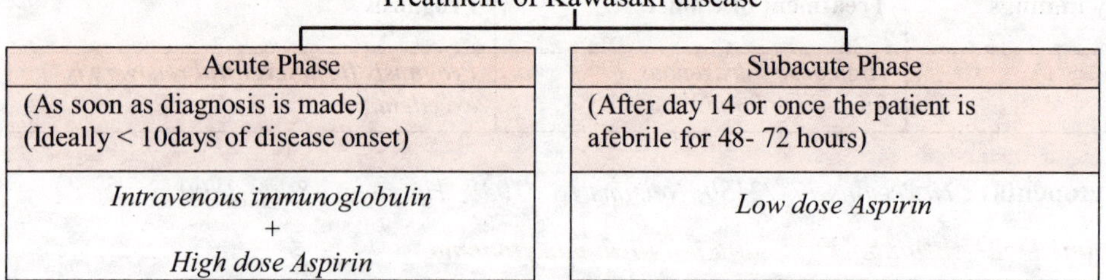

Corticosteroids are only recommended for patients who have persistent fever despite at least 2 doses of IVI G

46. Answer is A (IV Immunoglobulins): *Harrisons 18th/2800*

The treatment of choice in Kawasaki disease is intravenous immunglobulins

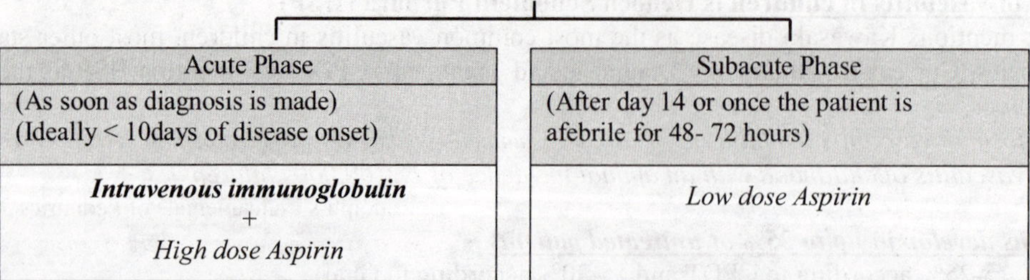

Corticosteroids are only recommended for patients who have persistent fever despite at least 2 doses of IVI G

47. Answer is A (Immunoglobulins) : *Harrison's 17th/2130; Nelson's 18th/1038; Harrison 18th/p 2800*

The treatment of choice for Kawasaki disease is intravenous immunoglobulins

Henoch Schonlein Purpura *(Refer Illustration -6 in Review Notes)*

48. Answer is A (Henoch Schonlein Purpura) *: Harrisons 17th/2128; Harrison 18th/p 2797*

Palpable Purpura (most commonly distributed over the buttocks and lower extremities), arthralgias, and abdominal pain are all charachteristic features of Henoch-Schonlein purpura. *Although H.S purpura is usually seen in a children and most patients range in age from 4-7 years, Harrisons text clearly mentions that this condition may also be seen in infants and adults.* ***The charachteristic clinical manifestation of palpable purpura, arthralgia and abdominal pain in this young adult suggest the diagnosis of H-S purpura.***

Henoch Schonlein Purpura : Anaphylactoid Purpura : Review

What is H. S. Purpura?

- H. S. Purpura is a vasculitis of ***small vessels***^{Q}
- The pathogenic mechanism for this vasculitis is ***iminune complex deposition***^{Q}
- The most common class of antibodies seen in immune complexes of H.S purpura is **IgA**^{Q}

How does H. S. Purpura Present?

Vasculitis

Vasculitis of Skin (cutaneous)	Vasculitis of Toints (Arthralgias)	Vasculitis of Gastrointesinal tract	Vasculitis of kidney
Palpable purpura^Q Most commonly distributed over the buttocks and lower extremity	• ***Polyarthralgias***^{Q} in absence of frank arthritis (Non deforming in nature) • Mainly involves large joints of the lower extremity • Joint involvement is often migratory	***Colicky Abdominal pain***^{Q} is the most charachteristic manifestation . *Other manifestations:* • Passage of blood & mucus per rectum • Nausea/vomiting • Diarrhea / constipation	***Mild glomerulonephritis***^{Q} leading to proteinuria, ***microscopic haematuria***^{Q} and RBC cast in urine are the charachteristic renal manifestation

49. Answer is A (Henoch Shonlein Purpura): *Repeat*

Presence of non-blanching palpable purpura (vasculitis of skin) and colicky abdominal pain (vasculitis of gastrointestinal tract) in a five-year-old child together with evidence of IgA deposition in immune complexes suggests the diagnosis of Henoch Scholein Purpura.

H. S. Purpura / Anaphylactoid Purpura

- **Small vessel vasculitis**^{Q} (ANCA – Negative^Q)
- Pathogenic mechanism of vasculitis is **immune complex deposition**^{Q}
- The most common class of Antibodies deposited in immune complexes is **IgA**^{Q}

- *Usually seen in children*^{Q}
  (Peak incidence in age of 4-7 years)
- May be seen in infants and adults^Q
  (Most common vasculitis in children^Q)

Characteristic Laboratory Features

- *ANCA Negative*^{Q}
- *Elevated serum IgA*^{Q}
- *Elevated ESR*^{Q}
- *Mild Leukocytosis and Normal Platelet count*^{Q}
- *No Thrombocytopenia* ^{Q}
  Purpura in H.S. Purpura is due to vasculitis and not due to thrombocytopenia
- Hematuria (RBC), Proteinuria and RBC cast (Glomerulonephritis) on Urinalysis
- Despite immune complex mechanism involved *serum complement levels are usually normal*^{Q}

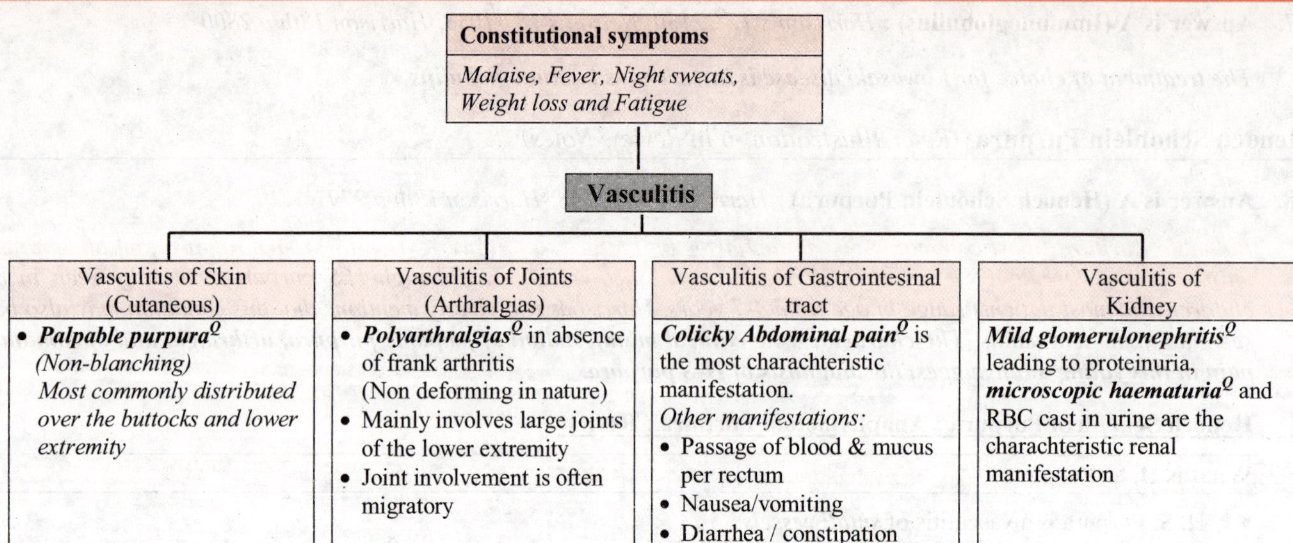

50. Answer is A (Thrombocytopenia) *; Harrison16th / 2010, 17th/2128; Harrison 18th/p 2797*

Purpura in Henoch Schönlein purpura is due to vasculitis and not thrombocytopenia. Platelet count is either normal or elevated.

<u>Henoch Schönlein Purpura</u> :

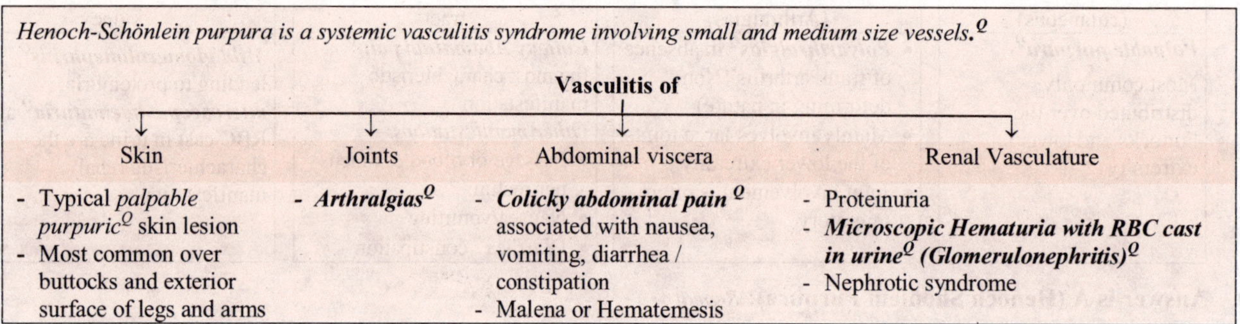

Remember:

- Usually seen in children (in fact *it is the most common small vessel vasculitis in children* [Q])
- Vasculitis is caused by immune complex deposition
- *Most common antibody seen in these immune complexes is 'IgA'*[Q] *(IgA levels are elevated)*[Q]
- *Platelet count is normal or elevated*[Q]
- Serum compliment levels are normal
- **Prognosis** : Is excellent and disease is self-limiting. Lasts about six weeks and resolves without sequelae.
- **Treatment** : Involves administration of ***glucocorticoids.*** [Q]

51. Answer is D (Thrombocytopenia): *Repeat*

Henoch Scholein Purpura is not associated with thrombocytopenia

52. Answer is A (Henoch Schonlein Purpura): *Harrison 17th /2128; Harrison's 18th*

Palpable Purpura (most commonly distributed over the buttocks and lower extremities), arthralgias, and abdominal pain are all charachteristic features of Henoch-Schonlein purpura. *Although H.S purpura is usually seen in children and most patients range in age from 4-7 years, Harrisons text clearly mentions that this condition may also be seen in infants and adults.* ***The charachteristic clinical manifestation of palpable purpura, arthralgia and abdominal pain in this young adult suggest the diagnosis of H-S purpura.***

Henoch Schonlein Purpura : Anaphylactoid Purpura : Review

What is H. S. Purpura?

- H. S. Purpura is a vasculitis of ***small vessels***[Q]
- The pathogenic mechanism for this vasculitis is ***iminune complex deposition***[Q]
- The most common class of antibodies seen in immune complexes of H.S purpura is **IgA**[Q]

How does H. S. Purpura Present?

Vasculitis

Vasculitis of Skin (cutaneous)	Vasculitis of Joints (Arthralgias)	Vasculitis of Gastrointesinal tract	Vasculitis of kidney
Palpable purpura[Q] Most commonly distributed over the buttocks and lower extremity	• ***Polyarthralgias***[Q] in absence of frank arthritis (Non deforming in nature) • Mainly involves large joints of the lower extremity • Joint involvement is often migratory	***Colicky Abdominal pain***[Q] is the most charachteristic manifestation. *Other manifestations:* • Passage of blood & mucus per rectum • Nausea/vomiting • Diarrhea / constipation	***Mild glomerulonephritis***[Q] leading to proteinuria, ***microscopic haematuria***[Q] and RBC cast in urine are the charachteristic renal manifestation

53. Answer is A (Thrombocytopenia) : *Repeat; Harrison 17th/2128; Harrison 18th/p 2797*

Purpura in 'Henoch Shonlein purpura' is due to vasculitis and not thrombocytopenia.

54. Answer is E (All of the above): *Current Rheumatology Diagnosis & Treatment 2nd/318;*

Abdominal pain, Intussusseption, Palpable Purpura and progression to end stage renal disease may all be seen in H.S. purpura

Abdominal pain is a characteristic manifestation of HSP (60-70% of patients)

Abdominal Manifestations

- *Colicky Abdominal pain*
- *Nausea, Vomiting, diarrhea or constipation*
- *Gastrointestinal bleeding*
- *Intussusception*

Intussusception may occur in H.S. purpura

Intussusception is rare in adults but may occur in children

HSP associated intussusception is usually ileoileal in contrast to idiopathic intussusception which is ileocolic

Palpable purpura is the most common manifestation of HSP.

Palpable purpura is seen in virtually all pediatric patients

HSP can lead to End stage Renal Disease

Although HSP is usually associated with mild Glomerulonephritis, patients may progress to end stage renal disease. *'Renal disease is more frequent and tends to be persistant in adults who have a higher risk than children of developing End-stage Renal Disease' – CRDT 2nd/318*

55. Answer is A (Blood in Stools) : *See Below and refer previous question; Harrison 17th/2128; Harrison 18th/p 2797*

Blood in stool (melena) and hematemesis are characteristically seen in Henoch Scholein Purpura as a manifestation of vasculitis of abdominal viscera.

56. Answer is C (Mesangial deposits of IgA): *Harrisons 17th/2128; Robins 7th/990; CMDT 2008/803,804,2009/ 749,750; Harrison 18th/p 2797*

Presence of non blanching rash (Purpura), swelling of knee (Arthralgia) along with haematuria (glomerulonephritis) suggests the diagnosis of Henoch- Schonlein purpura.

H.S purpura is characterized by deposition of IgA in the mesangial region (Robbins)

IgA deposition in Mesangium

IgA Nephropathy	H.S.Purpura
• Primarily as isolated renal disease	• Primarily a systemic disease with renal manifestations in 10-50% of patients Renal lesions are identical to those found in IgA Nephropathy
• Most common presenting complaint is an episode of gross hematuria Palpable purpura, arthralgias and abdominal colic are not characteristic and suggest Henoch-Scholein purpura	• Classically presents with palpable purpura, arthralgias and abdominal symptoms (colic). Renal manifestations include microscopic or gross hematuria.

57. Answer is C (IgA): *Harrison 16th/2010; Robbins 7th/650, 986-987; Harrison 17th/2128; Harrison 18th/p 2797*

The presumptive pathogenic mechanism for Henoch-Schönlein purpura is immune complex deposition on endothelium of blood vessels throughout the body and within glomerular mesangial regions.

IgA is the antibody class most often seen in the immune complexes and has been demonstrated in the renal biopsies of these patients' *- Harrison.*

58. Answer is C (IgA)

The most common class of antibodies deposited in immune complexes of Henoch Schonlein Purpura is IgA.

Behcet's Syndrome

59. Answer is C (Seen only in Tropics) : *Harrison 15th/ 1956; 16th/ 2014; Harrison 17th/2132; Harrison 18th/p 2801*

Behçet's syndrome is a multisystem disorder with a world wide distribution that mainly affects young adults. Recurrent aphthous ulceration is a sine-quo non for diagnosis.

Behçet's syndrome: *Review*

Behçet's syndrome is a multisystemic disorder of autoimmune etiology with vasculitis as the main pathologic lesion. Circulating antibodies to human oral mucus membranes are present in 50% of cases.
Diagnostic Criteria[Q]
Recurrent oral ulceration[Q] plus 2 of the following: 1. *Recurrent genital ulceration*[Q] 2. Eye lesion: iritis / posterior uveitis / optic neuritis 3. Skin lesion: folliculitis / erythema nodosum / acne / vasculitis 4. Pathergy test.
Features :
• ***World wide distribution***[Q] (not only seen in Tropics) • *Mainly affects **young adults***[Q] • *HLA-B_5 and HLA– DR_5 linked*[Q] / familial occurrence. • **"*Recurrent Aphthous ulceration*[Q] *is a sine quo non for diagnosis*"**[Q] • Pathergy test: Nonspecific skin inflammatory reactivity to any scratches or intradermal saline injection is a common and specific manifestation. • Arthritis: *Non deforming*[Q], and affects knees and ankles • Superficial and deep venous thrombosis: seen in 1/4 of patients • Central nervous system and gastrointestinal involvement may be present

60. Answer is A (Myocarditis): *Harrison 17th/2132; Current Rheumatology Diagnosis and Treatment 2nd/313; Harrison 18th/p 2801*

Myocarditis has not been mentioned as an association with Behcet's syndrome.

Behcet's syndrome may present with recurrent oral and genital ulceration, Thrombophlebitis and Erythema Nodosum (Skin lesions)

Behcet's syndrome

Behcet's syndrome is a chronic multisystem relapsing vascular inflammatory disease (vasculitis) of unknown origin

Behcet's disease is primarily a small vessel vasculitis but is can also involve large vessels both arteries and veins.

Behcet's disease is associated with HLA-B5 rather than HLA B27

- *Disease pf young people (20 par)* Q
- *Male's affected equally as females* Q

HLA B5 positive Q

Diagnostic criteria

Essential criteria plus two of the non essential criteria are required for diagnosis

Essential criteria

Recurrent oral Ulceration
• *Oral ulceration is the hallmark of disease* Q • *These are sin qua non for the diagnosis* • Types of Ulcers include - Minor Aphthous - Major Aphthous - Herpetiform ulcers • Features of oral ulcers - *Painful* Q - Shallow with a central yellowish necrotic base - Appear singly or in crops - Subside without leaving scars Q (persist for 1-2 weeks)

Non-Essential criteria

Recurrent Genital Ulcers
• Less common but more specific • Do not affect glans or urethra • Produce scars (scrotal scars)
Eye lesions : Uveitis
• Anterior Uveitis (Recurrent Hypopyon) • Posterior uveitis • Retinal vasculitis
Skin lesions
• Erythema nodosum • Pseudofolliculitis • Pseudopustular lesions • Acneiform nodules
Positive Pathergy Test
• Pathergy refers to hyperreactivity of skin to any intracutaneous injection or needle stick • Pathergy is characteristic feature of Behcet's although the mechanism is unknown • Pathergy test is said to be positive if a papule or pustule >2mm develops 24-48 hrs after needle prick to a depth of 5 mm.

Other Clinical Features

Arthritis
Non deforming Arthritis commonly affects knees and ankles
Thrombophlebitis : Vascular lesions
• Superficial or deep peripheral vein thrombosis (25% of patients) • Arterial thrombosis may be seen
Neurological involvement (5-10%)
Dural vein thrombosis may be seen
Pulmonary symptoms
Pulmonary artery vasculitis may occur and present with dyspnea, cough, chest pain, hemoptysis
Gastro intestinal involvement
Consists of mucosal ulceration of Gut similar to Crohn's disease

61. **Answer is B (Behcet's syndrome):** *Refer text below*

Recurrent bilateral Hypopyon is a characteristic feature of Behcet's syndrome.
Behcet's syndrome is also associated with thrombophlebitis which is therefore the single best answer of choice.

HLA – B27 associated uveitis *may also present with hypopyon but this is typically unilateral and not associated with thrombophlebitis.*

Cryoglobulinemia

62. **Answer is D (Strongly Positive Rheumatoid factor):** *Harrison 18th/2798; Wintrobe's Hematology 12th/Chapter 102 (p 2484); The manual of Dermatology (Springer) 2012/263; Other references with text*

Type I Cryoglobulinemia (simple cryoglobulinemia) is typically associated with Monoclonal IgM paraprotenemia producing a Hyperviscosity type syndrome. Type I Cryoglobulins rarely have Rheumatoid Factor Activity and do not activate complement in vitro (hence complement levels are usually normal).

'Monoclonal Cryoglobulins (Type I) rarely exhibit Rheumatoid Factor activity and do not interfere with complement mediated function in vitro'

— *'Cryoglobulins and Cryoglobulinemia' from Clinical Reviews in Allergy and Immunology: Vol 16, Number 3 (1998) page 249-264*

'Type I Cryoglobulins do not activate the complement cascade and are therefore associated with normal complement levels' – 'Primer on Rheumatic Disease' by Klippel (Springer) 13th/19

Mixed Cryoglobulinemias (Type II/Type III) are associated with Strongly Positive Rheumatoid Factors and Reduced Complement levels.
Hypocomplementemia occurs in 90% of patients with mixed cryoglobulinemias. *Rheumatoid factor is positive in 80-100% of patients with mixed cryoglobulinemia*

Cryoglobulinemia

- Cryoglobulins are immunoglobulins that precipitate as serum is cooled below core body temperature (below 37° C) and re-dissolve on re-warming.
- Cryoglobulinemia is characterized by the presence of cryoglobulins in the serum.
- Cryoglobulinemia is most commonly classified into three types in accordance with the Brouet Classification based on the components of the cryoprecipitate.
- Type I (Simple Cryoglobulinemia) and Type II, Type III (Mixed cryoglobulinemia)

Feature	Type I (Simple Cryoglobulinemia)	Type II (Mixed Cryoglobulinemia)	Type III (Mixed Cryoglobulinemia)
Cryoglobulin	Single Monoclonal	Mixed Monoclonal`	Mixed Polyclonal
Molecular composition	Monoclonal IgM or Monoclonal IgG Composed entirely of Monoclonal Immunoglobulins, usually IgM or IgG	Monoclonal IgM* (>IgG*) Polyclonal IgG Composed of Monoclonal Immunoglobulins usually IgM along with Polyclonal Immunoglobulin usually IgG	Polyclonal IgM and Polyclonal IgG Composed of polyclonal immunoglobulin of more than once isotype such as polyclonal IgM and polyclonal IgG
Rheumatoid Factor Activity	Rheumatoid factor activity is absent (rarely present) Monoclonal IgM in Type I Syndrome does not have Rheumatoid Factor Activity	Rheumatoid Factor activity is strongly positive Monoclonal IgM in Type II Syndrome has Rheumatoid Factor activity against IgG	Rheumatoid factor activity is positive Polyclonal IgM has Rheumatoid factor activity
Complement Activation in Vitro	Do not activate the complement cascade Complement levels normal	Activate the complement cascade Complement levels reduced	Activate the complement cascade Complement levels reduced.
Predominant clinical manifestation	Primarily related to Hyperviscosity and consequent thrombosis • Acrocyanosis • Retinal Hemorrhages • Raynaud's phenomenon with digital ulceration • Livido reticularis • Arterial reticularis • Arterial Thrombosis	Primarily related to vasculitis due to immune complex formation and activation of complement • Cutaneous vasculitis • Renal Glomerulonephritis • Neuropathy (Vasculitis) • Abdominal pain (mesenteric vasculitis) • Arthralgia & myalgia Mitzer's Triad: Purpura + Arthralgia + Weakness	
Associations	Lymphoproliferative Diseases • Multiple Myeloma • 'Waldenstroms Macroglobulinemia' • Monoclonal Gammopathy	• Chronic hepatitis C • Autoimmune disease • Sjogren's syndrome • CLL • NHL	Autoimmune Diseases • Systemic Lupus Erythematous • Rheumatoid Arthritis • Inflammatory Bowel Disease • Biliary Cirrhosis Chronic Infections • Viral (EBV, CMV, HIV, Hepatitis E) • Bacterial (Leprosy, Spirochetal, SBE) • Fungal • Parasitic

Hypersensitivity Vasculitis

63. Answer is C (Post-capillary venules): *Harrison's 17th/2128; Harrison 18th/p 2798*

Post-capillary venules are most commonly involved in Hypersensitivity vasculitis

Hypersensitivity vasculitis

- *Hypersensitivity vasculitis refers to small vessel vasculitis that is restricted to the skin and not associated with any other form of primary or secondary vasculitis.*

Implicit in the definition is that this condition is not associated with medium or large vessel disease at other sites, nor with small vessel disease in other organs (only skin)
Microscopic polyangitis affects the skin and also internal organs and hence is not considered part of hypersensitivity vasculitis

- *The typical histopathological feature of cutaneous vasculitis is the presence of leukocytoclastic vasculitis of small vessels.*

Vasculitis is charachterized by Leukocytoclasis – Harrison's
Synonyms for Hypersensitivity vasculitis include: cutaneous small vessels vasculitis, leucocytoclastic vasculitis, cutaneous leucocytoclastic angitis etc.

- *'Post-capillary venules are the most commonly involved vessels. Capillaries and arterioles may be involved less frequently' – Harrison*

American College of Rheumatology 1990 Criteria for the Classification of Hypersensitivity Vasculitis
• Age at disease onset > 16 years • Medication at disease onset • Palpable purpura • Maculopapular rash • Biopsy including arteriole and venule, showing granulocytes in a perivascular or extravascular location

For purposes of classification, hypersensitivity vasculitis may be diagnosed if the patient meets at least three of these five criteria.
Sensitivity = 71%; specificity = 83.9%.

Laboratory and Radiographic Work-up of Patients with Possible Hypersensitivity Vasculitis	
Complete blood cell count	Normal
Electrolytes	Normal
Liver function test	Normal
Urinalysis with microscopy	Normal
Erythrocyte sedimentation rate/CRP	Mild to moderate elevation in <50% of patients
Antinuclear antibody (ANA)	Negative
Rheumatoid factor	Negative
C3, C4	Normal
Antineutrophil cytoplasmic antibody (ANCA)	Negative
Antihepatitis B and C assays	Negative
Cryoglobulins	Negative
Chest radiography	Normal

Connective Tissue Disorders & Joint Disorders

64. Answer is B (SLE) : *Chandrasoma Taylor 3/ 985; Harrisons 16th/1961; Harrison 17th/2076; Harrison 18th/p 2727*

Anti double stranded DNA and anti smith antibodies are specific for SLE..

Antinuclear antibodies in Autoimmune diseases :

1. Anti double stranded DNA (anti dsDNA)	*SLE*
2. Anti histone antibodies	*Drug induced lupus erythematosis*
3. Anti Sm antibody[Q] (antibody to core[Q] protein of small nuclear ribonucleoprotein particles/smith antigen[Q])	*SLE*
4. SSA (Ro) } **antibodies to ribonucleo proteins antigens[Q]** **5. SSB (La)**	*Sjogren syndrome*
6. Antibodies of ribonucleoprotein antigen[Q] containing ULRNP	*Mixed connective tissue disease*
7. Anti DNA topoisomerase antibody (Scl 70)[Q]	*Systemic sclerosis (diffuse)*
8. Anti centromeric antibody[Q]	*Limited Scleroderma (crest)*
9. Histidyl-tRNA synthetase	*Inflammatory myopathy*
10. Anti mitochondrial antibody[Q]	*Primary biliary cirrhosis*

65. Answer is A (SLE): *Robbin's 7th/229: Harrison 17th/2076: Repeat*

Anti Ds DNA antibodies are specific for SLE

66. Answer is C (Anti Sm-Antibodies): *'Immunology: Core text with self assessment: Master Medicine Series' (2006)/120 (Q1); Interpretation of diagnostic tests 8th/1034; Harrison 17th/2076; Harrison 16th/1961; Harrison 18th/p 697*

Anti Smith Antibodies (Anti Sm) is found in 25 to 30% of SLE patients and is the most specific diagnostic test for SLE. *– Interpretation of diagnostic tests 8th/1034*
Anti Ds DNA is almost as specific as anti Sm antibodies but only when present in high titres.

Most sensitive stest for SLE	Anti nuclear antibodies
Most specific test for SLE	Anti Sm Antibody and Anti Ds DNA (Anti Sm Antibody > Anti Ds DNA)

Anti Sm antibodies have high specificity for SLE but low sensitivity being found in < 30% of patients with SLE
Anti Ds DNA is more sensitive than Anti Sm Antibodies being found in upto 70% of patients with SLE but it is almost equally specific than Anti Sm Antibodies when present in high titres. Low titres of Anti Ds DNA are less specific for SLE than low titres of Anti Sm Antibodies.

Antibody	Prevalence %	Clinical Utility
Anti-dsDNA	70	***High titres are SLE specific*** In some patients correlate with disease activity, nephritis, vasculitis
Anti-Sm	25	***Specific for SLE*** No definite clinical correlations

67. Answer is A (Antihistone antibodies) : *Robbin's 7th / 229, 235; Harrison 16th / 1961, 1967; 17th/2076 (Table 313-1); Harrison 18th/p 2726, (Table: 319.1)*

The best marker for Drug Induced Lupus are Antihistone Antibodies.
Drug induced is rarely associate with anti ds DNA and is commonly associated with antibodies to histone (antihistone antibodies): Harrison
Anti ds DNA Antibodis are rae but there is an extremely high frequency of antihistone antibodies' Robbins

Drug induced lupus

Syndrome of Lupus Erythymatosis like symptoms and positive ANA, that appears during therapy with certain medications and biological agent.

Differences from classical SLE

- Less predilection for females than SLE
- Rarely involves kidneys and brain (CNS involvement is rare[Q])
- Rarely associated with Anti-ds-DNA antibodies (Most common ANA are Antihistone Antibodies)
- Usually resolves (remits) after discontinuation of offending medication.

Note : Persons with HLA-D and 4 allele are of a greater risk of developing Lupus Erythematosus after administration of Hydalazine.

Drug associated with SLE (Drug Induced Lupus)	
Antiarrhythemics	Procainamide, disopyramide, propafenone
Antihypertensives	Hydralazine, Several ACE inhibitors and beta blockers
Antithyroid	Propylthiouracil
Antipsychotics	Chlopromazine and Lithium
Anticonvulsants	Carbamezapine and Phenytoin
Antibiotics	Isoniazid, Minocycline, Macrodantin
Diuretics	Hydrochlorthiazide
Antihyperlipidemics	Lovastatin, Simvastatin
Biologics	Interferon and TNF inhibitors

68. Answer is A (Antihistone Antibodies): *Robbins 7th/229*

Drug induced lupus has highest correleation with antihistone antibodies.
Antihistone Antibodies are positive in >95% of patients with drug induced lupus.

69. Answer is C (CREST syndrome): *Harrison 16th/1986; Harrison 17th/2100; Harrison 18th/p 697*

Anticentromere antibodies are characteristic of CREST syndrome.

Anticentromere antibodies are present in 40 - 80% of patients with limited cutaneous scleroderma or crest syndrome. Anticentromere antibodies are found in only about 2% to 5% of patients with diffuse cutaneous scleroderma, and rarely in other connective tissue disease.- Harrison 16th/1986

Systemic sclerosis subsets [Q]

Diffuse cutaneous	Limited cutatneous
Antipoisomerase - I antibody	Anticentromere antibody

Anti double stranded DNA and anti smith antibodies are specific for SLE.

Systemic Lupus Erythrmatosis (SLE)

70. Answer is A, B (ANA;Anti-dsDNA) : *Harrison 17th/2077; Harrison 18th/p 2728*

The revised ACR Criteria for diagnosis of SLE include presence of ANA, Anti-dsDNA, Leucocytopenia< 4000/microL, Lymphopenia< 4000/microL and Proteinuria > 0.5g /d.

Diagnostic criteria for systemic lupus erythematosus:

Criterion	Description
1. Malar rash	Fixed erythema, flat or raised, over the malar eminences
2. Discoid rash	Erythematous circular raised patches with adherent keratotic scaling and follicular plugging; atrophic scarring may occur
3. Photosensitivity	Exposure to ultraviolet light causes rash
4. Oral ulcers	Includes oral and nasopharyngeal ulcers, observed by physician
5. Arthritis	*Nonerosive arthritis* of two or more peripheral joints, with tenderness, swelling, or effusion
6. Serositis	Pleuritis or pericarditis documented by ECG or rub or evidence of effusion
7. Renal disorder	***Proteinuria >0.5 g/d*** or ≥3+, or cellular casts
8. Neurologic disorder	Seizures or psychosis without other causes
9. Hematologic disorder	Hemolytic anemia or ***Leukopenia (<4000/μL) or*** ***Lymphopenia (<1500μL) or*** ***Thrombocytopenia (<100,000μL)*** in the absence of offending drugs
10. Immunologic disorder	***Anti-dsDNA***, anti-Sm, and/or anti-phospholipid
11. Antinuclear antibodies	***An abnormal titer of ANA*** by immunofluorescence or an equivalent assay at any point in time in the absence of drugs known to induce ANAs

Note: ANA, antinuclear antibodies; dsDNA, double-strand DNA; ECG, electrocardiography.

If ≥4 of these criteria, well documented, are present at any time in a patient's history, the diagnosis is likely to be SLE. Specificity is ~95%; sensitivity is ~75%.

71. Answer is C (Polyserositis): *Harrison 17th/2077; Harrison 18th/p 2728*

Polyserositis is included as a diagnostic criteria for SLE and is the most characteristic feature of SLE amongst the options provided.

Uveitis is not a characteristic feature of SLE

Ocular manifestation include sicca syndrome, non specific conjunctivitis, episcleritis, retinal vasculitis and optic neuritis. Uveitis is not mentioned as an ocular manifestation of SLE.

Ocular manifestations are not characteristic of SLE and are not included in the diagnostic criteria for SLE.

Joint Deformity is not a characteristic feature of SLE

Arthritis is included amongst the diagnostic criteria for SLE, however arthritis in SLE is typically nor erosive and does not lead to joint deformities.

Cavitatory Lesion in lungs are not characteristic of SLE

Cavitatory Lesion in lungs are not characteristic of SLE

The most common pulmonary manifestation of SLE is pleuritis with or without pleural effusion.
Other Pulmonary manifestations include Interstitial fibrosis, intraalveolar hemorrhage and shrinking lung syndrome.

Diagnostic Criteria for Systemic Lupus Erythematous

Malar rash	Fixed erythema, flat or raised, over the malar eminences
Discoid rash	Erythematous circular raised patches with adherent keratitic scalling and follicular plugging; atrophic scarring may occur
Photosensitivity	Exposure to ultraviolet light causes rash
Oral ulcers	Includes oral and nasopharyngeal ulcers, observed by physician
Arthritis	Nonerosive arthritis of two or more peripheral joints, with tenderness, swelling, or effusion
Serositis	***Pleuritis or pericarditis documented by ECG or rub or evidence of effusion***
Renal disorder	Proteinuria >0.5g/d or ≥3+, or cellular casts
Neurologic disorder	Seizures or psychosis without other causes
Hematologic disorder	Hemolytic anemia or leucopenia (<4000/μL) or lymphonia (<1500/μL) or thrombocytopenia (< 100,000//μL) in the absence of offending drugs
Immunologic disorder	Anti-ds DNA, anti-Sm, and /or anti-phospholipid
Antinuclear antibodies	An abnormal titer of ANA by immunofluorescence or an equivalent assay at any point in time in the absence of drugs known to induce ANAs

72. Answer is C (Antinuclear antibody) : *Harrison's 15th/1925; 16th/1962, 1963; Harrison 17th/2076 (Table 313-1); Harrison 18th/p 2726, (Table: 319.1)*

The clinical features mentioned in the question suggest a diagnosis of SLE.
The best screening test for SLE is demonstration of anti-nuclear antibodies – *Harrison*

Sensitive test for SLE:	*Antinuclear antibodies (ANA)*^Q
Specific test for SLE:	*Anti ds DNA*^Q *and Anti Sm antibody*^Q

Clues to reaching the diagnosis of SLE in the given question:

	SLE	Patient in Question	Inference
Age / Sex	90% cases are women usually child bearing age	23 year old female	Consistent
Musculoskeletal complaints	All patients experience myalgias and arthralgias	Myalgias	Consistent
	Joint deformities are unusual	Arthralgias	
		No joint deformities	Consistent
Cardiopulmonary Complaints	Pericarditis is the most common manifestation	Pericarditis	Consistent
	Pleurisy and pleural effusion are common	Pleural effusion	Consistent

73. Answer is A (SLE): *Harrison 14th/1876; Harrison 15th/1921; Harrisons 16th/1962; 17th/2077; Harrison 18th/p 2728*

SLE is characterised typically by a non-erosive Arthritis (erosions are rare). *All other options mentioned in the question may have an erosive picture.*

Diagnostic criteria for arthritis in SLE includes
Non erosive arthritis involving two or more peripheral joints characterised by tenderness, swelling or effusion

74. Answer is D (Systemic Lupus Erythematosus): *Harrison 16th/1962; Harrison 17th/2077; Harrison 18th/p 2728*

SLE is characterised typically by a non-erosive Arthritis (erosions are rare). *All other options mentioned in the question may have an erosive picture.*

75. Answer is B (SLE): *Harrisons 17th/2077; Harrisons 16th/1962; Harrison 18th/p 2728*

Systemic Lupus Erythomatosis (SLE) is characterized by non erosive arthritis

Presence of Erosions on Joint X rays are rare and their presence suggests a non lupus inflammatory arthropathy such as Rheumatoid arthritis (Harrisons)

76. Answer is E (Joint Deformity): *Harrison 17th/2077; Harrison 18th/p 2728*

SLE is characterized by non erosive arthritis. Joint deformities may occur but these are rare and limited to hands & feet.
Presence of joint deformities should rasie the suspicion of a non lupus inflammatory arthropathy like RA, and hence joint deformities is the single best answer amongst the options provided.

77. Answer is A (SLE): *Harrison 17th/2078; Harrison 18th/p 2728*

Shrinking lung syndrome is a pulmonary manifestation of SLE.

Shrinking Lung Syndrome
Shrinking lung syndrome is a rare manifestation / complication of SLE and is characterized by diaphragmatic weakness or dysfunction.
Shrinking lung syndrome is associated with restrictive physiology and abnormalities of ventilation and the absence of overt parenchymal or vascular disease.
The restriction is due to weakness of muscles of respiration including the diaphragm – there is selective involvement of diaphragm & respiratory muscles.

78. Answer is A (SLE): *Robbins 7th / 229;*

Antibodies against double stranded DNA (Anti, ds DNA) and Sm antigen (Anti Sm) are highly specific and virtually diagnostic of SLE *– Robbins*

79. Answer is A (SLE): *Harrisons 17th/2077,2079; Harrisons 16th/1962,1964; Robbins 7th/228; Harrison 18th/p 2728, 2730*
Auto immune destruction of platelets or Immune Thrombocytopenia may be seen in variety of collagen vascular diseases but is most characteristic of SLE.

SLE is the single best answer of choice

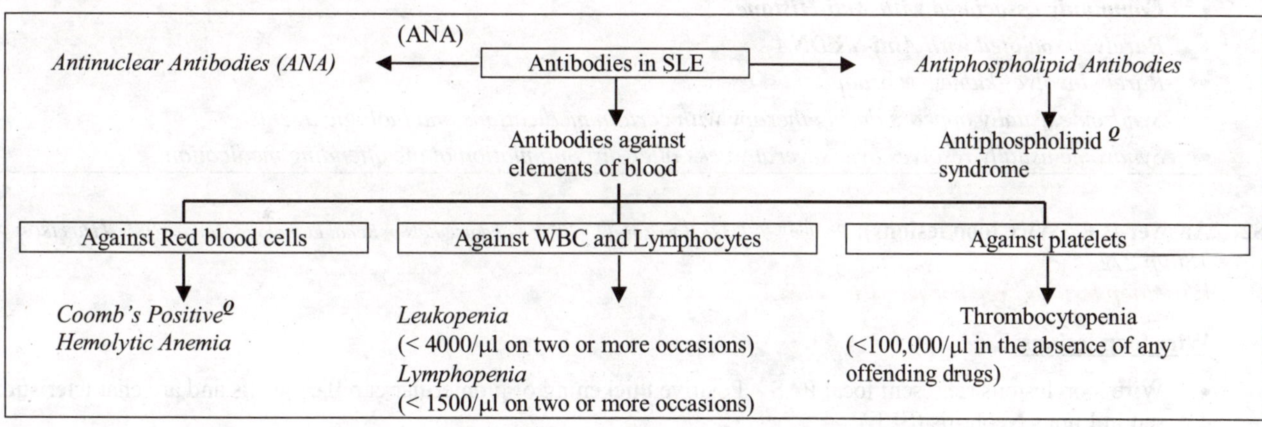

80. Answer is B (Penicillin): *Harrison's 17th/2083; 'Dubois Lupus Erythamatosus' 7th/871; Harrison 18th/p 2735*

Penicillin is not associated with drug induced Lupus.

Drugs reported to induce Lupus-Like disease and associated autoantibodies:

Agent	Risk	Agent	Risk
Antiarrhythmics		**Anticonvulsants**	
Procainamide (Pronestyl)	High	Carbamazepine (Tegretol)	Low
Quinidine (Quinaglute)	Moderate	Phenytoin (Dilantin)	Very low
Disopyramide (Norpace)	Very low	Trimethadone (Tridone)	Very low
Propafenone (Rythmol)	Very low	Primidone (Mysoline)	Very low
Amiodarone (Cordarone)	Very low	Ethosuxamide (Zarontin)	Very low
Antihypertensives		**Antithyroidals**	
Hydralazine (Apresoline)	High	Propylthiouracil (Propylthyracil)	Low
Methyldopa (Aldomet)	Low	**Anti-inflammatories**	
Captopril (Capoten)	Low	D-Penicillamine (Cuprimine)	Low

Acebutolol (Sectral)	Low	Sulfasalazine (Arunfidine)	Low
Enalapril (Vasotec)	Very low	Phenylbutazone (Butazolidin)	Very low
Clonidine (Catapres)	Very low	TNF-α inhibitors (Remicade)	Very low
Atenolol (Tenormin)	Very low	Mesalamine (Asacol)	Very low
Labetalol (Normodyne)	Very low	Zafirlukast (Accolate)	Very low
Pindolol (Visken)	Very low	**Diuretics**	
Minoxidil (Loniten)	Very low	Chlorthalidone (Hygroton)	Very low
Prazosin (Minipress)	Very low	Hydrochlorothiazide (DiuchlorH)	Very low
Lisinopril	Very low	**Antihyperlipidemics**	
Antipsychotics		Lovastatin (Mevacor)	Very low
Chlorpromazine (Thorazine)	Low	Simvastatin (Zocar)	Very low
Phenelzine (Nardil)	Very low	Atorvastatin (Lipitor)	Very low
Chlorprothixene (Taractan)	Very low	**Miscellaneous**	
Lithium carbonate (Eskalith)	Very low	Aminoglutethimide (Cytadren)	Very low
Perphanazine (Trilafon)	Very low	Interferorn –a (Wellferon) - β - γ	Very low
Antibiotics		Timolol eye drops (Timoptic)	Very low
Isoniazid (INH)	Low	Ticlopidine (Ticlid)	Very low
Minocycline (Minocin)	Low		
Nitroturantoin (Macrodantin)	Very low		

81. Answer is C (Renal involvement): *Harrison 17th/2083; Harrison 18th/p 2735*

Renal involvement is rare in Drug induced Lupus

Drug induced lupus is associated with Antihistone antibodies, rare anti ds DNA and serositis.

Drug induced Lupus: Features

- *Syndrome of Positive ANA with symptoms such as fever, malaise, arthritis, intense arthralgia/myalgia,* ***serositis*** *and / or rash (ANA usually appears before symptoms)*
- *Predominant in Caucasians*
- *Less female predilection than SLE*
- ***Commonly associated with Anti-Histone***
- ***Rarely associated with Anti- ds DNA***
- *Rarely involves kidney or brain*
- *Syndrome usually appears during therapy with certain medications and biologic agents*
- *Syndrome usually resolves over several weeks after discontinuation of the offending medication.*

82. Answer is C (Wire loop lesions): *Robbin's 7th/232; Harrison 17th/2077; Fundamentals of Renal Pathology (2006) 1st/85; Harrison 18th/p 2727*

Wire loop lesions are characteristic of SLE

Wire loop lesions:

- Wire loop lesions represent local PAS – Positive thickening of glomerular capillary walls and are characteristically sen in Lupus Nephritis (SLE)
- These lesions result from subendothelial deposits between endothelium and basement membrane. When extensive and confluent, these subendothelial deposits create a homogenous thickening of the capillary wall which can be seen in light microscopy as 'Wire loop lesion'
- Wire loop lesions are most characteristic of Lupus Nephritis Class IV or Diffuse Lupus Nephritis These may however also be seen in Class III (Focal Lupus Nephritis) and Class V (membranous) Lupus Nephritis.

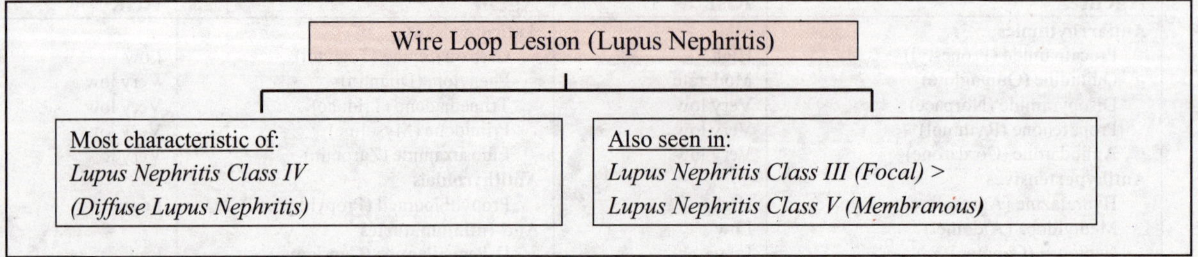

83. Answer is C (Diffuse Proliferative Glomerutonephritis); *Sternberg's Diagnostic surgical pathology 4th/1910,1911 Heptinstall's Pathology of the kidney 6th/546,547; Diseases of the kidney and Urinary Tract 8th/1688; Harrisons 17th/2076, 2077,2078; Harrisons 16th/1961,1963; Harrison 18th/p 2726, 2727, 2728*

Wire loop lesions are most charachteristic of diffuse proliferative glomerulonephritis (Class IV WHO) but may also be seen in focal proliferative glomerulonephritis (Class III WHO).

INTERNATIONAL SOCIETY OF NEPHROLOGY/RENAL PATHOLOGY CLASSIFICATION OF LUPUS NEPHRITIS (2003)

WHO CLASS	Nomenclature	Pathological Features
CLASS I	MINIMAL MESANGIAL LUPUS NEPHRITIS	Normal glomeruli by light microscopy, but mesangial immune deposits by immunofluorescence
CLASS II	MESANGIAL PROLIFERATIVE LUPUS NEPHRITIS	Purely mesangial hypercellularity of any degree or mesangial matrix expansion by light microscopy, with mesangial immune deposits.
CLASS III	FOCAL LUPUS NEPHRITIS	Active or inactive focal, segmental or global endo-or extracapillary glomerulonephritis involving <50% of all glomeruli, typically with focal subendothelial immune deposits, with or without mesangial alterations
CLASS IV	DIFFUSE LUPUS NEPHRITIS	Active or inactive diffuse, segmental or global endo-or extracapillary glomerulonephritis involving >50% of all glomeruli, typically with diffuse subendothelial immune deposits, with or without mesangial alterations. This class is divided into diffuse segmental (IV-S) lupus nephritis when>50% of the involved glomeruli have segmental lesions, and diffuse global (IV-G) lupus nephritis when > 50 % of the involved glomeruli have global lesions. Segmental is defined as a glomerular lesion that involves less than half of the glomerular tuft. ***This class includes cases with diffuse wire loop deposits but with little or no glomerular proliferation.***
CLASS V	MEMBRANOUS LUPUS NEPHRITIS	Global or segmental subepithelial immune deposits or their morphologic sequelae by light microscopy and by immunofluorescence or electron microscopy, with or without mesagial alterations Lupus nephritis may occur in combination with class III or IV in which case both will be diagnosed Class V lupus nephritis may show advanced sclerosis
CLASS VI	ADVANCED SCLEROTIC LUPUS NEPHRITIS	>90% of glomeruli globally sclerosed without residual activity

84. Answer is D (Anti – LA (SSB)): *Samter's Immunologic disease 6th/497; 'Systemic Lupus Erythematosis' 4th/894;*

Presence of Anti – LA (SSB) in SLE suggests concomitant Sjogren's syndrome. In SLE, patients with concomitant Sjogren's syndrome have a lower frequency of glomerulonephritis and a relatively good prognosis – Samter's Immunologic Diseases 6th/497

Factors associated with Adevrse Prognosis and High Risk of Renal Progression in Lupus Nephritis

Demographic

- *Black race*
- *Hispanic ethnicity*
- *Male gender*
- *Extremes of age at onset of SLE*
- *Limited access to health care*

Clinical

- *Hypertension*
- *Severe extrarenal (especially neuropsychiatric) lupus activity*
- *Failure to achieve remission or marked delay to renal remission*
- *Pregnancy*

Laboratory

- *Nephritic urinary sediment*
- *Azotemia*
- *Anemia*

Thrombocytopanea
Thrombotic microangiography (with or without anti-phospholipid antibodies)
Hypocomplementemia (especially falling levels)
High anti- DNA (especially rising titres)
Persistent severe nephritic syndrome (artherosclerotic and thrombotic diathesis)

Renal pathology

Contracted kidney size
Proliferative glomerulonephritis (WHO class III, IV)
Mixed membranous (V) and proliferative (III-IV) glomerulonephritis
Cellular crescents (>25% of glomeruli)
Fibrinoid necrosis (>25% of glomeruli)
Very high activity index
Moderate-to-high chronicity index
Combinations of active (cellular crescents) and chronic features (interstitial fibrosis)
Extensive subendothelial deposits

Note:
The presence of Anti-RO or Anti-La antibodies in a pregnant woman is associated with a chance of 'neonatal lupus' developing in the infant (1-5%)
This may present in the fetus as a congenital heart block or neonatal lupus rash.

85. Answer is B (Chloasma): *Behl/298;*

Non erythematous malar rash in a woman of child bearing age suggests diagnosis of chloasma.

Rash over face (MALAR)

- **Non erythematous**
  - *Chloasma*
- **Erythematous**
  - *SLE*
  - *Photosensitivity reaction*
  - *Contact dermatitis*

SLE	Chloasma	Photosensitive	Contact
Features of systemic[Q] involvement in history	No history suggestive of systemic involvement h/o Pregnancy	History of being exposed to sun for long time	History suggestive to contact with provocative agent
'Malar butterfly[Q] rash' Erythematous[Q]	'Light brown rash' Non-erythematous	Variable Erythematous	Variable Erythematous

86. Answer is B (Chloasma): *See previous question*

Patient has a characteristic 'brown' macule on cheek, with no history suggestive of any systemic involvement, with positive history of delivery of a baby suggesting pregnancy.

87. Answer is B (Sterility): *Harrison 14th/1876, 1877; 15th/1924; 16th/1966, 1967; Nelson 15th/660, 1436; Dutta 4th; ; Harrison 17th/2079, 2080; Harrison 18th/p2730, 2734*

Sterility is not a feature of SLE

- **Manifestations due to Lupus anticoagulant:**
  SLE is characterised by the presence of antiphospholipid antibodies in the form of 'Lupus anticoagulants' producing the Antiphospholipid syndrome.

Common obstetrical complications of antiphospholipid syndrome include:
1. *Recurrent thrombotic events[Q]*
2. *Thrombocytopenia[Q]*
3. ***Recurrent spontaneous abortions[Q]***
4. *IUGR[Q]*
5. *PIH (pregnancy induced Hypertension)[Q]*
6. *Placental abruption[Q]*

- **Hematological manifestations :**
  Most patients have *anemia of chronic disease*[Q]
  Small proportion of patients may have ***Coomb's positive hemolytic anemia***
- **Neurological complications:**
  Psychosis is a neurological manifestations with SLE[Q]

88. Answer is A (Bleeding disorders): *API Textbook of Medicine 8th/ed 306, 307; Harrison's 17th/ 732, 1579, 2082; 'Current Diagnosis and Treatment in Rheumatology' 2nd/219; Harrison 18th/p2734*

Antiphospholipid Antibody Syndrome is associated with thrombotic disorders and not bleeding disorders

Antiphospholipid Antibody syndrome (APLA) is primarily a disorder of coagulation resulting in a hypercoagulation state. ***Manifestations of Antiphospholipid Antibody syndrome including recurrent thrombosis and fetal loss result from the hypercoagulable state. Bleeding disorders are not seen.***

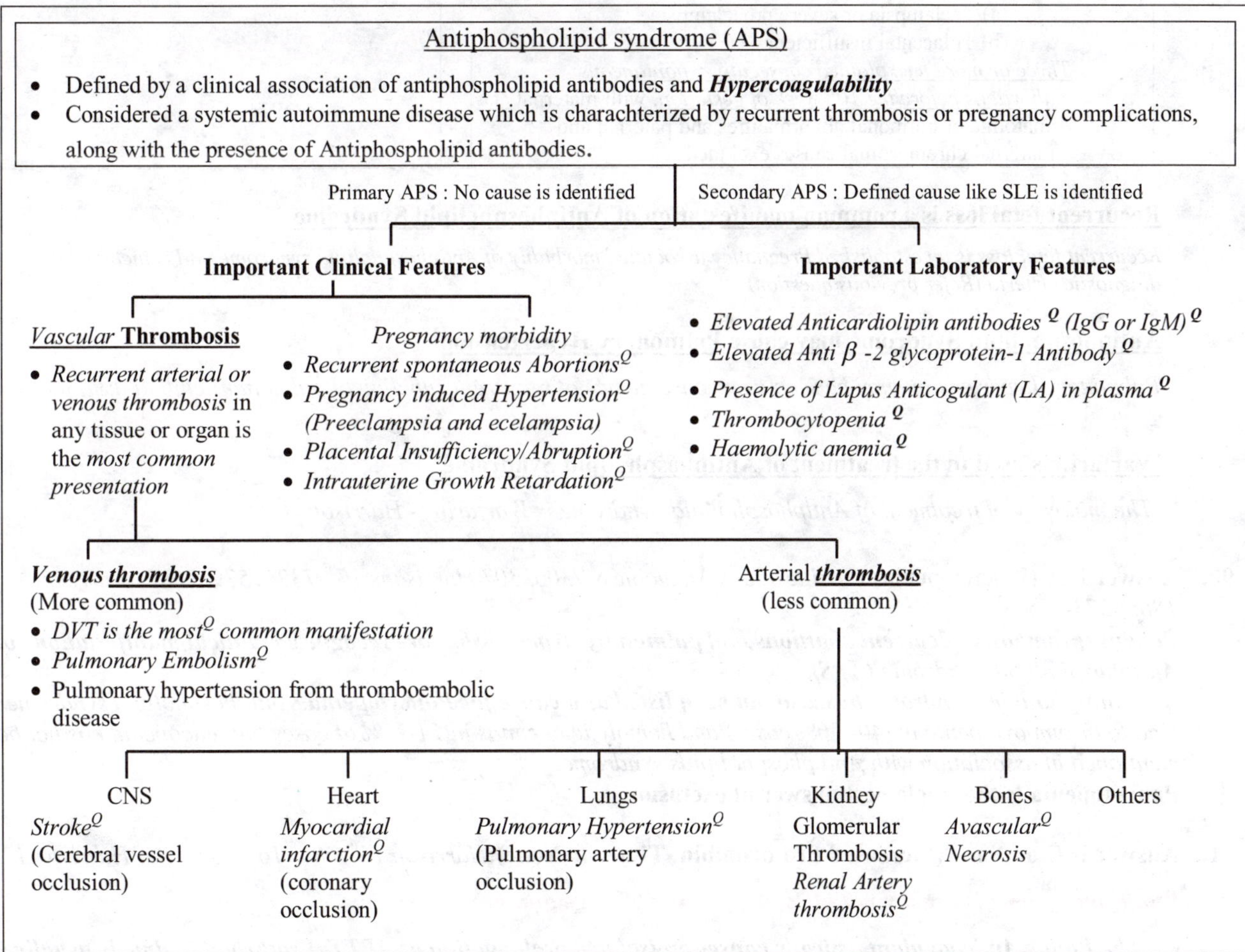

89. Answer is A (Single titre of Anticardiolipin is diagnostic): *API Textbook of Medicine 8th/ed 306, 307; Harrison's 17th/ 732, 1579, 2082; 'Current Diagnosis and Treatment 'Rheumatology' 2nd/219; Harrison 18th/p2734*

Single titre of anticardiolipin antibodies does not establish a diagnosis of APLAb syndrome
Laboratory criteria require anticardiolipin antibodies to be <u>present on 2 or more occasions</u> at least 12 weeks apart.
A Definite diagnosis of Antiphospholipid Syndrome requires at least one clinical criteria and one laboratory criteria to be met.

Diagnostic Criteria for Antiphospholipid Syndrome

Definitive Antiphospholipid Syndrome is said to be present if atleast one of the clinical criteria and one of the laboratory criteria are met

Clinical Criteria	Laboratory Criteria
• **Vascular Thrombosis (Arterial and/or Venous)** One or more clinical episodes of arterial, venous or small vessel thrombosis in any tissue or organ. • **Pregnancy morbidity** a. *One or more unexplained deaths* of a morphologically normal fetus at or *beyond the 10th week of gestation*, with normal fetal morphoology b. *One or more premature births* of a morphologically normal neonate *before the 34th week of gestation* because of: (a) eclampsia or severe preeclampsia (b) placental insufficiency c. *Three or more unexplained consecutive spontaneous abortions before the 10th week of gestation*, with maternal anatomic or hormonal abnormalities and paternal and maternal chromosomal causes excluded.	• **Anticardiolipin Antibody** of IgG and /or IgM isotype in serum or plasma *on 2 or more occasions, at least 12 weeks apart* • **Lupus anticoagulant** present in plasma, *on 2 or more occasions at least 12 weeks apart* • **Anti-β_2- glycoprotein-1 antibody** of IgG and or IgM isotype in serum or plasma, present *on 2 or more occasions, at least 12 weeks apart*

Recurrent fetal loss is a common manifestation of Antiphospholipid Syndrome

Recurrent fetal loss is an established Pregnancy associated morbidity of Antiphospholipid syndrome and is included in the diagnostic criteria (Refer previous question)

Antiphospholipid Syndrome may cause Pulmonary Hypertension

Pulmonary hypertension may be seen as a consequence of recurrent subclinical pulmonary emboli (Refer previous question)

Warfarin is used in the treatment of Antiphospholipid Syndrome

'The mainstay of treatment of Antiphospholipid Syndrome is Warfarin' - Harrison

90. Answer is A (Pancytopenia) : *API textbook Medicine 8th/306, 307 Harrisons 17th/732, 1579, 2082; Harrison 18th/p2734*

Venous thrombosis, recurrent abortions and pulmonary hypertension are recognized clinical manifestations of Antiphaspholipid Syndrome (APS).

Anti phospholipids syndrome has also not been listed as a cause for Pancytopenia*. Antiphospholipid syndrome may lead to thromboytopenia in (40- 50% cases) and hemolytic anemias in 14-25% of cases but leucopenia has not been mentioned in association with Anti phospholipids syndrome.*

Pancytopenia is the single best answer of exclusion.

91. Answer is C or None (Increased Prothrombin Time or None): *Harrison 15th/685; 16th/982, 685; Harrison 17th/1043*

Prothrombin time is usually not affected by Lupus Anticoagulant.

- ***The Lupus Anticoagulant typically causes an isolated prolongation of APTT. Prothrombin time is usually normal although slight prolongation in PT may also be observed***

  'Lupus anticoagulant should be suspected in cases of markedly prolonged PTT without clinical bleeding and normal or slightly elevated PT'- CMDT

- The presence of LA activity may predispose patients to **venous and arterial thromboembolism** and may cause mid trimester **abortions** – Harrisons 16th/685
- VDRL tests for syphillis are non specific tests, detecting anticardiolipin antibodies.
  Lupus anticoagulants are family of antiphospholipid antibodies of the same class and ***may give a false positive VDRL.***

Causes of false positive VDRL reactions:

Acute false positive (< 6 months)	Chronic false positive (≥ 6 months)
• Recent viral infection / immunization	• Aging
• Genital herpes	• Autoimmune disorders
• Human immunodeficiency virus	• SLE
• Malaria	• RA
• Parentral drug use	• Parentral drug use.

92. Answer is C (Thrombocytosis): *Dutta 5th/364; 4th/ 364*

Antiphospholipid syndrome is associated with thrombocytopenia and not thrombocytosis.

Common obstetric complications associated with antiphospholipid syndrome are:

1. Recurrent fetal loss[Q]
2. IUGR[Q]
3. Pregnancy associated hypertension[Q]
4. Placental abruption[Q]
5. Recurrent thrombotic events[Q]
6. Thrombocytopenia[Q] (and not thrombocytosis).

93. Answer is B (Aspirin + Low molecular weight Heparin): *Harrison's 17th/ 2082; Speroff's Clinical Gynaecological endocrinology & Infertility 7th/1083, 1084; Harrison 18th/p 2734*

The recommended treatment for women with recurrent pregnancy loss associated with antiphospholipid syndrome includes combined Aspirin and Heparin therapy.

'In pregnant SLE patients with Antiphospholipid antibodies and prior fetal loss, treatment with heparin (standard or low –molecular- weight) plus low dose aspirin has been shown in prospective controlled trials to increase significantly the proportion of live births'. – Harrison's 17th/2082

'Combined aspirin and heparin therapy has proven effectiveness and is the preferred treatment for women with recurrent pregnancy loss associated with antiphospholipid syndrome' - Speroff 7th/1084

Antiphospholipid syndrome in pregnancy

- The risk of pregnancy loss in women with APS and prior pregnancy loss may exceed 60%
- History of recurrent fetal loss in a pregnant woman with Antiphospholipid antibodies is an indication of treatment during pregnancy as these are identifiable and treatable immunologic disorders
- **Treatment options** include Antiplatelet agents such as Aspirin, Anticoagulants such as Heparin / LMWH, and corticosteroids
  Aspirin along with Heparin / LMWH *is the recommended treatment of choice.*
  Corticosteroids should be avoided if possible. If required to control maternal SLE, these should be used at the lowest effective doses for the shortest time required.

94. Answer is B (SLE): *Harrison, 15/1949; 16th/1991; ; Harrison 17th/2108; Harrison 18th/p 2771*

Bilateral parotid enlargement is not a feature of SLE.

Causes of Bilateral parotid enlargement

Viral infections	Metabolic causes	Endocrinal	Miscellaneous
• *Mumps*[Q]	• *Diabetes mellitus*[Q]	• Acromegaly	• Sarcoidosis
• *Influenza*[Q]	• *Hyper lipoproteinemia*	• Gonadal hypofunction	• Amyloidosis
• *Epstein barr virus*	• *Chronic pancreatitis*[Q]		• Sjogren syndrome
• *Coxackie virus A*	• *Cirrhosis*		
• *CMV*			
• *HIV*			

95. Answer is B (SLE): *Refer previous question*

Parotid enlargement is not a feature of SLE

96. Answer is B (Endocarditis) : *CMDT 2009/734; Not in Harrison*

Endocarditis has not been mentioned in the list for indications of corticosteroids i.e. SLE.

Indications for corticosteroids in SLE: *CMDT*		
1. *Thrombocytopenic purpura*[Q]	2. *Hemolytic anemia*[Q]	3. *Myocarditis*[Q]
4. *Pericarditis*[Q]	5. *Convulsions*[Q]	6. *Nephritis*[Q]

97. Answer is A (SLE) or (None): *William's 20th/ 701, 849; Harrison 15th/1212, 1388, 1394; Not in Harrison 16th & 17*

Low dose aspirin therapy has definite indication in preecclampsia, IUGR and post MI. There appears no rationale of using low dose aspirin for manifestation of SLE. Nevertheless low dose aspirin is of definite benefit in antiphospholipid antibody syndrome. SLE is thus the single best answer of exclusion here.

Low dose aspirin therapy markedly decreases thromboxane production but only partially blocks prostocyclin and prostaglandin E_2 production.

- ***Pre-ecalmpsia*:** In preeclamptic woman, thromboxane is increased and prostaglandin E_2 and prostacyclin are decreased, resulting in vasoconstriction and sensitivity to infused angiotensin II. Low dose aspirin as explained above enhances concentration of vasodilating prostanoids and restores refractoriness to infused angitensin II.
- ***Post MI*:** No confusions on this one. Low dose aspirin is advised to such patients.
- ***IUGR*:** Early antiplatelet therapy with low dose aspirin may prevent uteroplacental thrombosis, placental infarction, and idiopathic fetal growth retardation in women with a history of recurrent severe fetal growth restriction. - *Williams 20th/ 849*
  Further *Williams 21st/1212* says: "*Low dose aspirin & Dipyridamole are beneficial in reducing incidence of superimposed preeclampsia & growth restriction*".
- ***SLE*:** Arthralgias, arthritis, myalgias, fever and, mild serositis may improve on NSAID's including salicyclates. However there appears no rationale of using low dose aspirin therapy for the same. (*However low dose aspirin is beneficial in "Antiphospholipid antibody syndrome"*). – *William's 21st/1388, 1394*

Rheumatoid Arthritis and other Joint Arthritis

98. Answer is None or A (New bone formation) : *Harrison; 16th/2029, 2033; Harrison 17th/2150, 2155; Harrison 18th/p 2818, 2819*

Erythema, elevated ESR and prolonged morning stiffness lasting for more than one hour are all characteristic diagnostic criteria for inflammatory arthritis. New bone formation characterized by sclerosis and osteophyte formation is characteristic of osteoarthritis, a non inflammatory arthritis. Nevertheless, new bone formation may also be seen in inflammatory arthritis with progression of disease. ***New bone formation is the single best answer here, as it is not specific to inflammatory arthritis.***

Features of inflammatory arthritis : *Harrison 17th/2150*

Presence of some or all four cardinal signs of inflammation.	Systemic symptoms	Laboratory evidence of inflammation
i) *Erythema* ii) *Pain* iii) *Warmth* iv) *Swelling*	i) *Prolonged morning stiffness. Often lasting for several hours. (Non inflammatory arthritis are associated with intermittent stiffness. Stiffness usually lasts less than 1 hr.)* ii) *Fatigue* iii) *Fever* iv) *Weight Loss*	i) *Elevated ESR* ii) *Elevated C reactive protein* iii) *Thrombocytosis* iv) *Anemia of chronic disease.* v) *Hypoalbuminemia*

Inflammatory Arthritis	Non inflammatory arthritis
• *Infectious (Gonococcal, Tubercular)*	*Osteoarthritis*
• *Crystal induced (Gout, Pseudogout)*	*Osteonecrosis (Avascular necrosis)*
• *Immune related (Rheumatoid arthritis, SLE)*	*Traumatic arthritis*
• *Reactive (Rheumatic fever, Reiter's syndrome)*	*Tumor (villonodular synovitis)*
• *Idiopathic*	

99. Answer is D (C Reactive protein indicates better prognosis) : *Harrison; 16th/1973; Harrison 17th/2088;*

Persons who present with high titers of Rheumatoid factor, C Reactive protein and Haptoglobin have a worse prognosis than the individuals who present with Subcutaneous nodules or Radiographic evidence of erosions
–Harrison

Rheumatoid arthritis :

It is a chronic systemic inflammatory disease of unknown cause characterized by persistent involvement of synovial membrane of multiple joints and variety of systemic manifestations.

Diagnostic criteria :	
Morning stiffness:[Q]	Stiffness in and around joints lasting 1 hour before maximal improvement.
Arthritis:[Q]	• *Symmetrical*[Q], involving same joint areas on both sides of body simultaneously • *Multiple*[Q]: It commonly involves three or more joint areas, predominantly of the joint areas in hand (peripheral) [The 14 possible joint areas involved include bilateral PIP, MCP, Wrist, elbow, knee, ankle and MTP (*DIP are not involved*)]
Rheumatoid nodules[Q]:	
Serum Rheumatoid factor[Q]***:***	***An IgM antibody directed against the Fc fragment of IgG is present in sera of more than 75% of patients.***
Radiographic changes[Q]***:***	***Juxta articular osteoporosis***[Q], Joint erosion Narrowing of joint spaces.

100. Answer is B (Causes pleural effusion with low sugar) : *Harrison; 16th/1970, 1971*

Typically the pleural fluid contains very low levels of glucose[Q] *– Harrison; ; Harrison 17th/2087*

- *Pleuropulmonary manifestations include* ***'Pleuro-Pulmonary nodules'***[Q]*, Pleural disease, Interstitial fibrosis, Pneumonitis, Arteritis. Typically the pleural fluid contains very low levels of glucose*[Q]
- ***Enthesopathy*** *i.e. Inflammation of tendons and ligamentous attachments to bone, is characteristic of* ***Psoriatic*** *arthritis and not Rheumatoid Arthritis. – Harrison*
- *The Typical picture* ***of bilateral symmetrical inflammatory polyarthritis involving small and large joints in both upper and lower extremity with sparing of axial skeleton except the cervical spine "suggest the diagnosis of Rheumatoid Arthritis"*** *– Harrison*

Also remember

- Constitutional features indicative of the inflammatory nature of disease such as Morning stiffness **"support the diagnosis"**– *Harrison*
- Demonstration of subcutaneous nodules is **"Helpful diagnostic feature"**– *Harrison*
- Additionally, presence of Rheumatoid factor, Inflammatory synovial fluid and Radiographic findings. **"Substantiate the diagnosis"** *– Harrison*

101. Answer is A, B, E (PIP and DIP Joints involved equally; Pathology Limited to articular cartilage; 20 percent have extra articular manifestations) : *Harrison 17th/2083, 2085, 2087, 2086; Harrison 18th/p 2739, 2741, 2742*

Women are affected 3 times more commonly than men

'Women are affected approximately three time more often than men' Harrison's 17th / 2083.

Pathology is not limited to articular cartilage alone

'The majority of destruction occurs in juxtaposition to the inflamed synovium, or pannus, that spreads to cover the articular cartilage' Harrisn's 17th / 2085

The precise mechanism by which bone and cartilage destruction occurs has not been completely resolved. Although the synovial fluid contains a number of enzymes potentially able to degrade cartilage, the majority of destruction occurs in juxtaposition to the inflamed synovium, or pannus, that spreads to cover the articular cartilage. *The potential of the synovial inflammation to cause cartilage damage and bone erosions and subsequent changes in joint integrity is the hallmark of the disease*

PIP and DIP Joints are not involved equally (DIP joits are usually/typically spared)

'RA most often causes symmetric arthritis with characteristic involvement of certain specific joints such as the proximal interphalangeal and metacarpophalangeal joints. The distal interphalangeal joints are rarely involved'. - Harrison 17th/2086

Extra articular manifestations are seen in upto 40 percent of patients

'It is estimated that as many as 40% of patients may have extraarticular manifestations, and in ~15% these are severe' -Harrison's 17th/ 2087.

Rheumatoid nodules are seen in approximately 20% of patents

'Rheumotoid nodulels may develop in 20-30% of persons with RA' – Harrison's 17th/ 2087

102. Answer is C i.e. (Articular erosions on X ray): *Harrison's 17th/2077; Current Diagnosis & Treatment in Rheumatology 2nd/208; Harrison 18th/p 2728*

SLE is associated with non-erosive arthritis. Presence of articular erosions on X Ray suggests a diagnosis of Rheumatoid Arthritis

'Erosions on joint X-Rays are rare in SLE; their presence suggests a non-lupus inflammatory arthropathy such as Rheumatoid Arthritis' - Harrison 17th/2077

*'SLE may be confused with other connective tissue disease, especially Rheumatoid Arthritis. **SLE patients may have positive Rheumatoid Factor. The usual presentation of lupus arthritis is identical to that of Rheumatoid Arthritis, but SLE arthritis is rarely erosive.**' - Current Rheumatology 2nd/208*

103. Answer is D (Nephropathy): *Harrisons 16th/1972; Harrison 17th/2087; Harrison 18th/p 240*

Felty's syndrome consists of
- *Chronic rheumatoid arthritis*[Q]
- *Splenomegaly*[Q]
- *Neutropenia*[Q]

Anaemia or *thrombocytopenia* may be associated with Felty's syndrome.

104. Answer is A (Cervical): *Harrison; 16th/1971; Harrison 17th/2086; Harrison 18th/p 2738*

*Rheumatoid arthritis commonly involves the joints of hands, wrist, elbow, knees, ankle, and feet in a symmetrical manner. **Axial skeleton involvement is usually limited to Upper Cervical Spine**–Harrison 16th/1971*

105. Answer is A (Erosion): *Harrison 17th/2079; Harrison 18th/p 2728*

SLE is characterized by non erosive arthritis while bone erosions are characteristic in Rheumatoid Arthritis.

106. Answer is A > D (Antibody) > (Glycoprotien): *Harrisons 17th /2155, Davidsons 20th/ 1074; Harrison 18th/p 2825*

A Rheumatoid factor is an antibody (auto-antibody) of any immunoglobulin class directed against a specific region of the Fc fragment of human IgG. *- Davidson*

Rheumatoid Factor:

- A ***Rheumatoid Factors is an antibody*** (auto-antibody) *of any immunoglobulin class* (directed against Fc fragment of human IgG)
- *Rheumatoid factor in Rheumatoid Arthritis belongs to the IgM class*[Q] *(directed against Fc fragment of IgG)*[Q] (IgM Rheumatoid factor is positive in about 80% of patients with Rheumatoid arthritis *(Harrisons 17th/2155)*

  Note
  - Antibodies are glycoproteins and immunoglobulins are also glycoproteins
  - *A Rheumatoid factor is an antibody and because antibodies are glycoproteins, it would not be incorrect to say that Rheumatoid Factors are glycoproteins.*

    If Antibody / Auto- antibody is not provided amongst the options Glycoprotein would be the best correct answer.

107. Answer is E (IgM): *Harrison 17th/2088, 2155; Harrison 16th/1972, 1973; Harrison 18th/p 2825*

Rheumatoid factor is an IgM antibody directed against the Fc fragment of IgG

108. Answer is B (IgM): *Harrison 17th/2088, 2155; Harrison 16th/1972, 1973; Harrison 18th/p 2825*

Rheumatoid factor in Rheumatoid arthritis is an IgM antibody directed against the Fc fragment of IgG.

109. Answer is A (R. A. factor is associated with bad prognosis) :*Harrison; 16th/1972; Harrison 17th/2088; Harrison 18th/p 2825, 2746*

Rheumatoid factor is only of prognostic significance because patients with high titres tend to have more severe and progressive disease with extraarticular manifestations

- Rheumatoid factors are autoantibodies of IgM^Q type that react with FC portion of IgG^Q
- The presence of RA factor is not specific for R.A.
- The presence of Rheumatoid factor does not establish the diagnosis of RA

110. Answer is A (Inflammatory bowel disease): *Harrison 17th/2088;*

Enteropathic Arthrtis (Arthritis associated with inflammatory bowel disease) is a seronegative arthropathy that is characterized by the absence of Rheumatoid factor.

Causes of False Positive Rheumatoid factor
• ***SLE (Associated with a positive Coomb's test)***
• Sjogren syndrome
• Chronic Liver disease
• Sarcoidosis
• Interstitial Pulmonary Fibrosis
• Infectious mononucleosis
• ***Hepatitis B (Associated with HbsAg)***
• Tuberculosis
• Leprosy
• ***Syphilis (Associated with a positive VDRL)***
• Subacute bacterial endocarditis
• Visceral leishmaniasis
• Schistosomiasis
• Malaria

111. Answer is A (Anti - ccp Antibody) : *CMDT 2006 / 829; CMDT 09/727; Harrison 17th/2088; Harrison 18th/p 2825*

'Anti CCP antibodies are the most specific blood test for rheumatoid arthritis (specificity ~95%)' *- CMDT 09/727*

*Anti-cyclic citrullinated peptide (anti-CCP) antibody testing is particularly useful in the diagnosis of rheumatoid arthritis, **with high specificity,** presence early in the disease process, and ability to identify patients who are likely to have severe disease and irreversible damage. Anti-CCP antibodies have not been found at a significant frequency in other diseases to date, and are **more specific than rheumatoid factor for detecting rheumatoid arthritis**.*

- Oxford Journal of Medicine

112. Answer is A (Anti-CCP Antibodies): *Harrisons 18th/2745; CMDT 2006 / 829; CMDT 09/727; Harrison 17th/2088*

'Anti CCP antibodies are the most specific blood test for rheumatoid arthritis (specificity ~95%)' - CMDT 09/727

*Anti-cyclic citrullinated peptide (anti-CCP) antibody testing is particularly useful in the diagnosis of rheumatoid arthritis, **with high specificity,** presence early in the disease process, and ability to identify patients who are likely to have severe disease and irreversible damage. Anti-CCP antibodies have not been found at a significant frequency in other diseases to date, and are **more specific than rheumatoid factor for detecting rheumatoid arthritis**.*

- Oxford Journal of Medicine

113. Answer is D (Normocytic normochromic anaemia): *Harrison 15th/1933; Harrison 16th/1972; Harrison 17th/2088; Harrison 18th/p 2825*

'Normochromic, normocytic anaemia is frequently present in Rheumatoid arthritis. It is thought to reflect ineffective erythropoesis, large stores of iron are found in the bone marrow' *– Harrisons 17th/2088*

114. Answer is A (Mycoplasma) : *Harrisons 17th/2084, Harrisons 16th/1968; Harrison 18th/p 2825*

The true causative agent for Rheumatoid arthritis is not known. Mycoplasma has been suggested as a possible causative agent, and hence is the single best answer of choice

Possible causative agents suggested for Rheumatoid Arthritis	
Mycoplasma	*The organisms have only been suggested as possible*
Epstein Barr virus	*causative agents, but convincing evidence that these or any*
CMV	*other infectious agents cause RA has not emerged*
Parvovirus	
Rubella virus	

115. Answer is D (HLA-DR4): *Harrison 17th/2083; Emery and Rimoin's Principles and Practice of Medical Genetics 5th/1798; Rubin's Pathology 5th/1136; Harrison 18th/p 2741*

Rheumatoid arthritis is associated with multiple HLA-DR subtypes, but the strongest association has been reported with HLA DR4

'The class II MHC allele HLA DR4 and related alleles are knkwn to be major genetic risk factors for RA' – Harrison

HLA and Rheumatoid Arthirits

- Rheumatoid Arthritis is strongly associated with specific HLA class II markers (Rheumatoid Arthritis is only weakly associated with HLA class I marker)
- Rheumatoid Arthritis is associated with multiple HLA subtype encoded by the HLADRB1 gene

Multiple HLA subtypes that are associated with RA (HLA DRB1 gene)
HLA DR4 (strongest association in general)
HLA DR 1
HLA DR 6
HLA DR 9
HLA DR 10
HLA DR 14

- In different ethnic groups HLA DR1, HLA DR4, HLA DR6, HLA DR9, HLA-DR 10, HLA DR-14 molecules have been associated with RA.
- Certain HLA DR alleles may protect against development of RA.

HLADR Alleles that may protect against development of RA
HLA DR 2
HLA DR 3
HLA DR 5
HLA DR 7

116. Answer is B (HLA-B27 determine genetic susceptibility): *Reat text below; CMDT 2008/746,2009/752; Robbins 7th/1309*

HLA-B27 antigen is associated with seronegative spondyloarthropathies and not Rheumatoid Arthritis.

RA is associated with HLA DR alleles and may present with anemia, subcutaneous nodules and joint deformities.

HLA B 27 associated seronegative spondyloarthropathies
• *Ankylosing spondylitis*
• *Psoriatic arthritis*
• *Reactive arthritis (Reiter's syndrome)*
• *Enteropathic arthritis (Associated with Inflammatory Bowel disease)*
• *Undifferentiated spondyloarthropathy*

117. Answer is D (BAL) :*Harrisons 15th/1935; 16th/1974, 1975; Harrison 17th/2090; Harrison 18th/p 2747, 2478*

DMARDs: include agents that appear to have the capacity to alter the course of Rheumatoid Arthritis.

This includes:

DMARDs	
1.	Methotrexate[Q]
2.	*Gold* compounds[Q]
3.	*D-Penicillamine*
4.	Anti-malarials eg. *Chloroquines*[Q]
5.	Sulfasalazine
Methotrexate is the DMARD of choice.	

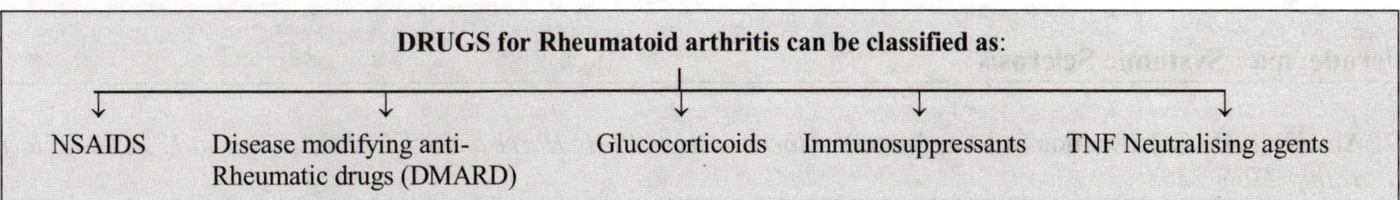

118. Answer is B (Rheumatoid arthritis) : *CMDT (Older editions);*

***Chrysotherapy (Gold salts)* :** are used as a *disease-modifying anti-rheumatic drugs* for patients who fail to improve on or who cannot tolerate methotrexate.

Indications	Contraindications
• Disease responding unfavorably to Conservative management • Erosive disease	• Previous gold toxicity • Significant renal dysfunction • Hepatic or hematopoietic dysfunction

Gold Preparations of choice:

- Intramuscular gold sodium thromalate or aurothioglucose
- Oral auranofin

  Intramuscular gold is used most often as it is more effective than oral gold[Q].

119. Answer is A (Mononeuritis Multiplex) : *Read text below*

Mononeuritis multiplex in Rheumatoid arthritis is due to nerve ischaemia from occlusion of vaso nervosum due to vasculitic change – *Harrison*

Indications of Steroids in Rheumatoid arthritis include:

1. On short term basis to tide over acute disabling episodes etc.
2. To manage serious extra-articular manifestations such as:
   a. Vasculitis: exemplified here by mononeuritis multiplex
   b. Pericarditis
   c. Perforating eye lesions etc.

120. Answer is C (Acetaminophen): *Turek's 6th/164*

The three major goasl of RA management includes reducing pain, reducing inflammation and preventing disability. Pain management (Analgesia) is not equivalent to inflammation control although they may be performed in concert. Acetaminophen does not inhibit platelet aggregation, therefore it is the analgesic of choice when bleeding tendencies are an issue. Acetaminophen is particularly useful for those with bleeding disorders such as bleeding ulcers or hemophilia and it has been termed appropriate for pain control (analgesia) in Rheumatoid Arthritis (Arthritis foundation). As the question is specifically directed for the 'analgesic of choice (pain control)', Acetaminophen is the single best answer of choice.

121. Answer is D (Raynaud's phenomenon): *CSDT 16th/828*

Raynaud's phenomenon is not a feature of JRA.

Systemic manifestation including fever, uveitis and nodules may all be seen in JRA.

Essentials of Diagnosis & Typical Features of JRA (CPDT)

Arthritis	Systemic features
• Non migratory monoarticular or polyatricular arthritis with a tendency to involve large joints or proximal interphalangeal joints lasting more than 3 months.	Systemic manifestations with ***Fever***, erythematous rashes, ***nodules***, leucocytosis and occasionally iridocyclitis ***(uveitis)***, pleuritis, pericarditis, anemia, fatigue and growth failure.

Scleroderma / Systemic Sclerosis

122. Answer is D (Calcification in Long bones) : *Harrison 15th/ 1941; Harrisons 16th/ 1983; Harrison 17th/2104; Harrison 18th/p 2766, 2767*

Scleroderma is associated with resorption of long bones and not their calcification.

Scleroderma (Systemic sclerosis) is a multisystemic disorder of unknown cause. It is characterized by fibrosis of the skin, blood vessels and visceral organs.

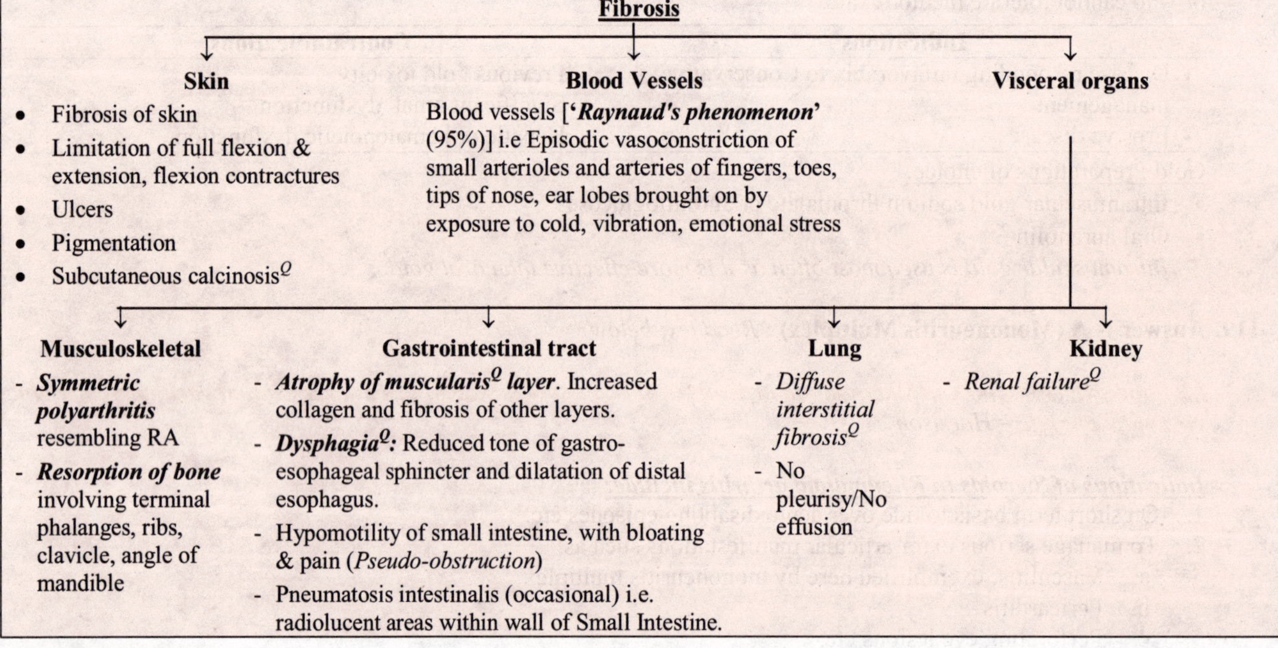

123. Answer is B (Systemic Sclerosis) : *Harrison 15th/1943; Harrisons 16th/1980; Harrison 17th/2096, 2097; Harrison 18th/p 2757, 2758*

Features of 'CREST' syndrome in association with antinuclear antibodies is sufficient to establish diagnosis of limited form of 'systemic sclerosis'

CREST Syndrome (Limited systemic sclerosis)

C	Calcinosis
R	Raynaud's syndrome
E	Esophageal dysmotility
S	Sclerodactyly
T	Telangiectasia

Antinuclear antibodies of 'Anticentromere' type are characteristic.

Remember:

Manifestations	Diffuse	Limited (CREST)
Skin involvement	Distal and proximal extremities, face, trunk	Distal to elbow, face
Raynaud's phenomenon	Onset within 1 year or at time of skin changes	May precede skin disease by years
Organ involvement	Pulmonary (interstitial fibrosis); Renal (renovascular hypertensive crisis) Gastrointestinal Cardiac	Gastrointestinal Pulmonary arterial hypertension after 10-15 years of disease in <10% of patients; Biliary cirrhosis
Antinuclear antibodies	Anti-topoisomerase 1	Anticentromere

124. Answer is C (Anticentromere antibodies are characteristic): *Harrison 17th/2097; Current Diagnosis & Treatment in Rheumatology 2nd/229; Harrison 18th/p 2758*

Antitopoisomerase antibodies (Scl 70) are characteristic of diffuse systemic sclerosis and not Anticentromere antibodies.

Subsets of systemic sclerosis (SSC): Limited cutaneous SSC versus diffuse cutaneous:

Features	Limited cutaneous SSc	Diffuse cutaneous SSc
Skin involvement	Limited to fingers, distal to elbows, face; slow progression	Diffuse: finger, extremities, face, trunk; rapid progression
Raynaud's phenomenon	Preceds skin involvement; associated with critical ischemia	Onset contemporaneous with skin involvement
Pulmonary fibrosis	May occur, moderate	Frequent, early and severe
Pulmonary arterial hypertension	Frequent, late, may be isolated	May occur, associated with pulmonary fibrosis
Scleroderma renal crisis	Very rare	Occurs in 15%; early
Calcinosis cutis	Frequent, prominent	May occur, mild
Characteristic autoantibodies	Anticentromere	Antitopoisomerase (Scl - 70)
Systemic symptoms	Infrequent systemic symptoms such as Arthralgias, weight loss and pulmonary symptoms	Significant systemic symptoms such as Arthralgias, weight loss and tendon friction rubs

125. Answer is B (Scleroderma) : *Harrison 15th/1941 & 1942; Harrisons 16th/1980, 1983; Harrison 17th/2101, 2102; Harrison 18th/p 2763, 2765*

The presence of tightness in fingers and dysphagia in a young female suggest a diagnosis of Scleroderma.

Diagnosis of scleroderma in this patient is suggested by:

- Evidence of fibrosis of skin : Tightness of fingers.
- Evidence of visceral involvement : Esophageal motility or dysphagia
- Epidemiological characteristic : Peak incidence of scleroderma is seen in ***women***[Q] during the 3rd to 5th decade

M : F	= 1 : 3
Peak age	= 3rd to 5th decade

126. Answer is E (More common in young patients): *Refer text below; Harrison 18th/p 2758*

Systemic sclerosis is primarily a disease of adults and the mean age of presentation is around 50 years.

Systemic sclerosis is not a disease of young individuals

The mean age of presentation of systemic sclerosis is 50 years – Current Diagnosis & Treatment in Rheumatology 2nd/228
The peak incidence of systemic sclerosis is 50-60 years – Robbins 7th/239
The most common age of onset in the range of 30-50 years – Harrison 17th/2097

Systemic sclerosis is more common in women

Like other connective tissue disorders systemic sclerosis shows a female predominance- Harrison 17th/2097
Systemic sclerosis is primarily a disease of women (female to male ratio is 3:1) – Robbin's 7th/239

Systemic sclerosis may present with Calcinosis, Sclerodactyly and hyperpigmentation

The skin of extremities and trunk may be darkly pigmented. Diffuse tanning in the absence of sun exposure may be a very early manifestation of skin involvement – Harrisons
Calcinosis and sclerodactyly are part of the 'Crest syndrome' in limited systemic sclerosis

CREST syndrome	
C	*Calcinosis*
R	*Raynauld's*
E	*Esophageal dysmotility*
S	*Sclerodactyly*
T	*Telengactasia*

127. Answer is B i.e. (Scleroderma): *Harrison's 17th/2096, 2101, Kelly's Essentials of Internal Medicine' 2nd /372, 373; Current Diagnosis & Treatment in Rheumatology 2nd/ 222, 223, 225; Harrison 18th/p 2757, 2762, 2763*

Pallor of extremities, followed by pain and cyanosis suggests a diagnosis of Reynaud's Phenomenon. Reynaud's phenomenon as the presenting manifestation is most strongly associated with scleroderma or systemic sclerosis.

Reynaud's Phenomenon and Scleroderma

- Reynaud's phenomenon (RP) is the clinical syndrome of episodic color change of the digits in response to cold and in some patients, emotional stress. *The typical sequence is pallor (arterial constriction) followed by cyanosis (vasospasm and desaturation) of hemoglobin.*
- Reynaud's Phenomenon is *may be associated with a variety of connective tissue disorders including SLE, Rheumatoid arthritis, scleroderma and dermatomyositis* (all options provided in question), ***however its association with scleroderma is exceptionally strong.***

- Reynaud's Phenomenon is associated with virtually every patient of scleroderma (or Systemic Sclerosis) (98-99%)

Feature	*Limited Scleroderma (59%)*	*Diffuse Scleroderma*
Reynaud's Phenomenon	*99%*	*98%*

- Reynaud's phenomenon is the ***presenting initial complaint in 70% of patient's with scleroderma***
- Reynaud's phenomenon precedes other symptoms of scleroderma briefly (< 2 years) in diffuse scleroderma while it precedes other symptoms by several years (>2 years) in the limited form (limited scleroderma)

Secondary causes of Raynaud Phenomenon:

Rheumatologic	**Hematologic disorders**
Systemic sclerosis (scleroderma) Systemic lupus erythematosus Rheumatoid arthritis Sjogren syndrome Dermatomyositis Polymyositis Vasculitis	Cryoglobulinemia Paraproteinemia Polycythemia Cold agglutinins
Mechanical	**Endocrine disorders**
Vibration injury Frostbite Thoracic outlet syndrome Vascular embolus or occlusion	Hypothyroidism Carcinoid syndrome Pheochromocytoma
Vasospasm	**Drugs**
Migraine headaches	Sympathomimetics drugs (decongestants, diet pills) Serotonin agonists (sumatriptan) Chemotherapeutic agents (bleomycin, cisplatin, carboplatin, vinvlastine) Ergotamine tartrate Caffeine Nicotine

Sjogren Syndrome

128. Answer is D (Systemic manifestations) : *Harrisons 16th/1992; Harrison 17th/2107, 2108; Harrison 18th/p 2770, 2771*

Although glandular manifestations in the form of dry eyes, dry mouth or parotid gland enlargement form the presenting features. Systemic manifestations may also be seen

Sjogren syndrome:

Sjogren's syndrome is a clinicopathologic entity characterized by *dry eyes* (keratoconjunctivitis sicca) and *dry mouth* (xerostomia) resulting from *immunologically mediated destruction of the lacrimal and salivary glands.*

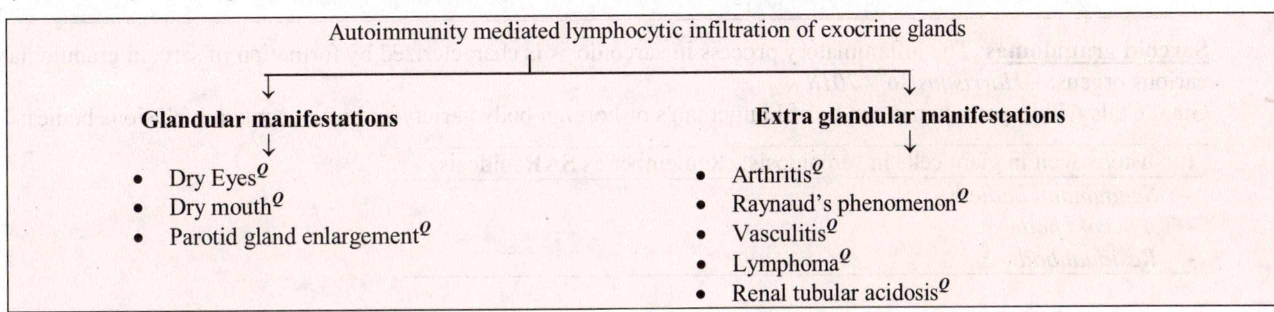

129. Answer is A (Midline granuloma): *Harrison, 15th/1947; Harrisons 16th/1990; CMDT 2002/ 741; Robbins Illustrated (Basis) 6th/ 225] ; Harrison 17th/2107 (Table 3171); Harrison 18th/p 2770 (Table: 324.1)*

Midline granuloma has no association with Sjogren Syndrome (Sicca Syndrome)
As a result of its tendency to cause 'dryness' Sjogren's syndrome is often referred to as 'Sicca' syndrome.
Being an autoimmune disorder this disorder is associated with a number of other disorders of autoimmune origin.
Rheumatoid arthritis, chronic active hepatitis and scleroderma are known autoimmune disorders that are often associated with Sjogren Syndrome.

These include:

Autoimmune disorders associated with Sjogren's syndrome:	
- Rheumatoid arthritis (***most common***)[Q]	- Chronic active hepatitis [Q]
- SLE [Q]	- Polymyositis
- Scleroderma [Q]	- Hashimoto's thyroditis
- Mixed connective tissue disease [Q]	- Interstitial pulmonary fibrosis.
- Primary biliary cirrhosis [Q]	- Sarcoidosis.
- Vasculitis	

What puzzles the question?

Sjogren is syndrome occurs as two types.

- ***Primary form*** **(Sicca syndrome)**- when it occurs as an *isolated disorder.*
- ***Secondary form*** – when it occurs in association with other *autoimmune disease.*

In the true sense it is not Sicca syndrome but the secondary form with which autoimmune disorders are associated. Nevertheless Midline granuloma remains the single best answer of exclusion.

Sarcoidosis

130. Answer is A (Sarcoidosis) : *Harrison; 16th/ 2017, 2018, 2023; Harrison 17th/2136, 2137; Harrison 18th/p 2807, 2808*

The presence of non-caseating granuloma, along with bilateral hilar lymphadenopathy, goes strongly in favour of a diagnosis of Sarcoidosis'.

Sarcoidosis: *Review*

Sarcoidosis is a chronic multisystem disorder of unknown cause characterized by accumulation of T lymphocytes and mononuclear phagocytes in various tissues of body

Non caseating **SAR**coid granulomas in affected organs

Lung (90%)	Lymph nodes (75-90%)	Skin	Others
• ***Interstitial lung disease***[Q] - Fibrosis of lung parenchyma • Pleura is involved in 1-5% of cases u/e ***pleural effusion***[Q] • *Cavitation* ***is rare***[Q]	• B/L hilar lymphadenopathy is the hallmark of sarcoidosis • Parotid enlargement B/e involvement is the vuli	• ***Erythema nodosum***[Q] • ***Lupus perenium***[Q] (purple blue shiny swollen lesions on nose, cheeks, lips, ears).	Eye – Uveitis Kidney (rare) – Renal hypercalcemia with or without hypercalcuria Skeletal – Arthritis Nervous system – Peripheral neuropathy. Heart – Cor pulmonle

Sarcoid granulomas: The inflammatory process in sarcoidosis is characterized by formation of sarcoid granulomas in various organs. – *Harrisons 16th/ 2018*

Giant Cells within granulomas can be of Langerhan's or Foreign body variety and often contain inclusions bodies:

Inclusions seen in giant cells in sarcoidosis. (Remember as **SAR**coidosis)
- ***Schaumann bodies***[Q]
- ***Asteroid bodies***[Q]
- ***Residual bodies***[Q]

131. Answer is C (VII Cranial N.): *Harrisons 16th/2021; Harrison 17th/2139; Harrison 18th/p 2809*

Neurological findings are observed in about 5% of patients with sarcoidosis. ***"Seventh nerve involvement with unilateral facial paralysis is most common. It occurs suddenly and is usually transient."*** –*H* 16th/ 2021

Other common involvement of neurosarcoid include:

- *Optic nerve dysfunction*
- *Papilledema*
- *Palate dysfunction*
- *Hearing abnormalities*
- *Chronic meningitis, hypothalamic and pituitary abnormalities.*

Syndromes in Acute sarcoidosis: *may present in the form of two syndromes*[Q] *(Harrisons 16th/2019)*

Heer fordt's syndrome[Q]	Löfgren's syndrome
• *Fever*[Q]	• Joint symptoms
• *B/l parotid enlargment*[Q]	• Erythema nodosum
• *Anterior uveitis*[Q]	• X-ray finding of bilateral hilar adenopathy
• *Facial nerve palsy (VIIth nerve)*[Q]	

132. Answer is A (Often cavitate):; *Harrison 16th/2020, 2023; Harrison 17th/2136, 2137; Harrison 18th/p 2807*

Cavitation is uncommon seen only in less than 5% of patients with sarcoidosis.

- Of individuals with **sarcoidosis** 90% have abnormal findings on chest x ray Sarcoidosis of the lung is primarily an interstitial lung disease in which the inflammatory process involves the alveoli, small bronchi and small blood vessels. **Cavitation is seen in <5% patients with sarcoidosis.**- Harrisons 16th-2020
- B/l hilar lymphadenopathy is the hallmark of disease – Harrisons 16th/2023

The three classic x-ray pattern of pulmonary sarcoidosis are		
• ***Type I***	:	*B/L hilar lymphadenopathy with no parenchymal changes*
• ***Type II***	:	*B/L hilar lymphadenopathy with diffuse parenchymal changes*
• ***Type III***	:	*Diffuse parenchymal change with no hilar lymphadenopathy.*

- Sarcoidosis has a variable course. Disease clears spontaneously in 50% of patients – *Harrisons 16th/2023*
- Tuberculin test may be negative due to the presence of skin anergy – *Harrisons 16th/2023*

133. Answer is A (CD4/CD8 counts in the blood) : *Harrison 16th/2017-2023; Not in Harrison 17th;*

The patient in question is suffering from sarcoidosis.

'While there is marked enhancement of no. of TH cells at the sites of disease the number of TH cells in the blood are normal' – Harrison

'Where as TH cells in the involved organs are proliferating at an enhanced rate the T cells in other sites such as blood are quiescent' - Harrison

It is the CD4 / CD8 counts in the affected organs which is an important ancillary aid in established the diagnosis of sarcoidosis and not the CD4 / CD8 count in the blood as specifically asked in the question.

Active sarcoidosis results from an exaggerated cellular immune response resulting in accumulation of large no. of T4 cells in the affected organs, where the ratio of CD4 to CD8 cells may be as high as 10:1.

Although CT of chest is also only rarely helpful, it may identify early fibrosis and active alveolitis and thus contribute to a diagnosis of sarcoidosis.

Diagnostic tests for sarcoidosis have often been asked

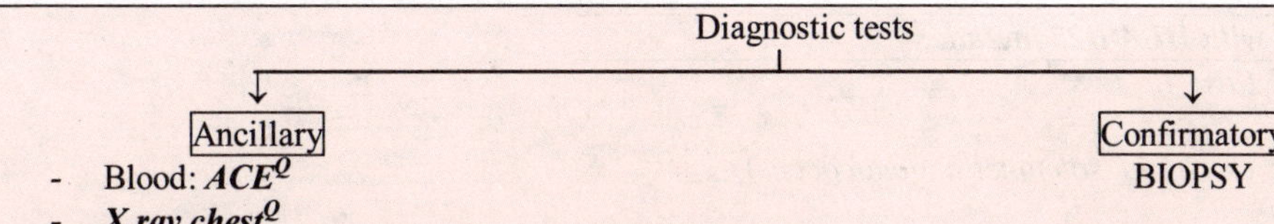

- Blood: ***ACE***[Q]
- ***X ray chest***[Q]
- ***Skin test for anergy***[Q]
- ***Gallium 67 etc.***[Q]

1. ***X-Ray chest***:
   - Bilateral hilar lymphadenopathy is the hallmark of disease
   - Parenchymal involvement may or may not be present ***(clear lung fields)***[Q]
   - ***Egg shell calcification of hilar nodes may be seen***[Q]
2. ***Kveim siltzbach test***[Q]***: Skin test***[Q]:
   - intradermal injection of a heat treated suspension of a sarcoidosis spleen extract.
3. ***Angiotensin converting enzyme (ACE) in blood***[Q]:
   - ACE is elevated in 2/3 of patients with sarcoidosis [Q] (60%) [Q]
   - ACE levels indicate activity of disease [Q]
   - ACE levels provide an important method of monitoring the course of disease.[Q]

   (The cells in granuloma release angiotensin converting enzyme into the serum)
4. ***Gallium 67 scan***: Gallium 67 lung scan is usually abnormal showing a pattern of diffuse uptake
5. ***Bronchoalveolar large:*** Lavage fluid is characterized by
   - increase in Lymphocytes[Q]
   - high CD4 / CD8 cell ratio[Q]
6. ***Biopsy***:
   - Biopsy is mandatory to make a definitive diagnosis of sarcoidosis
   - Characteristic finding is a typical non casseating granuloma[Q]
7. ***Lung function abnormalities***: Typical for interstitial lung disease.

134. Answer is D (Sarcoidosis): *Harrison 16th/2436; Current Rheumatology Diagnosis & Treatment 2nd/413*

Uveoparotid fever (Heerfordt syndrome) is seen in sarcoidosis

Uveoparotid fever / Uveoparotitis / Heerfordt syndrome:

- *Fever*
- *Parotid enlargement (also lacrimal gland enlargement, bilateral hilar adenopathy)*
- *Uveitis (Anterior uveitis)*
- *Facial Nerve Palsy (Cranial neuropathies)*

Seronegative Spondyloarthropathies

135. Answer is C (Rheumatoid arthritis): *Harrison 17th/2109; Harrison 18th/p 2774*

Rheumatoid arthritis is not a seronegative spondyloarthropathy.

Seronegative spondyloarthropathies

- *Ankylosing spondylitis*
- *Reactive Arthritis (and Reiter's syndrome)*
- *Psoriatic Arthritis and spondylitis*
- *Enteropathies Arthritis (Arthropathy of inflammatory bowel disease)*
- *Undifferentiated spondylorathropathy*

136. Answer is B i.e. (Ankylosing spondylitis): *Previous question;Repeat*

HLA B27 is typically associated with seronegative spondyloarthropathies like Ankylosing Spondylitis

Conditions associated with HLA B27 include:[Q]
1. *Ankylosing spondylitis*[Q]
2. *Reiter's syndrome*[Q]
3. *Reactive arthritis*[Q] *(yersonia, salmonella, gonococcus)*
4. *Psoriatic arthritis*[Q]
5. *Juvenile rheumatoid arthritis*[Q] *(not rheumatoid arthritis)*
6. *Acute anterior uveitis.*[Q]

137. Answer is C (Symmetrical Polyarthritis): *Multiple textbooks*

Seronegative spondyloarthropathies are usually associated with Asymmetrical Oligoarthritsis and not symmetrical polyarthritis.

The seronegative spondyloarthritis have the following in common:

- ***Negative RF***
- ***Strong association with HLA-B27 antigen***
- ***Oligoarthritis (asymmetrical)***
- ***Enthesitis*** *(inflammation at sites of insertion of fascia, ligament or tendon to bone)*
- *Inflammatory arthritis (axial and sacroiliac joints)*
- ***Extra-articular features (eyes, skin, genitourinary tract)***
- *Familial predisposition*

138. Answer is C (Rheumatoid Arthritis) : *C.M.D.T 2009 /752; Harrison 17th/2088*

Rheumatoid arthritis is a seropositive arthritis with autoantibodies against IgG present is in 75% of patients. It is not a seronegative arthritis.

The seronegative spondylo arthropathies include
- Ankylosing Spondylitis
- Psoriatic Arthritis
- Arthritis associated with Inflammatory bowel disease
- Reiter's syndrome *(Reactive arthritis)*

Characteristic features of these disorders are : *(CMDT 2009/752)*

- Onset usually before age 40
- Inflammatory Arthritis of spine or large peripheral joints or both
- Uveitis[Q]
- Absence of Auto antibodies in Serum (i.e. seronegative)
- Striking association with **HLA-B27**[Q]

139. Answer is A (HLA B_{27}) : *Harrison 14th /1781, 15th/1837; CMDT 2005/824*

Conditions associated with HLA B27 include: Q

7. Ankylosing spondylitis Q
8. Reiter's syndrome Q
9. Reactive arthritis Q *(yersonia, salmonella, gonococcus)*
10. Psoriatic arthritis Q
11. Juvenile rheumatoid arthritis Q *(not rheumatoid arthritis)*
12. Acute anterior uveitis. Q

140. Answer is A (Behcet's syndrome) : *Harrison 14th/1781; 15th/1956; 16th/2014 ; Harrison 17th/2132; Harrison 18th/p 2801*

Behcet's syndrome is associated with HLA B5 and HLA B51 – *Harrison 17th/2132*

Important conditions associated with certain HLA types

- **HLA B8** - Myasthenia Gravis Q
  - Hyper-thyroidism (Grave's) Q
- **DW4/DR4** - Rheumatoid arthritis Q
- **HLA DR3**:
  - Gluten sensitive enteropathy (Coeliac diseases) Q
  - Diabetes mellitus Type-I (this also has ***DR2 & DR4***) Q
  - Myasthenia Gravis (along with ***HLA B8***) Q

Also remember: ***Narcolepsy is associated with HLA DR2 and has exceptionally high relative risk of more than 100% i.e. 130%.*** Q

141. Answer is B and C (Pernicious Anemia and Behcet's syndrome): *Repeat*

HLA B 27 is not associated with pernicious anemia and Behcet's syndrome.
HLA B 27 is associated with seronegative spondyloarthropathies including Reiter's syndrome and Ankylosing spondylitis.

142. Answer is C (Indomethacin): *Harrison 17th/2112, 2114; 18th/p 2777, 2780; Other several standard textbooks*

Non steroidal anti-inflammatory drugs are the medications of choice in seronegative spondyloarthropathies. Indomethacin is the preferred NSAID for most of the seronegative spondyloarthropathies.

143. Answer is A (Psoriatic arthropathy): *Harrison 15th/1985, 2003 and CMDT 2005/ 826, 801, 802CMDT 09/754; Harrison 17th/2153;*

Psoriatic arthritis involves PIP, DIP and metacarpophalangeal joints, and may or may not involve the wrist.

- ***Involvement of DIP makes rheumatoid arthritis unlikely.*** *DIP is spared in rheumatoid arthritis.*
- ***Involvement of metacarpophalangeal joints makes osteoarthritis unlikely.*** *Metacarpophalangeal joints and carpometacarpal joint with the exception of base of thumb are spared in osteoarthritis.*

Remember

Osteoarthritis	Rheumatoid arthritis	Psoriatic arthritis
• Involvement of PIP, DIP and Ist carpometacarpal joint (base of thumb)	• Involvement of any small joints of the hand i.e. PIP, MCP, wrist.	• Involvement of PIP, DIP, MCP and wrist
• ***Sparing of MCP and wrist***	• ***Sparing of DIP***	• Sparing of any joint may or may not be present.

144. Answer is B (Reiter's syndrome): *Harrison 17th/2113, 2114; Kelley Essentials of Medicine 2nd/359; Current Rheumatology 2nd/183*

Arthropathy following recent travel suggests a probable diagnosis of Reactive arthritis secondary to organisms endemic in the zone of travel. The association of conjunctivitis (foreign body sensation in the eye) with arthritis suggests diagnosis of Reiter's syndrome.

Reiter's syndrome/Reactive Arthritis

Reiter's syndrome and Reactive arthritis are regarded as spectrum of same disease

- *Usually develops in young adults*
- *HLA B27 positive*
- *Features of seronegative spondyloarthropathy*

Usually follows gastroenteritis or genitourinary tract infection

Gastroenteritis (Shigella, Salmonella, Campylobacter or Yersenia) *(History of travel to endemic region may be positive)*

Genitourinary infection with Chlamydia trachomatis

Constitutional Symptoms
Fever, Fatigue, Malaise, Weight loss

Characteristic Triad

- *Arthritis*
- *Urethritis (and / or cervicitis)*
- *Conjunctivitis (and/or Uveitis)*

Additional Features

Mucocutaneous

- *Oral ulcers (superficial)*
- *Keratoderma blenorrhagica*
- *Circinate balanitis (glans lesions)*
- Dactylitis (sausage digits)
- Nail changes
  - onycholysis
  - hyperkeratosis
  - distal yellowish discolouration
- Enthesitis (Tendinitis & fascitis)

Rare features

- Cardiac conduction defects
- Aortic insufficiency
- Pleuropulmonary infiltrates
- Central or Peripheral nervous system lesions

145. Answer is A (Subcutaneous Nodules): *Harrison 17th/2114; Harrison 18th/p 2779*

Subcutaneous nodules are not a feature of Reactive Arthrtis/Reiter's syndrome.

Oral ulcers, circinate balanitis and keratoderma blennorrhagicum are characteristic mucocutaneous manifestations of Reactive arthritis.

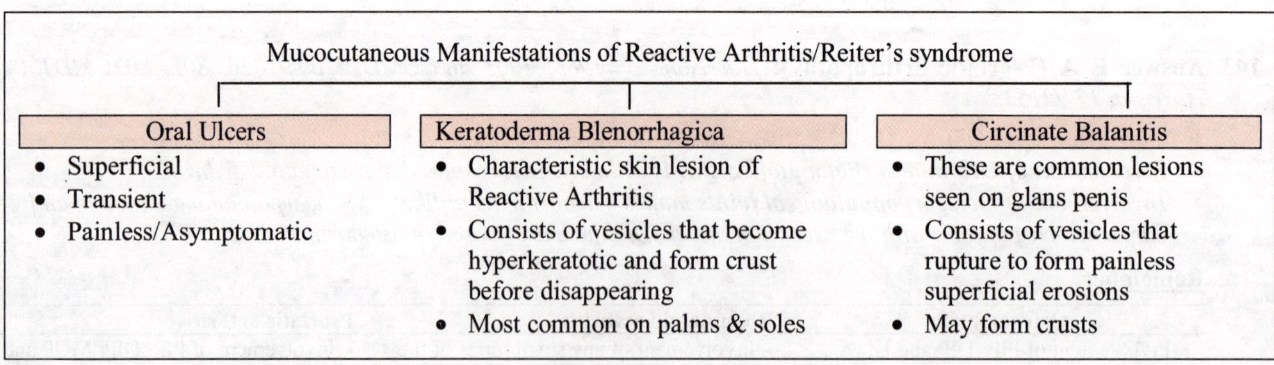

146. Answer is D (Chlamydia): *Harrison 17th/2113; 'Psoriatic and Reactive Arthritis 1st (2007)/123; Harrison 18th/p 2778, 2779*

Amongst the options provided Chlamydia is the most commonly implicated agent in Reactive arthritis.

'Chlamydia Trachomatis is by far the most common cause of urethritis and of reactive arthritis following urethritis.

– 'Psoriatic and Reactive Arthritis 1st (2007)/123

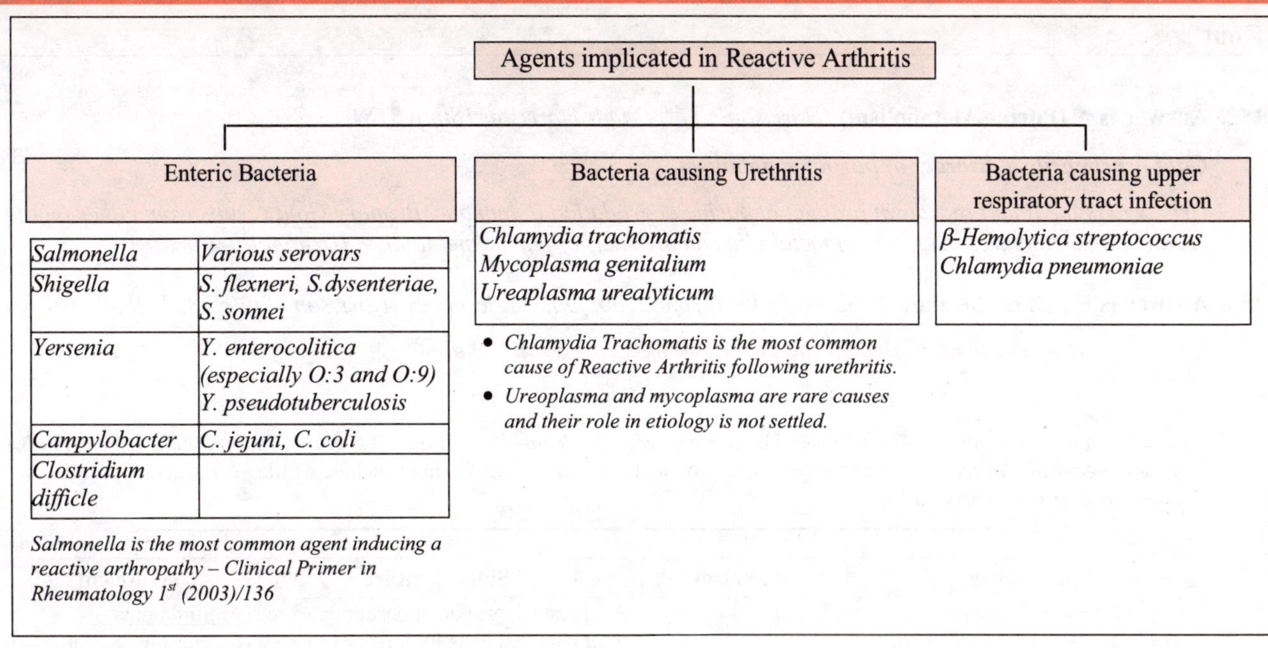

147. Answer is C (Reactive Arthritis): *Harrison's 18th/2779*

Keratoderma Blenorrhagica is the charachteristic skin lesion seen in patients with Reactive Arthritis.

*'**The charachteristic skin lesions in Reactive Arthritis, Keratoderma Blenorrhagica**, consist of vesicles that become hyperkeratotic, ultimately forming a crust before disappearing. In patients with HIV infection, these lesions are often extremely severe and extensive sometimes dominating the clinical picture'- Harrison's 18th/2779*

Osteoarthritis

148. Answer is D (Osteoarthritis) : *Harrison; 16th/2040, 2037; Harrison 17th/2158; Harrison 18th/p 2828*

Sparing of wrist and metacarpophalangeal joint with involvement of base of thumb (i.e. carpometacarpal joint) is very characteristic of 'osteoarthritis'.
Both DIP (Herbeden's nodes) and PIP (Bouchard's nodes) are involved in osteoarthritis. Q
***DIP** is the most common form of idiopathic O.A.* Q
Base of thumb (Ist carpometacarpal joint) is the 2nd most common site of involvement in idiopathic osteoarthritis Q

149. Answer is D (Metacarphalangeal joints) : *Harrison,; 16th/2040; Harrison 17th/2158; Harrison 18th/p 2828*

***Wrists and Metacarpophalangeal joints are generally not involved in Osteoarthritis** – Harrison 16th/2040*
Sparing of wrist and metacarpophalangeal joint with involvement of base of thumb (i.e. carpometacarpal joint) is very characteristic of 'osteoarthritis'.

150. Answer is A (Osteoarthritis) : *See previous question*

151. Answer is D (Distal interphalangeal joints) : *Harrison 16/2037, 2040; Harrison 17th/2158; Harrison 18th/p 2828*

Herbeden's nodes or bony enlargement of distal interphalangeal joints are the most common form of idiopathic osteoarthritis

Bouchard's nodes	Herbeden's nodes
Bony enlargement of PIP joint in osteoarthritis	Bony enlargement of DIP joint in osteoarthritis

Gout

152. Answer is A (Purine Metabolism): *Harrison's 17th/-2444; Harrison 18th/p 3181*

Gout is primarily a disorder of purine metabolism.

Uric acid is the final breakdown product of purine degradation in humans. Primary Gout results from either increased production or impaired excretion of metabolic end products of purine metabolism (Uric Acid)- Harrison

153. Answer is E (All of the above): *Harrison 17th/2165, 2166; Other references; Harrison 18th/p 2837, 2838*

Gout may present with all of the features mentioned as options in the above question.

Gout

A disorder of purine metabolism characterized by ***hyperuricaemia, deposition of mono – sodium urate- monohydrate crystals in joints and per-articular tissues***[Q] and recurrent attacks of acute synovitis. Late changes include cartilage degeneration, *renal dysfunction & uric acid urolithiasis*

Epidemiology	Pathology	Clinical Feature	Treatment
• Commoner in Caucasians • ***More wide spread in men than in women***[Q] (may be 20 :1) ***Usually men over the age of 30 years***[Q]; women are seldom affected *until after menopause.* Often there is a family history. • Sterotype patient is *obese, rubicund, hypertensive and fond of alcohol* and may be ***nudged into an attack by uncontrolled administration of diuretics or aspirin***[Q] • Common in Hypercurecemic patients • The rate of urate deposition in joint and articular destruction correlate with the duration and severity of hyperuricemia. The complications of gout correlate with both duration & severity of hyperuriacemia - ***Although the risk of developing clinical features of gout increases with increasing levels of serum uric acid, only a fraction of those with hyper uricaemia develop symptoms***[Q] - ***Any factor that causes either an abrupt increase or decrease in the serum urate levels may provoke an acute attack, the best correlations being factors that cause an abrupt fall***[Q]. ***Serum uric acid levels can be normal or low at the time of acute attack***[Q] - ***Despite these limitations, serum uric acid is almost always elevated at some time***[Q] and can be used to follow the cource of hypouricemic therapy.	<u>**Tophi**</u> • Tophi are nodular deposits of *monosodium urate monohydrate crystals*, with an associated *foreign body reaction*. It is deposited in minute clumps in connective tissue eg. - ***articular cartilage***[Q] - ***tendon (not muscle)***[Q] - ***bursae***[Q] - periarticular tissue - ***synovium & joints*** - pinnae (cartilage) of ear - ligaments - articular ends of bone - ***subcutaneous tissue***[Q] - kidney • Tophi may ulcerate through skin or destroy cartilage & periarticular bone	Acute attack is sudden onset of severe joint pain that lasts for a week or two. Usually comes out of blue but <u>may be precipitated by</u> - minor trauma - illness - unaccustomed exercise - alcohol - ACTCH - steroid withdrawl - hypouricemic therapy, drugs (pyri mol), MI, stroke - The ***commonest sites are metatarsophalangeal joint of big toe***[Q] > ankle & finger joints and olecranon bursae. - ***The skin is red, shiny, swollen, hot and extremely tender suggesting a cellulitis or septic arthritis***[Q] <u>Investigations</u> • ***Characteristic negatively birefringent monosodium urate crystals in the synovial fluid examined by polarizing microscopy is diagnostic***[Q]. • X- rays show only soft tissue swelling. Chronic gout may result in joint space narrowing & secondary OA • Tophi appear as characteristic ***punched out cysts or deep erosions with over hanging bony edges***[Q]**(Martel's or G' sign)**. These well defined erosions are larger & slightly further from joint margin than typical RA erosions.	<u>Antiinflammatory</u> • Mainstay of treatment during acute attack is administration of antinflammatory drug such as ***colchicine, NSAIDs (except aspirin) or glucocorticoids***[Q] • Glucocorticoids may be used. <u>Hypourecemics</u> • Probenecid or sulfin pyrazone can be used if renal function is normal. <u>Xanthine oxidase inhibitors</u> • Allopurinol, a xanthine oxidase inhibitor is usually preferred. ***These drugs should never be started in acute attack, and they should always be covered by an anti inflammatory preperations or colchicine; otherwise they may actually precipitate an acute attack***[Q]. ***In chronic tophaceous gout and in all patients with renal complications, allopurinol is drug of choice***[Q].

154. Answer is A (90% of cases are caused by over production of uric acid): *Harrison's 17th/2445, 2165, 2166; Current Diagnosis & Treatment in Rheumatology 2nd/ 345, 346; Harrison 18th/p 3181, 2837, 2838*

'Fewer than 5% of cases are caused by over production of uric acid'*- Current Rheumatology*
Most (~ 90%) cases of gout result from hyperuricemia secondary to decreased uric acid excretion by the kidneys and not from over production of uric acid.

Most patients with Gout have hyperuricemia due to decreased uric acid excretion by the kidney

- The underlying basis of gout is an increased total body urate pool.
- This is generally manifested as hypercuricemia and persistant hyperuricemia is the most important risk factor for gouty arthritis (Although hyperuricemia alone is not synonymous with gout)
- This hyperuricemia can result from increased urate production or decreased uric acid excretion by the kidneys or a combination of both mechanisms
- ***The most common mechanism of hyperuricemia in gout is a defect in the renal handing of uric acid (and not uric acid over production).***

'Over 90% of individuals with sustained hyper uricemia have a defect in the renal handling of uric acid' – Harrisons
'Fewer than 5% of patients with gout are hyper uricemic because of urate overproduction' – Current Rheumatology

Uric Acid levels may be normal at the time of an acute attack *- Harrisons 17th/2166*

Although most patients with acute gouty arthritis have associated hyperuricemia, elevated uric acid levels are not essential for the diagnosis of gout. This limits the value of serum uric acid determinations for the diagnosis of gout.

Gout is caused whenever, synovial fluid is supersaturated with uric acid, irrespective of serum concentration of uric acid. ***The serum levels of uric acid can be normal or even low at the time of an attack*** *and hence its determination is not diagnostic for gout.*

Gout is more common in Men than Women (Male > Female)
Gout presents predominantly in men
Women represent only 5-20% of all patients with gout

Definitive diagnosis of gout requires aspiration of synovial fluid

Definitive diagnosis of gout requires aspiration of the involved joint and demonstration of intracellular monosodium urate crystals in synovial fluid*. Under polarized light these are demonstrated as "strongly negative birefringent needle shaped crystals."*

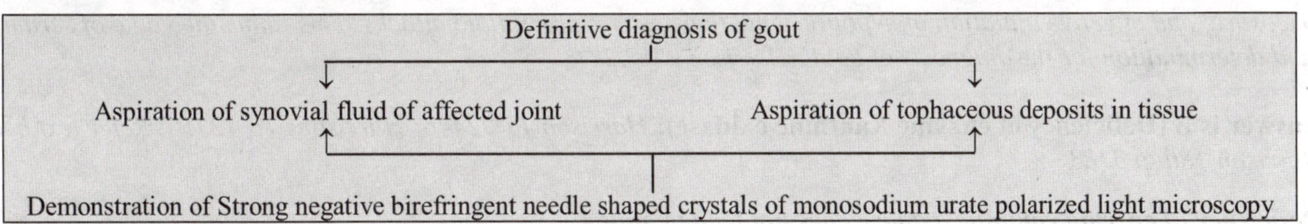

Tophi *are aggregates of monosodium urate monohydrate crystals that form in extra articular and articular structures and cause deformity and destruction of hard and soft tissue.*

155. Answer is D (Occurs more in females): *Harrison 17th/2165; Other references; Harrison 18th/p 2837*

Gout is more widespread in men than in women. Women represent only 5-20% of patients with gout. Women are seldom affected until after menopause.

156. Answer is B (Allopurinol should be started immediately): *Harrison's 18th*

Allopurinol should not be started immediately in acute attack of gout as it may precipitate acute symptoms.
The mainstay of treatment in acute gouty arthritis is the administration of anti inflammatory drugs such as NSAID, Cochicine and /or glucocorticoids.

Allopurinol should not be started immediately in Acute attack of Gout

Allopurinol should never be started in acute gout as it may actually precipitate an acute attack. Anti inflammatory drugs such as NSAIDs are the drugs of choice in acute gout.

Management of Gout

Acute Gout	Chronic Tophaceous Gout
Antiinflammatory drugs such as NSAIDs are the drugs of choice *Uricocurics such as Allopurinol should not be started in acute attacks as they may actually precipitate an acute attack*	Hypouricemic agents such as Allopurinol are the agents of choice in patients who already have tophi or chronic gouty arthritis Hypourecemic agents: **Xanthene oxidase inhibitors** • Allopurinol **Uricosuric agents** • Probenecid • Benzbromarone

Joint aspirate typically reveals strongly negative birefringent needle shaped crystals

Definitive diagnosis of gout requires aspiration of the involved joint and demonstration of intracellular monosodium urate crystals in synovial fluid. *Under polarized light these are demonstrated as "strongly negative birefringent needle shaped crystals."*

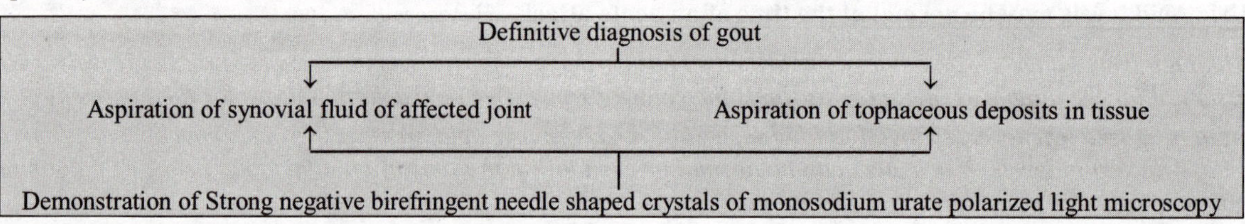

Tophi *are aggregates of monosodium urate monohydrate crystals that form in extra articular and articular structures and cause deformity and destruction of hard and soft tissue.*

Serum uric acid levels may be normal in Acute Gout

Gout is caused whenever; synovial fluid is supersaturated with uric acid, irrespective of serum concentration of uric acid. ***The serum levels of uric acid can be normal or even low at the time of an attack*** *and hence its determination is not diagnostic for gout.*

'Serum uric acid levels may be normal or low at the time of an acute attack, as inflammatory cytokines can be uricosuric and effective initiation of hypourecemic therapy can precipitate attacks. This limits the value of serum uric acid determination for the diagnosis of gout'- Harrison's 18th/2838

157. Answer is B (Deficiency of enzyme Xanthine oxidase): *Harrison 17th/2446; Harrisons 16th/2310; Refer text below; Harrison 18th/p 3183*

Deficiency of enzyme xanthine oxidase does not lead to gout.

Xanthine oxidase is the enzyme that is needed for synthesis of uric acid from purine. Deficiency of xanthine oxidase will result in decreased formation of uric acid and hence will not lead to gout, rather this shall prove protective in gout. Allopurinol is a xanthine oxidase inhibitor that mimic's the deficiency of xanthine oxidase and is actually used in treatment of gout.

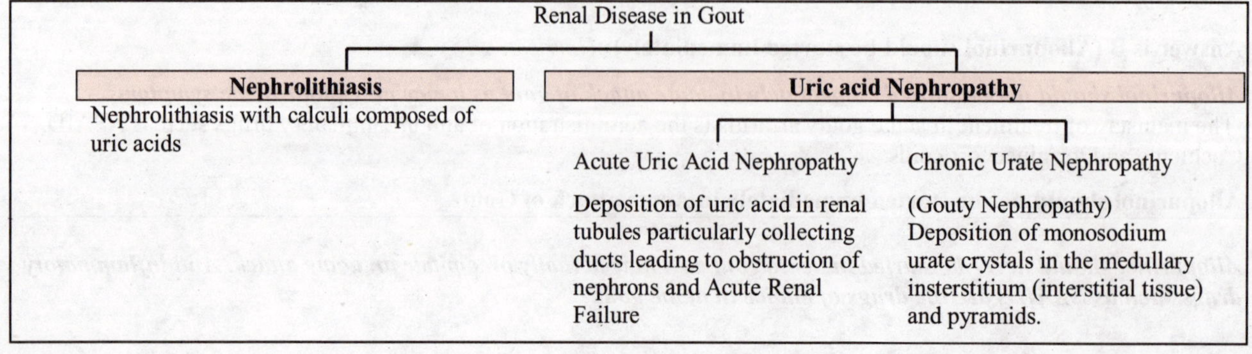

158. Answer is A (Abrupt increase in serum urate levels is more common a cause for acute gout than an abrupt fall in urate levels) : *Harrison, 15/ 1994, 2269, 2271, CMDT 2001/817; Harrison5 16th/2046 (Refer previous editions) ; Harrison 17th/2166 (Refer previous editions); Harrison 18th/p 2838*

Any factor that causes either an abrupt increase or decrease in the serum urate levels may provoke an acute attack, the best correlations being factors that cause an 'abrupt fall' *– Harrison, 15th*

- The vast ***majority of hyperuricemic patients are asymptomatic*** and are at no clinical risk because of it.
- *The higher the serum urate levels, the more likely is an individual is to develop gout – Harrison.*
  The rate of urate deposition in joint tissues and of articular destruction correlate with the duration and severity of hyperuricemia *– Harrison.*
  The complications of gout correlate with both duration of severity of hyperuricemia.
- Definitive diagnosis of gout requires aspiration of the involved joint and demonstration of intracellular monosodium urate crystals in synovial fluid polymorphonuclear leucocytes or tophaceous aggregates. ***Under polarized light these are demonstrated as "strongly negative birefringent needle shaped crystals."***

Remember: Serum uric acid levels may be normal or low at time of the acute attack – *Harrison 16th/2046*

159. Answer is B (Allopurinol is the treatment of choice in acute gout): *Harrison 17th/2165, 2166; 18th/p 2837, 2838*

Allopurinol should never be started in acute gout as it may actually precipitate an acute attack. Anti inflammatory drugs such as NSAIDs are the drugs of choice in acute gout.

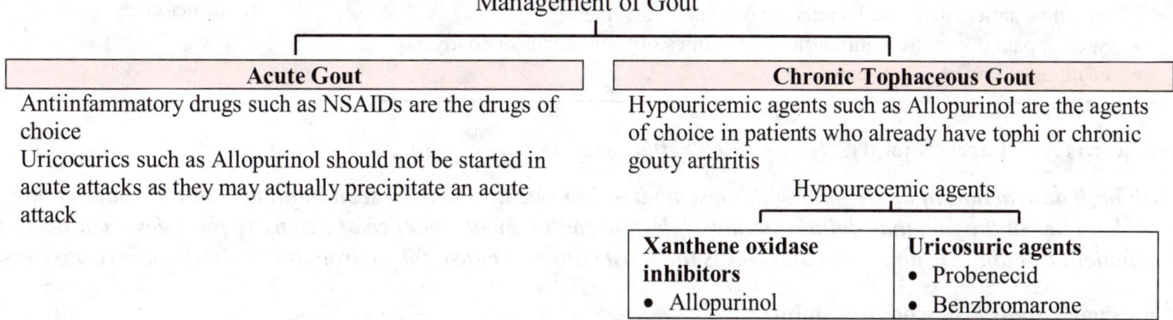

160. Answer is B (Raised uric acid in synovial fluid of joint) : *Harrison 16th/2046; Harrison 17th/2180, 2181; Harrison 18th/p 2855, 2856*

Definitive diagnosis of gout requires aspiration of the involved joint and demonstration of intracellular monosodium urate crystals in synovial fluid. *Under polarized light these are demonstrated as "strongly negative birefringent needle shaped crystals."*

Gout is caused whenever, synovial fluid is supersaturated with uric acid, irrespective of serum concentration of uric acid. ***The serum levels of uric acid can be normal or even low at the time of an attack*** and hence its determination is not diagnostic for gout.

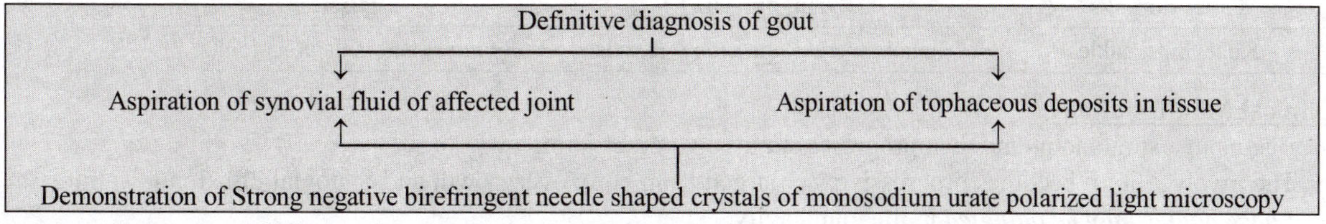

Tophi *are aggregates of monosodium urate monohydrate crystals that form in extra articular and articular structures and cause deformity and destruction of hard and soft tissue.*

161. Answer is C (Allopurinol): *Harrison 17th/2166; 16th/2046, 2047; Harrison 18th/p 2838, 2839*

Allopurinol should not be used in acute gout, as it may actually precipitate an acute attack.
Antiinflammatory drugs including NSAIDS (Naproxen) and Colchicine are effective in prociding rapid and safe pain relief.

Charcot's Joint

162. Answer is A (Charcot's joint): *Harrison 17th/2180, 2181; Mercer's 9th/814-817; Apley's 8th/89, 90, 213, 222, 508; Harrison 18th/p 2855, 2856*

Destructive arthritis and swollen joints in the absence ofpain suggest a diagnosis of neuropathic joint disease (Charcot joint). This is further supported by the fact that the patient isa diabetic, as diabetes is the most common cause of Charcot's joint.

<u>Neuropathic joint Disease/Charcot's joint</u>

It is progressive destructive arthritis arising from loss of pain sensation and proprioception (position sense).

Clinical Presentation

- Begins in a single joint & progress to involve other joints.
- Joint becomes progressively enlarged (swollen) from bony overgrowth and synovial effusion.
- Loose bodies may be palpated in the joint. Joint instability subluxation & crepitus occurs as the disease progresses.
- Patients complains of weakness, swelling, instability, laxity & progressive deformity usually involving knee or ankle. The markedly swollen joint is neither tender nor warm.
- The appearance suggest that movements would be agonizing and yet it is often painless. The paradox is diagnostic i.e. the amount of pain experienced is less than would be anticipated based on degree of joint involvement.
- Sudden pain occurs from intraarticular farctures of osteophytes or condyles
- Features of underlying disease

Radiological Features

- Similar to OA i.e. joint space narrowing, subchondrial bone sclerosis, osteophytes loose bodies and joint effusion. However charcot's joimt show more marked destructive and hypertrophic changes. The process is usually more rapid.
- Joint swelling and appearance of intraarticular calcification are further clues.

163. Answer is A (Charcot's joint):; *Harrison 16th/2060; Harrison 17th/2180, 2181; Harrison 18th/p 2855, 2856*

Although destruction of ankle joint with loose bodies and swelling may be seen in almost all the above condition, the clue here lies in the fact that 'joint is painless' despite radiological evidence of extensive joint destruction. Further, the patient is a diabetic and today diabetes is the most common cause for neuropathic joint disease (Charcot's joint)

<u>Charcoat's Joint / Neuropathic Joint:</u>

Neuropathic joint or charcoat's joint is a progressive destructive arthritis associated with loss of pain sensation, proprioception or both.

Disorder associated with neuropathic Joint disease / Charcot's joint	
- Diabetes mellitus^{Q}	- Amyloidosis^{Q}
- Tabes dorsalis^{Q}	- Leprosy^{Q}
- Meningomyelocoele or Synringomyelia	- Perineal muscular atrophy

<u>Joint involvement based on underlying joint disorder</u>

Tabes dorsalis^{Q}	Syringomyelia^{Q}	Diabetes^{Q}
Knee, hips, ankles	glenohumeral joint, elbow & wrist.	tarsal and metatarsal joints

<u>Clinical Manifestations:</u>

- Begins in a single joint and then progresses to involve other joints
- The involved joint becomes progressively enlarged from bony overgrowth and Synovial effusion (swelling).
- ***Loose bodies may be palpated*** in the joint cavity.
- Joint instability, Subluxation, crepitus occur as the disease progresses
- ***The amount of pain experienced by the patient is less than would be anticipated*** based on the degree of joint involvement (sudden pain may be experienced from intraarticular fractures of osteophytes or condyles).

164. Answer is D (Arthrogryposis multiple congenita): *Harrison 17th/2180; Harrison 18th/p 2856*

Arthrogryposis multiplex congenital is not associated with charcot's joint

Disorders associated with Neuropathic joint disease (Charcot's joint)	
Diabetes mellitus	*Amyloidosis*
Tabes dorsalis	*Leprosy*
Meningomyelocele	*Congenital indifference to pain*
Syringomyelia	*Peroneal muscular atrophy*

Polymyositis / Deratomyosistis

165. Answer is C (Ocular muscles): *Harrison 16th/2540; Harrison 17th/2696; Harrison 18th/p 2856*

***'Ocular muscles are almost never affected'** – Harrison.*

***Occular muscles are spared, even in advanced untreated cases** - Harrison*

Primary idiopathic polymyositis:

Condition of autoimmune[Q] etiology in which skeletal muscle[Q] is damaged by non suppurative inflammatory process[Q] dominated by Lymphocytic infiltration.[Q]

It is characterized by:

- Symmetrical weakness of proximal limb muscles especially hips and thigh (pelvic girdle) and later shoulder girdle.
- Weakness of flexor muscles of neck
- Involvement of striated muscles of pharynx (dysphagia)
- Involvement of respiratory muscles (late)

"Ocular muscles are almost never affected except in a rare case associated with myasthenia gravis."- Harrison
'Facial muscles are unaffected in Polymyositis'. – Harrison

166. Answer is B (Gottron's rash) : *Harrison, 15th/2524 and See previous question; Harrison 16th/2540; Harrison 17th/2696; Harrison 18th/p 3510*

Gottron's rash is a feature of dermatomyositis and is characterized by erythema of knuckles with raised violaceous scaly eruptions. No rash is seen in patients of polymyositis

Polymyositis is essentially a diagnosis of exclusion

Polymyositis is a subacute inflammatory myopathy affecting adults and rarely children who do not have

1. Rash[Q]
2. Involvement of extraocular or fascial muscles[Q]
3. Family history of neuromuscular disease
4. History of exposure to myotoxic drugs or toxins
5. Endocrinopathy
6. Neurogenic disease
7. Muscular dystrophy
8. Biochemical muscle disorder.

Dermatomyositis : is a distinctive entitiy identified by a characteristic rash, accompanying or more often preceding muscles weakness.

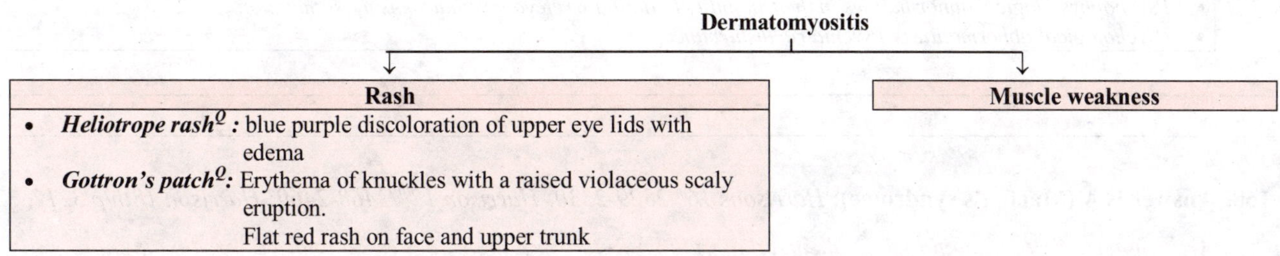

Fibromyalgia

167. Answer is D (SPECT studies have reduced blood flow to the thalamus): *Harrison 17th/2175; Harrison 18th/2849*

SPECT studies have shown reduced flow to the thalamus in patients with Fibromyalgia.
Fibromyalgia is more common in females and is associated with a decreased cortisol response to stress. Sleep EEG studies have shown disruption of Non REM (NREM) sleep.

SPECT studies in patients with fibrolyamgia have shown reduced blood flow to the thalamus

'***Single Photon Emission Computed Tomography (SPECT) imaging has demonstrated reduced blood flow to the thalamus****, caudate nucleus and pontinetectum which rae areas in the brain involved in signaling , integration and modulation of pain' – Harrison 17th/2175*

Fibromyalgia is more common in Females

'*Fibromyalgia is far more common in women than in men with a ratio of about 9:1' – Harrison 18th/2849*

Sleep Studies in Fibromyalgia have shown disruption of NREM sleep (Not REM sleep)
'*Sleep Electroencephalographic studies in patients with fibromyalgia have shown disruption of normal stage IV sleep [Non Rapid Eye Movement (NREM) sleep] by many repeated α-Wave intrusions' – Harrison 17th/2175*

Cortisol response to stress is decreased (and not increased) in patients with Fibromyalgia

'*Patients with fibromyalgia have a decreased cortisol response to stress. Low urinary free cortisol and a diminished corticotropin releasing hormone (CRH) suggests an abnormal hypothalamic – pituitary – adrenal axis'–Harrison 17th/2175*

Pathogenetic Features of Fibromyalgia
• *Disruption of normal stage 4 sleep [Non-rapid Eye Movement] (NREM) sleep*
Disturbed sleep has been implicated as a factor in pathogenesis, Nonrestorative sleep or awakening urefreshed has been observed in most patients with fibromyalgia.
• *Low levels of serotonin metabolites in cerebrospinal fluid (CSF)*
Deficiency of serotonin, a neurotransmitter that regulates pain and NREM sleep might be involved in the pathogenesis of Fibromyalgia
• *Reduced levels of Growth Hormone*
Growth hormone is important for muscle repair and strength. Growth hormone is secreted normally during stage 4 sleep, which is disturbed in patients with fibromyalgia. Reduction in Growth hormone may explain the extended period of muscle pain following excretion in these patients.
• *Increased levels of Neurotransmitter substance P in CSF*
Increased levels of substance P in CSF of fibromyalgia patients may contribute to spreading muscle pain.
• *Decreased cortisol response to stress and corticotropin releasing hormone (CRH)*
Patients with fibromyalgia have decreased cortisol response to stress Low urinary free cortisol and a diminished cortisol response to CRH suggests an abnormal Hypothalamic – Pituitary Adrenal axis.
• *Autonomic Dysfunction*
This may manifest as Orthostatic hypotension on tilt table testing, increased resting supine heart rates. May also account for dry eyes and mouth and the cold sesitivity and Raynaud's like symptoms in patients with fibromyalgia.
• *Reduced blood flow to thalamus, caudate nucleus and tectum on SPECT*
Reduced blood flow to above areas of brain, which are involved in signalling, integration modulation of pain may explain why fibromyalgia patients percieve stimuli such as heat or pressure as painful with less degree of stimulation than normal.
• *Psychophysiological abnormalities in their inability to inhibit irrelevant somatosensory stimulation.*
• *Psychological abnormalities / Psychiatric disturbances.*

Marfan's Syndrome

168. Answer is A (Marfan's syndrome): *Harrisons 16th/2329-2330; Harrison 17th/2468-2469; Harrison 18th/p 3212, 3213*

Arachnodactyly and ectopia lentis (dislocation of lens) in tall thin male suggests a charachteristic diagnosis of Marfan's syndrome.

Marfan Syndrome : Review

Marfan's syndrome is a genetic disorder of the connective tissue of the body manifested principally by changes in the skeleton, eye and cardiovascular system

Mutation in the fibrillary gene ♀ (15 q 21.1) ♀
↓
Loss of fibrillary fibre base for deposition of elastin
↓
Alteration in connective tissue in various parts of the body particularly in

Skeletal changes of marfans syndrome	Cardiovascular changes ♀	Ocular changes ♀
- *Patients are usually **tall** ♀* - *Have long limbs ♀* - *The ratio of upper segment to lower segment is usually 2 SDs below the mean for age, race & sex* - ***Arachnodactyly** (fingers are long and slender, spider like in appearance) ♀* - *Pectus Excavatum, Pectum Carinatum. ♀* - *Scoliosis, Kyphosis ♀*	- *Dmitral valve prolapse & ♀* - *Mitral valve progresses to Mitral valve Regurgitation* - *Aortic aneurysm occurs it can leads to Aortic Regurgitation* • Associated changes - *Spontaneous pneumothorax ♀* - *Inguinal & incisional hernias* - *Striae may occur over the shoulders & buttocks.*	- ***Dislocation of the lens ♀ (ectopia lentis)*** - *Elongation of globe (Myopia) ♀* - *Retinal detachment. ♀*

169. Answer is A (Ascending Aorta): *Echocardiography in Pediatric and Adult Congenital Heart Disease (Lippincott Williams) 2009/298; Mayo Clinic Internal Medicine Board Review' by Ghosh (Oxford Univ Press) 2010/330*

Marfan's syndrome most commonly involves the ascending aorta.

'Dilation of the ascending aorta at the level of aortic sinuses is the most common and charachteristic cardiovascular manifestation of Marfan's syndrome' - Echocardiography in Pediatric & Adult Congenital Heart Disease.

Most common cardiovascular Manifestations of Marfan's syndrome

The most common cardiovascular manifestations of Marfan's Syndrome are *Mitral valve prolapse* and *Dilation of Ascending Aorta*

Annula-Aortic Ectasia (Dilation of Ascending Aorta at level of aortic sinuses)	***Mitral Valve Prolapse*** ♀
• Annule aortic ectasia is a specific subgroup of aortic aneurysms affecting the root of aorta and the aortic annulus. This entity is charachteristic/typical of Marfan's syndrome *(Cystic Medial Necrosis ♀)* • Annuloaortic ectasia results in ***dilation of ascending aorta*** initially at level of aortic sinuses • May lead to Aortic Regurgitation, Ruptured Aneurysm and/or Aortic Dissection	• Mitral valve prolapse is usually progressive and leads to *Mitral Regurgitation* ♀

Major Cardiovascular Criteria for Marfan's
• *Dilation of ascending aorta with or without aortic regurgitation and atleast involving the sinus of valsava* • *Dissection of Ascending Aorta*

Minor Cardiovascular Criteria for Marfan's
• *Mitral valve prolapse with or without mitral regurgitation*

Wilson's Disease

170. Answer is B (Wilson's Disease): *Harrisons 17th/2449, 2450; Harrisons 16th/2313,2314; Harrison 18th/p 3188, 3189*

Psychiatric manifestations in the form of emotional lability along with neurological manifestations in the form of tremors and the characteristic 'Kayser Fleisher Rings' (golden brown discolouration of descemet's membrane) are diagnostic of Wilsons disease.

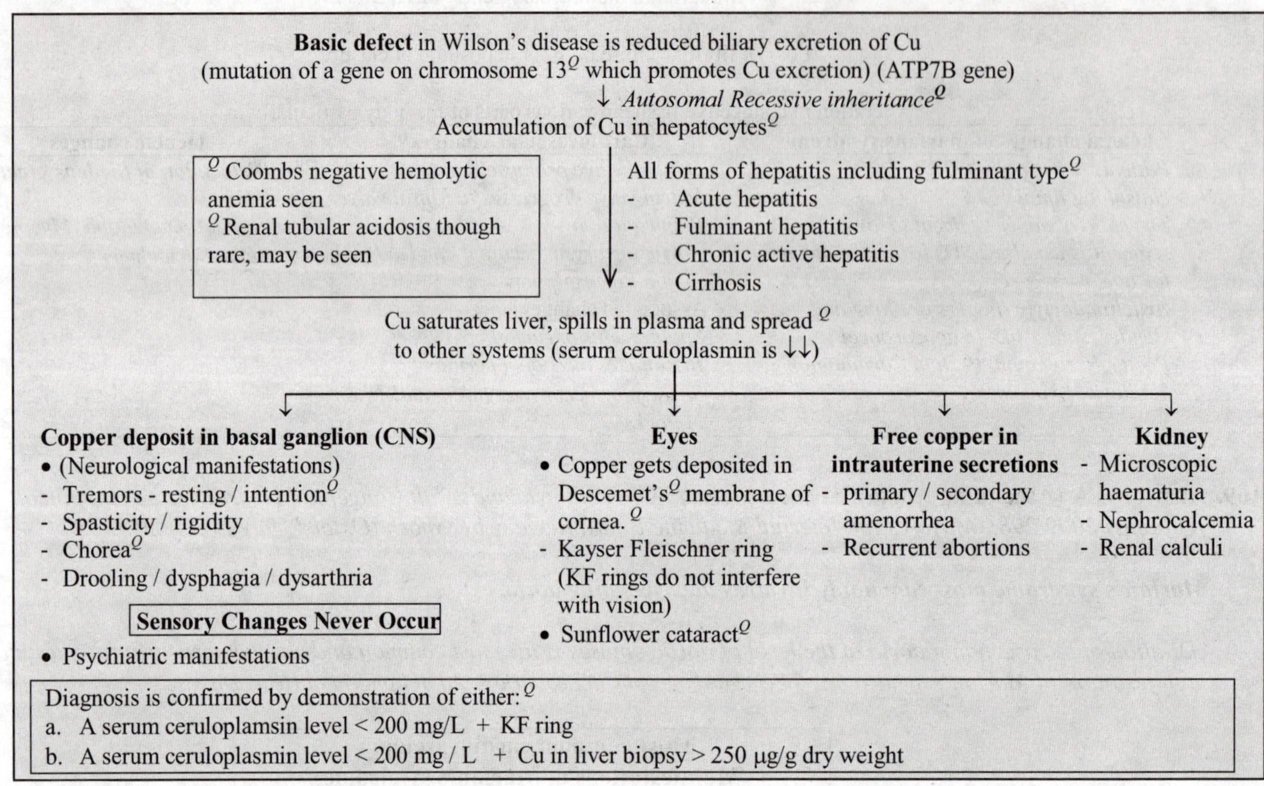

171. Answer is B (Testicular Atrophy): *Harrisons 17th/2449, 2450, 2451; Harrisons 16th/2313,2314; Harrison 18th/p 3188, 3189*

Testicular Atrophy is not documented as a feature of Wilson's disease.
Hemolytic Anemia, Chorea and Chronic active hepatitis are documented manifestations of Wilson's disease.

Hemolytic Anemia is a feature of Wilson disease

Hemolytic Anemia may occur in severe hepatic failure because large amounts of copper derived from Hepatocellular damage are released into the blood stream.

The association of hemolysis and liver disease makes Wilson's a likely diagnosis- Harrison

Chorea is a feature of Wilson's disease

Chorea is an established Neurological manifestation of wilson's disease

Chronic Active hepatitis is a feature of Wilson's disease

Wilson's disease may present as fatty change, acute hepatitis, chronic active hepatitis, cirrhosis or massive hepatic necrosis.

172. Answer is C (Urinary copper excretion is <100mg/day): *Harrisons 17th/2450; Harrisons 16th/2313,2314; Harrison 18th/p 3188, 3189*

Urine copper is an important diagnostic too. Symptomatic patients invariably have urine copper levels > 100 ur (>1.6 umol) per 24 hours.

Wilson's disease is an autosomal recessive disorder

It is caused by a mutation of a gene on chromosome 13^Q which promotes Cu excretion (ATP 7B gene)

<u>Symptomatic patients with Wilson's disease invariably have urinary copper excretion of >100 μg per 24 hours (>1.6 μmol /24 hr)</u>

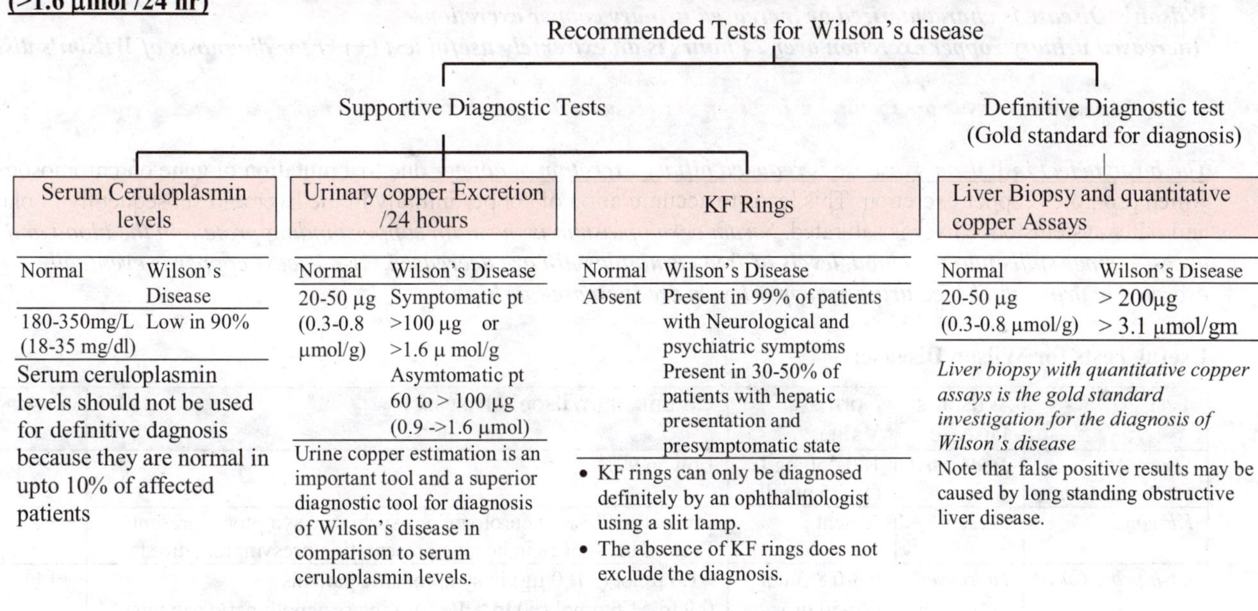

<u>Zinc is the treatment of choice for maintainance therapy in Wilson's disease</u>

Zinc is the treatment of choice in Wilson's disease for

- *Initial therapy in patients with hepatitis without decompensation*[Q]
- *Maintainance therapy*
- *Presymptomatic patient*
- *Pediatric patients*
- *Pregnant patients*

173. Answer is B (Low serum ceruloplasmin and high urinary copper) : *Harrison's 17th/2450; Harrison 18th/p 3189*

Wilson's disease is associated with low levels of serum ceruloplasmin and high urinary copper excretion.

<u>The basic defect in Wilson's disease is reduced biliary excretion of copper</u> due to a mutation of gene on chromosome 13 which promotes copper excretion. This leads to accumulation of copper initially in the liver and subsequently in plasma and other systems once liver is saturated. *Serum ceruloplasmin is the main copper binding protein in the blood and once excess copper spills into the blood, **levels of free ceruloplasmin are decreased.** Also excess copper is eventually excreted in urine and hence **urinary copper levels are increased or high.***

Useful Tests for Wilson Disease:

Test	Wilson's Disease	Normal Value	Comment (Wilson's Disease)	Usefulness
Serum ceruloplasmin	***Decreased***	180-350mg/L (18-35 mg/dL)	Low in 90%	+
KF rings	*Present*	Absent	Present in 99% if neurologic or psychiatric symptoms present Present in 30-50% in hepatic presentation/presymptomatic state	++
24-h urine Cu	***Increased***	0.3-0.8 μmol (20-50 μg)	>1.6 μmol (>100 μg) in symptomatic patients 0.9 to >1.6 μmol (60 to > 100 μg) in presymptomatic patients	+++
Liver Cu	*Increased*	0.3–0.8 μmol/g (20-50 μg)	>3.1 μmol (>200 μg) (obstructive liver disease can cause false-positive results)	++++
Haplotype analysis	*2 Matches*	0 Matches	2 Matches	++++ (Siblings only)

174. Answer is B (Increased urinary copper excretion): *Harrison 17th /2450*

Wilson's Disease is charachterized by increased urinary copper excretion.
Increased urinary copper excretion over 24 hours is an extremely useful test (+++) for diagnosis of Wilson's disease.

Wilson's disease is associated with low levels of serum ceruloplasmin and high urinary copper excretion

The basic defect in Wilson's disease is reduced biliary excretion of copper due to a mutation of gene on chromosome 13 which promotes copper excretion. This leads to accumulation of copper initially in the liver and subsequently in plasma and other systems once liver is saturated. *Serum ceruloplasmin is the main copper binding protein in the blood and once excess copper spills into the blood, **levels of free ceruloplasmin are decreased.** Also excess copper is eventually excreted in urine and hence **urinary copper levels are increased or high.***

Useful Tests for Wilson Disease:

Test	Wilson's Disease	Normal Value	Comment (Wilson's Disease)	Usefulness
Serum ceruloplasmin	***Decreased***	180-350mg/L (18-35 mg/dL)	Low in 90%	+
KF rings	*Present*	Absent	Present in 99% if neurologic or psychiatric symptoms present Present in 30-50% in hepatic presentation/presymptomatic state	++
24-h urine Cu	***Increased***	0.3-0.8 μmol (20-50 μg)	>1.6 μmol (>100 μg) in symptomatic patients 0.9 to >1.6 μmol (60 to > 100 μg) in presymptomatic patients	+++
Liver Cu	*Increased*	0.3–0.8 μmol/g (20-50 μg)	>3.1 μmol (>200 μg) (obstructive liver disease can cause false-positive results)	++++
Haplotype analysis	*2 Matches*	0 Matches	2 Matches	++++ (Siblings only)

175. Answer is A (Zinc): *Harrisons 17th/2451: Harrisons 16th/2313,2314; Harrison 18th/p 3188*

Presence of KF rings and decreased ceruloplasmin levels suggest the diagnosis of Wilson's disease.

The patient in question is presenting with intial hepatic disease without any evidence of hepatic decompensation.

Zinc is the therapy of choice for patients with hepatitis or cirrhosis without evidence of hepatic decompensation or neuropsychiatric symptoms.

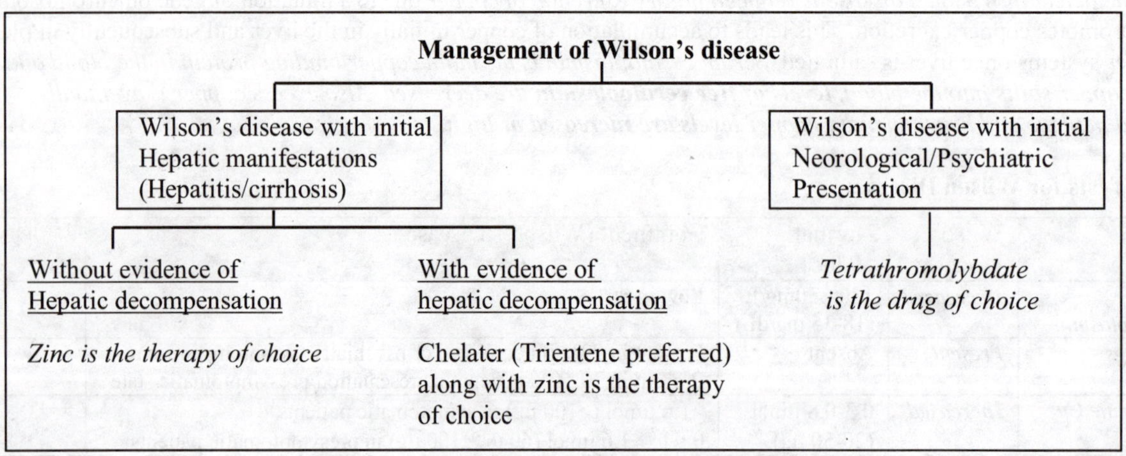

Recommended Anticopper Drugs for Wilson Disease

Disease Status	First Choice	Second Choice
Initial hepatic hepatitis,or cirrhosis without decompensation	Zinc	Trientine
Hepatic decompensation		
Mild	Trientine and zinc	Penicillamine and zinc
Moderate	Trientine and zinc	Hepatic transplantation
Severe	Hepatic transplantation	Trientine and zinc
Initial neurologic/psychiatric	Tetrathiomolybdate	Zinc
Maintenance	Zinc	Trientine
Presymptomatic	Zinc	Trientine
Pediatric	Zinc	Trientine
Pregnant	Zinc	Trientine

Hematochromatosis

176. Answer is A (Hemochromatosis): *Harrisons 16th/2288-2303; Harrisons 17th/2433; Harrison 17th/p 2432, 2433, 18th/p 3165, 3166*

The association of Arthritis, hyperpigmentation of skin and hypogonadism suggests the diagnosis of hematochromatosis.

Hematochromatosis (Disorder of iron storage)

Inappropriate increase in intestinal absorption results in deposition of excessive amounts of iron in parenchymal cells with eventual tissue damage and impaired function of organs

Serum iron ↑ed
% Transferrin saturation ↑ed
Serum ferritin ↑ed
Elevation in percent Transferrin saturation is the earliest phenotypic marker of herditary hemochromatosis[Q]

Liver	**Skin**	Pancreas	**Joints**	Heart	***Hypogonadism***
• Usually *first organ to be affected* • Hepatomegaly is seen in 95% of symptomatic patients • Cirrhosis may occur (Micronodular) • Hepatocellular carcinoma (30% of patients with cirrhosis). • It is the *most common cause of death in treated patients.*	• ***Excessive skin (Bronzing of skin) pigmentation*** is present in 90% of symptomatic patients • Usually diffuse and generalized. May be more pronounced on Face, Neck, Extensor aspect of forearm, dorsa of hands, lower legs and genitalia and ears • Usually results from increased melanin and iron in dermis	Involvement of pancreas *results in Diabetes mellitus* which is seen in 65% of symptomatic patients	• ***Arthropathy*** develops in 25-50% of patients • *The joints of hands especially the 2nd and 3rd MCP joints are the first to be involved* • Progressive polyarthritis involving wrist, knees, hips and ankles may also be seen	• Heart is involved in 15% of symptomatic patients • The most common manifestation is congestive heart failure • Cardiomyopathy and cardiac arrhythmias may be seen	• Results from impairment of Hypothalmo pituitary function by iron deposition which leads to decreased production of gonadotrophins.

Treatment of Haematochromatosis

Therapy of Haematochromatosis involves removal of excessive body iron and supportive treatment of damaged organs

Removal of Excessive Body iron
• ***Phlebotomy is the treatment of choice*** Iron removal is best accomplished by once or twice weekly phlebotomy of 500ml, - These should be continued until the serum ferritin level is < 50μg/L (May be required for 1-2 years) - Thereafter phlebotomies are performed at appropriate intervals to maintain ferritin levels between 50-100 μg/L (usually one phlebotomy every 3 months) • **Chelating agents** *(such as Desferoxamine) are alternative agents and indicated when anemia and hypoproteinemia are severe enough to preclude phlebotomy*

Alcohol consumption should be eleminated[Q] as it increases the risk of cirrhosis in hematochromatosis nearly ten fold.

The charachteristic clinical features of Haemochromatosis in order of frequency are[Q] :
• *Hepatomegaly (95%)* • *Skin pigmentation (90%)* • *Diabetes mellitus (65%)* • *Arthropathy (25-50%)* • *Cardiac disease (15%)* • *Hypogonadism*

177. Answer is D (Desferrioromine is treatment of choice): *Harrisons 16th/2288-2203; 17th /1764, 2433; 18th/2312*

The therapy of hematochromatosis involves removal of excess body iron.

Iron removal is best achieved by periodic phlebotomies which is the treatment of choice for Hematochromosis. *Chelating agents like desferoxamine are less effective and indicated when anemia or hypoproteinemia is severe enough to preclude phlebotomy.* ***Chelating agents are not the treatment of choice for Hematochromatosis.***

178. Answer is D (Increased Transferrin Saturation): *Harrisons 17th/2431,2432Mayo clinic Gastroenterology and Hepatology Board Review by Hauser 2nd/323; Clinical Laboratory medicine by Mc Clatchey 2nd/839; Harrison 18th/p 3164, 3165, 3166*

'A transferrin saturation of more than 45% is the earliest phenotypic abnormality in hereditary hematochromatosis'

- Hauser 2nd/3232

Transferrin saturation and measurement of unbound iron bindeng capacity are recommended for initial scrceening of individuals

Tests Recommended for screening for Hereditary Hematochromatosis

Transferrin Saturation	Iron binding capacity (Unbound /Unsaturated)
• *A transferrin saturation of more than 45% is the earliest phenotypic abnormality in hereditary hematochromatosis* • *Transferrin saturation is considered the best initial screening test for hereditary hematochromotosis* • Transferrin saturation has a high sensitivity of >90% in diagnosing hereditary hematochromatosis • Transferrin saturation is the ratio of serum iron to total iron binding capacity (SI/TIBC)	• *Unbound Iron binding capacity is an alternative screening test.* • *Unbound Iron binding capacity UIBC=TIBC-Serum Iron* • *Unbound iron binding capacity is decreased in hematochromatosis*

179. Answer is A (Iron binding capacity): *Harrisons 17th/2433; Harrison 18th/p 3165*

The presence of hyperpigmentation and diabetes (bronze diabetes) together with restrictive cardiomyopathy and cirrhosis suggests a diagnosis of hereditary hematochromatosis.

The best initial test to diagnose hereditary hematochromatosis are Transferrin saturation and unsaturated Iron binding capacity

As transferrin saturation is not provided amongst the options, Iron binding capacity is the single best answer of choice.

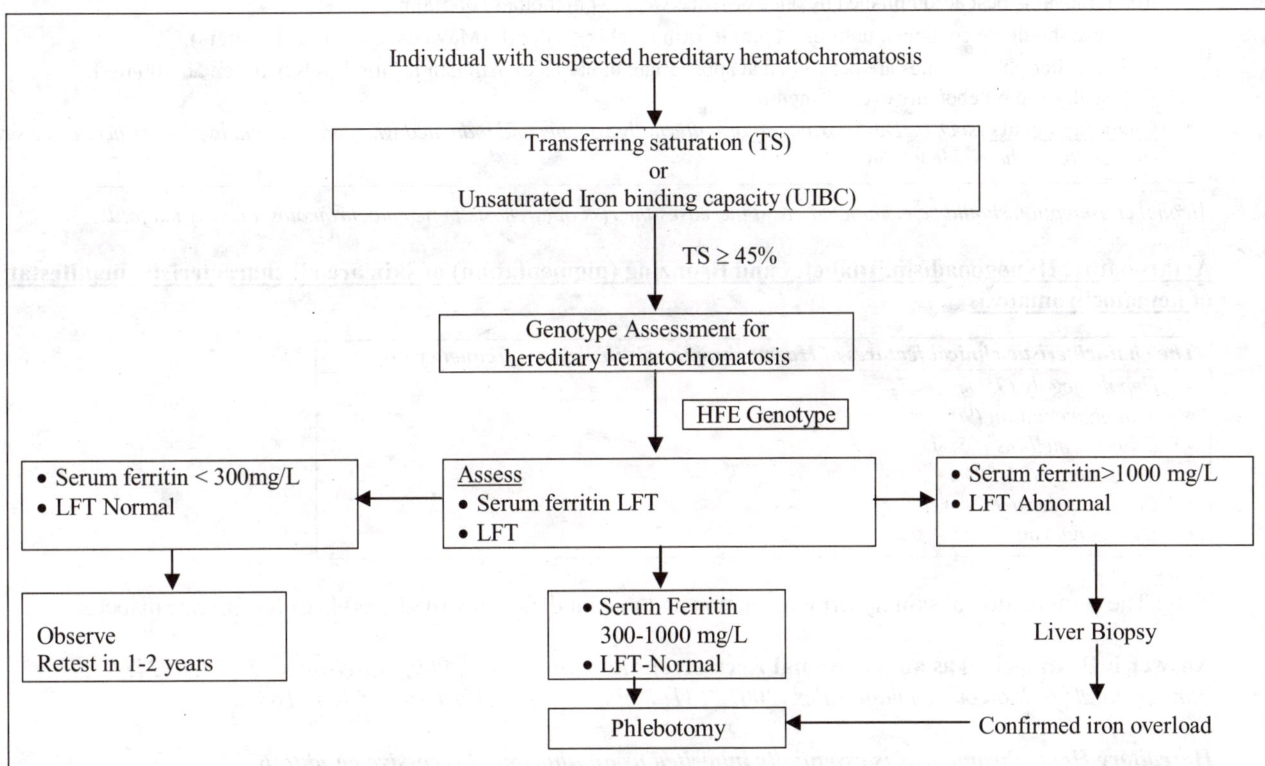

Note

Serum ferritin levels are a good index of body iron stores and are raised early during the cause of disease. Yet serum ferritin levels should not be used as initial screening test to detect hereditary hematochromatosis.

This is because serum ferritin also acts as an acute phase reactant and its levels are increased in variable infections and inflammatory conditions without iron overload. Also the serum concentration of ferritin may be increased in patients with hepatocellular injury as in viral hepatitis, alcoholic fatty liver disease or alcoholic liver diseases due to increased release from tissue cells.

180. Answer is C (Desferroxamine is the treatment of choice): *Harrisons 16th/2288-2203 , Harrisons 17th/ 2433; Harrison 18th/p 3166*

The therapy of hematochromatosis involves removal of excess body iron

Iron removal is best acieved by periodic phlebotomies which is the treatment of choice for Hematochromosis.

Chelating agents like desferoxamine are less effective and indicated when anemia or hypoproteinemia is severe enough to preclude phlebotomy (Harrison. ***Chelatingagents are not the treatment of choice for Hematochromatosis.***

181. Answer is D (Desferrioxamine is the treatment of choice): *Harrisons 17th/2433; Harrisons 16th/2288,2203; Harrison 18th/p 3166*

The treatment of choice for Hematochromatosis is removed of excess body iron by Phlebotomy and not with the use of chelating agents like desfernoxamine.

Phlebotomy is the treatment of choice in Hematochromatosis

Treatment of Haematochromatosis

Therapy of Haematochromatosis involves removal of excessive body iron and supportive treatment of damaged organs

Removal of Excessive Body iron
• ***Phlebotomy is the treatment of choice*** Iron removal is best accomplished by once or twice weekly phlebotomy of 500ml, - These should be continued until the serum ferritin level is < 50μg/L (May be required for 1-2 years) - Thereafter phlebotomies are performed at appropriate intervals to maintain ferritin levels between 50-100 μg/L (usually one phlebotomy every 3 months) • **Chelating agents** *(such as Desferoxamine) are alternative agents and indicated when anemia and hypoproteinemia are severe enough to preclude phlebotomy*

Alcohol consumption should be eleminated[Q] as it increases the risk of cirrhosis in hematochromatosis nearly ten fold

Arthropathy, Hypogonadism, Diabetes and Bronzing (pigmentation) of skin are all characteristic manifestation of hematochromatosis

The charachteristic clinical features of Haemochromatosis in order of frequency are[Q] :
• *Hepatomegaly (95%)* • *Skin pigmentation (90%)* • *Diabetes mellitus (65%)* • *Arthropathy (25-50%)* • *Cardiac disease (15%)* • *Hypogonadism*

Note: The combination of skin hyperpigmentation and insulin deficiency (diabetes) is called Bronze diabetes.

182. Answer is B (Inherited as an Autosomal Recessive) : *Robbins 7th/908, 909; Harrison's 17th/2430, 2431, 2432; Fundamentals of Molecular Diagnostics (2007)/131; Hurst 12th/859; Harrison 18th/p 3163, 3164*

Hereditary Hemochromatosis is essentially inherited as an autosomal recessive condition.

Hereditary Hemochromatosis is essentially an Autosomal Recessive condition

The most common form of hereditary hemochromatosis is related to mutations in *HFE gene*, which is a gene located on the short arm of chromosome 6 and is HLA linked

HFE related hereditary hemochromatosis (most common type) is inherited as an autosomal recessive condition

Hereditary Hemochromatosis

Type I (HFE Related)	Type II, III and IV (Non HFE related)
• Most common type • Inherited as an autosomal recessive condition	• Rare types of hemochromatosis • May be inherited as autosomal dominant conditions - *Type 2 is autosomal recessive* - *Type 3 is autosomal dominant* - *Type 4 is auto somal dominant*

Hereditary Hemochromatosis shows incomplete penetrance

Incomplete penetrance refers to the lack of disease symptoms in an individual despite the presence of pathological gene mutation

Expression of Hemochromatosis is variable and many HFE positive people neither have nor develop disease, thus displaying the phenomenon of incomplete penetrance

This suggests that other genetic and / or environmental factors modify the pathogenesis of disease

Hereditary Hemochromatosis is more common in Men

The clinical expression of disease is 5 – 10 times more common in men than women - Harrison

Phlebotomy is an effective management option but it does not lead to cure

'The therapy of hemochromatosis involves removal of excess body iron which is best accomplished by phlebotomy Phlebotomy is not curative and will be required at appropriate intervals to maintain ferritin levels (usually one phlebotomy every 3 months)' - Harrison

Miscellaneous

183. Answer is C (Cardiac Failure): *Harrison 17th /2147; 'Practical Cardiovascular Pathology by Burke (Lippincott - Williams) 2010/192; Cardiac Imaging. A Multimodelity Approach (Thieme) 2009/222; Rubin's Pathology 6th/1021; Rubin's Pathology 5th/249*

The most common cause of death in primary amylolosis is cardiac failure.

'Amyloid related cardiac disease is the most common cause of death in Primary Amyloidosis'- Rubin's pathology 6th/1021

Primary Amyloidosis is synonymous with light chain amyloidosis or AL-Amyloid disease.
Primary amyloidosis is primarily a consequence of plasma cell disorders and is the most common form of amyloidosis in the United States

- *The kidney is the most frequently involved organ (80%)Q*
- *The Heart is the second most frequently involved organ (≈40%) Q*
- *Cardiac dysfunction is the most frequent cause of death in Primary Amyloidosis Q*
- *Cardiac amyloidosis most frequently manifests as 'Restrictive cardiomyopathy Q*
- *Clinically significant cardiac involvement in Secondary Amyloidosis is Rare*

184. Answer is C (Positive antinuclear antibodies) : *Harrison 16/e, p 1489, 1490; CMDT 2006 / 464-465; Harrison 17th/1572; Harrison 18th/p 2071, 2072*

Raynaud's disease is the term applied for idiopathic Raynaud's phenomenon when secondary causes of the phenomenon have been excluded.
Presence of antinuclear antibodies points towards a secondary cause of Raynaud's phenomenon. ANA's are not associated with primary idiopathic Raynaud's disease.

The most common cause of Raynaud's phenomenon is Idiopathic Raynaud's disease.

- Raynaud's phenomenon/syndrome is an episodic vasopastic disorder characterized by digital colour change (white → Blue → Red), following exposure to cold and subsequent rewarming, or emotional stress.
- Idiopathic Raynaud's phenomenon is also known as Raynaud's disease.
- Raynaud's disease term is applied when secondary causes of Raynaud's phenomenon have been excluded.
- Over 50% of patient with Raynaud's phenomenon have Raynaud's disease. – Harrison

Raynaud's disease is more common in females

- 'Women are affected five times more often than men and the age of presentation is usually between 20-40 years'.

Raynaud's disease has a good prognosis

- 'Raynaud's disease is usually benign, causing mild disease appear to have the milder forms of Raynaud's Phenomenon.- *Harrison*

185. Answer is D (Coarctation of Aorta): *SOAP for Cardiology (2006) /100, 101; Moss and Adam's 7th/1288; Nelson's 18th/1900, 1901; Hurst 11th/ed 1809; Oski's Pediatrics 2nd/714; 'Pediatrics' Board Review Series 2nd/341*

Isolated upper extremity hypertension (200 / 140 mm Hg), together with absent/ diminished femoral pulses is a characteristic feature of coarctation of aorta.

Although coarctation of aorta does not commonly present with seizures, these may be seen as a consequence of severe hypertension (BP = 200/140) or complications like intracranial haemorrhage (from Berry aneurysms which are more common in patients with coarctation.

Coarctation of Aorta is the most likely diagnosis: Approach *(Nelson/Hurst)*

- The classic sign of coarctation of aorta is a disparity in pulsations and blood pressure in arms and legs. *The femoral, popliteal, posterior tibial and dorsalis pedis pulses are weak (or absent in upto 40% of patients) in contrast to bounding pulses in the arms and carotid vessels.*
- The blood pressure is the legs is lower than in the arms and *90% of patients with coarctation have hypertension in an upper extremity* greater than 95th perecentile for age

Age (yrs)	95th percentile (mm Hg)
> 1 yrs	*110 / 60*
1 – 5 yrs	*115 /75*
6 – 10 yrs	*125 /85*
11 – 18 yrs	*140 /90*

- *Severe hypertension* may be seen as a consequence of persistant hypertension in an individual who has not undergone corrective surgery for coarctation, and this usually *appears in the second or third decade of life (Hurst)*

A blood pressure of 200 /140 mm Hg in a 10 year old boy suggests severe hypertension (95th percentile at 10 years – 125/85)

- ***Children with severe / malignant hypertension may develop headaches, seizures and stroke (haemorrhage from Berry aneurysms which are more common in patients with coarctation).***

Takayasu Aortoarteritis may also present with severe hypertension and absent femoral pulses due to acquired midaortic coarctation but this is an uncommon presentation in Takayasu aortoarteritis (and hence not the single best answer of choice)

Takayasu arteritis (or non specific aortoarteritis) is a chronic vasculitis disease of medium and large sized arteries with a strong predilection for aortic arch and its branches.

This may lead to stenosis of the involved vessels and hence a picture of acquired coarctation. It may thus produce a clinical picture similar to that of coarctation with disparity in pulsations and blood pressure in arms & legs with hypertension depending on the site of the acquired stenosis.

However, this condition is *more common in women* and most *commonly affects the subclavican artery.* Hence it ***more commonly presents with*** claudication, along with unequal and ***reduced pulses / BP in the upper extremity*** than the lower extremity. Also *systemic symptoms are more common* is Takayasu than in coarctation. *Nevertheless Takayasu arteritis may affect the Thoracic or Abdominal aorta and present with absent lower limb pulses and upper extremity hypertension like coarctation of aorta.*

Takayasu arteritis can be picked as the answer if Coarctation of aorta is not provided amongst the options

Coarctation	Takayasu
• More common condition	• Less common condition
• More common in boys	• More common in girls (8 : 1 = F:M)
• Upper extremity hypertension	• Absent or decreased upper limb pulses (brachial / radial) and blood pressure difference between left and right arm is characteristic *('Reverse coarctation': Oski's Essential Pediatrics)*
• Bounding pulses in with arms and diminished / absent lower limb pulsations is characteristic	**Note** *Clinical picture similar to coarctation with absent lower limb pulsations and upper extremity hypertension may be seen if site of lesion is in the thoracic aorta / abdominal aorta (But this is not charachteristic).*
• Hypertension is frequent	• Hypertension is frequent

Renal Parenchymal Disease and Grandmal seizures do not present with isolated upper extremity hypertension and absent femoral pulses.

186. Answer is D (Polyarteritis nodosa): *Harrison 16th/1707,2007,2009; CMDT'06,460, API 8th.541; References alongside explanation*

Amongst the options provided renal artery stenosis is least likely to be seen in association with Polyarteritis nodosa.

- **Atherosclerosis and Fibromuscular disease**
  - Renal artery stenosis is produced predominantly by atherosclerotic occlusive disease (80% to 90% of patients) or fibromuscular dysplasia (10-15% of patients).- *CMDT'06 p 460*
  - The common cause of renal artery stenosis ***in the middle aged and elderly*** is an atheromatous plaque at origin of renal artery. *Harrison*
  - ***In younger women*** stenosis is due to intrinsic structural abnormalities of the arterial wall caused by a heterogenous group of lesions called 'fibromuscular dysplasia'. - *Harrison 16th/1707*
- **PAN or Takayasu arteritis ?**

  Harrison, CMDT do not mention PAN or Takayasu arteritis as a cause for renal artery stenosis.

  However, Takayasu arteritis is certainly a more common cause of renal artery stenosis than PAN.

  Takayasu arteritis (Aorto-arteritis) *is beleiveds to be the most common of renovascular hypertension in India and China. – Diseases of Kidney and Urinary Tract 8th/1279*

A number of research publications, however show Takayasu arteritis as a cause for renal artery stenosis.

Takayasu Arteritis	PAN
Takayasu arteritis (Aorto-arteritis) is the most common cause of renovascular hypertension in India and China.' – Diseases of kidney and Urinary Tract 8th/1279	Renal artery stenosis in a Case of PAN has only been described as an unusual association and published as a rare case report (single case) ***Reference:*** "PAN with renal Artery Stenosis": Indian Pediatrics Volume 41-Jan.17, 2004.

PAN

Although renal involvement is seen in upto 60% of patients with PAN its pathology does not involve renal artery stenosis.

The pathology involves arteritis without glomerulonephritis and is characterised by aneurysms of small and medium sized arteries. **Stenosis of main renal artery is an unusual association'.**

-Research paper, www. Indian paediatrics. net/Jan 2004/86.pdf

Causes of Renal artery stenosis : *API 8th/541; Renal Artery Stenosis : Diagnosis and Management - IHJ : May-June 2002, Vol. 54/No. 3*
1. Atherosclerosis 2. Fibromuscular dysplasia 3. Non specific Aorto arteritis 4. Takayasu arteritis and giant cell arteritis (Takayasu > Giant cell) 5. Antiphospholipid syndrome 6. Transplant renal artery stenosis 7. Renal artery embolism 8. Dissecting aneurysm of aorta 9. Radiation arteritis

187. Answer is C (Rectal biopsy): *Harrison 16th / 2028; Harrison 17th/2145; Harrison 18th/p 945*

Rectal biopsy is single best answer amongst the options provided.

'The systemic amyloidosis offer a choice of biopsy sites. Abdominal fat aspirates or renal or ***rectal biopsies*** *are often preferred'. – Harrison*

Biopsy site in systemic amyloidosis (CMDT)	Sensitivity
Rectal or gingival	80%
Bone marrow	50%
Abdominal fat aspirate	70 to 80%

188. Answer is A & B (Myesthenia gravis and Idiopathic thrombocytopenic purpura): *Harrison 16th/1929; 'Practical Transfusion Medicine' 2nd/151, 152;*

Idiopathic Thrombocytopenia purpura and M. Gravis are established indications for IVIG infusions

Clinical Indications for IVIG

Immunodeficiney States

Primary Immunodeficiency states
- Bruton's Hypogammaglobulinemia
- Severe combined Immunodeficiency (SCID)
- Primary Agammaglobulinemia
- X linked Agammaglobulinemia
- IgG – subclass deficiency
- Wiskott Aldrich Syndrome (Selected patients)*

Secondary Immunodeficiency States (Selected)
- Pediatric HIV
- CLL

Post Bone Marrow Transplantation

Prophylaxis against bacterial infection

Immunomodulation of Autoimmune Conditions
- Idiopathic / Immune Thrombocytopenic Purpura (ITP)
  (Certain other Autoantibody mediated cytopenias including post-transfusion purpura and neonatal cytopenias)
- Kawasaki disease
- G-B syndrome (& CIDP)
- Myaesthenia Gravis
- Multiple sclerosis
- Dermatomyositis
- Others

* Intravenous immunoglobulins may also be indicated in selected patients of Wiskott Aldrich Syndrome *(Harrison 17th/2060)*

In patinets with Wiskott Aldrich syndrome who lask a suitable donor, IVIG infusions may also be used to improve platelet count and reduce risk of serious hemorrhage.

189. Answer is D (Necrotizing vasculitis): *Refer text below*

Necrotizing vasculitis is characterized by inflammation and necrosis of blood vessels leading to tissue damage. This deiagnosis includes a braod spectrum of disorders and the most common immuno-process involves immune complexes and complement activation.

190. Answer is A, B and E (Kawasaki disease, GB syndrome and Myasthenia gravis): *Harriosn 17th/2044, 2059; Harrison 18th/p 2684*

191. Answer is A, B and E (Myathenia, I.T.P. and Guillian Barre syndrome): *Harrison 17th/663; 16th/617; Harrison 18th/p 887, 888*

192. Answer is D (PAN): *Refer previous question*

Immunoglobulin infusion are not indicated in PAN

Immunoglobulin infusions are indicated in Kawasaki disease and X linked Agammaglobulinemia and selected cases of Wiskott Aldrich Syndrome.

193. Answer is B (PAN): *Refer Previous question*

IV Immunoglobulins are not indicated in PAN

Kawasaki disease, GBS and Bruton's Hypogammaglobulinemia are established indications of IV Ig infusion.

194. Answer is B (Cholinergic crisis): *American society for Apharesis (ASFA) Guidelines for Therapeutic Apharesis – Official publication, Therapeutic Apharesis' JIACM vol- 8, No-3, 2007, p-233*

Plasmapharesis is not indicated in cholinergic crisis.

Myaesthenia Gravis (including Myaesthenic crisis) and Acute Inflammatory Demyelinating Polyradiculoneuropathics like GBS belong to category I indications for plasmapharesis.

Plasmapharesis in these disorders is standard and acceptable either as a primary therapy or a valuable first line adjunct therapy

Polymyositis belongs to category III indication for plasmapharesis.

Plasmapharesis is believed to be of benefit in these conditions (Category III) although existing evidence is insufficient to establish the efficacy of therapeutic plasmapharesis.

Therapeutic Plasma Exchange (TPE) / Plasmapharesis : Review

- TPE / plasmapharesis is an extracorporeal blood purification technique designed for removal of undesired large molecular weight substances from the plasma, such as pathogenic autoantibodies, immune complexes, cryoglobulins etc.
- The basic premise of TPE is that removal of these substances will reduce further damage and may permit reversal of the pathologic process
- Plasmapharesis has been used / trialled for the treatment of several diseases causing a lot of confusion on the actual indications and effectiveness of this procedures in various disorders.
- The American society of Apharesis (ASFA) and American Associations of Blood Banks (AABB) have issued guidelines for therapeutic application / indication of plasmapharesis / apharesis in various clinical disorders.

  They have classified the various indications of therapeutic apharesis (including plasmapharesis) into four different categories based on current evidence.

Category	Inference
Category I	Diseases for which Therapeutic Apharasis is standard and acceptable, either as primary therapy on valuable first line adjunct therapy
Category II	Diseases for which Therapeutic Apharesis is generally accepted but considered to be supportive or adjunctive to other, more definitive treatments, rather than a first line therapy
Category III	Diseases in which there is suggestion of benefit, however existing evidence is insufficient either to establish the efficacy of therapeutic aphaeresis or classify its risk-benefit ratio
Category IV	Disease in which evidence has not shown any benefit (should no longer be used as indications for plasmapharesis)

Disorders	Category
A. Hematological Diseases	Category
• *Thrombotic Thrombocytopenic Purpura (TTP)*	**I**
• *Post transfusion purpura*	**I**
• Myeloma with paraproteins / hyperviscosity	II
• Myeloma with Acute Renal failure	II
• Coagulation Factor Inhibitors	II
• Aplastic Anemia / Pure Red cell Aplasias	III
• Hemolytic disease of Newborn	III
• Platelet Alloimmunization	III
• Autoimmune Hemolytic Anemia	III
B. Neurological Disorders	Category
• ***Acute Inflammatory Demyclinating Poly radiculoneuropathy (AIDP) (including GB syndrome)***	***I***
• ***Chronic Inflammatory Demyelinating poly radiculoneuropathy (CIDP)***	***I***
• ***Myaesthenia Gravis (Myaesthenic crisis)***	***I***
• Lambert Eaten Syndrome	II
• Multiple Sclerosis - Acute Fulminant - Relapsing / Progressive	II / III II III
• Syndenham's chorea	II
• PANDAS	II
• Cryoglobulinemia with polyneuropathy	II
• Multiple Myeloma with Polyneuropathy	III
• POEMS syndrome	III

• ***Polymyositis / Dermatomyositis***	***III***
• Inclusion Body Myositis	III
• Rasmussen's Encephalitis	III
• Stiff man syndrome	III
Autoimmune / Rheumatic Diseases	Category
• Cryoglobulinemia	II
• Raynaud's phenomenon	III
• Vasculitis	III
• Scleroderma / Progressive Systemic Sclerosis	III
• Systemic Lupus Erythematosis (SLE)	III
Renal Diseases	Category
• Anti- Glomerular Basement Membrane Antibody disease (eg Goodpasture's disease)	I
• Rapidly Progressive Glomerulonephritis (RPGN)	II
• Hemolytic Urenic Syndrome	III
• Renal transplant - Prevention of Rejection / Presensitization - Treatment of Recurrent disease - Hyperacute Rejection	III III III IV
Metabolic Disease	Category
• Refusum's Disease (Phytonic Acid Storage Disease)	I
• Familial Hypercholesterolemia	II
• Acute Hepatic Failure	III
• Overdose poisoning	III

Endocrinology

ESSENTIAL REVISION NOTES

Multiple Endocrine Neoplasia (MEN) Syndromes

MEN I (Wermer's)

Characteristic Triad	Other Relatively Uncommon Manifestation
• ***Parathyroid Tumors*** • ***Pituitary Tumors*** • ***Pancreatic islet cell tumors***	• *Adrenal cortical hyperplasia* • *Pheochromocytomas (Rare)* • *Foregut carcinoid* • *Subcutaneous/Visceral Lipomas* • *Dermal (cutaneous) angiofibromas or collagenomas*

Charachteristic Triad of MEN I

Parathyroid tumors (Most Common)	Pancreatic endocrine tumors (Second Most Common)	Pituitary tumors (Third Most Common)
Hyperparathyroidism is the most common manifestation of MEN I -Harrison **Relative frequency of Tumors causing Hyperparathyroidism:** • *Parathyroid hyperplasia is the most common cause of hyperparathyroidism in MEN I* • *Parathyroid adenomas are less common than parathyroid hyperplasia and tend to occur in older patient or those with long standing disease.*	*Neoplasia of the pancreatic islets is the second most common manifestation of MEN I*[Q]. -Harrison **Relative frequency of Endocrine Tumors of Pancreatic Islets:** • *Pancreatic polypeptide (75 – 85%)* • *Gastrin (60%) (Gastrinomas /ZES)* • *Insulin (25 – 30%) (Insulinomas)* • *Glucagon (5 – 10%)(Glucagonoma)* • *VIP (3 – 5%) (VIPomas)* • *Somatostatin* (1 – 5%) (Somatostatinoma)	*Pituitary tumors are third most common tumors of MEN 1 and occur in more than half of patients with MEN 1* **Relative frequency of Pituitary Tumors:** • *Prolactinomas* are the most common pituitary tumors in MEN I • *Acromegaly* due to excessive growth hormone (GH) production is the second most common pituitary tumor in MEN I • *Cushing's syndrome*

VIPoma is synonymous with Verner Morrison syndrome or Water Diarrhea Syndrome or Pancreatic Cholera[Q].

Other Tumors in MEN I

- *Carcinoid tumours (foregut type: derived from lung, thymus, stomach or duodenum)*
- *Subcutaneous & visceral lipomas*
- *Cutaneous leiomyomas*
- *Skin angiofibromas or collagenomas*

Relative frequency of Endocrine Tumors of Pancreatic Islets in MEN I Syndromes

Gastrinomas > Insulinomas > Glucagonomas > VIPomos > Somatostainomas

8

Endocrinology

MEN II Syndrome

MEN II syndrome

- *Medullary Carcinoma Thyroid*
- *Pheocrhomocytoma*

\+

MEN II A	MEN II B
• *Parathyroid Adenoma or Hyperplasia* • *Cutaneous Lichen Amyloidosis* • *Hirschprung disease*	• *Mucosal neuromas* • *Gastrointestinal neuromas* • *Marfinoid features*

MEN I and MEN II

MEN I	MEN II	
	MEN II A	**MEN II B**
<u>Characteristic Manifestations</u> • Parathyroid hyperplasia or adenoma • Pancreatic tumors (Islet cell hyperplasia, adenoma, or carcinoma) • Pituitary hyperplasia or adenoma <u>Other less common manifestations</u> • Foregut carcinoid • Subcutaneous or visceral lipomas • Dermal angiofibromas or collagenomas	• MTC • Pheochromocytoma • Parathyroid hyperplasia or adenoma • Cutaneous lichen amyloidosis • Hischsprung disease • FMTC	• MTC • Pheochromocytoma • Mucosal and gastrointestinal neuromas • Marfanoid features

Disorders of Adrenal Cortex

Cushing's Syndrome

Causes of Cushing's syndrome

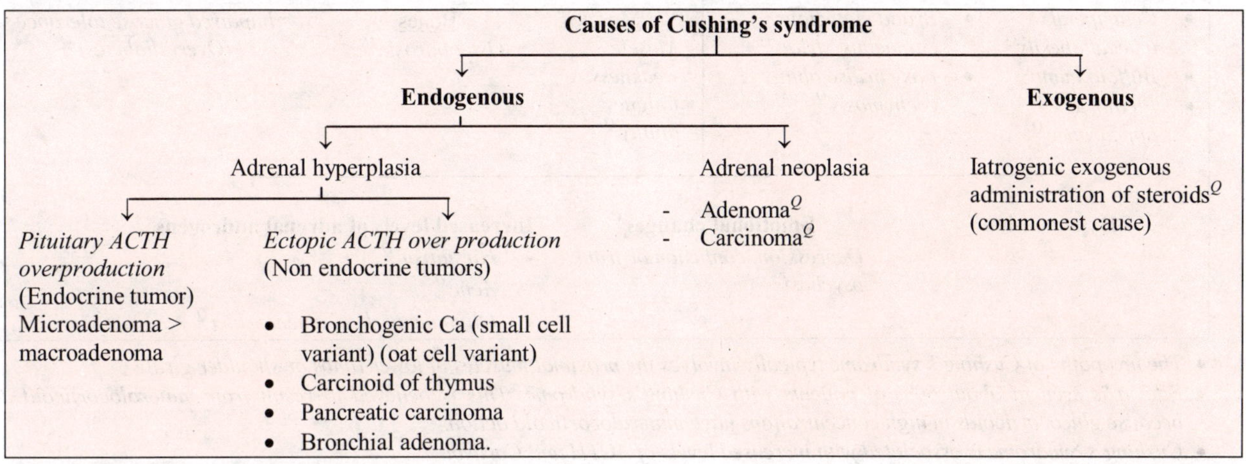

Endogenous Cushing's syndrome
Most common cause of endogenous Cushing's syndrome is adrenal hyperplasia from an ACTH secreting Pituitary Adenoma (Cushing's disease)

Exogenous Cushing's Syndrome
The most common cause of exogenous Cushing's syndrome is iatrogenic administration of steroids.

- *The most common overall cause of Cushing's syndrome is iatrogenic administration of steroids for a variety of reasons*
- *'Endogenous' Cushing's syndrome is most commonly associated with 'bilateral adrenal hyperplasia'*[Q]
- *Most common cause of Cushing's syndrome (endogenous) is a Pituitary microadenoma*[Q]*, which is less than 10 mm in diameter - Harrison*

Cushing's Disease and Cushing's Syndrome

Cushing's disease refers to increased production of Cortisol (↑ Cortisol) by Adrenals secondary to an ACTH producing tumor (↑ ACTH) in the pituitary gland.

Only an individual who has (increased cortisol due to) an ACTH producing pituitary tumor is defined as having Cushing's disease, whereas Cushing's syndrome refers to all causes of excess cortisol

Aetiological Approach to Cushing's syndrome

Elevated Cortisol with Elevated ACTH (↑ Cortisol + ↑ ACTH)	Elevated cortisol with Low ACTH (↑ Cortisol + ↓ ACTH)
• *ACTH producing Pituitary tumor* ***(Cushing's Disease)*** - *Pituitary Microadenoma* (Most common[Q]) - *Pituitary Macro adenoma* • *Ectopic ACTH producing tumors* - *Bronchogenic carcinoma (small cell or oat cell variant)* - *Carcinoid of thymus* - *Pancreatic carcinoma* - *Bronchial Adenoma*	• *Adrenal Adenoma* • *Adrenal Carcinoma* • *Exogenous steroid administration*

Clinical Manifestations of Cushing's syndrome

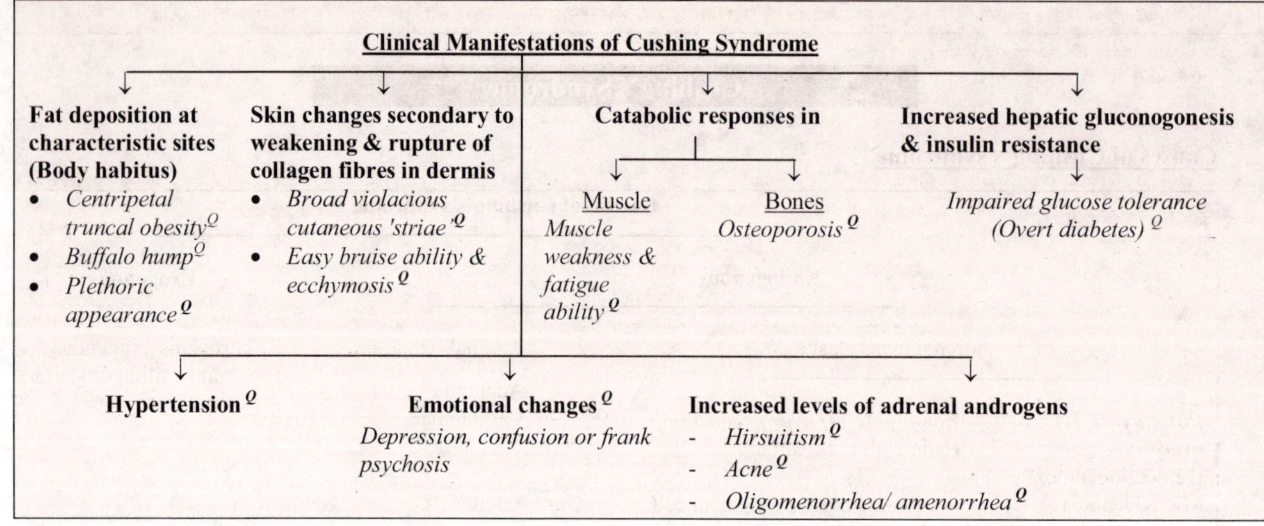

- *The myopathy of Cushing's syndrome typically involves the proximal muscles of lower limbs or shoulder girdle*
- *Edema is seen in about 60% of patients with Cushing's syndrome. This is believed to result from mineralocorticoid action, because glucocorticoids in high concentrations have mineralocorticoid action.*
- *Cushing's Syndrome is associated with increased levels of ACTH and Cortisol.*

Cushing's syndrome results from an excessive amount of corticosteroids secreted from the adrenal cortex (outer part) of the adrenal gland. Adrenaline is secreted from the adrenal medulla (inner part) of the gland and is not raised in Cushing's syndrome

- *Cushing's syndrome is associated with sustained / persistent hypertension and not episodic hypertension.*
- *Increased Adrenaline is not a feature of Cushing's syndrome. Increased adrenaline is a feature of adrenal medullary disorders like pheochromocytoma*
- *Increased urinary catecholamines are a feature of pheochromocytoma and not Cushing's disease*
- *Hypokalemia / hypochloremia and metabolic alkalosis are particularly present with ectopic ACTH production*

The ectopic production of CRH results in clinical, biochemical and radiologic feature indistinguishable from those caused by hypersecretion of pituitary ACTH. The Typical signs and symptoms of Cushing's syndrome may be absent or minimal with ectopic ACTH production and ***hypokalemic alkalosis*** *is a prominent manifestation.*

Diagnostic Protocol

- Serum cortisol estimation and assessment of Diurnal variation in serum levels of Cortisol

Loss of circadian rhythym – Loss of diurnal variation (8.00 AM & Mid night): API 7th/1072.
In normal individuals the serum levels of cortisol reach their lowest levels at midnight.
In patients with Cushings this diurnal variation is lost and serum levels of cortisol remain same throughout 24 hours.

- Those with increased cortisol levels are subjected to a ***dexamethasone supression test***.

Dexamethasone supression test : This is used to group etiology of Cushing's into the following:	
No response or failure of suppression	**Suppression positive (High dose)**
• Adrenal hyperplasia secondary to ACTH producing tumor • Adrenal neoplasia (adenoma or carcinoma)	• Adrenal hyperplasia secondary to ACTH secretion from the pituitary e.g. pituitary adenoma.

Aetiological approach to Cushing's syndrome with the help of ACTH levels

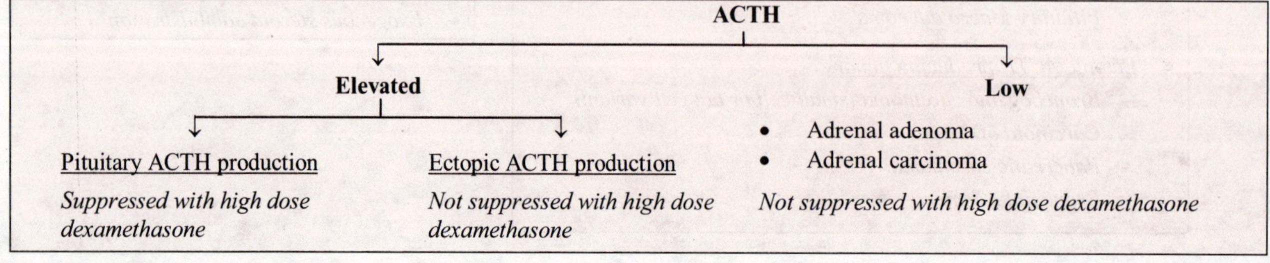

Hyperaldosteronism and Conn's Syndrome

Primary Hyperaldosteronism

Primary Hyperaldosteronism

Associated Adrenal Tumor	Without Associated Adrenal tumor
• *Adrenal Adenoma (Conn's syndrome)* • *Adrenal carcinoma (Rare cause)*	• *Bilateral Cortical Hyperplasia* *(Idiopathic Hyperoldosteronism/Nodular hyperplasia)*
The most common cause of Conn's syndrome is an aldosterone producing adrenal adenoma. *Most cases are unilateral[Q] with a small[Q] adenoma that may occur on either side.*	***The most common cause for primary Hyperaldosteronism is Bilateral Cortical Hyperplasia.*** *'These patients constitute 80% of patients with Primary Hyperaldosteronism' (Harrison)*

Conn's syndrome

This by defination refers to primary aldosteronism secondary to an aldosterone producing adrenal adenoma.

Primary Aldosteronism secondary to bilateral cortical hyperplasia is not defined as Conn's syndrome

The most common aldosterone producing adrenal tumor is a unilateral adrenal adenoma.

Adrenal carcinoma *is a rare cause of primary aldosteronism.*

Aldosterone producing adrenal tumor

Primary hyperaldosteronism 'Conn's syndrome'

↓

↑Aldosterone

↓

Increased exchange of intratubular Sodium with secreted Potassium ions

Increased exchange of Na^+ with K^+

Na^+ conservation[Q] ***(along with Water)***	***K^+ depletion***
• ***Hypernatermia[Q]*** *(Sodium Conservation)* • ***Hypertension[Q]*** *(diastolic & mild)* • *Polyuria and Polydipsia result from impaired urinary concentrating ability*	• ***Hypokalemia[Q]*** *(Potassium Excretion)* • ***Metabolic alkalosis[Q]*** • *Muscle weakness & fatigue[Q]*

Hypertension without Edema (Edema is typically absent)

'Patients with primary aldosteronism (Conn's syndrome) characteristically do not have edema since they exhibit an "escape" phenomenon from the sodium retaining aspects of mineralocorticoids' – Harrison

Conn's Syndrome is typically associated with low rennin levels

Hyposecretion of rennin that fails to increase appropriately in response to volume depletion is typical

Clinical Features
• *Muscle weakness & fatigue (hypokalemia)* • *Hypertension without edema* • *Polyuria & polydipsia*

Laboratory Features	
• *Hypokalemia* • *Hypernatremia* • *Metabolic alkalosis*	• *↑ Aldosterone* • *Low rennin.*

Conn's syndrome: Criteria For Diagnosis

Criteria for diagnosis of Conn's syndrome

Diagnostic criteria		
Diastolic hypertension without edema	**Hypersecretion of aldosterone** *that does not suppress appropriately in response to volume expansion*	**Low plasma rennin levels** Hyposecretion of rennin *that fails to increase appropriately in response to volume depletion.*

Adrenal Insufficiency (Addison's Disease)

Etiology Of Adrenal Insuficiency or Addison's Disease

Most common cause of Addison's disease in developing countries Q *(Including India)*	*Most common cause of Addison's disease in developed countries* Q
Tuberculosis	*Autoimmune disease (Idiopathic atrophy)*

Addison's disease: Review

Addison's disease or primary adrenocortical deficiency is characterized by primary inability of adrenals to elaborate sufficient quantities of adrenal cortical hormones

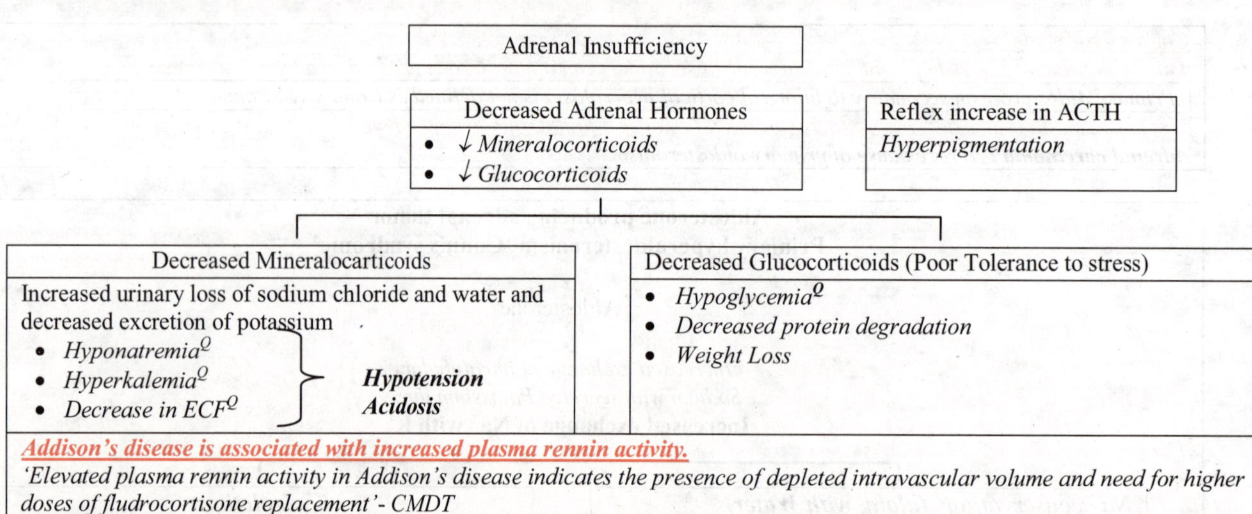

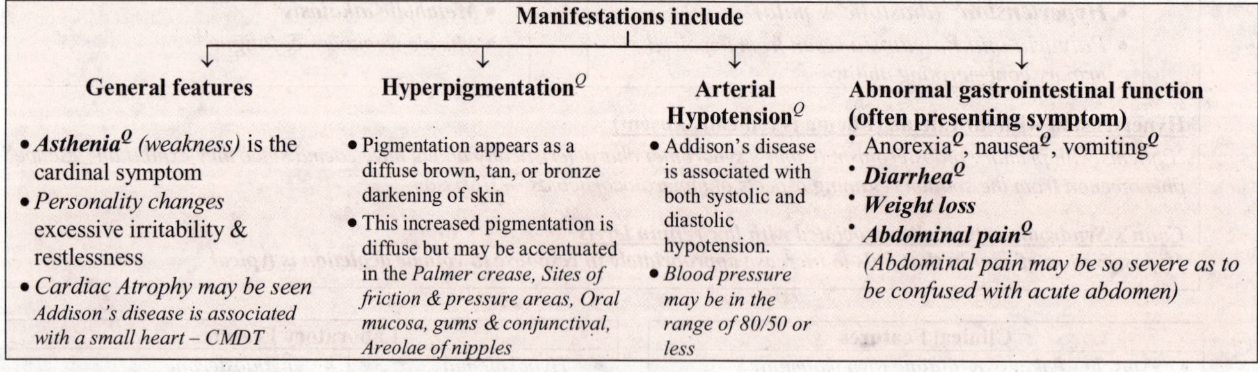

Abnormal Laboratory parameters in Addison's disease include:

Hyponatremia Q	• Loss of sodium in urine due to ↓ Aldosterone
Hyperkalemia Q	• Aldosterone deficiency, Impaired glomerular filtration, Acidosis
Hypercalcemia Q	• Unclear reason
Hypoglycemia Q	
Decreased chloride Q *and Decreased bicarbonate* Q *are also associated*	

Diagnosis of Addison's disease

The diagnosis of Adrenal insufficiency should be made only with ACTH stimulation testing **Cosyntropin stimulation test**

Addison's disease is associated with serum cortisol < 3 mcg/dl

Low plasma cortisol (<3 mcg/dl) at 8:00 AM is diagnostic especially if accompanied by simultaneous elevationof plasma ACTH level (usually > 200 pg/ml).

Diabetes Mellitus (Hyperglycemia)

Criteria for the Diagnosis of Diabetes Mellitus *(American Diabetic Association, 2011)*

Symptoms of Diabetes plus Random blood glucose concentration	*≥11.1 mmol/L (200 mg/dL) or*
Fasting plasma glucose	*≥7.0 mmol/L (126mg/dL) or*
HBAIC	*>6.5% or*
Two-hours plasma glucose (during an oral glucose tolerance test)	*≥11.1 mmol/L (200mg/dL)*

Note: In the absence of unequivocal hyperglycemia and acute metabolic decompensation, these criteria should be confirmed by repeat testing on a different day.

Differences between IDDM and NIDDM

Parameters	Type I (IDDM)	Type II (NIDDM)
Patho-physiological difference	• Results from complete or absolute lack of insulin caused by a **reduction in β cell mass.** Q • *Autoimmunity* Q is the major culprit - Autoantibodies are present Q in blood (against islet cells) - HLA DR3/DR4 are Q expressed in 95% of pt. - (Genetic factors are of low significance)	• Results from insufficient insulin secretion relative to glucose load 'or' '**insulin resistance**' i.e. inability of peripheral tissues to respond to insulin. • *Genetic factor* are the major culprit - No autoantibodies Q - No HLA association Q
Family History	Not significant (present in less than 15% of patients)	Significant (present in upto 90% of patients)
Age	< 40 years Q	> 40 years Q
Habitus	Non obese Q	Obese Q
Presentation	Patient present with **sudden onset** of osmotic symptoms in the form of polydipsia, Polyuria or symptoms of ketoacidosis	Patient present with a more **gradual/insidious onset** Q of **osmotic symptoms** (may not be present) Many of them may be **asymptomatic** Q and are recognized when they develop one of the macrovascular or microvascular symptoms of diabetes like delayed healing of wounds with atherosclerosis or gangrene or peripheral neuropathy etc.
Complication	• Ketoacidosis prone Q	• Ketoacidosis not prone Q (Non ketotic hyperglycemic coma)
Laboratory parameters	• Blood insulin is decreased • Blood glucagon High/ suppressible • Ketonuria: often present	• Insulin levels are normal or may be increased (explained by insulin resistance) • Blood glucagon High/ resistant • Not present
Pathology	• Early insulitis • Marked atrophy and fibrous • Beta cell depletion	• No insulitis • Focal atrophy and amyloid • Mild β cell depletion
Insulin/ C-peptide	• Low	• High
Treatment Protocol	**Nutrition therapy + Exercise** *(to coordinate and match the calorie intake with appropriate amount of insulin)* ↓ **Insulin**	**Nutrition therapy + Exercise** *(to reduce calorie intake, reduce hyperlipidemia and hypertension and promote weight loss)* ↓ **Oral hypoglycemia agents** (often sufficient) If not controlled ↓ Development of Complication (Pregnancy infection surgery) **Insulin** *(usually in complication)*

C – peptide used to distinguish Type I DM from Type II DM[Q]

Type I - DM (IDDM)[Q]	Type – II DM (NIDDM)[Q]
Results from complete / absolute lack of endogenous insulin secretion due to a reduction in β cell mass in pancreas • *Insulin levels are Reduced* • *C- peptide levels are Reduced*	Results from inability of peripheral tissues to respond to Insulin or 'Insulin Resistance' • *Insulin levels are actually increased* • *C- peptide levels are increased*

MODY: Maturity Onset Diabetes of the Young

- MODY is a group of nonn-insulin dependent diabetic syndrome defined by an early onset of diabetes (usually before age of 25 years) and an autosomal dominant inheritance.
- There is β cell dysfunction but in contrast to type II diabetes, obesity and / or insulin resistance is rare.

Diagnostic criteria that help establish diagnosis of MODY include:
• *Early diagnosis of diabetes – before age 25 years in at least one and ideally two family members.* • *Not insulin-dependent – shown by absence of insulin treatment 5 years after diagnosis or significant C-peptide in a patient on insulin treatment.* • *Autosomal dominant inheritance i.e. vertical transmission of diabetes through at least two generations (ideally three generation), with a similar phenotype in cousins or second cousins.* • *Rarely obese (obesity is not required for the development of diabetes)* • *Diabetes results from β-cell dysfunction (insulin levels are often in the normal range, though inappropriately low for the degree of hyperglycemia)*

Differentiating between Type I, Type II Diabetes Mellitus and MODY

	Type I	Type II	MODY
Age of onset	Predominantly young	Predominantly middle to old age	Predominantly young (usually < 25 years)
Family history	Not significant (uncommon)	Significant (Positive) Inheritance is Polygenic / Heterogenous ***Vertical transmission through successive generations is not essential for diagnosis***	Significant (Positive) Inheritance is Monogenic / Autosomal dominant ***Vertical transmission through at least two successive generation (ideally three) is essential for diagnosis.***
Risk of ketoacidosis	High	Low (Uncommon)	Low (Uncommon)
Insulin dependence	Insulin dependent	Non insulin dependent	Non insulin dependent
Obesity	Uncommon (may be present)	Common (may be absent)	Uncommon (may be present)
Pathophysiology	β cells dysfunction (Autoantibodies against β cells) No insulin resistance	β cell dysfunction Insulin resistance	β cell dysfunction No insulin resistance
Fasting 'C' peptide/ Insulin	Low	High	Low

Endocrine causes of Diabetes Mellitus

Endocrinopathies: Hyperglycemia or Diabetes
• *Cushing's syndromes (↑ed cortisol)* • *Acromegaly*[Q] *(↑ GH)* • *Glucagonoma*[Q] *(↑ Glucogen)* • *Pheochromocytoma*[Q] *(↑ catecholamines)* • *Hyperthyroidism*[Q] • *Somatostatinoma* • *Aldosteronoma*[Q]

Management of Uncontrolled Hyperglycemia

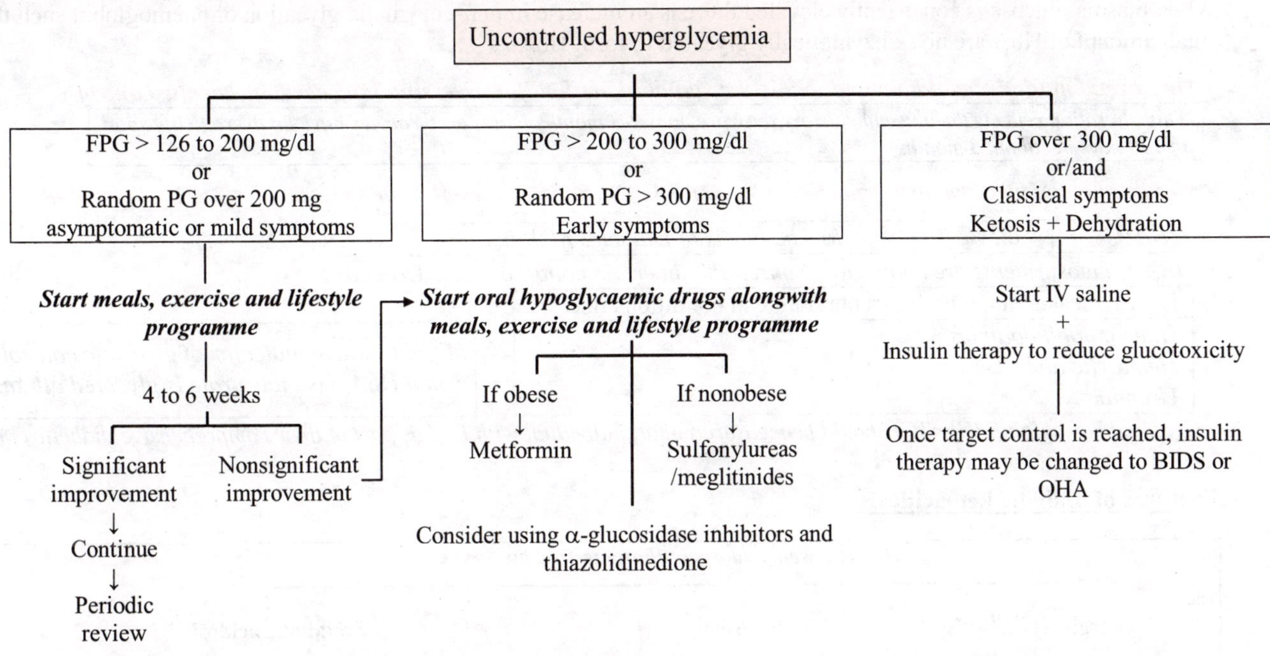

FPG, Fasting Plasma Glucose; OHA, Oral Hypoglycemic Agents; BIDS,

Antihypertensive drugs of choice in patients with diabeties

ACE inhibitors or angiotensin receptor blockers are the first line agents for management of hypertension in diabetics
These have no known adverse effects on glucose or lipid metabolism and minimize the development of diabetic nephropathy by reducing renal vascular resistance and renal perfusion pressure.

ACE inhibitors and Angiotensin Receptor Blockers are specifically indicated to reduce progression of renal disease.

Either ACE inhibitors or ARB's should be used to reduce the progression from microalbuminuria to macroalbuminuria, and the associated decline in GFR.
Drug specific benefit in diabetic nephropathy independent of blood pressure control has been shown only for ACE inhibitors and ARB's in patients with DM – Harrison

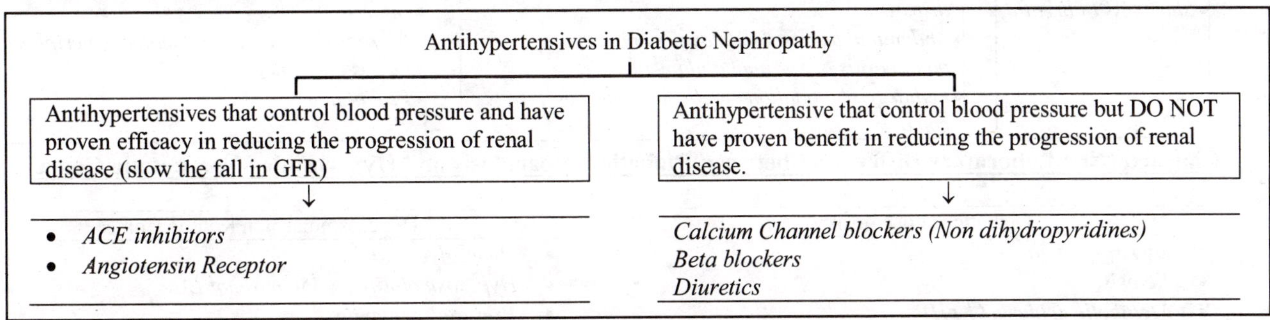

Defination of Terms: Normal and Impaired Glucose Tolerance and Overt Diabetes Mellitus

Definition	Fasting Plasma Glucose (FPG)		Plasma Glucose 2 hours after 75g oral glucose	
	mmol/l	mg/dl	mmol/l	mg/dl
Normal Glucose Tolerance	< 5.6	< 100	<7.8	<140
Impaired Glucose Tolerance	5.6 to 6.9	100-125 (<126)	7.8 – 11.1	140-199
Diabetes Mellitus	≥ 7	≥ 126	> 11.1	>200

Glycosylated Haemoglobin

When plasma glucose is consistently elevated there is an increase in non-enzymatic glycation of haemoglobin such that small amount of HbA are non-enzymatically glycated to form HbA_{1C}.

- ***Measurement of glycated haemoglobin is the standard method for assessing long-term glycaemic control***

This alteration reflects the glycemic history over previous 2-3 months (since erythrocytes have an average life span of 120 days i.e. about 3 months)

- ***Measurement of glycated haemoglobin is now a standard criterion for establishing the diagnosis of Diabetes Mellitus***

HBAIC	*>6.5% (Criterion for diagnosis of Diabetes Mellitus)*

- *HBAIC measurments are known to be unreliable in ertain conditions like Uremia*

HbA_{1C} measurement becomes unreliable in conditions like [Q]
Haemoglobinopathies [Q]
Hemolytic anemia [Q]
Uremia

*An alternative indicator of glycemic control when HbA_{1C} is inaccurate is **glycated albumin*** [Q]

- *Glycated hemoglobin (HbA1C) should be measured in all individual with DM as part of their comprehensive diabetic care*

Features of diabetic ketoacidosis

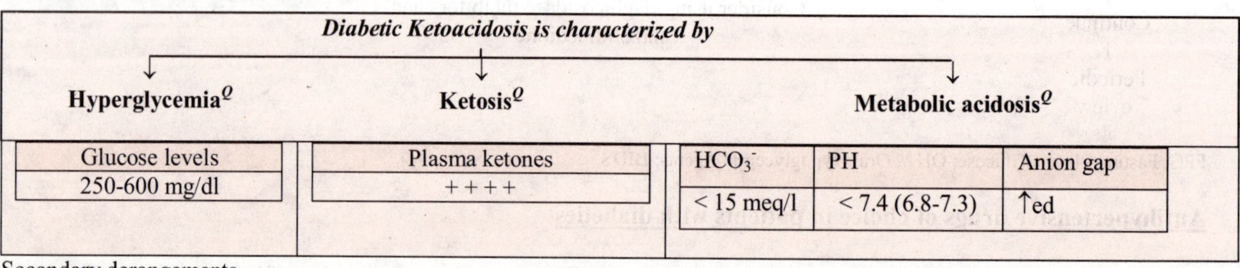

Diabetic Ketoacidosis is characterized by

Hyperglycemia[Q]

Glucose levels
250-600 mg/dl

Ketosis[Q]

Plasma ketones
+ + + +

Metabolic acidosis[Q]

HCO_3^-	PH	Anion gap
< 15 meq/l	< 7.4 (6.8-7.3)	↑ed

Secondary derangements

Sodium	125-135 meq/l	*For every 100 mg elevation of glucose in serum the Na concentration decreases by 3 meq.*

Manifestations of Diabetic Ketoacidosis

Symptoms	**Physical findings**	**Precipitating events**
• *Nausea/Vomiting* • *Thirst/Polyuria* • *Abdominal pain* • *Shortness of breath*	• *Tachycardia* • *Dehydration/hypotension* • *Tachypnea/Kussmaul respirations/respiratory distress* • *Abdominal tenderness (may resemble acute pancreatitis or surgical abdomen)* • *Lethargy/obtundation/cerebral edema/possibly coma*	• *Inadequate insulin administration* • *Infection (pneumonia/UTI/gastroenteritis/sepsis)* • *Infarction (Cerebral, coronary, mesenteric, peripheral)* • *Drugs (cocaine)* • *Pregnancy*

Characteristic Laboratory Differences between Diabetic Ketoacidosis and Hyperosmlar Non-ketotic Coma

Diabetic Ketoacidosis	Hyperosmolar non Ketotic Coma
• *Hyperglycemia*	• *Hyperglycemia*
• *Ketosis*	• *Hyperosmolality (> 350 mosmol/L)*
• ***Metabolic acidosis (↓pH)***	• ***Prerenal Azotemia***

The treatment of Choice for Diabetic Ketoacidosis is Insulin *(DKA cannot be reversed without Insulin)*

Dawn Phenomenon and Somogyi Phenomenon

What causes the "dawn phenomenon"?
The term dawn phenomenon describes a rise in, blood glucose that occurs during the early morning hours (between 5:00 and 8:00 Am), particularly among patients who have normal glucose levels throughout most of the night. The rise in glucose is thought to be due to several factors, including the following: • *The normal increase in the morning cortisol level* • *The cumulative effect of increased nocturnal growth hormone* • *Insulinopenia as a result of the length of time since the last injection* Strategies for managing the dawn phenomenon • Shift more aggressive insulin use to the evening and pre-bedtime hours, using a type of insulin that has a longer duration or peak of action, initiating insulin pump therapy • Not eating a carbohydrate snack at bedtime • Increasing the amount of vigorous physical activity in the evening hours. *The specific strategy or combination of strategies must be tailored to the individual.*

What is Somogyi phenomenon?
The *Somogyi phenomenon* is *rebound hyperglycemia after an incident of hypoglycemia.* This rebound is secondary to the release of counterregulatory hormones, which is the natural response to hypoglycemia. As tighter glucose control is maintained, there is an increased likelihood of hypoglycemia and, therefore, of the Somogyi phenomenon. If the hypoglycemia is recognized and treated promptly, rebound hyperglycemia is less like to occur. Thus, the Somogyi phenomenon is commonly reported more frequently at night because there is the greater likelihood of unrecognized and untreated hypoglycemia when the patient is asleep. **When should the Somogyi phenomenon be suspected?** The Somogyi phenomenon should be suspected when a person whose blood sugar is in excellent control begins to have intermittent high blood glucoses in the morning. *If that pattern is noted, blood glucose should be checked between 2:00 and 3:00 AM on several nights to determine whether hypoglycemia is occurring. If night time hypoglycemia can be documented the likely diagnosis is Somogyi phenomenon.* *This may require the dose or type of evening insulin or the time that the dose is given to be altered.*

Causes of early morning hyperglycemia in diabetics using insulin:

Causes	Frequency	Mechanism	Diagnosis	Treatment
Insufficient insulin	Most common	Inadequate night-time basal insulin dose	Blood glucose rises continuously throughout the night	↑ Night-time intermediate or long-acting insulin dose
Dawn phenomenon	Common	Early morning physiologic surge in growth hormone and cortisol	Blood glucose stable all night, then sharp rise early in the morning	Do not eat a carbohydrate snack at midnight
Somogyi effect	Least common	Excessive night-time basal insulin dose → hypoglycemia in the middle of the night → triggers release of counter-regulatory hormones	Hypoglycemia at 2-3 am*	↓ Night-time intermediate or long-acting insulin dose

*Patients with long-standing DM may not have symptoms of hypoglycemia (discomfort, tremors, sweating, etc) because of autonomic diabetic neuropathy.

Diabetic Nephropathy

Stages of diabetic nephropathy: (IDDM)

Year	Stage	Findings
0	I	Raised GFR, increase in Renal size and plasma flow
2	II	Thickening in glomerular capillary basement membrane
6-10	III	**Microalbuminuria**
10-15	IV	**Overt proteinuria, Clinical nephropathy,** *changes become irreversible.*
16-25	V	End stage renal disease.

- ***Microalbuminuria is the first clinically detectable sign of diabetic nephropathy***

Microalbuminuria	Overt proteinuria
30-300 mg/d in 24 hr urinary sample.	> 300 mg/d in 24 hr urinary sample.

- ***The most reliable indicator for diabetic nephropathy is presence of overt proteinuria.***
  Urinary protein > 550 mg/day in 3 consecutive samples confirms the diagnosis of overt proteinuria, reflects irreversible pathological changes in kidneys and confirms progression to end stage renal disease (diabetic nephropathy)

  Once nephropathy becomes overt the pathological changes are irreversible

- ***Pancreatic transplantation (or β-islet cell transplantation) may improve proteinuria in early stages.***

Pancreatic Trnaplantation may improve diabetic nephropathy (proteinuria)

Successful pancreatic transplantation results in normalization of blood glucose and glycosylated hemoglobin levels.

Complication that may be reversed/halled	Complications that do not appear to be reversed/halled
• *Diabetic nephropathy (microalbuminuria stage)* • *Diabetic Neuropathy*	• *Diabetic retinopathy* • *Peripheral vascular disease*

- **Microalbuminuria is associated with long term cardiovascular morbidity**
  'Both microalbuminuria and macroalbuminuria in individuals with DM are associated with increased risk of cardiovascular disease (morbidity)' – Harrison 17th/2287

- **Strict glycemic control may prevent or revert microalbuminuria**
  'With tight control of hyperglycemia and rigrous control of blood pressure the development of microalbuminuria may be prevented or reverted' – Harrison 13th/1312, Harrison 12th/1185

- **Angiotensin receptor blockers and ACE inhibitors are more effective than other drugs in slowing progression of diabetic nephropathy.**
  Blood pressure control with any agent is extremely important, but a drug specific benefit in diabetic nephropathy, independent of blood pressure control has only been shown for ACE inhibitors or Angiotensin receptor blockers.

- **Protein Restriction is helpful in diabetic nephropathy**
  Protein intake should be restricted in diabetic individuals with microalbuminuria and macroalbuminuria to modest levels

- **Urinary infection may cause false positive microalbuminuria**

- **Diabetic nephropathy does not protect against Diabetic Retinopathy**
  Diabetic nephropathy is usually associated with diabetic retinopathy. In fact, microvascular complications frequently present together, and, therefore, any patient with one microvascular condition should be carefully examined for other microavscular disease.

- **Blood pressure control tends to worsen after the development of diabetic nephropathy.**
  Therefore, tight blood pressure control in individuals with diabetic nephropathy is of prominent importance to avoid further deterioration of renal function.

Hypoglycemia

Endocrinal abnormalities causing altered glucose metabolism include two major categories:

Endocrine deficiency: Hypoglycemia	Other Selected causes of hypoglycemia
• *Decreased cortisol*[Q] *(Addison's disease)*	• *Hepatic congestion*[Q]
• *Decreased growth hormone*[Q]	• *Severe hepatitis*[Q]
• *Decreased glucagons*[Q]	• *Cirrhosis*[Q]
• *Decreased catecholamines*[Q] *(↓ epinephrine)*	• *Hypothermia*[Q]
	• *Glucose-6-phosphatase*[Q]

Tumors associated with Hypoglycemia

Tumors associated with hypoglycemia: *Harrisons 16th/e 2180*	
*1. **Insulinoma***	*3. Hepatoma*
2. Soft tissue sarcomas:	*4. Adrenocortical tumors*
• *Fibrosarcoma*	*5. Carcinoid*
• *Mesothelioma*	*6. Leukaemia/Lymphoma*
• *Rhabelomyosarcoma*	*7. Melanoma*
• *Liposarcoma.*	*8. Teratoma*

Approach to a patient with Hypoglycemia and Increased Insulin levels

- Normally Endogenous Insulin is secreted from β-cells of pancreas in the form of Pro-insulin
- This proinsulin is then broken down to Insulin and C- peptide such that *for each molecule of endogenous insulin, one molecule of C-peptide is produced.*
- C-peptide levels are thus increased whenever endogenous insulin is increased e.g. Insulinomas, Sulfonylureas, Autoimmune processes and in cases of Insulin resistance (type II DM).

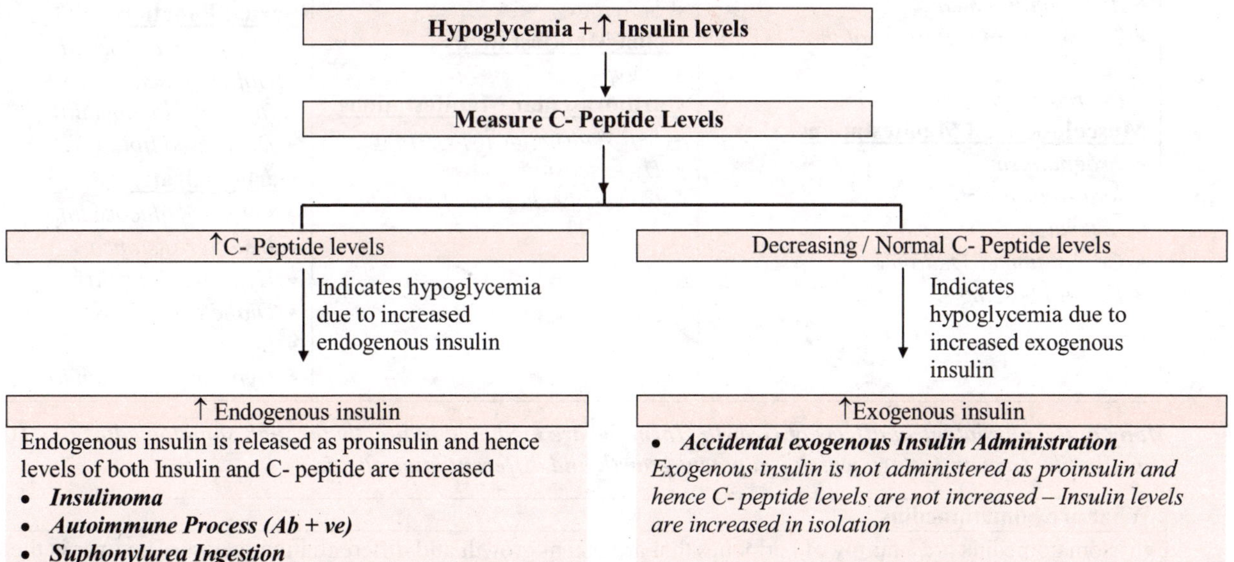

Biochemical Patterns In Patients With Various Causes Of Hyperinsulinemic Hypoglycemia

Diagnosis	Insulin	C Peptide	Proinsulin	Sulfonylurea	Insulin Antibody
Exogenous insulin	↑	↓	↓	-	-
Insulinoma, CHI	↑	↑	↑	-	-
Sulfonylurea	↑	↑	↑	+	-
Insulin autoimmune	↑	↑*	↑	-	+
Insulin receptor autoimmune+	±↑	↓	↓	-	-

**free C Peptide and proinsulin ↓. + Insulin receptor antibody +. CHI, Congenital hyperinsulinism.*

Disorders of Pituitary / Sexual Differentiation

Growth Hormone Hypersecretion (Acromegaly)

Growth Hormone Hypersecretion
IGF-1 Hypersecretion

- Acromegaly and Gigantism are clinical syndromes that result from hypersecretion of Growth Hormone (or somatamedins like IGF-1)

***Acromegaly** results in adults when excessive secretion of GH occurs following epiphyseal closure.*	**Gigantism** occurs is children when excessive secretion of GH occurs prior to epiphyseal closure as a result of increased linear bone growth

- The most common cause for Acromegaly is a Growth Hormone secreting pituitary adenoma[Q] (somatotrope adenoma)

Clinical manifestations of Acromegaly:

Local Tumor Effects	Sleep Disturbances	Visceral Manifestations
• *Visual field defects* • *Cranial nerve palsy (diplopia)* • *Headache* **Somatic Manifestations** • *Acral enlargement* • *Thickening of soft tissue of the hands/feet (increased ring/shoe size)* **Musculoskeletal Manifestations** • *Prognathism* • *Malocclusion* • *Arthralgias* • *Carpal tunnel syndrome* • *Frontal bossing*	• *Sleep apnea* • *Narcolepsy* **Skin Manifestations** • *Hyperhidrosis* • *Skin tags* **Colon Manifestations** • *Polyps* **Cardiovascular Manifestations** • *Left ventricular hypertrophy* • *Hypertension* *Congestive heart failure*	• *Macroglossia* • *Hepatomegaly* • *Splenomegaly* • *Thyroid enlargement* **Sexual Function** • *Menstrual abnormalities* • *Galactorrhea (hyperprolactinemia)* • *Decreased libido* **Carbohydrates** • *Impaired glucose intolerance* • *Insulin resistance* • *Hyperinsulinemia* • *Diabetes mellitus* • *Lipids* • *Hypertriglyceridemia*

Many of the physiological affects of Growth Hormone are mediated indirectly through somatomedins like IGF-1 (Insulin like Growth factor), which is a potent growth and differentiation factor.

What are Somatomedins

- Somatomedins are a family of harmones that are potent growth and differentiation factors. The liver is the major source of somatomedins like IGF-1 that mediates many of the physiological effects of Growth Hormone on target tissues.

Lack of Somatomedins causes Dwarfism

- Somatomedins are similar to insulin in molecular structure and are hence also known as *'Insulin like Growth factors'* (IGF) and these act on target tissue to increase protein synthesis by increasing the rate of uptake of amino acids. *Although GH exerts direct effects on target tissues, many of its physiological effects are mediated indirectly through somatomedins like IGF-1*

Hypersecretion of Growth hormone (gigantism in children; acromegaly in adults) is not associated with Mental Retardation

Diagnosis of Acromegaly

- IGF – I level
  Age and gender matched serum IGF-I level are elevated in Acromegaly.
  Elevated IGF-I levels are *primarily used as a screening test for Acromegaly and not as a confirmatory test.*

- Random GH Assay
  GH secretion is episodic and serum concentrations of GH may fluctuate from undetectable levels to significantly high levels during the day. *Due to pulsalilty of GH secretion, measurement of single random GH level is not useful for the diagnosis or exclusion of Acromegaly.*

- GH suppression test (Failure of GH suppression in response to Glucose load)
  The diagnosis of Acromegaly is confirmed by demonstrating the failure of GH suppression to <1 μg/L within 1-2 hours of an oral glucose load (75g).
  Infact, about 20% of patients exhibit a paradoxical rise in GH levels after glucose.

> - ***The diagnosis of Acromegaly is confirmed by demonstrating the failure of GH suppression after an oral glucose load.***
> - ***In patients with Acromegaly TRH can cause a paradoxical increase in GH secretion[Q] which is not observed in normal individuals.***

Nelson syndrome

- Nelson syndrome is a disorder characterized by rapid enlargement of a preexisting ACTH pituitary adenoma **after adrenalectomy.**
- *This syndrome occurs because following adrenalectomy, the suppressive effect of cortisol on ACTH secretion and tumor growth is removed resulting in increased ACTH secretion and tumor growth.*
- Patients with Nelson's syndrome present with hyperpigmentation and with manifestation of an expanding intrasellar mass lesion (visual field defects, headache, cavernous sinus invasion etc.)
- These tumors represent one of the most aggressive and rapidly growing of all pituitary tumors.
- ACTH levels are markedly elevated.
- Preoperative Radiotherapy may be indicated to prevent development of Nelson's syndrome after adrenelectomy.

Pituitary Apoplexy

Pituitary Apoplexy refers to the clinical syndrome of pan-hypopituitarism arising from hemorrhage or infarction of the pituitary gland.

Causes/Predisposing factors for Pituitary Apoplexy
• *Pre existing Pituitary Adenoma*
• *Pregnancy*
• *Post partum (Sheehan's syndrome)*
• ***Diabetes***
• ***Hypertension***
• ***Sickle cell anemia***
• *Acute shock*
• *Others (Internal Medicine 5th/1778)*   *Trauma, Carotid Angiography, Bleeding/Clotting disorders, Anticoagulant therapy, Radiation to pituitary tumor, Artificial Respiration.*

Hyperprolactinemia

Causes of Hyper-prolactinemia

Etiology of Hyperprolactinemia	
I. **Physiologic hypersecretion**	V. **Hypothalamic-pituitary stalk damage**
A. Pregnancy	A. Tumors
B. Lactation	- Craniopharyngioma
C. Chest wall stimulation	- Suprasellar pituitary mass extension
D. Sleep	- Meningioma
E. Stress	- Dysgerminoma
II. **Pituitary hypersecretion**	- Metastases
A. Prolactinoma	B. Empty sella
B. Acromegaly	C. Lymphocytic hypophysitis
III. **Systemic disorders**	D. Adenoma with stalk compression
A. Chronic renal failure	E. Granulomas
B. Hypothyroidism	F. Rathke's cyst
C. Cirrhosis	G. Irradiation
D. Pseudocyesis	H. Trauma
E. Epileptic seizures	- Pituitary stalk section
IV. **Drug-induced hypersecretion**	- Suprasellar surgery
Refer table below	

Drugs causing Hyper-Prolactinemia include:

- Dopamine receptor antagonists
  - Phenothiazine: chlorpromazine, periphenazine
  - Butyrophenones: haloperidol
  - Thioxanthenes
  - Metoclopramide
  - Resperidone
  - Sulpride
- Dopamine synthesis inhibitors: *α-Methyldopa*
- Catecholamine depletors: *Reserpine*
- Opiates
- H_2 antagonissts : *Cimetidine, ranitidine*
- Imipramines: *Amitriptyline, amoxapine*
- Serotonin-reuptake inhibitors: *Fluoxetine*
- Calcium channel blockers: *Verapamil*

Prolactinomas:

- Prolactinomas are the most common functional pituitary adenomas

> ***'Prolactinomas (Lactotroph Adenomas) are the most frequent type of hyperfunctioning pituitary adenomas, accounting for about 30% of all clinically recognized pituitary adenomas'*** *- Robbins*

- Most common cause of pituitary hormonal syndrome in adults
  'Pituitary adenomas are the most common cause of pituitary hormonal syndromes in adults – Harrison

- *'The functional tumors often produce clinical symptoms of endocrinopathies when they are still small (microadenomas) and restricted to sella. When a tumor grows outside the sella (macroadenoma) it compresses the optic chiasma and nerves and produces a variety of visual defects, the most common being a complete or incomplete bitemporal hemianopia'- API*

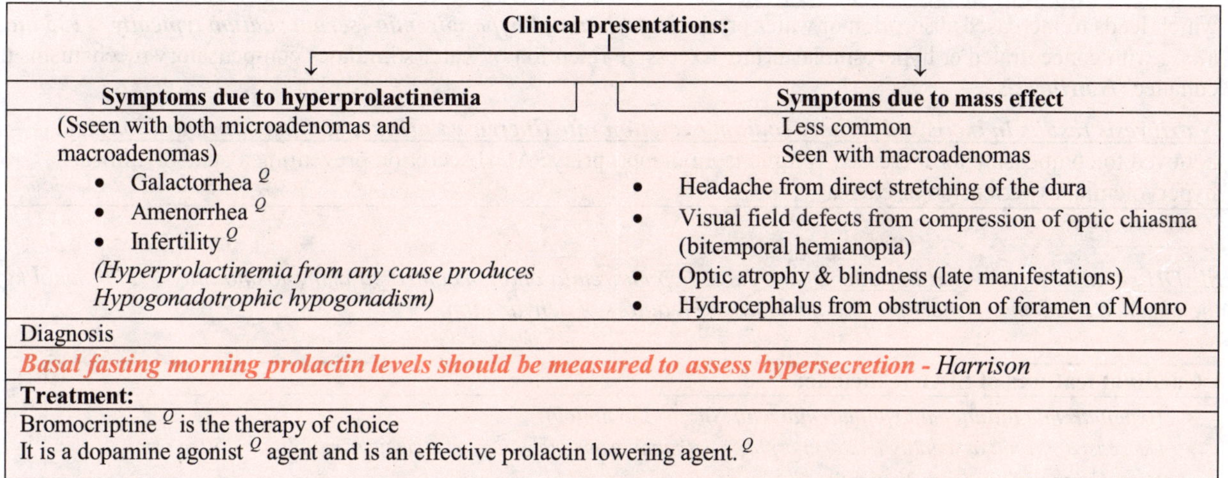

Clinical presentations:

Symptoms due to hyperprolactinemia	Symptoms due to mass effect
(Sseen with both microadenomas and macroadenomas) • Galactorrhea [Q] • Amenorrhea [Q] • Infertility [Q] *(Hyperprolactinemia from any cause produces Hypogonadotrophic hypogonadism)*	Less common Seen with macroadenomas • Headache from direct stretching of the dura • Visual field defects from compression of optic chiasma (bitemporal hemianopia) • Optic atrophy & blindness (late manifestations) • Hydrocephalus from obstruction of foramen of Monro

Diagnosis

Basal fasting morning prolactin levels should be measured to assess hypersecretion *- Harrison*

Treatment:

Bromocriptine [Q] is the therapy of choice
It is a dopamine agonist [Q] agent and is an effective prolactin lowering agent. [Q]

Microprolactinomas are more common than macroprolactinomas [Q]

Treatment of Symptomatic Prolactinomas

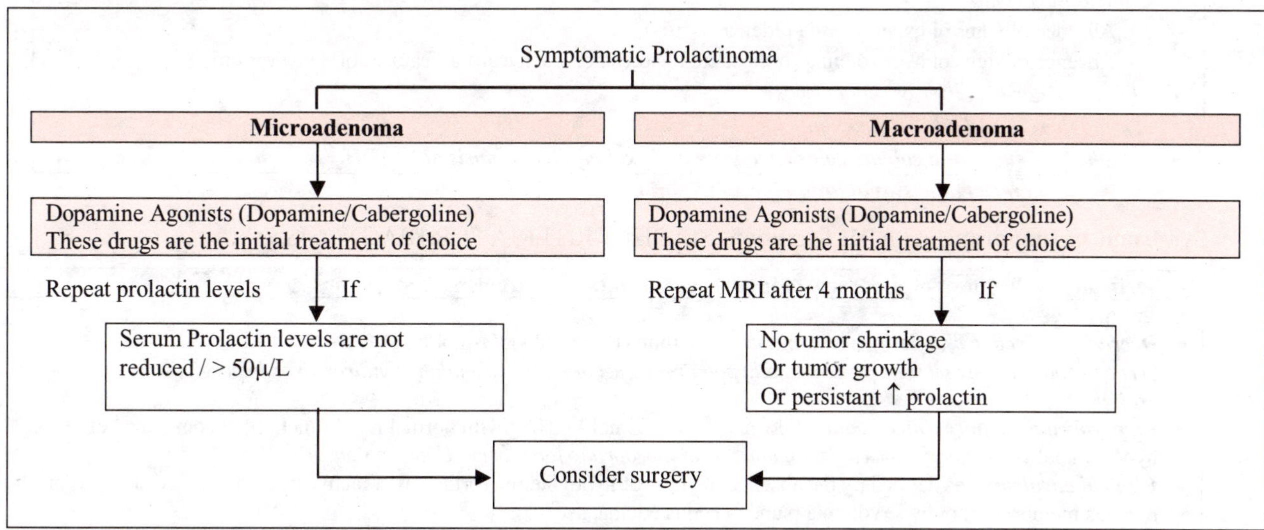

Sheehan's syndrome is post-partum infarction of the pituitary, leading to hypopituitarism.

Treatment of choice for Pan-Hypo-pituitarism

Multiple hormones must be replaced in patients with pan-hypopituitarism, but cortisol replacement is most important

Treatment consists of hormone replacement therapy including ***Glucocorticoids***, Thyroid hormone, Sex steroids, Growth hormone, Vasopressin, etc. Thus, multiple hormones must be replaced, but remember that Cortisol replacement is most important.

SIADH

8

Endocrinology

SIADH

- *The term SIADH is applied to conditions with vasopressin excess. Vasopressin excess is termed inappropriate as this increase occurs despite decreased plasma osmolality.*
- *Increased vasopressin acts on renal tubules, resulting in increased absorption of water (increased total body water), a concentrated urine*[Q] *and decreasing serum osmolality*[Q] *and hyponatremia* [Q].
- *Edema does not occur despite increased total body water* [Q] *(due to unknown reasons) – Clinical Euvolemia*[Q].

Syndrome of Inappropriate ADH Secretion (SIADH) is associated with increased secretion of vasopressin (ADH), which leads to increased absorption of water producing ***dilutional hyponatremia (serum sodium typically < 135 meq/l)*** along with concentrated or hyperosmolar urine. Excessive retention of water stimulates compensatory mechanisms that enhance ***'Natriuresis'***.

Natriuresis results in increased urinary sodium excretion rate (increased urinary sodium concentration) and is believed to compensate for increased volume from inappropriaye ADH secretion preventing a state of clinical hypervolemia, hypertension or edema.

SIADH should be suspected in patients who have hyponatremia and concentrated urine (osmolality > 300 mmol/kg) in the absence of edema, orthostatic hypotension and features of dehydration.

Cardinal features of SIADH include:

- ***Hyponatremia (dilutional hyponatremia with Na+ < 135 mmol/l)***
- *Decreased plasma osmolality (<280 m osm/kg) with inappropriately increased urine osmolality > 150 m osm).*
- ***High Urine sodium (over 20 meq/l)***
- *Low Blood urea Nitrogen < 10 mg/L*
- *Hypouricemia (<4 mg/dL)*
- *Clinical Euvolemia*
  - Absence of signs of hypervolemia (edema, ascitis)
  - Absence of signs of hypovolemia (orthostatic hypotension, tachycardia, features of dehydration)
- *Absence of cardiac, liver or renal disease*
- *Normal thyroid and adrenal function*
- ***A high BUN suggests a volume contracted state and excludes a diagnosis of SIADH.*** [Q]

SIADH is characterized by Euvolemic Hyponatremia.

Syndrome of Inappropriate ADH Secretion (SIADH): CRITERIA FOR DIAGNOSIS

Criteria for the diagnosis of syndrome of innapropriate antidiuretic hormone secretion

Essential

- ***Decreased effective osmolality*** of the extracellular fluid (P_{osm} < 275 mOsmol/kg H_2O).
  (*True hypoosmolality must be present and hyponatremia secondary to pseudohyponatremia or hyperglycemia must be excluded)*
  Inappropriate urinary concentration (Uosm > 100 mOsmol/kg H2O with normal renal function) at some level of hypoosmolality. *(Urinary concentration must be inappropriate for Plasma Hyposmolality)*
- ***Clinical euvolemia***, as defined by the absence of signs of hypovolemia (orthostasis, tachycardia, decreased skin rurgor, dry mucous membranes) or hypervolemia (subcutaneous edema, ascites).
- ***Elevated urinary sodium*** excretion while on normal salt and water intake.
- ***Absence of other potential causes of euvolemic hypoosmolality***: hypothyroidism, hypocortisolism (Addison's disease or pituitary adrenocorticotropic hormone [ACTH] insufficiency) and diuretic use.

Supplemental

- ***Abnormal water load test*** (inability to excrete at least 90% of a 20 mL/kg water load in 4 hours and/or failure to dilute Uosm to < 100 mOsmol/kg H_2O).
- ***Plasma AVP level inappropriately elevated*** relative to plasma osmolality.
- No significant correction of serum $[Na^+]$ with volume expansion but improvement after fluid restriction

Water loading test may be used to help diagnosis of SIADH

Water loading test is recognized as a 'supplemental criteria' in establishing a diagnosis of SIADH.

The 'Water Loading Test' is of value when there is uncertainity regarding the etiology of modest degrees hypo-osmolality in euvolemic patients but it does not add useful information if the plasma osmolality is < 275 mOsm/kg H_2O

Test Objective / Principle	Abnormal Water Loading Test Criteria
Fixed quantity of water is given to a patient and the amount of urine produced and changes in blood/urine osmolality are recorded. *Inability to excrete a normal water load (decreased urinary output) or failure to dilute urine is considered abnormal*	Abnormal water load *Inability to excrete* at least 90% of a 20ml/kg water load in 4 hours, and/or *Failure to dilute* urine (osm) to < 100 mOsm/kg H_2O.

Treatment of SIADH

- *The treatment of choice for SIADH is water restriction.*

  In Acute SIADH, the keystone of treatment is to restrict total fluid intake to less than the sum total of insensible losses and urinary output.
  If more rapid correction of hyponatremia is desired, the fluid restriction can be supplemented by intravenous infusion of hypertonic saline.

- ***The drug of choice for SIADH (when water restriction is unsuccessful) is demeclocycline.***
  [Q]*Demeclocycline (a tetracycline) acts as an ADH antagonist.*
  [Q]***Desmopressin has no role in the management of SIADH***
- **Vaptans are new FDA approved agents for treatment of SIADH**
  'Vaptans' are a new class of drugs that have emerged for treatment of hyponatremia. *These medications act as Vasopressin receptors antagonists blocking the action of AVP* in renal tubule, pituitary or smooth muscles depending upon receptor selectivity.

Conivaptan (Intravenous use)	*Tolivaptan (Oval use)*
Conivaptan is a combined V1/V2 receptor antagonist is *FDA approved for short-term intravenous use for treatment of hospitalized patients with SIADH.*	Tolivaptan is a V2 receptor antagonist that has received *FDA approval for oral use*

Causes of SIADH include:

Neoplasm		**Neurologic**	**Drugs**
Ca Lung Ca Duodenum Ca Pancreas Ca Ovary Ca Bladder, Ca Ureter	Thymoma Mesothelioma *Bronchial adenoma* [Q] Carcinoid Gangliocytoma Ewing's sarcoma	Guillain-Barré-syndrome Multiple sclerosis Delirium tremens Amyotrophic lateral sclerosis Hydrocephalus Psychosis Peripheral neuropathy	Vasopressin or DDAVP Chlorpropamide Oxytocin, high dose *Vincristine* [Q] Carbamazepine Nicotine Phenothiazines Cyclophosphamide Tricyclic antidepressants Monoamine oxidase inhibitors Serotonin reuptake inhibitors
Vascular			
Cerebrovascular occlusions, hemorrhage Cavernous sinus thrombosis			
Infections		**Metabolic**	**Congenital malformations**
Pneumonia, bacterial or viral *Abscess, lung* [Q] or brain Cavitation (aspergillosis) Tuberculosis, lung or brain Meningitis, bacterial or viral Encephalitis AIDS		Acute intermittent porphyria Pulmonary Asthma Pneumothorax Positive-pressure respiration	Agenesis of corpus callosum Cleft lip/palate Other midline defects **Head trauma (closed & penetrating)**

Diabetes Insipidus

Diabetes Insipidus *is a syndrome caused by either deficiency of vasopressin or resistance to action of vasopressin in passage of abnormally large volume of urine of low specific gravity.*

Nephrogenic Diabetes Insipidus *is charachterized by resistance of action of ADH on Renal tubules or unresponsiveness of renal tubules to the action of ADH or Renal Hyposensitivity to action of ADH.*

Central diabetes insipidus *is a syndrome caused by deficient secretion of AVP from the pituitary resulting in production of abnormality large volume of dilute urine.*

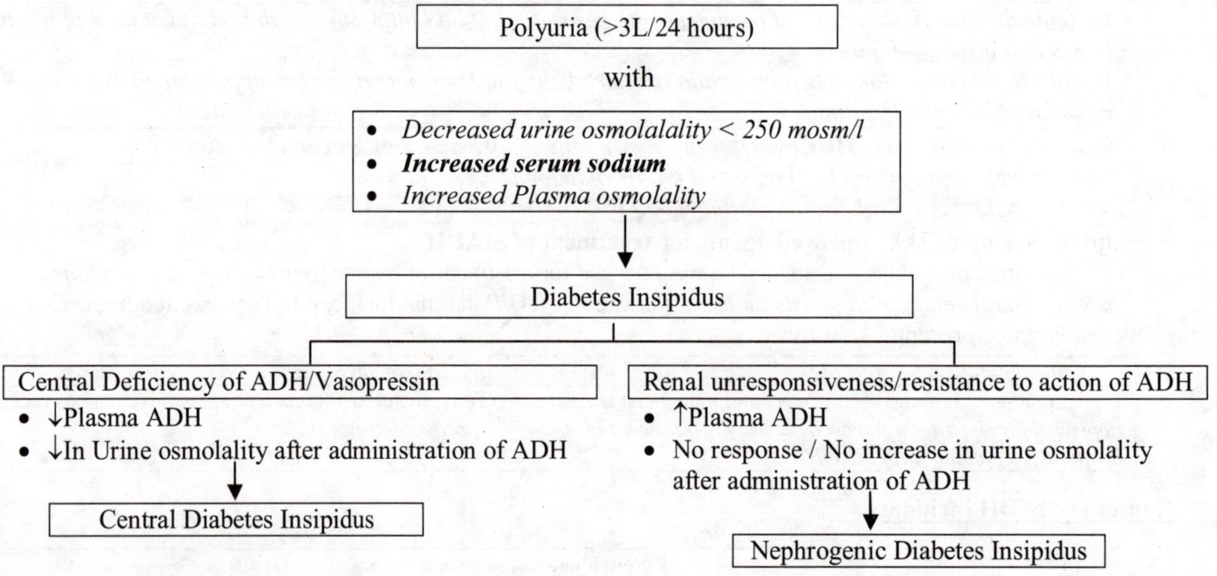

Clinical and Laboratory correlates in diabetes insipidus

1.	Passage of Large volume of urine	: 24 hr urine volume > 50 ml/kg body weight
2.	Passage of dilute urine	: **Urine osmolality** < 300 mosm/L

Effects on plasma osmolarity: (Normal serum osmolarity = 285-295 mosm/kg water).

Polyuria in DI results in a small decrease in plasma osmolarity and sodium concentration. These in turn stimulate thirst and a compensatory increase in water intake, which tend to bring the osmolarity towards normal.

Thus, the *serum osmolality may be normal or undergo a slight increase (because fluid from body is lost) however it never falls. Therefore we cannot expect osmolality of serum to be less than 285.*

Water deprivation test is often required to establish a diagnosis of Diabetes insipidus

Water deprivation test is indicated in patients with hypotonic polyuria (Uosm < 300 mosm/kg) and a plasma osmolality within the normal range (Posm = 275 – 295 mosm/kg) to establish the diagnosis of diabetes insipidus and differentiate central & nephrogenic forms.

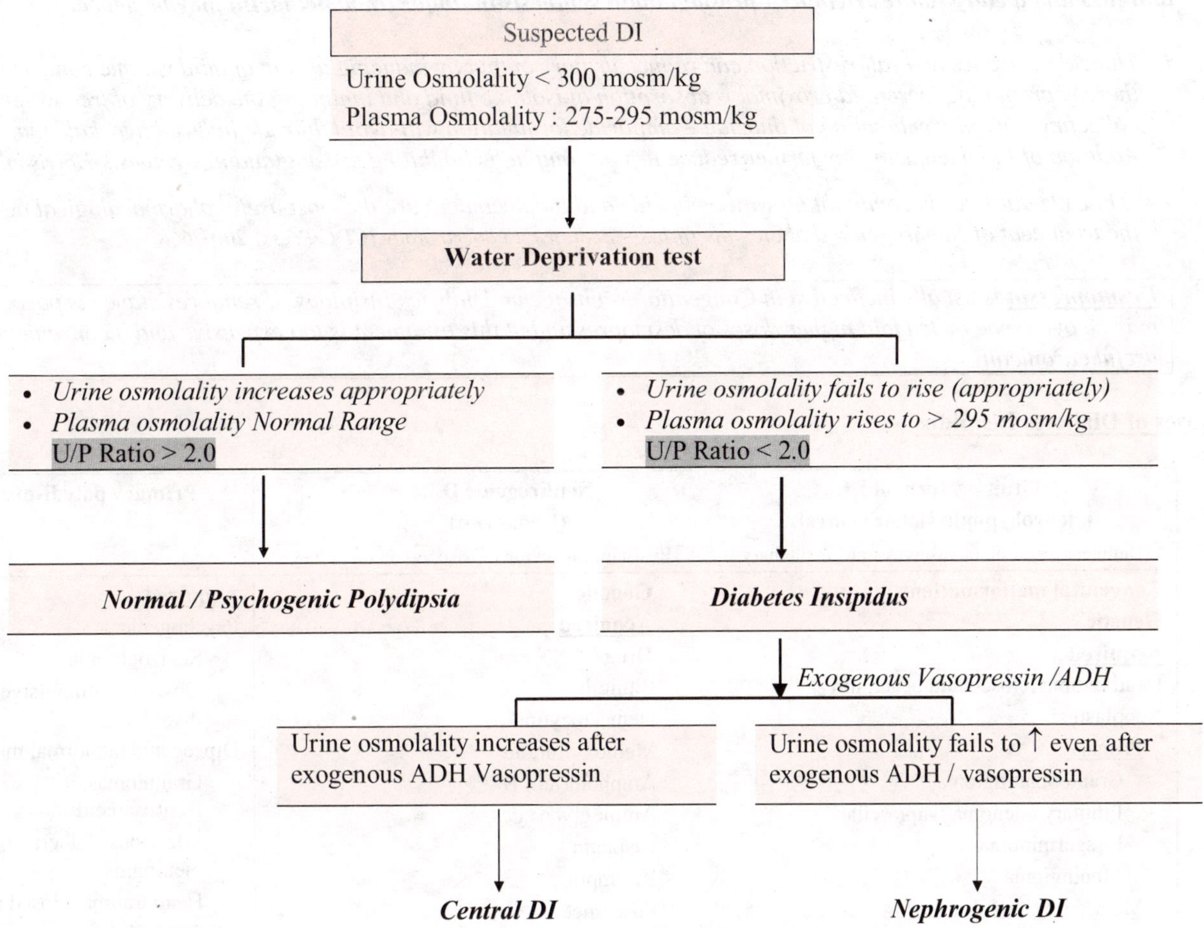

Water Deprivation Test should be performed when plasma osmolality is < 300 mosm/kg

- Water Deprivation Test is indicated in patients with hypotonic polyuria *(urine osmolality < 300 mosm /kg) and a plasma osmolality within the normal range (Plasma osmolality = 275 -295 mosm/kg)* to decide whether hypotonic polyuria is caused by Primary Polydipsia or Diabetes Insipidus

– 'Washington manual of Endocrinology' 2nd/22

- Low serum osmolality (< 270 mosm/kg) in a patient with hypotonic polyuria (Uosm < 300 mosm/kg) suggests a diagnosis of Psychogenic polydipsia and *water deprivation test is not always required*
- High serum osmolality (> 300 mosm/kg) in a patient with hypotonic polyuria (Uosm < 300 mosm /kg) suggests a diagnosis of Diabetes Insipidus and *water deprivation test in not always required*

'Water deprivation test should be performed when the plasma osmolality is < 300 mosm/kg'

– Partha's Fundamentals of Pediatrics 1st/504

'If initial serum osmolality is < 300 mosm/kg patient should undergo a water deprivation test to establish the diagnosis of Diabetes Insipidus and to defferentiatic central & Nephrogenic forms'

– Pediatric Endocrine Disorders 1st (2007) /295

Treatment of Central Diabetes Insipidus

Desmopressin is the drug of choice for Central / Neurogenic diabetes insipidus.

Treatment of Nephrogenic Diabetes Insipidus

The treatment of Nephrogenic Diabetes Insipidus is usually achieved through a combination of thiazide / amiloride diureties and dietary salt restriction. A prostaglandin synthesis inhibitor (indomethacin) may be added.

- *Thiazide diuretics and salt restriction can reduce urinary output by inducing a state of mild volume contraction thereby promoting increased proximal reabsorption of isotonic fluid and inhibiting the delivery of free water to the collecting duct. A combination of thiazide – amiloride formulation will avoid thiazide induced hypokalemia. Addition of Indomethacin may further reduce urinary output by inhibiting prostagländing synthesis-Harrison*
- *'Thiazide diuretics in combination with amiloride and indomethacin are the most useful pharmacological agents in the treatment of Nephrogenic diabetes insipidus'- Pediatric Endocrinology (CDC Press) 2007/668*

> ***Desmopressin*** *is usually ineffective in Congenital Nephrogenic Diabetes Insipidus. If renal resistance is partial, it may be overcome by ten fold higher doses of desmopressin but this treatment is too expensive and inconvenient to be useful chronically.*

Causes of Diabetes Insipidus

Pituitary form of DI **(Neurohypophysial or central)** Deficient secretion of vasopressin from pituitary	**Nephrogenic D.I.** **(Renal D.I.)** Resistance to action of vasopressin on kidney	**Primary polydispisa**
Congenital malformations **Genetic** **Acquired** Head trauma (closed and penetrating) Neoplasms Primary Craniopharyngioma Pituitary adenoma (suprasellar) Dysgerminoma Meningioma Metastatic (lung, breast) Hematologic (lymphoma, leukemia) Granulomas: Neurosarcoid Histiocytosis Xanthoma disseminatum Infectious: Chronic meningitis Viral encephalitis Toxoplasmosis Inflammatory:Lymphocytic Infundibuloneurohypophysitis Wegener's granulomatosis Lupus erythematous Scleroderma Chemical toxins: Tetrodotoxin, Snake venom Vascular:Sheehan's syndrome Aneurysm (internal carotid) Aortocoronary bypass Hypoxic encephalopathy Pregnancy (vasopressinase) Idiopathic	**Genetic** **Acquired** Drugs Lithium Demeclocyline Methoxyflurane Amphotericin B Aminoglycosides Cisplatin Rifampin Foscarnet Metabolic Hypercalcemia, hypercalcinuria Hypokalemia Obstruction (ureter or urethra) Vascular Sickle cell disease and trait Ischemia (acute tubular necrosis) Granulomas Neurosarcoid Neoplasms Sarcoma Infiltration Amyloidosis Pregnancy Idiopathic	**Acquired** Psychogenic Schizophrenia Obsesive-compulsive disorder Dipsogenic (abnormal thirst) Granulomas: Neurosarcoid Infectious: Tuberculous meningitis Head trauma (closed and penetrating) Demyelimation: Multiple sclerosis Drugs: Lithium Carbamazepine Idiopathic Iatrogenic

Psychogenic polydipsia and Distinction with Diabetes Insipidus

Psychogenic polydipsia: *Kumar & Clarke 5th/ 1058*

- Psychiatric disturbance characterized by excessive intake of water
- Plasma sodium and osmolality fall and urine produced is appropriately dilute
- Vasopressin levels become almost undetectable
- Characteristically the diagnosis is made by a water deprivation test. The initially low urine molarity gradually increases with the duration of water deprivation.

Approach to a patient with Polyuria: Diabetes insipidus , Psychogenic Polydipsia, Osmotic Diuresis

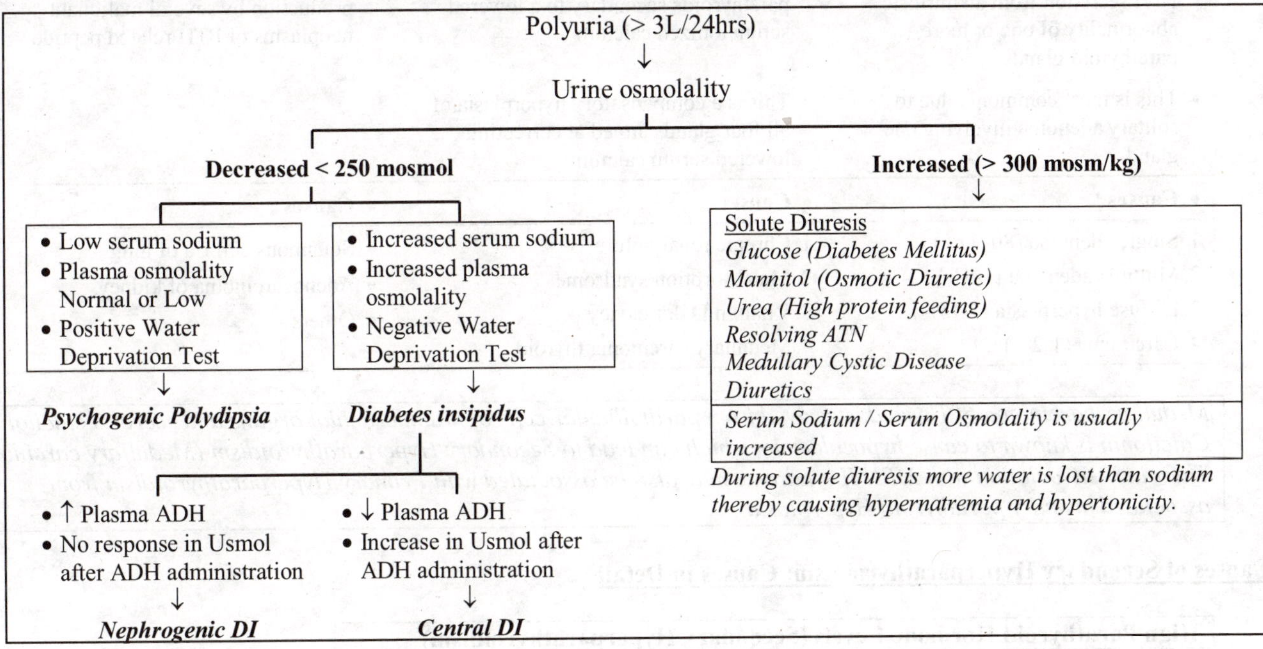

Laboratory differentiation of polyyuria

Laboratory Studies in Cases of Polyuria: Diabetic Insipidus (DI) versus Primary Polydipsia:

	Central DI	**Nephrogenic DI**	**Primary Polydipsia**
Serum Sodium	*Increased*	*Increased*	*Normal or decreased*
Plasma osmolality	*Increased or normal*	*Increased or normal*	*Decreased or normal*
Urine osmolality	*Decreased*	*Decreased*	*Decreased*
Urine osmolality during H_2O deprivation	*No change*	*No change*	*Increased*
Urine osmolality after dDAVP	*Increased*	*No change*	*Increased*
Plasma ADH	*Low*	*Normal to high*	*Low*

dDAVP= D-desaminoarginine vasopressin; ADH = antidiuretic hormone

Disorders of Calcium Metabolism

Hyperparathyroidism

- *The most common cause of primary hyperparathyroidism is a parathyroid adenoma.*
- *A single/solitary abnormal gland is the cause in approximately 80% of patients – Harrison*
- *The most common cause of primary hyperparathyroidism is a Solitary Parathyroid Adenoma* [Q]
- The abnormality of the gland is *usually a benign neoplasm or 'adenoma'* and rarely a parathyroid carcinoma.
- Adenomas are most commonly located in the *inferior parathyroid gland.* [Q]

Causes of hyperparathyroidism can be grouped into three categories

Primary hyperparathyroidism	Secondary hyperparathyroidism	Ectopic parathyroid hormone syndrome
• Elevated PTH due to increased PTH secretion from an intrinsic abnormality of one or more parathyroid glands • This is most commonly due to solitary adenoma involving one gland	• Excessive secretion of PTH by parathyroids secondary to a lowered serum ionized calcium • This is a compensatory hyperplasia of all four glands aimed at correcting lowered serum calcium	• Ectopic PTH syndrome results from the production by several malignant neoplasms of PTH related peptide
• **Causes**	• **Causes**	• **Causes**
1. Single adenoma (80-90%) 2. Multiple adenoma (1-4%) 3. Diffuse hyperplasia (3-15%) 4. Carcinoma (1-2%)	1. Chronic renal failure 2. Malabsorption syndrome 3. Vitamin D deficiency 4. Medullary carcinoma thyroid	• Squamous cell Ca of lung • Adenocarcinoma of kidney. • Others

Medullary carcinoma of Thyroid is derived from parafollicular cells of ultimobrachial organs and secretes calcitonin. Calcitonin is known to cause hypocalcemia, which can lead to Secondary Hyperparathyroidism (Medullary carcinoma Thyroid in association with MEN II syndrome may also be associated with Primary Hyperparathyroidism from associated primary parathyroid Hyperplasia).

Causes of Secondary Hyperparathyroidism: Causes in Detail

High Parathyroid Hormone Levels (Secondary Hyperparathyroidism)

Vitamin D deficiency or impaired 1, 25$(OH)_2$D production /action

- ***Nutritional vitamin D deficiency (Rickets/Osteomalacia)***
- ***Renal insufficiency with impaired 1, 25(OH)2D production***
- *Vitamin D resistance, including receptor defects*

Parathyroid hormone resistance syndromes

- *PTH receptor mutations*
- *Pseudohypoparathyroidism (G protein mutatins)*

Drugs

- *Calcium chelators*
- *Inhibitors of bone resorption (bisphosphonates, plicamycin)*
- *Altered vitamin D metabolism (phenytoin, ketoconazole)*

Miscellaneous causes

- *Acute pancreatitis*
- *Acute rhabdomyolysis*
- *Hungry bone syndrome after parathyroidectomy*
- *Osteoblastic metastases with marked stimulation of bone formation (prostate cancer)*

Clinical Presentation

There is a great variation in the manifestation of hyperparathyroidism

Manifestation may be with multiple signs and symptoms
- *Recurrent nephrolithiasis* [Q]
- *Peptic ulceration* [Q] *(abdominal pain)*
- *Extensive bone resorption*
- *Mental changes; Psychiatric manifestations.*

'Manifestation may be subtle and the disease many have a benign course with no symptoms and signs other than ***hypercalcemia*** *and elevated level of PTH'*

'Subtle presentation' may simulate 'asymptomatic hypercalcemia'

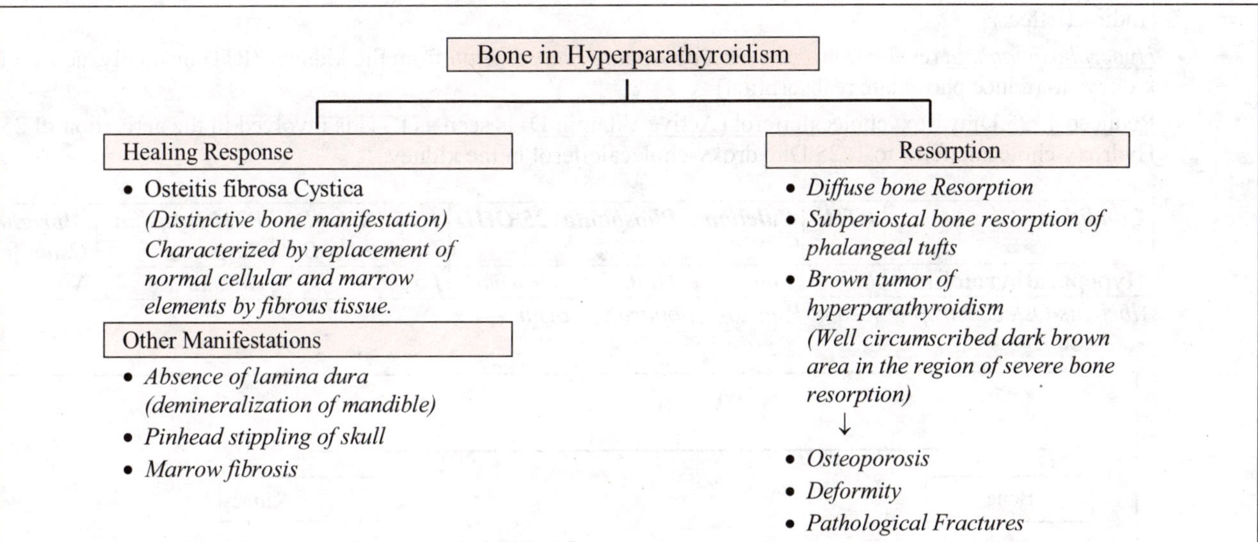

Diagnosis / Investigations

Condition	Serum Ca^{++}	Serum Phosphate	Serum PTH	Alk. Phosphate
Secondary Hyper- PTH	N or ↓ (Rarely ↑)	N (↓↑)	↑	N (↑)
Primary Hyper-PTH	↑	↓	↑	↑

Markers of hyperparathyroidism (↑ed PTH):

1. **Increased serum calcium:**
   - Stimulates Vit D which causes increased absorption of Ca^{++} from gut
   - Increased calcium reabsorption from tubules
   - Increases osteoblastic activity in bones and mobilizes calcium from bone into serum.
2. **Decreased serum phosphorus:**
   - PTH acts on tubules to increase excretion of phosphorus.
3. **Increased 24 hr urine calcium:**
   - Despite increased reabsorption of Ca^{++} in renal tubules urinary calcium is increased owing to increased filtration of calcium in glomerular filtrate.
4. **Increased Alkaline phosphatase:**
   - Increased resorption of bone leads to compensatory elevation of osteoblastic activity
5. **Radiological changes:**
   - Subperiosteal resorption of phalanges is characteristic (hand X Rays are always advised)
   - Bone resorption i.e. osteitis fibrosa et cystica (brown tumours)
   - 'Salt pepper' or 'pepper pot skull' appearance
   - Loss of lamina dura

The Rugger Jersey spine refers to band like osteosclerosis of the superior and inferior margin of the vertical body. Rugger Jersey Spine is characteristically seen in chronic renal failure due to secondary hyperparathyroidism or Renal osteodystrophy.

Hypoparathyroidism

Hypoparathyroidism

(Low calcium, High phosphate, Low 1, 25 Dihydroxycholecalciferol).

- Hypoparathyroidism is a disorder of mineral metabolism caused by diminished secretion of PTH from the parathyroid glands.
- *Hypocalcemia* results from *decreased mobilization* of calcium from bone, and *reduced renal reabsorption* of calcium (Direct effect) In addition, PTH deficiency results in impairment of renal 25 (OH) D-1-hydroxylase activity which limits serum calcitriol concentration and thereby *diminishes gastrointestinal calcium absorption* (Indirect effect)
- *Hyperphosphatemia* results from *increased phosphate reabsorption* from the kidneys (PTH normally, acts on the kidneys to reduce phosphate reabsorption)
- Reduced 1, 25 Dihydroxycholecalciferol (Active Vitamin D) is seen as PTH is involved in the activation of 25 Hydroxy-cholecalciferol to 1, 25 Dihydroxy-cholecalciferol in the kidney.

Condition	*PTH*	*Calcium*	*Phosphate*	*25 OHD*	*1'25 $(OH)_2$ D3 (Active Vit D3)*	*PTH Infusion Response*	*Albrights Osteodystrophy*
Hypoparathyroidism	*Low*	***Low***	***High***	*Normal*	*Low*	*Normal*	*No*

Albrights Osteodystrophy seen in Pseudo-hypoparthyroidism

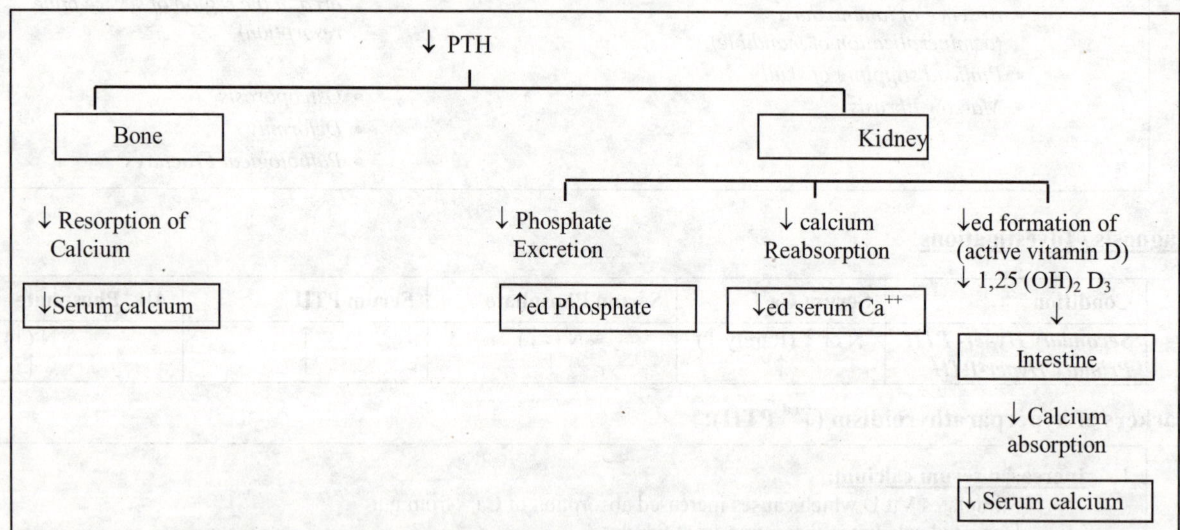

Pseudohypoparathyroidism

- This is a hereditary disorder associated with ***signs and symptoms of hypoparathyroidism despite an elevated PTH*** level *(Hence called pseudohypoparathyroidsm)*
- This is produced as a result of deficient end organ response to PTH
- The most common form of Pseudo hypoparathyroidism (PHP-1a) occurs in association with Albrights Hereditary Osteodystrophy and presents with distinctive skeletal and developmental defects

Laboratory Features	Distinctive skeletal & Development defects (Hereditary Albright's Osteodystrophy (AHO))
• *↑PTH* • *Hypocalcemia* } *features of* • *Hyperphosphatemia* } *hypoparathyroidism* • *Normal/Decreased response of urinary CAMP to PTH*	• *Short stature* • *Round face* • ***Brachydactyly*** *(short 4th/5th metacarpals and metacarpals)* • *Heterotopic calcification* • *Exostosis and Radius curves* • *Impairment in olfaction & taste*

Classification of Pseudo-hypoparathyroidism and Pseudo-pseudo-hypoparathyroidsm *(Harrison)*

Various diverse forms of Pseudohypoparathyroidism (PHP) are recognized based upon certain charachteristics like urinary cyclic AMP response to exogenous PTH, presence or absence of Albright's Hereditary Osteodystrophy (AHO) and assays of concentration of the $G_{S\alpha}$ subunit of the adenylate cyclase enzyme.

Type	Hypocalcemia, hyperphosphatemia	Response of Urinary cAMP to PTH	Serum PTH	Gsα Subunit Deficiency	AHO	Resistance to Hormones in Addition to PTH
PHP-Ia	Yes	↓	↑	Yes	Yes	Yes
PHP-Ib	Yes	↓	↑	No	No	No
PHP-II	Yes	Normal	↑	No	No	No
PPHP	No	Normal	Normal	Yes	Yes	±

Note

Pseudo Pseudo Hypoparathyroidism (PPHP) refers to a subset of patients who carry the abnormal GNAS1 mutation / $G_{S\alpha}$ subunit deficiency and have the distinctive skeletal features of Herediatary Albright's osteodystrophy, but do not show any evidence of endocrine or biochemical disturbance.

- ***The most common subtype of Pseudohypoparathyroidism (PHP-Ia) is typically associated with reduced / decreased cAMP production in response to exogenous PTH***

  Pseudohypoparathyroidism is associated with decreased formation of cyclic AMP and not decreased cyclic GMP or Inositol Triphosphate

- ***Pseudohypoparathyroidism(Ia) results from an inherited 'loss of function' mutation of the Gs_α subunit***

Gs_α inactivating mutation ('Loss of function')	*Pseudohypoparathyroidism(Ia)*

Taken from 'Principles & practice of Endocrinology and Metabolism' by Becher 3rd/595

Differential Diagnosis of conditions causing Hypocalcemia by key test results

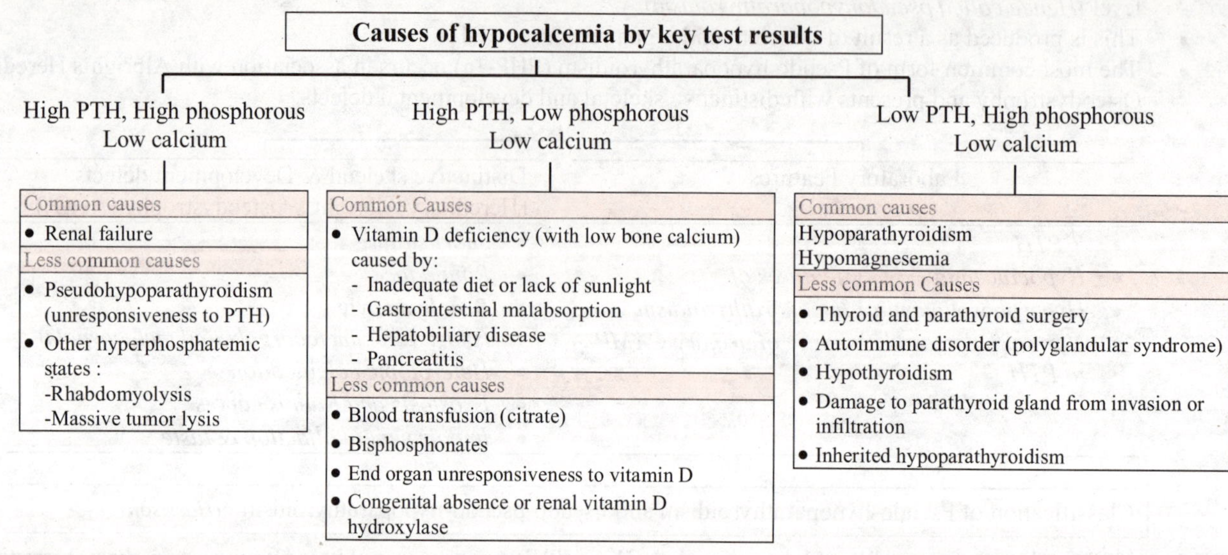

Differential Diagnosis of various conditions based on Key test results

	Serum Ca	Serum phosphorus	Alkaline phosphatase	PTH
• Osteomalacia (Rickets) (↓Vit. D)	↓	↓	↑	↑
• Primary hyperparathyroidism bone disease	↑	↓	↑	↑
• Bone disease in renal failure with secondary hyperparathyroidism	N/↓	↑	↑	↑
• Lytic bone neoplasms	N/↑	N/↑	N/↑	N
• ***Osteoporosis***	***N***	***N***	***N***	***N***
• Paget's disease	N	N	↑	N

Differential Diagnosis for Asymptomatic Hypercalcemia

The most likely cause of asymptomatic hypercalcemia in a patient aged 30 years is primary hyperparathyroidism. Familial hypocalciuric hypercalcemia is most often detected in the first ten years of life when hypercalcemia due to primary hyperparathyroidism is a rarity.

Both primary hyperthyroidism and familial hypocalciuric hypercalcemia may present with asymptomatic hypercalcemia.

The 'catch' in most questions lies in the 'age' of the patient

Primary hyperparathyroidism	Familial hypocalciuric hypercalcemia (F.H.H.) *(autosomal dominant)*
• The most common presentation in patients with primary hyperparathyroidism is '***asymptomatic' hypercalcemia***	• Affected individuals are discovered because of ***asymptomatic hypercalcemia***
• Commonly presents in ***third to fifth decade***	• Commonly presents in the ***first decade***

Hypercalcemia

Causes of Hypercalcemia:

Excessive PTH production
• *Primary hyperparathyroidism (adenoma, hyperplasia, rarely carcinoma)* • *Tertiary hyperparathyroidism (long-term stimulation of PTH secretion in renal insufficiency)* • *Ectopic PTH secretion (very rare)* • *Inactivating mutations in the CaSR **(Familial Hypercalciuric Hypercalcemia)*** • *Alterations in CaSR function **(Lithium therapy)***
Hypercalcemia of malignancy
• Overproduction of PTHrP (many solid tumors) • ***Lytic skeletal metastases (breast, myeloma)***
Excessive 1,25(OH)2D production
• Granulomatous diseases (sarcoidosis, tuberculosis, silicosis) • Lymphomas • Vitamin D intoxication
Primary increase in bone resorption
• Hyperthyroidism • Immobilization
Excessive calcium intake
• Milk-alkali syndrome • ***Total parenteral nutrition***
Other causes
• Endocrine disorders (adrenal insufficiency, pheochromocytoma, VIPoma) • Medications (thiazides, vitamin A, antiestrogens)

CaSR, calcium sensor receptor; FHH, familial hypocalciuric hypercalcemia; PTH, parathyroid hormone; PTHrP, PTH-related peptide.

Parathyroid related	Vitamin D related
• *Primary hyperparathyroidism* Q • ***Lithium therapy*** Q • Familial hypercalciuric hypercalcemia	• Vitamin D intoxication • Increased 1, 25 $(OH)_2$ D eg. *Sarcoidosis*Q***;*** other granulomatous ds. • Idiopathic hypercalcemia of infancy
Malignancy related	**Associated high bone turnover**
• Solid tumor with metastasis (Breast) • Solid tumor with paraneoplastic syndromes (Carcinoma Breast/Lung /Kidney etc.) • Hematological malignancies: ***Multiple myeloma***Q / Lymphoma / Leukemia • Pheochoromocytoma (rare) • MEN syndromes	• *Hyperthyroidism*Q • *Immobilization*Q • *Thiazides*Q • ***Vitamin A intoxication***Q • *Paget's disease* **Associated With *Renal Failure*Q** • Severe secondary hyper-parathyroidism • Aluminum intoxication • Milk Alkali syndrome

Q*Celiac disease is not a cause for hypercalcemia.*

Q*Hyperparathyroidism, Sarcoidosis and Milk alkali syndrome, may all lead to hypercalcemia.*

Q*Acute Pancreatitis is associated with hypocalcemia (not hypercalcemia)*

Q*Phenytoin toxicity is associated with hypocalcemia. Phenytoin desensitizes target tissues to vitamin D and produces hypocalcemia (Osteomalacia).*

Q*Primary hyperparathyroidism is a cause for hypercalcemia*Q *– Harrison*

Q*Multiple myeloma also causes hypercalcemia* Q *– Harrison*

Q*Sarcoidosis may be associated with Hypercalcemia (Hypercalciuria with or without hypercalcemia* is seenQ *– Harrison)*

Q*Tumorlysis syndrome is associated with Hypocalcemia*

Clinical Features of Hypercalcemia

Manifestations of Hypercalcemia

General	Renal feature	Bones	Abdomen	Cardiac	Calcification
• Anorexia • Nausea • Vomiting • Fatigue • Depression • Mental confusion (≅ altered sensorium)	• Polyuria* & Nocturia • Renal colic from stones	• Bone pain • When cause is hyperparathyroidism • Bone cysts • Brown tumors	• Abdominal pain (peptic ulceration) • Constipation	• Short QT interval in ECG & in some patients cardiac arrythmias	Ectopic calcification & chondrocalcinosis

* **Polyuria** results from effect of hypercalcemia on renal tubules reducing there concentrating ability a form of nephrogenic diabetes insipidus

Management of Hypercalcemia

Principles

- The first principle of treatment is to restore normal hydration [Q] as most hypercalcemia patients are dehydrated because of vomiting and polyuria etc.
- After rehydration has been achieved, saline can be administered
- Loop diuretics such as furosemide & ethacrynic acid can then be administered to depress tubular calcium resorption and enhance calcium excretion. ***Thiazide diuretics are not to be used.***
- Glucocorticoids have antitumor effect and are especially useful in hypercalcemia complicating malignancies.
- Dialysis is the treatment of choice for severe hypercalcemia complicating renal failure.
- Phosphate therapy - Correcting hypophosphatemia lower serum calcium sometimes strikingly.

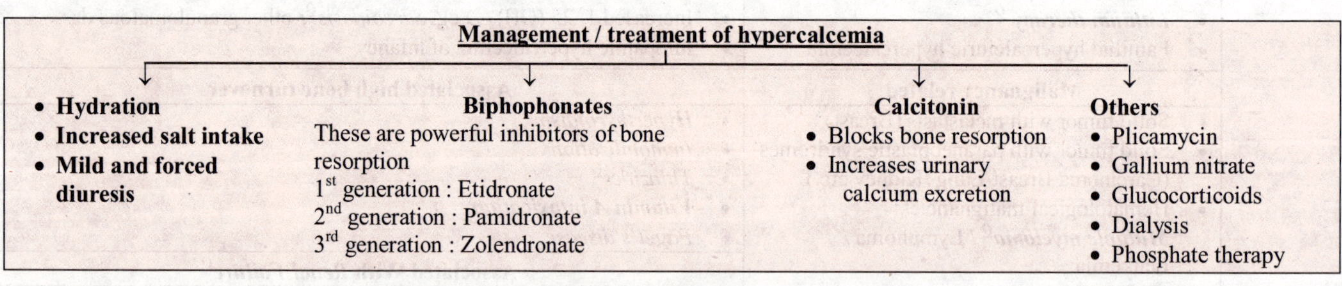

Onset of Action of Therapy for Severe Hypercalcemia

Immediate (Hours)	*Delayed (days)*
• *Hydration with **saline*** • *Loop diuretics **(Furosemide)** – once rehydrated* • *Calcitonin* • *Intravenous Phosphate* • ***Dialysis***	• ***Bisphosphonates*** • *Glucocorticoids* • *Gallium Nitrate*

Gallium Nitrate exerts s hypocalcemic effect by inhibiting calcium resorption from bone. Maximum hypocalcemic effect of gallium nitrate may take 3-4 days to appear and it is not often used now because of availability of superior alternatives.

Tumour Lysis Syndrome

Tumor lysis syndrome:

It is a clinical entity characterized by destruction of large number of rapidly proliferating neoplastic cells following chemotherapy.

Rapid lysis of tumor cells after chemotherapy **(Tumor Lysis Syndrome)**[Q]

- *Release of uric acid* [Q] from rapid turn-over nucleic acids.
  - Hyperuricemia[Q]
- Uric acid may precipitate in tubules, medulla and collecting duct
- ***Renal failure*** [Q]

- Release of intracellular Phosphate
  - Hyperphosphatemia[Q]
- Increased phosphate drives calcium into bone
  - Hypocalcemia [Q]
- Calcium phosphate may deposit in renal tubules
  - Renal failure
- Release of Intracellular Magnesium
  - Hypermagnesemia

- Release of intracellular Potassium
  - Hyperkalemia [Q]
- Predisposes to ***Arrhythmias*** [Q]
- ***Acidosis*** [Q] is also a feature and results in part from deranged oxidative metabolism
  -Lactic acidosis[Q]

Tumor Lysis Syndrome is associated with Hypocalcemia and not Hypercalcemia *Tumor Lysis Syndrome is also associated with Hyperuricemia, Hyperphosphatemia, Hyperkalemia and Acidosis.*

Management of Hypocalcemia

'Treatment of Hypocalcemia includes Calcium replacement with Vitamin D analogs along with Thiazide diuretics to prevent excess calcium excretion besides replenishing any decreases in magnesium and phosphate restriction'.

– Clinical Review for USMLE STEP – 2 (surgisphere) 2008/499

Management Stretegies in the management of Hypocalcemia

Increased Intake of Calcium

Oral calcium supplementation
- Calcium carbonate
- Calcium gluconate
- Calcium citrate
- Calcium lactate

Intravenous calcium supplementation
- Calcium chloride
- Calcium gluconate
- Calcium gluceptate

Enhanced Absorption of Calcium

Vitamin D / Vitamin D Analogs
- Vitamin D3 (Cholecalciferol)
- Vitamin D2 (Ergocalciferol)
- Calcitriol (1, 25 Dihydroxy Vitamin D3)
- Calcifediol (25 Hydroxy vitamin D3)
- Alfacalcidol (1α Hydroxyvitamin D3) (parenteral)

Reduce Excretion of Calcium in Urine

Thiazide Diuretics

Thiazide Diuretics have a hypocalciuric effect, and thereby reduce the amount of calcium excreted in urine.

Thiazide Diuretics must be used with caution

Vitamin D deficiency & Paget's Disease

Vitamin D deficiency (Rickets / Osteomalacia)

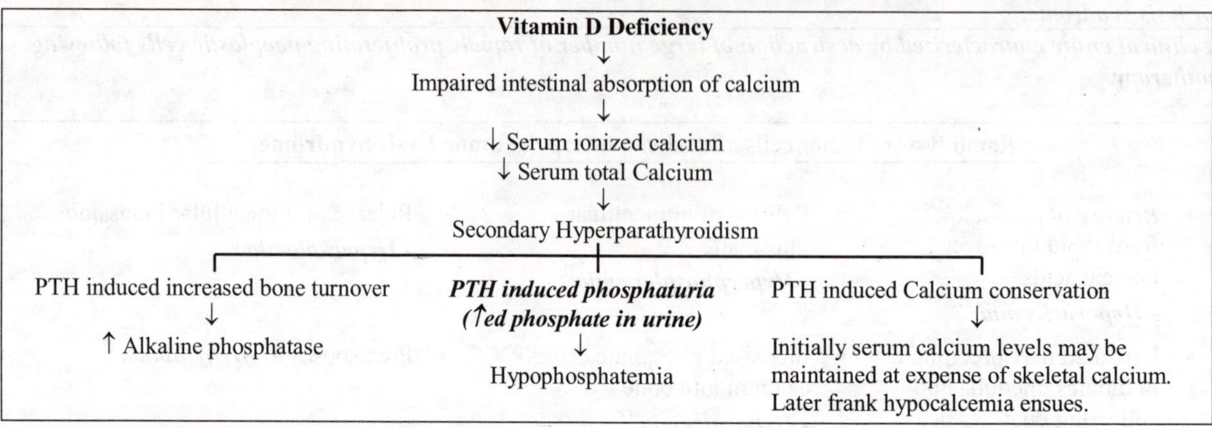

Rickets (or osteomalacia) is associated with hypophosphatemia due to PTH induced Phosphaturia (hyperphosphaturia). *Alkaline phosphatase levels are typically increased due to PTH induced increased bone turnover.*

Condition	Serum Ca	Serum phosphorus	Alkaline phosphatase	PTH
• Osteomalacia (Rickets) (↓Vit. D)	↓	↓	↑	↑

Paget's Diease

Over activity of osteoclasts causing widespread bone resorption
(Principal abnormality in Paget's disease)

↓

Compensatory increase in osteoblastic new bone formation
(Marked elevation of Alkaline phosphatase levels)

↓

Total bone volume may be maintained but the pagetic bone can be recognized as it is structurally disorganized and more susceptible to deformities and fractures.

Condition	Serum Ca	Serum phosphorus	Alkaline phosphatase	PTH
Paget's disease	N	N	Increase	N

Elevated alkaline phosphatase with normal serum Ca^{2+} and PO^{4-} is characteristic of Paget's disease.

'Serum calcium and phosphorus levels are normal in Paget's disease. Discovery of hypercalcemia even in presence of immobilization should prompt a search for another cause of hypercalcemia' – Harrisons

'Serum Alkaline phosphatase levels are markedly elevated reflecting the marked osteoblastic activity'-Chandrasoma Taylor

***Serum alkaline phosphatase** is the most valuable enzyme for assessment of bone disease and serves as an index of osteoblastic activity.*

Alkaline phosphatase level in metabolic bone disease

Increased	Normal
• *Paget's disease*	• *Hypoparathyroidism*
• *Rickets or osteomalacia* Q	• *Osteoporosis*
• *Hyperparathyroidism* Q	• *Multiple myeloma.*
• *Bone disease in renal failure* Q with secondary hyperparathyroidism	
• *Lytic bone neoplasms (levels may be normal)*	

Q***Levels of Alkaline phosphatase are higher in Pagets disease than in any other condition,*** *(except hereditary hypophosphatasia)*
Q*Serum Alkaline Phosphatase is usually normal in Multiple Myeloma even with extensive bone involvement because of absence of osetoblastic activity. – Harrison*

Osteoporosis

DISEASES ASSOCIATED WITH AN INCREASED RISK OF GENERALIZED OSTEOPOROSIS IN ADULTS :

Hypogonadal States	**Nutritional and gastrointestinal disorders**
Turner Syndrome Klinefelter syndrome Anorexia nervosa Hypothalmic amenorrhea Other primary or secondary hypogonadal states	Malnutrition Parenteral nutrition Malabsorption syndromes Gastrectomy Severe liver disease, especially biliary cirrhosis Pernicious anemia
Endocrine disorders	**Hematologic disorders / Malignancy**
Cushing's syndrome Hyperparathyroidism Thyrotoxicosis Insulin-dependent diabetes mellitus Acromegaly Adrenal insufficiency	Multiple disorders/malignancy Lymphoma and leukemia Malignancy-associated parathyroid hormone - related (PTHrP) production Mastocytosis Hemophilia Thalassemia
Selected inherited & Rheumatologic disorders	**Miscellaneous**
Osteogenesis imperfecta[Q] Marfan syndrome[Q] Hemochromatosis Hypophosphatasia[Q] Glycogen storage diseases Homocystinuria[Q] Ehlers-Danlos syndrome[Q] Porphyria Menkes' syndrome Epidermolysis bullosa Rheumatoid arthritis[Q] Ankylosing spondylitis	Immobilization[Q] Chronic obstructive pulmonary disease Pregnancy and lactation Scoliosis Multiple sclerosis Sarcoidosis Amyloidosis Alcoholism

DRUGS ASSOCIATED WITH AN INCREASED RISK OF GENERALIZED OSTEOPOROSIS IN ADULTS :

Glucocorticoids[Q] Cyclosporine Cytotoxic drugs Anticonvulsants Excessive alcohol	Excessive thyroxin Aluminium Gonadotropin-releasing hormone agonists[Q] Heparin Lithium

[Q]***Osteoporosis is seen with hyperthyroidism and not with hypothyroidism.***
[Q]***Osteoporosis is a feature of Hyperparathyroidism (not hypoparathyroidism).***
[Q]***Estrogen deficiency (Hypogonadal state)*** *is known to cause osteoporosis.*
[Q]***Cushing's syndrome*** is a known endocrine causes of osteoporosis.
[Q]*Fluorosis is associated with osteopetrosis and not osteoporosis*

Osteoporosis

- *Osteoporosis is defined as a reduction of bone mass or density, sufficient to increase the risk of fracture.*
- *Osteoporosis is usually asymptomatic until fracture occurs (**but serum Calcium is normal** [Q]).*
- *Serum parathyroid hormone, 25-(OH) D_2, Calcium, Phosphorus and Alkaline phosphatase are usually normal.*

Condition	Serum Ca	Serum phosphorus	Alkaline phosphatase	PTH
Osteoporosis	*N*	*N*	*N*	*N*

8

Endocrinology

Disorders of Thyroid Gland

Causes of Hypothyroidism and Hyperthyroidism

Causes of Hypothyroidism
Primary
• ***Autoimmune hypothyroidism**: **Hoshimoto's thyroiditis,** atrophic thyroiditis* • ***Iatrogenic:** ^{131}I treatment, subtotal or total thyroidectomy, external irradiation of neck for lymphoma or cancer* • ***Drugs**: Iodine excess (including iodine-containing contrast media and amiodarone), lithium, antithyroid drugs, p-aminosalicylic acid, interferon-α and other cytokines, aminoglutethimide* • ***Congenital hypothyroidism**: absent or ectopic thyroid gland, dyshormogenesis, TSH-R mutation* • ***Iodine deficiency*** • ***Infiltrative disorders**: amyloidosis, sarcoidosis, hemochromatosis, scleroderma, cystinosis, Riedel's thyroiditis* • *Overexpression of type 3 deoiodinase in infantile hemangioma*
Transient
• *Silent thyroiditis, including postpartum thyroiditis* • *Subacute thyroiditis* • *Withdrawal of thyroxine treatment in individuals with an intact thyroid* • *After 131I treatment or subtotal thyroidectomy for Grave's disease*
Secondary
• *Hypopituitarism: tumors, pituitary surgery or irradiation, infiltrative disorders, Sheehan's syndrome, trauma, genetic forms of combined pituitary hormone deficiencies* • *Isolated TSH deficiency or inactivity* • *Bexarotene treatment* • *Hypothalamic disease: tumors, trauma, infiltrative disorders, idiopathic*

Causes of Hyperthyroidism/ Thyrotoxicosis
Primary hyperthyroidism
• ***Grave's disease*** • ***Toxic multinodular goiter*** • *Toxic adenoma* • *Functioning thyroid carcinoma metastases* • *Activating mutation of the TSH receptor* • *Activating mutation of GSα (Mc-Cune Albright syndrome)* • ***Struma ovarii*** • *Drugs: iodine excess (Jod-Basedow phenomenon)*
Thyrotoxicosis without hyperthyroidism
• *Subacute thyroiditis* • *Silent thyroiditis* • *Other causes of thyroid destruction: amiodarone, radiation, infarction of adenoma* • *Ingestion of excess thyroid hormone (thyrotoxicosis factitia) or thyroid tissue*
Secondary hyperthyroidism
• *TSH-secreting pituitary adenoma* • *Thyroid hormone resistance syndrome: occasional patients may have features of thyrotoxicosis* • *Chrionic gonadotropin-secreting tumors* • *Gestational thyrotoxicosis*

Hypothyroidism (and Endemic Goitre) in sub-himalayan region is primarily due to deficiency of iodine.

[Q]The most common cause of neonatal hypothyroidism (congenital hypothyroidism) is thyroid gland dysgenesis (80-85%).
[Q]The most common of endemic goiter/hypothyroidism is iodine deficiency.

Approach to thyroid testing:

Because TSH change dramatically in response to alteration of free T_4 and T_3, a logical approach to thyroid testing is to determine first whether TSH is suppressed, normal or elevated – *Harrison*

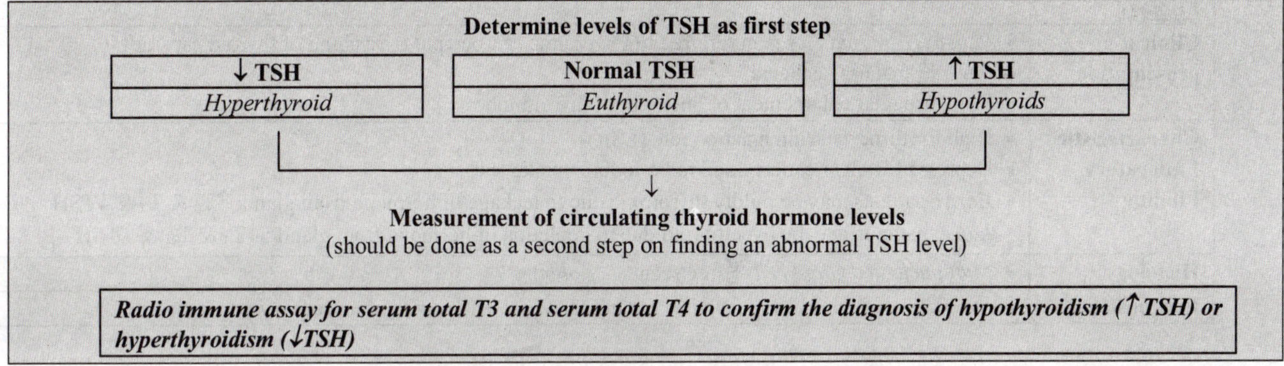

Laboratory Finding in Hypothyroidism

Primary Abnormalities

- *↓Total T4, ↓Free T4, ↓Free T4 Index*
- *↓Total T3; (↓free T3)*, ↓Free T3 Index*
- *↑TSH*
- *Positive TPO Antibodies (Autoimmune Throiditis, Hashiomato's Disease)*

Other Abnormalities

- ↑Cholesterol & Triglycerides
- ↑Creatine Phosphokinase (CPK)
- ↓Hb /Hct (Anemia is usually normocytic or macrocytic)
- ↑LDH
- ↑AST
- ↓Na

**Circulating unbound T3 (Free T3) levels may be normal in about 25% of patients reflecting adaptive diodinase responses to hypothyroidism. Free T3 measurements are therefore not indicated.*

The single most useful measurement for assessment of hypothyroidism is serum TSH[Q]. It is increased in primary hypothyroidism.

A normal TSH excludes primary (but not secondary) hypothyroidism. If the TSH is elevated an unbound T4 level is needed to confirm the presence of clinical hypothyroidism but T4 is inferior to TSH where used as a screening test.

Jod Basedow disease

Jod Basedow disease is synonymous with iodine-induced hyperthyroidism and may occur in patients with multinodular goitre after intake of large amount of iodine.

- In the diet
- In the form of radiographic contrast material
- In the form of drugs especially amiadarone

Thyrotoxicosis factitia :

Thyrotoxicosis produced due to ingestion of excessive amount of exogenous thyroid hormone is called Thyrotoxicosis factitia. Epidemics of thyrotoxicosis have been caused by consumption of ground beef contaminated with bovine thyroid gland.

Presentation is one of thyrotoxicosis with low or absent thyroid nucleotide uptake.

Wolff – Chaikoff effect:

Excess iodine transiently inhibits thyroid iodide organification. This phenomenon of iodine dependent transient supression of thyroid is called Wolff-Chaikoff effect.

DeQuervain's Thyroiditis, Granulomatous Thyroiditis or Subacute Thyroiditis or Giant cell Thyroiditis:

Origin / Etiology	• It is *viral in origin.* Q Symptoms usually follow an upper respiratory tract infection.
Clinical presentation	• *Pain over thyroid* Q or pain referred to lower jaw, ear, occiput (stretching of thyroid capsule) • *Fever* Q, malaise, asthenia • Firm, irregular enlargement of one or both thyroid lobes
Characteristic Laboratory Finding	• High Erythrocyte sedimentation rate (ESR) • Depressed RAIU i.e. decreased radio iodine uptake test • ***Early:*** patients may be mildly thyrotoxic due to leakage of hormone from gland: ↑T_3 & T_4 & ↓TSH ***Later:*** patients may be hypothyroid due to depletion of hormone from gland : ↓T_3 & T_4 & ↑TSH
Histology	• *Multinucleated Giant cells* Q are seen - *Robbins*
Prognosis	• *Disorder may smoulder for months but eventually subsides with return of normal function.*

De Quervain's Thyroiditis is viral in origin (and not autoimmune). *Symptoms usually follow an upper respiratory tract infection.* ***'DeQuervain's Thyroiditis is characterized by a depressed radioactive iodine uptake'.***

Hashimotas thyroiditis, ***also called chronic lymphocytic thyroiditis, is the most common form of thyroiditis. "The thyroid follicles are small and are lined by epithelial cells with abundant eosinophilic granular cytoplasm termed as Hurthle cells"*** - *Robbins 6th / 15*

Hurthle cells may be seen in :
• Hashimoto's Thyroiditis Q - *Robbins 6th / 1135* • Hurthle cell Thyroid adenoma Q - *Robbins 6th / 1141* • Follicular cell carcinomas Q - *Bailey 23rd / 728*

Hurthle cell tumors are a variant of Follicular neoplasms in which oxyphill or Hurthle / Ashkenazi cells predominate

Causes of High and Low Radioactive Iodine (RAIU)Uptake

High RAIU	Low RAIU
• ***Graves disease*** • ***Toxic nodule*** • *Autonomous nodular Goitre* • *Metastatic follicular thyroid carcinoma* • *HCG dependent hyperthyroidism of trophoblastic disease* • *TSH secreting pituitary adenoma*	• ***Subacute Thyroiditis*** - *De'Quervain's thyroiditis* - *Viral thyroiditis* • *Lymphocytic thyroiditis* • *Postpartum thyroiditis* • ***Exogenous hyperthyroidism*** *(Factitious hyperthyroidism)* • *Recent iodine load (eg contrast dye)*

Medullary Carcinoma thyroid :

It is a neuroendocrine carcinoma rising from parafollicular 'C' cells of thyroid. *Parafollicular 'C' cells are derived from neural crest and secrete calcitonin*

Medullary carcinoma should be suspected whenever :

a. ***High level of serum calcitonin*** Q *(> 0.08 ng/ml)*
b. ***Cervical lymph node*** are discovered at time of presentation. Q
- *Involvement of lymph nodes occurs early.* Q
- Thyroid and *blood born metastasis occurs early.* Q
c. ***Diarrhea*** Q is a presentation
d. ***Amyloid*** Q is present in stroma histologically.
e. ***MEN setting :*** Evidence of Pheochromocytoma / Hyperparathyroidism / Thyroid cancer in family. ***(Discovery of medullary carcinoma thyroid makes family surveillance advisable).*** Q
f. ***Hypocalcemia*** is associated: These cancers are ***associated with Hypocalcemia*** Q because calcitonin is secreted.

Medullary carcinoma thyroid is seen as
Sporadic: 80%
Familial: 20% (Non MEN setting / MEN II a / MEN II b)

Calcitonin: Screening test: Serum Calcitonin levels *fall after resection, & rise again if the tumor recurs,*

Treatment of Medullary Carcinoma Thyroid:
Total thyroidectomy + Resection of involved lymph nodes by radical / modified radical neck dissection.

Pheochromocytoma

What are Pheochromocytomas and what do they secrete

Pheochromocytomas are catecholamines secreting tumors of chromaffin cells derived from adrenal medulla or extradrenal sources (chromaffin cells in or about sympathetic ganglia.)

Adrenal	Extraadrenal
• *Most of them secrete Nor epinephrine in greater amount*	• *Most of them exclusively secrete Nor epinephrine*

• ***Most Pheochromocytomas contain and secrete both nor epinephrine and epinephrine.***

Most pheochromocytomas produce both norepinephrine and epinephrine and the percentage of norepinephrine is usually greater than in normal adrenal
'The ratio of norepinephrine to epinephrine is often as high as 20:1' – *Bailey (old edition)*

• ***Most extraadrenal pheochromocytomas secrete norepinephrine exclusively*** – *Harrison 16th/2148*

• Pheochromocytomas in association with MEN may rarely produce epinephrine alone.

Sites of Pheochromocytomas

Pheochromocytomas may be found in the adrenal gland, neck and mediastinum (along the sympathetic chain), abdomen (paraaortic) and urinary bladder

Sites of Pheochromocytomas
Adrenal Gland(Most common)
Head and neck
Thorax (Mediastinum)
Intra-abdominal (Para-aortic)
Bladder

Pheochromocytomas

Adrenal Pheochromocytomas *'Pheochromocytomas'*	**Extra-adrenal Pheochromocytomas** *'Paragangliomas'*
• *Adrenal Medulla (Most common site)*	*Extra-adrenal pheochromocytomas (Paragangliomas) are found where there is chromaffin tissue* • Along the *paraaortic sympathetic chain* • *Within organs of Zuckerkandl* (at the origin of inferior mesenteric artery) • *Along the sympathetic chain in the neck and mediastinum* • *In the wall of the urinary bladder*

Pheochromocytomas are also known as the 10 percent tumors

Pheoehromocytoma has been called the 10% tumor Q: 10% of tumor are

Bilateral Q
Extraadrenal Q
Familial
Malignant Q
Multiple Q
Occur in children Q

How does Pheochromocytoma Present?

- The most common manifestation is ***hypertension.*** [Q] Paroxysmal *Hypertension is the typical manifestation*
  The predominant clinical manifestation of pheochromocytoma is Hypertension.
  'The dominant sign is hypertension. Classically patients present with episodic hypertension but sustained hypertension is also common - Harrison's 18th/2962

<u>Pheochromocytoma is unique in presentation as it may present both with, Hypertension and hypotension</u>.   *Hypertension* occurs in paroxysms and is the most common manifestation   *Hypotension* occurs as ***'orthostatic hypotension'*** and it occurs as a consequence of diminished plasma volume and blunted sympathetic reflexes.

- ***The*** most common symptom is ***headache*** [Q]
- ***Pheochromocytomas are associated with Hypercalcemia and Constipation***
- ***Carbohydrate intolerance and elevated blood sugar (Hyperglycemia)***

Clinical Features Associated with Pheochromocytoma
• ***Headaches***
• ***Sweating attacks***
• *Palpitations and tachycardia*
• *Hypertension, sustained or paroxysmal*
• *Anxiety and panic attacks*
• *Pallor*
• *Nausea*
• *Abdominal pain*
• *Weakness*
• ***Weight loss***
• *Paradoxical response to antihypertensive drugs*
• *Polyuria and polydipsia*
• *Constipation*
• *Orthostatic* ***hypotension***
• *Dilated cardiomyopathy*
• *Erythrocytosis*
• *Elevated blood sugar*
• ***Hypercalcemia***

The most common symptoms in order of frequency during paroxysm are:	
- Headache	- Palpitation
- Vomiting	- Sweating
- Dyspnea	- Weakness
- Pallor	

Diagnosis of pheochromocytomas

- Pheochromocytomas and paragangliomas synthesize and store catecholamines which include norepinephrine (noradrenaline), epinephrine (adrenaline) and dopamine
- Pheochromocytomas are typically associated with elevated levels of plasma and urinary catecholamines and their metabolites such as VMA and metanephrines
- ***The most sensitive test for diagnosis of pheachromocytomas is measurement of fractionated metanephrines in urine and free metanephrine in plasma.***

<u>Biochemical and Imaging Methods Used for Pheochromocytoma and Paraganglioma Diagnosis</u>

Biochemical tests

Diagnostic Method	Sensitivity	Specificity
24-h urinary tests		
Vanillylmandelic acid	++	++++
Catecholamines	+++	+++
Fractionated metanephrines	++++	++
Total metanephrines	+++	++++
Plasma tests		
Catecholamines	+++	++
Free metanephrines	++++	+++

Imaging modalities

Diagnostic Method	Sensitivity	Specificity
CT	++++	+++
MRI	++++	+++
MIBG scintigraphy	+++	++++
Somatostatin receptor scintigraphy*	++	++
Dopa (dopamine) PET	+++	++++

*Particularly high in head and neck paragangliomas.
MIBG, metaiodobenzylguanidine; PET, positron emission tomography

Carcinoid Tumors and Carcinoid Syndrome

Carcinoid Syndrome

Typical Carcinoid Syndrome
- *Elevated levels of plasma serotonin*
- *Elevated levels of urinary **5HIAA***

↓

Typical carcinoid syndrome is charachteristic of Midgut carcinoids

Atypical Carcinoid Syndrome
- *Plasma serotonin levels are normal*
- *Plasma and urinary levels of 5HTP are increased* *(Urinary 5HIAA may be normal or mildly elevated)*

↓

Atypical carcinoid syndrome is charachteristic of foregut carcinoids

Midgut Carcinoids: Typical Carcinoid Syndrome
- Midgut tumors have high serotonin content are ***Argentaffin positive***[Q]
- Most frequently cause a 'typical' carcinoid syndrome when they metastize.
- Release serotonin and tachykinins (neuropeptide K. substance K, substances P)

Rarely secrete 5HTP or ACTH

- Metastatis to bone is uncommon (less common)

Foregut Carcinoids: Atypical Carcinoid Syndrome
- Foregut tumor have low serotonin content, are ***argentaffin negative but argyrophillic***[Q]
- Usually do not produce carcinoid syndrome but when they produce a carcinoid syndrome it is charachtristically usually an Atypical carcinoid syndrome

Occasionally secrete ACTH or 5HTP

- May metastize to bone
- Are often multihormonal

5HIAA, 5HT, 5HTP are metabolites of Tryptophan / Serotonin that may be elevated in carcinoid tumors.
- ***The diagnosis of typical carcinoid tumors is typically done by measurement of 5HIAA levels.***
- ***Elevated levels of urinary 5 HTP is suggestive of an atypical carcinoid syndrome***

Note that patients with atypical carcinoid syndrome may have elevated levels of 5HT, 5HTP and 5HIAA, but the presence of increased urinary 5HTP is most typical feature to suggest on Atypical carcinoid.

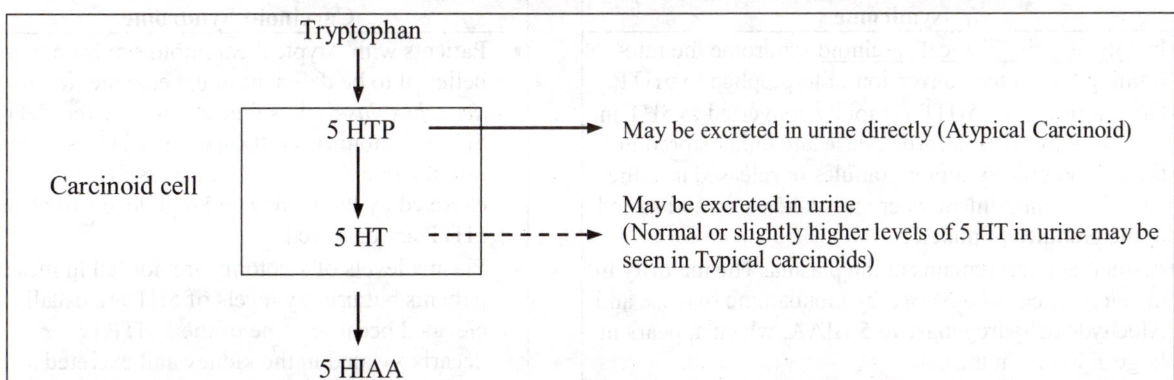

Vanillyl mandilic acid (VMA) *is the principal metabolite of catecholamines secreted by adrenal medulla. Elevated VMA levels in urine is a feature of increased catecholamine secreting tumors, typically pheochromocytomas (and not carcinoid tumors).*

8

Endocrinology

Diagnosis of Carcinoid Tumors *(Harrison)*

- The diagnosis of carcinoid syndrome relies on measurement of urinary or plasma serotonin or its metabolites in the urine.
- **Typical carcinoid syndrome** (high level of serotonin) is characterized by high levels of 5HIAA.
  The measurement of 5HIAA is most frequently used for typical carcinoid syndrome.

> *Most physicians' only use urinary 5HIAA levels / excretion rates however plasma and platelets serotonin levels if available provide additional information. Platelet serotonin levels (5-HT) are more sensitive than urinary 5HIAA levels but are not generally available.*

- **Atypical carcinoid syndromes** (low levels of serotonin) may have normal or minimally elevated 5HIAA levels.
- In such patient's urinary levels of other tryptophan metabolites such as 5HTP should be measured.

> *Elevated levels of urinary 5 HTP is suggestive of an atypical carcinoid syndrome*

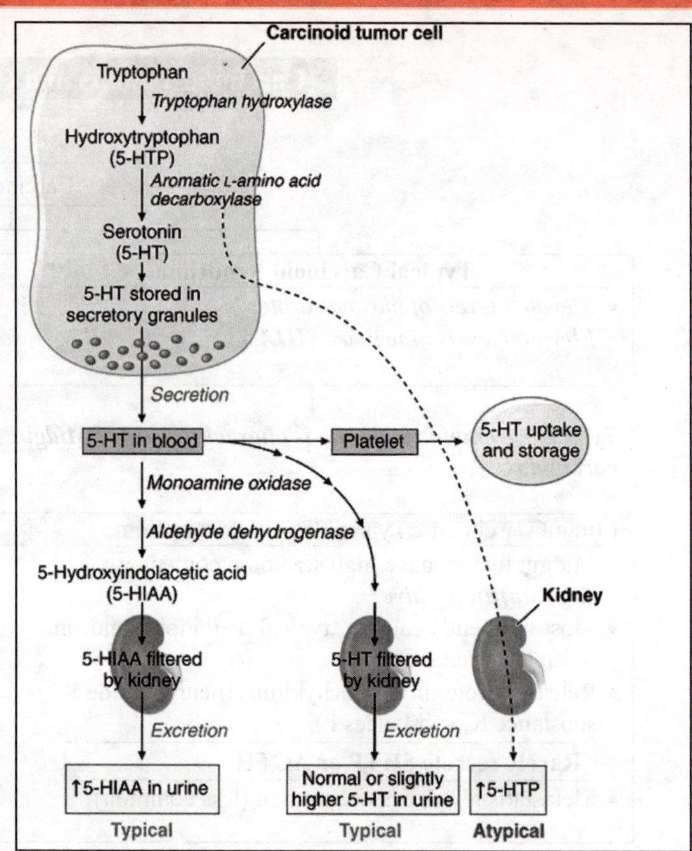

Typical VS Atypical Carcinoid syndrome

Patients with carcinoids may develop either a typical or atypical carcinoid syndrome

Most carcinoid tumors cause 'Typical' Carcinoid syndrome	Some carcinoid tumors cause on Atypical Carcinoid Syndrome
• In patients with Typical carcinoid syndrome the rate-limiting step is the conversion of tryptophan to 5HTP. • Once formed, the 5HTP is rapidly converted to 5HT in the tumor by dopa decarboxylase and either stored in the neurosecretory tumor granules or released into the vascular compartment where it is taken a up and stored in the granules of platelets. • A small amount remains in the plasma. The majority in the circulation is converted by monoamine oxidase and Aldehyde dehydrogenase to 5 HIAA, which appears in large amounts in the urine. • This is the typical pattern in argentaffin and argyrophilic tumors the midgut carcinoids which charachteristically secrete large amounts of serotonin (and comprise the majority of cases of carcinoid syndrome)	• Patients with Atypical carcinoid syndromes are believed to be deficient in the enzyme *'dopa decarboxylase'*; thus they cannot convert 5HTP to 5HT (serotonin) and the excess 5HTP is secreted into the blood stream. The excess 5HTP is excreted by the kidney and high levels of urinary 5HTP are observed • Plasma levels of serotonin are normal in these patients but urinary levels of 5HT are usually elevated because some of the 5 HTP is decarboxylated in the kidney and excreted as 5HT in the urine. • Levels of 5HIAA may be normal (or minimally elevated).

Carcinoid tumor location, Frequency of Metastases, and Association with the Carcinoid Syndrome

Site	Location (% of Total)	Incidence of Metastases	Incidence of Carcinoid Syndrome
Foregut			
Esophagus	<0.1	-	-
Stomach	4.6	10	9.5
Duodenum	2.0	-	3.4
Pancreas	0.7	71.9	20
Gallbladder	0.3	17.8	5
Bronchus, lung, trachea	*27.9*	5.7	13
Midgut			
Jejunum	1.8	}58.4	9
Ileum	*14.9*		9
Meckel's diverticulum	0.5	-	13
Appendix	*4.8*	38.8	<1
Colon	*8.6*	51	5
Liver	0.4	32.2	-
Ovary	1.0	32	50
Testis	<0.1	-	50
Hindgut			
Rectum	*13.6*	3.9	-

Site Specific incidence rate of Carcinoid Tumors

The reported anatomic distribution of carcinoid tumors varies widely amongst different textbooks depending on the source of data quoted.

Several textbooks including Schwartz and Sabiston, continue to mention Appendix as the most common site of gastrointestinal carcinoids however these incidence rates are based on old data before the 1970's and most studies thereafter report other locations as being more frequent. Results from Surveillance, Epidemiology and End Results (SEER) natural registry are now accepted as standard (Harrison.)

Based on PAN-SEER Data

- *The most common site of Carcinoid Tumors is Small Intestine*
- *The most common site wthin the small intestine is Ileum*
- *Rectum is the second most frequent site of Carcinoids after the ileum in accordance with the Pan SEER registry*
- *Small intestine and appendix together account for about 58% (≈60%) of gastrointestinal carcinoids according to the data from early SEER (1973-1991) and for about 51% of gastrointestinal carcinoids from the Pan SEER data*

Carcinoid site	Early SEER (1973-1991)	Late SEER (1992-1999)	Pan SEER (1973-1999)
Gastrointestinal tract	61.57	67.55	64.31
Esophagus	0.05	0.06	0.06
Stomach	3.55	5.85	4.61
Small intestine	28.82	28.22	28.54
Duodenum	1.94	3.83	2.80
Jejunum	2.11	1.48	1.81
Ileum	16.23	13.35	14.92
Not specified	7.86	8.74	8.26
Colon	9.48	7.62	8.62
Appendix	6.76	2.43	4.77
Rectum	9.44	18.54	13.61

Five year survival is > 60%.

The five survivals for all gstrointestinal carcinoids is getaer than 60 percent

5 Year Survival	Early SEER	Late SEER	Pan SEER
All Gastrointestinol Carcinoids	≈57%	≈68%	≈62.5%

Various Endocrinal Tumors of Pancreas

Pancreatic Endocrinal Tumor	Biologically active Peptides secreted
Zollinger Ellison Syndrome	Gastrin
VIPoma (Verner Morrison Syndrome, Pancreatic cholera, WDHA)	VIP
Glucagonoma	Glucagon
Insulinoma	Insulin
Somatostatinoma	Somatostatin
GRFoma	Growth hormone releasing hormone
ACTHoma	ACTH

Zollinger Ellison Syndrome

Zollinger Ellison Sydrome is characterized by unregulated secretion of gastrin leading to hypersecretion of gastric acid and the resulting manifestations.

'Gastrinomas' (non β cell tumour)Q
↓
Increased gastrin Q **secretion**
↓
Gastric acid hypersecretion Q
↓
Peptic ulceration Q
(And diarrhea)

Peptic ulceration Q

- *Most common manifestation*, **occuring in 90% of patient**
- *Most common site is duodenum (duodenal bulb)*
- Clinical situations that raise special suspicion include :
  a. ***Ulcers beyond the duodenal bulb (second part of duodenum and beyond) because these are unusual locations for ulcers in Peptic ulcer diseases.*** Q
  b. ***Ulcers refractory to standard medical therapy*** Q
  c. *Ulcers are recurrent* Q
  d. ***Ulcers presenting with frank complications.*** Q

Diarrhea Q

- *Is a common manifestation Q*
- *Etiology is multifactorial, and it may have a secretory component **as well.***

Presenting symptom in order of frequency

- Abdominal pain (70-100%)
- Diarrhea (37-73%)
- Gastroesophageal reflux disease (GERD) (30-35 years)

Observations in patients with peptic ulcer disease that should suggest a diagnosis of ZES

Observation that should suggest the diagnosis

- *Peptic ulcer disease (PUD) with diarrhea*
- *PUD in an unusual location or with multiple lesions*
- *PUD that is refractory to treatment or persistent*
- *PUD that is associated with findings suggestive of MEN I*
- *PUD without H. pylori infection.*

Chronic unexplained diarrhea should also suggest gastrinoma

Diagnosis of Zollinger Ellison Syndrome

STEP I	Assess fasting gastrin level	Gastrin levels are increased
STEP II	Assess acid secretion : BAO estimation	BAO is increased ; BAO / MAO is increased
STEP III	Perform provocative test if required.	i.v. secretin induces substantial increase in serum gastrin.

Zollinger Elision syndrome is characterized by an increased basal gastric acid output. The ratio of BAO to MAO (maximal acid output) is increased.

Gastrin provocative tests ***are used when acid secretory studies are not contributory*** **and include :**

- ***Secretin stimulation test*** ^{Q}***: most sensitive and specific*** ^{Q}
- ***Calcium infusion test***
- ***Standard meal test***

Secretin injection test is the most valuable provocative test in identifying patients with ZES

Histamine stimulation is not used and it does not bring about massive release of HCl in such patients.

Treatment of ZES:

PPIs are the treatment of choice for Zollinger - Ellison Syndrome and have decreased the need for total gastrectomy.

Remember :

- ***Most common*** site ^{Q} of gastrinoma is Duodenum (50-70%), (Pancreas 20-40%) - *Harrison*
- ***Most common*** hormone to be secreted besides gastrin is – ACTH ^{Q}
- ***Most common*** site of peptic ulcers produced is 1st part of Duodenum.
- ***Most valuable provocative test*** in identifying patients with ZES is the Secretin injection tests.
- Basal acid output is greater than 60 % of out put induced by maximal stimulation i.e. BAO > MAO ^{Q}

Pancreatic Cholera (VIPoma; 'Verner – Morrison Syndrome' or 'WDHA Syndrome')

- ***Pancreatic cholera is a Pancreatic endocrine tumor, most commonly of the Delta cells, characterized by net secretion of salt and water by gut***
- **Pancreatic cholera** results from excessive secretion of VIP from endocrine tumors i.e. VIPomas

'VIP' is an important neurotransmitter ubiquitously present in CNS and G.I. tract

ctions of VIP explain most features of the clinical syndrome. These include :

- Stimulation of small intestinal chloride secretion
- Effects on smooth muscle contractility
- Inhibition of acid secretion
- Vasodilatory effects

- **Pancreatic cholera is synonymous with 'Verner – Morrison Syndrome' or 'WDHA Syndrome'**
- ***Features of Pancreatic Cholera and/or WDHA Syndrome***

Features of Pancreatic cholera:

- *Severe watery diarrhea* ^{Q} / flushing / weight loss
- ***Hypokalemia*** ^{Q}
- ***Hypochlorhydria*** ^{Q}
- ***Hypercalcemia*** ^{Q} ***(not Hypocalcemia)***
- ***Hyperglycemia*** ^{Q}
- Inordinate fecal water and electrolyte loss

WDHA Syndrome
Watery **D**iarrhea
Hypokalemia
Achlorhydria

Insulinomas

- *Insulinomas are endocrine tumors of pancreas derived from Beta cells* ectopically secrete Insulin and result in Hypoglycemia

Classic presentation of ***insulinoma***: ***'Whipple's triad'***[Q] : - *Harrison 14th/589*

1. *Fasting hypoglycemia* [Q]
2. *Symptoms of hypoglycemia* [Q]
3. *Immediate relief after I.V. glucose administration* [Q]

- *They are generally small (>90% < 2 cm), usually single (90%) and usually benign (only 5-15% are malignant)*
- *The most common site of Insulinomas is the Pancreas.*

Insulinomas

Insulinomas are Endocrine tumors of the pancreas derived from Beta cells that ectopically secrete Insulin and result in Hypoglycemia

Average age of occurrence is 40-50 years

- *Generally Small* [Q] (>90% are < 2cm)
- *Usually single* [Q] (Not multiple in 90%)
- *Usually Benign* [Q] (5-15% are malignant)
- *Invariably occur in the pancreas* [Q] (Distributed equally in pancreatic Head, Body and Tail)

Symptoms due to Hypoglycemia

Most common symptoms are due to the effect of hypoglycemia on the central nervous system (Neuroglycemic Symptoms)

- Confusion
- Headache
- Disorientation
- Visual difficulties
- Irrational behavior (even coma)

Symptoms due to Excessive Catecholamine Release secondary to Hypoglycemia

- *Sweating*
- *Tremor*
- *Palpitation*

- *Insulinoma is characterised by an increase in weight (weight gain) and not by weight loss. Weight **gain may result from increased food ingested to combat symptoms of hypoglycemia.***

Diagnosis of Insulinomas

- *Diagnosis of Insulinoma requires demonstration of inappropriately high levels of plasma Insulin (and C-peptide) in the presence of documented hypoglycemia (Achieved by 72 hour fast test).*
- *Absolute values of Insulin or C- peptide are not reliable in establishing a diagnosis unless hypoglycemia is documented*

- ***The Gold standard test for diagnosis of Insulinoma is a supervised '72 hour fast' test The '72 hour fast test' allows demonstration of hypoglycemia, together will elevated levels of Insulin and C-peptide and thus becomes the most reliable – gold standard test for establishing a diagnosis of Insulinoma***

The '72 hour fast' test involves supervised fasting for upto 72 hours or until hypoglycemia can be documented
The test is considered positive if at any time when blood glucose levels drop to < 2.2mmol/l (40 mg/dl), the serum insulin levels are recorded to be greater than 6μU/ml. (and C- peptide levels > 100 pmol/l)

Metabolic Syndrome, Weight Gain & Obesity

Metabolic Syndrome:

Metabolic syndrome associated with Insulin Resistance (Insulin Resistance Syndrome)

- *Abdominal obesity (Waist circumference)*
- *Dyslipidemia*
  - *↑ Triglycerides*
  - *↓ HDL*
- *Hypertension*
- *Insulin Resistance*

Insulin Resistance States

Insulin Resistant states	
1. Obesity [Q]	6. Alstrom syndrome
2. Lipodystrophic states [Q]	7. Pineal hyperplasia syndrome
3. Ataxia - telengiectasia [Q]	8. Leprechaunism
4. Werners syndrome [Q]	9. Type A syndrome (absent or dysfunctional receptor)
5. Rabson Manden hall syndrome	10. Type B syndrome (antibody to insulin receptor)

Causes of weight gain (obesity):

Specific syndromes	Genetic syndromes
1. Cushing's syndrome [Q]	*1. Prader – willi syndrome*
2. Hypothyroidism [Q]	*2. Laurence Moom Biedl syndrome*
3. Insulinoma [Q]	*3. Ahistrom syndrome*
4. Craniopharyngioma and other disorders involving the hypothalamus	*4. Cohen syndrome*
	5. Carpenter syndrome

Causes of Weight Loss

Increased energy expenditure	Diminished food intake
Hyperthyroidism [Q] ***Pheochromocytoma*** [Q] *Extensive exercise* [Q]	*Cancer Infection* [Q] ***Uremia*** [Q] *Anorexia nervosa* [Q] ***Adrenal insufficiency*** [Q] *Hypercalcemia* *(Malignancy, Hyper PTH, sarcoidosis)* [Q] *Alzeimer's disease* [Q] *Depression* [Q]
Increased energy loss	
Diabetes mellitus [Q] *Malabsorption syndromes* [Q]	

Endocrine weight loss include
Hyperthyroidism
Diabetes mellitus
Pheochromocytoma
Adrenal insufficiency

RISKS OF OBESITY INCLUDE THE FOLLOWING:

A. **Cardiovascular disease :**
   - increased risk of *atherosclerosis* [Q]
   - increased risk of *hypertension* [Q]
   - increased risk of *sudden death* [Q]

B. **Pulmonary function :** *Sleep apnea* and *Right heart failure* [Q]

C. **Gall bladder disease :** Increased incidence of *Gall stones* [Q]

D. **Joint :** - Increased risk of *osteoarthritis* [Q] : partly due to added trauma of increased weight bearing
   -Increased incidence of *Gout* [Q] : due to impairment in urate clearance.

E. **Diabetes mellitus** : *Type II diabetes mellitus* [Q] is almost always seen in the obese.

F. **Cancer :** Increased incidence of
   - *Endometrial carcinoma* [Q]
   - *Post menopausal breast cancer* [Q]
   - *Prostate cancer* [Q]
   - *Colorectal carcinoma*

G. **Skin :** Increased incidence of *Acanthosis nigricans* [Q]

H. **Endocrine :**
   - *Insulin Resistance* [Q] : leading to Hyperinsulinemia is directly related to degree of obesity.
   - Growth hormone [Q] : secretions are reduced but IGF-I levels are normal thus growth is not affected.
   - *Testosterone level is reduced.* [Q]

8

Endocrinology

QUESTIONS

MEN Syndromes

1. A 20 year old male presented with chronic constipation, headache and palpitations. On examination he had marfanoid habitus, neuromas of tongue, medullated corneal nerve fibers and nodule of 2x2 cm size in the left lobe of thyroid gland. This patient is a case of :
   A. Sporadic medullary carcinoma of thyroid
   B. Familial medullary carcinoma of thyroid
   C. MEN IIA *(AI 2004)*
   D. MEN IIB
2. In MEN I, which is seen most commonly :
   A. Insulinoma *(AI 2007)*
   B. Gastrinoma
   C. Glucagonoma
   D. Somatostatinoma
3. MEN I syndrome is associated with all of the following, Except *(DNB 2012)*
   A. Pancreatic Tumors
   B. Parathyroid Tumors
   C. Pituitary Adenoma
   D. Medullary Carcinoma Thyroid
4. MEN I syndrome is most commonly associated with:
   A. Gastrinoma *(AI 2008)*
   B. Insulinoma
   C. Glucucagonoma
   D. Somatistatinoma
5. Type I MEN involves all, EXCEPT: *(AIIMS May 93)*
   A. Pancreas
   B. Adrenal
   C. Pituitary
   D. Parathyroid
6. A 36 year old female with symptoms of hyperparathyroidism, pituitary adenomas, islet cell tumor with cutaneous angiofibromas. What is the diagnosis?
   A. MEN 1 *(AIIMS Nov 07)*
   B. MEN 2A
   C. MEN 2B
   D. MEN 2C
7. All are associated with MEN 2 except:
   A. Pheochromocytoma *(AIIMS May 07)*
   B. Islet cell hyperplasia
   C. Medullary carcinoma thyroid
   D. Parathyroid adenoma
8. All of the following are features of MEN II a, except:
   A. Pituitary tumor *(AI 2001)*
   B. Pheochromocytoma
   C. Medullary ca thyroid
   D. Neuromas
9. All of the following are seen in MEN II B, Except:
   A. Hyperparathyroidism *(DNB June 2011)*
   B. Neuromas
   C. Pheochromocytoma
   D. Medullary Carcinoma Thyroid
10. Pancreatitis, pituitary tumor and pheochromocytoma may be associated with: *(AI 2004, 2005)*
    A. Medullary carcinoma of the thyroid
    B. Papillary carcinoma of the thyroid
    C. Anaplastic carcinoma of the thyroid
    D. Follicular carcinoma of the thyroid
11. A patient presents with intermittent headache. On examination there is hypertension and a thyroid nodule. Which of the following steps is to be taken next :
    A. Urine HIAA levels *(AIIMS Nov. 2000)*
    B. Urine VMA and aspiration of the thyroid nodule
    C. Ultrasound abdomen
    D. Echocardiography
12. A 25 year old young woman has recurrent episodes of headache and sweating. Her mother had renal calculi and died after having a neck mass. The physical examination reveals a thyroid nodule but no clinical sign of thyrotoxicosis. Before performing thyroid surgery, the surgeon should order : *(AIIMS Nov 02)*
    A. Measurement of thyroid hormones.
    B. Serial determinations of serum calcium, phosphorus protein and alkaline phosphatase.
    C. 24-hours urine test for 5 hydroxyindoleacetic acid excretion.
    D. Serial 24 hours test for catecholamines, metanephrines and vanillylamandelic acid excretion.

Disorders of Adrenal Cortex

Cushing's Syndrome

13. The most common cause of Cushing's syndrome is:
    A. Pituitary adenoma *(AI 1995)*
    B. Adrenal adenoma
    C. Ectopic ACTH
    D. Iatrogenic steroids
14. A common cause of Cushing syndrome is:
    A. Cancer producing ectopic ACTH
    B. Pituitary adenoma *(AIIMS May 93)*
    C. Adrenal tuberculosis
    D. None of the above
15. Intake of exogenous steroid causes: *(PGI June 97)*
    A. Addison's disease
    B. Cushing's syndrome
    C. Pheochromocytoma
    D. Conn's syndrome

16. Cushing syndrome is not a feature of : (AIIMS May 95)
A. Adrenal carcinoma
B. Oat cell carcinoma of lung
C. Medulloblastoma
D. Pituitary adenoma

17. All of the following are clinical features of Cushing's syndrome except : (DNB)
A. Insulin resistance
B. Menorrhagia
C. Violaceous striae
D. Centripetal obesity

18. All of the following are true about Cushing's syndrome, Except (PGI 08)
A. Red striae
B. Increased adrenaline
C. Proximal muscle weakness
D. Edema

19. Cushing syndrome is characterized by all except: (PGI June 98)
A. DM
B. HT
C. Proximal myopathy
D. Centripetal obesity
E. None (All are seen)

20. Features not seen in Cushing's Syndrome is : (AI 1997)
A. Hypoglycemia
B. Hypertension
C. Frank psychosis
D. Hypokalemia

21. All are features of Cushing's disease except: (AIIMS Nov 07)
A. Central obesity
B. Episodic hypertension
C. Easy bruising
D. Glucose intolerance

22. Cushing's disease is associated with: (AI 2008)
A. Increased ACTH and increased cortisol
B. Increased urinary Catecholamines
C. Increased ADH
D. Decreased ACTH and increased cortisol levels

23. About Cushing syndrome, true is: (PGI June 2000)
A. Low dose dexamethasone suppresses corticosone secretion
B. CA of adrenal is more common than adenoma
C. Pituitary adenoma size > 2 cm (usually)
D. ↑ ACTH secretion is the commonest endogenous cause

24. A patient with cushinoid features presents with hemoptysis; he shows no response to dexamethasone suppression test; most likely diagnosis here is: (AI 2001)
A. Adrenal hyperplasia
B. Adrenal adenoma
C. Ca lung with ectopic ACTH production.
D. Pituitary microadenoma

25. Lalloo, 50 years old, a chronic smoker, presents with history of hemoptysis. He was having truncal obesity and hypertension. He had an elevated ACTH level which was not suppressible with high dose dexamethasone. What would be the most probable diagnosis: (AIIMS Nov. 2000)
A. Bilateral adrenal hyperplasia
B. Adrenal adenoma
C. Pituitary tumour
D. Ectopic ACTH producing lung cancer

26. A chronic smoker presented with mild haemoptysis. He also gave a history of hypertension and obesity. Lab data showed raised ACTH levels, which were not suppressed by high dose dexamethasone. The cause for the Cushing's syndrome in the patient is : (AIIMS May 02)
A. MEN I
B. Pituitary adenoma
C. Adrenal cortical adenoma
D. Ectopic ACTH secreting tumor

27. The differentiating feature b/w Ectopic ACTH secretion and Cushing syndrome is: (AIIMS Dec 98)
A. Hypokalemic alkalosis
B. Clinical features of cushing syndrome
C. Hyperpigmentation
D. Hypertension

28. Which of the following is the earliest manifestation of Cushing 's syndrome? (AI 2004)
A. Loss of diurnal variation
B. Increased ACTH
C. Increased plasma Cortisol
D. Increased urinary metabolites of Cortisol

29. A 28 year old lady has put on weight (10 kg over a period of 3 years), and has oligomenorrhoea followed by amenorrohoea for 8 months. The blood pressure is 160/100 mm of Hg. Which of the following is the most appropriate investigation? (AI 2004)
A. Serum electrolytes
B. Plasma cortisol
C. Plasma testosterone and ultrasound evaluation of pelvis
D. T3, T4 and TSH

Hyperaldosteronism: Conn's Syndrome

30. Conn's syndrome is most commonly associated with: (AI 2008)
A. Cortical adenoma
B. Cortical hyperplasia
C. Cortical carcinoma
D. Pheochromocytoma

31. All of the following may be associated with primary aldosteronism, Except: (PGI June 05)
A. Adrenal adenoma
B. Adrenal hyperplasia
C. Von-Hippel-Lindau syndrome
D. Adrenal carcinoma

32. Conn's syndrome is associated with all, except : (AI 2002)
A. Hypertension
B. Muscle weakness

C. Hypokalemia
D. Edema

33. Increased Aldosterone leads to all except: *(AI 2009)*
A. Hypernatremia
B. Hypokalemia
C. Hypertension
D. Metabolic acidosis

34. NOT a feature of primary hyperaldosteronism is *(AIIMS Dec 94/ AI-1998)*
A. Pedal edema
B. Diastolic hypertension
C. Polyuria
D. Hypokalemia

35. In Conn's syndrome the following is true: *(PGI Dec 06)*
A. Diastolic HTN without oedema
B. Systolic HTN without oedema
C. Pseudotetany
D. Hyper K+

36. Excess Aldosterone is associated with all the following *except*: *(AI 1995)*
A. Hypokalemia
B. Hyperkalemia
C. Sodium retention
D. Hypertension

37. Excess Aldosterone is associated with all the following except: *(AI 1991)*
A. Hypokalemia
B. Hyperkalemia
C. Hypernatremia
D. Hypertension

38. Which is not a feature of primary hyperaldosteronism: *(AIIMS May 93)*
A. Hypokalemia
B. Hypertension
C. Hypernatremia
D. Increased rennin level

39. The following are feature of primary hyperaldosteronism: *(PGI June 97)*
A. Polyuria
B. Hypertensin
C. Hypokalemia
D. Hyperkalemia

40. True about Conn's syndrome (select two best options): *(PGI Dec 02)*
A. ↑K+
B. ↓K+
C. Proximal myopathy
D. ↑ed plasma rennin activity
E. Edema

41. True about primary aldosteronism (select three options): *(PGI June 05)*
A. Pedal oedema
B. Increased rennin
C. Increased Na+
D. Decreased K+
E. Hypertension

42. A young hypertensive patient has serum K^+ 2.8 meq/L and ↑aldosterone level with ↓ed plasma rennin activity. The likely cause is: *(PGI Dec 04)*
A. Renal artery stenosis
B. Ectopic ACTH syndrome
C. Diuretic therapy
D. Conn's syndrome
E. Liddle's syndrome

43. In primary adrenal hyperplasia, incorrect is: *(AIIMS May 94)*
A. Hypokalemia
B. Hyponatremia
C. Hypernatremia
D. Water retention

44. In primary adrenal hyperplasia, incorrect is *(AIIMS May 94)*
A. Hypokalemia
B. Hyponatremia
C. Hypernatremia
D. Water retention

45. All are features of Bartters syndrome, EXCEPT:– *(AIIMS Dec 95)*
A. Polyuria
B. Metabolic alkalosis
C. Periodic paralysis
D. Hypertension

Adrenal Insufficiency (Addison's Disease)

46. Most common cause of adrenal insufficiency in India is *(AIIMS May 94)*
A. Autoimmune
B. Surgery
C. Steroid withdrawal
D. Tuberculosis

47. Most common cause of Addison's Disease in India is: *(AIIMS Nov 2011)*
A. Autoimmune
B. Postpartum
C. HIV
D. Tuberculosis

48. Feature of addison's disease include all of the following except: *(DNB)*
A. Asthenia
B. Hyperpigmentation
C. Hypertension
D. Abdominal pain

49. Primary Adrenal Insufficiency causes all of the following, Except *(DNB 2012)*
A. Low Blood Pressure
B. Decrease in ECF
C. Decreased sodium potassium ratio
D. Increased protein breakdown

50. Chronic adrenal insufficiency is characterized by all of the following: *(AIIMS May 95)*
A. Excess pigmentation
B. Asthenia
C. Weight gain
D. Hypoglycemic episodes

51. Addisons disease is associated with all except:
A. Cardiac atrophy *(AIIMS May 07)*
B. Decreased diastolic B.P.
C. Serum cortisol < 3 mcg/dl
D. Low renin levels

52. Addison's disease is characterized by *all except:*
A. Hyperglycemia *(AI 1995)*
B. Hypotension
C. Hyperkalemia
D. Hyponatremia

53. Addison's disease is characterized by following except: *(PGI June 97)*
A. Hyperkalemia
B. Hypotension
C. Hyponatremia
D. Hypocalcemia

54. Which is NOT a clinical feature of Addison's disease:
A. Hypoglycemia *(AIIMS Feb 97)*
B. Hyponatremia
C. Hypocalcemia
D. Hyperkalemia

55. Regarding Addisonian pigmentation, all are true EXCEPT : *(AIIMS May 01)*
A. Involves moles and scars
B. Involves palmer creases
C. Does not involve oral mucosa
D. Decreased fibrosis

56. In addison's disease, most diagnostic test is:
A. Serum Na+, K+, rennin *(PGI Dec 97)*
B. Serum Na+, K+, saline suppression
C. Serum creatinine/urea ratio
D. ACTH stimulation test

Diabetes Mellitus (Hyperglycemia & Hypoglycemia)

57. Which type diabetes is HLA associated:
A. Type I diabetes *(AI 2002)*
B. Type II diabetes
C. Malnutrition related type disease
D. Pregnancy related type diabetes

58. A 45-year old woman visited her physician with complaints of increased appetite and thirst with increased frequency of urination. She also had the symptoms of diminished or impalpable pulses in the feet, besides gangrene of the feet. Her laboratory findings on the oral glucose tolerance test are as follows: *(AI 2004)*

Parameters	Fasting	1 hr	2 hr
Blood glucose (mg/dL)	155	270	205
Urine glucose	-ve	+++	++
Ketone bodies	-ve	-ve	-ve

Which of the following statements is not correct for the above mentioned case:
A. She was suffering from insulin dependent diabetes mellitus
B. She was suffering from non-insulin dependent diabetes mellitus
C. She was treated with oral hypoglycemic drugs only when diet and exercise could not control the pathological situation
D. Knowledge of family history of diabetes mellitus is useful in predicting the nature of the diabetes.

59. A 29 years old person is known diabetic on oral hypoglycemic agents since 3 years. He has lost weight and never had DKA. His grand father is diabetic but his father is nondiabetic. Which is the likely diagnosis: *(AI 2009)*
A. MODY
B. DM type I
C. DM type II
D. Pancreatic diabetes

60. A 29 years old person is known diabetic on oral hypoglycemic agents since 3 years. He has lost weight and never had DKA. His grand father and father both are diabetic. Which is the likely diagnosis:
A. MODY *(AI 2009)*
B. DM type I
C. DM type II
D. Pancreatic diabetes

61. All of the following statements about Type I Diabetes Mellitus are true, Except (select two options):
A. Family history is present in 90% cases
B. Dependent on insulin to prevent ketoacidosis
C. Time of onset is usually predictable *(PGI Dec 01)*
D. Autoimmune destruction of beta cells occur
E. Often occurs in children

62. All of the following are true about Type I DM, Except:
A. Family history is present in 90% of cases
B. Antibodies against β ells
C. Prone to Diabetic Ketoacidosis (DKA)
D. Insulin is required for management of DKA

63. In a patient with NIDDM which of the following condition is seen : *(AIIMS May 02)*
A. Ketosis commonly occurs on stopping treatment.
B. Hypertriglyceridmia never occurs
C. Pancreatic beta cells stop producing insulin
D. Increased levels of insulin in blood, may be seen

64. In diabetes all of the following statement are correct; except: *(PGI)*
A. Patients with type 2 diabetes never require insulin treatment
B. Maturity Onset Diabetes of the Young (MODY) is an autosomal recessive condition
C. The majority of type 2 diabetes patients die from cardiovascular disease

D. Weight loss is a common symptom of type 1 diseases
E. Recognized endocrine causes of diabetes include Acromegaly and Cushing's syndrome

65. An obese NIDDM patient present with FBS = 180 mg% and PPBS = 260 mg%. Initial management should include:
A. Glibenclamide
B. Diet therapy + exercise
C. Diet therapy + exercise + metformin
D. Insulin
E. Chlorpropamide

66. A 40 year old male patient is suffering from type II diabetes mellitus and hypertension. Which of the following antihypertensive drugs should not be used in such patients : *(AIIMS Nov 03)*
A. Lisinopril
B. Hydrochlorthiazide
C. Losartan
D. Trandolopril

67. Which of the following is not a test for diabetes mellitus *(AIIMS Nov 2010)*
A. Fasting blood glucose
B. Random blood glucose
C. D-Xylose test
D. Oral Glucose tolerance test

68. Which of the following findings can establish a diagnosis of Diabetes Mellitus: *(AIIMS Nov 2011)*
A. Fasting plasma glucose 100mg/dl and 2 hour prandial glucose 140 mg/dl
B. Fasting plasma glucose 125 mg/dl and 2 hour postprandial glucose 199 mg/dl
C. Symptoms of Diabetes plus random blood glucose of 190 mg/dl
D. Glycosylated Haemoglobin (HbA1C) > 6.5%

69. Impaired glucose tolerance on an oral GTT is indicated by: *(PGI Dec 02)*
A. Fasting plasma sugar > 126 mg/dl
B. Random blood sugar > 200mg/dl
C. Fasting blood sugar < 90 mg/dl
D. Fasting blood sugar < 140 mg/dl; two hours after glucose load > 200 mg/dl
E. 2 hrs after glucose load 140-200 mg/dl; fasting blood sugar < 126 mg/dl

70. A 42 year old male has strong positive Benedict's test, random blood sugar is > 163 mg%, fasting blood sugar is > 200mg%. Next line of investigation is:
A. Urine glucose charting 5 hourly
B. Oral GTT *(AIIMS June 99)*
C. Repeat benedict's test
D. 24 hr urine sugar estimation

71. At what value for one hour glucose challenge test will you recommend a standard glucose tolerance test:
A. 120 mg/dl *(AIIMS May 05)*
B. 140 mg/dl
C. 150 mg/dl
D. 160 mg/dl

72. HBAIC level in blood explains: *(AI 2004)*
A. Acute rise of sugar
B. Long terms status of blood sugar
C. Hepatorenal syndrome
D. Chronic pancreatitis

73. Diabetes control is best monitored by: *(PGI Dec 98)*
A. Serum glucose
B. Post prandial blood glucose
C. HbA1C
D. HbA2C

74. All are seen in DKA except: *(AIIMS Nov 07)*
A. Tachycardia
B. Dehydration
C. Bradycardia
D. Abdominal pain/tenderness

75. An obese lady aged 45 years, was brought to emergency in a semi comatose condition. The laboratory investigations showed K+ (5.8 mmol/L); Na+ (136 mmol/L); blood pH (7.1), HCO3 (12 mmol/L),' ketone bodies (350 mg/dl). The expected level of blood glucose for this lady is:
A. < 45 mg/dl. *(AIIMS May 03)*
B. < 120 mg/dl.
C. >180 mg/dl.
D. < 75 mg/dl.

76. Two most important test to be done in a comatose patient with blood glucose of 750mg/dl will be:
A. Serum creatinine *(PGI June 01)*
B. Serum sodium
C. CSF examination
D. Blood pH
E. Blood urea

77. A 35 years old man Ramu has fasting and post prandial blood sugar within normal limit but urine sugar is 3 plus (+++). The diagnosis is.
A. Renal Glycosuria *(AIIMS June 99)*
B. Pancreatic insufficiency
C. Alimentary glycosuria
D. High carbohydrate diet taken in the morning.

78. An obese patient presented in casualty in an unconscious state. His blood sugar measured 400 mg%, urine tested positive for sugar and ketones; drug most useful in management is:
A. Glibenclamide *(AI 2001, AIIMS 98)*
B. Troglitazone
C. Insulin
D. Chlorpropamide

79. Treatment of 42 year old obese man with blood glucose 450 mg, urine albumin 2+sugar 4+ketone 1+ is
A. Insulin *(AIIMS June 98)*
B. Glibenclamide
C. Glipizide
D. Metformin

80. If a patient with severe hyperglycemia is given IV insulin, which of the following can occur? *(AI 2009)*

A. Hypokalemia
B. Hyperkalemia
C. Hyponatremia
D. Hypernatremia

81. A diabetic patient with blood glucose of 600 mg/dL and Na 122 mEq/L was treated with insulin. After giving insulin the blood glucose decreased to 100 mg/dL. What changes in blood Na level is expected? *(AI 2002)*
A. Increase in Na^+ level
B. Decrease in Na^+ level
C. No change would be expected
D. Na^+ would return to previous level spontaneously on correction of blood glucose.

82. Increased insulin is charachterized by all of the following, except: *(DNB Dec 2009)*
A. Increased Glucagon secretion
B. Increased Intracellular potassium
C. Hypoglycemia
D. Enhanced fatty acid synthesis

83. Early morning hyperglycemia with increased blood glucose of 3.00 AM suggests: *(DNB)*
A. Insufficient Insulin
B. Dawn Phenomenon
C. Somogyi effect
D. None of the above

84. Which of the following statements about Dawn phenomenon is true: *(DNB)*
A. Morning hyperglycemia with midnight hypoglycemia
B. Morning hypoglycemia with midnight hyperglycemia
C. Morning hyperglycemia due to insufficient insulin
D. Morning hypoglycemia due to excess insulin

85. Which of the following are characteristic of diabetes mellitus: *(PGI June 03)*
A. Encephalopathy
B. Myelopathy
C. Neuropathy
D. Myopathy
E. Retinopathy

86. The characteristic and common presentation of diabetic neuropathy is: *(PGI Dec 98)*
A. Amyotrophy
B. Mononeuropathy
C. Symmetrical sensory neuropathy
D. Autonomic neuropathy

87. All are used in painful diabetic neuropathy, EXCEPT: *(AIIMS Dec 97)*
A. Phenytoin
B. Local use of capsicum
C. Dextroamphetamine
D. Amitrytline

88. Hypoglycemic unawareness that occurs in diabetic patients when transferred from oral hypoglycemics to insulin, is due to : *(AI 2000)*
A. Autonomic neuropathy
B. Insulin resistance
C. Lipodystrophy
D. Somogi phenomenon

89. A patient has IDDM diagnosed at age of 15 years. The most reliable indicator for diabetic nephropathy is *(AIIMS Nov 99)*
A. Urine albumin <50 mg per day in 3 consecutive samples
B. Urinary protein >550 mg per day for 3 consecutive samples
C. Development of diabetic retinopathy
D. Hematuria

90. Which of the following statements about diabetic nephropathy is true: *(PGI June 05)*
A. Microalbuminiuria is not an indicator of long term cardiovascular morbidity
B. Strict glycemic control cannot prevent microalbuminuria
C. β-islet cell/pancreatic transplantation can improve the proteinuria in early stage
D. Angiotensin receptor blockers have no additive advantage over other drugs except B.P. control
E. Protein restriction is not helpful

91. A 50 year old male with type 2 diabetes mellitus is found to have 24 hr urinary albumin of 250 mg. Which of the following drugs may be used to retard progression of renal disease: *(AIIMS Nov 04)*
A. Hydrochlorthiazide
B. Enalapril
C. Amiloride
D. Aspirin

92. The following statements are correct in relation to diabetic nephropathy: *(PGI 2007)*
A. The presence of microalbuminuria is associated with a reduction of cardiovascular risks in patient with diabetes
B. Progression of renal disease may be reduced by the use of calcium channel blockers
C. The development of diabetic nephropathy protects from diabetic retinopathy
D. False positive microalbuminuria may occur in the presence of urinary tract infections (UTI)
E. Blood pressure improves in the majority after the development of diabetic nephropathy

93. The most characteristric finding in diabetic nephropathy is: *(PGI June 99)*
A. Diffuse glomerulosclerosis
B. Nodular glomerulosclerosis
C. Armani-Ebstein reaction
D. Fibrin caps

94. Pathognomic factors involved in foot ulcers in DM include all, Except: *(PGI Dec 06)*
A. Trophic ulcers
B. Neuropathy
C. Microangiopathic changes in blood vessels
D. Macroangiopathy

95. Life threatening complications of diabetes mellitus are all except: *(AIIMS May 07)*
 A. Malignant otitis externa
 B. Rhinocerebral mucormycosis
 C. Emphesematous pyelonephritis
 D. Emphysematous appendicitis

96. In which of the following intensive management of diabetes needed except: *(AIIMS Nov 07)*
 A. Autonomic neuropathy causing postural hypotension
 B. Pregnancy
 C. Post kidney transplant in diabetic nephropathy
 D. DM with acute MI

97. Recombinant human insulin is made by
 A. CDNA from any eukaryote cell
 B. Genome of any eukaryote *(AIIMS June 2000)*
 C. CDNA of pancreatic cell
 D. Genome of pancreatic cell

98. If a patient with several hyperglycemia is given IV insulin, which of the following can occur? *(DNB)*
 A. Hypokalemia
 B. Hyperkalemia
 C. Hyponatremia
 D. Hypernatremia

99. Insulin resistance is seen in all, Except:
 A. Werner's syndrome
 B. Addison's disease *(AIIMS June 98)*
 C. Ataxia telengiectasia
 D. Lipodystrophy

100. Insulin resistance syndrome includes all of the following, Except: *(PGI June 06)*
 A. Dyslipidemia
 B. Hypertension
 C. Hyperuricemia
 D. Low HDL

101. Hypoglycemia is seen in *(AIIMS May 01)*
 A. Acromegaly
 B. Cushing's syndrome
 C. Hyperthyroidism
 D. Hypopitutarism

102. Hypoglycemia is associated with all, EXCEPT:
 A. Fibroma *(AIIMS Dec 97)*
 B. Soft tissue sarcoma
 C. Small cell carcinoma of lung
 D. Hepatocellular carcinoma

103. Hypoglycemia is a recognized feature of all of the following conditions, except : *(AI 2002)*
 A. Uremia
 B. Acromegaly
 C. Addison's disease
 D. Hepatocellular failure

104. A patient presents with symptoms of Hypoglycemia. Investigations reveal decreased blood glucose and increased Insulin levels. C-peptide assay is done which shows normal levels of C- peptide. The most likely diagnosis is: *(AI 2010)*
 A. Insulinoma
 B. Accidental sulfonylurea ingestion
 C. Accidental exogenous Insulin administration
 D. Accidental Metformin ingestion

105. Which of the following test is useful to distinguish between Insulinoma and Sulfonylurea related hypoglycemia: *(AIIMS May 08)*
 A. Antibody to Insulin
 B. Plasma – C- peptide level
 C. Plasma Insulin level
 D. Insulin- Glucose ratio

106. All of the following statements about Nesidioblastosis are true, Except: *(AI 2011)*
 A. Hypoglycemic episodes may be seen
 B. Occurs in adults more than children
 C. Histopathology shows hyperplasia of islet cells
 D. Diazoxide may be used for treatment

Disorders of Pituitary / Sexual Differentiation

Hyperprolactinemia and Anterior Pituitary Disorders

107. All are causes of hyperprolactinemia, *except*
 A. Bromocriptine *(AIIMS May 94)*
 B. Phenothiazine
 C. Methyldopa
 D. Metoclopramide

108. All of the following are associated with gigantism / acromegaly, except *(DNB)*
 A. Mental Retardation
 B. Hyperhydrosis
 C. Visceromegly
 D. Impaired Glucose Tolerance

109. A middle aged man noticed that he can no longer fit in his shoes and that his jaw was protruding and phalanges were enlarged. These effects are likely to be mediated by. *(DNB)*
 A. ACTH
 B. Somatomedins
 C. TRH
 D. TGF Beta

110. All of the following are known to cause hyperprolactenemia *except* : *(AI 1997)*
 A. Methyldopa
 B. Phenothiazines
 C. Bromocriptine
 D. Metoclopramide

111. Investigation of choice of hyper-prolactinemia:
 A. TRH estimation *(AIIMS Nov 93)*
 B. LH estimation
 C. Prolactin estimation
 D. Estradiol estimation

112. Which of the following is the most common type of pituitary adenoma? *(AIIMS May 05)*
A. Thyrotropinoma
B. Gonadotropinoma
C. Prolactinoma
D. Corticotropinoma

113. A 30 year old woman presented with secondary amenorrhoea for 3 years along with galactorrhoea. The most likely cause of her symptoms would be: *(AI 2004)*
A. Craniopharyngioma
B. Prolactinoma
C. Meningioma
D. Sub-arachnoid haemorrhage

114. Ramkali bai, a 35 year old female presented with one year history of menstrual irregularity and galactorrhea. She also had off-and-on headache. Her examination revealed bitemporal superior quadrantopia. Her fundus examination showed primary optic atropy. Which of the following is the most likely diagnosis in this case : *(AIIMS Nov 2004)*
A. Craniopharyngioma
B. Pituitary macroadenoma
C. Ophthalmic ICA aneurysm
D. Chiasmal glioma

115. In a lady with bilateral superior temporal quadrantopia, galactorrhea, the most probable cause is: *(AI 2009)*
A. Pituitary macroadenoma
B. Craniopharyngioma
C. Sheehan's syndrome
D. Pituitary hypophysitis

116. A young women with secondary amenorrhea and galactorrhea. MRI shows a tumour of < 10mm diameter in the pituitary fossa. Treatment is: *(PGI June 04)*
A. Hormonal therapy for withdrawal bleeding
B. Radiotherapy
C. Chemotherapy
D. Bromocriptine
E. Surgery

117. Confirmatory investigation for Acromegaly is: *(PGI June 01)*
A. Insulin induced GH suppression
B. Glucose induced GH suppression
C. Random GH assay
D. IGF – I level

118. Paradoxical response of GH release to TRH is seen in: *(AIIMS Dec 98)*
A. Prolactinoma
B. Acromegaly
C. Malnutrition
D. Pituitary adenoma

119. Nelson's syndrome is most likely seen after: *(AIIMS May 05)*
A. Hypophysectomy
B. Adrenalectomy
C. Thyroidectomy
D. Orchidectomy

120. All are associated with pituitary apoplexy except: *(AIIMS May 07)*
A. Hyperthyroidism
B. Diabetes mellitus
C. Sickle cell anemia
D. Hypertension

121. Which drug is essential in Sheehan's syndrome: *(AI 1996)*
A. Estrogen
B. Cortisone
C. Thyroxin
D. Growth hormone

122. A person sustains head trauma leading to transaction of pituitary stalk. All can be consequence of this, *except*: *(AIIMS Dec 97)*
A. SIADH
B. Diabetes mellitus
C. Diabetes insipidus
D. Hyperprolactinemia

123. A patient meets with an accident with resultant transaction of the pituitary stalk; what will NOT occur: *(AI 01)*
A. Diabetes mellitus
B. Diabetes insipidus
C. Hyperprolactinemia
D. Hypothyroidism

SIADH

124. SIADH secretion is seen in *all except* : *(AI 1994)*
A. Lung abscess
B. Interstitial Nephritis
C. Vinka alkaloids
D. Bronchial adenoma

125. SIADH is associated with the following drug : *(AI 2007)*
A. Vincristine
B. Erythromycin
C. 5 – FU
D. Methotrexate

126. SIADH is associated with : *(AIIMS Dec 97)*
A. Small cell carcinoma lung
B. Adeno carcinoma lung
C. Squamous cell carcinoma lung
D. Mixed cell tumor lung

127. All of the following statements about SIADH are true except: *(AIIMS Nov 2011)*
A. Serum sodium is low, typically < 135 meq/l
B. Urinary sodium excretion is low / normal
C. Water loading test may be used
D. Vaptans are new FDA approved agents for treatment of SIADH

128. Inappropriate ADH secretion is characterised by the following *except* : *(AI 2000)*
A. Hypo-osmolar urine
B. Water intoxication
C. Expanded fluid volume
D. Hypomagnesemia

Endocrinology 8

129. The syndrome of inappropriate antidiuretic hormone is characterized by the following :
   A. Hyponatremia and urine sodium excretion > 20 meq/l *(AI 2003)*
   B. Hypernatremia and urine sodium excretion > 20 meq/l
   C. Hyponatremia and hyperkalemia
   D. Hypernatremia and hypokalemia

130. A 35 year old man presents with vomitings and confusion. On examination Na^+ 120 m mol/L, K^+ 4.2 m mol/L, Uric acid 2 mg/dl. Patient is not edematous. The diagnosis is: *(AIIMS Nov 99)*
   A. Cerebral toxoplasmosis with SIADH
   B. Hepatic failure
   C. Severe dehydration
   D. Congestive heart failure

131. All are true regarding SIADH except: *(AIIMS Nov 93)*
   A. Increased level of ADH
   B. Urine hypoosmolar
   C. Hyponatremia
   D. Adequate hydration status

132. Which of the following statements is true about SIADH: *(AI 1991)*
   A. Hypovolemic Hyponatremia
   B. Euvolemic Hyponatremia
   C. Hypervolemic Hyponatremia
   D. Hypervolemic Hypernatremia

133. Which of the following is the drug of choice for the treatment of inappropriate anti-diuretic hormone secretion: *(AIIMS Nov 05)*
   A. Frusemide
   B. Hydrochlorothiazide
   C. Spironolactone
   D. Demeclocycline

134. Which drug is not used in SIADH: *(AI 1996)*
   A. Fludrocortisone
   B. Demeclocycline
   C. Desmopressin
   D. Hypertonic saline

Diabetes Insipidus/Psychogenic Polydypsia/Polyuria

135. Hyponatremia may be seen in all of the following conditions *except* : *(AI 1997)*
   A. Glucocorticoid deficiency
   B. SIADH
   C. Diabetes insipidus
   D. Hypothyroidism

136. All of the following conditions are known to cause diabetes insipidus, *except* : *(AIIMS May 04)* *(AI 2005)*
   A. Multiple sclerosis
   B. Head injury
   C. Histiocytosis
   D. Viral encephalitis

137. Choose the best Lab value for a patient with central diabetes insipidus : *(AI 2000)*

	Urinary Osmolality	&	Serum Osmolality
A.	50		300
B.	500		260
C.	50		260
D.	500		100

138. A 33 year old lady presents with polydipsia and polyuria. Her symptoms started soon after a road traffic accident 6 months ago. The blood pressure is 120/80mm Hg with no postural drop. The daily Na 130mEq/L, K 3.5 mEq/L, urea 15 mg/dL, sugar 65 mg/dL. The plasma osmolality is 268 mosmol/L and urine osmolality 45 mosmol/L. The most likely diagnosis is: *(AIIMS Nov 02)*
   A. Central diabetes insipidus
   B. Nephrogenic diabetes insipidus
   C. Resolving acute tubular necrosis
   D. Psychogenic polydipsia

139. In a patient if administration of exogeneus vasopressin does not increase the osmolality of urine the likely cause is *(DNB June 2009)*
   A. SIADH
   B. Psychogenic polydipsia
   C. Renal Hyposensitivity to ADH
   D. ADH Deficiency

140. Which of the following is true about nephrogenic diabetes insipidus *(DNB June 2011)*
   A. Renal tubule is unresponsive to ADH
   B. There is central decrease in secretion of ADH
   C. Serum sodium is low
   D. Urine osmolality is increased after administration of ADH

141. A 33 year old lady presents with polydipsia and polyuria. Her symptoms started soon after a road trafic accident 6 months ago. The blood pressure is 120/80 mm Hg with no postural drop. The daily urinary output is 6-8 liters. Investigation showed, Na 130 mEq/L, K.3.5 mEq/L, urea 15 mg/dL, sugar-65 mg/dL. The plasma osmolality is 268 mosmol/L and urine osmolality 45 mosmol/L. The most likely diagnosis is:
   A. Central diabetes insipidus. *(AIIMS Nov 02)*
   B. Nephrogenic diabetes insipidus.
   C. Resolving acute tubular necrosis.
   D. Psychogenic polydipsia.

142. Which of the following statements about Diabetes Insipidus is true: *(AI 2011)*
   A. Urine osmolality should be > 300 mosm/L
   B. Plasma osmolality should be < 280 mmol/L
   C. Water deprivation test is required
   D. Plasma osmolality should be > 300 mosm/L prior to H_2O Deprivation

143. A patient following head injury was admitted in intensive care ward with signs of raised intracranial pressure. He was put on ventilator and atarted on intravenous fluids and diuretics. Twenty four hours

later his urine output was 3.5 litres, serum sodium 156 mEq/l and urine osmolality of 316 mOsm/kg. The most likely diagnosis based on these parameters is
A. High output due to diuretics *(AIIMS Nov 04)*
B. Diabetes insipidus
C. Too much infusion of normal saline
D. Cerebral salt retaining syndrome

144. Primary Hyperaldosteronism can be diagnosed by all of the following criteria, except: *(AIIMS Nov 2011)*
A. Diastolic Hypertension without edema
B. Hyperaldosteronism which is not supressed by volume expansion
C. Low Plasma Renin Activity
D. Metabolic Acidosis

145. In a woman with polyuria of 6L/day, which are the 2 most important investigations to be done:
A. Water deprivation test *(PGI Dec 01)*
B. Water loading
C. Plasma and urine osmolality
D. Plasma osmolality
E. Skull X-ray

146. Mainstay of treatment of Nephrogenic Diabetes Insipidus is: *(DNB)*
A. Desmopressin
B. Thiazide / Amiloride diureties and salt restriction
C. Desmopressin and salt restriction
D. Vasopressin and salt restriction

147. Mainstay of treatment of Neurogenic (central) Diabetes Insipidus is *(DNB)*
A. Desmopressin
B. Vasopressin
C. Terlipressin
D. Amidodarone

Disorders of Calcium Metabolism

Hyperparathyroidism

148. Most common cause of hyperparathyroidism:
A. Iatrogenic *(AIIMS Nov 93)*
B. Medullary carcinoma thyroid
C. Parathyroid adenoma
D. Parathyroid hyperplasia

149. Most common cause of primary hyperparathyroidism is: *(AI 1997)*
A. Solitary adenoma
B. Chief cell hyperplasia
C. Multiple adenoma
D. Werner's syndrome

150. The commonest cause of primary hyperparathyroidism is : *(AIIMS May 95)*
A. Carcinoma parathyroid
B. Solitary adenoma of parathyroid
C. Chronic renal failure
D. Hyperplasia of the parathyroid

151. A common cause of Primary hyperparathyroidism is:
A. Multiple parathyroid adenomas *(AI 1995)*
B. Solitary parathyroid adenoma
C. Adrenal hyperplasia
D. Ectopic PTH production

152. Asymptomatic hypercalcemia in a 30 year old young male is due to : *(AI 2000; AIIMS June 99)*
A. Occult primary malignancy
B. Primary Hyperparathyroidism
C. Familial hypocalciuria
D. Hyper-nephroma

153. All are TRUE about hyperparathyroidism, Except:
A. Commonly occurs after thyroidectomy
B. May cause hypercalcemia
C. Solitary adenoma is the most common cause
D. None of the above

154. Subtle presentation of hyperparathyroidism is:
A. Psychiatric manifestation
B. Neprocalcinosis *(AIIMS Dec 97)*
C. Abdominal pain
D. Asymptomatic hypercalcemia

155. Which of the following is associated with secondary hyperparathyroidism *(AIIMS Dec 94)*
A. Parathyroid adenoma
B. Marked hypercalcemia
C. Chronic renal failure
D. Parathyroidectomy relieves the symptoms

156. Secondary Hyperparathyroidism is seen in all of the following, Except *(AIIMS Nov 2010)*
A. Rickets
B. Osteomalacia
C. Osteoporosis
D. Renal failure

157. Secondary Hyperparthyroidism is seen in all of the following, Except *(DNB)*
A. Chronic Renal Failure
B. Parathyroid adenoma
C. Vitamin D Deficiency
D. Medullary Carcinoma Thyroid

158. A 45 year old man, known case of chronic renal failure develops rugger jersy spine. The probable cause it :
A. Aluminium intoxication *(AI 2000)*
B. Secondary hyperparathyroidism
C. Osteoporosis
D. Osteomalacia

159. A 45 year old man, known case of chronic renal failure develops rugger jersey spine. The probable cause is
A. Aluminium intoxication *(AIIMS 93)*
B. Secondary hyperparathyroidism
C. Osteoporosis
D. Osteomalacia

160. Rugger jersey spine is seen in: *(PGI June 98)*
A. Myeloma
B. TB spine
C. CRF
D. Ankylosing spondylitis

161. In hyperparathyroidism all are seen except: *(PGI Dec 98)*
   A. Osteopetrosis
   B. Osteoporosis
   C. Cysts
   D. Brown tumor

162. Tufting of the terminal phalanges is seen in : *(AI 1995)*
   A. Hypoparathyroidism
   B. Hyperparathyroidism
   C. Hyperthyroidism
   D. Hypothyroidism

163. Not a marker for hyperparathyroidism is :
   A. Increase in serum calcium
   B. Increase in 24 hour urinary calcium excretion
   C. Decrease in serum calcitonin *(AIIMS June 98)*
   D. Subperiosteal resorption of phalanges

164. Low calcium and high phosphate is seen in: *(AI 2010)*
   A. Hyperparathyroidism
   B. Hypoparathyroidism
   C. Hyperthyroidism
   D. Hypothyroidism

165. All of the following statements about Pseudohypoparathyroidism are true, except: *(AI 2010)*
   A. ↓ Serum PTH
   B. ↓ Serum calclum
   C. ↑ Serum Phosphate
   D. Albreight's Hereditary osteodystrophy

166. Which of the following statements about Pseudohypoprathyroidism is true: *(AI 2011)*
   A. Caused by 'Gain of function' inherited mutation in Gsα subunit
   B. Decreased formation of cyclic GMP is observed
   C. Decreased formation of Inositol triphosphate is observed
   D. Decreased formation of c-AMP is observed

167. A patient has hyperphosphatemia with short metacarpals and associated cataract. The diagnosis is: *(PGI June 99)*
   A. Pseudohypoparathyroidism
   B. Hypophophatasia
   C. Hyperparathyroidism
   D. Osteomalacia

168. True about pseudohypoparathyroidism: *(PGI Dec 02)*
   A. Heterotopic calcification
   B. ↑ed Ca2+
   C. ↓ed PO4
   D. ↑ed PTH
   E. ↑ed response of urinary CAMP on PTH

169. A patient presents with low serum calcium, high phosphorus and elevated PTH. Which of the following investigations is least contributory to establish a diagnosis: *(AI 2011)*
   A. Vitamin D levels
   B. Serum creatinine levels
   C. Cyclic AMP response to PTH
   D. Urine myoglobin

Hypercalcemia and Related Disorders

170. Hypercalcemia is not seen in: *(AI 1995)*
   A. Lithium therapy
   B. Chronic renal failure
   C. Multiple myeloma
   D. Vitamin A deficiency

171. Hypercalcemia is associated with all Except: *(AI 2009)*
   A. Hyperparathyroidism
   B. Sarcoidosis
   C. Milk alkali syndrome
   D. Celiac disease

172. Hypercalcemia is seen in all, *except:* *(AIIMS June 99)*
   A. Acute pancreatitis
   B. Parathyroid adenoma
   C. Breast cancer
   D. Hodgkin's lymphoma

173. All are causes of hypercalcemia, *except:* *(AIIMS Dec 97)*
   A. Thyrotoxicosis
   B. Sarcoidosis
   C. Vitamin A toxicity
   D. Phenytoin toxicity

174. All are causes of hypercalcemia, except: *(AIIMS Dec 95)*
   A. Thyrotoxicosis
   B. Sarcoidosis
   C. Vitamin A toxicity
   D. Phenytoin toxicity

175. Hypercalcemia is seen in all except: *(AIIMS June 99)*
   A. Acute pancreatitis
   B. Parathyroid adenoma
   C. Breast cancer
   D. Hodgkin's lymphoma

176. Hypercalcemia is seen in all except: *(AIIMS May 93)*
   A. Acute pancreatitis
   B. Hypervitaminosis D
   C. Addison's disease
   D. Hyperparathyroidism

177. Hypercalcemia is not a feature of one of the following conditions : *(AI 1997)*
   A. Primary hyperparathyroidism
   B. Multiple myeloma
   C. Tumourlysis syndrome
   D. Sarcoidosis

178. Hypercalcemia is NOT seen in: *(AIIMS Dec 94)*
   A. Primary hyperparathyroidism
   B. Tumor lysis syndrome
   C. Multiple sclerosis
   D. Sarcoidosis

179. Causes of Hypercalcemia include all of the following except *(DNB 2010)*
   A. Multiple myeloma
   B. Lytic skeletal metastasis
   C. Total parentral nutrition
   D. Acute Pancreatitis

180. Hypercalcemia is caused by all except: *(PGI Dec 03)*
   A. Thyrotoxicosis
   B. Vit. D intoxication
   C. Sarcoidosis
   D. Furosemide
   E. Thiazide

181. Abnormalities of bone metabolism is associated with excess of which vitamins (select two best options): *(PGI June 02)*
   A. Vitamin A
   B. Thiamine
   C. Vitamin B12
   D. Vitamin D
   E. Tocoferol

182. Most common cause of hypercalcemic crisis is: *(AIIMS May 93)*
   A. Carcinoma breast
   B. Parathyroid hyperplasia
   C. Parathyroid adenoma
   D. Paget's disease

183. Surgical causes of hyper Ca^{2+}: *(PGI Dec 06)*
   A. Hyperparathyroidism
   B. MEN
   C. Hyperparathyroidism
   D. Pheochromocytoma
   E. All of the above

184. Increased serum calcium is seen in all except: *(PGI Dec 01)*
   A. Myxedema
   B. Multiple myeloma
   C. Sarcoidosis
   D. Primary hyperparathyroidism
   E. Hyperthyroidism

185. Hypercalciuria is seen in: *(PGI June 2000)*
   A. Hyperparathyroidism
   B. Vit. D intoxication
   C. Sarcoidosis
   D. All

186. A 55 year old man, a chronic smoker is brought to emergency with history of polyuria, polydipsia, nausea and altered sensorium for last two days. He had been diagnosed as having squamous cell carcinoma of lung two months prior to this. On examination, he was lethargic and confused. An ECG was normal except for a narrowed QT interval. Which one of the following is the most likely metabolic abnormality? *(AIIMS Nov 03)*
   A. Hypernatremia
   B. Hypercalcemia
   C. Hypokalemia
   D. Hyponatremia

187. Which of the following is not a feature of hypercalcemia *(AI 06)*
   A. Diarrhoea
   B. Polyuria
   C. Depression
   D. Vomiting

188. Treatment of hypercalcemia includes, all, *except*: *(AIIMS Dec 97)*
   A. Gallium nitrate
   B. Plicamycin
   C. Etidronate
   D. Rizol

189. All of the following may be used to treat hypercalcemia, except:
   A. Normal saline with forced diuresis with chlorthiazide
   B. Plicamycin
   C. Gallium nitrate
   D. Mitramycin
   E. Bisphosphonates

190. Treatment of Hypercalcemia (select two options): *(PGI Dec 04)*
   A. Calcitonin
   B. Gallium nitrate
   C. Orthophosphate
   D. Thyroxin

191. All of the following are true about Hypercalcemia, except: *(PGI June 04)*
   A. Management of primary cause
   B. Malignancy may cause hypercalcemia
   C. IV fluid with furosemide is given
   D. Pamidronate is not effective

192. All are used in treatment of hypercalcemia, except: *(AIIMS May 93)*
   A. Phosphate
   B. Mithramycin
   C. Vitamin D in high dose
   D. Any of the above

193. All of the following may be used to treat Acute Hypercalcemia Except:
   A. Hydration with saline
   B. Calcitonin
   C. Biphosphonates
   D. Gallium Nitrate

194. A 75 year old lady with fracture neck of femur presents with two days history of altered sensorium and decreased urinary output. Serum calcium is 15.5 mg dl, Urea is 140 mg/dl, Creatinine is 2 mg/dl. All of the following are useful for immediate management of Hypercalcemia, Except: *(AIIMS Nov 2010)*
   A. Normal saline
   B. Furosemide
   C. Dialysis
   D. Bisphosphonates

195. All of the following agents may be used in the management of Chronic Hypocalcemia, except: *(AI 2012)*
   A. Etidronate
   B. Thiazides
   C. Elemental calcium
   D. Vitamin D analogs

196. Raised calcium and phosphorous seen in: *(PGI June 02)*
   A. CRF
   B. Vitamin D intoxication
   C. Hyperparathyroidism
   D. Pseudohypoparathyroidism

197. Hypocalcemia with hyperphosphatemia are seen in: *(PGI Dec 2000)*
   A. CRF
   B. Pseudohypoparathyroidism

C. Vit. D deficiency
D. Magnesium deficiency

198. Hypophophatemia is seen in: *(PGI Dec 02)*
A. Pseudohypoparathyroidism
B. CRF
C. Rickets
D. Hyperparathyroidism
E. Respiratory acidosis

199. Hypophosphatemia is seen in all except: *(AI 2007)*
A. Acute renal failure
B. Resolving phases of diabetic ketocidosis
C. Respiratory alkalosis / COPD
D. Chronic alcoholism

Vitamin D deficiency & Paget's Disease

200. Which of the following is not seen in Vitamin D deficiency: *(PGI Dec 01)*
A. Increased alkaline phosphate
B. Decreased phosphate in urine
C. Hypophosphatemia
D. Decreased serum calcium

201. A patient Shweta with raised serum alkaline phosphatase and raised parathormone level along with low calcium and low phosphate level is likely to have
A. Primary hyperparathyroidism *(AIIMS June 99)*
B. Paget's disease
C. Osteoporosis
D. Vitamin D deficiency

202. True about rickets: *(PGI June 01)*
A. Hyperphosphatemia
B. Hypophosphatemia
C. Hypophosphaturia
D. Decreased alkaline phosphatase

203. All of the following are seen in ricket's except:
A. Bow legs *(AIIMS May 03)*
B. Gunstock deformity
C. Pot belly
D. Cratio tabes

204. Which is not *true* of hypocalcaemia: *(AI 1995)*
A. Can occur in hypoparathyroidism
B. Latent tetany is seen
C. Prolonged QT intervala
D. Inverse relation with Mg^{++} levels

205. During a routine check up, a 67-year-old man is found to have a level of serum alkaline phosphatase three times the upper limit of normal. Serum calcium and phosphorus concentrations and liver function test results are normal. He is asymptomatic. The most likely diagnosis is : *(AIIMS Nov 99)*
A. Metastatic bone disease
B. Primary hyperparathyroidism
C. Paget's disease of bone
D. Osteomalacia

206. Increased alkaline phosphate in seen in : *(AI 1999)*
A. Multiple myeloma
B. Primary hyperparathyroidism
C. Chronic renal failure
D. Osteoporosis

207. Alkaline phosphatase is elevated in all, EXCEPT:
A. Rickets *(AIIMS Dec 97)*
B. Osteomalacia
C. Hypoparathyroidism
D. Hypophosphatemia

208. Raised serum alkaline phosphatase is seen in all, Except: *(AIIMS Dec 94)*
A. Paget's disease
B. Multiple myeloma
C. Osteomalacia
D. Hyperthyroidism

Osteoporosis

209. Osteoporosis is seen in all the following *except:*
A. Thyrotoxicosis *(AI 1994)*
B. Rheumatoid arthritis
C. Hypoparathyroidism
D. Steroid therapy

210. All are causes of Osteoporosis, *except* :
A. Thyrotoxicosis *(AI 2000)*
B. Hypothyroidism
C. Chronic heparin therapy
D. Old age

211. Osteoporosis may be seen in all *except*:
A. Hyperparathyroidism *(AI 1998)*
B. Hypoparathyroidism
C. Thyrotoxicosis
D. Heparin administration

212. Osteoporosis is caused by *all except:* *(AI 1996)*
A. Sarcoidosis
B. Old age
C. Hypoparathyroidism
D. Steroid therapy

213. Osteoporosis is seen in : *(AI 1994)*
A. Thyrotoxicosis
B. Cushing's disease
C. Menopause
D. All of the above

214. All of the following are the known causes of osteoporosis except : *(AI 06)*
A. Fluorosis
B. Hypogonadism
C. Hyperthyroidism
D. Hyperparathyroidism

215. The most common manifestation of osteoporosis is:
A. Compression fracture of the spine *(AI 1994)*
B. Asymptomatic, detected incidentally by low serum Calcium
C. Bowing of legs
D. Loss of weight

Tumour Lysis Syndrome

216. Tumor Lysis Syndrome causes all of the following except *(DNB)*
   A. Hypercalcemia
   B. Hyperuricemia
   C. Hypermagnesemia
   D. Hyperkalemia
217. Features of tumor lysis syndrome are: *(PGI Dec 2000)*
   A. Hypocalcemia
   B. Hypophosphatemia
   C. Alkalosis
   D. Hypokalemia
218. Features of tumor lysis syndrome (select three best options): *(PGI June 06)*
   A. Hyperuricemia
   B. Hypercalcemia
   C. Hyperphosphatemia
   D. Hypernatremia
   E. Hyperkalemia
219. True about tumor lysis syndrome are A/E: *(PGI Dec 03)*
   A. Hyperuricemia
   B. Hypercalcemia
   C. Hyperkalemia
   D. Hyperphosphatemia
   E. Hypocalcemia
220. All of the following are seen in Tumor Lysis Syndrome, except: *(AIIMS May 09; AIIMS Nov 03)*
   A. Hyperkalemia
   B. Hypercalcemia
   C. Hyperuricemia
   D. Hyperphosphatemia
221. Tumor lysis syndrome is associated with all of the following laboratory feature except: *(AIIMS Nov 03)*
   A. Hyperkalemia
   B. Hypercalcemia
   C. Hyperuricemia
   D. Hyperphosphatemia

Disorders of Thyroid Gland

222. Hypothyroidism may be caused by *(DNB)*
   A. Lithium
   B. Hematochromatosis
   C. Scleroderma
   D. All of the above
223. Which of the following conditions is associated with Hypothyroidism: *(AI 2011)*
   A. Hoshimoto's Thyroiditis
   B. Grave's Disease
   C. Toxic Multinodular Goiter
   D. Struma ovary
224. Hypothyroidism in sub-himlayan region is due to deficiency of *(DNB 2010)*
   A. Iron
   B. Iodine
   C. Copper
   D. Selenium
225. Which of the following is not associated with hypothyroidism *(DNB)*
   A. Low T3
   B. High TSH
   C. High Triglycerides
   D. Low cholesterol
226. All of the following are features of thyrotoxicosis, EXCEPT- *(AIIMS June 99)*
   A. Diastolic murmur
   B. Soft non ejection systolic murmur
   C. Irregularly, irregular pulse
   D. Scratching sound in systole
227. Dancing carotid is seen in : *(AIIMS Dec 98)*
   A. Thyrotoxicosis
   B. Hypothyroidism
   C. AV Fistula
   D. Blow out carotid
228. Thyroid carcinoma associated with hypocalcemia is *(AIIMS Dec 94)*
   A. Follicular carcinoma
   B. Medullary carcinoma
   C. Anaplastic carcinoma
   D. Papillary carcinoma
229. The best marker to diagnose thyroid related disorder is *(AI 2004)*
   A. T3
   B. T4
   C. TSH
   D. Thyroglobulin
230. The Lab investigation of patient shows ↓T3, ↓T4, & ↓TSH. It cannot be : *(AI 2000)*
   A. Primary hypothyroidism
   B. Pan-hypopinitarism
   C. Liver disease
   D. None of the above
231. The occurrence of hyperthyroidism following administration of supplemental iodine to subjects with endemic iodine deficiency goiter is known as: *(AI 2004)*
   A. Jod-Basedow effect
   B. Wolff-Chaokoff effect
   C. Thyrotoxicosis factitia
   D. De Quervain's thyroiditis
232. The occurrence of hyperthyroidism following administration of supplemental iodine to subjects with endemic iodine deficiency goiter is known as: *(AI 2012, 04)*
   A. Jod-Basedow effect
   B. Wolff-Chaokoff effect
   C. Thyrotoxicosis factitia
   D. De Quervain's thyroiditis
233. All of the following are true about amiadarone induced thyroid dysfunction except? *(AI 2004)*
   A. Hyperthyroidism is common in iodine deficient areas
   B. Hypothyroidism is more common in men
   C. Amiodarone inhibits deiodinase activity
   D. Amiodaraone therapy is associated with initial reduction of serum T4 levels

234. In Thyrotoxicosis, β-blockers do *not* control: (AI 1994)
A. Anxiety
B. Tremors
C. Tachycardia
D. Oxygen consumption

235. All of the following are associated with Thyroid storm, Except : (AI 2002)
A. Surgery for thyroiditis
B. Surgery for thyrotoxicosis
C. Stressful illness in thyrotoxicosis
D. I^{131} therapy for thyrotoxicosis

236. Most common cause of Thyroiditis is: (AI 2000)
A. Reidl 's Thyroiditis
B. Subacute Thyroditis
C. Hashimoto's Thyroiditis
D. Viral Thyroiditis

237. A patient presents with B/L proptosis, heat intolerance and palpitations; most unlikely diagnosis here would be (AI 2001)(AI 2000)
A. Hoshimoto's thyroiditis
B. Thyroid adenoma
C. Diffuse thyroid goitre
D. Reidel's thyroiditis

238. All the following are true of DeQuervan's Thyroiditis *except* (AI 1996)
A. Pain
B. Increased ESR
C. Increased radioactive iodine uptake
D. Fever

239. Not a feature of dequervan's disease: (AI 2002)
A. Autoimmune in etiology
B. ↑ESR
C. Tends to regress spontaneously
D. Painful & associated with enlargements of thyroid

240. 'Hurthle cells' are seen in (AI 1995)
A. Agranulomatous Thyroiditis
B. Hashimoto's Thyroiditis
C. Papillary carcinoma of the thyroid
D. Thyroglossal cyst

241. The most common presentation of endemic goiter is (AI 1996)
A. Hypothyroid
B. Diffuse goiter
C. Hyperthyroid
D. Solitary nodule

242. Decreased Radio iodine uptake is / are seen in (select two options): (PGI Dec 2000)
A. Toxic multinodular goiter
B. Grave's disease
C. Subacute thyroiditis
D. Factitious thyroiditis

243. Needle biopsy of solitary thyroid nodule in a young woman with palpable cervical lymph nodes on the same sides demonstrates amyloid in stroma of lesion. Likely diagnosis is (AI 2002)
A. Medullary carcinoma thyroid
B. Follicular carcinoma thyroid
C. Thyroid adenoma
D. Multi nodular goitre

244. Screening method for medullary carcinoma thyroid is : (AI 1997)
A. Serum calcitonin
B. S. calcium
C. S. alkaline phosphate
D. S. acid phosphatase

245. FNAC is useful in all the following types of thyroid carcinoma *except* (AI 1995)
A. Papillary
B. Follicular
C. Anaplastic
D. Medullary

246. A 26 year woman presents with a palpable thyroid nodule, and needle biopsy demonstrates amyloid in the stroma of the lesion. A cervical lymph node is palpable on the same side as the lesion. the preferred treatment should be : (AI 2002)
A. Removal of the involved node, the isthmus, and the enlarged lymph node
B. Removal of the involved lobe, the isthmus, a portion of the opposite lobe, and he enlarged lymph node.
C. Total thyroidectomy and modified neck dissection on the side of the enlarged lymph node.
D. Total thyroidectomy and irradiation of the cervical lymph nodes.

Endocrine Tumors

247. Pheochromocytoma predominantly secretes (AIIMS Nov 01)
A. Epinephrine
B. Norepinephrine
C. Dopamine
D. DOPA

248. Extraadrenal Pheochromocytoma predominantly secretes: (PGI June 03)
A. Epinephrine
B. Norepinephrine
C. Dopamine
D. DOPA

249. Which of the following urinary metabolites are most sensitive for diagnosis of pheochromocytomas (DNB)
A. VMA
B. Metanephrines
C. 5HIAA
D. 5HTP

250. All of the following are increased in pheochromocytomas, except (DNB 2012)
A. Vinyl Mandelic Acid (VMA) (DNB)
B. Metanephrines
C. 5HIAA
D. Catecholamines

251. Pheochromocytomas are known to arise from all of the following, except: (PGI 09)
A. Adrenal gland
B. Mediastinum

C. Neck
D. Abdomen
E. Chest wall

252. All of the following are features of phaeochromocytoma *except* : (AI 2002)
A. Hypertensive paroxysm
B. Headache
C. Orthostatic hypotension
D. Wheezing

253. All are clinical features of pheochromocytoma, *except* :
A. Increased hematocrit (AIIMS Feb 97)
B. Orthostatic hypotension
C. Low cortisol level
D. Impaired glucose tolerance

254. All of the following are seen in pheochromocytoma, Except (DNB 2010)
A. Headache
B. Sweating episodes
C. Weight loss
D. Hypocalcemia

255. The predominant symptom / sign of pheochromocytoma is (DNB 2012)
A. Sweating
B. Weight loss
C. Orthostatic hypotension
D. Episodic Hypertension

256. Somatostatin is secreted by : (AIIMS Feb 97)
A. D-cell
B. A-cell
C. B-cell
D. D1-cell

257. Weight loss may be seen in all of the following *except* :
A. Uremia (AI 1998)
B. Pheochromacytoma
C. Adrenal insufficiency
D. Insulinoma

258. The triad originally described by Zollinger Ellison syndrome is characterized by: (AI 2002)
A. Peptic ulceration, gastric hypersecretion, non beta cell tumour
B. Peptic ulceration, gastric hypersecretion, beta cell tumour
C. Peptic ulceration, achlorhydria, non beta cell tumour
D. Peptic ulceration, achlorhydria, beta cell tumour

259. Gold standard test for diagnosis of Insulinoma is:
A. '72 hour' fast test (AI 2009)
B. Plasma Glucose levels < 3 mmol/l
C. Plasma Insulin levels > 6μU/ml
D. C- peptide levels < 50 p mol/e

260. Which of the following tests is not used in the diagnosis of insulinoma (AI 2011)
A. Fasting blood glucose
B. Xylose test
C. C- peptide levels
D. Insulin /Glucose Ratio

261. Carcinoid tumour is most common in
A. Esophagus (AIIMS May 04)
B. Stomach
C. Jejunum
D. Appendix

262. All of the following statements about carcinoid syndrome are true except (DNB)
A. Atypical carcinoid syndrome is usually produced by foregut carcinoids
B. Plasma serotonin levels are normal in Atypical carcinoid syndrome
C. Midgut carcinoids have high serotonin content
D. Foregut carcinoids are usually argentaffin positive

263. All of the following may be raised in carcinoid syndrome, Except (DNB 2012)
A. 5HIAA
B. 5HT
C. 5HTP
D. VMA

264. Diagnosis of carcinoid tumors is done by: (DNB)
A. 5HIAA
B. DHEA
C. VMA
D. Metanephrines

265. Which of the following is most likely to be raised in patients with Atypical carcinoids (DNB)
A. 5 HIAA
B. 5 HTP
C. VMA
D. Metanephrines

266. All of the following about Gastrointestinal Carcinoid tumors are true, Except: (AI 2010)
A. Small intestine and appendix account for almost 60% of all gastrointestinal carcinoid.
B. Rectum is spared
C. 5 year survival for carcinoid tumors is >60%
D. Appendicial carcinoids are more commin in females than males.

267. Carcinoid syndrome produces valvular disease primarily of the (AIIMS May 04)
A. Venous valves
B. Tricuspid valve
C. Mitral valve
D. Aortic valve

Weight Gain & Obesity

268. Weight gain occurs in all, *except* :
A. Pheochromocytoma (AIIMS June 97, 99)
B. Cushing's syndrome
C. Hypothyroidism
D. Insulin secreting tumor

269. All cause weight gain, *except* : (AIIMS Sept 96)
A. Diabetes mellitus
B. Cushing's syndrome
C. Hypothyroidism
D. Insulin secreting tumour

270. Obesity is not a feature of : *(AIIMS May 95)*
   A. Hypothyroidism
   B. Adrenal insufficiency
   C. Hypogonadism
   D. Cushing's syndrome

271. Weight gain is seen in all except: *(AIIMS June 99)*
   A. Pheochromocytoma
   B. Insulinoma
   C. Myxoedema
   D. Cushing's disease

272. Weight loss may be seen in all of the following except : *(AI 1998)*
   A. Uremia
   B. Pheochromacytoma
   C. Adrenal insufficiency
   D. Insulinoma

273. Obesity is associated with all of the following *except*: *(AI 1997)*
   A. Osteoarthritis
   B. Hypertension
   C. Gall stones
   D. Pancreatitis

Miscellaneous

274. All of the following statements about Galactorrhea are true, Except:
   A. May be Bilateral
   B. Associated with lactation
   C. Associated with Prolactinomas
   D. All statements are true

275. Estimation of the following hormones is useful while investigating a case of gynaecomastia *except* : *(AI 2004)*
   A. Testosterone
   B. Prolactin
   C. Estradiol
   D. Lutenizing hormone

276. A combination of gynaecomastia, decreased serum testosterone and LH in a male patient is seen in: *(AIIMS Dec 97)*
   A. Testicular failure
   B. Sertoli cell tumor
   C. Gonadotrophins
   D. Androgen resistant state

277. The karyotype of patient with androgen insensitivity syndrome is : *(AI 2005)*
   A. 46XX
   B. 46XY
   C. 47XXY
   D. 45XO

278. A baby girl presents with bilateral inguinal masses, thought to be hernias but are found to be testes in the inguinal canals. Which karyotype would you expect to find in the child : *(AIIMS Nov 2004)*
   A. 46, XX
   B. 46, XY
   C. 47, XXY
   D. 47, XYY

279. A 21 year old woman presents with complaints of primary amenorrhoea. Her height is 153 cms, weight is 51 kg. She has well developed breasts. She has no pubic or axillary hair and no hirsuitism. Which of the following is the most probable diagnosis? *(AI 2004)*
   A. Turner's syndrome
   B. Stein-Leventhal syndrome
   C. Premature ovarian failure
   D. Complete androgen insensitivity syndrome

280. A 15 year old female presents with primary amenorrhoea. Her breasts are Tanner 4 but she has no axillary or pubic hair. The most likely diagnosis is : *(AI 06)*
   A. Turner's syndrome
   B. Mullerian agensis
   C. Testicular feminization syndrome
   D. Premature ovarian failure

281. The diagnosis of a patient presenting with familial Polyostosis, Precocious puberty and Pigmentation is: *(AI 1995)*
   A. Tuberous sclerosis
   B. McCune Albright syndrome
   C. Klinefelter syndrome
   D. SLE

282. All of the following are associated with hypergonadotrophic hypogonadism in males, Except: *(AI 2010)*
   A. Viral orchitis
   B. Klinefelter's syndrome
   C. Kallman's syndrome
   D. Noonan syndrome

283. Which of the following is the most common cause of hypergonadotrophic hypogonadism in males: *(AI 2010)*
   A. Viral Orchitis
   B. Klinefelter's syndrome
   C. Kallman's Syndrome
   D. Noonan Syndrome

284. Endocrinal causes of Carpal Tunnel syndrome include all of the following, Except *(AI 2009)*
   A. Diabetes Mellitus
   B. Hypothyroidism
   C. Acromegaly
   D. Addison's disease

285. Hirsuitism is caused by all, Except: *(AI 2009)*
   A. Cushing's syndrome
   B. Hyperthyroidism
   C. Hyperprolactinemia
   D. Acromegaly

286. Which of the following is not associated with diarrhea *(DNB 2011)*
   A. Diabetes Mellitus
   B. Hypercalcemia
   C. Hyperthyroidism
   D. Carcinoids

287. ACTH is produced by which of the following Bronchogenic carcinomas *(DNB)*
   A. Adenocarcinoma
   B. Small cell carcinoma
   C. Squamous cell carcinoma
   D. Branchoalveolar carcinoma

ANSWERS, REFEARENCES, EXPLANATIONS AND RELEVANT HIGH YIELD FACTS

MEN Syndromes

1. **Answer is D (MEN IIB)**; *Harrison 16th/2231; Harrison 17th/2359; Harrison 18th/p 3073*

The association of medullary carcinoma thyroid & pheochromocytoma, with mucosal neuromas and marfinoid habitus is designated 'MEN IIB' – *Harrison 15th/2187.*

- *Mucosal neuromas and marfinoid habitus are the most distinctive features of MEN IIB and are recognized in childhood. – Harrison*
- *True Neuromas are present on the tip of tongue, under the eyelids and throughout the gastrointestinal tract and are tree neuromas distinct from neurofibromas.*

MEN I	MEN II	
	MEN II A	MEN II B
Characteristic Manifestations • Parathyroid hyperplasia or adenoma • Pancreatic tumors (Islet cell hyperplasia, adenoma, or carcinoma) • Pituitary hyperplasia or adenoma Other less common manifestations • Foregut carcinoid • Subcutaneous or visceral lipomas • Dermal angiofibromas or collagenomas	• MTC • Pheochromocytoma • Parathyroid hyperplasia or adenoma • Cutaneous lichen amyloidosis • Hischsprung disease • FMTC	• MTC • Pheochromocytoma • Mucosal and gastrointestinal neuromas • Marfanoid features

2. **Answer is B (Gastrinoma):***Harrison 16th / 2232; Harrison 17th/2358, 2359; Harrison 18th/p 3072, 3073*

Amongst the options provided Gastrinomas are the most common association with MEN 1.

Gastrinomas > Insulinomas > Glucagonomas > VIPomos > Somatostainomas

MEN 1

Parathyroid tumors (Most Common)	Pancreatic endocrine tumors (Second Most Common)	Pituitary tumors (Third Most Common)
Hyperparathyroidism is the most common manifestation of MEN I -Harrison	***Neoplasia of the pancreatic islets is the second most common manifestation of MEN I***[Q]. -Harrison	*Pituitary tumors are third most common tumors of MEN 1 and occur in more than half of patients with MEN 1*
Relative frequency of Tumors causing Hyperparathyroidism :	**Relative frequency of Endocrine Tumors of Pancreatic Islets :**	**Relative frequency of Pituitary Tumors :**
Parathyroid hyperplasia *is the most common cause of hyperparathyroidism in MEN I* **Parathyroid adenomas** *are less common than parathyroid hyperplasia and tend to occur in older patient or those with long standing disease.*	Pancreatic polypeptide (75 – 85%) ***Gastrin (60%) (Gastrinomas /ZES)*** Insulin (25 – 30%) (Insulinomas) Glucagon (5 – 10%)(Glucagonoma) VIP (3 – 5%) (VIPomas) Somatostatin (1 – 5%) (Somatostatinoma)	**Prolactinomas** are the most common pituitary tumors in MEN I **Acromegaly** due to excessive growth hormone (GH) production is the second most common pituitary tumor in MEN I **Cushing's** syndrome

VIPoma is synonymous with Verner Morrison syndrome or Water Diarrhea Syndrome or Pancreatic Cholera[Q]**.**

Other Tumors in MEN I

- *Carcinoid tumours (foregut type : derived from lung,thymus,stomach or duodenum)*
- *Subcutaneous & visceral lipomas*
- *Cutaneous leiomyomas*
- *Skin angiofibromas or collagenomas*

3. **Answer is D (Medullary Carcinoma Thyroid)**

Medullary Carcinoma Thyroid is a feature of MEN II syndrome. These tumors are not seen in MEN I syndrome.

Parathyroid Tumors, Pancreatic islet cell tumors and Pituitary Tumors are typical of MEN I Syndrome.

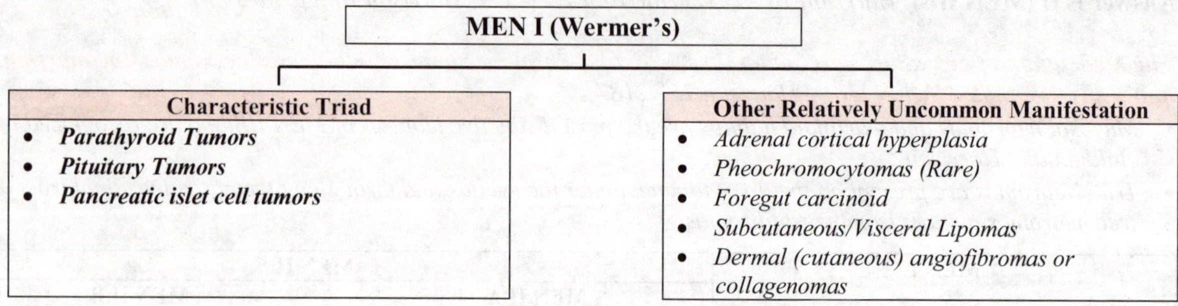

4. **Answer is A (Gastrinoma):** *Harrisons 16th/ 2232; 17th/2358, 2359; Refer previous question; Harrison 18th/p 3073*

Amongst the options provided Gastrinomas are the most common association with MEN-I

Gastrinomas > Insulinomas > Glucagonomas > VIPomos > Somatostainomas

5. **Answer is B (Adrenal):** *Harrison 16th/2231; Harrison's 17th/2359; Harrison 18th/p 3073*

Adrenal tumors are not a characteristic feature of MEN I syndrome.
Tumors of parathyroid, pituitary and pancreas are characteristic of MEN I syndrome.

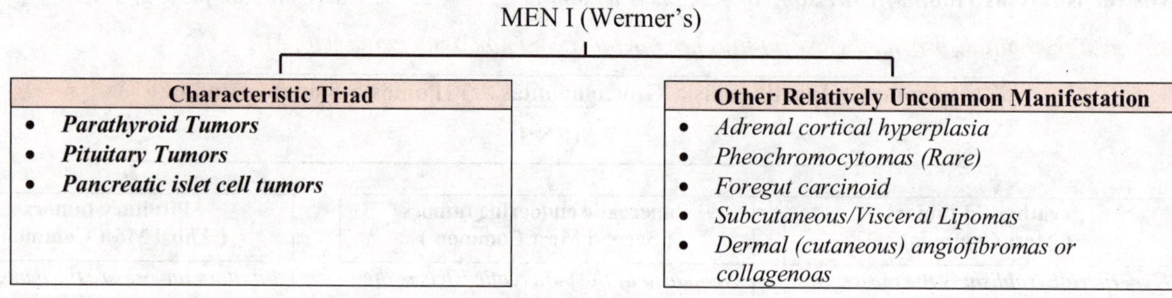

6. **Answer is A (MEN I):** *Harrison 17th/2359; Harrison 18th/p 3073*

Association of Parathyroid, Pancreatic and Pituitary tumors along with adrenal cortical hyperplasia and cutaneous angiofibromas suggests a diagnosis of MEN I syndrome.

7. **Answer is B (Islet cell hyperplasia):** *Harrison 16th/2231; Harrison 17th/2359; Harrison 18th/p 3073*
Pituitary islet cell tumors/hyperplasia are associated with MEN- I syndromes and not with MEN II syndromes.

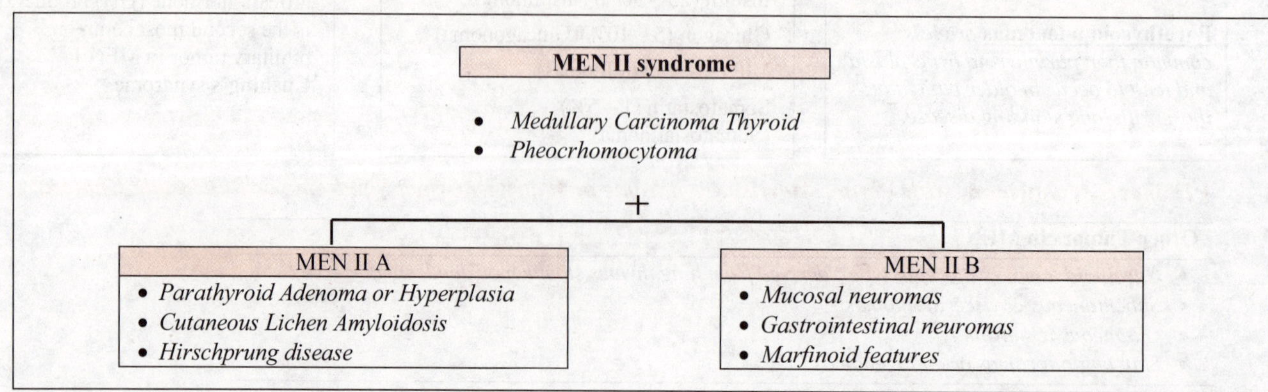

8. Answer is A (Pituitary Tumor): *Harrison 16th/2231;; Robbin's 5th/1170; Harrison 17th/2359; Harrison 18th/p 3073*

Both pituitary tumor (MEN I) and neuromas (MEN IIb) are not part of MEN IIa.
Pituitary tumor is the single best answer of exclusion here in view of the fact that MEN IIb syndromes are more similar to MEN IIa than MEN I syndromes.

'While MEN IIb is very similar to MEN IIa, MEN I is distinctly different from the MEN II syndromes'*-Harrison*

- Medullary Ca thyroid and Pheochromocytoma are features of MEN IIa
- *Mucosal and GI ganglioneuroma are a features of MEN II b and not MEN II a.*
- *Pituitary adenoma are not a feature of any of the MEN II syndromes. They are seen in MEN I only.*

9. Answer is A (Hyperparthyroidism): *Harrison 16th/2231; Harrison's 17th/2359*

Hyperparathyroidism is not seen in MEN II B syndromes.

Hyperparathyroidism (Parathyroid Hyperplasia or adenoma) is seen in MEN I and MEN II A.

10. Answer is A (Medullary Carcinoma of Thyroid); *Harrison 16th/2231; 17th/2358; Harrison 18th/p 3072, 3073*
Out of all the histological variants of carcinoma thyroid it is the medullary variant that is associated with multiple endocrinal neoplastic syndromes and hence is the answer here.
(No confusion regarding the answer)

What puzzles the situation? is the fact that the combination of pancreatitis, pituitary tumor and pheochromocytoma, suggests a diagnosis of MENI syndrome. MEN I has been mentioned to be associated with C cell hyperplasia, and not Medullary carcinoma thyroid. Medullary thyroid carcinomas is a feature of MEN II syndromes.
Justification: Medullary carcinoma thyroid arises from parafollicular C cells. C cell hyperplasia thus, may be regarded as a precursor of Medullary carcinoma thyroid.
If present in the options, C cell hyperplasia would have been a more correct answer, however in its absence, Medullary thyroid carcinoma is certainly the option of choice

MEN SYNDROMES (Broad Perspective)

<table>
<tr><th rowspan="2">MEN I (WERMER'S)</th><th colspan="2">MEN II</th></tr>
<tr><td colspan="2">Characterized by association of
- Medullary carcinoma thyroid &
- Pheochromocytoma</td></tr>
<tr><td rowspan="2">Characterized by tumors of
1. Parathyroid
2. Pituitary
3. Pancreatic islet cells
- Zollinger Ellison syndrome (gastrin)
- Insulinoma (Insulin)
- Glucagonoma (Glucagen)
- Verner morrison or watery diarrhea syndrome (pancreatic cholera)</td><td>II A</td><td>II B</td></tr>
<tr><td>When associated with hyper-parathyroidism</td><td>When associated with mucosal neuromas and marfinoid habitus</td></tr>
</table>

11. Answer is B (Urine VMA and aspiration of the thyroid nodule) : *Refer previous question; Harrison 17th/2361; Harrison 18th/3075, 3076*

Intermittent headache *(most common symptom of Phaeochromocytoma)* and presence of Thyroid Nodule point towards the occurrence of Phaeochromocytoma with Medullary Carcinoma Thyroid suggesting a diagnosis of MEN II syndrome.
Next logical step to be taken is to confirm the provisional diagnosis and hence the following investigations are recommended.

For diagnosis of phaeochromocytoma	For diagnosis of Medullary Ca Thyroid
Demonstrate excretion of Catecholamine metabolites in urine such as VMA, Metanephrine or free Catecholamines.	**Aspiration of thyroid nodule**

12. Answer is D (Serial 24 hours test for catecholamines, metanephrines and vanillylamandelic acid excretion) : *Harrison 16th/ 2150; Bailey 24th/ 802/819; Harrison 17th/2361, Love & Bailey 24th/809, 819; Harrison 18th/p 3076*

'Pheochromocytoma, must be excluded by measurement of urinary catecholamines levels in all cases before embarking upon thyroid surgery to avoid the potential hazards of this condition' – *Bailey*

Essays employed for diagnosis of pheochromocytoma include those for:
1. Vanillyl mandelic acid (VMA) 2. Metanephrines 3. Free catecholamines

<u>The patient in question is a case of inherited Men II a syndromes</u>

The presence of 'headache and sweating' in a patient with thyroid nodule warrants prompt investigation for a possible pheochromocytoma as part of MEN II syndrome, more so in a patient with a positive family history (as suggested by presence of renal calculi and thyroid nodule in mother).

Pheochromocytoma secrete large amounts of catecholamines, the secretion of which is further increased during surgery. This may result in large swings in blood pressure and arrhythmias, and increases the risk of surgical mortality. Stabie α adrenergic blockage is essential before embarking on thyroid surgery.

<u>Excluding other options</u>:

Measurement of thyroid hormones	5-HIAA urinary estimation	Serum calcium, phosphorus alkaline phosphatase
• Medullary carcinoma thyroid is usually euthyroid, the levels of thyroid hormone remaining unaltered (Pt. in question has no clinical signs of thyrotoxicosis) • Medullary Ca thyroid is assayed by measuring calcitonin level in blood. • Calcitonin levels may aid in diagnosis of MCT but offer no specific advantage to surgeons prior to surgery	This is done for the diagnosis of carcinoid syndrome (not associated MEN II a)	These may aid in diagnosis of hyperparathyroidism a part of MEN II a but again offer no specific advantage to surgeons prior to surgery on thyroid.

Disorders of Adrenal Cortex

Cushing's Syndrome

13. Answer is D (Iatrogenic steroids): *Harrison 16th/2135; Harrison 17th/2254 (336.2); Harrison 18th/p 2945*

"The most common cause of Cushing's syndrome is Iatrogenic administration of steroids for a variety of reasons." *-Harrison*

<u>Causes of Cushing's syndrome</u>

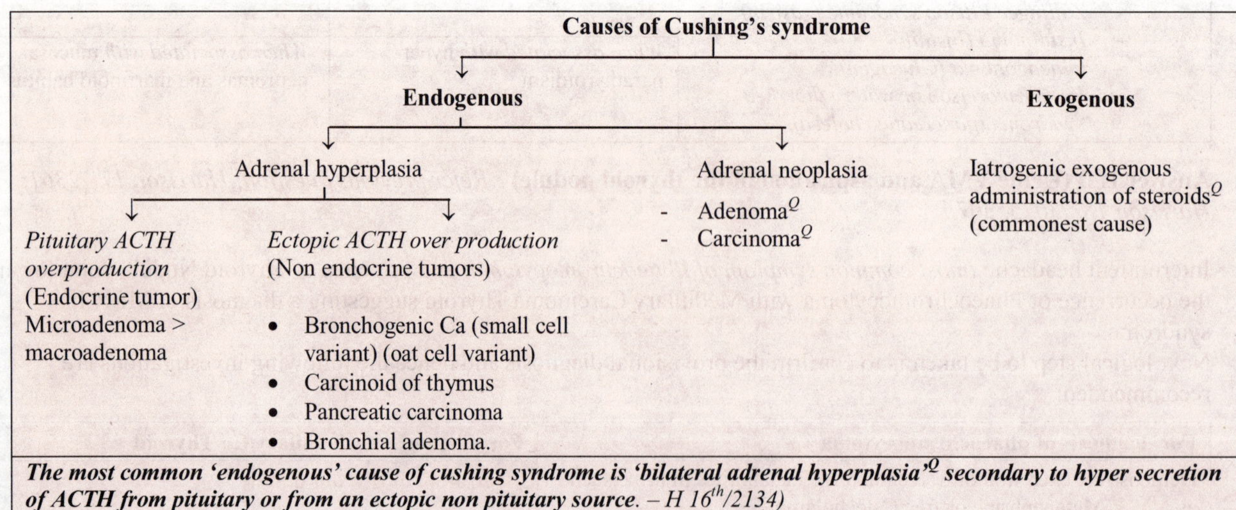

14. Answer is B (Pituitary adenoma): *Harrison's 17th/2254; Harrison 18th/p 2945*

ACTH producing pituitary adenoma are the most common cause of endogenous Cushing syndrome.

Cushing's Syndrome

Endogenous Cushing's Syndrome	Exogenous Cushing's Syndrome
Most common cause of endogenous Cushing's syndrome is an ACTH secreting pituitary adenoma (Cushing's disease)	*The most common cause of exogenous Cushing's syndrome is iatrogenic administration of steroids.*

15. Answer is B (Cushing's syndrome): *Harrison 17th/2255; Harrison 18th/p 2945*

The most common cause of Cushing's syndrome is iatragenic administration of steroids for a variety of reasons.

- Harrison

16. Answer is C (Medulloblastoma) : *Harrison 16th/2134; Harrison 17th/2254-2255; Harrison 18th/p 2945, 2946*

Meduloblastoma is not associated with Cushing's syndrome

Tumors associated with Cushing Syndrome

Non-endocrine tumors	Endocrine Tumors
• Bronchogenic Ca (small cell or oat cell variant) • Carcinoid of thymus • Pancreatic carcinoma. • Bronchial adenoma.	Pituitary adenomas

17. Answer is B (Menorrhagia): *Harrison 16th/2135; Harrison 17th/2255; Harrison 18th/p 2945, 2946*

Cushing syndrome is associated with amenorrhea or oligomenorrhea and not with menorrhagia.

'In women increased levels of adrenal androgens can cause oligommorrhea or amenorrhea' *– Harrisons*

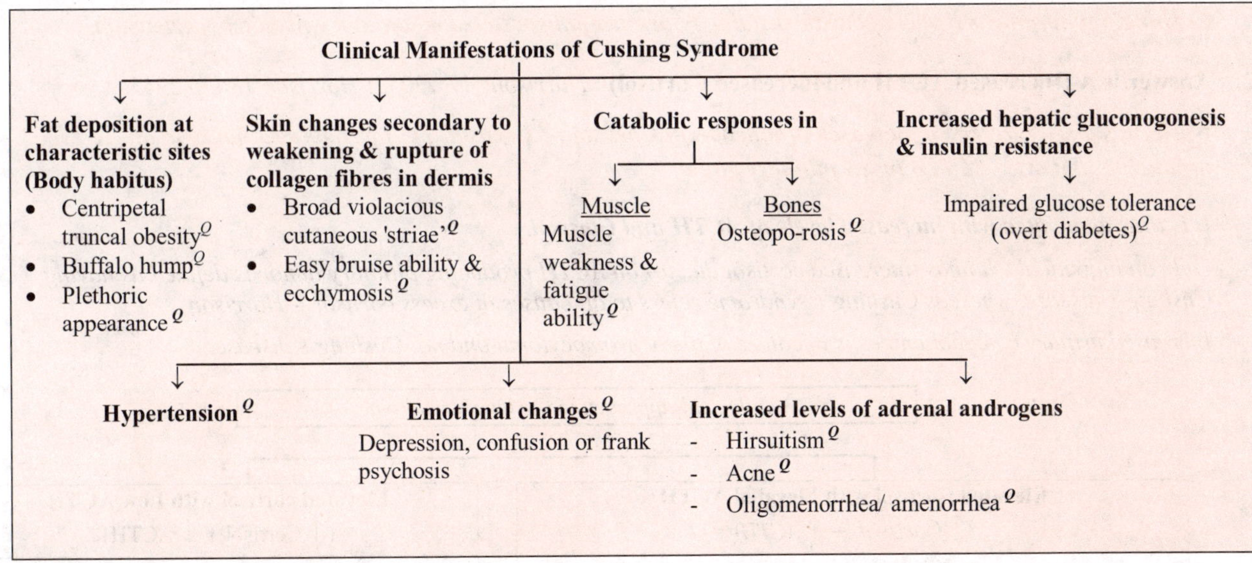

Hypokalemia / hypochloremia and metabolic alkalosis are particularly present with ectopic ACTH production.

18. Answer is B (Increased adrenaline): *Harrison's 17th/2255; William's Endocrinology 11th/463; 18th/2945, 2946, 2947*

Increased Adrenaline is not a feature of Cushing's syndrome

Cushing's syndrome results from an excessive amount of corticosteroids secreted from the adrenal cortex (outer part) of the adrenal gland. Adrenaline is secreted from the adrenal medulla (inner part) of the gland and is not raised in Cushing's syndrome. Increased adrenaline is a feature of adrenal medullary disorders like pheochromocytoma.

Red striae may be seen in Cushing Syndrome

Red or purplish 'violaceous' striae are typical of Cushing's syndrome – William's Endocrinology

Proximal muscle weaknes may be seen in Cushing's syndrome

'The myopathy of Cushing's syndrome typically involves the proximal muscles of lower limbs or shoulder girdle'
– William's Endocrinology

Edema may be seen in Cushing's syndrome *(Harrison 17th/2255)*

Edema is seen in about 60% of patients with Cushing's syndrome. This is believed to result from mineralocorticoid action, because glucocorticoids in high concentrations have mineralocorticoid action.

19. **Answer is E (None – All are seen):** *Refer previous question*

Cushing's syndrome may be associated with all features mentioned in the question.

20. **Answer is A (Hypoglycemia):** *Harrison 16th/ 2135; Harrison 17th/2255; Harrison 18th/p 2945*

Cushing's syndrome is characterised by Hyperglycemia and not Hypoglycemia.

- Cushing's syndrome is characterised by **Hyperglycemia**. Increased hepatic gluconeogenesis and insulin resistance causes increase in blood glucose.
- **Hypertension** is common, & emotional changes may be profound, ranging from irritability & emotional liability to severe depressions, confusion or even **frank psychosis**.
- **Hypokalemia**, hypochloremia and metabolic alkalosis may be seen.

21. **Answer is B (Episodic Hypertension):** *Harrison 17th/2255; Harrison 18th/p 2945*

Cushing's syndrome is associated with sustained / persistent hypertension and not episodic hypertension.

22. **Answer is A (Increased ACTH and increased Cortisol) :** *Harrisons 17th/2255; Harrison 18th/p 2945*

Cushing's disease refers to increased production of Cortisol (↑ Cortisol) by Adrenals secondary to an ACTH producing tumor (↑ ACTH) in the pituitary gland.

It is thus associated with increased levels of ACTH and Cortisol.

Only an individual who has (increased cortisol due to) an ACTH producing pituitary tumor is defined as having Cushing's disease, whereas Cushing's syndrome refers to all causes of excess cortisol' - Harrison

Increased urinary catecholamines is a feature of pheochromocytoma and not Cushing's disease.

Aetiological Approach to Cushing's syndrome

Elevated Cortisol with Elevated ACTH (↑ Cortisol + ↑ ACTH)	**Elevated cortisol with Low ACTH** (↑ Cortisol + ↓ ACTH)
• *ACTH producing Pituitary tumor* ***(Cushing's Disease)*** - *Pituitary Microadenoma* (Most common[Q]) - *Pituitary Macro adenoma* • *Ectopic ACTH producing tumors* - *Bronchogenic carcinoma (small cell or oat cell variant)* - *Carcinoid of thymus* - *Pancreatic carcinoma* - *Bronchial Adenoma*	• *Adrenal Adenoma* • *Adrenal Carcinoma* • *Exogenous steroid administration*

23. Answer is D (Increased ACTH secretion is the commonest endogenous cause): *Harrison 17th/2254, 2255; 18th/2945, 2946*

The most common endogenous cause of Cushing's syndrome is increased ACTH secretion by a pituitary adenoma.

In Cushing syndrome low dose dexamethasone fails to suppress cortisol secretion

'In normal subjects administration of supraphysiological doses of glucocorticoid results in suppression of ACTH and hence of cortisol secretion. In Cushing's syndrome of whatever cause there is failure of this suppression when low doses of synthetic glucocorticoid dexamethasone are given'. – Oxford Textbook of Medicine 4th/246

Carcinoma of Adrenal is not more common than Adrenal Adenoma as a cause for Cushing's syndrome

'Adrenal Adenoma are responsible for about the same number of cases as Adrenal Carcinomas'. – Oxford Textbook

'Adrenal Neoplasms are usually unilateral and about half are malignant' – Harrison

The size of pituitary Adenoma is usually < 1 cm and not > 2 cm

Most common cause of Cushing's syndrome (endogenous) is a Pituitary microadenoma which is less than 10 mm in diameter - Harrison

24. Answer is C (Ca lung with ectopic ACTH production); *Harrison 16th/2136 17th/2256; Harrison 18th/p 2946, 2947*

Lack of suppression to dexamethasone challenge (ACTH producing tumor) and presence of hemoptysis (Carcinoma lung) in a patient with Cushinoid features suggests a diagnosis of Carcinoma lung with ectopic ACTH secretion.

As a method of diagnostic workup of any patient with suspected Cushings we screen the patient with plasma cortisol levels at 8:00 a.m. in the morning. Those with increased cortisol levels are subjected to a ***dexamethasone supression test***. This is used to group etiology of cushings into the following:

No response or failure of suppression	Suppression positive (High dose)
• Adrenal hyperplasia secondary to ACTH producing tumor • Adrenal neoplasia (adenoma or carcinoma)	• Adrenal hyperplasia secondary to ACTH secretion from the pituitary e.g. pituitary adenoma.

In the given question there is lack of suppression to dexamethasone challenge so option (d) is out.
Out of the choices remaining the presence of hemoptysis points towards the diagnosis of carcinoma lung with ectopic ACTH.

Aetiological approach to Cushing's syndrome with the help of ACTH levels

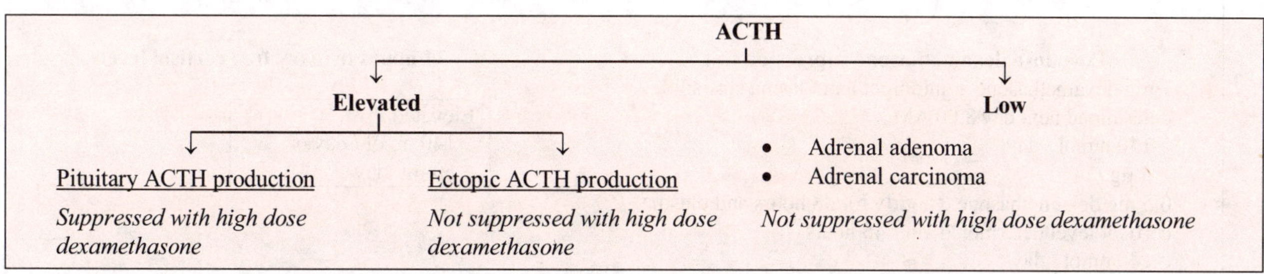

25. Answer is D (Ectopic ACTH producing lung cancer) : *Harrison 16th/2136; 17th/2256; Chandrsoma Taylor 3rd/868; Harrison 18th/p 2946, 2947*

Truncal obesity, hypertension and elevated ACTH levels suggest a diagnosis of Cushing's syndrome.
Elevated ACTH level not suppressible by high dose Dexamethasone indicate the diagnosis of Cushing's syndrome due to Ectopic ACTH production.

26. Answer is D (Ectopic ACTH secreting tumor) : *Harrison; 16th/2136; 17th/2256; Harrison 18th/p 2946, 2947*

Raised ACTH levels not suppressible by high dose dexamethosone in the backdrop of chronic smoking and hemoptysis lead us to a diagnosis of ectopic ACTH secretion from a bronchogenic carcinoma.

27. Answer is A (Hypokalemic alkalosis); *Harrison 16th/2134, 2135; 17th/2255; 2256; 2257; 18th/p 2945, 2946, 2947*

'Hypokalemia, hypochloremia and metabolic alkalosis are present particularly with ectopic production of ACTH' *– Harrison 16th/2135*

"The ectopic production of CRH results in clinical, biochemical and radiologic feature indistinguishable from those caused by hypersecretion of pituitary ACTH. The Typical signs and symptoms of Cushing's syndrome may be absent or minimal with ectopic ACTH production and ***hypokalemic alkalosis*** *is a prominent manifestation." – Harrison*

28. Answer is A (Loss of Diurnal variation) :; *API 7th / 1072; Harrison 16th/2136, 2136; 17th/2256; Harrison 18th/p 2946*

"Owing to circadian variability plasma cortisol and to a certain extent ACTH determinations are not meaningful when determined in isolation, but the absence of normal fall of plasma cortisol at midnight (Loss of diurnal variation) is consistent with Cushing's syndrome" *– Harrison 15th / 2092*

From the statement above, options of increased ACTH and increased plasma cortisol are ruled out as desirable early manifestation of Cushing's syndrome.

We are then left with the options of loss of diurnal variation and increased urinary metabolites of cortisol.

Although 'free cortisol' in urine is used as a screening test for Cushing's syndrome, no mention has been made about use of 'increased metabolites of cortisol in urine' for the same purpose. Secondly, manifestation in ***serum level*** *of cortisol are certain to precede changes* ***in urine*** *and hence loss of diurnal variation in serum cortisol is certain to be the earliest manifestation of Cushing's syndrome amongst the options provided.*

Diagnostic Protocol

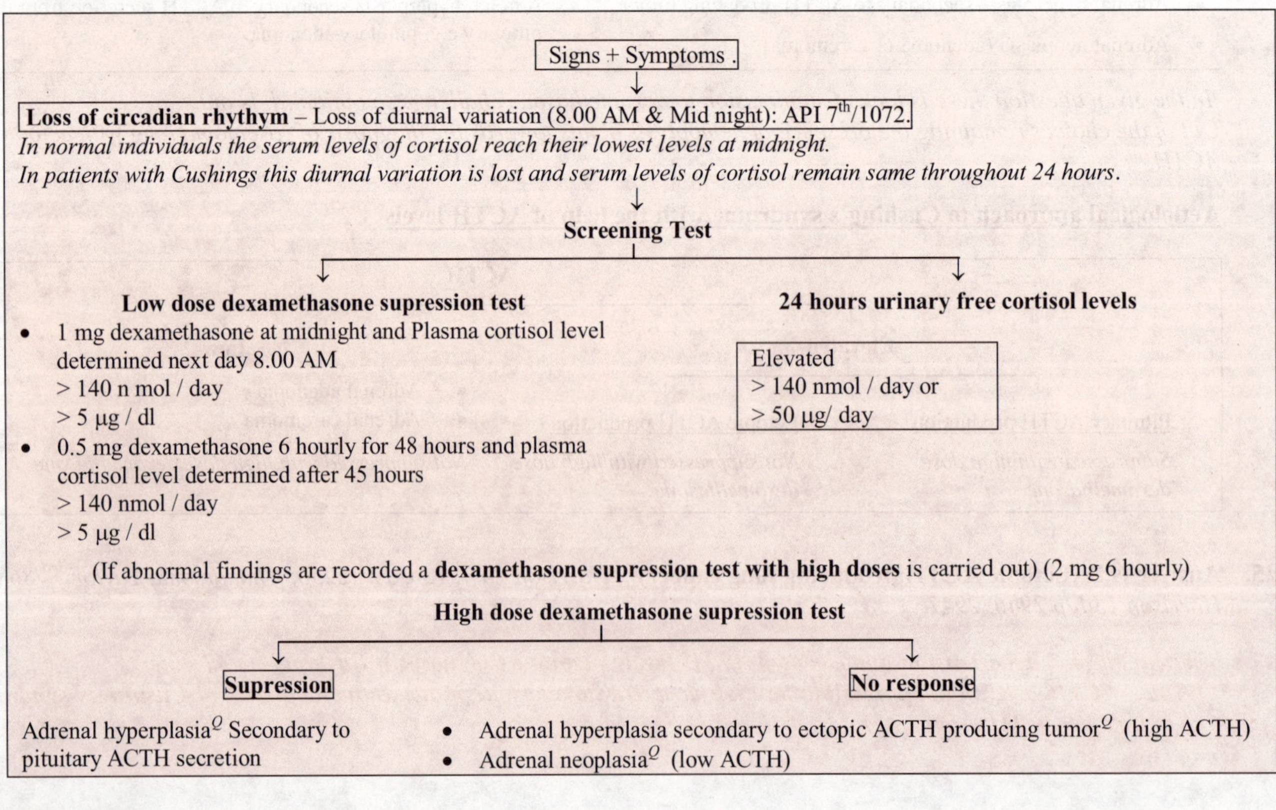

29. Answer is B (Plasma cortisol) : *API Medicine 7th /1058;*

As all features in the presentation are consistent with a diagnosis of Cushing's Syndrome and there are no points to doubt / disfavour our diagnosis, plasma cortisol would be the most appropriate investigation which would confirm our diagnosis.

The clinical presentation of patient in question gives us the following leads:

1. Weight gain (10 kg)
2. Hypertension (160/100) (both systolic and diastolic hypertension for a 28 year old lady)
3. Menstrual irregularities in the form of oligomenorrhea followed by amenorrhea.

The above presentation leaves us to consider two possible diagnosis:

a. Cushing's syndrome
b. Hypothyroidism

Cushing's Syndrome

Signs and symptoms of presentation in decreasing order	
1. Typical habitus (centripetal obesity)^{Q}	8. Personality changes^{Q}
2. Increased body weight : **Weight gain** ^{Q}	9. Echymosis^{Q}
3. Fatiguability and weakness^{Q}	10. Proximal myopathy^{Q}
4. Hypertension^{Q} (> 150/90 mm Hg)	11. Edema^{Q}
5. Hiruitism^{Q}	12. Polyuria / Polydipsia
6. **Amenorrhea**^{Q}	13. Hypertrophy of clitoris
7. Broad violoceous cutaneous stria^{Q}	

Hypothyroidism: Although hypothyroidism may also present with all features in the question, the points which go against its probable diagnosis are :

1. *Presence of both systolic and diastolic hypertension as against mild diastolic hypertension expected in hypothyroidism.*
2. *Presence of oligomenorrhea followed by amenorrheo as against menorrhagia initially which is a much more common form of menstrual irregularity in hypothyroidism.*

Signs and symptoms of Hypothyroidism:

	System	Symptom / Sign
1.	Skin	Dry scaly skin ^{Q} Loss of hair ^{Q} from scalp and body Generalized oedema ^{Q} – initially pitting Brittle nails
2.	ENT	Hoarseness of voice^{Q} and slowness of speech^{Q} : impaired hearing^{Q}
3.	Gastrointestinal tract	Constipation^{Q} Weight gain^{Q} & loss of appetite^{Q} Bradycardia^{Q}
4.	Cardiovascular system	Mild diastolic hypertension^{Q} Breathlessness^{Q} Cold intolerance^{Q}
5.	Neurological	Physical and mental slowness^{Q}, lethargy and somnalence^{Q} Delayed tendon reflexes^{Q} Paraestheseas
6.	Female reproductive system	Menorrhagia^{Q} (Later oligomenorrheo and amenorrheo) Galactorrhea^{Q} (d/t hyperprolactinemia^{Q} due to high TRH)
7.	Miscellaneous	Carpal tunnel syndrome^{Q} Serous cavity effusion^{Q}

Hyperaldosteronism : Conn's Syndrome

30. Answer is A (Cortical adenoma): *Harrisons 16th/ 2138, 17th/ 2260, API Textbook of Medicine 8th /1023;18th/2949*

Conn's syndrome by defination refers to primary aldosteronism secondary to an aldosterone producing adrenal adenoma. The most common aldosterone producing adrenal tumor is a unilateral adrenal adenoma.

***Adrenal carcinoma** is a rare cause of primary aldosteronism. Primary Aldosteronism secondary to bilateral cortical hyperplasia is not defined as Conn's syndrome.*

Primary Aldosteronism

Associated Adrenal Tumor	Without Associated Adrenal tumor
• Adrenal Adenoma (Conn's syndrome) • Adrenal carcinoma (Rare cause)	• Bilateral Cortical Hyperplasia (Idiopathic Hyperoldosteronism)/Nodular hyperplasia)
According to Harrisons 17th edition **the most common cause of Conn's syndrome is an aldosterone producing adrenal adenoma.** Most cases are unilateral[Q] with a small[Q] adenoma which may occur on either side.	*According to Harrisons 17th edition the most common cause for primary Hyperaldosteronism is Bilateral cortical Hyperplasia. 'These patients constitute 80% of patients with Primary Hyperaldosteronism' (Harrison)*

31. Answer is C (Von-Hippel-Lindau syndrome): *Harrison 17th/2260; Harrison 18th/p 2949*

Von Hippel Lindau syndrome is not associated with primary aldosteronism.

Primary Aldosteronism

Associated with Adrenal tumor	**Without an Adrenal tumor**
• Adrenal Adenoma (Conn's syndrome) - Unilateral - Small • Adrenal Carcinoma (Rare)	• Bilateral nodular cortical hyperplasia/Idiopathic hyperaldosteronism
Adrenal Adenoma is the most common tumor associated with Primary Aldosteronism[Q]	*This is the most common cause of Primary Aldosteronism[Q]*

32. Answer is D (Edema): *Harrison, 16th/2139; Harrison 17th/2260; Harrison 18th/p 2950*

'Patients with primary aldosteronism (Conn's syndrome) characteristically do not have edema since they exhibit an "escape" phenomenon from the sodium retaining aspects of mineralocorticoids' – *Harrison 16th/2139.*

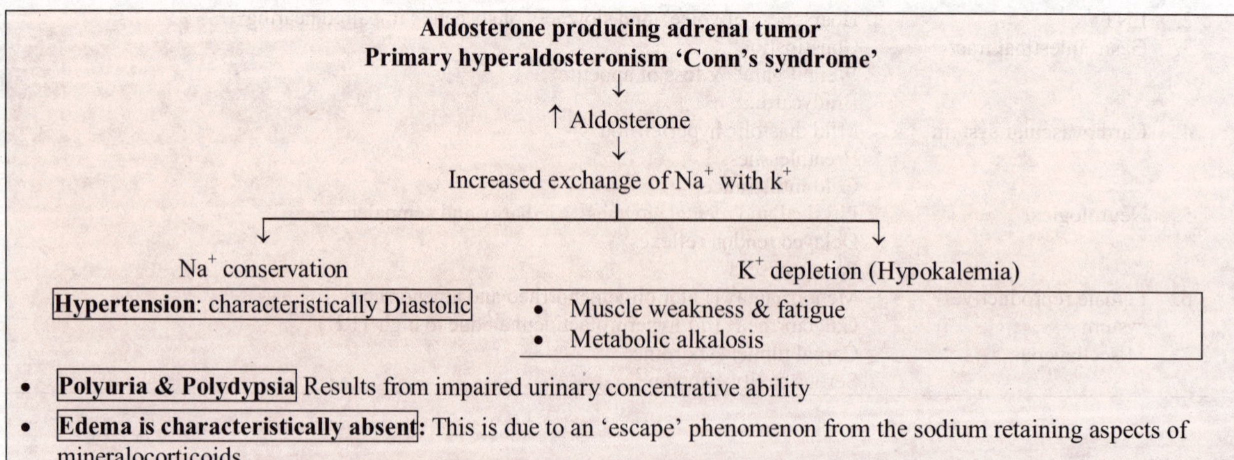

33. Answer is D (Metabolic acidosis): *Harrison, 16th/2139; Harrison 17th/2260; Harrison 18th/p 2950*

Increased Aldosterone is associated with metabolic alkalosis and not metabolic acidosis.

Hypokalemia (potassium excretion), Hypernatremia (sodium conservation) and hypertension (characteristically diastolic) may all be seen with increased aldosterone.

34. Answer is A (Pedal edema): *Ref previous question; Harrison 16th/2138, 2139; 17th/2260; Harrison 18th/p 2950*

'Patients with primary aldosteronism (Conn's syndrome) characteristically do not have edema since they exhibit an "escape" phenomenon from the sodium retaining aspects of mineralocorticoids' *– Harrison 16th/2139.*

Conn's syndrome: Manifestations

Clinical	Laboratory
1. Muscle weakness & fatigue (hypokalemia)	1. Hypokalemia
2. Hypertension without edema	2. Metabolic alkalosis
3. Polyuria & polydipsia	3. Hypernatremia
	4. ↑ Aldosterone
	5. Low rennin.

Criteria for diagnosis of Conn's syndrome

- **Diastolic hypertension without edema**
- **Hypersecretion of aldosterone** *that does not suppress appropriately in response to volume expansion*
- **Low plasma rennin levels** Hyposecretion of rennin *that fails to increase appropriately in response to volume depletion.*

35. Answer is A (Diastolic hypertension without edema): *Refer previous question*

Conn's syndrome is characterized by diastolic hypertension without edema.

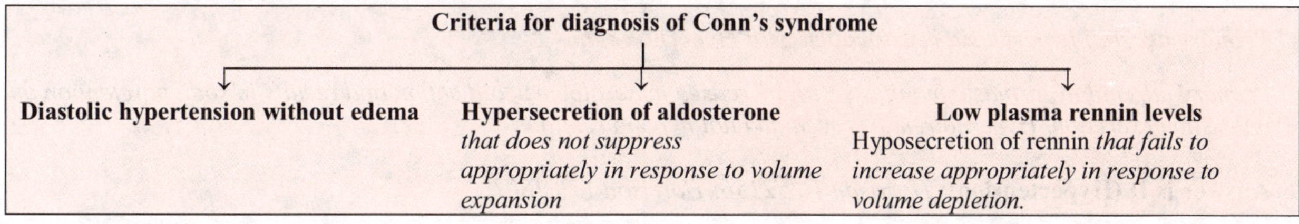

36. Answer is B (Hyperkalemia): *Harrison 16th/2138, 2139; Harrison 17th/2260; Harrison 18th/p 2950*

Excess Aldosterone is associated with Hypokalemia and not Hyperkalemia

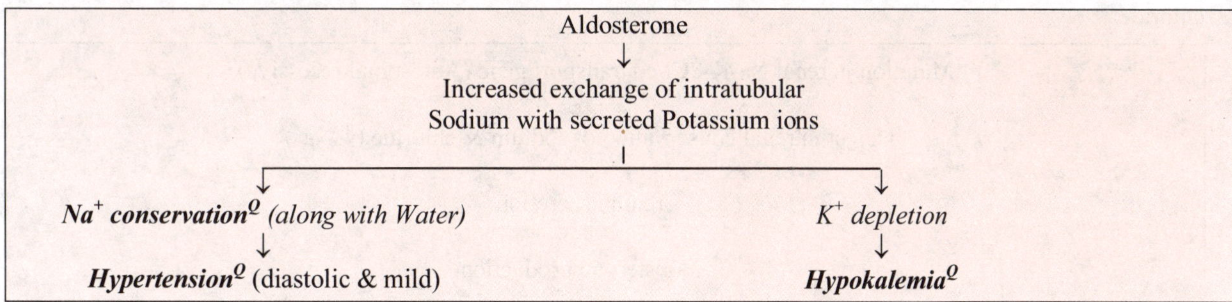

37. Answer is B (Hyperkalemia): *Refer previous question*

Excess Aldosterone levels are associated with Hypokalemia due to K+ depletion and not hyperkalemia.

38. Answer is D (Increased Renin levels): *Refer previous question*

Primary Aldosteronism (Conn's syndrome) is characteristically associated with low rnnin levels and not increased renin levels.

Hypokalemia, Hypertension and Hypernatremia are characteristic features of Conn's syndrome.

39. Answer is D (Hyperkalemia): *Refer previous question*

Primary Hyperaldosteronism is associated with hypokalemia and not hyperkalemia.

40. Answer is B and C (↓ K+ and Proximal myopathy): *Refer previous question*

Conn's syndrome is associated with hypokalemia and muscle weakness (proximal myopathy)

Patients with Conn's syndrome characteristically do not have edema, and Plasma rennin activity is typically low (decreased).

41. Answer is C, D and E (Increased Na^+, Decreased K^+ and Hypertension): *Refer previous question*

Primary Aldosteronism (Conn's syndrome) is associated with Hypertension, Hypernatremia (↑Na+) and Hypokalemia (↓K+)

Edema is characteristically absent and plasma rennin levels are decreased (low).

42. Answer is D (Conn's syndrome): *Refer previous question*

Increased Aldosterone levels (Hyperaldosteronism) in the presence of hypertension hypokalemia and decreased rennin activity suggests a diagnosis of Conn's syndrome.

43. Answer is B (Hyponatremia): *Refer previous question*

Primary Adrenal hyperplasia lead to Primary Aldosteronism or increased Aldosterone secretion. ***This is associated with sodium conservation with water retention and potassium excretion (Hypokalemia).***

44. Answer is B (Hyponatremia) : ***Read text below***

Primary adrenal hyperplasia is associated with Hypernatremia.

Primary adrenal hyperplasia manifests with increased mineralocorticoid action and results in sodium retention and potassium excretion. Hypernatremia is seen and not hyponatremia.

45. Answer is D (Hypertension): *Harrison 16th/2156; Harrison 17th/1801*

'Bartter's syndrome is associated with normal to low blood pressure' *– Harrison.*

Bartters syndrome: Review

It is characterized by a defect in sodium-potassium co transport resulting in defective renal conservation of sodium and chloride.

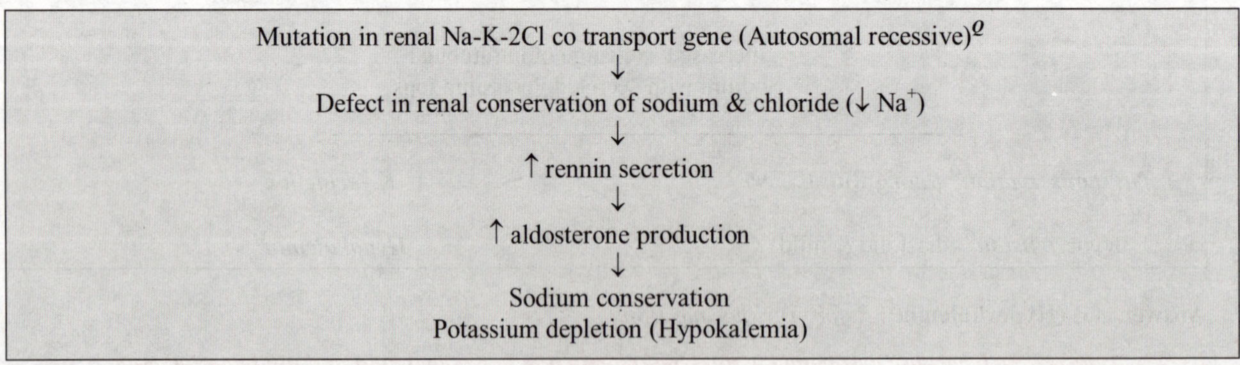

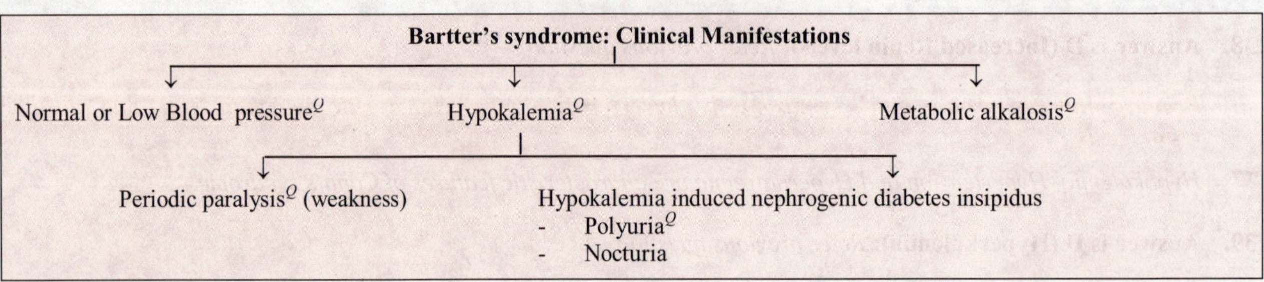

Adrenal Insufficiency (Addison's Disease)

46. Answer is D (Tuberculosis): ***API 7th/1073; Harrison 16th/2141***

'The commonest cause of adrenal insufficiency (Addison's disease) in underdeveloped countries is Tuberculosis, followed by autoimmune disorders.' – *API*

Most common cause of Addison's disease in developing countries	Most common cause of Addison's disease in developed countries
Tuberculosis	Autoimmune disease (Idiopathic atrophy)

47. Answer is D (Tuberculosis): *API 7th/1073; Harrison 16th/2141*

'The commonest cause of adrenal insufficiency (Addison's disease) in underdeveloped countries is Tuberculosis, followed by autoimmune disorders.' – API

Most common cause of Addison's disease in developing countries	Most common cause of Addison's disease in developed countries
Tuberculosis	*Autoimmune disease (Idiopathic atrophy)*

48. Answer is C (Hypertension): *Harrison 16th/2142; Harrison 17th/2263; Harrison 18th/p 2956, 2957*

Addison's disease is associated with hypotension & not hypertension.

'Arterial hypotension with postural accentuation is frequent and blood pressure may be in the range of 80/50 mmHg or less' – *Harrison 16th/2142*

Addison's disease: Review

Addison's disease or primary adrenocortical deficiency is characterized by primary inability of adrenals to elaborate sufficient quantities of adrenal cortical hormones

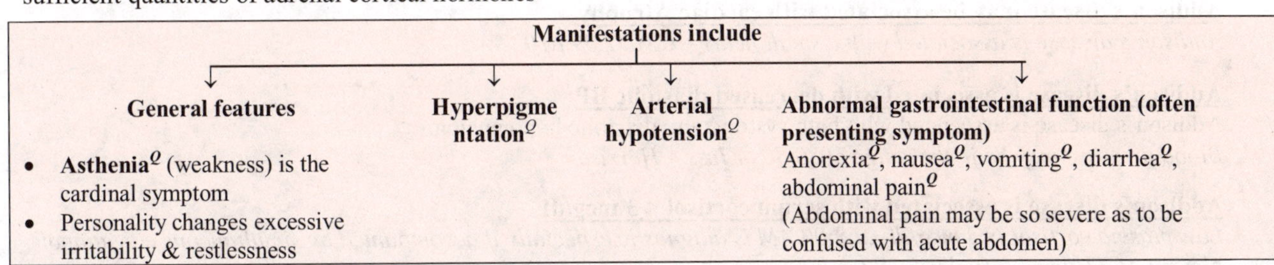

49. Answer is D (Increased protein breakdown): *Basic Medical Endocrinology 4th (Academic Press)/76; Parth Pathophysiology (Lippincot Williams) 2009/1000*

Increased protein breakdown is a feature of increased amounts of glucocorticoids (Cortisol excess; Cushing's) and is not seen in glucocorticoid deficient states like Adrenal insufficiency.

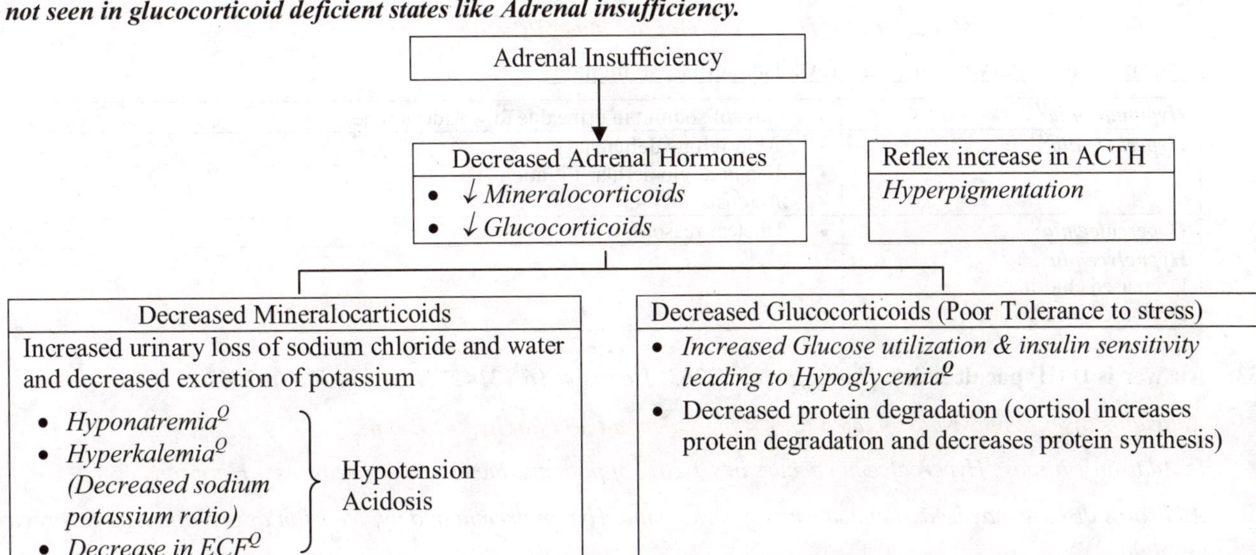

50. Answer is C (Weight gain): *Refer previous question*

Adrenal insufficiency is associated with weight loss and not weight gain.
Weight gain is a feature of Cushing's syndrome or Adrenal hyperfunction and not of Adrenal insufficiency.

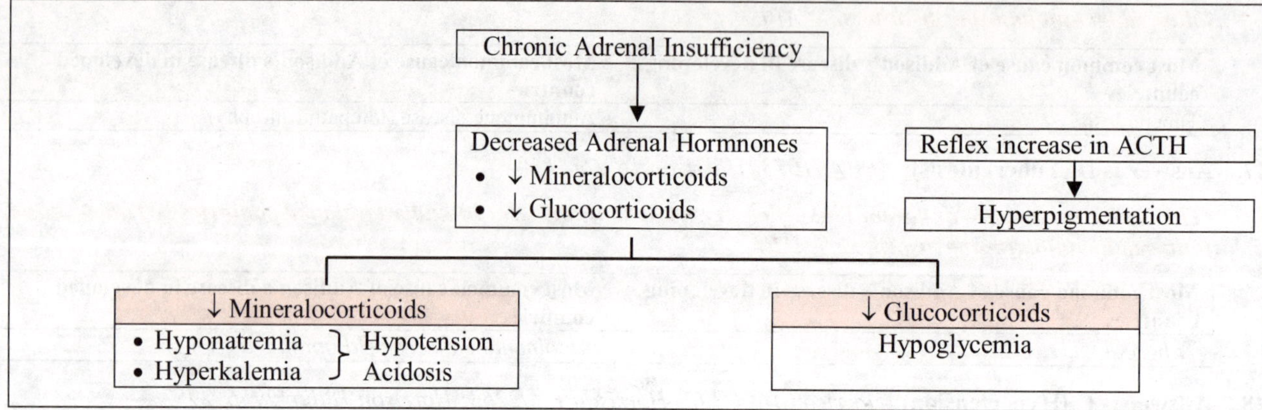

51. Answer is D (Low Renin levels): *CMDT 2008/1003,2009/1022; Harrison 17th/2263, 2264; Harrison 18th/p 2957*

Addison's disease is associated with increased plasma rennin activity.

'Elevated plasma renin activity in Addison's disease indicates the presence of depleted intravascular volume and need for higher doses of fludrocortisone replacement'- CMDT

Addison's disease may be associated with cardiac Atrophy
Addison's disease is associated with a small heart – CMDT 09 p1022

Addison's disease is associated with decreased diastolic BP
Addison's disease is associated with both systolic and diastolic hypotension.
Blood pressure may be in the range of 80/50 or less – Harrison

Addison's disease is associated with serum cortisol < 3 mcg/dl
Low plasma cortisol (<3 mcg/dl) at 8:00 AM is diagnostic especially if accompanied by simultaneous elevationof plasma ACTH level (usually > 200 pg/ml).

52. Answer is A (Hyperglycemia) : *Harrison 15th/2097; Harrison 16th / 2142; CMDT 2009/ 1022; Harrison 17th/2263; Harrison 18th/p 2956, 2957*

Addison's disease is associated with Hypoglycemia, not hyperglycemia

Abnormal Laboratory parameters in Addison's disease include:

Hyponatremia[Q]	• Loss of sodium in urine due to ↓ Aldosterone
Hyperkalemia[Q]	• Aldosterone deficiency • Impaired glomerular filtration • Acidosis
Hypercalcemia[Q]	• Unclear reason
Hypoglycemia[Q] Decreased chloride[Q] Decreased bicarbonate[Q]	

53. Answer is D (Hypocalcemia): *Harrisons 17th/2263; Harrison 16th/2142; Harrison 18th/p 2967*

Addison's disease may be associated with Hypercalcemia and not hypocalcemia.

In Addison's disease Hypercalcemia occurs in 10-20% of patients due to unclear reasons – Harrison

Addison's disease may be associated with Hyperkalemia, Hyponatremia and hypotension as explained in the previous question.

54. Answer is C (Hypocalcemia): *Refer previous question. Harrison 17th/2263*

Addison's disease is associated with Hypercalcemia and not Hypocalcemia

55. Answer is C (Does not involve oral mucosa) :*Harrison 16th/2142, 302; 15th/322, 2098, 2099; Harrison 17th/2263*

Addison's disease pigmentation may involve the oral mucosa.

Pigmentation in Addison's disease

In Addison's disease pigmentation appears as a diffuse brown, tan, or bronze darkening of skin
This increased pigmentation is diffuse but may be accentuated in the

- *Palmer crease*
- *Sites of friction & pressure areas*
  - *knuckles, elbows, knees, nail beds*
  - *belt brassier line, buttocks*
- *Scars*
- *Oral mucosa, gums & conjunctival*
- *Areolae of nipples*

56. Answer is D (ACTH stimulation test): *Harrison 17th/2264; 18th/2957; CMDT 2008/1004,CMDT2009/1022*

The diagnosis of Adrenal insufficiency should be made only with ACTH stimulation testing *– Harrison's*

ACTH stimulation test / Cosyntropin stimulation test

- Synthetic ACTH (Cosyntropin) is given parentrally in a dose of 250 μg (or 0.25 mg)
- Serum is obtained for cortisol between 30 to 60 minutes after Cosyntropin is administered
- Cortisol levels should be greater than 495 mmol/L (> 18μg/dL)
- Cortisol levels >495 exclude the diagnosis of Addison's disease while cortisol levels < 495 suggest a possible diagnosis of Adrenal insufficiency (primary or secondary).

Diabetes Mellitus (Hyperglycemia & Hypoglycemia)

57. Answer is A (Type I Diabetes): *Harrison; 16th/2156; Harrison 17th/2279; Harrison 18th/p 2973*

95% of Type I IDDM patients express either HLA DR3 or HLA DR4 or the heterozygous HLA DR3/DR4 configuration. No HLA association is seen with Type II Diabetes Mellitus or NIDDM. *- Harrison*

Diabetes Mellitus: Review *(Robbins / Harrison)*

Parameters	Type I (IDDM)	Type II (NIDDM)
Patho-physiological difference	• Results from complete or absolute lack of insulin caused by a **reduction in β cell mass.** Q • *Autoimmunity* Q is the major culprit - Autoantibodies are present Q in blood (against islet cells) - HLA DR3/DR4 are Q expressed in 95% of pt. - (Genetic factors are of low significance)	• Results from insufficient insulin secretion relative to glucose load 'or' **'insulin resistance'** i.e. inability of peripheral tissues to respond to insulin. • *Genetic factor* are the major culprit - No autoantibodies Q - No HLA association Q
Family History	Not significant (present in less than 15% of patients)	Significant (present in upto 90% of patients)
Age	< 40 years Q	> 40 years Q
Habitus	Non obese Q	Obese Q
Presentation	Patient present with **sudden onset** of osmotic symptoms in the form of polydipsia, Polyuria or symptoms of ketoacidosis	Patient present with a more **gradual/insidious onset** Q of **osmotic symptoms** (may not be present) Many of them may be **asymptomatic** Q and are recognized when they develop one of the macrovascular or microvascular symptoms of diabetes like delayed healing of wounds with atherosclerosis or gangrene or peripheral neuropathy etc.
Complication	• Ketoacidosis prone Q	• Ketoacidosis not prone Q (Non ketotic hyperglycemic coma)

Laboratory parameters	• Blood insulin is decreased • Blood glucagon High/ suppressible • Ketonuria: often present	• Insulin levels are normal or may be increased (explained by insulin resistance) • Blood glucagon High/ resistant • Not present
Pathology	• Early insulitis • Marked atrophy and fibrous • Beta cell depletion	• No insulitis • Focal atrophy and amyloid • Mild β cell depletion
Insulin/ C-peptide	• Low	• High
Treatment Protocol	**Nutrition therapy + Exercise** *(to coordinate and match the calorie intake with appropriate amount of insulin)* ↓ **Insulin**	**Nutrition therapy + Exercise** *(to reduce calorie intake, reduce hyperlipidemia and hypertension and promote weight loss)* ↓ **Oral hypoglycemia agents** (often sufficient) If not controlled ↓ Development of Complication (Pregnancy infection surgery) **Insulin (usually in confenation)**

58. Answer is A (She was suffering from insulin dependent diabetes mellitus) *: Read text below*
Harrison 17th/2281; API 7th/ 1105, CMDT 2004 1149; Harrison 18th/p 2974, 2975

The patient in question is suffering from non insulin dependent diabetes mellitus i.e. type II DM.

Before proceeding with the explanation to this question you need to be clear with the distinguishing characteristics between type I & type II DM. Reread explanation to the previous questions on DM.

<u>Points which favour a diagnosis of non insulin dependant diabetes mellitus (type 2) in this question:</u>

1. Age > 40 yrs (45 yrs)
2. Complication in the form of impalpable pulses in feet, gangrene at presentation hint to the possibility of occult disease which is likely to have been present for some time prior to diagnosis.
   Note: This type of diabetes goes unrecognised for many years because the hyperglycemia develops gradually and in the early stages it is often not severe enough for the patient to notice any feature of developing complications. The presence of the microvascular complications of diabetes at presentation e.g. peripheral neuropathy hypertension, atherosclerosis dyslipidemia points in favour of a diagnosis of long standing undetected type II D.M.
3. Absence of Ketonuria: Ketonuria is a feature of type – I diabetes.

<u>As depicted in the comparative analysis:</u>

- Family history (genetic tendency) is more important in type II disease and is useful in predicting the nature of diabetes.
- Protocol for management of type II diabetes involves diet control and exercise as the primary management, followed by oral hypoglycemics and still further by insulin if pathological situations can not be controlled.

59. Answer is C > A (DM type II > MODY): *CMDT 2007/1222; 'Clinical Endocrinology and Diabetes Mellitus' by Sachdev & Gupta 1st/916; 'Hand book of Diabetes' by Williams 3rd/72*

Positive family history, absence of DKA and management on oral hypoglycemic agents (non insulin dependence) suggests a possible diagnosis of Type II DM or MODY. Although weight loss and young age of presentation is more consistent with MODY, absence of Diabetes in father makes MODY an unlikely diagnosis as MODY is inherited as an autosomal dominant condition and vertical transmission through atleast two generations is required for its diagnosis.

Type II DM is the single best answer of exclusion amongst the options provided

	Type I	Type II	MODY
Age of onset	Predominantly young	Predominantly middle to old age	Predominantly young (usually < 25 years)
Family history	Not significant (uncommon)	Significant (Positive) <u>Inheritance is Polygenic / Heterogenous</u> ***Vertical transmission through successive generations is not essential for diagnosis***	Significant (Positive) <u>Inheritance is Monogenic / Autosomal dominant</u> ***Vertical transmission through at least two successive generation (ideally three) is essential for diagnosis.***

Risk of ketoacidosis	High	Low (Uncommon)	Low (Uncommon)
Insulin dependence	Insulin dependent	Non insulin dependent	Non insulin dependent
Obesity	Uncommon (may be present)	Common (may be absent)	Uncommon (may be present)
Pathophysiology	β cells dysfunction (Autoantibodies against β cells) No insulin resistance	β cell dysfunction Insulin resistance	β cell dysfunction No insulin resistance
Fasting 'C' peptide/ Insulin	Low	High	Low

60. Answer is A>C (MODY > DM type II): *CMDT 2007/1222,2009/1054; 'Clinical Endocrinology and Diabetes Mellitus' by Sachdev and Gupta 1st/916; Refer previous question*

Onset of non insulin dependent Diabetes at a young age (≈ 26 years), absence of obesity and DKA and positive family history with evidence of vertical transmission of diabetes through two generations (possible autosomal dominant inheritance) suggests the diagnosis of MODY.

MODY: Maturity Onset Diabetes of the Young

- MODY is a group of non insulin dependent diabetic syndrome defined by an early onset of diabetes (usually before age of 25 years) and an autosomal dominant inheritance.
- There is β cell dysfunction but in contrast to type II diabetes, obesity and / or insulin resistance is rare.

Diagnostic criteria that help establish diagnosis of MODY include:

- *Early diagnosis of diabetes – before age 25 years in at least one and ideally two family members.*
- *Not insulin-dependent – shown by absence of insulin treatment 5 years after diagnosis or significant C-peptide in a patient on insulin treatment.*
- *Autosomal dominant inheritance i.e. vertical transmission of diabetes through at least two generations (ideally three generation), with a similar phenotype in cousins or second cousins.*
- *Rarely obese (obesity is not required for the development of diabetes)*
- *Diabetes results from β-cell dysfunction (insulin levels are often in the normal range, though inappropriately low for the degree of hyperglycemia)*

61. Answer is A & C (Family history is present in 90% cases and Time of onset is usually predictable): *Harrison 17th/2275, 2276, 2277; Oxford textbook of Medicine/360; Harrison 18th/p 2968, 2969*

Family history is present in about 15% of patients with type I DM and time of onset is not predictable.

Type I Diabetes often occurs in children *(Oxford textbook)*

'Type I Diabetes is the most severe form of diabetes with acute onset often in children' – Oxford Textbook of Medicine
Median age of diagnosis of Type I DM is 12 years
As many as 25% of cases are now diagnosed under the age of 5 years.

Family History is present in about 15% of cases of Type I DM *(Harrison 17th)*

'Most individuals with type I DM do not have a first degree relative with this disorder' – Harrison 17th/2280
The risk of developing type I D.M. is 3-9% if the parent has type I DM.
The risk of developing type I D.M. is 5-15% if a sibling has type I DM.

Percent of cases with positive family history in Type I DM ≈ 10-15%
Percent of cases with positive family history in Type II DM ≈ 90%

Type I DM is associated with auto immune destruction of Beta cells
Pathogenesis of type I DM involves autoimmune destruction of Beta cells mediated by T cells and humoral mediators, resulting in absolute insulin deficiency – Robbins 7th/1204

Diabetic Ketoacidosis is dependant on Insulin
Diabetic ketoacidosis is a serious complication of Type I DM and requires insulin for reversal.
'Diabetic ketoacidosis cannot be reverted without insulin' – Harrison

Time of onset of Type I DM cannot be predicted

62. Answer is A (Family history is present in 90% of cases): *Refer previous question*

A strong family history (≈90%) is a feature of type II DM and not type I DM. Family history may be present in only about 15% cases of type I DM.

63. Answer is D (Increased levels of insulin in blood may be seen):*Harrison 16th/2157; Harrison 17th/2280, 2281, 2282*

Increased levels of insulin in blood may be seen in patients with type II DM or NIDDM.

- The prominent mechanism involved in pathogenesis of NIDDM is 'insulin resistance' i.e. the decreased ability of insulin to act effectively on peripheral tissues. This insulin resistance is relative and supra normal levels of insulin are still capable of normalizing blood glucose. In ***NIDDM (type II DM) insulin secretion initially increases in response to insulin resistance to maintain normal glucose levels in blood. Thus increased levels of insulin in blood may be seen in patients with NIDDM or type II DM.***
- Pancreatic β cells respond by an initial increase in insulin secretion. They are however unable to maintain there hyperinsulinemia for long and gradually as the disease progresses insulin levels decline.
  Secretion of insulin from β cells may thus decrease but it never stops completely.
- Ketosis or diabetic ***Ketoacidosis*** is an acute metabolic complication of diabetes mellitus. ***It is typically seen in patients of type I D.M*** or IDDM who either are untreated, inadequately treated or have stopped treatment-*API 7th/1113*
- Individuals with DM may have several forms of dyslipidemia
  Dyslipidemias are more frequent in type II DM or NIDDM
  The most common patterns of dyslipidemia is hypertriglyceredemia & reduced HDL cholestrol–*Harrison 16th/2167.*

64. Answer are A and B (Patients with type 2 diabetes never require insulin treatment) and (Maturity Onset Diabetes of the Young (MODY) is an autosomal recessive condition): *Refer text below*

Patients with type 2 diabetes may require insulin treatment
MODY is inherited as an Autosomal dominant condition.

Patients with type 2 diabetes may require insulin treatment

Patients with type 2 diabetes are initially managed with diet and exercise, with or without oral hypoglycaemic agents. After varying lengths of time, the majority of patients end up on insulin treatment secondary to pancreas β-cell failure.

MODY is inherited as an Autosomal dominant condition

Maturity onset diabetes of the young is a monogenic form of diabetes (i.e. caused by a mutation in a single gene) and it is an autosomal dominant not recessive conditions

Cardiovascular disease is the main cause of mortality in diabetes

'Cardiovascular disease remains the main cause of mortality in subjects with diabetes, as up to 80% of patients die of this condition'.

Weight loss is common in tytpe 1 diabetes

Type 1 diabetes subjects usually present with a short history of weight loss.

Acromegaly and Cushing's syndrome are recognized endocrine causes of diabetes.

Endocrinopathies associated with diabetes mellitus	
Acromegaly	*Pheochromocytoma*
Cushing's	*Hyperthyroidism*
Glucagonoma	*Somatostatinoma*
Aldosteronoma	

65. Answer is B >C (Diet therapy + exercise > Diet therapy + exercise + metformin): *Harrison 17th/2299; Clinical Endocrinology & Diabetes Mellitus by Sachdev & Gupta/940; Harrison 18th/p 2995*

The initial management of an asymptomatic type II DM with fasting blood glucose < 200mg/dl should include dietry/ life style modification and exercise. Oral hypoglycemics (Metformin) should be added if blood glucose level are not controlled with diet and exercise.

As the question has specifically asked about the initial therapy in this case, 'option B' with diet and exercise is the better choice of the two.

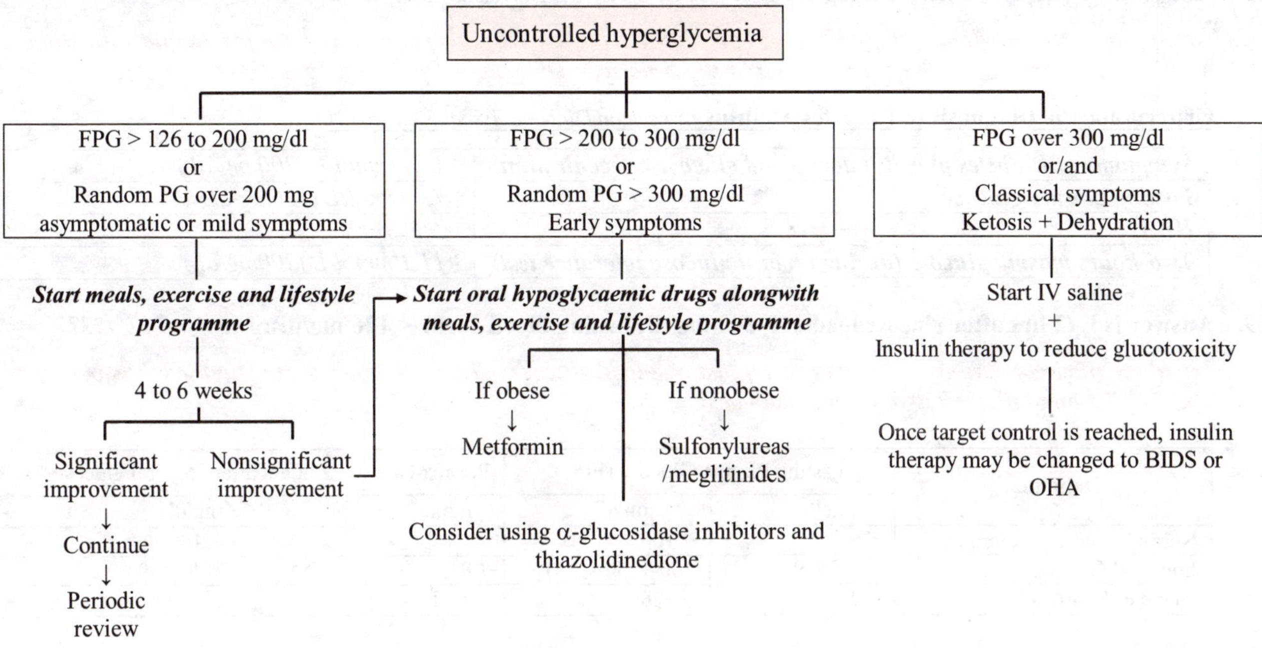

FPG, Fasting Plasma Glucose; OHA, Oral Hypoglycemic Agents; BIDS,

66. Answer is B (Hydrochlorthiazide) : *Harrison 16th/1479, 2160; K.D.T 4th/543, 5th/532*

Hydrochlorthiazide is not a preferred agent for the treatment of hypertension in diabetics as it causes unfavorable alteration in glucose and lipid profile of the patient.
'Hyperglycemia and hyperlipidemia have been reported with the use of diuretics as antihypertensives' *– KDT*

Antihypertensive drugs in diabetics:
*'**ACE inhibitors or angiotensin receptor blockers** are the first line agents for management of hypertension in diabetics' – Harrison 16th/ 1479*
Lisinopril & Trandalopvil are examples of ACE inhibitors while Losartan is an angiotensin receptor blocking agent. These have no known adverse effects on glucose or lipid metabolism and minimize the development of diabetic nephropathy by reducing renal vascular resistance and renal perfusion pressure.
What puzzles the situation:
In Diabetic patient with hypertension multiple agents are usually needed to achieve good blood pressure control. The average diabetic patient will require at least three medications to achieve appropriate control. *While ACE inhibitors/ angiotensin receptor blockers will form an essential component of the regimen, Thiazide diuretics may also be used as an additional agent. Thus diuretics though not preferred agents for treatment of hypertension in diabetics, may well be used as conjunctive agents and are a possible treatment modality. Nevertheless they are the single best answer to exclude amongst the options provided here.*

67. Answer is C (D-Xylose test): *Harrison's 17th/2275, 2277*

The D-Xylose test is a test for assessment of proximal small intestinal mucosal function. D- Xylose test is used to assess carbohydrate malabsorption and is not a test for assessment of Diabetes mellitus
Fasting blood glucose, Random blood glucose and Oral Glucose Tolerance test are all used for assessment of diabetes mellitus.

Criteria for the diagnosis of Diabetes Mellitus
Symptoms of diabetes plus ***random blood glucose*** *concentration ≥ 11.1 mmol/L (200 mg/dL) or*
Fasting plasma glucose *≥ 7.0 mmol/L (126 mg/dL) or*
Two-hour plasma glucose ≥ 11.1 mmol/L (200 mg/dL) during an ***oral glucose tolerance test.***

68. Answer is D (Glycosylated Haemoglobin (HbA1C) > 6.5%): *Harrisons 18th/2970*

Glycosylated Haemoglobin (HbA1C) values of > 6.5% represents an independent criteria for diagnosis of Diabetes Mellitus in accordance with the criteria set by the American Diabetic Association, 2011.

Criteria for the Diagnosis of Diabetes Mellitus *(American Diabetic Association, 2011)*

Symptoms of Diabetes plus Random blood glucose concentration	*≥11.1 mmol/L (200 mg/dL) or*
Fasting plasma glucose	*≥7.0 mmol/L (126mg/dL) or*
HBAIC	*>6.5% or*
Two-hours plasma glucose (during an oral glucose tolerance test)	*≥11.1 mmol/L (200mg/dL)*

69. Answer is E (2 hrs after glucose load 140-200 mg/dl; fasting blood sugar < 126 mg/dl): *Harrison 17th/2277*

Impaired glucose tolerance is indicated by a fasting glood glucose < 126 g/dl and plasma glucose levels between 140 and 200, 2 hours after a 75g oral glucose load.

Definition	Fasting Plasma Glucose (FPG)		Plasma Glucose 2 hours after 75g oral glucose	
	mmol/l	mg/dl	mmol/l	mg/dl
Normal Glucose Tolerance	< 5.6	< 100	<7.8	<140
Impaired Glucose Tolerance	5.6 to 6.9	100-125 (<126)	7.8 – 11.1	140-199
Diabetes Mellitus	≥ 7	≥ 126	> 11.1	>200

70. Answer is B (Oral GTT): *Harrison 17th/2277*

Oral glucose tolerance test (Oral GTT) should be performed when the diagnosis of diabetes is in doubt

The patient in question has a random blood glucose of 163 mg/dl which is lower than the required level (200 mg/dl) to consider diabetes.

He however has a fasting blood glucose level of 200mg/dl which is well above the desired level (126 mg/dl) to consider diabetes. Although fasting blood glucose is the more reliable test for identifying DM, and diabetes may be diagnosed with a fasting blood glucose > 126mg/dl such diagnosis should not be made if only a single fasting blood glucose meets the criterion.

The next best step is either to repeat the test on a different day (preferred) or perform an oral GTT.

As the option of repeating 'fasting blood glucose' is not provided in the question, performing an oral GTT becomes the single best answer of exclusion.

Criteria for the diagnosis of diabetes mellitus

- *Symptoms of diabetes plus random blood glucose concentration ≥ 11.1 mmol/L (200mg/dL)*
- *Fasting plasma glucose ≥ 7.0 mmol/L (126 mg/dL) or*
- *Two-hour plasma glucose ≥ 11.1 mmol/L (200 mg/dL) during an oral glucose tolerance test.*

Note: In the absence of unequivocal hyperglycemia and acute metabolic decompensation, these criteria should be confirmed by repeat testing on a different day.

71. Answer is B (140 mg/dl): *'Manual of Laboratory and Diagnostic Test' 8th/350*

A serum blood glucose value greater than 140 mg/dl at one hour in an 'one hour glucose challenge test' is termed suspicious and requires a formal/standard glucose tolerance test.

One hour glucose challenge test (O' Sullivan test)

The one hour glucose challenge test (O' Sullivan test) is done to detect gestational diabetes and screen non symptomatic pregnant women.

This test is the recommended screening test by the American College of Obstetricians and Gynaecologists (ACOG)

The test (One step approach)
An oral glucose load of 50g is administered and blood is examined for glucose levels one hour after administration.

Reference values
A plasma glucose level of ≥140 mg/dl 1 hour after challenge is considered suspicious.

Implication
Patients with a positive 1 hour glucose challenge test should undergo the standard 3 hour, 100 gm oral GTT for pregnant women.

Note:
The standard oral GTT for pregnant women is a 3 hour test.
The standard oral GTT for individuals other than pregnant women is a 2 hour test.

72. Answer is B (Long term status of blood sugar): *Harrison 16th/2171; Harrison 17th/2296; Harrison 18th/p 2992*

'Measurement of glycated haemoglobin is the standard method for assessing long term glycaemic control
Harrison 16th/ 2172

When plasma glucose is consistently elevated there is an increase in non enzymatic glycation of haemoglobin – small amount of HbA are nonenzymatically glycated to form HbA_{1C}.

This alteration reflects the glycemic history over previous 2-3 months (since erythrocytes have an average life span of 120 days i.e. about 3 months)

Remember:

HbA_{1C} measurement becomes unreliable in conditions like [Q]
- Haemoglobinopathies [Q]
- Hemolytic anemia [Q]
- Uremia [Q]

An alternative indicator of glycemic control when HbA_{1C} is inaccurate is : glycated albumin [Q]
(glycation of other proteins such as albumin occurs)

73. Answer is C (HbA_{1C}): *Harrison 17th/2296; Harrison 16th/2171, 2172; Harrison 18th/p 2992*

Measurement of glycate hemoglobin (HbA1C) is the standard method for assessing long term glycemic control.

Glycated hemoglobin (HbA1C) should be measured in all individual with DM as part of their comprehensive diabetic care. – Harrison 17th/2296

74. Answer is C (Bradycardia): *Harrison 16th/2159; Harrison 17th/2283*

Diabetic ketoacodosis (DKA) is associated with tachycardia and not bradycardia.

Manifestations of Diabetic Ketoacidosis

- **Symptoms**
  - *Nausea/Vomiting*
  - *Thirst/Polyuria*
  - *Abdominal pain*
  - *Shortness of breath*
- **Precipitating events**
  - *Inadequate insulin administration*
  - *Infection (pneumonia/UTI/gastroenteritis/sepsis)*
  - *Infarction (cerebral, coronary, mesenteric, peripheral)*
  - *Drugs (cocaine)*
  - *Pregnancy*
- Physical findings
  - ***Tachycardia***
  - ***Dehydration/hypotension***
  - *Tachypnea/Kussmaul respirations/respiratory distress*
  - ***Abdominal tenderness (may resemble acute pancreatitis or surgical abdomen)***
  - *Lethargy/obtundation/cerebral edema/possibly coma*

75. Answer is C (> 180 mg/dL); *Harrison 16th/2159, 2160; Harrison 17th/2283, 290; Harrison 18th/p 2976, 2977*

'The patient in question is a case of diabetic Ketoacidosis.

Diabetic Ketoacidosis is associated with serum glucose levels between 250-300 mg/dl' – *Harrison*

Features of diabetic ketoacidosis

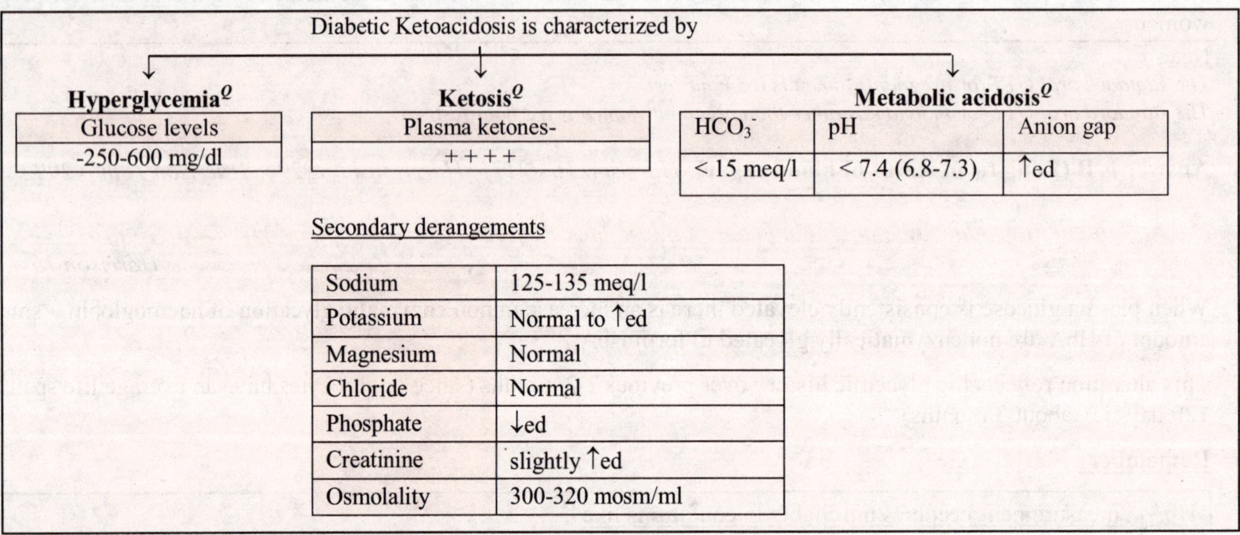

Diabetic Ketoacidosis is characterized by

Hyperglycemia[Q]

Glucose levels
-250-600 mg/dl

Ketosis[Q]

Plasma ketones-
++++

Metabolic acidosis[Q]

HCO_3^-	pH	Anion gap
< 15 meq/l	< 7.4 (6.8-7.3)	↑ed

Secondary derangements

Sodium	125-135 meq/l
Potassium	Normal to ↑ed
Magnesium	Normal
Chloride	Normal
Phosphate	↓ed
Creatinine	slightly ↑ed
Osmolality	300-320 mosm/ml

Note: *For every 100 mg elevation of glucose in serum the Na concentration decreases by 3 meq.*

76. Answer is A and D (Serum creatinine and Blood pH): *Harrison 17th; Harrison 18th/p 2977, 2979*

Presence of blood glucose of 750mg/dl in a comatose patient suggests a possible diagnosis of non ketotic hyperglycemic coma or diabetic ketoacidosis. Amongst the options provided estimation of blood pH will help establish a diagnosis of diabetic ketoacidosis while estimation of serum creatinine will help in establishing a diagnosis of hyperosmolar non ketotic coma as prerenal azotema is a characteristic feature of the latter.

Characteristic Laboratory Feature

Diabetic Ketoacidosis

- *Hyperglycemia*
- *Ketosis*
- ***Metabolic acidosis (↓ pH)***

Ketosis is not provided amongst the options and hence estimation of pH is the single best option

Hyperosmolar non Ketotic Coma

- *Hyperglycemia*
- *Hyperosmolality (> 350 mosmol/L)*
- ***Prerenal Azotemia***

Osmolality is not provided amongst the options and hence serum creatinine (Azotemia) estimation is the single best option.

77. Answer is A (Renal Glycosuria): *Harrison 15th/2315*

'Renal glycosuria' is characterized by urinary excretion of glucose at normal concentration of glucose in blood'.

Patient in question is testing positive for urinary glucose despite normal levels of both fasting and postprandial glucose in blood. This thus leads us to the diagnosis of renal glycosuria.

78. Answer is C (Insulin) .; *Harrison 16th/2158, 2159, 2160; Harrison 17th/2284; Harrison 18th/p 2978*

'Diabetic ketoacidosis cannot be reverted without insulin' – *Harrison*

The patient in the above question is a definite case of ***diabetic Ketoacidosis***, as suggested by *increased blood sugar (Diabetes)* and presence of *sugar & ketones in urine (ketoacidosis)* in an *obese* (type I) diabetic.

Diabetic ketoacidosis cannot be reverted without insulin. – *Harrison 14th/ 2073*

Remember:

Apart from diabetes the only other common ketoacidotic state is ***alcoholic ketoacidosis.***

Alcoholic ketoacidosis is invariably associated with hypoglycemia.

A plasma glucose estimation usually is required to delineate such patients. Most patients have a plasma glucose, levels of less than 150 mg/dl. Hyperglycemia may occur but is usually mild, & rarely if ever exceeds 300 mg/dl. It is important to know this distinction as, in contrast to diabetic acidosis this syndrome is rapidly reversed by the intravenous administration of glucose.

79. Answer is A (Insulin): *Refer previous question*

Presence of sugar and ketones in urine and the presence of hyperglycemia (400 mg Glucose) suggests a diagnosis of Diabetic ketoacidosis. The treatment of choice in Diabetic ketoacidosis is Insulin.

80. Answer is A (Hypokalemia): *Ganong 22nd/338*

Insulin causes K^+ to enter cells with a resultant lowering of extracellular K^+ concentration (Hypokalemia)

Relation of Insulin to Potassium *(Ganong 22nd/338)*

- Insulin causes K^+ to enter cells with a resultant lowering of the extracellular K^+ concentration (*Hypokalemia*)
- Infusion of insulin and glucose significantly lower the plasma K^+ level in normal individual (*Hypokalemia*)
- Infusion of insulin and glucose is very effective for the temporary relief of hyperkalemia
- The reason for intracellular migration of K^+ is still uncertain. However it is belived to result from increase in the activity of Na^+ - K^+ ATPase in cell membranes so that more K^+ is pumped into cells

81. Answer is A (Increase in Na+ level) *: Schwartz Pre-Test /Q.62; Harrison 17th/2283; Harrison 18th/p 2977*

A rise in the extracellular fluid concentration of a substance that does not diffuse passively across cell membranes (eg. glucose or urea) causes an increase in effective osmotic pressure, a transfer of water from cells and dilutional hyponatremia. ***For each 100 mg/dl rise in blood glucose above normal, the serum sodium level falls approximately 3 meq/L.*** *Alternatively, for every 100 mg/dl fall in blood glucose level serum Na^+ would increase by 3 meq/L. Thus if blood glucose falls from 600-100 i.e. by 500 mg/dl therefore serum Na^+ would increase by 15 meq/L*

82. Answer is A (Increased Glucagon secretion): *Refer text below*

Insulin Inhibits glucogon release by pancreatic alpha cells.

Insulin facilitates increased cellular uptake glucose into most tissues (insulin sensitive tissues) with a resultant lowering of serum glucose (Hypoglycemia). Insulin enhance fatty acid synthesis and inhibits lipolysis.

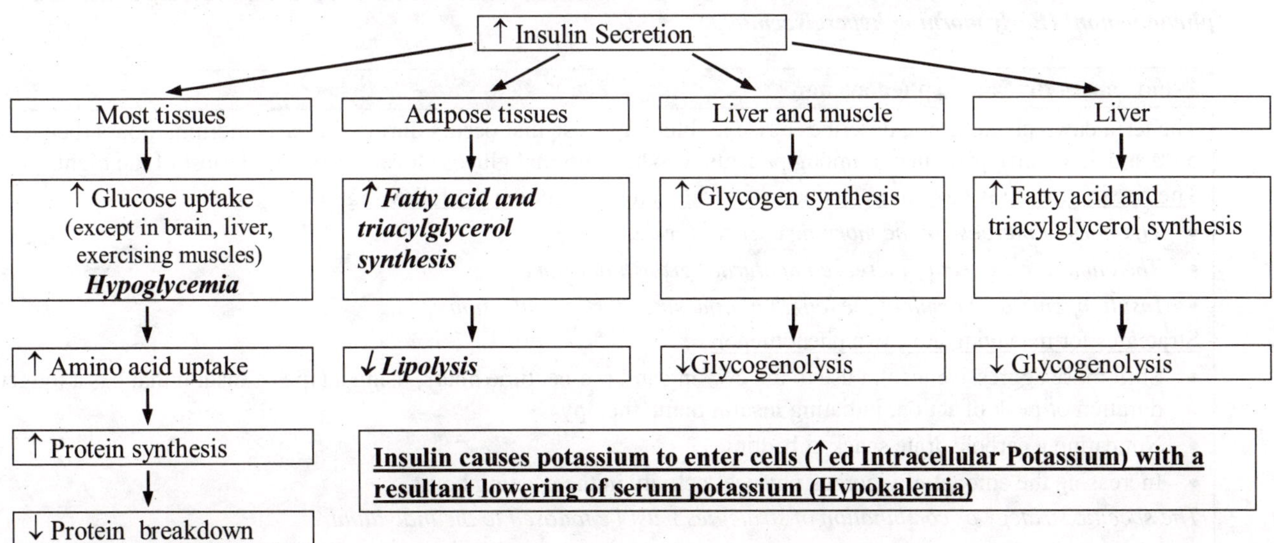

83. Answer is A (Insufficient Insulin): *NMS medicine case book by Tilak Shah (Lippincott Williams) 2008/299*

Early morning hyperglycemia with increased blood glucose at 3.00 Am typically suggests inadequate night time insulin dose (insufficient insulin).

Dawn phenomenon also presents with early morning hyperglycemia but blood glucose is typically stable (normal) at 3.00AM. If insufficient insulin is not provided amongst the options. Dawn phenomenon may be selected as the ***Answer*** *by exclusion since several textbooks do not make a distinction between Dawn phenomenon and insufficient insulin and include insufficient night time insulin as a mechanism for Dawn phenomenon.*

Causes of early morning hyperglycemia in diabetics using insulin:

Causes	Frequency	Mechanism	Diagnosis	Treatment
Insufficient insulin	Most common	Inadequate night-time basal insulin dose	Blood glucose rises continuously throughout the night	↑ Night-time intermediate or long-acting insulin dose
Dawn phenomenon	Common	Early morning physiologic surge in growth hormone and cortisol	Blood glucose stable all night, then sharp rise early in the morning	Do not eat a carbohydrate snack at midnight
Somogyi effect	Least common	Excessive night-time basal insulin dose → hypoglycemia in the middle of the night → triggers release of counter-regulatory hormones	Hypoglycemia at 2-3 am*	↓ Night-time intermediate or long-acting insulin dose

*Patients with long-standing DM may not have symptoms of hypoglycemia (discomfort, tremors, sweating, etc) because of autonomic diabetic neuropathy.

84. Answer is C (Morning hyperglycemia due to insufficient insulin):

Dawn phenomenon typically refers to early morning hyperglycemia with stable blood glucose levels all night (no Hypoglycemia at night)
Although typically Dawn phenomenon is caused by early morning physiological surge of counter regulatory hormones such as cortisol, and growth hormone, inadequate night time insulin may also contribute to the 'Dawn phenomenon' (Early morning hyperglycemia).

What causes the "dawn phenomenon"?

The term dawn phenomenon describes a rise in, blood glucose that occurs during the early morning hours (between 5:00 and 8:00 Am), particularly among patients who have normal glucose levels throughout most of the night.

The rise in glucose is thought to be due to several factors, including the following:

- *The normal increase in the morning cortisol level*
- *The cumulative effect of increased nocturnal growth hormone*
- *Insulinopenia as a result of the length of time since the last injection*

Strategies for managing the dawn phenomenon

- Shift more aggressive insulin use to the evening and pre-bedtime hours, using a type of insulin that has a longer duration or peak of action, initiating insulin pump therapy
- Not eating a carbohydrate snack at bedtime
- Increasing the amount of vigorous physical activity in the evening hours.

The specific strategy or combination of strategies must be tailored to the individual.

What is Somogyi phenomenon?
The *Somogyi phenomenon* is *rebound hyperglycemia after an incident of hypoglycemia.* This rebound is secondary to the release of counterregulatory hormones, which is the natural response to hypoglycemia. As tighter glucose control is maintained, there is an increased likelihood of hypoglycemia and, therefore, of the Somogyi phenomenon. If the hypoglycemia is recognized and treated promptly, rebound hyperglycemia is less like to occur. Thus, the Somogyi phenomenon is commonly reported more frequently at night because there is the greater likelihood of unrecognized and untreated hypoglycemia when the patient is asleep. **When should the Somogyi phenomenon be suspected?** The Somogyi phenomenon should be suspected when a person whose blood sugar is in excellent control begins to have intermittent high blood glucoses in the morning. *If that pattern is noted, blood glucose should be checked between 2:00 and 3:00 AM on several nights to determine whether hypoglycemia is occurring. If night time hypoglycemia can be documented the likely diagnosis is Somogyi phenomenon.* *This may require the dose or type of evening insulin or the time that the dose is given to be altered.*

85. Answer is C and E (Neuropathy and Retinopathy): *Harrison 17th/2285; Harrison 18th/p 2980*

Neuropathy and Retinopathy are characteristic complication of Diabetes Mellitus.

Characteristic complications of DM	
Microvascular	*Macrovascular*
Retinopathy	*Peripheral vascular disease*
Neuropathy	*Coronary Artery Disease*
Nephropathy	*Cerebrovascular disease*

86. Answer is C (Symmetrical sensory neuropathy): *Harrison 17th/2289; Harrison 18th/p 2984*

The most common form of diabetic neuropathy is distal symmetric sensory polyneuropathy

'The most common form of diabetic neuropathy is distal symmetric polyneuropathy. It most frequently presents with distal sensory loss. - Harrison 17th/2289

87. Answer is C (Dextroamphetamine):; *Harrison 16th/2166; Harrison 17th/2289; Harrison 18th/p 2984*

Dextroamphetamine has not been mentioned as an agent for treatment of painful diabetic neuropathy.

Chronic painful diabetic neuropathy is difficult to treat.

Common agents	**Other agents**
• Tricyclic antidepressants (***Amitryptiline****, Desipramine, Nortriptyline*) • *NSAID'S (avoid in renal dysfunction)* • *Gabapentin*	- ***Phenytoin*** - Carbamazapine - Mexilitine - ***Capsacin cream***

88. Answer is A (Autonomic neuropathy): *CMDT 2003/1183; CMDT 2009/1075-1076, Harrison 17th/2289, 2307; 16th/2182; Harrison 18th/p 2984*

Hypoglycemic unawareness *refers to a loss of warning symptoms that alert individuals to the presence of hypoglycemia and prompt them to eat and abort the episode.*

Hypoglycemic unawareness can be attributed to two factors :

a. ***Autonomic neuropathy***
b. *Loss of catecholamine response to hypoglycemia :* This means that patients with repeated attacks of hypoglycemia lose their capacity to release epinephrine and norepinephrine in response to hypoglycemia. (increase release of glucogon in response to hypoglycemia is lost very early in type 1 Diabetes Mellitus.)

Thus type I patients overtreated with insulin may be unaware of critically low levels of blood glucose because of an adaptive blunting of their alarm systems owing to repeated episodes of hypoglycemia.

89. Answer is B (Urinary protein > 550 mg/day for 3 consecutive sample): *Harrison 15th/2121 & 2122 (Not elaborated in Harrison 16th) Harrison 17th/2288, Robinsons 7th/992; Harrison 18th/p 2982, 2983*

The most reliable indicator for diabetic nephropathy is presence of overt proteinuria.

Urinary protein > 550 mg/day in 3 consecutive samples confirms the diagnosis of overt proteinuria, reflects irreversible pathological changes in kidneys and confirms progression to end stage renal disease (diabetic nephropathy)

This is evident from the following lines from Harrisons text:

- *Once overt proteinuria is present there is steady state decline in G.F.R. and ~50% of individuals reach end stage renal disease in 7-10 days.*
- *Once nephropathy becomes overt the pathological changes are irreversible.*

Microalbuminuria	Overt proteinuria
30-300 mg/d in 24 hr urinary sample.	> 300 mg/d in 24 hr urinary sample.

Stages of diabetic nephropathy: (IDDM)

Year	Stage	Findings
0	I	Raised GFR, increase in Renal size and plasma flow
2	II	Thickening in glomerular capillary basement membrane
6-10	III	**Microalbuminuria**
10-15	IV	**Overt proteinuria, Clinical nephropathy,** *changes become irreversible.*
16-25	V	End stage renal disease.

90. Answer is C (β-islet cell/pancreatic transplantation can improve the proteinuria in early stage): *Harrison 17th/2288; Pancreatic Transplantation by Carry & Shapira 1st/334; Harrison 18th/p 2982, 2983*

Pancreatic transplantation (or β-islet cell transplantation) may improve proteinuria in early stages.

Pancreatic Trnaplantation may improve diabetic nephropathy (proteinuria)
Successful pancreatic transplantation results in normalization of blood glucose and glycosylated hemoglobin levels.

Successful Pancreatic Transplantation

Complication that may be reversed/halled	Complications that do not appear to be reversed/halled
• *Diabetic nephropathy (microalbuminuria stage)* • *Diabetic Neuropathy*	• *Diabetic retinopathy* • *Peripheral vascular disease*

Microalbuminuria is associated with long term cardiovascular morbidity
'Both microalbuminuria and macroalbuminuria in individuals with DM are associated with increased risk of cardiovascular disease (morbidity)' – Harrison 17th/2287

Strict glycemic control may prevent or revert microalbuminuria
'With tight control of hyperglycemia and rigrous control of blood pressure the development of microalbuminuria may be prevented or reverted' – Harrison 13th/1312, Harrison 12th/1185

Angiotensin receptor blockers and ACE inhibitors are more effective than other drugs in slowing progression of diabetic nephropathy.

Blood pressure control with any agent is extremely important, but a drug specific benefit in diabetic nephropathy, independent of blood pressure control has only been shown for ACE inhibitors or Angiotensin receptor blockers.

Protein Restriction is helpful in diabetic nephropathy

Protein intake should be restricted in diabetic individuals with microalbuminuria and macroalbuminuria to modest levels. – Harrison 17th/2289

91. Answer is B (Enalapril): *Harrison 17th/2288; Harrison 18th/p 2983*

ACE inhibitors and Angiotensin Receptor Blockers are specifically indicated to reduce progression of renal disease.

Either ACE inhibitors or ARB's should be used to reduce the progression from microalbuminuria to macroalbuminuria, and the associated decline in GFR.

Drug specific benefit in diabetic nephropathy independent of blood pressure control has been shown only for ACE inhibitors and ARB's in patients with DM – Harrison

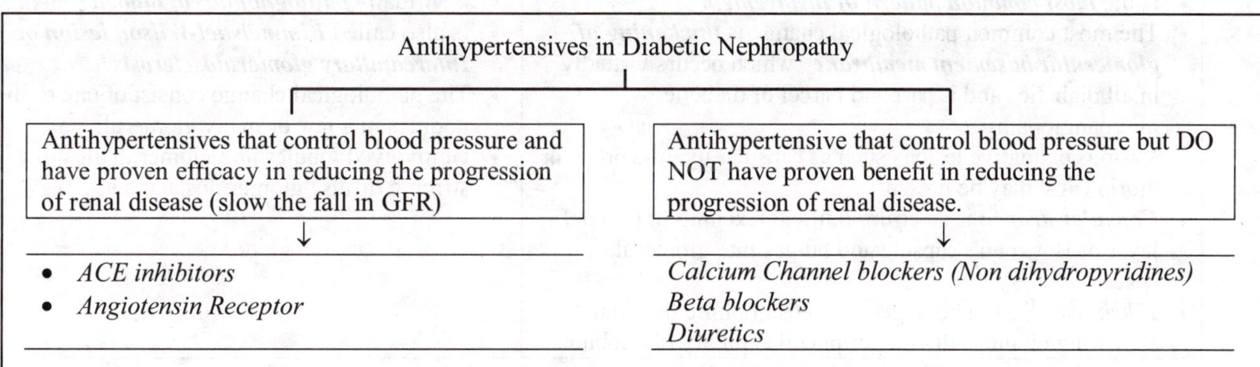

92. Answer is D (False positive microalbuminuria may occur in the presense of urinary tract infections (UTI)
Harrison's 17th/2287, 2288; Internal Medicine 5th/859,860; Harrison 18th/p 2982

Urinary infection is the major cause of false positive microalbuminuria

Urinary infection may cause false positive microalbuminuria

UTI should be ruled out in any individulas who has a positive microalbuminuria result. Patients are advised to have the urine collection first thing in the morning as exercise can cause microalbuminuria in the absence of renal disease.

Potential important causes of false positive microalbuminuria
• *UTI*
• *Exercise*
• *Menstruation,*
• *Pregnancy,*
• *Febrile illness*
• *Congestive heart failure*

The presence of microalbuminuria significantly increases the risk of cardiovascular disease and does not decrease the risk.

Calcium channel-blockers are not proven to reduce progression of renal disease.

Progression of renal disease can be reduced by ACE Inhibitors and Angiotensin Receptor Blockers (ARB)

Diabetic nephropathy does not protect against Diabetic Retinopathy

Diabetic nephropathy is usually associated with diabetic retinopathy. In fact, microvascular complications frequently present together, and, therefore, any patient with one microvascular condition should be carefully examined for other microavscular disease.

Blood pressure control tends to worsen after the development of diabetic nephropathy.

Therefore, tight blood pressure control in individuals with diabetic nephropathy is of prominent importance to avoid further deterioration of renal function.

93. Answer is B (Nodular glomerulosclerosis) : *Harsh Mohan 4th / 662; Robbibs 7th/992*

The most characteristic lesion in Diabetic Nephropathy is Nodular glomerulosclerosis.

Nodular glomerulosclerosis is virtually pathognomic[Q] of diabetes mellitus- Robbins

Glomerular Lesions in Diabetes	
Diffuse glomerulosclerosis :	**Nodular glomerulosclerosis**
• Is the ***most common pattern of involvement***[Q] • The most common pathological change is ***thickening of glomerular basement membrane***[Q] which occurs virtually in all diabetics and is part and parcel of diabetic microangiopathy • Various exudative lesions such as capsular hyaline drops or 'fibrin caps' may be present • ***Capsular drop***[Q] : is an eosinophilic thickening of parietal layer of Bowman's capsule and bulges into glomerular space • ***Fibrin caps***[Q] : is a homogeneous eosinophilic material appearing on the wall of a peripheral capillary of a lobule	• Is virtually ***pathognomic***[Q] ***of diabetes mellitus*** • Is also called ***Kimmelstiel-Wilson lesion*** *or* ***Intercapillary glomerulosclerosis***[Q] • The pathological change consist of one or more nodules in a few or many glomeruli • Uninvolved lobules and glomeruli all show striking diffuse glomerulosclerosis

94. Answer is C (Microangiopathic changes in blood vessels): *Harrison 17th/2292; Harrison 18th/p 2987*

Macroangiopathic changes in blood vessels in the form of peripheral arterial disease contribute to the generation of foot ulcers and non microangiopathic changes.

Pathogenic Factors in generation of foot ulcers in DM
• *Neuropathy (Peripheral Sensory neuropathy): Trophic changes*
• *Abnormal Foot Biomechanics (d/t disordered propioception and sensorimotor neuropathy)*
• *Peripheral Arterial disease (Macroangiopathy) and poor wound healing*
• *Autonomic neuropathy (anhidrosis and altered superficial blood flow in foot)*

95. Answer is D (Emphysematous Appendicitis): *Harrisons 16th/186, 189, 1720*

Emphysematous Appendicitis has not been listed as a fatal complication of diabetes mellitus.

Malignant Otitis Externa is a potential life threatening complication of Diabetes

'Invasive otitis externa, also known as malignant otitis externa or necrotizing otitis externa is an aggressive and life threatening disease that occurs predominantly in elderly diabetics and other immunocompromised patients'

-Harrison 16th/189

Rhinocereberal Mucormycosis is a potential life threatening complication of Diabetes

'Rhinocerebral mucormycosis is an invasive life threatening fungal infection that usually develops in diabetic patients and immunocompromised patients' - Harrison 16th/186

Emphysematous Pyelonephritis is a potential life threatening complication of Diabetes

Emphysematous pyelonephritis is usually characterized by rapidly progressive clinical course, with accumulation of fermentative gases in the kidney and perinephritic tissues. This condition almost always occurs in diabetic patients and surgical resection of the involved tissue and antimicrobial therapy is usually needed to prevent a fatal outcome- Harrison 16th/1720

96. Answer is D (DM with Acute MI): *Harrison 16th/2166, 2167, 2173; Harrison 17th/2290, 2296; Harrison 18th/p 2985*

Cardiovascular disease is increased in patient with Diabetes, but there is no evidence to suggest that improved glycemic control with intensive management reduces cardiovascular complications in DM.

'Proof that improved glycemic control reduces cardiovascular complications in DM is lacking; in fact it is possible that macrovascular complications may be unaffected or even worsened by such therapy' – Harrison 16th/2167

Indications for Intensive Diabetes Management

- *Otherwise healthy adults with either type 1 or 2 diabetes (selected adolescents and older children)*
- ***Purposeful, therapeutic attempt to avoid or lessen microvascular complications***
- ***All pregnant women with diabetes; all women with diabetes who are planning pregnancy***
- *Management of labile disease*
- *Availability of health care professionals with appropriate expertise*
- ***Patients who have had kidney transplantation for diabetic nephropathy***

Autonomic Neuropathy is a microvascular complication and intensive management for glycemic control should be pursued to improve nerve conduction (Harrison 16th/2166)
'Impaired glycemic control (intensive management) should be the primary goal.' – Harrison 17th/2290

97. Answer is C (CDNA of pancreatic cell) *Harrison 17th/390, 2297; Harrison 18th/p 2993*

98. Answer is A (Hypokalemia): *Ganong 22nd/338*

Insulin causes K^+ to enter cells with a resultant lowering of extracellular K^+ concentration (Hypokalemia)

Relation of Insulin to Potassium (Ganong 22nd/338)

- Insulin causes K^+ to enter cells with a resultant lowering of the extracellular K^+ concentration (Hypokalemia)
- Infusion of insulin and glucose significantly lower the plasma K^+ level in normal individual (Hypokalemia)
- Infusion of insulin and glucose is very effective for the temporary relief of hyperkalemia
- The reason for intracellular migration of K^+ is still uncertain. However increase the activity of Na^+ - K^+ ATPase in cell membranes so that more K^+ is pumped into cells.

99. Answer is B (Addison's disease) : *Harrison 16th/2158, 2153; KDT 5th/244, 245*

Insulin resistance (diabetes mellitus) occurs in Cushing's syndrome and not in Aaddison's disease.

Endocrinopathies associated with diabetes mellitus	
Acromegaly	Pheochromocytoma
Cushing's	Hyperthyroidism
Glucagonoma	Somatostatinoma
Aldosteronoma	

Insulin Resistant states - *Table from Harrisons 14th/e 2079*Q	
1. Obesity Q	6. Alstrom syndrome
2. Lipodystrophic states Q	7. Pineal hyperplasia syndrome
3. Ataxia - telengiectasia Q	8. Leprechaunism
4. Werners syndrome Q	9. Type A syndrome (absent or dysfunctional receptor)
5. Rabson Manden hall syndrome	10. Type B syndrome (antibody to insulin receptor)

100. Answer is C (Hyperuricemia): *Harrison's 17th/1506, 1507*

Hyperuricemia is not a feature of Insulin resistance metabolic syndrome.

Insulin resistance syndrome refers to the metabolic syndrome associated with insulin resistance. Besides insulin resistance, the associated manifestations of the syndrome include hypertension, dyslipidemia (↑ Triglycerides & ↓ HDL) and obesity.

Metabolic syndrome associated with Insulin Resistance (Insulin Resistance Syndrome)
• *Abdominal obesity (Waist circumference)* • *Dyslipidemia* - ↑ *Triglycerides* - ↓ *HDL* • *Hypertension* • *Insulin Resistance*

101. Answer is D (Hypopituitarism): *Harrison 16th/ 2180; Harrison 17th/2308; Harrison 18th/p 3007*

Acromegaly, Cushing's syndrome and Hyperthyroidism are all associated with Hyperglycemia

Hypopituitarism is associated with hypoglycemia.

Endocrinal abnormalities causing altered glucose metabolism include two major categories:

Endocrinopathies: Hyperglycemia	Endocrine deficiency: Hypoglycemia
• Cushing's syndromes (↑ed cortisol) • Acromegaly Q (↑ GH) • Glucagonoma Q (↑ Glucogen) • Pheochromocytoma Q (↑ catecholamines) • Hyperthyroidism Q • Somatostatinoma • Aldosteronoma Q	• Decreased cortisol Q (Addison's disease) • Decreased growth hormone Q • Decreased glucagons Q • Decreased catecholamines Q (↓ epinephrine)

102. Answer is C (Small cell Ca of lung) :; *Harrison 16th/2180; Harrison 17th/2305; Harrison 18th/p 3003*

Small cell carcinoma is associated with hyperglycemia, as a result of production of cushing's syndrome.

Tumors associated with hypoglycemia: *Harrisons 16th/e 2180*	
1. Insulinoma 2. Soft tissue sarcomas : • Fibrosarcoma • Mesothelioma • Rhabelomyosarcoma • Liposarcoma.	3. Hepatoma 4. Adrenocortical tumors 5. Carcinoid 6. Leukaemia/Lymphoma 7. Melanoma 8. Teratoma

103. Answer is B (Acromegaly) *Harrison 16th/2180; Harrison 17th/2305; Harrison 18th/p 3003*

Acromegaly is associated with Hyperglycemia and not Hypoglycemia.

Selected causes of hypoglycemia

A. Hormone deficiencies:	***B. Enzyme defects:***
• Hypopituitarism Q • Adrenal insufficiency (addison's disease) Q • Catecholamine deficiency Q • Glucagon deficiency Q	• Glucose-6-phosphatase Q **C. Liver disease:** • Hepatic congestion Q • Severe hepatitis Q • Cirrhosis Q • Hypothermia Q

104. Answer is C (Accidental exogenous Insulin administration): *Harrison's 17th/2309; Harrison 18th/p 3003*

Normal / Reduced levels of C- peptide in the presence of increased insulin suggest a diagnosis of exogenous insulin administration as the cause of hypoglycemia.

Approach to a patient with Hypoglycemia and Increased Insulin levels: Role of C- peptide Assay

- Normally Endogemous Insulin is secreted from β-cells of pancreas in the form of Pro-insulin
- This proinsulin is then broken down to Insulin and C- peptide such that *for each molecule of endogenous insulin, one molecule of C-peptide is produced.*

C-peptide levels are thus increased whenever endogenous insulin is increased e.g. Insulinomas, Sulfonylureas, Autoimmune processes and in cases of Insulin resistance (type II DM).

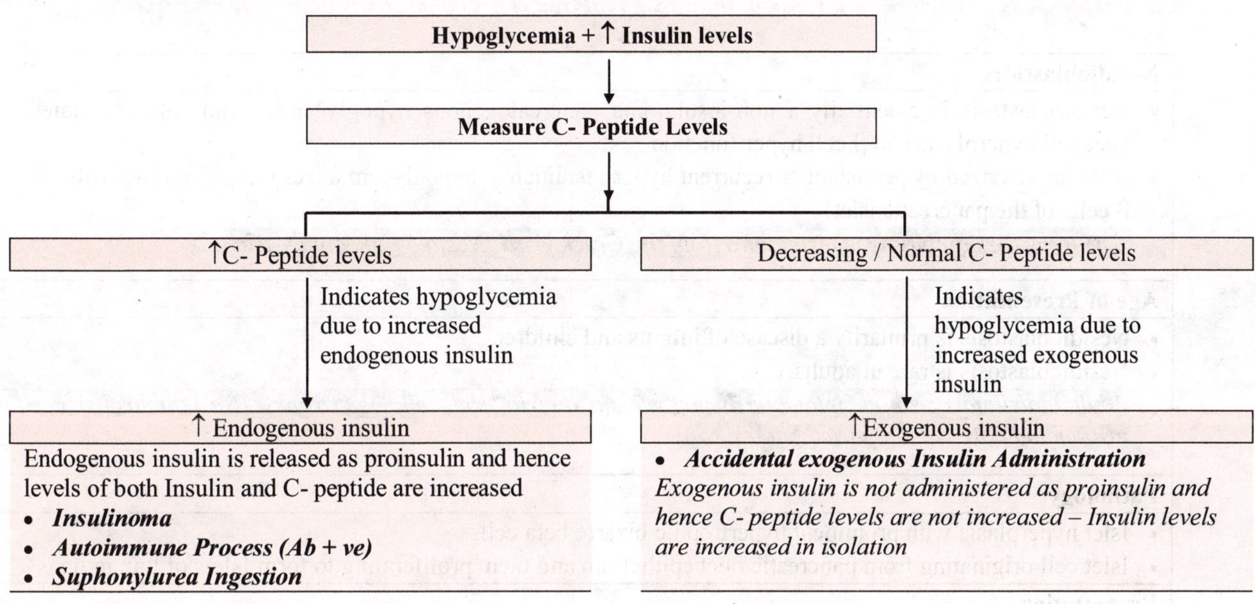

Note

C – peptide can also be used to distinguish Type I DM from Type II DM[Q]

Type I - DM (IDDM)[Q]	Type – II DM (NIDDM)[Q]
Results from complete / absolute lack of endogenous insulin secretion due to a reduction in β cell mass in pancreas **Hence** • *Insulin levels are Reduced* • *C- peptide levels are Reduced*	Results from inability of peripheral tissues to respond to Insulin or 'Insulin Resistance' **Hence** • *Insulin levels are actually increased* • *C- peptide levels are increased*

105. Answer is None (None of the above): *Harrison's 17th/2354, 2355; Williams Endocrinology 11th/1521,1522*

Insulinomas and Sulfonylureas, both produce endogenous hyperinsulinemia <u>leading to the same biochemical pattern.</u> These can only be distinguished by directly measuring the drug concentration of sulfonylureas in the plasma

'It is necessary to screen the plasma for sulphonylureas and other insulin secretagogues (repaglinide, nateglinide) at the time of hypoglycemia since these produce an insulin, C- peptide,, proinsulin and glucose pattern, indistinguishable from that produced by an insulinoma' - Harrison

Biochemical Patterns In Patients With Various Causes Of Hyperinsulinemic Hypoglycmia

Diagnosis	Insulin	C Peptide	Proinsulin	Sulfonylurea	Insulin Antibody
Exogenous insulin	↑	↓	↓	-	-
Insulinoma, CHI	↑	↑	↑	-	-
Sulfonylurea	↑	↑	↑	+	-
Insulin autoimmune	↑	↑*	↑	-	+
Insulin receptor autoimmune[+]	±↑	↓	↓	-	-

*free C Peptide and proinsulin ↓. [+] Insulin receptor antibody +. CHI, Congenital hyperinsulinism.

106. Answer is B (Occurs in adults more than children) : *Nelson's 18th/1652; 'Endocrine Tumors' by Clarke (American Cancer-Society) 2003 /162; 'Surgical pathology of Endocrine and Neuroendocrine Tumors' by Ashraf Khan (Springer, 2009) 1st/145; 'Clinical Endocrinology' by Grossman (Wiley-Blackwell, 1998) /538; 'Advanced Imaging of the Abdomen' by Skucas (Springer, 2006) /556; 'Gastrointestinal Oncology' by Jankowski, Kerr, Fong (Blackwell, 2008) /621*

Nesidioblastosis is primarily a disease of infants & children. This condition is extremely rare in adults.

Nesidioblastosis
• Nesidioblastosis is essentially a non-insulinoma pancreatogenous hypoglycemic syndrome associated with islet cell hyperplasia and β cell hyper function • It is characterized by persistant or recurrent hyper insulinemic hypoglycemia (resulting from hyperplasia of the β cells of the pancreatic islet) *The term 'Nesidioblastosis' originates from the Greek word 'Nesidion' meaning' islet.*
Age of Presentation
• Nesidioblastosis is primarily a disease of infants and children • Nesidioblastosis is rare in adults *Adult individuals with symptomatic hypoglycemia due to islet cell hypertrophy (Nesidioblastosis) without insulinoma have been reported but are rare*
Pathology
• Islet hyperplasia with prominent hypertrophic bizarre beta cells • Islet cell originating from pancreatic duct epithelium and then proliferating to form Islets of Langerhans
Presentation
• Symptomatic Hypoglycemia with endogenous hyperinsulinemia
Treatment
• Medical Treatment with diazoxide and /or chlorthiazide or with long acting somatostatin should be tried *In infants with hyperinsulinism due to nesidioblastosis and adults with islet hyperplasia (nesidioblastosis) treatment should be instituted with diazoxide and chlorthiazide or with long acting somatostatin – Clinical Endocrinology* • Surgical treatment should be considered only if above medical treatment if above medical treatment fails *Subtotal Pancreatectomy (80% removal of pancreases) should be tried initially* *Total Pancreatectomy may be required in severe cases*

Disorders of Pituitary / Sexual Differentiation

Hyperprolactinemia and Anterior Pituitary Disorders

107. Answer is A (Bromocriptine): *KDT 5th/218; Harrison 16th/2085; Harrison 17th/2204, 2205; Harrison 18th/ 2887, 2888*

Bromocriptine is a potent dopamine agonist. It decreases prolactin release from pituitary by activating inhibitory dopaminergic receptors on lactotrope cells, a strong anti-galactopoietics action.

All others are known to cause increased Prolactin.

Drugs causing Hyper-Prolactinemia include:

A. Dopamine receptor antagonists - Phenothiazine: chlorpromazine, periphenazine - Butyrophenones: haloperidol - Thioxanthenes - Metoclopramide - Resperidone - Sulpride	B. Dopamine synthesis inhibitors: *α-Methyldopa* C. Catecholamine depletors: *Reserpine* D. Opiates E. H_2 antagonissts : *Cimetidine, ranitidine* F. Imipramines: *Amitriptyline, amoxapine* G. Serotonin-reuptake inhibitors: *Fluoxetine* H. Calcium channel blockers: *Verapamil*

108. Answer is A (Mental Retardation): *Harrison's 18th/2894; Williams Textbook of Endocrinology*

Hypersecretion of Growth hormone (gigantism in children; acromegaly in adults) is not associated with Mental Retardation

Growth Hormone Hypersecretion
IGF-1 Hypersecretion

- Acromegaly and Gigantism are clinical syndromes that result from hypersecretion of Growth Hormone (or somatamedins like IGF-1)

***Acromegaly** results in adults when excessive secretion of GH occurs following epiphyseal closure.*	**Gigantism** occurs is children when excessive secretion of GH occurs prior to epiphyseal closure as a result of increased linear bone growth

- The most common cause for Acromegaly is a Growth Hormone secreting pituitary adenoma[Q] (somatotrope adenoma)

Clinical manifestations of Acromegaly:

Local Tumor Effects • *Visual field defects* • *Cranial nerve palsy (diplopia)* • *Headache* **Somatic Manifestations** • *Acral enlargement* • *Thickening of soft tissue of the hands/feet (increased ring/shoe size)* **Musculoskeletal Manifestations** • *Prognathism* • *Malocclusion* • *Arthralgias* • *Carpal tunnel syndrome* • *Frontal bossing* **Skin Manifestations** • *Hyperhidrosis* • *Skin tags* **Colon Manifestations** • *Polyps* **Cardiovascular Manifestations** • *Left ventricular hypertrophy* • *Hypertension* • *Congestive heart failure*	**Sleep Disturbances** • *Sleep apnea* • *Narcolepsy* **Visceral Manifestations** • *Macroglossia* • *Hepatomegaly* • *Splenomegaly* • *Thyroid enlargement* **Sexual Function** • *Menstrual abnormalities* • *Galactorrhea (hyperprolactinemia)* • *Decreased libido* **Carbohydrates** • *Impaired glucose intolerance* • *Insulin resistance* • *Hyperinsulinemia* • *Diabetes mellitus* • *Lipids* • *Hypertriglyceridemia*

109. Answer is B (Somatomedins): *Harrison's 18th/2871-2894*

Many of the physiological affects of Growth Hormone are mediated indirectly through somatomedins like IGF-1 (Insulin like Growth foactor) which is a potent growth and differentiation factor.

Increased shoe size, Prognathism (protruding jaw) and enlarged phalanges in a middle aged man suggest a diagnosis of Growth Hormone oversecretion or Acromegaly. Growth Hormone exerts several effects through induction of somatomedins (like IGF), a family of hormones secreted in the blood by the liver and other tissues.

What are Somatomedins

Somatomedins are a family of harmones that are potent growth and differentiation factors. The liver is the major source of somatomedins like IGF-1 that mediates many of the physiological effects of Growth Hormone on target tissues.

Somatomedins are similar to insulin in molecular structure and are hence also known as *'Insulin like Growth factors'* (IGF) and these act on target tissue to increase protein synthesis by increasing the rate of uptake of amino acids.

Although GH exerts direct effects on target tissues, many of its physiological effects are mediated indirectly through somatomedins like IGF-1

Lack of Somatomedins cause dwarfism[Q]

110. Answer is C (Bromocriptine) : *KDT 5th/217, 382; Harrison 16th/2085; Harrison 17th/ 2205; Harrison 18th/p 2887*

Bromocriptine is a potent dopamine agonist. It decreases prolactin release from pituitary by activating inhibitory dopaminergic receptors on lactotrope cells, a strong anti-galactopoietics action.

Etiology of Hyperprolactinemia	
I. **Physiologic hypersecretion** A. Pregnancy B. Lactation C. Chest wall stimulation D. Sleep E. Stress II. **Pituitary hypersecretion** A. Prolactinoma B. Acromegaly III. **Systemic disorders** A. Chronic renal failure B. Hypothyroidism C. Cirrhosis D. Pseudocyesis E. Epileptic seizures IV. **Drug-induced hypersecretion** *Ref. previous question*	V. **Hypothalamic-pituitary stalk damage** A. Tumors - Craniopharyngioma - Suprasellar pituitary mass extension - Meningioma - Dysgerminoma - Metastases B. Empty sella C. Lymphocytic hypophysitis D. Adenoma with stalk compression E. Granulomas F. Rathke's cyst G. Irradiation H. Trauma - Pituitary stalk section - Suprasellar surgery

111. Answer is C (Prolactin estimation): *Harrison 17th/2205, 2206; Harrison 18th/p 2888*

Basal fasting morning prolactin levels should be measured to assess hypersecretion *- Harrison*

112. Answer is C (Prolactinoma): *Robbins 7th/1160;*

'Prolactinomas (Lactotroph Adenomas) are the most frequent type of hyperfunctioning pituitary adenomas, accounting for about 30% of all clinically recognized pituitary adenomas' *- Robbins*

113. Answer is B (Prolactinoma): *Harrison 16th/2086; Harrison 17th/ 2206; Harrison 18th/p 2889*

Menstrual cycle disturbance in the form of amenorrhea along with galactorrhea suggests a diagnosis of hyperprolactinemia.
Amongst the options provided the tumor most likely to produce above endocrine manifestation is a prolactinoma.

Prolactinomas: Most common functional pituitary adenomas [Q]
Most common cause of pituitary hormonal syndrome in adults

Clinical presentations:

Symptoms due to hyperprolactinemia
(More common seen with both microadenomas and macroadenomas)
- Galactorrhea [Q]
- Amenorrhea [Q]
- Infertility [Q]

(Hyperprolactinemia from any cause produces Hypogonadotrophic hypogonadism)

Symptoms due to mass effect
Less common
Seen with macroadenomas
- Headache
- Visual field defects (bitemporal hemianopia)
- Optic atrophy & blindness (late manifestations)

Treatment: Bromocriptine [Q] is the therapy of choice
It is a dopamine agonist [Q] agent and is an effective prolactin lowering agent. [Q]

Microprolactinomas are more common than macroprolactinomas [Q]

Craniopharyngiomas: these tumors arise from remnants of Rathke's pouch. [Q] Although craniopharyngiomas may also produce hyper prolactinemia, purely endocrinal manifestations in the form of galactorrhea and amenorrhea are unlikely with craniopharyngiomas.

These tumors present mostly in childhood with features of raised ICT and visual abnormalities.

Meningiomas and SAH will not produce symptoms of hyperprolactinemia alone.

114. Answer is B (Pituitary macroadenoma): *Harrison 16th/2081; API 7th/864; see previous question; Harrison 17th/2206; Harrison 18th/p 2889*

Presence of long standing endocrinopathies (menstrual irregularities and galactorrhea) in an adult suggests a diagnosis of pituitary adenoma over craniopharyngiomas as the latter are primarily tumours of childhood. Visual field defects and optic atrophy suggest local mass effects which are associated with 'macroadenomas' and hence the most likely diagnosis is a pituitary macroadenoma.

Note :

'Pituitary adenomas are the most common cause of pituitary hormonal syndromes in adults – Harrison

'The functional tumors often produce clinical symptoms of endocrinopathies when they are still small (microadenomas) and restricted to sella. When a tumor grows outside the sella (macroadenoma) it compresses the optic chiasma and nerves and produces a variety of visual defects, the most common being a complete or incomplete bitemporal hemianopia'- API

As the tumor progresses it may result in optic atrophy and blindness.

Optic gliomas occur mainly in childhood and presentation is usually with visual loss and not endocrinal manifestations.

Opthalmic ICA aneurysm is unlikely to present with long standing endocrinopathies over a year prior to appearance of visual symptoms.

Craniopharyngiomas can be excluded as in the previous question.

115. Answer is A (Pituitary Macroadenoma): *Refer text below*

Presence of galactorrhea (hyperprolactinemia) and bitemporal superior quadrantopia (visual field defect) is consistent with a diagnosis of pituitary macroadenoma. Both non secretory pituitary Macroadenoma and prolactin secreting Macroadenoma (Large Prolactinoma) may produce the above manifestation.

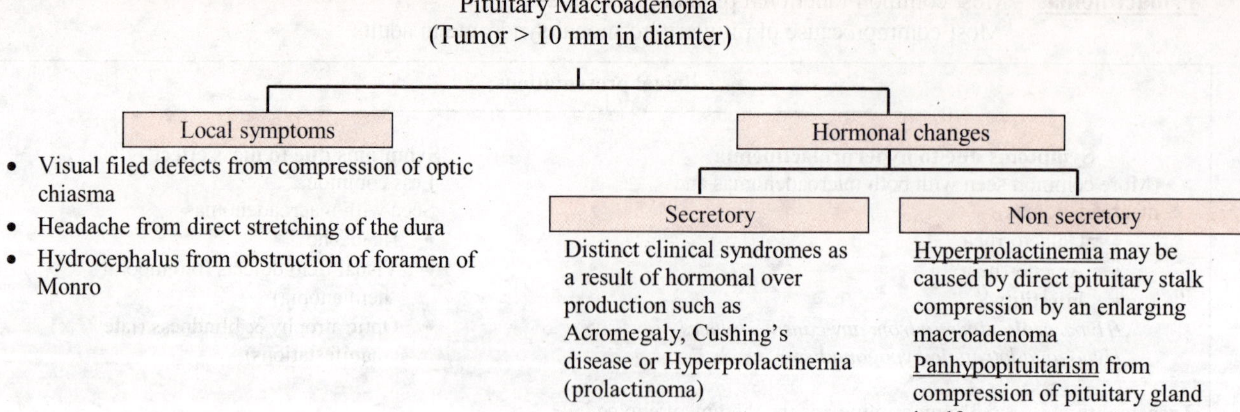

Craniopharyngioma *may also produce visual filed defects, along with galactorrhea due to enhanced prolactin secretion. However this symptom complex is more common and more characteristic of pituitary macroadenomas which is the single best answer of choice.*

116. Answer is D (Bromocriptine): *Harrison 17th/2206; Harrison 18th/p 2890*

Secondary Amenorrhea and galactorrhea in a young women with evidence of microadenoma (tumor ≤ 10mm) in the pituitary fossa suggest a diagnosis of prolactinoma.

Oral dopamine agonists (Dopamine or Cabergoline) are the treatment of choice for patients with prolactinomas.

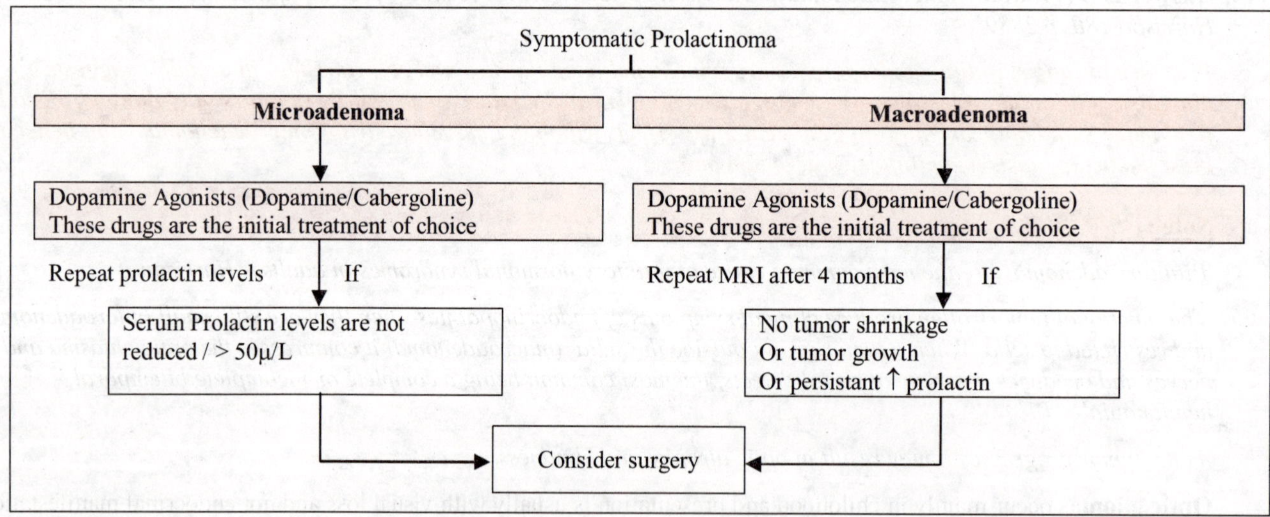

117. Answer is B (Glucose induced GH suppression): *Harrison 17th/2210; Harrison 18th/p 2894*

The diagnosis of Acromegaly is confirmed by demonstrating the failure of GH suppression after an oral glucose load.

Diagnosis of Acromegaly

- IGF – I level
  Age and gender matched serum IGF-I level are elevated in Acromegaly.
  Elevated IGF-I levels are *primarily used as a screening test for Acromegaly and not as a confirmatory test.*

- Random GH Assay
  GH secretion is episodic and serum concentrations of GH may fluctuate from undetectable levels to significantly high levels during the day. *Due to pulsalilty of GH secretion, measurement of single random GH level is not useful for the diagnosis or exclusion of Acromegaly.*

- <u>GH suppression test (Failure of GH suppression in response to Glucose load)</u>
  The diagnosis of Acromegaly is confirmed by demonstrating the failure of GH suppression to <1 µg/L within 1-2 hours of an oral glucose load (75g).
  Infact, about 20% of patients exhibit a paradoxical rise in GH levels after glucose.

118. Answer is B (Acromegaly): *Harrison 16th/2090*

In patients with Acromegaly TRH can cause a paradoxical increase in GH secretion which is not observed in normal individuals.

'About 60% of patients with GH secreting tumors (Acromegaly) may exhibit paradoxical GH response to TRH administration'- Harrison 16th/2090

119. Answer is B (Adrenalectomy): *Harrison 16th/2094, 2138; Harrison 17th/2214; Basic Clinical Endocrinology (Lange) 7th/162; Harrison 18th/p 2899*

Adrenalectomy predisposes to development of Nelson's syndrome.

<u>Nelson syndrome</u>

- Nelson syndrome is a disorder characterized by rapid enlargement of a preexisting ACTH pituitary adenoma **<u>after adrenalectomy</u>.**
- *This syndrome occurs because following adrenalectomy, the suppressive effect of cortisol on ACTH secretion and tumor growth is removed resulting in increased ACTH secretion and tumor growth.*
- Patients with Nelson's syndrome present with hyperpigmentation and with manifestation of an expanding intrasellar mass lesion (visual field defects, headache, cavernous sinus invasion etc.)
- These tumors represent one of the most aggressive and rapidly growing of all pituitary tumors.
- ACTH levels are markedly elevated.
- Preoperative Radiotherapy may be indicated to prevent development of Nelson's syndrome after adrenelectomy.

120. Answer is A (Hyperthyroidism): *Harrison 17th/2198; Harrison 18th/p 2879*

Hyperthyroidism is not mentioned as a cause of pituitary apoplexy.

<u>Pituitary Apoplexy</u>

Pituitary Apoplexy refers to the clinical syndrome arising from hemorrhage or infarction of the pituitary gland.

Causes/Predisposing factors for Pituitary Apoplexy
• *Pre existing Pituitary Adenoma* • *Pregnancy* • *Post partum (Sheehan's syndrome)* • ***Diabetes*** • ***Hypertension*** • ***Sickle cell anemia*** • *Acute shock* • *<u>Others</u> (Internal Medicine 5th/1778)* *Trauma, Carotid Angiography, Bleeding/Clotting disorders, Anticoagulant therapy, Radiation to pituitary tumor, Artificial Respiration.*

121. Answer is B (Cortisone): *Harrison 15th/ 2033; (Not elaborated in Harrison 16th) ; Harrison 17th/ 2199, 2200; Harrison 18th/p 2880, 2882*

"Multiple hormones must be replaced in patients with pan-hypopituitarism, but cortisol replacement is most important"^{Q} *– Harrison 14th /1994*

Sheehan's syndrome is post-partum infarction of the pituitary, leading to hypopituitarism.

Treatment consists of hormone replacement therapy including ***Glucocorticoids***, Thyroid hormone, Sex steroids, Growth hormone, Vasopressin, etc. Thus, multiple hormones must be replaced, but remember that Cortisol replacement is most important.

122. Answer is B (Diabetes mellitus): *Refer text below*

Insulin is a pancreatic hormone, not under the control of pituitary. Transection of the pituitary stalk would therefore in no way affect glucose levels or lead to diabetes mellitus.

123. Answer is A (Diabetes Mellitus): *Repeat*

Insulin is a pancreatic hormone, not under the control of pituitary. Transection of the pituitary stalk would therefore in no way affect glucose levels or lead to diabetes mellitus.

SIADH

124. Answer is B (Interstitial nephritis) : *Harrison 16th/2102; Nelson 17th/ 200, 202; 17th/ 2222; Harrison 18th/p 2908*

SIADH is not associated with interstitial nephritis

Causes of SIADH include:

Neoplasm		**Neurologic**	**Drugs**
Ca Lung	Thymoma	Guillain-Barré-syndrome	Vasopressin or DDAVP
Ca Duodenum	Mesothelioma	Multiple sclerosis	Chlorpropamide
Ca Pancreas	*Bronchial adenoma* [Q]	Delirium tremens	Oxytocin, high dose
Ca Ovary	Carcinoid	Amyotrophic lateral sclerosis	*Vincristine* [Q]
Ca Bladder,	Gangliocytoma	Hydrocephalus	Carbamazepine
Ca Ureter	Ewing's sarcoma	Psychosis	Nicotine
		Peripheral neuropathy	Phenothiazines
			Cyclophosphamide
			Tricyclic antidepressants
			Monoamine oxidaseinhibitors
			Serotonin reuptake inhibitors
Infections		**Metabolic**	**Congenital malformations**
Pneumonia, bacterial or viral		Acute intermittent porphyria	Agenesis of corpus callosum
Abscess, lung [Q] or brain		Pulmonary	Cleft lip/palate
Cavitation (aspergillosis)		Asthma	Other midline defects
Tuberculosis, lung or brain		Pneumothorax	
Meningitis, bacterial or viral		Positive-pressure respiration	
Encephalitis			
AIDS			
Vascular		**Head trauma (closed & penetrating)**	
Cerebrovascular occlusions, hemorrhage			
Cavernous sinus thrombosis			

125. Answer is A (Vincristine):*Harrison 16th / 2102; Harrison 17th/ 2222*

Vincristine is known to cause SIADH.

Drugs associated with SIADH : *Harrison 16th / 2102*
• *Vasopressin or desmopressin* • *Chlorpropamide* • *Oxytocin, high dose* • ***Vincristine*** • *Carbamezapine* • *Nicotine* • *Phenothiazines* • *Cyclophosphamide* • *Tricyclic antidepressants* • *MAO inhibitors* • *Serotonin reuptake inhibitors*

126. Answer is A (Small cell Ca of lung): *Harrison 16th/507; 17th/ 2222; Nelson 17th/200-202; Harrison 18th/p 2908*

Small cell Ca of lung causes SIADH due to ectopic secretion of ADH.

127. Answer is B (Urinary sodium excretion is low / normal): *Harrisons 18th/2908, 2909, 2910; Harrisons 17th/2222; CMDT 2007/891; 'Spiral Manul of Endocrinology and Metabolism' by Lavin (4th)/70-74; 'Disease of kdney and Urinary Tract' by Shrier (Lippincott Williams) 8th/2220; 'Renal and Electrolyte Disorders' by Shrier (Lippincott Williams) 2010/40*

SIADH is typically characterized by high urinary sodium (Increased rate of excretion of sodium).

Syndrome of Inappropriate ADH Secretion (SIADH) is associated with increased secretion of vasopressin (ADH), which leads to increased absorption of water producing ***dilutional hyponatremia (serum sodium typically < 135 meq/l)*** along with concentrated or hyperosmolar urine. Excessive retention of water stimulates compensatory mechanisms that enhance ***'Natriuresis'***.

Natriuresis results in increased urinary sodium excretion rate (increased urinary sodium concentration) and is believed to compensate for increased volume from inappropriaye ADH secretion preventing a state of clinical hypervolemia, hypertension or edema.

SIADH is associated low serum sodium levels (<135 meq/l) and High urinary sodium

Cardinal features of SIADH include:

• ***Hyponatremia (dilutional hyponatremia with Na+ < 135 mmol/l)***
• *Decreased plasma osmolality (<280 m osm/kg) with inappropriately increased urine osmolality > 150 m osm).*
• ***High Urine sodium (over 20 meq/l)***
• *Low Blood urea Nitrogen < 10 mg/L*
• *Hypouricemia (<4 mg/dL)*
• *Clinical Euvolemia*
  - Absence of signs of hypervolemia (edema, ascitis)
  - Absence of signs of hypovolemia (orthostatic hypotension, tachycardia, features of dehydration)
• *Absence of cardiac, liver or renal disease*
• *Normal thyroid and adrenal function*
• ***A high BUN suggests a volume contracted state and excludes a diagnosis of SIADH.*** [Q]

Water loading test may be used to help diagnosis of SIADH

Water loading test is recognized as a 'supplemental criteria' in establishing a diagnosis of SIADH.

The 'Water Loading Test' is of value when there is uncertainity regarding the etiology of modest degrees hypo-osmolality in euvolemic patients but it does not add useful information if the plasma osmolality is < 275 mOsm/kg H_2O

Test Objective / Principle	Abnormal Water Loading Test Criteria
Fixed quantity of water is given to a patient and the amount of urine produced and changes in blood/urine osmolality are recorded. *Inability to excrete a normal water load (decreased urinary output) or failure to dilute urine is considered abnormal*	Abnormal water load *Inability to excrete* at least 90% of a 20ml/kg water load in 4 hours, and/or *Failure to dilute* urine (osm) to < 100 mOsm/kg H_2O.

Vaptans are new FDA approved agents for treatment of SIADH

'Vaptans' are a new class of drugs that have emerged for treatment of hyponatremia. *These medications act as Vasopressin receptors antagonists blocking the action of AVP* in renal tubule, pituitary or smooth muscles depending upon receptor selectivity.

Conivaptan (Intravenous use)	*Tolivaptan (Oval use)*
Conivaptan is a combined V1/V2 receptor antagonist is *FDA approved for short-term intravenous use for treatment of hospitalized patients with SIADH.*	Tolivaptan is a V2 receptor antagonist that has received *FDA approval for oral use*

Syndrome of Inappropriate ADH Secretion (SIADH): Concept Review

Criteria for the diagnosis of syndrome of innapropriate antidiuretic hormone secretion
Essential
• ***Decreased effective osmolality*** of the extracellular fluid (P_{osm} < 275 mOsmol/kg H_2O). *(True hypoosmolality must be present and hyponatremia secondary to pseudohyponatremia or hyperglycemia must be excluded)* ***Inappropriate urinary concentration*** (Uosm > 100 mOsmol/kg H2O with normal renal function) at some level of hypoosmolality. *(Urinary concentration must be inappropriate for Plasma Hyposmolality)*
• ***Clinical euvolemia***, as defined by the absence of signs of hypovolemia (orthostasis, tachycardia, decreased skin rurgor, dry mucous membranes) or hypervolemia (subcutaneous edema, ascites).
• ***Elevated urinary sodium*** excretion while on normal salt and water intake.
• ***Absence of other potential causes of euvolemic hypoosmolality***: hypothyroidism, hypocortisolism (Addison's disease or pituitary adrenocorticotropic hormone [ACTH] insufficiency) and diuretic use.
Supplemental
• ***Abnormal water load test*** (inability to excrete at least 90% of a 20 mL/kg water load in 4 hours and/or failure to dilute Uosm to < 100 mOsmol/kg H_2O).
• ***Plasma AVP level inappropriately elevated*** relative to plasma osmolality.
• No significant correction of serum [Na^+] with volume expansion but improvement after fluid restriction

Differential Diagnosis of Hyponatremia Based on Clinical Assessment of Extracellular Fluid Volume (ECFV)

Clinical Findings	Type 1, Hypervolemic	Type II, Hypervolemic	Type III, Hypervolemic	SIADH Euvolemic
History				
CHF, cirrhosis, or nephrosis	Yes	No	No	No
Salt & water loss	No	Yes	No	No
ACTH- cortisol deficiency and/or nausea and vomatiting	No	No	Yes	No
Physical examination				
Generalized edema, ascites	Yes	No	No	No
Postrual hypotension	May be	May be	May be[a]	No
Laboratory				
BUN, creatinine	High-normal	High-normal	Low-normal	Low-normal
Uric acid	High-normal	High-normal	Low-normal	Low-normal
Serum potassium	Low-normal	Low-normal	Normal	Normal
Serum albumin	Low-normal	High-normal	Normal	Normal
Serum cortisol	Normal-high	Normal-high	Low	Normal
Plasma renin activity	High	High	Low	Low
Urinary sodium (Meq unit of time)	Low	Low	High	***High***

128. Answer is A (Hypo-osmolar urine): *Harrison16th/2102, 2103; Harrison 17th/ 2222; Harrison 18th/p 2908, 2909*

SIADH is characterized by increased vasopressin release leading to increased absorption of water producing a concentrated or hyperosmolar urine.

SIADH

- *The term SIADH is applied to conditions with vasopressin excess. Vasopressin excess is termed inappropriate as this increase occurs despite decreased plasma osmolality.*
- *Increased vasopressin acts on renal tubules, resulting in increased absorption of water (increased total body water), a concentrated urine[Q] and decreasing serum osmolality[Q] and hyponatremia [Q].*
- *Edema does not occur despite increased total body water [Q] (due to unknown reasons) – Clinical Euvolemia[Q].*

SIADH should be suspected in patients who have hyponatremia and concentrated urine (osmolality > 300 mmol/kg) in the absence of edema, orthostatic hypotension and features of dehydration.

Diagnosis is supported by finding of blood urea nitrogen, serum uric acid, creatinine, etc. in low normal or subnormal range [Q] (as can be expected from hypervolumia).

Increased action of ADH causes increased reabsorption of water, and resulting expanded fluid volume & water intoxication, and this also explains fall in conc. of serum electrolytes such as Mg^{2+}.

129. Answer is A (Hyponatremia and urine sodium excretion > 20 meq/l) : *Harrison 17th/ 2222; CMDT 2007/891; CMDT 2009/770; Harrison 18th/p 2908, 2909*

Cardinal features of SIADH include:

- *Hyponatremia (dilutional hyponatremia with Na+ < 135 mmol/l)*
- *Decreased plasma osmolality (<280 m osm/kg) with inappropriately increased urine osmolality > 150 m osm).*
- *Urine sodium over 20 meq/l*
- *Low Blood urea Nitrogen < 10 mg/L*
- *Hypouricemia (<4 mg/dL)*
- *Clinical Euvolemia*
  - Absence of sign of hypervolemia (edema, ascitis)
  - Absence of signs of hypovolemia (orthostatic hypotension, tachycardia, features of dehydration)
- *Absence of cardiac, liver or renal disease*
- *Normal thyroid and adrenal function*

A high BUN suggests a volume contracted state and excludes a diagnosis of SIADH. Q

130. Answer is A (Cerebral toxoplasmosis with SIADH): *Harrison/CMDT; Refer previous question*

The patient in question satisfies all the diagnostic features of SIADH, leaving no doubt as regards the diagnosis.

	Laboratory parameters in patient	Normal values	SIADH CRITERIA
1.	Serum Na^+: 120 mmol/l i.e. Hyponatremia	(137-145 mmol/l)	< 135 mmol/l
2.	Uric acid: 2 mg/dl i.e. Hypouricemia	2.5-8.5 mg/dl	< 4 mg/dl
3.	Serum K^+: 4.2 mmol i.e. Normokalemia	3.5-4.5 mmol/l	3.5-4.5 mmol/l

Edema does not occur in SIADH despite hypervolumia. The patient in question has distinctly been mentioned as 'non edematous', thus providing us with an important lead to the answer.

131. Answer is B (Hyposmolar urine): *Harrison 17th/2222; Harrison 18th/p 2910*

SIADH is characterized by an inappropriately increased urine osmolality (Hyperosmolar urine) in the presence of decreased plasma osmolality.

132. Answer is B (Euvolemic Hyponatremia): *Harrison 17th/2223; Harrison 18th/p 2909*

SIADH is characterized by Euvolemic Hyponatremia.

Hyponatremia

Hypovolemic Hyponatremia

In hypovolemic hyponatremia both Total body sodium and Total body water (TBW) are reduced such that sodium is two to greater extent than TBW

- TBW ↓
- Sodium ↓↓

Hypervolemic Hyponatremia

In Hypervolemic Hyponatremia both total body sodium and TBW are increased such that increase in TBW is greater than increase in sodium.

- TBW ↑↑
- Sodium ↑

Euvolemic Hyponatremia (SIADH)

In Euvolemic Hyponatremia total body sodium is normal but total body water is increased.

- TBW ↑
- Sodium No change (normal)

133. Answer is D (Demeclocycline): *Harrison 17th/2223; Katzung 10th/249; Harrison 18th/p 2910*

The treatment of choice for SIAPH is water restriction.

The drug of choice for SIAPH (when water restriction is unsuccessful is demeclocycline). Demeclocycline *(a tetracycline) acts as an ADH antagonist.*

134. Answer is C (Desmopressin) :; *Harrison 16th/2103; Harrison 17th/ 2223; Harrison 18th/p 2910*

Desmopressin has no role in the management of SIADH.

- ***In Acute SIADH, the keystone of treatment is to restrict total fluid intake* to less than the sum total of insensible losses and urinary output.**
- *If more rapid correction of hyponatremia is desired*, the fluid restriction can be supplemented by intravenous infusion of ***hypertonic saline***.
- In chronic SIADH, the hyponatremia can be minimized by treatment with ***demeclocycline or fludrocortisone***.

Diabetes Insipidus/Psychogenic Polydypsia/Polyuria

135. Answer is C (Diabetes insipidus):; *Harrison 16th/ 255, 2099; Harrison 17th/ 2218-2219; Harrison 18th/p 2904, 2905*

Diabetes insipidus is associated with hyper-natremia (due to free water loss), and not hyponatremia

All other conditions are associated with hyponatremia

Causes of Hyponatremia:

I. Pseudohyponatremia		
Normal plasma osmolality 1. Hyperlipidemia 2. Hyperproteinemia 3. Posttransurethral resection of prostate/bladder tumor	***Increased plasma osmolality*** 1. Hyperglycemia 2. Mannitol	
II. Hypoosmolal hyponatremia		
Primary Na+ loss (secondary water gain)	***Primary water gain (secondary Na+ loss)***	***Primary Na+ gain (exceeded by secondary water gain)***
1. Integumentary loss : sweating, burns 2. Gastrointestinal loss : vomiting, tube drainage, fistula, obstruction, diarrhea 3. Renal loss: diuretics, osmotic diuresis, hypoaldosteronism, salt-wasting nephropathy, postobstructive diuresis, nonoliguric acute tubular necoris.	1. Primary polydipsia 2. Decreased solute intake (e.g. beer potomania) 3. AVP release due to pain, nausea, drugs 4. Syndrome of inappropriate AVP secretion 5. Glucocorticoid deficiency 6. Hypothyroidism 7. Chronic renal insufficiency	1. Heart failure 2. Hepatic cirrhosis 3. Nephrotic syndrome

136. Answer is A (Multiple sclerosis) : *Harrison; 16th/ 2099; CMDT. 2009 page, 970, Harrison 17th/ 2218; Harrison 18th/p 2905*

Multiple sclerosis has not been mentioned as a cause for diabetes insipidus.

Diabetes insipidus *is a syndrome caused by either deficiency of vasopressin or resistance to action of vasopressin in passage of abnormally large volume of urine of low specific gravity.*

Causes of diabetes insipidus

Pituitary form of DI (Neurohypophysial or central) Deficient secretion of vasopressin from pituitary	**Nephrogenic D.I. (Renal D.I.)** Resistance to action of vasopressin on kidney	**Primary polydispisa**
Congenital malformations **Genetic** **Acquired** Head trauma (closed and penetrating) Neoplasms Primary Craniopharyngioma Pituitary adenoma (suprasellar) Dysgerminoma Meningioma Metastatic (lung, breast) Hematologic (lymphoma, leukemia)	**Genetic** **Acquired** Drugs Lithium Demeclocyline Methoxyflurane Amphotericin B Aminoglycosides Cisplatin Rifampin Foscarnet Metabolic	**Acquired** Psychogenic Schizophrenia Obsesive-compulsive disorder Dipsogenic (abnormal thirst) Granulomas: Neurosarcoid Infectious: Tuberculous meningitis Head trauma (closed and penetrating)

Granulomas: Neurosarcoid Histiocytosis Xanthoma disseminatum Infectious: Chronic meningitis Viral encephalitis Toxoplasmosis Inflammatory:Lymphocytic Infundibuloneurohypophysitis Wegener's granulomatosis Lupus erythematous Scleroderma Chemical toxins: Tetrodotoxin, Snake venom Vascular:Sheehan's syndrome Aneurysm (internal carotid) Aortocoronary bypass Hypoxic encephalopathy Pregnancy (vasopressinase) Idiopathic	Hypercalcemia, hypercalcinuria Hypokalemia Obstruction (ureter or urethra) Vascular Sickle cell disease and trait Ischemia (acute tubular necrosis) Granulomas Neurosarcoid Neoplasms Sarcoma Infiltration Amyloidosis Pregnancy Idiopathic	Demyelimation: Multiple sclerosis Drugs: Lithium Carbamazepine Idiopathic Iatrogenic

137. Answer is A (Urinary osmolality 50, serum osmolality 300) : *Nelson / 1575;; Harrison 16th/ 2098; CMDT 2009/970; CMDT 2003/1075; Harrison 17th/ 2219; Nelson 16th/2099, 1575; Harrison 18th/p 2905*

The only option which shows hypo-osmolar urine, along with a normal to greater serum osmolality is option A and so thus it is the answer here.

Central diabetes insipidus is a syndrome caused by deficient secretion of AVP from the pituitary resulting in production of abnormality large volume of dilute urine.

Clinical and Laboratory correlates in diabetes insipidus

1.	Passage of Large volume of urine	: 24 hr urine volume > 50 ml/kg body weight
2.	Passage of dilute urine	: **Urine osmolality** < 300 mosm/L

Effects on plasma osmolarity: (Normal serum osmolarity = 285-295 mosm/kg water).

Polyuria in DI results in a small decrease in plasma osmolarity and sodium concentration. These in turn stimulate thirst and a compensatory increase in water intake, which tend to bring the osmolarity towards normal.
Thus, the *serum osmolality may be normal or undergo a slight increase (because fluid from body is lost) however it never falls. Therefore we cannot expect osmolality of serum to be less than 285. Thus serum osmolality of 300 as in the question above is compatible with mild rise in serum osmolality as seen in diabetes insipidus.*

138. Answer is D (Psychogenic Polydipsia): *Harrison's Manual of Medicine 17th/277; Clinical Laboratory Medicine by Mc Clatchey 2nd/382; Harrison 18th/p 346*

Association of decreased urinary osmolality with decreased plasma osmolality along with reduced serum sodium suggests the diagnosis of Primary Polydipsia.

Laboratory differentiation of polyyuria

Laboratory parameters	Psychogenic Polydipsia	Diabetes insipidus	Nephrogenic diabetes insipidus	Osmotic Diuresis
Serum Na	N or ↓	↑	↑	N or ↑
Posm	N, ↓	↑	↑	N, ↑
Uosm	↓	↓	↓	↑
Plasma ADH	↓	↓	↑	↑
Uosm after ADH	Increase	Increase	Nil	Slight increase

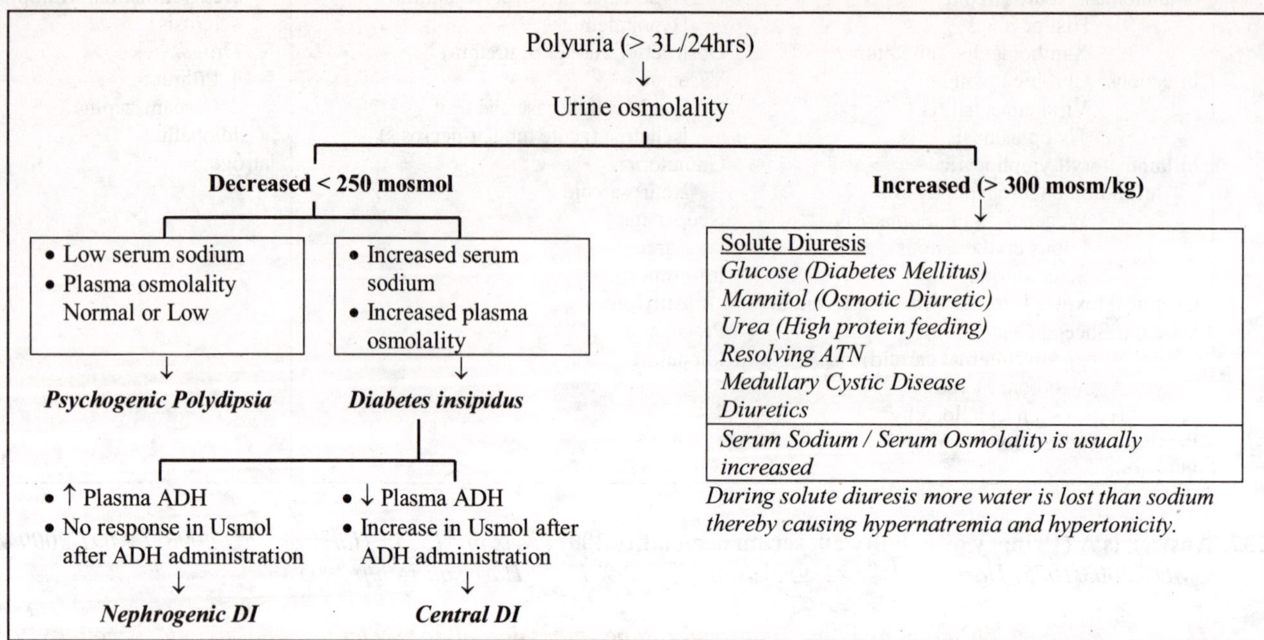

139. Answer is C (Renal Hyposensitivity to ADH): *Ref text below*

Failure of urine osmolality to rise even after administration of exogenous ADH/vasopressin suggests a diagnosis of Nephrogenic Diabetes Insipidus due resistance to action of vasopressin on the Renal tubule (Renal Hyposensitivity to ADH).

Feature	*Psychogenic Polydipsia*	*Central Diabetes Insipidus (ADH Deficiency)*	*Nephrogenic Diabetes Insipidus (Renal Hyposensitivity to ADH)*
Urinary osmolality after administration of ADH/vasopressin	*Increases*	*Increases*	*Nil (Urinary osmolality fails to rise even after exogenous ADH/ vasopression)*

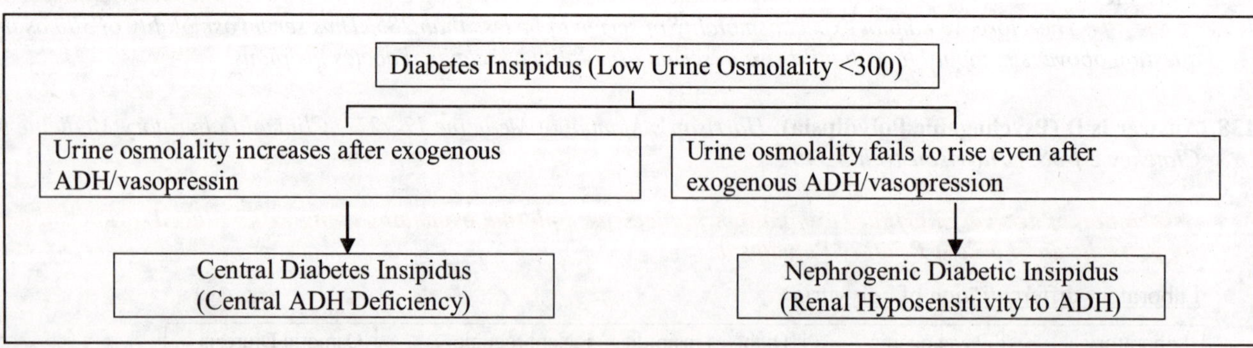

140. Answer is A (Renal tubule is unresponsive to ADH): *Refer text below*

Nephrogenic Diabetes Insipidus is charachterized by resistance of action of ADH on Renal tubules or unresponsiveness of renal tubules to the action of ADH or Renal Hyposensitivity to action of ADH.

Serum sodium is typically high (increased), urine osmolality is low and fails to increase after exogenous administration of ADH /vasopression.

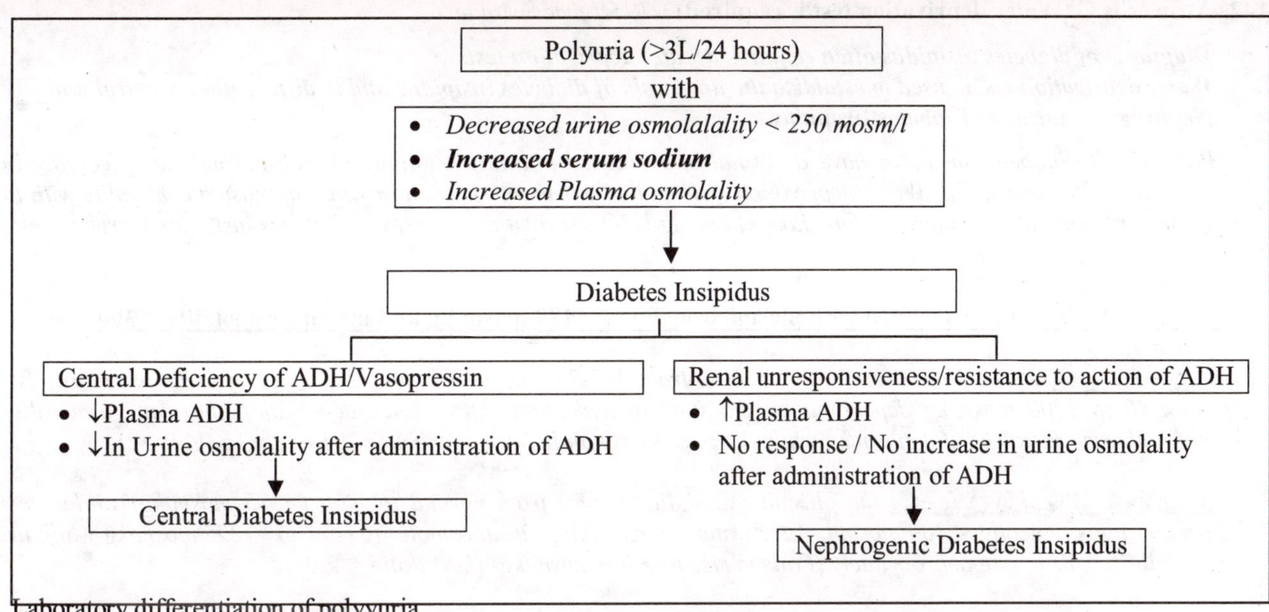

Laboratory differentiation of polyyuria

Laboratory parameters	Psychogenic Polydipsia	Diabetes insipidus	Nephrogenic diabetes insipidus	Osmotic Diuresis
Serum Na	N or ↓	↑	↑	N or ↑
Posm	N, ↓	↑	↑	N, ↑
Uosm	↓	↓	↓	↑
Plasma ADH	↓	↓	↑	↑
Uosm after ADH	Increase	Increase	Nil	Slight increase

141. Answer is D (Psychogenic polydipsia) :; *Harrison 16th/251, 255, 2098, 2099; Harrison 17th/ 2219; Harrison 18th/p 2904*

All of the options provided may present with polyuria & polydipsia but only Psychogenic polydipsia presents with associated decreased serum and urine osmolality.

Laboratory diagnostic parameters amongst conditions provided.

Diabetes insipidus (Nephrogenic / central)	*Resolving ATN (Diuretic phase of renal failure)*	*Psychogenic polydypsia*
• Serum osmolarity (N or ↑) • Urinary osmolarity ↓	• Serum osmolarity ↑ed (↑ed serum Na^+) • Urinary osmolarity ↓ed	Serum osmolarity ↓ed Urine osmolarity ↓ed

Laboratory parameters for patient in question

Parameter	Normal value	Patient in question	Inference
Serum Sodium (Na)	136-145 meq/L	130 meq/l	Decreased
Serum potassium (K)	3.5-5.0 meq/L	3.5 meq/l	Normal
Serum Osmolality	285-295 mmol/kg	208 mosm/kg	**Decreased**
Urine Osmolality	350-1000 mosmol/kg	45 mosm/L	**Decreased.**

Thus the only viable answer amongst the options that satisfies decreased serum and urine osmolality is psychogenic polydypsia.

Psychogenic polydipsia: *Kumar & Clarke 5th/ 1058*

- Psychiatric disturbance characterized by excessive intake of water
- Plasma sodium and osmolality fall and urine produced is appropriately dilute
- Vasopressin levels become almost undetectable
- Characteristically the diagnosis is made by a water deprivation test. The initially low urine molarity gradually increases with the duration of water deprivation.

142. Answer is C (Water deprivation test is required) : *References with text*

Diagnosis of diabetes insipidus often requires a water deprivation test.
Water deprivation test is used to establish the diagnosis of diabetes insipidus and to differentiate Central and Nephrogenic forms of Diabetes Insipidus.

Patients with diabetes insipidus have a normal or increased plasma osmolality (> 280 mosm/l) and decreased urine osmolality (<300mosm/l). 'Water deprivation test' typically demonstrates an increase in plasma osmolality with failure of urinary osmolality to increase (no change) during H2O deprivation in cases of diabetes insipidus thereby suggesting the diagnosis.

8

Diabetes Insipidus is associated with plasma osmolality > 280 mosm/kg and urinary osmolality < 300 mosm /kg

In normal subjects the plasma osmolality ranges from 275-295 mosm /kg while the range of urine osmolality is wide, from 40 to 1000 mosm/kg depending on the state of hydration. After water deprivation the urine osmolality will normally rise to exceed 800 mosm/kg while the plasma osmolality remains below 295 mosm/kg (U/P >2)

In Diabetes Insipidus subjects *the plasma osmolality ranges from normal to high (>275 mosm/kg) while the urine osmolality is typically < 300 mosm/l. After water deprivation plasma osmolality rises to > 295 mosm/kg while urinary osmolality fails to rise appropriately (Fails to rise to >300 mosm/kg) (U/P Ratio < 2.0)*

Endocrinology

Water deprivation test is often required to establish a diagnosis of Diabetes insipidus

Water deprivation test is indicated in patients with hypotonic polyuria (Uosm < 300 mosm/kg) and a plasma osmolality within the normal range (Posm = 275 – 295 mosm/kg) to establish the diagnosis of diabetes insipidus and differentiate central & nephrogenic forms.

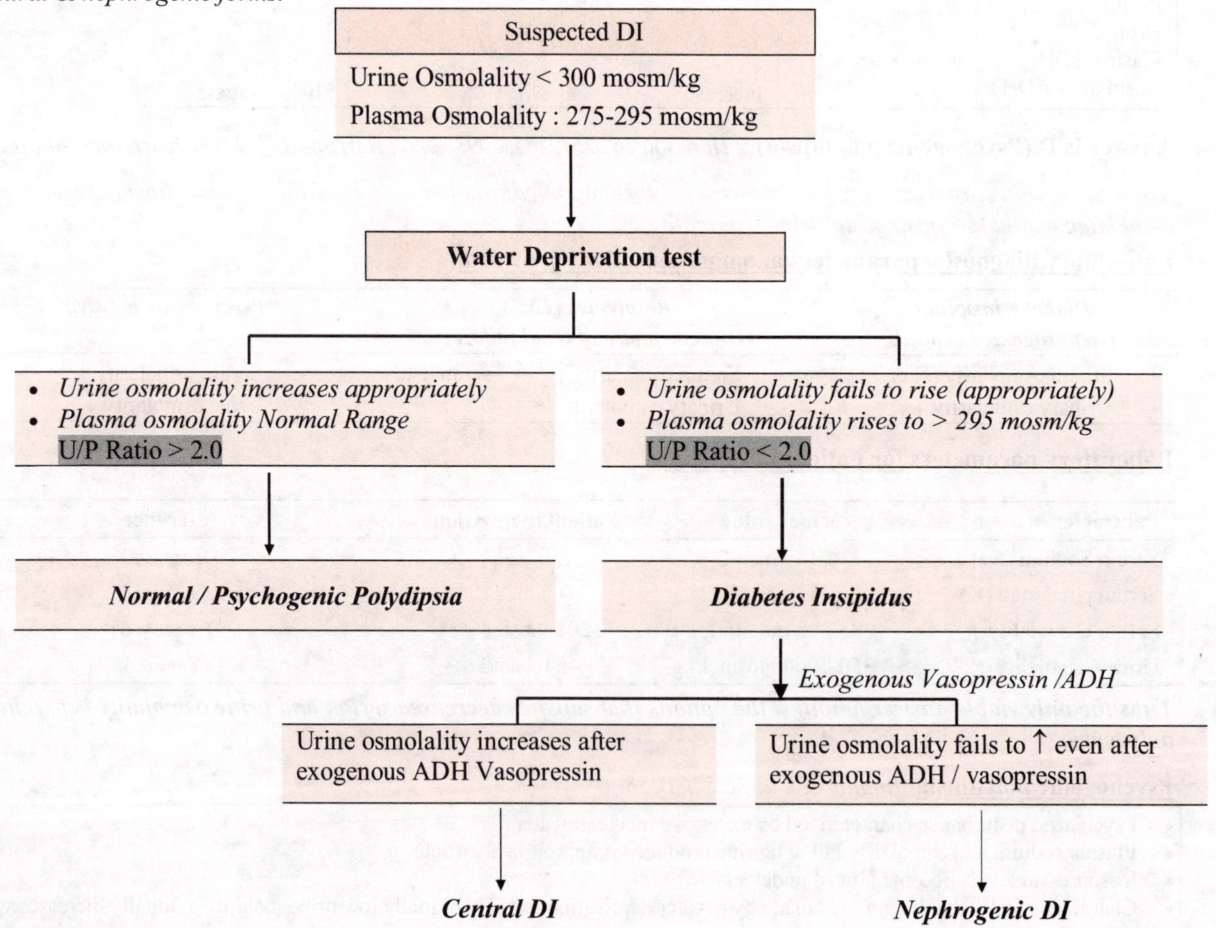

Water Deprivation Test should be performed when plasma osmolality is < 300 mosm/kg

- Water Deprivation Test is indicated in patients with hypotonic polyuria *(urine osmolality < 300 mosm /kg) and a plasma osmolality within the normal range (Plasma osmolality = 275 -295 mosm/kg)* to decide whether hypotonic polyuria is caused by Primary Polydipsia or Diabetes Insipidus

– 'Washington manual of Endocrinology' 2nd/22

- Low serum osmolality (< 270 mosm/kg) in a patient with hypotonic polyuria (Uosm < 300 mosm/kg) suggests a diagnosis of Psychogenic polydipsia and *water deprivation test is not always required*
- High serum osmolality (> 300 mosm/kg) in a patient with hypotonic polyuria (Uosm < 300 mosm /kg) suggests a diagnosis of Diabetes Insipidus and *water deprivation test in not always required*

'Water deprivation test should be performed when the plasma osmolality is < 300 mosm/kg'

– Partha's Fundamentals of Pediatrics 1st/504

'If initial serum osmolality is < 300 mosm/kg patient should undergo a water deprivation test to establish the diagnosis of Diabetes Insipidus and to defferentiatic central & Nephrogenic forms'

– Pediatric Endocrine Disorders 1st (2007) /295

Laboratory Studies in Cases of Polyuria: Diabetic Insipidus (DI) versus Primary Polydipsia:			
	Central DI	**Nephrogenic DI**	**Primary Polydipsia**
Plasma osmolality	*Increased or normal*	*Increased or normal*	*Decreased or normal*
Urine osmolality	*Decreased*	*Decreased*	*Decreased*
Urine osmolality during H_2O deprivation	*No change*	*No change*	*Increased*
Urine osmolality after dDAVP	*Increased*	*No change*	*Increased*
Plasma ADH	*Low*	*Normal to high*	*Low*

dDAVP= D-desaminoarginine vasopressin; ADH = antidiuretic hormone

143. Answer is A (High output due to diuretics): *Refer previous question*

Presence of high urine osmolality >300 (316 mosmol/Kg) along with increased serum Na suggest a diagnosis of solute diuresis.

The patient inquestion has sustained head injury and mannitol is often used insuch cases to reduce the intracranial pressure. Solute diuresis secondary to use of mannitol (diuretic) explains the parameters of the patient in question.

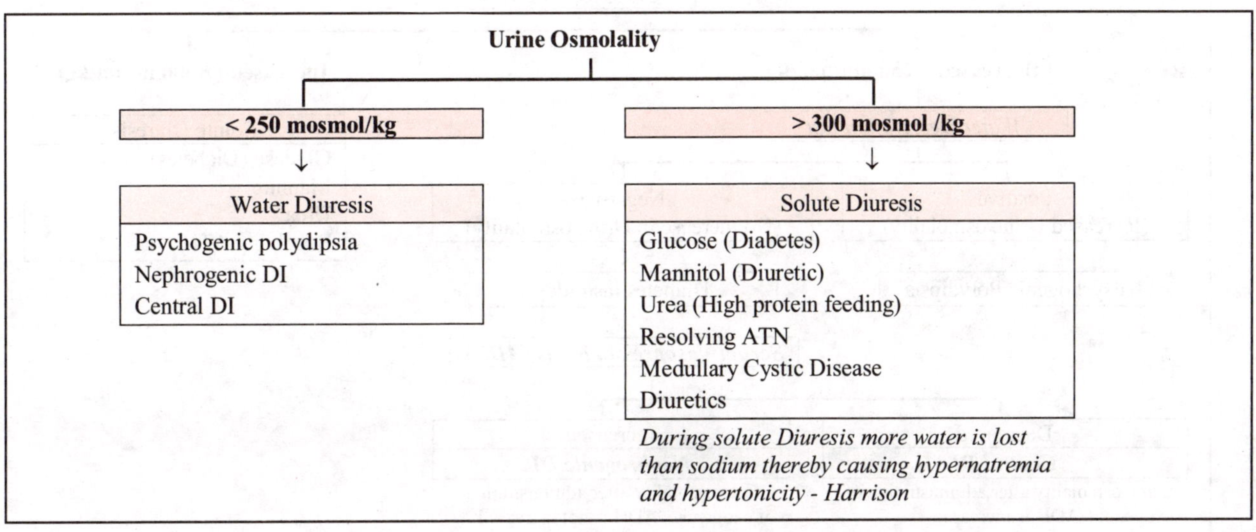

144. Answer is D (Metabolic Acidosis): *Harrisons 17th/2260; Manual of Endocrinology & Metabolism 4th/150*

Primary hyperaldosteronism is associated with metabolic alkalosis and not metabolic acidosis.

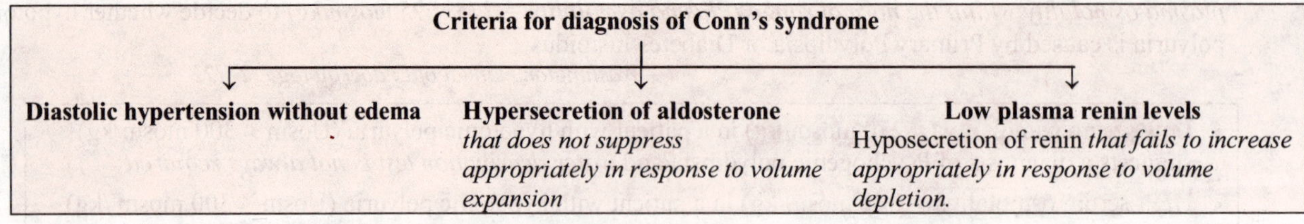

Classic Triad of Biochemical Criteria for diagnosis of Primary Hyperaldoteronism
• *Hypokalemia with inappropriate kaliuresis (Metabolic alkalosis)* • *Suppressed plasma renin activity* • *Elevated Aldosterone levels* that do not fall appropriately in response to volume expansion or sodium load

Taken from Manual of Endocrinology & Metabolism 4th/150

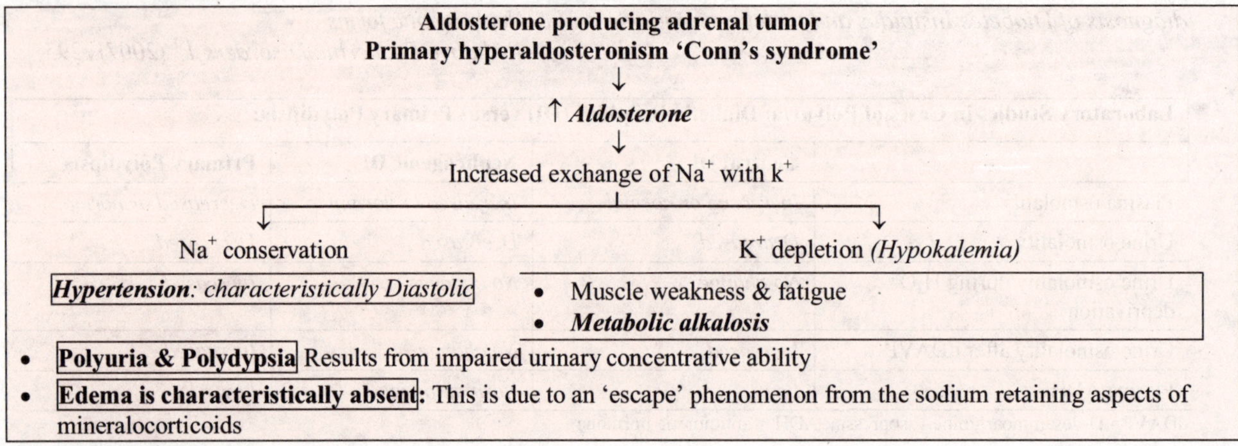

145. Answer is A and C (Water Deprivation test and Plasma and Urine Osmolality): *Harrisons 17th/274; 18th/p 340*

The important investigations in a patient with polyuria include estimation of urine osmolality, water deprivation test and plasma vasopressin (ADH) levels.

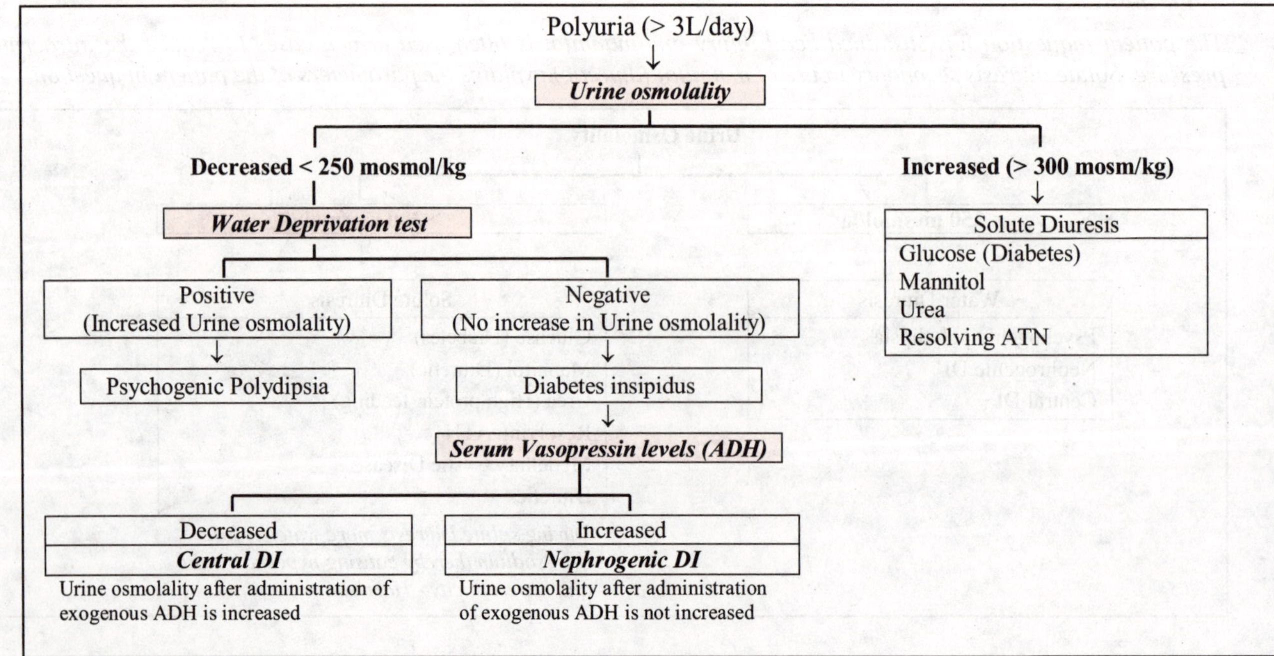

146. Answer is B (Thiazide / Amiloride diuretics and salt restriction): *Conn's Current Therapy (Elsevier)2012/693; Harrison's 18th/2964*

The treatment of Nephrogenic Diabetes Insipidus is usually achieved through a combination of thiazide / amiloride diureties and dietary salt restriction. A prostaglandin synthesis inhibitor (indomethacin) may be added.

- *Thiazide diuretics and salt restriction can reduce urinary output by inducing a state of mild volume contraction thereby promoting increased proximal reabsorption of isotonic fluid and inhibiting the delivery of free water to the collecting duct. A combination of thiazide – amiloride formulation will avoid thiazide induced hypokalemia. Addition of Indomethacin may further reduce urinary output by inhibiting prostaglanding synthesis-Harrison*
- *'Thiazide diuretics in combination with amiloride and indomethacin are the most useful pharmacological agents in the treatment of Nephrogenic diabetes insipidus'- Pediatric Endocrinology (CDC Press) 2007/668*

__Desmopressin__ is usually ineffective in Congenital Nephrogenic Diabetes Insipidus. If renal resistance is partial, it may be overcome by ten fold higher doses of desmopressin but this treatment is too expensive and inconvenient to be useful chronically.

147. Answer is A (Desmopressin): *Harrison's 18th/2906*

Desmopressin is the drug of choice for Central / Neurogenic diabetes insipidus.

Disorders of Calcium Metabolism

Hyperparathyroidism

148. Answer is C (Parathyroid Adenoma): *Refer previous question*

The most common cause of primary hyperparathyroidism is a single / solitary parathyroid adenoma.

149. Answer is A (Solitary adenoma) :; *Harrison 16th/2252; Harrison 17th/ 2380; Harrison 18th/p 3099*

The most common cause of primary hyperparathyroidism is a Solitary Parathyroid Adenoma Q
Adenomas are most commonly located in the *inferior parathyroid gland.* Q

150. Answer is B (Solitary adenoma of parathyroid): *Harrison 16th/2252; Harrison 17th/ 2380; Harrison 18th/p 3099*

Most common cause of primary hyperparathyroidism is parathyroid adenoma.

151. Answer is B (Solitary parathyroid adenoma) : *Harrison 16th/2252; Harrison 17th/ 2380; Harrison 18th/p 3099*

The most common cause of primary hyperparathyroidism is a parathyroid adenoma.
A single/solitary abnormal gland is the cause in approximately 80% of patients - Harrison
The abnormality of the gland is ***usually a benign neoplasm or 'adenoma'*** and rarely a parathyroid carcinoma.

152. Answer is B (Primary Hyperparathyroidism) : *Harrison 16th/2257; Harrison 17th/ 2380; Harrison 18th/p 3099*
The most likely cause of asymptomatic hypercalcemia in a patient aged 30 years is primary hyperparathyroidism. Familial hypocalciuric hypercalcemia, is most often detected in the first ten years of life when hypercalcemia due to primary hyperparathyroidism is a rarity.

Both primary hyperthyroidism and familial hypocalciuric hypercalcemia may present with asymptomatic hypercalcemia.

The 'catch' in the above question lies in the 'age' of the patient

Primary hyperparathyroidism	Familial hypocalciuric hypercalcemia (F.H.H.) *(autosomal dominant)*
• The most common presentation in patients with primary hyperparathyroidism is ***'asymptomatic' hypercalcemia***	• Affected individuals are discovered because of ***asymptomatic hypercalcemia***
• Commonly presents in ***third to fifth decade***	• Commonly presents in the ***first decade***

153. Answer is A (Commonly occurs after thyroidectomy): *Harrison's 17th/2380; 16th/2252; Harrison 18th/p 3099*

Thyroidectomy may lead to hypoparathyroidism and not hyperparathyroidism due to inadvertent removal of the parathyroid glands.

154. Answer is D (Asymptomatic hypercalcemia) :*Harrison; 16th/2252; API Medicine 6th/1100; Harrison 17th/ 2382; 18th/ 3102*

There is a great variation in the manifestation of hyperparathyroidism

Manifestation may be with multiple signs and symptoms	'Manifestation may be subtle and the disease many have a benign course with no symptoms and signs other than **hypercalcemia** and elevated level of PTH'
• Recurrent nephrolithiasis [Q] • Peptic ulceration [Q] (abdominal pain) • Extensive bone resorption • Mental changes; Psychiatric manifestations.	

In view of the above facts from Harrison the best option to consider a 'subtle presentation' should probably be 'asymptomatic hypercalcemia'

155. Answer is C (Chronic renal failure): *Chandrasoma Taylor 3rd/ 858-865; Harrison 17th/ 2388; Harrison 18th/p 3109*

Conditions leading to decrease in serum calcium levels cause a compensatory increase in secretion of PTH resulting in secondary hyperparathyroidism. Amongst the options provided chronic renal failure is one such cause of secondary hyperparathyroidism

Causes of hyperparathyroidism can be grouped into three categories

Primary hyperparathyroidism	Secondary hyperparathyroidism	Ectopic parathyroid hormone syndrome
• Elevated PTH due to increased PTH secretion from an intrinsic abnormality of one or more parathyroid glands • This is most commonly due to solitary adenoma involving one gland	• Excessive secretion of PTH by parathyroids secondary to a lowered serum ionized calcium • This is a compensatory hyperplasia of all four glands aimed at correcting lowered serum calcium	• Ectopic PTH syndrome results from the production by several malignant neoplasms of PTH related peptide
• **Causes**	• **Causes**	• **Causes**
1. Single adenoma (80-90%) 2. Multiple adenoma (1-4%) 3. Diffuse hyperplasia (3-15%) 4. Carcinoma (1-2%)	1. Chronic renal failure 2. Malabsorption syndrome 3. Vitamin D deficiency 4. Medullary carcinoma thyroid	• Squamous cell Ca of lung • Adenocarcinoma of kidney. • Others

In most cases, serum calcium levels are corrected towards normal as a result of compensatory increase in serum PTH levels. Serum calcium levels thus may be low or normal but are not elevated.

Condition	Serum Ca^{++}	Serum Phosphate	Serum PTH	Alk. Phosphate
Secondary hyperparathyroidism	N or ↓ (Rarely ↑)	N (↓↑)	↑	N (↑)
Primary hyperparathyroidism (solitary adenoma)	↑	↓	↑	↑

156. Answer is C (Osteoporosis): *Harrison's 17th/287; Harrison 18th/p 362*

Osteoporosis is neither associated with hypocalcaemia nor with secondary Hyperparathyroidism

	Serum Ca	Serum phosphorus	Alkaline phosphatase	PTH
• Osteomalacia (Rickets) (↓Vit. D)	↓	↓	↑	↑
• Primary hyperparathyroidism bone disease	↑	↓	↑	↑
• Bone disease in renal failure with secondary hyperparathyroidism	N/↓	↑	↑	↑
• Lytic bone neoplasms	N/↑	N/↑	N/↑	N
• ***Osteoporosis***	***N***	***N***	***N***	***N***
• Paget's disease	N	N	↑	N

High Parathyroid Hormone Levels (Secondary Hyperparathyroidism)

Vitamin D deficiency or impaired 1, $25(OH)_2D$ production /action

- ***Nutritional vitamin D deficiency (Rickets/Osteomalacia)***
- ***Renal insufficiency with impaired 1, 25(OH)2D production***
- *Vitamin D resistance, including receptor defects*

Parathyroid hormone resistance syndromes

- *PTH receptor mutations*
- *Pseudohypoparathyroidism (G protein mutatins)*

Drugs

- *Calcium chelators*
- *Inhibitors of bone resorption (bisphosphonates, plicamycin)*
- *Altered vitamin D metabolism (phenytoin, ketoconazole)*

Miscellaneous causes

- *Acute pancreatitis*
- *Acute rhabdomyolysis*
- *Hungry bone syndrome after parathyroidectomy*
- *Osteoblastic metastases with marked stimulation of bone formation (prostate cancer)*

157. Answer is B (Parathyroid adenoma): *Chandrasoma Taylar 3rd/858-865*

Parathyroid Adenomas are associated with Primary Hyperparathyroidism and not Secondary Hyperparathyroidism.

Hyperparathyroidism

Primary Hyperparathyroidism

- Elevated PTH due to increased PTH secretion from an intrinsic abnormality of one or more parathyroid glands
- This is most commonly due to solitary adenoma involving one gland
- **Causes**

  5. *Single adenoma (80-90%)*
  6. *Multiple adenoma (1-4%)*
  7. *Diffuse hyperplasia (3-15%)*
  8. *Carcinoma (1-2%)*

Secondary Hyperparathyroidism

- Excessive secretion of PTH by parathyroids secondary to a lowered serum ionized calcium
- This is a compensatory hyperplasia of all four glands aimed at correcting lowered serum calcium
- **Causes**

  5. *Chronic renal failure*
  6. *Malabsorption syndrome*
  7. *Vitamin D deficiency*
  8. *Medullary carcinoma thyroid*

Medullary carcinoma of Thyroid is derived from parafollicular cells of ultimobrachial organs and secretes calcitonin. Calcitonin is known to cause hypocalcemia which can lead to Secondary Hyperparathyroidism (Medullary carcinoma Thyroid in association with MEN II syndrome may also be associated with Primary Hyperparathyroidism from associated primary parathyroid Hyperplasia).

158. Answer is B (Secondary hyperparathyroidism): *CMDT 2001/1126, 1127; CMDT 2009/1009; Harrison 15th/1985 fig 320-6; Harrison 17th/ 2388; Harrison 18th/p 3109*

Rugger jersey spine results from osteosclerosis, which occurs in the setting of secondary hyperparathyroidism in chronic renal failure.

In chronic renal failure, hyperphosphatemia and decreased renal production of active vit. D, initially produce a decrease in ionized calcium. This stimulates the parathyroid glands causing secondary hyperparathyroidism.
The bone disease resulting in this setting is known as *Renal Osteodystrophy*. Patients with renal osteodystrophy may have ectopic calcifications around joints or in soft tissues. They may exhibit X-Ray changes of osteopenia, osteitis fibrosa, or **osteosclerosis**; alone or in combination.

Osteosclerosis of vertebral bodies is known as "Rugger jersey spine".

159. Answer is B (Secondary Hyperparathyroidism): *Essential Radiology 2nd/373, 374; Rubin's Pathology 5th/1116*

Rugger Jersey Spine is characteristically found in secondary hyperparathyroidism (Renal osteodystrophy in CRF).

160. Answer is C (CRF): *Essential Radiology 2nd/373, 374*

The Rugger Jersey spine refers to band like osteosclerosis of the superior and inferior margin of the vertical body. Rugger Jersey Spine is characteristically seen in chronic renal failure due to secondary hyperparathyroidism or Renal osteodystrophy.

161. Answer is A (Osteopetrosis): *Harrison 17th/2382, 2393; Harrison 18th/p 3102, 3103*

Hyperparathyroidism is associated with osteoporosis and not with osteopetrosis.

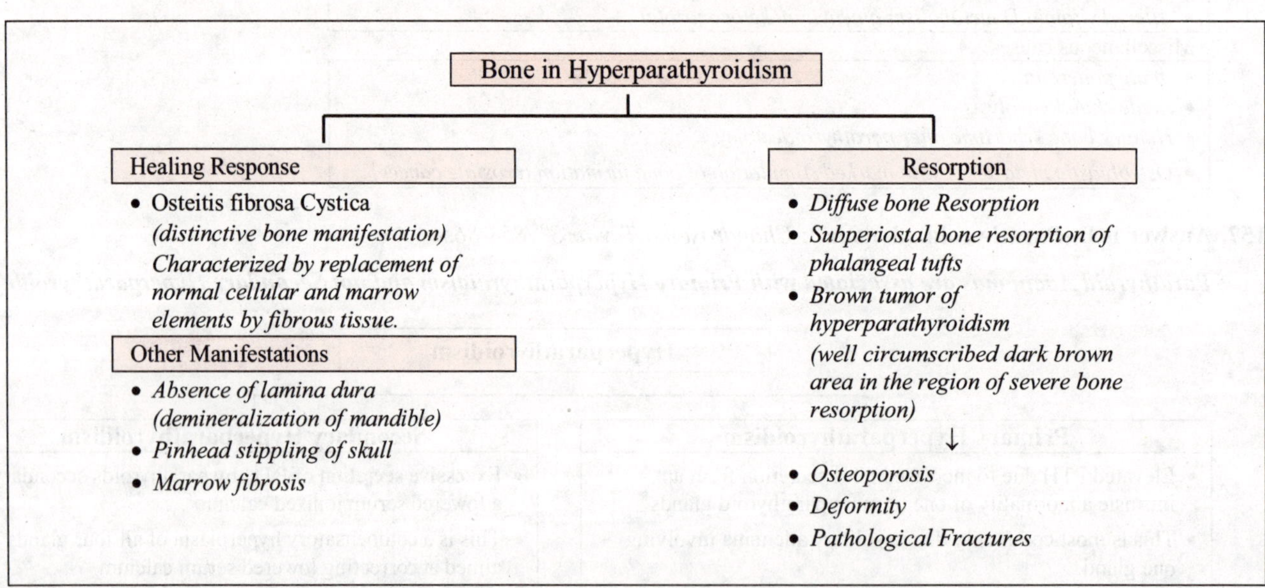

162. Answer is B (Hyperparathyroidism) : *Harrison 17th/ 2382-2383; Harrison 18th/p 3102, 3103*

163. Answer is C (Decrease in serum calcitonin) : *Read text below ; Harrison 17th/ 2382-2383; Chandrasoma Taylor 3rd/859; Harrison 18th/p 3102, 3103*

Serum calcitonin is no marker for hyperparathyroidism. *It antagonizes the actions of parathyroid hormone and may be used as a modality of treatment of hypercalcemia secondary to hyperparathyroidism.*

Markers of hyperparathyroidism (↑ed PTH):

1. **Increased serum calcium:**
   - Stimulates Vit D which causes increased absorption of Ca^{++} from gut
   - Increased calcium reabsorption from tubules
   - Increases osteoblastic activity in bones and mobilizes calcium from bone into serum.
2. **Decreased serum phosphorus:**
   - PTH acts on tubules to increase excretion of phosphorus.
3. **Increased 24 hr urine calcium:**
   - Despite increased reabsorption of Ca^{++} in renal tubules urinary calcium is increased owing to increased filtration of calcium in glomerular filtrate.
4. **Increased Alkaline phosphatase:**
   - Increased resorption of bone leads to compensatory elevation of osteoblastic activity
5. **Radiological changes:**
   - Subperiosteal resorption of phalanges is characteristic (hand X Rays are always advised)
   - Bone resorption i.e. osteitis fibrosa et cystica (brown tumours)
   - 'Salt pepper' or 'pepper pot skull' appearance
   - Loss of lamina dura

8

164. Answer is B (Hypoparathyroidism): *Harrisons 17th/2391; Other References*

Low calcium and high phosphate is seen in Hypoparathyroidism.

Condition	*PTH*	*Calcium*	*Phosphate*	*25 OHD*	*1'25 (OH)$_2$ D3 (Active Vit D3)*	*PTH Infusion Response*	*Albrights Osteodystrophy*
Hypoparathyroidism	*Low*	*Low*	*High*	*Normal*	*Low*	*Normal*	*No*

Albrights Osteodystrophy seen in Pseudo-hypoparthyroidism

Hypoparathyroidism *(Low calcium, High phosphate, Low 1, 25 Dihydroxycholecalciferol).*

- Hypoparathyroidism is a disorder of mineral metabolism caused by diminished secretion of PTH from the parathyroid glands.
- *Hypocalcemia* results from *decreased mobilization* of calcium from bone, and *reduced renal reabsorption* of calcium (Direct effect) In addition, PTH deficiency results in impairment of renal 25 (OH) D-1-hydroxylase activity which limits serum calcitriol concentration and thereby *diminishes gastrointestinal calcium absorption* (Indirect effect)
- *Hyperphosphatemia* results from *increased phosphate reabsorption* from the kidneys (PTH normally, acts on the kidneys to reduce phosphate reabsorption)
- Reduced 1, 25 Dihydroxycholecalciferol (Active Vitamin D) is seen as PTH is involved in the activation of 25 Hydroxy-cholecalciferol to 1, 25 Dihydroxy-cholecalciferol in the kidney.

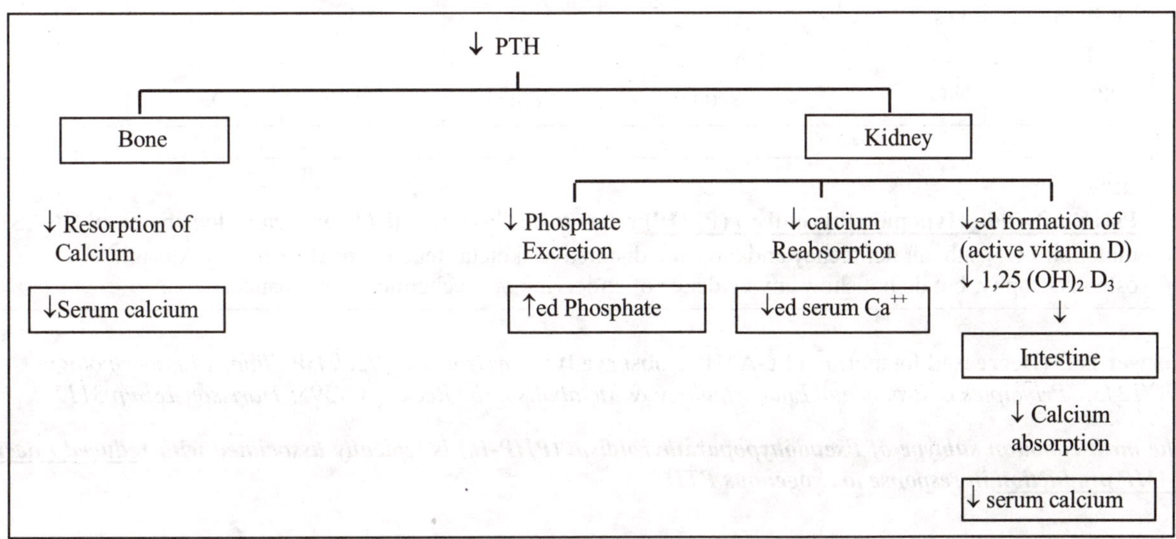

Endocrinology

165. Answer is A (↓ Serum PTH): *Harrison's 17th/-2394; Harrison 18th/p 3117*

Pseudohypoparathyroidism is associated with increased serum PTH levels.

Pseudohypoparathyroidism

- This is a hereditary disorder associated with ***signs and symptoms of hypoparathyroidism despite an elevated PTH*** level *(Hence called pseudohypoparathyroidsm)*
- This is produced as a result of deficient end organ response to PTH
- The most common form of Pseudo hypoparathyroidism (PHP-1a) occurs in association with Albrights Hereditary Osteodystrophy and presents with distinctive skeletal and developmental defects

Laboratory Features	Distinctive skeletal & Development defects (Hereditary Albright's Osteodystrophy (AHO))
• *↑ PTH* • *Hypocalcemia* } *features of hypoparathyroidism* • *Hyperphosphatemia* } • *Normal/Decreased response of urinary CAMP to PTH*	• *Short stature* • *Round face* • ***Brachydactyly*** *(short 4th/5th metacarpals and metacarpals)* • *Heterotopic calcification* • *Exostosis and Radius curves* • *Impairment in olfaction & taste*

Classification of Pseudo-hypoparathyroidism and Pseudo-pseudo-hypoparathyroidsm *(Harrison)*

- Various diverse forms of Pseudohypoparathyroidism (PHP) are recognized based upon certain charachteristics like urinary cyclic AMP response to exogenous PTH, presence or absence of Albright's Hereditary Osteodystrophy (AHO) and assays of concentration of the $G_{5\alpha}$ subunit of the adenylate cyclase enzyme.

Type	Hypocalcemia, hyperphosphatemia	Response of Urinary cAMP to PTH	Serum PTH	Gsα Subunit Deficiency	AHO	Resistance to Hormones in Addition to PTH
PHP-Ia	Yes	↓	↑	Yes	Yes	Yes
PHP-Ib	Yes	↓	↑	No	No	No
PHP-II	Yes	Normal	↑	No	No	No
PPHP	No	Normal	Normal	Yes	Yes	±

Note

Pseudo Pseudo Hypoparathyroidism (PPHP) refers to a subset of patients who carry the abnormal GNAS1 mutation / $G_{S\alpha}$ subunit deficiency and have the distinctive skeletal features of Herediatary Albright's osteodystrophy, but do not show any evidence of endocrine or biochemical disturbance.

166. Answer is D (Decreased formation of c-AMP is observed) : *Harrison's 17th/2394; William's Endocrinology 11th/1243; 'Principles & Practice of Endocrinology & Metabolism' by Becker 3rd/595; Harrison 18th/p 3117*

The most common subtype of Pseudohypoparathyroidism (PHP-Ia) is typically associated with reduced / decreased cAMP production in response to exogenous PTH

Pseudohypoparathyroidism is associated with decreased formation of cyclic AMP and not decreased cyclic GMP or Inositol Triphosphate

- The Gs family of G-proteins use the activation of adenylate cyclase as the next step in signal transduction, to produce cyclic AMP
- Pseudohypoparathyroidism(Ia) is associated with '***loss of function***' mutation of Gs_{α} subunit, and hence results in decreased formation of cyclic AMP

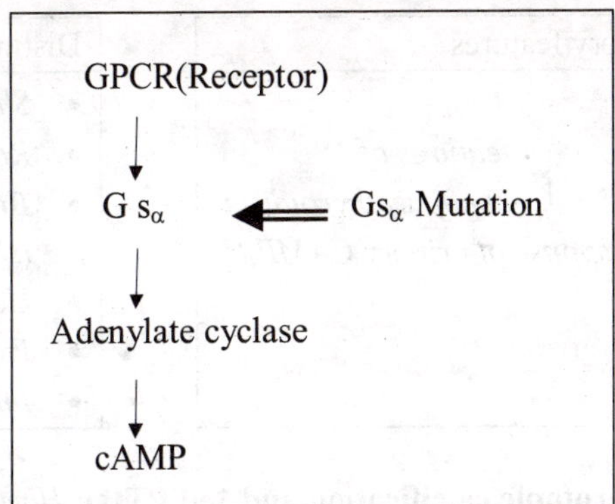

Pseudohypoparathyroidism is associated with reduced urinary c-AMP response to PTH

The term '*Pseudohypoparathyroidism*' describes a heterogeneous syndrome characterized by *biochemical Hypoparathyroidism (Hypocalcemia & Hyperphosphatemia) with paradoxical increased plasma levels of PTH.* This is caused by peripheral unresponsiveness to the biological action of PTH or PTH resistance.

Although several subtypes of *Pseudohypoparathyroidism* are identified, the most common subtype of PHP (PHP Ia) is characterized by *deficient urinary cyclic AMP response to administration of exogenous PTH.* Failure of cAMP production in these patients after PTH infusion is believed to result from a defect in cyclic AMP mediated signal transduction from a Gs_{α} Loss of function' mutation as depicted in the figure (previous heading)

'The measurement of cyclic AMP in urine following an infusion of synthetic PTH is now used to establish a diagnosis of PTH resistance' - William's Endocrinology 11th/1243

Pseudohypoparathyroidism is associated with a 'loss of function' inherited G s_{α} mutation.

Endocrine diseases can result from either 'loss' or 'gain' of gene function (acquired or inherited)

Pseudohypoparathyroidism(Ia) results from an inherited 'loss of function' mutation of the Gs_{α} subunit

Gs_{α} activating mutation ('Gain of function')	Gs_{α} inactivating mutation ('Loss of function')
• *Acromegaly* • *Pituitary corticotroph Adenoma* • *Mc.Cune Albright syndrome* • *Hyperfunctioning Thyroid Adenomas* • *Endocrine ovarian neoplasms*	• *Pseudohypoparathyroidism(Ia)*

Taken from 'Principles & practice of Endocrinology and Metabolism' by Becher 3rd/595

167. Answer is A (Pseudohypoparathyroidism): *Harrison 17th/2394, 2395; Harrison 18th/p 3117, 3118*

The presence of hyperphosphatemia (↑Serum phosphate) along with characteristic brachydactyly suggests the diagnosis of pseudohypoparathyroidism.

Cataract may be seen as a result of hypoparathyroidism.

Pseudohypoparathyroidism

- This is a hereditary disorder associated with symptoms and signs of hypoparathyroidism despite an elevated PTH level (pseudohypoparathyroidism)
- This is produced as a result of deficient end organ response to PTH.

Pseudohypoparathyroidism

Laboratory features	Distinctive skeletal & developmental defects
• *↑PTH* • *Hypocalcemia* } *features of* • *Hyperphosphatemia* } *hypoparathyroidism* • *Normal/Decreased response of urinary CAMP to PTH*	• *Short stature* • *Round face* • ***Brachydactyly*** *(short 4th/5th metacarpals and metacarpals)* • *Heterotopic calcification* • *Exostosis and Radius curves* • *Impairment in olfaction & taste*

168. Answer is A and D (Heterotopic calcification and ↑ed PTH): *Harrison 17th/2394; Harrison 18th/p 3117*

Pseudohypoparathyroidism is associated with elevated PTH and signs of ineffective PTH action i.e. ↓ Serum Ca^{++} and ↑ed serum PO_4^-.

The response of urinary cAMP to PTH is decreased/normal and Heterotopic ossification may be characteristically seen.

169. Answer is A (Vitamin D levels): *Multiple References; Harrison's 17th/2391; Chandrasoma Taylor 3rd/965; William's Endocrinology; Harrison 18th/p 3112, 3113*

Vitamin D deficiency is associated with hypophosphatemia and not hyperphosphatemia

Renal failure (↑ serum creatinine), Pseudohypoparathyroidism (↓CAMP response to PTH) and increased urinary myoglobin (crush syndrome; tissue injury) may all be associated with combination of hypocalcemia, hyperphosphatemia and elevated PTH levels

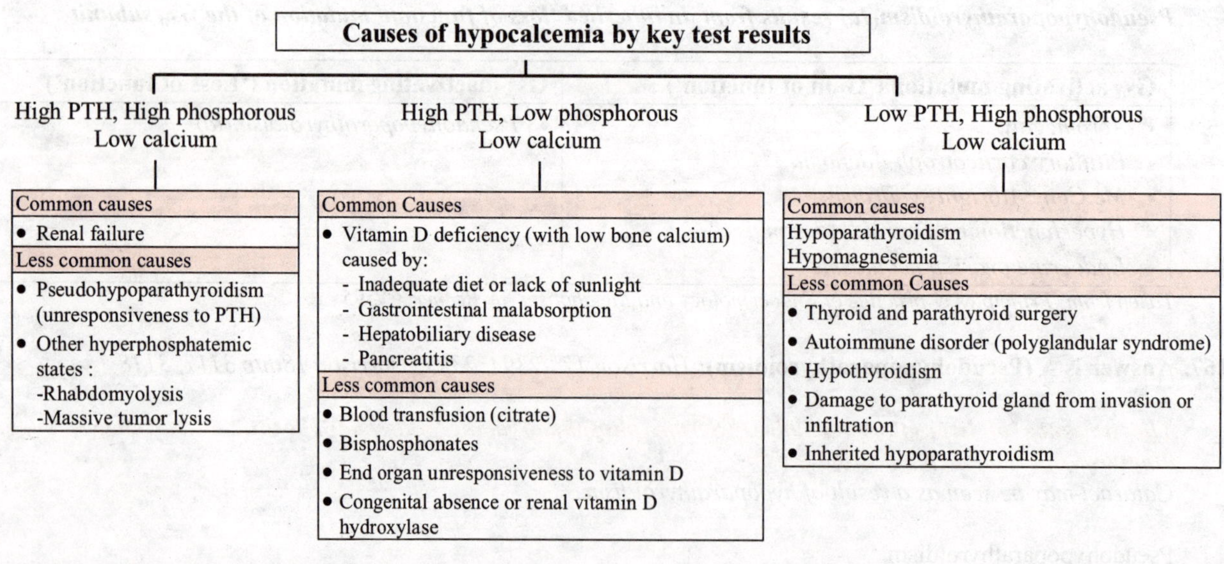

Hypercalcemia and Related Disorders

170. Answer is D (Vitamin A deficiency): *Harrison 16th/ 2252; Harrison 17th/ 2380, 286; Harrison 18th/p 360, 3099*

Hypercalcemia is seen with Vit. A intoxication (not deficiency) due to associated high bone turnover.

Causes of hypercalcemia:

Parathyroid related	Vitamin D related
• *Primary hyperparathyroidism* Q • ***Lithium therapy*** Q • Familial hypercalciuric hypercalcemia	• Vitamin D intoxication • Increased 1, 25 $(OH)_2$ D eg. *Sarcoidosis*Q; other granulomatous ds. • Idiopathic hypercalcemia of infancy
Malignancy related	**Associated high bone turnover**
• Solid tumor with metastasis (Breast) • Solid tumor with paraneoplastic syndromes (Carcinoma Breast/Lung /Kidney etc.) • Hematological malignancies: ***Multiple myeloma***Q / Lymphoma / Leukemia • Pheochoromocytoma (rare) • MEN syndromes	• *Hyperthyroidism*Q • *Immobilization*Q • *Thiazides*Q • ***Vitamin A intoxication***Q • *Paget's disease* **Associated With *Renal Failure*Q** • Severe secondary hyper-parathyroidism • Aluminum intoxication • Milk Alkali syndrome

171. Answer is D (Celiac disease): *Harrison 17th/ 2380, 286; Harrison 18th/p 360, 3099*

Celiac disease is not a cause for hypercalcemia.

Hyperparathyroidism, Sarcoidosis and Milk alkali syndrome, may all lead to hypercalcemia.

172. Answer is A (Acute Pancreatitis) : *; Harrison 16th/2252; Refer previous question; 17th/ 2380, 286; 18th/360, 3099*

Pancreatitis is associated with hypocalcemia.

173. Answer is D (Phenytoin toxicity) : *; Harrison 16th/2252, 17th/ 2380, 286; Harrison 18th/p 360, 3099*

Phenytoin toxicity is associated with hypocalcemia. Phenytoin desensitizes target tissues to vitamin D and produces hypocalcemia (Osteomalacia).

174. Answer is D (Phenytoin toxicity): *Repeat*

Phenytoin toxicity is associated with hypocalcemia.

175. Answer is A (Acute Pancreatitis): *Repeat*

Acute Pancreatitis is associated with hypocalcemia and not hypercalcemia.

176. Answer is A (Acute Pancreatitis): *Repeat*

Acute Pancreatitis is associated with hypocalcemia and not hypercalcemia.

177. Answer is C (Tumourlysis syndrome) : *Harrison; 16th/2252, 581; 17th/ 2380, 286, 1736; Harrison 18th/p 360, 3099*

Tumorlysis syndrome is associated with Hypocalcemia

- *Primary hyperparathyroidism is a cause for hypercalcemia*Q *– Harrison*
- *Multiple myeloma also causes hypercalcemia* Q *– Harrison*
- *Sarcoidosis : Hypercalciuria with or without hypercalcemia* is seenQ *-- Harrison*

Tumor lysis syndrome *:*

It is a clinical entity characterized by destruction of large number of rapidly proliferating neoplastic cells following chemotherapy.

Rapid lysis of tumor cells after chemotherapy **(Tumor Lysis Syndrome)**[Q]

• ***Release of uric acid*** [Q] from rapid turn-over nucleic acids. • Uric acid may precipitate in tubules, medulla and collecting duct • ***Renal failure*** [Q]	• Release of intracellular Phosphate ***- Hyperphosphatemia***[Q] • Increased phosphate drives calcium into bone ***- Hypocalcemia*** [Q] • Calcium phosphate may deposit in renal tubules ***- Renal failure***	• Release of intracellular Potassium ***- Hyperkalemia*** [Q] • Predisposes to ***Arrythmias*** [Q] • ***Acidosis*** [Q] is also a feature and results in part from deranged oxidative metabolism ***-Lactic acidosis***[Q]

178. Answer is B (Tumor Lysis Syndrome): *Repeat*

Tumor Lysis syndrome is associated with hypocalcemia and not hypercalcemia.

179. Answer is D (Acute pancreatitis): *Harrison's 18th/360, 361, 362*

Acute Pancreatitis is a miscellaneous cause for Hypocalcemia (not hypercalcemia).

Note that Hypercalcemia may cause Acute Pancreatitis but Acute Pancreatitis causes hypocalcemia[Q]***.***

Multiple myeloma, Lytic skeletal metastasis and excessive calcium intake from Total Parentral Nutrition are all established causes of Hypercalcemia

Causes of Hypercalcemia:

Excessive PTH production
• Primary hyperparathyroidism (adenoma, hyperplasia, rarely carcinoma) • Tertiary hyperparathyroidism (long-term stimulation of PTH secretion in renal insufficiency) • Ectopic PTH secretion (very rare) • Inactivating mutations in the CaSR (FHH) • Alterations in CaSR function (lithium therapy)
Hypercalcemia of malignancy
• Overproduction of PTHrP (many solid tumors) • ***Lytic skeletal metastases (breast, myeloma)***
Excessive 1,25(OH)2D production
• Granulomatous diseases (sarcoidosis, tuberculosis, silicosis) • Lymphomas • Vitamin D intoxication
Primary increase in bone resorption
• Hyperthyroidism • Immobilization
Excessive calcium intake
• Milk-alkali syndrome • ***Total parenteral nutrition***
Other causes
• Endocrine disorders (adrenal insufficiency, pheochromocytoma, VIPoma) • Medications (thiazides, vitamin A, antiestrogens)

CaSR, calcium sensor receptor; FHH, familial hypocalciuric hypercalcemia; PTH, parathyroid hormone; PTHrP, PTH-related peptide.

180. Answer is D (Furosemide): *Harrison 17th/2380; Harrison 18th/p 3099*

Thiazide diuretics cause hypercalcemia while loop diuretics (furosemide) cause hypocalcemia.

Furosemide is a loop diuretic that is characteristically associated with hypocalcemia and not hypercalcemia.

181. Answer is A and D (Vitamin A and Vitamin D): *Refer previous question*

Hypercalcemia is associated with Vitamin A intoxication due to increased / high bone turnover and Vitamin D intoxication.

182. Answer is A (Carcinoma Breast): *Surgical Oncology 1st (2003)/601; Basic and Clinical Endocrinology 7th/880*

The most common cause of hypercalcemic crisis is malignancy. Hypercalcemic crisis due to primary hyperparathyroidism is rare – Surgical Oncology 1st (2003)/601

Amongst the options provided, carcinoma breast is the single best answer of choice.

Hypercalcemic Crisis

- Hypercalcemic crisis refers to the presence of severe hypercalcemia and is defined arbitrarily as a total calcium > 14mg/dl (> 3.5 mmol/l)
- The most common cause of hypercalcemic crisis is malignancy and the most common cause is believed to be unregulated secretion of PTH related protein (PTHrP)

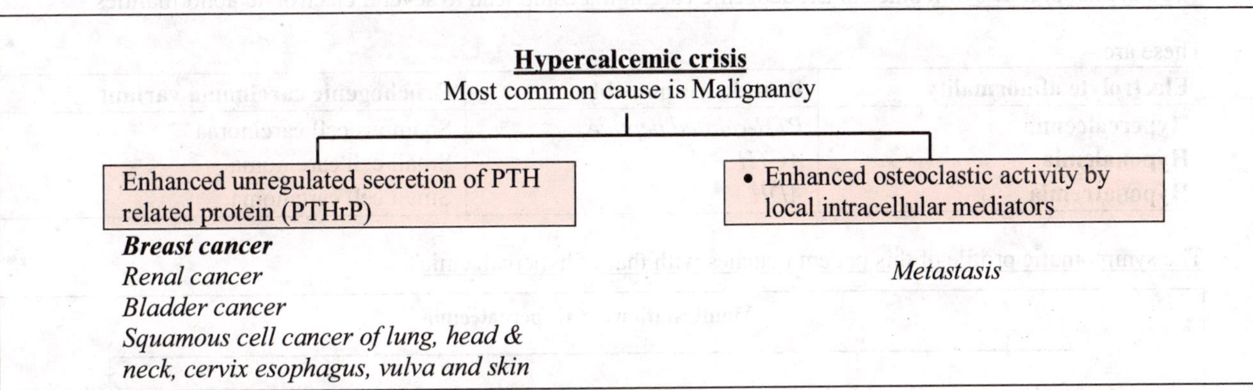

183. Answer is E (All of the above): Harrison 17th/2380; Manual of Nephrology 7th/64, 65; *Harrison 18th/p 3100*

Hypercalcemia may be associated with MEN type I and type II, Hyperparathyroidism and Hyperthyroidism. Pheochromocytoma is also described as a rare cause of hypercalcemia and usually causes hypercalcemia in association with MEN syndrome.

184. Answer is A (Myxoedema): *Refer previous question*

Hypercalcemia is a feature of Hyperthyroidism and not hypothyroidism (Myxoedema)

185. Answer is D (All of the above): *Refer text below*

Hypercalciuria may be associated with Vitamin D intoxication (hypervitaminosis D), Sarcoidosis and hyperparathyroidism.

Causes of Hypercalciuria-associated Nephrolithiasis in Children and Adults

- Idiopathic hypercalciuria
- Increased intestinal calcium absorption
  - ***Granulomatous disease e.g. sarcoidosis***
  - ***Hypervitaminosis D***
  - Milk alkali syndrome
- Increased bone resorption
  - Immobilization e.g. paraplegia and quadriplegia
  - High animal protein diet
  - Systemic acidosis e.g. distal renal tubular acidosis
  - Adrenocorticotrophic hormone or cortisol excess
  - Primary hyperparathyroidism

- Decreased renal calcium reabsorption
  - Barret's syndrome
  - Chronic loop diuretic administration
  - X-linked hypercalciuria nephrolithiasis
  - Familial hypocalcemic hypercalciuria
- Systemic disease associated with chronic hypercalcemia
  - Williams syndrome
  - ***Primary hyperparathyroidism***

186. Answer is B (Hypercalcemia) : *Harrison 16th/ 2252;; Kumar & Clark 5th/ 1060; Harrison 17th/ 2380, 286; 18th/p 361, 3100*

Presence of a shortened QT interval along with a history of polyuria and altered sensorium in a patient with squamous cell carcinoma suggest a diagnosis of hypercalcemia secondary to paraneoplastic syndrome.

The **Paraneoplastic syndromes** in Broncogenic carcinoma could lead to several electrolyte abnormalities.

These are –

Electrolyte abnormality	Peptide responsible	Brochogenic carcinoma variant
Hypercalcemia	*PTH-related peptide*	Sqamous cell carcinoma
Hypokalemia	*ACTH*	Small cell carcinoma
Hyponatremia	*ADH*	Small cell carcinoma

The symptomatic profile of this patient matches with that of hypercalcemia

Manifestations of Hypercalcemia

General	Renal feature	Bones	Abdomen	Cardiac	Calcification
• Anorexia • Nausea • Vomiting • Fatigue • Depression • Mental confusion (≅ altered sensorium)	• Polyuria* & Nocturia • Renal colic from stones	• Bone pain • When cause is hyperparathyroidism • Bone cysts • Brown tumors	• Abdominal pain (peptic ulceration) • Constipation	• Short QT interval in ECG & in some patients cardiac arrythmias	Ectopic calcification & chondrocalcinosis

* **Polyuria** results from effect of hypercalcemia on renal tubules reducing there concentrating ability a form of nephrogenic diabetes insipidus

187. Answer is A (Diarrhea): *Harrison 16th/2252 (Repeat), Refer previous question; Harrison 17th/ 2380, 286; 18th/3100*

Hypercalcemia is associated with constipation (and not diarrhea).

*Hypercalcemia from any cause can result in fatigue, **depression,** mental own fusion, anorexia, nausea, **vomiting, constipation,** reversible renal tubular defects, **increased urination** (polyuria) a short QT interval and in some patients cardiac arrhythmias. - Harrison 16th/ 2252*

188. Answer is D (Rizol) : *; Harrison 16th/2261; Harrison 17th/ 2389, 2390, 286; Harrison 18th/p 361, 3111, 3112*

Rizol is the commercial name for cotrimoxale. It is not used in treatment of hypercalcemia.

Rizol = Trimethoprim & Sulphamethazole – Drug index

Management / treatment of hypercalcemia

	Biphophonates	Calcitonin	Others
• **Hydration** • **Increased salt intake** • **Mild and forced diuresis**	These are powerful inhibitors of bone resorption 1st generation : Etidronate 2nd generation : Pamidronate 3rd generation : Zolendronate	• Blocks bone resorption • Increases urinary calcium excretion	• Plicamycin • Gallium nitrate • Glucocorticoids • Dialysis • Phosphate therapy

Principles

- The first principle of treatment is to restore normal hydration [Q] as most hypercalcemia patients are dehydrated because of vomiting and polyuria etc.
- After rehydration has been achieved, saline can be administered
- Loop diuretics such as furosemide & ethacrynic acid can then be administered to depress tubular calcium resorption and enhance calcium excretion. ***Thiazide diuretics are not to be used.***
- Glucocorticoids have antitumor effect and are especially useful in hypercalcemia complicating malignancies.
- Dialysis:is the treatment of choice for severe hypercalcemia complicating renal failure.
- Phosphate therapy - Correcting hypophosphatemia lower serum calcium sometimes strikingly.

189. Answer is A (Normal saline with forced diuresis with Thiazides): *Refer text*

Thiazide diuretics should not be used in cases of hypercalcemia as these may themselves cause hypercalcemia.

190. Answer is A and B (Calcitonin and Gallium Nitrate): *Harrison 17th/2390; Harrison 18th/p 3113*

Calcitonin and Gallium Nitrate may be used in treatment of hypercalcemia.

191. Answer is D (Pamidronate is not effective): *Harrison 17th/2370; Harrison 18th/p 3112*

Pamidronate is a second generation biphosphonate that is approved for intravenous use in the treatment of hypercalcemia.

192. Answer is C (Vitamin D in high doses): *Harrison 17th/2390, 2386; Harrison 18th/p 3113, 3108*

Vitamin D administration is associated with hypercalcemia and hence it cannot be used in the treatment of hypercalcemia.

193. Answer is D (Gallium Nitrate): *Harrison 16th/2262, 2263; CMDT 2008/1450;*

Gallium Nitrate exerts s hypocalcemic effect by inhibiting calcium resorption from bone. Maximum hypocalcemic effect of gallium nitrate may take 3-4 days to appear and it is not often used now because of availability of superior alternatives.

Gallium nitrate is the single best answer of exclusion.

Treatment of Hypercalcemia	Onset of Action
Hydration with Saline	*Hours*
Forced diuresis (saline + loop diuretic)	*Hours*
Calcitonin	*Hours*
Intravenous phosphate	*Hours*
Pheomycin / Mithromycin	*Hours*
Dialysis	*Hours*
Biphosphonates	*Days (1 to 2 days)*
Glucocorticoids	*Days*
Gallium Nitrate	*Days (3-4 days)*

194. Answer is D (Bisphosphonates): *Harrison's 17th/2390; Harrison 18th/p 3112*

Bisphosphonates have a delayed onset of action beginning after days and are not recommended in patients with renal failure. Bisphosphonates is the single best answer by exclusion.

Onset of Action of Therapy for Severe Hypercalcemia

Immediate (Hours)	***Delayed (days)***
• *Hydration with **saline*** • *Loop diuretics **(Furosemide)** – once rehydrated* • *Calcitonin* • ***Dialysis***	• ***Bisphosphonates***

195. Answer is A (Etidronate): *Greenspan's Endocrinology 8th/316; Clinical Review of USMLE Step 2 (Surgisphere) 2008/499; Spiral Manual of Endocrinology & Metabolism 4th/360, 361*

Etidronate is a first generation bisphosphonate, used for the management of Hypercalcemia (not used for Hypocalcemia).

'Treatment of Hypocalcemia includes Calcium replacement with Vitamin D analogs along with Thiazide diuretics to prevent excess calcium excretion besides replenishing any decreases in magnesium and phosphate restriction'.

– Clinical Review for USMLE STEP – 2 (surgisphere) 2008/499

Management Stretegies in the management of Hypocalcemia

Increased Intake of Calcium	Enhanced Absorption of Calcium	Reduce Excretion of Calcium in Urine
Oral calcium supplementation • Calcium carbonate • Calcium gluconate • Calcium citrate • Calcium lactate ***Intravenous calcium supplementation*** • Calcium chloride • Calcium gluconate • Calcium gluceptate	***Vitamin D / Vitamin D Analogs*** • Vitamin D3 (Cholecalciferol) • Vitamin D2 (Ergocalciferol) • Calcitriol (1, 25 Dihydroxy Vitamin D3) • Calcifediol (25 Hydroxy vitamin D3) • Alfacalcidol (1α Hydroxyvitamin D3) (parenteral)	***Thiazide Diuretics*** Thiazide Diuretics have a hypocalciuric effect, and thereby reduce the amount of calcium excreted in urine. Thiazide Diuretics must be used with caution

196. Answer is B (Vitamin D intoxication): *Harrison 17th/2371; Harrison 18th/p 3089*

Vitamin D intoxication is associated with both hypercalcemia and hyperphosphatemia

Chronic Renal Failure is associated with hyperphosphatemia and hyporcalcemia

Hyperparathyroidism is associated with hypercalcemia and hypophosphatemia

Pseudohypoparathyroidism is associated with hypocalcemia and hyperphosphatemia

Causes of Hyperphosphatemia

I. Impaired renal phosphate excretion
- *A. Renal insufficiency*
- *B. Hypoparathyroidism*
  - *1. Developmental*
  - *2. Autoimmune*
  - *3. After neck surgery or radiation*
  - *4. Activating mutations of the calcium-sensing receptor*
- *C. Parathyroid suppression*
  - *1. Parathyroid-independent hypercalcemia*
    - *a. **Vitamin D or Vitamin A intoxication***
    - *b. Sarcoidosis, other granulomatous disease*
    - *c. Immobilization, osteolytic metastases*
    - *d. Milk-alkali syndrome*
  - *2. Severe hypermagnesia or hypomagnesemia*
- *D. Pseudohypoparathyroidism*
- *E. Acromegaly*
- *F. Tumoral calcinosis*
- *G. Heparin therapy*

II. Massive extracellular fluid phosphate loads
A. Rapid administration of exogenous phosphate (intravenous, oral, rectal)
B. Extensive cellular injury or necrosis
1. Crush injuries
2. Rhabdomyolysis
3. Hyperthermia
4. Fulminant hepatitis
5. Cytotoxin therapy
6. Severe hemolytic anemia
C. Transcellular phosphate shifts
1. Metabolic acidosis
2. Respiratory acidosis

197. Answer is A and B (CRF and Pseudohypoparathyroidism): *Harrison 16th/1655, 2267*

CRF and Pseudohypoparathyroidism are associated with Hypocalcemia and Hyperphosphatemia

Hypocalcemia with Hyperphosphatemia (Common Causes)
• *Chronic Renal Failure*
• *True Hypoparathyroidism*
• *Pseudo hypoparathyroidism*
• *Tumor lysis syndrome*
• *Rhabdomyolysis*

198. Answer is C and D (Ricket's and Hyperparathyroidism): *Harrison 17th/2370; Harrison 18th/p 3087*

Hypophosphatemia may be seen in X-linked Hypophoaphatemic Rickets and in Hyperparathyroidism.

Causes of Hypophosphatemia:

I. Reduced renal tubular phosphate reabsorption	
A. PTH/PTHrP – dependant	
1. Primary hyperparathyroidism	3. PTHrP dependant hypercalcemia of malignancy
2. Secondary hyperparathyroidism	4. Familial hypocalciuria hypercalcemia
a. Vitamin D deficiency/resistance	
b. Calcium starvation/malabsorption	
c. Bartter syndrome	
d. Autosomal recessive renal hypercalciuria with hypomagnesemia	
B. PTH/PTHrP independent	
1. Genetic hypophosphatemia	3. Other systemic disorders
a. ***X-linked hypophophatemic rickets***	a. Poorly controlled diabetes mellitus
b. Dent disease	b. Alcoholism
c. Autosomal dominant hypophophatemic rickets	c. Hyperaldosteronism
	d. Hypomagnesemia
d. Fanconi syndrome(s)	e. Amyloidosis
e. Cystinosis	f. Hemolytic uremic syndrome
f. Wilson disease	g. Renal transplantation or partial liver resection
g. McCune-Albright syndrome (fibrous dysplasia)	h. Rewarming or induced hyperthermia
	4. Drugs or toxins
h. Idiopathic hypercalciuria (absorptive subtype)	a. Ethanol
	b. Acetazolamide, other diuretics
i. Hereditary hypophosphatemia with hypercalciuria (Bedouins)	c. High-dose estrogens or glucocorticoids
	d. Heavy metals (lead, cadmium)
2. Tumor-induced osteomalacia	e. Toluene, N-methyl formamide
	f. Cisplatin, ifosfamide, foscarnet, rapamycin
	g. Calcitonin, pamidronate

II. Impaired intestinal phosphate absorption
A. Aluminium-containing antacids
B. Sevalamer
III. Shifts of extracellular phosphate into cells
A. Intravenous glucose
B. Insulin therapy of prolonged hyperglycemia or diabetic ketoacidosis
C. Catecholamines (epinephrine, dopamine, albuterol)
D. Acute respiratory alkalosis
E. Gram negative sepsis, toxic shock syndrome
F. Recovery from starvation or acidosis
G. Rapid cellular proliferation
1. Leukemic blast crisis
2. Intensive erythropoietin, other CSF therapy
IV. Accelerated net bone formation
A. Following parathyroidectomy
B. Treatment of Vitamin D deficiency, Paget disease
C. Osteoblstic metastases

199. Answer is A (Acute renal failure): *Harrison 16th / 2243, 1650; CMDT 2006 / 882, 881, 1230,CMDT2009/782*

Renal insufficiency is associated with hyperphosphatemia due to impaired renal phosphate excretion.

- **Acute renal failure:** '*Mild Hyperphosphatemia is an almost invariable complication of Acute Renal Failure. Severe hyperphosphatemia may develop in highly catabolic patients or following rhabdomyolysis, hemolysin or tumor lysis.' – Harrison 16th / 1650*
- **Diabetic ketoacidosis** *or Metabolic acidosis from any other causes may be associated with hyperphosphatemia from transcellular phosphatic shifts.*
  However resolving phases of diabetic ketoacidosis are associated with hypophosphatemia and not hyperphosphatemia. *This is a result of insulin therapy for diabetic ketoacidosis.*

Causes of hyperphosphatemia (*Harrison / CMDT*)
Metabolic acidosis (Lactic acidosis / Diabetic Ketoacidosis)

Causes of hypophosphatemia (*Harrison*)
Insulin therapy of diabetic ketoacidosis or prolonged hyperglycemia.

Laboratory values in DKA / *Harrison 6th / 323 - 324*
Phosphate values are : decreased (large changes occurs during treatment of DKA

Also note that total body stores of phosphorus (Also potassium, sodium, chloride, magnesium) are reduced in DKA, but are not accurately reflected by their levels (serum values may be increased) because of dehydration and hyperglycemia. – Harrison

- **Respiratory alkalosis** is associated with ***hypophosphatemia*** by causing intracellular shift of phosphorus into cells.

Hypophosphatemia	Hyperphosphatemia
• Metalbolic alkalosis	• Metabolic acidosis
• Respiratory alkalosis	• Respiratory acidosis

- **Chronic alcoholism / Alcoholism** *is known to cause* ***hypophosphatemia****. – Harrison 16th / 881*
  Severe hypophosphatemia is common and multifactorial in alcoholic patients.
  Chronic alcohol use results in a decrease in the renal threshold of phosphate excretion.' – CMDT
- **Patients with COPD and Asthma** *commonly have* ***hypophosphatemia****.*
  This is attributed to xanthine derivatives causing shifts of phosphate intracellularly and the phosphaturic effects of beta – adrenergic agonists, loop diuretics, xanthine derivatives and corticosteroids. – CMDT 2006 / 88

Vitamin D deficiency & Paget's Disease

200. Answer is B (Decreased phosphate in urine): *Harrison 17th/2376; Harrison 18th/p 3094*

Vitamin D deficiency is associated with PTH induced phosphaturia or increased phosphate in urine.

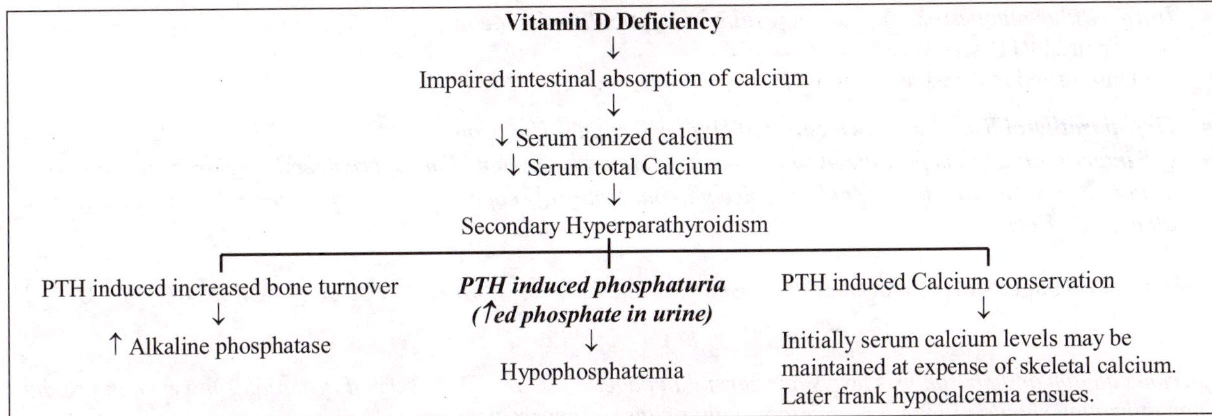

201. Answer is D (Vitamin D deficiency) : *Chandrasoma Taylor 3rd/ 965*

	Serum Ca	Serum phosphorus	Alkaline phosphatase	PTH
• Osteomalacia (Rickets) (↓Vit. D)	↓	↓	↑	↑
• Primary hyperparathyroidism bone disease	↑	↓	↑	↑
• Bone disease in renal failure with secondary hyperparathyroidism	N/↓	↑	↑	↑
• Lytic bone neoplasms	N/↑	N/↑	N/↑	N
• Osteoporosis	N	N	N	N
• Paget's disease	N	N	↑	N

202. Answer is C (Hypophosphaturia): *Refer previous question*

Rickets (or osteomalacia) is associated with hypophosphatemia due to PTH induced Phosphaturia (hyperphosphaturia)
Alkaline phosphatase levels are typically increased due to PTH induced increased bone turnover.

203. Answer is B (Gunstock deformity): *OP Ghai 6th/128-129; Nelson 17th/186, 188*

Gunstock deformity is a feature of malunion following supracondylar fracture of humerus or fracture of either condyle.
Gunstock deformity is not usually seen with rickets

Features of Rickets

- *Growth Retardation*
- *Craniotabes* *(Earliest manifestation of Rickets due to softening of skull bones)*
- *Bossing* *(Bossing of Frontal and Parietal skull bones)*
- *Caput Quadratum* *(Square appearance of head)*
- *Rachitic Rosary* *(Prominent costochondral junctions)*
- *Harrison sulcus* *(Horizontal depression along lower border of chest corresponding to insertion and inward pull of diaphragm)*
- *Pigeon Breast* *(Anterior protrusion of sternum)*
- *Deformities of long bones & spine*
  - *Knock knees*
  - *Bow eyes*
  - *Coxa vera*
  - *Lumbar lardosis*
- *Broad / Widened physis*
- *Irregular metaphyseal margin*
- *Cupping of metaphysis*

204. Answer is D (Inverse relation with Mg^{++} levels) : *Harrison 16th/ 2264; 17th/ 286, 2391, 2393; 18th/361, 3113, 3114, 3115*

Magnesium levels usually bear a direct, not an inverse, relationship with serum Ca^{++} levels. Severe hypo-magnesemia is associated with hypocalcemia.

- ***Intracellular magnesium deficiency results in Hypocalcemia due to*** :
  - Impaired PTH secretion
  - Diminished responsiveness to PTH
- ***Hypoparathyroidism is a known cause of Hypocalcemia*** *- Harrison*
- ***QT interval on ECG is prolonged in Hypocalcemia*** *and is shortened in hypercalcemia – Harrison*
- ***Tetany*** *is a recognized feature of hypocalcemia, but it may also occur with hypomagnesemia and respiratory alkalosis – Harrison*

205. Answer is C (Paget's disease of bone) : *Chandrasoma Taylor 3rd/ 965; Harrison 16th/ 2279; 17th/ 2409, 2410; 18th/3137, 3138*

Elevated alkaline phosphatase with normal serum Ca^{2+} and PO^{4-} is characteristic of Paget's disease.

'Serum calcium and phosphorus levels are normal in paget's disease. Discovery of hypercalcemia even in presence of immobilization should prompt a search for another cause of hypercalcemia' – Harrisons
'Serum Alkaline phosphatase levels are markedly elevated reflecting the marked osteoblastic activity'-Chandrasoma Taylor

Paget's disease of bone is characterized by the following pathological process:

Over activity of osteoclasts causing widespread bone resorption
(principal abnormality in Paget's disease)
↓
Compensatory increase in osteoblastic new bone formation
(Marked elevation of Alkaline phosphatase levels)
↓
Total bone volume may be maintained but the pagetic bone can be recognized as it is structurally disorganized and more susceptible to deformities and fractures.

Condition	Serum Ca	Serum phosphorus	Alkaline phosphatase	PTH
Paget's disease	N	N	Increase	N

206. Answer is B & C (Primary hyperparathyroidism & Chronic renal failure):
Kumar & Clarke 5th/646; Harrison 17th/ 2380

Serum alkaline phosphatase is the most valuable enzyme for assessment of bone disease and serves as an index of osteoblastic activity.

Alkaline phosphatase level in metabolic bone disease

Increased	Normal
• *Paget's disease* • *Rickets or osteomalacia* Q • *Hyperparathyroidism* Q • *Bone disease in renal failure* Q with secondary hyperparathyroidism • *Lytic bone neoplasms (levels may be normal)*	• *Hypoparathyroidism* • *Osteoporosis* • *Multiple myeloma.*

"Levels of Alkaline phosphatase are higher in Pagets disease than in any other condition, *(except hereditary hypophosphatasia)"* Q

207. Answer is C (Hypoparathyroidism) : *Chandrasoma Taylor 3rd/965*

Raised alkaline phosphatase levels are associated with hyperparathyroidism and not with hypoparathyroidism.
Serum alkaline phosphatase levels may be raised in hyperparathyroidism depending upon degree of involvement of bone. Q

208. Answer is B (Multiple Myeloma): *Harrison 16th/659*

Multiple Myeloma is not associated with elevated serum alkaline phosphatase.

Serum Alkaline Phosphatase is usually normal (in Multiple Myeloma) even with extensive bone involvement because of absence of osetoblastic activity. – Harrison

Osteoporosis

209. Answer is C (Hypoparathyroidism) :; *Harrison 16th/ 2271; Harrison 17th/ 2400; Harrison 18th/p 3124*

Osteoporosis as associated with hyperparathyroidism (not hypoparathyroidism).

DISEASES ASSOCIATED WITH AN INCREASED RISK OF GENERALIZED OSTEOPOROSIS IN ADULTS :

Hypogonadal States	**Nutritional and gastrointestinal disorders**
Turner Syndrome Klinefelter syndrome Anorexia nervosa Hypothalmic amenorrhea Other primary or secondary hypogonadal states	Malnutrition Parenteral nutrition Malabsorption syndromes Gastrectomy Severe liver disease, especially biliary cirrhosis Pernicious anemia
Endocrine disorders	**Hematologic disorders / Malignancy**
Cushing's syndrome Hyperparathyroidism Thyrotoxicosis Insulin-dependent diabetes mellitus Acromegaly Adrenal insufficiency	Multiple disorders/malignancy Lymphoma and leukemia Malignancy-associated parathyroid hormone - related (PTHrP) production Mastocytosis Hemophilia Thalassemia
Selected inherited & Rheumatologic disorders	**Miscellaneous**
Osteogenesis imperfecta[Q] Marfan syndrome[Q] Hemochromatosis Hypophosphatasia[Q] Glycogen storage diseases Homocystinuria[Q] Ehlers-Danlos syndrome[Q] Porphyria Menkes' syndrome Epidermolysis bullosa Rheumatoid arthritis[Q] Ankylosing spondylitis	Immobilization[Q] Chronic obstructive pulmonary disease Pregnancy and lactation Scoliosis Multiple sclerosis Sarcoidosis Amyloidosis Alcoholism

DRUGS ASSOCIATED WITH AN INCREASED RISK OF GENERALIZED OSTEOPOROSIS IN ADULTS :

Glucocorticoids[Q] Cyclosporine Cytotoxic drugs Anticonvulsants Excessive alcohol	Excessive thyroxin Aluminium Gonadotropin-releasing hormone agonists[Q] Heparin Lithium

210. Answer is B (Hypothyroidism) : *Harrison 16th/ 2271; Harrison 17th/ 2400; Harrison 18th/p 3124*

Osteoporosis is seen with hyperthyroidism and not with hypothyroidism.
Chronic heparin therapy, *thyrotoxicosis* and *old age* are all causes of osteoporosis

211. Answer is B (Hypoparathyroidism) :; *Harrison 16th/2271; Harrison 17th/ 2398-2400; Harrison 18th/p 3122-3124*

Osteoporosis is caused by hyperparathyoroidism and not by hypoparathyroidism

212. Answer is C (Hypoparathyroidism) : *Harrison 16th/ 2271; Harrison 17th/ 2398-2400; Harrison 18th/p 3122-3124*

Osteoporosis is a feature of Hyperparathyroidism (not hypoparathyroidism).

213. Answer is D (All of the above) :, *Harrison 16th/ 2271; Harrison 17th/ 2398-2400; Harrison 18th/p 3122-3124*

Estrogen deficiency (Hypogonadal state) *is known to cause osteoporosis. The most frequent estrogen deficient state is the cessation of ovarian function at the time of* ***menopause.***
Thyrotoxicosis and ***Cushing's syndrome*** are known endocrine causes of osteoporosis.

214. Answer is A (Fluorosis): *Harrison 16th/410, 2271; Harrison 17th/ 449, 2400; Harrison 18th/p 3124*

Fluorosis is associated with 'Osteosclerosis' and not with osteoporosis. *Hypogonodism, Hyperthyrodism and Hyperparathyrodism are all known causes for osteoporosis.*

215. Answer is A (Compression fracture of the spine) : *CMDT 2002/1166,2009/1013; Harrison 17th/ 2400; Harrison 18th/p 3124*

It most commonly presents as backache of varying degrees of severity. This backache is due to spontaneous fracture or collapse of vertebra.

- *Osteoporosis is defined as a reduction of bone mass or density, sufficient to increase the risk of fracture.*
- *Osteoporosis is usually asymptomatic until fracture occurs* ***(but serum Calcium is normal*** [Q]*).*
- *Serum parathyroid hormone, 25-(OH) D_2, Calcium, Phosphorus and Alkaline phosphatase are usually normal.*

Tumour Lysis Syndrome

216. Answer is A (Hypercalcemia): *Harrison's 18th/2274; Critical Case Nephrology (Elsevier) 2008/53*

Tumor Lysis Syndrome is associated with Hypocalcemia and not Hypercalcemia.

Rapid lysis of tumor cells after chemotherapy **(Tumor Lysis Syndrome)**[Q]

↓	↓	↓
• *Release of uric acid* [Q] from rapid turn-over nucleic acids. ***- Hyperuricemia***[Q]	• Release of intracellular Phosphate ***- Hyperphosphatemia***[Q]	• Release of intracellular Potassium ***- Hyperkalemia*** [Q]
• Uric acid may precipitate in tubules, medulla and collecting duct	• Increased phosphate drives calcium into bone ***- Hypocalcemia*** [Q]	• Predisposes to ***Arrhythmias*** [Q]
• ***Renal failure*** [Q]	• Calcium phosphate may deposit in renal tubules ***- Renal failure*** • Release of Intracellular Magnesium ***- Hypermagnesemia***	• ***Acidosis*** [Q] is also a feature and results in part from deranged oxidative metabolism ***-Lactic acidosis***[Q]

217. Answer is A (Hypocalcemia): *Harrison 17th/1736; Refer previous question; Harrison 18th/p 2274*

Tumor Lysis syndrome is associated with Hypocalcemia.

Tumor Lysis Syndrome is also associated with Hyperphosphatemia, Hyperkalemia and Acidosis.

Rapid lysis of tumor cells after chemotherapy **(Tumor Lysis Syndrome)**[Q]

- ***Release of uric acid*** [Q] from rapid turn-over nucleic acids- ***Hyperuricemia***
- Uric acid may precipitate in tubules, medulla and collecting duct
- ***Renal failure*** [Q]

- Release of intracellular Phosphate - ***Hyperphosphatemia***[Q]
- Increased phosphate drives calcium into bone - ***Hypocalcemia*** [Q]
- Calcium phosphate may deposit in renal tubules ***- Renal failure***
- Release of Intracellular Magnesium ***- Hypermagnesemia***

- Release of intracellular Potassium - ***Hyperkalemia*** [Q]
- Predisposes to ***Arrythmias*** [Q]
- ***Acidosis*** [Q] is also a feature and results in part from deranged oxidative metabolism ***-Lactic acidosis***[Q]

218. Answer is A, C and E (Hyperuricemia, Hyperphosphatemia and Hyperkalemia): *Refer previous questions*

Tumor Lysis Syndrome is associated with Hyperuricemia, Hyperphosphatemia and Hyperkalemia.

219. Answer is B (Hypercalcemia): *Harrison's 17th/1736; Refer previous question; Harrison 18th/p 2274*

Tumor Lysis syndrome is characterized with hypocalcemia and not hypercalcemia.

220. Answer is B (Hypercalcemia): *Harrison 17th/2380, 286, 1736; Harrison 18th/p 360, 2274, 3100*

Tumor lysis syndrome is associated with Hypocalcemia and not Hypercalcemia

Tumor lysis syndrome:

It is a clinical entity characterized by destruction of large number of rapidly proliferating neoplastic cells following chemotherapy.

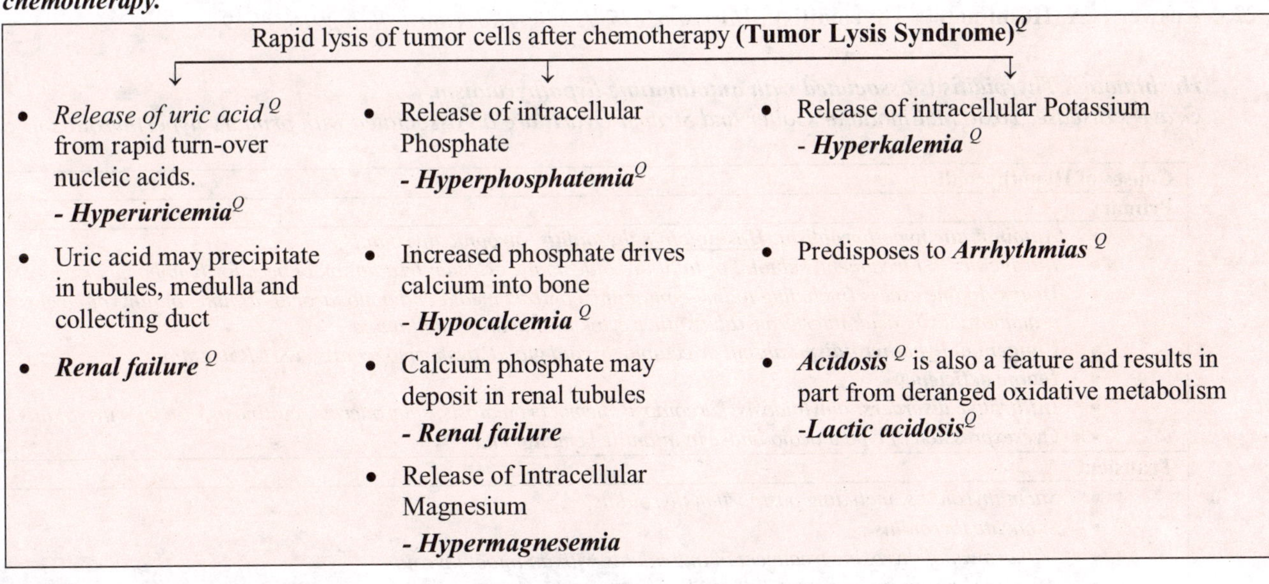

221. Answer is B (Hypercalcemia): *Repeat; Refer previous question*

Tumor Lysis Syndrome is associated with hypocalcemia and not hypercalcemia.

Disorders of Thyroid Gland

222. Answer is D (All of the above): *Harrison's 18th/2918*

Hypothyroidism may be caused by drugs like Lithium and /or Infiltrative disorders like Scleroderma and Hematochromatosis.

Causes of Hypothyroidism

Primary
• Autoimmune hypothyroidism: Hashimoto's thyroiditis, atrophic thyroiditis • Iatrogenic: ^{131}I treatment, subtotal or total thyroidectomy, external irradiation of neck for lymphoma or cancer • ***Drugs: iodine excess (including iodine-containing contrast media and amiodarone), lithium, antithyroid drugs, p-aminosalicylic acid, interferon- and other cytokines, aminoglutethimide, sunitinib*** • Congenital hypothyroidism: absent or ectopic thyroid gland, dyshormonogenesis, TSH-R mutation • Iodine deficiency • *Infiltrative disorders:* ***amyloidosis****, sarcoidosis,* ***hemochromatosis****,* ***scleroderma****, cystinosis, Riedel's thyroiditis* • Overexpression of type 3 deoiodinase in infantile hemangioma
Transient
• Silent thyroiditis, including postpartum thyroiditis • Subacute thyroiditis • Withdrawal of thyroxine treatment in individuals with an intact thyroid • After ^{131}I treatment or subtotal thyroidectomy for Graves' disease
Secondary
• Hypopituitarism: tumors, pituitary surgery or irradiation, infiltrative disorders, Sheehan's syndrome, trauma, genetic forms of combined pituitary hormone deficiencies • Isolated TSH deficiency or inactivity • Bexarotene treatment • Hypothalamic disease: tumors, trauma, infiltrative disorders, idiopathic

TSH, thyroid-stimulating hormone; TSH-R, TSH receptor.

223. Answer is A (Hoshimoto's Thyroiditis) : *Harrison's 17th/2230; Harrison 18th/p 2918, 2919*

Hoshimoto's Thyroiditis is associated with autoimmune hypothyroidism.
Grave's disease, Toxic Multinodular Goiter and Struma Ovarii are all associated with primary hyperthyroidism

Causes of Hypothyroidism
Primary
• ***Autoimmune hypothyroidism****: **Hashimoto's thyroiditis,** atrophic thyroiditis* • ***Iatrogenic:*** *^{131}I treatment, subtotal or total thyroidectomy, external irradiation of neck for lymphoma or cancer* • ***Drugs****: Iodine excess (including iodine-containing contrast media and amiodarone), lithium, antithyroid drugs, p-aminosalicylic acid, interferon-α and other cytokines, aminoglutethimide* • ***Congenital hypothyroidism****: absent or ectopic thyroid gland, dyshormogenesis, TSH-R mutation* • ***Iodine deficiency*** • ***Infiltrative disorders****: amyloidosis, sarcoidosis, hemochromatosis, scleroderma, cystinosis, Riedel's thyroiditis* • *Overexpression of type 3 deoiodinase in infantile hemangioma*
Transient
• *Silent thyroiditis, including postpartum thyroiditis* • *Subacute thyroiditis* • *Withdrawal of thyroxine treatment in individuals with an intact thyroid* • *After 131I treatment or subtotal thyroidectomy for Grave's disease*
Secondary
• *Hypopituitarism: tumors, pituitary surgery or irradiation, infiltrative disorders, Sheehan's syndrome, trauma, genetic forms of combined pituitary hormone deficiencies* • *Isolated TSH deficiency or inactivity* • *Bexarotene treatment* • *Hypothalamic disease: tumors, trauma, infiltrative disorders, idiopathic*

Causes of Hyperthyroidism/ Thyrotoxicosis
Primary hyperthyroidism
• ***Grave's disease*** • ***Toxic multinodular goiter*** • *Toxic adenoma* • *Functioning thyroid carcinoma metastases* • *Activating mutation of the TSH receptor* • *Activating mutation of GSα (Mc-Cune Albright syndrome)* • ***Struma ovarii*** • *Drugs: iodine excess (Jod-Basedow phenomenon)*
Thyrotoxicosis without hyperthyroidism
• *Subacute thyroiditis* • *Silent thyroiditis* • *Other causes of thyroid destruction: amiodarone, radiation, infarction of adenoma* • *Ingestion of excess thyroid hormone (thyrotoxicosis factitia) or thyroid tissue*
Secondary hyperthyroidism
• *TSH-secreting pituitary adenoma* • *Thyroid hormone resistance syndrome: occasional patients may have features of thyrotoxicosis* • *Chrionic gonadotropin-secreting tumors* • *Gestational thyrotoxicosis*

224. Answer is B (Iodine): *Park 20th/540*

Hypothyroidism (and Endemic Goitre) in sub-himalayan region is primarily due to deficiency of iodine.

'Dietary iodine deficiency is widely prevalent in many parts of India, especially the sub-Himalayan region and is the principal cause of endemic goiter. Where the deficiency is severe, goiter, hypothyroidism and endemic cretinism is common'-'Pediatrics: A concise Test' by kabra Elsevier 2007/2

> *ºThe most common cause of neonatal hypothyroidism (congenital hypothyroidism) is thyroid gland dysgenesis (80-85%).*
> *ºThe most common of endemic goiter/hypothyroidism is iodine deficiency.*

225. Answer is D (Low cholesterol): *Harrison 17th /2231; Koda Kimble and Young's Applied Therapeutics (2012)/1189*

Hypothyroidism is associated with increased cholesterol (Hypercholesterolemia) and not with low cholesterol (Hypocholesterolemia).

> A normal TSH excludes primary (but not secondary) hypothyroidism. If the TSH is elevated an unbound T4 level is needed to confirm the presence of clinical hypothyroidism but T4 is inferior to TSH where used as a screening test.

Laboratory Finding in Hypothyroidism

Primary Abnormalities

- *↓Total T4, ↓Free T4, ↓Free T4 Index*
- *↓Total T3; (↓free T3)*, ↓Free T3 Index*
- *↑TSH*
- *Positive TPO Antibodies (Autoimmune Throiditis, Hashiomato's Disease)*

Other Abnormalities

- ↑Cholesterol & Triglycerides
- ↑Creatine Phosphokinase (CPK)
- ↓Hb /Hct (Anemia is usually normocytic or macrocytic)
- ↑LDH
- ↑AST
- ↓Na

*Circulating unbound T3 (Free T3) levels may be normal in about 25% of patients reflecting adaptive diodinase responses to hypothyroidism. Free T3 measurements are therefore not indicated.

226. Answer is A (Diastolic murmur) *: Harrison 16th/1423; Harrison 17th/2234; Harrison 18th/p 2923*

Thyrotoxicosis is associated with a systolic murmur. It is not associated with any diastolic murmur.

Cardiovascular manifestations of thyrotoxicosis: *Harrison 16th/1423; 2114*

Hyperthyroidism

Increased atrial irritability
- *Sinus tachycardia*[Q]
- *Palpitations*[Q]
- *Supraventricular tachycardia*[Q]
- *Atrial fibrillation*[Q]

High cardiac output
(Hyperthyroidism causes an increase in total body metabolism and O_2 consumption that indirectly increases work load on the heart)
- *Bounding pulse*[Q]
- *Wide pulse pressure*[Q]
- *Hyperdynamic precordium*[Q]
- *Increased intensity of first heart sound and the pulmonic component of second heart sound and a third sound (S_3)*[Q]
- *Aortic systolic murmur*[Q]
- *Means lerman scratch*[Q]

- **Sinus tachycardia**[Q] *is the* ***most common***[Q] *manifestation of Thyrotoxicosis.*
- **Midsystolic murmur**[Q] *heard best at left sternal border with or without* ***Systolic ejection click.***
- **Means lerman scratch**[Q]**:** *It is a systolic scratchy sound heard at the 2nd left intercostal space during expiration. It is thought to result from rubbing of hyperdynamic pericardium against the pleura*
- Angina and heart failure may be precipitated by hyperthyroidism in patients with underlying heart disease.

227. Answer is A (Thyrotoxicosis) *: Kundu 3rd/357; Harrison 16th/2108*

Dancing carotids may be seen in
• Aortic regurgitation
• Thyrotoxicosis

228. Answer is B (Medullary Carcinoma)

Medullary carcinoma of thyroid secretes calcitonin and this causes reduction in calcium levels.

229. Answer is C (TSH) *: Harrison; 16th/2108; 2208-2209*

The enhanced sensitivity and specificity of TSH assays have greatly improved laboratory assessment of thyroid function *– Harrison*

With rare exceptions a normal TSH level excludes a primary abnormality of thyroid function. *– Harrison*

Approach to thyroid testing:

Because TSH change dramatically in response to alteration of free T_4 and T_3, a logical approach to thyroid testing is to determine first whether TSH is suppressed, normal or elevated – *Harrison*

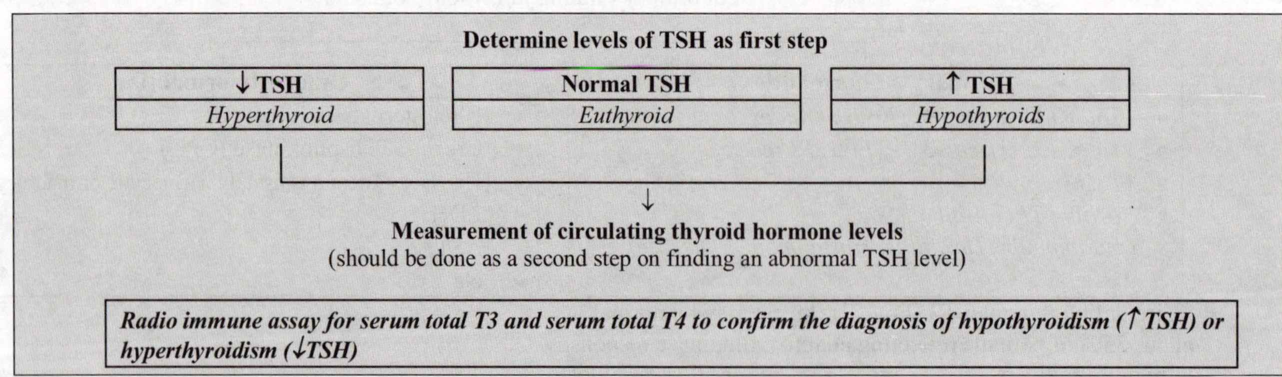

230. Answer is A (Primary hypothyroidism) : *Harrison 16th/2108, 2109; 17th/2231*

The single most useful measurement for assessment of hypothyroidism is serum TSH[Q]***. It is increased in primary hypothyroidism.***

Primary hypothyroidism is characterised by inability to synthesize enough thyroid hormone (↓T_3 and ↓T_4). This leads to compensatory hypersecretion of TSH (↑ TSH).
Overall picture thus is : *↓ T3, ↓T4 and ↑ TSH.*

231. Answer is A (Jod-Basedow effect) *CMDT 2004 / 1093; Harrison 16th/2121; Harrison 17th/2241; CDMT 2005/1102,2009/982; Harrison 18th/p 2932*

Contrast agents and other iodine containing substance should be avoided because of risk of inducing the 'Jod – Basedow effect' characterized by enhanced production of thyroid hormone by autonomous nodules' *- Harrison*

Jod Basedow disease is synonymous with iodine induced hyperthyroidism and may occur in patients with multinodular goitre after intake of large amount of iodine.

- in the diet
- in the form of radiographic contrast material
- in the form of drugs especially amiadarone

Thyrotoxicosis factitia :

Thyrotoxicosis produced due to ingestion of excessive amount of exogenous thyroid hormone is called Thyrotoxicosis factitia. Epidemics of thyrotoxicosis have been caused by consumption of ground beef contaminated with bovine thyroid gland.
Presentation is one of thyrotoxicosis with low or absent thyroid nucleotide uptake.

Wolff – Chaikoff effect: *Harrison 15th / 2062, 2073, 2076; Harrison 16th/2117, 2106*

Excess iodine transiently inhibits thyroid iodide organification. This phenomenon of iodine dependent transient supression of thyroid is called Wolff-Chaikoff effect.

De Quervon's thyroiditis is same as subacute thyroiditis, granulomatosus thyroiditis or viral thyroiditis.

232. Answer is A (Jod-Basedow effect): *CMDT 2004 / 1093; Harrison 16th/2121; Harrison 17th/2241; CDMT 2005/1102,2009/982*

Contrast agents and other iodine containing substance should be avoided because of risk of inducing the 'Jod – Basedow effect' characterized by enhanced production of thyroid hormone by autonomous nodules' *- Harrison*

JodBasedow disease

JodBasedow disease is synonymous with iodine-induced hyperthyroidism and may occur in patients with multinodulargoitre after intake of large amount of iodine.

Increased intake of iodine:

- In the diet
- In the form of radiographic contrast material
- In the form of drugs especially amiadarone

Thyrotoxicosis factitia:

Thyrotoxicosis produced due to ingestion of excessive amount of exogenous thyroid hormone is called Thyrotoxicosis factitia. Epidemics of thyrotoxicosis have been caused by consumption of ground beef contaminated with bovine thyroid gland.
Presentation is one of thyrotoxicosis with low or absent thyroid nucleotide uptake.

Wolff – Chaikoff effect:

Excess iodine transiently inhibits thyroid iodide organification. This *phenomenon of iodine dependent transient supression of thyroid is called Wolff-Chaikoff effect.*

De Quervain's thyroiditis is same as subacute thyroiditis, granulomatosus thyroiditis or viral thyroiditis.

233. Answer is B (Hypothyroidism is more common in men): *Harrison 15th / 2076; 16th/2119; Harrison 17th/2239, 2240; Harrison 18th/p 2929, 2930*

'Amiadarone associated hypothyroidism is more common in women and individual with positive TPO antibodies'
– Harrison 15th / 2076

Amiadarone is a class III antiarrythmic agent structurally related to thyroid hormone and containing very high amount of iodine.

Mechanism of action*[Q]**: *Amiadorone* ***inhibits deiodinase activity. [Q]

Initiation of Amiadarone treatment

↓
- Inhibitory effect of iodine on T_4 release
- Wolff Choikoff effect: Excess iodine transiently inhibit thyroid iodide organification

Transient decrease in T4 levels (Hypothyroidism)

↓
- Escape from Wolff Choikoff effect (most individuals escape from iodide dependent supression of thyroid)
- Inhibition of deiodination (deiodination is required for conversion of T_4 to T_3.)

- Enhanced T_4 levels
- Decreased T_3 levels / increased rT_3
- Elevated TSH levels (TSH levels normalize or are slightly suppressed after about 1-3 months)

Amiadarone associated hypothyroidism:

Involves an inability of thyroid to escape from high iodine load. Consequently ***amiadarone associated hypothyroidism is more common in women*** and in individuals with positive TPO[Q].

Amiadarone associated hyperthyroidism:

Two types of Amiadarone induces thyrotoxicosis (AIT) are seen –

AIT – Type I	AIT - Type II
Associated with an underlying thyroid abnormality - preclinical gravis - multinodular goitre	Associated with individuals with no intrinsic thyroid abnormality
Thyroid hormone synthesis becomes excessive as a result of increased iodine exposure - Jod basedow phenomenon	Thyrotoxicosis results from drug induced lysosomal activation leading to destruction thyroiditis. This can resolve spontaneously or can occasionally lead to hypothyroidism
Increased vascularity is seen on color-flow dopler scan	Decreased vascularity is seen on color flow dopler scan
IL_6 levels are marginally raised.	IL_6 levels are markedly raised.

234. Answer is D (Oxygen consumption): *Harrison 14th / 2024; KDT 5th/130 (Not elaborated in later editions); Harrison 17th/2236; Harrison 18th/p 2926*

Betablockers do not correct the underlying metabolic abnormalities (i.e. does not affect the oxygen consumption[Q]). This is why propanolol should only be used as an adjunctive therapy.

Advantages of Propanolol	Limitations of Propanolol (β blocking)
• **Propanolol alleviates such adrenergic manifestations as** - Sweating - *Tremor* [Q] - *Tachycardia* [Q] - Palpitations - *Nervousness (Anxiety)* [Q]	• **β-blockers do not significantly affect the thyroid status.** [Q] It reduces to some extent the conversion of T_4 to T_3 • **β-blockers do not correct the underlying metabolic abnormalities**

235. Answer is A (Surgery for thyroiditis) : *Bailey and Love 24th/796; CMDT 2003/1104;CMDT 2009/988 Harrison 17th/2237; Harrison 18th/p 2927*

Thyroid storm occurs in a thyrotoxic patient who has been inadequately prepared for thyroidectomy.

All options other than thyroiditis mentioned as options reflect a thyrotoxic state under stress and may lead to thyroid storm. Thyroiditis may not be necessarily associated with thyrotoxicosis. Infact many forms of thyroiditis have associated hypothyroidism and hence these patients are unlikely to develop thyroid storm when taken for surgery.

Thyroid storm is an extreme form of thyroitoxicosis that may occur with a variety of conditions:

Conditions that may lead to thyroid storm in thyrotoxic patients
Stressful illness
Thyroid surgery
Radioactive iodine administration

236. Answer is C (Hashimoto's Thyroiditis) : *Harrisson 16th/2110; 17th/2239; CMDT-2001/1121; CMDT 2003/1105-1106, CMDT 2009/989; Harrison 18th/p 2929*

Hashimotas thyroiditis, also called chronic lymphocytic thyroiditis, is the most common form of thyroiditis.

237. Answer is D (Reidel's thyroiditis) : *Bailey & Love 23rd/733, 719; Harrison; 16th/2119; 17th/2239;Harrison 18th/p 2929*

Reidel's thyroiditis is usually a consistantly hypothyroid condition.

The patient in the given question is presenting with symptoms of Hyperthyroidism. The condition, most unlikely to produce the picture is the one where hyperthyroidism is not a feature, not even transient. Reidel's thyroiditis is one such consistently hypothyroid condition.
Thyrotoxicosis is usual with thyroid adenoma and diffuse thyroid goitre and Hashimoto's thyroiditis can present with transient hyperthyroidism.

- **Hashimoto's Thyroiditis (Auto immune):** In this variant, ***mild hyperthyroidism may be present initially***, although hypothyroidism is inevitable. Hypothyroidism may develop rapidly or extremely slowly. The initial phase of hyperthyroidism may account for the symptoms in the given patient.
- **Thyroid adenoma, diffuse toxic goitre or Grave's disease, toxic nodular goitre, toxic nodule:** All are causes of thyrotoxicosis & explain the symptoms of thyrotoxicosis in the above patient. *733/L&B*
- **Riedle's thyroiditis** is a very rare disease wherein , the thyroid tissue is replaced by cellular fibrous tissue.

  The goitre may be unilateral or bilateral & is very hard and fixed. ***This condition presents with features of hypothyroidism. Hyperthyroidism is not manifested, not even transiently.*** The differential diagnosis is from an anaplastic carcinoma & can be made with certainity only by biopsy.
- **Diffuse thyroid goitre :** Most commonly presents with a euthyroid status however patients may present with hyperthyroidism.

238. Answer is C (Increased radioactive Iodine uptake) : *Repeat; Bailey & Love 23rd/733; 24th/804; Harrison 16th/2118; 17th/2238; Harrison 18th/p 2928*

'DeQuervain's Thyroiditis is characterized by a depressed radioactive iodine uptake'.

DeQuervain's Thyroiditis, Granulomatous Thyroiditis or Subacute Thyroiditis or Giant cell Thyroiditis:

Origin / Etiology	• It is *viral in origin.*Q Symptoms usually follow an upper respiratory tract infection.
Clinical presentation	• *Pain over thyroid* Q or pain referred to lower jaw, ear, occiput (stretching of thyroid capsule) • *Fever* Q, malaise, asthenia • Firm, irregular enlargement of one or both thyroid lobes
Characteristic Laboratory Finding	• High Erythrocyte sedimentation rate (ESR) • Depressed RAIU i.e. decreased radio iodine uptake test • ***Early:*** patients may be mildly thyrotoxic due to leakage of hormone from gland: $\uparrow T_3$ & T_4 & $\downarrow$TSH ***Later :*** patients may be hypothyroid due to depletion of hormone from gland : $\downarrow T_3$ & T_4 & $\uparrow$TSH
Histology	• *Multinucleated Giant cells* Q are seen - *Robbins*
Prognosis	• *Disorder may smoulder for months but eventually subsides with return of normal function.*

239. Answer is A (Autoimmune etiology) : *Harrison 15th/2074; 16th/2118; Refer previous questions; Harrison 17th/2238; Harrison 18th/2928*

De Quervain's Thyroiditis is viral in origin (and not autoimmune). *Symptoms usually follow an upper respiratory tract infection.*

240. Answer is B (Hashimoto's Thyroiditis) : *Robbins 6th /1135; Bailey 23rd /728; 24th/803, 804*

"The thyroid follicles are small and are lined by epithelial cells with abundant eosinophilic granular cytoplasm termed as Hurthle cells" *- Robbins 6th / 1135*

Hurthle cells may be seen in :
• Hashimoto's Thyroiditis Q *- Robbins 6th / 1135* • Hurthle cell Thyroid adenoma Q *- Robbins 6th / 1141* • Follicular cell carcinomas Q *- Bailey 23rd / 728*

"Hurthle cell tumors are a variant of Follicular neoplasms in which oxyphill or Hurthle / Ashkenazi cells predominate"
- Bailey

8

241. Answer is B (Diffuse Goiter) : *Bailey & Love 22nd / 511 ; Robbins 6th / 1138*

'Euthyroid state is generally the rule' *– Robbins*

<u>**Endemic goiter :**</u> occurs in geographical areas where the soil, water and food supply contains only low levels of iodine. The lack of the iodine leads to decreased synthesis of thyroid hormones and a compensatory increase in TSH, which in turn leads to follicular cell hypertrophy and hyperplasia and goitrous enlargement - Diffuse hyperplastic goitre.
'Euthyroid state is generally the rule' 'Rare patients are hyperthyroid'

Endocrinology

242. Answer is C and D (Subacute thyroiditis and Factitious thyroiditis): *Harrison 17th/2229; Mayo Clinic Internal Medicine Concise Textbook (2007)/181; Harrison 18th/p 2917*

Subacute Thyroiditis and Facititious thyroiditis are associated with decreased radioiodine uptake.

High RAIU	Low RAIU
• ***Graves disease*** • ***Toxic nodule*** • *Autonomous nodular Goitre* • *Metastatic follicular thyroid carcinoma* • *HCG dependent hyperthyroidism of trophoblastic disease* • *TSH secreting pituitary adenoma*	• ***Subacute Thyroiditis*** - *Dequervain's thyroiditis* - *Viral thyroiditis* • *Lymphocytic thyroiditis* • *Postpartum thyroiditis* • ***Exogenous hyperthyroidism*** *(Factitious hyperthyroidism)* • *Recent iodine load (eg contrast dye)*

243. Answer is A (Medullary Carcinoma thyroid) : *Bailey 23rd/731, 732; CMDT 2002/1142; CMDT 2003/1088-1089; Robbins 5th/1141; CMDT 2009/997*

Presence of thyroid nodule along with palpable cervical lymph nodes and amyloid histologically is clearly indicative of Medullary variety of Carcinoma Thyroid.

<u>**Medullary Carcinoma thyroid**</u> **:**
It is a neuroendocrine carcinoma rising from parafollicular 'C' cells of thyroid

Parafollicular 'C' cells are derived from neural crest and secrete calcitonin.

Medullary carcinoma should be suspected whenever :
a. ***High level of serum calcitonin***Q are discovered b. ***Cervical lymph node*** are discovered at time of presentation. Q - *Involvement of lymph nodes occurs early.* Q - Thyroid and *blood born metastasis occurs early.* Q c. ***Diarrhea***Q is a presentation d. ***Amyloid***Q is present in stroma histologically. e. ***MEN setting :*** Evidence of Pheochromocytoma / Hyperparathyroidism / Thyroid cancer in family. ***(Discovery of medullary carcinoma thyroid makes family surveillance advisable).***Q *f.* ***Hypocalcemia*** is associated: These cancers are ***associated with Hypocalcemia***Q because calcitonin is secreted.

<u>**Medullary carcinoma thyroid is seen as**</u> **-**
a. Sporadic : 80%
b. Familial : 20% - Non MEN setting / MEN II a / MEN II b

244. Answer is A (Serum Calcitonin): *Bailey 23rd/ 731; Bailey 24th/801, 802*

Medullary Carcinoma Thyroid are tumors of para-follicular 'C' cells derived from the neural crest, & are not derived from the cells of thyroid follicles. ***Since these para-follicular 'C' cells secrete Calcitonin^{Q}, high level of serum Calcitonin (> 0.08 ng/ml) are found.*** These levels fall after resection, & will rise again if the tumor recurs, making it the ***ideal candidate for screening tests***.
Also note : These cancers are ***associated with Hypocalcemia***^{Q} because calcitonin counteracts parathormnone.

245. Answer is B (Follicular) : *Bailey 23rd / 716*

FNAC is the investigation of choice in discrete thyroid swellings.
FNAC cannot distinguish between a Follicular Adenoma and a Follicular Carcinoma as this distinction is dependant not on cytology but on histological criteria such as capsular and vascular invasion. FNAC thus cannot be used to diagnose Follicular carcinomas.

Conditions that may be diagnosed by FNAC are :
1. Papillary carcinoma
2. Medullary carcinoma
3. Anaplastic carcinoma
4. Lymphoma
5. Thyroiditis
6. Colloid nodules

246. Answer is C (Total Thyroidectomy and Modified neck dissection on the side of enlarged lymph node) :

Presence of thyroid nodule along with palpable cervical lymph nodes and amyloid histologically is clearly indicative of Medullary variety of Carcinoma Thyroid.

Treatment of Medullary Carcinoma Thyroid :
Total thyroidectomy + Resection of involved lymph nodes by radical / modified radical neck dissection.

Endocrine Tumors

247. Answer is B (Norepinephrine): *Harrison 16th / 2148, 2149; Harrison 17th/2270; Harrison 18th/p 2963*

Most Pheochromocytomas contain and secrete both nor epinephrine and epinephrine.
'The ratio of norepinephrine to epinephrine is often as high as 20:1' *– Bailey (old edition)*

Pheochromocytomas are catecholamines secreting tumors of chromaffin cells derived from adrenal medulla or extradrenal sources (chromaffin cells in or about sympathetic ganglia.)

Adrenal	Extraadrenal
• *Most of them secrete Nor epinephrine in greater amount*	• *Most of them exclusively secrete Nor epinephrine*

248. Answer is B (Norepinephrine): *Harrison's 16th/2148*

Most extraadrenal pheochromocytomas secrete norepinephrine exclusively *– Harrison 16th/2148*

Most pheochromocytomas produce both norepinephrine and epinephrine and the percentage of norepinephrine is usually greater than in normal adrenal.
Most Extraadrenal pheochromocytoma secrete norepinephrine exclusively.
Pheochromocytomas in association with MEN may rarely produce epinephrine alone.

249. Answer is B (Metanephrines): *Harrison's 18th/2963*

The most sensitive test for diagnosis of pheochromocytomas is measurement of fractionated metanephrines in urine and free metanephrines in plasma.

Biochemical and Imaging Methods Used for Pheochromocytoma and Paraganglioma Diagnosis

Biochemical tests

Diagnostic Method	Sensitivity	Specificity
24-h urinary tests		
Vanillylmandelic acid	++	++++
Catecholamines	+++	+++
Fractionated metanephrines	++++	++
Total metanephrines	+++	++++
Plasma tests		
Catecholamines	+++	++
Free metanephrines	++++	+++

Imaging modalities

Diagnostic Method	Sensitivity	Specificity
CT	++++	+++
MRI	++++	+++
MIBG scintigraphy	+++	++++
Somatostatin receptor scintigraphy*	++	++
Dopa (dopamine) PET	+++	++++

*Particularly high in head and neck paragangliomas.
MIBG, metaiodobenzylguanidine; PET, positron emission tomography

250. Answer is C (5HIAA): *Harrison's 18th/2063*

5HIAA levels are elevated in carcinoid syndrome and not in pheochromocytoma.

Pheochromocytomas (and paragangliomas)

- Pheochromocytomas and paragangliomas synthesize and store catecholamines which include norepinephrine (noradrenaline), epinephrine (adrenaline) and dopamine
- Pheochromocytomas are typically associated with elevated levels of plasma and urinary catecholamines and their metabolites such as VMA and metanephrines
- *The most sensitive test for diagnosis of pheachromocytomas is measurement of fractionated metanephrines in urine and free metanephrine in plasma.*

251. Answer is E (Chest wall): *William's Endocrinology 11th/510*

Pheochromocytomas are not found in the chest wall

Pheochromocytomas may be found in the adrenal gland, neck and mediastinum (along the sympathetic chain), abdomen (paraaortic) and urinary bladder.

Sites of pheochromocytoma

- *Adrenal gland (most common)*
- *Head and Neck*
- *Thorax (mediastinum)*
- *Intra abdominal (paraaortic)*
- *Bladder*

Pheochromocytomas

Adrenal Pheochromocytomas
'Pheochromocytomas'

- *Adrenal Medulla (Most common site)*

Extra-adrenal Pheochromocytomas
'Paragangliomas'

Extra-adrenal pheochromocytomas (Paragangliomas) are found where there is chromaffin tissue

- Along the *paraaortic sympathetic chain*
- *Within organs of Zuckerkandl* (at the origin of inferior mesenteric artery)
- *Along the sympathetic chain in the neck and mediastinum*
- *In the wall of the urinary bladder*

252. Answer is D (Wheezing): *Harrison 15th / 2106; 17th / 2270-71; 16th/2149 : Not elaborated); 18th/2962, 2963*

Wheezing has not been mentioned as a symptom of Pheochromocytoma.

The most common symptoms in order of frequency during paroxysm are:	
- Headache	- Palpitation
- Vomiting	- Sweating
- Dyspnea	- Weakness
- Pallor	

- The most common manifestation is ***hypertension.*** Q It most commonly occurs in paroxysms i.e. Paroxysmal Hypertension
- The most common symptom is ***headache*** Q
- ***Orthothostatic Hypotension*** Q : is seen as a consequence of diminished plasma volume & blunted sympathetic reflexes.

Pheochromocytoma has been called the 10% tumor Q: 10% of tumor are		
- bilateral Q	- familial	- multiple Q
- extraadrenal Q	- malignant Q	- occur in children

253. Answer is C (Low cortisol level) : *Harrison 16th / 2149, 2150; Harrison 17th/2270-2271; Harrison 18th/p 2962, 2963*

Pheochromocytoma is not associated with low cortisol levels.

- Pheochromocytoma is unique in presentation as it may present both with, Hypertension and hypotension.
    - Hypertension occurs in paroxysms and is the most common manifestation
    - Hypotension occurs as ***'orthostatic hypotension'*** and it occurs as a consequence of diminished plasma volume and blunted sympathetic reflexes.
- ***Carbohydrate intolerance:*** Over half of patients have impaired carbohydrate tolerance due to suppression of insulin and stimulation of hepatic glucose output.
- Hematocrit: An ***elevated hematocrit*** may be secondary to diminished plasma volume.

254. Answer is D (Hypocalcemia): *Harrison's 18th/2965*

Pheochromacytomas may be associated with hypercalcemia and are not associated with hypocalcemia.

Clinical Features Associated with Pheochromocytoma

- ***Headaches***
- ***Sweating attacks***
- *Palpitations and tachycardia*
- *Hypertension, sustained or paroxysmal*
- *Anxiety and panic attacks*
- *Pallor*
- *Nausea*
- *Abdominal pain*
- *Weakness*
- ***Weight loss***
- *Paradoxical response to antihypertensive drugs*
- *Polyuria and polydipsia*
- *Constipation*
- *Orthostatic hypotension*
- *Dilated cardiomyopathy*
- *Erythrocytosis*
- *Elevated blood sugar*
- ***Hypercalcemia***

255. Answer is D (Episodic Hypertension): *Harrison's 18th/2962; Robbins Basic Pathology (Elsvier) 2012/761*

The predominant clinical manifestation of pheochromocytoma is Hypertension. The classical manifestation of Hypertension in pheochromocytoma is 'Episodic Hypertension' which is the single best answer amongst the options provided.

'The dominant sign is hypertension. Classically patients present with episodic hypertension but sustained hypertension is also common - Harrison's 18th/2962

The predominant clinical manifestation of pheochromocytoma is Hypertension but Sustained Hypertension is more common than Paroxysmal Hypertension.

'The predominant clinical manifestation of pheochromocytoma is hypertension. In majority of patients (2/3rd) the hypertension occurs in the form of chronic sustained elevation in blood pressure. In clinical practice isolated paroxysmal episodes of hypertension occur in fewer thn half of patients with pheochromocytoma'-Robbins

'Hypertension present in more thn 90% of patient is the most common physical finding in pheochromocytoma. It is usually severe, refractory to conventional therapy. Despite the association of pheochromocytoma with paroxysms, only 25 to 40% of patients truly experience Paroxysmal hypertension' – Washington Manual of Endocrinology

'Hypertension is the most common feature and occurs in more than 90% of patients. It is usually sustained and may be without definitive crises resembling essential hypertension. Unstable Blood Pressure is usually present and many patients with sustained hypertension also have distinct paroxysms'

-Tumor Marker Physiology, Pathobiology technology and Clinical applications (American Association of Clinical Chemistry) 2002/344

256. Answer is A (D-cell) *: Ganong 20th/e 339; Harrison 17th/1857; Harrison 18th/p 2440, 2441*

Pancreatic cell		Hormone secreted
Alpha cells	:	Glucagon
Beta cells	:	Insulin
Delta cells	:	Somatostatin

257. Answer is D (Insulinoma); *Harrison 16th/ 2227; Harrison 17th/2354; Harrison 18th/p 3066*

Insulinoma is characterised by an increase in weight (weight gain) and not by weight loss.

Weight gain may result from increased food ingested to combat symptoms of hypoglycemia.

Classic presentation of ***insulinoma*** : ***'Whipple's triad'***Q : *- Harrison 14th/589*	
1.Fasting hypoglycemia Q	*3. Immediate relief after I.V. glucose administration* Q
2 Symptoms of hypoglycemia Q	

Causes of weight loss include:

A. Increased energy expenditure	**C. Diminished food intake**
1. Hyperthyroidism Q	*1. Cancer* Q
*2. **Pheochromocytoma*** Q	*2. Infection* Q
3. Extensive exercise Q	*3. **Uremia*** Q
B. Increased energy loss	*4. Anorexia nervosa* Q
1. Diabetes mellitus Q	*5. **Adrenal insufficiency*** Q
2. Malabsorption syndromes Q	*6. Hypercalcemia(malignancy, Hyper PTH, sarcoidosis)* Q
	7. Alzheimer's disease Q
	8. Depression Q

258. Answer is A (Peptic Ulceration, Gastric Hypersecretion, Non β Cell Tumour): *Harrison16th/ 2227, 17th/1868; Harrison 18th/p 2455*

Zollinger Ellison Syndrome is characterised by peptic ulceration due to gastrin hyper secretion by a non beta cell tumor.

Zollinger Ellison Syndrome

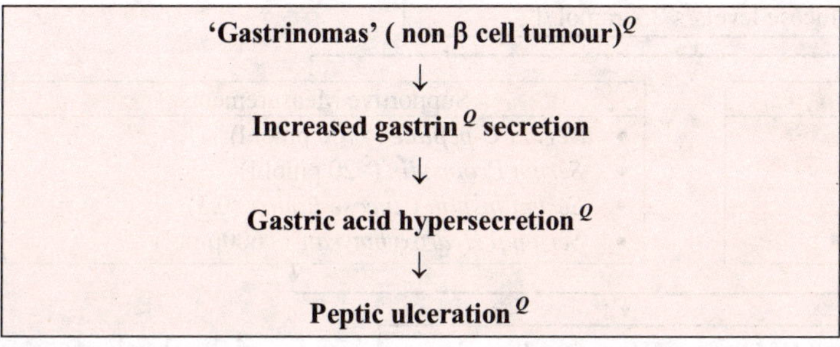

Remember :

- ***Most common*** site Q of gastrinoma is Duodenum (50-70%), (Pancreas 20-40%) *- Harrison*
- ***Most common*** hormone to be secreted besides gastrin is – ACTH Q
- ***Most common*** site of peptic ulcers produced is 1st part of Duodenum.
- ***Most valuable provocative test*** in identifying patients with ZES is the Secretin injection tests.
- Basal acid output is greater than 60 % of out put induced by maximal stimulation i.e. BAO > MAO Q

259. Answer is A ('72 hour' fast test): *Harrison's 17th/2354, 2355, Oxford Textbook of Medicine 4th/365, 366, 'Clinical Endocrinology' by Grossmann 2nd/534; Harrison 18th/p 3066, 3067*

The Gold standard test for diagnosis of Insulinoma is a supervised '72 hour fast' test

Diagnosis of Insulinoma requires demonstration of inappropriately high levels of plasma Insulin (and C- peptide) in the presence of documented hypoglycemia (Achieved by 72 hour fast test).

Absolute values of Insulin or C- peptide are not reliable in establishing a diagnosis unless hypoglycemia is documented

The '72 hour fast test' allows demonstration of hypoglycemia, together will elevated levels of Insulin and C-peptide and thus becomes the most reliable – gold standard test for establishing a diagnosis of Insulinoma

Diagnosis of Insulinoma: '72 hour fast' test

- The diagnosis of Insulinoma requires the demonstration of an inappropriately elevated plasma insulin (and C-peptide) at the time of hypoglycemia
- The '72 hour fast' test involves supervised fasting for upto 72 hours or until hypoglycemia can be documented (<2.2 mmol/L or < 40 mg/dl)
- The test is considered positive if at any time when blood glucose levels drop to < 2.2mmol/l (40 mg/dl), the serum insulin levels are recorded to be greater than 6μU/ml. (and C- peptide levels > 100 pmol/l)
- *Studies indicate that 100% of patient with insulinoma will be detected after a supervised 72 hour fast and hence this test is considered the gold standard test*

First 24 hours :	*70-80% of patients with insulinoma can be detected*
Upto 48 hours :	*98% of patients with insulinoma can be detected*
By 72 hours:	*100% of patients with insulinoma can be detected*

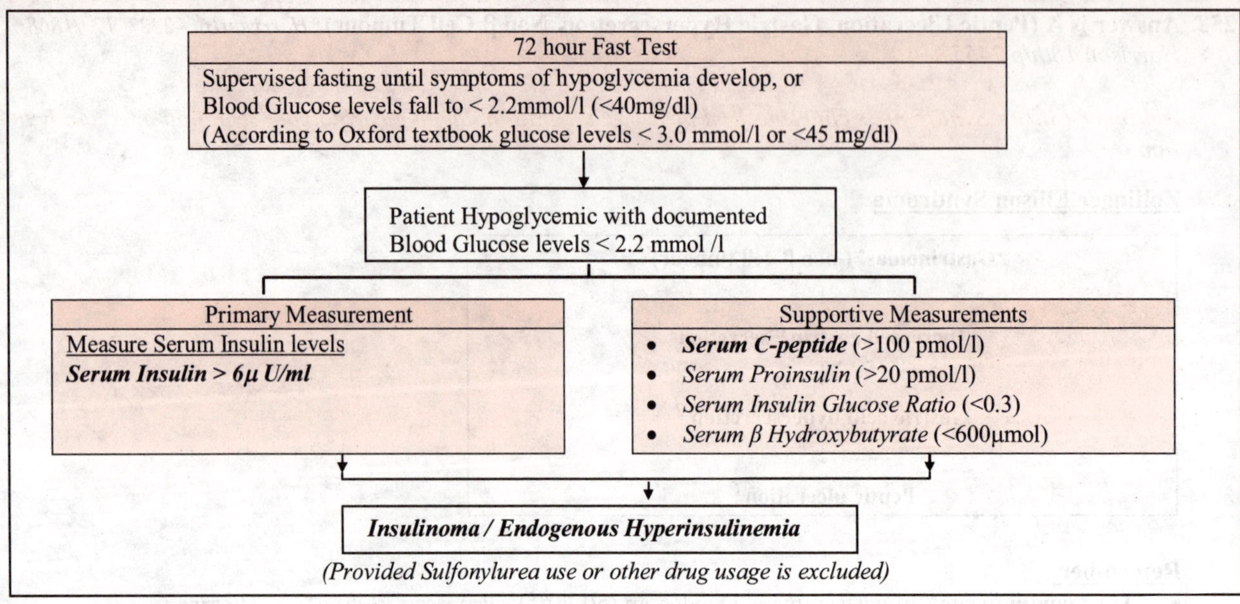

260. Answer is B (Xylose test) : *Harrison's 17th/ 2354 ; Harrison 18th/p 3066, 3067*

Xylose test is used in the diagnosis of malabsorption due to intestinal mucosal disease. This test is not used for the diagnosis of Insulinomas

Fasting blood glucose, C- peptide levels and Insulin Glucose Ratio are all used in the diagnosis of Insulinomas.

Diagnosis of Insulinomas

- *Serum insulin levels (fasting)*
- *Serum glucose levels (fasting)*
- *Serum C- peptide levels (Elevated)*
- *Serum proinsulin levels (Elevated)*
- *Insulin / Glucose Ratio (> 0.3)*
- *Plasma β-Hydroxybulyrate (Decreased)*

Serum insulin levels > 6μU/ml when blood glucose in < 40 mg/dl

The most reliable test is a fast upto 72 hours with serum glucose, C-peptide and insulin levels measurements every 4-8 hours

261. Answer is D (Appendix); *Harrison 16th/ 2223; Harrison 17th/2349; Harrison 18th/p 3058*

Among the given option the most common site of carcinoid tumour is appendix.

Carcinoid tumor location, Frequency of Metastases, and Association with the Carcinoid Syndrome

Site	Location (% of Total)	Incidence of Metastases	Incidence of Carcinoid Syndrome
Foregut			
Esophagus	<0.1	-	-
Stomach	4.6	10	9.5
Duodenum	2.0	-	3.4
Pancreas	0.7	71.9	20
Gallbladder	0.3	17.8	5
Bronchus, lung, trachea	*27.9*	5.7	13
Midgut			
Jejunum	1.8	} 58.4	9
Ileum	*14.9*		9
Meckel's diverticulum	0.5	-	13
Appendix	*4.8*	38.8	<1
Colon	*8.6*	51	5
Liver	0.4	32.2	-
Ovary	1.0	32	50
Testis	<0.1	-	50
Hindgut			
Rectum	*13.6*	3.9	-

262. Answer is D (Foregut carcinoids are usually argentaffin positive): *Harrison's 18th/3058*

Foregut tumors (carcinoids) have low serotonin levels and are argentaffin negative.

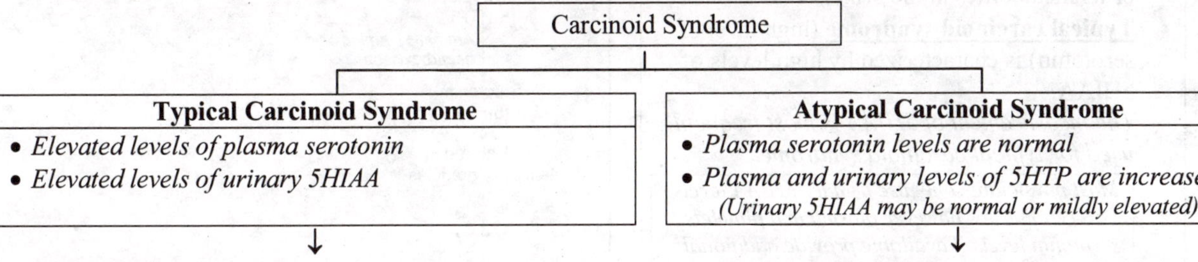

Typical carcinoid syndrome is charachteristic of Midgut carcinoids

Atypical carcinoid syndrome is charachteristic of foregut carcinoids

Midgut Carcinoids: Typical Carcinoid Syndrome	Foregut Carcinoids: Atypical Carcinoid Syndrome
• Midgut tumors have high serotonin content are ***Argentaffin positive***[Q] • Most frequently cause a 'typical' carcinoid syndrome when they metastize. • Release serotonin and tachykinins (neuropeptide K. substance K, substances P) **Rarely secrete 5HTP or ACTH** • Metastatis to bone is uncommon (less common)	• Foregut tumor have low serotonin content, are ***argentaffin negative but argyrophillic***[Q] • Usually do not produce carcinoid syndrome but when they produce a carcinoid syndrome it is charachtristically usually an Atypical carcinoid syndrome **Occasionally secrete ACTH or 5HTP** • May metastize to bone • Are often multihormonal

263. Answer is D (VMA): *Harrison's 18th/2962, 3058, 3063*

5HIAA, 5HT, 5HTP are metabolites of Tryptophan / Serotonin that may be elevated in carcinoid tumors.

Vanillyl mandilic acid (VMA) *is the principal metabolite of catecholamines secreted by adrenal medulla. Elevated VMA levels in urine is a feature of increased catecholamine secreting tumors, typically pheochromocytomas (and not carcinoid tumors).*

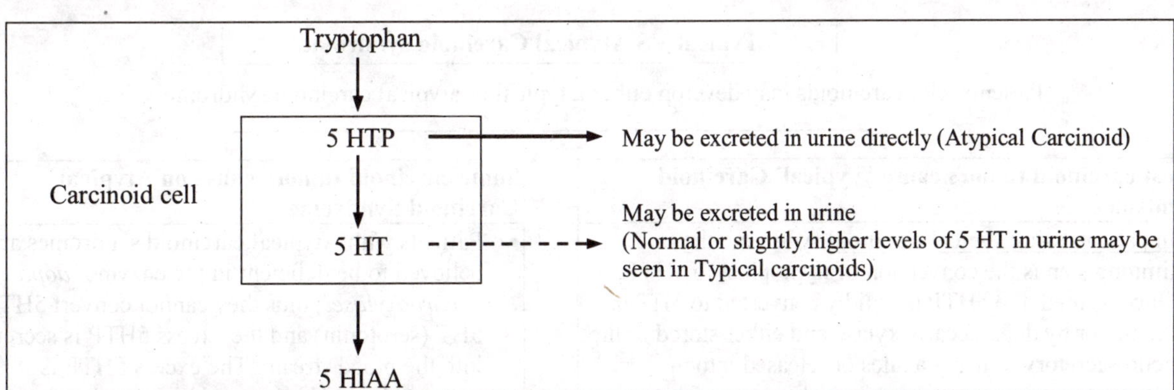

264. Answer is A (5HIAA): *Harrison's 18th/3058, 3063*

The diagnosis of typical carcinoid tumors is done by measurement of 5HIAA levels.

Diagnosis of Carcinoid Tumors *(Harrison)*

- The diagnosis of carcinoid syndrome relies on measurement of urinary or plasma serotonin or its metabolites in the urine.
- **Typical carcinoid syndrome** (high level of serotonin) is characterized by high levels of 5HIAA.
  The measurement of 5HIAA is most frequently used for typical carcinoid syndrome.

  Most physicians' only use urinary 5HIAA levels / excretion rates however plasma and platelets serotonin levels if available provide additional information. Platelet serotonin levels (5-HT) are more sensitive than urinary 5HIAA levels but are not generally available.
- **Atypical carcinoid syndromes** (low levels of serotonin) may have normal or minimally elevated 5HIAA levels.
- In such patient's urinary levels of other tryptophan metabolites such as 5HTP should be measured.

  Elevated levels of urinary 5 HTP is suggestive of an atypical carcinoid syndrome

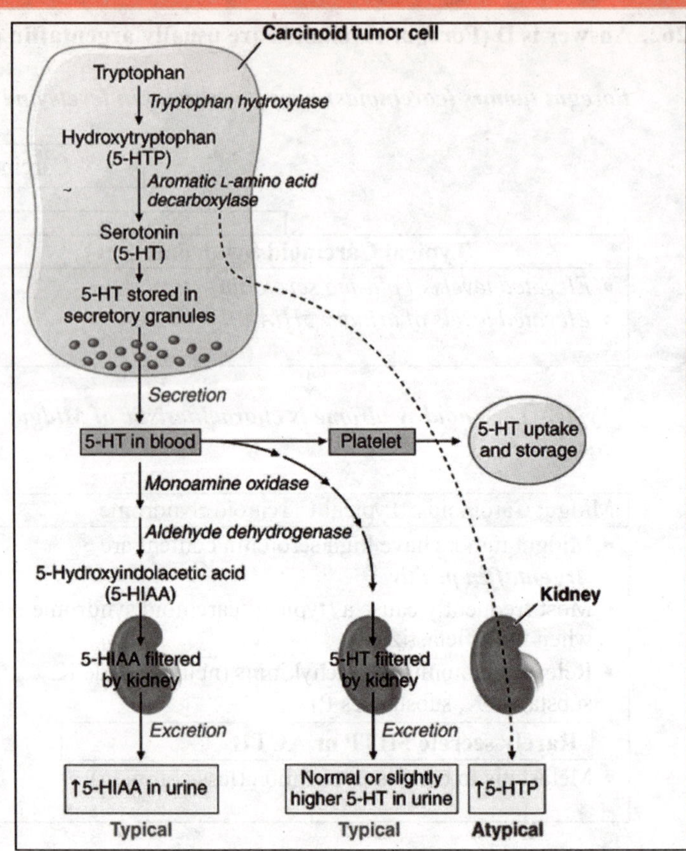

265. Answer is B (5 HTP): *Harrison's 18th ; Devita*

Elevated levels of urinary 5 HTP is suggestive of an atypical carcinoid syndrome

Note that patients with atypical carcinoid syndrome may have elevated levels of 5HT, 5HTP and 5HIAA, but the presence of increased urinary 5HTP is most typical feature to suggest on Atypical carcinoid.

Typical VS Atypical Carcinoid syndrome

Patients with carcinoids may develop either a typical or atypical carcinoid syndrome

Most carcinoid tumors cause 'Typical' Carcinoid syndrome	Some carcinoid tumors cause on Atypical Carcinoid Syndrome
• In patients with Typical carcinoid syndrome the rate limiting step is the conversion of tryptophan to 5HTP. Once formed, the 5HTP is rapidly converted to 5HT in the tumor by dopa decarboxylase and either stored in the neurosecretory tumor granules or released into the vascular compartment where it is taken a up and stored in the granules of platelets. A small amount remains in the plasma. The majority in the circulation is converted by monoamine oxidase and Aldehyde dehydrogenase to 5 HIAA, which appears in large amounts in the urine. This is the typical pattern in orgentaffin and argyrophilic tumors the midgut carcinoids which charachteristically secrete large amounts of serotonin (and comprise the majority of cases of carcinoid syndrome)	• Patients with Atypical carcinoid syndromes are believed to be deficient in the enzyme *'dopa decarboxylase'*; thus they cannot convert 5HTP to 5HT (serotonin) and the excess 5HTP is secreted into the blood stream. The excess 5HTP is excreted by the kidney and high levels of urinary 5HTP are observed • Plasma levels of serotonin are normal in these patients but urinary levels of 5HT are usually elevated because some of the 5 HTP is decarboxylated in the kidney and excreted as 5HT in the urine. • Levels of 5HIAA may be normal (or minimally elevated).

266. Answer is B (Rectum is spared): *Harrison 17th/2350, 2351; Sleisenger and Fordtran's Gastrointestinal & Liver diseases 8th/609; SEER National Registry Database Official Publication.; Harrison 18th/p 3061, 3062*

Rectum is not spared from carcinoids.

'Rectum is a common site of carcinoids (19% of all carcinoids) and the incidence appears to be rising'

– Sleisenger and Fordtran's 8th/609

Rectum is a common site of carcinoid tumors (It is not spared)

Rectum is a common site of carcinoid tumors in the gastrointestinal tract accounting for almost 19% of all carcinoid tumors of the GI tract in the late SEER registry (1992-1999).

It is the second most frequent site of Carcinoids after the ileum in accordance with the Pan SEER registry (1973-1999).

Carcinoid site	Early SEER (1973-1991)	Late SEER (1992-1999)	Pan SEER (1973-1999)
Gastrointestinal tract	61.57	67.55	64.31
Esophagus	0.05	0.06	0.06
Stomach	3.55	5.85	4.61
Small intestine	28.82	28.22	28.54
Duodenum	1.94	3.83	2.80
Jejunum	2.11	1.48	1.81
Ileum	16.23	13.35	14.92
Not specified	7.86	8.74	8.26
Colon	9.48	7.62	8.62
Appendix	6.76	2.43	4.77
Rectum	9.44	18.54	13.61

Small intestine and appendix account for almost 60% of gastrointestinal carcinoids

Small intestine and appendix together account for about 58% (≈60%) of gastrointestinal carcinoids according to the data from early SEER (1973-1991) and for about 51% of gastrointestinal carcinoids from the Pan SEER data (1973-1999)

Although the statement (option A) is not entirely correct in view of the late SEER registry and/or the Pan SEER data, this may be accepted as a 'true statement' for the purpose of the question.

Site Specific incidence rate of Carcinoid Tumors

The reported anatomic distribution of carcinoid tumors varies widely amongst different textbooks depending on the source of data quoted.

Several textbooks including Schwartz and Sabiston, continue to mention Appendix as the most common site of gastrointestinal carcinoids however these incidence rates are based on old data before the 1970's and most studies thereafter report other locations as being more frequent. Results from Surveillance, Epidemiology and End Results (SEER) natural registry are now accepted as standard (Harrison.)

Five year survival is > 60%.

The five survival for all gstrointestinal carcinoids is getaer than 60 percent

5 Year Survival	Early SEER	Late SEER	Pan SEER
All Gastrointestinol Carcinoids	≈57%	≈68%	≈62.5%

Appendecial carcinoids are more common in females

'Appendecial carcinoids are more coomon in females. Two of Three cases of appendecial carcinoids are females.' - Sleisenger & Fordtradn 8th/609

The evaluation of carcinoid tumors by Pan-SEER (1973-1999) reveals a slight overall female predominance in all type of carcinoid tumors (55%).

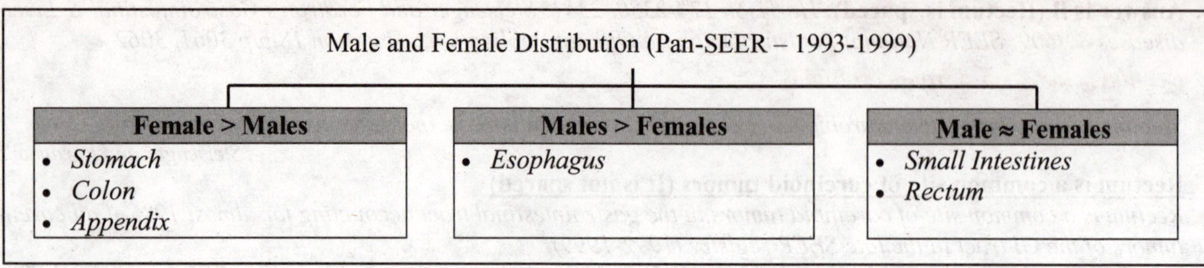

267. Answer is B (Tricuspid valve); *Harrison 16th/ 2224; Harrison 17th/2351; Harrison 18th/p 3062*

The most common site of involvement is the – Ventricular surface of Tricuspid valve.

'Cardiac manifestations in carcinoid syndrome are due to fibrosis involving the endocardium, primarily on the right side although left side lesions also occur. Dense fibrous deposits are most commonly on the ventricular aspect of the tricuspid valve and less commonly on the pulmonary valve cusps.' – Harrison 16th

They can result in either constriction of valves (stenosis) or fixation of valves in open (regurgitation)

- Abnormality produced due to *tricuspid valve involvement – Tricuspid regurgitation* [Q]
- Abnormality produced due to *pulmonary valve involvement – Pulmonary stenosis* [Q]

Weight Gain & Obesity

268. Answer is A (Pheochromocytoma): *Harrison 16th/ 234, 424, 425, 426; Harrison 15th/ 481; Harrison 17th/ 255, 2269; Harrison 18th/p 2963*

Pheochromocytoma causes weight loss.

Causes of weight gain (obesity):

Specific syndromes	Genetic syndromes
1. *Cushing's syndrome* [Q]	1. *Prader – willi syndrome*
2. *Hypothyroidism* [Q]	2. *Laurence Moom Biedl syndrome*
3. *Insulinoma* [Q]	3. *Ahistrom syndrome*
4. *Craniopharyngioma and other disorders involving the hypothalamus*	4. *Cohen syndrome*
	5. *Carpenter syndrome*

269. Answer is A (Diabetes mellitus) : *Harrison 16th/ 234; Harrison 17th/ 255, 2269; Harrison 18th/p 2963*

Endocrine and metabolic causes of weight loss include
1. Hyperthyroidism
2. Diabetes mellitus
3. Pheochromocytoma
4. Adrenal insufficiency

270. Answer is B (Adrenal insufficiency) : *See previous question*

271. Answer is A (Pheochromocytoma): *Harrison 17th/255, 2269; Harrison 18th/p 2963*

Pheochromocytoma is associated with weight loss and not weight gain.

272. Answer is D (Insulinoma) : *Harrison 16th/234 (t36-1), 2227*

Insulinoma is characterised by an increase in weight (weight gain)

Weight gain may result from increased food ingested to combat symptoms of hypoglycemia.

Classic presentation of ***insulinoma*** consists of ***'Whipple's triad'*** [Q]: *- Harrison 14th/589*

1. *Fasting hypoglycemia* [Q]
2. *Symtoms of hypoglycemia* [Q]
3. *Immediate relief after I.V. glucose administration* [Q]

Causes of weight loss include:

A. Increased energy expenditure	C. Diminished food intake
1. Hyperthyroidism Q	*1. Cancer* Q
2. ***Pheochromocytoma*** Q	*2. Infection* Q
3. Extensive exercise Q	*3.* ***Uremia*** Q
B. Increased energy loss	*4. Anorexia nervosa* Q
1. Diabetes mellitus Q	*5.* ***Adrenal insufficiency*** Q
2. Malabsorption syndromes Q	*6. Hypercalcemia (malignancy, Hyper PTH, sarcoidosis)* Q
	7. Alzeimer's disease Q
	8. Depression Q

273. Answer is D (Pancreatitis): *Harrison 16th/426, 427; Harrison 17th/ 255, 469, 470; Harrison 18th/p 629, 631*

Pancreatitis has no association with obesity.

RISKS OF OBESITY INCLUDE THE FOLLOWING :

A. **Cardiovascular disease :**
- increased risk of *atherosclerosis* Q
- increased risk of *hypertension* Q
- increased risk of *sudden death* Q

B. **Pulmonary function :** *Sleep apnea* and *Right heart failure* Q

C. **Gall bladder disease :** Increased incidence of *Gall stones* Q

D. **Joint :**
- Increased risk of *osteoarthritis* Q : partly due to added trauma of increased weight bearing
- Increased incidence of *Gout* Q : due to impairment in urate clearance.

E. **Diabetes mellitus** : *Type II diabetes mellitus* Q is almost always seen in the obese.

F. **Cancer :** Increased incidence of
- *endometrial carcinoma* Q
- *post menopausal breast cancer* Q
- *prostate cancer* Q
- *colorectal carcinoma*

G. **Skin :** Increased incidence of *Acanthosis nigricans* Q

H. **Endocrine :**
- *Insulin Resistance* Q : leading to Hyperinsulinemia is directly related to degree of obesity.
- Growth hormone Q : secretions is reduced but IGF-I levels are normal thus growth is not affected.
- *Testosterone level is reduced.* Q

Miscellaneous

274. Answer is B (Associated with lactation): *Harrison 17th/2205; Harrison 18th/p 2888*

Galactorrhea is defined as inappropriate secretion of milk containing fluid from the breast. Secretion of milk during lactation is physiological / appropriate and hence can not be termed as Galactorrhea.

Galactorrhea may be Bilateral

Galactorrhea may arise either unilaterally or bilaterally – *Harrison*

Galactorrhea may be associated with Prolactinomas

'Prolactinomas are the most common pathological cause of Galactorrhea in adolescent of both sexes'.

- Current Pediatrics 18th/124

275. Answer is B (Prolactin): *Harrison 16th/2192, 2193; Harrison 17th/2318; Harrison 18th/p 3019*

Gynaecomastia does not result from either excess or deficiency of prolactin.

Gynaecomastia may result from deficient testosterone or increased estrogen.

'Prolactin' *causes synthesis of milk in the female breast, and its excess results in galactorrhea. It also opposes the action of pituitary gonadotrophins on the gonads and may thus result in hypogonadism and amenorrhea.*

Gynaecomastia does not result from either excess or deficiency of prolactin.

Endocrine work up for Gynaecomastia includes:

1. *Measurement of serum androstenedione or 24hr urinary 17 ketosteroids* (usually elevated in feminizing adrenal states)
2. *Measurement of plasma **estradiol** and hcG.*
3. *Measurement of plasma **LH** and **testosterone***

276. Answer is B (Sertoli cell tumour) : *Harrison 15th/2171; (Refer Harrison 15th)*

Decreased levels of Leutenizing hormone and testosterone suggest a disorder of increased primary estrogen production such as Sertoli cell tumors provided hypogonadotrophic hypergonadism has been excluded. Because hypogonadotrophic hypogonadism has not been mentioned in the options, the answer of choice is Sertoli cell tumor.

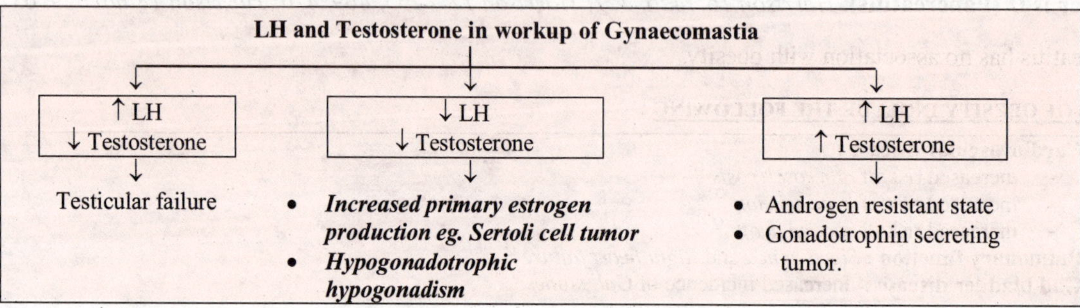

277. Answer is B (46XY) : *Harrison 16th/2218; Harrison 17th/ 2344; Harrison 18th/p 3019*

Individual with 'androgen insensitivity syndrome' are XY individuals (male karyotype) with a female phenotype. *Mutation in the androgen receptor causes resistance to androgen action and the androgen insensitivity syndrome results.*

278. Answer is B (46 XY) : *Harrison 16th/2218; Harrison 17th/ 2344; Harrison 18th/p 3051, 3053*

This is a case of testicular feminization syndrome or complete androgen sensitivity syndrome. *The characteristic feature as explained in the previous question is that phenotypically they present as females while genotypically they are males with an **XY karyotype.***
'Most patients present with an inguinal hernia containing testes in childhood or with primary amenorrhea in adulthood'.- Harrison

279. Answer is D (Complete androgen insensitivity syndrome) *Harrison 16th/2218; Harrison 17th/2344*

The patient in question presents as a 21 year old women (truly feminine appearance) with well-developed breasts, no hiruitism, no pubic or axillary hair with primary amenorrhea. All features thus mentioned lead to a diagnosis of complete androgen insensitivity.

Complete androgen insensitivity syndrome : syn: complete testicular feminization:
(Common form of male pseudohermaphroditism)

A 46 XY karyotypic male presents with a truly feminine appearance with complaints of primary amenorrhea (third most common cause of primary amenorrhea after gonadal dysgenesis and congenital absence of vagina)

- Mature breast development
- Habitus and distribution of body fat are female in character
- Scalp hair is that of normal women and facial hair is absent (no hiruitism)
- External genitalia is unambiguously female and clitoris is normal
- Internal genitalia : All internal genitalia are absent except testes that contain normal leydig cells and seminiferous tubules but without spermatogenesis.

Also remember:

- *The testes may be located in the abdomen, along the course of inguinal canal or in the labia majora (undescended testes)* [Q]
- *The major complication of undescended testes in this disorder is the development of tumors.* [Q]

Turner's Syndrome : Gonadal dysgenesis

A phenotypic female presents with primary amenorrhea. Pubic and axillary hair remain sparse and *breasts are infantile (patient in question has mature breasts)*

Stein Leventhal syndrome: Polycystic ovarian disease: *Harrison 15th / 2163*
This is *characterized by Hirsuitism (patient in question has no hiruitism)* along with amenorrhea / oligomenorrhea, obesity and infertility.

Premature ovarian failure: Presents with *secondary amenorrhea* and not primary amenorrhea.

280. Answer is C (Testicular feminization syndrome): *Harrison 16th/2218, Refer previous question, http://www.mcg.edv/pediatric/ccivotebook/chapter3/tanner.htm; Harrison 17th/ 2344; Harrison 18th/p 3051, 3053*

Presence of well developed breast (tanner stage 4) with scanty axillary or pubic hair in a phenotypic 'female' with primary amenorrhea (? no uterus) suggests the diagnosis of Testicular feminization syndrome.

Testicular Feminization Syndrome / Complete Androgen Insensitivity :	*– Harrison 16th*
• Resistance to androgens due to mutation in androgen receptors • Genotype is XY • Phenotype is **female**	XY Genotype Resistance to androgens due to mutation in androgen receptors Female Phenotype and Female psychosexual development • Normal breast (tanner stage 4 or 5) • Short vagina but no uterus (primary amenorrhea) • ***Scanty pubic and axillary hair***

Tanner stage 4 breasts indicate well developed breasts

Tanner Stage	Stage of develop	Pubic Hair	Breasts
Stage 1	Early adolescence (10 - 13 years)	Preadolescent	Preadolescent
Stage 2		Sparse, straight	Small mound
Stage 3	Middle adolescence (12 - 14 years)	Dark, curl	Bigger, no contour separation
Stage 4		Coarse, curly, abundant	Secondary mound of areola
Stage 5	(14 - 17 years)	Triangle; medial thigh	Nippler projects; areola part of breast

281. Answer is B (McCune Albright syndrome); *Stedman's /1760; 16th/2284; Harrison 17th/ 2413; Harrison 18th/p 3142*

McCune Albright syndrome'
• *Polyostotic form of fibrous dysplasia*
• *Cutaneous pigmentation*
• *Endocrine dysfunction, especially Precocious puberty in girls.*

The triad of symptoms in the question thus characterizes McCune Albright syndrome and hence is the answer.

282. Answer is C (Kallman's syndrome): *Harrison's 17th/2316, 2317; Harrison 18th/p 3017, 3018*

Kallman's syndrome is associated with hypogonadotrophic hypogonadism and not hypergonadotrophic hypogonadism

Kallman's syndrome is an X-Linked disorder *characterized by deficiency of GnRH with a resultant decrease in FSH and LH levels producing an isolated Hypogonadotrophic Hypogonadism.* Kallman's syndrome may be seen in both men and women but is more common in men. It is typically also associated with agenesis or hypoplasia of the olfactory bulb producing anosmia or hyposmia.

Klinefelter's syndrome – Noonan syndrome and viral orchitis *may all be associated with hypergonadotrophic hypogonadism in men.* These disorders are associated with primary testicular dysfunction (gonadal failure) and result in high gonadotrophin levels *(hypergonadotrophic)* since the thalamus and pituitary function normally.

Causes of Hypergonadotrophic Hypogonadism in Males (Primary Testicular Failure)
• ***Klinefelter's syndrome***
• ***Noonan syndrome (Nelson's)***
• *Cryptorchidism*
• ***Testicular Infections (Infectious orchitis)***
• *Testicular Trauma or Torsion*
• *Cancer chemotherapy and Radiation*
• *Anorchia syndrome (testicular agenesis)*
• *Myotonic Dystrophy (testicular atrophy)*

283. Answer is B (Klinefelter's syndrome): *Harrison's 17th/2317; Manual of Endocrinology and Metabolism (Lippincott Williams) 4th/291; NMS Medicine 6th/437; Nelson' 17th/2379, 2380; Pediatric Endocrine disorders 1st (2001) / 131; Harrison 18th/p 3018*

Klinefelter's syndrome is the most common cause of hypergonadotrophic hypogonadism in males

'*Klinefelter's syndrome is the commonest cause of male hypergonadotrophic hypogonadism among primary gonadal disorders'* – *Pediatric Endocrine Disorders*

'*Klinefelter's syndrome constitutes the most common cause of mole hypogonadism'*

- Spiral Manual of Endocrinology and Metabolism

284. Answer is D (Addison's disease): *CMDT 2008/716*

Addison's disease is not associated with carpal tunnel syndrome

Endocrinal Causes of Carpal Tunnel Syndrome
• *Acromegaly (CMDT)*
• *Hypothyroidism (Myxoedema) (Harrison's)*
• *Hyperparathyroidism (CMDT)*
• *Diabetes Mellitus (Harrison's')*

285. Answer is B (Hyperthyroidism): *Harrison's 17th/301; Harrison 18th/p 381*

Hyperthyroidism is not associated with Hirsuitism

Cushing's Syndrome, Hyperprolactinemia and Acromegaly are established endocrinal causes of Hirsuitism.

Causes of Hirsutism:

Gonadal hyperandrogenism	
Ovarian hyperandrogenism	
Polycystic ovary syndrome/functional ovarian hyperandrogenism	
Ovarian steroidogenic blocks	
Syndromes of extreme insulin resistance	
Ovarian neoplasms	
Adrenal hyperandrogenism	
Premature adrenarche	
Functional adrenal hyperandrogenism	
Congenital adrenal hyperplasia (nonclassic and classic)	
Abnormal cortisol action/metabolism	
Adrenal Neoplasms	
Other endocrine disorders	
Cushing's syndrome Hyperprolactinemia Acromegaly	
Peripheral androgen overproduction	
Obesity	*Idiopathic*
Pregnancy-related hyperandrogenism	
Hyperreactio luteinalis	*Thecoma of pregnancy*
Drugs	
Androgens	*Oral contraceptives containing androgenic progestins*
Minoxidil	*Phenytoin*
Diazoxide	*Cyclosporine*
True hermaphroditism	

286. Answer is B (Hypercalcemia): *Harrison 17th /2380, 286; Harrison's 18th/313; Diarrhea' by Guandalini (springer, 2011)/359*

Hypercalcemia is typically associated with constipation (and not diarrhea).

Diabetes Mellitus, Hyperthyroidism and Carcinoids are all established causes of 'Endocrinal Diarrhea'.

Causes of Endocrinal Diarrhea *('Diarrhea' by Guondolini (Springer, 2011/359))*
Neoplastic causes
• Carcinoid syndrome • Gastrinoma • Somatostatinoma • VIPoma • Medullary carcinoma of thyroid • Mastocytosis*
Non-neoplastic causes

• Diabetes mellitus
• Thyroid disorders
  - Thyrotoxicosis
  - Hypothyroidism
• Adrenal gland disorders
  - Addison's disease
  - Autoimmune polyglandular syndromes type I and II
• X-linked immune deficiency with polyendocrinopathy and diarrhea (IPEX)

287. Answer is B (Small cell carcinoma): *Robbins 7th/762*

Small cell carcinomas are the most common bronchogenic carcinomas associated with paraneoplastic syndrome and ectopic hormone production including ACTH.

ACTH may also be uncommonly produced by non small cell variants including adenocarcinoma and squamous carcinomas, but small cell carcinoma is the most common source of ectopic ACTH.

'Small cell carcinoma lung (>50%) is by for the most common cause of ectopic ACTH production followed by Thymic carcinoids (15%), islet cell tumors (10%), bronchial carcinoids (10%), other carcinoids (5%) and pheochromocytomas (2%) - Harrison's 18th/829

Ectopic ACTH Production (Bold)
• *Small cell carcinoma (50) Lung* • *Thymic carcinoids (15%)* • *Islet cell tumors (10%)* • *Bronchial carcinoid (10%)* • *Other carcinoids (5%)* • *Pheochromocytomas (2%)*

NOTES

Nervous System

ESSENTIAL REVISION NOTES

Headache

Migraine and Cluster Headache

Migraine	Cluster Headache
• *Lateralised* Q, usually frontotemporal may be generalised • *All age groups* Q are affected • *Females* Q are affected more than males • *Family history present* Q • Presentation : Pain - *often preceded by aura* Q - *builds up gradually* Q - may lasts for *several hours* Q or longer - usually *throbbing* Q but may be dull - onset is *after awakening* Q*&quietened by sleep* Q • Associated symptoms include : - *nausea, vomiting, diarrhea* Q - *photophobia and visual disturbance* Qin the form of *photopsia and fortification spectra* Q - *paraestheisias with tingling and numbness* Q - other *focal neurological symptoms* Qsuch as clumsiness *and weakness* Q.	• *Lateralized* Q, *periorbital* Q or less commonly temporal • All ages *above 10 yrs* Q with *peak at 30-50 yrs* Q • *Male preponderance* Q (90%). Men affected 7-8 times more than females. • *Hereditary factors usually absent* Q • Presentation: Pain (periodic attacks 1-2/day) - begins *without warning* Q - reaches *crescendo within 5 minutes*Q - lasts for *45 minutes*Q - *excruciating, deep, explosive* pain but only *rarely pulsatile* Q - commonly *awakens the patients from sleep*Q • Associated symptoms : These are typical and characteristic : Q - *homolateral lacrimation* Q - *reddening of eye*Q - *nasal stuffiness*Q - *Ptosis* Q, *and* - *nausea* Q

Cluster headache affects predominantly males. Men are affected 3 times more often than women. *Harrison 17th/101*

Common Migraine and Classical Migraine

Common Migraine (Migraine without aura)	Classical Migraine (Migraine with aura)
• This is characterized by headache with autonomic system dysfunction (eg. pallor & nausea, vomiting), but without stereotypical neurological or ophthalmic features as in classical migraine • Premonitory features include changes in mood frequent yawning or nonspecific prodromal symptoms like loss of concentration • Headache starts anywhere in the cranium and is pounding or throbbing • It usually spreads to involve one half or even the whole head. • During the attack which lasts from hours to a day or more patient is frequently photophobia and phonophobic and seeks relief in quiet dark environment, or through sleep.	• This is characterized by headache heralded by a visual aura which lasts about 20 minutes. • Visual aura may consist of bright or dark spots, zig zags, heat haze distortions, fig san puzzle defects scintillating scotoma, tunnel vision or fortification spectra which may progress to homonymous hemianopia. • The headache follows the aura and is usually hemicranial opposite the hemianopia. • During the attacK patient has associated nausea and photophobia.

Basilar Type Migraine (subtype of migraine with aura)

- Basilar type migraine describes recurrent attacks of migraine with aura in which symptoms suggest a brainstem origin ***(including vertigo & ataxia)***
- ***The onset of Basilar type migraine is typically before 30 years ofage*** and peaks during adolescence
- ***There is a distinct female preponderance*** with girls more frequently affected than boys in a ratio of 3:1 *(majority of sufferers are girls)*
- ***Family history of migraine is frequent***
- ***Unlike other types of migraine headache may be occipital in origin***

9

Nervous System

Management of Migraine

The drugs of choice for management of acute attack of Migaine are Triptans *(e.g. Sumatriptan)*

Triptans

- Triptans are selective agonists at 5HT 1B/1D Receptors
- A variety of Triplans are now available for the management of acute migraine

Triptans

Fast Acting

- *Rizatriptan*
- *Eletriptan*
- *Sumatriptan*
- *Zolmipriptan*
- *Almotriptan (relatively slower)*

Slow Acting / Better tolerability

- *Naratriptan*
- *Frovatriptan*

These agents have longer half life

- *Rizatriptan and Electriptan are the most efficacious of the triptans currently available in the US'. - Harrison*

Efficacy appears to be related more to t max (time to peak plasma levels) than to the potency half life or bioavailability

- Almatriptan, Noratriptan and Fravotriptan are somewhat slower in onset and better tolerated.

Treatment of Acute Migraine

Drugs

Simple Analgesics
Acetaminophen, aspirin, caffeine
NSAIDs
Naproxen
Ibuprofen
Tolfenamic acid
5-HT$_1$ Agonists
Oral
Ergotamine
Ergotamine 1 mg, Caffeine 100 mg
Naratriptan
Rizatriptan
Sumatriptan
Frovatriptan
Almotriptan
Eletriptan
Zolmitriptan
Nasal
Dihydroergotamine
Sumatriptan
Zolmitriptan
Parenteral
Dihydroergotamine
Sumatriptan

Dopamine Antagonists
Oral
Metoclopramide
Prochlorperazine
Parenteral
Chlorpromazine
Metoclopramide
Prochlorperazine
Other
Oral
Acetaminophen, 325 mg, *plus* dichloralphenazone, 100 mg, *plus* isometheptene, 65 mg
Nasal
Butorphanol
Parenteral
Narcotics

Preventive Treatment of Migraine (Chronic migraine)

Drugs

Pizotifen
Beta blocker
Propranolol
Tricyclics
Amitriptyline
Dothiepin
Nortriptyline
Anticonvulsants
Topiramate
Valproate
Gabapentin
Serotonergic drugs
Methysergide
Flunarizine
No convincing evidence from controlled trials
Verapamil
Controlled trials demonstrate *no effect*
Nimodipine
Clonidine
SSRIs: fluoxetine

Tension Headache :

- Is a chronic head pain syndrome characterised by tight band like discomfort
- Headaches is usually ***generalised***may be most intense about the neck or back of the head.
- Patients frequently complain of poor concentration and other vague non specific symptoms
- May be ***exacerbated by emotional stress***, fatigue, noise or glare.
- It is not associated with focal neurological symptoms.

Aphasia

Aphasias *are disorders of understanding, thought and word finding and represent a lesion in the dominant (usually left) hemisphere*

	Broca's apahasia	Wernicke's apahsia
Lesion site^{Q}	• Lesion in Broca's area (inferior frontal gyrus) *Dominant Hemisphere*	• Lesion lies in Wernicke's area (supramarginal gyrus) of the parietal lobe and upper part of temporal lobe *(Dominant Hemisphere)*
Cause^{Q}	• Lesion is due to occlusion of superior br. of middle cerebral artery	• Lesion is due to occlusion of inferior division of middle cerebral artery.
Comprehension	• Comprehension is preserved (except grammar)	• Comprehension is impaired
Fluency^{Q}	• Decreased Speech is not fluent, laboured, dysarthric, and interrupted with many word-finding pauses. It is telegraphic but informative	• Preserved or increased: Speech is fluent but is highly paraphasic and associated with neologisms (Jagron Ahasia)
Naming^{Q}	• Impaired	• Impaired
Repetition^{Q}	• Impaired	• Impaired
Neologism^{Q}	• Absent	• Present
Insight	• Insight into condition is preserved	• Not preserved

Aphasia occur when the lesion lies in the dominant (usually left) hemisphere
Repetition is impaired in both Broca's and Wernicke's aphasias
Senseless, fluent speech suggests a diagnosis of 'Wernicke's' Aphasia

Anomic aphasia: Remember:

Most common language disturbance seen in - Head trauma = Anomic Apahsia^{Q}
Most common language disturbance seen in - Metabolic encephalopathy = Anomic Apahsia^{Q}
Most common language disturbance seen in - Alzheimer's disease = Anomic Apahsia^{Q}

• Defect in hearing:	Deafness
• Defect in understanding:	Receptive aphasia / Sensory aphasia
• Defect in thought and word finding:	Motor / Expressive aphasia
• Defect in voice production:	Dysphonia
• Defect in articulation:	Dysarthric

UMN vs LMN lesions

UMN	*LMN*
1. ***Power***: *Decreased* *Weakness*; Q (Muscle groups or Limbs being affected & not individual muscles Q) 2. ***Tone*** : Hypertonia = *Clasp knife spasticity* Q 3. ***Wasting / Atrophy***: Minimal, if present and due to disuse atrophy. 4. ***Reflexes*** *Superficial Reflexes* : Lost Q *Deep reflexes* : Brisk/Exaggerated Q *Clonus* : May be + nt Q *Plantar* : Extensor Q 5. ***Fasciculations***: Absent Q 6. ***Reaction of degeneration in muscles***: absent Q	1. ***Power***: Very much decreased *Weakness* (severe) due to paralysis of individual muscles. Q 2. ***Tone***: Flaccidity (Hypotonia) Q 3. ***Wasting / Atrophy***is marked (cardinal feature) Q 4. ***Reflexes*** *Superficial reflexes* : Lost Q *Deep reflexes* : Exaggerated Q *Clonus* : Absent Q *Plantar* : Flexor or no response Q 5. ***Fasciculations*** : Present Q 6. ***Reaction of degeneration in muscles*** : Present Q

Bulbar Palsy and Pseudobulbar Palsy

Paralysis of Speech and Swallowing

Bulbar Palsy	Pseudobulbar Palsy
LMN paralysis from a lesion of the bulb (medulla) or its nerves (IX, X and XII)	***UMN paralysis*** from a lesion that is neither in the bulb (medulla) or its nerves (IX, X or XIIth)
Anatomistsvisualized the medulla asa bulb like expansion of the spinal cord and hence referred to the medulla as 'the bulb'	

	Bulbar	Pseudobulbar
Dysarthria	***Yes***	***Yes***
Dysphagia	***Yes***	***Yes***
Movement of palate		
Voluntary	*No*	*No*
Gag reflex	*No*	*Yes*
Respiratory impairment	*Yes*	*No*
Jaw jerk	***Hypoactive***	***Hyperactive***
Emotional lability	***No***	***Yes***
Intellectual impairment	*No*	*Yes*

Jaw jerk is exaggerated in supranuclear lesions that are above the mid pons.

Exaggerated Jaw Jerk

Jaw jerk is exaggerated in supranuclear lesions that are above the mid pons
Jaw Jerk is helpful in localization of the lesion to the brainstem.
It depends on the mesencephalic tract of the 5th cranial nerve, which mediates proprioceptive information from jaw muscles.

Common cause of exaggerated jaw jerk include

- *Neurodegenerative diseases with generalized loss of cortical inhibition*
- ***Pseudobulbar palsy***
- ***Motor neuron disease***
- ***Multiple sclerosis***

Shock associated with spinal cord injury

Acute Spinal Cord Injury

Spinal Shock	Neurogenic Shock
• *Refers to flaccidity and loss of reflexes seen after spinal cord injury.* • The 'shock' here is to the 'injured cord', which makes it appear completely functionless although all areas are not necessary destroyed. • The duration of spinal shock is variable.	• Produced as a result of loss of sympathetic tone. • It results from impairment of the descending sympathetic pathways in the spinal cord. • Classical picture of Neurogenic shock is hypotension without tachycardia or cutaenous vasoconstriction.
• *Complete Motor Paralysis* • *Flaccidity (Flacid Paralysis)* • *Areflexia* • *Anaesthesia* • *Bladder Involvement (Usually areflexic bladder with Urinary retention)*	• *Hypotension* • *Bradycardia* • *Skin hyperaemia and warmth*
The true mechanism of spinal shock after spinal cord injury is not known	*The mechanism of neurogenic shock after spinal cord injury is believed to be disruption of sympathetic flow with preserved and unopposed vagal (parasympathetic) tone*

Pyramidal Tract versus Extra-Pyramidal Tract Lesions

Features	Pyramidal Tract	Extra Pyramidal Tract
Structure involved	*Includes the Corticospinal tract*	*Includes the basal ganglia and cerebellum*
Muscle tone	***Spasticity (clasp-knife rigidity)***	***Plastic (cogwheel rigidity)***
Distribution of hyper tonus	*Flexors of arm and extensors of leg*	*Generalised*
Shortening and lengthening reaction	*Present*	*Absent*
Involuntary movements	***Absent***	***Present***
Tendon reflexes	***Exaggerated***	***Normal***
Babinski sign	***Positive***	***Negative***
Paralysis	*Of voluntary movements*	*No paralysis*

Sensations carried by Posterior Column

Sensations Transmitted by Posterior / Dorsal Column
• ***Fine Touch*** (Sensations requiring fine gradients of intensity / high degree of localization • *Fine Pressure* (Fine degrees of judgement of pressure intensity) • *Vibration* • *Joint Position Sense*

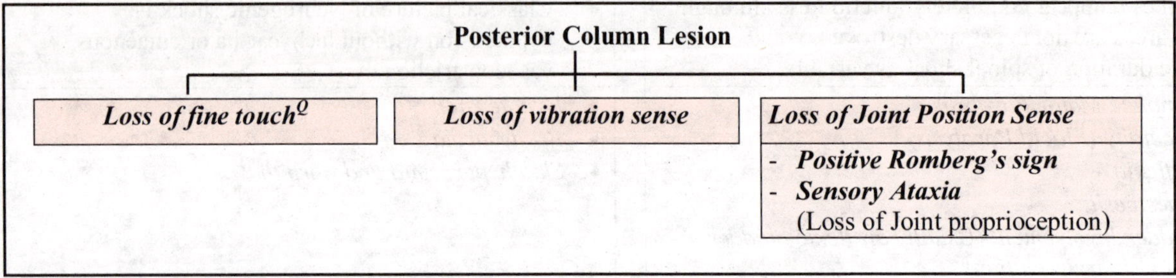

Sensations Transmitted by Anterolateral Column / Spinothalamic Tract[Q]

Sensations Transmitted by Anterolateral Column / Spinothalamic Tract[Q]	
• *Crude Touch*[Q] • *Crude pressure*[Q]	Anterior Spinothalamic tract (ventral)
• *Pain (Pin Prick)* [Q] • *Temperature*[Q]	*Lateral Spinothalamic Tract*

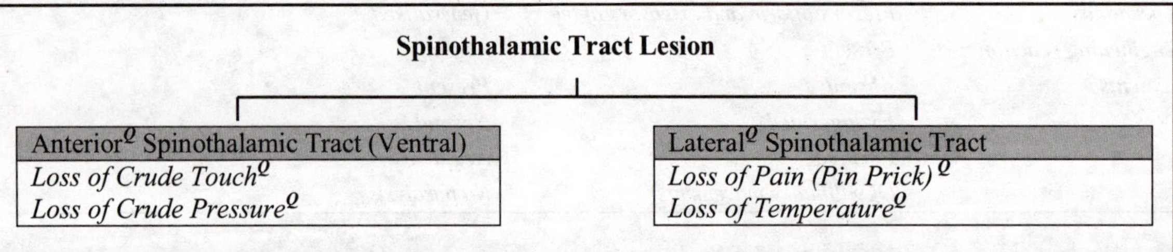

Ventrolateral cordotomy *is a surgical procedures in which the spinal anterolateral ascending system for transmission of nociception (pain) known as the spinothalamic tract is interrupted for the relief of severe, intractible pain* (cancer pain) not responding to any other conventional measures of pain control***Pain sensations from the right leg are carried via the contralateral Lateral Spinothalamic tract. Ventrolateral cordotomy (surgical procedure of ablating selected pain conducting tracts) of the Left Spinothalamic Tract should effectively relieve pain from the right lower extremity.***

Brown-Sequard Syndrome

Brown-Sequard Syndrome (Hemisection of spinal cord) is characterized by lesions of the ipsilateral posterior column and contralateral spinothalamic tract

Brown Sequard Syndrome
(Hemisection of the cord)

Sensations lost on the same side as the lesion	***Motor power is lost on the same side as that of the lesion***	***Sensation lost on the opposite side of lesion***
Sensations transmitted by the posterior column are lost on the same side ***Ipsilateral posterior column involvement***[Q] • *Vibration* • *Joint position (proprioception)*[Q] • *Fine touch*	Motor power controlled by the corticospinal tract is lost on the same side of the lesion ***Ipsilateral corticospinal tract involvement***[Q] • *Loss of voluntary motor power* • *Planter Extensor Response (Positive Babiniski Reflex)* • *Brisk* tendon jerks	Sensations transmitted by the anterolateral spinothalamic tracts are lost on the opposite side ***Contralateral spinothalamic tract involvement***[Q] • *Touch (Crude touch)* • *Pain* • *Temperature*
Fibers from the posterior column ascend in the spinal cord uninterrupted upto the medulla where they decussate (cross-over)	*Unilateral Segmental signs, such as radicular pain, muscle atrophy, or loss of a deep tendon reflex may be seen*	*Fibers from the spinothalamic tract ascend in the spinal cord on the contralateral side after having crossed over at their respective spinal levels*

The pyramidal tract (corticospinal tract) is involved on the same side (ipsilateral pyramidal tract features), which also explains the ipsilateral planter extensor response.
The spinothalamic tract is involved on the contralateral side since fibres of the spinothalamic tract ascends in the spinal cord after having crossed at their respective spinal levels.
The Posterior column is involved on the ipsilateral side

Syringomyelia

- Refers to cavitatory expansion of central canal of spinal cord by chronic progressive destruction of it's grey & white matter.[Q]
- The most commonly involved regions are the '*Lower cervical*' and '*upper thoracic*'.[Q]
- Since the disease usually starts at the base of the posterior horns of the lower cervical spinal cord, it tends to involve the sensory fibres, which cross the midline to form the spinothalamic tract.
- As these fibres carry the sensations for temperature & pain, one of the *earliest signs of disease is an inability to differentiate or appropriate 'Hot and Cold' sensations on the inner side of forearm and hand.*
- *Thermo-anaesthesia*usually precedes the *Analgesia* while *Touch sensitivity is usually preserved* (This leads to Multiple burns and non healing ulcers over the hands and forearms)
- Also note that this particular form of "sensory loss" to temperature & pain with sparing of touch, is described as ***'Dissociate Anaesthesia'***[Q] and is considered as the "***True Hallmark of the disease***"[Q].

Syringomyelia
Disease in which the central canal of the spinal cord becomes enlarged
(Usually in the cervical or upper thoracic levels)

Sensory Features (Early)	**Motor Features (Late)**
• ***Dissociative sensory loss***[Q] *(Loss of pain and temperature with preserved proprioception / touch)* • ***Segmental***[Q] *(confined to a limited number of segments)* • ***Bilateral***[Q] *(since location is central)*	• ***Weakness and Atrophy typically of small muscles of the hand*** due to degeneration of motor neurons in the anterior horn of spinal cord. (Weakness if present is usually more marked in arms than in legs – *central cord syndrome*)

Syringomyeliais characterized by ***bilateral, segmental, dissociative*** sensory loss with ***atrophy & weakness of small muscles of the hand***

Distinguishing features between Extramedullary and Intramedullary Compression of the spinalcord

(Harrisons / API medicine / Paul Bracis – Localization in clinical neurology / Fuller)

Features	*Extra medullary*	*Intramedullary*
Pathological process	*Arise outside the spinal cord (extradural and intradural) and produce symptoms by compressing nerve roots, spinal cord or its vascular supply*	*Arise within the substance of the spinal cord and produce symptoms by invading the spinal cord tracts and grey matter.* Nerve root symptoms are not seen
Pain • **Radicular /Root pain** • *Diffuse burning pain (Funicular)* • **Vertebral pain (Midline back pain)**	 **Common** *Uncommon* **Common**	 **Rare** *Common* **Uncommon**
Motor Weakness **(Corticospinal tract involvement)** *(UMN signs)*	**Occurs early** *Lower extremity is involved earlier than upper extremity* *(Leg fibres in the cortico spinal tract are more superficial/lateral and hence involved early)*	**Occurs late** *Upper extremity is involved earlier than lower extremity* *(Leg fibres are more superficial / lateral and hence involved late)*
Sacral sensations	**Lost (No sacral sparing)** *(Sacral fibres are located outmost within the laminated arrangement of the spinothalamic tract and hence involved early)*	**Spared (sacral sparing)** *(Sacral fibres are located outermost and hence spared)*
Paraesthesias	*Less common* *(Ascending progression)*	*More common* *(Descending prgression)*
Dissociative Anaesthesia	*Absent*	*Present*
Lhermite's sign	*Present*	*Absent*
Autonomic *Bladder Bowel involvement* *(Sphincter abnormalities)*	*Late*	*Early with caudal lesions* *(conus/cauda equina)*
CSF Proteins	**CSF proteins are markedly raised** *in extradural lesion and raised in intradural extra medullary lesions*	**CSF proteins are usually normal** *(May be raised eg conus medullaris lesion)*
Myelogram	*Classic signs* *'Meniscus sign' in intadural tumors* *'Brush border sign' in extradural tumors*	*Classic sign* *'Expansion sign' of the cord is diagnostic of syringomylia*
Imaging / X-ray / CT	*Bony changes or changes in inter vertebral discs are frequent*	*Bony changes/Disc changes are infrequent*

Sacral sparing is a feature of intramedullary tumors and not extramedullary tumors.

'With extramedullary tumors there is early loss of sacral sensations (lateral spinothalamic tract). Intramedullary lesions spare sensations in the perenial and sacral areas (sacral sparing)' - Harrisons

Signs and Symptoms Differentiating Between Lesions of the Conus Medullaris and Cauda Equina

Features	**Conus Medullaris**	**Cauda Equina**
Site of Injury	• Sacral Spinal Cord (conus) + Lumbosacral nerve roots	• Lumbosacral nerve roots (alone)
Nature of lesion (UMN/LMN)	• UMN + LMN *Mixture of UMN paralysis (conus) and LMN paralysis (LS nerve roots)*	• LMN *LMN paralysis alone as cord is not involved*
Babinski	• ***Extensor /Positive (due to UMN lesion)***	***Flexor /Negative (May be absent)***
Tendon Reflexes	• ***Only Ankle Reflex is absent (Knee reflex may be exaggerated)***	***Both Ankle Reflex and Knee reflex may be absent***
Pain (spontaneous)	• Minimal • Not common or severe • Bilateral and Symmetric • In perineum or thighs	• Significant • May be most prominent symptoms, Severe unilateral or asymmetric • In perineum, thighs legs, or back, distribution of sacral nerves • Radolar in type,
Sensory defect	• ***Saddle distribution*** • Bilateral, usually symmetric • Dissociation of sensation may be seen	• ***Saddle distribution*** • May be unilateral and asymmetric • No dissociation of sensation
Motor loss	• Symmetric • Not marked • Fasciculation may be present • Atrophy may occur	• Asymmetric • More marked, • Usually no fasciculations • Atrophy may occur,
Bladder and rectal symptoms	• Early and marked	• Late and less marked
Trophic changes	• Decubti common	• Decubti less marked
Sexual functions	• Erecton and ejaculation impaired	• Less marked impairment
Onset	• Sudden and bilateral	• Gradual and unilateral

Consus Medullaris lesions are associated with absent ankle jerk alone. Knee jerk (Patellar Reflex) is not absent.

Conus medullaris is associated with early and marked bladder involvement.

Loss of bladder control is an early and marked feature of conus medullaris.

Feature	Conus Medullaris	Cauda Equina syndrome	GBS	AMLS
Bladder Involvement	**Early and Marked** *'Bladder dysfunction is a prominent feature and comes early in the course of disease'*	**Late and less marked** *'Bladder involvement is a late presentation in cauda-equina syndrome*	**Uncommon** *'If bladder dysfunction a prominent feature and comes early in the course, diagnostic possibilities other than GBS should be considered*	**Absent /uncommon** 'Even in late stages of the illness bowel and bladder functions are preserved'

Causes of spastic paraplegia:

Spinal cord compression	***Cervical spondylosis*** *Cervical or thoracic disc* *Metastatic tumor* *Primary tumor (meningioma, neurofibroma etc)* *Infective (epidural abscess, spinal TB etc)* *Epidural haematoma*
Inflammatory disorders	*Multiple sclerosis* *Idiopathic transverse myelitis* *Sarcoidosis* *Infections (lyme, zoster, TB, AIDS)*
Degenerative disorders	***Motor neuron disease*** *Syringomyelia*
Vascular	*Spinal cord infarction* *Vasculitis, systemic lupus erythematosus etc* *Spinal AVM*
Trauma	*Cord contusion, laceration or transaction* *Displaced vertebral fracture or disc* *Traumatic epidural haematoma*
Metabolic/Nutritional	***B12 deficiency (subacute combined degeneration)***
Rare hereditary conditions	*Friedreich's ataxia* *Hereditary spastic paraparesis*
Parasagittal brain lesions	*Meningioma* *Cerebral venous sinus thrombosis* *Congenital spastic diplegia*

Beevor's Sign (Thoracic Cord Lesion)

- Beevor's sign refers to upward movement of the umbilicus when the abdominal ***muscle contracts***
- Beevor's sign represents a consequence to a *Thoracic Cord lesion*
- *Lesions at T9-T10* paralyze the lower- but not the – upper abdominal muscles resulting in *an upward movement of the umbilicus* when the abdominal muscle contracts

Anterior Spinal Artery Thrombosis / Syndrome

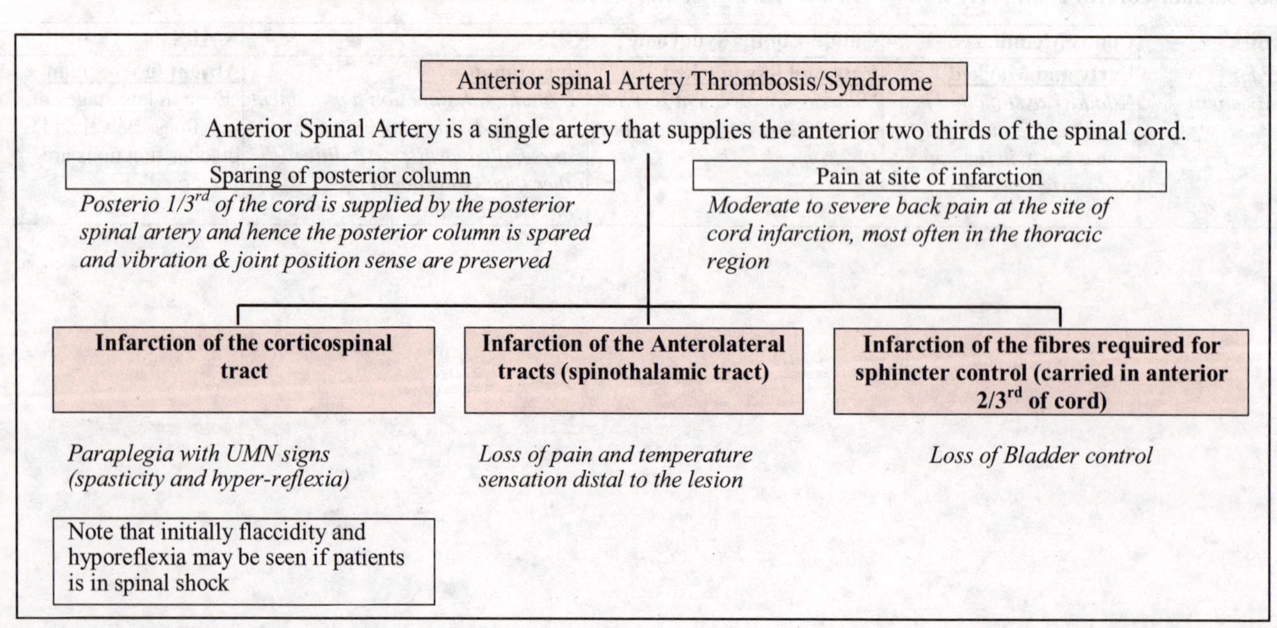

Motor Neuron Disease

This encompasses disorders that predominantly or exclusively affect *the upper motor neurons* (Neurons that lie in the cerebral cortex and project through the corticospinal / corticobulbar tract) or *lower motorneurons* (Neurons that lie in the anterior horn cell of the spinal cord or motor cranial nuclei that lie in the brainstem) *or both.*

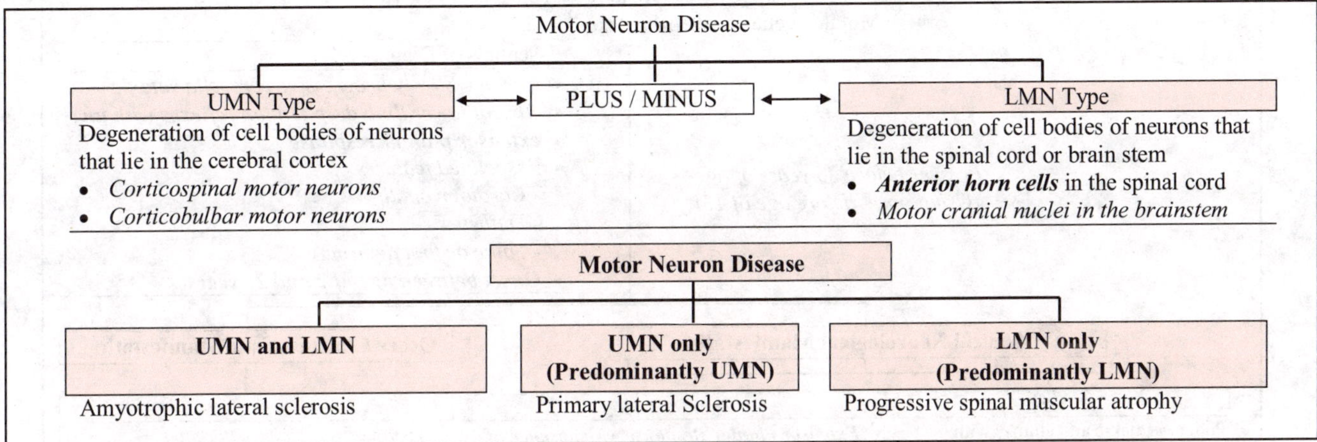

***Spinomuscular Atrophy* is a form of motor neuron disease that affects the lower motor neuron (Anterior horn cells) only.**
***Amyotrophic lateral sclerosis* involves degeneration of both upper motor neurons (corticospinal motor neurons originating in layer five of the motor cortex) and Lower motor neurons (*Anterior horn cells in the spinal cord* or their homologues)**

Manifestations are variable and depend on the neurons involved

Upper Motor Neurons Manifestations (UMN)	Lower Motor Neurons Manifestations (LMN)
Corticospinal Tract Involvement (UMN of Limbs)	***Lower motor neurons of Limbs involved***
• Hyperactive tendon reflexes • Spasticity / spastic resistance to passive movements.	• Weakness - Asymmetric - Insidious - Distal to proximal • Progressive wasting and atrophy of muscles [Q] • Fasciculations or spontaneous twitchings
Corticobulbar Tract Involvement (UMN to bulbar muscles)	***Lower motor neurons of bulbar muscles involved***
• Dysarthria • Exaggeration of emotion involuntary excess weeping/ laughing (pseudobulbar affect)	• Difficulty in chewing - Swallowing • Movements of face and tongue

Criteria often used to exclude Motor Neuron Disease

Motor neuron diseases can be excluded remembering the following parameters
1. **NO** sensory deficit. Deficit is purely motor.
2. **NO** bladder bowel involvement
3. **NO** impairment of cognitive function
4. **NO** involvement of ocular muscles. Ocular motility is spared until very late.

Ocular muscles are usually not involved in motor neuron disease.
Fasciculation is a visible or palpable twitch within a single muscle due to spontaneous discharge of one motor unit ***Disease of motor neurons are associated with fasciculations***

Friadreich's Ataxia

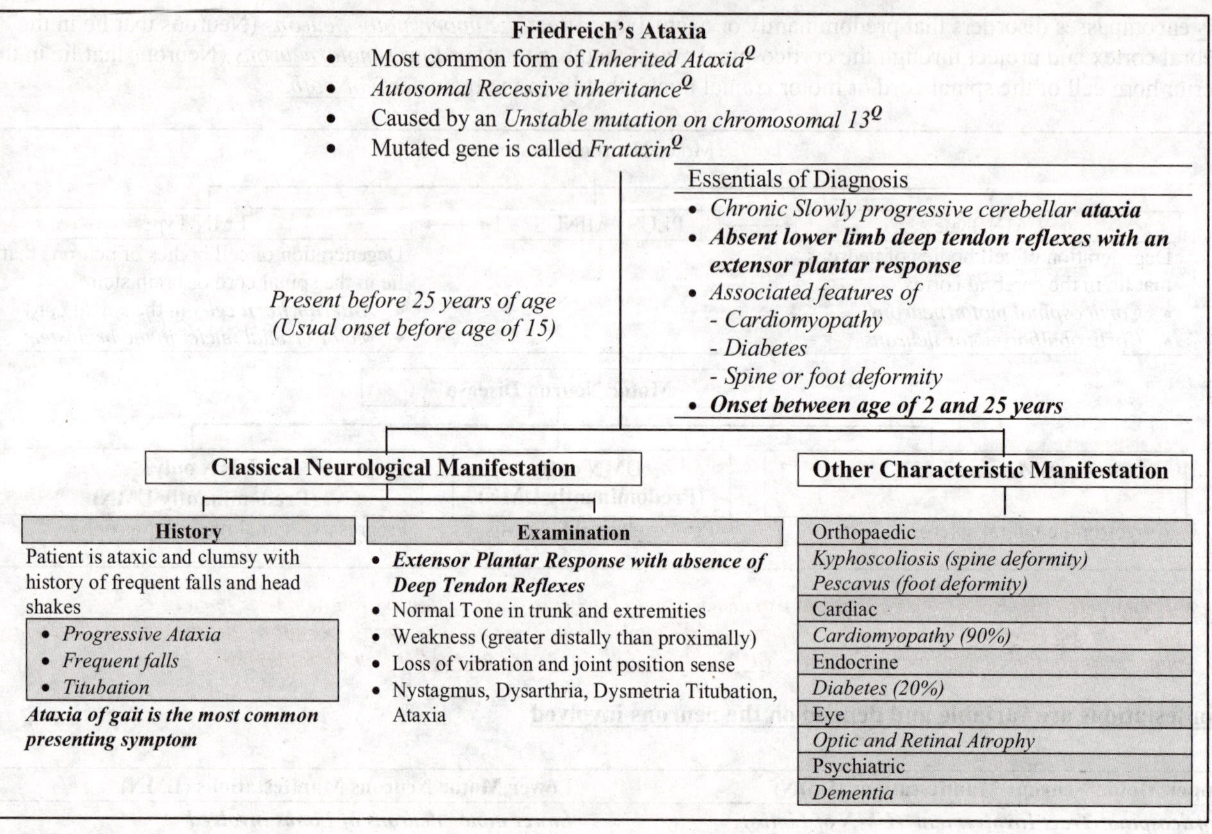

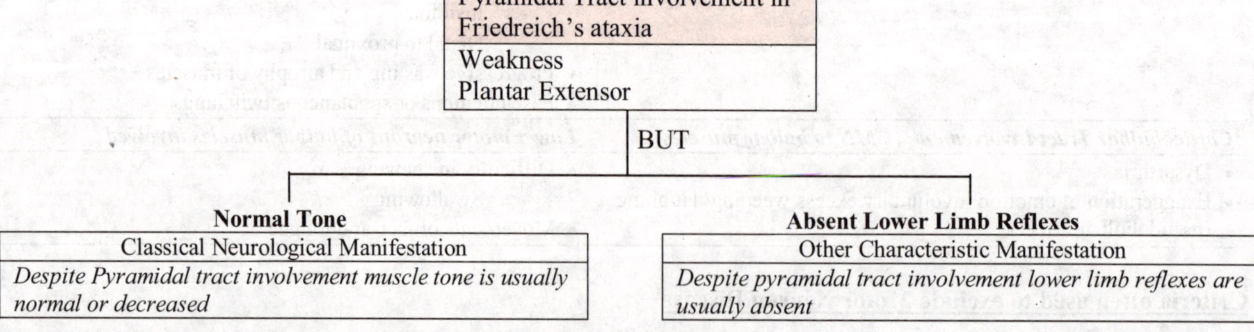

- *Friedreich's Ataxia is characteristically associated with an extensor plantar response but absent lower limb reflexes.* [Q]
- *Lower limb reflexes are characteristically absent (in most patients) and not brisk.* [Q]
- *Cardiomyopathy is a common association seen in up to 90% of patients*[Q]
- *Diabetes mellitus may be associated in up to 25% of cases*[Q]
- *Progressive ataxia is the most common presenting symptom*[Q].
  'In most patients ataxia of gait and stance is the first manifestation of the disease'
- *The first pathological changes in Friedreich's ataxia are thought to occur in the dorsal root ganglia with loss of large sensory neurons*[Q]

Subacute Combined Degeneration Of Cord

This *is a condition of the spinal cord characterized by demyelination of its neurons due to deficiency of Vit B_{12}, which results in defective/ deficient myelination.*

Such demyelination occurs predominantly in
• *Posterior column of spinal cord* • *Pyramidal tract of spinal cord*

Subacute Combined Degeneration of Cord (SACD) is caused by vitamin B_{12} dificiency

Subacute Combined Degeneration of Cord

Degeneration/Demyelination of Posterior column of lower cervical & upper thoracic region This is where changes commence.	**Degeneration/Demyelination of Lateral columns (corticospinal tracts)** Their involvement follows the involvement of post.columns.
• Paraesthaesias, consisting of tingling & numbness and that of pins & needles [Q] • Loss of vibration sense [Q] • Position sense is involved to a lesser extent. [Q] • Ataxic gait [Q]	1. Motor defects such as weakness and spasticity [Q] 2. *Increased deep tendon reflexes, clonus* [Q] 3. Plantar extensor [Q] 4. Spastic gait (Note that gait is initially ataxic but later becomes both spastic and ataxic. [Q] *(at an early stage patellar & achilles reflexes may be diminished, increased or absent).*

Presence of a combination of hematological manifestations (anemia) and neurological manifestation (posterior column dysfunction) suggest a diagnosis of Vit. B_{12} deficiency.

'Tabes dorsalis'

(Parenchymatous manifestation of tertiary stage of syphyllis)

Characterised by demyelination and degenration of posterior nerve roots and posterior column of cord

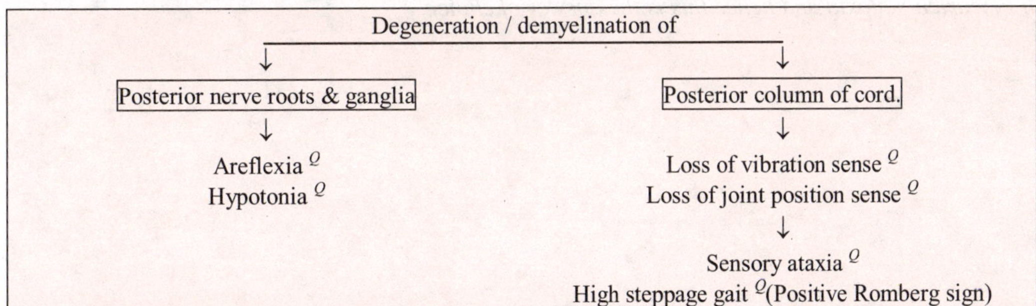

Tabes Dorsalis
• *Tabes dorsalis I a late manifestation of syphilis that presents as symptoms and signs of demyclination of the posterior column, dorsal roots and dorsal root ganglia* • *The charachteristic symptoms of Tabes are fleeting and repetitive lancinating pains, primarily in the legs and less often in the back thorax, abdomen, arms and face.* • *Ataxia of the legs and gout due to loss of position sense with wide based gate (seen in <50% of patients)* • *Paresthesis, bladder disturbance and acute abdominal pain with vomiting (visceral crisis) occur in 15-30% of patients* • *Trophic joint degeneration (charcot's joints) and perforating ulceration of feet can result from loss of pain sensation* • *The cardinal neurological signs of tabes are loss of reflexes in legs impaired position and vibratory sense.* • *Romberg's sign and bilateral Argyll Robertson pupils.*

Associated with an Atonic bladder [Q] and Argyll Robertson pupil [Q]

9

Comparitive Features of Freidrich's ataxia, SACD and Tabes Dorsalis

Disorder	Pyramidal tract involvement	Posterior column involvement	Deep tendon reflexes	Planter	Associations	
					Neurological	Others
Friedrich's ataxia (genetic)	Present	Present	Areflexia[Q] (Areflexia despite corticospinal involvement) [Q]	Extensor	- Wide based ataxia - Nystagmus - Dysarthria - Dysmetria	- Cardiomyopathy - Optic atrophy - Skeletal abnormality - Diabetes mellitus
SACD (↓ B_{12})	Present	Present	Exaggerated usually[Q] (May be decreased increased or absent)	Extensor	Spastic gait (initially ataxic)	Low serum B_{12}megaloblastic anemia
Tabes dorsalis (tertiary syphilis)	Absent	Absent	Areflexia[Q]	Absent	Argyll Robertson pupil	Atonic bladder

Pyramidal tract may be involved in Friedrich's ataxia or SACD but is usually not involved in Tabes Dorsalis

Absent deep tendon reflexes despite corticospinal tract involvement with an extensor plantar reflex is characteristic of Friedrich's ataxia.

Reflexes are *usually exaggerated in SACD while they are diminished / absent (areflexia) in Tabes Dorsalis and Freidrich's Ataxia*

Friedrich's ataxia	SACD
• Deep tendon reflex are characteristically absent • Planter response is extensor	• Increased deep tendons reflexes / clonus • Extensor planter [At an early stage the patellar and achillis reflexes may be diminished increased or absent]

Thus although both Friedrich's ataxia and SACD may present with absent ankle jerk, this feature is more characteristic and consistent with Friedrich's ataxia and hence this is the answer of choice.

Cerebrovascular Stroke: Causes and Sites

- ***The most common cause of cerebrovascular accidents is embolism.***

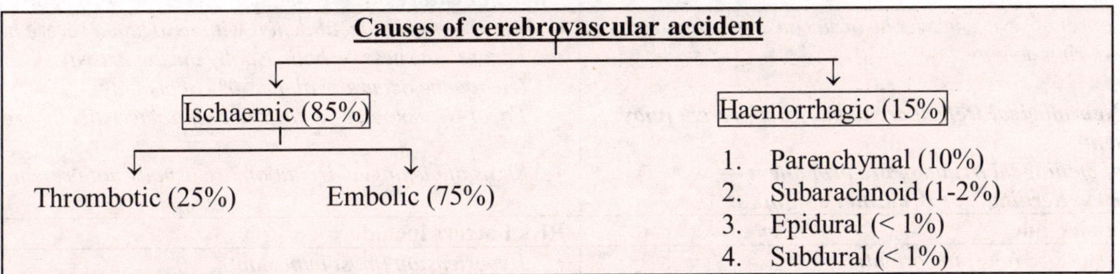

- ***An intracerebral parenchymal haemorrhage constitutes the most common form of intracranial haemorrhage.***

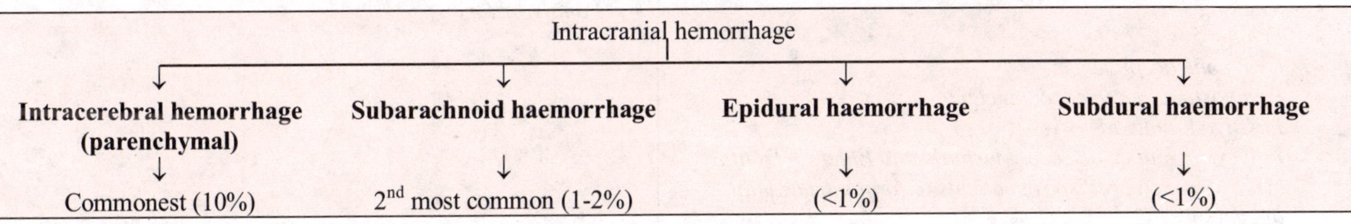

- ***An intracerebral bleed (parenchymal) invariably results from rupture of small perforating arteries or arterioles as a result of Hypertension.***

Intracerebral (parenchymal haemorrhage)	Subarachnoid haemorrhage
• Most common type of intracranial haemorrhage [Q] • Most common cause is hypertension [Q] causing rupture of small perforating arteries or arterioles [Q] • Most common site is Putamen [Q] (basal ganglia)	• Second most common cause of intracranial haemorrhage [Q] • Most common cause is spontaneous rupture of saccular aneurysm i.e. Berry aneurysm [Q] (excluding trauma) • Most common site of berry aneurysm is anterior circulation of 'circle of Willis' [Q]

- ***The putamen (Basal ganglia) is the most common site for hypertensive haemorrhage***

The most common sites of hypertensive haemorrhage are :

1. The ***basal ganglia*** (***putamen***, thalamus and adjacent deep white matter)- ***commonest***
2. *Deep cerebellum*
3. *Pons*

The most common site of hypertensive haemorrhage within basal ganglia is the Putamen.

- ***The most common cause of subarachnoid haemorrhage is rupture of a saccular aneurysm*** *(excluding head trauma)*

Most common cause of subarachnoid haemorrhage is rupture of a saccular aneurysm[Q]
Most common cause of subarachnoid haemorrhage is rupture of a Berry aneurysm[Q]
Most common cause of subarachnoid haemorrhage is rupture of 'Circle of Willis' aneurysm[Q].

Saccular aneurysms are synonymous with Berry Aneurysms and most commonly occur in the anterior circulation on the Circle of Willis

- ***Most common site of saccular aneurysms is the anterior circulation on the circle of Willis***
  About 80-90% of berry aneurysms occur in the anterior circulation on the circle of Willis.
  Posterior circulation as in vertebral artery is a very uncommon location for berry aneurysm.

Location of Berry Aneurysms : (*In order of frequency of occurrence*)

- *Anterior communicating - Ant. cerebral junction (29%).*
- *Post communicating - Internal carotid junction (28%).*
- *Middle cerebral bifurcation (18%).*
- *Intracranial carotid bifurcation (8%)*
- *Vertebrobasilar* **or basilar bifurcation** (3%)

- ***Berry aneurysms (Saccular aneurysms) are believed to arise from a defect in the tunica media of the involved vessel.***

Differences between presentation of Subarachnoid Haemorrhage and Hypertensive Intracerebral Haemorrhage

Subarachnoid Haemarrhage	Intracerebral Haemorrhage (Intraparcnchymal)
Clinical Features	**Clinical Features**
• *Abrupt onset of severe headache or unconsciousness or both usually during activity* • ***Focal Neurological Defecit are usually not present (may be present)*** • ***Signs of meningeal irritation are prominent (Stiff neck, Kerning's or Brudzinki's sign)***	• *Abrupt onset of focal deficit with associated severe headache or unconsciousness or both usually during activity. (Headache occurs in about 50% of pts only).* • *Focal Neurological defects are characteristically present* • *Signs of meningeal irritation are usually not present*
Risk Factors include	**Risk Factors include**
• *Aneurysmal size (most important)* • *Prior aneurysmal SAH* • *Hypertension* • *Smoking* • *Female Sex* • *Oral contraceptive use* • *Psychostimulant use (cocaineQ)* • *Positive Family history* • *Polycystic kidney disease, Marfan's and Ehlers – Donlos syndrome also predispose patients to form intracranial aneurysms*	• *Hypertension (most important)* • *Smoking* • *Alcohol* • *Family history*
CT scan	**CT scan**
Evidence of ***blood in Sylvian fissure*** *or between the frontal lobes or in the basal cistern or in the cerebral ventricles*	Evidence of intraparenchymal hematoma
Presence of sudden onset headache, meningeal signs in the form of neck stiffness and absence of focal neurological defecit suggests the diagnosis of subarachnoid haemorrhage. Presence of blood in sylvian fissure on the CT scan further confirms the diagnosis of SAH.	***Hypertensive hemorrhage*** *almost always occurs while the patient is* ***awake*** *and sometimes when stressed. It generally presents as* ***severe headache*** *along with abrupt onset of* ***focal neurological deficit****. The focal deficit typically worsens steadily and is associated with a diminishing level of consciousness and signs of increased ICP, such as headache & vomiting.*

Classical Clinical Presentation of Subarachanoid Hemorrhage

Clinical manifestation of Subarachnoid haemorrhage:

- ***Sudden transient loss of consciousness*** (occurs in nearly half of the patients)
- ***Excruciating severe headache:*** presenting complaint in 45% of cases (***worst headache of patient's life***) more common upon regaining consciousness when loss of consciousness is associated
- ***Neck stiffness***, Photophobia &vomiting:*Signs of Meningeal Irritation are common associations*
- ***Focal neurological deficit: uncommon.***
  'Sudden headache in the absence of focal neurological deficit is the hallmark of aneurysmal rupture.' Q
- ***Associated prodromal symptoms*** (suggest location of progressively enlarging unruptured aneurysm)
  - *Third cranial nerve palsy: aneurysm at junction of PCA & ICA*
  - *Sxith nerve palsy: aneurysm in cavernous sinus*
  - *Occipital and posterior cervical pain: inferior cerebellar artery aneurysm (Ant. or Post.)*
  - *Pain behind the eye: MCA aneurysm*
- ***Sentinel Bleeds***:'Aneurysms may undergo small ruptures or leaks, so called sentinel bleeds.'

Investigations

- Non contrast CT scan:
  *Investigation of choice*Q *(Lumbar puncture is not indicated prior to an imaging procedure)*
  Evidence of ***blood in Sylvian fissure*** *or between the frontal lobes or in the basal cistern or in the cerebral ventricles*
- CSF picture:
  *The hallmark of aneurysmal rupture is blood in CSF*Q*:Xanthochromic spinal fluid*Q
  (Lumbar puncture should be performed if the CT scan fails to establish the diagnosis of SAH and no mass lesion or obstructive hydrocephalus is found to establish the presence of subarachnoid blood)

Localization of Stroke: Clinical Features

Paracentral Lobule Lesions

The paracentral lobule is located on the medial frontal lobe and is involved in anterior cerebral artery occlusion. The involvement of paracentral lobule leads to contralateral lower limb weakness and urinary incontinence.

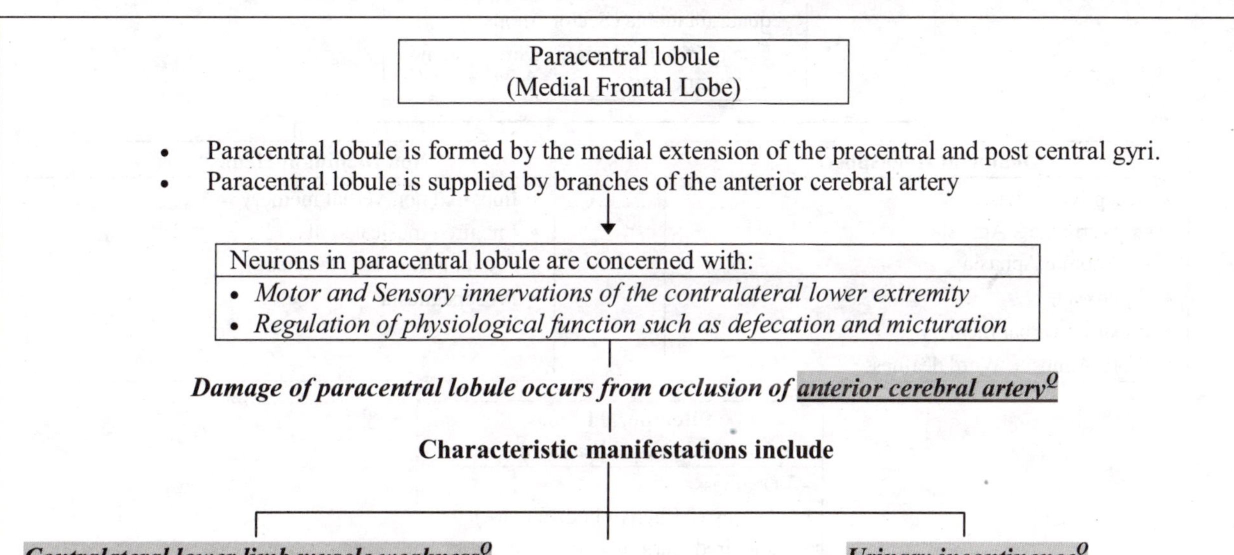

Features of Parietal lobe lesions

Unilateral Parietal Lobe

- Contralateral hemisensory loss
- Astereognosis
- Agraphaesthesia
- Contralateral homonymous Lower quadrantanopia
- Asymmetry of optokinetic Nystagmus (OKN)
- Sensory Seizures
- Mild hemiparesis

Dominant Hemisphere

- Dysphasia/Aphasia
- Dyscalculia
- Dyslexia
- Apraxia (Bilateral Apraxia)
- Agnosia (Textile Agnosia)
- Gerstmann Syndrome

Non Dominant Hemisphere

- Neglect of contralateral side (Hemineglect)
- Extinction phenomenon (contralateral)
- Spatial disorientation
- Constructional apraxia
- Dressing apraxia
- Anosagnosia

*[Q]**Hemineglect or neglect of contralateral side is a feature of Parietal lobe lesion (Non dominant hemisphere)***

[Q]Aphasia and Inferior quadrantic anopsia are features of dominant (left) parietal lobe injury.

[Q]Acalculia is a feature of Dominant parietal lobe lesion.

Features of Temporal lobe lesions

Unilateral Temporal Lesion

- Contralateral homonymous upper quadrantanopia (Sector Anopsia)
- Complex hallucinations (Smell, sound, vision, memory)

Dominant Hemisphere

- Receptive asphasia
  - Wernicke's Aphasia
  - Anomic Aphasia
- Dyslexia
- Impaired verbal memory
- Word Agnosia, Word deafness

Non Dominant Hemisphere

- Impaired non-verbal memory
- Impaired musical skills (Tonal perception) (Amusia)
- Prosopagnosia

Bitemporal lesions
(Additional Features)

- Deafness
- Apathy (Affective in difference)
- Impaired learning and Memory
- Amnesia, Korsakoff syndrome
  Kluver Bucy syndrome

Q Wernicke's Aphasia is a feature of Temporal lobe lesion
Q Contralateral superior homonymous quadrantopia is a feature of Temporal lobe lesion
Q Auditory hallucinations is a feature of Temporal lobe lesion

The Medial Temporal Lobe

The medial temporal lobe is most characteristically associated with memory.
Unilateral dominant lesions produce disorders of verbal memory (Auditory amnesia).
Unilateral nondominant lobe lesions produce disorders of non verbal memory (visual amnesia), and
Bilateral lesions produce Antegrade amnesia.

Lesions of Medial Temporal lobe

Unilateral lesion affecting Dominant Lobe (Left)	Unilateral lesion affecting Non dominant lobe (Right)	Bilateral lobe involvement
Verbal Memory loss (Auditory Amnesia)	*Non Verbal Memory loss (e.g. Visual Amnesia)*	*Antegrade Amnesia* *Loss of new learning and recent memory*

Urinary incontinence is primarily a feature of frantal lobe lesion.

Anterior Cerebral Artery Lesion

Anterior Cerebral Artery

Anterior Cerebral Artery supplies the medial surface of the cerebral cortex as far as the parietooccipital sulcus and a strip of about 1 inch wide on the adjoining lateral surface.
It also supplies the frontal pole and the corpus callosum.

Paracentral lobule and adjoining sensory motor cortex on the 1 inch wide strip over the lateral hemisphere

- Motor
  - ***Paralysis of contralateral leg and foot***[Q]
- Sensory
  - Cortical sensory loss over toes foot and leg.
  - ***Urinary incontinence***[Q] ***(paracentral lobule)***

Supplemental motor cortex (Medial Surface of posterior frontal lobe)

Reappearance of primitive reflexes that are normally present only in infants

Frontal Reflex Signs
- Grasp Reflex
- Suck Reflex
- Rooting Reflex
- Snout Reflex
- Gegenhalton-Paratonic rigidly

Frontal cortex near the leg motor area

Impairment of gait and stance (Gait Apraxia)

Prefrontal cortex (Frontal Pole) and Uncertain localization

Cognitive and Behavioral impairment
- Abulia (Akinetic mutism)
- Apathy
- Euphoria, Disinhibition or Distractibility
- Slowness, Delay
- Lock of spontaneity

Corpus Callosum

Dyspraxia of left limbs
Tactile Aphasia of left limbs

A lesser degree of paresis of the opposite arm is also seen in lesions of the anterior cerebral artery because fibers descending to corona radiata are involved by deep branches

Middle Cerebral Artery Lesion

The sensory motor cortex is located on the lateral surface of the cerebral hemisphere and is supplied by middle cerebral artery.Occlusion of the middle cerebral artery thus produces contralateral hemiplegia and contralateral hemisensory loss.

Pure Motor Hemiplegia

Deep branches of the middle cerebral artery or the lenticulostriate branches supply the internal capsule (posterior limb) Motor tracts are densely packed in this region and hence occlusion of deep branches or lenticulostrials branches leads to Dense Hemiplegia / Pure motor Hemiplegia

Middle Cerebral Artery

Middle cerebral Artery supplies most of the lateral aspect of the cerebral hemispheres chiefly of the frontal, parietal and temporal lobes (cortical or superficial branches)

Frontal lobe

Lesions affect most of the frontal lobe except the medial aspect is lobule and supplemental Motar area on the medial surface of posterior frontal lobe

Features

- *Contra lateral* Hemiparesis primarily involving face and upper limb > lower limb
  (D/t motor cortex lesion)
- *Conjugate gaze preference*, away from paresis towards the side of lesion
  (D/t Frontal eye field)
- *Broca's Aphasia*
  (D/t involvement of Broca's area)
- *Cognitive and Behavioral impairment*
  Mutism and Apathy may be associated

> Note that because Paracentral lobule is not involved in middle cerebral artery occlusion there is no associated sphincter disturbance of the bladder and bowel (No urinary incontinence)
> Paracentral lobule is supplied by the anterior cerebral Artery

Parietal lobe

Lesions affect most of the Parietal lobe

Features

Contralateral hemianaesthesia primarily involving face and upper limb >lower limb (d/t involvement of sensory cortex)
(Loss of pain, touch, vibration, joint position, two point discrimination etc)

- *Astereognosis*
- *Agraphaesthesia*
- *Asymmetry of optokinetic nystagmus*

Dominant	Non Dominant
• Aphasia (conduction) • Apraxia • Alexia • Aacalculia • Agnosia • Right to left confusion • Gerstmann syndrome	• Heminglect of contralateral side • Spatial disorientation • Anosognosia • Constructional and dressing Aprexia • Apractagnosia

Temporal lobe

Lesions affect most of the temporal lobe except the medial temporal lobe

Features

- Hallucinations
- Anomic Aphasia
- Word Agnosia
- Word Deafness

> Note that memory is not impaired because memory is storedd mainly in the medial part of temporal lobe and hippocampus which is not supplied by the middle cerebral artery.

Visual sings include Contra lateral Homonymous Hemianopia because both superior quadrant (temporal lobe) and inferior quadrant (parietal lobe) is involved.

Anterior Choroidal Artery Lesion

Anterior choroidal artery supplies the posterior limb of Internal capsule (and not anterior limb of internal capsule).

'Anterior choroidal artery arises from the internal carotid artery and supplies the posterior limb of internal capsule. The complete syndrome of anterior choroidal artery occlusion consists of contralateral hemiplegia hemianesthesia (hypoesthesia) and homonymous hemianopia'- Harrison's 17th/2524

Anterior Choroidal Artery Occlusion

Anterior Choroidal Artery arises from the Supraclinoid Internal Carotid Artery

Territories Supplied / Involved (Areas Involved)

- ***Posterior Limb of Internal Capsule***
- *Optic Tract*
- *Lateral Geniculate Body*
- *Cerebral Peduncle*
- *Choroid Plexus*

<u>Areas of Perfusion may include</u>

- Medial temporal lobe / uncus
- Medial Globus pallidus
- Lateral Thalamus
- Posterior paraventricular corona radiata region

Typical Syndrome / Complete Syndrome (Most Common Syndrome)

Hemiplegia (Contralateral)
Hemianesthesia / Hypoesthesia (Contralateral)
Homonymous Hemianopia (Contralateral)

<u>Posterior Cerebral Artery Lesion</u>

*The posterior Cerebral Artery supplies the **<u>midbrain</u>**, **<u>thalamus</u>**, lateral geniculate bodies, posterior portion of choroid plexus, occipital lobes, inferior and medial aspect of the **<u>temporal lobe</u>** and posterior inferior areas of the parietal lobe.*

Occlusion of the Posterior Cerebral Artery usually results in two common clinical syndromes depending on the areas involved

P1 Syndrome

Occlusion of the *<u>proximal segment of PCA</u>* from its origin to its union with the posterior communicating artery

<u>P1 syndrome present primarily with the following signs</u>

- ***Midbrain signs***
- ***Thalamic signs***
- *Subthalamic signs*

P2 Syndrome

Occlusion of the *<u>distalsegment of PCA</u>* distal to the junction of PCA with the posterior communicating artery

<u>P2 syndrome presents primarily with the following signs</u>

- ***Temporal lobe signs***
- *Occipital lobe signs*

The focal neurological signs vary according to the site of the hemorrhage

Basal ganglia	Thalamus	Pons	Cerebellum
Arteries involved	Arteries involved	Arteries involved	Arteries involved
Medial & lateral striate branches of Middle cerebral artery.	Perforating branches of posterior cerebral artery	Basilar artery	Cerebellar arteries - Superior cerebellar - Ant. inferior - Post. Inferior
Manifestations	Manifestations	Manifestations	Manifestations
• Contralateral hemiparesis is the sentinel sign • Paralysis may worsen until the affected limbs become flaccid or extend rigidly • When haemorrhage is large signs of brainstem compression may appear - Coma - Cheyne Stokes respiration - Dilated & fixed ipsilateral pupil - Decerebrate rigidity	• Hemisensory loss involving all modalities • Contralateral hemiparesis ***sensory loss > motor loss*** • Several typical ocular disturbances: - down & inward deviation of eyes - unequal pupils with loss of light reflex - skew deviation with eye opp. haemorrhage deviated down and medially - I/L horners syndrome - Absence of convergence - Paralysis of vertical gaze - Retraction nystagmus • Contralateral pain syndrome (Deferne-Roussy syndrome) • Aphasias	• Quadriplegia • Deep coma • Decerebrate rigidity Q • Pinpoint pupil that react to light • Impairment of reflex eye movement on head turning (doll's head or occulocephalic maneuver) • Hyperapnea • Hypertension • Hyperhydrosis	• Occipital headache • Vomiting • Gain ataxia • Dizziness or vertigo • Ocular changes - paresis of conjugate gaze - forced deviation of eyes to opposite side - I/L 6th nerve palsy • Dysarthria • Dysphagia • Stupor & coma if brainstem compression occurs

Remember :

Abnormal movement	Site of lesion
1. *Chorea*	• *Caudate nucleus and Putamen (striatum)*
2. *Athetosis*	• *Lentiform nucleus (Globus pallidus)*
3. *Hemiballismus*	• *Subthalamic nucleus 3*
4. *Parkinsonism*	• *Substantia nigra*

Cerebral Lateralization

Categorical Hemisphere (Dominant Hemisphere)	Representative Hemisphere (Non-Dominant Hemisphere)
The cerebral hemisphere for: • Sequential – Analytic process - Mathematical calculations - Logical decision making • Language (Aphasias) - *Expressive / Motor (Braco's)* - *Sensory / Receptive (Wernicke's)*	**The cerebral hemisphere for:** • Visuo-spatial processing - to identify familiar objects by touch, smell, sight, taste or feel • Analyzing the emotional context of a conversion

Dyscalculi is a feature of categorical/dominant hemisphere involvement or left lobe involvement

Visuospatial defects, Anosognosia and Spatial dysgraphia are all features of non dominant / representative hemisphere involvement or right lobe involvement

Categorical Dominant Hemisphere Lesion (Sequential Analytical Process & Language)	Representative Non-Dominant Hemisphere lesion (Visuospatial processing)
• ***Dysphasia / Aphasia*** *(difficulty with words)* - *Expressive / Motor (Braco's)* - *Sensory / Receptive (Wernicke's)* • ***Dyslexia*** *(difficulty with words)* • ***Dysgraphia*** *(difficulty with drawing)* • ***Dyscalculia*** *(difficulty with calculations)* • ***Dyspraxia*** *(difficulty to perform complex motor tasks)*	• ***Neglect*** of contralateral side • ***Spatial disorientation*** • ***Anosognosia*** • ***Dressing Apraxia*** (*Apraxia is a misnomer*) *(Problem results from visuospatial disorientation of body parts to clothing)* • ***Constructional Apraxia*** (Apraxia is a misnomer) *(Inability to copy complex shapes due to visuospatial disorientation)* • ***Astereognosis*** • ***Afferent Dysgraphia*** (*Spatial Dysgraphias*) • ***Impaired musical skills*** (tonal perception) • Impaired non-verbal memory

Senseless fluent speech most closely suggests a diagnosis of Aphasia (Wernicke's aphasia) which results from damage to the categorical or dominant hemisphere

Lateral Medullary Syndrome

Vessel occlusion that result in Lateral Medullary syndrome:

- *Vertebral (most common)*
- *Posterior inferior cerebellar (2nd most common)*
- *Superior, middle or Inferior lateral medullary arteries*

'Most cases result from ipsilateral vertebral artery occlusion; in the reminder occlusion of posterior inferior cerebellar artery is responsible' – Harrison

Embolic occlusion or thrombosis of the fourth segment is responsible for this syndrome [Q]

Structures involved in lateral medullary syndrome or Wallenberg Syndrome (Posterior Inferior Cerebellar Artery lesion)

- *Spinal nucleus of Trigeminal Nerve and it's tract (Vth Nerve)*
- *Vestibular Nuclei (VIII nerve)*
- *Fibres of IXth and Xth nerve*
- *Nucleus Ambiguous (IX, Xth and XIth nerve)*
- *Nucleus tractus solitarus*
- *Descending sympathetic fibres from the cerebellum*
- *Restiform body or Base of inferior cereballar peduncle*
- *Olivocerebellar fibres*
- *Cuneate and Gracilis nuclei*
- *Spinothalamic tract*

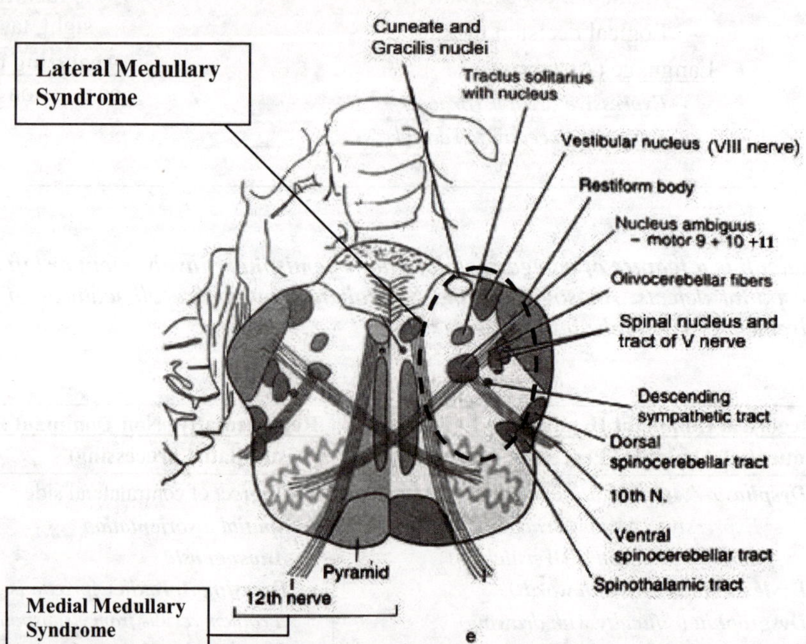

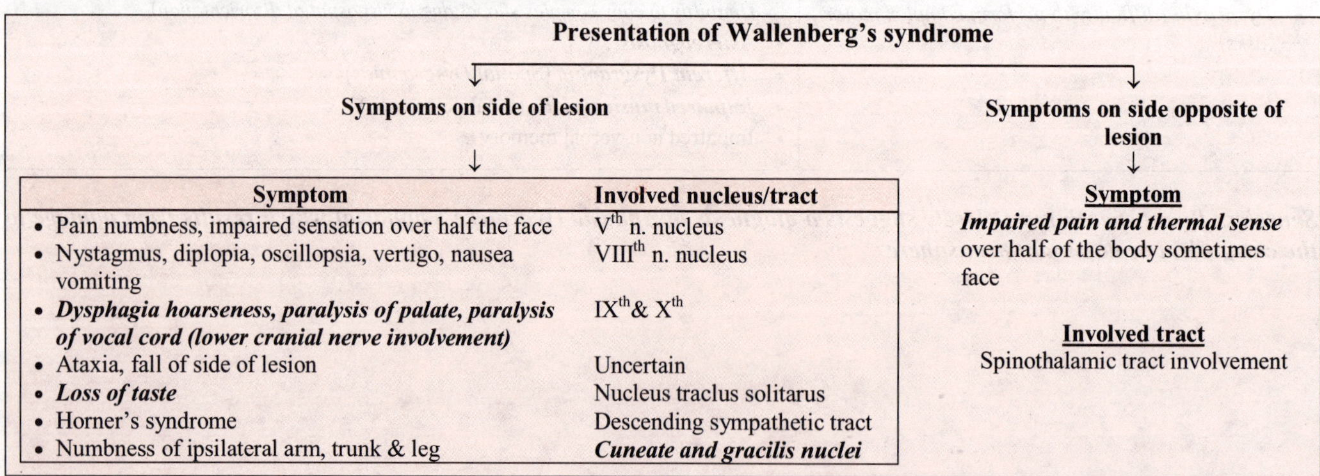

Presentation of Wallenberg's syndrome

Symptoms on side of lesion

Symptom	Involved nucleus/tract
• Pain numbness, impaired sensation over half the face	V^{th} n. nucleus
• Nystagmus, diplopia, oscillopsia, vertigo, nausea vomiting	VIIIth n. nucleus
• ***Dysphagia hoarseness, paralysis of palate, paralysis of vocal cord (lower cranial nerve involvement)***	IXth & X^{th}
• Ataxia, fall of side of lesion	Uncertain
• ***Loss of taste***	Nucleus traclus solitarus
• Horner's syndrome	Descending sympathetic tract
• Numbness of ipsilateral arm, trunk & leg	***Cuneate and gracilis nuclei***

Symptoms on side opposite of lesion

Symptom

Impaired pain and thermal sense over half of the body sometimes face

Involved tract

Spinothalamic tract involvement

Pain and temperature sense are lost over opposite side of lesion due to involvement of spinothalamic tract.
Horner's syndrome forms part of the constellation of manifestations seen in lateral medullary syndrome or Wallenberg syndrome. It is produced as a result of infarction of the descending sympathetic tract.

Cranial Nerves involved in Lateral Medullary Syndrome

Lateral Medullary Syndrome involves the spinal nucleus of the trigeminal nerve and its tract (CN V); vestibular nuclei (CN VIII), Nucleus ambiguous (IX, X, XI) and fibers of the cranial nerves IX and X.

Cranial Nerves involved in Lateral Medullary syndrome V, VIII, IX, X, XI

Cranial Nerve XII is involved in medial medullary syndrome and not in lateral medullary syndrome.

Medial Medullary Syndrome

Ipsilateral 12th nerve palsy and contralateral pyramidal tract signs (paralysis) are features of medial medullary syndrome.

Medial Medullary Syndrome (Dejerine's Anterior Bulbar Syndrome)

- The medial medullary syndrome is caused by occlusion of the anterior spinal artery or the paramedian branches of the vertebral artery.
- The affected area usually includes the following structures:
  - Medial lemniscus
  - Pyramid
  - Rootlets of the hypoglossal nerve or its nucleus within the medulla
- The neurologic signs resulting from the involvement of these areas are as follows:
  - Contralateral loss of kinesthesia and discriminative touch resulting from involvement of the medial lemniscus.
  - Contralateral paralysis, of the upper motor neuron type (weakness, hyperactive reflexes, Babinskis sign, clonus, and spasticity) with sparing of the face caused by involvement of the pyramid
  - Lower motor neuron paralysis of the homolateral half of the tongue (weakness, atrophy, and fibrillation) and deviation of the protruded tongue to the atrophic side caused by involvement of the hypoglossal nucleus or nerve

The medial medullary syndrome may occur bilaterally resulting in bilateral upper motor neuron weakness or paralysis (with facial sparing), bilateral paralysis of the tongue of the lower motor neuron type, and bilateral loss of kinesthesia and discriminative touch.

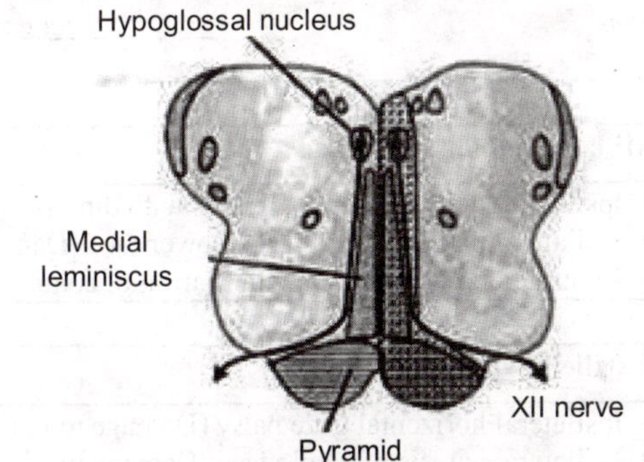

Medial Medullary Syndrome

- Paralysis of homolateral half of tongue (lower motor neuron type)
- Contralateral paralysis (upper motor neuron type)
- Contralateral loss of kinesthesia and discriminative touch

Midbrain Syndromes:

	Symptoms and Signs	Structures involved
Weber's syndrome	• Ipsilateral oculomotor nerve palsy • Contralateral hemiplegia including face	• Oculomotor nerve • Corticospinal and corticobulbar tracts
Benedikt's syndrome	• Ipsilateral oculomotor nerve palsy • Contralateral hemiparesis including face • Contralateral intention tremor	• Oculomotor nerve • Corticospinal and corticobulbar tracts • Red nucleus
Claude's syndrome	• Ipsilateral oculomotor nerve palsy • Contralateral hemiataxia and hemiasynergia	• Oculomotor nerve • Red nucleus and brachium conjunctivum
Parinaud's syndrome	• Bilateral vertical palsy • Bilateral paralysis of convergence	• Superior colliculus • Superior colliculus

Benedict's syndrome also known as dorsal mid brain syndrome results from a lesion in the midbrain tegmentum / red nucleus. It is not a pontine syndrome.

In benedict's syndrome injury to the ***red nucleus*** midbrainresults in ***ipsilateral occulomotor palsy***and ***contralateral tremor ,chorea and athetosis.*** – *Harrison*

Pontine syndromes

Ventral pontine syndrome (Millard Gubler syndrome)	***Lower dorsal pontine syndrome (Foville's syndrome)***	***Upper dorsal pontine syndrome (Raymond Ceston syndrome)***
Caused by paramedian infarction of pons	*Caused by lesion in dorsal tegmentum of lower pons*	*Caused by obstruction of long circumferential branches of basilar artery*

Millard Gubler syndrome
▪ Ipsilateral paresis of lateral rectus with diplopia (Damage to abducent fasciculus / nucleus spared) ▪ Ipsilateral paresis of upper and lower face (Damage to 7th cranial nerve) ▪ Contralateral hemiplegia with sparing of contralateral face(Damage to corticospinal tract)

Faville's syndrome
▪ Ipsilateral horizontal gaze palsy (Damage to nucleus of abducent nerve and paramedian pontine reticular formation.) ▪ Ipsilateral paresis of whole face (Damage to nucleus and fibers of 7th nerve) ▪ Contralateral hemiplegia with sparing of Contralateral face(Damage to corticospinal tract)

Raymond Ceston syndrome / Upper dorsal pontine syndrome
Caused by obstruction of long circumferential branches of basilar artery and results in : ▪ Ipsilateral ataxia and coarse intention tremor (damage to superior and middle cerebellar peduncle) ▪ Ipsilateral paralysis of muscles of mastication and sensory loss in face (damage to sensory and motor nuclei and tracts of CN V) ▪ Contralateral loss of sensory modalities in the body (damage to spinothalamic tract and medial leminiscus) ▪ Contralateral hemiparesis of face and body (damage to corticospinal tract) may occur with ventral extension of lesion. ▪ Horizontal gaze palsy may occur (as in lower dorsal pontine syndrome)

Locked – In – syndrome:Bilateral ventral pontine lesion (Able to communicate only by vertical eye movement and blinking but otherwise is completely immobile)
▪ Occurs in patients will bilateral ventral pontine lesion[Q]. ▪ Its most common cause is pontine infarction. ▪ Patient - Is quadriplegic (bilateral damage to corticospinal tract in ventral pons - Is unable to speak and incapable of facial movements (involvement of corticobulbar tracts) - Has limited Horizontal eye movements (bilateral involvement of nucleiand fibres of 6th CN) - Has intact vertical eye movements and blinking (supranuclear ocular motor pathways are spared) - Has preserved consciousness (reticular formation is not damaged)

Features of Pontine Stroke

Features of pontine stroke
• Sudden onset • Deep coma with ***quadriplegia*** (usually occurs over a few minutes) • ***Pinpoint pupils*** (1mm pupils) that react to light. • Loss of reflex eye movements and corneal responses (There is impairment of reflex horizontal eye movements evoked by head turningi.e doll's head or oculocephalic maneuver or by irrigation of the ears with ice water). • Decrebrate rigidity / Posturing • Hyperpnea / Hyperventilation • Severe Hypertension • Ocular bobbing • Excessive Sweating / Hyperhidrosis • ***Hyperpyrexia,*** (*Neurology Secrets 4th Ed.*)

Seizures and Epilepsy

Classification of seizures:

Partial seizures	Primarily generalized seizures	Unclassified seizures
• Simple partial seizures (with motor, sensory, autonomic, or psychic signs) • Complex partial seizures • Partial seizures with secondary generalization	• Absence (petitmal) • Tonic-clonic (grandmal) • Tonic • Atonic • Myoclonic	• Neonatal seizures • Infantile spasms

Characteristic features of Absence seizures / Petitmal seizures:

Clinical Hallmarks

- Almost always begin in childhood and cease by age of 20.
- Sudden brief lapses of consciousness without loss of postural control
- Seizure typically lasts only for seconds. Impairment is so brief that patient may be unaware of it.
- Consciousness returns as suddenly as it was lost i.e. Inset and termination of attack, both are abrupt.
- Usually accompanied by subtle bilateral motor signs such as
  - Rapid blinking of eye lids
  - Chewing movements
  - Small amplitude, clonic movements of hands
- There is no postictal confusion(*Absence of postictal confusion is characteristic of Absence Seizures)*
- The seizure can occur hundreds of times per day.
- First clued to absence seizure is often unexplained 'day dreaming' and a decline in school performance recognized by a teacher.

Electrophysiological hallmark

- Electrophysiological hallmark of typical absence seizure is a generalized symmetric, 3 Hz spike and wave discharge that begins and ends suddenly superimposed on a normal EEG background.
- Hyperventilation tends to provoke these electrographic discharges and even the seizures themselves.

Absence Seizures must primarily be differentiated from Complex Partial Seizures and Day dreaming

Clinical data	Absence	Complex partial	Daydreaming
Frequency/day	***Multiple***	***Rarely over 1-2***	***Mutiple; situation-dependent***
Duration	*Frequently< 10 sec (Rarely longer than 30 sec)*	*Average duration ober 1 min, 10 sec*	*Seconds to minutes; rarely more rarely less*
Aura	***Never***	***Frequently***	***No***
Eye blinking	*Common*	*Occasionally*	*No*
Automatism	*Common*	*Frequently*	*No*
Postictal impairment	***None***	***Frequently***	***No***
Seizures activated by			
Hyperventilation	*Very frequently*	*Occassionally*	*No*
Photic	*Frequently*	*Rarely*	*No*
EEG			
Ictal	*Generalized spike and wave*	*Usually unilateral or bilateral temporal frontal discharges*	*Normal*
Interictal	*Usually normal*	*Variable; may be spikes or sharp waves in frontal or temporal lobes*	*Normal*

- *Day-dreaming is usually not associated with automatism while automatism is common in seizures.*
- *Day-dreaming can often be 'broken' with stimulation while seizures can usually not be 'broken'.*
- *Day-dreaming usually occurs when child is tired /bored or involved in a monotonous activity but seizures can start abruptly at any time (for example in the middle of a sentence).*

9

Juvenile Myoclonic Epilepsy

Juvenile Myoclonic epilepsy is a generalized seizure disorder (not a focal seizure disorder) classified as an epilepsy syndrome. *Epilepsy syndromes are disorders in which epilepsy is a predominant feature and there is sufficient evidence to suggest a common underlying mechanism*

Juvenile Myoclonic Epilepsy

- ***It is a generalized seizure disorder***
- Typically seen in the juvenile age group (12-18 years) or early adolescence.
- Family history of epilepsy is common
- Most frequent in morning after awakening
- Can be provoked by sleep deprivation
- Typical Seizures include generalized myoclonic seizures (Bilateral myoclonic jerks that may be single or repetitive)
- Association with generalized tonic clonic seizures and absence seizures is seen

Myoclonic seizures (most frequent in the morning) *Tonic clonic seizures (seen in upto 90% of patients)* *Absence seizures (in about one third of patients)*

- Consciousness is usually preserved 9unless myoclonus is especially severe)
- Typical EEG shows a 4-6 seconds irregular ***spike and wave pattern*** (this is enhanced by a stimulation)
- Condition is considered benign but complete remission is uncommon
- Seizures respond well to anticonvulsant medications
- ***Valproic acid is the drug of choice in Juvenile Myoclonic epilepsy***
  'Majority ofpatients respond dramatically to valproate – Nelson.

Treatment of Juvenile Myoclonic Epilepsy

Antiepileptic Drugs in the treatment sequence of Juvenile Myoclonic Epilepsy (JME)	
First choice	*Valproate, Lamotrigine*
Second choice	*Levetivacetam, Clonazepam*
Consider	*Topiramate, Zonisamide, Pnenobarbitol, Primidone (Felbamate may also be effective againts JME)*

Taken from 'Current Management in Child Neurology' by Maria 4th/127, 163

Note Q ***CarbamezapineQ and PhenytoinQ may aggravate myoclonus in juvenile myoclonic epilepsy.***

Subacute Sclerosing PanEncephalitis

SSPE is characteristically associated with myoclonic jerks or seizures.

'The hallmark of second stage of SSPE is massive myoclonus.' – Nelson 18th/1335

Subacute Sclerosing Panencephalitis (SSPE)

- *SSPE is a chronic complication of measles with a delayed onset and an outcome that is nearly always fatal*
- *This is considered a 'slow virus infection' and is believed to result from persistant infection with an altered measles virus that is harboured intracellularly in CNS for several years.*

Stage I (Initial stage)	Subacute changes in behaviour or school performance including irritability, reduced attention, temper outbursts.
Stage II (Second stage)	Outbursts believed to result from extension of inflammatory process to deeper structures in the brain ***Massive Myoclonus is the hallmark of this stage.*** ***Involuntary movements and repetitive mycoclonic jerks are seen*** Consciousness is maintained
Stage III (Third state)	Believed to result from damage/destruction of deeper centres in blood ganglia Involuntary movements disappear and are replaced by choreoathetosis, immobility, dystonia &lead pipe rigidity. Sensorium deteriorates and dementia, stupor or coma may be seen.
Stage IV (Final stage)	Believed to result from damage to critical centres in the brain that support breathing, heart rate & blood pressure Death soon ensues

Post-traumatic Epilepsy

The term post traumatic epilepsy should be used if seizures occur after first week post injury (within several weeks to months) and are recurrent

Post traumatic epilepsyis diagnosed in a person who presents with two or more episodes of ***late post traumatic seizures***

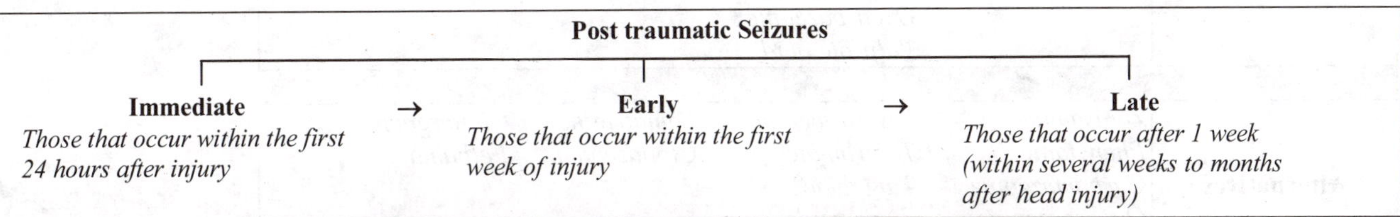

Subtypes of Neonatal Seizures

Subtypes of Neonatal Seizures
1. **Subtle (commonest subtype)**
2. *Clonic (Focal /Multifocal)*
3. *Tonic (Focal / Generalized)*
4. *Myoclonic (Focal / Multifocal / Generalized)*

'Subtle seizures are the most common sub-type, comprising about half of all seizures in term and premature new borns' *- Cloherty*

Adverse Risk Factors Predicting Risk of developing 'Epilepsy' after Febrile Seizures

Adverse Risk Factors for developing later 'Epilepsy' after Febrile Seizures

Three Major Risk Factors (Blueprints Pediatrics / Pediatric secrets)	**Additional Factors**
• *Complex Febrile seizures* - *Focal seizures* - *Prolonged (≥15min)* - *Repetitive (Recur within 24 hours)* • *Preexisting Neurodevelopmental abnormalities* - *Neurological Disorder* - *Developmental Delay* • *Close Family History of Epilepsy* *Epilepsy in first degree relatives/ siblings*	• *History of first seizure under age of 1 year (Before 12 months of age)* • *Short duration of fever prior to seizures* • *Number of febrile seizures*
Complex febrile seizures, Neurodevelopmental abnormalities and Positive family history of epilepsy are the threemajor risk factors for future epilepsy after febrile seizures.	*Early age of onset (before 12 months of age) is accepted as an adverse risk factor for future epilepsy however this has not been included as a major risk factor in certain standard textbooks and may be selected as the single best answer by exclusion if other three major risk factors are present as options*

9

Nervous System

Selection of Antiepileptic Drugs:

Agents	**Primary Generalized Tonic-Clonic**	**Partial[a]**	**Absence**	**Atypical Absence, Myoclonic, Atonic**
First-Line	*Valproic acid* *Lamotrigine* *Topiramate*	*Carbamazepine* *Phenytoin* *Lamotrigine* *Oxcarbazepine* *Valproic acid*	*Valproic acid* ***Ethosuxamide***	*Valproic acid* *Lamotrigine* *Topiramate*
Alternatives	*Zonisamide[b]* *Phenytoin* *Carbamazepine* *Oxcarbazepine* *Phenobarbital* *Primidone* *Felbamate*	*Levetiracetam[b]* *Topiramate* *Tiagabine[b]* *Zonisamide[b]* *Gabapentin*[3]* *Phenobarbital* *Primidone*	*Lamotrigine* *Clonazepam*	*Clonazepam* *Felbamate*

[a]Includes simple partial, complex partial, and secondarily generalized seizures.
[b]As adjunctive therapy.

- *Carbamazepine is the most effective drug for complex partial seizures*
- *The first line drugs for absence seizures include Valproic Acid and Ethosuxamide.*
  Ethosuxamide is generaly accepted as the primary drug of choice for the treatment of Absence seizures (Petitmal).
- *Valproate and Lamotrigine and Topiramate are the agents of first choice in cases of Generalized Tonic Clonic Seizures, atypical absence, myoclonic and atonic seizures*

Anticonvulsant therapy therapy for status epilepticus

First choice drugs	Second choice drugs	Alternative / Add on drugs
Diazepam (I.V.)	*Phenytoin (I.V.)*	*General Anaesthetic e.g.*
Clonozepam (I.V.)	*Phenobarbitone (I.V. I.M.)*	*Thiopentone sodium (KDT)*
Lorazepam (I.V.)		

Thiopentone sodium can occasionally be used for rapid control of convulsions – KDT

Adverse Effects of Phenytoin and Valproate

Side Effects of Valproate	Side effects of phenytoin:
1. Hepatotoxicity : - asymptomatic rise in serum transaminases is seen-KDT - Fulminant hepatitis may be seen	1. **Hy**perplasia of gums
2. Weight gain	2. **Hy**perglycemia
3. Hyper ammonemia	3. **Hi**rsutism
4. Gastric Irritation : Anorexia, vomiting	4. **Hy**persensitivity reaction
5. Thrombocytopenia	5. **Hy**dantoin syndrome is foetus : during pregnancy
6. Transient alopecia	6. Megaloblastic anemia
7. Ataxia, tremors and sedation may be seen	7. Osteomalacia
8. Use during pregnancy may cause neural tube defects	8. **Lymphadenopathy** - *(Harrison 15th /2364)* (**Pseudolymphoma**)
	9. Neurological symptoms like dizziness, ataxia, incordination, confusion, diplopia

Drugs causing Lymphadenopathy–*Harrisons*

Lymphadenopathy 'Pseudolymphoma' is a complication associated with use of phenytoin and is not seen with valproate.

Phenytoin Q
Primidone Q

Alzheimer's Disease

- ***Dementia from Alzheimer's disease (Dementia of Alzheimer's Type) is the classical proto-type of cortical dementias.***
  Alzheimer's dementia is the most common cortical dementia.
  Alzheimer's Disease is the most common cause of Dementia in elderly.

- ***Alzheimer's disease predominantly affects the temporoparietal cortex although frontal lobe is also frequently involved***
  'Alzheimer's disease predominantly affects the temporo-parietal cortex' – Alzheimer's Disease by Terry

- *The most important risk factors for Alzheimer's disease are old age and a positive family history–Harrison*

Risk factors for Alzheimer's Disease

Factors associated with increased risk of Alzheimer's disease	Factors associated with decreased risk of Alzheimer's disease
• Increasing Age [Q] • Female sex [Q] • Lower educational attainment [Q] • Family history of dementia [Q] • Numerous environmental factors eg. Al, Hg, Viruses & Prions. • Several genetic factors - *Amyloid Precursor Protein on chromosomes 21* - *Adult with trisomy 21 (Down's)* [Q]*-Harrison*	• *Post menopausal estrogen use* • *NSAID's use*

***Adults with trisomy 21 (Down's) consistently develop the Neuropathologic hallmarks of Alzheimer's disease if they survive beyond age 40** - Harrisons*

Point mutation on APP gene on chromosome 21 produces early onset autosomal-dominant AD. Presumably extra dose of APP gene on chromosome 21 is the initiating cause of AD in adult Down's syndrome–Harrisons

- ***A Histopathological diagnosis of Alzheimer's disease is made in cases of progressive dementia when β amyloid plaques (Neuritic/Senile plaques) co-occur with Neurofibrillary Tangles.***

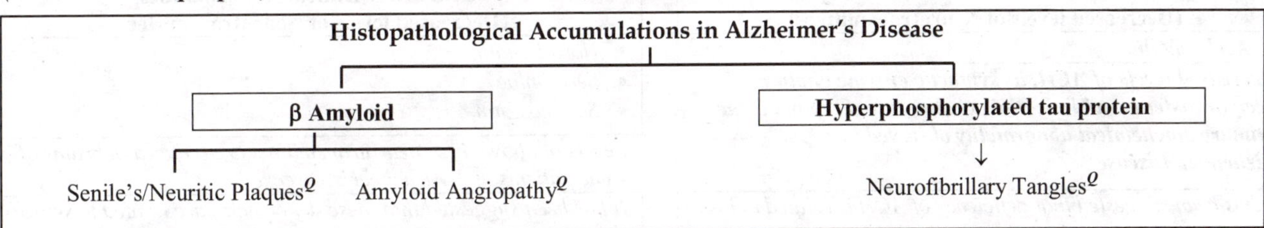

β Amyloid Plaques (Extracellular)	Neurofibrillary Tangles (Intracellular)
• β Amyloid ***Neuritic Plaques are formed by extracellular accumulation of beta amyloid*** deposits within the neutropil • 'Neuritic' or 'Senile' β-amyloid plaques are an early histopathological sign of Alzheimer's disease (that occur rarely in healthy subjects) • The amyloid β-protein accumulated in single neuritic plaques is toxic to surrounding structures and adjacent neurons. • ***Clinicopathological studies have shown that amyloid burden does not directly correlate with severity or duration of dementia.***	• Neurofibrillary tangles are formed by ***intracellular accumulation of hyperphosphorylated microtubule binding protein 'tau'.*** • NFT's occur in many neurodegenerative diseases and /or a group of diseases called 'taupathies'. These include Frontotemporal dementia, Pick's disease etc. *The cooccurance of β-amyloid plaques with NFT's suggests a diagnosis of AD.* • The NFT's are toxic to the neurons and neurons with NFT's eventually die and degenerate leaving a residual '*ghost tangle*', in the extracellular space reminding of the pyramidal cell body in which it was initially formed. • ***Clinicopathological studies have shown that dementia correlates more strongly with NFT's than with senile plaques (β-amyloid)***

Neurofibrillary Tangles are Intracellular Accumulations
• Neurofibrillary Tangles are *intracellular accumulations* of ***hyperphosphorylated microtubule binding protein 'tau'.***
• Paired helical filaments of tau protein (NFTs) form intracellularly within the soma and proximal dendrites of neurons.
• *These cytoskeletal protein tangles (NFTs),* initially impede cellular metabolism and axosplasmic transport leading to impaired synaptic function and *eventually to neuronal death.*
• *These neurofibrillary tangles may be seen as extracellular tangles after degeneration of the neuron as evidence of the neuronal cell's demise*
Neurofibrillary Tangles are intracellular accumulations that may appear extracellularly after degeneration of neuron (neuronal death)

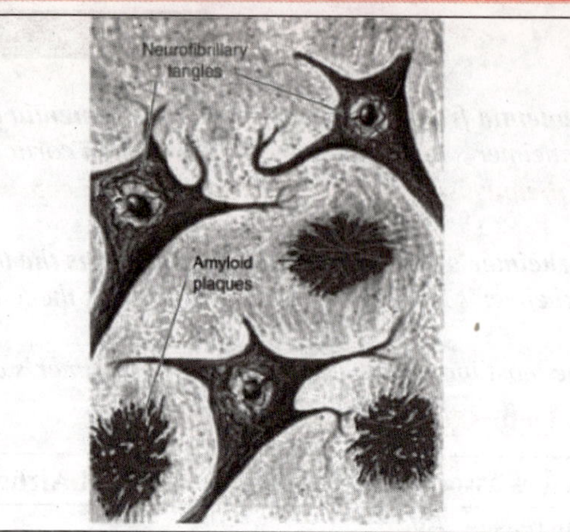

9

Topographical Distribution of NFTs in Alzheimer's disease

Neuro fibrillary Tangles (NFT): Density distribution in Alzheimer's disease
• ***Entorhinal cortex – Hippocampus*** – Amygdala interconnections (*most vulnerable*)
• Limbic and Temporal cortical areas (*next most severely involved*)
• ***Association areas of the neocortex***

'Lateral geniculate body' is usually not affected

- ***The most important biochemical abnormality in Alzheimer's disease is the decrease in cortical levels of Acetylcholine***

Biochemical Abnormalities in Alzheimer's Disease

Primary Bichemical Abnormality (Decreased levels of Neurotransmitters)
• *Acelylcholine*

Decreased levels of ACH, its synthetic enzyme choline acetyltransferase and nicotinic cholinergic receptors is the primary biochemical abnormality observed in Alzheimer'Disease

It has been suggested that deficiency of ACH is related to loss of memory / dementia in patients with AD

Other Biochemical Abnormalities (Decreased levels of Neurotransmitters)
• *Noradrenaline* • *Serotonine* • *Somatostatin*

Levels of above three neurotransmitters are reduced in brains of some patients with Alzheimer's Disease

It has been suggested that these deficiencies are related to sensory disturbance and aggressive behavior in patient with AD

Dopamine deficiency is not a feature of Alzheimer's disease.

Alzeimer's Disease: Review:

Clinically	Pathologically		Biochemically
	Gross [Q]	**Microscopic**	
• Subtle onset memory loss followed by • Slowly progressive dementia over several years	• Diffuse atrophy of cerebral cortex • Secondary enlargement of ventricular system	• ***Neuritic plaques***[Q] containing β amyloid • ***Neurofibrillary*** [Q] ***tangles*** • ***Amyloid angiopathy*** accumulation of β amyloid in arterial walls of cerebral blood vessels.	• Decrease in cerebral cortical levels of acetyl choline [Q] (choline acety transferase (CAT) and nicotinic cholinergic receptors are also reduced) [[Q] Reduction in ACH is related to degeneration of nucleus basalis of meynert [Q]]

'Lewy bodies' are characteristically seen in idiopathic Parkinson's disease (and not in Alzheimer's disease).

Parkinsonism

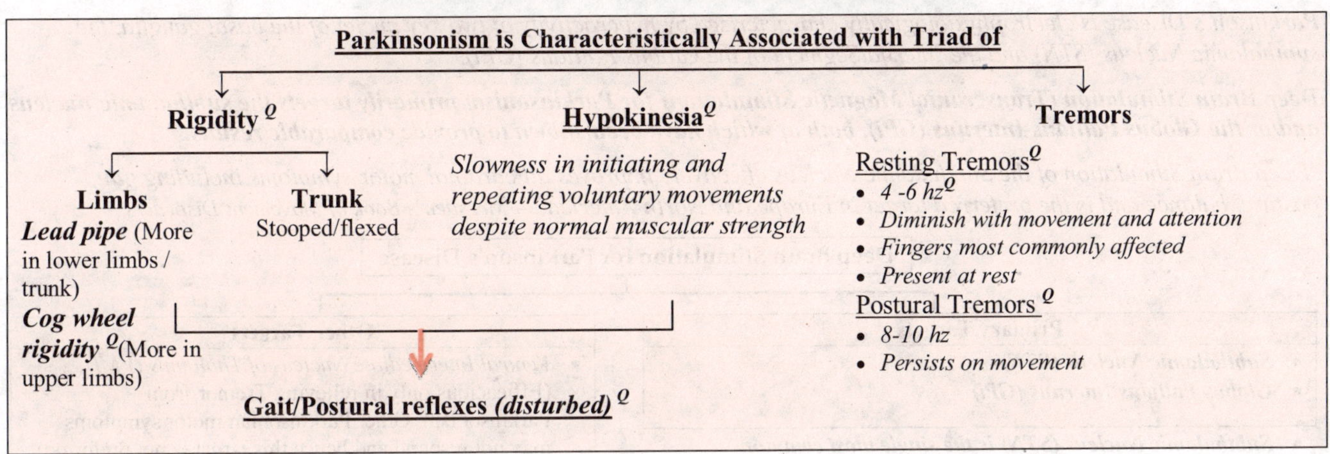

- *Parkinsonism is caused by a disturbance in nigrostriatal naurons of the substantia nigra.* [Q]
- *Parkinson's Disease is electrophysiologically characterized by hyperactivity of two key nuclei of the basal ganglia, the subthalamic Nucleus (STN) and the InternalSegment of the Globus Pallidus (GPi)*
- *The main biochemical charachteristic of Parkinson's disease is the reduction of neurotransmitter and the dopamine synthesizing enzyme system including* ***Tyrosine Hydroxylase (TH)*** *and Tetrahydrobiopterin (BH_4) Cofactor in nigrostriatal neurons.*

Phenylalanine —(Phenylalanine Hydroxylase)→ Tyrosine —(***Tyrosine Hydroxylase***; Rate limiting step)→ ***DOPA*** —(DOPA Decarboxylase)→ Dopamine

Once approximately 80% of these neurons degenerate, the nigrostriatal tract cannot synthesize adequate dopamine and Parkinson's disease symptoms appear

- *Several Toxins including manganese Q have been implicated in the pathogenesis of Parkinson's Disease*

Toxins Implicated in Parkinsonism *(Harrison)*	
• *Manganese (Mn)* • *MPTP (1 Methyl - 4 Phenyl – 1, 2, 3, 6 tetrahydropyridine)* • *Carbonmonoxide* • *Carbondisulphide*	• *Cyanide* • *Hexane* • *Methanol*

- *Parkinsonism is typically charachterized by a triad of Rigidity, Bradykinesia and Tremor at rest*

Triad of Parkinsonism.
2. Rigidity
3. Bradykinesia
4. Tremor at rest,

- *Tremor is typically at rest* [Q] *with frequency 4 - 6 Hz.*[Q]
- Rigidity, Hypokinesia and loss of postural Reflexes result in a characteristic disturbance of gait and posture

• *Difficulty in maintaining balance* • *Slow to start walking* • *Shortened stride* • *Rapid small steps (tendency to run): festinating gait*	• *Reduced arm swing* • *Difficulty in stopping suddenly* • *Impaired balance on turning* • *Small Handwriting*

- *Masked expressionless facies* [Q]
- *Slurred indistinct speech* [Q]
- *Normal intelligence* [Q]
- *Emotional lability* [Q]
- *A depressed mood is common and an impairment of cognitive functions sometimes amounting to frank dementia is frequently evident in advanced cases - this explains the memory loss present in the patient*
- *Tendon reflexes are unaltered* [Q] *(Normal deep tendon reflexes)* [Q]
- *Plantar reflex is typically flexor* [Q] *(Negative Babiniski)* [Q]

Deep Brain Stimuation for Parkinsonism

Parkinson's Disease is electrophysiologically characterized by hyperactivity of two key nuclei of the basal ganglia, the subthalamic Nucleus (STN) and the InternalSegment of the Globus Pallidus (GPi).

Deep Brain Stimulation (Transcranial Magnetic Stimulation) for Parkinsonism primarily targets the subthalamic nucleus and/or the Globus Pallidus Internus (GPi), both of which have been shown to provide comparable results.

'Deep Brain Stimulation of the Subthalamic Nucleus effectively improves all cardinal motor symptoms including gait, posture, balance and is the preferred target in Europe and North America'. – Marsden's Book of Movement Disorders

Deep Brain Stimulation for Parkinson's Disease

Primary Targets

- ***Subthalamic Nucleus (STN)***
- ***Globus Pallidus Internus (GPi)***

- ***Subthalamic Nucleus (STN) is the single most common preferred site*** *for Deep Brain Stimulation in patients with Parkinsonism.*
- ***Globus Pallidus Internus (GPi) is the second most common site*** for Deep Brain Stimulation in patients with Parkinsonism and provides comparable results to DBS of STN.
- ***Subthalamic nucleus and Globus Pallidus Internus both provide comparable efficacy*** (Believed to be equally effective)

Other Targets

- *Ventral Intermediate Nucleus of Thalamus (VMI)* (Efficacious only in relieving Tremor from Parkinsonism. Other Parkinsonian motor symptoms may not respond and hence this target is not preferred)
- *Pedunculopantine Nucleus* (DBS of Pedunculopontine nucleus may be beneficial for patients with advanced parkinsonism and predominant axial symptoms, postural instability and gait disturbance. Results are however still limited to only a few patients)

Treatment of Drug Induced Extrapyramidal Symptoms/Signs

Central anticholinergics are the only drugs effective in phenothiazine / drug induced extrapyramidal symptoms

Central anticholinergics include

1. *Trihexphenidyl: Most commonly used drug (Benzhexol)*
2. *Procyclidine*
3. *Biperidin*
4. *Benztropine.*

All antipsychotics have potent dopamine blocking action. Dopaminergic blockage in basal ganglia results in deficiency of dopamine, which controls muscle tone and coordinates movements.
This is turn shift the balance between the inhibitory dopaminergic system and excitatory cholinergic system, towards excitatory levels and results in dystonias.
Balance can thus be restored by suppression of the unopposed excitatory cholinergic system (Administration of central anticholinergics).

Characteristic features ofCerebellar disease and Parkinsonism

Cerebellar Disease

Nystagmus
Scanning speech/Dysarthria
Hypotonia
Past pointing
Pendular knee jerks
Dysdiadokinesia
Truncal ataxia
Intention tremor
Loss of coordination

Positive Romberg's test
Positive Heel – Shin test
Positive Finger Nose test

Parkinson's disease

Rigidity
Hypokinesia/Akinesia
Tremor
Loss of postural Reflexes

Huntington's Chorea

- *Huntington's disease is a degenerative* Q *brain disorder that is genetically determined.* Q
- *Huntington's disease is inheried as an autosomal dominant disorder*

  Huntingtons Disease: Inheritance and genetics:

  The minimum chance of getting disease in a child with one affected parent is 1:2 and with both affected parents is 3:4

Chance of getting disease in a child

If one parent is affected	If both parents are affected
Minimum chance of getting the disease in a child would be 50 percent or 1 in 2 (1:2)	*Minimum chance of getting the disease in a child would be 75 percent or 3 in 4 (3:4)*

Genetic abnormality responsible for Huntington's disease is a CAG trimucleotide expansion on a gene called 'Huntingtin' which is localized on chromosome 4.

HD is not caused by a point mutation but by a Triplet Repeat Expansion mutation.

- The age of onset of Huntington's disease depend on the sex of the parent and on the age of onset in the parent

  Individual who inherit the disease from the father usually have an early onset of disease

  Individual who inherit the disease from the mother usually have a late onset of disease

Mean age of onset of HD: 40-50 years
Mean age of juvenile onset of HD < 20 years

Effect of parental sex in Huntington's disease

Characteristic manifestations include

Gene inherited from father

- Individuals who inherit the gene from their father usually have an *early onset disease*
- **Effect of Anticipation** is exhibited strongly

  'Anticipation' means that successive generations develop the disease at an earlier age than their parent

  When gene is inherited from father the phenomenon of Anticipation is exhibited strongly.
- **Effect of CAG trimucleotide Expansion**

  Onset of disease depends on length of CAG trinucleotide (onset is inversely related to length of trinucleotide).

  CAG repeats tend to expand significantly more when passed from father to child.

Gene inherited from mother

- Individuals who inherit disease from the mother usually have a *late onset disease*
- **Effect of Anticipation** is less characteristic

  Anticipation means that successive generations develop the disease at an earlier age than the parent

  When gene is inherited from motor, the phenomenon of 'Anticipation' may be exhibited but this phenomenon is less marked or less characteristic.
- **Effect of CAG trinucleotide Expansion**

  Onset of disease depends on length of CAG trinucleotide

  CAG repeats tend to expand more slowly when disease is passed from mother to child

- ***'The reported abnormality in Huntington's disease suggests a relative under activity of neurons containing gamma-aminobutyric acid (GABA) and acetylcholine'*** *– CMDT*
- *'There is **severe loss of striatal neurons**, the most dramatic changes being found in the caudate nucleus' – Robbins (Caudate nucleus is part of striatum)*
- ***Memory loss is frequently not impaired until late in the disease,*** *although attention judgement & executive functions may be seriously deficient at an early stage.*

Age of onset :	Neuropathologically :	Clinical Hallmarks :
It's usual age of onset in *4th or 5th decade* Q	Neuropathologically the disease predominantly strikes the *striatum* Q*&atrophy of caudate nucleus* is seen Q	• *Chorea* Q • *Behavioural disturbance* Q • *Dementia* Q

9

Nervous System

Normal Pressure Hydrocephalus

Normal Pressure Hydrocephalus

This is a communicating hydrocephalus with a aqueduct of sylvius caused by obstruction to normal flow of CSF over the cerebral convexities and delayed absorption into the venous system. *The CSF opening pressure is in the high normal range (Hence called Normal Pressure Hydrocephalus).*

Characteristic Clinical Triad
- ***Abnormal Gait (Ataxic or Apractic)***
- ***Dementia (Usually mild or moderate)***
- ***Urinary Incontinance***

Neuroimaging	CSF Picture
Enlarged lateral ventricles Q (Hydrocephalus) Q with little or No Cortical-Atrophy Q	• Pressure : High **normal** range (Hence called NPH) Q • Protein : Normal Q • Sugar : Normal Q • Cell count : Normal Q

Supranuclear Gaze Palsy

Steel Richardson syndrome

Nature of disorder

Is a degenerative disorder where in there occurs loss of neurons in parts of our CNS which are involved with maintenance of posture & equilibrium, namely the Mid brain, Pons, Basal ganglion and cerebellum.

The clinical features are characteristic

"Progressive supranuclear palsy should be considered whenever a middle aged or elderly person-person presents with history of repeated falls and has an extrapyramidal syndrome accompanied by nuchal dystonia and paralysis of voluntary down gaze"

Factors which distinguish this from Parkinson's

a. *Marked impairment of voluntary downward gaze and horizontal gaze.* Q
b. *Extended rather than flexed dystonic posturing* Q
c. *Absence of tremor* Q
d. Poor response to antiparkinsonian medication

Pseudotumor cerebri

It is a benign self-limiting disorder with a favorable outcome.

Characteristic features:	Causes include :
Elevated intracranial pressure (*intracranial hypertension*) with : • ***Normal or Small sized ventricular system*** Q • ***No focal neurological signs*** Q • **Papilledema** Q (enlarged blind spot in visual fluid). • **Normal CSF findings** Q • **Normal CT scan, MRI and isotope brain scan** • Excessive slow-wave activity on ECG	• *High doses of vitamin A* Q • Outdated Tetracycline • Quinolones • *Withdrawal of corticosteroid therapy* Q • *Addison's disease* Q • SLE • *Hypoparathyroidism* Q

There are no focal neurological signs in pseudotumor cerebri. Therefore, Pseudotumor Cerebri does not present with convulsions.

Wernicke's Disease and Delirium Tremens

Wernicke's Disease

- Wernicke's disease is seen in *Alcoholic*[Q] patients with *chronic thiamine deficiency*[Q].
- *Wernicke's Disease is charachterized by he clinical triad of Global Confusion, Ophthalmoplegia and Ataxia*

Triad of Wernicke's encephalopathy (Thiamine deficiency in alcoholics)
• *Ophthalmoplegia (Third & Sixth Nerve palsies & Nystagmus are typical)* • *Ataxia* • *Confusion (Global confusion)*

- *Principle sites within the brain that are affected in this syndrome include Mamillary bodies, Periventricular Grey Matter and Thalamus*

Principle Sites of Involvement in Wernicke's Korsakoff Syndrome
• Mammillary bodies *(Petechial haemorrhages are characteristic)* • Thalamus *(Dorsomedial Nucleus)* • Periaqueductal Grey Matter *(Periventricular lesions around the Third ventricle, Aqueduct and Fourth ventricle)*

[Q]***Small pelicheal Haemorrhages in the mamillary bodies are characteristic of Wernicke's disease***, a complication of chronic alcoholism and thiamine deficiency. Neither Vascular stroke, Pyridoxine deficiency, Lwey body disease nor Cluster headaches present with haemorrhages in the mamillary bodies. – Kaplan & Saddock's Study Guide (2007)/Q 5.10

Hippocamous is not involved in Wernicke's Korsakoff syndrome.

- ***The Amnestic effect in Wernicke's Korsakoff Syndrome is related to lesions in the dorso-medial nuclei of the thalamus.***

'Lesions in the dorsomedial nucleus of the thalamus seem to be the best correlate of the memory disturbance and confabulation'

'The amnestic defect is related to lesions in the dorso-medial nuclei of the thalamus' – Harrison's 18th/2260

Delirium Tremens

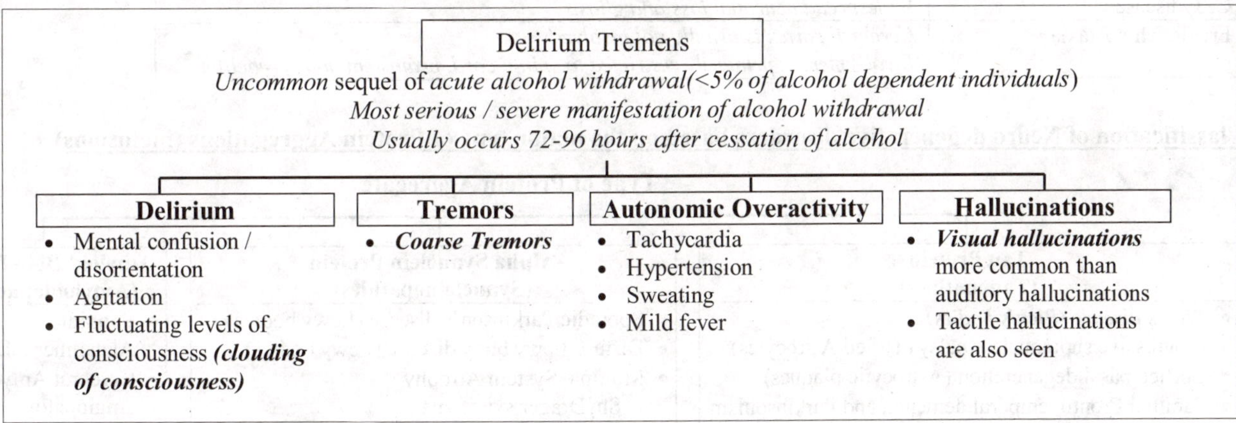

Down's Syndrome and Memory Loss

Down Syndrome is associated with memory impaiment

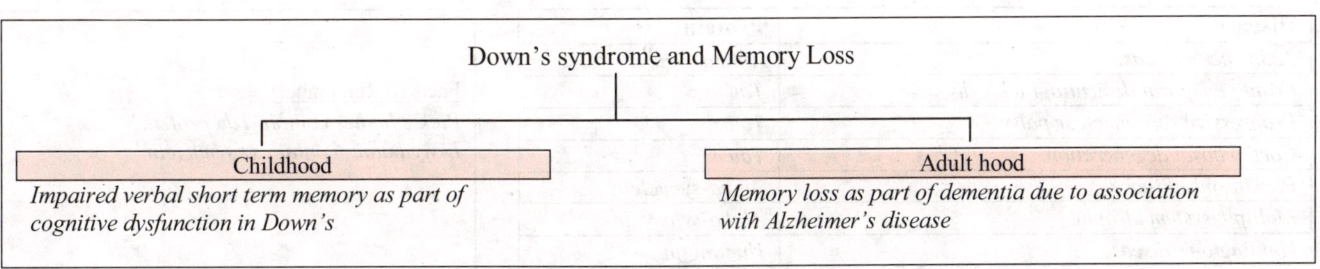

Classification of Dementias

Classification of Dementias

Cortical Dementias	Subcortical Dementias	Mixed Dementias (Dementias with Cortical & Subcortical Features)
• ***Alzheimer's Dementia*** • *Fronto-temporal dementia (Pick's disease)* • *Dementia due to Creutzfeldt-Jakob disease* • *Dementia due to Chronic Subdural Hematoma*	• ***Parkinson's Disease*** • *Huntington's Disease* • *Multiple Sclerosis* • ***Progressive Supranuclear Palsy*** • ***Dementia due to HIV***	• *Vascular dementias (Multi-infarct dementia)* • *Vascular Dementia (Post-stroke)* • *Lewy body variant of Alzheimer's* • *Lewy body dementia* • *Dementia due to Fragile-X-associated tremor/ataxia syndrome*

Predominant site affected in Dementias

Predominant Site Affected in Cortical Dementias

Alzheimer's Disease	Pick's Disease
• *Temporo-Parietal Cortex (Predominant)* • Frontal lobe may also be involved	• *Fronto-temporal cortex*[Q]

Condition	Anatomical Feature
Frontotemporal dementia	***Regional Atrophy of temporal and/or frontal lobe***
Alzheimer's disease	*Diffuse cerebral atrophy*
PML	*Widespread demyelinating lesions of cerebral cortex*
C. J. disease	*Widespread neuronal loss and gliosis*
Friedreich's Ataxia	*Cerebral cortex is usually not involved.* *Involvement is primarily restricted to spinal cord, brainstem and cerebellum.*

Classification of Neuro degenerative disorders based on the major type of Protein Aggregations (inclusions)

Type of Protein Aggregate

Tau Protein (Tauopathies)	Alpha Synuclein Protein (Synucleinopathies)	Amyloid Beta Protein (Amyloidopathies)
• ***Pick's disease (Pick's bodies)*** • Progressive supranuclear palsy (Tufted Astrocytes) • Cortico basal degeneration (Astrocytic plaques) • Familial Fronto temporal dementia and Parkinsonism linked to chromosome 17 (FTDP-17)	• Sporadic Parkinson's disease (Lewy bodies) • Diffuse Lewy body disease (Lewy bodies) • Multiple System Atrophy - ShyDrager syndrome - Striatonigral degeneration - Olivopontocerebellar atrophy	• Sporadic Alzheimer's Disease • Cerebral Amyloid Angiopathy

Protein Aggregations in Major Dementias and Related Cognitive Disorders:

Disease	Protein
Alzhiemer's disease	*A-beta, Tau*[Q]
Fronto temporal dementia, Pick's disease	*Tau*
Progressive supranuclear palsy	*Tau*
Corticobasal degeneration	*Tau*
Parkinson's disease	*Alpha-synuclein*
Multiple system atrophy	*Alpha-synuclein*
Huntington's disease	*Huntingtin*
Prion disease	*Prion protein*
Spinocerebellar ataxia	*Ataxin*

Facts to Remember:
Pick's bodies contain Tau protein[Q]
Lewy bodies contain α synuclein[Q]

CNS Infections

Normal CSF evaluation

Common C.S.F values	
• C.S.F. pressure	• 50-180 mm H_2O
• C.S.F. volume	• 150 ml
• C.S.F. glucose	• 40-70 mg/dl
• Total protein	• 15-50 mg/dl
• C.S.F. RBC	• 0
• C.S.F. leucocytes	• < 5 micro/litre
Total Differential • Lymphocytes • Monocytes • Neutrophils	 • 60-70% • 30-50% • None
• C.S.F. pH	• 7.1-7.34

C.S.F Glucose is 40-70 mg/dl which is about 2/3 of plasma glucose (80-120 mg/dl): *Harrison*

CSF changes in Infection of CNS:

Parameters (Normal values)	Bacterial Meningitis	Tuberculous Meningitis	Viral Meningitis
Pressure	Raised	Raised	Raised
Gross appearance	Turbid	Clear (may clot)	Clear
Protein (Normal: 20-50 mg/dL)	High	Very High	Slightly high
Glucose (40-70 mg/dL)	Very Low	Low	Normal
Chloride (116-122 μg/dL)	Low	Very Low	Normal
Cells < 5/microlit	Neutrophils	Pleocytosis (Lymphocytes and Neutrophils in CSF)	Lymphocytosis

(Pleocytosis is the presence of both Neutrophils and Lymphocytes in CSF)

9

Nervous System

Tubercular Meningitis

Classic CSF Abnormalities in Tubercular Meningitis

Classic CSF abnormalities in Tuberculosis Meningitis :*Harrison*
• *Elevated opening pressure*
• *Elevated protein concentration (Range of 1 to 5 g/L or 10 to 500mg/dL)*
• *Decreased glucose concentration (Range of 1.1 to 2.2 mmol/L or 20 to 40 mg/dL)*
• *Lymphocytic pleocytosis (10 to 500 cells / μL)* *Mononuclear cells (except early infection when PMN cells are seen)* Q
• *Chloride level : usually reduced.*

Classical Radiological Features (CT/MRI) in Tubercular Meningitis

Classical Radiological Features (CT/MRI) in Tubercular Meningitis
• ***Basal exudates / Obliteration of Basal cisterns*** *(Tubercular Exudates are primarily located in the vicinity of basal cisterns that are obscured by presence of inflammatory tissue exudate.* *Subarachnoid space is involved by the exudate i.e. subarachnoiditis is present)* Q
• *Abnormal Leptomeningeal Enhancement* (Usually most pronounced in the basal cisterns) (Involvement is *mainly of the leptomeninges i.e. Pia-arachnoid; Duramater is usually spared.)* Q
• ***Hydrocephalus*** (Usually communicating although non-communicating may also be seen)
• ***Ischemic / Vasculitic Infarcts*** (Basal ganglia and / or Internal capsule)
• *Tuberculomas* (Granulomas)
• *Calcification* is commonly seen in the meninges at the base of the brain.
• *Ventriculitis* may be seen, but it is not common

The pathological hallmark of Tubercular Meningitis is predominant involvement of basal cisterns that are observed by the presence of basal inflammatory tissue exudate.

'The triad of CT features (Thalamic infarction, Basal cistern enhancement and Hydrocephalus) is diagnostic of Tubercular Meningitis' – Journal of Indian Medical Association

Bacterial meningitis (Pneumococcal meningitis)

Bacterial Meningitis ***is characterized by polymorphonuclearleucocytosis, high protein concentration and low sugars.CSF proteins are increased and glucose levels are characteristically decreased.***

Cerebrospinal Fluid (CSF) Abnormalities in Bacterial Meningitis

Opening pressure	> 180 mmH_2O
White blood cells	10μL; neutrophils predominate
Red blood cells	Absent in nontraumatic tap
Glucose	< 2.2 mmol/L (<40 mg/dL)
CSF/serum glucose	< 0.4
Protein	> 0.45 g/L (> 45 mg/dL)
Gram's stain	Positive in > 60%
Culture	Positive in > 80%
Larex agglutination	May be positive in patients with meningitis due to S. pneumoniae, N. meningitis, H. Influenzae type B, E.coli, group B streptococci
Limulus lysate	Positive in cases of gram-negative meningitis
PCR	Detects bacterial DNA

Pneumococci are the most common cause of recurrent meningitis in the setting of CSF leaks

'Streptococcus Pneumoniae is the most common cause of recurrent meningitis due to cerebrospinal fluid leaks'

- Infections of the CNS 3rd/354; Mayo Clinic 8th/567

Viruses causing encephalitis and meningoencephalitis

- *The most common cause of sporadic* **viral encephalitis is HSV-I**

The most common cause of sporadic viral encephalitis [Q]	*HSV-I*
The most common cause of epidemic viral encephalitis [Q]	*Arbovirus*
The most common cause of viral ***meningitis*** *is* [Q]	*Enterovirus*

- ***HSV type 2 is a common cause of aseptic meningitis, however encephalitis following HSV type 2 has not been mentioned.***
- *Japanese encephalitis virus* is an arbovirus and is one of the most common causes of encephalitis outbreaks.
- ***Enteroviruses are the most common cause of viral meningoencephalitis.***
- ***Viruses causing Encephalitis***

Common	Less common	Rare
• Arboviruses e.g. Japanese – B encephalitis virus • Enterovirus • HSV – I • Mumps	• CMV • EBV • HIV • Measles • Varicella Zoster	• Adenovirus • Influenza • Para influenza (Nipahvirus) • Rabies • Rubella • CTFV (Colarado tick fever virus) • LCMV (Lymphocytic choriomeningitis virus)

Nipah virus: is a new member of the paramyxo virus family.
New cases of viral encephalitis are constantly appearing as evidenced by the recent outbreaks of 300 cases of encephalitis with 40% mortality rate in Malaysia caused by Nipah virus (paramyxovirus family).

Herpes Simplex Encephalitis

Focal findings in a patient with encephalitis should always raise the possibility of HSV encephalitis.

Herpes Simplex Encephalitis: Characteristic Anatomic Localization

- HSV encephalitis has a charachteristic neuroanatomic pattern of involvement affecting primarily the temporal lobe and inferior frontal lobe (cingulate gyrus).

The virus preferentially involves the temporal lobes and often the frontal lobes (especially the cingulate gyrus)
(In most cases the involvement is unilateral, but contralateral involvement may also be seen and patient may present with asymmetric bilateral temporal lobe involvement)

- Herpes Encephalitis is also often haemorrhagic although not always
- This characteristic neuroanatomic pattern of involvement in Herpes Simplex Encephalitis can help in specifically suggesting the diagnosis of HSV encephalitis on MR scans.

MRI Scan Features of H.S.V. Encephalitis

- ***Hyperintensity on T2- weighted sequences*** (T2 prolonging lesions) within the medial temporal lobes (insula) and inferior frontal lobes (cingulate gyrus region)(Note: Hypointensity is seen on T1 weighted images)
- ***Enhancement of lesions with contrast***. Enhancement of the meninges, cortex and white matter (Enhancement means that blood brain barrier has broken down and that the process is biologically active)

CT	*Temporoparietal areas of low absorption, mass effect and control enhancement*
EEG	*Periodic temporal lobe spikes on a background of slow or low amplitude activity on EEG*

Hyperintensity in the temporal lobe and inferior frontal lobe on T2 weighted images with contrast enhancement is a charachteristic neuroanatomic pattern of involvement in Herpes simplex Encephalitis and in the presence of suggestive clinical features (fever / focal seizures) specifically suggests the diagnosis of HSV Encephalitis

The drug of choice for treatment of HSV Encephalitis is ACYCLOVIR

Condition	Drug of choice
Herpes simplex Encephalitis	***Acyclovir***
Neonatal herpes simplex [Q]	*Acyclovir* [Q]
Herpes simplex Keratitis [Q]	*Trifluridine / Vidarabine* [Q]
Herpes simplex Oro-labialis	Pencicyclovir

Neurocysticercosis

- ***Neurocysticercosis is the most common parasitic infestation of the cns in an immune-competent host***

> *"The most common parasitic infestation to affect the non-immunosuppressed host is neurocysticercosis, a disorder caused by the larval form of taenia solium" – Cecil*

- *Cysticercosis is infection with the larval stage (cysticercus) of T. sollum.*

These cysts are located in order of frequency in:
a. *CNS (Neurological manifestations are the most common) - Harrison's*
b. *Subcutaneous tissue*
c. *Striated muscle*
d. *Globe of the eye*

- *The most common clinical manifestation of Neurocysticercosis is Epilepsy*

> *"These is wide variety of presentation of Neurocysticercosis depending on the intensity of the infestation, the localization of cystecerci and the degree of inflammatory reaction.* ***Epilepsy (seizure activity) is the most common manifestation occurring in upto 50% cases*** *- API text book of Medicine*

- ***Brain Parcnchyma is the most common site of neurocysticercosis.***

'The ventricular system is the second most common site of neurocysticercosis.

Most comon sites of Nurocysticercosis :
Parenchymatous > intrventricular > subarachnoid > spinal > orbital.

- *The most common findings on brain imaging is* ***Paenchymal brain calcifications***

> *The lesion of neurocysticereosis is readily visualized by MRI or CT Scan.*
> ***Paenchymal brain calcifications are the most common findings.*** *- Harrison*

- *Albendazole is the drug of choice for treatment of Neurocysticercosis*

> *Albendazole and Proziquantel are both effective in treatment*
> *Albendazole is preferred. (DOC is Albendazole)*
> ***Niclosamide is ineffective for Neurocysticercosis***

- ***Anticonvulsants (antiepileptics)*** should be given during drug treatment and probably for an indefinite time afterwards.
- ***Corticosteroids*** may be used during the acute phase of cysticercotic encephalitis, if intracranial hypertension is present. (*It is used for the prevention of development of hydrocephalus, and does not have much role once hydrocephalus is already present.*)

Prions and Prion associated diseases

- **Prions are infectious proteins *devoid of any nucleic acid (RNA or DNA)*** Q
  *(Prions are the only known infectious agents that are devoid of nucleic acid*Q*)*
- Prion diseases result from the accumulation of the *abnormal prion protein 'Pr P*^{SC}*'*Q
- Prions are most *resistant to physical and chemical agents such as heat, irradiation and formaline*Q.
- They are sensitive to proteasesQ (contain protein) but resistant to nucleasesQ (do not contain nucleic acid)
- The diseases caused by Prions include diseases in human & animals

Prion diseases

Human	Animals
• *Creutzfeldt Jakob disease*Q • *Gerstmann – Straussier Scheinker disease*Q • *Fatal Familial Insomnia*Q • *Kuru*Q	• *Scrapie (sheep)* Q • *Bovine Spongiform Encephalopathy (cattle)* Q • *Mink Encephalopathy (Mink)* Q • *Chronic Wasting Disease (Mule, Deer, Elk)* Q • *Feline Spongiform Encephalopathy (Cats)* Q • *Exotic lingulate encephalopathy (kudu, nyala or oryx)*

Q*The sporadic form of CJD is the most common prion disorder in humans*

- Prion Diseases share several distinguishing hallmarks

Hallmarks of Prion Diseases
• The disease *is confined to the Nervous system*Q (Although agent may be recoverable from other organs) • The basic features are *Neurodegeneration and Spongiform*Q changes • Amyloid plaques may be present • Clinical illness is preceded by *a long incubation period*Q (months to decades) • Onset of clinical illness is followed by *chronic progressive disease*Q (weeks to years) • The disease is *always fatal*Q with *no known cases of remission*Q or recovery • The host shows *no inflammatory response and no immune response*Q - *Agents do not appear to be antigenic*Q - No production of interferon is elicited - *There is no effect on host B cell or T cell function* - *Immunosupression of the host has no effected on pathogenesis*

Creutzfeldt-Jacob disease : Review

Nature of illness : *Heritable, degenerative, infectious disease.*
• Creutzfeldt- Jacob disease is the most common prion disease (infectious) in humans [Q] • It is a neurodegenerative disease with major pathological changes confined to CNS [Q] – *Harrisons 16th / 2496* • The prion concept explains how this disease can manifest both a heritable [Q] as well as an infectious illness. [Q]
Clinical manifestations :
• Non specific prodromal symptoms : Fatigue, sleep disturbance, weight loss, headache, malaise, ill defined pain • Dementia [Q] (deficit in higher cortical functions) : Memory loss, impaired judgement, decline in intellectual function • Myoclonus [Q]: Most patients (90%) exhibit myoclonus at some time throughout illness. *'Myoclonus is a very common manifestation of C-J disease. 'Most patient (90%) with CJD exhibit myoclonus that appears at various times throughout the illness'* – Harrisons. • Cerebellar signs visual impairment may occur
Characteristic ECG finding [Q]:
• Paroxysm of high voltage and slow waves
Treatment
• There is no specific treatment.

Approach to the Diagnosis of Creutzfeldt Jakob Disease

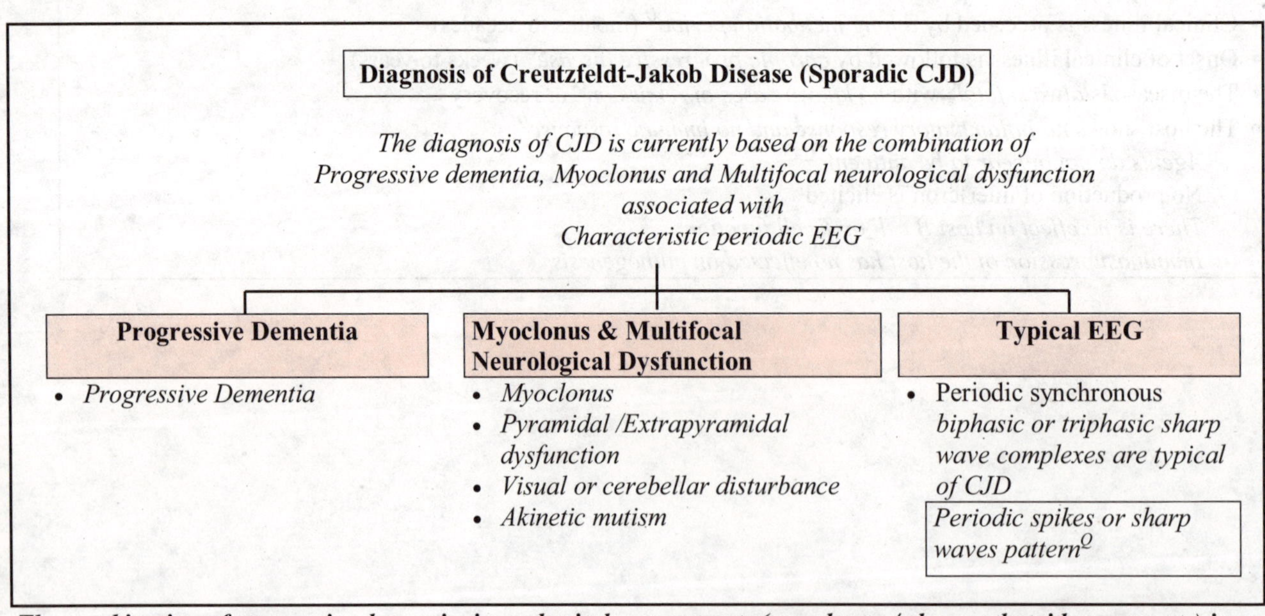

Diagnosis of Creutzfeldt-Jakob Disease (Sporadic CJD)

The diagnosis of CJD is currently based on the combination of Progressive dementia, Myoclonus and Multifocal neurological dysfunction associated with Characteristic periodic EEG

Progressive Dementia
- *Progressive Dementia*

Myoclonus & Multifocal Neurological Dysfunction
- *Myoclonus*
- *Pyramidal /Extrapyramidal dysfunction*
- *Visual or cerebellar disturbance*
- *Akinetic mutism*

Typical EEG
- Periodic synchronous *biphasic or triphasic sharp wave complexes are typical of CJD*

Periodic spikes or sharp waves pattern[Q]

The combination of progressive dementia, irregular jerky movements (myoclonus / choreoathetoid movements) in association with a characteristic EEG pattern (periodic sharp biphasic waves) suggests a diagnosis Creutzfeldt Jakob Disease.

CNS Tumors

Most common Cenral Nervous Tumors

Gliomas *(Most common)*
Astrocytomas (includes Glioblastoma multiforme)
Ependymomas
Oligodendrogliomas

Most common intracranial tumors in adults is
Glioblastoma multiforme (Glioma)
(Grade IV Astrocytoma)

Most common intracranial tumor in children is
Cerebellar Astrocytoma (Glioma)

Glial tumors in decreasing order of frequency amongst adults

- Astrocytomas (Most common): *Glioblastoma multiforme is the most common type of Astrocytoma*
- Ependymoma
- Oligodendroglioma

Most Common Primary intracranial Neoplasms in adults	
Glioblastoma Multiforme (Type of Gliomastrocytoma)	*20%*
Meningioma	*15%*

Most common Primary Intracranial Neoplasms in adults	
Astrocytomas (Type of Glioma and includes Glioblastoma Multiforma)	*≈30%*
Meningiomas	*15%*

Most common Primary Intracranial Neoplasms in adults	
Gliomas (includes Astrocytomas, Ependymomas and oligodendrogliomas)	*>50%*
Menengioma	*15%*

Most common Posterior Fossa Tumors in Children

Cerebellar Astrocytomas are the most common posterior fossa tumors in children.
Medulloblastoma are the second most common posterior fossa tumors in children and the most common malignant posterior fossa tumors in children.

Most Common Posterior Fossa Tumors in Children

Cerebellar Astrocytomas are the most common posterior fossa tumors In children
Most Cerebellar Astrocytomas are benign.

Medulloblastomas and other primitive neuroectodermal tumors (PNET) are the most common malignant posterior fossa tumors in children
Most medulloblastomas are malignant

Although CPDT and Nelson's textbook mention an equal incidence of cerebellar astrocytoma and medulloblastoma in the posterior fossa in children, most other standard textbooks mention cerebellar astrocytomas as the most common posterior fossa tumors in children.

Facts to Remember :

- *The most common tumors in children are : Leukaemia*
- *The most common solid tumours in children are: CNS tumors*
- *The most common site of brain tumors in children is Infratentorial (cerebellar)*
- *The most common site of brain tumors in neonates is supratentorial*
- *The most common CNS tumors in children are Glial tumors*

Glial tumors
• *Astrocytomas* • *Oligodindrogliomas* • *Ependymomas*

Note

- ***Glial tumors as a group are more common than medulloblastomas***
- *If a question asks about the most common brain tumor in children, and it does not have astrocytoma as an option, but it has 'glioma' as an option, mark Glioma in preferance to Medulloblastoma. (Astrocytoma is also a ' glioma').*
- *When based on histology the prevalence of Medulloblastomas and Juvenile Pilocytic astrocytoma / cerebellar astrocytomas has been mentioned as equal in most textbooks* ***Yet Cerebellar astrocytomas are accepted as the most common posterior fossa tumors in children***

- ***Astrocytoma (Cerebellar)***
  - *Most common posterior fossa tumor in children is Cerebellar Astrocytoma.*[Q]
  - *Therefore most common brain tumor in children is also Cerebellar Astrocytoma.*[Q]
  - *Astrocytoma also has the best prognosis in children.*[Q]
  - *Therefore tumor with best prognosis in children is also Astrocytoma.*[Q]
- ***Medulloblastoma***
  - *The second most common posterior fossa tumor in children.*[Q]
  - *Tumor which spreads along CSF pathways is medulloblastoma.*[Q]
  - *Tumor which is capable of metastasising to extracranial sites is medulloblastoma.*[Q]
  - *Medulloblostoma is highly radiosensitive.*[Q]
- ***Brain Stem Gliomas :***
  - *These are the third most frequent post. fossa tumors in children*[Q]
- ***Craniopharyngioma :***
  - *These are the most common supratentorial tumor in children.*[Q]

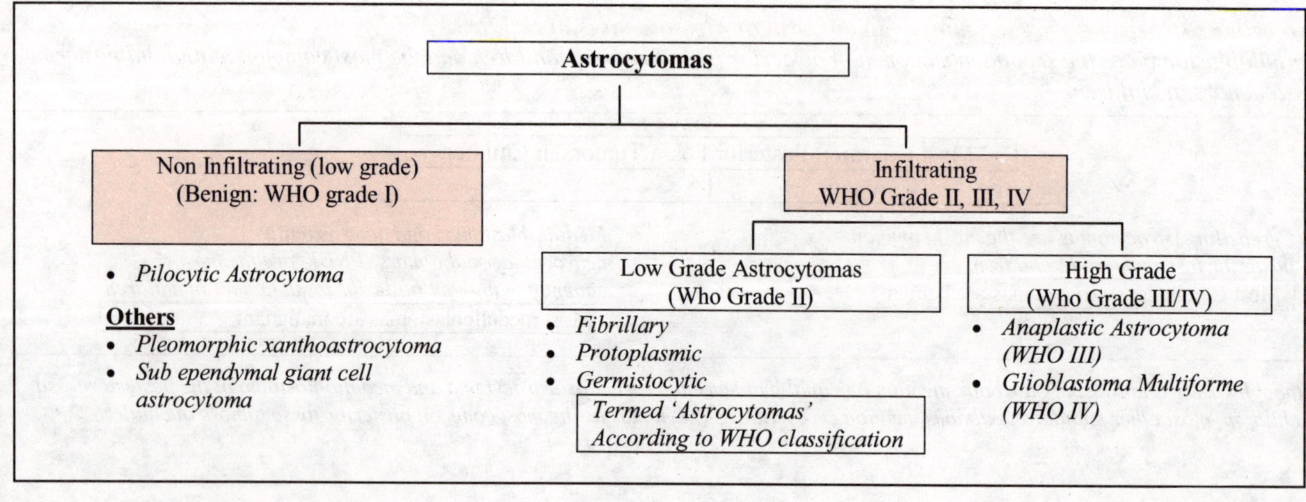

Cerebellar Astrocytomas

- ***The predominant group of astrocytomas in childhood are low grade astrocytomas*** *(Nelsons)*
  Juvenile Pilocytic Astrocytoma (JPA) is the most common astrocytoma in children[Q]
  Juvenile Pilocytic Astrocytoma is a **low grade tumor and is classified as a WHO grade I tumor**
- ***Cerebellar Astrocytomas (JPA) do not show any clear gender predelection***[Q]*(i.e, Equally common in males and females)* (From WHO classification of tumors of CNS)
- ***Cerebellar Astrocytomas (Juvenile JPA) most commonly develop during the first two decades of life***[Q](WHO classification of Tumors of CNS)
- ***Cerebellar Astrocytomas have a good prognosis*** *With complete surgical resection the overall survival for Juvenile Pilocytic Astrocytomas approaches 80% - 100%*

Medulloblastomas

- *The second most common posterior fossa tumor in children.* [Q]
- *Tumor which spreads along CSF pathways is medulloblastoma.* [Q]
- *Tumor which is capable of metastasising to extracranial sites is medulloblastoma.* [Q]
- *Medulloblostoma is highly radiosensitive.* [Q]

> ***Medulloblastomas are highly radiosensitive tumors of the Central Nervous system and more radiosensitive than all gliomas (Astrocytoma, Eperdymoma, Glioblastoma Multiforme)***
> *'Medulloblastoma is the most radiosensitive of all gliomas whereas Glioblastomas are the least radiosensitive'*
> *– Current Guidelines for Management of Cancer (1986)/289*

- *Medulloblastomas are classified as Primitive Neuroectodermal Tumors (PNET)*

> *Medulloblastoma were originally classified as 'gliomas' but are now classified as primitive neuroectodermal Tumors (PNET)*

Radiosensitive Brain Tumors in Children
• *Medulloblastomas and other PNET (Most radiosensitive)* • *Gliomas (low grade astrocytoma), ependymoma* • *Pineal blastoma* • *Craniopharygnioma* • *Germ cell tumors (pure germinoma-highly radiosensitive)*

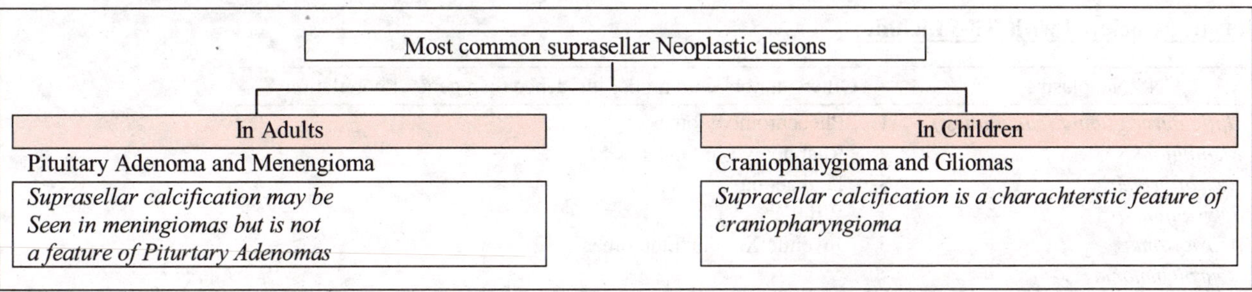

The most common neoplasm in the central Nervous System (CNS malignancy) in HIV positive patients is primary CNS Lymphoma.

9

Nervous System

Neurofibromatosis

Neurofibromatosis

Oculoneurocutaneous syndrome characterized by multisystem involvement

Neurofibromatosis I (NF1) Peripheral Neurofibromatosis (Von Recklinghausen's syndrome)	Neurofibromatosis II (NF II) Central Neurofibromatosis (Bilateral Acoustic Neurofibromatosis)
• Most prevalent type (90%) • Recognized to be related to abnormality of chromosome 17 (NFI gene) • Transmitted as an ***Autosomal Dominant disorder*** Diagnostic Criteria for NF1 Diagnosed when any two of the following are present 1. Six more *café-au-lait* macules over 5 mm in greatest diameter in prepubertal individuals and over 15 mm in greatest diameter in post-pubertal individuals. 2. Axillary or inguinal freckling 3. Two or more iris *Lisch nodules* 4. Two or more ***neurofibromas*** or one plexiform neurofibroma 5. A distinctive osseous lesion such as sphenoid dysplasia or cortical thinning of long bone, with or without pseudoarthrosis. 6. Optic gliomas. 7. A first degree relative with NFI whose diagnosis was based on the aforementioned criteria.	• Less prevalent type (10%) recognized to be related to abnormality of chromosome 22 (NF2 gene) • Transmitted as an ***Autosomal dominant disorder*** Diagnostic Criteria for NF2 Diagnosed when any one of the following is present. 1. ***Bilateral eighth nerve masses consistent with acoustic neuromas*** as demonstrated by CT scanning or MRI 2. A parent, sibling, or child with NF-2 and either 3. unilateral eight nerve mass or any two of the following: - Neurofibroma - Meningioma - Glioma - Schwannoma - ***Juvenile posterior subcapsular opacity*** *Bilateral acoustic neuromas are the most distinctive tumors in patients with NF-2.*
Note ***Scoliosis****is the most common orthopaedic manifestation of NF1* although it is not specific enough to be included as a diagnostic criteria – *Nelson 18th/2483*	Note ***Posterior subcapsular lens opacities (cataract)*** *are identified in ~ 50% of patients with NF2 – Nelson 18th/2484*

The commonest tumor in neurofibromatosis I is optic nerve glioma. Optic gliomas are present in approximately 15% of patients with NFI and its presence is included as one of the criteria in establishing its diagnosis.

Neoplasms associated with NF-I include:

CNS Neoplasms		Others tumors with higher incidence than general population	
1.	***Optic nerve glioma (commonest)***	1.	Pheochromocytomas
2.	*Meningiomas*	2.	Rhabdomyosarcomas
3.	*Neurofibromas*	3.	Leukaemia
4.	*Schwannomas*	4.	Wilm's
5.	*Astrocytomas*	5.	Juvenile Xanthogranulomas
6.	*Neurolemmomas*		

Neurofibromatosis II is recognized to be related to an abnormality on chromosome 22. Bilateral Accoustic Neuromas (schwannomas) are the most charachteristic tumors associated with NF2 while Juvenile posterior subcapsular cataracts are the one of the most charachteristic ocular manifestations of NF2.

Von-Hippel Lindau Syndrome

- *Von Hippel Lindau disease (VHL) is a rare autosomal disease characterised by abnormal angiogenesis with benign and malignant tumors that affect* ***multiple sites***
- *Craniospinal Hemangioblastomas are considered the hallmark tumors in Von-Hippel Lindau disease (VHL)*
  Hemangioblastomas in VHL are often multiple and most frequently found in the cerebellum, spinal cord and brainstem

Von Hippel Lindau Syndrome

Autosomal dominant syndrome

Characteristic Tumors/Cysts	Other tumors / Cysts
Hemagioblastomas *-Cerebellar hemangioblastoma* -Retinal hemangioblastoma -Spinal hemangioblastoma	• ***Renal cell carcinoma / hypernephroma*** • ***Pheochromocytoma*** • *Pancreatic endocrine tumors* • *Adrenal carcinomas* • *Benign cysts in Kidney, epidydimis, Liver or pancreas*

Polycythemia is a characteristic associated feature in VHL due to erythropoietin production by hemangioblastoma and/or Renal cell carcinoma

Clinical spectrum includes:

Haemangiomas		Tumors	Cysts	Polycythemia
Capillary haemangiomas of retina or optic nerve head.	*with or without*	Haemangioblastoma: - Cerebellum - Spinal cord - Medulla or pons Renal carcinoma Pheochromocytoma	Renal Pancreatic Hepatic Epidydimal Ovarian Pulmonary	

Cerebellar hemangioblastoma is a benign neoplasm that occurs either sporadically or as part of Von Hippel - Lindau disease

Clinically presentation is with:

- *Cerebellar dysfunction*
- *Hydrocephalus*
- *Polycythemia (the tumor produces erythropoetin).*[Q]

Diagnostic Criteria for Von-Hippel-Lindau Disease

• *Central nervous system and retinal hemangioblastoma*	• *Hemangioblastoma and at least one of the following:* - *Renal, pancreastic, hepatic, epididymal cyst* - *Pheochromocytoma* - *Renal cancer*	• *Family history and at least one of the following* - *Hemangioblastoma* - *Visceral changes* - *Pheochromocytoma* - *Renal cancer*

'The most common CNS manifestation of VHL is the charachteristic cerebellar hemangioblastoma.

- *Tumors in Von Hippel Lindau syndrome are charcateristically Infratentorial.*

Neurocutaneous Syndromes	Location
Neurofibromatosis 1 (NF1)	*Supratentorial and Infratentorial*
Neurofibromatosis II (NF II)	*Supratentorial and Infratentorial*
Sturge-Weber Syndrome	*Supratentorial*
Von-Hippel Lindau Syndrome (VHL)	***Infratentorial more than Supratentorial***
Tuberous Sclerosis (Bournville's Disease)	*Supratentorial (Primarily Supratentorial)*

Tumors in Von Hippel Lindau syndrome are rarely found supratentorially'

Tuberous Sclerosis

The presence of hypopigmented macules in the background of seizures and mental retardation suggests the diagnosis of Tuberous Sclerosis.

Tuberous Sclerosis

Autosomal Dominant[Q] Neurocutaneous Disorder

Cutaneous Features

- **Hypopigmented macules/Ash-leaf spots**[Q]
  - Seen in >90% of cases
  - Are small, ovoid, scattered and variable in number
  - Larger lesions are known as 'Ash-leaf' spots as these may have jagged edges resembling a 'leaf'
- **Shagreen Spots**[Q]
  - Roughened, raised, leathery lesions with an orange peel consistency
- **Adenoma Sebacium**[Q]
  - Facial skin hamartoma that develops in early childhood (~ 4-6 years of age)
  - Appears as tiny red nodules over nose and cheeks resembling acne
- ***Facial Angiofibromas / Ungual Fibromas***
  Facial angiofibromas may seen ungula fibromas are more common in toes
- **Café- au- lait spots**
  These may be seen occasionally

Neurological Features

- **Seizures**[Q]
  - *Seizures are the most common presenting symptom*
  - *Infantile spasms may be the presenting feature during infancy*
- **Mental Retardation**[Q]
  - Mental Retardation occurs in upto 50% of patients referred to tertiary care
  - Patients with seizures are more prone to mental retardation

The charachteristic brain lesion is a cortical 'Tuber'. The most common neurological manifestations include seizures, cognitive impairment and behavioral abnormalities including autism.

Other Features

- **Renal Lesions**
  Renal cysts or angiomyolipomas may occur (Hematuria /obstruction)
- **Cardiac Lesions**
  Rhabdomyomas of the heart may occur
- **Pulmonary Lesions**
  Lymphagiomyomatosis is the classical pulmonary lesion
  Rarely cystic lung disease may occur
- **Eye lesions**
  Retinal Hamartomas may occur
- **Skeletal lesions**
  Cystic rarefaction of the bones or the fingers or toes.

T. S. 'Classical Triad' described includes Seizures, Mental Retardation and Adenoma Sebacium (occurs in <33% patients)
T.S should be suspected in any child presenting with unexplained seizures who shows hypopigmented cutaneous macules.

Characteristic Triad of Tuberous Sclerosis
• *Epilepsy/Seizures*[Q]
• *Mental Retardation / Subnormal Intelligence*[Q]
• *Adenoma Sebacium*[Q]

[Q]Tuberous Sclerosis is charachteristically (but not always) associated with Sub-ependymal Giant Cell Astrocytomas

Subependymal Giant cell Astrocytomas (SEGCA)

- *Subependymal Giant cell Astrocytomas are low grade non filtrating (benign) variants of astrocytomas.*
- *They are characteristically (but not always) associated with tuberous sclerosis*

  Occur most frequently in patients with autosomal dominant phakomatosis tuberous sclerosis[Q]
- ***The most common site of SEGCA is the ependymal wall of lateral ventricle near the foramen of munro and these tumors tend to grow towards the foramen of munro (leading to obstructive hydrocephalus)***
- *Pathologically lesions are composed of Giant cells*
- *Candle dripping radiographic appearance is characteristic*
- *These tumors predominantly occur is children (1st decade)*
- *These tumors are essentially benign*
- *Total Gross resection is the treatment of choice*

Most common site of subependymal giant cell astrocytoma is the ependymal wall of lateral ventricle near the foramen of Munro.

Sturge weber syndrome

It results from the **anomalous** development of **primordial vascularbed** during early stages of cerebral vascularization. The leptomeninges are richly vascularized and the brain beneath becomes **atrophied** and **calcified**, particularly in molecular layer of cortex.

Clinical manifestations	
Cutaneous	**Neurological features**
Facial nevus (Port-wine stain) • Present at birth • Tends to be unilateral • Always involves upper face and eyelid • May involve lower face, & mucosa of mouth and pharynx.	1. Seizures (hallmark) • Present in most patients during first year of life • Typically focal tonic clonic and contralateral to the side of facial nevus 2. Hemiparesis • Associated with slowly developing hemiparesis in most cases. 3. Mental retardation 4. Buphthalmos and glaucoma of the ipsilateral eye are common.
Diagnostic hallmarks	
Skull radiograph	**CT Scan**
Intracranial calcification in the occipitoparietal region - Railroad track appearance - Serpentine appearance	- Unilateral cortical atrophy - Ipsilateral dilatation of lateral ventricle. - Extent of calcification.

<u>Sturge Weber syndrome may be associated with leptomeningeal angiomatosis but it is not associated with an increased risk of developing true brain tumors.</u>

Sturge Weber Syndrome

- *Port wine nevus over the trigeminal distribution*
- *Ipsilateral leptomeningial angiomatosis*
- *Contralateral hemiparesis*
- *Seizures*
- *Mental Retardation*
- *Congenital Glaucoma*

<u>Characteristic Features of Benign Extramedullary Spinal Tumors:</u>

Characteristic	**Meningioma**	Schwannoma	Neurofibroma
Age of presentation	*5th-7th decade*	5th decade	4th decade
Spinal level predominance	*Thoracic (80%)*	All levels evenly	Cervical (66%)
Multiplicity	*1 to 2%*	Rare unless NF2 associated	Common
Proportion or primary spinal tumors	*25%*	~33%	3.5%
Gender predominance	*Female (75-80%)*	None	None
Associations	More commonly psammomatous or transitional histologies	NF2, merlin/schwannomin gene on chromosome 22	NF1, neurofibromin gene on chromosome 17

NF1, neurofibromatosis type 1; NF2, neurofibromatosis type 2

<u>Spinal meningiomas</u>

'The typical clinical scenario of intraspinal meningiomas is a <u>middle aged woman</u> with signs and symptoms of <u>cord or nerve root compression</u>. The <u>dorsal (Thoracic) spine</u> is most commonly involved. At MRI scan, the tumor typically appears as a <u>well-circumscribed</u> lesion iso-intense or slightly hypotense to the spinal cord. On T1 and T2 sequences with <u>homogenous gadolinium (contrast) enhancement</u>' – Learning Musculoskeletal Imaging (Springer) 2010/101

Meningiomas are typically characterized by isointense homogenous contrast enhancement.

Disorders of Nerve / Neuropathies

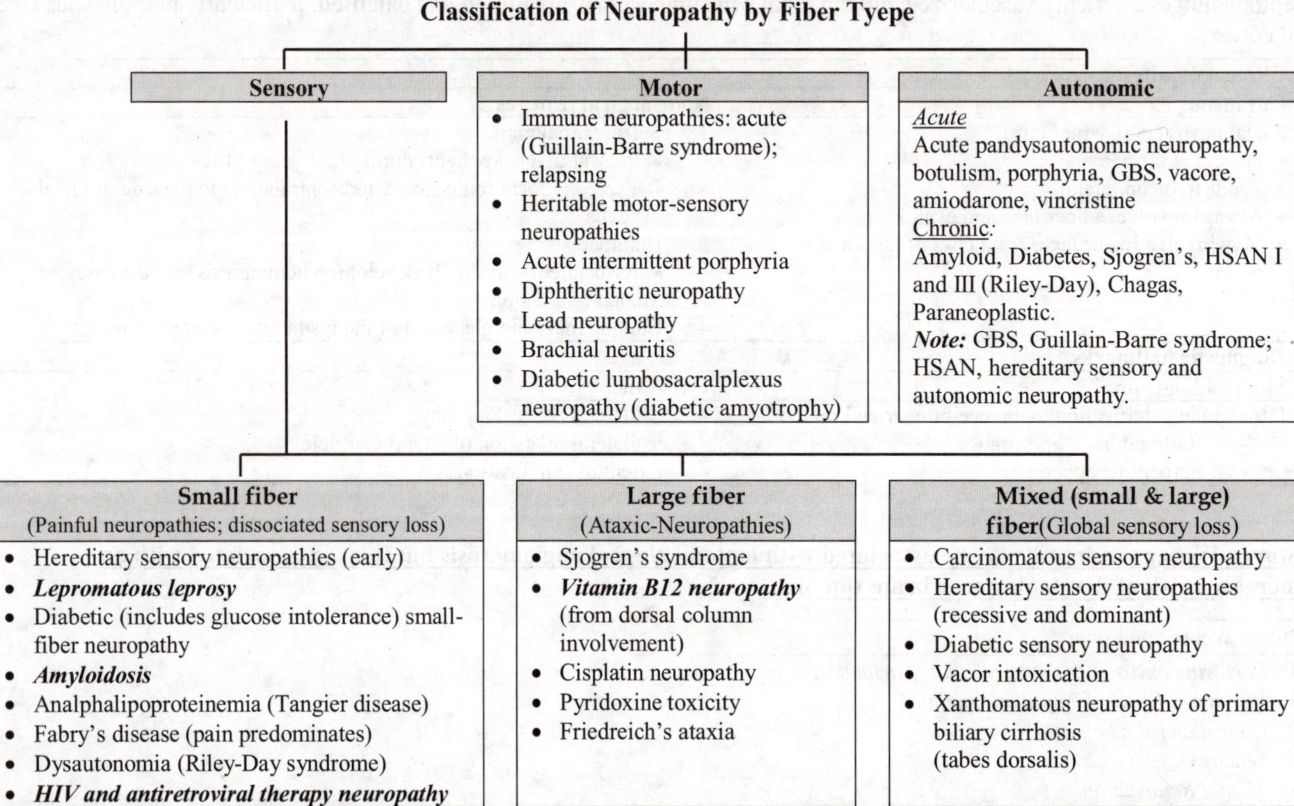

Vitamin B12 deficiency associated neuropathy is primarily a 'Large Fiber' neuropathy arising from dorsal column involvement.
Lepromatous Leprosy (Hansen's Disease), HIV associated neuropathy and Amyloidosis associated neuropathy are all classified as 'Small-Fiber' neuropathies.

Symptoms, Signs and Tests in Peripheral Neuropathy

Type of Neuropathy	Symptoms	Signs
Large fiber	• ***Numbness*** • ***Tingling*** • *"Pins and needles"* • *Poor balance*	• *Decreased Vibration* • *Decreased Joint-position sense* • *Decreased Reflexes*
Small fiber	• ***Pain:*** *burning, shock-like, stabbing, prickling, shooting, lancinating* • *Allodynia*	• *Decreased Pin prick* • *Decreased Temperature sensation*
Motor	• *Cramps* • *Weak grip* • *Footdrop* • *Twitching*	• *Reduced Strength* • *Reduced Reflexes*
Autonomic	• *Decreased or increased sweating* • *Dry eyes, mouth,* • *Erectile dysfunction* • *Gastroparesis/diarrhea* • *Faintness, light-headedness*	• *Orthostasis* • *Unequal pupil size* • *Resting tachycardia*

Q *Burning pain is a characteristic feature of small –fiber neuropathies*
Q *Tingling and Numbness* is a feature of large fiber neuropathies while *foot drop & twitching* are features of motor neuropathies

Autonomic Neuropathy

Causes of Autonomic Neuropathy

Autonomic Neuropathies

Acute / Subacute Autonomic Neuropathies	Chronic Peripheral Autonomic Neuropathies
1. Subacute autoimmune autonomic ganglionopathy (AAG) a) Subacute paraneoplastic autonomic neuropathy b) Guillain-Barré syndrome c) Botulism d) Porphyria e) Drug induced autonomic neuropathies-stimulants, drug withdrawal, vasoconstrictor, vasodilators, beta-receptor antagonists, beta-agonists f) Toxic autonomic neuropathies g) Subacute cholinergic neuropathy	1. Distal small fiber neuropathy 2. Combined sympathetic and parasympathetic failure a) Amyloid b) Diabetic autonomic neuropathy c) Autoimmune autonomic ganglionopathy (paraneoplastic and idiopathic) d) Sensory neuronopathy with autonomic failure e) Familial dysautonomia (Riley-Day syndrome) f) Diabetic, uremic, or nutritional deficiency g) Dysautonomia of old age 3. Disorders of reduced orthostatic intolerance-reflex syncope, POTS, associated with prolonged bed rest, associated with space flight, chronic fatigue

Clinical presentation of Autonomic Neuropathy

Autonomic Neuropathy

Cardiovascular AutonomicNeuropathy	Gastrointestinal Autonomic Neuropathy	Genitourinary Autonomic Neuropathy
• ***Resting tachycardia*** • *Loss of Heart Rate Variability* • ***Orthostatic Hypotension*** • ***Silent Myocardial Infarction*** • *Reduced response to Valsalva maneuver, Sustained exercise and Medications (atropine & propanalol)* • *Prolonged QT interval/dysrhythmias* • *Hypoglycemic unawareness/lack of diaphoresis (sweating) and tremulousness* • *Sudden death*	• *Gastroparesis*	• *Neurogenic bladder* • *Sexual dysfunction / Impotence*

Common causes of Neuropathic / Trophic ulcers

Common Causes of Trophic/Neuropathic Ulcers

Peripheral Nerve involvement	Spinal Cord involvement
• *Diabetic Neuropathy* • *Peripheral Neuropathy from other cause* • ***Leprotic Neuropathy*** • *Hereditary Sensory neuropathy*	• ***Syringomyelia*** • *Tabes dorsalis* • *Transverse myelitis* • ***Prolapsed intervertebral disc*** • *Cervical spondylosis* • *Spinal cord trauma*

Diabetic Neuropathy

Diabetic neuropathy may be of several types including distal symmetric sensory neuropathy, autonomic neuropathy and diabetic mananeuropathy

Diabetic Neuropathy

- Diabetes Meelitus is the most common cause of peripheral neuropathy in developed countries

Diabetes is associated with several types of Neuropathy

- Distal symmetric sensory or sensorimotor polyneuropathy (DSPN)
- Autonomic Neuropathy
- Diabetic Radiculoplexus Neuropathy (diabetic omyotrophy or Brunse Garland syndrome)
- Diabetic mononeuropathies or multiple mononeuropathies

- *Diabetic Distal symmetric sensory and senorimotor polyneuropathy (DSPN) is the most common form of diabetic polyneuropathy*[Q]
- *The most common diabetic mononeuropathy at wrist is median neuropathy*[Q]
- *The most common diabetic mononeuropathy at the elbow is ulnar mononeuropathy*[Q]
- The most common diabetic cranial mononeuropathy is VIIth nerve palsy[Q] (followed by third nerve, sixth nerve and less frequently fourth nerve)

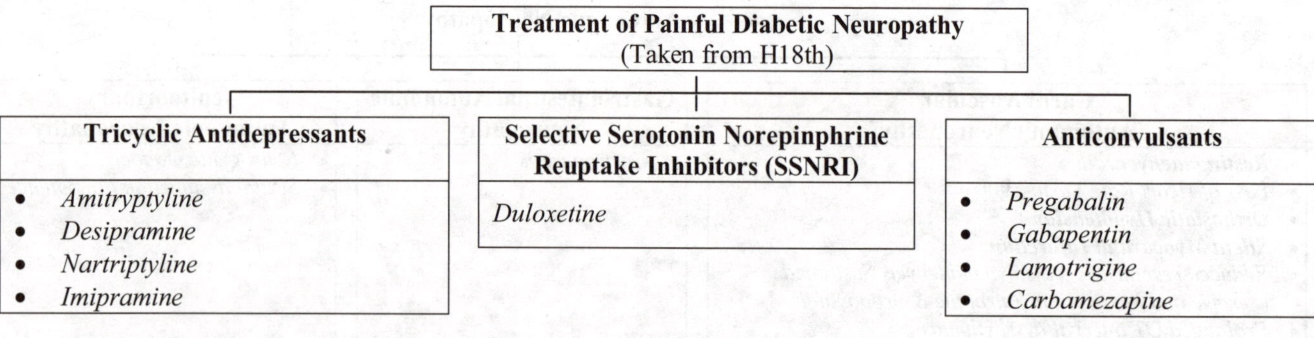

Two agents, Duloxetine and Pregabalin have been approved by the U.S. FDA for pain associated with diabetic neuropathy - Harrison's 18th

Treatment of Trigeminal Neuralgia

Carbamezapine is the most commonly employed drug of first choice against Trigeminal Neuralgia.

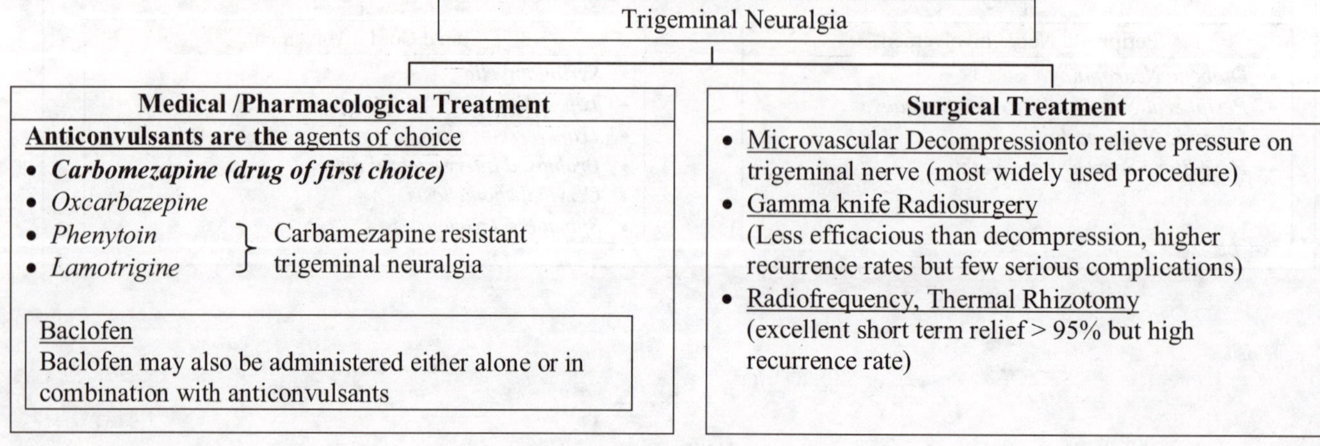

Conditions that may cause Sensorimotor Neuropathies

Polyneuropathy associated with Sensorimotor neuropathies (Harrison)	
Systemic Disease	
Diabetes mellitus	***Sensory, Sensorimotor, Motor***
Uremia	Sensorimotor
Porphyria (3 types)	Sensorimotor
Vitamin deficiency excluding B12	Sensorimotor
Chronic liver disease	Sensory or Sensorimotor
Primary systemic amyloidosis	Sensorimotor
Chronic obstructive lung disease	Sensory or Sensorimotor
Malabsorption (sprue, celiac disease)	Sensory or Sensorimotor
Carcinoma (sensorimotor)	Sensorimotor
Carcinoma (demyelinating)	Sensorimotor
Multiple Myeloma, lytic type	Sensory, Motor or Sensorimotor
MGUS	
IgA	Sensorimotor
IgG	Sensorimotor
IgM	Sensorimotor or Sensory
Cryoglobulinemia	***Sensorimotor***
Drugs	
Amiodarone (antiarrhythmic)	Sensorimotor
Aurothioglucose (antirheumatic)	Sensorimotor
Isoniazid	***Sensorimotor***
Metronidazole (antiprotozoal)	Sensory or Sensorimotor
Misonidazole (radiosensitizer)	Sensory or Sensorimotor
Environmental Toxins	
Arsenic (herbicide; insecticide)	***Sensorimotor***
Diptheria toxin	Sensorimotor
γ-Diketone hexacarbons (solvents)	Sensorimotor
Organophosphates	Sensorimotor
Thallium (rat poison)	Sensorimotor

Cisplatin and Pyridoxine are associated with predominantly sensory neuropathies.

Pure motor neuropathy:

Disorders affecting any level of 'the motor unit' can result in purely motor neuropathy without sensory disturbance.

The affections include- anterior horn cell, motor axon, neuromuscular junction

Pure motor neuropathies

1. Lower motor neuron form of amyotrophic lateral sclerosis [Q]
2. Poliomyelitis [Q]
3. Hereditary spinal muscular atrophy
4. Adult variant of Hexosaminidase deficiency
5. Lead intoxication [Q]
6. Dapsone intoxication [Q]
7. Acute intermittent porphyria (occasionally)
8. Neuromuscular Junction disorder :
   Lambert Eaton Myasthenia syndrome [Q]
   Tick bite paralysis [Q]

Neuropathies with predominant Motor symptoms
[Sensory component is subclinical but readily demonstrable electro diagnostically]

1. Hereditary motor sensory neuropathy
2. GBS or Acute inflammatory demyelinating polyneuropathy [Q]
3. CIPD [Q]

Porphyria :'The peripheral neuropathy is due to axonal degeneration and ***primarily affects motor neurons***[Q]. *Sensory changes such as paraesthesias and loss of sensations are less prominent. (Neuropathy: M or SM*

Arsenic *produces a mixed sensory and motor polyneuritis manifestating as numbness and tingling in a 'stocking – glove' distribution, distal weakness and quadriplegia*

[Q]***The Most common case of mononeuritis multiplex in India is Leprosy or Hansen's disease***

Demyelinating Versus Axonal Neuropathies

The primary function of myelin is to increase axonal conduction velocity without a significant increase in axonal diameter. This function is achieved by a process of *saltatory conduction*, in which nerve impulses jump between electrically excitable regions of the axon, called nodes of Ranvier located between elctrically insulated areas ensheathed by myelinating Schwann cells.

A demyelinating process disrupts the normal saltatory conduction along some axons within the nerve *slowing the conduction velocity* of these axons. As demyelination becomes more profound, conduction through some areas is blocked completely (*conduction block*), functionally disconnecting the motor neuron from the innervated muscle resulting in weakness.

In axonal neuropathies the conduction velocity is typically either preserved or only midly reduced.

Electrophysiologic Features: Axonal Degenaration vs. Segmental Demylination

Features	Axonal Degeneration	Segmental Demylination
Motor Nerve Conduction Studies		
CMAP amplitude	Decreased	Normal (except with CB)
Distal latency	Normal	Prolonged
Conduction velocity	***Normal***	***Slow***
Conduction block	***Absent***	***Present***
Temporal dispersion	Absent	Present
F wave	Normal or Absent	Prolonged or Absent
H reflex	Normal or Absent	Prolonged or Absent
Sensory Nerve Conduction Studies		
SNAP amplitude	Decreased	Normal
Distal latency	Normal	Prolonged
Conduction velocity	Normal	Slow
Needle EMG		
Spontaneous activity		
Fibrillations	Present	Absent
Fasciculation	Present	Absent
Motor unit potentials		
Recruitment	Decreased	Decreased
Morphology	Long duration / polyphasic	Normal

Charcot joint : Neuropathic joint

Neuropathic joint disease (Charcot's joint) is a progressive destructive arthritis associated with loss of pain sensation, proprioception or both. Without these protective reflexes joints are subject to repeated trauma, resulting in progressive cartilage and bone damage.

Disorders associated with Neuropathic joint disease/Charcot's joint	
▪ Diabetes Mellitus	• Amyloidosis
▪ Tabes Dorsalis	• Leprosy
▪ Meningomyelocele	• Congenital indifference to pain
▪ Syringomyclia	• Peroneal muscular atrophy (Charcot-Marie Tooth disease)

Diabetes mellitus is the most common cause for Neuropathic joint disease Q

Distribution of joint involvement Q

Condition Q	Most commonly affected joints Q
Tabes dorsolis	Knees, hips and ankles
Syringomyelia	Glenohumeral joint (Shoulder), elbow and wrist
Diabetes mellitus	Tarsal and Tarsometatarsal joint

Guillain Barre Syndrome

Guillain – Barre Syndrome

Acute Autoimmune Fulminant Demyelinating Polyradiculopathy

(Usually occurs 1-3 weeks after an acute infections process usually gastrointestinal or respiratory (70% cases)

Fever and constitutional symptoms are absent at onset[Q]

Nerve Conduction Studies

Show evidence of Demyelination

CSF studies

Show evidence of ***Albumin cytological dissociation***[Q]
(Increased CSF protein without increased cell count

Motor	Sensory	Autonomic

• Rapidly evolving motor paralysis
• ***Ascending (usually)***
• Areflexic (Reflexes Diminished or absent)
• Symmetric (Weaknes is usually symmetric)
• ***Flaccid***
• Sphincter tone is normal
• Facial Nerve and other cranial nerves may be involved.
Bulbar muscles may be involved with difficulty in swallowing, speech etc.
• Life threatening respiratory paralysis requiring ventilation may be seen.
	• Sensory disturbance may or may not be present in GBS and a ***distinct sensory level is not seen***.
	• Mild sensory involvement
	- Cutaneous sensory deficits (e.g. loss of pain and temperature sensation) are usually ***mild****(Harrison's)* ***or absent****(Current Neurology)*
	- Sensory symptoms such as paraesthesias, tingling etc may be prominent *(but objective sensory loss* on clinical *examination is mild/absent*.
	• Bladder dysfunction is uncommon. It is usually transient and seen only in severe cases *(If Bladder disturbance is prominent and comes early diagnostic possibilities other that GBS should be considered)*.
		• Autonomic involvement is common
		• May occur even in patients whose GBS is otherwise mild
		• Manifestations include
		  • Loss of vasomotor control (Fluctuation in B.P / Postrual Hypotension)
		  • Cardiac dysrhythmias

Prognosis

Recovery is usually remarkable in GBS, although all patients may not recover fully.

Approximately 85% of patients with GBS achieve a full functional recovery within several months to a year-*Harrison 15th/2509*

Treatment

Treatment includes intravenous immunoglobulins (IVIG) or plasmapharesis both of which are equally effective (treatment should be initiated as early as possible as immunotherapy is believed to be no longer effective if initiated 2 weeks after first motor symptoms).

Treatment of GBS

IV immunoglobulins and /or plasmapharesis

- Treatment should be initiated as soon after diagnosis as possible (Each day counts. Immunotherapy may not be effective if initited 2 weeks after the first motor symptom)[Q]
- ***Either High dose IV Immunoglobulins or plasmapharesis may be initiated as they are equally effective for typical GBS***[Q]

  Anecdotal data has suggested that IVIg may be preferable to plasmapharesis for the AMAN and MFS variants of GBS
- A combination of both therapies is not significantly better than either alone[Q]
- The lack of noticeable improvement after a course of IVIg or plasmaphoresis is not an indication to treat with alternate therapy.
- If the patient has already reached a plateau stage, than treatment is probably no longer indicated.
- IVIg is often the initial therapy chosen of its ease of administration and good safetyrecord

Supportive Therapy

- Patients require monitoring in critical care setting
- ~30% of patients with GBS require ventilator assistance
- Particular attention should be given to vital capacity, early consideration of tracheostomy (after 2 week of intubation) and chest physiotherapy.
- Monitor CVS status, nutrition and skin care.

Glucocorticoids have not been found to be effective in Guillan-Barre Syndrome.

Botulinism

Botulism

Botulism is caused by Botulism toxin, which is the most toxic substance known

Food Borne Botulism	Wound Botulism	Infant Botulism	Iatrogenic Botulism
Caused by ingestion of food contaminated by Botulinum toxin (canned food)	*Caused by Wounds contaminated with Clostridium Botulinum spores*	*Caused by absorption of toxin prodced in situ by toxigenic Clostridia colonizing the intestine of children < 1year*	*Results from injection of toxin*

Botulism is caused by toxin's inhibition of Acetylcholine Release at the neuromuscular junction through an enzymatic mechanism

Typical Manifestations

- Symmetric Cranial Nerve Palsies (marks the onset)
  - **Diplopia**
  - **Dysarthria**
  - **Dysphonia**
  - **Dysphagia**
  - Ptosis & facial nerve palsies
  - Pupillary reflexes are depressed and pupils are dilated & fixed

  Extraocular muscle paralysis manifests as blurred vision or diplopia and an inability to accomodate for near vision
- Flaccid Descending completely symmetric paralysis of voluntary muscles
  (Extent of paralysis, from cranial nerves only to quadriplegia dependes on toxin dose). Upper extremities are affected first followed by respiratory muscles and finally lower extremity paralysis.
- Deep tendon reflexes are preserved initially though they progressively disappear.

  Gag reflex is lost early
- Autonomic Dysfunction
  - Dry mouth
  - Constipation
  - Urinary retention

  Anticholinesgic features are typical
- **Sensorium is typically preserved**
  Patients usually exhibit no cognitive defects
- **Patients are usually afebrile**
  Fever is typically absent, except in some cases of wound botulinum
- Sensory findings are generally absent

Gastrointestinal manifestations of food borne botulism

- Nausea, vomiting, abdominal pain may precede or follow onset of paralysis.
- Incubation period from ingestion of toxin to onset of symptoms is usually 18-36 hours but may range from few hours to several days.

The most common cause of death in untreated botulism is from respiratory failure (airway obstuction from pharyngeal muscle paralysis and inadequate tidal volume resulting from paralysis of diaphragm and accessory resp.muscles)

Cardinal Feature of Botulism

- ***Cranial Nerve Palsies****with prominent bulbar palsy (4 '**D**'s of Bulbar Palsy)*
  (Diplopia, Dysarthria, Dysphonia, Dysphagia, Ptosis, Loss of Accomodation, Fixed / Dilated pupils)
- ***Descending motor paralysis***
  (Extent of paralysis from a few cranial nerves only to quadriperesis depends on dose of toxin)
- ***Symmetry of symptoms/signs***
- ***A clear sensorium***
- ***Absence of fever***
- ***Lack of sensory findings***

Important causes of Descending Motor Paralysis

- Botulinum [Q]
- Diphtheria [Q]
- Polio

Facial Nerve Palsy

Lower motor neuron	Upper motor neuron
Lesion of facial nerve or its nucleus in the pons	Lesion of intracranial portion proximal to pontine nucleus
Common causes of affection	**Common causes of affection**
• Bell's palsy • Pontine vascular accidents • Lesion in cerebellopontine angle • Herpetic infection (Ramsay Hunt syndrome) • Lesion in its course through temporal bone • Parotid tumors	• Cerebrovascular accidents • Demyelination • Tumors
Presentation (There is loss of muscles of facial expression)	**Presentation**
• *Ipsilateral face is involved* • *Absence of furrowing of face on the same side* • *Inability to close the ipsilateral eye (*on attempted closure the eyeball rolls upwards-**Bell's phenomenon)** • *Flattening of the nasolabial folds* • *Drooping of the angle of the mouth* • Deviation of mouth towards **opposite side***	*Contralateral face is involved* ***Upper motor neuron VII nerve palsy causes contralateral facial muscle paresis that is worse in the lower facial muscles. With UMN lesion the forehead is relatively spared.*** *This is a unique feature seen only with facial nerve. The part of facial nerve supplying the upper half of face has bilateral cortical representation and thus in a unilateral UMN lesion the upper half of face escapes paresis.*

Topographical Testing of Facial Nerve Function

Shirmer's test	Stapedial Reflex test (Acoustic Reflex Testing)	Taste Testing Electrogustometry	Salivary flow Rate
• Shirmer's test for lacrimation evaluates the integrity of the *greater superficial petrosalnerve* (GSPN) by comparing the amount of tearing produced on the involved side with the normal side • Greater superficial petrosal nerve is the first branch of facial nerve that arises from the geniculate ganglion and carries preganglionic parasympathetic fibers destined for lacrimal gland	• Stapedial Reflex test is used to evaluate the *stapedius branch of facial nerve* • A lesion of the facial nerve proximal to the stapedius branch disrupts the are <u>Persistance or Return of stapedius reflex provides prognostic value</u> Restoration of stapedius reflex within 3 weeks of onset of facial palsy indicates functional recovery.	• Taste testing is used *to test integrity of chorda tympani branch of facial nerve* that carries taste sensation to anterior 2/3rd of tongue.	• Salivary flow rates may also be used to assess integrity of chorda lympani branch of facial nerve • Reduction of salivation to less thn 25% of normal is considered significant

Topographical Test for Facial Nerve Function	Branch / Nerve assessed
Shirmer's test	*Greater Superficial Petrosal Nerve (GSPN)*
Stapedial Reflex /Accoustic Reflex	*Stapedial branch (Branch to stapedius)*
Electrogustometry (Taste testing)	*Chorda Tympani Branch*
Salivary Flow Rate	*Chorda Tympani Branch*

Syndromes Associated with Facial Palsy

Syndrome	Feature
Ramsay Hunt Syndrome^Q *(Herpes Zoster Oticus)*	Facial palsy due to reactivation of Herpes zoster in geniculate ganglion with vesicular eruption in the external ear
Melkerson – Rosenthal Syndrome^Q	Rare neuromyocutaneous disorder charachterized by triad of Recurrent facial palsy' (cheilitis granulomatosa) and fissured tongue (lingua plicata)
Heerfordt's Syndrome^Q *(Uveoparotoid fever)*	Facial palsy in association with sarcoidosis (Facial palsy with uveitis. Iritis, parotid enlargement & fever)
Bell's Palsy	Idiopathic Facial N.palsy
Frey's Syndrome (Gustatary sweating) Gusatory Lacrimation Crocodiletears	Results from damage to parasympathetic fibers of facial nerve, which regenerates in a misdirected manner. Stimuli that promote parotid gland secretion result in sweating or flushing over areas of the foci during mastication
Mobius syndrome	Congenital bilateral facial palsy with several other cranial nerve involvement
Albers shonberg syndrome	Facial nerve palsy with osteopetrosis

Myaesthenia Gravis

Myaesthenia Gravis

Etiology:
Autoimmune disorders mediated by specific Anti ACH receptor antibodies.
Fundamental defect:
Decrease in number of available ACH receptors at post-synaptic muscle membrane.
Age / Sex:
All ages are affected Most prevalent in women in twenties/ thirties and men in fifties & sixties. Women are affected more frequently than men[Q]. (3 : 2)
Features:
Weakness: in characteristic distribution as elaborated below Fatigability: Weakness increases on repeated use and may improve following rest or sleep A variable course marked by remissions and exacerbations (Remissions are rarely complete or permanent)
Association:
Thymic abnormalities and Thymomas *(Neoplastic)* Autoimmune disorders:*Rheumatoid Arthritis, SLE, Perenicious anemia, hyperthyroidism, ulcerative colitis, polymyositis etc.*

The primary defect in Myaesthenia gravis is decreased transmission across the myoneural junction due to decrease in the number of Acetylcholine receptors.Despite the muscle weakness, deep tendon reflexes are preserved

Suspect Myaesthenia gravis in a case of weakness with fatiguability, without loss of reflexes & impairment of sensations

Characteristics Distribution of Weakness

Craniofacial muscle weakness

- Lids and extraocular muscles : diplopia and ptosis are common early complaints
- Facial weakness :
  produces snarling expression on attempt to smile weakness in chewing
- Speech:
  Nasal timbre due to weakness of palate dysarthric mushy quality due to tongue weakness
- Difficulty in swallowing and nasal regurgitation or aspiration of liquids or food due to weakness of palate, tongue & pharynx.
- Muscles of neck particularly extensors are frequently involved.

Limb muscles

- Affected in 85% of cases
- Proximal weakness
- Usually symmetric but may be asymmetric

Weakness of Respiratory muscles (crises)

- If weakness of respiratory muscles becomes so severe so as to require respiratory assistance the patient is said to be in crisis.
- Crisis is often precipitated by unrelated infections or systemic disorders.

Thymic Abnormalities and Myasthenia Gravis (MG)

Myasthenia Gravis patients have a high incidence of thymic abnormalities Thymus is abnormal in about 75% of patients

65% of patients have a Hyperplastic Thymus[Q]	***10% of patienthave Thymomas[Q]***

Thymus *is believed to play a role in the autoimmune dysfunction in M.G and thymectomy has shown significant improvement in upto 85% of patients with MG (35% achieve drug free remission).*

Investigations for Myesthenia Gravis

Edrophonium test / Tensilon test	Acetylcoline Receptor antibodies
• *Highly sensitive test with 85% sensitivity in ocular and 95% sensitivity in systemic myasthenia-Kanski* • Diagnosis is highly probable if test in unequivocally positive • An initial dose of 2mg of edrophonium is given intravenously. If improvement occurs the test is considered positive and terminated. If there is no change an additional 8mg are given intravenously.	• Sensitivity of 80-90% in *systemic* myasthenia - CMDT • Highly specific and presence of Anti ACH Receptor Antibodies is virtually diagnostic of M. gravis 85% positive in generalized M.G. 50% positive in ocular M.G. Definitive if positive Negative test does not exclude M.G. 40% of Antiantibody negative patients have Anti-Musk antibodies.
Repetitive nerve stimulation / Electrodiagnostic test	**Single fiber electromyography**
• Helpful diagnostic evidence • Best when weak muscles/ proximal ms. groups are tested • Amplitude of evoked muscle end potential is measured - No change in normal patients - Reduction by > 10-15 % in myasthenic patients.	• Demonstrates blocking and jitter with normal fiber density • *Most sensitive diagnostic test for MG with sensitivity of greater than 95%* • *Confirmatory but not specific* • Often performed in conjunction with repetitive nerve stimulation test (Oxford handbook)

Single Fiber Electromyography (SFEMG) is the single most sensitive assay of neuromuscular function dysfunction in myasthenia gravis

[Q]*Single most sensitive test for diagnosis of Myasthenia Gravis: SFEMG*

[Q]*Single most specific test for diagnosis of Myasthenia Gravis: AChR antibodies*

Note

Conventional (EMG) is not a sensitive diagnostic test for MG. The conventional needle EMG is usually normal in patients with MG although certain findings may indicate probability of MG. Conventional EMG evaluation in MG serves mostly in excluding other causes of weakness like motor neuron disease, neuropathy or myopathy

Test	Generalized MG (sensitivity)	Ocular MG (sensitivity)
AchR antibodies (ACHR Antibodies)	80%	60%
Repetitive Nerve stimulation (RNS)	75%	48%
Single Fiber EMG (SFEMG)	99%	97%
Edrophonium (Tensilon) test	95%	85%

Taken from 'Neuromuscular Junction Disorder's: Diagnosis & Treatment (2003) /109

Recommendations for Thymectomy in patients with Myasthenia Gravis

Treatment recommendations for Thymectomy in patients with MG.[Q]

Patients with Thymomas

Thymectomy should be carried out in all patients who have thymomas[Q]

(Thymectomy in thymonas is necessary because of the possibility of local tumor spread although most thymomas are benign)

Patients without Thymomas

Thymectomy should be carried out in all patients with **generalizedMG** who are between the ages of **puberty** and **at least 55 years**

Thymectomy not clearly recommended for[Q]*:*

- Children (< puberty)
- Elderly > 55 years
- Localized M.G with weakness limited to extra ocular muscles
- Patients with MUSK antibody positive Myaesthenia gravis.

Clinical Syndromes Associated with Thymomas

Paraneoplastic Immunologic Syndromes associated with both benign and malignant thymomas occur frequently, do not affect prognosis and may not reverse following thymectomy.

Charachteristic Syndromes

- ***Myaesthenia Gravis (most common)***[Q]
- ***Acquired Hypogammaglobulinemia (10%)*** [Q]
- *Pure Red Cell Aplasia* [Q]

Rare Syndromes / Associated Diseases

- ***Ectopic Cushing's Syndrome***
- Autoimmune Thyroiditis / Grave's Disease
- Connective Tissue Disorders / Vasculitis
  - Polymyositis / Dermatamyositis
  - Granulomatous myocarditis
  - SLE
  - Rheumatoid Arthritis
  - Sjogren's syndrome, Scleroderma
  - Churg- Strauss syndrome, Microscopic polyangitis, Isolated Pauci- immune crescenteric glomenulonephritis
- Optic neuritis / Limbic encephalitis
- Hypertrophic Osteoarthropathy
- Pernicious anemia
- Pemphigus
- Panhypopituarism
- Ulcerative colitis
- Addison's disease

Lambert Eaten Myasthenic Syndrome and Myasthenia Gravis

Lambert Eaten Myasthenia Syndrome	Myasthenia Gravis
What it is & Associations	**What it is & Associations**
• Paraneoplastic syndrome • Associated with - Small cell carcinoma lung - Certain autoimmune diseases	• Autoimmune disorder • Associated with - Thymomas - Certain autoimmune diseases
Defect	**Defect**
• Presynaptic disorder • Antibodies to calcium channels (P/Q type) • Decrease in presynaptic release of Acetylcholine at Neuromuscular junction is the fundamental defect	• Postsynaptic disorder • Antibodies against ACH Receptors • Decrease in number of ACH Receptors at post synaptic muscle membrane is the fundamental defect
Presentation	**Presentation**
• Onset usually after 40 years • Men > Women (5: 1) • ***Proximal limb muscles and muscles of trunk are the most commonly involved muscles*** Proximal limb muscles >> extraocular & lid muscles • ***No fatiguability / Incremental response*** ***Repeated stimulation causes increased muscle strength*** • Reflexes : Hyporeflexia or absent reflexes • Autonomic changes such as dry mouth and impotence are associated	• Onset Often < 40 years • Women > Men (4: 3) • Craniofascial muscles particularly lids and ***extraocular muscles are the most commonly involved.*** Extraocular & lid muscles > proximal limb muscles • ***Fatiguability / Decremental response*** ***Repeated stimulation causes decreased muscle strength*** • Reflexes : Intact • No associated autonomic changes
Diagnosis	**Diagnosis**
• Repeated nerve stimulation : incremental response • Radioimmune assay : Antibodies against P/Q Ca^{2+} channels • *Tensilon test : Negative* (mildly positive in some)	• Repeated nerve stimulation : Decremental • Radioimmune assay : - Anti ACHR antibody response - Anti-Musk antibodies • ***Tensilon test : Characteristically Positive***

Lambert Eaten Myaesthenic syndrome presents with an incremental response to repeated electrical stimulation

The Muscular Dystrophies

Type	Inheritance pattern	Chromosomal or genomic defect	Missing or abnormal gene product	Incidence (i.e. frequency with respect to live births)	Age of onset	Clinical features	Prognosis
Duchenne	X-linked 30% sporadic	Xp21.2	Dystrophin absent	20-30/ 100 000 boys	2nd-3rd year	onset in pelvic girdle, pseudohypertrophy of calves	rapidly progressive, most patients die by age 25
Becker	X-linked	Xp21.2	Dystrophin abnormal	3/100 000 boys	1st (-4th) decade	same as in Duchene muscular dystrophy, but milder; sometimes cardiomyopathy	ambulatory till age 15 or later, death in 4th or 5th decade or later
Mery-Dreifuss	X-linked, rarely autosomal dominant	Xp28	Emerin	1/100 000	childhood adolescence	scapuloperoneal dystrophy, contractures, and cardiopathy may be prominent	ambulatory till 3rd decade or for entire life; cardiac arrhythmia a frequent cause of death
Facio-scapulo humeral dystrophy (Duchenne-Landouzy-Dejerine)	Autosomal dominant	4q35	Homebox gene	5/100 000	childhood to young adulthood	weakness of facial, shoulder girdle, and calf muscles	practically normal life expectancy
Scapulo-peroneal dystrophy	Autosomal dominant, autosomal recessive, or sporadic	Unknown	Unknown	rare	childhood to adulthood	weakness of shoulder girdle and dorsiflexors of the feet and toes	usually normal life expectancy
Limb girdle dystrophy	Autosomal recessive, autosomal dominant or sporadic	5q, 13q, 15q	Unknown	rare	childhood to adulthood	mainly proximal weakness of pelvic or shoulder girdle	depending on type, premature death or only minor disability or into old age
Oculopharyngeal dystrophies	Autosomal dominant	Unknown	Unknown	rare	middle age	oculofaciobulbar paresis	often premature death due to dystrophagia and aspiration pneumonia
Congenital dystrophies (for variants)	Autosomal recessive	Unknown	Unknown	rare	at birth	depending on type: involvement of muscles, eye, and brain: contractures, arthrogryposis multiplex	ranging from mild disability to severe meantal retardation
Steinertmyotonic dystrophy	Autosomal dominant	19q13.3	Protein kinase	13.5/100000, prevalence 5/100 000	young adulthood, rarely congenital, earlier age of onset in each successive generation ("anticipation")	mainly distal weakness, faciobulbar paresis, myotonia, cataracts	age of significant disability depends on age of onset, usually middle age; premature death
Distal myopathies (Welander type, Markesbery- Griggs, Finnish variant)	Autosomal dominant	unknown	Unknown	rare	middle age	mainly distal atrophy and weakness	only minor disability into old age
Distal myopathies (Nonaka and Miyoshi types)	Autosomal recessive	Miyoshi: 2p12-14 Nonaka: unknown	Unknown	rare	adolescene to young adulthood	mainly distal weakness	progression to inability to walk

Duchenne Muscular Dystrophy (PseudoHypertrophic Muscular Dystrophy)

- Duchenne muscular dystrophy is the most common hereditary neuromuscular disease affecting all races and ethnic groups.
- Inheritance : X linked recessive
- Abnormal gene lies on Chromosome 21 (Xp21)
- Missing or defective gene product is : Dystrophin

  Dystrophin is part of Dystrophin – Glycoprotein sarcolemmal complex and this protein deficiency leads to secondary loss of sarcoglycans and dystroglycans resulting in weakness of sarcolemma, causing membrane tears and muscle fibre necrosis
- Presentation occurs between ages 3 and 5 [disorder does not present at birth or in infancy[Q]]

Clinical manifestations:

- Gower's sign is positive[Q]
- Pseudohypertrophy of calf is seen[Q] (muscle is replaced by fat & connective tissue)
- Loss of muscle strength is progressive. [Q]
- Proximal muscles and neck flexors are involved more. [Q]
- Leg involvement is more severe than arm involvement.
- Contractures of heel cords and iliotibial band occurs (by age of 6 years)
- Progressive scoliosis develops.

Complications:

Chest deformity[Q] (scoliosis) [Q]:

Impairs pulmonary function[Q]

By age of 16 and 18 years patients are predisposed to serious pulmonary fatal infections.

Cardiac:

Cardiomyopathy [Q] and CHF may be seen

Cardiac cause of death is uncommon

Intellectual impairment :

is common[Q] (IQ is one SD below the mean)

Remember:

Onset [Q]	*Before age of 5* [Q]
Confined to wheel chair *Inability to walk*	*After age of 12* [Q]
Respiratory failure	*In second or third decade (after 16-18 years)* [Q]

Laboratory diagnosis:

- *Serum creatinephosphokinase (CK)* [Q] : elevated (20-100 times)
- *EMG :* features of myopathy
- *Muscle biopsy*[Q] :
  - Definitive diagnosis established on basis of dystrophin deficiency in biopsied muscle tissue
  - Groups of necrotic and regenerating muscle fibres are seen.

Treatment:

- Glucocorticoids (Prednisolone) have been tried.
- Significant alteration in the progression of disease has been seen with **prednisolone.**

Oculopharyngeal muscular dystrophy

Characterized by

Progressive external ophthalmoplepia

- Slowly progressive ptosis
- Limitation of eye movements
- Sparing of pupillary reactions for light and accomodation

'Patients usually do not complain of diplopia in contrast to patients having conditions with a more acute onset of ocular muscle weakness such as M. gravis'- Harrison

Pharyngeal muscle weakness

- Progressive dysphagia
- May become debilitating and result in pooling of seretions and repeated episodes of aspiration

Facio-Scapulo-Humeral Dystrophy

Facio-Scapulo-Humeral Dystrophy

- Autosomal Dominant (Positive Family History[Q])
- Abnormal gene 4q (4q35 deletion)
- Childhood to young adulthood (may be delayed to 5th decade)
- Mild ↑ CPK (Normal Dystrophy)

Clinical Sign

- Weakness preferentially affects the facial and shoulder girdle muscles
  - Unable to whistle
  - Unable to smile
  - Unable to fully close their eyes
- Extraocular muscles are typically spared
- Pelvic girdle weakness may be present (20%)
- Usually asymmetric at onset

Orthopaedic Manifestations

- Winging of scapula (Scapular winging contracture may be present)
- Winging of scapula becomes more evident when the patient attempts to elevate the arms laterally

Prognosis

- Life expectancy is normal
- Respiratory insufficiency is rare

Extramuscular manifestations

These occur with variable frequency and include mental impairment, hearing loss, retinal vasculopathy and cardiac involvement.

Myotonia Dystrophica

- It is the most common adult muscular dystrophy.[Q]
- Myotonic dystrophy is an autosomal dominant disorder. [Q]
- The disorder is transmitted by a mutation in an 'unstable trinucleotide repeat sequence' in a gene at 19q 133
- Muscle atrophy selectively involves type I fibres only. [Q] (in 50% of cases)
- Myopathy in Myotonia is unique in the sense that it is ***typically distal*** in contrast to other myopathies which are mostly proximal. [Q]
- Myotonia usually appears by the age of 5 years [Q], and causes a slow relaxation of hand grip following a forced voluntary closure.

Progressive Muscular Dystrophies & Defective Gene / Protein

Duchenne and Becker's	Limb girdle	Emery-Dreifuss	Myotonic dystrophy	Fascio-scapulo humeral	Oculopharyngeal
Dystrophin[Q]	Myotilin Laminin A/c Caveolin - 3 ***Calpain - 3*** ***Dysferlin*** ***γ,α,β,γ sarcoglycans*** Telethonin Fukutin related protein Titin TRIM 32 gene	Emerin Laminins	▪ (DM1) Unstable expansion of a CTG trinucleatide repeat in a serine threonine protein kinase gene (named DMPK) on chromosome 19q 13.3 ▪ (DM2) DNA expansion of a CcTG repeat in the ZNF9 gene on chromosome 3q 13.3 - q24	Deletion distal 4q	Expansion poly A RNA binding protein.

9

Nervous System

Congenital Myopathies

These are a group of rare disorders distinguished from muscular dystrophies by the presence of specific histochemical and structural abnormalities in muscle.

Most of these are characterized by :
- *Onset in early life (primarily disorders of infancy & childhood, but may present in adulthood)*
- *Non progressive or slowly progressive course*
- *Proximal or generalized muscle weakness*
- *Hypotonia*

Disease and Inheritance	Gene and Locus	Clinical Findings	Pathologic Findings
Central core disease; *Autosomal-dominant*	Ryanodine receptor-1 (RYR1) gene; 19q 13.1	Early-onset hypotonia and non progressive weakness; associated skeletal deformities; may develop malignant hyperthermia	Cytoplasmic cores are lightly eosinophilic and distinct from surrounding sarcoplasm; Found only in type 1 fibers, which usually predominate, best seen on NADH stain
Nemaline myopathy; *Autosoma-dominant or Autosomal-recessive*	Autosomal-dominant (NEM1) – Tropomyosin 3 (TPM3) gene; Autosomal-recessive (NEM2) – nebulin (NEB) gene; 2q22 Autosomal-dominant or recessive – skeletal muscle actin, α chain (ACTA1) gene; 1q42.1	Weakness, hypotonia and delayed motor development in childhood; may also be seen in adults; usually nonprogressive; involves proximal limb muscles most severely; skeletal abnormalities may be present	Aggregates of subsarcolemmal spindle shaped particles (nemaline rods); occur predominantly in type 1 fibers; derived from Z-band material (α-actinin) and best seen on modified Gomori stain
Myotubular myopathy (Centronuclear); *X-linked (MTM1), Autosomal recessive, or Autosomal-dominant*	X-linked-myotubularin (MTM1) gene; Xq28	X-linked form presents in infancy with prominent hypotonia and poor prognosis; autosomal forms have limn weakness and are slowly progressive; autosomal recessive form is intermediate in severity and prognosis	Abundance of centrally located nuclei involving the makority of muscle fibers; central nuclei are usually confined to type I fibers, which are small in diameter, but can occur in both fiber types

Other uncommon types include minicore myopathy, fingerprint body myopathy and sarcotubular myopathy.

Inverted champagne bottle appearance of lower limbs

Inverted champagne bottle appearance of lower limbs is produced as a result of greater wasting of distal musculature in comparison to proximal musculature.

Charcoal Movie Tooth disease (CMT) or peroneal muscular Atrophy (Synonym for CMT) is classically associated with an inverted champagne bottle appearance of lower limbs

Inverted Champagne bottle appearance of lower limbs

- ***Sensorimotor Neuropathy causing distal muscular atrophy*** eg Charcot MarieTooth disease or Peroneal Muscular Atrophy
- *Chronic Venous insufficiency leading to lipodermotosclerosis of distal limb (Davidson , CMDT)*

Polymyositis

Primary idiopathic Polymyositis

Condition of autoimmune[Q] etiology in which skeletal muscle[Q] is damaged by non-suppurative inflammatory process[Q] dominated by Lymphocytic infiltration. [Q]

It is a subacute inflammatory myopathy and mimics many other myopathies.

It is characterized by:

- *Symmetrical weakness of proximal limb muscles especially hips and thigh (pelvic girdle) and later shoulder girdle.*
- *Weakness of flexor muscles of neck (Head drop: difficulty in holding up the head)*
- *Involvement of striated muscles of pharynx (dysphagia)*
- *Involvement of respiratory muscles (late)*
- *Tendon reflexes are preserved but may be absent in severely weakened or atrophic muscles' – Harrison*

Its diagnosis is essentially established as a disgnosisd of exclusion.

- **Polymyositis should be considered in adults and rarely in children who DO NOT HAVE any of the following:**

Patients with Polymyositis DO NOT HAVE

- ***Rash***
- ***Involvement of extraocular and facial muscles***

Involvement of extraocular and facial muscles excludes a diagnosis of Polymyositis

Ocular muscles are almost never affected except in a rare case associated with myasthenia gravis

Facial muscles are unaffected in Polymyositis

- *Family history of a neuromuscular disease*
- *History of exposure to myotoxic drugs or toxins*
- *Endocrinopathy*
- *Neurogenic disease*
- *Muscular dystrophy*
- *Biochemical muscle disorder (deficiency of a muscle enzyme)*

Dermatomyositis

Dermatomyositis is a distinctive entitiy identified by a characteristic rash, accompanying or more often preceding muscles weakness.

Dermatomyositis

Rash	Muscle weakness
• ***Heliotrope rash[Q] :*** blue purple discoloration of upper eye lids with edema • ***Gottron's patch[Q]:*** Erythema of knuckles with a raised violaceous scaly eruption. Flat red rash on face and upper trunk	

Cutaneous features of Dermatomyositis

Cutaneous feature	Description
Heliotrope Rash[Q]	Periocular or facial erythema and edema with pink/purple /blue (heliotrope) hue *(blue purple discoloration on upper eye lids with edema)*
Gottren's Papules[Q] (Gottren's sign)	Violaceous papules over the knuckles *Erythema of the knuckles with a raised violaceous scaly eruption*
'V' sign	*Erythematous rash over other body surfaces such as anterior chest (often in a V form)*
Shawl sign	*Erythematous rash over other body surfaces including the upper trunk, neck, back & shoulders (shawl pattern)*
Periungual Telengiectasias[Q]	*Dilated capillary loops at the base of fingernails*
Mechanic's hands[Q]	*Irregular, thickened, distorted cuticles, with rough and cracked areas over the lateral and palmar areas of fingers with irregular dirty horizontal lines resembling mechanic's hand.*
Calcinosis Cutis[Q]	*Presence of hard calcium deposits in the skin*

Differences Between Polymyositis and Dematomyositis

	Polymyositis	Dermatomyositis
Age of onset	*> 18 yr*	*Adulthood and childhood*
Familial associations	*No*	*No*
Extramuscular manifestations	*Yes*	*Yes*
Associated conditions		
Connective tissue diseases	*Yes*	*Scleroderma and mixed connective tissue disease (overlap syndromes)*
Systemic autoimmune diseases	*Frequent*	*Infrequent*
Malignancy	*No*	*Yes, in upto 15% of cases*
Viruses	*Yes*	*Unproven*
Drugs	*Yes*	*Yes, rarely*
Parasites and bacteria	*Yes*	*No*
Pathogenic mechanism	*T cell*	*Immune complex*
Skin Rash/ Dermatitis	***No***	***Yes***
Pharyngeal muscle involvement	***Yes***	***Yes***
Proximal muscle involvement	***Yes***	***Yes***
Ocular muscle involvement	***No***	***No***
Facial muscle involvement	***No***	***No***

Myositis Specific Antibodies (MSA)

- Myositis Specific antibodies are autoantibodies, usually directed against intracellular ribonucleoproteins that are involved in protein translation.
- *The three best described Myositis Specific Antibodies (MSA) are Anti-Jo-1(directed to t-RNA histidyl-synthetase), Anti-Mi-2 and Anti – SRP (Anti Signal Recognition Particle)*
- The sensitivity of these antibodies is believed to be low
- Specific MSA are however associated with certain clinical features and prognosis.

M.S.A	Association	Clinical Features	Prognosis
Anti-Jo-1	*Polymyositis (30% sensitive)*	• Relatively Acute Onset • Predicts deforming arthritis, Reynaud's Phenomenon and Pulmonary fibrosis	• *Moderate* • Moderate Response to therapy but persistent disease
Anti-Mi-2	*Dermatomyositis (5%) sensitive*	• Relatively Acute Onset • Predicts classical dermatomyositis rash ('V' sign, Shawl sign) and cuticular over growth	• *Good* • Good response to therapy and good prognosis
Anti- SRP	*Polymyositis / Dermatomyositis (< 5% sensitive)*	• Very Acute onset • Predicts severe weakness, palpitations (no rash)	• *Poor* • Poor response to therapy and poor prognosis

Episodic Weakness & Channellopathies

Channelopathies: Refers to a group of disorders caused by affection of muscle membrane excitability.

Causes of Episodic generalized weakness

Electrolyte disturbances

- ***Hypokalemia***
- Hyperkalemia
- ***Hyponatremia***
- Hypernatremia
- ***Hypophosphatemia***
- ***Hypercalcemia***
- Hypermagnesemia

Muscle disorders

- Channelopathies (periodic paralysis)
- Metabolic defect of muscle
  - Impaired carbohydrate or fatty acid utilization
  - Abnormal mitochondrial function

Neuromuscular junction disorder

- Myaesthenia gravis
- Lambert – Eaten Myaesthenic syndrome

Central nervous system disorders

- Transient ischaemic attacks of the brainstem
- Transient global cerebral ischemia
- Multiple sclerosis

Neurologic Channelopathies :

Category	Disorder	Channel type
Ataxias	Episodic ataxia –1	K
	Episodic ataxia – 2	Ca
	Spinocerebellar ataxia - 6	Ca
Migraine	Familial hemiplegic migraine	Ca
Epilepsy	Benign neonatal familial convulsions	K
	Generalised epilepsy with febrile convulsions plus	Na
Periodic paralysis	Hyperkalemic periodic paralysis	Na
	Hypokalemic periodic paralysis	Ca
Myotonia	Myotonia congenital	Cl
	Paramyotonia congenital	Na
Deafness	Jorvell and Lange-Nielsen syndrome (deafness, prolonged QT interval, and arrhythmia)	K
	Autosomal dominant progressive deafness	K

Spinocerebellar ataxia – 6 is classified as meurological channelopathy but not spinocerebellar ataxia – 1

Spontaneous (Non Traumatic CSF Leaks)

Spontaneous (Non Traumatic CSF Leaks)

High Pressure Leaks

- ***Elevated Intracranial Pressure***
  - *Hydrocephalus*
  - *Intracranial Tumors*
- *Benign Intracranial Hypertension **(Pseudotumor cerebri)***

Normal Pressure Leaks

- ***Empty Sella syndrome***
- *Congenital anomalies*
  - ***Encephalocele***
  - *Meningocele*
  - *Focal olfactory Atrophy*
  - *Cribriform Plate Defects*
- *Osteomyelitis (skull base)*
- *Connective Tissue Disorder*
  - *Marfan's syndrome*
  - *Ehler's Danlos syndrome*
  - *Osteogenesis Imperfecta*

Head Injuries & Miscellaneous

Glasgow Coma Scale

Eye Opening		Verbal Response		Motor Response	
Response	*Score*	*Response*	*Score*	*Response*	*Score*
Spontaneous	*4*	*Oriented & Converses*	*5*	*Obeyes command*	*6*
To verbal stimuli	*3*	*Disoriented / confused and converses*	*4*	*Localizes pain*	*5*
To pain	*2*	*Inappropriate words*	*3*	*Withdraws to pain*	*4*
Nil	*1*	*Incomprehensible words*	*2*	*Abnormal flexion (decorticate rigidity)*	*3*
		No response	*1*	*Extension response*	*2*
				Nil	*1*

Note :

The maximum score is 15

The minimum score is 03

Decorticate rigidity is not seen as a manifestation of uncal herniation. All other features form part of the spectrum.

'Herniation or coning' is said to be occurring when part of the brain is forced through a rigid hole.

Uncal herniation			Central herniation		
The uncus and the temporal lobe are forced through the cerebellar tentorium (tentorium that separates the cerebrum from the cerebellum)			The diencephation i.e. the thalamus and related structures that lie between upper brainstem and cerebral hemispheres are forced through the tentorium.		
What happens			**What happens**		
Sequential compression occurs of the - Ipsilateral third nerve - Contralateral brainstem (later) - Whole brainstem (eventually)			Sequential compression occurs of the - Upper midbrain (first) - Pons (later) - Medulla (finally)		
Physical signs			**Physical signs**		
Early	***Later***	***Still later***	***Early***	***Later***	***Still later***
• I/L dilated pupils • Signs of supra xentorial mass lesions	• I/L hemiplegia • Progressive ptosis & third n palsy • Cheyne- stokes respiration	• Tetraparesis • B/e fixed dilated pupils • Erratic respiration • Death	• Errotic respiration • Small reactive pupils. • Increased limb tone • Bilateral extensor plantar	• Cheyne stokes respiration • Decorticate rigidity	• Fixed dilated pupils • Decerebrate posturing

Source of hemorrhage in various types of intracranial hemorrhage

Source of hemorrhage in various types of intracranial hemorrhage

Epidural hemorrhage	Subdural hemorrhage	Subarachnoid hemorrhage	Intracerebral hemorrhage
Most commonly caused by rupture of middle meningeal artery[Q] (br. of maxillary artery)	*Most commonly caused by rupture of superior cerebral veins[Q] (Bridging veins that connect the cerebral cortex to superior saggital sinus)*	*Most commonly caused by rupture of saccular aneurysms[Q] (Berry aneurysms are the most common saccular aneurysms involved[Q])*	*Most commonly caused by rupture of lenticulostriate branch of middle cerebral artery[Q].*

Subdural hemorrhage is caused by the rupture of bridging veins that connect the brain and the dural sinuses (cortical bridging veins)

Most common cause of extradural hemorrhage is *Rupture of middle meningeal artery.*

Chronic Subdural Hematoma

Gradual accumulation of blood in subdural space and classically presenting 3 weeks after the initial bleed. (Chronic)

Pathogenesis

Rupture of bridging veins

Repeated cycles of recurrent bleeding into subdural space and resorption of the resultant hematoma.

Chronic subdural haematoma is the common in conditions of cerebral atrophy notably old age and alcoholism. Minor trauma leads to a little insignificant bleeding in subdural space that goes unnoticed. As the blood breaks down over the next few weeks or months, fluids are drawn into subdural space because the breakdown products are hyperosmolol and membrane forms. ***This collection gradually enlarges and compresses the brain producing focal neurological defects mimicking tumor.***

Risk Factors

- *Elderly age, Coagulopathy, Alcoholism, Epilepsy, Metastatic Carcinoma,* Birth trauma and child abuse are risk factors in infants

Clinical Features

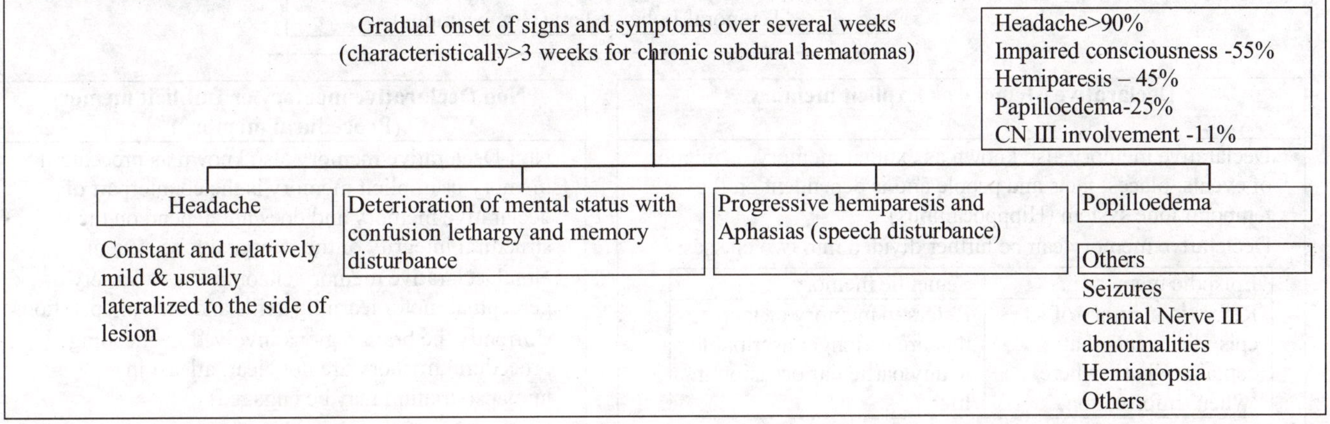

Gradual onset of signs and symptoms over several weeks (characteristically>3 weeks for chronic subdural hematomas)

Headache>90%
Impaired consciousness -55%
Hemiparesis – 45%
Papilloedema-25%
CN III involvement -11%

- Headache
  - Constant and relatively mild & usually lateralized to the side of lesion
- Deterioration of mental status with confusion lethargy and memory disturbance
- Progressive hemiparesis and Aphasias (speech disturbance)
- Popilloedema
- Others
  - Seizures
  - Cranial Nerve III abnormalities
  - Hemianopsia
  - Others

Diffuse Axonal Injury (DAI)

- *DAI represents the presence of wide spread axonal damage (white matter) in both hemispheres, secondary to severe head injury*
- *DAI results from application of severe acceleration / deceleration or angular rotational to the brain which* **results in injuries to the axons by a shearing force (shear injuries)**

Pathobiological Features

- *Focal (irreversible) disruption of axons (white matter) at multiple places in both hemisphers (occurs at the moment of injury) –* **white matter tears**
- *These white matter tears* **may be haemorrhagic or non-haemorrhagic**
- *When non-haemorrhagic they are edematous (Non-haemorrhagic lesions are not detected by CT scan but may be recognized on MRI as it picks up edema)*

Frequent location of tears

- **The most frequent location of tears is in the lobar white matter at the junction of grey and white matter***)*
  - *Frontal / Temporal lobe >Parietal lobe / Occipital lobes*
  - **Basal ganglia**
  - *-Cerebellum*
  - *-Internal / External capsule*
- **Corpus Callosum** *(Second most commonly involved location)*
- *Brain stem (third most commonly involved location)*

Clinical presentation

Clinical presentations may however range from symptoms of concussion to coma

Loss of consciousness is a common finding[Q] *and* DAI is the commonest cause of post traumatic vegetative state[Q]

Raised intracranial tension may or may not be associated[Q]

Diagnosis

- Many of these injuries are likely to go undetected by any imaging modality[Q]
- *DAI may be recognized on CT scan and MRI (MRI > CT scan)*

CT scan	*MRI*
CT scan can usually detect only those lesions that are large and haemorrhagic *CT scan often fails to recognize DAI lesions because most lesions are small and non haemorrhagic* (CT is often normal[Q])	*MRI is more sensitive than CT scan for detecting DAI* *MRI can recognize smaller lesion than CT scan and also non haemorrhagic lesions from associated edema*

A normal CT scan in light of a neurologically devastated patient following head injury is a classic finding in Diffuse Axonal injury[Q]

Prognosis: *Diffuse Axonal injury carries an extremely* poor prognosis[Q]

Hippocampus and Memory

- *The Hippocampus is essential to forming new memories for fasts and general information (sementic memory) and also for life experiences (episodic memory). But the hippocampus does not appear to play a role in precedureal memory, the kind of memory we draw upon while riding bike or using a tool*
- *With Hippocampal lesions long term memory that has already been consolidated (transformed and stored) may be retained*
- *With Hippocampal lesions new short-term memory may be acquired*
- *With Hippocampal lesion newly acquired short term memory is not consolidated and transformed into long term memory (antegrade amnesia)*
- *With Hippocampal lesions previous memory that has not been fully consolidated prior to lesion is lost (retrograde amnesia)*

Classification of Memory Based on Anatomy of Temporal Lobe system (Hippocampus)

Declarative Memory or Explicit memory

- Declarative memory also known as explicit memory, is memory of events, places, facts and people and is dependent on the temporal lobe system (Hipppocampus)
- Declerative memory can be further divided into two classes.

Episodic memory	Sementic memory
Refers to memory of episodic events that contain 'what' 'where' 'when' information	Refers to memory or facts that are no longer ascribable to any particular occasion in life

- Lesions of the temporal lobe such as hippocampus are known to greatly impair patient's ability to learn new facts, concepts vacobulary and knowledge about the world

Non Declarative memory or Imblicit memory (Procedural memory)

- Non-Declarative memory also known as procedural memory or implicit memory is the counterpart of declarative memory and does not depend on the structural integrity of the temporal lobe system.
- Non Declarative memory encompasses a variety of perceptual motor learning skills and mental operations
- Currently the brain regions involved in encoding procedural memory are not clear, atleast in humans(striatum may be engaged)

Temporal (Time based) classification of memory

Short term memory

Newly formed memories
(Over a time course of seconds or hours)

Patients with Hippocampal lesions may acquire new memories for a <u>short term</u> but are not able to transform them into long term memories

They tend to have amnesia for recent events, though they may retain memory acquired a very long time ago since such memory has already been consolidated

Long term memories

Memories from events acquired over course of weeks, months or years

Long term memories refers to relatively permanent storage of information resulting from transformation and consolidation of sensory inputs

Hippocampal lesion

Antegrade Amnesia

Hippocampal lesions do not allow consolidation / transformation of newly acquired short-term memories to long-term memories producing leairning defects.

The impairment is centered on declarative knowledge and non-declarative learning is rarely impaired.

Retrograde Amnesia

Hippocampal lesions may result in loss of memory immediately before sustaining the lesion. The information from the time closest to the point of injury is most likely to be lost (memory which has not been consolidated)

Hippocampal lesions primarily affect Declarative or Explicity memory.

Narcolepsy

Narcolepsy is a common sleep disorder charachterized by excessive daytime sleepiness, cataplexy (episodes of muscle weakness triggered by emotions), hypnagogic hallucinations and sleep paralysis.

Narcolepsy (classic Tetrad)
1. Excessive day-time somnolence 2. Sudden weakness or loss of muscle tone without loss of consciousness often elicited by emotion (cataptexy) 3. Hallucination at sleep onset (Hypnagogic Hallucination) or upon awakening (Hypnopompic Hallucination) 4. Muscle Paralysis upon awakening

Pathology /Pathogenesis
Most important cause of narcolepsy is believed to be deficiency of neuropeptide Hypocretin (orexin) produced in Hypothalamus

Autoimmune
All narcoleptics with cataplexy are positive for HLA DQB1 (0602)

Narcolepsy in humans is caused by deficiency of hypocretin (Orexin) a neurotransmitter produced in the Hypothalamus. *'Recently several convergent lines of evidence suggest that the hypothalamic neuropeptide hypocretin (orexin) is involved in the pathogenesis of Narcolepsy' - Harrison's 18th/220*

Argyll Robertson Pupil (ARP)

- The Argyll Robertson Pupil (ARP) refers to a *small (miotic), irregular pupil, with an absent light reflex (both direct and consensual) and normal accommodation reflex (normal near reflex)*. This phenomenon is often called *Light Near dissociation.*
- The ARP results from a lesion involving fibers that pass from pretectal area of the midbrain to the Edinger – Westphal nucleus. However only the rostrally placed fibers subserving the light reflex are involved while the more caudally located fibers responsible for near vision / accommodation are unaffected.

The ARP was first described in neuro-syphillis, but this may be seen in several conditions affecting the midbrain including Encephalitis, CVA, M.S. etc

- ARP shares several features with Adie's Tonic pupil from which it must be differentiated.

Comparison between Argyll-Robertson pupil and Adie's pupil:

Features	**ARP**	**Adie's**
Vision	*Good*	*Good*
Pupil	*Constricted*	*Dilated*
Laterality	*Bilateral; may be unilateral*	*Unilateral; may become bilateral*
Effect of Illumination	*Nil*	*Larger in bright light*
Light reflex (Direct and consensual)	*Absent*	*Absent/poor*
Near reflex (Accomodation)	*Brisk*	*Tonic*
Atropine	*No mydriasis*	*Mydriasis*
Miotic	*Constrict*	*Constrict with very weak solution*
Lesion	*Pretectal*	*Ciliary ganglion*

9

Nervous System

Horner's Syndrome

Clinical Finding In Horner's Syndrome

Classical Triad	Other Signs of Horner's Syndrome
• ***Miosis*** • ***Ptosis*** • ***Anhidrosis***	• ***Apparent Enophthalmos****(d/t narrow palpebral fissure)* • Anisocoria • ***Heterochromia of iris*** • Dilation lag (slow dilation of pupil after lights are dimmed) • Increased accommodative amplitude or accommodative paresis • Transient ocular Hypotonia and conjunctival Hyperemia

Anhidrosis *is absent in lesions at the level of internal carotid artery or above sudomotor and vasomotor fibers to the face follow the external carotid artery at the bifurcation.*

Horner's Syndrome from lesion of sympathetic Pathway below bifurcation of carotic artery	Horner's syndrome from lesion of sympathetic pathway above bifurcation of carotid artery
• Ptosis • Miosis • ***Anhidrosis***	• Ptosis • Miosis ***(Anhidrosis is absent)***

Clinical Findings in Horner's Syndrome (Taken from *Localization in Clinical Neurology (Lippincott Williams) 2011/208;*

- *Ipsilateral mild (usually < 2 mm) ptosis* (due to denervation of the Muller's muscle of the upper eyelid)
- *Reverse Ptosis or 'Upside down ptosis'* (due to sympathetic denervation to the lower eyelid retractors)
- ***Apparent enophthalmos***
- ***Miosis***
- *Anisocoria* due to ipsilateral miosis
- *Dilation lag* (slow dilation of the pupil after lights are dimmed)
- *Increased accommodative amplitude or accommodative paresis* (Patients hold the near card closer to read)
- *Transient (acute phase) ocular hypotony and conjunctival hyperemia*
- ***Heterochromia of the iris***
- *Variable ipsilateral facial* ***anhidrosis***
- Ipsilateral straight hair in some congenital cases (usually congenital but rarely acquired)
- Rarely neurotrophic corneal endothelial failure with pain and stromal edema (rare).
- Ipsilateral nasal obstruction with contralateral rhinorrhea with infantile cases (rare).

Most common causes of Horner's Syndrome in Adults Based on Lesion Location

Central (First order)	Preganglionic (Second order)	Postganglionic (Third order)
Hypothalamus Stroke Tumor Brainstem Stroke ***(lateral medullary infarction)*** Demyelination***(multiple sclerosis)*** Tumor Spinal cord (cervicothoracic) Trauma Syringomyelia Tumor (intramedullary) Demyelination ***(multiple sclerosis)*** Myelitis Arteriovenous malformation	Cervical spine disease Brachial plexus injury Pulmonary apical lesion Apical lung tumor Mediastinal tumors Cervical rib Trauma Iatrogenic jugular or subclavian cannulation, chest tube, thoracic surgery Subclavian artery aneurysm Thyroid tumors	Superior cervical ganglion Trauma Jugular venous ectasia Iatrogenic (surgical neck dissection) Internal carotid artery Dissection Aneurysm Trauma Arteritis Tumor Skull base lesion Nasopharyngeal carcinoma Lymphoma Cavernous sinus lesion Tumors Pituitary tumor Inflammation Thrombosis Carotid aneurysm Cluster headache

Horner's syndrome is associated with Lateral Medullary Syndrome or Wallenberg Syndrome and not with Medial Medullary Syndrome.

Multiple Sclerosis

- *Multiple Sclerosis is a chronic disease characterized by inflammation, demyelination, gliosis (scarring) and neuronal loss*
- *The course can be relapsing – remitting or progressive*
- *The clinical manifestations of M.S. are diverse and vary depending on the site and severity of demyelinating lesions within the CNS*

Lesions are disseminated in time and space (Typically occur at different times and different CNS locations)

- *The onset of symptoms may be abrupt or insidious*
- *The lesions may be anywhere in the CNS including the* ***spinal cord***

Sensory Symptoms

- *Paresthesias, Dystheseas Hypestheseas*
- *Sensory impairment and sensory level indicate spinal cord as site of lesion*
- *Pain (anywhere) is seen upto 50%*

Motor Weakness

Usually UMN type and associated with

- *Spasticity*
- *Hyperreflexia*
- *Babiniski sign +ve*

Occasionally tendon reflex may be lost if an MS lesion disrupts the afferent reflex fibres

Visual Symptoms/Signs

- **Optic Neuritis***is typical (usually unilateral but may be bilateral)*
- **Diplopia** may result from internuclear *ophthalmoplegia (INO) or from palsy of 6th CN (Rarely IIIrd/IVth CN)*
- **Visual Blurring***may result from Optic Neuritis or Diplopia*

Bladder Bowel Involvement

- *Bladder dysfunction is seen in > 90% of MS patients*
- *May include Detrusor Hyper-reflexia or Detrusor sphincter dyssynergia*
- *Constipation > Fecal urgency or incontinence*

Sexual Disfunction

Ataxia/Dysarthria

Ataxia usually manifests as cerebellar tremors.

Facial weakness

Usually due to lesion in pons.

Vertigo

From brainstem lesion.

Cognitive Dysfunction and Depression

Fatigue

Experienced by >90% of patients.

Ancillary Symptoms

- *Heat sensitivity* (Uhtoff's symptom)
- *Lhermitte's symptom*
- *Paroxysmal symptoms*
- *Trigeminal neuralgia Hemifacial spsm Glossophoryngeal neuralgia*

Initial Symptoms of MS

The most common earliest presenting features of multiple sclerosis are transient sensory defects followed by visual disturbances due to optic neuritis.

Symptom	*Percent of Cases*	*Symptom*	*Percent of Cases*
Sensory loss	*37*	*Lhermitte's*	*3*
Optic neuritis	*36*	*Pain*	*3*
Weakness	*35*	*Dementia*	*2*
Paresthesias	*24*	*Visual loss*	*2*
Diplopia	*15*	*Facial palsy*	*1*
Ataxia	*11*	*Impotence*	*1*
Vertigo	*6*	*Myokymia*	*1*
Paroxysmal attacks	*4*	*Epilepsy*	*1*
Bladder	*4*	*Falling*	*1*

Interferon Beta should be considered in patients with Relapsing / Remitting MS (RRMS) and Secondary Progressive MS (SPMS) with superimposed relapses.
Interferon Beta reduces the attack rate in M.S. patients and also improves disease severity measures and disease burden.

Therapy (Treatment) of Multiple Sclerosis

Treatment with Disease Modifying Agents that reduce the biological activity of Multiple Sclerosis

Seven such agents are approved by the U.S. FDA

- *Interferon Beta-1a (IFN-β-1a) (Avonex)*
- ***Interferon Beta -1a** (IFN-β-1a) (Rebif)*
- ***Interferon Beta-1b** (IFN-β-1b) (Betaseron)*
- ***Glatiramer Acetate** (Copaxone)*
- *Natalizumab (Tysabri)*
- *Fingolimod (Gilenya)*
- *Mitoxantrone (Novantrone)*

Cladribine (Leustatin) is the eighth agent currently awaiting FDA approval

Treatment of Acute Attacks

(Acute Exacerbations or Initial Demyelinating Episodes)

- Glucocorticoids
- Plasma exchange

(Plasma exchange may benefit patients with fulminant attacks of demyelination that are unresponsive to glucocorticoids)

Off Label Treatment options for Relapsing /Remitting MS and Secondary Progressive M.S.

- *Azathioprine*
- *Methotrexate*
- *Cyclophosphamide*
- *Intravenous Immunoglobulin*
- *Methylprednisolone*

Features of Cerebellar Disease

Features of Cerebellar Disease / Dysfunction

- *Dysmetria (Inaccuracy of movement, disturbance of role, range & force of movement)*
- *Dysarthria (Ataxic dysarthria results from disruption of timing, force, range and direction of movement needed to maintain normal articulation)*
- *Ataxi (unsteady to stand or sit without support)*
- *Incoordination*

  Pastpointing
  Intention tremor (Inability to coordinate fine motor activity)
  Dysdiadokinesia (Inability to perform rapid lternating movements)

- *Hypotonia*
- *Cerebellar Nystagmus*

Kluver Bucy Syndrome

Kluver Bucy Syndrome is caused due to bilateral ablation of Amygdala

Features of K.B. syndrome (Experimented on animals)

1. *Is not afraid of anything*
2. *Has extreme curiosity about everything*
3. *Forgets rapidly*
4. *Has tendency to place everything in its mouth and sometimes even tries to eat solid object*
5. *Often has a sex drive so strong that it attempts to copulate with immature animals of the wrong sex or even animals of different species.*

Criteria for Brain Death/Brainstem death

The definition of Brain stem death requires simultaneous demonstration that the patient has irreversibly lost the capacity of consciousness (Coma) and the capacity to breathe (Apnoea) both of which are dependent on intact brainstem.

Clinical assessment of the integrity of Brainstem has two components including assessment of the integrity of brainstem mediated cranial nerve reflexes and the Apnea test.

Deep Unresponsive Coma	Absence of all Brainstem Cranial Reflexes	Complete Aponea in pressure of hypercarbia (Absence of Brainstem Respiratory Reflex)
Patients with brain death show the deepest coma possible with total unresponsiveness to all stimuli. • No spontaneous movement • No response to external stimuli (Verbal/ Deep pain)	All reflexes mediated by cranial nerve must be absent • Absent Pupillary Light reflex (CN II, III) (*Pupils are usually midsized but may be enlarged but they should not be small*) • Absent Corneal Reflex (CN V, VII) • Absent Vestibulocochlear Reflex (CN III, IV, VI, VIII) (No eye movement in response to caloric irrigation of ears) • Absent Oculocephalic Reflex (Absent Doll's eye reflex) Eyes will move with the head (No occular movements on rapid turning of head). • Absent Gag Reflex (CNIX, X) • Absent Tracheal Cough Reflex (CNX) • Absent Central Motor Response to Pain (CN V, VII) (No response to deep somatic stimulation).	• No respiratory effort in response to hypercarbia needs to be demonstrated to show that aponea is due to brainstem (medullary) damage • Absent respiratory movement during disconnection from the ventilator with the PaCO2 > 60 mm Hg is required for the test to be valid

Cranial nerve reflexes in Brain Stem Death testing:

Reflex	Cranial nerves	Notes
Pupillary light reflex	II, III	Use bright light source (not ophthalmoscope) in a dimmed environment. Look for both direct and consensual reaction. Important reflex that integrates at level of midbrain
Corneal reflex	V, VII	Stroke cornea with gauze, whilst gently holding eyes open; avoid trauma to cornea. The various nuclei of V are found throughout the whole length of the brainstem, whilst that of VII (facial nerve) is in the upper medulla.
Central response to deep somatic stimulation	V, VII	Apply deep pressure stimulation centrally (e.g. supra-orbital ridge) and peripherally (e.g. nail bed). Look for central motor response in the distribution of the facial nerve. Peripheral stimulation may illicit peripheral spinal reflexes.
Cold caloric vestibulo-ocular reflex	III, IV, VI, VIII	Check patency of external auditory canal with auroscope. Flex head to 30° (or apply 30° head up tilt if cervical spine injury is suspected). Slowly irrigate canal with 50mL ice-cold water over 60s. Observe for nystagmus for a further 30s. Contra-indicated in trauma-related otorrhea. The nuclei of III and IV lie within the midbrain, whilst those of VI and VIII are in the medulla.
Oculocephalic reflex (Doll's eye reflex)	VIII, III, VI	Rapid lateral movement of the head normally results in eye deviation to the contralateral side, testing brainstem gaze mechanism. In brainstem death eyes remain in a fixed position within the orbit.
Gag reflex	IX, X	Stimulate uvula under direct vision with throat spatula, observing for contraction of soft palate. The nuclei of IX and X lie in the medulla.
Tracheal cough reflex	X	Expose patient to umblicus. Stimulate trachea to level of carina by introduction of sterile suction catheter down endotracheal tube. Observe for cough response

QUESTIONS

Headache

1. A 45-year old man presents with a daily headache. He describes two attacks per day over the past 3 weeks. Each attack lasts about an hour and awakens the patient from sleep. The patient has noted associated tearing and reddening of his right eye as well as nasal stuffiness. The pain is deep, excruciating, and limited to the right side of the head. The neurologic examination is nonfocal. The most likely diagnosis of this patient's headache is :
   A. Migraine headache *(AIIMS Nov 99)*
   B. Cluster headache
   C. Tension headache
   D. Brain tumour
2. Cluster headache is characterized by all, **except**:
   A. Affects predominantly females. *(AI 2005)*
   B. Unilateral headache.
   C. Onset typically in 20-50 years of life.
   D. Associated with conjunctival congestion.
3. A female has episodic, recurrent headache in left hemicranium with nausea and parasthesia on right upper and lower limbs is most probably suffering from : *(AIIMS June 2000)*
   A. Migraine
   B. Glossopharyngeal neuralgia
   C. Herpes zoster infection of trigeminal Nerve
   D. Brain tumour
4. A female aged 30, presents with episodic throbbing headache for past 4 yrs. It usually involves one half of the face and is associated with nausea and vomiting. There is no aura. Most likely diagnosis is:
   A. Migraine *(AI 2001)*
   B. Cluster headache
   C. Angle closure glaucoma
   D. Temporal arteritis
5. A woman complains of headache associated with paresthesias of the right upper and lower limb: likely diagnosis is: *(AI 2001)*
   A. Trigeminal neuralgia
   B. Glossopharyngeal neuralgia
   C. Migraine
   D. Cluster headache
6. Ophthalmoplegic migraine means: *(AIIMS May 03)*
   A. When headache is followed by complete paralysis of the IIIrd and VI nerve on the same side as the hemicrania.
   B. When the headache is followed by partial paralysis of the IIIrd nerve on the same side as the hemicrania with out any scotoma.
   C. Headache associated with IIIrd, IVth and VIth nerve paralysis.
   D. Headache associated with optic neuritis
7. A woman has bilateral headache that worsens with emotional stress; she has two children, both doing badly in school; diagnosis is *(AI 2001)*
   A. Migraine
   B. Cluster headache
   C. Tension headache
   D. Trigeminal neuralgia
8. A 64 year old lady Kamla complains of severe unilateral headache on the right side and blindness for 2 days. On examination there is a thick cord like structure on the lateral side of the head. The ESR is 80 mm/hr in the first hour. The most likely diagnosis is : *(AIIMS May 01)*
   A. Temporal arteritis
   B. Migraine
   C. Cluster headache
   D. Sinusitis
9. A 35 year old Lady Malti has unilateral headache, nausea, vomiting and visual blurring. The diagnosis is: *(AIIMS June 99)*
   A. Cluster headache
   B. Glaucoma
   C. Subarachnoid haemorrhage
   D. Posterior fossa cyst.
10. A young girl presents with repeated episodes of throbbing occipital headache associated with ataxia and vertigo. The family history is positive for similar headaches in her mother. Most likely diagnosis is:
    A. Vestibular Neuronitis *(AI 2011)*
    B. Basilar migraine
    C. Cluster headache
    D. Tension headache
11. All of the following statements about treatment of migraine are true, Except *(DNB 2012)*
    A. Narotriptan has slower onset and longer t1/2 than sumatriptan
    B. Rizatriptan is more efficacious than sumatriptan
    C. Sumatriptan is a selective 5-HT 1B/1D agonist
    D. Sumatriptan is used for chronic migraine
12. What is drug of choice for acute attack of migraine-
    A. Methysergide *(AIIMS May 95)*
    B. Caffeine
    C. Amitryptiline
    D. Sumatriptan
13. All of the following agents are used for prophylaxis of migraine, Except *(AI 2010)*
    A. Propanalol
    B. Valproate
    C. Topiramate
    D. Ethosuxamide

Aphasias

14. Motor aphasia refers to defect in : *(AI 1998)*
   A. Peripheral speech apparatus
   B. Verbal expression
   C. Auditory comprehension
   D. Verbal comprehension

15. Lesion in inferior frontal gyrus causes:
   A. Defect in articulation *(AIIMS Dec 97)*
   B. Incomprehension of written language
   C. Incomprehension of spoken language
   D. Motor aphasia

16. All of the following are true about Broca's aphasia except :
   A. Lesion lies in frontal lobe
   B. Fluency is impaired
   C. Neologisms are absent
   D. Repetition is preserved

17. A patient being evaluated for aphasia is unable to repeat sentences correctly or to name objects properly. However, the patient's speech is effortless and melodic. There are frequent errors in word choice and obvious difficulties in comprehension. The remainder of the patient's neurologic examination is normal. Damage in which area of the brain would account for this type of aphasia: *(AIIMS Nov 99)*
   A. Posterior temporal and parietal lobes, dominant hemisphere
   B. Frontal and parietal lobes, dominant hemisphere
   C. Prefrontal and frontal regions, dominant hemisphere
   D. Posterior parietal and temporal lobes, nondominant hemisphere

18. Which of the following speech indicates damage to the categorical hemisphere: *(AIIMS May 08)*
   A. Normal speech
   B. Increased speech
   C. Decreased speech
   D. Senseless, fluent speech

Clinical Neurology & Diseases of Spinal Cord

UMN vs LMN lesions & Motor Neuron DIsease

19. UMN lesion is characterised by : *(AI 1999)* *(AIIMS 1994)*
   A. Weakness & spasticity
   B. Fasciculations
   C. Rigidity
   D. Localised muscle atrophy

20. With which one of the following Lower motor neuron lesions are associated?
   A. Flaccid paralysis
   B. Hyperactive stretch reflex
   C. Spasticity
   D. Muscular incordination.

21. Fasciculations are seen in: *(AI 1995, 96)*
   A. Motor neuron disease
   B. Duchenne's muscular dystrophy
   C. Polymyositis
   D. None of the above

22. Fasciculation is seen in: *(PGI Dec 03)*
   A. UMN type of lesion
   B. LMN type of lesions
   C. Myoneural junction
   D. Peripheral neuropathy

23. Bulbar paralysis refers to: *(PGI Dec 03)*
   A. LMN lesion
   B. UMN lesion
   C. Paralysis of cranial nerve IX to XII
   D. Paralysis of cranial nerve III to XII

24. All of the following are features of Pseudobulbar palsy, except: *(AI 1991)*
   A. Dysarthria
   B. Dysphagia
   C. Emotional lability
   D. Hypoactive jaw jerk

25. Which among the following does not cause exaggerated jaw jerk: *(PGI June 99)*
   A. Multiple sclerosis
   B. Motor neurone disease
   C. Pseudobulbar palsy
   D. Syringomyelia

26. All are features of pyramidal tract lesion, Except :
   A. Involuntary movement *(AIIMS Sept 96)*
   B. Positive Babinski's sign
   C. Spasticity
   D. Increased deep tendon reflexes

27. Which of the following represents the site of lesion in Motor Neuron disease: *(AI 2010)*
   A. Anterior Horn cells
   B. Peripheral Nerve
   C. Spinothalamic Tract
   D. Spinocerebellar tract

28. Which is pathgnomonic for motor neuron disease :
   A. Fasciculation *(AIIMS Dec 95)*
   B. Bladder, bowel involvement
   C. Pseudohypertrophy
   D. Sensory loss in patchy manner

29. Spinomuscular atrophy is seen in lesion of:
   A. Anterior horn *(PGI Dec 98)*
   B. Peripheral nerve
   C. Neuromuscular junction
   D. Any of the above

30. Amyotrophic lateral sclerosis involve: *(PGI June 03)*
   A. Anterior horn cell
   B. Posterior horn cell

C. Dorsal root ganglia
D. Ventral root ganglia
E. Myoneural junction

31. A middle aged man presents with progressive atrophy and weakness of hands & forearms. On examination he is found to have slight spasticity of the legs, generalized hyper-reflexia and increased signal in the cortico-spinal tracts on T2 weighted MRI. The most likely diagnosis is : *(AIIMS Nov 04)*
A. Multiple sclerosis
B. Amyotrophic lateral sclerosis
C. Subacute combined degeneration
D. Progressive spinal muscular atrophy

32. Motor neuron disease, TRUE is : *(AIIMS May 94)*
A. Sensory involvement
B. Ocular motility is spared
C. Involvement of anterior and lateral columns of spinal cord
D. Intellectual improvement

33. Fasciculations are seen in: *(AI 1995)*
A. Motor neuron disease
B. Duchenne's muscular dystrophy
C. Polymyositis
D. None of the above

Spinal Cord Disorders

General and Fine touch

34. Which of the following sensation are transmitted by the Dorsal Tract/ Posterior column: *(AI 2008)*
A. Fine touch
B. Pain
C. Temperature
D. All of the above

35. Which of the following is not affected by a lesion in posterior column of spinal cord:
A. Romberg's sign *(PGI Jun 05)*
B. Temperature sense
C. Vibration sense
D. Ataxia

36. Which is not affected in lesion of posterior column of spinal cord? *(PGI June 07)*
A. Romberg's sign
B. Temperature sense
C. Vibration sense
D. Ataxia

37. A ventrolateral cordotomy is performed to produce relief of pain from the right leg. It is effective because it interrupts the: *(AI 2012)*
A. Left Dorsal Column
B. Left Lateral Spinothalamic tract
C. Right Lateral Spinothalamic tract
D. Right Corticospinal tract

38. Type of sensation lost on same side in Brown sequard syndrome is: *(AIIMS Nov 93)*
A. Pain
B. Touch
C. Proprioception
D. Temperatiure

39. 1. All of the following are true about Brown Sequard Syndrome, except: *(AIIMS Nov 2011)*
A. Ipsilateral Pyramidal Tract Features
B. Contralateral Spinothalamic Tract Features
C. Contralateral Posterior Column Features
D. Ipsilateral Planter Extensor

40. The following are components of Brown Sequard syndrome except : *(AI 2007)*
A. Ipsilateral extensor plantar response
B. Ipsilateral pyramidal tract involvement
C. Contralateral spinothalamic tract involvement
D. Contralateral posterior column involvement

41. Which of the following statements about Brown Sequard Syndrome is true: *(PGI 2009)*
A. Ipsilateral loss of temperature
B. Contralateral loss of pain
C. Contralateral loss of vibration
D. Bilateral Segmental signs

42. Which of the following is not a feature of extramedullary tumour: *(AI 2008)*
A. Early Corticospinal signs and paralysis
B. Root pain or midine Back –pain
C. Abnormal CSF
D. Sacral sparing

43. Clinical features of Conus Medullaris syndrome include all of the following Except: *(AI 2008)*
A. Plantar Extensor
B. Absent knee & ankle jerks
C. Sacral anesthesia
D. Lower sacral & coccygeal involvement

44. Clinical Features of conus medullaris include all of the following except *(DNB 2012)*
A. Extensor Plantar Reflex
B. Saddle anesthesia
C. Late Bladder involvement
D. Bilateral and usually symmetric sensory loss

45. Early loss of bladder control is seen in *(DNB 2012)*
A. Conus Medullaris
B. Cauda Equina
C. Gullain Barre Syndrome
D. Amyotrophic Lateral Sclerosis

46. Hypotension in Acute Spinal Cord Injury is due to :
A. Loss of Sympathetic tone *(AIIMS Nov. 06)*
B. Loss of Parasympathetic tone
C. Vasovagal Attack
D. Orthostatic Hypotension

47. Spinal shock is characterized by (select three best options): *(PGI June 03)*
A. Spasticity

B. Wasting
C. Sensory loss
D. Urinary retention
E. Areflexia

48. Spinal shock is characterized by all of the following, Except : *(PGI 09)*
A. Spastic paralysis
B. Flaccid paralysis
C. Urinary Bladder involvement
D. Areflexia
E. Sensory loss

49. Cervical cord injury does not cause: *(PGI June 99)*
A. Horner's syndrome
B. Loss of sensation over face
C. Spasticity of foot
D. Wasting with fasciculations of lower limb

50. An unconscious patient is brought to the Emergency Department with suspected cervical cord injury. Which of the following clinical signs is not suggestive of cervical spinal cord injury. *(PGI June 97)*
A. Flaccidity
B. Increased Rectal sphincter Tone
C. Diaphragmatic Breathing
D. Priapism

51. Which of the following signs is not suggestive of a cervical spinal cord injury : *(AIIMS Nov. 05)*
A. Flaccidity
B. Increased rectal sphincter tone
C. Diaphragmatic breathing
D. Priapism

52. Spastic paraplegia is caused by all, except: *(AI 2009)*
A. Vitamin B12 deficiency
B. Cervical spondylosis
C. Lead poisoning
D. Motor neuron disease

53. Causes of Acute Flaccid Paralysis include: *(PGI June 08)*
A. Poliomyelitis
B. Tick paralysis
C. AIDP (Acute Inflammatory Demyelinating Polyneuropathy)
D. ADEM (Acute Disseminated Encephalamyelitis)
E. All of the above

54. A patient involved in a road traffic accident presents with quadriparesis, sphincter disturbance, sensory level up to the upper border of sternum and a respiratory rate of 35/minute.The likely level of lesion is : *(AI 2010)*
A. C1-C2
B. C4-C5
C. T1-T2
D. T3-T4

55. A patient with traumatic paraplegia due to injury of the thoracic cord of 'T3 level' is observed to have a blood pressure of 210/120. What should be the initial management? *(AI 2012)*
A. Subcutaneous LMWH
B. Steroids
C. Nifedipine
D. Normal saline/Dextrose

56. Beevor's Sign is seen in: *(AIIMS May 09)*
A. Abdominal muscle
B. Facial muscle
C. Respiratory muscle
D. Hand muscle

57. Beevor's sign indicates a lesion in the : *(PGI 05)*
A. Thoracic cord
B. Cervical cord
C. Cauda Equina
D. Conus Medullaris

58. Anterior spinal Artery thrombosis is characterized by all, except: *(PGI Dec 2000)*
A. Loss of pain & touch
B. Loss of vibration sense
C. Loss of power in lower limb
D. Sphincter dysfunction

59. All of the following may cause metaststic tumour causing spinal cord compressions except: *(AI 1998)*
A. Lung carcinoma
B. Breast carcinoma
C. Lymphoma
D. Meningioma

Friadreich's Ataxia

60. A 12-year-old boy presents to the Outpatient department with history of progressively increasing difficulty in walking and frequent falls. Physical examination reveals an ataxic gait and nystagmus. All deep tendon reflexes were observed to be absent while the plantar response was 'Extensor'. What is the most likely diagnosis? *(AI 2012)*
A. Friedreich's Ataxia
B. Subacute Combined Degeneration of Cord (SACD)
C. Becker's Muscular Dystrophy
D. Tabes Dorsalis

61. All of the following are features of Friadreich's Ataxia, Except: *(AI 1992)*
A. Prograssive Ataxia is the most common presentation
B. Cardiomyopathy is a common association
C. Diabetes mellitus may be associated
D. Extensor plantar with brisk lower limb reflexes.

62. Bilateral loss of ankle jerk and extensor plantar response is seen in: *(AIIMS Dec 98)*
A. Amyotrophic lateral sclerosis
B. Freidrich's ataxia
C. Tabes dorsalis
D. Lead poisoning

63. Features of Friedreich's Ataxia include all of the following except: *(AI 1992)*

A. Progressive weakness
B. Absent lower limb reflexes
C. Increased tone in lower limbs
D. Extensor plantar Response

64. Pyramidal tract involvement with absent ankle jerk is seen in : *(AIIMS May 01)*
A. Frederick's ataxia
B. Subacute combined degeneration of the spinal cord
C. Lathyrism
D. Tabes dorsalis

65. Absent ankle jerk and extensor plantar response is found in: *(PGI June 98)*
A. Friederich's ataxia
B. Tabes dorsalis
C. SACD
D. Vit B deficiency

66. Which of the following regions of the spinal cord is involved first in Friedreich's Ataxia: *(AI 1991)*
A. Dorsal Root ganglion
B. Spinal tracts
C. Peripheral nerve
D. Cerebellum

67. Earliest presentation of Friedrich's ataxia is- *(AIIMS Nov 93)*
A. Ataxia
B. Seizures
C. Optic atrophy
D. Stuttering

SACD & Tabes Dorsalis

68. Vitamin B12 deficiency can give rise to all of the following, **except**: *(AI 2005)*
A. Myelopathy.
B. Optic atrophy.
C. Peripheral neuropathy.
D. Myopathy.

69. Subacute Combined Degeneration of Cord is caused due to deficiency of? *(DNB June 2012)*
A. Vitamin B_1
B. Vitamin B_5
C. Vitamin B_6
D. Vitamin B_{12}

70. 65 year old man presents with anaemia and posterior column dysfunction, the likely cause is: *(AIIMS May 95)*
A. B_1-deficit
B. B_{12}-deficit
C. SSPE
D. Multiple sclerosis

71. All are true about subacute combined degeneration of spinal cord except : *(AI 1999)*
A. Due to deficiency of vitamin B_{12}
B. Posterior column involvement
C. Corticospinal involvement
D. Absent deep tendon reflexes

72. Which of the following is not true about Tabes Dorsalis *(DNB)*
A. Seen in Neurosypillis
B. Deep tendon reflexes are brisk
C. Loss of vibration sense
D. Acute abdominal pain and visceral symptoms

73. Subacute combined degeneration due to Vit B12 deficiency mainly involves: *(PGI Dec 03)*
A. Peripheral nerve
B. Corticospinal tract
C. Posterior column
D. Spinocerebellar tract
E. Spinothalamic tract

74. All are features of tabes dorsalis, ***except*** : *(AIIMS Dec 97)*
A. Ataxia
B. Argyll Robertson's pupil
C. Bladder disturbances
D. Hyperreflexia

Syringomyelia

75. Features of syringomyelia include all of the following, Except : *(PGI 09)*
A. Dissociative sensory loss
B. Bilateral involvement
C. Segmental sensory loss
D. Wasting of small muscles of hand
E. Ascending weakness

76. Painless burn in hand is a characteristic feature of : *(AI 1999)*
A. Syringomgelia
B. Thalamic syndrome
C. Cord compression
D. Systemic-lupus-erthromatosis

Cerebrovascular Diseases & Aphasias

Cerebrovascular Stroke: Causes and Sites

77. Cerebral Ischemia occurs when cerebral blood flow is less than: *(AI 2012)*
A. 10 ml/100g / minute
B. 20 ml/100g / minute
C. 40 ml/ 100g/minute
D. 50 ml/100g/minute

78. Most common cause of cerebrovascular accident is : *(AIIMS 96)*
A. Embolism
B. Arterial thrombosis
C. Venous thrombosis
D. Haemorrhage

79. Commonest cause of cerebrovascular accident is : *(AI 98)*
A. Arterial thrombosis
B. Venous thrombosis
C. Embolism
D. Tumour

80. Most common cause of stroke in young women in India among OCP users: *(PGI Dec 98)*
A. Cortical vein thrombosis

B. Moyamoya disease
C. Atherosclerosis
D. HT

81. Most common cause of intracranial haemorrhage is: *(AIIMS Nov 98)*
A. Sub arachnoid haemorrhage
B. Intracerebral hemorrhage
C. Subdural haemorrhage
D. Extradural haemorrhage

82. The commonest cause of Intracerebral Bleed is: *(AI 1995)*
A. Thrombocytopenia
B. Diabetes
C. Hypertension
D. Berry aneurysm

83. The commonest cause of Intracerebral Bleed is: *(AI 1995)*
A. Thrombocytopenia
B. Diabetes
C. Hypertension
D. Berry aneurysm

84. The most common location of hypertensive intracranial hemorrhage is: *(AI 2006)*
A. Subarachnoid space
B. Basal ganglia
C. Cerebellum
D. Brainstem

85. Which of the following is the most common location of hypertensive hemorrhage? *(AI 1994, 2003)*
A. Pons
B. Thalamus
C. Putamen/external capsule
D. Subcortical white matter

86. The most common site for hypertensive bleed is? *(DNB Dec 2010)*
A. Pons
B. Putamen
C. Frontal lobe
D. Thalamus

87. Which of the following is the most common location of hypertensive hemorrhage? *(AIIMS Nov 02)*
A. Pons
B. Thalamus
C. Putamen/external capsule
D. Cerebellum

88. The most common location of hypertensive intracranial hemorrhage is: *(AI 2006)*
E. Subarachnoid space
F. Basal ganglia
G. Cerebellum
H. Brainstem

89. The most common intracranial site of hypertensive aemorrhage is: *(AIIMS May 07)*
A. Basal ganglia
B. Brainstem
C. Cerebellum
D. Hippocampus

90. The common cause of subarachnoid hemorrhage is: *(AI 2006)*
A. Arterio-venous malformation
B. Cavernous angioma
C. Aneurysm
D. Hypertension

91. The most common cause of subarachnoid hemorrhage is: *(DNB)*
A. Arteriovenous malformation
B. Cavernous angioma
C. Aneurysm
D. Hypertension

92. Most common cause of subarachnoid hemorrhage is: *(AIIMS Nov 98) (AI 1999)*
A. Hypertension
B. A.V. malformation
C. Berry aneurysm
D. Tumours

93. Commonest cause of subarachnoid haemorrhage is: *(AI 1998)*
A. Rupture of circle of Willis aneurysm
B. Rupture or vertebral artery aneurysm
C. Rupture of venecomitants of corpus striatum
D. Rupture of dural sinusis

94. Berry aneurysm is caused by: *(AIIMS May 2011)*
A. Degeneration of internal elastic lamina
B. Degeneration of tunica media
C. Degeneration of muscular layer
D. Degeneration of external elastic lamina

95. Which is least common site of berry aneurysm: *(AIIMS Dec 95)*
A. Basilar artery
B. Vertebral artery
C. Anterior cerebral artery
D. Posterior cerebral artery

96. The most common site of Berry aneurysm is:
A. Junction of anterior communicating artery with anterior cerebral artery *(AI 1994)*
B. Junction of posterior communicating artery with internal carotid artery
C. Bifurcation of middle cerebral artery
D. Vertebral artery

97. A patient with suspected subarachnoid haemorrhage presents with blood isolated in the fourth ventricle on a CT scan. Aneurysmal rupture is likely to have resulted from: *(AI 2012)*
A. Posterior Inferior Cerebellar Artery Aneurysm
B. Anterior Communicating Artery Aneurysm
C. Posterior Communicating Artery Aneurysm
D. Basilar Artery Tip Aneurysm

98. Which of the following is the most common cause of late neurological deterioration in a case of cerebrovascular accident : *(AIIMS Nov. 2000)*
A. Rebleeding
B. Vasospasm
C. Embolism
D. Hydrocephalus

99. A patient known to have mitral stenosis and atrial fibrillation presents with acute onset of weakness in the left upper limb which recovered completely in two weeks. The most likely diagnosis is:

A. Transient Ischemic Attack *(AI 2010)*
B. Ischemic stroke
C. Hemorrhagic stroke
D. Vasculitis

100. 'Duret Hemorrhages' are seen in : *(AIIMS May 08)*
A. Brain
B. Kidney
C. Heart
D. Lung

Subarachnoid Haemorrhage

101. A 45 years old hypertensive male presented with sudden onset severe headache, vomiting and neck stiffness. On examination he didn't have any focal neurological deficit. His CT scan showed blood in the Sylvain fissure. The probable diagnosis is:
A. Meningitis *(AIIMS May 03)*
B. Ruptured aneurysm
C. Hypertensive bleed.
D. Stroke

102. A 45 year old male patient presented in the casualty with two hours history of sudden onset of severe headache associated with nausea and vomiting on clinical examination the patient had necks stiffness and right sided ptosis. Rest of the neurological examination was normal. What is the clinical diagnosis : *(AIIMS Nov 03)*
A. Hypertensive brain haemorrhage
B. Migraine
C. Aneurysmal subarachnoid haemorrhage
D. Arteriovenous malformation haemorrhage

103. A nondiabetic, non hypertensive adult male develops sudden severe headache with altered sensorium, likely diagnosis is : *(AI 1999)*
A. Brain tumour
B. Sub arachnoid haemorrhage
C. Encephalitis
D. Meningitis

104. A young female presents with severe headache and neck stiffness of abrupt onset. She says, she has never had such severe headache before. She also complains of associated nausea and photophobia. Likely diagnosis is: *(AIIMS May 09)*
A. Subarachnoid hemorrhage (SAH)
B. Migraine
C. Viral Encephalitis
D. Hydrocephalus

105. Sudden excruciating headache is most characteristic of *(PGI Dec 01)*
A. SAH
B. Aneurysmal bleeding
C. Epilepsy
D. Intracerebral hemorrhage
E. Hysteria

106. A patient presented with thunder clap headache followed by unconsciousness and progressive III cranial nerve palsy. Which of the following is the most likely diagnosis: *(AIIMS Nov 2010)*
A. Extradural Hemorrhage
B. Aneurysmal Subarachnoid hemorrhage
C. Basilar migraine
D. Cluster Headache

107. A 25-year-old male had severe headache followed by unconsciousness. CSF tap revealed red blood cells. Most likely diagnosis is : *(AIIMS Dec 94)*
A. Subdural hematoma
B. Embolism
C. Tumour
D. Ruptured aneurysm

108. A 45 years old hypertensive male presented with sudden onset severe headache, vomiting and neck stiffness. On examination he didn't have any focal neurological deficit. His CT scan showed blood in the Sylvain fissure. The probable diagnosis is:
A. Meningitis *(AIIMS May 03)*
B. Ruptured aneurysm
C. Hypertensive bleed.
D. Stroke

Localization of Stroke: Clinical Features

109. A lesion in the paracentral lobule causes:
A. Contralateral foot weakness *(PGI June 99)*
B. Seizures only
C. Migraine
D. Cognitive loss

110. A lesion in the paracentral lobule causes:
A. Contralateral foot weakness *(PGI June 97)*
B. Memory impairment
C. Brocas aphasia
D. Cognitive loss

111. All of the following are features of temporal lobe lesions Except: *(AIIMS Dec 94)*
A. Wernicke's Aphasia
B. Contralateral homonymous superior quadrantanopia
C. Auditory hallucinations
D. Hemineglect

112. Lesions of the medial temporal lobe may produce (select three options) *(PGI June 99)*
A. Visual Amnesia
B. Auditory Amnesia
C. Antegrade Amnesia
D. Apraxia

113. In a Right handed person, left parietal lobe injury may be associated with all of the following except.
A. Aphasia *(AI 1992)*
B. Acalculia
C. Urinary incontinence
D. Inferior quadrantic Anopsia

114. In a right handed person, left temporoparietal lobe injury leads to all, Except: *(AIIMS June 98)*
A. Wernicke's Aphasia
B. Urinary Incontinence
C. Acalculia
D. Superior quadrantic Anopsia

115. Anterior cerebral artery occlusion can cause:
A. Urinary retention *(AIIMS May 93)*
B. Contralateral lower leg weakness
C. Hemianaesthesia of opposite side of face
D. Hemianopia

116. Hemiplegia is commonly associated with infarction of the area of distribution of the:
A. Anterior cerebral artery *(AI 1994)*
B. Middle cerebral artery
C. Posterior cerebral artery
D. Anterior communicating artery

117. All of the following are true about anterior choroidal artery syndrome except: *(AI 2011)*
A. Hemiparesis
B. Hemisensory loss
C. Homonymous Hemianopia
D. Involvement of anterior limb of internal capsule

118. Which of the following is not a usual feature of right middle cerebral artery territory infarct :
A. Aphasia. *(AIIMS Nov 02) (AIIMS May 03)*
B. Hemiparesis.
C. Facial weakness.
D. Dysarthria.

119. Which of the following is not a usual feature of right middle cerebral artery territory infarct:
A. Aphasia. *(AIIMS Nov 02)*
B. Hemiparesis.
C. Facial weakenss.
D. Dysarthria.

120. Which of the following sites is not involved in a posterior cerebral artery infarct: *(AI 2011)*
A. Midbrain
B. Thalamus
C. Temporal lobe
D. Anterior Cortex

121. Memory impairment occurs in embolism of posterior cerebral artery because of damage to :*(AIIMS Dec 94)*
A. Hipppocampal gyrus
B. Superior temporal gyrus
C. Prefrontal gyrus
D. Angular gyrus

122. A 45 years male presents with hypertension. He has sudden abnormal flinging movements in right upper and lower limbs. Most likely site of haemorrhage is :
A. Substantia nigra *(AI 2001)*
B. Caudate nuclei
C. Pons
D. Subthalmic nuclei

123. A hypertensive individual had a sudden headache and became unconscious within a few minutes. On regaining consciousness, there was complete flaccid hemiplegia with no involvement of upper face, absence of tendon reflexes and a positive Babinski sign. Which one of the following arteries could have ruptured : *(AIIMS Nov 03)*
A. Lateral striate branch of middle cerebral
B. Medial striate branch of anterior cerebral
C. Posterolateral branch from posterior cerebral
D. Posterior choroidal branch of posterior cerebral

124. All of the following Neurophysiological defects are likely to result from right lobe involvement, except:
A. Visuospatial defects *(AIIMS May 08)*
B. Anosognosia
C. Dyscalculi
D. Spatial Dysgraphia

125. Which of the following speech indicates damage to the categorical hemisphere: *(AIIMS May 08)*
A. Normal speech
B. Increased speech
C. Decreased speech
D. Senseless, fluent speech

126. All of the following are features of Millard Gubler Syndrome, Except : *(AIIMS May 08)*
A. 5th cranial nerve palsy
B. 6th cranial nerve palsy
C. 7th cranial nerve palsy
D. Contralateral hemiplegia

127. Third nerve palsy with pupillary sparing is seen in all except: *(AIIMS May 95)*
A. Hypertension
B. Aneurysm of posterior communicating artery
C. Diabetes mellitus
D. Craniopharyngioma

128. Which of the following structure is most likely to be compressed by an aneurysm of the posterior communicating artery: *(AIIMS May 08)*
A. Occulomotor nerve
B. Optic nerve
C. Trochlear nerve
D. Hypophysis cerebri

129. Most common nerve involved in intracranial aneurysm is : *(AI 1998)*
A. Trochlear
B. VII
C. VIII
D. Occulomotor

130. Damage to Auditory Cortex on one side causes:
A. Hearing loss and impaired tonal discrimination on the contralateral side *(DNB)*
B. Hearing loss and impaired tonal discrimination on the ipsilateral side
C. No noticeable hearing loss or loss of tonal discrimination
D. Impaired localization of sound on the ipsilateral side

Lacunar infarcts

131. Lacunar infarcts are caused by : *(AI 2001)*
   A. Lipohyalinosis of penetrating arteries
   B. Middle carotid artery involvement
   C. Emboli to anterior circulation
   D. None of the above

132. Lacunar infarcts may manifest all of the following except: *(PGI)*
   A. Pure sensory weakness
   B. Pure motor weakness
   C. Ataxia paresis
   D. Dysarthria
   E. Quadriparesis

133. All of the following manifestations may be associated with lacunar infarcts, except: *(PGI)*
   A. Pure motor loss
   B. Pure sensory loss
   C. Ataxia
   D. Dysarthria
   E. Quadriplegia

Carotid Stenosis

134. Which is true about carotid stenosis: *(PGI June 2000)*
   A. Ipsilateral hemiplegia by embolism of MCA
   B. Bruit indicates severity of stenosis
   C. Common in External carotid artery
   D. Aspirin reduces risk of TIA

135. Investigation of choice for screening of proximal internal carotid artery stenosis is : *(AIIMS June 2000)*
   A. Doppler flow USG
   B. CT substraction angiography
   C. MRI
   D. Angiography (DSA)

Lateral Medullary Syndrome and Other Brain Stem Syndromes

136. Lateral medullary syndrome is caused by thrombosis of: *(AIIMS Dec 95)*
   A. Anterior inferior cerebral artery
   B. Posterior inferior cerebellar artery
   C. Vertebral artery
   D. Basilar artery

137. Lateral Medullary Syndrome is most frequently due to: *(DNB)*
   A. Vertebral Artery
   B. Posterior Inferior Cerebellar Artery (PICA)
   C. Anterior Inferior Cerebellar Artery (AICA)
   D. Basilar Artery

138. Lesion of posterior inferior cerebellar artery at brain involves/affects: *(PGI Dec 03)*
   A. Spinal tract of trigeminal nerve
   B. Tractus Solitarus
   C. Spinothalamic tract
   D. Corticospinal tract

139. Wallenberg's syndrome does not involve: *(PGI June 99)*
   A. IX
   B. X
   C. XI
   D. XII

140. Lateral Medullary Syndrome involves all of the following cranial nerves, Except: *(DNB)*
   A. Vth CN
   B. IXth CN
   C. Xth CN
   D. XII CN

141. All are features of Wallenberg's syndrome, Except:
   A. Ipsilateral loss of pain and temperature
   B. Ipsilateral loss of taste sensation *(AIIMS Feb 97)*
   C. Ipsilateral loss of posterior column sensations
   D. Ipsilateral involvement of lower cranial nerves

142. Abdul Khan presents with pain, numbness and impaired sensation over half of the face along with ataxia, nystagmus, dysphagia and hoarseness of voice. His pain and thermal sensations over opposite half are impaired). Horner's syndrome is present. Likely cause of the disease is thrombosis of which vessel?
   A. AICA (Anterior inferior cerebellar artery)
   B. PICA (Posterior inferior cerebellar artery)
   C. Basilar *(AIIMS Nov 01)*
   D. Pontine vessels

143. Lateral medullary syndrome (Wallenberg syndrome) is characterized by all, Except : *(AIIMS June 97)*
   A. Giddiness
   B. Dysphagia
   C. Crossed hemianaesthesia
   D. Horner's syndrome is rare

144. Clinical features of medial medullary syndrome (select two options) *(PGI June 05)*
   A. Ipsilateral numbness of arm, trunk
   B. Horner's syndrome
   C. Ipsilateral 12th nerve palsy
   D. Contralateral pyramidal tract sign

145. Which of the following is a features of Medial Medullary Syndrome, except: *(PGI June 07)*
   A. Ipsilateral numbness of face and trunk
   B. Horner's syndrome
   C. Ipsilateral ataxia
   D. Contralateral paralysis

146. All of the following are true about Weber's syndrome. Except *(DNB 09, 12)*
   A. Ipsilateral occulomotor nerve palsy
   B. Diplopia
   C. Contralateral hemiplagia
   D. Ipsilateral facial nerve palsy

147. Benedikt's syndrome, all are true except :
   A. Contralateral tremor *(AI 2007)*
   B. 3rd nerve palsy
   C. Involvement of the penetrating branch of the basilar artery
   D. Lesion at the level of the pons

148. Millard Gubler syndrome includes the following except *(AI 2007)*
A. 5th nerve palsy
B. 6th nerve palsy
C. 7th nerve palsy
D. Contralateral hemiparesis

149. Pontine Stroke is associated with all except : *(AI 2007)*
A. Bilateral pin point pupil
B. Pyrexia
C. Vagal palsy
D. Quadriparesis

Others

150. The only thrombolytic agent approved for the treatment of acute ischemic stroke is : *(AIIMS May 04)*
A. Tissue Plasminogen activator
B. Streptokinase
C. Urokinase
D. Pro-urokinase

151. The only thrombolytic agent approved for the treatment of acute ischemic stroke is: *(AIIMS Nov 03)*
A. Tissue Plasminogen activator
B. Streptokinase
C. Urokinase
D. Pro-urokinase

152. Which one of the following agents has been associated with hemorrhagic stroke? *(AI 2006)*
A. Phenylpropanolamine
B. Terfenadine
C. Quinidine
D. Fenfluramine

Seizures and Epilepsy

153. Absence seizures are seen in: *(AIIMS Dec 98)*
A. Grand mal epilepsy
B. Myoclonic epilepsy
C. Petitmal epilepsy
D. Hyperkinetic child

154. Absence seizures are characterized on EEG by: *(AI 2003)*
A. 3 Hz spike & wave
B. 1-2 Hz spike & wave
C. Generalized poly spikes
D. Hypsarrythmia

155. A child presents with short episodes of vacant stare several times a day. The vacant episode begins abruptly and the child remains unresponsive during the episode. There is no associated history of aura or postictal confusion and the child is otherwise normal. The likely diagnosis is *(AI 2010)*
A. Grandmal seizures
B. Absence seizures
C. Complex partial seizures
D. Day dreaming

156. All of the following are features of absence seizures *except:* *(AIIMS May 05)*
A. Usually seen in childhood
B. 3-Hz spike wave in EEG
C. Postictal confusion
D. Precipitation by hyperventilation

157. All of the following are features of juvenile Myoclonic epilepsy, EXCEPT *(AIIMS May 04)*
A. Myoclonus on awakening
B. Generalized tonic-clonic seizures
C. Automatism
D. Absence seizures

158. All of the following are true about Juvenile Mycoclonic epilepsy, except: *(PGI Dec 03)*
A. Focal seizures
B. Generalized seizures
C. Myoclonus
D. Responses to sodium valproate
E. Spike and waves in EEG

159. Myoclonic seizure typically seen in: *(PGI Dec 98)*
A. SSPE
B. Cerebellar lesion
C. Pontine lesion
D. Thalamic lesion

160. Which of the following drugs is not used in Juvenile Myoclonic Epilepsy (JME): *(AI 2010)*
A. Topiramate
B. Zonisamide
C. Carbamezapine
D. Valproate

161. The term post traumatic epilepsy refers to seizures occurring *(AIIMS Nov 02)*
A. Within moments of head injury.
B. Within 7 days of head injury.
C. Within several weeks to months after head injury.
D. Many years after head injury

162. Commonest type of seizure in newborn: *(AI 08)*
A. Clonic
B. Tonic
C. Subtle
D. Myoclonic

163. All of the following factors are associated with a substantially greater risk of developing epilepsy after febrile seizures, Except *(AI 2010)*
A. Complex Febrile seizures
B. Early age of onset
C. Developmental abnormalities
D. Positive family History of Epilepsy

164. All of the following drugs are used for managing status epilepticus except : *(AIIMS Nov. 04)*
A. Phenytoin
B. Diazepam
C. Thiopentone sodium
D. Carbamazepine

165. All of the following drugs are used for managing status epilepticus except : *(AIIMS May 06)*
A. Phenytoin
B. Diazepam
C. Thiopentone sodium
D. Carbamzepine

9

Nervous System

166. Ethosuxamide is the drug of choice for: *(AI 2010)*
A. Generalized Tonic clonic seizures
B. Complex partial seizures
C. Absence seizures
D. Myoclonic seizures

167. The drug of choice for absence seizure *(AIIMS Nov. 06)*
A. Valproate
B. Gabapentin
C. Carbamezapine
D. Phenytoin

168. Generalized Tonic clonic status epilepticus, Rx of choice: *(PGI Dec 03)*
A. Ethosuxamide
B. Sodium valproate
C. Lamotrigene
D. Lorazepam
E. Vigabatrin

169. A 15 year old boy with epilepsy on treatment with combination of valproate and phenytoin has good control of seizures. Levels of both drugs are in the therapeutic range. All of the following adverse effects can be attributed to valproate except : *(AI 2004)*
A. Weight gain of 5 kg
B. Serum alanine aminotransaminase 150 IU/L
C. Rise in serum ammonia level by 20μg/dL
D. Lymphadenopathy

170. A patient who is being treated for temporal lobe epilepsy (complex partial seizures) and who is having recurrent seizures on his chronic regimen of carbamazepine is given phenobarbital as a second drug. However, the seizures increase in frequency. What is the probable reason for the apparent deleterious effect of adding phenobarbital:
A. Intracerebral bleeding from worsening bone marrow suppression *(AIIMS Nov 99)*
B. Decreased carbamazepine level
C. Decreased stability of CNS neuronal membranes
D. Hypokalemia

171. All of the following are true about delirium tremens, except: *(AI 2011)*
A. Visual Hallucinations
B. Tremors
C. Ophthalmoplegia
D. Clouding of consciousness

Dementias & Extrapyramidal Disorders

Alzheimer's Disease

172. All of the following cause subcortical dementia, Except: *(AIIMS May 09)*
A. Alzheimer's disease
B. Porkinsonism
C. HIV encephalopathy
D. Progressive Supranuclear palsy

173. Which of the following is predominantly involved in Alzheimer's dementia: *(AIIMS May 08)*
A. Frontal cortex
B. Temporo-Parietal cortex
C. Fronto-Parietal cortex
D. Franto-Temporal cortex

174. All of the following are known predisposing factors for Alzheimer's disease except : *(AI 1999)*
A. Down-syndrome
B. Low education level
C. Smoking
D. Female sex

175. A chromosomal anomaly associated with Alzheimer's dementia is: *(AI 2001)*
A. Trisomy 18
B. Patau syndrome.
C. Trisomy 21
D. Turners syndrome

176. All of the following neurotransmitter deficiencies are observed in Alzheimer's disease, Except *(DNB)*
A. Acetylcholine
B. Serotonine
C. Noradrenaline
D. Dopamine

177. Which of the following is the most important neurotransmitter deficient in the cortex of patients with Alzheimer's Disease *(DNB 2012)*
A. Acetylcholine
B. Serotonin
C. Dopamine
D. Noradrenaline

178. Alzheimer's Disease is associated with : *(AI 1999)*
A. Delerium
B. Delusion
C. Dementia
D. Depression

179. Which of the following is not seen in early onset Alzheimer's Disease: *(AIIMS Nov 2011)*
A. Aphasia
B. Apraxia
C. Acalculia
D. Agnosia

180. Which of the following statements about the pathology in Alzheimer's disease is not true:
A. Neuritic Plaques are formed of amyloid protein
B. Neurofibrillary tangles (NFT) are made of tau protein *(AIIMS Nov 2011)*
C. NFTs appear extracellularly before intracellular appearance
D. Number of NFTs correlates with dementia

181. Which of the following areas of brain is most resistant to Neurofibrillary tangles in Alzheimer's disease: *(AI 2012)*
A. Entorhinal cortex
B. Hippocampus /Temporal lobe
C. Lateral Geniculate Body

D. Visual Association area

182. The following is not a feature of Alzheimer's disease:
A. Neurofibrillary tangles *(AI 2004)*
B. Senile (neuritic) plaques
C. Amyloid Angiopathy
D. Lewy bodies

183. An 80 year old female presents with progressive loss of memory, difficulty in recalling names, difficulty in speech and inability to perform desired tasks.Which of the following pathological features is likely to be found along with neurofibrillary tangles : *(AIIMS May 09)*
A. Beta Amyloid
B. Lewy bodies
C. Ceramidase
D. Pick's bodies

184. Which of the following enzymes is believed to be deficient in Parkinsonism? *(DNB)*
A. DOPA Decarboxylase
B. Tyrosine Hydroxylase
C. Phenylalanine Hydroxylase
D. Dopamine oxidase

185. **273.Which of the following metal ions is associated with secondary** Parkinsonisms: *(DNB June 2012)*
A. Mangnese (Mn)
B. Magnesium (Mg)
C. Selenium (Se)
D. Molybednum (Mo)

Parkinsonism

186. Which of the following is ***not*** seen in Parkinsonism:
A. Preserved postural reflexes
B. Hypokinesia *(AI 1996) (AIIMS Sept 1996)*
C. Rigidity
D. Static tremors

187. Dinesh, a 56 yr aged man presents with complaints of slowness of movements, postural instability, tremors, rigidity and memory loss. Most likely diagnosis is :
A. Multi infarct dementia *(AI 2001)*
B. Alzheimer's disease
C. Parkinsonism
D. None of the above

188. In parkinsonism what is not present: *(AIIMS May 94)*
A. Tremors at rest
B. Past pointing
C. Akinesia
D. Rigidity

189. Parkinsonism is characterised by all of the following characteristic features except :
A. Rigidity *(AI 1997)*
B. Akinesia
C. Tremors at rest
D. Past pointing

190. Transcranial Magnetic Stimulation of which part of the brain has been shown to reduce frequency of symptoms in Parkinsonism: *(AI 2012)*
A. Striatus
B. Globus Pallidus Externus
C. Subthalamic nucleus
D. Putamen

191. Which of the following is the most commonly used site for Transcranial Magnetic Stimulation to reduce frequency of Parkinsonism symptoms: *(AI 2012)*
A. Striatus
B. Globus Pallidus
C. Subthalamic Nucleus
D. Putamen

192. Drug of choice in phenothiazine-induced Dystonia is:
A. Diphenhydramine *(AI 1996)*
B. Metoclopramide
C. Trifluperamide
D. Benztropine

Huntington's Chorea

193. Huntington's disease is due to the loss of :
A. Nigrostriatal dopaminergic neurons
B. Intrastriatal cholinergic neurons *(AIIMS May 04)*
C. Intrastriatal GABAergic neurons
D. Intrastriatal cholinergic and GABAergic neurons

194. All are true about Huntington's disease except:
A. Chorea *(AI 2001)*
B. Behavioral disturbance
C. Early onset of memory loss
D. Cog-wheel rigidity.

195. A family consist of husband, wife and 2 children. Wife's father has Huntington's chorea. Which statement is true: *(AIIMS Nov 99)*
A. Chance of getting disease in child is 1:4
B. Can occur upto age of 50
C. If wife does not get disease till age 50 children are not affected.
D. Huntington's chorea is due to point mutation in gene.

Normal Pressure Hydrocephalus

196. A patient presents with ataxia, urinary incontinence and dementia. The likely diagnosis is: *(AI 2010)*
A. Alzheimer's Disease
B. Parkinson's disease
C. Steel Richardson syndrome
D. Normal Pressure Hydrocephalus

197. Triad of normal-pressure hydrocephalus includes :
A. Tremor, aphasia dementia *(AI 1999)*
B. Ataxia, aphasia, gait disorder
C. Gait disorder, urinary incontinence, dementia
D. Gait disorder, urinary incontinence, lower cranial nerve palsy

198. Normal pressure Hydrocephalus is characterized by *all except:* *(AI 1996) (AI 1997)*
A. Aphasia
B. Dementia
C. Ataxia
D. Urinary incontinence

Supranuclear Gaze Palsy

199. An elderly man presents with features of dementia, ataxia, difficulty in downward gaze and a history of frequent falls. Likely diagnosis is:
A. Parkinsons disease *(AI 2001) (AIIMS May 01)*
B. Progressive supranuclear gaze palsy
C. Alzheimers disease
D. None of the above.

200. A 76 year old male comes with a history of frequent falls and difficulty in looking downwards and laterally. The diagnosis is : *(AIIMS May 01)*
A. Alzheimer's disease
B. Supranuclear palsy
C. Amyotropic lateral sclerosis
D. Oculomotor nerve palsy

201. A 45-year-old man presents with history of frequent falls. He has difficulty in looking down also. What is the most probable diagnosis : *(AIIMS Nov. 2000)*
A. Normal pressure hydrocephalus
B. Parkinson's disease
C. Alzheimer's disease
D. Progressive supranuclear palsy

Pseudotumor Cerebri

202. All the following are features of Pseudotumor Cerebri *except :* *(AI 1996)*
A. Normal-sized ventricles on CT scan
B. Increased protein in CSF
C. Papilledema
D. Absence of focal neurological deficit

203. All the following are features of Pseudotumor cerebri *except:* *(AI 1994)*
A. Increased intracranial tension
B. Convulsions
C. Papilledema
D. Normal CT scan

Others

204. Pick's body in pick's disease is: *(AI 2008)*
A. Tau protein
B. Alpha synuclein
C. Beta synuclein
D. A β amyloid

205. Localised regional cerebral atrophy is seen in:
A. Alzheimer's disease *(PGI Dec 02)*
B. Frontotemporal dementia
C. PML
D. C.J. disease
E. Friedreich's ataxin

206. All are feature of Wernicke's encephalopathy, Except: *(AIIMS Feb 97) (AIIMS Dec 95)*
A. Cogwheel rigidity
B. Alteration in mental function
C. Ophthalmoplegia
D. Ataxia

207. Which of the following is not involved in Wernicke's Korsakoff psychosis: *(AI 2012)*
A. Mamillary body
B. Thalamus
C. Periventricular Grey matter
D. Hippocampus

208. Which of the following sites is responsible for the amnestic defect in Wernicke's Korsakoff syndrome:
A. Mamillary body *(AI 2012)*
B. Thalamus
C. Periventricular Grey matter
D. Hippocampus

209. Memory impairment is most likely to occur in:
A. Downs Syndrome *(AIIMS Nov 99)*
B. Alkaptonuria
C. Attention deficit disorder
D. Conduct disorder

210. Which of the following is a cause of reversible dementia? *(AI 2005)*
A. Subacute combined degeneration.
B. Picks disease.
C. Creutzfeldt – Jakob disease.
D. Alzheimer's disease.

CNS Infections

211. CSF glucose level is *(AIIMS June 2000)*
A. Half the plasma glucose
B. 2/3 plasma glucose
C. 1/3 plasma glucose
D. Same as plasma glucose

212. Which of the following is not seen in Tubercular meningitis *(DNB June 2011)*
A. Low sugar
B. High protein
C. Low opening pressure
D. Lymphocytic ploeocytosis

213. The CSF findings in TB meningitis are all the following *except:* *(AI 1995)*
A. Raised protein
B. Low sugar
C. Low chloride
D. High RBC count

214. A ten yr old girl presents with fever convulsion, neck rigidity. CSF - Findings are protein 150 mg, Sugar 40 mg, chloride 50 µg/dl with lymphadenopathy:
A. Viral Meningitis *(AIIMS Dec 98)*
B. Pyogenic Meningitis *(AIIMS June 99)*

C. Cryptococcal Meningitis
D. Tubercular Meningitis

215. Which of the following is the classical CSF finding seen in TBM? *(AI 2007)*
A. Increased protein, decreased sugar, increased lymphocytes
B. Increased protein, sugar and lymphocytes
C. Decreased protein, increased sugar and lymphocytes
D. Increased sugar, protein and neutrophils

216. A 25 years old lady with history of fever for 1 month presents with headache and ataxia. Brain imaging shows dilated ventricles and significant basal exudates. Which of the following will be the most likely CSF finding: *(AIIMS Nov 2011)*
A. Lymphocytosis, Low Glucose, High protein
B. Lymphocytosis, Normal Glucose, High protein
C. Lymphocytosis, Low Glucose, Normal protein
D. Neutrophillia, Low glucose, Low Protein

217. Characteristic finding in CT in a TB case is : *(AI 2001)*
A. Exudate seen in basal cistern
B. Hydrocephalus is non communicating
C. Calcification commonly seen in umbellium
D. Ventriculitis is a common finding

218. Basal exudates, infarcts and hydrocephalus are findings observed in Brain imaging studies. The most likely diagnosis is: *(AI 2012)*
A. Tubercular meningitis
B. Viral meningitis
C. Herpes encephalitis
D. Cerebral Malaria

219. True about C.S.F. finding in pyogenic meningitis is: *(AI 1998)*
A. Protein ↑, sugar ↓
B. Protein ↓, sugar ↑
C. Chloride ↑, protein ↓
D. ↓Protein, ↓sugar

220. Pneumococcal meningitis is associated with the following CSF findings: *(AI 2012)*
A. Pleocytosis with low protein and low sugar
B. Pleocytosis with high protein and low sugar
C. Lymphocytosis with low protein and low sugar
D. Lymphocytosis with high protein and low sugar

221. True about CSF finding in pyogenic meningitis is:
A. CSF contains no organisms *(AI 1995)*
B. ↓ Chloride, ↓ Glucose
C. ↑ Glucose, ↑ protein
D. ↑ Chloride, ↓ glucose

222. The drug of choice in Cryptococcal Meningitis is:
A. Pentostatin *(AI 1995)*
B. Amphotericin B
C. Clotrimazole
D. Zidovudine

223. Neurological complications of meningitis include all of the following, except:
A. Seizures. *(AIIMS Nov 02)*
B. Increased intra-cranial pressure.
C. Cerebral hamartoma.
D. Subdural effusions.

224. Which of the following agents is most commonly associated with recurrent meningitis due to CSF leaks: *(AI 2010)*
A. Meningococci
B. Pneumococci
C. Hemophilus Influenza
D. E. Coli

225. Subdural empyema is most commonly caused by:
A. H influenza *(AI 2000)*
B. Staphylococcus aureus
C. Streptococcus pneumoniae
D. E. Coli

226. Which of the following viruses is not a common cause of viral encephalitis? *(AI 2004)*
A. Herpes simplex virus type 2
B. Japanese encephalitis virus
C. Nipah virus
D. Cytomegalovirus

227. Which of the following is the most common cause of meningoencephalitis in children: *(AI 2010)*
A. Mumps
B. Arbovirus
C. HSV
D. Enterovirus

228. Commonest cause of sporadic encephalitis is:
A. Japanese B Virus *(AIIMS May 04)*
B. Herpes Simplex Virus *(AI 2003)*
C. Human Immunodeficiency Virus
D. Rubeola Virus

229. A young male develops fever, followed by headache, confusional state, focal seizures and right hemiparesis. The MRI performed shows bilateral frontotemporal hyper intense lesion. The most likely diagnosis is: *(AI 2004)*
A. Acute pyogenic meningitis
B. Herpes simplex encephalitis
C. Neurocysticercosis
D. Carcinomatous meningitis

230. A 25 year old person presents with acute onset of fever and focal seizures. MRI scan shows hyperintensity in the temporal lobe and frontal lobe with enhancement. The most likely diagnosis is:
A. Meningococcal Meningitis *(AI 2010)*
B. Herpes simplex Encephalitis
C. Japanese Encephalitis
D. –

231. The drug of choice in Herpes Simplex Encephalitis is:
A. Acyclovir *(AI 1994)*
B. Zidovudine
C. Amantadine
D. Vidarabine

232. Which of the following is the most common central nervous system parasitic infection?
A. Echinococcosis. *(AIIMS May 03)*
B. Sparganosis.
C. Paragonimiasis.
D. Neurocysticercosis.

233. Commonest presentation of neurocysticercosis is:
A. Seizures *(AI 2003)*
B. Focal neurological deficits
C. Dementia
D. Radiculopathy

234. Which of the following is the most common location of intracranial neurocysticercosis :
A. Brain parenchyma *(AIIMS Nov. 05)*
B. Subarachnoid space
C. Spinal cord
D. Orbit

235. True statement about neurocysticercosis is:
A. Seizures due to neurocysticercosis are resistant to anti epileptic drugs *(AI 2001)*
B. Albendazole is superior to praziquantel in the treatment of above condition
C. Common presentation is 6th CN palsy and hemiparesis.
D. Steroids are used in the management of hydrocephalus.

236. Treatment of Neurocysticercosis includes all of the following except : *(AI 1998)*
A. Prazequentil
B. Albendazole
C. Niclosamide
D. Flubendazole

237. All of the following statements are true regarding central nervous system infections, EXCEPT :
A. Measles virus is the causative agent for subacute sclerosing pan encephalitis (SSPE)
B. Cytomegalo virus causes bilateral temporal lobe hemorrhagic infarction *(AIIMS Nov 04)*
C. Prions infection causes spongiform encephalopathy
D. JC virus is the causative agent for progressive multifocal leucoencephalopathy

238. Which of the following statements about Prions is true: *(AI 2008)*
A. They are infectious proteins
B. They are made up of bacteria and virus
C. They have rich nuclear material
D. They can be cultured in cell free media

239. Prions include: *(AIIMS Nov 07)*
A. DNA and RNA
B. Only RNA
C. Proteins
D. Only DNA

240. Which one of the following is not a prion associated disease : *(AI 2005)*
A. Scrapie
B. Kuru
C. Creutzfeldt-Jakob disease
D. Alzheimer's disease

241. Fatal familial insomnia is associated with :
A. Prion disease *(AI 1999)*
B. Degenerative disease
C. Neoplastic disease
D. Vascular disease

242. A 60 year old man with progressive dementia of recent onset presents with intermittent irregular jerky movemets. EEG shows periodic sharp biphasic waves. The most likely diagnosis is: *AI-2011*
A. Alzheimer's disease *(AIIMS Nov 2010)*
B. Creutzfeldt Jakob disease
C. Lewy body dementia
D. Herpes Simplex Encephalitis

243. All of the following statements about Creutzfeldt-Jakob disease are true, EXCEPT : *(AIIMS May 04)*
A. It is a neurodegenerative disease
B. It is caused by infectious proteins
C. Myoclonus is rarely seen
D. Brain biopsy is specific for diagnosis

244. Seizures may be the presenting feature in all of the following, Except *(DNB 2012)*
A. Cryptococcus meningitis
B. Toxoplasmosis
C. CMV
D. Entamoeba Histolytica

CNS Tumors

245. Most common Intracranial neoplasm in adults is:
A. Meningioma *(AIIMS May 93)*
B. Astrocytoma
C. Posterior fossa tumor
D. Ganglioneuroma

246. Most common intracranial tumour is:
A. Meningioma *(AIIMS May 94)*
B. Glioma
C. Cranipharyngioma
D. Metastasis

247. Which of the following is the most common type of Glial tumors? *(AI 06)*
A. Astrocytomas
B. Medulloblastomas
C. Neurofibromas
D. Ependymomas

248. In children most common posterior fossa tumour is:
A. Meningiomas *(AIIMS Dec 95)*
B. Astrocytoma
C. Medulloblastoma
D. Glioblastoma multiforme

249. Which of the following statements about cerebellar astrocytomas in paediatric age group is False:
   A. These are usually Low grade tumors
   B. These tumors have a good prognosis
   C. These are more commonly seen in the 1st and 2nd decades *(AI 2008)*
   D. These tumours are more common in females
250. Most common site of sub ependymal astrocytoma (giant cell): *(AIIMS Nov 07)*
   A. Trigone of lateral ventricle
   B. Foramen of Munro
   C. Temporal horn of lateral ventricle
   D. 4th ventricle
251. Tumor with best prognosis is: *(AIIMS May 94)*
   A. Ependymoma
   B. Medulloblastoma
   C. Cerebellar astrocytoma
   D. Glioblastoma multiforme
252. All of the following tumors may be malignant except: *(AI 1997)*
   A. Glioma
   B. Astrocytoma
   C. Hemangioblastoma
   D. Ependymoma
253. Most radiosensitive brain tumor is: *(AIIMS Sept 96)* *(AI 1997)*
   A. Ependymoma
   B. Medduloblastoma
   C. Glioblastoma multiforme
   D. Astrocytoma
254. Which of the following brain tumors does not spread via CSF? *(AI 2004)*
   A. Germ cell tumors
   B. Medulloblastoma
   C. CNS Lymphoma
   D. Craniopharyngoma
255. A 6 year old boy has been complaining of headache, ignoring to see the objects on the sides for four months. On examination, he is not mentally retarded, his grades at school are good, and visual acuity is diminished in both the eyes. Visual charting showed significant field defect. CT scan of the head showed suprasellar mass with calcification. Which of the following is the most probable diagnosis? *(AIIMS Nov 04)*
   A. Astrocytoma
   B. Craniopharyngioma
   C. Pituitary adenoma
   D. Meningioma
256. Which of the following statements about neuroblastoma is not true *(AI 2009)*
   A. Most common extracranial solid tumor in childhood
   B. > 50% present with metastasis at time of diagnosis
   C. Lung metastasis are common
   D. Often encase aorta and its branches at time of diagnosis
257. All the following are true of Craniopharyngioma *except* *(AI 1994)*
   A. Derived from Rathke's pouch
   B. Contains epithelial cells
   C. Present in sella or infra-sellar location
   D. Causes visual disturbances
258. A 30-year-old male complains of loss of erection; he has low testosterone and high prolactin level in blood; What is the likely diagnosis: *(AI 2001)*
   A. Pituitary adenoma
   B. Testicular failure
   C. Cranio pharyngioma
   D. Cushing's syndrome
259. Which of the following is the most common CNS tumor associated with HIV infection? *(DNB 2012)*
   A. Lymphoma
   B. Glioma
   C. Astrocytoma
   D. Medulloblastoma
260. Which of the following is the most common false localizing neurological sign in assessing brain tumors. *(DNB 2010)*
   A. Seizures
   B. Unilateral papilloedema
   C. Abnormal unilateral pupil
   D. Diplopia
261. The characteristic feature of a frontal lobe tumor is: *(AI 1994)*
   A. Abnormal gait
   B. Aphasia
   C. Distractibility
   D. Antisocial behavior
262. A young female patient with long history of sinusitis presented with frequent fever along with personality changes and headache of recent origin. The fundus examination revealed papilledema. The most likely diagnosis is : *(AIIMS Nov. 04)*
   A. Frontal lobe abscess
   B. Meningitis
   C. Encephalitis
   D. Frontal bone osteomyelitis
263. All of the following statements about Neurofibromatosis are true, Except: *(AI 2009)*
   A. Autosomal Recessive Inheritance
   B. Cutaneous neurofibromas
   C. Cataract
   D. Scoliosis
264. All of the following are seen in Neurofibromtosis, Except *(DNB 2011)*
   A. Lisch nodules
   B. Axillary Freckling
   C. Shagreen Patch
   D. Caffe-au-lait spots
265. Which of the following is the most common tumor associated with type I neurofibromatosis?
   A. Optic nerve glioma. *(AIIMS May 03)*
   B. Meningioma.

C. Acoustic Schwannoma.
D. Low grade astrocytoma.

266. Neurofibromatosis type-II is associated with (select three options): *(PGI Dec 2000)*
A. B/L acoustic schwannoma
B. Multiple café-au-lait spots
C. Chromosome-22
D. Lisch nodule
E. Posterior subcapsular lenticular cataract

267. Neurofibromatosis I is most commonly associated with: *(AIIMS Nov 07)*
A. Brain stem gliomas
B. Optic pathway glioma
C. Sub ependymal pilocytic astrocytoma
D. Glioblastoma multiforme

268. All of the following may be associated with Von Hippel Lindau syndrome, except: *(AI 2009)*
A. Retinal and cerebellar hemangioblastomas
B. Gastric carcinoma
C. Pheochromocytoma
D. Renal cell carcinoma

269. Hemangioblastoma associated with VHL are most commonly seen in *(DNB 2012)*
A. Cerebellum
B. Liver
C. Kidney
D. Pancreas

270. In Von Hippel-Lindau Syndrome, the retinal vascular tumours are often associated with intracranial hemangioblastoma. Which one of the following regions is associated with such vascular abnormalities in this syndrome? *(AI 2005)*
A. Optic radiation.
B. Optic tract.
C. Cerebellum.
D. Pulvinar

271. CNS tumor seen in Von Hippel Lindau syndrome is:
A. Meningioma *(PGI Dec 99)*
B. Cerebellar hemangioblastoma
C. CNS lymphoma
D. Glioma

272. Which of the following statements about Von-Hippel Lindau syndrome is true: *(AI 2012)*
A. Multiple tumors are rarely seen
B. Craniospinal hemangioblastomas are common
C. Supratentorial lesions are common
D. Tumors of Schwann cells are common

273. All of the following tumors are malignant except:
A. Glioma *(AI 1997)*
B. Astrocytoma
C. Hemangioblastoma
D. Ependymoma

274. A child presents to the clinic with history of seizures and mental retardation. Clinical examination reveals multiple hypopigmented macules. What is the likely diagnosis: *(AI 2010)*
A. Tuberous Sclerosis
B. Neurofibromatosis
C. Sturge Weber Syndrome
D. Linear epidermal nevus syndrome

275. The diagnosis of a patient presenting with Seizures, Mental retardation and Sebaceous adenoma is:
A. Hypothyroidism *(AI 1995)*
B. Tuberous sclerosis
C. Toxoplasmosis
D. Down syndrome

276. Triad of Tuberous Sclerosis includes all, except:
A. Epilepsy *(AI 2009)*
B. Adenoma sebacium
C. Low intelligence
D. Hydrocephalus

277. Brain tumor is associated with A/E: *(PGI Dec 99)*
A. Tuberous sclerosis
B. Von hippel landau syndrome
C. Neurofibromatosis
D. Sturge Weber syndrome

278. What is NOT a feature of Sturge Weber syndrome :
A. Rail track appearance *(AIIMS Dec 94)*
B. Hemiatrophy of the brain
C. Convulsion
D. Empty sella

279. A middle aged female presents with prolonged history of back pain followed by slowly progressive weakness of both lower limbs, spasticity and recent onset difficulty in micturation. On neurological examination there is evidence of dorsal myelopathy. MRI scan of spine shows a well-defined mid-dorsal intradural homogenous contrast enhancing mass lesion. The likely diagnosis is: *(AIIMS Nov 2011)*
A. Intradural Lipoma
B. Dermoid cyst
C. Epidermoid cyst
D. Spinal meningioma

Disorders of Nerve / Neuropathies

280. All are true about peripheral-neuropathy except :
A. Glove and stocking anaesthesia
B. Proximal muscle weakness *(AI 1999)*
C. Nerve-conduction deficit
D. Decreased reflexes

281. All can cause peripheral neuropathy, except :
A. Uraemia *(AIIMS June 97)*
B. HIV
C. Chronic liver disease
D. Hypothyroidism

282. All of the following are classified as 'Small fiber' neuropathies' except: *(AI 2012)*
A. Vitamin B12 deficiency
B. HIV Induced
C. Hansen's disease
D. Amyloidosis

283. Small fiber neuropathy presents as: *(PGI June 08)*
A. Burning pain
B. Tingling & Numbness
C. Foot drop
D. Twitching

284. All of the following are associated with Autonomic Neuropathies, Except *(DNB 2009)*
A. Diabetes
B. Amyloid
C. Hyperthyroidism
D. Botulinism

285. All of the following are feature of autonomic neuropathy, Except: *(AIIMS May 08)*
A. Resting Tachycardia
B. Silent Myocardial Infarction
C. Orthostatic Hypotension
D. Bradycardia

286. Which of the following types of neuropathy are seen in Diabetes *(DNB 2010)*
A. Distal symmetric sensory neuropathy
B. Autonomic neuropathy
C. Mononeuropathy
D. All of the above

287. The most common form of diabetic neuropathy is
A. Distal symmetric sensory neuropathy *(DNB)*
B. Distal symmetric sensory and motor neuropathy
C. Autonomic neuropathy
D. Distal Motor neuropathy

288. Which of the following drugs is used for painful diabetic neuropathy *(DNB June 2011)*
A. Duloxetine
B. Pregabalin
C. Amitriptyline
D. All of the above

289. Drug of choice for Trigeminal Neuralgia is: *(DNB)*
A. Chlorpromazine
B. Carbamezapine
C. Gabapentin
D. Fluoxetine

290. Polyneuropathy may be seen in all of the following, except: *(PGI)*
A. Vitamin deficiency
B. Osteoporosis
C. DM
D. Myxoedema
E. Amyloidosis

291. Neuropathy is not seen in: *(PGI June 03)*
A. Tuberculosis
B. SLE
C. Diabetes Mellitus
D. Polyarteritis nodosa
E. Sarcoidosis

292. Sensorimotor neuropathy may be caused by all, except: *(PGI Dec 02)*
A. DM
B. Lead poisoning
C. Arsenic
D. Isoniazid
E. Cryoglobulinemia

293. Predominantly sensory neuropathy is/are caused by:
A. Cisplatin *(PGI June 01)*
B. Pyridoxine excess
C. Suramin
D. Diptheria
E. Guillian-Barre syndrome

294. All of the following can cause neuropathies with predominant motor involvement except: *(AI 2004)*
A. Acute inflammatory demyelinating polyneuropathy
B. Acute intermittent porphyria
C. Lead intoxication
D. Arsenic intoxication

295. All of the following are predominant motor neuropathy except :
A. Acute inflammatory demylinating poly radiculoneuropathy
B. Porphyric neuropathy *(AIIMS May' 06)*
C. Lead intoxication
D. Arsenic intoxication

296. Most common cause of mononeuritis multiplex in India is *(AIIMS Nov 08)*
A. Hansen's disease
B. Rheumatoid arthritis
C. Tuberculosis
D. PAN

297. Pure motor paralysis is seen in : *(AI 2000)*
A. Polio
B. Gullien Barre syndrome
C. Diabetes mellitus
D. Sub-Acute Combined Degeneration

298. All cause ascending motor paralysis except :
A. Diabetes mellitus *(AI 2000)*
B. Diphtheria
C. Gullien Barre syndrome
D. Porphyria

299. Trophic ulcers are seen in all, Except: *(PGI Dec 2000)*
A. Leprosy
B. Syringomyelia
C. Polio
D. All of the above (seen in all)

300. All of the following can lead to trophic ulcers in the fingers EXCEPT- *(AIIMS Nov 2000)*
A. Cervical disc prolapse
B. Subacute combined degeneration of spinal cord
C. Leprosy
D. Syringomyelia

301. Dying back neuropathy is seen in all except :
A. Diabetic Neutropathy *(AI 2008)*
B. Arsenic neuropathy
C. Porphyria
D. Gullian Bare syndrome (GBS)

302. All of the following are true about Guillain Barre Syndrome (GBS), Except: *(AI 2010)*
A. Ascending paralysis
B. Flaccid paralysis
C. Sensory level
D. Albumino-Cytological Dissociation

303. All the following are features of Guillain-Barre syndrome *except:* *(AI 1996)*
A. Predominant motor involvement
B. Facial nerve involvement
C. Absence of pleocytosis in CSF
D. Bladder bowel involvement

304. All of the following statements about Guillain – Barre Syndrome are true, Except *(DNB Dec 2011)*
A. Inflammatory
B. Demyelinating
C. Descending
D. Cranial Nerve Involvement

305. All are true regarding G.B. syndrome, Except :
A. Predominant motor involvement *(AI 1996)*
B. Absence of pleocytosis in CSF
C. Residual disability if treatment delayed
D. Sparing of bladder function *(AIIMS June 97)*

306. All of the following statements regarding treatment of GBS are true, Except: *(DNB)*
A. Corticosteroids may be used for early recovery and prevent long hospital stay
B. High dose intravenous immunoglobulin (IVIg) can be initiated
C. Plasmapbaresis can be done
D. High dose intravenous immunoglobulins and plasmapharesis are equally effective

307. Conduction velocity of nerve is reduced in all of the following conditions, except: *(AI 2012)*
A. Acute Motor Axonal Neuropathy (AMAN)
B. Acute Inflammatory Demyelinating Neuropathy (AIDP)
C. Hereditary Sensory Motor Neuropathy (HSMN)
D. Multifocal Motor Neuropathy

308. A child presents with ascending flaccid paralysis. There is subsequent respiratory muscle involvement. CSF examination shows albuminocytological dissociation. Treatment of choice is : *(AIIMS May 02)*
A. Cycloserine
B. Oral prednisolone
C. I.V. methyl prednisolone
D. I.V. immunoglobins

309. An 18-year-old male presented with acute onset descending paralysis of 3 days duration. There is also a history of blurring of vision for the same duration. On examination, the patient has quadriparesis with are flexia. Both the pupils are non-reactive. The most probable diagnosis is : *(AIIMS May' 06)*
A. Poliomyelitis
B. Botulism
C. Diphtheria
D. Porphyria

310. All of the following are features of Botulism except:
A. Cranial nerve palsies *(DNB June 2011)*
B. Descending paralysis
C. Fever
D. Clear Sensorium

311. Acute onset of blurred vision and absent pupillary response with rapidly progressive descending muscular weakness manifesting as quadriparesis in an afebrile 20 year old male with preserved sensorium is
A. Porphyria *(DNB)*
B. Botulism
C. Polio
D. Diphtheria

312. A 45-year-old female presents to the outpatient clinic with symptoms of pain, fatigue and weakness in both lower limbs. She gives history of paralysis affecting both lower limbs in childhood from which she made good functional recovery. Which of the following is the most likely suspected diagnosis: *(AI 2012)*
A. Post Polio syndrome
B. Polymyositis
C. Muscular Dystrophy
D. Neuropathy

313. Charcot's Joint includes all of the following except :
A. Syringomyelia *(AIIMS Nov. 06)*
B. Leprosy
C. Diabetes
D. Arthrogryposis Multiplex Congenita

314. After a minor head injury a young patient was unable to close his left eye and had drooling of saliva from left angle of mouth. He is suffering from:
A. VIIth nerve injury *(AIIMS May 03)*
B. Vth nerve injury
C. IIIrd nerve injury
D. Combined VIIth and IIIrd nerve injury

315. TRUE regarding upper motor neuron VIIth nerve paralysis is: *(AIIMS Dec 95)*
A. Ipsilateral upper face paresis
B. Ipsilateral lower face paresis
C. Contralateral upper face paresis
D. Contralateral lower face paresis

316. Shirmer's test is done for *(DNB Dec 2011)*
A. Occulomotor nerve
B. Optic nerve
C. Facial nerve
D. Hypoglossal nerve

317. Shirmer's test is used to assess *(DNB 2012)*
A. Greater superficial petrosal nerve
B. Stapedial branch
C. Chorda tympani nerve
D. Stylohyoid branch

318. **Herpes zoster in geniculate ganglion causes:**
A. Bell's palsy (DNB 2010)
B. Ramsay Hunt syndrome
C. Merkelson Rosenthal syndrome
D. Frey's syndrome

Disorders of Muscles / Myopathies

Myaesthenia Gravis

319. Myaesthenia gravis is associated with: (PGI Dec 01)
A. Decreased acetylcholine at nerve endings
B. Decreased myosin
C. Absent troponin C
D. Decreased myoneural junction transmission

320. All are clinical features of myasthenia gravis, EXCEPT: (AIIMS Feb 97)
A. Spontaneous remission
B. Absent deep tendon reflexes
C. Proximal muscle involvement
D. Worsen by exertion

321. A 45 year old woman, presenting with the history of diplopia and dysphagia worsening as the day progresses, can be diagnosed to have : (AIIMS Nov. 05)
A. Thyrotoxciosis
B. Myasthenia gravis
C. Muscular dystrophy
D. Brain tumor

322. The most sensitive test for the diagnosis of myasthenia Gravis is (AI 2005)
A. Elevated ACH Receptor Antibodies (ACHR Antibodies)
B. Repetitive Nerve Stimulation test (RNS)
C. Positive Edrophonium test (Tensilon test)
D. Single Fiber Electromyography (SFEMG)

323. A thirty five year old female has proximal weakness of muscles, ptosis and easy fatigability. The most sensitive test to suggest the diagnosis is: (AI 2011)
A. Muscle Biopsy
B. CPK levels
C. Edrophonium test
D. EMG

324. A Thirty five year old female has proximal weakness of muscles, ptosis and easy fatigability. The most sensitive test to suggest the diagnosis is: (AI 2011)
A. Muscle Biopsy
B. CPK levels
C. Edrophonium test
D. Single fiber EMG

325. Which of the following statements about Lambert Eaten Myaesthenic syndrome is true: (AI 2009)
A. Tensilon test is positive
B. Extraocular muscles are most commonly involved
C. Incremental response to repeated electrical stimulation
D. Associated with adenocarcinoma of lung

326. Which one of the following is correct regarding Eaton-Lambert syndrome- (AIIMS Nov 04)
A. It commonly affects the ocular muscle
B. Neostigmine is the drug of choice for this syndrome
C. Repeated electrical stimulation enhances muscle power in it.
D. It is commonly associated with adenocarcinoma of lung

327. All of the following may be associated with Thymoma, Except: (AI 2010)
A. SIADH
B. Myaesthenia Gravis
C. Hypogammaglobulinemia
D. Cushing's syndrome

328. Thymomas may be associated with all of the following, Except (DNB)
A. Myaesthania Gravis
B. Hypergammaglobulinemia
C. Panhypopituitarism
D. SLE

329. Thymoma is associated with: (AI 2000)
A. Myasthenia gravis
B. Scleroderma
C. Oesophageal atrasia
D. Hyper-gammaglobulinemia

330. Thymoma can be associated with all, EXCEPT:
A. Superior mediastinum syndrome
B. Myasthenia gravis (AIIMS Dec 95)
C. Hypergammaglobulinemia
D. Pure red cell aplasia

331. Which of the following is not associated with Thymomas: (AI 2001)
A. Red cell aplasia
B. Myasthenia gravis
C. Hypergammaglobulinemia
D. Compression of the superior mediastinum

332. Thymoma is associated with: (AI 2008)
A. Myasthenia gravis
B. Hypergammaglobulinemia
C. SLE
D. Multiple sclerosis

333. In myasthenia gravis, correct statement regarding thymectomy is : (AI 2001)
A. Should be done in all cases
B. Should be done in cases with ocular involvement only
C. Not required if controlled by medical management
D. Should be done only in cases that are associated with thymoma

334. Drug of choice for myasthenia gravis: *(PGI Dec 99)*
A. Gallamine
B. Succinylcholine
C. tubocurare
D. Pyridostigmine

Muscular Dystrophies & Myopathies

335. Dystrophic gene mutation leads to : *(AIIMS May 03)*
A. Myasthenia gravis
B. Motor neuron disease
C. Poliomyelitis
D. Duchenne muscular dystrophy

336. A young adult presents with proximal weakness of upper limbs, features of facial palsy and winging of scapula. The most likely diagnosis is: *(AI 2012)*
A. Facio-Scapulo-Humeral Dystrophy
B. Limb-Girdle Dystrophy
C. Scapuloperoneal Dystrophy
D. Duchene Muscular Dystrophy

337. Duchenne Muscular Dystrophy is a disease of:
A. Neuromuscular junction *(AI 2004)*
B. Sarcolemmal proteins
C. Muscle contractile proteins
D. Disuse atrophy due to muscle weakness.

338. In Duchenne's muscular dystrophy, which muscle is not involved : *(AIIMS Feb 97)*
A. Gastrocnemius
B. Vastus medialis
C. Brachioradialis
D. Infraspinatus

339. Gene for myotonic dystrophy is coded on chromosome number : *(AI 1999)*
A. 19
B. 20
C. 21
D. 24

340. Which of the following is not a Limb Girdle Dystrophy
A. Sarcoglycan dystrophy *(AIIMS Nov. 06)*
B. Dystrophin dystrophy
C. Dysferlin dystrophy
D. Calpain dystrophy

341. Which of the following is not a Limb Girdle Dystrophy: *(AIIMS Nov 2011)*
A. Sarcoglycan dystrophy *(AIIMS Nov. 06)*
B. Dystrophin dystrophy
C. Dysferlin dystrophy
D. Calpain dystrophy

342. All are congenital myopathies EXCEPT :
A. Centralcore myopathy *(AIIMS Nov 01)*
B. Nemaline myopathy
C. Z band myopathy
D. Centronuclear myopathy

343. All are Congenital Myopathies, Except:
A. Central-core Myopathy *(AIIMS Nov 01)*
B. Nemaline Myopathy *(AIIMS May 2011)*
C. Z band Myopathy
D. Centro-nuclear Myopathy

344. Inverted Champaign bottle muscle atrophy occurs in:
A. Peroneal muscular atrophy *(AIIMS May 93)*
B. Duchenne's muscular dystrophy
C. Progressive muscular atrophy
D. Amyotrophic lateral stenosis

Polymyositis

345. Which of the following antibodies is specific for myositis: *(AIIMS Nov 08)*
A. Anti – Jo-1
B. Anti – Scl-70
C. Anti - Sm
D. Anti- ku

346. Primary idiopathic polymyositis does not involve:
A. Pelvic girdle muscles *(AIIMS-97)*
B. Neck muscles
C. Ocular muscles
D. Pharyngeal muscle

347. Which one of the following clinical findings excludes the diagnosis of polymyositis? *(AI 06)*
A. Neck muscle involvement
B. Extraocular muscle involvement
C. Dysphagia
D. Abdominal muscle involvement

348. Which is NOT a feature of polymyositis?
A. Pharyngeal muscle involvement
B. Gottron's rash *(AIIMS-97)*
C. Proximal muscle involvement
D. Pain in limbs

349. In idiopathic polymyositis, following are seen except:
A. Ocular muscles are not involved *(PGI June 97)*
B. Pharyngeal muscles involved
C. Cutaneous manifestations
D. Proximal limb muscles invariably involved

350. All of the following are feature of dermatomyositis, Except: *(AIIMS Nov 09)*
A. Salmon Patch
B. Gottron's patch
C. Mechanic finger
D. Periungual telengiectasias

351. True about polymyositis is: *(PGI June 99)*
A. Ocular muscle involvement
B. Pharyngeal involvement
C. Muscle atrophy
D. Brisk reflexes common

352. Muscular weakness due to deficiency of magnesium is enhanced by presence of: *(PGI June 97)*
A. Hyperkalemia

B. Metabolic alkalosis
C. Metabolic acidosis
D. Hypernatremia

Episodic Weakness & Channellopathies

353. Episodic generalized weakness can occur due to all of the following acute electrolyte disturbances, except : *(AIIMS May 06)*
A. Hypokalemia
B. Hypocalcemia
C. Hyponatremia
D. Hypophastemia

354. Episodic weakness is seen in all of the following, Except: *(DNB Dec 2011)*
A. Eaten Lambert Sndrome
B. Hypokalemia
C. Hypercalcemia
D. Hyperglycemia

355. All of the following are associated with 'Episodic' weakness, except: *(AI 2012)*
A. Channelopathy
B. Lambert Eaten Syndrome
C. Hyperphosphatemia
D. Hyperkalemia

356. Episodic generalized weakness is associated with all except: *(PGI June 03)*
A. ↓K+
B. Lambert Eaton Syndrome
C. Myasthenia Gravis
D. Tuberculosis
E. Multiple sclerosis

357. All of the following are neurologic channelopathies, *except* : *(AIIMS May 04)*
A. Hypokalemic periodic paralysis
B. Episodic ataxias
C. Familial hemiplegic migraine
D. Huntington's disease

358. All of the following are neurologic channelopathies *except* : *(AI 2005)*
A. Hypokalemic periodic paralysis
B. Episodic ataxia type 1
C. Familial hemiplegic migraine
D. Spinocerebellar ataxia 1

Head Injuries & Miscellaneous

359. According to the Glasgow Coma Scale (GCS), a verbal score of 1 indicates: *(AI 2005)*
A. No response
B. Inappropriate words
C. Incomprehensible sounds
D. Disoriented response

360. Which of the following is not a component of Glasgow Coma Scale? *(AI 2006)*
A. Eye opening
B. Motor response
C. Pupil size
D. Verbal response

361. A head injured patient, who opens eyes to painful stimulus, is confused and localizes to pain. What is the Glassgow coma score : *(AIIMS Nov. 05)*
A. 7
B. 9
C. 11
D. 13

362. Total score in Glasgow Coma Scale of a conscious person is: *(AI 2006)*
A. 8
B. 3
C. 15
D. 10

363. A person with 'Inappropriate speech' evaluated by the 'Glasgow Coma Scale' will have a verbal score of: *(AI 2012)*
A. 4
B. 3
C. 2
D. 1

364. The cause of systemic secondary insult to injured brain include all of the following except : *(AIIMS May' 06)*
A. Hypercapnia
B. Hypoxaemia
C. Hypotension
D. Hypothermia

365. In a patient with head injury damage in the brain is aggravated by *(AI 2010)*
A. Hyperglycemia
B. Hypothermia
C. Hypocapnia
D. Serum osmolality

366. APACHE II Score includes: *(PGI June 08)*
A. Age
B. PaO_2
C. Chronic Medical Condition
D. Respiratory Rate
E. BP
F. All of the above

367. Best prognostic factor for head injury is : *(AI 2007)*
A. Glasgow coma scale
B. Age
C. Mode of injury
D. CT

368. Subdural haematoma most commonly results from rupture of *(AIIMS May 93)*
A. Middle meningeal artery
B. Superior cerebral veins
C. Saccular aneurysms
D. Lenticulostriate branch of middle cerebral artery

369. Subdural haematoma most commonly results from: *(AIIMS May 04)*
A. Rupture of intracranial aneurysm
B. Rupture of cerebral AVM
C. Injury to cortical bridging veins
D. Hemophilia

370. A 62 year old diabetic female patient presented with history of progressive right-sided weakness of one-month duration. The patient was also having speech dificulty. Fudus examination showed papilledema. Two months ago, she also had a fall in her bathroom and struck her head against a wall. The most likely clinical diagnosis is: *(AIIMS Nov 04)*
A. Alzheimer's disease
B. Left parietal glioma
C. Left MCA territory stroke
D. Left chronic subdural haematoma

371. A elderly female presented with history of progressive right-sided weakness and speech difficulty. She gives a history of a fall in her bathroom two months back. The most likely clinical diagnosis is : *(AI 91)*
A. Progressive supranuclear palsy
B. Left cerebral tumor
C. Left sided stroke
D. Left chronic subdural haematoma

372. A 24- year old man falls on the ground when he is struck in the right temple by a baseball. While being driven to the hospital, he lapses into coma. He is unresponsive with the dilated right pupil when he reaches the emergency department. The most important step in initial management is: *(AI 2002)*
A. Craniotomy
B. CT scan of the head
C. X-ray of the skull and cervical spine
D. Doppler ultrasound examination of the neck

373. A pt is brought to the emergency as a case of head injury, following a head on collision road traffic accident. His BP is 90/60 mmHg. Tachycardia is present. Most likely diagnosis is: *(AI 2001)*
A. EDH
B. SDH
C. Intracranial hemorrhage
D. Intraabdominal bleed

374. The earliest manifestations of increased intracranial pressure following head injury is : *(AI 2005)*
A. Ipsilateral papillary dilatation
B. Contralateral papillary dilatation
C. Altered mental status
D. Hemiparesis

375. Transtentorial uncal herniation causes all except : *(AIIMS May 01)*
A. Ipsilateral dilated pupils
B. Ipsilateral hemiplegia
C. Cheyne stokes respiration
D. Decorticate rigidity

376. All of the following are used to decrease intracranial pressure, Except : *(AIIMS Sept 96)*
A. Frusemide
B. Mannitol
C. Steroid
D. Hyperventilation

377. A patient presents with unilateral painful ophthalmoplegia. Imaging revealed an enlargement of cavernous sinus on the affected side. The likely diagnosis is: *(AIIMS May 08)*
A. Gradenigo syndrome
B. Covernous sinus thrombosis
C. Tolosa-Hunt Syndrome
D. Orbital Pseudotumor

378. Non-noxious stimuli perceived as pain is termed as: *(AIIMS May 08)*
A. Allodynia
B. Hyperalgesia
C. Hyperesthesia
D. Hyperpathia

379. Spontaneous CSF leaks may be associated with all, Except: *(AIIMS Nov 08)*
A. Increased Intracranial Tension
B. Pseudotumor cerebri
C. Empty Sella Syndrome
D. Encephalocele

380. All of the following statements about Diffuse Axonal Injury (DAI) are true Except: *(AI 2008)*
A. Caused by shearing force
B. Predominant white matter haemorrhages, in basal ganglion and corpus callosum
C. Increased Intracranial tension is seen in all cases
D. Most common at junction of grey and white matter

Miscellaneous

381. The first center that gets activated for voluntary skilled movments is: (DNB)
A. Neocortex
B. Hypothalamus
C. Basal ganglia
D. Cerebellum

382. The most important area involved in planning and organizing complex sequential skilled movements is *(DNB 2012)*
A. Primary Motor Area
B. Premotor Area
C. Supplementary motor Area
D. Primary sensory Area

383. Hippocampus lesion affects: *(DNB June 2010)*
A. Implicit memory
B. Procedural memory
C. Non-declarative memory
D. Explicit memory

384. Hippocampus lesion affects: *(DNB)*
A. Short term memory
B. Long term memory
C. Transformation of short-term memory to long-term memory
D. Implicit memory

385. Which of the following is the most important part of brain involved in Narcolepsy *(DNB)*
A. Neocortex

B. Hypothalamus
C. Hippocampus
D. Pons

386. All of the following statements about Argyll Robertson Pupil are correct, Except: *(AI 2011)*
A. Near Reflex Normal
B. Direct light Reflex Absent
C. Consensual Light Reflex Normal
D. Visual Acuity Normal

387. Impotence is a feature of which of the following :
A. Multiple sclerosis *(AIIMS Nov. 2000)*
B. Poliomyelitis
C. Amyotropic lateral sclerosis
D. Meningitis

388. All of the following clinical findings are seen in Horner's syndrome, Except: *(AIIMS May 2011)*
A. Miosis
B. Anhidrosis
C. Heterochromia of iris
D. Apparent Exophthalmos

389. Which of the following drugs is not recommended for the treatment of Multiple Sclerosis:
A. Interferon β-1a *(AIIMS Nov 2011)*
B. Interferon β-1b
C. Glatiramer Acetate
D. Mycophenolate

390. Horner's syndrome may be caused by all of the following, Except *(AIIMS Nov 2010)*
A. Carotid Artery Aneurysm
B. Medial Medullary Syndrome
C. Iatrogenic
D. Multiple Sclerosis

391. Multiple Sclerosis is associated with all of the following, Except *(DNB 2012)*
A. Hydrocephalus
B. Optic Neuritis
C. Spasticity
D. Spinal cord involvement

392. Which of the following is the most common initial presenting feature of multiple sclerosis: *(DNB)*
A. Optic Neuritis
B. Cerebellar Ataxia
C. Internuclear ophthalmoplegia
D. Diplopia

393. Which of the following is used in the treatment of Multiple Sclerosis:
A. Interferon Alpha *(AIIMS Nov. 2006)*
B. Interferon Beta
C. Infliximab
D. Interferon gamma

394. EEG is usually abnormal in all of the following, except : *(AI 2005)*
A. Subacute sclerosing panencephalitis.
B. Locked – in state.
C. Creutzfoldt – Jackob disease
D. Hepatic encephalopathy

395. A symmetric high-voltage, triphasic slow wave pattern is seen on EEG in the following :
A. Hepatic encephalopathy *(AIIMS May' 06)*
B. Uremic encephalopathy
C. Hypoxic encephalopathy
D. Hypercarbic encephalopathy

396. Burst Supression pattern on EEG is typically seen in:
A. Anoxic Encephalopathy *(DNB 2012)*
B. Absence seizures
C. SSPE
D. Herpes Simplex Encephalitis

397. Burst – suppression EEG pattern is seen in all of the following, Except? *(DNB 2012)*
A. Hypoxic ischemic encephalopathy
B. Phenobarbital administration to lower ICP in traumatic brain injury
C. Severe Hypothermia
D. Creutzfeldt Jacob disease

398. Metabolic encephalopathy presents with :
A. Broca's aphasia *(AIIMS June 99)*
B. Anomic aphasia
C. Transcortical sensory aphasic
D. Transcortical motor aphasia

399. All of the following are true about manifestations of vitamin E deficiency, except: *(AI 2005)*
A. Hemolytic anemia.
B. Posterior column abnormalities.
C. Cerebellar ataxia.
D. Autonomic dysfunction.

400. Spinal segment in knee jerk include all of the following except : *(AI 1997)*
A. L1
B. L2
C. L3
D. L4

401. Lesions of the lateral cerebellum cause all of the following, Except *(AI 2010)*
A. Incoordination
B. Intention tremor
C. Resting tremor
D. Ataxia

402. All the following are features of cerebellar disease ***except:*** *(AI 1996)*
A. Intention tremors
B. Past pointing
C. Hypertonia
D. Ataxia

403. Dysmetria is due to lesion of *(DNB June 2010)*
A. Midbrain
B. Pons
C. Medulla
D. Cerebllum

404. "Prosopagnosia" is characterised by : *(AI 1999)*
A. Inability to read
B. Inability to identify faces
C. Inability to write
D. Inability to speak

405. Following sensory impairments occur in extensive damage to primary somatosensory area of cerebral cortex, EXCEPT: *(AIIMS Dec 94)*
A. Pressure
B. Sensory localization
C. Exact weight determination
D. Pain

406. Lesion in which of the following structure leads to Kluver-Bucy syndrome: *(AIIMS May 04)*
A. Amygdala
B. Hippocampus
C. Hypothalamus
D. Temporal lobe

407. Extrapyramidal symptoms are seen in all EXCEPT:
A. Paralysis agitans *(AIIMS Nov. 2000)*
B. Carbon monoxide poisoning
C. Cerebrovascular accident
D. Multiple sclerosis

408. Criteria for Brainstem death includes: *(AI 2012)*
A. Positive Doll's eye Reflex
B. Absent pupillary light reflex and delated pupils
C. Pinpoint pupils
D. Positive vestibulo-ocular reflex

409. Which test is not useful in a patient with history of Syncopal attack?
A. Electrophysiological testing *(AIIMS Nov. 06)*
B. Tilt Table testing
C. PET Scan
D. Holter monitoring

410. Which of the following cranial structures are insensitive to pain: *(AI 2009)*
A. Dural sheath surrounding vascular sinuses
B. Choroid Plexus
C. Falx cerebri
D. Middle meningeal Artery

ANSWERS, REFERENCES, EXPLANATIONS AND RELEVANT HIGH YIELD FACTS

Headache

1. **Answer is B (Cluster headache):** *Q No. 5 (Neurological disorders) pretest Harrison 15th; 16th/93; 17th/ 101; 18th/122*

"Cluster headaches, which can cause excruciating hemicranial pain, are notable for their occurance during characteristic episodes. Usually attacks occur during a 4 to 8 week period in which the patient experiences. One to three severe brief headaches daily. There may then be a prolonged pain -free interval before the next episode. Men between ages 20 and 50 are most commonly affected. The unilateral pain is usually associated with lacrimation, eye reddening, nasal stuffiness, ptosis, and nausea. During episodes alcohol may provoke the attacks. Even though the pain caused by brain tumors may awaken a patient from sleep, the typical history and normal neurological examination do not mandate evaluation for a neoplasm of the CNS." – Harrison Pretest

Migraine	Cluster Headache
• *Lateralised* Q, usually frontotemporal may be generalised • *All age groups* Q are affected • *Females* Q are affected more than males • *Family history present* Q • Presentation : Pain - *often preceded by aura* Q - *builds up gradually* Q - may lasts for *several hours* Q or longer - usually *throbbing* Q but may be dull - onset is *after awakening* Q & *quietened by sleep* Q • Associated symptoms include : - *nausea, vomiting, diarrhea* Q - *photophobia and visual disturbance* Q in the form of *photopsia and fortification spectra* Q - *paraestheisias with tingling and numbness* Q - other *focal neurological symptoms* Q such as clumsiness *and weakness* Q.	• *Lateralized* Q, *periorbital* Q or less commonly temporal • All ages *above 10 yrs* Q with *peak at 30-50 yrs* Q • *Male preponderance* Q (90%). Men affected 7-8 times more than females. • *Hereditary factors usually absent* Q • Presentation: Pain (periodic attacks 1-2/day) - begins *without warning* Q - reaches *crescendo within 5 minutes* Q - lasts for *45 minutes* Q - *excruciating, deep, explosive* pain but only *rarely pulsatile* Q - commonly *awakens the patients from sleep* Q • Associated symptoms : These are typical and characteristic : Q - *homolateral lacrimation* Q - *reddening of eye* Q - *nasal stuffiness* Q - *Ptosis* Q, *and* - *nausea* Q

2. **Answer is A (Affects predominantly females) :** *Harrisons 16th/93; Harrison 17th/101; Harrison 18th/p 122*

Cluster headache affects predominantly males. Men are affected 3 times more often than women. Harrison 17th/101

3. **Answer is A (Migraine):** *Harrison 15th/ 73; Harrison 16th/90, 91; Harrison 17th/ 96, 97; Harrison 18th/p 114, 115*

Migraine is a syndrome of episodic recurrent throbbing *headache, more often unilateral, which is associated with nausea vomiting, photophobia or phonophobia. Parastheasis with tingling and numbness and focal neurological deficits are often associated. Aura may or may not be present.*

4. **Answer is A (Migraine):** *Harrison 14th/ 70, 71; Harrison 15th/ 73, 79; 16th/88, 93, 90, 91; Harrison 17th/ 96, 97; Harrison 18th/p 114, 115*

Episodic unilateral throbbing headache in a 30 year old female with associated nausea and vomiting suggests a diagnosis of migraine. Aura may or may not be present. Infact 80% of patients with migraine have migraine without aura and 15-20% have migraine with aura.

Common Migraine (Migraine without aura)	Classical Migraine (Migraine with aura)
• This is characterized by headache with autonomic system dysfunction (eg. pallor & nausea, vomiting), but without stereotypical neurological or ophthalmic features as in classical migraine • Premonitory features include changes in mood frequent yawning or nonspecific prodromal symptoms like loss of concentration • Headache starts anywhere in the cranium and is pounding or throbbing • It usually spreads to involve one half or even the whole head. • During the attack which lasts from hours to a day or more patient is frequently photophobia and phonophobic and seeks relief in quiet dark environment, or through sleep.	• This is characterized by headache heralded by a visual aura which lasts about 20 minutes. • Visual aura may consist of bright or dark spots, zig zags, heat haze distortions, fig san puzzle defects scintillating scotoma, tunnel vision or fortification spectra which may progress to homonymous hemianopia. • The headache follows the aura and is usually hemicranial opposite the hemianopia. • During the attach patient has associated nausea and photophobia.

5. **Answer is C (Migraine) :** *Harrison 16th/90, 91; Harrison 17th/ 96, 97; Repeat ; Harrison 18th/p 114, 115*

6. **Answer is B (When the headache is followed by partial paralysis of the IIIrd nerve on the same side as the hemicrania with out any scotoma.):** *Parson 19th/ 147 (18th/ 269): New edition does not mention this*

*'Occasionally people who suffer from ordinary migraine have attacks in which, **without any scotoma**, the headache is followed by partial paralysis of the third nerve **(ophthalmoplegic migraine)** on the same side as hemicrania. Slight ptosis, diplopia, and sluggishness of the pupillary reactions continue for some hours and gradually disappear.'- Parson*

Variants of migraine depending on the accompanying neurological deficit: - *'Kanski'*

Focal migraine	Is characterized by transient dysphagia, hemisensory symptoms or even focal weakness in addition to other symptoms of migraine.
Migraine sine migraine	Is characterized by episodic visual disturbances without headache. Elderly patients with a history of classical migraine are typically affected
Retinal migraine	Is characterized by acute transient unilateral loss of vision. This may occur in middle aged persons without past history of migraine.
Ophthalmoplegic migraine	Is rare and typically starts before the age of loycars. It is characterized by a recurrent transient third nerve palsy which begins after the headache.
Familial hemiplegic migraine	Is characterized by a failure of full recovery of focal neurological features after an attack of migraine subsides.
Basilar migraine	Occurs in children. It is characterized by a typical migrainous aura associated with numbness and tingling of lips and extremities which is often bilateral Ataxia of gait and speech also occurs, with occasional impairment of consciousness.

7. **Answer is C (Tension headache):** *Harrison 15th/ 73; Harrison 16th/88; 17th/ 100, 101; 18th/p 120, 121, 122*

*Tension type headache is a generalized headache that occurs in patients subjected to stress anxiety and depression. **The patient in question has distinctly generalised type of headache worsening with stress (children doing badly in school). This suggests a diagnosis of tension headache.***
More so the symptomatology of cluster headache, migraine and trigeminal neuralgia is quiet distinct from that mentioned above.

Tension Headache :
- Is a chronic head pain syndrome characterised by tight band like discomfort
- Headaches is usually ***generalised*** may be most intense about the neck or back of the head.
- Patients frequently complain of poor concentration and other vague non specific symptoms
- May be ***exacerbated by emotional stress***, fatigue, noise or glare.
- It is not associated with focal neurological symptoms.

8. Answer is A (Temporal Arteritis): *Harrison 15th/ 72, 73, 74, 75; 17th/ 96;Elaborated in chapter on connective tissue.; Harrison 18th/p 114*

The symptom and the laboratory examination of the patients almost confirms the diagnosis of temporal arteritis. *Always suspect temporal arteritis in an elderly patient who presents with headache, visual symptoms (blindness), malaise, fever, weakness with or without pain or tenderness over temporal artery (thick cord like structure) and a raised ESR.*

9. Answer is B (Glaucoma): *Harrison 15th/ 78, 16th/93; 17th/ 96; Kanski 4th/ 211; Harrison 18th/p 114*

Presence of visual blurring and female sex suggest a diagnosis of glaucoma over cluster headache amongst the options provided.
The major diagnostic dilemma lies between Glaucoma and Cluster headache.
Points favouring a diagnosis of Glaucoma over cluster headache are:

- ***Female patient*** (Glaucoma is about four times more common in females while 80% of patients with cluster headache are males)
- ***Visual blurring*** (Visual blurring is a feature of Glaucoma. Cluster headache has ocular features mainly limited to reddening of eye and homolateral lacrimation but vision has not been mentioned as being affected.

10. Answer. is B (Basilar migraine) : *'Current Diagnosis & Treatment in Neurology' (LANGE)1st/66; Pediatric ENT (Springer, 2008) /473; 'Vertigo & Disequilibrium: A practical guide to diagnosis and management' by Weber (Thieme); 'Handbook of Headache (Lippincott- Williams)' 2nd/214*

Repeated episodes of throbbing occipital headache in association with ataxia and vertigo in a young female with a positive family history of headache suggest a diagnosis of basilar migraine.

'Dizziness, vertigo and ataxia heralding an intense throbbing (occipital) headache are typical features of basilar type migraine' – Headache in Children & Adolescents 2nd/22

'Diagnosis of Basilar Migraine is suggested by age, female gender, positive family history and attacks of headache with vertiginous aura provoked by usual migraine triggers' – 'Practical Neurology' by Biller 3rd/15

Basilar Type Migraine (subtype of migraine with aura)

- Basilar type migraine describes recurrent attacks of migraine with aura in which symptoms suggest a brainstem origin ***(including vertigo & ataxia)***
- ***The onset of Basilar type migraine is typically before 30 years of age*** and peaks during adolescence
- ***There is a distinct female preponderance*** with girls more frequently affected than boys in a ratio of 3:1 *(majority of sufferers are girls)*
- ***Family history of migraine is frequent***
- ***Unlike other types of migraine headache may be occipital in origin***

Diagnostic criteria have been suggested for the diagnosis of Basilar type migraine, but the information provided in the question is insufficient to establish 'Basilar Type Migraine' on the basis of criterion. ***Nevertheless the information provided does suggest a likely diagnosis of Basilar Migraine which is the single best answer amongst the options provided.***

11. Answer is D (Sumatriptan is used for chronic migraine): *Harrison 18th /118, 119*

Selective oral 5HT Receptor agonists (Triptans) are all used for the management of acute attacks of migraine. Triptans are not used in the management of chronic migraine (preventive treatment).

Triptans

- Triptans are selective agonists at 5HT 1B/1D Receptors
- A variety of Triptans are now available for the management of acute migraine

Triptans

Fast Acting	Slow Acting / Better tolerability
• *Rizatriptan* • *Eletriptan* • *Sumatriptan* • *Zolmitriptan* • *Almotriptan (relatively slower)*	• *Naratriptan* • *Frovatriptan* *These agents have longer half life*

- *Rizatriptan and Eletriptan are the most efficacious of the triptans currently available in the United States' - H18th*

Efficacy appears to be related more to t max (time to peak plasma concentration) than to the potency, half life or bioavailability

- Almatriptan, Naratriptan and Fravotriptan are somewhat slower in onset and better tolerated.

Treatment of Acute Migraine

Drugs

Simple Analgesics
Acetaminophen, aspirin, caffeine
NSAIDs
Naproxen Ibuprofen Tolfenamic acid
5-HT$_1$ Agonists
Oral
Ergotamine Ergotamine 1 mg, Caffeine 100 mg Naratriptan Rizatriptan Sumatriptan Frovatriptan Almotriptan Eletriptan Zolmitriptan
Nasal
Dihydroergotamine Sumatriptan Zolmitriptan
Parenteral
Dihydroergotamine Sumatriptan

Dopamine Antagonists
Oral
Metoclopramide Prochlorperazine
Parenteral
Chlorpromazine Metoclopramide Prochlorperazine
Other
Oral
Acetaminophen, 325 mg, *plus* dichloralphenazone, 100 mg, *plus* isometheptene, 65 mg
Nasal
Butorphanol
Parenteral
Narcotics

Preventive Treatment of Migraine (Chronic migraine)

Drugs

Pizotifen
Beta blocker
Propranolol
Tricyclics
Amitriptyline Dothiepin Nortriptyline
Anticonvulsants
Topiramate Valproate Gabapentin
Serotonergic drugs
Methysergide Flunarizine
No convincing evidence from controlled trials
Verapamil
Controlled trials demonstrate *no effect*
Nimodipine Clonidine SSRIs: fluoxetine

12. **Answer is D (Sumatriptan):** *Harrison 17th/ 98, 99; Harrison 18th/p 117, 118, 119*

    The drug of choice for an acute attack of migraine is Sumatriptan

13. **Answer is D (Ethosuxamide):** *Harrison's 17th/-102; Harrison 18th/p 122, 123*

    Ethosuxamide is not used for the prophylaxis of migraine.

    Propanalol, valproate and topiramate are all commonly used agents for prophylaxis in migraine

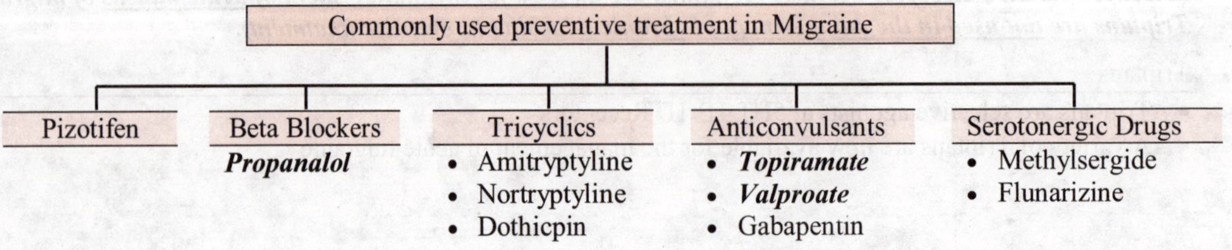

Aphasia

14. Answer is B (Verbal expression): *Ref: Fuller's neurological examination 2nd/ 10;*

Motor aphasia also known as expressive aphasia is a disorder of thought and word finding resulting in inadequate verbal expression.

• Defect in hearing:	Deafness
• Defect in understanding:	Receptive aphasia / Sensory aphasia
• Defect in thought and word finding:	Motor / Expressive aphasia
• Defect in voice production:	Dysphonia
• Defect in articulation:	Dysarthric

15. Answer is D (Motor aphasia): *Harrison 15th/ 141; Harrison 16th/146, 147*

Broca's aphasia (Motor aphasia/Expressive aphasia)	Wernicke's aphasia (Receptive aphasia, Sensory aphasia)
Inferior frontal gyrus (Dominant hemisphere)	Supramarginal gyrus of partial lobe Upper part of temporal lobe

Aphasia occur when the lesion lies in the dominant (usually left) hemisphere

16. Answer is D (Repetition is preserved): *Fuller 2nd/ 11; Harrisons 14th/135,136; 16th/146, 147; 17th/ 164; 18th/p 204*

Repetition is impaired in both Broca's and Wernicke's aphasias.

Aphasias are disorders of understanding, thought and word finding.

	Broca's apahasia	Wernicke's apahsia
Lesion site[Q]	• Lesion in Broca's area (inferior frontal gyrus)	• Lesion lies in Wernicke's area (supramarginal gyrus) of the parietal lobe and upper part of temporal
Cause[Q]	• Lesion is due to occlusion of superior br. of middle cereb. art.	• Lesion is due to occlusion of inferior division of middle cerebral artery.
Comprehension	• Comprehension is preserved (except grammar)	• Comprehension is impaired
Fluency[Q]	• Decreased : speech is not fluent, laboured, dysarthric, and interrupted with many word finding pauses. It is telegraphic but informative	• Preserved or increased : Speech fluent but is highly paraphasic and associated with neologisms (Jagron Ahasia)
Naming[Q]	• Impaired	• Impaired
Repetition[Q]	• Impaired	• Impaired
Neologism[Q]	• Absent	• Present
Insight	• Insight into condition is preserved	• Not preserved

Anomic aphasia : Remember :

Most common language disturbance seen in - Head trauma = Anomic Apahsia[Q]
Most common language disturbance seen in - Metabolic encephalopathy = Anomic Apahsia[Q]
Most common language disturbance seen in - Alzheimer's disease = Anomic Apahsia[Q]

17. Answer is A (Posterior temporal and parietal lobes, dominant hemisphere): *Ref: Fuller 2nd/ 14, 13; Harrison 17th/164; Harrison 18th/p 204*

*Aphasias are disorders of understanding, thought and word finding and represent a lesion in the **dominant (usually left) hemisphere.** The patient in question represents a case of sensory / receptive **Wernicke's aphasia and hence a lesion in the temporal and parietal lobe** of the dominant hemisphere.*

18. Answer is D (Senseless, fluent speech): *Harrison's 17th/164; Ganong 22nd/273;* Harrison 18th/p 204

Senseless fluent speech most closely suggests a diagnosis of Aphasia (Wernicke's aphasia) which results from damage to the categorical or dominant hemisphere

Senseless, fluent speech suggests a diagnosis of 'Wernicke's' Aphasia. Such disorders of speech represent a lesion is the categorical or dominant hemisphere

Cerebral Lateralization

Categorical Hemisphere (Dominant Hemisphere)	Representative Hemisphere (Non-Dominant Hemisphere)
The cerebral hemisphere for: • Sequential – Analytic process - Mathematical calculations - Logical decision making • Language (Aphasias)	**The cerebral hemisphere for:** • Visuo-spatial processing - to identify familiar objects by touch, smell, sight, taste or feel • Analyzing the emotional context of a conversion

9

Nervous System

Clinical Neurology & Diseases of Spinal Cord

UMN vs LMN lesions & Motor Neuron DIsease

19. Answer is A (Weakness and Spasticity): *Harrison 15th/ 119-20, Harrison 16th/134; Harrison 17th/148; 18th/p 182*

Spasticity is a characteristic of U.M.N. lesion. Fasciculations, hypotonia and muscle atrophy are features of LMN, & not UMN palsy

UMN	*LMN*
1. ***Power*** *: Decreased* *Weakness*; Q (Muscle groups or Limbs being affected & not individual muscles Q) 2. ***Tone*** : Hypertonia = *Clasp knife spasticity* Q 3. ***Wasting / Atrophy*** : Minimal, if present and due to disuse atrophy. 4. ***Reflexes*** *Superficial Reflexes* : Lost Q *Deep reflexes* : Brisk/Exaggerated Q *Clonus* : May be + nt Q *Plantar* : Extensor Q 5. ***Fasciculations*** : Absent Q 6. ***Reaction of degeneration in muscles*** : absent Q	1. ***Power*** : Very much decreased *Weakness* (severe) due to paralysis of individual muscles. Q 2. ***Tone***: Flaccidity (Hypotonia) Q 3. ***Wasting / Atrophy*** is marked (cardinal feature) Q 4. ***Reflexes*** *Superficial reflexes* : Lost Q *Deep reflexes* : Exaggerated Q *Clonus* : Absent Q *Plantar* : Flexor or no response Q 5. ***Fasciculations*** : Present Q 6. ***Reaction of degeneration in muscles*** : Present Q

20. Answer is A (Flaccid paralysis): *Refer previous question; Harrison 16th/134; Harrison 17th/148; Harrison 18th/p 182*

Lower motor neuron lesions are characteristically associated with weakness of muscles (paralysis) with decreased tone (flaccidity) i.e. flaccid paralysis.

21. Answer is A (Motor neuron disease): *Ref: Harrisons 15th/ 119; 16th/134; Harrison 17th/148; Harrison 18th/p 182*

Fasciculation is a visible or palpable twitch within a single muscle due to spontaneous discharge of one motor unit. Disease of motor neurons are associated with fasciculations' *- Harrison's*

22. Answer is B (LMN type of lesion): *Harrisons 17th/148; Harrison 16th/134; Harrison 18th/p 182*

Fasciculations is a feature of Lower Motor neuron lesions especially in anterior horn cell disease.

23. Answer is A and C (LMN lesion and Paralysis of cranial nerve IX to XII): *Refer text below*

Bulbar paralysis refers to Lower motor neuron paralysis of medullary (bulbar) cranial nerves IX to XII.

Paralysis of Speech and Swallowing

Bulbar Palsy	Pseudobulbar Palsy
LMN paralysis from a lesion of the bulb (medulla) or its nerves (IX, X and XII)	***UMN paralysis*** from a lesion that is neither in the bulb (medulla) or its nerves (IX, X or XIIth)

Anatomists visualized the medulla as a bulb like expansion of the spinal cord and hence referred to the medulla as 'the bulb'

24. Answer is D (Hypoactive jaw jerk): *Clinical Neurology 6th/40*

Pseudobulbar palsy is associated with a hyperactive or exaggerated jaw jerk and not a hypoactive jaw jerk.

Comparison of Bulbar and Pseudobulbar Palsy

	Bulbar	Pseudobulbar
Dysarthria	***Yes***	***Yes***
Dysphagia	***Yes***	***Yes***
Movement of palate		
Voluntary	*No*	*No*
Gag reflex	*No*	*Yes*
Respiratory impairment	*Yes*	*No*
Jaw jerk	***Hypoactive***	***Hyperactive***
Emotional lability	***No***	***Yes***
Intellectual impairment	*No*	*Yes*

25. Answer is D (Syringomyelia): *Harrison 17th/2594; Neurological Examination by Schwartzman (2006)/51*

Jaw jerk is exaggerated in supranuclear lesions that are above the mid pons.
Suringomyelia is a lesion of the spinal cord placed distal to the brainstem (or mid pons) and hence does not lead to an exaggerated jaw jerk.

Exaggerated Jaw Jerk

Jaw jerk is exaggerated in supranuclear lesions that are above the mid pons
Jaw Jerk is helpful in localization of the lesion to the brainstem.
It depends on the mesencephalic tract of the 5th cranial nerve which mediates proprioceptive information from jaw muscles.

Common cause of exaggerated jaw jerk include

- *Neurodegenerative diseases with generalized loss of cortical inhibition*
- ***Pseudobulbar palsy***
- ***Motor neuron disease***
- ***Multiple sclerosis***

26. Answer is A (Involuntary movement): *Textbook of practical physiology 2nd/275; Harrison's 17th/147,148 Harrison's 16th/134; Harrison 18th/p 181, 182*

Involuntary movement is a feature of Extra pyramidal Tract involvement and not pyramidal tract involvement

Features	Pyramidal Tract	Extra Pyramidal Tract
Structure involved	*Includes the Corticospinal tract*	*Includes the basal ganglia and cerebellum*
Muscle tone	***Spasticity (clasp-knife rigidity)***	***Plastic (cogwheel rigidity)***
Distribution of hyper tonus	*Flexors of arm and extensors of leg*	*Generalised*
Shortening and lengthening reaction	*Present*	*Absent*
Involuntary movements	***Absent***	***Present***
Tendon reflexes	***Exaggerated***	***Normal***
Babinski sign	***Positive***	***Negative***
Paralysis	*Of voluntary movements*	*No paralysis*

27. Answer is A (Anterior Horn cells): *Harrison's 17th/148, 2572, 2573; Fundamental's of Neurology: An Illustrated Guide (2005) /154; Harrison 18th/p 182, 3345, 3346, 3347*

Motor neuron disease is associated with degeneration of anterior horn cells in the spinal cord.

Peripheral nerves, spinothalamic tract and spinocerebellar tract are not involved in motor neuron diseases.

Motor Neuron Disease encompasses disorders that predominantly or exclusively affect *the upper motor neurons* (Neurons that lie in the cerebral cortex and project through the corticospinal / corticobulbar tract) or *lower motor neurons* (Neurons that lie in the anterior horn cell of the spinal cord or motor cranial nuclei that lie in the brainstem) *or both.*

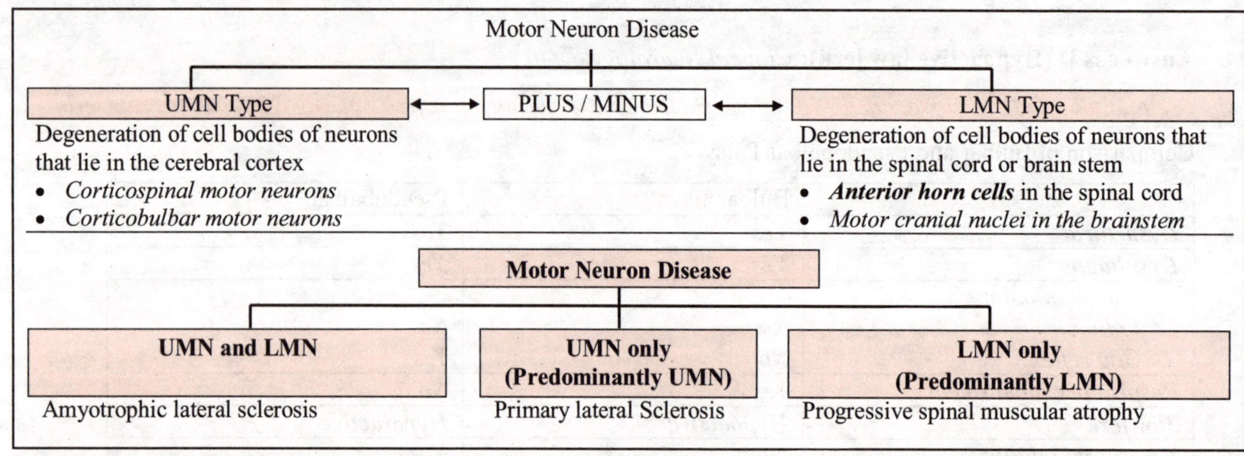

Isolated Anterior Horn Cell Disorders (Mostly infectious or genetic)

- Polio Virus Infection (or other Enteroviruses)
- Motor Neuron Disease (Spinal Muscular Atrophy Subtypes-Genetic SMA)
  - *Infantile SMA (Werdnig – Hoffman)*
  - *Intermediate / Childhood SMA (Kugelberg- Welander)*
  - *Adult SMA (Aran – Duchenne)*

Amyotrophic Lateral Sclerosis (UMN + LMN type motor neuron disease) is associated with simultaneous degeneration of anterior horn cells and the neurons of the corticospinal and /or corticobulbar tract.

28. Answer is A (Fasciculation): *Ref: Harrisons 15th/ 2412; Harrison 16th/2424, 2425; Harrison 17th/148, 2572, 2573; Harrison 18th/p 182, 3345, 3346, 3347*

Spontaneous twitchings of motor neurons or fassiculations are a characteristic feature of motor neuron disease affecting the lower motor neurons.

Motor neuron disease is characterized by degeneration of motor neurons, either upper motor neuron or lower motor neuron or both.

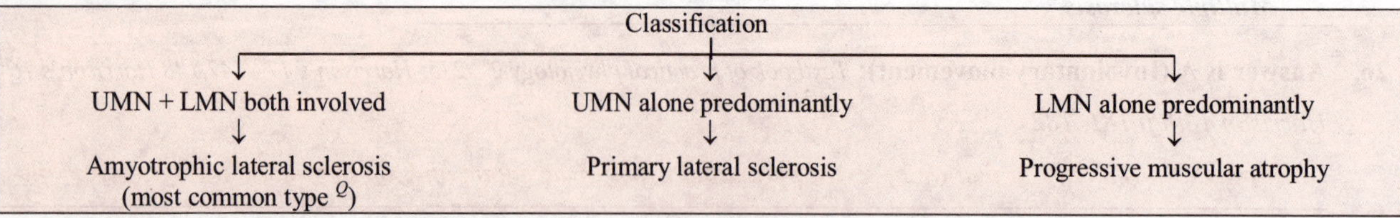

Manifestations are variable and depend on the neurons involved

Upper Motor Neurons Manifestations (UMN)	Lower Motor Neurons Manifestations (LMN)
Corticospinal Tract Involvement (UMN of Limbs)	***Lower motor neurons of Limbs involved***
• Hyperactive tendon reflexes • Spasticity / spastic resistance to passive movements.	• Weakness - Asymmetric - Insidious - Distal to proximal • Progressive wasting and atrophy of muscles ϱ • Fasciculations or spontaneous twitchings

Corticobulbar Tract Involvement (UMN to bulbar muscles)	Lower motor neurons of bulbar muscles involved
• Dysarthria • Exaggeration of emotion involuntary excess weeping/ laughing (pseudobulbar affect)	• Difficulty in chewing - Swallowing • Movements of face and tongue

29. Answer is A (Anterior horn cells): *Harrison 17th/2572, 2573; Harrison 18th/p 3345-3347*

Spinomuscular Atrophy is a form of motor neuron disease that affects the lower motor neuron (Anterior horn cells) only.

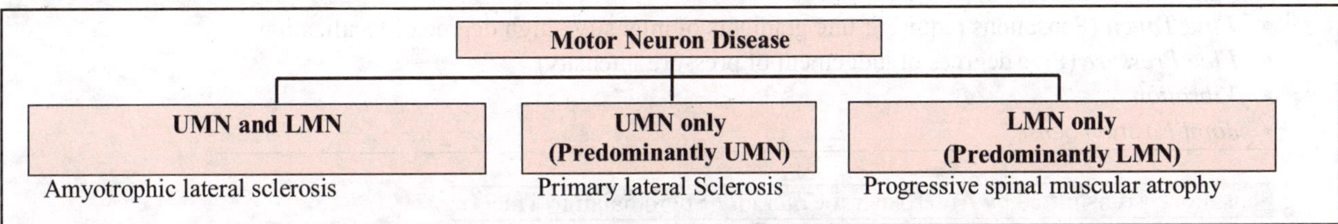

The site of LMN lesion in LMN type motor neuron disease is the anterior horn cell.

30. Answer is A (Anterior Horn Cells): *Harrison 17th/2572; Harrison 18th/p 3345*

Amyotrophic lateral sclerosis involves degeneration of both upper motor neurons (corticospinal motor neurons originating in layer five of the motor cortex) and Lower motor neurons (Anterior horn cells in the spinal cord or their homologues)

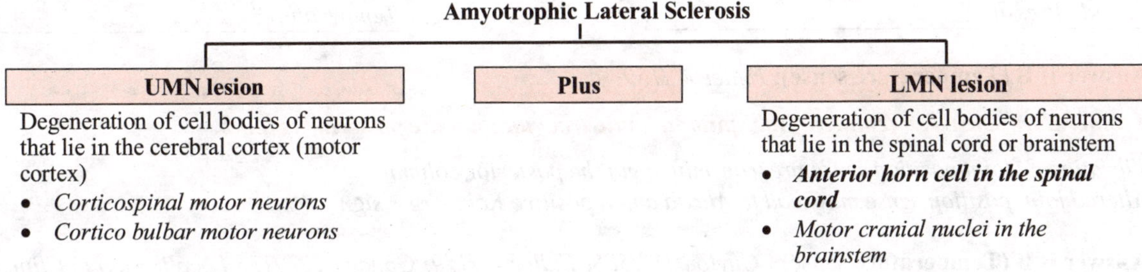

31. Answer is B (Amyotrophic lateral sclerosis) : *Harrison 16th/2424, 2425; Harrison 2572, 2573; 18th/p 3345-3347*

The presence of both lower motor neuron features (progressive atrophy and weakness of hands and forearms) and upper motor neuron features (spasticity and hyper reflexer, in the patient leads us to the diagnosis of Amyotrophic lateral sclerosis. Increased signal in the corticospinal tracts on T2 weighted MRI is characteristic MRI finding.

32. Answer is B (Ocular motility is spared): *Ref: Harrisons 15th/ 2412; Harrison 2573; Harrison 18th/p 3346-3347*

Ocular muscles are usually not involved in motor neuron disease.

Motor neuron diseases can be excluded remembering the following parameters
1. **NO** sensory deficit. Deficit is purely motor.
2. **NO** bladder bowel involvement
3. **NO** impairment of cognitive function
4. **NO** involvement of ocular muscles. Ocular motility is spared until very late.

33. Answer is A (Motor neuron disease): *Ref: Harrisons 15th/ 119; 16th/134; Harrison 17th/148; Harrison 18th/p 182*

Fasciculation is a visible or palpable twitch within a single muscle due to spontaneous discharge of one motor unit
***Disease of motor neurons are associated with fasciculations** - Harrison's 14th / 119*

Spinal Cord Disorders

General and Fine touch

34. Answer is A (Fine Touch): *Ganong 22nd /138; Guyton 11th/588;*

Fine touch is transmitted through the Dorsal /Posterior column

Sensations Transmitted by Posterior / Dorsal Column
• ***Fine Touch*** (Sensations requiring fine gradients of intensity / high degree of localization
• *Fine Pressure* (Fine degrees of judgement of pressure intensity)
• *Vibration*
• *Joint Position Sense*

Sensations Transmitted by Anterolateral Column / Spinothalamic Tract[Q]
• *Crude Touch*[Q]
• *Crude pressure*[Q]
• *Pain (Pin Prick)*[Q]
• *Temperature*[Q]

Anterior[Q] Spinothalamic Tract (Ventral)	Lateral[Q] Spinothalamic Tract
Crude Touch[Q]	*Pain (Pin Prick)*[Q]
Crude Pressure[Q]	*Temperature*[Q]

35. Answer is B (Temperature sense): *Fuller 4th/159*

Temperature sense is a feature of the spinothalamic tract and not the posterior column.

Vibration & Joint position sense are transmitted via the posterior column.

Altered joint position sense may lead to Ataxia and a positive Romberg's sign.

36. Answer is B (Temperature sense) : *Guyton 11th/588; Fuller 4th/159; Ganong 22nd/138 Localization in Clinical Neurology 5th/106*

Temperature sense is transmitted through the Anterolateral /Spinothalamic tract and is not affected by lesions in the posterior column of the spinal cord

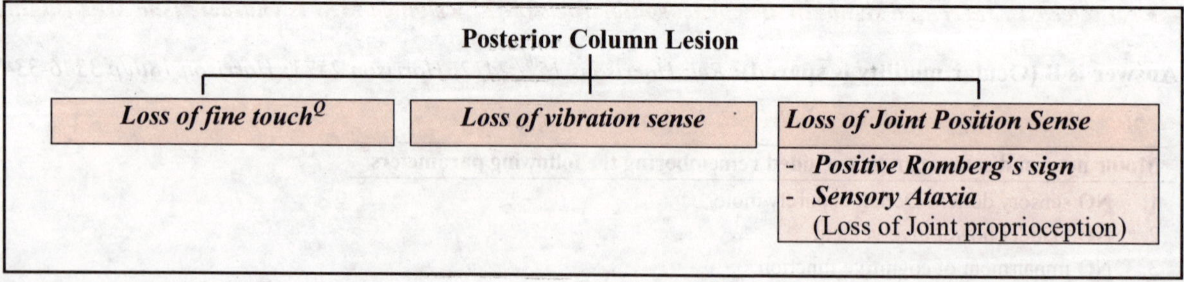

37. Answer is B (Left Lateral Spinothalamic tract): *Ganong 23rd/179 (Q1); 'Bonica's Management of Pain' 4th/Chapter 'Neurosurgical Operations on the Spinal Cord'*

Pain sensations from the right leg are carried via the contralateral Lateral Spinothalamic tract. Ventrolateral cordotomy (surgical procedure of ablating selected pain conducting tracts) of the Left Spinothalamic Tract should effectively relieve pain from the right lower extremity.

Ventrolateral Cordotomy

- *Ventrolateral cordotomy is a surgical procedures in which the spinal anterolateral ascending system for transmission of nociception (pain) known as the spinothalamic tract is interrupted for the relief of severe, intractible pain* (cancer pain) not responding to any other conventional measures of pain control.

> Ventrolateral cordotomy can be performed by both, percutaneous and open surgical techniques.

- Ventrolateral cordotomy has been shown to be most effective in the treatment of intermittent shooting pain and evoked pain such as allodynia and hyperpathia, which is *essentially mediated by the Lateral Spinothalamic Tract.*
- The optimal candidate for such a procedure is a patient with unilateral severe pain (usually with malignant cancer) not adequately treated with less invasive measures.
- Fibres carrying sensation of 'pain' decussate (cross obliquely) to the opposite side within the spinal cord (over one to five segments) and ascend in the contralateral white column as the Lateral spinothalamic Tract.

> *The **Left** spinothalamic tract carries sensation of pain from the **Right** side of the body.*

- ***Cordotomy (ventrolateral) therefore aims to interrupt the lateral spinothalamic tract ascending contralaterally to the painful side.***

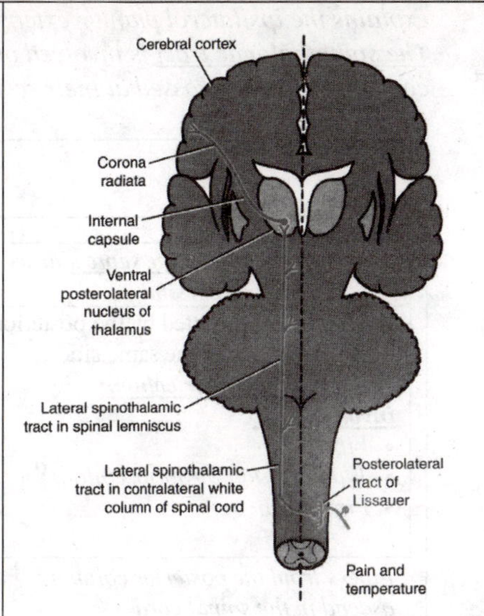

Fibres carrying sensation of 'pain' decussate (cross obliquely) to the opposite side within the spinal cord and ascend in the contralateral white column as the Lateral Spinothalamic Tract.

38. Answer is C (Proprioception): *Harrison's 17th/157, 2589; 16th/144, 2441; Harrison 18th/p 191, 3367; Fuller 4th/173;*

Proprioception is lost on the same side of lesion in Brown Sequard Syndrome.

Brown sequard syndrome or hemisection of the cord is associated with loss of posterior column sensations (vibration joint position sense, proprioception, fine touch) on the same side of lesion.

Sensations transmitted by the anterolateral column or spinothalamic tract (pain, touch, temperature) are lost on the opposite side of lesion

Brown Sequard Syndrome (Hemisection of the cord)

Sensations lost on the same side as the lesion	Motor power is lost on the same side as that of the lesion	Sensation lost on the opposite side of lesion
Sensations transmitted by the posterior column are lost on the same side Ipsilateral posterior column involvement • *Vibration* • *Joint position (proprioception)*[Q] • *Fine touch*	(Ipsilateral corticospinal tract involvement)[Q]	Sensations transmitted by the anterolateral spinothalamic tracts are lost on the opposite side Contralateral spinothalamic tract involvement • *Touch (Crude touch)* • *Pain* • *Temperature*

39. Answer is C (Contralateral Posterior Column Features): *Repeat*

Brown-Sequard Syndrome (Hemisection of spinal cord) is characterized by lesions of the ipsilateral posterior column (and not contralateral posterior column).

<u>The pyramidal tract (corticospinal tract)</u> is involved on the same side (ipsilateral pyramidal tract features), which also explains the ipsilateral planter extensor response.
<u>The spinothalamic tract</u> is involved on the contralateral side since fibres of the spinothalamic tract ascends in the spinal cord after having crossed at their respective spinal levels.

Brown Sequard Syndrome
(Hemisection of the cord)

<u>Sensations lost on the same side</u> as the lesion	***Motor power is lost on the same side as that of the lesion***	***<u>Sensation lost on the opposite side</u> of lesion***
Sensations transmitted by the posterior column are lost on the same side ***<u>Ipsilateral posterior column involvement</u>***[Q] • *Vibration* • *Joint position (proprioception)*[Q] • *Fine touch*	Motor power controlled by the corticospinal tract is lost on the same side of the lesion ***<u>Ipsilateral corticospinal tract involvement</u>***[Q] • *Loss of voluntary motor power* • *Planter Extensor Response (Positive Babiniski Reflex)* • *Brisk* tendon jerks	Sensations transmitted by the anterolateral spinothalamic tracts are lost on the opposite side ***<u>Contralateral spinothalamic tract involvement</u>***[Q] • *Touch (Crude touch)* • *Pain* • *Temperature*
Fibers from the posterior column ascend in the spinal cord uninterrupted upto the medulla where they decussate (cross-over)		*Fibers from the spinothalamic tract ascend in the spinal cord on the contralateral side after having crossed over at their respective spinal levels*

40. Answer is D (Contralateral posterior column involvement): *Harrison 16th /2440, 144; 17th/157, 2589; 18th/191, 3367*

***Brown – Sequard syndrome or hemisection of the spinal cord leads to loss of joint position and vibratory sense (posterior column movement) on the ipsilateral side and not on the contralateral side.** – Harrison 16th / 2441, 144*

Brown sequard syndrome: Hemisection of spinal cord
• Ipsilateral involvement of corticospinal tract : ipsilateral loss of motor power. • Ipsilateral involvement of posterior column : ipsilateral loss of joint position and vibratory sense. • Contralateral involvement of spinothalamic tract : contralateral loss of joint position and vibratory sense.

Segmental signs such as radicular pain muscle atrophy or loss of deep tendon reflexes arc unilateral (Lower motor neuron signs at level of lesion).

41. Answer is B (Contralateral loss of pain): *Harrison 17th/2589; Harrison 18th/p 3367*

Brown-Sequard Hemicord Syndrome is associated with contralateral loss of pain and temperature sense

Brown-Sequard Hemicord Syndrome
• *Ipsilateral Weakness (corticospinal tract)* • *Ipsilateral Loss of joint position and vibratory sense (posterior column),* • *Contralateral Pain and temperature sense (spinothalamic tract) one or two levels below the lesion* • *Unilateral Segmental signs, such as radicular pain, muscle atrophy, or loss of a deep tendon reflex*

42. Answer is D (Sacral sparing): *Harrisons 17th /2589, 2590; Harrison 18th/p 3367*

Sacral sparing is a feature of intramedullary tumors and not extramedullary tumors.

'With extramedullary tumors there is early loss of sacral sensations (lateral spinothalamic tract). Intramedullary lesions spare sensations in the perenial and sacral areas (sacral sparing)' - Harrisons

<u>Distinguishing features between Extramedullary and Intramedullary Compression of the spinal cord</u>

(Harrisons / API medicine / Paul Bracis – Localization in clinical neurology / Fuller)

Features	*Extra medullary*	*Intramedullary*
Pathological process	*Arise outside the spinal cord (extradural and intradural) and produce symptoms by compressing nerve roots, spinal cord or its vascular supply*	*Arise within the substance of the spinal cord and produce symptoms by invading the spinal cord tracts and grey matter.* Nerve root symptoms are not seen
Pain • **Radicular /Root pain** • *Diffuse burning pain (Funicular)* • **Vertebral pain (Midline back pain)**	 **Common** *Uncommon* **Common**	 **Rare** *Common* **Uncommon**
Motor Weakness **(Corticospinal tract involvement)** *(UMN signs)*	**Occurs early** *Lower extremity is involved earlier than upper extremity* *(Leg fibres in the cortico spinal tract are more superficial/lateral and hence involved early)*	**Occurs late** *Upper extremity is involved earlier than lower extremity* *(Leg fibres are more superficial / lateral and hence involved late)*
Sacral sensations	**Lost (No sacral sparing)** *(Sacral fibres are located outmost within the laminated arrangement of the spinothalamic tract and hence involved early)*	**Spared (sacral sparing)** *(Sacral fibres are located outermost and hence spared)*
Paraesthesias	*Less common* *(Ascending progression)*	*More common* *(Descending prgression)*
Dissociative Anaesthesia	*Absent*	*Present*
Lhermite's sign	*Present*	*Absent*
Autonomic *Bladder Bowel involvement* *(Sphincter abnormalities)*	*Late*	*Early with caudal lesions* *(conus/cauda equina)*
CSF Proteins	**CSF proteins are markedly raised** *in extradural lesion and raised in intradural extra medullary lesions*	**CSF proteins are usually normal** *(May be raised eg conus medullaris lesion)*
Myelogram	*Classic signs* *'Meniscus sign' in intadural tumors* *'Brush border sign' in extradural tumors*	*Classic sign* *'Expansion sign' of the cord is diagnostic of syringomylia*
Imaging / X-ray / CT	*Bony changes or changes in inter vertebral discs are frequent*	*Bony changes/Disc changes are infrequent*

43. Answer is B (Absent knee and Ankle Jerks) : *Principles of Surgical patient care 2nd /501, De Jong's Neurological examination 6th/578, Neurological Examination by Schwartzman (2006)/175, Principles and practic of Pediatric oncology by Pizzo, Poplach 5th/1220;*

Consus Medullaris lesions are associated with absent ankle jerk alone. Knee jerk (Patellar Reflex) is not absent.

– Dejong's 6th/518

Signs and Symptoms Differentiating Between Lesions of the Conus Medullaris and Cauda Equina

Features	**Conus Medullaris**	**Cauda Equina**
Site of Injury	• Sacral Spinal Cord (conus) + Lumbosacral nerve roots	• Lumbosacral nerve roots (alone)
Nature of lesion (UMN/LMN)	• UMN + LMN *Mixture of UMN paralysis (conus) and LMN paralysis (LS nerve roots)*	• LMN *LMN paralysis alone as cord is not involved*
Babinski	• ***Extensor /Positive (due to UMN lesion)***	***Flexor /Negative (May be absent)***
Tendon Reflexes	• ***Only Ankle Reflex is absent (Knee reflex may be exaggerated)***	***Both Ankle Reflex and Knee reflex may be absent***

Pain (spontaneous)	• Minimal • Not common or severe • Bilateral and Symmetric • In perineum or thighs	• Significant • May be most prominent symptoms, Severe unilateral or asymmetric • In perineum, thighs legs, or back, distribution of sacral nerves • Radolar in type,
Sensory defect	• ***Saddle distribution*** • Bilateral, usually symmetric • Dissociation of sensation may be seen	• ***Saddle distribution*** • May be unilateral and asymmetric • No dissociation of sensation
Motor loss	• Symmetric • Not marked • Fasciculation may be present • Atrophy may occur	• Asymmetric • More marked, • Usually no fasciculations • Atrophy may occur,
Bladder and rectal symptoms	• Early and marked	• Late and less marked
Trophic changes	• Decubti common	• Decubti less marked
Sexual functions	• Erecton and ejaculation impaired	• Less marked impairment
Onset	• Sudden and bilateral	• Gradual and unilateral

44. Answer is C (Late Bladder involvement): *Principles of Surgical patient care 2nd /501, De Jong's Neurological examination 6th/578, Neurological Examination by Schwartzman (2006)/175, Principles and practic of Pediatric oncology by Pizzo, Poplach 5th/1220*

Conus medullaris is associated with early and marked bladder involvement.

Signs and Symptoms Differentiating Between Lesions of the Conus Medullaris and Cauda Equina

Features	Conus Medullaris	Cauda Equina
Plantar (Babinski) *Tendon Reflexes*	• ***Extensor /Positive (due to UMN lesion)*** • Only Ankle Reflex is absent (Knee reflex may be exaggerated)	***Flexor /Negative (May be absent)*** Both Ankle Reflex and Knee reflex may be absent
Sensory defect	• Saddle distribution • ***Bilateral, usually symmetric*** • Dissociation of sensation may be seen	• Saddle distribution • ***May be unilateral and asymmetric*** • No dissociation of sensation
Bladder symptoms	• ***Early and marked***	• ***Late and less marked***

45. Answer is A (Conus Medullaris): *Harrison's 18th*

Loss of bladder control is an early and marked feature of conus medullaris.

Feature	Conus Medullaris	Cauda Equina syndrome	GBS	AMLS
Bladder Involvement	**Early and Marked** *'Bladder dysfunction is a prominent feature and comes early in the course of disease'*	**Late and less marked** *'Bladder involvement is a late presentation in cauda-equina syndrome*	**Uncommon** *'If bladder dysfunction a prominent feature and comes early in the course, diagnostic possibilities other than GBS should be considered*	**Absent /uncommon** 'Even in late stages of the illness bowel and bladder functions are preserved'

46. Answer is A (Loss of sympathetic tone) : *Advanced Trauma Life Support (ATLS) Manual 7th / 73, 181; Harrison 16th / 1605; Harrison 17th/2588, 2589; Harrison 18th/p 3366, 3367*

Spinal cord injury may produce hypotension due to loss of sympathetic tone. - ATLS 7th / 73

Interruption of sympathetic vasomotor input after a high cervical spinal cord injury may result in neurogenic shock.
- Harrison

Shock associated with spinal cord injury

Neurogenic Shock	Spinal Shock
• *Produced as a result of loss of sympathetic tone.* • It results from impartment of the descending sympathetic pathways in the spinal cord. • Classical picture of Neurogenic shock is *hypotension without tachycardia or cutaenous vasoconstriction.*	• *Refers to flaccidity and loss of reflexes seen after spinal cord injury.* • The 'shock' here is to the 'injured cord' which makes it appear completely functionless although all areas are not necessary destroyed. • The duration of spinal shock is variable.

47. **Answer is C, D and E (Sensory loss, Urinary retention and Areflexia):** *Refer text below; Harrison 17th/2708; Current Critical Care Diagnosis and Treatment 3rd/691;*

Spinal shock is associated with sensory loss, areflexia and urinary retention.

Spinal shock is defined as total loss of motor and sensory function below the level of lesion with areflexia, and flaccidity occurring immediately after spinal cord injury.

Features of spinal shock
• Complete motor paralysis (loss of all voluntary movements) • Flaccidity • Areflexia • Sensory loss with anaesthesia to all modalities

Spinal shock is usually associated with Urinary Retention

The urinary bladder becomes areflexic during spinal shock and urinary retention develops in most cases. Following the spinal shock phase reflex detrusor activity reappears – Textbook of Neurogenic Bladder (2004)/180

Acute Spinal Cord Injury

Spinal Shock	Neurogenic Shock
• *Flaccid Paralysis* • *Areflexia* • *Anaesthesia*	• *Hypotension* • *Bradycardia* • *Skin hyperaemia and warmth*
The true mechanism of spinal shock after spinal cord injury is not known	*The mechanism of neurogenic shock after spinal cord injury is believed to be disruption of sympathetic flow with preserved and unopposed vagal (parasympathetic) tone*

48. **Answer is A (Spastic paralysis): Repeat**

Spinal Shock is associated with Flaccid paralysis and not Spastic paralysis

Spinal shock
• *Flaccid Paralysis (complete motor paralysis)* • *Areflexia* • *Sensory loss (anesthesia to all modalities)* • *Bladder Involvement (usually areflexic bladder with urinary retention)*

49. **Answer is B and D (Loss of sensation over face and Wasting with fasciculations of lower limb):** *Harrison 17th/2588; Harrison 18th/p 3367*

Cervical cord injury is not associated with loss of sensations over face. Cervical cord injury may be associated with wasting and fasciculations over the limbs but not on the lower limbs.

Cervical Cord Injury

UMN features below the site of lesion	LMN features at site of lesion	Horner's syndrome
Lower limbs will show signs of UMN lesions and not LMN lesions	*Upper limbs may show signs of LMN lesion at the site of transaction*	Horner's syndrome may be seen in cervical cord lesions
Wasting and fasciculations are signs of LMN lesion and are not seen in the lower limbs in a patient with cervical injury	***Wasting and fasciculations are signs of LMN lesion and may be seen in the upper limbs in patient with cervical cord injury.***	

50. **Answer is B (Increased Rectal sphincter Tone):** *'Accident and Emergency' by Dolan and Holt 1st (2000)/135; 'Emergency medicine' Board Review 5th/169*

Cervical cord injury is suggested by a decrease in tone of the Rectal Sphincter and not by an increased tone of the rectal sphincter

Findings that indicate a cervical cord injury (in an unconscious patient)

- ***Flaccid Paralysis with Areflexia (Spinal shock)***
- *Flaccid Rectal sphincter or decreased tone of the rectal sphincter*
- *Hypotension with bradycardia (Neurogenic shock)*
- ***Diaphragmatic Breathing***
- ***Priapism (Autonomic transaction)***
- *Ability to flex but not extend the elbow*
- *Response on eliciting painful stimuli above the clavicle but not below the clavicle*

51. **Answer is B (Increased Rectal Sphincter tone):** *Repeat*

Cervical spinal cord injury is associated with a decreased rectal sphincter tone (and not an increased rectal sphincter tone).

52. **Answer is C (Lead poisoning):** *Neurology by Anish Bahra/68; Oxford Handbook of tropical Medicine 2nd/436*

Lead poisoning is the single best answer of exclusion.

Although there are a few isolated case reports that implicate lead poisoning as a cause of spastic paraplegia, such reports are not confirmed and hence lead poisoning remains the single best answer of exclusion.

Cord compression due to Cervical spondylosis, subacute combined degeneration of cord due to vitamin B12 deficiency, and motor neuron disease involving the UMN's are all established cause for spastic paraplegia.

Causes of spastic paraplegia:

Spinal cord compression	***Cervical spondylosis*** *Cervical or thoracic disc* *Metastatic tumor* *Primary tumor (meningioma, neurofibroma etc)* *Infective (epidural abscess, spinal TB etc)* *Epidural haematoma*
Inflammatory disorders	*Multiple sclerosis* *Idiopathic transverse myelitis* *Sarcoidosis* *Infections (lyme, zoster, TB, AIDS)*
Degenerative disorders	***Motor neuron disease*** *Syringomyelia*
Vascular	*Spinal cord infarction* *Vasculitis, systemic lupus erythematosus etc* *Spinal AVM*
Trauma	*Cord contusion, laceration or transaction* *Displaced vertebral fracture or disc* *Traumatic epidural haematoma*

Metabolic/Nutritional	*B12 deficiency (subacute combined degeneration)*
Rare hereditary conditions	*Friedreich's ataxia* *Hereditary spastic paraparesis*
Parasagittal brain lesions	*Meningioma* *Cerebral venous sinus thrombosis* *Congenital spastic diplegia*

53. Answer is E (All of the above): *Multiple References; Refer table*

Poliomyelitis, Tick paralysis, AIDP, and ADEM may all present with Acute Flaccid Paralysis

Muscle (acute myopathies)	**Nerve Roots (acute polyradiculopathies):**
- Inflammatory myopathy (polymyositis, dermatomyositis) - Rhabodmyolysis - Acute alcoholic necrotizing myopathy - Periodic paralyses (hypokalemia, hyperkalemia) - Metabolic derangements (hypophosphatemia, hypokalemia, hypermagnesemia)	- ***Acute Inflammatory Demyelinating Polyneuropathy (Guillain Barre syndrome)*** - Lyme disease - Sarcoidosis - HIV & oher viruses (CMV, *West Nile etc.*) **Anterior Horn cell (motor neuron diseases):** - ***Poliomyelitis*** - Anterior spinal artery syndrome
Neuromuscular Junction	**Spinal cord (corticospinal tract diseases):**
- Myasthenia gravis - Botulism - ***Tick paralysis*** - Other biotoxins (tetadotoxin, ciguatoxin) - Organophosphate toxicity (can also cause neuropathy) - Lambert-Eaton Myasthenic Syndrome (LEMS)	- Inflammatory (transverse myelitis) - Suacute combined degeneration (B_{12} deficiency) - Spinal cord infarction - Other myelopathies (spondylosis, epidural abscess or hematoma)
Nerve (acute neuropathies)	**Brain**
- Diphtheria - Porphyria - Drugs & Toxins (arsenic, thallium, lead, gold chemotherapy – cisplatin/vincristine) - Vasculitis - Pareneoplastic syndromes and Paraproteinemias - Multifocal motor neuropathy	- Pontine lesions (e.g., central pontine myelinolysis, pontine infarct or bleed) - ***Acute Disseminated Encephalamyelitis (ADEM)*** - Multifocal lesions (multiple metastases,multiple infarcts or haemorrhages e.g., DIC, TTP, bacterial endocarditis).

54. Answer is B (C4-C5): *Harrisons 17th/2588; 'The Cervical Spine' by Clarke (Lippincott-Williams) 4th/ 181; Refer text below; Harrison 18th/p 3367*

Presence of quadriparesis, sensory level up to the upper border of sternum together with an increased respiratory rate suggests a lesion of cervical spine at C4-C5 level

Localization of lesion to cervical level C3-C4

The level of lesion in the above presentation can be localized to Cervical C4-C5 segments with the help of clues provided in the form of motor involvement (quadriparesis), sensory level and the affection of respiratory function.

Quadriparesis (Motor level)

Presence of quadriparesis (affection of all four limbs) suggests that the lesion is located in the cervical spine (The lesion may be located either at C1-C2 or C4-C5)

Lesions of thoracic spine (T1-T2 or T3-T4) will only affect the two lower limbs and produce paraparesis or paraplegia, but not quadriparesis

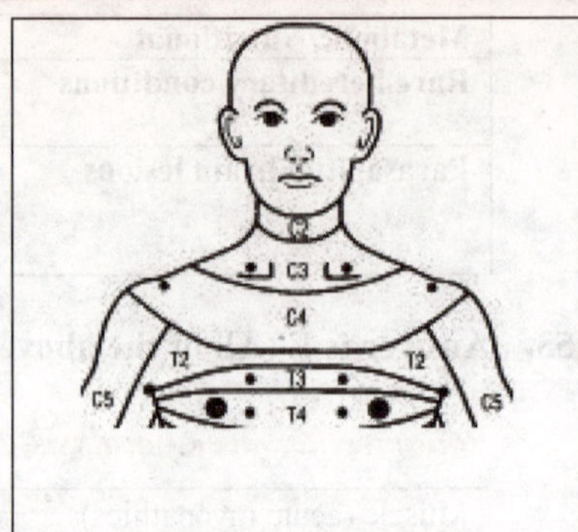

Sensory level

C4 dermatome covers the area just below the clavicle

Sensory loss up to the upper border of sternum is consistent with a cervical lesion at C4 level *(refer figure)*

Lesion at C1-C2 is unlikely as this would cause complete loss of sensation below the head(C1) or below the Occiput(C2)

> *The C2 dermatome covers the occiput and the top part of the neck.*
> *The C3 dermatome covers the lower part of the neck to the clavicle*
> *The **C4 dermatome covers the area just below the clavicle***

Respiratory Rate

Lesion at C4-C5 level is consistent with preserved respiratory function and an increased respiratory rate

'Injuries at C4 level may present with adequate function of the diaphragm secondary to innervations from a preserved C3 segment. The respiratory rate is increased and the patient compensates by using auxiliary muscles like sternomastoid, trapezius and platysma' - 'The Cervical Spine' by Clarke (Lippincott-Williams) 4th/ 181

> *Lesions above C3(C1-C2) result in a total loss of ventilatory function and requires immediate respiratory support / mechanical ventilation*

55. Answer is C (Nifedipine): *Disease of kidney & Urinary Tract/1416; Medical Management of Adults with Neurological Diabetes/11; Spine and Spinal Cord Trauma: Evidence Based Management Chapter 46*

Presence of accelerated hypertension with blood pressures in excess of 200/100 mm Hg in a patient with high thoracic spinal cord injury (above T6) suggests a diagnosis of Autonomic Dysreflexia. Urgent management of the hypertensive crisis is paramount to prevent complications such as retinal haemorrhage, seizures, hypertensive encephalopathy or an intracerebral haemorrhage.

Oral Clonidine and/or Nifedipine are the most commonly used pharmacological agents to control hypertensive crisis in patients with autonomic dysreflexia

Autonomic Dysreflexia (AD) (Hypertensive Crisis following Spinal Cord injury above T6)

What is Autonomic Dysreflexia
Autonomic Dysreflexia (AD) is a syndrome of sympathetic overactivity that typically affects patient with spinal cord injury above or proximal to the upper thoracic level (T6 or above) due to unopposed sympathetic nervous system impulses. This is an acute medical emergency that occurs in patients whose spinal cord injury lies above the greater splanchnic outflow from thoracolumbar preganglionic sympathetic neurons (T6 or above). This results from interruption of normal feedback mechanism in the sympathetic pathway. *Patients with spinal cord injury below T8 are rarely affected by this condition.*
When does Autonomic Dysreflexia occur
Autonomic Dysreflexia is traditionally/historically believed to occur 4-6 months after the spinal cord injury (After the phase of spinal shock resolves) However recently AD has also been reported in early phases after SCI
How does Autonomic Dysreflexia Present
The most characteristic presentation of AD is sudden increase in Blood Pressure (Accelerated Hypertension) *often in excess of 200mm Hg systolic and 100 mm Hg diastolic.* *It is important to note that normal resting Blood Pressure in patients with spinal cord injury is often 80 to 90 mmHg, and a systolic blood pressure of 130 mm Hg may be an early sign of autonomic dysreflexia*

Features of Autonomic Dysreflexia	
• *Hypertension* (Paroxysmal; Accelerated) • Headache (most common symptom during a paroxysm of Hypertension) • *Bradycardia* • Other symptom / signs	
Above the level of lesion	Below the level of lesion
• Feeling of Doom • Facial Flushing • Nasal congestion • Diaphoresis/Sweating • Piloerection	Cool clammy skin (Due to vasoconstriction)

• Complications of Hypertension

• Seizures • Retinal haemorrhage	• Hypertensive encephalopathy	• Intracerebral haemorrhage

Bradycardia in association with hypertension is another typical feature of AD and this results primarily from vagal compensation. Bradycardia is however present in only 50% of the cases.

What are the Triggering factors for AD

Autonomic Dysreflexia can be triggered by any painful/noxious stimulus in the dermatomes (skin), muscles or viscera below the level of cord injury.

Bladder Distension is the single most common inciting stimuli

Trigger Stimuli / Inciting stimuli for AD

- Distension of Bladder (Due to obstructed urine outflow from spasm/kinked Foley's catheter)
- Bowel impaction (Constipation)
- Irritation from skin lesions (Dermatomes)
  - Insect bites, pressure sores, constrictive clothing, localized wounds or ingrowing toe nails
- Labour and pregnancy
- Gynecological instrumentation and/or patients with SCI undergoing surgery

What is the treatment of AD

Treatment of Autonomic Dysreflexia

- Prevention of Trigger Factors
- Management of Hypertensive crisis

Prevention of Trigger Factors

- Avoid Bladder Distension (leading cause) (prompt catheterization)
- Avoid Fecal Impaction (Second leading cause) (Manual evacuation, anal sphincter block, bowel programs)
- Evaluate & treat for skin lesions (Pressure sores/Ingrowing toe nails)

Anti-cholinergic Medicines are recommended

Management of Hypertensive crisis

- Patient should be brought in a sitting position with legs dangling to take advantage of natural orthostosis.
- Pharmacological management with oral/transdermal medicine should be initiated
  - Transdermal Nitroglycerine
  - ***Oral Clonidine***
  - ***Oral Nifedipine***
  - Oral Phenoxybenzamine
  - Oral Prazocin
- Pharmacological management with intravenous medicines may be considered in cases of hypertensive crises or encephalopathy or intraoperative hypertension
  - Nitroprusside
  - *Diazoxide*
  - Trimethaphan
  - Fenoldopam

56. Answer is A (Abdominal muscle) : *Harrison's 17th/2589; Harrison 18th/p 3367*

Beevor's sign is seen in relation to abnormal abdominal muscle contraction

Beevor's Sign (Thoracic Cord Lesion)
• Beevor's sign refers to upward movement of the umbilicus when the abdominal ***muscle contracts***
• Beevor's sign represents a consequence to a *Thoracic Cord lesion*
• *Lesions at T9-T10* paralyze the lower- but not the – upper abdominal muscles resulting in *an upward movement of the umbilicus* when the abdominal muscle contracts

57. Answer is A (Thoracic cord): *Harrison's 17th/2589; Harrison 18th/p 3367*

Beevor's sign result from a lesion in the Thoracic cord (T9 – T10)

58. Answer is B (Loss of vibration sense): *Current Diagnosis & Treatment in Neurology 1st/268, 270*

Anterior spinal artery thrombosis does not involve the posterior column and hence vibration sense and joint positions sense (proprioception) are preserved.

Anterior spinal Artery Thrombosis/Syndrome

Anterior Spinal Artery is a single artery that supplies the anterior two thirds of the spinal cord.

Sparing of posterior column

Posterio 1/3rd of the cord is supplied by the posterior spinal artery and hence the posterior column is spared and vibration & joint position sense are preserved

Pain at site of infarction

Moderate to severe back pain at the site of cord infarction, most often in the thoracic region

Infarction of the corticospinal tract

Paraplegia with UMN signs (spasticity and hyper-reflexia)

Note that initially flaccidity and hyporeflexia may be seen if patients is in spinal shock

Infarction of the Anterolateral tracts (spinothalamic tract)

Loss of pain and temperature sensation distal to the lesion

Infarction of the fibres required for sphincter control (carried in anterior 2/3rd of cord)

Loss of Bladder control

59. Answer is D (Meningioma): *Read text below : Harrison 16th/2441; 14th/2383; Harrison 15th/2427*

Meningiomas are not listed as a cause of metastatic tumors causing spinal cord compression.

Tumors causing compression of spinal cord, include the following two major categories:

A. **Retroperitoneal tumors** which extend via, intervertebral foramen into the spinal cord and thus cause compression. Examples include : Lymphoma, sarcomas.

B. **Those which metastasize to the spine** : These are *most common from the breast, lung, prostate, kidney Lymphomas and plasma cell dyscrasias (multiple myeloma)[Q]*

Remember :

- Most common site for metastasis to spine is : *thoracic segment* [Q]
- Most common site for metastasis to spine from CA prostate and CA ovary is *sacral and Lumber vertebra.*[Q]

Friadreich's Ataxia

60. Answer is A (Friedreich's Ataxia): *Harrison 18th/3338; Harrison's 17th/2510, 2570; Harrison 16th/2422, 2423; CMDT 2008/883; Current Diagnosis and treatment in Neurology/238,239; Clinical Neurology by Goetz 2nd/742,743*

History of ataxic gait and frequent falls in a young boy (<25 years of age) together with classical findings of absent deep tendon reflexes with an extensor plantar response suggests a typical diagnosis of Friedreich's ataxia.

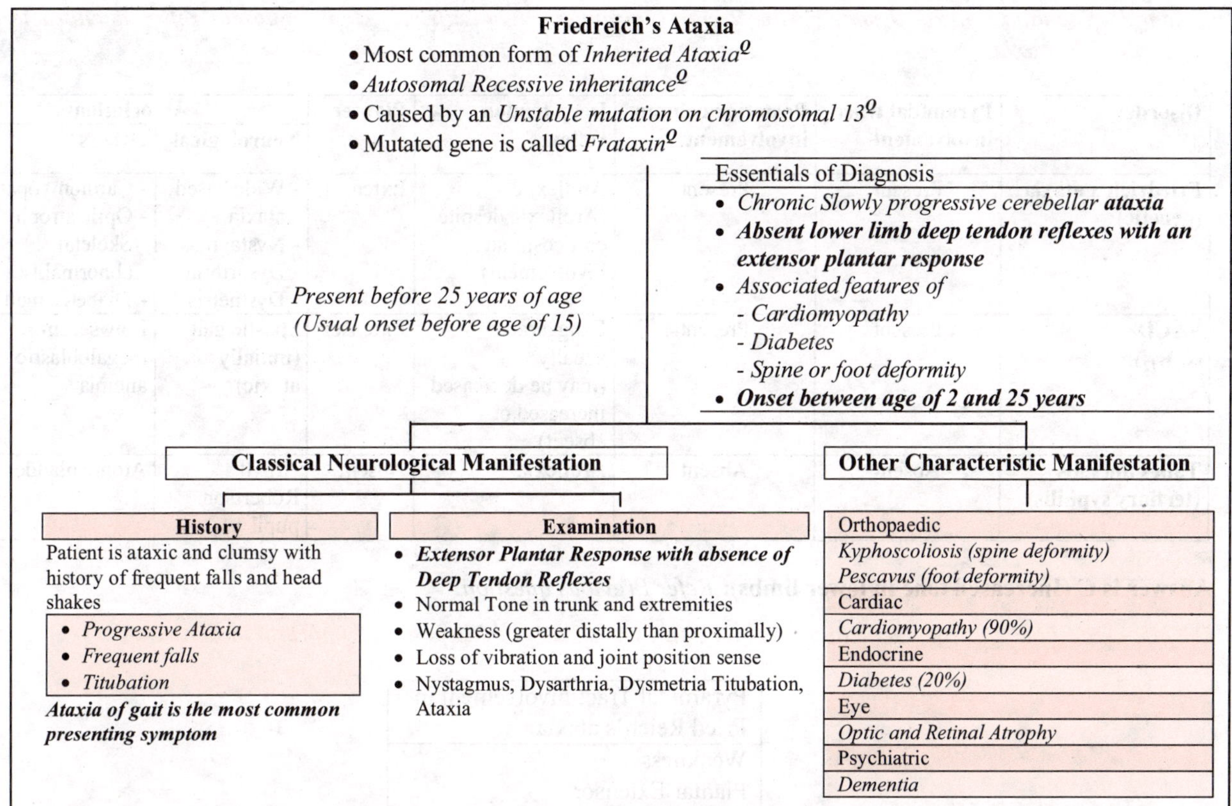

Disorder	Pyramidal tract involvement	Posterior column involvement	Deep tendon reflexes	Planter	Associations	
					Neurological	Others
Friedrich's ataxia (genetic)	Present	Present	Areflexia[Q] (Areflexia despite corticospinal involvement)[Q]	Extensor	- Wide based ataxia - Nystagmus - Dysarthria - Dysmetria	- Cardiomyopathy - Optic atrophy - Skeletal abnormality - Diabetes mellitus
SACD (↓ B_{12})	Present	Present	Exaggerated usually[Q] (May be decreased increased or absent)	Extensor	Spastic gait (initially ataxic)	Low serum B_{12}megaloblastic anemia
Tabes dorsalis (tertiary syphilis)	Absent	Absent	Areflexia[Q]	Absent	Argyll Robertson pupil	Atonic bladder

61. Answer is D (Extensor plantar with brisk lower limb reflexes): *Harrison's 17th/2510; Harrison's 16th; CMDT 2008/883; Current Diagnosis and treatment in Neurology/238,239; Clinical Neurology by Goetz 2nd/742,743; Harrison 18th/p 2570, 3343*

Friedreich's Ataxia is characteristically associated with an extensor plantar response but absent lower limb reflexes.

Lower limb reflexes are characteristically absent (in most patients) and not brisk.

Cardiomyopathy is a common association seen in up to 90% of patients
Diabetes mellitus may be associated in up to 25% of cases
Progressive ataxia is the most common presenting symptom.

62. Answer is B (Friedrich's ataxia): *Ref: See below; Harrison 16th/2422, 2423; Harrison 17th/2570;Harrison 18th/ 3343*

Absent deep tendon reflexes despite corticospinal tract involvement with an extensor plantar reflex is characteristic of Friedrich's ataxia.

Disorder	Pyramidal tract involvement	Posterior column involvement	Deep tendon reflexes	Planter	Associations	
					Neurological	Others
Friedrich's ataxia (genetic)	Present	Present	Areflexia[Q] (Areflexia despite corticospinal involvement) [Q]	Extensor	- Wide based ataxia - Nystagmus - Dysarthria - Dysmetria	- Cardiomyopathy - Optic atrophy - Skeletal abnormality - Diabetes mellitus
SACD (↓ B_{12})	Present	Present	Exaggerated usually[Q] (may be decreased increased or absent)	Extensor	Spastic gait (initially ataxic)	Low serum B_{12} megaloblastic anemia
Tabes dorsalis (tertiary syphilis)	Absent	Absent	Areflexia[Q]	Absent	Argyll Robertson pupil	Atonic bladder

63. Answer is C (Increased tone in lower limbs): *Refer Previous question*

Despite pyramidal tract involvement muscle tone in Friedreich's ataxia is usually normal or decreased

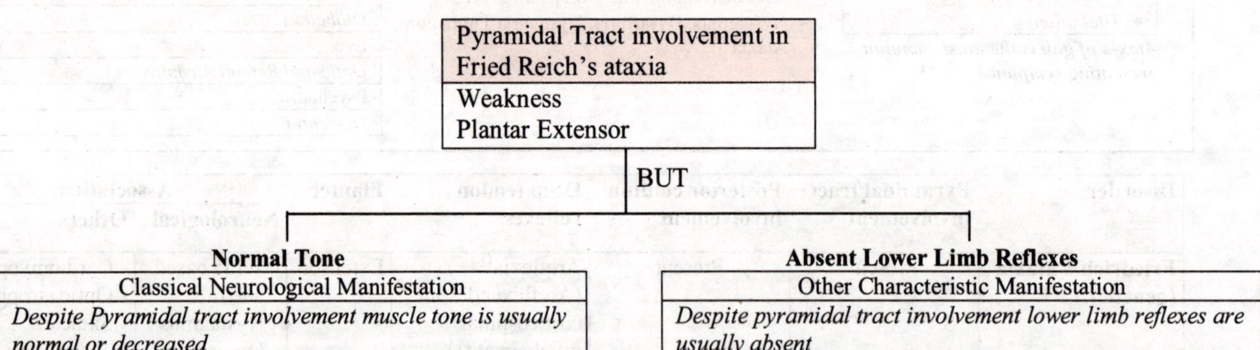

64. Answer is A (Friedrich's ataxia): *Harrison 15th/ 1410, 1432; Harrison 16th/2422, 2446; Harrison 17th/ 2570; Harrison 18th/p 3343*

Absent deep tendon reflexes despite corticospinal tract involvement with an extensor plantar reflex is characteristic of Friedrich's ataxia.

Pyramidal tract may be involved in Friedrich's ataxia or SACD amongst the options provided.
Reflexes amongst these two conditions present the following picture

Friedrich's ataxia	SACD
• Deep tendon reflex are characteristically absent • Planter response is extensor	• Increased deep tendons reflexes / clonus • Extensor planter [At an early stage the patellar and achillis reflexes may be diminished increased or absent]

Thus although both Friedrich's ataxia and SACD may present with absent ankle jerk, this feature is more characteristic and consistent with Friedrich's ataxia and hence this is the answer of choice.

65. Answer is A (Friedreich's Ataxia): *Repeat*

Absent ankle jerk with extensor planter response is characteristic of Friedreich's ataxia.

66. Answer is A (Dorsal Root Ganglion): *Clinical Neurology by Goetz 2nd/742*

The first pathological changes in Friedreich's ataxia are thought to occur in the dorsal root ganglia with loss of large sensory neurons- *Clinical Neurology by Goetz*

Pathological Changes in Friedreich's Ataxia

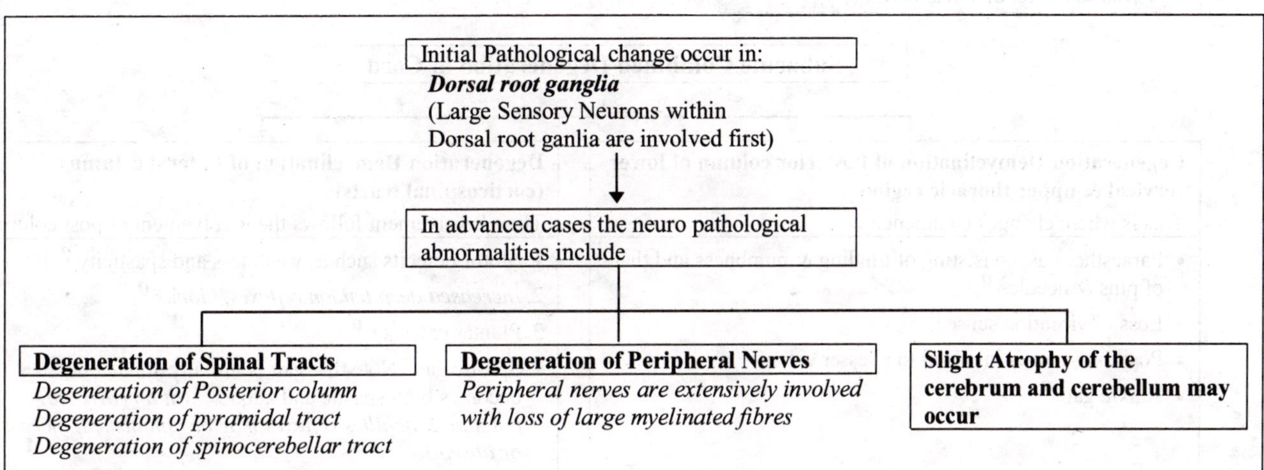

67. Answer is A (Ataxia): *Harrison's 17th/2570; Harrison's 16th/2422; Clinical Neurology by Goetz 2nd/742; Harrison 18th/p 3343*

In most patients ataxia of gait and stance is the first manifestation of the disease.- Clinical Neurology by Goetz 2nd/742

Friedreich's ataxia presents with progressive staggering gait, frequent falling and titubation- Harrison

Note:

The first pathological changes in Friendreich's Ataxia are thought to occur is dorsal root ganglia with loss of large sensory neurons.

SACD & Tabes Dorsalis

68. Answer is D (Myopathy) : *Harrison 16th/2404; 17th/2595; API 7th; Harrison 18th/p 3374*

Vitamin B12 deficiency does not produce myopathy. All other neurological manifestations may be seen with vitamin B_{12} deficiecny.

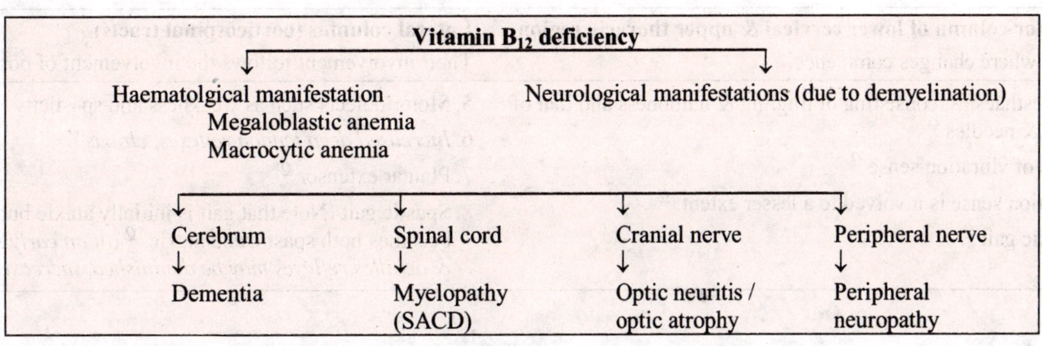

9

69. Answer is D (Vitamin B_{12}): *Harrison's 18th/3374*

Subacute Combined Degeneration of Cord (SACD) is caused by vitamin B_{12} dificiency.

Subacute Combined Degeneration Of Cord is a condition of the spinal cord characterized by demyelination of its neurons due to deficiency of Vit B_{12}, which results in defective/ deficient myelination.

Such demyelination occurs predominantly in
• Posterior column of spinal cord • Pyramidal tract of spinal cord

Subacute Combined Degeneration of Cord

Degeneration/Demyelination of Posterior column of lower cervical & upper thoracic region This is where changes commence.	**Degeneration/Demyelination of Lateral columns (corticospinal tracts)** Their involvement follows the involvement of post columns.
• Paraesthaesias, consisting of tingling & numbness and that of pins & needles Q • Loss of vibration sense Q • Position sense is involved to a lesser extent. Q • Ataxic gait Q	1. Motor defecits such as weakness and spasticity Q 2. *Increased deep tendon reflexes, clonus* Q 3. Plantar extensor Q 4. Spastic gait (Note that gait is initially ataxic but later becomes both spastic and ataxic. Q *(at an early stage patellar & achilles reflexes may be diminished, increased or absent).*

70. Answer is B (B_{12} deficiency): *Harrison 17th/ 25695; Read text below; Harrison 18th/p 3374*

Presence of a combination of hematological manifestations (anemia) and neurological manifestation (posterior column dysfunction) suggest a diagnosis of Vit. B_{12} deficiency.

71. Answer is D (Absent deep tendon reflexes): *Harrison 14th/ 2456, 2388; 15th/ 2432; 16th/2446; 17th/2595; Harrison 18th/p 3374*

Deep tendon reflexes are increased and clonus may be present in patients with subacute combined degenration of cord.

Subacute Combined Degeneration Of Cord is a condition of the spinal cord characterized by demyelination of its neurons due to deficiency of Vit B_{12} which results in defective/ deficient myelination.

Such demyelination occurs predominantly in
- Posterior column of spinal cord - Pyramidal tract of spinal cord

Subacute Combined Degeneration Of Cord is characterized by involvement of:

Posterior column of lower cervical & upper thoracic region This is where changes commence.	**Lateral columns (corticospinal tracts)** Their involvement follows the involvement of post columns.
• Paraesthaesias, consisting of tingling & numbness and that of pins & needles Q • Loss of vibration sense Q • Position sense is involved to a lesser extent. Q • Ataxic gait Q	5. Motor defects such as weakness and spasticity Q 6. *Increased deep tendon reflexes, clonus* Q 7. Plantar extensor Q 8. Spastic gait (Note that gait is initially ataxic but later becomes both spastic and ataxic. Q *(at an early stage patellar & achilles reflexes may be diminished, increased or absent).*

72. Answer is B (Deep tendon reflexes are brisk): *Harrison 18th /3375*

Tabes dorsalis is characterized by areflexia ***resulting from degeneration, demyelination of posterior nerve root and ganglia.***

Tabes Dorsalis

- Tabes Dorsalis is a parenchymatous manifestation of tertiary stage of Syphilis 9Late manifestation of Syphilis)
- Tabes dorsalis presents as symptoms and signs of demyelination of the posterior column, dorsal roots and dorsal root ganglia

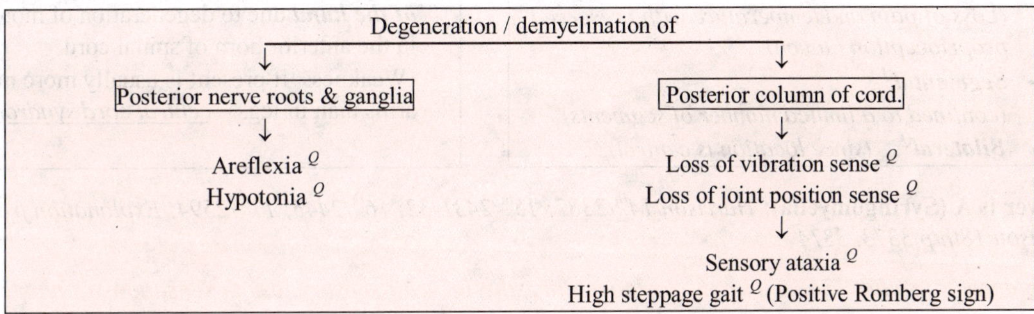

- The charachteristic symptoms of Tabes are fleeting and repetitive lancinating pains, primarily in the legs and less often in the back thorax, abdomen, arms and face.
- Ataxia due to loss of position sense with wide based gate (seen in <50% of patients)
- Paresthesis, bladder disturbance and ***acute abdominal pain with vomiting (visceral crisis)*** occur in 15-30% of patients
- Trophic joint degeneration (charcot's joints) and perforating ulceration of feet can result from loss of pain sensation
- The cardinal neurological signs of Tabes are loss of reflexes in legs, impaired position and vibratory sense, Positive Romberg's sign, Atonic Bladder and Bilateral Argyll Robertson pupils.

Argyll Robertson pupil Q

- Loss of light reflex Q
- Accommodation reflex present (ARP) Q
- Pupil is small, irregular and does not respond to mydriatics

QTabes Dorsalis is associated with an Atonic Bladder

73. Answer is B and C (Corticospinal tract and Posterior column): *Harrison 17th/2595; Refer previous question; Harrison 18th/p 3374*

Subacute combined degeneration of cord primarily involves the posterior column and the corticospinal tract (lateral tracts).

Peripheral neuropathy may be associated with SACD due to vitamin B12 deficiency, but it is not characteristic of SACD.

74. Answer is D (Hyperreflexia): *Harrison 15th/ 2432; Harrison 17th/ 2595; API / 778; Harrison 18th/p 3375*

Tabes dorsalis is characterized by areflexia resulting from degeneration, demyelination of posterior nerve root and ganglia.

Syringomyelia

75. Answer is E (Ascending weakness): Refer text below

Ascending weakness is not a typical feature of syringomyelia

Syringomyelia is characterized by ***bilateral, segmental, dissociative*** sensory loss with ***atrophy & weakness of small muscles of the hand.***

Syringomyelia

Disease in which the central canal of the spinal cord becomes enlarged

(Usually in the cervical or upper thoracic levels)

Sensory Features (Early)	Motor Features (Late)
• ***Dissociative sensory loss***[Q] *(Loss of pain and temperature with preserved proprioception / touch)* • ***Segmental***[Q] *(confined to a limited number of segments)* • ***Bilateral***[Q] *(since location is central)*	• ***Weakness and Atrophy typically of small muscles of the hand*** due to degeneration of motor neurons in the anterior horn of spinal cord. (Weakness if present is usually more marked in arms than in legs – central cord syndrome)

76. Answer is A (Syringomyelia): *Harrison 14th/2387; 15th/2431-32; 16th/2445; 17th/2594; Explanation from API; Harrison 18th/p 3373, 3374*

Syringomyelia is characterized by 'dissociative anaesthesia' with sensory loss to sensations of temperature and pain while sensation of 'touch' is preserved. This leads to multiple burns and non healing ulcers over the hand and forearms.

Syringomyelia

Syringomyelia is a cavitatory expansion of central canal of spinal cord caused by chronic progressive destruction of it's grey & white matter. [Q]

- The most commonly involved regions are the '*Lower cervical*' and '*upper thoracic*'. [Q]
- Since the disease usually starts at the base of the posterior horns of the lower cervical spinal cord, it tends to involve the sensory fibres, which cross the midline to form the spinothalamic tract.
- As these fibres carry the sensations for temperature & pain, one of the *earliest signs of disease is an inability to differentiate or appropriate 'Hot and Cold' sensations on the inner side of forearm and hand.*
- *Thermo-anaesthesia* usually precedes the *Analgesia* while *Touch sensitivity is usually preserved* (This leads to Multiple burns and non healing ulcers over the hands and forearms)
- Also note that this particular form of "sensory loss" to temperature & pain with sparing of touch, is described as ***'Dissociate Anaesthesia'***[Q] and is considered as the "***True Hallmark of the disease***"[Q].

Cerebrovascular Diseases & Aphasias

Cerebrovascular Stroke: Causes and Sites

77. Answer is B (20 ml/100g / minute): *Harrison's 18th/3271; 'Neurotrauma and Critical care of the Brain' (Thieme) 2009/30*

Cerebral blood flow < 20 ml / 100g tissue per minute causes cerebral ischemia without infarction *(Harrison's 18th/3271)*

Critical Cerebral Blood Flow	Effects
• ≤ 20 ml/100 gm/minute	• ***Cerebral Ischemia without infarction*** (*Reversible unless prolonged for* **several hours or days**) • Clinical syndrome of TIA • Consciousness is usually lost as the brain tissue loses the capacity to make neurotransmitter substances and coma ensues • *Damage is Reversible*
• ≤ 16-18 ml / 100 gm / minute	• Cerebral Infarction within one hour
• ≤ 10 ml / 100 gm / minute	• Cerebral Infarction within several minutes • Membrane integrity is lost • Biochemical cascade of neuronal destruction becomes irreversible
• Zero ml / 100 gm / minute	• Death of Brain tissue within 4 – 6 minutes

78. Answer is A (Embolism): *Ref: Harrison 15th/ 2370; Harrison 16th/ 2373; Harrison 17th/ 2513, 2514; 18th/3270, 3271*

The most common cause of cerebrovascular accidents is embolism.

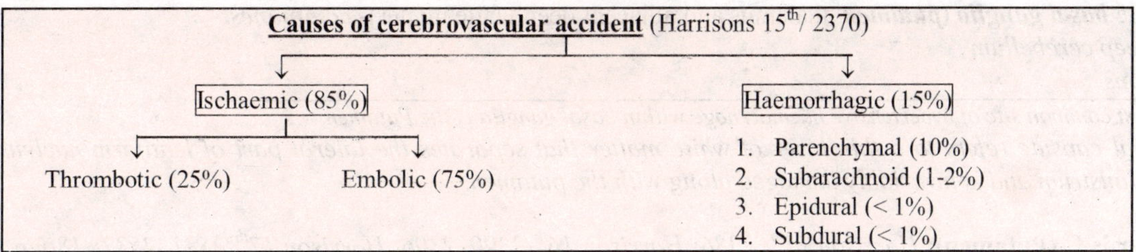

Harrisons 16th has not classified ischaemic strokes into thrombotic and embolic events but into Atherosclerosis (4%), cardioembolic (17%), & others (64%). Nevertheless even others (64%) include most commonly embolic events other than those of cardiac origin such as 'artery to artery embolic strokes' etc. and hence the answer stays the same.

79. Answer is C (Embolism): *Harrison 15th/ 2371; 16th/2373; 17th/ 2513, 2514; See previous question; 18th/3270, 3271*

The most common cause of cerebrovascular accidents is embolism.

80. Answer is A (Cortical vein thrombosis): *Harrison 17th/2520; Harrison 18th/p 3278*

Young women on OCPs are predisposed to stroke due to venous thrombosis of lateral saggital sinus or small cortical veins (cortical vein thrombosis)

'Venous sinus thrombosis of the lateral or saggital sinus or small cortical veins (cortical vein thrombosis) occurs as complication of oral contraceptive use, pregnancy and postpartum period, inflammatory bowel disease, intracranial infections (meningitis) and dehydration' - Harrison

81. Answer is B (Intracerebral haemorrhage): *Harrison 15th/ 2386; Harrison 16th/2387; 17th/ 2531; 18th/p 3294*

An intracerebral parenchymal haemorrhage constitutes the most common form of intracranial haemorrhage.

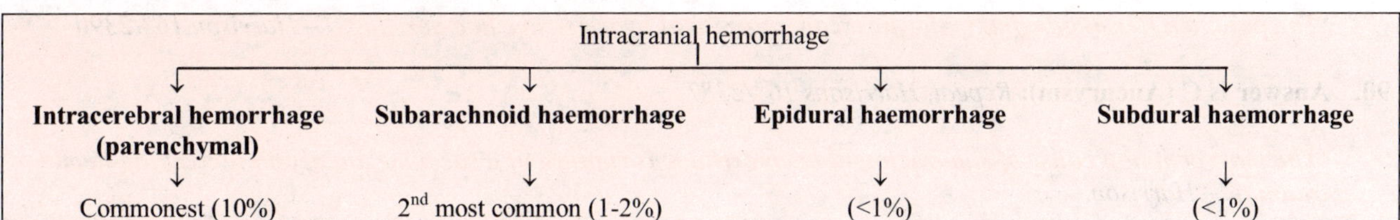

82. Answer is C (Hypertension): *Ref: Harrison 17th/ 2531; See below; Harrison 18th/ 3294*

An intracerebral bleed (parenchymal) invariably results from rupture of small perforating arteries or arterioles as a result of Hypertension.

Intracerebral (parenchymal haemorrhage)	Subarachnoid haemorrhage
• Most common type of intracranial haemorrhage [Q]	• Second most common cause of intracranial haemorrhage [Q]
• Most common cause is hypertension [Q] causing rupture of small perforating arteries or arterioles [Q]	• Most common cause is spontaneous rupture of saccular aneurysm i.e. Berry aneurysm [Q] (excluding trauma)
• Most common site is Putamen [Q] (basal ganglia)	• Most common site of berry aneurysm is anterior circulation of 'circle of Willis' [Q]

83. Answer is C (Hypertension): *Ref: Harrison 17th/ 2531; Harrison 18th/ 3294*

An intracerebral bleed (parenchymal) invariably results from rupture of small perforating arteries or arterioles as a result of Hypertension.

84. Answer is B (Basal ganglia): *Repeat; Harrison 15th/ 2386; Harrison 16th/2390, 2396; Harrison 17th/2531, 2532*

The basal ganglia is the most common site of hypertensive haemorrhage

The most common site of hypertensive haemorrhage within basal ganglia is the Putamen.

The most common sites of hypertensive haemorrhage are :

1. The ***basal ganglia*** (***putamen***, thalamus and adjacent deep white matter)- ***commonest***
2. *Deep cerebellum*
3. *Pons*

The most common site of hypertensive haemorrhage within basal ganglia is the Putamen.
External capsule refers to a thin layer of white matter that separates the lateral part of lentiform nucleus (putamen) from claustrum and is invariably damaged along with the putamen.

85. Answer is C (Putamen): *Harrison 15th/ 2386; Harrison 16th/2390, 2396; Harrison 17th/2531, 2532; 18th/p 3294*

'The putamen is the most common site for hypertensive haemorrhage' - Harrison's

86. Answer is C (Putamen): *Harrison 15th/ 2386; Harrison 16th/2390, 2396; Harrison 17th/2531, 2532*

The putamen (Basal Ganglia) is the most common site for hypertensive haemorrhage
External capsule refers to a thin layer of white matter that separates the lateral part of lentiform nucleus (putamen) from claustrum and is invariably damaged along with the putamen.

87. Answer is C (Putamen): *Harrison 15th/ 2386; Harrison 16th/2390, 2396; Harrison 17th/2531, 2532; 18th/p 3294*

'*The putamen (basal ganglia) is the most common site of hypertensive haemorrhage'* *– Harrison*

88. Answer is B (Basal ganglia): *Repeat; Harrison 15th/ 2386; 16th/2390, 2396; 17th/2531, 2532; 18th/p 3294*

'*The putamen (basal ganglia) is the most common site of hypertensive haemorrhage'* *– Harrison 16th/2390*

89. Answer is A (Basal ganglia): *Repeat; Harrison 15th/ 2386; Harrison 16th/2390, 2396; 17th/2531, 2532; 18th/p 3294*

'*The putamen (basal ganglia) is the most common site of hypertensive haemorrhage'* *– Harrison 16th/2390*

90. Answer is C (Aneurysm): *Repeat, Harrisons 16th/2387*

'The most common cause of subarachnoid haemorrhage is rupture of a saccular aneurysm (excluding head trauma)' *– Harrison.*

Previously asked frequently as follows: *(Excluding hand trauma)*
Most common cause of subarachnoid haemorrhage is rupture of a saccular aneurysm[Q]
Most common cause of subarachnoid haemorrhage is rupture of a Berry aneurysm[Q]
Most common cause of subarachnoid haemorrhage is rupture of 'Circle of Willis' aneurysm[Q].
(Saccular aneurysms are synonymous with Berry Aneurysms and most commonly occur in the anterior circulation on the Circle of Willis).

91. Answer is C (Aneurysm): *Repeat, Harrisons 16th/2387*

The most common cause of subarachnoid haemorrhage is rupture of a saccular aneurysm
(Saccular aneurysms are synonymous with Berry Aneurysms or 'Circle of Willi's aneurysms' and most commonly occur in the anterior circulation on the Circle of Willis).

92. Answer is C (Berry aneurysm): *Harrison 14th/ 2345; AI-Medicine, 17th/ 1726; 15th/ 2388; 16th/2387, 2388; 18th/ 2262*

Most common cause of "subarachnoid Haemorrhage" is spontaneous rupture [Q] ***of saccular aneurysms*** [Q] ***(excluding trauma).***
Most common cause of "intracerebral Haemorrhage" is *Hypertension* [Q] due to rupture of small *perforating arteries or Arterioles.* [Q]

93. Answer is A (Rupture of circle of Willis aneurysm): *Harrison 15th/ 2388, 2385; 16th/2387,2388; 17th/1726; 18th/2262*

Most common cause of subarachnoid haemorrhage is ruptured saccular aneurysms.
Most common site of saccular aneurysms is the anterior circulation on the circle of Willis

94. Answer is B (Degeneration of tunica media): *Robbins 8th/1297, 1298; Harrison 15th/2388; Harrison 17th/1727; Porth Pathology (2009)/475, 1268*

Berry aneurysms (Saccular aneurysms) are believed to arise from a defect in the tunica media of the involved vessel. Berry aneurysms represent developmental anomalies predisposed by a congenital defect in the media of the involved vessel.

'Saccular aneurysms (Berry aneurysms) develop over time because of an underlying defect in the media of vessel'.
– Robbins 8th/1297

Berry aneurysms represent developmental anomalies predisposed by a congenital defect in the media of the involved vessel

- Berry aneurysms are *saccular in appearance (saccular aneurysms)* presenting as out pouching of the vessel wall involving only a portion of the circumference *(resembles a 'berry' attached to a twig of the arterial tree)*
- Berry aneurysms are rare in childhood but increase in frequency in young adults and middle life. *They are therefore not congenital anomalies but develop over the years from developmental defects of the 'media' of the arterial wall* at the bifurcation of arteries. These may however be predisposed by a congenital defect in the media of the involved vessel.
- *'In the past, most berry aneurysm were thought to be congenital in origin arising from focal defects in the 'media' and gradually developing over the years as arterial pressure, first weakens and subsequently balloons out the vessel wall.* ***Recent studies however suggest that these intracranial aneurysms probably result from hemodynamically induced degenerative vascular injury to the tunica media'.***
- Berry aneurysms *typically occur at branch points in arterial walls* and tend to arise at branch sites within the 'circle of Willis'.
- *About 80-90% of berry aneurysms occur in the anterior circulation on the circle of Willis.*

Location of Berry Aneurysms : (*In order of frequency of occurrence***)**

- *Anterior communicating - Ant. cerebral junction (29%).*
- *Post communicating - Internal carotid junction (28%).*
- *Middle cerebral bifurcation (18%).*
- *Intracranial carotid bifurcation (8%)*
- *Vertebrobasilar* **or basilar bifurcation** (3%)

95. Answer is B (Vertebral artery): *Harrison 15th/ 2388, API 6th/ 759; 16th/2388; Harrison 17th/ 1727; 18th/2262*

About 85% (Harrison) to 90% (Robbins) aneurysms occur in the Anterior circulation, on the circle of Willis.

Posterior circulation as invertebral artery is a very uncommon location for berry aneurysm.

In order of frequency of occurrence the location of

- Anterior communicating - Ant. cerebral junction **(29%).**
- Post communicating - Internal carotid junction (28%).
- Middle cerebral bifurcation (18%).
- Intracranial carotid bifurcation (8%)
- **Vertebrobasilar or basilar bifurcation** (3%)

96. Answer is A (Junction of Anterior communicating artery with Anterior cerebral artery): *Harrison 15th/ 2388; Harrison 16th/2388; Robbin's 6th/ 1311; Harrison 17th/ 1727; Harrison 18th/p 2262*

About 85% (Harrison) to 90% (Robbins) aneurysms occur in the Anterior circulation*, on the circle of Willis. Posterior circulation as invertebral artery is a very uncommon location for berry aneurysm.*

9

Nervous System

97. Answer is A (Posterior Inferior Cerebellar Artery Anurysm): *References with text*

Blood isolated to the fourth ventricle suggets a rupturted Posterior Inferior Cerebellar Artery (PICA) Aneurysm.

'The diagnosis is usually obvious on CT. Blood isolated to the fourth ventricle suggests a ruptured posterior inferior cerebellar artery anurysm' – Plum & Posner's Diagnosis of Stupor & Coma (Oxford) 4th/145

'Subarachnoid Haemorrhage involving blood only from the fourth ventricle is almost diagnostic of Vertebral artery – PICA aneurysm' – Surgery of the Craniovertebral Junction (Thieme) 1998/323

'PICA aneurysm should be suspected when there is little blood in the cisterns supratentorially compared with the cisterna magna, around the brainstem and in the fourth ventricle' – Atlas of Neurosurgical Technique (Thieme) 2006/182

'Ruptured PICA aneurysm almost always coexist with intraventricular haemorrhage in the fourth ventricle and Hydrocephalus' – Intracranial Malformation & Aneurysms (Springer) 2008/189

Posterior Inferior Cerebellar Artery Aneurysm

- Represents 1% to 3% of all intracranial aneurysm
- When a posterior inferior cerebellar artery (PICA) aneurysm ruptures, the patient *may present with hemorrhage isolated to the posterior fossa and/or fourth ventricle*; hemorrhage may extend to the cerebellum.

Most frequent presentation of PICA origin aneurysms

- Subarachnoid haemorrhage (SAH), and
- Intraventricular haemorrhage (4th ventricle), with
- Acute ***Hydrocephalus***.
  (The cerebellum may be involved)

PICA aneurysms lie in the close proximity to the fourth ventricle. Blood from the aneurysms enters the ventricular system (fourth ventricle) through either the foramen of Luschka or Magendie.

- Both PICAs need to be studied in all angiograms performed to rule out an intracranial aneurysm; this can be done by refluxing contrast into the contralateral vertebral artery or by injecting each vertebral artery individually.
- Conventional angiography fails to demonstrate an intracranial aneurysm in 5% of all patients with spontaneous subarachnoid hemorrhage.

Neuroradiology Companion: Methods, Guidelines, and Imaging Fundamentals *by Castillo (Lippincott Williams & Wilkins) 3rd/ 104*

Aneurysms and Vascular Malformations:

Condition	Comments
Anterior communicating artery aneurysm	*Approximately 30% to 35% of intracranial aneurysms.* Rupture results in hemorrhage in the gyrirecti, anterior interhemispheric fissure, septum pellucidum, and frontal horns of the lateral ventricles.
Posterior communicating artery aneurysm	*Approximately 30% to 35% of intracranial aneurysms.* Rupture tends to result in diffuse subarachnoid hemorrhage, but bleeding may be concentrated in the basilar cisterns.
Middle cerebral artery bifurcation aneurysm	*Approximately 20% of intracranial aneurysms.* Rupture results in hemorrhage in the sylvian fissure, frontal opercula and basilar cisterns.
Basilar artery tip aneurysm	*Approximately 5% of intracranial aneurysms.* Rupture results in hemorrhage in the basilar cisterns and posterior position of the third ventricle.
Posterior inferior cerebellar artery aneurysm	*Approximately 1% to 3% of intracranial aneurysms.* ***Rupture may produce hemorrhage isolated to the posterior fossa or fourth ventricle***
Post traumatic aneurysm	*Less than 1% of intracranial aneurysm.* Common sites include the intracavernous portion of the internal carotid artery; the distal part of the anterior cerebral artery; and distal branches of the middle cerebral artery.

CT can predict aneurysm location based on the pattern of blood in ~78% of cases (but mostly for MCA and A-comm aneurysms)

('Clinical Imaging: An Atlas of Differential Diagnosis' by Eisenberg (Lippincott Williams & Wilkins) 5th/1376)

- Blood predominantly in anterior interhemispheric fissure (± blood in lateral ventricles) or within the gyrus rectus suggests a-comm aneurysm
- Blood predominantly in 1 sylvian fissure is compatible with p-comm or MCA aneurysm on that side
- Blood predominantly in the prepontine or penduncular cistern suggets a basilar apex or SCA aneurysm.
- Blood predominantly within ventricles:
  1) Blood primarily in 4th and 3rd ventricle: suggests lower posterior fossa source, such as PICA aneurysm or VA dissection
  2) Blood primarily in the 3rd ventricle suggets a basilar apex aneurysm

98. Answer is B (Vasospasm): *Ref: Harrison 15th/ 2388, Harrison 16th/ 2389; Harrison 17th/ 1727; Harrison 18th/p 2262*

Vasospasm : *Narrowing of the arteries at the base of the brain following SAH occurs regularly. This vasospasm causes symptomatic ischemia and infarction in approximately 30% of patients and* ***is the major cause of delayed morbidity or death.*** *Sign of ischemia appear 4 to 14 days after the haemorrhage, most frequently at about 7 days – Harrisons 16th/ 2309*

Four major causes of delayed neurological deficit
Rerupture
Hydrocephalus
Vasospasm
Hyponatremia

99. Answer is B (Ischemic stroke): *Harrison's 17th/2516, Transient Ischemic Attacks' by Chaturredi (2004)/ 3 ; Hand book of cerebrovascular diseases 2nd/ 32, 33; Harrison 18th/p 3274*

The acute onset of focal neurological defecit in a patient with atrial fibrillation suggest cardioembolic event leading to an ischemic stroke.

Although complete recovery after strokes is unusual, it may be seen in the first few weeks of onset of symptoms, in cases of minor strokes. Such cases with complete recovery are also referred to as cases of ***Reversible Ischemic Neurological defecit or 'RIND'****. Contemprory cross-sectional brain* ***studies have shown these cases of reversible neurological defecit to represent minor ischemic strokes*** *(This terminology is now infrequently used.)*

Transient Ischemic Attacks (TIA's) by definition show complete recovery in less than 24 hours (<24 hrs). Since the defecit of this patient recovered in two weeks, TIA cannot be selected as the answer of choice. 'RIND' is not provided amongst the options, however since cases of 'RIND' have been shown to represent minor ischemic strokes, an 'ischemic stroke' is the single best answer of choice.

Designation	Duration of Defecit
Transient Ischemic Attack (TIA)	Complete recovery in < 24 hours
Reversible Ischemic Neurological Defecit (RIND) (*Represent minor ischemic strokes*)	Complete recovery after 24 hours but < 3 weeks (< 1 week by some) (*There is some controversy regarding the definition of RIND in terms of its end point and some define the end of RIND period as one week*

Reversible Ischemic Neurological Defecit (RIND): Ischemic Stroke with complete Recovery

- Reversible Ischemic Neurological Defecit (RIND) ***refers to an ischemic stroke*** charachterized by a *focal neurological defecit that persist for > 24 hours but clears completely within three weeks* (although some define the end period of RIND as one week).
- RIND lies in the middle of the spectrum of ischemic cerebrovascular syndromes between TIA's at one end and Completed stroke at the other end
- ***Contemporary cross sectional brain imaging studies have shown that cases with 'RIND' represent minor ischemic strokes and this terminology is now infrequently used.***
- *Nevertheless, the existence of this terminology explains that these are cases of ischemic strokes where focal neurological defecit may completely recover in the first few weeks.*

Note: Atrial fibrillation is one of the most common causes of cardioembolic ischemic stroke and cardioembolism is responsible for upto 20% of all Ischemic syndromes

100. Answer is A (Brain): *'Handbook of Clinical Neurology' by Young (Elsevier) /85; 'Fundamentals of Diagnostic Radiology' by Brant & Helms 3rd/73; 'Vascular Neurology: Questions & Answers' (2008) /Q 479 p-266*

The term 'Duret Hemorrhage' is used for all secondary mechanically induced hemorrhages within the brainstem

Nervous System

9

Duret Hemorrhages

- Duret hemorrhages refer to *secondary mechanically induced* hemorrhages *within the brainstem*
- They are believed to result from damage to perforating branches of the basilar artery as a result of mechanical injury during trans-tentorial herniation of brainstem
- Duret hemorrhages are usually found in the ventral and paramedian upper brainstem (mesencephalon & pons) after transtentorial and subfalcine herniations due to supra-tentorial mass lesions
- During transtentorial herniations when the uncus slides under the tentorium, the midbrain is stretched. This ruptures small perforating vessels and produces hemorrhages.
- Duret hemorrhages are typically diagnosed on CT scan on MRI of the brain (as midline lesions) and carry a poor prognosis.

Subarachnoid Haemorrhage

101. Answer is B (Ruptured Aeurysm): *Harrison's 18th/2388, 2389; 87; Harrison's 17th/1726, 1727, 1728; 96; Diagnostic Criteria in Neurology by lerner 1st/13; Current Diagnosis and Treatment in Neurology 1st/126-137*

Presence of sudden onset headache, meningeal signs in the form of neck stiffness and absence of focal neurological deficit suggests the diagnosis of subarachnoid haemorrhage. Presence of blood in sylvian fissure on the CT scan further confirms the diagnosis of SAH.

The most common cause of SAH is rupture of an intracranial saccular aneurysm which is the single best answer of choice.

Subarachnoid Haemarrhage	Intracerebral Haemorrhage (Intraparcnchymal)
Clinical Features	**Clinical Features**
• *Abrupt onset of severe headache or unconsciousness or both usually during activity*	• *Abrupt onset of focal deficit with associated severe headache or unconsciousness or both usually during activity. (Headache occurs in about 50% of pts only).*
• ***Focal Neurological Defecit are usually not present (may be present)***	• *Focal Neurological defects are characteristically present*
• ***Signs of meningeal irritation are prominent (Stiff neck, Kerning's or Brudzinki's sign)***	• *Signs of meningeal irritation are usually not present*
Risk Factors include	**Risk Factors include**
• *Aneurysmal size (most important)* • *Prior aneurysmal SAH* • *Hypertension* • *Smoking* • *Female Sex* • *Oral contraceptive use* • *Psychostimulant use (cocaineQ)* • *Positive Family history* • *Polycystic kidney disease, Marfan's and Ehlers – Donlos syndrome also predispose patients to form intracranial aneurysms*	• *Hypertension (most important)* • *Smoking* • *Alcohol* • *Family history*
CT scan	**CT scan**
*Evidence of **blood in Sylvian fissure** or between the frontal lobes or in the basal cistern or in the cerebral ventricles*	Evidence of intraparenchymal hematoma

102. Answer is C (Aneurysmal subarachnoid hemorrhage): *Harrison 16th/ 2388, 2389; Harrison 17th/ 1727*

The patient is presenting with classical features of a subarachnoid haemorrhage from rupture of saccular (Berry) aneurysms. *'Sudden headache in the absence of focal neurological deficit is the hallmark of aneurysmal rupture'.* Q *Neck stiffness & vomiting are common associations.*

***Focal neurological deficit** according to the area involved is an important characteristic of both hypertensive haemorrhage and in haemorrhage from arteriovenous malformations. Neck stiffness is not seen in either.*

Clinical manifestation of Subarachnoid haemorrhage :

- Sudden transient loss of consciousness (occurs in nearly half of the patients)
- Excruciating severe headache: presenting complaint in 45% of cases (worst headache of patient's life) more common upon regaining consciousness when loss of consciousness is associated
- Neck stiffness & vomiting: are common associations
- Focal neurological deficit: uncommon.

  ***'Sudden headache in the absence of focal neurological deficit is the hallmark of aneurysmal rupture.'** [Q]*
- Associated prodromal symptoms (suggest location of progressively enlarging unruptured aneurysm)
  - Third cranial nerve palsy: aneurysm at junction of PCA & ICA
  - Sxith nerve palsy: aneurysm in cavernous sinus
  - Occipital and posterior cervical pain : inferior cerebellar artery aneurysm (Ant. or Post.)
  - Pain in c behind the eye: MCA aneurysm
- 'Aneurysms may undergo small ruptures or leaks, so called sentinel bleeds.'

Investigations

- Non contrast CT scan: Investigation of choice[Q] (Lumbar puncture is not indicated prior to an imaging procedure)
- CSF picture: The hallmark of aneurysmal rupture is blood in CSF[Q] : Xanthochromic spinal fluid[Q]

  (Lumbar puncture should be performed if the CT scan fails to establish the diagnosis of SAH and no mass lesion or obstructive hydrocephalus is found to establish the presence of subarachnoid blood)

103. Answer is B (Subarachnoid Haemorrhage): *Harrison 14th/ 2345, Harrison 15th/ 2388, Harrison 17th /1727*

Sudden severe headache with altered sensorium indicates haemorrhage as the likely vascular event in this patient.The patient is a non diabetic & non hypertensive, thereby indicating that he has no risk factor to account for the weakening of small perforating vessels, that could lead to their rupture and an intracerebral haemorrhage. The haemorrhage is thus a spontaneous one.

Most likely diagnosis therefore is spontaneous rupture of a saccular aneurysm or 'Subarachnoid H'rrage'.

104. Answer is A (Subarachnoid Hemorrhage): *Harrison's 17th/1727; 'A Guide to Neurological Disorders' (Thieme) 2007/303*

Abrupt onset of severe headache with signs of meningeal irritation including neck stiffness and photophobia is characteristic of subarachnoid hemorrhage.

Typical Clinical Presentation of Aneurismal SAH

- *Sudden (Abrupt), Severe Headache (Worst Headache of life)*
- *Nausea, Vomiting*
- *Photophobia, Neck stiffness (Meningeal Irritation)*
- *Third Nerve Palsy (frequent finding) or other nerve palsies*
- *Loss of consciousness*

105. Answer is A and B (Subarachnoid haemorrhage and Aneurysmal bleed): *Harrison 17th/1726-1728, 95*

Sudden onset excruciating headache is most characteristic of subarachnoid hemorrhage.
SAH most often results from an aneurysmal bleed due to rupture of a saccular or berry aneurysm and hence aneurismal bleeding is also included in the list of options.

106. Answer is B (Aneurysmal subarachnoid hemorrhage): *Repeat*

Thunderclap Headache (sudden onset severe headache reaching maximum intensity < 1 min) together with third cranial nerve palsy and unconsciousness suggest a diagnosis of aneurysmal subarachnoid hemorrhage

Thunderclap Headache *is defined as high intensity headache of abrupt onset that reaches maximum intensity in less than 1 minute. **Subarachnoid hemorrhage is the most common secondary cause of thunderclap headache** although it may be seen with several other conditions including migraine (Thunder clap migraine). The diagnosis is suggested by clues in the history and physical examination. **The presence of an associated third nerve palsy (subarachnoid aneurysm) and unconsciousness following the sudden severe headache suggests a diagnosis of SAH in the above question.***

107. Answer is D (Ruptured aneurysm): *Harrison 15th/ 2388; Harrison 17th/ 1727*

***Severe headache, brief period of unconsciousness** and blood in C.S.F. is a classical feature of **subarachnoid hemorrhage**.*

108. Answer is B (Ruptured aneurysm): *Ref: Harrison 16th/ 2388, 2389; Harrison 17th/ 1727; See previous question*

*This is a case of **subarachnoid hemorrhage** resulting from rupture of a saccular (berry) aneurysm.*

Localization of Stroke: Clinical Features

109. Answer is A (Contralateral foot weakness): *Neuroanatomical bases of clinical neurology (2001)/125*

Paracentral lobule lesions are associated with contra lateral lower extremity weakness and urinary incontinence.

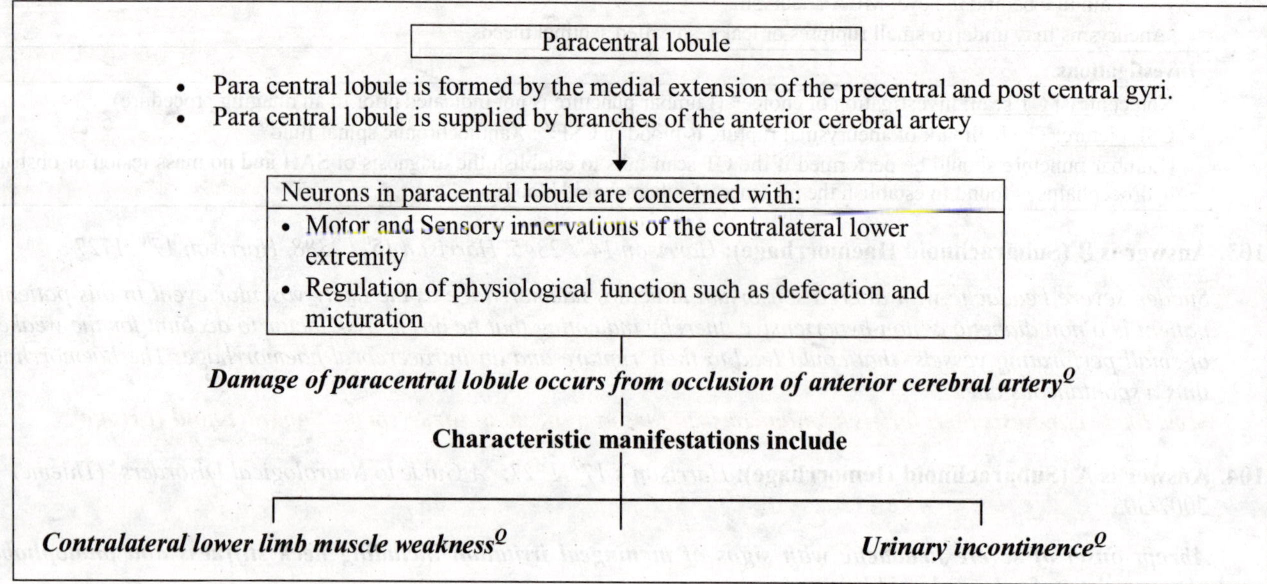

110. Answer is A (Contralateral foot weakness): *Gray's 38th/114; Harrison 17th/2524; Harrison 18th/p 3285*

The paracentral lobule is located on the medial frontal lobe and is involved in anterior cerebral artery occlusion. The involvement of paracentral lobule leads to contralateral lower limb (foot) weakness and urinary incontinence.

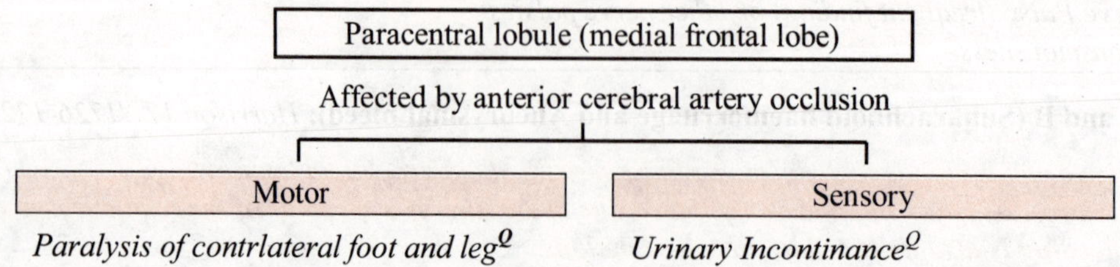

111. Answer is D (Hemi neglect): *Davidson's 20th/1152; Neurology 4th/376*

Hemineglect or neglect of contralateral side is a feature of Parietal lobe lesion (Non dominant hemisphere) and is not a feature of temporal lobe lesion.

Wernicke's Aphasia contralateral superior homonymous quadrantopia and auditory hollucinations are all features of temporal lobe lesions.

Features of Temporal lobe lesions

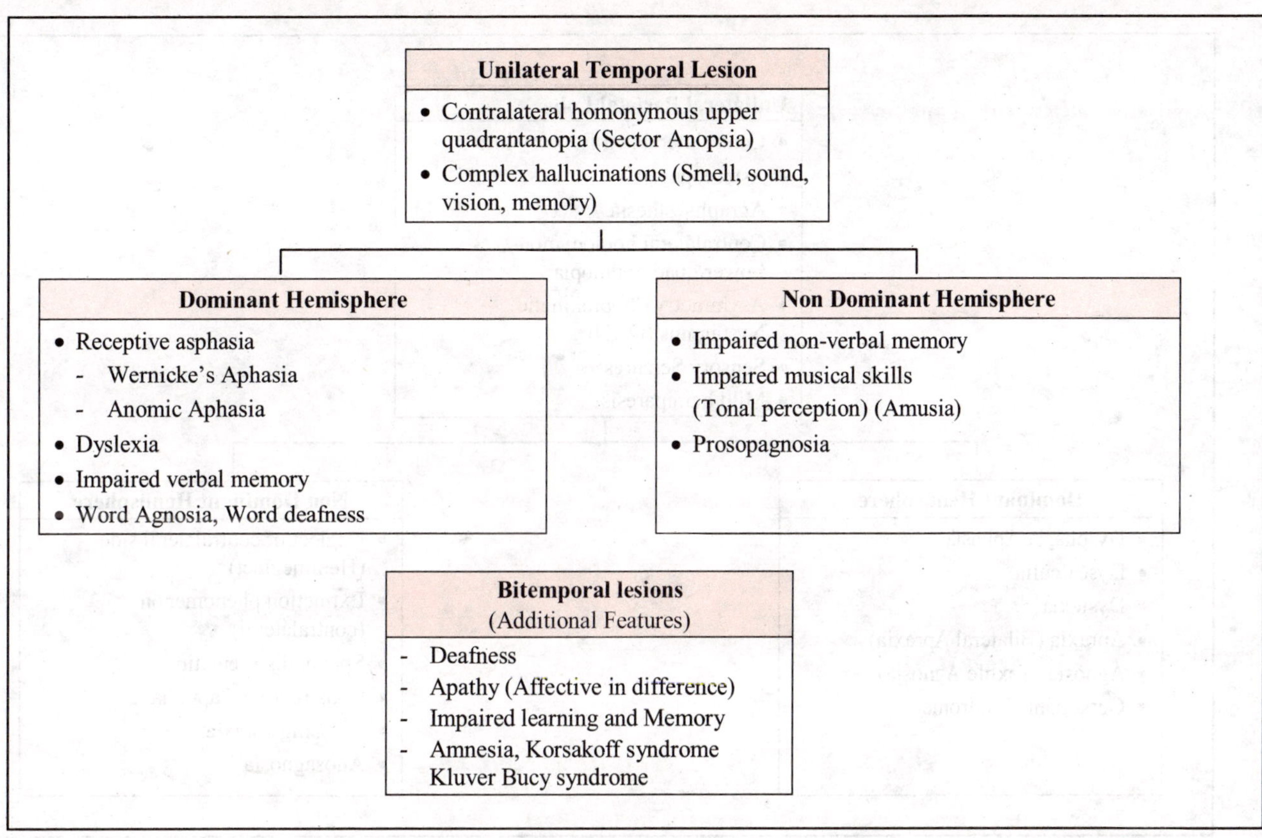

112. Answer is A, B, C (Visual Amnesia, Auditory, Antigrade Amnesia): *Memory 1st (2004)/76, 77*

The medial temporal lobe is most characteristically associated with memory. Unilateral dominant lesions produce disorders of verbal memory (Auditory amnesia). Unilateral nondominant lobe lesions produce disorders of non verbal memory (visual amnesia) and bilateral lesions produce Antegrade amnesia.

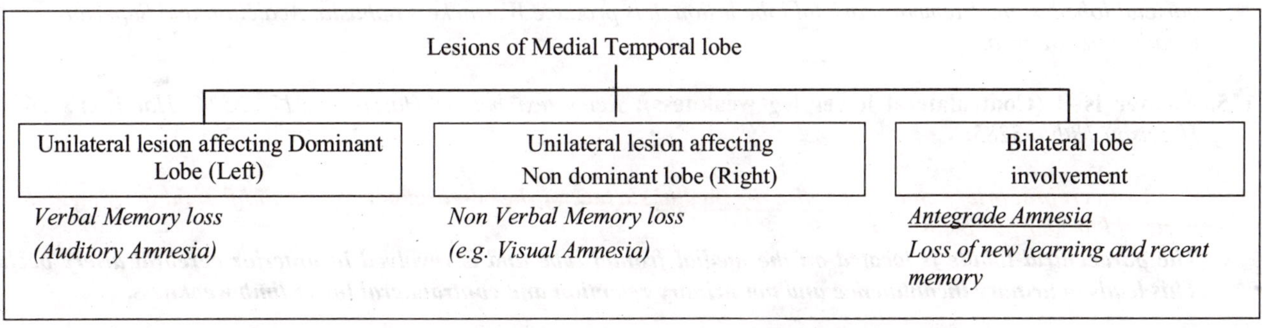

113. Answer is C (Urinary incontinence): *Davidson's 20th/1152; Neurology 4th/376*

Urinary incontinence is a feature of frontal lobe lesion and not parietal lobe lesion.
Aphasia, Acalculia and Inferior quadrantic anopsia are all features of dominant (left) parietal lobe injury.

Features of Parietal lobe lesions

Unilateral Parietal Lobe

- Contralateral hemisensory loss
- Astereognosis
- Agraphaesthesia
- Contralateral homonymous Lower quadrantanopia
- Asymmetry of optokinetic Nystagmus (OKN)
- Sensory Seizures
- Mild hemiparesis

Dominant Hemisphere

- Dysphasia/Aphasia
- Dyscalculia
- Dyslexia
- Apraxia (Bilateral Apraxia)
- Agnosia (Textile Agnosia)
- Gerstmann Syndrome

Non Dominant Hemisphere

- Neglect of contralateral side (Hemineglect)
- Extinction phenomenon (contralateral)
- Spatial disorientation
- Constructional apraxia
- Dressing apraxia
- Anosagnosia

114. Answer is B (Urinary Incontinence): Refer previous question

Urinary incontinence is primarily a feature of frantal lobe lesion.

Wernicke's aphasia and superior quadrantic anopsia are features of temporal lobe lesion and Acalculia is a feature of parietal lobe lesion. A temporoparietal lobe lesion thus produce Wernicke's aphasia, Acalculia and Superior Quadrantic Anopsia.

115. Answer is B (Contralateral lower leg weakness): *Refer text below; Harrison's 17th/2524: Harrison's 16th/2382; Harrison 18th/p 3285*

Anterior cerebral artery chiefly supplies the medial surface of the cerebral cortex (medial frontal lobe, medial parietal lobe, corpus callosum)

The paracentral lobule is located on the medial frontal lobe and is involved in anterior cerebral artery occlusion. This leads to urinary incontinence and not urinary retention and contralateral lower limb weakness.

Hemianaesthesia of opposite side of face is caused by involvement of the lateral surface of sensory cortex in the parietal lobe (middle cerebral Artery)

Hemionopia (Homonymous) is caused by involvement of the occipital lobe (position cerebral Artery).

Anterior Cerebral Artery

Anterior Cerebral Artery supplies the medial surface of the cerebral cortex as far as the parietooccipital sulcus and a strip of about 1 inch wide on the adjoining lateral surface. It also supplies the frontal pole and the corpus callosum.

Paracentral lobule and adjoining sensory motor cortex on the 1 inch wide strip over the lateral hemisphere

- Motor
  - ***Paralysis of contralateral leg and foot***[Q]
- Sensory
  - Cortical sensory loss over toes foot and leg.
  - ***Urinary incontinence***[Q] ***(paracentral lobule)***

Supplemental motor cortex (Medial Surface of posterior frontal lobe)

Reappearance of primitive reflexes that are normally present only in infants

Frontal Reflex Signs
- Grasp Reflex
- Suck Reflex
- Rooting Reflex
- Snout Reflex
- Gegenhalton-Paratonic rigidly

Frontal cortex near the leg motor area

Impairment of gait and stance (Gait Apraxia)

Prefrontal cortex (Frontal Pole) and Uncertain localization

Cognitive and Behavioral impairment
- Abulia (Akinetic mutism)
- Apathy
- Euphoria, Disinhibition or Distractibility
- Slowness, Delay
- Lock of spontaneity

Corpus Callosum

Dyspraxia of left limbs

Tactile Aphasia of left limbs

A lesser degree of paresis of the opposite arm is also seen in lesions of the anterior cerebral artery because fibers descending to corona radiata are involved by deep branches

116. Answer is B (Middle cerebral artery): *Ref: Harrison 16th/ 2381; Harrison 17th/ 2523, 2524, 2525; Harrison 18th/p 3284, 3285*

The sensory motor cortex is located on the lateral surface of the cerebral hemisphere and is supplied by middle cerebral artery. ***Occlusion of the middle cerebral artery thus produces contralateral hemiplegia and contralateral hemisensory loss.***

Middle Cerebral Artery

Middle cerebral Artery supplies most of the lateral aspect of the cerebral hemispheres chiefly of the frontal, parietal and temporal lobes (cortical or superficial branches)

Pure Motor Hemiplegia

Deep branches of the middle cerebral artery or the lenticulostriate branches supply the internal capsule (posterior limb) Motor tracts are densely packed in this region and hence occlusion of deep branches or lenticulostrials branches leads to Dense Hemiplegia / Pure motor Hemiplegia

Frontal lobe	Parietal lobe	Temporal lobe
Lesions affect most of the frontal lobe except the medial aspect is lobule and supplemental Motar area on the medial surface of posterior frontal lobe	Lesions affect most of the Parietal lobe	Lesions affect most of the temporal lobe except the medial temporal lobe

Features	Features	Features
• Contra lateral Hemiparesis primarily involving face and upper limb > lower limb (D/t motor cortex lesion) • Conjugate gaze preference, away from paresis towards the side of lesion (D/t Frontal eye field) • *Broca's Aphasia* *(D/t involvement of Broca's area)* • *Cognitive and Behavioral impairment* *Mutism and Apathy may be associated*	Contralateral hemianaesthesia primarily involving face and upper limb >lower limb (d/t involvement of sensory cortex) (Loss of pain, touch, vibration, joint position, two point discrimination etc) • *Astereognosis* • *Agraphaesthesia* • *Asymmetry of optokinetic nystagmus*	• Hallucinations • Anomic Aphasia • Word Agnosia • Word Deafness

ℓNote that because Paracentral lobule is not involved in middle cerebral artery occlusion there is no associated sphincter disturbance of the bladder and bowel (No urinary incontinence)
Paracentral lobule is supplied by the anterior cerebral Artery

Dominant	Non Dominant
• Aphasia (conduction) • Apraxia • Alexia • Aacalculia • Agnosia • Right to left confusion • Gerstmann syndrome	• Hemineglect of contralateral side • Spatial disorientation • Anosognosia • Constructional and dressing Aprexia • Apractagnosia

ℓNote that memory is not impaired because memory is storedd mainly in the medial part of temporal lobe and hippocampus which is not supplied by the middle cerebral artery.

Visual sings include Contra lateral Homonymous Hemianopia because both superior quadrant (temporal lobe) and inferior quadrant (parietal lobe) is involved.

117. Answer is D (Involvement of anterior limb of internal capsule): *Harrison's 17th/2524; Practical Neuroimaging in Stroke (Saunders, 2009) /44; Harrison 18th/p 3285*

Anterior choroidal artery supplies the posterior limb of Internal capsule (and not anterior limb of internal capsule).

'Anterior choroidal artery arises from the internal carotid artery and supplies the posterior limb of internal capsule. The complete syndrome of anterior choroidal artery occlusion consists of contralateral hemiplegia hemianesthesia (hypoesthesia) and homonymous hemianopia' - Harrison's 17th/2524

Anterior Choroidal Artery Occlusion

Anterior Choroidal Artery arises from the Supraclinoid Internal Carotid Artery

Territories Supplied / Involved (Areas Involved)	Typical Syndrome / Complete Syndrome (Most Common Syndrome)
• ***Posterior Limb of Internal Capsule*** • *Optic Tract* • *Lateral Geniculate Body* • *Cerebral Peduncle* • *Choroid Plexus* **Areas of Perfusion may include** • Medial temporal lobe / uncus • Medial Globus pallidus • Lateral Thalamus • Posterior paraventricular corona radiata region	***Hemiplegia (Contralateral)*** ***Hemianesthesia / Hypoesthesia (Contralateral)*** ***Homonymous Hemianopia (Contralateral)***

118. Answer is A (Aphasia): *Harrison 15th/ 2373, 2374, 2375; Harrison 16th/ 2381; Harrison 17th/ 2523, 2524; Harrison 18th/p 3284*

Aphasia is a manifestation of dominant parietal lobe involvement. *Dominant hemisphere is right handed person is left hemisphere and thus a* ***right middle cerebral artery infarct indicates 'Non Dominant Partial Lobe' involvement. Apahsia will not be a manifestation because an infarction in middle cerebral artery distribution on the right side will affect the non dominant parietal lobe (left parietal lobe).***

Clinical manifestations of Middle cerebral artery involvement

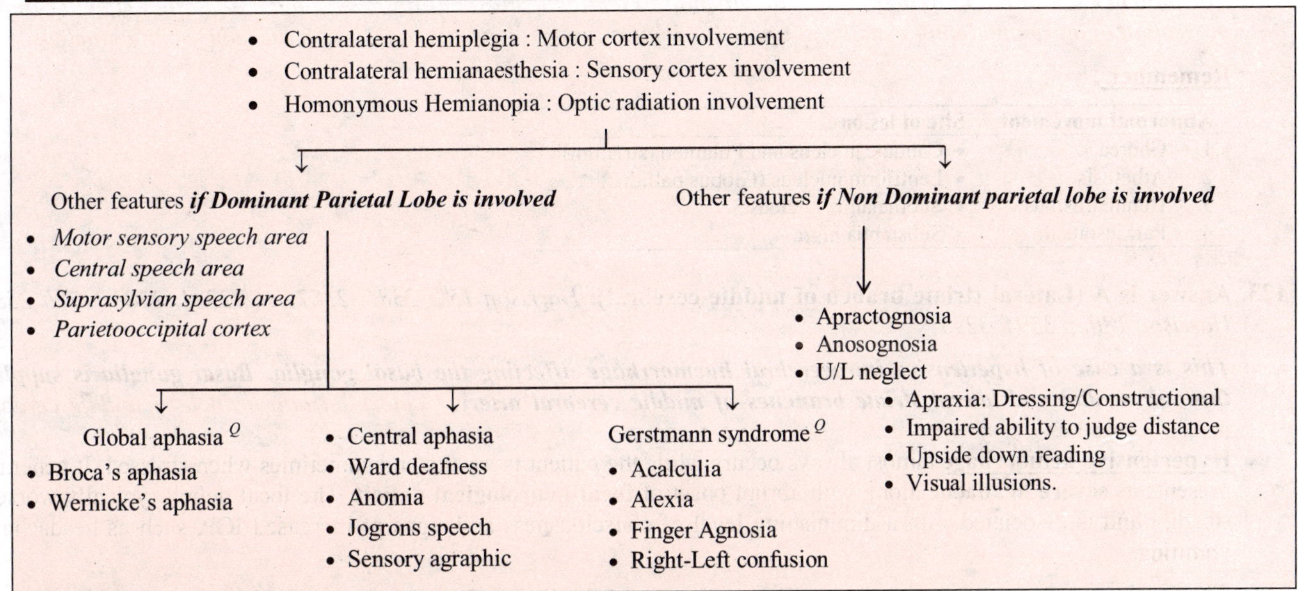

***Dysathria is common because of facial weakness** – Harrisons*

119. Answer is A (Aphasia): *Refer Previous question;*

Right middle cerebral artery supplies the right cerebral hemisphere which is the non dominant hemisphere. Aphasia is a feature of involvement of the dominant hemisphere (Wernicke's area-Temporal lobe) of the dominant hemisphere. A lesion of the non dominant Wernieke's area does not lead to Aphasia.

Note that in up to 95% of all people the dominant hemisphere is the left hemisphere

120. Answer is D (Anterior Cortex) : *Harrison's 17th/2525; Harrison 18th/p 3286, 3287*

Anterior Cortex (Frontal lobe) is not involved in posterior cerebral artery infarct

Posterior Cerebral Artery Infarcts

*The posterior Cerebral Artery supplies the **midbrain**, **thalamus**, lateral geniculate bodies, posterior portion of choroid plexus, occipital lobes, inferior and medial aspect of the **temporal lobe** and posterior inferior areas of the parietal lobe.*

Occlusion of the Posterior Cerebral Artery usually results in two common clinical syndromes depending on the areas involved

P1 Syndrome

Occlusion of the *proximal segment of PCA* from its origin to its union with the posterior communicating artery

P1 syndrome present primarily with the following signs

- ***Midbrain signs***
- ***Thalamic signs***
- *Subthalamic signs*

P2 Syndrome

Occlusion of the *distal segment of PCA* distal to the junction of PCA with the posterior communicating artery

P2 syndrome presents primarily with the following signs

- ***Temporal lobe signs***
- *Occipital lobe signs*

9

Nervous System

9

121. Answer is A (Hippocampal gyrus): *Ref: Harrison 15th/ 2374, Harrison 16th/ 2385; Harrison 17th/ 2526; Harrison 18th/p 3287*

'Medial temporal lobe and Hippocampal involvement may cause an acute disturbance in memory particularly of it occurs in the dominant hemisphere' – Harrisons 16th

122. Answer is D (Subthalmic Nucleus): *Harrison 14th/ 114, 15th/ 125-26; 16th/139; 17th/2563; Harrison 18th/p 3332*

The patient's abnormal movement is 'Hemiballismus'. Hemiballismus manifests as sudden and often violent flinging movement of a proximal limb usually an arm. Hemiballismus develops due to lesion in the subthalamic nucleus.

Remember :

Abnormal movement	Site of lesion
1. Chorea	• Caudate nucleus and Putamen (striatum)
2. Athetosis	• Lentiform nucleus (Globus pallidus)
3. Hemiballismus	• Subthalamic nucleus 3
4. Parkinsonism	• Substantia nigra

123. Answer is A (Lateral striate branch of middle cerebral): *Harrison 15th/ 2386, 2387; 16th/2381, 2383; 17th// 2532; Harrison 18th/p 3294, 3295*

This is a case of hypertensive intracerebral haemorrhage affecting the basal ganglia. Basal ganglia is supplied through medial and lateral striate branches of middle cerebral artery. Lateral striate branch of middle cerebral artery is thus the site of rupture

Hypertensive hemorrhage almost always occurs while the patient is **awake** and sometimes when stressed. It generally presents as **severe headache** along with abrupt onset of **focal neurological deficit**. The focal deficit typically worsens steadily and is associated with a diminishing level of consciousness and signs of increased ICP, such as headache & vomiting.

The focal neurological signs vary according to the site of the hemorrhage

Basal ganglia	Thalamus	Pons	Cerebellum
Arteries involved	Arteries involved	Arteries involved	Arteries involved
Medial & lateral striate branches of Middle cerebral artery.	Perforating branches of posterior cerebral artery	Basilar artery	Cerebellar arteries - Superior cerebellar - Ant. inferior - Post. Inferior
Manifestations	Manifestations	Manifestations	Manifestations
• Contralateral hemiparesis is the sentinel sign • Paralysis may worsen until the affected limbs become flaccid or extend rigidly • When haemorrhage is large signs of brainstem compression may appear - Coma - Cheyne Stokes respiration - Dilated & fixed ipsilateral pupil - Decerebrate rigidity	• Hemisensory loss involving all modalities • Contralateral hemiparesis ***sensory loss > motor loss*** • Several typical ocular disturbances: - down & inward deviation of eyes - unequal pupils with loss of light reflex - skew deviation with eye opp. haemorrhage deviated down and medially - I/L horners syndrome - Absence of convergence - Paralysis of vertical gaze - Retraction nystagmus • Contralateral pain syndrome (Deferne-Roussy syndrome) • Aphasias	• Quadriplegia • Deep coma • Decerebrate rigidity Q • Pinpoint pupil that react to light • Impairment of reflex eye movement on head turning (doll's head or occulocephalic maneuver) • Hyperapnea • Hypertension • Hyperhydrosis	• Occipital headache • Vomiting • Gain ataxia • Dizziness or vertigo • Ocular changes - paresis of conjugate gaze - forced deviation of eyes to opposite side - I/L 6th nerve palsy • Dysarthria • Dysphagia • Stupor & coma if brainstem compression occurs

124. Answer is C (Dyscalculi): *'High yield Neuroanatomy' by Fix 4th/144, 146; 'Lecture Notes in Neurology' by Ginsberg 9th/14, 15, 16; Davidson's 21st/1136;*

Dyscalculi is a feature of categorical/dominant hemisphere involvement or left lobe involvement
Visuospatial defects, Anosognosia and Spatial dysgraphia are all features of non dominant / representative hemisphere involvement or right lobe involvement

Categorical Dominant Hemisphere Lesion (Sequential Analytical Process & Language)	Representative Non-Dominant Hemisphere lesion (Visuospatial processing)

• ***Dysphasia / Aphasia*** *(difficulty with words)*
  - *Expressive / Motor (Braco's)*
  - *Sensory / Receptive (Wernicke's)*
• ***Dyslexia*** *(difficulty with words)*
• ***Dysgraphia*** *(difficulty with drawing)*
• ***Dyscalculia*** *(difficulty with calculations)*
• ***Dyspraxia*** *(difficulty to perform complex motor tasks)*
	• ***Neglect*** of contralateral side
	• ***Spatial disorientation***
	• ***Anosognosia***
	• ***Dressing Apraxia*** *(Apraxia is a misnomer)*
	(Problem results from visuospatial disorientation of body parts to clothing)
	• ***Constructional Apraxia*** (Apraxia is a misnomer)
	(Inability to copy complex shapes due to visuospatial disorientation)
	• ***Astereognosis***
	• ***Afferent Dysgraphia*** *(Spatial Dysgraphias)*
	• ***Impaired musical skills*** (tonal perception)
	• Impaired non-verbal memory

125. Answer is D (Senseless, fluent speech): *Harrison's 17th/164; Ganong 22nd/273*

Senseless fluent speech most closely suggests a diagnosis of Aphasia (Wernicke's aphasia) which results from damage to the categorical or dominant hemisphere

Senseless, fluent speech suggests a diagnosis of 'Wernicke's' Aphasia. Such disorders of speech represent a lesion is the categorical or dominant hemisphere

Cerebral Lateralization

Categorical Hemisphere (Dominant Hemisphere)	Representative Hemisphere (Non-Dominant Hemisphere)

The cerebral hemisphere for:
• Sequential – Analytic process
  - Mathematical calculations
  - Logical decision making
• Language (Aphasias)
  - *Expressive / Motor (Braco's)*
  - *Sensory / Receptive (Wernicke's)*
	The cerebral hemisphere for:
	• Visuo-spatial processing
	  - to identify familiar objects by touch, smell, sight, taste or feel
	• Analyzing the emotional context of a conversion

126. Answer is A (5th Cranial nerve palsy): *Anatomic Basis of Neurologic Diagnosis (Thieme) 2009/272*

5th cranial nerve palsy is not a feature of Millard Gubler Syndrome

Millard Gubler Syndrome *(Ventral Pons Syndrome)*
• *Ipsilateral VIIth Nerve palsy* • *Ipsilateral VIth Nerve Palsy* • *Contralateral Hemiplegia*

Millard-Gubler syndrome

Millard-Gubler syndrome results from a lesion in the ventral pons and presents with the following three charachteristic signs and symptoms:

- **Ipsilateral facial paralysis** (due to interruption of the facial nerve)
- **Ipsilateral lateral rectus palsy** (due to interrusption of the abducens nerve)
- **Contralateral hemiplegia** (due to interruption of the corticospinal tract)

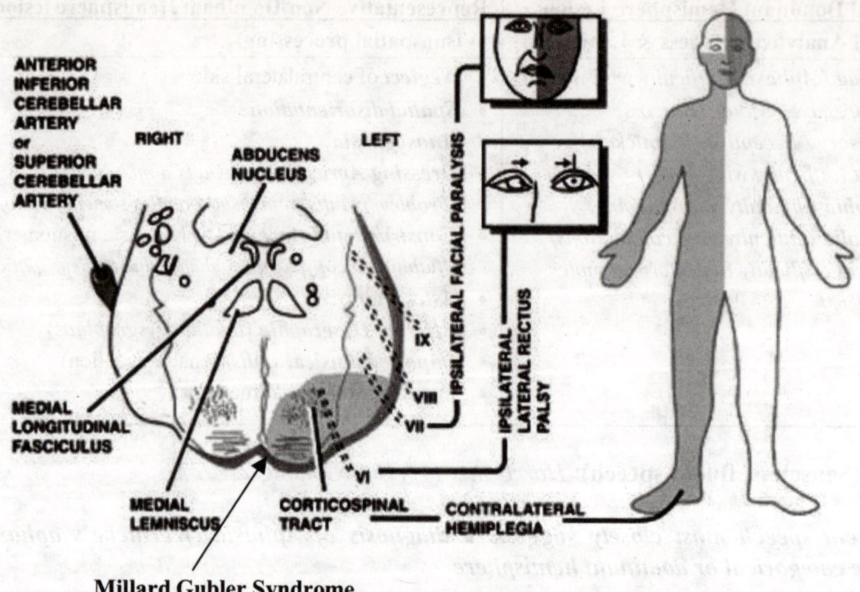

Millard Gubler Syndrome

127. Answer is B (Aneurysm of posterior communicating artery): *Ref: Harrison 16th/ 174; Harrison 17th/ 193; Harrison 18th/p 238*

If the pupil is entirely normal, with all other components of an occulomotor palsy present aneurysm is so rare that an angiogram is seldom indicated. *- Harrison*

Isolated pupil-sparing occulomotor palsy

Most cases are thought to result from microvascular infarction of the nerve. Somewhere along its course from the brainstem to the orbit

Major risk factors are:
• Diabetes • Hypertension • Vascular disease

Major presentation is with pain.
Spontaneous recovery over a period of months is the rule.

128. Answer is A (Occulomotor nerve): *Harrison's 17th/1727; Controversies in Neurological Surgery (Thieme) 2006/79; Hand book of Clinical Neurology' by Toole (Elsevier)/17; Harrison 18th/p 2262*

The occulomotor nerve courses in close relationship to the posterior communicating artery and is frequently compressed by an enlarging aneurysm of the posterior communicating artery

- The occulomotor nerve(III rd C.N) courses through the inter-pedicular cistern in close relationship to the posterior communicating artery
- Growth of an aneurysm may injure the nerve by direct compression or the aneurysm may rupture into the nerve
- The commonest cause of third nerve palsy in cases of SAH is direct compression of the nerve by an enlarging or ruptured aneurysm

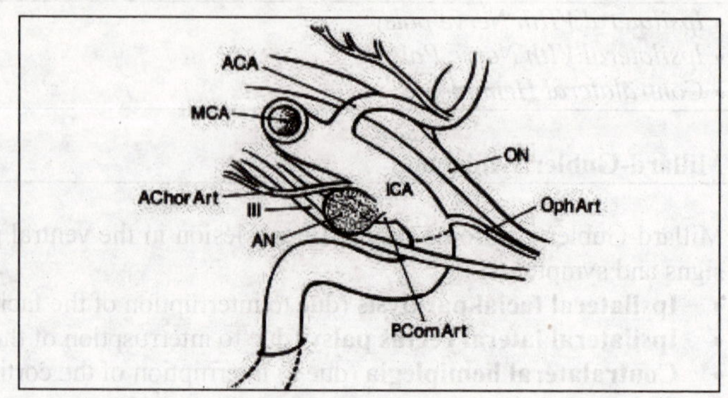

129. Answer is D (Occulomotor nerve): *Harrison 14th/ 2345, Harrison 15th/ 2388; Harrison 16th/2386; Harrison 17th/ 1727; Harrison 18th/p 2262*

Progressively enlarging unruptured aneurysms most commonly involve the occulomotor nerve.
This usually occurs from an expanding aneurysm at junction of post communicating artery and internal carotid artery. Otherwise however, remember : the most common nerve to be involved with raised I.C.T. is the abducent nerve or VIth cranial nerve" (false localizing sign)

130. Answer is C (No noticeable hearing loss or loss of tonal discrimination) : *Otolaryngology: Basic science & Clinical Review (Thieme)2006/354; 'Cognitive Neuroscience' 2010/23*

Unilateral destruction of primary auditory cortex does not cause hearing loss or impaired tonal discrimination because the pathways are bilateral.

Cortical Auditory Areas: Auditory Cortex

- The primary auditory cortex of the human brain is located in the superior portion of the temporal lobe in 'Heschl's gyri'. These gyri are hidden within the sylvian fissure and are not visible on the convexity of the brain.

In the cytoarchitectural map of human brain, primary auditory cortex corresponds to 'Broadman's area' 41 and 42

- Unlike most other sensory systems, in which information from one side of the body projects solely to the contralateral hemisphere, the auditory system is organized so that there are both ipsilateral and contralateral projections from each ear to the brain.

Therefore each auditory cortex (temporal lobe) receives auditory input from both ears.
Auditory information received at right ear (or left ear) projects to both, the left and the right hemisphere.

Damage to Auditory Cortex

Unilateral Damage to Primary Auditory Cortex	Bilateral Damage to Primary Auditory Cortex
Unilateral destruction of primary auditory cortex does not cause hearing loss or impaired tonal discrimination because the pathways are bilateral. *If primary cortex of the right hemisphere is damaged, primary cortex of the left hemisphere can still process sounds from both ears.*	Bilateral distruction of primary auditory cortex causes severe hearing loss and impaired tonal discrimination.

What type of defects may be observed after damage to one auditory cortex

Inactivation of one auditory cortex may induce sound localization defects from the contralateral ear
'Sound localization of sounds that are contralateral to the damaged hemisphere may be impaired'
- Otolaryngology: Basic Science and Clinical Review
'The ability to perceive the location of sound becomes poorer for the contralateral side of space.
- Cognitive Neuroscience

Lacunar infarcts

131. Answer is A (Lipohyalinosis of penetrating arteries): *Harrison 14th/ 2326; Harrison 16th/ 2378; Harrison 17th/ 2519; Harrison 18th/p 3276*

'Lacunar infarcs are small infarcts in deep white matter of hemisphere or brainstem caused as a result of lipohyalinosis of penetrating arteries'

Lacunar infarction (small-vessel stroke):

- The term lacunar infarction refers to infarction following atherothrombotic or lipohyalinotic occlusion of small arteries (30 to 300 μm) in the brain. Occlusion of such small penetrating arteries are now termed as small vessel strokes.
- Lacunar infarcts are not confined to middle carotid artery distributions. The MCA stem, arteries comprising circle of Willis, basilar and vertebral arteries all give to rise to penetrating branches (30μm – 300μm) that penetrate the deep grey and white matter of cerebrum or brain stem.
- Each of these vessels can occlude by
  - Atherothrombotic disease at its origin
  - Development of lipohyalinotic thickening
- Thrombosis of these vessels cause small infarcts referred to as lacunes.
- Hypertension and age are the principal risk factors.

132. Answer is E (Quadriparesis): *Current Diagnosis and Treatment in Neurology 1st/107; Harrison 17th/2519, 2520; Harrison 18th/p 3276, 3278*

Quadriparesis or Quadriplegia are not associated with lacunar infarcts.

Lacunar Infarcts

- Lacunar infarcts are small vessel strokes caused by occlusion of a single penetrating artery that supplies one of the deep structures in brain such as the internal capsule, corona radiate, basal ganglia, thalamus and brainstem.
- These are usually caused by Lipohyalinosis of penetrating arteries from longstanding hypertension, atherosclerosis or diabetes
- Several distinct syndromes are associated with lacunar infarcts.

Distinct clinical syndromes associated with lacunar infarcts.

Clinical Syndrome	Features
Pure motor Hemiparesis	• Most common lacunar syndrome • Results from infarction of contralateral internal capsule (may also be seen with infarcts in corona radiate and pons) • The face, arm and leg are equally affected • There is no sensory loss, homonymous hemianopia, Aphasia or hemineglect
Pure sensory stroke	• Infarction almost always involves the thalamus • Sensory loss is present throughout the contralateral side, but various partial hemisensory syndrome can occur. • Sensation is usually decreased for all sensory modalities, and no other neurologic deficits are present. • Patient often complains of abnormal spontaneous sensation, such as "pins-and-needles" or skin tightness.
Sensorimotor stroke	• Infarcts involve both internal capsule and thalamus
Ataxic Hemiparesis	• Contralateral weakness and limb ataxia • Weakness and ataxia present on the same side with the ataxia usually more severe than the weakness. • Most commonly occurs in the pons, the internal capsule or the corona radiata
Dysarthria Clumsiness Syndrome	• Prominent dysarthria and ataxia of the upper limb • Facial weakness, dysphagia and varying degrees of weakness in the arm and leg • Associated with infarction in the internal capsule or the pons.

133. Answer is E (Quadriplegia): *Refer previous question*

Quadriplegia/Quadriparesis are not associated with lacunar infarcts.

Carotid Stenosis

134. Answer is D (Aspirin reduces risk of TIA): *Harrison 17th/2517, 2520, 2523*

Antiplatelet therapy (including Aspirin) is recommended for medical therapy in patients with asymptomatic carotid stenosis to reduce the risk of TIA's.

Carotid artery stenosis is not common in the External Carotid Artery

Carotid Artery stenosis is common at the bifurcation of the common carotid artery and internal carotid artery. –Harrison

Embolism in the Middle Cerebral Artery does not lead to ipsilateral hemiplegia

Embolic material can dislodge from a plaque at the bifurcation of the common carotid artery and occlude a more distal middle cerebral artery. However such occlusion will lead to contralateral hemiplegia and not ipsilateral hemiplegia.

Bruit does not always indicate the severity of lesion

Bruit may be associated with tight stenotic lesions, but as the stenosis grows tighter and flow distal to the stenosis gets reduced, the bruit becomes fainter and may disappear when complete occlusion is imminent.

135. Answer is A (Doppler flow USG): *Ref: Harrison 15th/ 2237*

'Stenosis at the origin of the internal carotid Artery can be identified and quantified reliably by ultrasonography that combines B mode ultrasound image with a Doppler ultrasound assessment of flow velocity.'

Lateral Medullary Syndrome and other Brain Stem Syndromes

136. Answer is C > B (Vertebral artery > Posterior inferior cerebellar artery): *Ref: Harrison 16th/ 2385; Harrison 17th/ 2526; Harrison 18th/p 3288, 3289*

'Most cases result from ipsilateral vertebral artery occlusion; in the reminder occlusion of posterior inferior cerebellar artery is responsible' *– Harrison*

Vessel occlusion that result in Lateral Medullary syndrome:

- Vertebral (most common)
- Posterior inferior cerebellar (2nd most common)
- Superior, middle or Inferior lateral medullary arteries

Vertebral artery	Posterior inferior cerebellar artery
• The vertebral artery consists of four segments. The fourth segment courses upward to joint the other vertebral artery to form the basilar artery. Only this segment gives rise to branches that supply the brainstem and cerebellum. • Embolic occlusion or thrombosis of the fourth segment is responsible for this syndrome Q	• Posterior inferior cerebellar artery in its proximal part supplies the lateral medulla and in its distal branches the inferior surface of cerebellum

137. Answer is A > B (Vertebral Artery > Posterior Inferior Cerebellar Artery): *Harrison 16th/ 2385; 17th/ 2526*

'Most cases result from ipsilateral vertebral artery occlusion; in the reminder occlusion of posterior inferior cerebellar artery is responsible' *– Harrison*

138. Answer is A, B and C: *Harrison's 17th/2383; Functional Neuronatomy 2nd/99; Harrison 18th/p 3288, 3289*

Posterior Inferior cerebellar Artery (PICA) lesions cause lateral medullary Syndrome or Wallenberg Syndrome

Wallenberg Syndrome involves the spinal tract of trigeminal nerve, tractus solitarus and the spinothalamic tract

Corticospinal tract is not involved in Wallenberg syndrome or lesions of the Posterior Inferior carebullar Artery (PICA)

Structures involved in lateral medullary syndrome or Wallenberg Syndrome (Posterior Inferior Cerebellar Artery lesion)

- *Spinal nucleus of Trigeminal Nerve and it's tract (Vth Nerve)*
- *Vestibular Nuclei (VIII nerve)*
- *Fibres of IXth and Xth nerve*
- *Nucleus Ambiguous (IX, Xth and XIth nerve)*
- *Nucleus tractus solitarus*
- *Descending sympathetic fibres from the cerebellum*
- *Restiform body or Base of inferior cereballar peduncle*
- *Olivocerebellar fibres*
- *Cuneate and Gracilis nuclei*
- *Spinothalamic tract*

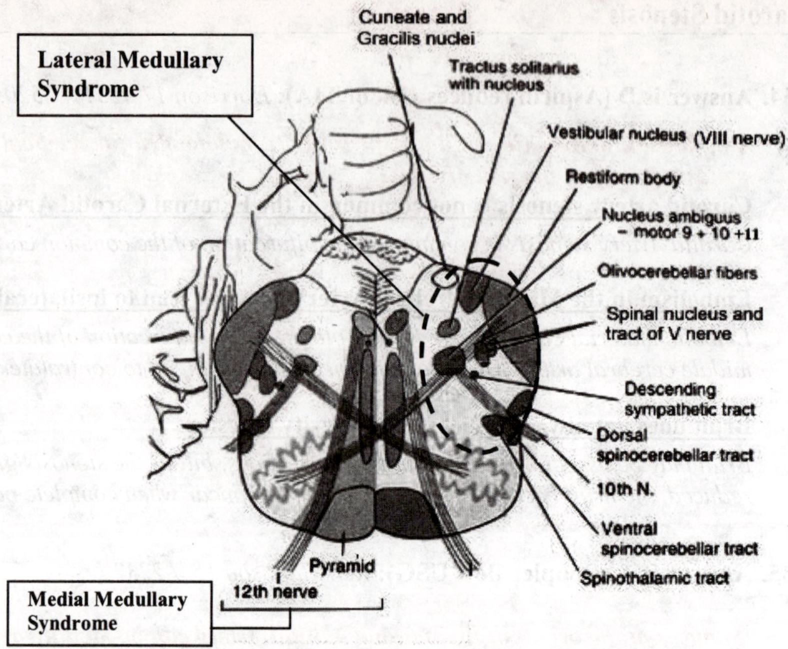

139. Answer is D (XII): *Harrison's 17th/2383; Snell's Neuroanatomy 6th/190; Harrison 18th/p 3288, 3289*

Cranial Nerve XII is involved in medial medullary syndrome and not in lateral medullary syndrome.

Issuing fibres of cranial nerve IX and X are involved directly while cranial part of spinal accessory nerve (XI) may be affected because of the involvement of nucleus ambiguous

Nucleus Ambiguous is involved in Lateral Medullary Wallenberg syndrome

Nucleus ambiguous consists of large motor neurons and is situated deep within the reticular formation.
The emerging nerve fibres joint the glosso pharyngeal (IX), vagus (X) and cranial part of the accessory nerve (XI) and are distributed to voluntary muscles.

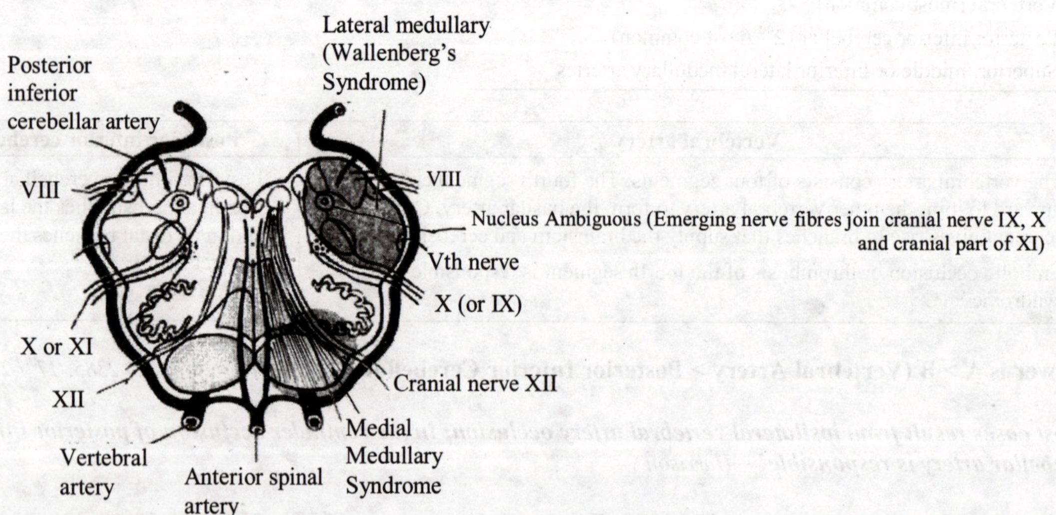

140. Answer is D (XII CN): *Harrison's 17th/2383; Functional Neuronatomy 2nd/99*

Cranial Nerve XII is involved in the Medial medullary syndrome and not in Lateral medullary syndrome.

Lateral Medullary Syndrome involves the spinal nucleus of the trigeminal nerve and its tract (CN V); Vestibular nuclei (CN VIII); Nucleus Ambiguous (IX, X, XI) and fibers of the cranial nerves IX and X.

Cranial Nerves involved in Lateral Mediallary syndrome: V, VIII, IX, X, XI

141. Answer is A (Ipsilateral loss of pain and temperature): *Ref: Harrison 16th/ 2385; Harrison 17th/ 2526, 2527; Harrison 18th/p 3288, 3289*

Pain and temperature sense are lost over opposite side of lesion due to involvement of spinothalamic tract.

Presentation of Wallenberg's syndrome

Symptoms on side of lesion

Symptom	Involved nucleus/tract
• Pain numbness, impaired sensation over half the face	V^{th} n. nucleus
• Nystagmus, diplopia, oscillopsia, vertigo, nausea vomiting	VIIIth n. nucleus
• ***Dysphagia hoarseness, paralysis of palate, paralysis of vocal cord (lower cranial nerve involvement)***	IXth & X^{th}
• Ataxia, fall of side of lesion	Uncertain
• ***Loss of taste***	Nucleus traclus solitarus
• Horner's syndrome	Descending sympathetic tract
• Numbness of ipsilateral arm, trunk & leg	***Cuneate and gracilis nuclei***

Symptoms on side opposite of lesion

Symptom

Impaired pain and thermal sense over half of the body sometimes face

Involved tract

Spinothalamic tract involvement

142. Answer is B (Posterior inferior cerebellar artery): *Ref: Harrison 15th/ 2376, 16th/ 2384, 2385; 17th/ 2526, 2527; Harrison 18th/p 3288, 3289*

The patient in question is presenting with symptoms typical of lateral medullary syndrome or wallenberg syndrome. *Amongst the options provided occlusion of post inferior cerebellar artery is the most common cause of this syndrome.*

'Most cases result from ipsilateral vertebral artery occlusion; in the reminder occlusion of posterior inferior cerebellar artery is responsible' *– Harrison 16th/ 2385*

Vessel occlusion that result in Lateral Medullary syndrome:
- Vertebral (most common)
- Posterior inferior cerebellar (2nd most common)
- Superior, middle or Inferior lateral medullary arteries

Lateral medullary syndrome (Wallenberg syndrome):
• Vertigo
• Numbness of ipsilateral face and contralateral limbs
• Diplopia
• Dysphagia
• Dysarthria
• Ataxia
• Hoarseness
• Ipsilateral Horner's syndrome

143. Answer is D (Horner's syndrome is rare): *Ref: Harrison 16th/ 2385; Harrison 17th/ 2526; Harrison 18th/p 3288*

Horner's syndrome forms part of the constellation of manifestations seen in lateral medullary syndrome or Wallenberg syndrome. It is produced as a result of infarction of the descending sympathetic tract.

144. Answer is B and C (Horner's syndrome and Ipsilateral 12th nerve palsy): *Harrison's 17th/2383; Functional Neuroanatomy 2nd/99; Harrison 18th/p 3288, 3289*

Ipsilateral 12th nerve palsy and contralateral pyramidal tract signs (paralysis) are features of medial medullary syndrome.

Ipsilateral Horner's Syndrome and Ipsilateral numbness of arm and trunk are characteristic features of lateral medullary syndrome and are not seen in medial medullary syndrome.

Medial Medullary Syndrome (Dejerine's Anterior Bulbar Syndrome)

- The medial medullary syndrome is caused by occlusion of the anterior spinal artery or the paramedian branches of the vertebral artery.
- The affected area usually includes the following structures:
  - Medial lemniscus
  - Pyramid
  - Rootlets of the hypoglossal nerve or its nucleus within the medulla
- The neurologic signs resulting from the involvement of these areas are as follows:
  - Contralateral loss of kinesthesia and discriminative touch resulting from involvement of the medial lemniscus.
  - Contralateral paralysis, of the upper motor neuron type (weakness, hyperactive reflexes, Babinskis sign, clonus, and spasticity) with sparing of the face caused by involvement of the pyramid
  - Lower motor neuron paralysis of the homolateral half of the tongue (weakness, atrophy, and fibrillation) and deviation of the protruded tongue to the atrophic side caused by involvement of the hypoglossal nucleus or nerve

The medial medullary syndrome may occur bilaterally resulting in bilateral upper motor neuron weakness or paralysis (with facial sparing), bilateral paralysis of the tongue of the lower motor neuron type, and bilateral loss of kinesthesia and discriminative touch.

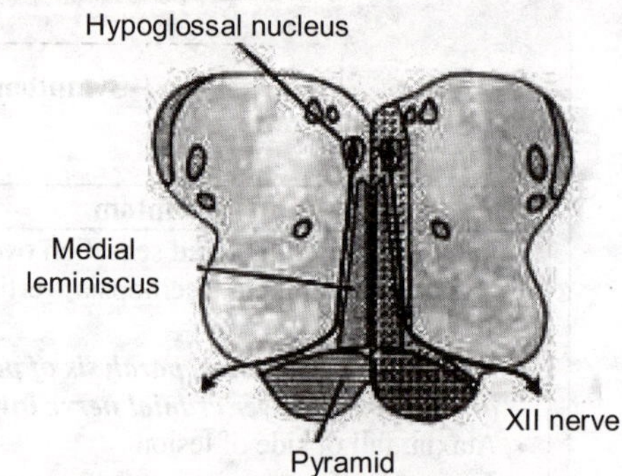

Medial Medullary Syndrome
- Paralysis of homolateral half of tongue (lower motor neuron type)
- Contralateral paralysis (upper motor neuron type)
- Contralateral loss of kinesthesia and discriminative touch

---

145. Answer is D (Contralateral paralysis): *Harrison's 17th/2383; Refer previous question; Harrison 18th/p 3288, 3289*

Contralateral paralysis is a feature of medial medullary syndrome due to involvement of pyramidal tract.

Ipsilateral numbness of face and trunk, lpsilateral horner's syndrome and Ipsilateral Ataxia are characteristic features of lateral medullary syndrome and not medial medullary syndrome.

146. Answer is D (Ipsilateral facial nerve palsy): *Handbook of Neurology by Oishi (World Scientific) 1997/80*

Weber's syndrome is 'midbrain' syndrome charachterized by Ipsilateral Occulomotor Nerve Palsy (Opthalmoplegia / Diplopia) and Contralateral Hemiplegia.

Midbrain Syndromes

	Symptoms and Signs	Structures involved
Weber's syndrome	• ***Ipsilateral oculomotor nerve palsy*** • ***Contralateral hemiplegia including face***	• *Oculomotor nerve* • *Corticospinal and corticobulbar tracts*
Benedikt's syndrome	• Ipsilateral oculomotor nerve palsy • Contralateral hemiparesis including face • Contralateral intention tremor	• Oculomotor nerve • Corticospinal and corticobulbar tracts • Red nucleus
Claude's syndrome	• Ipsilateral oculomotor nerve palsy • Contralateral hemiataxia and hemiasynergia	• Oculomotor nerve • Red nucleus and brachium conjunctivum
Parinaud's syndrome	• Bilateral vertical palsy • Bilateral paralysis of convergence	• Superior colliculus • Superior colliculus

147. Answer is D (Lesion at the level of the pons): *Harrison 16th / 174; Harrison 17th/ 193; Neurology secrets 4th / 138; Harrison 18th/p 238*

Benedict's syndrome also known as dorsal mid brain syndrome results from a lesion in the midbrain tegmentum / red nucleus. It is not a pontine syndrome.

In benedict's syndrome injury to the ***red nucleus*** midbrain results in ***ipsilateral occulomotor palsy*** and ***contralateral tremor ,chorea and athetosis.*** *– Harrison 16th 174*

Benedikt's syndrome / Dorsal midbrain syndrome
• The dorsal midbrain syndrome or Benedikt's syndrome results from a lesion in the red nucleus or tempmentum of midbrain. • It is caused by occlusion of the paramedian / penetrating branches of the basilar or posterior cerebral artery or both.
Signs include
• Ipsilateral occulomotor paresis / ptosis and dilated pupil (damage to fascicle of 3rd CN including parasympathetic fibres) • Contralteral involuntary movement – tremor , chorea , athetosis (damage to red nucleus interrupts fibers from opposite cerebellar hemisphere) • Contralateral hemiparesis may be present if lesion extends ventrally (damage to descending corticospinal tract) • Contralateral hemianaesthesia may be present if lesion extends laterally (damge to spinothalamic tract and medial meniscus)

Other Midbrain syndromes in association with injury to fascicle / nucleus of CN III: *Harrison 17th/ 193*

Weber's syndrome *(Injury to cerebral peduncle)*	***Nothnagel's syndrome*** *(Injury to superior cerebellar peduncle)*	***Claude's syndrome*** *(Injury to red nucleus + superior cerebellar peduncle)*
• Ipsilateral occulomotor palsy • Contralatral hemiparesis	• Ipsilateral occulomotor palsy. • Contralatral cerebellar ataxia	• Ipsilateral occulomotor pasly • Contralateral cerebellar ataxia tremor, chorea, athetosis (Benedikt's + nothnogel's)

148. Answer is A (5th nerve palsy): *Harrison 16th / 175; Harrison 17th/ 193; Harrison 18th/p 239*

5th cranial nerve palsy is not a feature of Millard Gubler syndrome.

Millard Gubler syndrome from ventral pontine injury is associated with lateral rectus weakness(6th CN Involvement), ipsilateral facial palsy (7th nerve palsy) and contralateral hemiparesis. – Harrison 16th / 175

Pontine syndromes

Ventral pontine syndrome (Millard Gubler syndrome)	***Lower dorsal pontine syndrome (Foville's syndrome)***	***Upper dorsal pontine syndrome (Raymond Ceston syndrome)***
Caused by paramedian infarction of pons	*Caused by lesion in dorsal tegmentum of lower pons*	*Caused by obstruction of long circumferential branches of basilar artery*

Millard Gubler syndrome	**Faville's syndrome**
▪ Ipsilateral paresis of lateral rectus with diplopia (damage to abducent fasciculus / nucleus spared)	▪ Ipsilateral horizontal gaze palsy (damage to nucleus of abducent nerve and paramedian pontine reticular formation.)
▪ Ipsilateral paresis of upper and lower face (damage to 7th cranial nerve)	▪ Ipsilateral paresis of whole face (damage to nucleus and fibers of 7th nerve)
▪ Contralateral hemiplegia with sparing of contralateral face (damage to corticospinal tract)	▪ Contralateral hemiplegia with sparing of Contralateral face (damage to corticospinal tract)

Raymond Ceston syndrome / Upper dorsal pontine syndrome

Caused by obstruction of long circumferential branches of basilar artery and results in :

- Ipsilateral ataxia and coarse intention tremor (damage to superior and middle cerebellar peduncle)
- Ipsilateral paralysis of muscles of mastication and sensory loss in face. (damage to sensory and motor nuclei and tracts of CN V)
- Contralateral loss of sensory modalities in the body (damage to spinothalamic tract and medial leminiscus)
- Contralateral hemiparesis of face and body (damage to corticospinal tract) may occur with ventral extension of lesion.
- Horizontal gaze palsy may occur (as in lower dorsal pontine syndrome)

Locked – In – syndrome: Bilateral ventral pontine lesion

(Able to communicate only by vertical eye movement and blinking but otherwise is completely immobile)

- Occurs in patients will bilateral ventral pontine lesion[Q].
- Its most common cause is pontine infarction.
- Patient
  - Is quadriplegic (bilateral damage to corticospinal tract in ventral pons
  - Is unable to speak and incapable of facial movements (involvement of corticobulbar tracts)
  - Has limited Horizontal eye movements (bilateral involvement of nucleiand fibres of 6th CN)
  - Has intact vertical eye movements and blinking (supranuclear ocular motor pathways are spared)
  - Has preserved consciousness (reticular formation is not damaged)

149. Answer is C (Vagal palsy) :*Harrison 16th / 1630, 239; Harrison 17th/ 2528, 2529, 2530;*

Vagal palsy is not a recognized feature of pontine stroke

Features of pontine stroke

- Sudden onset
- Deep coma with ***quadriplegia*** (usually occurs over a few minutes)
- ***Pinpoint pupils*** (1mm pupils) that react to light.
- Loss of reflex eye movements and corneal responses (There is impairment of reflex horizontal eye movements evoked by head turning i.e doll's head or oculocephalic maneuver or by irrigation of the ears with ice water).
- Decerebrate rigidity / Posturing
- Hyperpnea / Hyperventilation
- Severe Hypertension
- Ocular bobbing
- Excessive Sweating / Hyperhidrosis
- ***Hyperpyrexia,*** (*Neurology Secrets 4th Ed.*)

Hyperpyrexia and intracerebral haemorrhage ; Harrison 16th / 164

- *A fever of > 41.5^{0}C (>1067^{0}F) is called hyperpyrexia.*
- This extraordinary high fever can develop in patients with severe infections, but ***most commonly occurs in patients with central nervous system (CNS) haemorrhages.***

Others

150. Answer is A (Tissue plasminogen activator): *Harrison 15th/ 2382, 2383; Harrison 16th/ 2374; Harrison 17th/ 2515; Harrison 18th/p 3272, 3273*

Recombinant Tissue plasminogen Activator (RtPA) is the only thrombolytic agent that is approved for the treatment of acute ischaemic stroke

The use of all other thrombolytics except Recombinant Tissue plasminogen activator has been stopped because of associated high rates of intracranial hemorrhage.

'The National Institute of Neurological disorders and recombinant tPA stroke study showed a clear benefit of intravenous rtPA in selected patients with Acute stroke' *– Harrisons 16th/ 2374*

The use of thrombolysis has always been an issue of controversy in the management of ischaemic strokes. The theoretical advantage of these agents in clearing arterial occlusions has to be weighed against the risk of intracranial haemorrhage.

'Despite an increased incidence of symptomatic intracerebral bleed, treatment with intravenous rtPA within 3 hours of onset of ischaemic stroke improved clinical outcome' *– Harrison 17th/ 2515.*

Guidelines of administration of intravenous recombinant tPA for acute ischaemic stroke

Indications	Contraindications
• Clinical diagnosis of stroke • Onset of symptoms to time of drug administration ≤ 3 h • CT scan showing no hemorrhage or edema of > 1/3 of the MCA territory. • Age ≥ 8 years • Consent by patient or surrogate	• Sustained BP > 185/110 despite treatment • Platelets < 100,000; • HCT < 25%; glucose < 50 or > 400 mg/dL. • Use of heparin within 48 h and prolonged PTT, or elevated INR. • Rapidly improving symptoms • Prior stroke or head injury within 3 months; prior intracranial hemorrhage. • Major surgery in preceding 14 days • Minor stroke symptoms • Gastrointestinal bleeding in preceding 21 days. • Recent myocardial infarction • Coma or stupor.

151. Answer is A (Tissue plasmiogen Activator): *Harrison's 17th/2515; Harrison's 16th/2374; Harrison 18th/p 3272, 3273*

Recombinant Tissue plasminogen Activator (RtPA) is the only thrombolytic agent that is approved for the treatment of acute ischaemic stroke

The use of all other thrombolytics except Recombinant Tissue plasminogen activator has been stopped because of associated high rates of intracranial hemorrhage.

152. Answer is A (Phenylpropanolamine): *KDT 5th/115*

'Many reports associating PPA use for weight loss with haemorrhagic stroke amongst women appeared in USA.
-KDT 5th/115

None of the other agents has been mentioned to be associated with any risk of haemorrhagic stroke.

Phenylpropanolamine

- *Chemically and pharmacologically similar to ephedrine*
- *Used in oral cold/decongesant combination remedies*
- *Used as an apetitic suppressant[Q]*

PPA and Haemorrhagic stroke: 'Haemorrhagic stroke Project':

- *Many reports associating PPA use for weight loss with haemorhagic stroke appeared in USA.*
- *A case control study 'Haemorrhagic Stroke Project' was undertaken. Study showed only a marginally increased risk, but also revealed a strong association when 3 day exposure preceding stroke was considered.*
- *The FDA has concluded that indications for which PPA is used do not warrant the excess risk (though marginal) and has recommended discontinuation of PPA containing products.*

Seizures and Epilepsy

153. Answer is C (Petitmal epilepsy): *Harrison 16th/ 2357, 15th/ 2354; Harrison 2498, 2499; Harrison 18th/p 3251, 3252*

Absence seizures are synonymous with Petitmal epilepsy

Classification of seizures:

Partial seizures	Primarily generalized seizures	Unclassified seizures
• Simple partial seizures (with motor, sensory, autonomic, or psychic signs) • Complex partial seizures • Partial seizures with secondary generalization	• Absence (petitmal) • Tonic-clonic (grand mal) • Tonic • Atonic • Myoclonic	• Neonatal seizures • Infantile spasms

154. Answer is A (3 Hz spike and wave): *CMDT 2002/ 1006; Harrison 16th/ 2358; Harrison 2499; Harrison 18th/p 3252*

EEG in absence seizures shows bursts of bilaterally synchronous and symmetric 3 Hz spike and wave activity.

Characteristic features of Absence seizures / Petitmal seizures:

Clinical Hallmarks
• Almost always begin in childhood and cease by age of 20. • Sudden brief lapses of consciousness without loss of postural control • Seizure typically lasts only for seconds. Impairment is so brief that patient may be unaware of it. • Consciousness returns as suddenly as it was lost i.e. Inset and termination of attack, both are abrupt. • Usually accompanied by subtle bilateral motor signs such as - Rapid blinking of eye lids - Chewing movements - Small amplitude, clonic movements of hands • There is no postictal confusion • The seizure can occur hundreds of times per day. • First clued to absence seizure is often unexplained 'day dreaming' and a decline in school performance recognized by a teacher.
Electrophysiological hallmark
• Electrophysiological hallmark of typical absence seizure is a generalized symmetric, 3 Hz spike and wave discharge that begins and ends suddenly superimposed on a normal EEG background. • Hyperventilation tends to provoke these electrographic discharges and even the seizures themselves.

155. Answer is B (Absence seizures): *Nelson's 18th/2462, Pediatric Epilepsy 3rd/329,330, 175;*

Presence of multiple short episodes of vacant stare (absence) in an otherwise normal child with no history of aura or postictal confusion suggests the diagnosis of typical absence seizures.

Absence seizures versus Day dreaming

Absence seizures can easily be confused with episodes day dreaming however there are certain clues that can help differentiate these two conditions

- Day dreaming is usually not associated with automatism while automatism is common in seizures.
- Day dreaming *can often be 'broken' with stimulation while seizures can usually not be 'broken'.*
- Day dreaming usually *occurs when child is tired /bored or involved in a monotonous activity but seizures can start abruptly at any time (for example in the middle of a sentence).*

Abrupt onset of vacant episodes and the fact that the child remains unresponsive during the episode (cannot be broken) favours a diagnosis of absence seizures in this child.

Absence seizures versus complex partial seizures

Complex partial seizures are frequently associated with aura and postictal confusion. Absence of these features favours a diagnosis of 'Absence seizures'

Absence seizures must primarily be differentiated from complex partial seizures and Day dreaming

Clinical data	Absence	Complex partial	Daydreaming
Frequency/day	***Multiple***	***Rarely over 1-2***	***Mutiple; situation-dependent***
Duration	*Frequently < 10 sec (Rarely longer than 30 sec)*	*Average duration ober 1 min, 10 sec*	*Seconds to minutes; rarely more rarely less*
Aura	***Never***	***Frequently***	***No***
Eye blinking	*Common*	*Occasionally*	*No*
Automatism	*Common*	*Frequently*	*No*
Postictal impairment	***None***	***Frequently***	***No***
Seizures activated by			
Hyperventilation	*Very frequently*	*Occassionally*	*No*
Photic	*Frequently*	*Rarely*	*No*
EEG			
Ictal	*Generalized spike and wave*	*Usually unilateral or bilateral temporal frontal discharges*	*Normal*
Interictal	*Usually normal*	*Variable; may be spikes or sharp waves in frontal or temporal lobes*	*Normal*

156. Answer is C (Postictal confusion): *Harrison's 17th/2499; Harrison's 16th/2357, 2358; CMDT 2008/843; Current Diagnosis and treatment in Neurology 1st/51; Refer previous question; Harrison 18th/p 3252*

Absence of postictal confusion is characteristic of Absence Seizures

Absence seizures are usually seen in childhood, are precipitated by hyperventilation and a 3 Hz spike and wave discharge on EEG is the Electrophysiological hallmark of absence seizures.

157. Answer is C (Automatism): *Harrison 15th 2356; 16th/2359; 17th/ 2500; Harrison 18th/p 3253*

Automatism is not seen in Juvenile myoclonic epilepsy

Juvenile myoclonic epilepsy is an epilepsy syndrome. Epilepsy syndromes are disorders in which epilepsy is a predominant feature and there is sufficient evidence to suggest a common underlying mechanism.

It is characterized by:

- Appearance in early adolescence
- Bilateral myoclonic jerks that may be single or repetitive
- Most frequent in morning after awakening
- Can be provoked by sleep deprivation
- Consciousness is usually preserved unless myoclonus is specially severe
- Association with generalized tonic-clonic seizures and absence seizure is seen
- Benign condition although complete remission is uncommon
- Seizure responds well to appropriate anticonvulsant medication
- Family history of epilepsy is common
- Treatment is with valproate [Q]

158. Answer is A (Focal seizures): *Harrison 17th/2500; Nelson 18th/242; Harrison 18th/p 3253*

Juvenile Myoclonic epilepsy is a generalized seizure disorder and not a focal seizure disorder

Juvenile Myoclonic Epilepsy

- ***It is a generalized seizure disorder***
- Typically seen in the juvenile age group (12-18 years)
- Seizures include generalized myoclonic seizures, generalized tonic clonic seizures and absence seizures
  - ***Myoclonic seizures (most frequent in the morning)***
  - *Tonic clonic seizures (seen in upto 90% of patients)*
  - *Absence seizures (in about one third of patients)*
- Consciousness is usually preserved.
- Typical EEG shows a 4-6 seconds irregular ***spike and wave pattern*** (this is enhanced by a stimulation)
- Condition is considered benign but complete remission is uncommon
- ***Valproic acid is the drug of choice in Juvenile Myoclonic epilepsy***
  'Majority ofpatients respond dramatically to valproate – Nelson.

159. Answer is A (SSPE): *Harrison 17th/2635; Nelson 18th/1335; Harrison 18th/p 3428*

Subacute sclerosing Panencephalitis is characteristically associated with myoclonic jerks or seizures.

'The hallmark of second stage of SSPE is massive myoclonus.' – Nelson 18th/1335

Subacute Sclerosing Panencephalitis (SSPE)

- SSPE is a chronic complication of measles with a delayed onset and an outcome that is nearly always fatal
- This is considered a 'slow virus infection' and is believed to result from persistant infection with an altered measles virus that is harboured intracellularly in CNS for several years.

Stage I (initial stage)	:	Subacute changes in behaviour or school performance including irritability, reduced attention, temper outbursts.
Stage II (Second stage)	:	Outbursts believed to result from extension of inflammatory process to deeper structures in the brain ***Massive Myoclonus is the hallmark of this stage.*** ***Involuntary movements and repetitive mycoclonic jerks are seen*** Consciousness is maintained
Stage III (Third state)	:	Believed to result from damage/destruction of deeper centres in blood ganglia Involuntary movements disappears and are replaced by choreoathetosis, immobility, dystonia and lead pipe rigidity. Sensorium deteriorates and dementia, stupor or coma may be seen.
Stage IV (Final stage)	:	Believed to result from damage to critical centres in the brain that support breathing, heart rate & blood pressure Death soon ensues

160. Answer is C (Carbamezapine): *Current Management in Child Neurology 4th/127,163; Goodman & Gillman's Manual of Pharmacology.*

Carbamezapine is not indicated in the treatment of Juvenile Myoclonic Epilepsy. Carbamezapine (and phenytoin) may aggravate myoclonus in juvenile myoclonic epilepsy.

Antiepileptic Drugs in the treatment sequence of Juvenile Myoclonic Epilepsy (JME)	
First choice	*Valproate, Lamotrigine*
Second choice	*Levetivacetam, Clonazepam*
Consider	*Topiramate, Zonisamide, Pnenobarbitol, Primidone* *(Felbamate may also be effective againts JME)*

Taken from 'Current Management in Child Neurology' by Maria 4th/127, 163

Note
Carbamezapine[Q] and Phenytoin[Q] may aggravate myoclonus in juvenile myoclonic epilepsy.

161. Answer is C (Within several weeks to months often head injury): *Textbook of Traumatic Brain Injury (2008)/309; Brain Injury Medicine (2006)/306*

The term post traumatic epilepsy should be used if seizures occur after first week post injury (within several weeks to months) and are recurrent

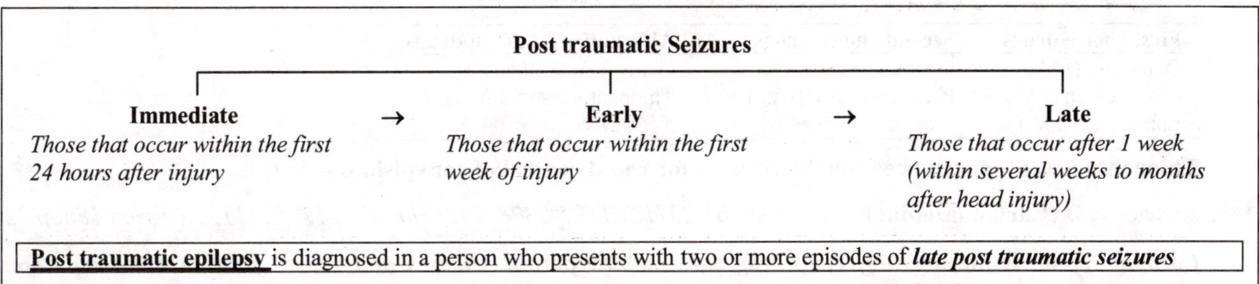

Post traumatic epilepsy is diagnosed in a person who presents with two or more episodes of ***late post traumatic seizures***

162. Answer is C (Subtle seizure): *Manual of Neonatal Care by Cloherty 6th/484.*

'Subtle seizures are the most common sub-type, comprising about half of all seizures in term and premature new borns' *- Cloherty*

Subtypes of Neonatal Seizures
1. **Subtle (commonest subtype)**
2. *Clonic (Focal /Multifocal)*
3. *Tonic (Focal / Generalized)*
4. *Myoclonic (Focal / Multifocal / Generalized)*

163. Answer is B or None (Early age of onset or None) : *Nelson's 18th/2458, Blueprints Pediatrics 5th/238, Pediatric Secrets 4th (2005)/486*

Early age of onset is the single best answer by exclusion.

Complex febrile seizures, Neurodevelopmental abnormalities and Positive family history of epilepsy are the three major risk factors for future epilepsy after febrile seizures.

Early age of onset (before 12 months of age) is accepted as an adverse risk factor for future epilepsy however this has not been included as a major risk factor in certain standard textbooks and hence is the single best answer by exclusion.

Adverse Risk Factors for Developing later 'Epilepsy' after Febrile Seizures

Three Major Risk Factors (Blueprints Pediatrics / Pediatric secrets)	**Additional Factors**
• *Complex Febrile seizures* - *Focal seizures* - *Prolonged (≥15min)* - *Repetitive (Recur within 24 hours)* • *Preexisting Neurodevelopmental abnormalities* - *Neurological Disorder* - *Developmental Delay* • *Close Family History of Epilepsy* - *Epilepsy in first degree relatives/ siblings*	• *History of first seizure under age of 1 year (Before 12 months of age)* • *Short duration of fever prior to seizures* • *Number of febrile seizures*

164. Answer is D (Carbamazepine) : *Harrison 16th/2371; Harrison 17th/ 2511; KDT 5th/378, 342; Harrison 18th/p 3262*

Carbamazepine is the most effective drug for complex partial seizures and shares first choice drug status with phenytoin for generalized tonic clonic seizures and simple partial seizures. It is however not indicated in status epilepticus.

Anticonvulsant therapy therapy for status epilepticus : *(KDT 5th/378)*

First choice drugs	Second choice drugs	Alternative / Add on drugs
Diazepam (I.V.) Clonozepam (I.V.) Lorazepam (I.V.)	Phenytoin (I.V.) Phenobarbitone (I.V. I.M.)	General Anaesthetic e.g. Thiopentone sodium *(KDT 5th/342)*

Thiopentone sodium can occasionally be used for rapid control of convulsions – *KDT*

9

165. Answer is D (Carbamazepine) : *Harrison 16th/2371; KDT 5th/378, 342; Harrison 17th/ 2511; Harrison 18th/p 3262*

Carbamazepine is the most effective drug for complex partial seizures and shares first choice drug status with phenytoin for generalized tonic clonic seizures and simple partial seizures. It is however not indicated in status epilepticus.

166. Answer is C (Absence seizures): *Harrisons 17th/2507, 2508, 2509; Goodman & Gillman's Manual of Pharmacology (2007)/327; Harrison 18th/p 3262, 3263, 3266*

Ethosuxamide is primary agent for the treatment of Absence seizures (Petitmal).

'Ethosuxamide is particularly effective in the treatment of absence seizures, but it is not useful for generalized tonic clonic seizures or partial seizures' - Harrisons 17th/ 2509

'Ethosuxamide is a primary agent for the treatment of Absence seizures' -Goodman & Gillman

Selection of Antiepileptic Drugs:

Agents	**Primary Generalized Tonic-Clonic**	**Partial[a]**	**Absence**	**Atypical Absence, Myoclonic, Atonic**
First-Line	*Valproic acid* *Lamotrigine* *Topiramate*	*Carbamazepine* *Phenytoin* *Lamotrigine* *Oxcarbazepine* *Valproic acid*	*Valproic acid* ***Ethosuxamide***	*Valproic acid* *Lamotrigine* *Topiramate*
Alternatives	*Zonisamide[b]* *Phenytoin* *Carbamazepine* *Oxcarbazepine* *Phenobarbital* *Primidone* *Felbamate*	*Levetiracetam[b]* *Topiramate* *Tiagabine[b]* *Zonisamide[b]* *Gabapentin*[3]* *Phenobarbital* *Primidone*	*Lamotrigine* *Clonazepam*	*Clonazepam* *Felbamate*

[a]Includes simple partial, complex partial, and secondarily generalized seizures.
[b]As adjunctive therapy.

167. Answer is A (Valproate) : *Harrison 16th / 2367; Harrison 17th/ 2507; Harrison 18th/p 3262*

The first line drugs for absence seizures includes valproic acid and Ethosuxamide.
As Ethosuxamide is not provided in the options valproic acid is the undisputed single correct answer of choice.

168. Answer is D (Lorazepam): *Repeat; Harrison 16th / 2367; Harrison 17th/ 2507; KDT 5th/378, 342; 18th/p 3262*

Although Valproate and Limotrigine are the agents of first choice in cases of Generalized Tonic Clonic Seizures, they are not the preferred agents if the patient presents in status epilepticus. ***The patient in question is presenting in status epilepticus hence the initial agents of choice is Lorazepam.***

First choice drugs in status epilepticus
Diazepam (I.V.)
Clonozepam (I.V.)
Lorazepam (I.V.)

169. Answer is D (Lymphadenopathy): *Harrison 15th 375; 16th/2368; 17th/ 2508 (table); 18th/p 3263(Table: 369.9)*

Lymphadenopathy 'Pseudolymphoma' is a complication associated with use of phenytoin and is not seen with valproate.

Side Effects of Valproate	Side effects of phenytoin:
1. Hepatotoxicity : - asymptomatic rise in serum transaminases is seen-KDT - Fulminant hepatitis may be seen	1. **H**yperplasia of gums
2. Weight gain	2. **H**yperglycemia
3. Hyper ammonemia	3. **H**irsutism
4. Gastric Irritation : Anorexia, vomiting	4. **H**ypersensitivity reaction
5. Thrombocytopenia	5. **H**ydantoin syndrome is foetus : during pregnancy
6. Transient alopecia	6. Megaloblastic anemia
7. Ataxia, tremors and sedation may be seen	7. Osteomalacia
8. Use during pregnancy may cause neural tube defects	8. **Lymphadenopathy** - *(Harrison 15th /2364)* **(Pseudolymphoma)**
	9. Neurological symptoms like dizziness, ataxia, incordination, confusion, diplopia

Drugs causing Lymphadenopathy - *Harrisons*

Phenytoin [Q]
Primidone [Q]

170. Answer is B (Decreased Carbamazepine levels): *KDT 5th/ 372; Harrison 17th/ 2508 (table see dru); Harrison 18th/p 3264(Table: 369.9)*

Phenobarbitone is a microsomal enzyme inducer so administration of phenobarbitone induces the metabolism of carbamazepine and reduces its level in blood.

171. Answer is C (Ophthalmoplegia): *Harrison's 17th/2278; Lecture Notes in Neurology (Blackwell) 8th/162; Current Diagnosis & Treatment in Neurology 1st/516, 517; 'Clinical Neuropsychology of Alcoholism' (1994)/39; Other References;*

Ophthalmoplegia is a feature of Wernicke's syndrome (Encephalopathy) and is not a feature of Delirium Tremens

Clouding of consciousness, Coarse Tremors and Visual Hallucinations may all be seen in Delirium Tremens

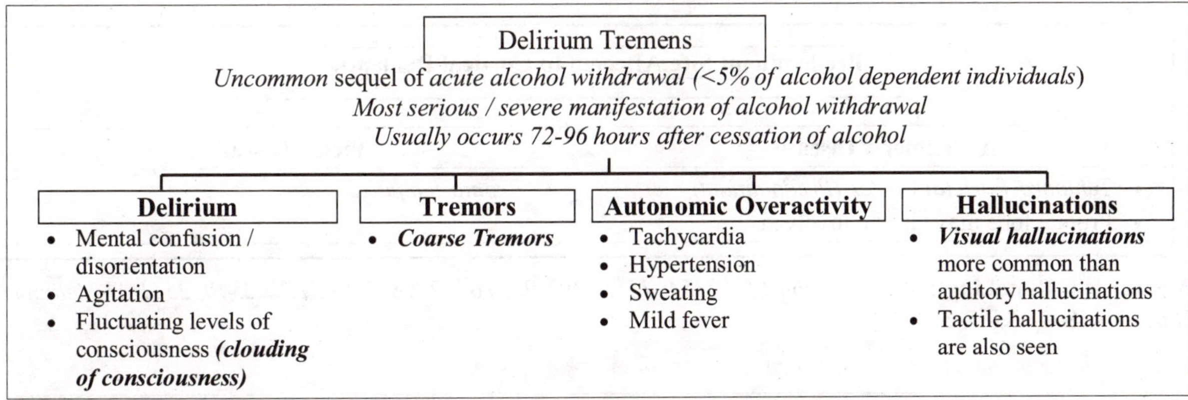

Ophthalmoplegia is a feature of Wernicke's Encephalopathy and not Delirium Tremens

Triad of Wernicke's encephalopathy (Thiamine deficiency in alcoholics)
• *Ophthalmoplegia (Third & Sixth Nerve palsies & Nystagmus are typical)*
• *Ataxia*
• *Confusion (Global confusion)*

Dementias & Extrapyramidal Disorders

Alzheimer's Disease

172. Answer is A (Alzheimer's disease): *'The American Psychiatric Publishing Text book of Psychiatry' 5th/323*

Dementia from Alzheimer's disease (Dementia of Alzheimer's Type) is the classical proto-type of cortical dementias. *Alzheimer's dementia is the most common cortical dementia.*

Classification of Dementias

Cortical Dementias	Subcortical Dementias	Mixed Dementias (Dementias with Cortical & Subcortical Features)
• ***Alzheimer's Dementia*** • *Fronto-temporal dementia (Pick's disease)* • *Dementia due to Creutzfeldt-Jakob disease* • *Dementia due to Chronic Subdural Hematoma*	• ***Parkinson's Disease*** • *Huntington's Disease* • *Multiple Sclerosis* • ***Progressive Supranuclear Palsy*** • ***Dementia due to HIV***	• *Vascular dementias (Multi-infarct dementia)* • *Vascular Dementia (Post-stroke)* • *Lewy body variant of Alzheimer's* • *Lewy body dementia* • *Dementia due to Fragile-X-associated tremor/ataxia syndrome*

173. Answer is B (Temporo-Parietal cortex): *Robbins 7th/1386; 'Alzheimer's Disease' by D. Terry (Lippincott-Wiliams) 2nd/1999*

Alzheimer's disease predominantly affects the temporoparietal cortex although frontal lobe is also frequently involved

'Alzheimer's disease predominantly affects the temporo-parietal cortex' – Alzheimer's Disease by Terry
'Regional deficits are most prominent in the temporo-parietal cortex' – Alzheimer's Disease by Terry

Predominant Site Affected in Cortical Dementias

Alzheimer's Disease	Pick's Disease
• *Temporo-Parietal Cortex (Predominant)* • Frontal lobe may also be involved	• *Fronto-temporal cortex*[Q]

174. Answer is C (Smoking): *Ref: Harrison 14th/ 2354; 15th/ 2392-93; 16th/ 2398, 2399; 17th/ 2540, 2541 AI-Medicine; Harrison 18th/p 3305, 3306*

Smoking has not been mentioned as a risk factor for Alzheimer's disease.

Factors associated with increased risk of Alzheimer's disease
• Increasing Age [Q] • Female sex [Q] • Lower educational attainment [Q] • Family history of dementia [Q] • Numerous environmental factors eg. Al, Hg, Viruses & Prions. • Several genetic factors - amyloid precursor protein on chromosomes 21 - adult with trisomy 21 (Down's) [Q] *-Harrison*

Factors associated with decreased risk of Alzheimer's disease
• *Post menopausal estrogen use* • *NSAID's use*

The most important risk factors for Alzheimer's disease are old age and a positive family history–Harrison 16th/ 2398

175. Answer is C (Trisomy 21): *Harrison 14th/ 2350, Harrison 15th/ 2393, Harrison 16th/ 2398; Harrison 17th/2541, 2542; Harrison 18th/p 3307*

Adults with trisomy 21 (Down's) consistently develop the Neuropathologic hallmark's of Alzheimer's disease if they survive beyond age 40 - *Harrisons*
Several genetic factors are known to play important roles in pathogenesis of at least some cases of Alzheimers disease. Trisomy 21 is one of them.
Point mutation on APP gene on chromosome 21 produces early onset autosomal dominant AD. Presumably extra dose of APP gene on chromosome 21 is the initiating cause of AD in adult Down's syndrome–Harrisons16th/ 2399

176. Answer is D (Dopamine): *Harrison's 18th/3306-3307; Guide to Alzheimer's Disease (Harward Health Publications) 2009/11*

Dopamine deficiency is not a feature of Alzheimer's disease.
The most important biochemical abnormality in Alzheimer's disease is the decrease in cortical levels of Acetylcholine

Biochemical Abnormalities in Alzheimer's Disease

Primary Bichemical Abnormality (Decreased levels of Neurotransmitters)	**Other Biochemical Abnormalities (Decreased levels of Neurotransmitters)**
• *Acelylcholine*	• *Noradrenaline* • *Serotonin* • *Somatostatin*
Decreased levels of ACH, its synthetic enzyme choline acetyltransferase and nicotinic cholinergic receptors is the primary biochemical abnormality observed in Alzheimer'Disease	*Levels of above three neurotransmitters are reduced in brains of some patients with Alzheimer's Disease*
It has been suggested that deficiency of ACH is related to loss of memory / dementia in patients with AD	*It has been suggested that these deficiencies are related to sensory disturbance and aggressive behavior in patient with AD*

Dopamine deficiency is not a feature of Alzheimer's disease.

177. Answer is A (Acetylcholine): *Harrison's 18th/3306*

The most important biochemical abnormality in Alzheimer's disease is the decrease in cortical levels of Acetylcholine

*'Biochemically Alzheimer's disease is associated with a decrease in the cortical levels of several proteins and neurotransmitters **especially acetylcholine**, its synthetic enzyme choline-acetyl-transferase, and nicotinic cholinergic receptors. Reduction of acetylcholine is related in part to degeneration of cholinergic neurons in the nucleus basalis of Meynert (NBM) that projects through the cortex. There is also noradrenergic and serotonergic depletion due to degeneration of brainstem nuclei such as the locus ceruleus and dorsal raphe' - Harrison's 18th/3306, 3307*

178. Answer is C (Dementia): *Read text below, Harrison 16th/ 2398; Harrison 17th/ 2536; Harrison 18th/p 3300*

Alzheimer's Disease is the most common cause of Dementia in elderly.

Clinically, AD most often presents with subtle onset of memory loss followed by slowly progressive dementia that has a course of several years.

179. Answer is None (All are seen) > Agnosia: *Kaplan and Sadock's Synopsis of Psychiatry 10th (2007)/342*

Aphasia, Apraxia, Acalculia and Agnosias may all be seen in Alzheimer's Dementia.

'Agnosia' in Alzheimer's disease usually presents late in the disease and is not included in the ICD-10 Diagnostic criteria for dementia in Alzheimer's disease <u>with early onset</u> and hence may be selected as the single best answer by exclusion.

Dementia in Alzheimer's Disease with Early Onset (ICD-10 criterion)

1. The criteria for dementia in Alzheimer's Disease must be met, and the age at onset must be less than 65 years.
2. In addition atleast one of the following requirements must be met:
   a) evidence of relatively rapid onset and progression
   b) in addition to memory impairment there must be:
- *Aphasia (Amnesia or sensory)*
- *Agraphia*
- *Alexia* (indicating the presence of temporal, parietal or frontal lobe involvement)
- *Acalculia or*
- *Apraxia*

180. Answer is C (NFTs appear extracellularly before intracellular appearance): *Harrisons 17th/2541; Harrisons 18th/3306; Basic Clinical Neuroscience (Lippincott Williams) 2008/310; 'Neurodegenerative Diseases' by Lang & Ludolph (Cambridge) 2005/452, 453*

NFTs are typically seen intracellularly within the soma and proximal dendrites of neurons.

Neurofibrillary Tangles (NFTs) are intracellular accumulations of hyperphosphorylated 'tau' proteins.

Neurofibrillary Tangles are Intracellular Accumulations

- Neurofibrillary Tangles are *intracellular accumulations* of ***hyperphosphorylated microtubule binding protein 'tau'.***
- Paired helical filaments of tau protein (NFTs) form intracellularly within the soma and proximal dendrites of neurons.
- *These cytoskeletal protein tangles (NFTs),* initially impede cellular metabolism and axosplasmic transport leading to impaired synaptic function and *eventually to neuronal death.*
- *These neurofibrillary tangles may be seen as extracellular tangles after degeneration of the neuron as evidence of the neuronal cell's demise*

Neurofibrillary Tangles are intracellular accumulations that may appear extracellularly after degeneration of neuron (neuronal death)

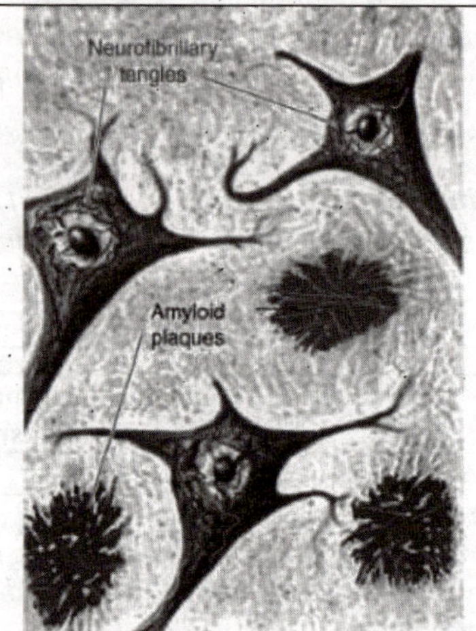

Histopathological Hallmarks of Alzheimer's Disease

β Amyloid Plaques (Extracellular)	**Neurofibrillary Tangles (Intracellular)**
• β Amyloid ***Neuritic Plaques are formed by extracellular accumulation of beta amyloid*** deposits within the neutropil • 'Neuritic' or 'Senile' β-amyloid plaques are an early histopathological sign of Alzheimer's disease (that occur rarely in healthy subjects) • The amyloid β-protein accumulated in single neuritic plaques is toxic to surrounding structures and adjacent neurons. • ***Clinicopathological studies have shown that amyloid burden does not directly correlate with severity or duration of dementia.***	• Neurofibrillary tangles are formed by ***intracellular accumulation of hyperphosphorylated microtubule binding protein 'tau'.*** • NFT's occur in many neurodegenerative diseases and /or a group of diseases called 'taupathies'. These include Frontotemporal dementia, Pick's disease etc. *The cooccurance of β-amyloid plaques with NFT's suggests a diagnosis of AD.* • The NFT's are toxic to the neurons and neurons with NFT's eventually die and degenerate leaving a residual '*ghost tangle*', in the extracellular space reminding of the pyramidal cell body in which it was initially formed. • ***Clinicopathological studies have shown that dementia correlates more strongly with NFT's than with senile plaques (β-amyloid)***

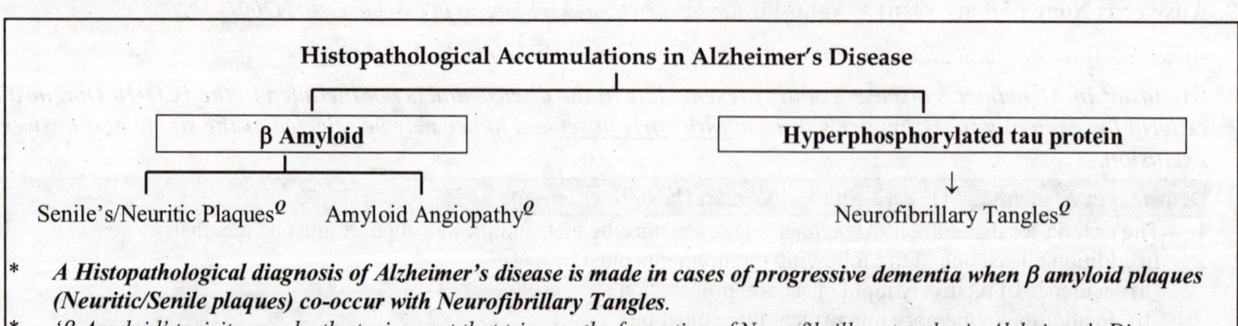

181. Answer is C (Lateral Geniculate Body): *'The Neuropathology of Dementia' (Cambridge) 1997/7; 'The topographical and neuroanatomical distribution of Neurofibrillary tangles and Neuritic Plaques in the Cerebral cortex of patients with Alzheimer's Disease' – Cerebral Cortex (1991): (1): 103-116*

'Lateral geniculate body' is the least commonly affected area amongst the options provided.

'Neurofibrillary tangles are region specific occuring predominantly in the Hippocampus, Entorhinal cortex and association areas of the Neocortex'- 'The Neuropathology of Dementia' (Cambridge) 1997/7

'Not even a single neuron with Neurofibrillary Tangles (NFT) was seen in the Lateral Geniculate Bodies' – Distribution of Alzheimer's Neurofibrillary tangles (Taken from 'Alzheimer's Disease' by George Parry (2006)/55)

Neuro fibrillary Tangles (NFT): Density distribution in Alzheimer's disease
• ***Entorhinal cortex – Hippocampus*** – Amygdala interconnections (*most vulnerable*) • Limbic and Temporal cortical areas (*next most severely involved*) • ***Association areas of the neocortex***

Topographical Distribution of NFTs in Alzheimer's disease

'The spatiotemporal pattern of progression of NFTs in Alzheimer's disease is steriotypical and predictable. Briefly, the neurofibrillary degeneration starts in the aliocortex of medial temporal lobe (entorhinal cortex and hippocampus) and spreads to the associative neocortex, relatively sparing the primary sensory and primary motor and visual cortex.'

Enterohinal cortex, Hippocampus and Associative areas of neocortex are primarily involved.

Taken from 'Neuropathological Alterations in Alzheimer's Disease'; Perspectives in Medicine 2011 (www.perspectivesinmedicine.cshlp.org/content/i/i/a006189.full.pdf+html)

Braak and Braak distinguished six stages to explain topographical distribution and progression of NFT.

Stage I	The first NFTs consistently appear in the ***Transentorhinal (perihilar) region along with Entorhinal cortex*** proper
Stage II	NFTs appear in the CA 1 region of the ***Hippocampus***
Stage III	NFTs appear in the ***Limbic structures*** such as the subiculum of Hippocampal formation
Stage IV	NFTs appear in the Amygdala, Thalamus & Claustrum
Stage V	NFTs appear in all isocortical areas with the affection of ***Associative areas***
Stage VI	NFTs appear in primary sensory, motor and visual areas *(Primary sensory, motor and visual area are considered most resistant)*

These six stages can be summarized into three for the purpose of understanding, namely: Entorhinal, Limbic and Isocortical

182. Answer is D (Lewy bodies): *Harrison 15th/ 2396; Harrison 16th/2403; Harrison 17th/ 2540, 2541, 2542; Robbin's 6th*

'Lewy bodies' are characteristically seen in idiopathic parkinsons disease (and not in Alzheimer's disease).

Alzheimer's disease is the most common cause of dementia in the Western world and is characterized by the following clinical, pathological and biochemical triad.

Clinically	Pathologically		Biochemically
	Gross Q	**Microscopic**	
• Subtle onset memory loss followed by • Slowly progressive dementia over several years	• Diffuse atrophy of cerebral cortex • Secondary enlargement of ventricular system	• ***Neuritic plaques*** Q containing β amyloid • ***Neurofibrillary*** Q ***tangles*** • ***Amyloid angiopathy*** accumulation of β amyloid in arterial walls of cerebral blood vessels.	• Decrease in cerebral cortical levels of acetyl choline Q (choline acety transferase (CAT) and nicotinic cholinergic receptors are also reduced) [Q Reduction in ACH is related to degeneration of nucleus basalis of meynert Q]

Lewy bodies are not mentioned as feature of Alzheimer's disease.

'Lewy bodies' *are intraneuronal, intracytoplasmic, eosinophilic inclusions that have a dense core surrounded by a pale halo. They are composed by Neurofilaments and contain epitopes recognized by antibodies against neurofilament proteins, Ubiqutin and α-synuclein (presynaptic protein)*

They are characteristically seen in idiopathic parkinsons disease (and not in Alzheimer's disease)

Diffuse Lewy body disease	Dementia + Large number of lewy bodies in cortical neurons + No other pathological findings
Diffuse Lewy body variant of Alzheimer's disease (and not in Alzheimer's disease)	Dementia + Large number of Lewy bodies in cortical neurons + Neurofibrillary tangles and amyloid plaques.

183. Answer is A (Beta Amyloid): *Harrison's 17th/ 2540, 2541; Harrison 18th/p 3305, 3306*

Beta- Amyloid protein is associated with Alzheimer's disease along with Neurofibrillary tangles

Progessive loss of cognitive function (loss of memory), aphasias (difficulty in recalling names), impaired language (difficulty in speech) and apraxia (inability to perform desired tasks) together with the presence of Neurofibrillary tangles suggest a diagnosis of cortical dementia of the Alzheimer's type.
Pathological features of Alzheimer's disease include Neurofibrillary tangles (NFT) and Neuritic plaques containing beta amyloid proteins.

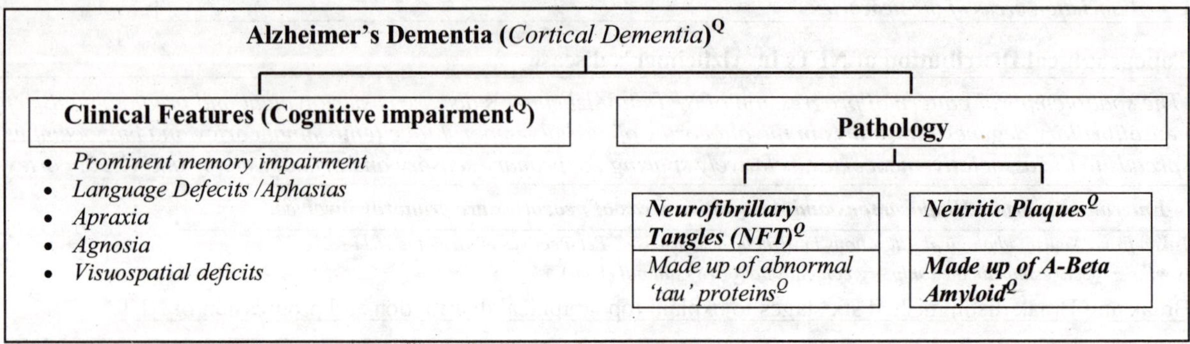

184. Answer is B (Tyrosine Hydroxylase): *Parkinson' Disease. Methods and Protocols (Springer) 2001/157; 'Clinical Neurology for Psychiatrists' by Kaufmann (Elsevier) 2007/409*

Tyrosine Hydroxylase is the most important (critical) enzyme, deficiency which leads to Parkinson's disease

The main biochemical charachteristic of Parkinson's Disease is the reduction of neurotransmitter and the dopamine synthesizing enzyme system including Tyrosine Hydroxylase (TH) and Tetrahydrobiopterin (BH_4) Cofactor in nigrostriatal neurons.

'The loss of Tyrosine Hydroxylase represents the critical failure in Parkinson's Disease because this enzyme is the rate limiting enzyme dopamine synthesis. *With a deficiency of tyrosine hydroxylase the ever-shrinking pool of nigrostriatal tract neurons cannot sustain the essential synthetic pathway. Once approximately 80% of these neurons degenerate, the nigrostriatal tract cannot synthesize adequate dopamine and Parkinson's disease symptoms appear'*
- 'Clinical Neurology for Psychiatrits'.

	Phenylalanine Hydroxylase		***Tyrosine Hydroxylase***		DOPA Decarboxylase	
Phenylalanine	⟶	Tyrosine	⟶	***DOPA***	⟶	Dopamine
			Rate limiting step			

185. Answer is A (Mangnese (Mn)): *Harrison's 18th/3318; Goldfrank's Toxicoogic Enurgencies 9th/159, Handbook of Atypical Parkinsonism (Cambridge Univ. Press) 2011/102*

Manganese ion exposure is implicated in the free radical damage of the basal ganglia causing Parkinsonism.

Toxins Implicated in Parkinsonism *(Harrison)*

- ***Manganese (Mn)***
- *MPTP (1 Methyl - 4 Phenyl – 1, 2, 3, 6 tetrahydropyridine)*
- *Carbonmonoxide*
- *Carbondisulphide*
- *Ctanide*
- *Hexane*
- *Methanol*

Toxins reported to induce Parkinsonism: (Handbook of Atypical Parkinsonism)	
• *Betel nut (plus antipsychotics)*	• ***Manganese***
• *Carbon monoxide*	• *Maneb (Manganese Ethylene-Bis-Dithiocarbamate)*
• *Contrast agent for cardiac catheterization*	• *Mercury*
• *Cyanide*	• *Methanol*
• *Ethanol intoxication, ethanol withdrawal*	• *Methcathinone (manganese ephedrone)*
• *Ethylene glycol*	• *MPTP (1-methyl-4-phenyl-1,2,3,6-tetrahydropyridine)*
• *Herbicides (paraquat, diquat, glyphosate)*	• *Organic solvents (carbon disulfide, n-hexane, toluene, trichloroethylene)*
• *Heroin*	• *Organophosphate insecticide poisoning*
• *Hydrogen sulfide*	• *Petroleum products*
• *Kava-kava*	

Parkinsonism

186. Answer is A (Preserved postural reflexes): *Ref: Harrison 15th/ 2399; 16th/ 2406, 2407; 2550, 2551*

In Parkinsonism, the postural reflexes are not preserved.

There is difficulty in maintaining balance. The posture is stooped, and the attitude is flexed.

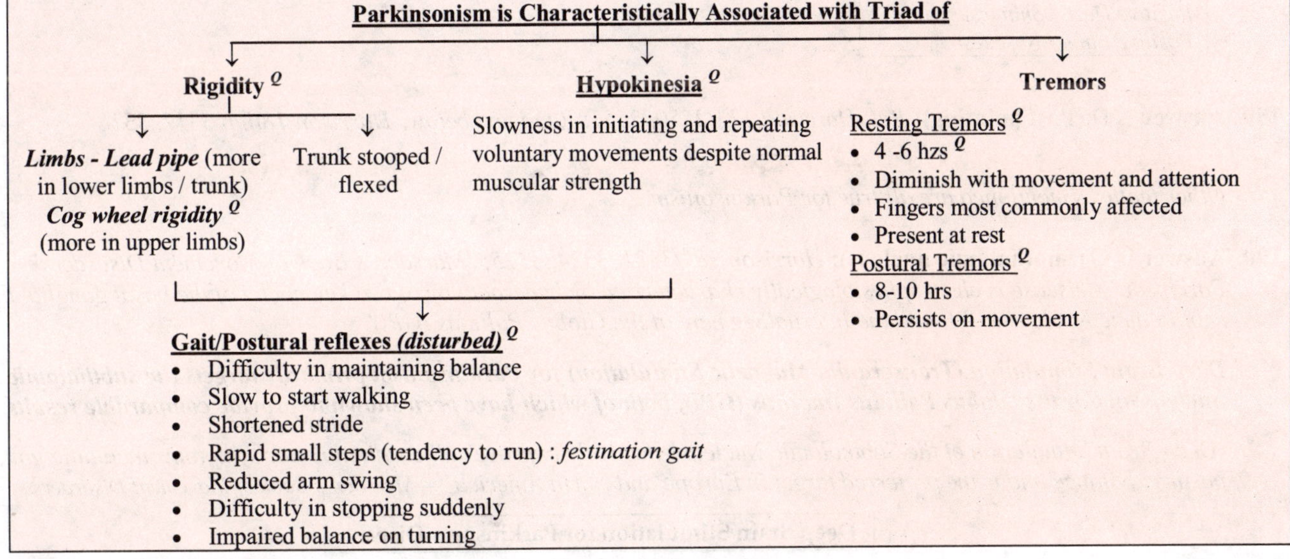

187. Answer is C (Parkinsonism): *Ref: Harrison 14th/ 2356; 15th/2399; 16th/2406, 2407; 17th/2550; API 6th/ 791; 18th/3317*

Patient is present with the characteristic triad of Parkinsonism.

Triad of Parkinsonism.
2. Rigidity
3. Bradykinesia
4. Tremor at rest,

- A characteristic disturbance of gait and posture is seen - this explains slowness of movements
- A depressed mood is common and an impairment of cognitive functions sometimes amounting to frank dementia is frequently evident in advanced cases - this explains the memory loss present in the patient

Parkinsonism : *Quick Revision :*

- Parkinsonism is caused by a disturbance in *substantia nigra.* Q
- Tremor is typically *at rest* Q with frequency *4 - 6 Hz.* Q
- Tendon *reflexes are unaltered* Q (Normal deep tendon reflexes) Q
- *Plantar reflex is typically flexor* Q (Negative Babiniski) Q
- Gait is *festinating gait* Q
- Small handwriting Q
- Normal intelligence Q
- Emotional ability Q
- Masked expressionless facies Q
- Slurred indistinct speech Q

188. Answer is B (Past pointing): *Harrison's 17th/2550,2551; Harrison's 16th/2407, 2408; Harrison 18th/p 3317, 3318*

Past pointing is a feature of cerebellar disease and is not a feature of Parkinsonism.

Characteristic features of Cerebellar disease and Parkinsonism

Cerebellar Disease	Parkinson's disease
Nystagmus	*Rigidity*
Scanning speech/Dysarthria	*Hypokinesia/Akinesia*
Hypotonia	*Tremor*
Past pointing	*Loss of postural Reflexes*
Pendular knee jerks	
Dysdiadokinesia	
Truncal ataxia	
Intention tremor	
Loss of coordination	
Positive Romberg's test	
Positive Heel – Shin test	
Positive Finger Nose test	

189. Answer is D (Past pointing): *Ref: Harrison 17th/2550, 2551; Read text below; Harrison 18th/p 3317, 3318*

Past pointing is a feature of 'Cerebellar disease'. *It is not seen in an extrapyramidal syndrome.*
Other features mentioned are all true for Parkinsonism.

190. Answer is C (Subthalamic nucleus): *Harrison 18th/3321, 3324, 3325; 'Marsden's Book of Movement Disorders' Parkinson's Disease is electrophysiologically characterized by hyperactivity of two key nuclei of the basal ganglia, the subthalamic Nucleus (STN) and the InternalSegment of the Globus Pallidus (GPi).*

Deep Brain Stimulation (Transcranial Magnetic Stimulation) for Parkinsonism primarily targets the subthalamic nucleus and/or the Globus Pallidus Internus (GPi), both of which have been shown to provide comparable results.

'Deep Brain Stimulation of the Subthalamic Nucleus effectively improves all cardinal motor symptoms including gait, posture, balance and is the preferred target in Europe and North America'. – Marsden's Book of Movement Disorders

Deep Brain Stimulation for Parkinson's Disease

Primary Targets

- ***Subthalamic Nucleus (STN)***
- ***Globus Pallidus Internus (GPi)***

- ***Subthalamic Nucleus (STN) is the single most common preferred site*** *for Deep Brain Stimulation in patients with Parkinsonism.*
- ***Globus Pallidus Internus (GPi) is the second most common site*** for Deep Brain Stimulation in patients with Parkinsonism and provides comparable results to DBS of STN.
- ***Subthalamic nucleus and Globus Pallidus Internus both provide comparable efficacy*** (Believed to be equally effective)

Other Targets

- *Ventral Intermediate Nucleus of Thalamus (VMI)* (Efficacious only in relieving Tremor from Parkinsonism. Other Parkinsonian motor symptoms may not respond and hence this target is not preferred)
- *Pedunculopantine Nucleus* (DBS of Pedunculopontine nucleus may be beneficial for patients with advanced parkinsonism and predominant axial symptoms, postural instability and gait disturbance. Results are however still limited to only a few patients)

191. Answer is C (Subthalamic Nucleus): *Harrison's 18th/3325; Operative Neuromodulation Volume II (Springer) 2007/180; Mardsen's Book of movement Disorders (Oxford) 2012/298*

Subthalamic Nucleus is widely accepted as the preferred site for Deep Brain Stimulation (Transcranial Magnetic Stimulation) for patients with Parkinsonism.

Deep Brain Stimulation for Parkinson's Disease (Taken from Operative Neuromodulation)
• Deep Brain Stimulation has become a standard therapy for patients with advanced Parkinson's Disease • ***Although clinical efficacy of both GPi and STN stimulation is comparable it has become widely accepted to prefer STN over GPi*** • The Rationale for STN targeting include: (i) The stimulation energy required to gain maximum clinical improvement seem to be lower for STN than for GPi (ii) STN stimulation seems to have more prominant and stable effects on L-DOPA responsive off-period symptoms in the long term.

'*Subthalamic Nucleus Stimulation effectively improves all cardinal motor symptoms including gait, posture and balance and is the preferred target in Europe and North America' – Mardsen's Book of MOvement Disorders (Oxford) 2012/298*

Note: *STN stimulation bears a higher risk of cognitive and neuropsychiatric behavioural complications in comparison to GPi stimulation.* *GPi stimulation may be preferred over STN stimulation for patients with pre-existing conditions like depression.*

Deep Brain Stimulation for Parkison's Disease: *Review*
What is Deep Brain Stimulation (DBS)
• DBS is a relatively new procedure that uses an implantable electrode into a specific target in the brain and is attached to a programmable pulse generator. The pulse generator is implanted in a pocket below the clavicle and connected to the DBS electrode in the Brain. (The pulse generation is just like a cardiac pacemaker but the wire goes to the specific site in the brain)
What is the principle of DBS in Parkinson's Disease
• *Parkinson's disease* is characterized by loss of dopaminergic input to the striatium, which has been shown to be *associated with hyperactivity of two key nuclei within the basal ganglia, namely the subthalamic nucleus and the Globus Pallidus Internus.* Dopaminergic dennervation in PD leads to increased firing of neurons in the STN and GPi resulting in excessive inhibition of the thalamus, reduced activation of the cortical motor systems and development of Parkinsonian Features. • *DBS is believed to reduce the neuronal overactivity of the STN and/or the GPi and thereby improve features of PD.*
What specific regions in the brain are targetted by DBS
There are three brain targets that have been FDA approved for use in Parkinson's Disease for Deep Brain Stimulation • *Subthalamic nucleus (STN): Most preferred & commonly used target* • *Globus pallidus Internus (GPi): Effective target (Results comparable with STN)* • *Thalamus (Ventral Intermediate Nucleus): Only effective in relieving Tremor (not preferred anymore)*
What are the indications for DBS (Ideal candidate)
• The procedure is primarily indicated for patients who suffer disability from levodopa induced motor complications that cannot be satisfactorily controlled with drug manipulation. Symptoms that improve DBS are essentially the same individual symptoms that improve with levodopa (dopamine) with the exception of medication refractory tremor and dyskinesias. • DBS provides effective relief from all cardinal dopaminergic motor symptoms including gait, posture and balance. Improves tremor, rigidity bradykinesia. It provides dramatic result with respect to "off" time and dyskinesias but does not improve features that fail to respond to levodopa. It does not prevent the development or progression of non-dopaminergic features such as freezing, falling and dementia. *DBS does not improve cognitive (thinking ability).* • Decrease the dose of medications required (in many but not all cases)

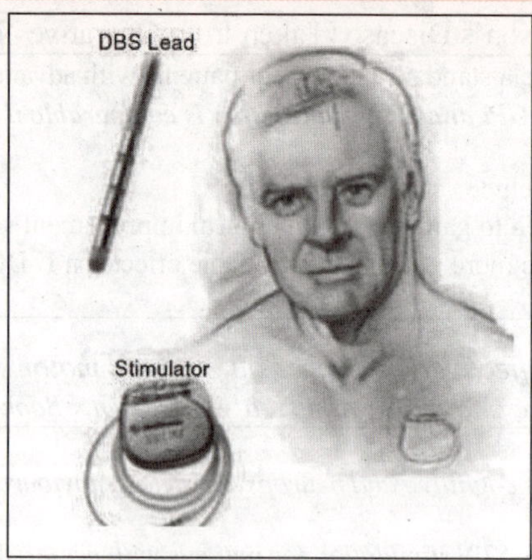

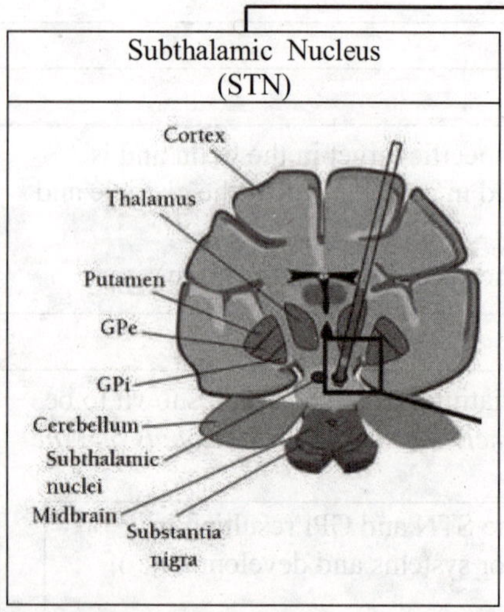

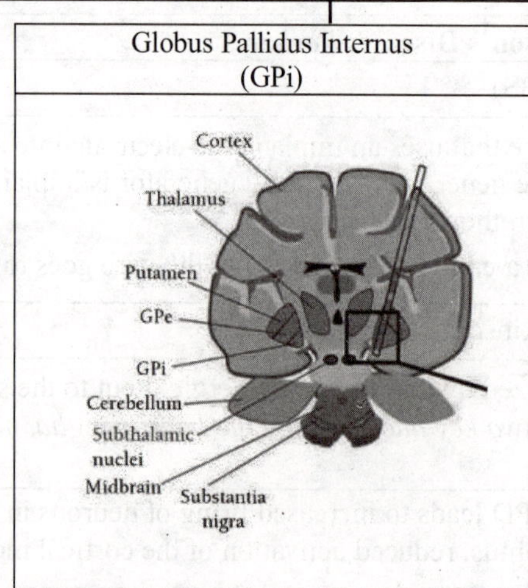

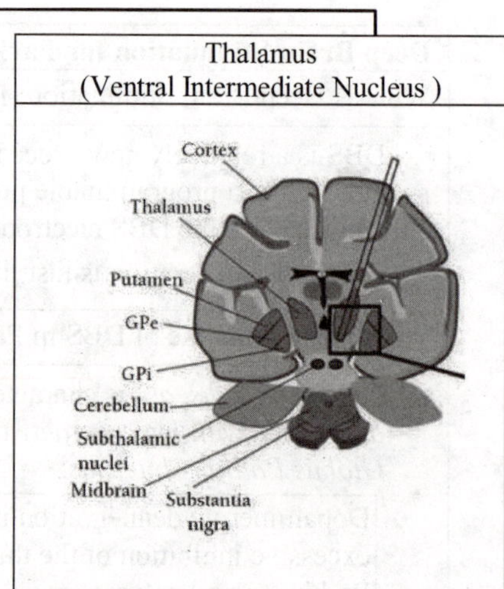

192. Answer is D (Benztropine): *Ref: KDT 4th / 401; KDT 5th / 397; Other references;*

'Central anticholinergics (eg. Benztropine) are the only drugs effective in phenothiazine / drug induced extrapyramidal symptoms' – KDT

Central anticholinergics include
1. Triherphenidyl : Most commonly used drug (Benzhexol)
2. Procyclidine
3. Biperidin
4. Benztropine.

All antipsychotics have potent dopamine blocking action. Dopaminergic blockage in basal ganglia results in deficiency of dopamine, which controls muscle tone and coordinates movements.

This is turn shift the balance between the inhibitory dopaminergic system and excitatory cholinergic system, towards excitatory levels and results in dystonias.

Balance can thus be restored by suppression of the unopposed excitatory cholinergic system (Administration of central anticholinergics).

Huntington's Chorea

193. Answer is D (Intrastrial cholinergic and GABAergic neurons): *CMDT 2003 / 979, CMDT 2005/ 980; Harrison 15th / 2397; Robbin's 7th / 1394; Harrison 16th /2415; Harrison 17th / 2561, 2562; Harrison 18th/p 3330*

'The reported abnormality in Huntington's disease suggests a relative under activity of neurons containing gamma-aminobutyric acid (GABA) and acetylcholine' *– CMDT 2005 / 980*

*'There is **severe loss of striatal neurons**, the most dramatic changes being found in the caudate nucleus' – Robbins 7th / 1394 (Caudate nucleus is part of striatum)*

194. Answer is C (Early onset memory loss): *Harrison 14th/ 2354, Harrison 15th/ 2397, Harrisons 16th/ 2415 (Refer earlier editions also); Harrison 17th/ 2561, 2562; Harrison 18th/p 3330*

'Memory loss is frequently not impaired until late in the disease' *– Harrison*

Huntington's disease is : a *degenerative* Q brain disorder that is *genetically determined.* Q *Autosomal dominant* Q

Age of onset :	Neuropathologically :	Clinical Hallmarks :
It's usual age of onset in *4th or 5th decade* Q	Neuropathologically the disease predominantly strikes the *striatum* Q & *atrophy of caudate nucleus* is seen Q	• *Chorea* Q • *Behavioural disturbance* Q • *Dementia* Q

Memory loss is frequently not impaired until late in the disease, although attention judgement & executive functions may be seriously deficient at an early stage.
Involvement of extrapyramidal system (caudate nucleus) may explain ***cog wheel rigidity.***

195. Answer is C > B (If wife does not get disease by age of 50 years children are not affected > can occur upto age of 50): *Harrison's 17th/251,2562; Practical Neurology 2nd/354; Principles of molecular medicine 2nd; Harrison 18th/p 3330*

Huntington's disease is an autosomal dominant condition and presence of a single affected allele is sufficient for expression of disease
The age of onset of Huntington's disease depends on the sex of the parent.
Individuals who inherit disease from the father usually have an early onset of disease (juvenile onset) while individuals who inherit the disease from the mother usually have a late onset disease (4th or 5th decade)

The 'mother' in the question has an affected 'father'. If the mother would have inherited the disease from her father she should have presented with an early onset disease (should present at a significantly earlier age than 50 years and almost definitely by the age of 50.
If she does not develop symptoms till age of 50 years she is unlikely to have inherited the diseases from her father, hence her children will not be affected.

Huntingtons Disease: Inheritance and genetics:

Huntington's disease is inherited as an autosomal dominant disease
The minimum chance of getting disease in a child with are affected parent is 1:2 and not 1:4

Chance of getting disease in a child

If one parent is affected	If both parents are affected
Minimum chance of getting the disease in a child would be 50 percent or 1 in 2 (1:2)	*Minimum chance of getting the disease in a child would be 75 percent or 3 in 4 (3:4)*

Genetic abnormality responsible for huntington's for huntington's disease is a CAG trimucleotide expansion on a gene called 'Huntingtin' which is localized on chromosome 4.

HD is not caused by a point mutation but by an Triplet Repeat Expansion mutation.

The age of onset of Huntington's disease depend on the sex of the parent and on the age of onset in the parent

Individual who inherit the disease from the father usually have an early onset of disease
Individual who inherit the disease from the mother usually have a late onset of disease

Mean age of onset of HD: 40-50 years
Mean age of juvenile onset of HD < 20 years

Effect of parental sex in Huntington's disease

Characteristic manifestations include

Gene inherited from father	Gene inherited from mother
• Individuals who inherit the gene from their father usually have an *early onset disease*	• Individuals who inherit disease from the mother usually have a *late onset disease*
• **Effect of Anticipation** is exhibited strongly 'Anticipation' means that successive generations develop the disease at an earlier age than their parent *When gene is inherited from father the phenomenon of Anticipation is exhibited strongly.*	• **Effect of Anticipation** is less characteristic Anticipation means that successive generations develop the disease at an earlier age than the parent *When gene is inherited from motor, the phenomenon of 'Anticipation' may be exhibited but this phenomenon is less marked or less characteristic.*
• **Effect of CAG trimucleotide Expansion** Onset of disease depends on length of CAG trinucleotide (onset is inversely related to length of trinucleotide). *CAG repeats tend to expand significantly more when passed from father to child.*	• **Effect of CAG trinucleotide Expansion** Onset of disease depends on length of CAG trinucleotide *CAG repeats tend to expand more slowly when disease is passed from mother to child*

Normal Pressure Hydrocephalus

196. Answer is D (Normal Pressure Hydrocephalus): *Harrison's 17th/2546; Harrison 18th/p 3313*

Abnormal gait (Ataxia), Urinary incontinence and Dementia constitute the charachteristic triad for Normal Pressure Hydrocephalus.

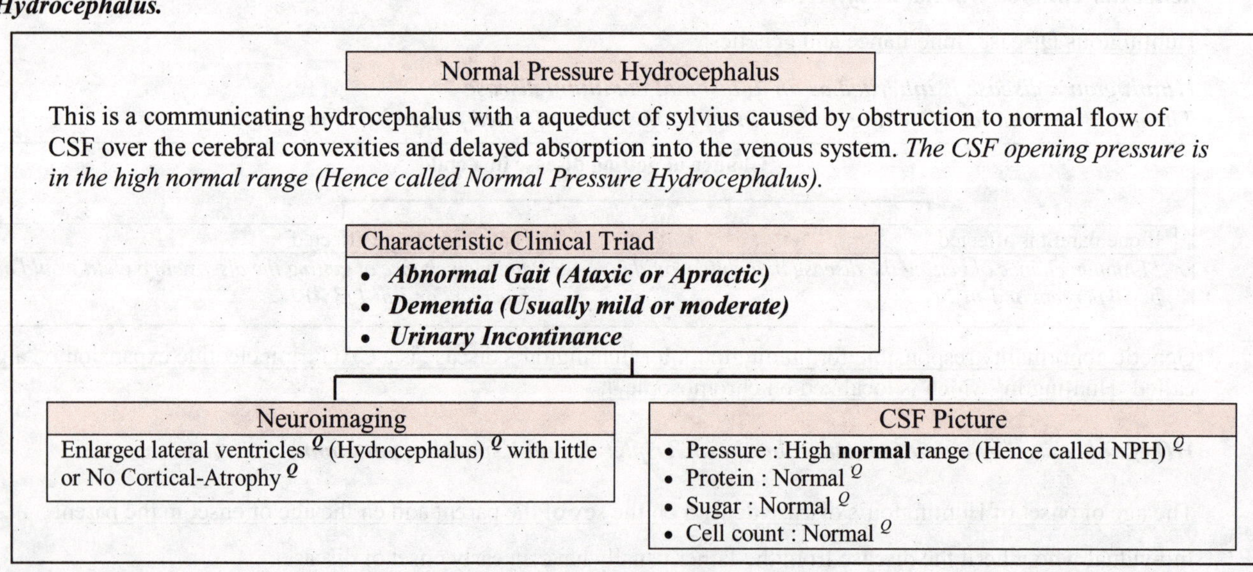

Normal Pressure Hydrocephalus

This is a communicating hydrocephalus with a aqueduct of sylvius caused by obstruction to normal flow of CSF over the cerebral convexities and delayed absorption into the venous system. *The CSF opening pressure is in the high normal range (Hence called Normal Pressure Hydrocephalus).*

Characteristic Clinical Triad
- ***Abnormal Gait (Ataxic or Apractic)***
- ***Dementia (Usually mild or moderate)***
- ***Urinary Incontinance***

Neuroimaging	CSF Picture
Enlarged lateral ventricles [Q] (Hydrocephalus) [Q] with little or No Cortical-Atrophy [Q]	• Pressure : High **normal** range (Hence called NPH) [Q] • Protein : Normal [Q] • Sugar : Normal [Q] • Cell count : Normal [Q]

197. Answer is C (Gait disorder, Urinary incontinence & Dementia): *Harrison 14th/ 2353, 15th/ 23961; 16th/2403; 17th/2546; Harrison 18th/p 3313*

<u>**Normal Pressure Hydrocephalus (NPH)**</u> is a communicating hydrocephalus with a patent aqueduct of sylvius, caused by obstruction to normal flow of CSF over the cerebral convexities and delayed absorption into the venous system.

Clinical triad	Neuroimaging	CSF picture
• Abnormal gait [Q] • Dementia [Q] • Urinary incontinence [Q]	Enlarged lateral ventricles [Q] (Hydrocephalus) [Q] with little or No Cortical-Atrophy [Q]	• Pressure : High **normal** range (Hence called NPH) [Q] • Protein : Normal [Q] • Sugar : Normal [Q] • Cell count : Normal [Q]

198. Answer is A (Aphasia): *Harrison 15th/ 2393; Harrison 16th/2403; Harrison 17th/2546; Harrison 18th/p 3313*

Ataxia, Urinary incontinence & Dementia constitute the characteristic triad of Normal Pressure Hydrocephalus.

Supranuclear Gaze Palsy

199. Answer is B (Supranuclear gaze palsy): *Harrison 14th/2360; 15th/2403; 16th/2402; 17th/2559; 18th/p 3311, 3312*

Progressive supranuclear palsy should always be considered when a middle aged/elderly persons presents with a history of repeated falls, & difficulty in downward or horizontal gaze.

Steel Richardson syndrome

Nature of disorder
Is a degenerative disorder where in there occurs loss of neurons in parts of our CNS which are involved with maintenance of posture & equilibrium, namely the Mid brain, Pons, Basal ganglion and cerebellum.
The clinical features are characteristic
"Progressive supranuclear palsy should be considered whenever a middle aged or elderly person-person presents with history of repeated falls and has an extrapyramidal syndrome accompanied by nuchal dystonia and paralysis of voluntary down gaze"
Factors which distinguish this from Parkinson's
a. *marked impairment of voluntary downward gaze and horizontal gaze.* [Q] b. *extended rather than flexed dystonic posturing* [Q] c. *absence of tremor* [Q] d. poor response to antiparkinsonian medication

200. Answer is B (Supranuclear palsy): *Ref: Harrison 17th/ 2561, 2562; See previous question; Harrison 18th/p 3311, 3312*

201. Answer is D (Progressive supranuclear palsy): *Ref: Harrison 17th/2529; See previous question; Harrison 18th/p 3311, 3312*

Pseudotumor cerebri

202. Answer is B (Increased protein in CSF): *Ghai 5th/ 404, 6th/530, 121; Harrison 15th/ 171; 16th/87; 17th/ 105, 188; Harrison 18th/p 126, 233*

Pseudotumor cerebri is associated with a normal CSF picture.

Pseudotumor cerebri

It is a benign self-limiting disorder with a favorable outcome.

Characteristic features:	Causes include :
Elevated intracranial pressure (*intracranial hypertension*) with : • ***Normal or Small sized ventricular system*** [Q] • ***No focal neurological signs*** [Q] • **Papilledema** [Q] (enlarged blind spot in visual fluid). • **Normal CSF findings** [Q] • **Normal CT scan, MRI and isotope brain scan** • Excessive slow-wave activity on ECG	• *High doses of vitamin A* [Q] • Outdated Tetracycline • Quinolones • *Withdrawal of corticosteroid therapy* [Q] • *Addison's disease* [Q] • SLE • *Hypoparathyroidism* [Q]

203. Answer is B (Convulsions): *Ghai 5th/ 404, Ghai 6th/530, 121; Harrison 15th/ 171; Harrison 16th/87; 17th/ 105, 188; Harrison 18th/p 126, 233*

There are no focal neurological signs in pseudotumor cerebri. Therefore, Pseudotumor Cerebri does not present with convulsions.

Seizures are produced due to focal neurological electrical abnormalities that may or may not involve the whole brain. In any case, these always start in a localized area of the brain.

Others

204. Answer is A (Tau protein) : *Harrison's 17th/2545; Neurodegenerative Diseases by Beal, Lang & Ludolph (2003) /188; Handbook of Medical Psychiatry by Soares (2003) / 105, 106; Harrison 18th/p 3311*

Classic Pick's bodies stain positive with silver and tau-Harrison17th/ 2545

Classification of Neuro degenerative disorders based on the major type of Protein Aggregations (inclusions)

Type of Protein Aggregate

Tau Protein (Tauopathies)	Alpha Synuclein Protein (Synucleinopathies)	Amyloid Beta Protein (Amyloidopathies)
• ***Pick's disease (Pick's bodies)*** • Progressive supranuclear palsy (Tufted Astrocytes) • Cortico basal degeneration (Astrocytic plaques) • Familial Fronto temporal dementia and Parkinsonism linked to chromosome 17 (FTDP-17)	• Sporadic Parkinson's disease (Lewy bodies) • Diffuse Lewy body disease (Lewy bodies) • Multiple System Atrophy - ShyDrager syndrome - Striatonigral degeneration - Olivopontocerebellar atrophy	• Sporadic Alzheimer's Disease • Cerebral Amyloid Angiopathy

Protein Aggregations in Major Dementias and Related Cognitive Disorders:

Disease	Protein
Alzhiemer's disease	*A-beta, TauQ*
Fronto temporal dementia, Pick's disease	*Tau*
Progressive supranuclear palsy	*Tau*
Corticobasal degeneration	*Tau*
Parkinson's disease	*Alpha-synuclein*
Multiple system atrophy	*Alpha-synuclein*
Huntington's disease	*Huntingtin*
Prion disease	*Prion protein*
Spinocerebellar ataxia	*Ataxin*

Facts to Remember :

Pick's bodies contain Tau protein Q

Lewy bodies contain α synucleinQ

205. Answer is B (Frontotemporal dementia): *Harrison 17th/2544; Harrison 18th/p 3310*

Fronto-temporal dementia is characterized by localized or regional atrophy of the temporal and or frontal lobe.

'The distinguishing anatomical hallmark of Frontotemporal dementia is a marked lobar atrophy (regional atrophy) of temporal and/or frontal lobe' – Harrison 17th/2544

Condition	Anatomical Feature
Frontotemporal dementia	***Regional Atrophy of temporal and/or frontal lobe***
Alzheimer's disease	*Diffuse cerebral atrophy*
PML	*Widespread demyelinating lesions of cerebral cortex*
C. J. disease	*Widespread neuronal loss and gliosis*
Friedreich's Ataxia	*Cerebral cortex is usually not involved.* *Involvement is primarily restricted to spinal cord, brainstem and cerebellum.*

206. Answer is A (Cogwheel rigidity): *Harrison 15th/ 2496; Harrison 16th/1636; Harrison 17th/2546, 2547; 18th/p 3313*

Wernicke's disease is seen in *Alcoholic*[Q] patients with *chronic thiamine deficiency*[Q].

The characteristic **clinical triad** is that of :

Global confusion
Ophthalmoplegia
Ataxia

207. Answer is D (Hippocampus): *Harrison 18th/2260; Handbook of Dementia (John Wiley & Sons) 2003/204; Robbins Pathology 8th/1328*

Hippocamous is not involved in Wernicke's Korsakoff syndrome.
Mamillary bodies, Periventricular Grey Matter and Thalamus may all be involved in Wernicke's Korsakoff syndrome.

Principle Sites of Involvement in Wernicke's Korsakoff Syndrome
• Mammillary bodies *(Petechial haemorrhages are characteristic)*
• Thalamus *(Dorsomedial Nucleus)*
• Periaqueductal Grey Matter *(Periventricular lesions around the Third ventricle, Aqueduct and Fourth ventricle)*

[Q]Small pelicheal Haemorrhages in the mamillary bodies are characteristic of Wernicke's disease, a complication of chronic alcoholism and thiamine deficiency. Neither Vascular stroke, Pyridoxine deficiency, Lwey body disease nor Cluster headaches present with haemorrhages in the mamillary bodies. – Kaplan & Saddock's Study Guide (2007)/Q 5.10

208. Answer is B (Thalamus): *Harrison 18th/2260; Robbin's 8th/1328*

The Amnestic effect in Wernicke's Korsakoff Syndrome is related to lesions in the dorso-medial nuclei of the thalamus.

'Lesions in the dorsomedial nucleus of the thalamus seem to be the best correlate of the memory disturbance and confabulation' - Robbins

'The amnestic defect is related to lesions in the dorso-medial nuclei of the thalamus' – Harrison's 18th/2260

209. Answer is A (Down's syndrome) : *Harrisons 17th/2541,2542; Harrison 18th/p 3307*

Down Syndrome is associated with memory impairment.

Adults with trisomy 21 (Down's) consistently develop the neuropathologic hallmark's of Alzheimer's disease of they survive beyond 40 years of age – Harrison's

The most noble aspect is down's syndrome is marked mental retardation, relatively poor expressive language and impaired verbal short term memory' – Child and Adolescent Psychiatry

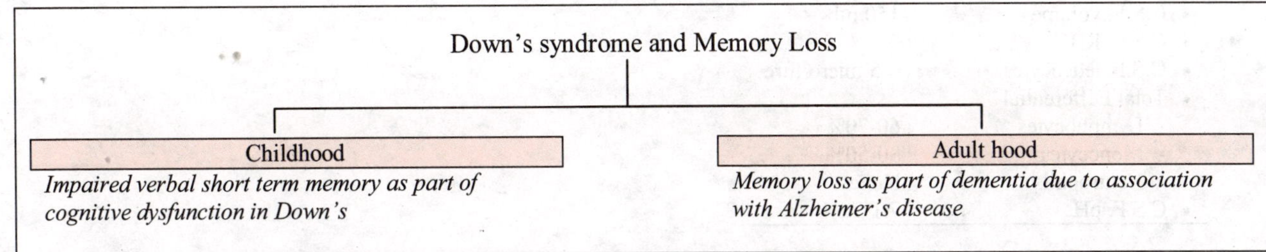

210. Answer is A (Subacute combined degeneration) : *Harrison 16th/2395, 2396; Harrison 17th/2538 (Table 365-3); Harrison 18th/p 3302 (Table: 371.3)*

'Subacute combined degeneration' is caused by vitamin B_{12} deficiency. Vitamin deficiencies including vitamin B_{12} deficiency constitute potentially reversible causes of dementia.

Differential Diagnosis of Dementia:

Potentially Reversible dementia	**Irreversible dementias**
Vitamin deficiencies Thiamine (B1): Wernicke's encephalopathy B12 (pernicious anemia) Nicotinic acid (pellagra) Endocrine and other organ failure Hypothyroidism Adrenal insufficiency and Cushing's syndrome Hypo-and hyperparathyroidism Renal failure Liver failure Pulmonary failure Alcoholism Drug Psychiatric Depression (pseudodementia) Schizophrenia Conversion reaction	Alzheimers Vascular dementia : • Multi infarct • Diffuse white matter disease (Binswanger's) Parkinsons disease Degenerative Hutington's disease Pick's disease Dementia with Lewy bodies Progressive supranuclear palsy (Steel Richardson syndrome) Multisystem degeneration (Shy-Drager syndrome) Hereditary ataxias (some forms) Motor neuron disease [amyotrophic lateral sclerosis (ALS); some forms] Frontotemporal dementia Cortical basal degeneration Multiple sclerosis
Chronic Infections	**Chronic Infections**
Neurosyphilis Tuberculosis, fungal, protozal **Whipples disease**	HIV Papovirus (progressive multifocal leukoencephalopathy) Prion (Creutzfeldt-Jakob and Gerstmann-Straussler-Scheinker diseases)
Head trauma and diffuse brain damage	**Head trauma and diffuse brain damage**
Chronic subdural haemorrhage Normal pressure hydrocephalus	Dementia pugilistica Postanoxia
Toxic disorders	**Toxic disorders**
Drug, medication, and narcotic poisoning Heavy metal intoxication	Dialysis dementia Organic toxins
Neoplastic	**Neoplastic**
Primary brain tumor Metastatic brain tumor	Paraneoplastic limbic encephalitis

CNS Infections

211. Answer is B (2/3 of plasma glucose): *Ref: Harrison 15th/; Harrison 16th/ Appendix B (reference values);*

C.S.F Glucose is 40-70 mg/dl which is about 2/3 of plasma glucose (80-120 mg/dl): *Harrison 17th/Appendix A-11(Table 6)*

Common C.S.F values	
• C.S.F. glucose	: 40-70 mg/dl
• C.S.F. pressure	: 50-180 mm H_2O
• Total protein	: 15-50 mg/dl
• C.S.F. volume	: 150 ml
• C.S.F. RBC	: 0
• C.S.F. leucocytes	: < 5 micro/litre
• Total Differential	
- Lymphocytes	: 60-70%
- Monocytes	: 30-50%
- Neutrophils	: None
• C.S.F. pH	: 7.1-7.34

212. Answer is D (High RBC count): *Ref: Chandrasoma Taylor 3rd/ 915*

CSF cell count in Tubercular meningitis is characterized by an increase in the total cell count with a predominance of mononuclear cells or Lymphocytes. RBC count holds no relevance.

CSF changes in Infection of CNS :

Parameters (Normal values)	Bacterial Meningitis	Tuberculous Meningitis	Viral Meningitis
Pressure	Raised	Raised	Raised
Gross appearance	Turbid	Clear (may clot)	Clear
Protein (Normal : 20-50 mg/dL)	High	Very High	Slightly high
Glucose (40-70 mg/dL)	Very Low	Low	Normal
Chloride (116-122 µg/dL)	Low	Very Low	Normal
Cells < 5/microlit	Neutrophils	Pleocytosis	Lymphocytosis

(Pleocytosis is the presence of both neutrophils and Lymphocytes in CSF)

213. Answer is C (Low opening pressure) : *Harrison's 18th/3414; Chardasoma Jaylor 3rd/915*

Tubercular meningitis is associated with a Raised (High) Opening pressure.

Tubercular Meningitis is characterized by Lymphocytic Pleocytosis, Low Glucose and High Proteins within the CSF.

CSF changes in Infection of CNS:

Parameters (Normal values)	Bacterial Meningitis	Tuberculous Meningitis	Viral Meningitis
Pressure	Raised	Raised	Raised
Gross appearance	Turbid	Clear (may clot)	Clear
Protein (Normal: 20-50 mg/dL)	High	Very High	Slightly high
Glucose (40-70 mg/dL)	Very Low	Low	Normal
Chloride (116-122 µg/dL)	Low	Very Low	Normal
Cells < 5/microlit	Neutrophils	Pleocytosis (Lymphocytes and Neutrophils in CSF)	Lymphocytosis

(Pleocytosis is the presence of both Neutrophils and Lymphocytes in CSF)

The pathological hallmark of Tubercular Meningitis is predominant involvement of basal cisterns that are observed by the presence of basal inflammatory tissue exudate.

214. Answer is D (Tubercular meningitis): *Harrison 17th/ 2642; Harrison 18th/p 3436*

Elevated CSF protein and decreased sugar and chloride levels alongwith characteristic clinical features of meningitis suggest a diagnosis of Tubercular meningitis.

Typical CSF features of Tubercular Meningitis are :

- Cells : *Mononuclear cells* (except *early infection when PMN cells are seen*) [Q]
- Protein : Increased *above 40 mg/100 ml.* [Q]
- Sugar : Usually reduced to *less than 2/3rd of blood sugar* [Q].
- Chloride level : usually *reduced.*

Important points about TBM :

- In TBM, the exudate is mainly basal (*basal brain is involved*) [Q]
- Subarachnoid space is involved by the exudate (i.e. *subarachnoiditis is present*) [Q].
- Involvement is *mainly of the leptomeninges i.e. Pia-arachnoid. (Duramater is usually spared.)* [Q]

215. Answer is A (Increased protein, Decreased sugar, Increased Lymphocytes): *Harrison 16th / 2487; Harrison 17th/2642; Harrison 18th/p 3436*

Tuberculous meningitis is associated with elevated protein concentration decreased glucose concentration and Lymphocytic pleocytosis.

Classic CSF abnormalities in Tuberculosis Meningitis : Harrison
• Elevated opening pressure
• Elevated protein concentration (Range of 1 to 5 g/L or 10 to 500mg/dL)
• Decreased glucose concentration (Range of 1.1 to 2.2 mmol/L or 20 to 40 mg/dL)
• Lymphocytic pleocytosis (10 to 500 cells / μL)

216. Answer is A (Lymphocytosis, Low Glucose, High protein) : *Harrison 18th/3414; Chandrasoma Taylor 3rd/915*
Presence of significant basal exudates, together with dilated ventricles (hydrocephalus) in a young female with prolonged history of fever and headache suggests a diagnosis of Tubercular Meningitis.

Tubercular Meningitis is characterized by Lymphocytic Pleocytosis, Low Glucose and High Proteins within the CSF.

The pathological hallmark of Tubercular Meningitis is predominant involvement of basal cisterns that are observed by the presence of basal inflammatory tissue exudate.

CSF changes in Infection of CNS :

Parameters (Normal values)	Bacterial Meningitis	Tuberculous Meningitis	Viral Meningitis
Pressure	Raised	Raised	Raised
Gross appearance	Turbid	Clear (may clot)	Clear
Protein (Normal: 20-50 mg/dL)	High	Very High	Slightly high
Glucose (40-70 mg/dL)	Very Low	Low	Normal
Chloride (116-122 μg/dL)	Low	Very Low	Normal
Cells < 5/microlit	Neutrophils	Pleocytosis (Lymphocytes and Neutrophils in CSF)	Lymphocytosis

(Pleocytosis is the presence of both Neutrophils and Lymphocytes in CSF)

217. Answer is A (Exudate seen in Basal Cisterns): *Ref: Cranial MRI & CT, Lee Rao & Zimmer Man – 4th/ 479*

CSF proteins are increased and glucose levels are characteristically decreased.

- *Basal Cisterns* are most frequently affected, although often sylvian cisterns and other subarachnoid spaces may be involved. The Basal Cisterns are obscured by presence of inflammatory tissue exudate.
- *Hydrocephalus* is communicating & is usually persistent i.e. it does not improve even if ATT is given.
- *Calcification* is commonly seen in the meninges at the base of the brain.
- *Ventriculitis* may be seen, but it is not common.

218. Answer is A (Tubercular meningitis): *'Brain Imaging Studies: Case Review Series' by Arora (Jaypee) 2007/86; Journal of the Indian Medical Association, volume 100, Issue 7-12 (2002); Harrison 17th/Chapter 381 & 382*

Basal exudates, hydrocephalus and ischemic infarcts are classical features of Tubercular Meningitis.
'The triad of CT features (Thalamic infarction, Basal cistern enhancement and Hydrocephalus) is diagnostic of Tubercular Meningitis' – Journal of Indian Medical Association

Classical Radiological Features (CT/MRI) in Tubercular Meningitis
• ***Basal exudates*** / *Obliteration of Basal cisterns* (Tubercular Exudates are primarily located in the vicinity of basal cisterns)
• *Abnormal Leptomeningeal Enhancement* (Usually most pronounced in the basal cisterns)
• *Communicating* ***Hydrocephalus*** (Usually communicating although non-communicating may also be seen)
• ***Ischemic / Vasculitic Infarcts*** (Basal ganglia and / or Internal capsule)
• *Tuberculomas* (Granulomas)

219. Answer is A (Protein ↑, sugar ↓): *Harrison 14th/ 2424; 15th/ 2464; 16th/2474 t; 17th/2625 (Table 376-2) ; Harrison 18th/p 3414 (Table: 381.2)*

CSF proteins are increased and glucose levels are characteristically decreased.

CSF Protein	CSF Glucose
Is elevated in all cases bacterial meningitis, sometimes to an extreme degree This is presumed to be due to - disruption of blood brain barrier - generation of protein by leucocytes and microorganisms	Is decreased in most patients with bacterial meningitis. It is usually less than 40 mg/dl.

220. Answer is B (Pleocytosis with high protein and low sugar): *Harrison 18th/3414; Chandrasoma Taylor 3rd/915*

Bacterial meningitis (Pneumococcal meningitis) is characterized by polymorphonuclear leucocytosis, high protein concentration and low sugars.
Pleocytosis refers to presence of increased numbers of both neutrophils and lymphocytes, and is more typical of Tubercular meningitis, however for the purpose of this question, pleocytosis with high protein and low sugar is the single best answer amongst the options provided.

Cerebrospinal Fluid (CSF) Abnormalities in Bacterial Meningiti

Opening pressure	> 180 mmH_2O
White blood cells	10μL; neutrophils predominate
Red blood cells	Absent in nontraumatic tap
Glucose	< 2.2 mmol/L (<40 mg/dL)
CSF/serum glucose	< 0.4
Protein	> 0.45 g/L (> 45 mg/dL)
Gram's stain	Positive in > 60%
Culture	Positive in > 80%
Larex agglutination	May be positive in patients with meningitis due to S. pneumoniae, N. meningitis, H. Influenzae type B, E.coli, group B streptococci
Limulus lysate	Positive in cases of gram-negative meningitis
PCR	Detects bacterial DNA

CSF changes in Infection of CNS:

Parameters (Normal values)	Bacterial Meningitis	Tuberculous Meningitis	Viral Meningitis
Pressure	Raised	Raised	Raised
Gross appearance	Turbid	Clear (may clot)	Clear
Protein (Normal: 20-50 mg/dL)	High	Very High	Slightly high
Glucose (40-70 mg/dL)	Very Low	Low	Normal
Chloride (116-122 μg/dL)	Low	Very Low	Normal
Cells < 5/microlit	Neutrophils	Pleocytosis (Lymphocytes and Neutrophils in CSF)	Lymphocytosis

221. Answer is B (↓ Chloride, ↓ Glucose): *Chandrasoma Taylor 3rd/ 915; Harrison 16th/2474; 17th/2625(376-2) ; Harrison 18th/p 3414 (Table: 381.2)*

CSF Features	Pyogenic meningitis
Pressure	↑
Gross	Turbid
Protein	High
Glucose Q	*Very low* Q
Chloride Q	*Low* Q
Cells	Neutrophils

222. Answer is B (Amphotericin B): *Harrison 15th/ 1175; Harrison 16th/1184; 17th/1253; Harrison 18th/p 1650*

Amphotericin B is the drug of choice for Cryptococcosis

Treatment of Cryptococcosis:

Neural (Meningo-encephalitis)	Extraneural
iv Amphotericin B ± Flucytosine for 2 weeks ↓ followed by Fluconazole (oral) OD	iv Amphotericin B ± Flucytosine

9

Nervous System

9

223. Answer is C (Cerebral hamartoma): *Harrison 15th/ 2464, 2481; O.P. Ghai Pediatrics 5th/ 393;*

Cerebral hamartoma is a benign, neoplastic condition and is not associated with meningitis.

Complications of Meningitis
1. *Hydrocephalus*
2. *Cranial nerve involvement*
3. *Seizures*
4. *Subdural effusions*
5. *Subdural empyema*
6. *Cerebral herniation d/t increased ICT.*

224. Answer is B (Pneumococci): *Nelson 18th/2514; 'Infections of the Central Nervous System' 3rd/354; 'Mayo Clinic Internal Medicine Review' 8th/567*

Pneumococci are the most common cause of recurrent meningitis in the setting of CSF leaks

'Streptococcus Pneumoniae is the most common cause of recurrent meningitis due to cerebrospinal fluid leaks'
- Infections of the CNS 3rd/354; Mayo Clinic 8th/567

***'Congenital or Acquired CSF leak** across a mucocutaneous barrier such as cranial or midline facial defects (cribriform plate) and middle ear (stapedial foot plate) or inner ear fistulas (oval window, internal auditory canal, cochlear aqueduct) or CSF leakage through a rupture of meninges due to basal skull fractures into the cribriform plate or paranasal sinus **is associated with an increased risk of pneumococcal meningitis'.** - Nelson 18th/2514*

225. Answer is C (Streptococcus pneumoniae): *Harrison 14th/ 2430; 15th/ 2469; 16th/2487; 17th/2638; 18th/p 3432*

Aerobic and Anaerobic streptococci are the most common aetiological agents for subdural emphyema.

H. influenzae is the most common causative organism in Children, and not in Adults.
Subdural Empyema is a collection of pus in the space between he dura and arachnoid.
In most cases a single organism is responsible, but many cultures are sterile because patients are often receiving anti-microbial therapy.

The major pathogens include
1. Aerobic and anaerobic Streptococci (about 50%)
2. Staph (about 12-16%)
3. Aerobic gram -ve bacilli (3-10%)
4. Other anaerobes (5%)

226. Answer is A (Herpes simplex virus type 2) : *Harrison 15th/ 2475; 16th/2477t, 2480; 17th/2628; 18th/p 3419, 3420*

HSV type 2 is a common cause of aseptic meningitis, however encephalitis following HSV type 2 has not been mentioned.

Viruses causing encephalitis:

Common	Less common	Rare
• Arboviruses e.g. Japanese – B encephalitis virus • Enterovirus • HSV – I • Mumps	• CMV • EBV • HIV • Measles • Varicella Zoster	• Adenovirus • Influenza • Para influenza (Nipahvirus) • Rabies • Rubella • CTFV (Colarado tick fever virus) • LCMV (Lymphocytic choriomeningitis virus)

- *Japanese encephalitis virus* is an arbovirus and is one of the most common causes of encephalitis outbreaks.
- *Nipah virus:* is a new member of the paramyxo virus family.
  New cases of viral encephalitis are constantly appearing as evidenced by the recent outbreaks of 300 cases of encephalitis with 40% mortality rate in Malaysia caused by Nipah virus (paramyxovirus family).

227. Answer is D (Enterovirus): *Nelson's 18th/2521*

Enteroviruses are the most common cause of viral meningoencephalitis.

Arboviruses, HSV and Mumps virus are all important agents associated with viral meningoencephalitis, but Enteroviruses are the most commonly associated agents and the answer of choice.

'Enteroviruses are the most common cause of viral meningoencephalitis' - Nelson's 18th/2521

228. Answer is B (Herpes simplex encephalitis): *Harrison 15th/ 2475; 16th/2480, 1036; 17th/2630; Harrison 18th/p 3421*

The most common cause of sporadic viral encephalitis is HSV-I

The most common cause of sporadic viral encephalitis Q	HSV-I
The most common cause of epidemic viral encephalitis Q	Arbovirus
The most common cause of viral **meningitis** is Q	Enterovirus

229. Answer is B (Herpes simplex encephalitis): *Harrison 15th/ 2476; 16th/2480, 2481; 17th/2631; 18th/p 3422, 3423*

Focal findings in a patient with encephalitis should always raise the possibility of HSV encephalitis.

Since the patient in question is presenting with focal findings, HSV encephalitis is the most likely clinical diagnosis.

The patient in question is presenting with two groups of clinical manifestations

Clinical manifestations common to all viral encephalitis
- Fever
- Altered level of consciousness/ confusional state
- Headache

Focal findings
- Focal seizures
- Right sided hemiparesis
- Frontoparital hyper intense lesion on MRI

According to *Harrison 15th / 2476: Harrison 17th/ 2631*

Focal findings in a patient with encephalitis should always raise the possibility of HSV encephalitis.

Examples of focal findings include:

MRI	Areas of increased signal intensity in the frontotemporal, cingulate or insular region of brain on MRI (T2 weighted spinecho MRI)
CT	Temporoparietal areas of low absorption, mass effect and control enhancement
EEG	Periodic temporal lobe spikes on a background of slow or low amplitude activity on EEG

Since the patient in question is presenting with focal findings, HSV encephalitis is the most likely clinical diagnosis.

MRI findings in other options provided in question:

Condition	**MRI findings**
Neurocysticercosis	Multiple cystic lesions with enhancement on MRI
Acute pyogenic meningitis	Diffuse meningeal enhancement on MRI
Carcinoma meningitis	Nodular tumor deposits in the meninges or diffuse meningeal enhancement on MRI.

230. Answer is B (Herpes simplex Encephalitis): *Teaching Atlas of Brain Imaging 2nd/ 159 'MRI of Brain and spine' by Scott W. Atlas 4th/930 'Radiology secrets' 2nd/10 Harrison's 17th/1099; Harrison 18th/p 1458*

Hyperintensity in the temporal lobe and inferior frontal lobe on T2 weighted images with contrast enhancement is a charachteristic neuroanatomic pattern of involvement in Herpes simplex Encephalitis and in the presence of suggestive clinical features (fever / focal seizures) specifically suggests the diagnosis of HSV Encephalitis

'Suspect Herpes Simplex Encephalitis in the setting of T2 prolonging lesions with enhancement in the temporal lobe in a patient presenting with altered mental status, seizures and /or fever'- Teaching Atlas of Brain Imaging '2nd / 159

9

Herpes Simplex Encephalitis: Characteristic Anatomic Localization

- HSV encephalitis has a charachteristic neuroanatomic pattern of involvement affecting primarily the temporal lobe and inferior frontal lobe (cingulate gyrus).

The virus preferentially involves the temporal lobes and often the frontal lobes (especially the cingulate gyrus) (In most cases the involvement is unilateral, but contralateral involvement may also be seen and patient may present with asymmetric bilateral temporal lobe involvement)

- Herpes Encephalitis is also often haemorrhagic although not always
- This characteristic neuroanatomic pattern of involvement in Herpes Simplex Encephalitis can help in specifically suggesting the diagnosis of HSV encephalitis on MR scans.

MRI Scan Features of H.S.V. Encephalitis
• ***Hyperintensity on T2- weighted sequences*** (T2 prolonging lesions) within the medial temporal lobes (insula) and inferior frontal lobes (cingulate gyrus region) (Note: Hypointensity is seen on T1 weighted images) • ***Enhancement of lesions with contrast***. Enhancement of the meninges, cortex and white matter (Enhancement means that blood brain barrier has broken down and that the process is biologically active)

231. Answer is A (Acyclovir): *Harrison 15th/ 1094 (t-524.76); 16th /1041t; 17th/2632, 2633; Harrison 18th/p 3425, 3425*

The drug of choice in Herplex Simplex encephalitis is Acyclovir.

Condition	Drug of choice
Herpes simplex Encephalitis	***Acyclovir***
Neonatal herpes simplex Q	*Acyclovir* Q
Herpes simplex Keratitis Q	*Trifluridine / Vidarabine* Q
Herpes simplex Oro-labialis	Pencicyclovir

232. Answer is D (Neurocysticercosis): *Refer below*

"The most common parasitic infestation to affect the non immuno suppressed host is neurocysticercosis, a disorder caused by the larval form of taenia solium" *– Cecil*

233. Answer is A (Seizures): *CMDT 2002/ 1528; Harrison's 15th/ 1508; 16th/2487; 17th/2637; Harrison 18th/p 3431*

"These is wide variety of presentation of Neurocysticercosis depending on the intensity of the infestation, the localization of cystecerci and the degree of inflammatory reaction. ***Epilepsy (seizure activity) is the most common manifestation occurring in upto 50% cases*** *- API text book of Medicine 6th/784*

Cysticercosis is infection with the larval stage (cysticercus) of T. sollum.

These cysts are located in order of frequency in :
a. **CNS (Neurological manifestations are the most common)** *- Harrison's 15th/1249*
b. Subcutaneous tissue
c. Striated muscle
d. Globe of the eye

234. Answer is A (Brain Parenchyma): *Harrison 16th/2487; Harrison 17th/ 2638; Unusual manifestations of neurocystiurcosis in MR Imaging; Analysis of 172 cases' : Link : www. scielo. http;//www.scielo.br/scielo.php?script=sci arttext&=S004-282X2003000 400002; Harrison 18th/p 3431*

The lesion of neurocysticereosis is readily visualized by MRI or CT Scan. ***Paenchymal brain calcifications are the most common findings.*** *- Harrison 16th/2487*

Brain Parcnchyma is the most common site of neurocysticercosis. 'The ventricular system is the second most common site of neurocysticercosis. *-Above reference*

Most comon sites of Nurocyslicercosis : 'Unusual manifestation of Neurocysticerosis' (Reference as above)
Parenchymatous > intrventricular > subarachnoid > spinal > orbital.

235. Answer is B (Albendazole is superior to praziquantel in the treatment of above condition): *Katzung 8th/ 905*

*Although Albendazole and Praziquantel are both effective in treatment , **albendazole is the drug of choice.***

- ***Albendazole is preferred for the following reasons***:
  - Albendazole penetrates the subarachnoid space better than Praziquantel
  - Albendazole course of treatment is shorter (1 week) than that of praziquantel (2 weeks)
  - Albendazole is cheaper
  - Co-administration of albendazole and steroid (to treat inflammation) results in increased albendazole absorption, whereas combined use of prazaquantel and a steroid greatly decreases plasma levels of praziquantel.
- ***Anticonvulsants (antiepileptics)*** should be given during drug treatment and probably for an indefinite time afterwards. - *CMDT 2001/1458*
- ***Corticosteroids*** are used during the acute phase of cysticercotic encephalitis, if intracranial hypertension is present. (*It is used for the prevention of development of hydrocephalus, and does not have much role once hydrocephalus is already present.*)

236. Answer is C (Niclosamide): *CMDT 2001/ 1458; Harrisons 14th/ 1225; Harrison 15th/ 1193, 1248-49; 16th/1274; CMDT 2003/ 1458; Harrison 17th/1338; Harrison 18th/p 1762*

Niclosamide is ineffective for Neurocysticercosis
Albendazole and Proziquantel are both effective in treatment
Albendazole is preferred. (DOC is Albendazole)

237. Answer is B (Cytomegalovirus causes bilateral temporal lobe haemorphic infarction) : *Harrison 16th/2484, 2485, 1050; Harrison 17th/2631, 2635; Robbins 7th/1380, 346; Harrison 18th/p 3427, 3428*

CNS manifestation of CMV include meningoencephalitis and retinits. Haemorrhagic infarctions have not been mentioned as any feature of CMV retinitis.

All other options mentioned are true as explained below:

Progressive multifocal leukoencephalopathy (PML)	Subacute sclerosing panencephalitis (SSPE)	Spongiform encephalopathy
• Progressive disorder characterized pathologically by multifocal areas of demyelination disturbed throughout CNS. • JV virus (Human papovirus) grows in human glial cells and is found in oligodendrocytes of patients of PML. – Ananthnarayan 7th/562	• Progressive disorder characterized by demyelination of CNS • Associated with a chronic infection of brain tissue with measles virus. – Harrisons	• 'Disorders characterized by pongioform change' i.e. intracellular vacuoles in neurons and glia • Associated with infection with Prion proteins. - *Robbins*

238. Answer is A (They are infectious proteins): *Ananthnarayanan 7th/567; Harrisons 16th/2495; Jawetz 24th/581*

Prions are infectious proteins devoid of any nucleic acid - *Harrisons*

Prions and Prion associated diseases

- **Prions are infectious proteins** ***devoid of any nucleic acid (RNA or DNA)***[Q]
  (Prions are the only known infectious agents that are devoid of nucleic acid[Q]*)*
- Prion diseases result from the accumulation of the *abnormal prion protein 'Pr P*^{SC}*'*[Q]
- Prions are most *resistant to physical and chemical agents such as heat, irradiation and formaline*[Q].
- The diseases caused by Prions include diseases in human & animals

Prion diseases

Human
- *Creutzfeldt Jakob disease*[Q]
- *Gerstmann – Straussier Scheinker disease*[Q]
- *Fatal Familial Insomnia*[Q]
- *Kuru*[Q]

Animals
- *Scrapie (sheep)*[Q]
- *Bovine Spongiform Encephalopathy (cattle)*[Q]
- *Mink Encephalopathy (Mink)*[Q]
- *Chronic Wasting Disease (Mule, Deer, Elk)*[Q]
- *Feline Spongiform Encephalopathy (Cats)*[Q]

9 Nervous System

- Prion Diseases share several distinguishing hallmarks

Hallmarks of Prion Diseases
• The disease *is confined to the Nervous system*[Q] (Although agent may be recoverable from other organs)
• The basic features are *Neurodegeneration and Spongiform*[Q] changes
• Amyloid plaques may be present
• Clinical illness is preceded by *a long incubation period*[Q] (months to decades)
• Onset of clinical illness is followed by *chronic progressive disease*[Q] (weeks to years)
• The disease is *always fatal*[Q] with *no known cases of remission*[Q] or recovery
• The host shows *no inflammatory response and no immune response*[Q]
- *Agents do not appear to be antigenic*[Q]
- No production of interferon is elicited
- *There is no effect on host B cell or T cell function*
- *Immunosupression of the host has no effected on pathogenesis*

239. Answer is C (Proteins): *Harrison's 16th/2495; Ananthnarayanon 7th/567; Jawetz 24th/581*

Prions are infectious proteins devoid of any nucleic acid (RNA or DNA)

240. Answer is D (Alzheimer's disease): *Harrison 16th/2496;17th/ 2647 (Table 378-2); 18th/p 3442 (Table: 383.2)*

Alzheimer's disease is the most common cause of dementia in the Western World. It is not classified as a Prion disease.

Prion Diseases :

Humans	Animals
Kuru	Scrapic (sheep)
Creutzfeldt Jacob disease (CJD)	Bovine spongioform encephalopathy – BSE (cattle)
Gerstamann – Straussler – Scheinker disease (GSS)	Transmissable Mink encephalopathy – TME (Mink)
Fatal Familial insomnia	Chronic wasting disease – CWD (Mule, deer, elk)
	Feline spongioform encephalopathy – FSE (Cats)
	Exotic lingulate encephalopathy (kudu, nyala or oryx)

The sporadic form of CJD is the most common prion disorder in humans.

241. Answer is A (Prion Disease): *Ref: Harrison 14th/ 2451; 15th/ 2486; 16th/ 2495; 17th/2647 (Table 378-2) ; Harrison 18th/p 3442 (Table: 383.2)*

Fatal familial insomnia is one of the commonly caused prion disease.

PRIONS refer to a class of proteinacious infectious particles without any detectable nucleic acid i.e. 'virus like particles without the nucleic acid components'. – *Ananthnarayan 6th / 416*
As can be expected they are sensitive to proteases[Q] (contain protein) but resistant to nucleases[Q] (do not contain nucleic acid) as well as to heat & UV rays.

The most commonly caused prion diseases include :
1. Kuru [Q]
2. Creutzfeildt - Jakob disease [Q]
3. Gestermann - Straussler - Scheinker syndrome [Q]
4. *Fatal familial insomnia* [Q]

242. Answer. is B (Creutzfeldt Jakob disease) : *Harrison's 17th/ 2649; Diagnostic Criteria in Neurology 1st (2006)/29; Current Diagnosis and Treatment in Neurology 1st/478,479; Harrison 18th/p 3444, 3445*

The combination of progressive dementia, irregular jerky movements (myoclonus / choreoathetoid movements) in association with a characteristic EEG pattern (periodic sharp biphasic waves) suggests a diagnosis Creutzfeldt Jakob Disease.

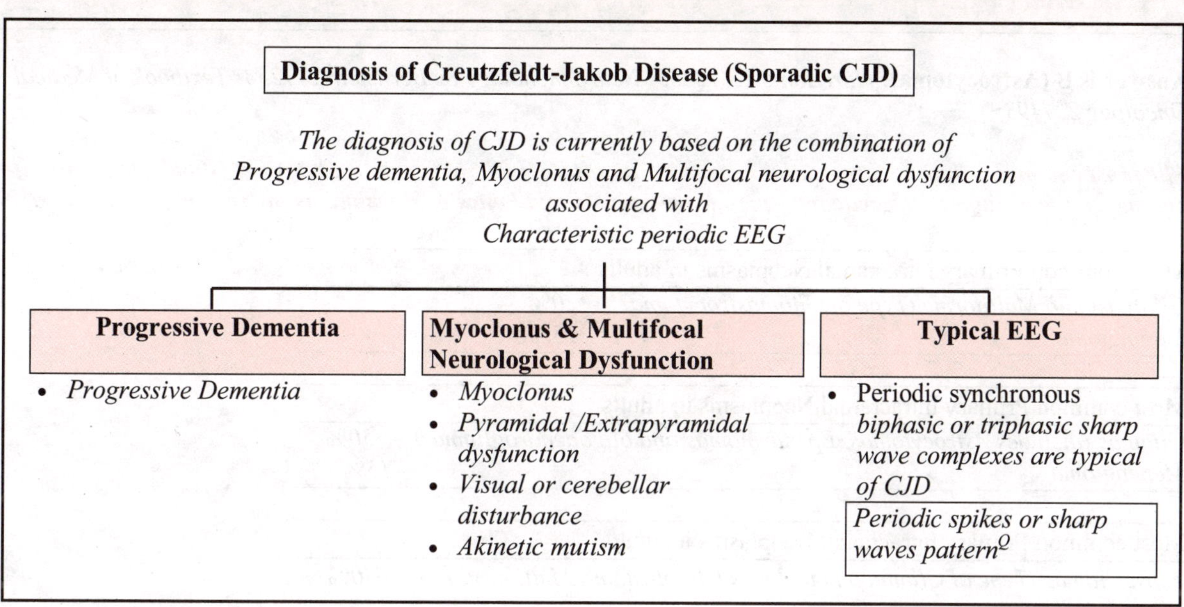

243. Answer is C (Myoclonus is rarely seen): *Ref: Harrison 16th/ 2499; Harrison 17th/2649, 2650;CMDT 2005/ 1327 Harrison 18th/p 3444, 3445, 3447*

'Myoclonus is a very common manifestation of C-J disease. 'Most patient (90%) with CJD exhibit myoclonus that appears at various times throughout the illness' – Harrisons.

Creutzfeldt-Jacob disease : Review

Nature of illness : *Heritable, degenerative, infectious disease.*
• Creutzfeldt- Jacob disease is the most common prion disease (infectious) in humans Q • It is a neurodegenerative disease with major pathological changes confined to CNS Q – *Harrisons 16th/ 2496* • The prion concept explains how this disease can manifest both a heritable Q as well as an infectious illness. Q
Clinical manifestations :
• Non specific prodromal symptoms : Fatigue, sleep disturbance, weight loss, headache, malaise, ill defined pain • Dementia Q (deficit in higher cortical functions) : Memory loss, impaired judgement, decline in intellectual function • Myoclonus Q: Most patients (90%) exhibit myoclonus at some time throughout illness. • Cerebellar signs visual impairment may occur
Characteristic ECG finding Q:
• Paroxysm of high voltage and slow waves
Treatment
• There is no specific treatment.

244. Answer is D (Entamoeba Histolytica): *Child Neurology 7th/517, Oxford Textbook of Medicine 'Infection' 5th (2012)/661 'Surgical Diseases in Tropical countries by Sood (Jaypee) 1996/8*

Amoebiasis is the least likely cause of seizures amongst the options provided.

Seizures may occur in Entamoeba Histolytica infections that cause an Amoebic Brain abscess however; Amoebic Brain Abscess due to Entamoeba Histolytica is a rare feature. This may occur from spread of infection from the bowel to a site within the CNS but this is remarkably rare. The presenting features of amoebic brain abscess are similar to other infective abscesses and brain tumors and may include seizures. Majority of such cases are however discovered postmortem.

CNS Tumors

245. Answer is B (Astrocytoma): *Harrison's 18th/2453; Neuroonchology by Bernstein 2nd/254; Textbook of Medical Oncology 2nd/493;*

The most common primary intracranial neoplasms in adults is Glioblastoma multifarme. Glioblastoma multiforme belongs to the group of astrocytic tumors or astrocytomas and hence astrocytoma is the single best answer of choice

Most Common Primary intracranial Neoplasms in adults	
Glioblastoma Multiforme (Type of Gliomastrocytoma)	*20%*
Meningioma	*15%*

Most common Primary Intracranial Neoplasms in adults	
Gliomas (includes Astrocytomas, Ependymomas and oligodendrogliomas)	*>50%*
Menengioma	*15%*

Most common Primary Intracranial Neoplasms in adults	
Astrocytomas (Type of Glioma and includes Glioblastoma Multiforma)	*≈30%*
Meningiomas	*15%*

246. Answer is B (Gliomas): *Harrisons 16th/2453; Neurooncology by Bernstein 2nd/254; Textbook of Medical oncology 2nd/493*

Gliomas are the most common primary intracranial neoplasms of the central system

Gliomas *(Most common)*
Astrocytomas (includes Glioblastoma multiforme)
Oligodendrogliomas
Ependymomas

Most common intracranial tumors in adults is
Glioblastoma multiforme (Glioma)
(Grade IV Astrocytoma)

Most common intracranial tumor in children is
Cerebellar Astrocytoma (Glioma)

247. Answer is A (Astrocytomas): *Harrisons 16th/2453*

Astrocytic tumors (Astrocytomas) are the most common types of glial tumors.

Glial tumors in decreasing order of frequency

- Astrocytomas (Most common)
  Glioblastoma multiforme is the most common type of Astrocytoma
- Ependymoma
- Oligodendroglioma

248. Answer is B (Astrocytoma): *CMDT 16th/899; High yield Nueroantomy 3rd/52; BRS Neuroanatomy 4th/87*

Cerebellar Astrocytomas are the most common posterior fossa tumors in children.
Medulloblastoma are the second most common posterior fossa tumors in children and the most common malignant posterior fossa tumors in children.

Most Common Posterior Fossa Tumors in Children	
Cerebellar Astrocytomas are the most common posterior fossa tumors In children	*Medulloblastomas and other primitive neuroectodermal tumors (PNET) are the most common malignant posterior fossa tumors in children*
Most Cerebellar Astrocytomas are benign.	Most medulloblastomas are malignant

Although CPDT and Nelson's textbook mention an equal incidence of cerebellar astrocytoma and medulloblastoma in the posterior fossa in children, most other standard textbooks mention cerebellar astrocytomas as the most common posterior fossa tumors in children.

249. Answer is D (These tumors are more common in females) : *Nelsons 18th /2130, 2131; WHO classification of Tumours of the Central Nervous System (2007) /14.*

Cerebellar Astrocytomas do not show any clear gender predilection and are equally common in both males & females.

- ***The predominant group of astrocytomas in childhood are low grade astrocytomas*** *(Nelsons)*
  Juvenile Pilocytic Astrocytoma (JPA) is the most common astrocytoma in children[Q]
  Juvenile Pilocytic Astrocytoma is a **low grade tumor and is classified as a WHO grade I tumor**
- ***Cerebellar Astrocytomas (JPA) do not show any clear gender predeliction***[Q] *(i.e, Equally common in males and females)* (From WHO classification of tumors of CNS)
- ***Cerebellar Astrocytomas (Juvenile JPA) most commonly develop during the first two decades of life***[Q] (WHO classification of Tumors of CNS)
- ***Cerebellar Astrocytomas have a good prognosis***

With complete surgical resection the overall survival for Juvenile Pilocytic Astrocytomas approaches 80% - 100%

Facts to Remember :

- The most common tumors in children are : Leukaemia
- The most common solid tumours in children are: CNS tumors
- The most common site of brain tumors in children is Infratentorial (cerebellar)
- The most common site of brain tumors in neonates is supratentorial
- The most common CNS tumors in children are Glial tumors

Glial tumors
• *Astrocytomas*
• *Oligodindrogliomas*
• *Ependymomas*

Note

- **Glial tumors as a group are more common than medulloblastomas**
- If a question asks about the most common brain tumor in children, and it does not have astrocytoma as an option, but it has 'glioma' as an option, *mark* Glioma in preferance to Medulloblastoma. (Astrocytoma is also a ' glioma').
- When based on histology the prevalence of Medulloblastomas and Juvenile Pilocytic astrocytoma / cerebellar astrocytomas has been mentioned as equal in most textbooks **Yet Cerebellar astrocytomas are accepted as the most common posterior fossa tumors in children**

- ***Astrocytoma (Cerebellar)***
  - *Most common posterior fossa tumor in children is Cerebellar Astrocytoma.*[Q]
  - *Therefore most common brain tumor in children is also Cerebellar Astrocytoma.*[Q]
  - *Astrocytoma also has the best prognosis in children.*[Q]
  - *Therefore tumor with best prognosis in children is also Astrocytoma.*[Q]
- ***Medulloblastoma***
  - *The second most common posterior fossa tumor in children.*[Q]
  - *Tumor which spreads along CSF pathways is medulloblastoma.*[Q]
  - *Tumor which is capable of metastasising to extracranial sites is medulloblastoma.*[Q]
  - *Medulloblostoma is highly radiosensitive.*[Q]
- ***Brain Stem Gliomas :***
  - *These are the third most frequent post. fossa tumors in children*[Q]
- ***Craniopharyngioma :***
  - *These are the most common supratentorial tumor in children.*[Q]

250. Answer is B (Foraman of munro): *Neurology in clinical practice 4th/1428; Neuro-ancology by Bernstein (2000)*

Most common site of subependymal giant cell astrocytoma is the ependymal wall of lateral ventricle near the foramen of munro.

Subependymal Giant cell Astrocytomas (SEGCA)

- *Subependymal Giant cell Astrocytomas are low grade non filtrating (benign) variants of astrocytomas.*
- *They are characteristically (but not always) associated with tuberous sclerosis*

Occur most frequently in patients with autosomal dominant phakomatosis tuberous sclerosis[Q]

- ***The most common site of SEGCA is the ependymal wall of lateral ventricle near the foramen of munro and these tumors tend to grow towards the foramen of munro (leading to obstructive hydrocephalus)***
- *Pathologically lesions are composed of Giant cells*
- *Candle dripping radiographic appearance is characteristic*
- *These tumors predominantly occur is children (1st decade)*
- *These tumors are essentially benign*
- *Total Gross resection is the treatment of choice*

251. Answer is C (Cerebellar Astrocytomas): *Nelsons 18th/2130; Textbook of medical Oncology 2nd/494*

Most cerebellar astrocytomas are histologically Juvenile pilocytic astrocytomas.
Juvenile pilocystic astrocytomas are benign and non infiltrating astrocytomas with an excellent prognosis (95% 5 year survival with surgery alone)

Ependymomas are also histologically benign but carry a worse prognosis than cerebellar astrocytomas with (80% 5 year survival rate)
Medulloblastomas and **Glioblastoma Multiforme** are malignant tumors with a poor prognosis.

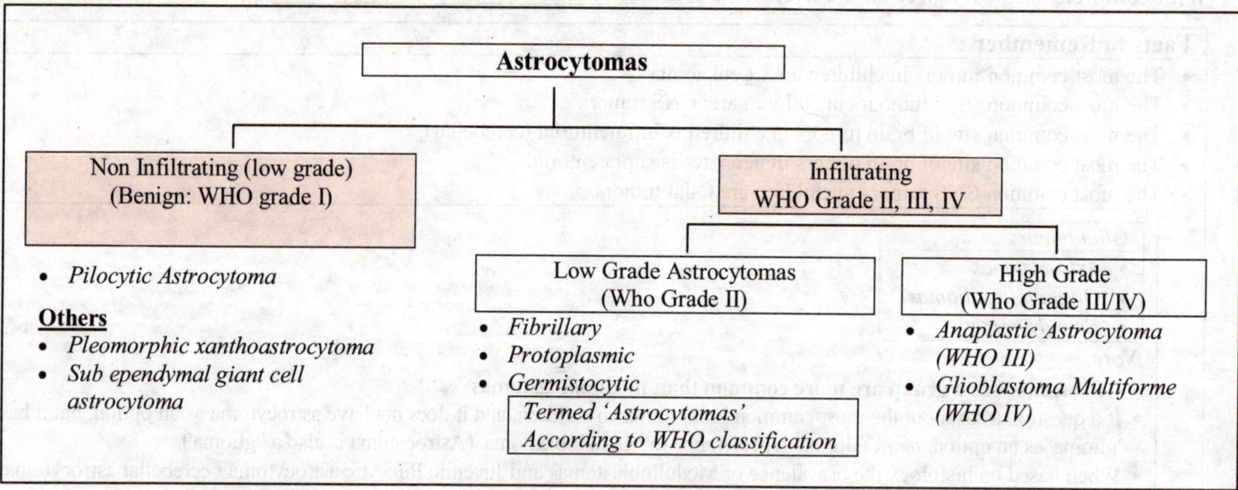

252. Answer is C (Hemangioblastoma) : *Chandrasoma Taylor 2nd / 933*

Cerebellar hemangioblastoma is a benign neoplasm that occurs either sporadically or as part of Von Hippel - Lindau disease - *Chandrasoma Taylor 2nd/933*

Clinically presentation is with:
- Cerebellar dysfunction
- Hydrocephalus
- Polycythemia (the tumor produces erythropoetin).[Q]

253. Answer is B (Medulloblastomas): *Principles of Cancer treatment (1981)/876; Current Guidelines for Management of Cancer (1986)/289*

Medulloblastomas are highly radiosensitive tumors of the Central Nervous system and more radiosensitive than all gliomas (Astrocytoma, Eperdymoma, Glioblastoma Multiforme)

'Medulloblastoma is the most radiosensitive of all gliomas whereas Glioblastomas are the least radiosensitive'
– Current Guidelines for Management of Cancer (1986)/289

NOTE
Medulloblastoma were originally classified as 'gliomas' but they are now classified as primitive neuroectodermal Tumors (PNET)

Radiosensitive Brain Tumors in Children

- *Medulloblastomas and other PNET (Most radiosensitive)*
- *Gliomas (low grade astrocytoma), ependymoma*
- *Pineal blastoma*
- *Craniopharygnioma*
- *Germ cell tumors (pure germinoma-highly radiosensitive)*

254. Answer is D (Craniopharyngioma): *Text book on Clinical and radiation Oncology*

'Certain brain tumors such as medulloblastomas, primitive neurectodermal tumors, anaplastic ependymomas, choroid plexus carcinoma, pineoblastomas germ cell tumors and lymphomas may involve the CSF, leptomeningis of the brain or spinal cord'.

Thus all tumors except craniopharyngiomas mentioned as options may involve CSF.

255. Answer is B (Craniopharygioma): *Harrison's 17th/2201, 2607; 16th/2080, 2081, 2457; Harrison 18th/p 2883, 3389*

Presence of headache, visual field defects and suprasellar calcification suggests a diagnosis of suprasellar neoplastic lesions.

The most common suprasellar neoplastic lesion in children (6 years) associated with suprasellar calcification is craniopharyngioma which is the single best answer of choice.

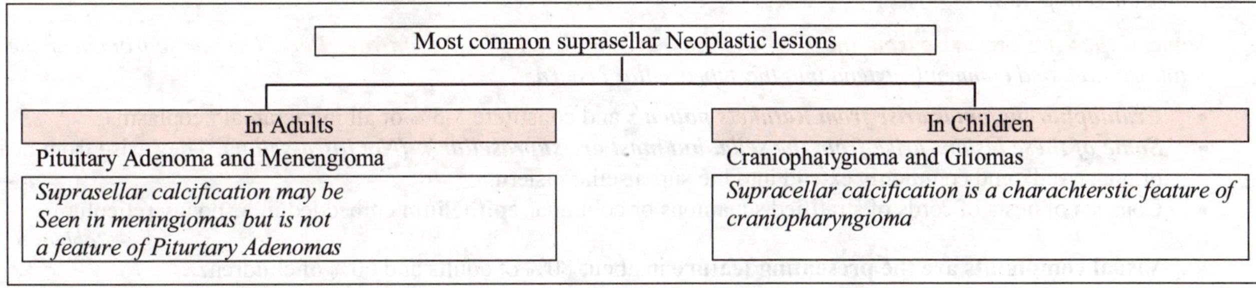

Presence of suprasellar calcification in pediatric age group (6 years old child) suggest the diagnosis of craniopharyngioma.

256. Answer is C (Lung Metastasis is common) : *Nelson's 18th/2138; Robbins 7th/500, 501; Ghai 6th/573; 'Neuroblastoma' by Pochedly (1990) / 154*

***Lung metastasis are rare in neuroblastoma** - Nelson*

Neuroblastoma is the most common extracranial solid tumor in childhood

Neuroblastoma is the second most common solid malignancy of childhood after brain tumors which makes it the most common extracranial solid tumor in childhood

Most common solid tumor in childhood: Brain tumors[Q]
Most common extracranial solid tumor in childhood: Neuroblastoma[Q]
Most common intra abdominal solid tumor in childhood: Neuroblastoma[Q]

Metastasis is present in > 50% of patients at the time of diagnosis

'Metastasis is present in 60- 70% of patients at the time of diagnosis' - Ghai 6th /573

Metastasis to Lungs is Rare (uncommon)

'Lung metastasis is rare occurring in < 3% of cases' – Nelson 18th / 2138

Common sites of metastasis in Neuroblastoma

- Long bones – skull, bone marrow
- Liver
- Lymph nodes
- Skin

Often Encases Aorta and its branches at time of diagnosis

'Encasement of abdominal aorta and inferior vena cava by tumor is common'- 'Neuroblastoma' by Pochedly (1990)/154

'Some neuroblastomas are sharply demarcated with a fibrous pseudocapsule but others are far more infiltrative and invade surrounding strictures including the kidney, renal vein, I V C and envelop the aorta' - Robbins 7th / 501

'Wilm's tumor does not encase the aorta whereas encasement is characteristic of neuroblastoma'

- Radiology Illustrated (2003) / 209

Note

Although encasement of aorta is likely to occur late in disease neuroblastomas are already metastatic (stage IV disease) at presentation in > 50% of patients. Hence encasement of aorta may be often found at the time of diagnosis.

Remember

Feature	Neuroblastoma	Wilm's Tumor
Common tumor	Most common intraabdominal solid tumor in children	Most common renal tumor in children
At the time of Diagnosis	Already metastatic in greater than 50% of patients	Generally confined to the kidney
Lung Metastasis	Rare	Common
Encasement of Aorta	Characteristic	Uncommon
Calcification	Common	Rare

257. Answer is C (Present in sella or infrasellar location): *Harrison 15th/2034; 16th/2081, 2457; 17th/2201Robbins 6th/1129; Harrison 18th/p 2883*

Some of these lesions arise from the sella, but most are suprasellar Q (Not infra-sellar). *They arise from near the pituitary stalk and commonly extend into the supra sellar cistern.*

- ***Craniopharyngiomas arise from Rathke's pouch Q*** and constitute 3-5% of all intracranial neoplasms.
- ***Some of these lesions arise from the sella, but most are suprasellar Q (Not infra-sellar)***. They arise from near the pituitary stalk and commonly extend into the supra sellar cistern.
- Consists of nests of cords of stratified squamous or columnar **epithelium** embedded in a spongy reticulum *– Robbins 6th/1129*
- **Visual complaints are the presenting feature** in about 80% of adults and 60% of children.

258. Answer is A (Pituitary adenoma): *Harrison 14th/ 1975, Harrison 15th/ 2038; 17th/2206; Harrison 18th/p 2889*

Pituitary adenomas produce excess prolactin which causes hypogonadism, decreased levels of testosterone and explains loss of erection.

Pituitary adenomas (Prolactinomas) lead to an excess of prolactin. This inhibits hypothalamic release of LHRH resulting in defective LH & FSH secretion. Defective LH & FSH secretion in turn result in decreased levels of estrogen in females & testosterone in males. This is how prolactin excess can cause hypogaonadism

In men prolactin excess can cause	In females prolactin excess can cause
Decreased Libido, impotence	Irregular mensus (amenorrhea)
Infertility.	Infertility despite regular mensus.

This explains this 30 year old male's complaints of loss of erection & his low testosterone & high prolactin levels.
Testicular failure *explains both loss of erection and low testosterone levels but not the high prolactin levels*

259. Answer is A (Lymphoma): *Harrison's 18th/1566*

The most common neoplasm in the central Nervous System (CNS malignancy) in HIV positive patients is primary CNS Lymphoma.

'Primary CNS Lymphoma is the most common neoplasm of the CNS in HIV positive patients'.

- 'Radiology of AIDS' (Springer 2001)/69

'Primary CNS Lymphoma is the most common CNS opportunistic malignancy in patients with HIV infection'.
-Spiral Manual of Allergy & Immunology 4th/439

Lymphomas in HIV / AIDS

Three main types /categories of Lymphomas are seen in patients with HIV infection

Immunoblastic Lymphomas (60%)	Small Non-cleaved cell Lymphoma (Burkitt's Lymphoma ~20%)	Primary CNS Lymphoma (~20%)
• ***Immunoblastic Lymphomas are the most common Lymphomas seen in patients with AIDS*** • The majority of these are Diffuse Large B-cell Lymphomas (DLBCL)	• Burkitt's type lymphomas in patients with AIDS • *In contrast to African Burkitt's Lymphoma where 97% of the cases contain EBV genome, only 50% of HIV associated Burkitt's Lymphoma are EBV positive.*	• Primay CNS Lymphoma account for 20% of lymphomas in patient with AIDS • ***This is however the most common CNS tumor/Lymphoma*** seen in patients with HIV/AIDS

260. Answer is D (Diplopia): *Merrst's Neurology 12th/373; Essential Neurology (John Wiley & Sons) 2009/44*

Sixth Nerve Palsy (Abducent; Lateral Rectus) producing double vision (diplopia) is the most common false localizing sign because of its long intracranial course.

'A right sided brain tumor can produce either a right sided or a left sided sixth nerve palsy as an initial sign. Thus left sided sixth nerve palsy in a right-sided brain tumor represents the infamous 'false localizing sign'.

'The most common false localizing sign is a sixth nerve palsy (diplopia). The nerve is particularly vulnerable because of its long course' - Merritt's Neurology

Brain Tumors

Generalized features (Non-Localizing signs)	Localizing /Focal signs	False Localizing Signs
Generalized symptoms like headache (most common generalized sign), nausea, vomiting, vertigo, dizziness and non specific mental and cognitive abnormalities represent generalized features of brain tumors that do not help localize the tumor to a particular part of brain.	• The presence of a tumor impairs the function of the part of the brain where it resides • The nature of evolving focal neurological defect / focal seizures serves as localizing signs for tumors in various parts of brain • ***Unilateral papillaedema, abnormal unilateral pupil, specific aphasia, agnosias etc. can localize the tumor to a particular part of the brain.***	• Neurological signs that reflect dysfunction, distant from the actual part of the brain involved are called ***False localizing signs*** • *False localizing signs are generally produced from raised ICT and/or shift and compression of brain remote from the primary site.* • *The most common false localizing sign is sixth nerve palsy (Lateral Rectus Palsy producing Diplopia).* The sixth CN is especially vulnerable because of its long intracranial course.

False Localizing signs (Brain tumors causing Raised ICT are known to produce false localizing signs)

1. Sixth Nerve Palsy (Lateral pectus palsy) producing diplopia is the most common false localizing sign produced by compression of the abducent nerve as it passes over the petrous ridge.
2. Ventricular dilation above midline in CSF obstructive lesions or posterior fossa lesions may produce false localizing signs
   - *Intellectual and Behavioral changes suggestive of primary frontal pathology*
   - *An interference with vertical eye movement (impaired up-gaze) which are programmed in the upper midbrain because of the dilation of posterior part of 3rd ventricle and aqueduct*
3. Ipsilateral hemiparesis may represent a false localizing sign when a herniating uncus compresses the contralateral cerebral peduncle against the tentorium.
4. Cortical blindness or hemianopia may occur from compression of posterior cerebral arteries with occipital infarction from herniation through the tentorial notch.
5. Tinnitus may present as a false localizing sign as this may result from raised ICP of any cause.
6. Hydrocephalus may lead to presonality changes, gait abnormalities and urinary incontinence suggesting false localizing signs.

261. Answer is D (Antisocial behaviour): *Harrison 14th/ 140; 16th/152; 17th/170;*

Antisocial behaviour is a characteristic feature of frontal disinhibition syndrome produced from frontal lobe damage

A tumor of the frontal lobe is likely to damage the pre-frontal network. This presents as two relatively distinct syndromes.

Frontal abulic syndrome	**Frontal disinhibition syndrome**
- Loss of initiative, creativity and curiosity	- Socially disinhibited and shows severe impairment of judgement, insight and foresight.
- Pervasive emotional apathy and blandness	- Patient cannot learn from experience and displays inappropriate behavior without experiencing emotional pain, guilt or regret ***'Antisocial behavior'***. Q

262. Answer is A (Frontal lobe abscess) : *Read text below*

Development of headache, fever and papilledema in the setting of sinusitis suggest an infective pathology causing raised introcranial tension. Further, presence of personality changes suggest a mass lesion affecting the frontal lobe. A brain abscess typically presents as an expanding intracranial mass lesion, and the presence of personality changes limits such a mass lesion to the frontal lobe. A frontal lobe abscess thus explains the presence of an infectious mass lesion causing personality changes.

263. Answer is A (Autosomal Recessive inheritance): *Nelsons 18th/ 2483,2484,2485*

Neurofibromatosis is inherited as an autosomal dominant condition

Neurofibromatosis

Oculoneurocutaneous syndrome characterized by multisystem involvement

Neurofibromatosis I (NF1) Peripheral Neurofibromatosis (Von Recklinghausen's syndrome)	Neurofibromatosis II (NF II) Central Neurofibromatosis (Bilateral Acoustic Neurofibromatosis)
• Most prevalent type (90%) • Recognized to be related to abnormality of chromosome 17 (NFI gene) • Transmitted as an ***Autosomal Dominant disorder*** Diagnostic Criteria for NF1 Diagnosed when any two of the following are present 1. Six more *café-au-lait* macules over 5 mm in greatest diameter in prepubertal individuals and over 15 mm in greatest diameter in post-pubertal individuals. 2. Axillary or inguinal freckling 3. Two or more iris *Lisch nodules* 4. Two or more ***neurofibromas*** or one plexiform neurofibroma 5. A distinctive osseous lesion such as sphenoid dysplasia or cortical thinning of long bone, with or without pseudoarthrosis. 6. Optic gliomas. 7. A first degree relative with NFI whose diagnosis was based on the aforementioned criteria.	• Less prevalent type (10%) recognized to be related to abnormality of chromosome 22 (NF2 gene) • Transmitted as an ***Autosomal dominant disorder*** Diagnostic Criteria for NF2 Diagnosed when any one of the following is present. 1. ***Bilateral eighth nerve masses consistent with acoustic neuromas*** as demonstrated by CT scanning or MRI 2. A parent, sibling, or child with NF-2 and either 3. unilateral eight nerve mass or any two of the following: - Neurofibroma - Meningioma - Glioma - Schwannoma - ***Juvenile posterior subcapsular opacity*** *Bilateral acoustic neuromas are the most distinctive tumors in patients with NF-2.*
Note ***Scoliosis*** *is the most common orthopaedic manifestation of NF1* although it is not specific enough to be included as a diagnostic criteria – *Nelson 18th/2483*	Note ***Posterior subcapsular lens opacities (cataract)*** *are identified in ≃ 50% of patients with NF2* *– Nelson 18th/2484*

264. Answer is C (Shgreen Patch): *Nelson's 18th/ 2483-2484-2485*

Shagreen Patch is seen in Tuberous Sclerosis and not in Neurofibromatosis
Lisch Nodules, Axillary Freckling and Caffe-au-lait spots are seen in Neurofibromotosis

Shagreen Patch are seen in Tuberous Sclerosis
Shagreen Spots[Q] are *roughened, raised, leathery lesions with an orange peel consistency seen as cutaneous manifestations of Tuberous sclerosis*

265. Answer is A (Optic Nerve Glioma): *Nelson 17th/ 2016; 18th/2483, 2484; Diagnostic Neuroradiology; Anne G. Osborn, 1994*

The commonest tumor in neurofibromatosis I is optic nerve glioma. Optic gliomas are present in approximately 15% of patients with NFI and its presence is included as one of the criteria in establishing its diagnosis.

Neoplasms associated with NF-I include:

CNS Neoplasms	Others tumors with higher incidence than general population
1. Optic nerve glioma (commonest)	1. Pheochromocytomas
2. Meningiomas	2. Rhabdomyosarcomas
3. Neurofibromas	3. Leukaemia
4. Schwannomas	4. Wilm's
5. Astrocytomas	5. Juvenile Xanthogranulomas
6. *Neurolemmomas*	

266. Answer is A, C, E: *'Orbital Tumors: Diagnosis Treatment (2004)/199; Nelsons 17th/2016*

Neurofibromatosis II is recognized to be related to an abnormality on chromosome 22. Bilateral Accoustic Neuromas (schwannomas) are the most charachteristic tumors associated with NF2 while Juvenile posterior subcapsular cataracts are the one of the most charachteristic ocular manifestations of NF2.

Lisch nodules and multiple café –au-lait spots are feature of Neurofibromatosis 1 (NF-1) and not Neurofibromatosis II (NF-2)

Neurofibromatosis

Oculoneurocutaneous syndrome characterized by multisystem involvement

Neurofibromatosis I (NF1)

Peripheral Neurofibromatosis
(Von Recklinghausen's syndrome)

- Most prevalent type (90%)
- Recognized to be related to abnormality of chromosome 17 (NFI gene)
- Transmitted as an Autosomal Dominant disorder

Diagnostic Criteria for NF1

Diagnosed when any two of the following are present

8. Six more ***café-au-lait*** macules over 5 mm in greatest diameter in prepubertal individuals and over 15 mm in greatest diameter in post-pubertal individuals.
9. Axillary or inguinal freckling
10. Two or more iris ***Lisch nodules***
11. Two or more neurofibromas or one plexiform neurofibroma
12. A distinctive osseous lesion such as sphenoid dysplasia or cortical thinning of long bone, with or without pseudoarthrosis.
13. Optic gliomas.
14. A first degree relative with NFI whose diagnosis was based on the aforementioned criteria.

Neurofibromatosis II (NF II)

Central Neurofibromatosis
(Bilateral Acoustic Neurofibromatosis)

- Less prevalent type (10%) recognized to be related to abnormality of chromosome 22 (NF2 gene)
- Transmitted as an autosomal dominant disorder

Diagnostic Criteria for NF2

Diagnosed when any one of the following is present.

4. ***Bilateral eighth nerve masses consistent with acoustic neuromas*** as demonstrated by CT scanning or MRI
5. A parent, sibling, or child with NF-2 and either unilateral eight nerve mass or any two of the following:
   - Neurofibroma
   - Meningioma
   - Glioma
   - Schwannoma
   - ***Juvenile posterior subcapsular opacity***

Bilateral acoustic neuromas are the most distinctive tumors in patients with NF-2.

267. Answer is B (Optic Nerve Glioma): *Rudolph's Pediatrics 21st/2399; Child Neurology 7th/777*

Optic Gliomas are the most common intracranial tumors in Neurofibromotosis 1.

Optic Gliomas are present in about 15 to 25% of patient with NF-1 and its presence is included as one of the criteria in establishing its diagnosis (Diagnostic criteria in NF1)

Optic Gliomas are the most common intracranial tumors of Neurofibromatosis 1- Child Neurology

268. Answer is B (Gastric carcinoma): *Harrison 17th/2607; Harrison Endocrinology 1st/395; Harrison 18th/p 2360*

Gastric carcinoma are not associated with Von Hippel Lindau syndrome.

Von Hippel Lindau Syndrome

Autosomal dominant syndrome

Characteristic Tumors/Cysts	Other tumors / Cysts
Hemagioblastomas - Cerebellar hemangioblastoma - Retinal hemangioblastoma - Spinal hemangioblastoma	• ***Renal cell carcinoma / hypernephroma*** • ***Pheochromocytoma*** • *Pancreatic endocrine tumors* • *Adrenal carcinomas* • *Benign cysts in Kidney, epidydimis, Liver or pancreas*

Polycythemia is a characteristic associated feature in VHL due to erythropoietin production by hemangioblastoma and/or Renal cell carcinoma

269. Answer is A (Cerebellum)

Hemangioblastomas associated with Von-Hippel–Lindau Disease are most commonly seen in the cerebellum.

'The hallmark lesion of Von-Hippel-Lindau (VHL) disease is the hemangioblastoma. These are most commonly seen in the cerebellum but occasionally seen in the medulla oblongata (most common brainstem site), spinal cord and supratentorially in the optic nerves and cerebral hemispheres' - *MRI of the Brain and spine (Lippincott).*

'The most common CNS manifestation of VHL is the charachteristic cerebellar hemangioblastoma. Approximately 60-80% of VHL patients ultimately develop a CNS Hemangioblastoma. ***Three quarters of these are cerebellar in location*** *with the majority of the remaining hemangioblastomas located in the spinal cord. Hemangioblastomas of the cerebral hemisphere account for only a small minority of lesions'* - *Oncology of CNS Tumors (Springer) 2010/377*

Diagnostic Criteria for Von-Hippel-Lindau Disease

Central nervous system *and* *Retinal Hemangioblastoma*	*Hemangioblastoma and at least one of the following:* • *Renal, pancreastic, hepatic, epididymal cyst* • *Pheochromocytoma* • *Renal cancer*	*Family history and at least one of the following* • *Hemangioblastoma* • *Visceral changes* • *Pheochromocytoma* • *Renal cancer*

270. Answer is C (Cerebellum) : *Kanski 5th/719*

Von Hipple-Lindau Syndrome is associated with haemangioblastomas of cerebellum, spinal cord, medulla or pons.

Von Hippel – Lindau Syndrome : *Review*
Von Hipple Lindau Syndrome is a life threatening phakomastosis characterized by capillary haemoangiomas of retina or optic nerve head.

Clinical spectrum includes:

Haemangiomas		Tumors	Cysts	Polycythemia
Capillary haemiangiomas of retina or optic nerve head.	*with or without*	Haemangioblastoma: - Cerebellum - Spinal chord - Medulla or pons Renal carcinoma Pheocrhomocytoma	Renal Pancreatic Hepatic Epidydimal Ovarian Pulmonary	

271. Answer is B (Cerebellar Hemangioblastomas): *Harrison 17th/2607; Harrison 18th/p 2360*

Von Hippel Lindau syndrome is associated with retinal, cerebellar and spinal hemangioblastoma.

Von Hippel Lindau Syndrome

Autosomal dominant syndrome

Characteristic Tumors/Cysts	Other tumors / Cysts
Hemagioblastomas - Cerebellar hemangioblastoma - Retinal hemangioblastoma - Spinal hemangioblastoma	• ***Renal cell carcinoma / hypernephroma*** • ***Pheochromocytoma*** • *Pancreatic endocrine tumors* • *Adrenal carcinomas* • *Benign cysts in Kidney, epidydimis, Liver or pancreas*

Polycythemia is a characteristic associated feature in VHL due to erythropoietin production by hemangioblastoma and/or Renal cell carcinoma

272. Answer is B (Craniospinal hemangioblastomas are common): *'Current Diagnosis & Treatment in Neurology' (2008)/149; Harrison's 18th/2360; 'NORD' Guide to Rare Disorders (Lippincott Williams) 2003/265*

Multiple Craniospinal Hemangioblastoma (Infratentorial) are characteristic of Von-Hippel Lindau syndrome.

Von-Hippel-Lindau syndrome is associated with multiple tumors

*'Von Hippel Lindau disease (VHL) is a rare autosomal disease characterised by abnormal angiogenesis with benign and malignant tumors that affect **multiple sites'*** *– Harrisons*

*'CNS Hemangioblastomas are often **multiple**' – 'NORD' Guide to rare Disorders*

Craniospinal Hemangioblastomas are common while tumors of Schwann cells are Rare

Craniospinal Hemangioblastomas are considered the hallmark tumors in Von-Hippel Lindau disease (VHL)
Hemangioblastomas in VHL are often multiple and most frequently found in the cerebellum, spinal cord and brainstem

Von Hippel Lindau Syndrome

Autosomal dominant syndrome

Characteristic Tumors/Cysts	Other tumors / Cysts
Hemagioblastomas (Cranio-spinal) • *Cerebellar hemangioblastoma* • *Retinal hemangioblastoma* • *Spinal* hemangioblastoma	• ***Renal cell carcinoma / hypernephroma*** • ***Pheochromocytoma*** • *Pancreatic endocrine tumors* • *Adrenal carcinomas* • *Benign cysts in Kidney, epidydimis, Liver or pancreas*

Polycythemia is a characteristic associated feature in VHL due to erythropoietin production by hemangioblastoma and/or Renal cell carcinoma

Clinical spectrum includes:

Haemangiomas		Tumors	Cysts	Polycythemia
Capillary haemiangiomas of retina or optic nerve head.	*with or without*	Haemangioblastoma: - Cerebellum - Spinal cord - Medulla or pons Renal carcinoma Pheochromocytoma	Renal Pancreatic Hepatic Epidydimal Ovarian Pulmonary	

Tumors in Von Hippel Lindau syndrome are charcateristically Infratentorial.

Tumors in Von Hippel Lindau syndrome are rarely found supratentorially'

- 'Pattern Recognition Neuroradiology' (Cambridge) 2011/26

Neurocutaneous Syndromes	Location
Neurofibromatosis 1 (NF1)	*Supratentorial and Infratentorial*
Neurofibromatosis II (NF II)	*Supratentorial and Infratentorial*
Sturge-Weber Syndrome	*Supratentorial*
Von-Hippel Lindau Syndrome (VHL)	***Infratentorial more than Supratentorial***
Tuberous Sclerosis (Bournville's Disease)	*Supratentorial (Primarily Supratentorial)*

273. Answer is C (Hemangioblastoma): *Chandrasoma Taylor 2nd/ 933;*

Cerebellar hemangioblastoma is a benign neoplasm that occurs either sporadically or as part of Von Hippel - Lindau disease - *Chandrasoma Taylor 2nd/ 933*

Clinically presentation is with :
- Cerebellar dysfunction Q - Hydrocephalus - Polycythemia (the tumor produces erythropoietin). Q

274. Answer is A (Tuberous Sclerosis): *Oski's Pediatrics 4th/861, CPDT 19th/715, Nelson's 18th/2485, 2486*

The presence of hyopigmented macules in the background of seizures and mental retardation suggests the diagnosis of Tuberous Sclerosis.

Often hypopigmented macules are the initial clue to tuberous sclerosis, a neurocutaneous disorder inherited in an autosomal dominant manner. ***Any child with unexplained seizures should be examined carefully for cutaneous clues, particularly hypopigmented macules****. The hypopigmented lesions are small, ovoid and scattered and their number varies.' – Oski's Pediatrics 4th/861*

The off white hypomelonotic macules are seen more easily in tanned or dark skinned individuals. The macules often are oval or 'ash leaf' in shape and follow dermatomes. ***In infancy the presence of these macules accompanied by seizures is virtually diagnostic of Tuberous Sclerosis'*** *– CPDT 19th/715*

Tuberous Sclerosis

Autosomal Dominant^Q Neurocutaneous Disorder

Cutaneous Features

- **Hypopigmented macules/Ash-leaf spots^Q**
  - Seen in >90% of cases
  - Are small, ovoid, scattered and variable in number
  - Larger lesions are known as 'Ash-leaf' spots as these may have jagged edges resembling a 'leaf'
- **Shagreen Spots^Q**
  - Roughened, raised, leathery lesions with an orange peel consistency
- **Adenoma Sebacium^Q**
  - Facial skin hamartoma that develops in early childhood (~ 4-6 years of age)
  - Appears as tiny red nodules over nose and cheeks resembling acne
- ***Facial Angiofibromas / Ungual Fibromas***
  Facial angiofibromas may seen ungula fibromas are more common in toes
- **Café- au- lait spots**
  These may be seen occasionally

Neurological Features

- **Seizures^Q**
  - *Seizures are the most common presenting symptom*
  - *Infantile spasms may be the presenting feature during infancy*
- **Mental Retardation^Q**
  - Mental Retardation occurs in upto 50% of patients referred to tertiary care
  - Patients with seizures are more prone to mental retardation

The charachteristic brain lesion is a cortical 'Tuber'. The most common neurological manifestations include seizures, cognitive impairment and behavioral abnormalities including autism.

Other Features

- **Renal Lesions**
  Renal cysts or angiomyolipomas may occur (Hematuria /obstruction)
- **Cardiac Lesions**
  Rhabdomyomas of the heart may occur
- **Pulmonary Lesions**
  Lymphagiomyomatosis is the classical pulmonary lesion
  Rarely cystic lung disease may occur
- **Eye lesions**
  Retinal Hamartomas may occur
- **Skeletal lesions**
  Cystic rarefaction of the bones or the fingers or toes.

T. S. 'Classical Triad' described includes Seizures, Mental Retardation and Adenoma Sebacium (occurs in <33% patients)
T.S should be suspected in any child presenting with unexplained seizures who shows hypopigmented cutaneous macules.

275. Answer is B (Tuberous Sclerosis): *Ref: Read text below; Nelson 17th/ 2017; 18th/2483, 2484*

Neurological features of seizures and mental retardation together with cutaneous manifestations in the form of sebaceous adenomas are characteristic of the neurocutaneous syndrome of Tuberous sclerosis.

Tuberous sclerosis

It is genetically determined autosomal dominant, neuro-cutaneous syndrome characterized by :

Skin (Cutaneous) Involvement	Neurological Features	Benign Neoplasms
• *Adenoma sebacium* ^{Q}: facial angiofibroma. • *Ash-leaf* ^{Q} shaped hypopigmented macules • *Shagreen patches* ^{Q}: yellowish thickening of skin over Lumbosacral region of back. • *Depigmented Nevi* ^{Q}	• *Epilepsy* ^{Q}, Seizures • *Mental retardation* ^{Q} • *Hydrocephalus* ^{Q} • Subependymal nodules ^{Q} with calcification on neuroimaging is characteristic. ^{Q}	• Rhabdomyoma of myocardium ^{Q} • Angiomyoma of kidney / liver / pancreas ^{Q}/ adrenals. • Ependymomas ^{Q} and Childhood Subependymal giant cell Astrocytoma. ^{Q}

276. Answer is D (Hydrocephalus): *Harrison 17th/2607; CPDT 16th/757; Harrison 18th/p 3390*

The characteristic triad in tuberous sclerosis includes epilepsy, mental retardation and Adenoma Sebacium

Characteristic Triad of Tuberous Sclerosis
• *Epilepsy/Seizures*^{Q}
• *Mental Retardation / Subnormal Intelligence*^{Q}
• *Adenoma Sebacium*^{Q}

277. Answer is D (Sturge Weber Syndrome): *Harrison 17th/2607; Current Neurology 1st/554, 555; Harrison 18th/p 2360, 3389, 3390*

Sturge Weber Syndrome is not associated with brain tumors

Von Hippel Lindau Syndrome, Neurofibromatosis and Tuberous sclerosis may all be associated with brain tumors

Brain Tumors associated with various syndrome

Von Hippel Lindau syndrome	Tuberous sclerosis	Neurofibromatosis
Retinal, Cerebellar and spinal hemangioblastomas	*Ependymomas and childhood astrocytomas*	Patients with NFI are at increased risk of developing *optic pathway gliomas, ependymomas, meningiomas and astrocytomas* while NF2 patients are at increased risk of *Schwannomas*

Sturge Weber syndrome may be associated with leptomeningeal angiomatosis but it is not associated with an increased risk of developing true brain tumors.

Sturge Weber Syndrome

- *Port wine nevus over the trigeminal distribution*
- *Ipsilateral leptomeningial angiomatosis*
- *Contralateral hemiparesis*
- *Seizures*
- *Mental Retardation*
- *Congenital Glaucoma*

278. Answer is D (Empty sella): *Ref: Nelson 17th/ 2017*

The clinical hallmark in the form of convulsions, Rail road tract appearance on X-ray and unilateral cortical atrophy (hemiatrophy) on CT scan are diagnosis of Sturge-Weber syndrome.

Sturge weber syndrome

It results from the **anomalous** development of **primordial vascular bed** during early stages of cerebral vascularization. The leptomeninges are richly vascularized and the brain beneath becomes **atrophied** and **calcified**, particularly in molecular layer of cortex.

Clinical manifestations	
Cutaneous	**Neurological features**
Facial nevus (Port-wine stain) • Present at birth • Tends to be unilateral • Always involves upper face and eyelid • May involve lower face, & mucosa of mouth and pharynx.	1. Seizures (hallmark) • Present in most patients during first year of life • Typically focal tonic clonic and contralateral to the side of facial nevus 2. Hemiparesis • Associated with slowly developing hemiparesis in most cases. 3. Mental retardation 4. Buphthal most and glaucoma of the ipsilateral eye are common.
Diagnostic hallmarks	
Skull radiograph	**CT Scan**
Intracranial calcification in the occipitoparietal region - Railroad track appearance - Serpentine appearance	- Unilateral cortical atrophy - Ipsilateral dilatation of lateral ventricle. - Extent of calcification.

279. Answer is D (Spinal meningioma): *'Meningiomas: Diagnosis, Treatment and Outcome' by Lee (Springer) 2009/530, 531, 532; 'Spine Radiosurgery (Thieme) 2008/113, 114; 'Spinal Cord and Spinal Column Tumors (Thieme) 2006*

The clinical picture and MRI findings of an intradural, contrast-enhancing lesion in the dorsal spine are typical of spinal meningiomas.

'The typical clinical scenario of intraspinal meningiomas is a middle aged woman with signs and symptoms of cord or nerve root compression. The dorsal (Thoracic) spine is most commonly involved. At MRI scan, the tumor typically appears as a well-circumscribed lesion iso-intense or slightly hypotense to the spinal cord. On T1 and T2 sequences with homogenous gadolinium (contrast) enhancement' – Learning Musculoskeletal Imaging (Springer) 2010/101

Meningiomas are typically characterized by isointense homogenous contrast enhancement.

Epidermoid cyst, Dermoid cysts and Lipomas do not show contrast enhancement.

Characteristic Features of Benign Extramedullary Spinal Tumors:

Characteristic	**Meningioma**	Schwannoma	Neurofibroma
Age of presentation	*5th-7th decade*	5th decade	4th decade
Spinal level predominance	*Thoracic (80%)*	All levels evenly	Cervical (66%)
Multiplicity	*1 to 2%*	Rare unless NF2 associated	Common
Proportion or primary spinal tumors	*25%*	~33%	3.5%
Gender predominance	*Female (75-80%)*	None	None
Associations	More commonly psammomatous or transitional histologies	NF2, merlin/schwannomin gene on chromosome 22	NF1, neurofibromin gene on chromosome 17

NF1, neurofibromatosis type 1; NF2, neurofibromatosis type 2

Spinal Meningiomas: Review

- Spinal meningiomas are believed to *originate from arachnoid cap cells of neural crest* or mesodermal origin (meningiomthelial cells).
- Spinal meningiomas are *primarily intradural tumors*, although extradural meningiomas have been reported in 3-15% of cases.

Majority of spinal meningiomas are extramedullary intradural tumors. [Q]

- Spinal meningiomas are the second most common spinal intradural tumors after nerve sheath tumors *(Schwannomas)*

Schwannomas are the most common intradural spinal tumors.

- Spinal meningiomas are rare in children and are primarily believed to be tumors of Adults. Spinal meningiomas can be found at any age but they are most commonly seen in the 5th to 7th decade. The mean age of diagnosis is ~50 years. Most spinal meningiomas occur in woman (75-85%)

Spinal meningiomas are most commonly seen in middle aged females [Q]

- Spinal meningiomas may be seen in the cervical spine, thoracic spine or the lumbar spine, but are most frequently seen in the thoracic spine.

Within the spinal axis, meningiomas are most frequently seen in the thoracic/dorsal spine (70-80%)

- Most meningiomas are slow growing benign tumors, however higher grade tumors with more aggressive behaviour compose as many as 10% of all meningiomas.
- *The most common and initial symptom of intraspinal meningiomas is 'pain'*. This is followed by variable degree of neurological deterioration, causing defects depending on tumor location.

Symptoms and Signs of Intraspinal Meningiomas

Pain *(most common and initial symptom)*

↓ Delay between pain and neurological deterioration depends on rate of growth of tumor

Neurological Deterioration

Nerve root compression	**Spinal cord compression**	**Symptoms due to compression of vasculature**
• Exiting N. roots: Radicular pain • Dorsal roots: loss of sensation • Ventral root: motor defect	• Corticospinal tract compression: Upper motor neuron defects with spastic paresis (Myelopathy) • Spinothalamic tract compression: Compromise of pain & temperature • Posterior column compression: Compromise of position & vibration sense	Compression of radicular arteries or anterior spinal arteries may lead to compromise of the function of cord in the Watershed zones that are distant from the tumor.

Impairment of Autonomic pathways are generally uncommon but bowel or bladder involvement can occur as late findings with meningiomas

Nervous System 9

- MRI is the investigation of choice for diagnosis of spinal meningiomas

  At MRI the tumor typically appears as a ***well-circumscribed lesion*** iso-intense or slightly hypo-intense to the spinal cord on T1 and T2 weighted images. MRI typically shows ***intense and near homogenous enhancement after contrast (homogenous gadolinium enhancement)***

  The 'dural tail sign' consisting of dural enhancement adjacent to dural attachment may be seen in spinal meningiomas but this is not specific to meningiomas and may be seen in other conditions like metastasis, sarcoidosis, lymphomas etc.

Disorders of Nerve / Neuropathies

280. Answer is B (Proximal Muscle Weakness): *Harrisons 14th/ 2458, 15th/ 2500; 16th/2502, 2503; 17th/2651; 18th/p 3448*

Symptoms and findings in Peripheral neuropathy whether motor or sensory are generally symmetric and 'graded distally' & not proximally.

Involvement of the peripheral nerve explains both, defects in conduction as well as decreased reflexes.

281. Answer is D (Hypothyroidism): *Harrisons 16th/ 2504 t; 17th/2653; Harrison 18th/p 3450 (Table: 384.1)*

All options mentioned are associated with peripheral neuropathy however hypothyroidism is the single best answer as it is the one with which peripheral neuropathy is least likely.

Condition	Association with neuropathy
Diabetes mellitus	Common
Uraemia	Sometimes
HIV	Sometimes
Hypothyroidism	Rare

282. Answer is A (Vitamin B12 deficiency): *Harrison 17th/2653*

Vitamin B12 deficiency associated neuropathy is primarily a 'Large Fiber' neuropathy arising from dorsal column involvement.

Lepromatous Leprosy (Hansen's Disease), HIV associated neuropathy and Amyloidosis associated neuropathy are all classified as 'Small-Fiber' neuropathies.

Classification of Neuropathy by Fiber Tyepe

Sensory

Motor
- Immune neuropathies: acute (Guillain-Barre syndrome); relapsing
- Heritable motor-sensory neuropathies
- Acute intermittent porphyria
- Diphtheritic neuropathy
- Lead neuropathy
- Brachial neuritis
- Diabetic lumbosacralplexus neuropathy (diabetic amyotrophy)

Autonomic

<u>*Acute*</u>
Acute pandysautonomic neuropathy, botulism, porphyria, GBS, vacore, amiodarone, vincristine

<u>Chronic</u>:
Amyloid, Diabetes, Sjogren's, HSAN I and III (Riley-Day), Chagas, Paraneoplastic.

Note: GBS, Guillain-Barre syndrome; HSAN, hereditary sensory and autonomic neuropathy.

Small fiber
(Painful neuropathies; dissociated sensory loss)
- Hereditary sensory neuropathies (early)
- ***Lepromatous leprosy***
- Diabetic (includes glucose intolerance) small-fiber neuropathy
- ***Amyloidosis***
- Analphalipoproteinemia (Tangier disease)
- Fabry's disease (pain predominates)
- Dysautonomia (Riley-Day syndrome)
- ***HIV and antiretroviral therapy neuropathy***

Large fiber
(Ataxic-Neuropathies)
- Sjogren's syndrome
- ***Vitamin B12 neuropathy*** (from dorsal column involvement)
- Cisplatin neuropathy
- Pyridoxine toxicity
- Friedreich's ataxia

Mixed (small & large) fiber
(Global sensory loss)
- Carcinomatous sensory neuropathy
- Hereditary sensory neuropathies (recessive and dominant)
- Diabetic sensory neuropathy
- Vacor intoxication
- Xanthomatous neuropathy of primary biliary cirrhosis (tabes dorsalis)

283. Answer is A (Burning pain): *Harrison's 17th/2652;*

Burning pain is a characteristic feature of small –fiber neuropathies

Tingling and Numbness is a feature of large fiber neuropathies while *foot drop & twitching* are features of motor neuropathies

Symptoms, Signs and Tests in Peripheral Neuropathy

Type of Neuropathy	Symptoms	Signs
Large fiber	• ***Numbness*** • ***Tingling*** • *"Pins and needles"* • *Poor balance*	• *Decreased Vibration* • *Decreased Joint-position sense* • *Decreased Reflexes*
Small fiber	• ***Pain**: burning, shock-like, stabbing, prickling, shooting, lancinating* • *Allodynia*	• *Decreased Pin prick* • *Decreased Temperature sensation*
Motor	• *Cramps* • *Weak grip* • *Footdrop* • *Twitching*	• *Reduced Strength* • *Reduced Reflexes*
Autonomic	• *Decreased or increased sweating* • *Dry eyes, mouth,* • *Erectile dysfunction* • *Gastroparesis/diarrhea* • *Faintness, light-headedness*	• *Orthostasis* • *Unequal pupil size* • *Resting tachycardia*

284. Answer is C (Hyperthyroidism): *Harrison 17th /1764; Harrison's 18th/3353*

Hyperthyroidism is not associated with an autonomic neuropathy.
Thyroid Hormones interact with the sympathetic branch of the autonomic nervous system and stimulate /simulate increased activity of sympathetic nervous system. Hyperthyroidism however is not associated with an autonomic neuropathy.

Autonomic Neuropathies

Acute / Subacute Autonomic Neuropathies	Chronic Peripheral Autonomic Neuropathies
Subacute autoimmune autonomic ganglionopathy (AAG) *a) Subacute paraneoplastic autonomic neuropathy* *b) Guillain-Barré syndrome* ***c) Botulism*** *d) Porphyria* *e) Drug induced autonomic neuropathies-stimulants, drug withdrawal, vasoconstrictor, vasodilators, beta-receptor antagonists, beta-agonists* *f) Toxic autonomic neuropathies* *g) Subacute cholinergic neuropathy*	1. Distal small fiber neuropathy 2. Combined sympathetic and parasympathetic failure ***a) Amyloid*** *b)* ***Diabetic*** *autonomic neuropathy* *c) Autoimmune autonomic ganglionopathy (Paraneoplastic and idiopathic)* *d) Sensory neuronopathy with autonomic failure* *e) Familial dysautonomia (Riley-Day syndrome)* *f) Diabetic, uremic, or nutritional deficiency* *g) Dysautonomia of old age* 3. Disorders of reduced orthostatic intolerance-reflex syncope, POTS, associated with prolonged bed rest, associated with space flight, chronic fatigue

285. Answer is D (Bradycardia) : *Morgan's 4th/804, 805; 'Stoelting's Anesthesia' 5th/375; 'Clinical Adult Neurology'3rd/423*

Autonomic neuropathy is associated with tachycardia and not bradycardia.

Autonomic Neuropathy

Cardiovascular AutonomicNeuropathy	Gastrointestinal Autonomic Neuropathy	Genitourinary Autonomic Neuropathy
• ***Resting tachycardia*** • *Loss of Heart Rate Variability* • ***Orthostatic Hypotension*** • ***Silent Myocardial Infarction*** • *Reduced response to Valsalva maneuver, Sustained exercise and Medications (atropine & propanalol)* • *Prolonged QT interval/dysrhythmias* • *Hypoglycemic unawareness/lack of diaphoresis (sweating) and tremulousness* • *Sudden death*	• *Gastroparesis*	• *Neurogenic bladder* • *Sexual dysfunction / Impotence*

286. Answer is D (All of the above): *Harrison's 18th/3457, 3458*

Diabetic neuropathy may be of several types including distal symmetric sensory neuropathy, autonomic neuropathy and diabetic manoneuropathy

Diabetic Neuropathy

- Diabetes Meelitus is the most common cause of peripheral neuropathy in developed countries

Diabetes is associated with several types of Neuropathy

- *Distal symmetric sensory or sensorimotor polyneuropathy (DSPN)*
- *Autonomic Neuropathy*
- *Diabetic Radiculoplexus Neuropathy (diabetic amyotrophy or Brunse Garland syndrome)*
- *Diabetic mononeuropathies or multiple mononeuropathies*

- *Diabetic Distal Symmetric Sensory and Senorimotor Polyneuropathy (DSPN) is the most common form of diabetic polyneuropathy[Q]*
- *The most common diabetic mononeuropathy at wrist is median neuropathy[Q]*
- *The most common diabetic mononeuropathy at the elbow is ulnar mononeuropathy[Q]*
- *The most common diabetic cranial mononeuropathy is VIIth nerve palsy[Q]*
  (*Followed by third nerve, sixth nerve and less frequently fourth nerve)*

287. Answer is B (Distal Symmetric Sensory and Motor Neuropathy): *Harrison's 18th/3457, 3458*

Diabetic Distal Symmetric Sensory and Sensorimotor Polyneuropathy (DSPN) is the most common form of Diabetic Neuropathy.

288. Answer is D (All of the above): *Harrison's 18th/2984*

Duloxetine, Pregabalin and /or Amitriptyline may all be used for treatment of painful diabetic neuropathy.

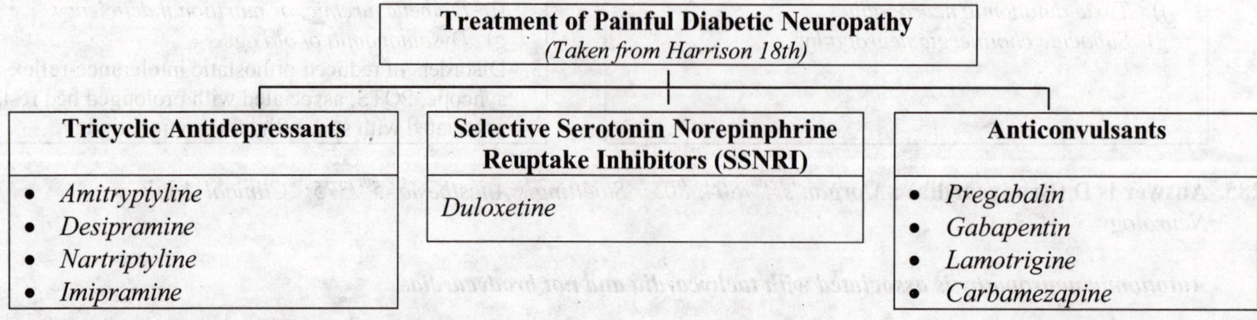

Two agents, Duloxetine and Pregabalin have been approved by the U.S. FDA for pain associated with diabetic neuropathy - Harrison's 18th

289. Answer is B (Carbamezapine): *Harrison's 18th/3360, 336*

Carbamezapine is the most commonly employed drug of first choice against Trigeminal Neuralgia.

Trigeminal Neuralgia

Medical /Pharmacological Treatment	Surgical Treatment
Anticonvulsants are the agents of choice • ***Carbamezapine (drug of first choice)*** • *Oxcarbazepine* • *Phenytoin* } Carbamezapine resistant trigeminal neuralgia • *Lamotrigine* Baclofen Baclofen may also be administered either alone or in combination with anticonvulsants	• Microvascular Decompression to relieve pressure on trigeminal nerve (most widely used procedure) • Gamma knife Radiosurgery (Less efficacious than decompression, higher recurrence rates but few serious complications) • Radiofrequency, Thermal Rhizotomy (Excellent short term relief > 95% but high recurrence rate)

290. Answer is B (Osteoporosis): *Harrison 16th/2504, 2505*

Osteoporosis is not associated with polyneuropathy

Vitamin deficiency, diabetes, amyloidosis and myxoedema may all be associated with polyneuropathy.

Condition	Polyneuropathy
Vitamin deficiency excluding B12	• *Sensorimotor polyneuropathy*
Vitamin B12 deficiency	• *Sensory polyneuropathy*
Diabetes Mellitus	• *Sensory polyneuropathy or sensori motor polyneuropathy (rarely motor neuropathy alone)*
Amyloidosis (rare)	• *Sensorimotor polyneuropathy*
Myxoedema (rare)	• *Sensory polyneuropathy*

291. Answer is A (Tuberculosis): *Harrison 16th/2504, 2505*

Tuberculosis is not mentioned as a cause of peripheral neuropathy

Diabetic Mellitus, SLE, PAN and sarcoidosis may all cause peripheral neuropathies.

***SLE** can cause a distal symmetric sensory or sensorimotor neuropathy and rarely monouritis multiplex.*

– Current Neurology 1st/318

***Sarcoidosis** may cause a diffuse sensorimotor neuropathy - Current Neurology 1st/318*

***PAN** may be associated with mononeuropathy multiplex – Current Neurology 1st/318*

292. Answer is B (Lead poisoning): *Harrison 16th/2504, 2505*

Inorganic lead poisoning is not associated with a sensorimotor neuropathy
Inorganic lead poisoning is primarily associated with a pure motor neuropathy. Selective motor neuropathy with wrist drop is characteristic of lead poisoning.

Conditions that may cause Sensorimotor Neuropathies

Polyneuropathy associated with Sensorimotor neuropathies (Harrison)	
Systemic Disease	
Diabetes mellitus	***Sensory, Sensorimotor, Motor***
Uremia	Sensorimotor
Porphyria (3 types)	Sensorimotor
Vitamin deficiency excluding B12	Sensorimotor
Chronic liver disease	Sensory or Sensorimotor
Primary systemic amyloidosis	Sensorimotor
Chronic obstructive lung disease	Sensory or Sensorimotor

Malabsorption (sprue, celiac disease)	Sensory or Sensorimotor
Carcinoma (sensorimotor)	Sensorimotor
Carcinoma (demyelinating)	Sensorimotor
Multiple Myeloma, lytic type	Sensory, Motor or Sensorimotor
MGUS	
IgA	Sensorimotor
IgG	Sensorimotor
IgM	Sensorimotor or Sensory
Cryoglobulinemia	***Sensorimotor***
Drugs	
Amiodarone (antiarrhythmic)	Sensorimotor
Aurothioglucose (antirheumatic)	Sensorimotor
Isoniazid	***Sensorimotor***
Metronidazole (antiprotozoal)	Sensory or Sensorimotor
Misonidazole (radiosensitizer)	Sensory or Sensorimotor
Environmental Toxins	
Arsenic (herbicide; insecticide)	***Sensorimotor***
Diptheria toxin	Sensorimotor
γ-Diketone hexacarbons (solvents)	Sensorimotor
Organophosphates	Sensorimotor
Thallium (rat poison)	Sensorimotor

293. Answer is A and B (Cisplatin and Pyridoxine excess): *Harrison 16th/2505(t)*

Cisplatin and Pyridoxine are associated with predominantly sensory neuropathies.

294. Answer is D (Arsenic intoxication): *Harrisons 15th/ 2503, 2506, 2594; 16th/2505, 2509, 2577; 17th/2653 (379-3)*

"Arsenic produces a sensory and motor polyneuritis manifestating as numbness and tingling in a 'stocking – glove' distribution, distal weakness and quadriplegia" *– Harrison 15th/ 2594, 2503*

Pure motor neuropathy: Disorders affecting any level of 'the motor unit' can result in purely motor neuropathy without sensory disturbance.

The affections include- anterior horn cell, motor axon, neuromuscular junction

Pure motor neuropathies
1. Lower motor neuron form of amyotrophic lateral sclerosis Q
2. Poliomyelitis Q
3. Hereditary spinal muscular atrophy
4. Adult variant of Hexosaminidase deficiency
5. Lead intoxication Q
6. Dapsone intoxication Q
7. Acute intermittent porphyria (occasionally)
8. Neuromuscular junction disorder : Lambert Eaton Myasthenia syndrome Q; Tick bite paralysis Q

Neuropathies with predominant Motor symptoms [Sensory component is subclinical but readily demonstrable electro diagnostically]
1. Hereditary motor sensory neuropathy
2. GBS or Acute inflammatory demyelinating polyneuropathy Q
3. CIPD Q

295. Answer Di.e. (Arsenic intoxication): *Harrison 16th / 2505, 2509, 2578; 17th/2653*

Arsenic intoxication is associated with a mixed sensory motor form of neuropathy and not predominantly motor neuropathy.

Lead *(H16th / 2578)*: '*Chronic subclinical exposures are associated with demyelinating peripheral neuropathy, mainly motor'*. (Neuropathy : M>S or M)

Porphyria (*H16th/ 2305)* 'The peripheral neuropathy is due to axonal degeneration and ***primarily affects motor neurons***Q. *Sensory changes such as paraesthesias and loss of sensations are less prominent.(Neuropathy: M or SM)*

<u>**Acute inflammatory demyelinating polyradiculoneuropathy (GBS) (*H16th/ 2509*)**</u>: *'Motor Sensory Polyneuropathy with predominant motor symptoms and signs.'. 'Manifests as rapidly developing areflexic motor paralysis with or without sensory symptoms'- Harrison.*

Pure motor Neuropathies	
Lower Motor form of Amyotrophic Lateral Sclerosis	Pure motor
Poliomyelitis	Pure motor
Hereditary Spinal Muscular Atrophics	Pure motor
Adult variant of Hexosaminidase A deficiency	Pure motor
Neuromuscular junction disorders	Pure motor
Lambert : Eaton Myasthenic syndrome	
Tick bite paralysis	
Dapsone Intoxication (H/16th/2505)	Pure motor
Predominantly Motor Neuropathies	
Lead Intoxication (H 16th / 2578)	Predominantly motor or ***Pure Motor*** (M>S or M)
Porphyria (H 16th / 2578)	Predominantly motor (sensory changes less prominent)
Acute Inflammatory Demyelinating Polyradiculoneuropathy	Predominantly motor (subclinical sensory component).
CIDP (H 16th / 2509)	Predominantly motor

296. Answer is A (Hansen's disease): *Neurological Practice: an Indian Perspective by Walia (2005)/591 'Clinical Neurophysiology' 2nd (2006)*

The most common case of mononeuritis multiplex in India is Leprosy or Hansen's disease

Though the incidence and prevalence of leprosy has been gradually reducing, Leprosy continues to be the most common case of treatable peripheral neuropathy in India. The characteristic presentation of Leprous neuropathy is mononeuritis multiplex although it may present as a mononeuritis or symmetric polyneuropathy

297. Answer is A (Polio): *Harrisons 14th/ 2466, Harrison 15th/ 2506; 16th/2509; 17th/2573; Harrison 18th/p 3347*

Poliomyelitis affects the anterior horn cells and causes a pure motor neuropathy.

298. Answer is B (Diphtheria): *See text below*

Diptheria is associated with a descending motor paralysis. *All other options mentioned in the question give rise to ascending motor paralysis.*

Important causes of descending motor paralysis.
• Botulinum Q
• Diphtheria Q
• Polio

These three causes of descending motor paralysis need to be remembered as they are frequently asked and help to answer several questions by exclusion.

299. Answer is C (Polio): *Refer previous question*

Polio is associated with a pure motor neuropathy. There is no sensory involvement in polio and hence trophic ulcers are not seen in polio.

300. Answer is B (Subacute combined degeneration of cord): *Harrison's 16th/2509; Localization in clinical Neurology 5th/106*

Subacute combined degeneration of cord (SACD) is associated with dysfunction of posterior column and corticospinal tract but spinothalamic tracts are preserved.

Pain temperature and crude touch sensations remain intact in SACD because of the preservation of spinothalamic tract and hance trophic or neuropathic ulcers are not seen in SACD.

Common Causes of Trophic/Neuropathic Ulcers

Peripheral Nerve involvement	Spinal Cord involvement
• *Diabetic Neuropathy* • *Peripheral Neuropathy from other cause* • ***Leprotic Neuropathy*** • *Hereditary Sensory neuropathy*	• ***Syringomyelia*** • *Tabes dorsalis* • *Transverse myelitis* • ***Prolapsed intervertebral disc*** • *Cervical spondylosis* • *Spinal cord trauma*

301. Answer is D (GBS) : *Diagnostic Neuropathology by Vinters, Farrell and Mischel (1998) /12; Acute Rheumatic and Immunological diseases by Mandell (1994) / 486, 487; Harrison 16th/2504, 2505.*

The two basic pathological processes of pathogenesis in neuropathy include Axonal degenetration and Demyelination. ***Neuropathy associated with Axonal degeneration is often called 'dying back neuropathy' as degeneration usually proceeds from distal to proximal. Neuropathy associated with Diabetes mellitus, Porphyria and Arsenic are primarily caused by axonal degeneration and represent examples of dying back neuropathy.***
GBS is primarily a demyelinating neuropathy and is the single best answer of choice.

Pathology of Neuropathy

Axonal Degeneration (Retrograde) (Dying Back Neuropathy)	Demyelination
• Retrograde Axonal Degeneration is one type of classical response of nerve to an insult and consists of degeneration of axon from distal to proximal *(Referred to as 'Dying back neuropathy')* • This type of degeneration is *most commonly seen after toxic and metabolic injuries* (Since the distal axon is the portion farthest from the cell body it is most vulnerable to toxic and metabolic derangements) ***Neuropathies resulting from Toxins (eg Arsenic) and Metabolic derrangements (Diabetes, Porphyria) are pathologically caused by axonal degeneration (Refer Harrison 16th/2504, 2505) and may hence be grouped as dying back neuropathies.***	• Demyelination is another type of response of nerve to an insult. • Such demyelination is associated with a ' conduction block' which results from failure of nerve conduction across the demyelinated segment and results in a rapid onset type neuropathy (weakness) • Neuropathies resulting from demyelination do not have a distal to proximal progression and may occur either distally or proximally depending on the location of the demyclinated segment of the nerve ***The primary pathological process in GBS is demyelination*** *(although associated axonal degeneration may be present)* ***and hence it represents an example of Demyelinating neuropathies and not a type of dying back neuropathy***

302. Answer is C (Sensory level):*Harrison's 17th/2667,2668,2669, 2670;Current Diagnosis & Treatment in Neurology(2008)/302-3; Harrison 18th/p 3473, 3474, 3475, 3476, 3477*

Guillion Barre syndrome is not associated with a distinct sensory level.

Sensory involvement in GBS is mild. Although sensory symptoms (tingling / paraesthesias) may be prominent, cutaneous sensory deficits (eg loss of pain and temperature sensations) are usually mild (Harrison's) or even absent (Current Neurology).

Guillain – Barre Syndrome

Acute Autoimmune Fulminant Demyelinating Polyradiculopathy

(Usually occurs 1-3 weeks after an acute infections process usually gastrointestinal or respiratory (70% cases)

Fever and constitutional symptoms are absent at onset[Q]

Nerve Conduction Studies	**CSF studies**
Show evidence of Demyelination	Show evidence of ***Albumin cytological dissociation***[Q] (Increased CSF protein without increased cell count

Motor	**Sensory**	**Autonomic**
• Rapidly evolving motor paralysis • ***Ascending (usually)*** • Areflexic (Reflexes Diminished or absent) • Symmetric (Weaknes is usually symmetric) • ***Flaccid*** • Sphincter tone is normal • Facial Nerve and other cranial nerves may be involved. Bulbar muscles may be involved with difficulty in swallowing, speech etc. • Life threatening respiratory paralysis requiring ventilation may be seen.	• Sensory disturbance may or may not be present in GBS and a ***distinct sensory level is not seen.*** • Mild sensory involvement - <u>Cutaneous sensory deficits</u> (e.g. loss of pain and temperature sensation) are usually ***<u>mild</u> (Harrison's) or <u>absent</u>*** *(Current Neurology)* - Sensory symptoms such as paraesthesias, tingling etc may be prominent *(but objective sensory loss* on clinical *examination is mild/absent.* • Bladder dysfunction is uncommon. It is usually transient and seen only in severe cases *(If Bladder disturbance is prominent and comes early diagnostic possibilities other that GBS should be considered).*	• Autonomic involvement is common • May occur even in patients whose GBS is otherwise mild • <u>Manifestations include</u> • Loss of vasomotor control (Fluctuation in B.P / Postrual Hypotension) • Cardiac dysrhythmias

Prognosis

Recovery is usually remarkable in GBS, although all patients may not recover fully.

Approximately 85% of patients with GBS achieve a full functional recovery within several months to a year-*Harrison 15th/2509*

Treatment

Treatment includes intravenous immunoglobulins (IVIG) or plasmapharesis both of which are equally effective (treatment should be initiated as early as possible as immunotherapy is believed to be no longer effective if initiated 2 weeks after first motor symptoms).

303. Answer is D (Bladder bowel involvement): *Harrison 14th/2462; 15th/ 2507; 16th/2513-2515; 17th/2667-2670; API 6th/ 835; Harrison 18th/p 3473-3477*

Bladder bowel involvement is rare in G. B. syndrome. *Bladder dysfunction may occur in severe cases but is usually transient. 'If bladder dysfunction is prominent and comes early possibilities other than GBS should be considered'.*

- Harrison

<u>Guillain Barré syndrome (GBS)</u> is an autoimmune disease characterized by acute demyelinating polyneuropathy.

It has several distinctive features, which are so often asked. These include :

Aetiology		
Preceding evidence of a viral infection [Q] such as that with - Herpes group : CMV / EBV - Campylobacter jejuni gastroenteritis - Lymphoma / Lupus Erythematosus		
Clinical manifestation		
Predominant motor involvement	Sensory disturbance	Autonomic
• Paraplegia / Quadriplegia • Proximal muscles affected more than the	• *Sensory **disturbance** may or may not be present* : Cutaneous sensory deficits (eg. loss of pain and temperature sensation)	• *Autonomic involvement* characterized by Postural hypotension, episodes of

distal ones • Ascending pattern of paralysis • *Cranial nerve involvement* Q *:* The commonest involvement is bilateral Facial and then Bulbar muscles. The patient has difficulty in swallowing, speech, etc. • *Areflexia* Q *:* Deep tendon reflexes usually disappear within the first few days of onset.	when present are usually mild. • **Bladder & Bowel rarely involved** Q **:** Bladder dysfunction may occur in severe cases but is usually transient - If bladder dysfunction is a prominent feature and comes early, possibilities other than GBS should be considered.	hypotension or hypertension and tachycardia.

CSF Findings	Nerve Conduction Studies
- *CSF shows albumino-cytological dissociation* Q. i.e. Increased proteins with normal cells - ***CSF Pleocytosis** with cells above 50/mm^3 is against the diagnosis of GBS.* - API / 35	Nerve conduction studies show *demyelination* i.e. slow conduction velocity, distal latency, conduction block

Prognosis
- ***Recovery is usually remarkable*** in GBS, although all patients may not recover fully. - ***Approximately 85% of patients with GBS achieve a full functional recovery within several months to a year.***-*Harrison 15th/2509*

304. Answer is C (Descending): *Harrison's 18th/3473-3476*

Guillain Barre Syndrome is typically an 'ascending' (not descending) neuropathy.

*Guillan Barre Syndrome is typically an acute **inflammatory demyelinating** polyneuropathy. The usually pattern is an **ascending paralysis** and **cranial nerve involvement is common**.*

The typical/most common variant of GBS is Acute Inflammatory Demyelinating Polyneuropathy (AIDP).

Diagnostic Features of Acute Inflammatory Demyelinating Polyneuropathy (AIDP)

I. Required for Diagnosis
1. Progressive weakness of variable degree from mild paresis to complete paralysis 2. ***Generalized hyporeflexia or areflexia*** Q
II. Supportive of Diagnosis
1. Clinical Features a) Symptom progression: Motor weakness rapidly progresses initially but ceases by 4 weeks. Nadir attained by 2 weeks in 50%, 3 weeks 80%, and 90% by 4 weeks. b) Demonstration of relative limb ***symmetry*** Q regarding paresis. c) Mild to moderate sensory signs. d) Frequent cranial nerve involvement: Facial (cranial nerve VII) 50% and typically bilateral but asymmetric; occasional involvement of cranial nerves XII, X, and occasionally III, IV, and VI as well as XI. e) Recovery typically begins 2–4 weeks following plateau phase. f) Autonomic dysfunction can include tachycardia, other arrhythmias, postural hypotension, hypertension, other vasomotor symptoms. g) A preceding gastrointestinal illness (e.g., diarrhea) or upper respiratory tract infection is common. 2. Cerebrospinal Fluid Features Supporting Diagnosis a. Elevated or serial elevation of CSF protein. b. CSF cell counts are <10 mononuclear cell/mm^3. 3. Electrodiagnostic Medicine Findings Supportive of Diagnosis a) 80% of patients have evidence of NCV slowing/conduction block at some time during disease process. b) Patchy reduction in NCV attaining values less than 60% of normal. c) Distal motor latency increase may reach 3 times normal values. d) F-waves indicate proximal NCV slowing. e) About 15–20% of patients have normal NCV findings. f) No abnormalities on nerve conduction studies may be seen for several weeks.
III. Findings Reducing Possibility of Diagnosis
1. Asymmetric weakness 2. Failure of bowel/bladder symptoms to resolve 3. Severe bowel/bladder dysfunction at initiation of disease 4. Greater than 50 mononuclear cells/mm3 in CSF 5. Well-demarcated sensory level
IV. Exclusionary Criteria
1. Diagnosis of other causes of acute neuromuscular weakness (e.g., myasthenia gravis, botulism, poliomyelitis, toxic neuropathy). 3. Abnormal CSF cytology suggesting carcinomatous invasion of the nerve roots

NCV, nerve conduction velocity.

305. Answer is C (Residual disability if treatment is delayed): *Harrisons 15th/ 2507; 16th/2513, 2515; 17th/2667-2670; Harrison 18th/p 3473-3477*

In Guillain-Bare syndrome 85% of the patients achieve a full functional recovery within several months to years. *Recovery is usually remarkable in GBS although all patients may not recover fully*

- **'<u>Bladder dysfunction</u>** may occur in severe cases but is usually transient.' (This makes us presume that bladder is most often spared then it is involved)
  Infact Harrison goes on to state that 'If bladder dysfunction is a prominent feature and comes early in the course possibilities other than GBS should be considered particularly spinal cord disease.
- **<u>CSF finding</u>** is characteristic consisting of:
  Elevated protein level (100 to 1000 mg/dl) without accompanying pleocytosis albuminocytological dissociation (increased protein/ no increase in cells)
  Note that CSF is normal when symptoms are present for less than 48 hrs. Protein is usually elevated by the end of first week
- GBS evolves as rapidly developing areflexic **'predominantly motor paralysis'.** They may have a sensory component which is often subclinical. Usual pattern is an ascending paralysis.

306. Answer is A (Corticosteroids may be used for early recovery and prevent long hospital stay): *Harrison 17th /1764; Harrison's 18th/2312*

Glucocorticoids have not beam found to be effective in Guillan-Barre Syndrome.
'Glucocorticoids have not been found to be effective in GBS' -Harrison's 18th/3477

Treatment of GBS

IV immunoglobulins and /or plasmapharesis	Supportive Therapy
• Treatment should be initiated as soon after diagnosis as possible *(Each day counts) (Immunotherapy may not be effective if initited 2 weeks after the first motor symptom)* Q • ***Either High dose IV Immunoglobulins or plasmapharesis may be initiated as they are equally effective for typical GBS*** Q *Anecdotal data has suggested that IVIg may be preferable to plasmapharesis for the AMAN and MFS variants of GBS* • *A combination of both therapies is not significantly better than either alone* Q • *The lack of noticeable improvement after a course of IVIg or plasmapharesis is not an indication to treat with alternate therapy.* • *If the patient has already reached a plateau stage, than treatment is probably no longer indicated.* • *IVIg is often the initial therapy chosen of its ease of administration and good safety record.*	• Patients require monitoring in critical care setting • ~30% of patients with GBS require ventilator assistance • Particular attention should be given to vital capacity, early consideration of tracheostomy (after 2 week of intubation) and chest physiotherapy. • Monitor CVS status, nutrition and skin care.

307. Answer is A (Acute Motor Axonal Neuropathy (AMAN)): *Current Diagnosis & Treatment in Neurology (LANGE)/6; Harrison 18th/3452, 3473*

Preserved conduction velocity (No/minimal reduction in conduction velocity) is a feature of <u>Axonal neuropathies</u>.
Acute Motor Axonal Neuropathy (AMAN) is pure axonal neuropathy characterized by normal motor conduction velocity.

<u>Demyelinating neuropathies</u> are typically associated with reduced conduction velocities.
AIDP, HSMN and MMN are all demyelinating neuropathies characterized by reduced conduction velocity on nerve conduction studies.

Demyelinating Versus Axonal Neuropathies

The primary function of myelin is to increase axonal conduction velocity without a significant increase in axonal diameter. This function is achieved by a process of *saltatory conduction*, in which nerve impulses jump between electrically excitable regions of the axon, called nodes of Ranvier located between elctrically insulated areas ensheathed by myelinating Schwann cells.

A demyelinating process disrupts the normal saltatory conduction along some axons within the nerve *slowing the conduction velocity* of these axons. As demyelination becomes more profound, conduction through some areas is blocked completely (*conduction block*), functionally disconnecting the motor neuron from the innervated muscle resulting in weakness.

In axonal neuropathies the conduction velocity is typically either preserved or only midly reduced.

Electrophysiologic Features: Axonal Degenaration vs. Segmental Demylination

Features	Axonal Degeneration	Segmental Demylination
Motor Nerve Conduction Studies		
CMAP amplitude	Decreased	Normal (except with CB)
Distal latency	Normal	Prolonged
Conduction velocity	***Normal***	***Slow***
Conduction block	***Absent***	***Present***
Temporal dispersion	Absent	Present
F wave	Normal or Absent	Prolonged or Absent
H reflex	Normal or Absent	Prolonged or Absent
Sensory Nerve Conduction Studies		
SNAP amplitude	Decreased	Normal
Distal latency	Normal	Prolonged
Conduction velocity	Normal	Slow
Needle EMG		
Spontaneous activity		
Fibrillations	Present	Absent
Fasciculation	Present	Absent
Motor unit potentials		
Recruitment	Decreased	Decreased
Morphology	Long duration / polyphasic	Normal

308. Answer is D (I.V. Immunoglobins): *Nelson 16th/ 1893; Harrisons 15th/ 2508; 16th/2516; 17th/2670; API 6th/ 835; Harrison 18th/p 3477*

The characteristic clinical presentation and CSF finding lead us to the diagnosis of GBS

Either high does intravenous immunoglobulins or plasmapharesis can be initiated as they are equally effective.

– Harrison's

Glucocorticoids have not been found to be effective in GBS – Harrisons

Steroids do not reduce the duration but may increase the risk of infection and worsen the problem. Steroids should be considered contraindicated in the treatment of GB syndrome – API 6th/ 835

309. Answer is B (Botulism) : *Harrison 16th / 843, 2305, 832, 1144; 17th/901; CMDT 2006 /1410; 18th/1200-1201*

The clinical picture of the patient in question is consistent with a diagnosis of botulism.

***Symmetric descending paralysis** is characteristic. Dizziness, **Blurred vision** and dry mouth are common. Ptosis is frequent. **The pupillary reflexes may be depressed and fixed or dilated pupils are noted** in half of patients.*

- Regarding clinical manifestations of Botulism;Harrison 16th / 843

Characteristics of Botulism : *CMDT 2006 / 1410; Harrison 16th / 843*

- History of recent ingestion of home canned or smoked food or injection of drug.
- Symmetric descending paralysis with prominent bulbar palsy

  4 '**D**' of Bulbar palsy:
  - '**D**'iplopia
  - '**D**'ysarthria
  - '**D**'ysphonia
  - '**D**'ysphogia

- Pupils are fixed and dilated in most cases - *CMDT*
  'Ptosis, cranial nerve palsies with impairment of extraocular muscles and fixed dilated pupils are characteristic signs' - *CMDT*
- Normal sensory examination normal sensorium (not confused)
- Afebrile (Temperature remains normal)[Q]
  (Because Botulism is not an 'infection' but on 'intoxication' manifestation are due to the effect of toxin. Patient remains without fever until secondary infection is acquired).

Diphteria Poliomyelitis, & Porphyria may all present with descending paralysis and bulbar palsy but fixed dilated pupils are characteristic of Botulism.

310. Answer is C (Fever): *Harrison's 18th/1200,1201; Irwin Rippe's Intensive Care Medicine 6th/1136, 1137*

Patients with Botulism are usully afebrile *and have a clear sensarium (alert and oriented).*
Cranial nerve palsies with a flaccid, descending, completely symmetric paralysis is typical of Botulism.

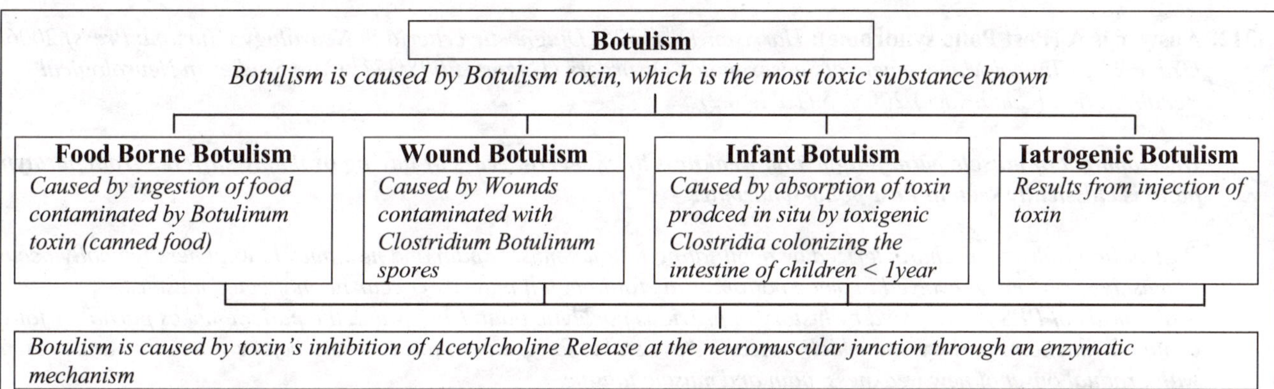

Typical Manifestations

- <u>Symmetric Cranial Nerve Palsies</u> (marks the onset)
  - **D**iplopia
  - **D**ysarthria
  - **D**ysphonia
  - **D**ysphagia
  - Ptosis & facial nerve palsies
  - Pupillary reflexes are depresed and pupils are dilated & fixed

  Extraocular muscle paralysis manifests as blurred vision or diplopia and an inability to accomodate for near vision
- <u>Flaccid Descending completely symmetric paralysis of voluntary muscles</u>
  (Extent of paralysis, from cranial nerves only to quadriplegia dependes on toxin dose). Upper extremities are affected first followed by respiratory muscles and finally lower extremity paralysis.
- <u>Deep tendon reflexes are preserved initially though they progressively disappear.</u>

  Gag reflex is lost early
- <u>Autonomic Dysfunction</u>

  Dry mouth
  Constipation
  Urinary retention

  Anticholinesgic features are typical
- <u>**Sensorium is typically preserved**</u>
  Patients usually exhibit no cognitive defects
- <u>**Patients are usually afebrile**</u>
  Fever is typically absent, except in some cases of wound botulinum
- <u>Sensory findings are generally absent</u>

Gastrointestinal manifestations of food borne botulism

- Nausea, vomiting, abdominal pain may precede or follow onset of paralysis.
- Incubation period from ingestion of toxin to onset of symptoms is usually 18-36 hours but may range from few hours to several days.

The most common cause of death in untreated botulism is from respiratory failure (airway obstuction from pharyngeal muscle paralysis and inadequate tidal volume resulting from paralysis of diaphragm and accessory resp. muscles)

311. Answer is B (Botulism): *Harrison's 18th/1200-1201; Irwind Rippe's Intensive Care Medicine 6th/1136, 1137*

Sudden onset of blurred vision, absent pupillary reflexes (fixed / dilated pupil with lack of accomodation), symmetric descending paralysis progressing to qudriparesis and preserved sensorium suggest a diagnosis of Botulism.

Cardinal Feature of Botulism
• ***Cranial Nerve Palsies*** *with prominent bulbar palsy (4 '**D**'s of Bulbar Palsy)* *(**D**iplopia, **D**ysarthria, **D**ysphonia, **D**ysphagia, Ptosis, Loss of Accomodation, Fixed / Dilated pupils)*
• ***Descending motor paralysis*** *(Extent of paralysis from a few cranial nerves only to quadriperesis depends on dose of toxin)*
• ***Symmetry of symptoms/signs***
• ***A clear sensorium***
• ***Absence of fever***
• ***Lack of sensory findings***

312. Answer is A (Post Polio syndrome): *Harrison 18th/1595; Diagnostic criteria in Neurology (Humana Press) 2006/195 (Table 21); Clinical Management of Sensorimotor Disorders (Thieme) 2008/371; Case Studies in Neurological Rehabilitation (Cambridge) 2008/75 (Table 6.2)*

Development of muscle pain, fatigue and weakness after several years of having probably suffered from paralytic polio is classically seen in Post-polio-syndrome.

Post-polio syndrome is characterized by debilitating fatigue, muscle pain and new muscle weakness typically occuring in muscles previously involved in acute poliomyelitis (although it may also occur in unaffected muscles).
A diagnosis of PPS is suggested by history of previous paralytic polio from which the patient makes partial or fairly complete function recovery and which typically stays stable for greater than 15 years before worsening and presenting with gradual onset of new weakness, pain and muscle fatigue.

Consensus Workshop Diagnostic Criteria for Post-Polio Syndrome

- History of paralytic polio with partial or fairly complete neurologic and functional recovery.
- A period of neurological and functional stability of at least 15 years.
- Development of new muscle dysfunction (After a period of functional stability of at least 15 years)
  - ***Muscle weakness***
  - Muscle atrophy
  - ***Muscle pain***
  - ***Fatigue***
- Neurological examination compatible with prior poliomyelitis
  - Lower motor lesion
  - Decreased or absent tendon reflexes
  - No sensory loss
  - Compatible findings on electromyogram and/or magnetic resonance imaging

Taken from 'Diagnostic Criteria in Neurology' (Humana Press) 2006/195 (table 21)

Signs and Symptoms of PPS
• ***Fatigue*** that may be debilitating and worsens as the day progress
• New joint and ***muscle pain***
• New ***weakness in muscles*** affected by polio; unaffected muscles are also affected. (The new weakness may be more prominent on one side of the body).
• New dyspnea and other respiratory problems
• *Severe cold intolerance*, even with mild cold exposure. This causes the muscle weakness to worsen, the arms or legs to become pale or cyanotic, and the extremities to feel cold to touch. The patient may say, "It's so cold it hurts".
• Muscle spasms and cramps that are sometimes severe and painful
• *Difficulty swallowing* and increased risk of choking
• Difficulty falling asleep and waking frequently during the night
• Anxiety, anger, frustration, and emotional outbursts due to loss of ability
• Disturbed sleep, sleep apnea

313. Answer is D (Arthrogryposis multiplex congenita) : *Harrison 16th / 2060; Harrison 17th/2180 (Table 330.2); Harrison 18th/p 2856(Table: 336.2)*

***Syringomyelia, Leprosy and diabetes are all common causes for Neuropathic / Charcot joint disease. Arthrogryposis multiplex congenita comprises** a non progressive condition characterized by multiple joint contractures found throughout the body at birth. Charcot joint has not been mentioned in association with Arthrogryposis multiplex.*

Charcot joint : Neuropathic joint - *Harrison 16th / 2060; Harrison 17th/2180*

Neuropathic joint disease (Charcot's joint) is a progressive destructive arthritis associated with loss of pain sensation, proprioception or both. Without these protective reflexes joints are subject to repeated trauma, resulting in progressive cartilage and bone damage.

Disorders associated with Neuropathic joint disease/Charcot's joint	
▪ Diabetes Mellitus	• Amyloidosis
▪ Tabes Dorsalis	• Leprosy
▪ Meningomyelocele	• Congenital indifference to pain
▪ Syringomyclia	• Peroneal muscular atrophy (Charcot-Marie Tooth disease)

***Diabetes mellitus is the most common cause for Neuropathic joint disease** Q*

Distribution of joint involvement Q

Condition Q	Most commonly affected joints Q
Tabes dorsolis	Knees, hips and ankles
Syringomyelia	Glenohumeral joint (Shoulder), elbow and wrist
Diabetes mellitus	Tarsal and Tarsometatarsal joint

314. Answer is A (VII nerve injury): *API medicine 6th/ 730; Dhingra 3rd/ 123 (2nd/ 99)*

Inability to close the eye and drooling of saliva from the same side of the mouth is characteristic of VII nerve palsy (U/L)

Lower motor neuron	Upper motor neuron
Lesion of facial nerve or its nucleus in the pons	Lesion of intracranial portion proximal to pontine nucleus
Common causes of affection	**Common causes of affection**
• Bell's palsy • Pontine vascular accidents • Lesion in cerebellopontine angle • Herpetic infection (Ramsay Hunt syndrome) • Lesion in its course through temporal bone • Parotid tumors	• Cerebrovascular accidents • Demyelination • Tumors
Presentation (There is loss of muscles of facial expression)	**Presentation**
• *<u>Ipsilateral</u> face is involved* • *Absence of furrowing of face on the same side* • *Inability to close the ipsilateral eye* (on attempted closure the eyeball rolls upwards-**Bell's phenomenon)** • *Flattening of the nasolabial folds* • *Drooping of the angle of the mouth* • Deviation of mouth towards **opposite side***	*<u>Contralateral face</u> is involved* The lower half of the face is involved as in lower motor neuron palsy where as the **upper half of the face is spared** as it has B/L innervation.

315. Answer is D (Contralateral lower face paresis): *Ref: Fuller 2nd/ 85; Macleods clinical examination, 10th/ 206*

Upper motor neuron VII nerve palsy causes contralateral facial muscle paresis that is worse in the lower facial muscles. With UMN lesion the forehead is relatively spared.

This is a unique feature seen only with facial nerve. The part of facial nerve supplying the upper half of face has bilateral cortical representation and thus in a unilateral UMN lesion the upper half of face escapes paresis.

316. Answer is C (Facial nerve): *Khurana 4th/366; Yanoff 2nd/254; 'Atlas of Surgery of Facial Nerve' by Grewal (JP) 2012/ ch-4*

Shirmer's test is done to assess the lacrimation function of the Facial Nerve (Greater Superficial Petrosal Nerve).

Topographical Testing of Facial Nerve Function

Shirmer's test	Stapedial Reflex test (Acoustic Reflex Testing)	Taste Testing Electrogustometry	Salivary flow Rate
• Shirmer's test for lacrimation evaluates the integrity of the *Greater Superficial Petrosal Nerve* (GSPN) by comparing the amount of tearing produced on the involved side with the normal side • Greater Superficial Petrosal Nerve *is the first branch of facial nerve* that arises from the geniculate ganglion and carries preganglionic parasympathetic fibers destined for lacrimal gland (and glands within nasal and palatal mucosa)	• Stapedial Reflex test is used to evaluate the *stapedius branch of facial nerve* • A lesion of the facial nerve proximal to the stapedius branch disrupts the arc Persistance or Return of stapedius reflex provides prognostic value *Restoration of stapedius reflex within 3 weeks of onset of facial palsy indicates functional recovery.* *Persistance of stapedial reflex in Bell's palsy indicates good prognosis*	• Taste testing is used *to test integrity of chorda tympani branch of facial nerve* that carries taste sensation to anterior 2/3rd of tongue.	• Salivary flow rates may also be used to assess integrity of *chorda lympani branch of facial nerve* • Reduction of salivation to less than 25% of normal is considered significant

317. Answer is A (Greater superficial petrosal nerve): *Previous question*

Shirmer's test is done to assess the integrity of Greater Superficial Petrosal Nerve (Branch of Facial Nerve) by assessing the Lacrimation function.

Topographical Test for Facial Nerve Function	Branch / Nerve assessed
Shirmer's test	*Greater Superficial Petrosal Nerve (GSPN)*
Stapedial Reflex *Accoustic Reflex*	*Stapedial branch (Branch to stapedius)*
Electrogustometry (Taste testing)	*Chorda Tympani Branch*
Salivary Flow Rate	*Chorda Tympani Branch*

318. Answer is B (Ramsay Hunt sSyndrome): *Harrison's 18th/3362, 3363; 'Atlas of Surgery of Facial Nerve' by Grewal (Jp)2012/ Ch.13*

Herpes Zoster of geniculate ganglion causes Ramsay Hunt Syndrome.

'The Ramsay Hunt Syndrome is caused by reactivation of Herpes Zoster in the geniculate ganglion and consists of a severe facial nerve palsy associated with a vesicular eruption in the external auditory canal and sometimes in the pharynx and other parts of the cranial integument'- Harrison

Syndromes Associated with Facial Palsy

Syndrome	Feature
Ramsay Hunt Syndrome[Q] *(Herpes Zoster Oticus)*	Facial palsy due to reactivation of Herpes zoster in geniculate ganglion with vesicular eruption in the external ear
Melkerson – Rosenthal Syndrome[Q]	Rare neuromyocutaneous disorder charachterized by triad of Recurrent facial palsy, Cheilitis granulomatosa and fissured tongue (lingua plicata)
Heerfordt's Syndrome[Q] *(Uveoparotoid fever)*	Facial palsy in association with sarcoidosis (Facial palsy with Uveitis/Iritis, parotid enlargement & fever)
Bell's Palsy	Idiopathic Facial N.palsy
Frey's Syndrome *(Gustatary sweating)* *Gusatory Lacrimation* *Crocodile tears*	Results from damage to parasympathetic fibers of facial nerve, which regenerates in a misdirected manner. *Stimuli that promote parotid gland secretion result in sweating or flushing over areas of the foci during mastication*
Mobius syndrome	Congenital bilateral facial palsy with several other cranial nerve involvement
Albers shonberg syndrome	Facial nerve palsy with osteopetrosis

Disorders of Muscles / Myopathies

Myaesthenia Gravis

319. Answer is D (Decreased Myoneural junction transmission): *Harrison 17th/2672, 2673; Harrison 18th/p 3480, 3481*

The primary defect in Myaesthenia gravis is decreased transmission across the myoneural junction due to decrease in the number of Acetylcholine receptors.

'The fundamental defect is Myaesthenia gravis is a decrease in the number of Acetylcholine Receptors at the postsynaptic muscle membrane, which results in decreased efficiency of neuromuscular transmission' – Harrison

320. Answer is B (Absent deep tendon reflexes): *Harrison 15th/1516, 16th/2519; 17th/2673; Harrison 18th/p 3480, 3481*

***'Despite the muscle weakness, deep tendon reflexes are preserved'** – Harrison 16th/2519; Harrison 17th/ 2673*

'Suspect Myaesthenia gravis in a case of weakness with fatiguability, without loss of reflexes & impairment of sensations' – Harrison

Myaesthenia Gravis : Review :

Etiology :
Autoimmune disorders mediated by specific Anti ACH receptor antibodies.
Fundamental defect :
Decrease in number of available ACH receptors at post synaptic muscle membrane.
Age / Sex :
All ages are affected Most prevalent in women in twenties/ thirties and men in fifties & sixties. Women are affected more frequently than men[Q]. (3 : 2)
Features :
Weakness : in characteristic distribution as elaborated below Fatiguability: Weakness increases on repeated use and may improve following rest or sleep A variable course marked by remissions and exacerbations (remissions are rarely complete or permanent)
Association :
Thymic abnormalities and Thymomas (Neoplastic) Autoimmune disorders : Rheumatoid Arthritis, SLE, Perenicious anemia, hyperthyroidism, ulcerative colitis, polymyositis etc.

Characteristics Distribution of Weakness

Craniofacial muscle weakness	**Limb muscles**	**Weakness of Respiratory muscles (crises)**
• Lids and extraocular muscles : diplopia and ptosis are common early complaints • Facial weakness : produces snarling expression on attempt to smile weakness in chewing • Speech: Nasal timbre due to weakness of palate dysarthric mushy quality due to tongue weakness • Difficulty in swallowing and nasal regurgitation or aspiration of liquids or food due to weakness of palate, tongue & pharynx. • Muscles of neck particularly extensors are frequently involved.	• Affected in 85% of cases • Proximal weakness • Usually symmetric but may be asymmetric	• If weakness of respiratory muscles becomes so severe so as to require respiratory assistance the patient is said to be in crisis. • Crisis is often precipitated by unrelated infections or systemic disorders.

321. Answer is B (Myaesthenia Gravis): *Harrison 16th/2519, 2531; Harrison 17th/2673; Harrison 18th/p 3481*

*'**Fatiguability**' and '**Weakness**' in the typical distribution of 'extraocular muscles **(diplopia)** and muscle of 'palate, tongue and pharynx' **dysphagia** suggests the characteristic diagnosis of myaesthenia gravis.*

Other options are easy to exclude

Muscular dystrophy (occulopharyngeal)	Thyrotoxicosis	Brain tumor
• No fatiguability • No diplopia (see below)	• No fatiguability • Marked systemic symptoms of thyrotoxicosis	• No fatiguability • Focal neurological signs

Ocutopharyngeal muscular dystrophy

Characterized by

Progressive external ophthalmoplepia	Pharyngeal muscle weakness
• Slowly progressive ptosis • Limitation of eye movements • Sparing of pupillary reactions for light and accomodation ***'Patients usually do not complain of diplopia in contrast to patients having conditions with a more acute onset of ocular muscle weakness such as M. gravis'- Harrison***	• Progressive dysphagia • May become debilitating and result in pooling of seretions and repeated episodes of aspiration

322. Answer is D (Single Fiber Electromyagraphy (SFEMG)) : *Harrison's 17th/ 2674; Merritt's Neurology 12th/389; Kanski 5th/654; Adult Neurology 2nd/299; Other References with Text; Harrison 18th/p 3481*

Single Fiber Electromyography (SFEMG) is the single most sensitive assay of neuromuscular function dysfunction in myasthenia gravis

'SFEMG is the single most sensitive assay of neuromuscular function dysfunction in myasthenia gravis having a sensitivity of greater than 95% when applied to clinically affected muscle' – Merrit's Neurology 12th(2009) /389

'Single fiber electromyography is the most sensitive diagnostic test for MG, but abnormalities are not specific'.
– 'Neuromuscular Junction Disorders: Diagnosis & Treatment (2003)/109

'Single fiber EMG is the most sensitive electrophysiological test for myasthenia gravis'
- Adult Neurology' 2nd (Blackwell publishing) /299

Test	Generalized MG (sensitivity)	Ocular MG (sensitivity)
AchR antibodies (ACHR Antibodies)	80%	60%
Repetitive Nerve stimulation (RNS)	75%	48%
Single Fiber EMG (SFEMG)	99%	97%
Edrophonium (Tensilon) test	95%	85%

Taken from 'Neuromuscular Junction Disorder's: Diagnosis & Treatment (2003) /109

Edrophonium test / Tensilon test	Acetylcoline Receptor antibodies
• *Highly sensitive test with 85% sensitivity in ocular and 95% sensitivity in systemic myasthenia -Kanski* • Diagnosis is highly probable if test in unequivocally positive • An initial dose of 2mg of edrophonium is given intravenously. If improvement occurs the test is considered positive and terminated. If there is no change an additional 8mg are given intravenously.	• Sensitivity of 80-90% in *systemic* myasthenia - CMDT • Highly specific and presence of Anti ACH Receptor Antibodies is virtually diagnostic of M. gravis 85% positive in generalized M.G. 50% positive in ocular M.G. Definitive if positive Negative test does not exclude M.G. 40% of Anti antibody negative patients have Anti-Musk antibodies.

Repetitive nerve stimulation / Electrodiagnostic test	Single fiber electromyography
• Helpful diagnostic evidence • Best when weak muscles/ proximal ms. groups are tested • Amplitude of evoked muscle end potential is measured - No change in normal patients - Reduction by > 10-15 % in myasthenic patients.	• Demonstrates blocking and jitter with normal fiber density • *Most sensitive diagnostic test for MG with sensitivity of greater than 95%* • *Confirmatory but not specific* • Often performed in conjunction with repetitive nerve stimulation test (Oxford handbook)

323. Answer is C (Edrophonium test) : *Harrison's 17th/ 2354; 'Myasthenia Gravis & Related Disorders' by Kaminski 2nd/134 ; Harrison 18th/p 3481*

Edrophonium test is the most sensitive test to suggest the diagnosis of myasthenia gravis amongst the options provided

Proximal weakness of muscles, ptosis and easy fatigability suggests a diagnosis of Myasthenia Gravis. Edrophonium (Tensilon) test is a highly sensitive test with 85% sensitivity in ocular and 95% sensitivity in systemic myasthenia. The diagnosis of MG is highly probable if Edrophonium test is unequivocally positive.

> **Note**
> *Conventional (EMG) is not a sensitive diagnostic test for MG. The conventional needle EMG is usually normal in patients with MG although certain findings may indicate probability of MG. Conventional EMG evaluation in MG serves mostly in excluding other causes of weakness like motor neuron disease, neuropathy or myopathy*

EMG in Myasthenia Gravis

Conventional EMG *'EMG'*	Single Fiber EMG *'SFEMG'*
• ***Not a sensitive diagnostic test for myasthenia gravis*** • Performed to exclude other causes of weakness like motor neuron disease, myopathies and neuropathies	• ***Most sensitive diagnostic test for myasthenia gravis*** • Performed as a confirmatory (but not specific) test for neuromuscular junction dysfunction or myasthenia gravis

324. Answer is D (Single fiber EMG) : *Merritt's Neurology 12th/389; Harrison's 17th/2674; Adult Neurology 2nd/299; Harrison 18th/p 3481*

Single Fiber EMG is the single most sensitive diagnostic test for Myasthenia Gravis.

Proximal weakness of muscles, ptosis and easy fatigability in this 35 years old female suggests a diagnosis of Myasthenia Gravis.

Edrophonium test and Single Fiber EMG are both sensitive diagnostic tests for myasthenia gravis. Single fiber EMG is reported as the single most sensitive test for diagnosis of neuromuscular dysfunction in myasthenia gravis, and is the single best answer of choice.

> *Single most sensitive test for diagnosis of Myasthenia Gravis: SFEMG*
> *Single most specific test for diagnosis of Myasthenia Gravis: AChR antibodies*

325. Answer is C (Incremental response to repeated electrical stimulation): *Harrison's 16th/2521; Harrison's 17th/2674, API 7th/915; CMDT 2009; Delong's Neurological Examination 6th/625; Harrison 18th/p 3481 ; Harrison 18th/p 3481*

Lambert Eaten Myaesthenic syndrome presents with an incremental response to repeated electrical stimulation.

Lambert Eaten Myasthenia Syndrome	Myasthenia Gravis
What it is & Associations	**What it is & Associations**
• Paraneoplastic syndrome • Associated with - Small cell carcinoma lung - Certain autoimmune diseases	• Autoimmune disorder • Associated with - Thymomas - Certain autoimmune diseases
Defect	**Defect**
• Presynaptic disorder • Antibodies to calcium channels (P/Q type) • Decrease in presynaptic release of Acetylcholine at Neuromuscular junction is the fundamental defect	• Postsynaptic disorder • Antibodies against ACH Receptors • Decrease in number of ACH Receptors at post synaptic muscle membrane is the fundamental defect
Presentation	**Presentation**
• Onset usually after 40 years • Men > Women (5: 1) • ***Proximal limb muscles and muscles of trunk are the most commonly involved muscles*** Proximal limb muscles >> extraocular & lid muscles • ***No fatiguability / Incremental response Repeated stimulation causes increased muscle strength*** • Reflexes : Hyporeflexia or absent reflexes • Autonomic changes such as dry mouth and impotence are associated	• Onset Often < 40 years • Women > Men (4: 3) • Craniofascial muscles particularly lids and ***extraocular muscles are the most commonly involved.*** Extraocular & lid muscles > proximal limb muscles • ***Fatiguability / Decremental response Repeated stimulation causes decreased muscle strength*** • Reflexes : Intact • No associated autonomic changes
Diagnosis	**Diagnosis**
• Repeated nerve stimulation : incremental response • Radioimmune assay : Antibodies against P/Q Ca^{2+} channels • *Tensilon test : Negative* (mildly positive in some)	• Repeated nerve stimulation : Decremental • Radioimmune assay : - Anti ACHR antibody response - Anti-Musk antibodies • ***Tensilon test : Characteristically Positive***

326. Answer is C (Repeated electrical stimulation enhances muscle power): *Harrison 16th/2521, Harrison 17th/2674; CMDT 2005/2003 API 7th/915; Harrison 18th/p 3481*

'Patients with Lambert – Eaten myaethenic syndrome show incremental rather than decremental response on repeated nerve stimulation' *– Harrison 17th/2674*
'Muscle response to stimulation of its motor nerve increases remarkably if nerve is stimulated repeatedly even in muscles that are clinically weak' *- CMDT*

Lambert Eaten Myasthenia Syndrome commonly involves proximal limb muscles and muscles of trunk
Extraocular muscles are the most commonly involved in Myaesthenia Gravis and not in Lambert Eaten Myasthenia Syndrome

Neostigmine is not considered the drug of choice
Plasmapharesis and immunosuppression form mainstay of treatment
3, 4 Diaminopyridine is the drug of choice for enhancement of neuromuscular transmission.
Pyridostigmine (or Neostigmine) may be sympatomatically helpful but their response is variable – *Harrison & CMDT*

Lambert Eaten Myasthenia Syndrome is associated with small cell carcinoma of lung

Lambert Eaten Myasthenia Syndrome is associated with small cell carcinoma of lung and not adenocarcinoma

327. Answer is A (SIADH): *Harrison's 17th/2060; Harrison's 16th/313, 574, 1946; Manual of Clinical Oncology 6th/409; Rubin's Pathology 5th/931;*

Syndrome of Inappropriate ADH secretion (SIADH) has not been mentioned in association with Thymomas.

Clinical Syndromes Associated with Thymomas

Paraneoplastic Immunologic Syndromes associated with both benign and malignant thymomas occur frequently, do not affect prognosis and may not reverse following thymectomy.

Charachteristic Syndromes	Rare Syndromes / Associated Diseases
• ***Myaesthenia Gravis (most common)***[Q] • ***Acquired Hypogammaglobulinemia (10%)*** [Q] • *Pure Red Cell Aplasia* [Q]	• ***Ectopic Cushing's Syndrome*** • Autoimmune Thyroiditis / Grave's Disease • Connective Tissue Disorders / Vasculitis - Polymyositis / Dermatamyositis - Granulomatous myocarditis - SLE - Rheumatoid Arthritis - Sjogren's syndrome, Scleroderma - Churg- Strauss syndrome, Microscopic polyangitis, Isolated Pauci- immune crescenteric glomenulonephritis • Optic neuritis / Limbic encephalitis • Hypertrophic Osteoarthropathy • Pernicious anemia • Pemphigus • Panhypopituarism • Ulcerative colitis • Addison's disease

328. Answer is B (Hypergammaglobulinemia): *Harrison 17th /2060; Manual of clinical oncology 6th/409. Robbin's Pathology 5th/931*

Thymoms may be associated with Hypogammaglobulinemia and not with Hypergammaglobulinemia.

Immune status with Thymoma
• T-cell number & cell medicated immunity are usually intact [Q] • These patients are very *deficient in circulating B lymphocytes*[Q] & pre B cell in the bone marrow *Hypogammaglobulinemia*[Q] usually occurs relatively late in adult life. • Bacterial infection & diarrhea usually reflect this antibody deficiency.[Q] • Frequently have *eosinopenia*[Q] • May develop *Red cell (Erythroid) Aplasia.*[Q]

Thymoma is associated with Hypogammaglobulinemia and not with hypergammaglobulinemia

329. Answer is A (Myaesthenia Gravis): *Harrisons 17th/chapter e/2/XVIII,2673,2675; Harrison 18th/p 3480, 3483*

Thymoma is most commonly associated with myaesthenia gravis which is the single best answer of choice

330. Answer is C (Hypergammoglobutinemia): *Rubin's Pathology 5th/931; Harrison's 17th/2060, 626,627,668; Harrison's 16th/313, 574, 1946*

Thymomos are associated with Hypogammoglobulinemia and not hypergammaglobulinemia.

331. Answer is C (Hypergammoglobulinemia): *Harrison's 17th/2060, 626,627,668; Harrison's 16th/1746*

Thymoma is associated with Hypogammaglobulinemia and not with hypergammaglobulinemia

332. Answer is A (Myasthenia Gravis): *Harrisons 17th/Chapter e12/ XVIII; 2673 2675; Harrison 18th/p 3480, 3483*

About 30% of patients with thymomas have Myasthenia gravis and Myasthenia gravis patients have a high incidence of thymic abnormalities - Harrisons 17th

Thymic Abnormalities and Myasthenia Gravis (MG) and Recommendations for Thymectomy

Myasthenia Gravis patients have a high incidence of thymic abnormalities Thymus is abnormal in about 75% of patients

65% of patients have a Hyperplastic Thymus[Q]	**10% of patient have Thymomas[Q]**

***Thymus** is believed to play a role in the autoimmune dysfunction in M.G and thymectomy has shown significant improvement in upto 85% of patients with MG (35% achieve drug free remission).*
Thymectomy is therefore recommended as a form of treatment for MG.

Treatment recommendations for Thymectomy in patients with MG.[Q]

Patients with Thymomas	*Patients without Thymomas*
Thymectomy should be carried out in all patients who have thymomas[Q] *(Thymectomy in thymonas is necessary because of the possibility of local tumor spread although most thymomas are benign)*	Thymectomy should be carried out in all patients with **generalized MG** who are between the ages of **puberty** and **at least 55 years**

Thymectomy not clearly recommended for[Q]:
- Children (< puberty)
- Elderly > 55 years
- Localized M.G with weakness limited to extra ocular muscles
- Patients with MUSK antibody positive Myaesthenia gravis.

333. Answer is A (Should be done in all cases) : *Harrison 15th/2519; 16th/2522; 17th/2675; CMDT 2001/1024; 2003/1002; Harrison 18th/p 3483, 3484*

- ***Thymectomy should be carried out in all patient with generalized Myasthenia gravis*** between the ages of puberty and 55 years of age – *Harrison 17th/2675*
- ***Thymectomy should be considered in all patients with generalised M. gravis*** younger than 60 years of age.
- ***Done even in those case, controlled by medical treatment***: The advantage of thymectomy is that it offers the possibilities of long term benefit. It may diminish or even eliminate the need for continuing medical treatment. This is why it is done even in those cases, controlled by medical treatment.
- ***Done in those cases also, where thymoma is not associated:*** 85% of patients without a Thymoma, also experience improvement after thymectomy. 55% to an extent that they may achieve drug free remission. This is why thymectomy is done in those cases also, where thymoma is not associated.

  Only 10% of patients with M. Gravis have an associated thymoma. [Thymus is abnormal in approximately 75% but in the majority (65%), the thymus is only hyperplastic and does not have a tumor]
- ***Thymectomy is not indicated if weakness is restricted to extraocular muscles*** – *CMDT 2001 pg.1024*

334. Answer is D (Pyridostigmine): *Harrison 17th/2675-2676; Harrison 18th/p 3483*

Pyridostigmine is the most widely used anticholinesterase medication in Myaesthenia Gravis. Pyridostigmine's the single best answer of choice amongst the options provided.

Muscular Dystrophies & Myopathies

335. Answer is D (Duchenne Muscular Dystrophy) : *Harrison 16th/2527; Harrison 17th/2683; Nelson 17th/2061; Harrison 18th/p 3492*

Duchenne muscular dystrophy is caused by a mutation in the gene responsible for producing dystrophin.

Progressive Muscle Dystrophies

Type	Inheritance	Defective gene/Protein	Onset age	Clinical features	Other Organ systems involved
Duchenne	XR	Dystrophin	Before 5 years	Progressive weakness of girdle muscles Unable to walk after age 12 Progressive kyphoscoliosis Respiratory failure in second or third decade	Cardiomyopathy Mental impairment
Becker	XR	Dystrophin	Early childhood to adult	Progressive weakness of girdle muscles Able to walk after age 15 Respiratory failure may develop by fourth decade	Cardiomyopathy
Limb –girdle	AD/AR	Several	Early childhood to early adult	Slow progressive weakness of shoulder and hip girdle muscles	Cardiomyopathy
Emery-Dreifuss	XR/AD	Emerin/Lamins A/C	Childhood to adult	Elbow contractures humeral and peroneal weakness	Cardiomyopathy
Congenital	AR	Several	At birth or within first few month	Hypotonia, contractures , delayed milestones Progression to respiratory failure in some, static course in others	CNS abnormalities (hypomyelination malformation) Eye abnormalities
Myotonic (DM1, DM2)	AD	DM1 : Expansion CTG repeat DM2 : Expansion CCTG repeat	Usually second decade may be infancy if mother affected (DM1 only)	Slowly progressive weakness of face, shoulder girdle and foot dorsiflexion Preferential proximal weakness in DM2	Cardiac conduction defects, mental impairments cataracts, frontal baldness, gonadal atrophy
Facioscapu-lohumeral	AD	Deletion, Distal 4q	Before age 20	Slowly progressive weakness of face, shoulder girdle and foot dorsiflexion	Deafness, Coat's (eye) disease
Oculopharyngeal	AD	Expansion, poly A-RNA binding protein	5th to 6th decade	Slowly progressive weakness of extraocular, pharyngeal and limb muscles	-

336. Answer is A (Facio-Scapulo-Humeral Dystrophy): *Current Diagnosis & Treatment in Neurology (2008)/385*

Weakness preferentially affecting the facial and shoulder girdle (proximal weakness of upper limb) together with winging of scapula in a young adult suggests a diagnosis of facio-scapulo-humeral dystrophy.

Facio-Scapulo-Humeral Dystrophy

- Autosomal Dominant (Positive Family History^Q^)
- Abnormal gene 4q (4q35 deletion)
- Childhood to young adulthood (may be delayed to 5th decade)
- Mild ↑ CPK (Normal Dystrophy)

Clinical Sign

- Weakness preferentially affects the facial and shoulder girdle muscles
  - Unable to whistle
  - Unable to smile
  - Unable to fully close their eyes
- Extraocular muscles are typically spared
- Pelvic girdle weakness may be present (20%)
- Usually asymmetric at onset

Orthopaedic Manifestations

- Winging of scapula (Scapular winging contracture may be present)
- Winging of scapula becomes more evident when the patient attempts to elevate the arms laterally

Prognosis

- Life expectancy is normal
- Respiratory insufficiency is rare

Extramuscular manifestations

These occur with variable frequency and include mental impairment, hearing loss, retinal vasculopathy and cardiac involvement.

Disease	Age at Diagnosis	Inheritance pattern	Abnormal gene	Life Expectancy	Signs	Orthopaedic Manifestations	Laboratories
Duchenne muscular dystrophy (DMD)	2-6 yrs	X-linked recessive (½ have new mutation)	Xp21	~20-30yr	Late walker, calf pseudohypertrophy, Meryon and Gower signs, mild mental retardation	Contractures: equinovarus, knee flexion, hip flexion-abduction, wheelchair dependance, scoliosis	↑↑ CK ↓↓dystrophin
Limb-Girdle dystrophy	2nd to 3rd decade of life	Autosomal recessive and dominant forms	Many	Wide range	Weakness of pelvic or shoulder girlde muscles	Similar to DMD, milder	↑ CK, Normal dystrophin
Facioscapulohumeral dystrophy	2nd decade of life	Autosomal dominant	4q	Normal	Facial and shoulder girdle weakness, expresisonaless face	Scapular winging contractures	Mild ↑ CPK, Normal dystrophin
Scapulo-peroneal dystrophy	Childhood to Adulthood	Autosomal dominant, Autosomal recessive, or sporadic	Unknown	Usually normal life expectancy	Weakness of shoulder girdle and dorsiflexors of the feet and toes	Weakness of shoulder girdle and dorsiflexors of the feet and toes	Abnormal gene product unknown

The muscular dystrophies:

Type	Inheritance pattern	Chromosomal or genomic defect	Missing or abnormal gene product	Incidence (i.e. frequency with respect to live births)	Age of onset	Clinical features	Prognosis
Duchenne	X-linked 30% sporadic	Xp21.2	dystrophin absent	20-30/ 100 000 boys	2nd-3rd year	onset in pelvic girdle, pseudohypertrophy of calves	rapidly progressive, most patients die by age 25
Becker	X-linked	Xp21.2	dystrophin abnormal	3/100 000 boys	1st (-4th) decade	same as in Duchene muscular dystrophy, but milder; sometimes cardiomyopathy	ambulatory till age 15 or later, death in 4th or 5th decade or later

Mery-Dreifuss	X-linked, rarely autosomal dominant	Xp28	emerin	1/100 000	childhood adolescence	scapuloperoneal dystrophy, contractures, and cardiopathy may be prominent	ambulatory till 3rd decade or for entire life; cardiac arrhythmia a frequent cause of death
Facio-scapulo humeral dystrophy (Duchenne-Landouzy-Dejerine)	autosomal dominant	4q35	homebox gene	5/100 000	childhood to young adulthood	weakness of facial, shoulder girdle, and calf muscles	practically normal life expectancy
Scapulo-peroneal dystrophy	autosomal dominant, autosomal recessive, or sporadic	unknown	unknown	rare	childhood to adulthood	weakness of shoulder girdle and dorsiflexors of the feet and toes	usually normal life expectancy
Limb girdle dystrophy	autosomal recessive, autosomal dominant or sporadic	5q, 13q, 15q	unknown	rare	childhood to adulthood	mainly proximal weakness of pelvic or shoulder girdle	depending on type, premature death or only minor disability or into old age
Oculopharyngeal dystrophies	autosomal dominant	unknown	unknown	rare	middle age	oculofaciobulbar paresis	often premature death due to dystrophagia and aspiration pneumonia
Congenital dystrophies (for variants)	autosomal recessive	unknown	unknown	rare	at birth	depending on type: involvement of muscles, eye, and brain: contractures, arthrogryposis multiplex	ranging from mild disability to severe meantal retardation
Steinertmyotonic dystrophy	autosomal dominant	19q13.3	protein kinase	13.5/100000, prevalence 5/100 000	young adulthood, rarely congenital, earlier age of onset in each successive generation ("anticipation")	mainly distal weakness, faciobulbar paresis, myotonia, cataracts	age of significant disability depends on age of onset, usually middle age; premature death
Distal myopathies (Welander type, Markesbery- Griggs, Finnish variant)	autosomal dominant	unknown	unknown	rare	middle age	mainly distal atrophy and weakness	only minor disability into old age
Distal myopathies (Nonaka and Miyoshi types)	autosomal recessive	Miyoshi: 2p12-14 Nonaka: unknown	unknown	rare	adolescene to young adulthood	mainly distal weakness	progression to inability to walk

337. Answer is B (Sarcolemmal protein) : *Harrison 15th / 2530; Nelson 17th / 2061; Harrison 16th/2527; Harrison 17th/2683 (2684-fig 382-6); Harrison 18th/p 3491-3494(Table: 387.6)*

Duchenne muscular dystrophy is caused by a mutation in the gene responsible for producing dystrophin.
Dystrophin is 'subsarcolemmal protein' (Nelson) localized to the inner surface of the sarcolemma of the muscle fibre. *Harrison 17th/2683*

Dystrophin is part of Dystrophin – Glycoprotein sarcolemmal complex and this protein deficiency leads to secondary loss of sarcoglycans and dystroglycans resulting in weakness of sarcolemma, causing membrane tears and muscle fibre necrosis

9

Duchenne muscular dystrophy : Review (pseudohypertrophic muscular dystrophy)

- Duchenne muscular dystrophy is the most common hereditary neuromuscular disease affecting all races and ethnic groups.
- Inheritance : X linked recessive
- Presentation occurs between ages 3 and 5 [disorder does not present at birth or in infancy[Q]]

Clinical manifestations:

- Gower's sign is positive[Q]
- Pseudohypertrophy of calf is seen[Q] (muscle is replaced by fat & connective tissue)
- Loss of muscle strength is progressive. [Q]
- Proximal muscles and neck flexors are involved more. [Q]
- Leg involvement is more severe than arm involvement.
- Contractures of heel cords and iliotibial band occurs (by age of 6 years)
- Progressive scoliosis develops.

Complications:

Chest deformity[Q] (scoliosis) [Q]:
Impairs pulmonary function[Q]
By age of 16 and 18 years patients are predisposed to serious pulmonary fatal infections.

Cardiac:
Cardiomyopathy [Q] and CHF may be seen
Cardiac cause of death is uncommon

Intellectual impairment :
is common[Q] (IQ is one SD below the mean)

Remember:

Onset [Q]	*Before age of 5* [Q]
Confined to wheel chair *Inability to walk*	*After age of 12* [Q]
Respiratory failure	*In second or third decade (after 16-18 years)* [Q]

Laboratory diagnosis:

- *Serum creatinephosphokinase (CK)* [Q] : elevated (20-100 times)
- *EMG :* features of myopathy
- *Muscle biopsy*[Q] :
  - Definitive diagnosis established on basis of dystrophin deficiency in biopsied muscle tissue
  - Groups of necrotic and regenerating muscle fibres are seen.

Treatment:

- Glucocorticoids (Prednisolone) have been tried.
- Significant alteration in the progression of disease has been seen with **prednisolone.**

338. Answer is B & D (Vastus medialis & infraspinatus): *Ghai 6th/548;*

Vastus medialis and infracpinatus are answers of exclusion as they have not been mentioned in the list of muscles involved in Ghai's text.

'The calf muscles (gastronemius), glutei deltoid, serratus anterior, brachioradialis and tongue muscles appear large (pseudohypertrophy).

Sternal head of pectoralis major and supraspinatus are atrophied.- Ghai

339. Answer is A (Chromosome19) : *Harrison 14th/2475, 15th/2532; 17th/2686; AI-Medicine; Harrison 18th/p 3498*

The disorder is transmitted by a mutation in an 'unstable trinucleotide repeat sequence' in a gene at 19q 133.

Myotonia Dystrophica :

- It is the most common adult muscular dystrophy.[Q]
- Myotonic dystrophy is an autosomal dominant disorder. [Q]
- The disorder is transmitted by a mutation in an 'unstable trinucleotide repeat sequence' in a gene at 19q 133
- Muscle atrophy selectively involves type I fibres only. [Q] (in 50% of cases)
- Myopathy in Myotonia is unique in the sense that it is ***typically distal*** in contrast to other myopathies which are mostly proximal. [Q]
- Myotonia usually appears by the age of 5 years [Q], and causes a slow relaxation of hand grip following a forced voluntary closure.

340. Answer is B (Dystrophin dystrophy) : *Harrison 16th / 2528,2531; Harrison 17th/2682, 2683; Harrison 18th/p 3492, 3493, 3494*

Calpain - J, Sarcoglycans (γ,α,β and γ) and dysferlin are all examples of defective gene / locus in Limb girdle dystrophies. Dystrophin is associated with Duchenne's and Becker's type of muscular dystrophics and is not associated with Limb girdle dystrophies.

The Limb girdle muscular dystrophies (LGMD) typically manifest with progressive weakness of pelvic and shoulder girdle musculature. Respiratory insufficiency from weakness of diaphragm and cardiomyopathy may occur. However unlike Duchenne dystrophies (Dystrophin) intellectual function remains intact. - Harrison

Progressive Muscular dystrophies & defective gene / protein

Duchenne	**Becker's**	**Limb girdle**	**Emery-Dreifuss**	**Myotonic dystrophy**	**Fascio-scapulo humeral**	**Oculo-pharyngeal**
Dystrophin[Q]	Dystrophin[Q]	Myotilin Laminin A/c Caveolin - 3 ***Calpain - 3*** ***Dysferlin*** ***γ,α,β,γ sarcoglycans*** Telethonin Fukutin related protein Titin TRIM 32 gene	Emerin Laminins	▪ (DM1)Unstable expansion of a CTG trinucleatide repeat in a serine threonine protein kinase gene (named DMPK) on chromosome 19q 13.3 ▪ (DM2) DNA expansion of a CcTG repeat in the ZNF9 gene on chromosome 3q 13.3 - q24	Deletion distal 4q	Expansion poly A RNA binding protein.

341. Answer is B (Dystrophin dystrophy): *Harrison 16th / 2528,2531; Harrison 17th/2682, 2683*

Calpain - J, Sarcoglycans (γ, α, β and γ) and dysferlin are all examples of defective gene / locus in Limb girdle dystrophies.
Dystrophin is associated with Duchenne and Becker's type of muscular dystrophics and is not associated with Limb girdle dystrophies.

The Limb girdle muscular dystrophies (LGMD) typically manifest with progressive weakness of pelvic and shoulder girdle musculature. Respiratory insufficiency from weakness of diaphragm and cardiomyopathy may occur. However unlike Duchenne dystrophies (Dystrophin) intellectual function remains intact. - Harrison

Progressive Muscular Dystrophies & Defective Gene / Protein

Duchenne and Becker's	**Limb girdle**	**Emery-Dreifuss**	**Myotonic dystrophy**	**Fascio-scapulo humeral**	**Oculopharyngeal**
Dystrophin[Q]	Myotilin Laminin A/c Caveolin - 3 ***Calpain - 3*** ***Dysferlin*** ***γ,α,β,γ sarcoglycans*** Telethonin Fukutin related protein Titin TRIM 32 gene	Emerin Laminins	▪ (DM1) Unstable expansion of a CTG trinucleatide repeat in a serine threonine protein kinase gene (named DMPK) on chromosome 19q 13.3 ▪ (DM2) DNA expansion of a CcTG repeat in the ZNF9 gene on chromosome 3q 13.3 - q24	Deletion distal 4q	Expansion poly A RNA binding protein.

342. Answer is C (Z band Myopathy) : *Harrison 16th/2533; Harrison 17th/2688; Robbins 7th/1340; Harrison 18th/p 3499*

Z band myopathy is not classified as a congenital myopathy.

Congenital Myopathy: These are a group of rare disorders distinguished from muscular dystrophies by the presence of specific histochemical and structural abnormalities in muscle.

Most of these are characterized by :

- Onset in early life (primarily disorders of infancy & childhood, but may present in adulthood)
- Non progressive or slowly progressive course
- Proximal or generalized muscle weakness
- Hypotonia

Congenital Myopathies:

Disease and Inheritance	Gene and Locus	Clinical Findings	Pathologic Findings
Central core disease; autosomal-dominant	Ryanodine receptor-1 (RYR1) gene; 19q 13.1	Early-onset hypotonia and non progressive weakness; associated skeletal deformities; may develop malignant hyperthermia	Cytoplasmic cores are lightly eosinophilic and distinct from surrounding sarcoplasm; Found only in type 1 fibers, which usually predominate, best seen on NADH stain
Nemaline myopathy; autosoma-dominant or autosomal-recessive	Autosomal-dominant (NEM1) – Tropomyosin 3 (TPM3) gene; Autosomal-recessive (NEM2) – nebulin (NEB) gene; 2q22 Autosomal-dominant or recessive – skeletal muscle actin, α chain (ACTA1) gene; 1q42.1	Weakness, hypotonia and delayed motor development in childhood; may also be seen in adults; usually nonprogressive; involves proximal limb muscles most severely; skeletal abnormalities may be present	Aggregates of subsarcolemmal spindle shaped particles (nemaline rods); occur predominantly in type 1 fibers; derived from Z-band material (α-actinin) and best seen on modified Gomori stain
Myotubular (centronuclear) myopathy; X-linked (MTM1), autosomal recessive, or autosomal-dominant	X-linked-myotubularin (MTM1) gene; Xq28	X-linked form presents in infancy with prominent hypotonia and poor prognosis; autosomal forms have limn weakness and are slowly progressive; autosomal recessive form is intermediate in severity and prognosis	Abundance of centrally located nuclei involving the makority of muscle fibers; central nuclei are usually confined to type I fibers, which are small in diameter, but can occur in both fiber types

Other uncommon types include minicore myopathy, fingerprint body myopathy and sarcotubular myopathy.

343. Answer is C (Z band Myopathy): *Harrison 16th/2533; Harrison 17th/2688; Robbins 7th/1340*

Z band myopathy is not classified as a congenital myopathy.

Nemaline myopathy, Central-core myopathy and Centro-nuclear (Myotubular) myopathy are all examples of congenital myopathies

Congenital Myopathies

These are a group of rare disorders distinguished from muscular dystrophies by the presence of specific histochemical and structural abnormalities in muscle.

Most of these are characterized by :

- *Onset in early life (primarily disorders of infancy & childhood, but may present in adulthood)*
- *Non progressive or slowly progressive course*
- *Proximal or generalized muscle weakness*
- *Hypotonia*

Disease and Inheritance	Gene and Locus	Clinical Findings	Pathologic Findings
Central core disease; *Autosomal-dominant*	Ryanodine receptor-1 (RYR1) gene; 19q 13.1	Early-onset hypotonia and non progressive weakness; associated skeletal deformities; may develop malignant hyperthermia	Cytoplasmic cores are lightly eosinophilic and distinct from surrounding sarcoplasm; Found only in type 1 fibers, which usually predominate, best seen on NADH stain
Nemaline myopathy; *Autosoma-dominant or Autosomal-recessive*	Autosomal-dominant (NEM1) – Tropomyosin 3 (TPM3) gene; Autosomal-recessive (NEM2) – nebulin (NEB) gene; 2q22 Autosomal-dominant or recessive – skeletal muscle actin, α chain (ACTA1) gene; 1q42.1	Weakness, hypotonia and delayed motor development in childhood; may also be seen in adults; usually nonprogressive; involves proximal limb muscles most severely; skeletal abnormalities may be present	Aggregates of subsarcolemmal spindle shaped particles (nemaline rods); occur predominantly in type 1 fibers; derived from Z-band material (α-actinin) and best seen on modified Gomori stain
Myotubular myopathy (Centronuclear); *X-linked (MTM1), Autosomal recessive, or Autosomal-dominant*	X-linked-myotubularin (MTM1) gene; Xq28	X-linked form presents in infancy with prominent hypotonia and poor prognosis; autosomal forms have limn weakness and are slowly progressive; autosomal recessive form is intermediate in severity and prognosis	Abundance of centrally located nuclei involving the makority of muscle fibers; central nuclei are usually confined to type I fibers, which are small in diameter, but can occur in both fiber types

Other uncommon types include minicore myopathy, fingerprint body myopathy and sarcotubular myopathy.

344. Answer is A (Peroneal muscular Atrophy): *'Pretest physical Diagnosis' 6th/Q370/256; Harrison's 16th/2510*

Inverted champagne bottle appearance of lower limbs is produced as a result of greater wasting of distal musculature in comparison to proximal musculature.

Charcoal Movie Tooth disease (CMT) or peroneal muscular Atrophy (Synonym for CMT) is classically associated with an inverted champagne bottle appearance of lower limbs

Inverted Champagne bottle appearance of lower limbs

- ***Sensorimotor Neuropathy causing distal muscular atrophy*** eg Charcot Marie Tooth disease or Peroneal Muscular Atrophy
- *Chronic Venous insufficiency leading to lipodermotosclerosis of distal limb (Davidson 20th/1227, CMDT 2008/27)*

Polymyositis

345. Answer is A(Anti-Jo-1): *The Washington Manual Rheumatology Subspecialty Consult (2003)/ 31, 32; Rheumatology: Diagnosis & Therapeutics 2nd/87*

Anti-Jo-1 Antibodies (Antibodies to histidyl - tRNA) are the most common and most clinically assayed Myositis Specific Antibodies (MSA)

Myositis Specific Antibodies (MSA)

- Myositis Specific antibodies are autoantibodies, usually directed against intracellular ribonucleoproteins that are involved in protein translation.
- *The three best described Myositis Specific Antibodies (MSA) are Anti-Jo-1(directed to t-RNA histidyl-synthetase), Anti-Mi-2 and Anti – SRP (Anti Signal Recognition Particle)*
- The sensitivity of these antibodies is believed to be low
- Specific MSA are however associated with certain clinical features and prognosis.

M.S.A	Association	Clinical Features	Prognosis
Anti-Jo-1	*Polymyositis (30% sensitive)*	• Relatively Acute Onset • Predicts deforming arthritis, Reynaud's Phenomenon and Pulmonary fibrosis	• *Moderate* • Moderate Response to therapy but persistent disease
Anti-Mi-2	*Dermatomyositis (5%) sensitive*	• Relatively Acute Onset • Predicts classical dermatomyositis rash ('V' sign, Shawl sign) and cuticular over growth	• *Good* • Good response to therapy and good prognosis
Anti- SRP	*Polymyositis / Dermatomyositis (< 5% sensitive)*	• Very Acute onset • Predicts severe weakness, palpitations (no rash)	• *Poor* • Poor response to therapy and poor prognosis

346. Answer is C (Ocular muscles): *Harrison, 14th/1896, 1897 and 15th/2524; Harrison 16th/2540; Harrison 17th/2696; Harrison 18th/p 3510*

'Ocular muscles are almost never affected' – Harrison.

Occular muscles are spared, even in advanced untreated cases *– Harrison*

Primary idiopathic polymyositis:

Condition of autoimmune[Q] etiology in which skeletal muscle[Q] is damaged by non suppurative inflammatory process[Q] dominated by Lymphocytic infiltration.[Q]

It is characterized by:

- Symmetrical weakness of proximal limb muscles especially hips and thigh (pelvic girdle) and later shoulder girdle.
- Weakness of flexor muscles of neck
- Involvement of striated muscles of pharynx (dysphagia)
- Involvement of respiratory muscles (late)

"Ocular muscles are almost never affected except in a rare case associated with myasthenia gravis."- Harrison
'Facial muscles are unaffected in Polymyositis'. - Harrison

347. Answer is B (Extraocular muscle involvement): *Harrisons 16th/2540; Harrison 17th/2696; 18th/p 3509, 3510*

Involvement of extraocular and facial muscles excludes a diagnosis of Polymyositis. – Harrison

Polymyositis

- It is a subacute inflammatory myopathy and mimics many other myopathies.
- Its diagnosis is essentially established as a disgnosisd of exclusion.
- **Polymyositis should be considered in adults and rarely in children who DO NOT HAVE any of the following :**

DO NOT HAVE

- ***Rash***
- ***Involvement of extraocular and facial muscles***
- Family history of a neuromuscular disease
- History of exposure to myotoxic drugs or toxins
- Endocrinopathy
- Neurogenic disease
- Muscular dystrophy
- Biochemical muscle disorder (deficiency of a muscle enzyme)

348. Answer is B (Gottron's rash): *Harrison, 15th/2524 and See previous question; Harrison 16th/2540; 17th/2696;*

Gottron's rash is a feature of dermatomyositis and is characterized by erythema of knuckles with raised violaceous scaly eruptions. No rash is seen in patients of polymyositis.

Dermatomyositis : is a distinctive entitiy identified by a characteristic rash, accompanying or more often preceding muscles weakness.

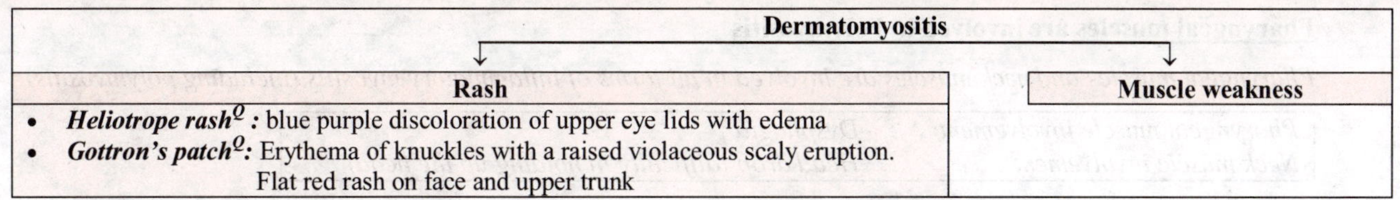

349. Answer is C (Cutaneous manifestation): *Harrison 17th/2696; Harrison 16th/2540*

Cutaneous manifestations (Rash) are a feature of Dermatomyositis and are characteristically absent in Polymyositis.

	Polymyositis	Dermatomyositis
Age of onset	*> 18 yr*	*Adulthood and childhood*
Familial associations	*No*	*No*
Extramuscular manifestations	*Yes*	*Yes*
Associated conditions		
Connective tissue diseases	*Yes*	*Scleroderma and mixed connective tissue disease (overlap syndromes)*
Systemic autoimmune diseases	*Frequent*	*Infrequent*
Malignancy	*No*	*Yes, in upto 15% of cases*
Viruses	*Yes*	*Unproven*
Drugs	*Yes*	*Yes, rarely*
Parasites and bacteria	*Yes*	*No*
Pathogenic mechanism	*T cell*	*Immune complex*
Skin Rash/ Dermatitis	***No***	***Yes***
Pharyngeal muscle involvement	***Yes***	***Yes***
Proximal muscle involvement	***Yes***	***Yes***
Ocular muscle involvement	***No***	***No***
Facial muscle involvement	***No***	***No***

350. Answer is A (Salmon Patch): *Harrisons 17th/2696*

Salmon patch is not a feature of dermatomyositis

Cutaneous features of dermatomyositis

Cutaneous feature	Description
Heliotrope Rash^Q	Periocular or facial erythema and edema with pink/purple /blue (heliotrope) hue *(blue purple discoloration on upper eye lids with edema)*
Gottren's Papules^Q (Gottren's sign)	Violaceous papules over the knuckles *Erythema of the knuckles with a raised violaceous scaly eruption*
'V' sign	*Erythematous rash over other body surfaces such as anterior chest (often in a V form)*
Shawl sign	*Erythematous rash over other body surfaces including the upper trunk, neck, back & shoulders (shawl pattern)*
Periungual Telengiectasias^Q	*Dilated capillary loops at the base of fingernails*
Mechanic's hands^Q	*Irregular, thickened, distorted cuticles, with rough and cracked areas over the lateral and palmar areas of fingers with irregular dirty horizontal lines resembling mechanic's hand.*
Calcinosis Cutis^Q	*Presence of hard calcium deposits in the skin*

351. Answer is B and C (Pharyngeal involvement and Muscle atrophy): *Harrison 17th/2696; Harrison 16th/2540; Harrison 18th/p 3510*

Polymyositis is associated with involvement of pharyngeal muscles and muscle atrophy may be seen if severe weakness is left untreated.

Pharyngeal muscles are involved in Polymyositis

Pharyngeal muscles and neck muscles are involved in all forms of inflammatory myositis (including polymyositis)

Pharyngeal muscle involvement	:	*Dysphagia*
Neck muscle involvement	:	*Head drop (difficulty in holding up the head)*

Muscle atrophy may be seen in Polymyositis

'Severe weakness if untreated is almost always associated with muscle wasting (atrophy) – Harrison

Ocular muscles are not involved in Polymyositis

'Ocular muscles are characteristically spared even in advanced untreated cases. If these muscles are involved, the diagnosis of inflammatory myopathy should be questioned'. - Harrisons

Tendon Reflexes are usually preserved (normal) but these are not brisk/exaggerated

'Tendon reflexes are preserved but may be absent in severely weakened or atrophic muscles' – Harrison

352. Answer is C (Metabolic acidosis): *Harrison 17th/2372/ 2373;*

Episodic Weakness & Channellopathies

353. Answer is B (Hypocalcemia): *Harrison 16th / 137 (table 21-2); Harrison 17th/150 (Table 23-2)*

Episodic generalized weakness is associated with hypercalcemia and not Hypocalcemia.

Causes of Episodic generalized weakness

Electrolyte disturbances
• ***Hypokalemia***
• Hyperkalemia
• ***Hyponatremia***
• Hypernatremia
• ***Hypophosphatemia***
• ***Hypercalcemia***
• Hypermagnesemia

Muscle disorders
• Channelopathies (periodic paralysis)
• Metabolic defect of muscle
- Impaired carbohydrate or fatty acid utilization
- Abnormal mitochondrial function
Neuromuscular junction disorder
• Myaesthenia gravis
• Lambert – Eaten Myaesthenic syndrome
Central nervous system disorders
• Transient ischaemic attacks of the brainstem
• Transient global cerebral ischemia
• Multiple sclerosis

354. Answer is D (Hyperglycemia): *Harrison 17th /150*

Hyperglycemia is not associated with episodic weakness.
Hypercalcemia, Hypokalemia and Lambert-Eaten syndrome may all be associated with episodic generalized weakness (Refer table in previous question)

355. Answer is C (Hyperphosphatemia): *Harrison 17th/150 (Table 23-2)*

Hypophosphatemia is associated with 'Episodic' generalized weakness and not Hyperphosphatemia.
Channelopathies, Hyperkalemia and Lambert-Eaten syndrome may all be associated with episodic generalized weakness (Refer table in previous question)

356. Answer is D (Tuberculosis): *Harrison 17th/150*

Tuberculosis is not associated with Episodic Generalized Muscular Weakness.

357. Answer is D (Huntington's disease): *Harrison 15th/ 2345-2350, Harrisons 16th/ 2415, 2536; Harrison 2478 (Table360-1); Harrison 18th/p 3225 (Table: 366.1)*

Huntington's disease is not a channelopathy.

Huntington's disease is an autosomal dominant disorder caused by mutations in the Huntington's gene on the short arm of chromosome 4, specifically in an expanding and unstable polyglutamine repeat sequence (CAG). The gene encodes for protein 'Huntington' which is present in all neurons.

Channelopathies: Refers to a group of disorders caused by affection of muscle membrane excitability.

Neurologic Channelopathies :

Category	Disorder	Channel type
Ataxias	Episodic ataxia –1 Episodic ataxia – 2 Spinocerebellar ataxia - 6	K Ca Ca
Migraine	Familial hemiplegic migraine	Ca
Epilepsy	Benign neonatal familial convulsions Generalised epilepsy with febrile convulsions plus	K Na
Periodic paralysis	Hyperkalemic periodic paralysis Hypokalemic periodic paralysis	Na Ca
Myotonia	Myotonia congenital Paramyotonia congenital	Cl Na
Deafness	Jorvell and Lange-Nielsen syndrome (deafness, prolonged QT interval, and arrhythmia) Autosomal dominant progressive deafness	K K

358. Answer is D (Spinocerebellar Ataxia 1): *Harrisons 15th/2321; Harrisons 16th/2339; Harrison 17th/2478; Refer previous question. Harrison 18th/p 3225*

Spinocerebellar ataxia – 6 is classified as meurological channelopathy bit not spinocerebellar ataxia – 1

Head Injuries & Miscellaneous

359. Answer is A (No response): *Fuller*

On trying to rouse the patient by asking a simple question, no response is given a score of 1 under the GCS scale.

Glasgow coma scale:

Eye opening		Best verbal response		Best motor response	
Response	**Score**	**Response**	**Score**	**Response**	**Score**
Spontaneously	4	Oriented and Converses	5	Obeys commands	6
To verbal stimuli	3	Disoriented and converses	4	Localises pain	5
To pain	2	Inappropriate words	3	Flexion- withdrawal to pain	4
Never	1	Incomprehensible words	2	Abnormal flexion (decorticate rigidity)	3
		No response	1	Abnormal extensive obsturing	2
				No response	1

Maximum score is Q : 15
Minimum score is Q : 03

360. Answer is C (Pupil size): *Fuller; Bailey Love 24th/601*

The Glasgow Coma Scale records three parameters namely, 'Eye opening', 'Best motor response' and 'Best verbal response'. Pupil size is not part of the GCS System.

Nervous System

9

Glasgow Coma Scale

Eye Opening	
Response	*Score*
Spontaneous	*4*
To verbal stimuli	*3*
To pain	*2*
Nil	*1*

Verbal Response	
Response	*Score*
Oriented & Converses	*5*
Disoriented / confused and converses	*4*
Inappropriate words	*3*
Incomprehensible words	*2*
No response	*1*

Motor Response	
Response	*Score*
Obeyes command	*6*
Localizes pain	*5*
Withdraws to pain	*4*
Abnormal flexion (decorticate rigidity)	*3*
Extension response	*2*
Nil	*1*

Note :

The maximum score is 15
The minimum score is 03

361. Answer is C (11): *Harrison 16th/2451; Harrison 17th/2601 (Table 373.2); Harrison 18th/p 3381 (Table: 378.1)*

A head injury patient who opens eyes to painful stimulus (2), is confused (4) and localizes pain (5) has a GCS 'Glasgow coma scale' score of 11.

GCS

Eye opening	
Nil	1
To pain	2
To command	3
Spontaneous	4

Best verbal response	
Nil	1
Incomprehensible sounds	2
Inappropriate words	3
Disoriented / confused	***4***
Oriented	5

Best motor response	
Nil	1
Abnormal extension posturing	2
Flexion posturing	3
With draws (flexion)	4
Localizes pain	***5***

362. Answer is C (15): *Fuller; Bailey & Love 24th/601;*

Aconscious person has spontaneous eye opening (3), is oriented and converses (5) and obeys commands (6).

The total GCS score for a conscious person therefore is 15.

Eye opening	*Spontaneous*	*4*
Verbal Response	*Oriented / converses*	*5*
Motor Response	*Obeys commands*	*6*
TOTAL GCS SCORE		*15*

363. Answer is B (3): *Harrison 18th/3381*

Use of Inappropriate words (Inappropriate speech) carries a score of '3' under the 'Verbal Response' according to the Glasgow Coma scale.

Glasgow Coma Scale

Eye Opening	
Response	Score
Spontaneous	4
To verbal stimuli	3
To pain	2
Nil	1

Verbal Response	
Response	Score
Oriented & Converses	5
Disoriented / confused and converses	4
Inappropriate words	3
Incomprehensible words	2
No response	1

Motor Response	
Response	Score
Obeyes command	6
Localizes pain	5
Withdraws to pain	4
Abnormal flexion (decorticate rigidity)	3
Extension response	2
Nil	1

Note :

The maximum score is15

The minimum score is 03

364. Answer is D (Hypothermia): *Harrison 16th / 1634, 1632 1631; Harrison 17th/1722*

Hypothermia is known to have neuro protective effects and may even be used as a modality of management of refractory elevated intracranial pressure.

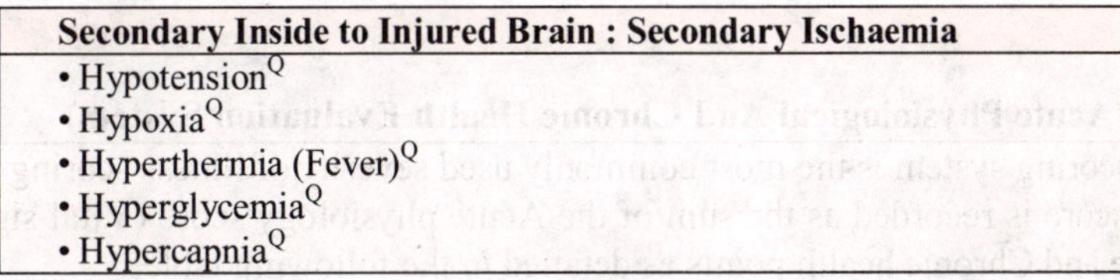

Secondary Inside to Injured Brain : Secondary Ischaemia
• Hypotension[Q] • Hypoxia[Q] • Hyperthermia (Fever)[Q] • Hyperglycemia[Q] • Hypercapnia[Q]

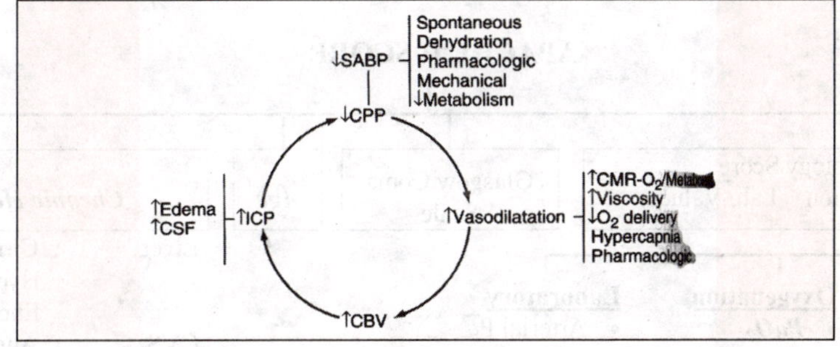

Hypotension and Hypoxia initiate the 'ischaemic cascade' by reducing delivery of substrates principally oxygen and glucose there by interfering with cellular function.

Hypercapnia causes cerebral vasodilatation, increases cerebral blood flow and intracranial pressure and worsens cerebral perfusion and hence contributes to the ischemic cascade - *Harrison 16th / 1632*

Hyperthermia (fever) and hyperglycemia contribute to secondary insult by increasing cellular metabolism and hence the requirement of essential substrates outstripping the compensatory process.

Hypothermia has a neuroprotective role. "Hypothermia is sometimes used for refractory elevated Intracranial pressure". *Harrison 16th / 1634*

365. Answer is A >C (Hyperglycemia > Hypocapnia): *Harrisons 17th/1722, 1723 'Key Topics in Critical care' 2nd/164 'Trauma: Contemporary Principles & Therapy' (Lippincott) 2007/284; Harrison 18th/p 2257, 2258*

Both hyperglycemia and hypocapnia may aggravate a head injury.

Hyperglycemia is probably the better answer here because hyperglycemia has been shown to be associated with increased mortality in patients with head injury. Hyperglycemia has also been distinctly mentioned in Harrison's text

Secondary Brain Injury : Factors causing aggrevation of brain injury

- *Hypotension*
- *Hypoxia / Hypoxemia*
- *Hypercapnia (also hypocapnia)*
- *Hyperthermia*
- *Hyperglycemia*

Hyperglycemia is associated with a poor outcome after traumatic brain injury and has been shown to be associated with increased mortality. Hyperglycemia injures the microvasculature and worsens ischemia

'Fever (Hyperthermia) and hyperglycemia both worsen experimental ischemia and have been associated with worsened clinical outcome after stroke and head trauma. A reasonable goal is to maintain the serum glucose level at < 7.8 mmol/l (< 140 mg/dl) although some have suggested that even tighter control is warranted. The use of iv insulin is encouraged for control of hyperglycemia as this allows better regulation of serum glucose levels than subcutaneous insulin'-Harrison

Hypocapnia (pCO_2 < 30 mm Hg) produces vasoconstriction reducing cerebral blood volume and cerebral blood flow. *In the past hypocapnia was often therapeutically induced through controlled hyperventilation in an attempt to reduce intracranial pressure.* ***Recent studies however show that prolonged reduction in cerebral blood flow may increase***

potential for ischemia within injured areas of the brain and thus a poor outcome. Hypocapnia is therefore no longer recommended

Hypercapnia causes cerebral vasodilatation which in the trauma victims may increase intracranial pressure and cause exacerbation of mass effect

366. Answer is F (All of the above): *Harrison's 17th/1674; Harrison 18th/p 2197*

APACHE II score includes Age, GCS, Physiological parameters (BP, Respiratory Rate, PaO_2) and chronic medical conditions.

APACHE II SCORE (Acute Physiological And Chronic Health Evaluation System)

- The APACHE II scoring system is the most commonly used severity of illness scoring system in North America
- The APACHE II score is recorded as the sum of the Acute physiology score (Vital signs, oxygenation, laboratory values), GCS, Age and Chronic health points as detailed in the following table.

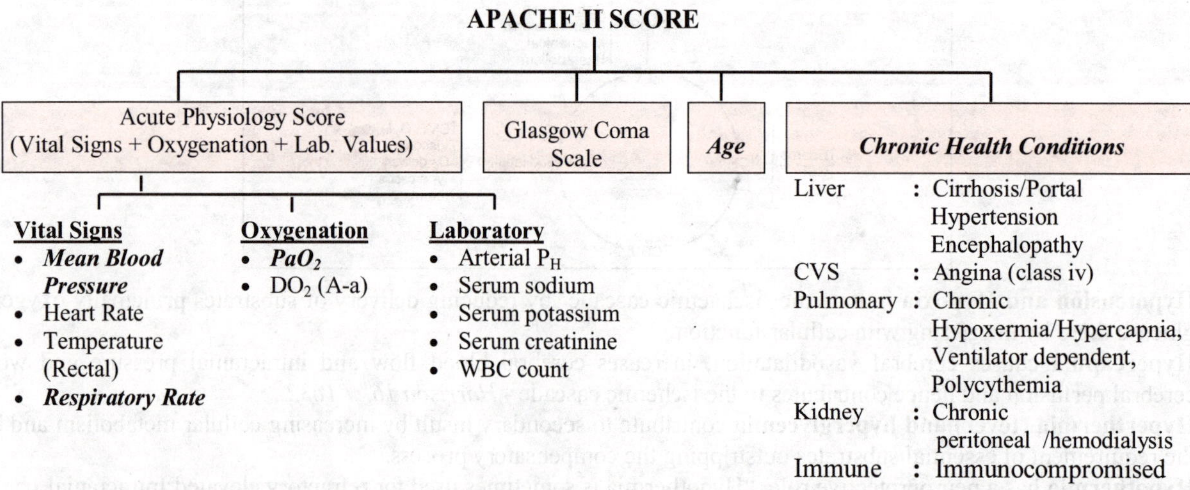

367. Answer is A (Glasgow coma scale): *Harrison 16th / 2450, 2451; Harrison 17th/2601; ATLS course Manual 6th Ed.; Harrison 18th/p 3381*

Amongst the option provided GCS is the single best answer of choice.

Determining the patient prognosis after TBI (Traumatic Brain Injury) is difficult and complex.

- Several independent variables have been identified that correlate with severity.
- ***Most studies have indicated Glasgow Coma Scale in the field and at arrival at the emergency department as a highly predictive indicator of prognosis.***

Harrison 17th / 2601

In severe head injury eye opening, the best motor response and verbal output have been found to be roughly predictive of outcome.
There have been summarized using the Glasgow coma scale.

Coma score = E + M + V

- Patient scoring 3 or 4 have an 85% chance of dying or remaining vegetative.
- Patients scoring 11 or above have only a 5 – 10% chance of dying or remaining vegetative.
- Intermediate scores correlate with proportional chances of recovery.

Other Poor prognosis indicators : Harrison	
• Older age • Increase ICP • Hypoxia & Hypotension	• CT evidence of compression of cisterns / midline shift • Delayed evacuation of large intracerebral hemorrhage • Carrier status for apolipoprotein E-4 allele

368. Answer is C (Injury to cortical bridging veins): *Bailey 24th/598; Bailey 23rd/*

Subdural Haemorrhage results from rupture of bridging veins that run from the cortex to dural sinuses.
The superior cerebral veins that bridge the cortex to superior saggital sinus are most commonly involved.

Source of hemorrhage in various types of intracranial hemorrhage

Epidural hemorrhage	Subdural hemorrhage	Subarachnoid hemorrhage	Intracerebral hemorrhage
Most commonly caused by rupture of middle meningeal artery[Q] (br. of maxillary artery)	*Most commonly caused by rupture of superior cerebral veins[Q] (Bridging veins that connect the cerebral cortex to superior saggital sinus)*	*Most commonly caused by rupture of saccular aneurysms[Q] (Berry aneurysms are the most common saccular aneurysms involved[Q])*	*Most commonly caused by rupture of lenticulostriate branch of middle cerebral artery[Q].*

369. Answer is C (Injury to cortical bridging veins): *Bailey & Love 24th/ 598, 23rd/ 550*

Subdural hemorrhage is caused by the rupture of bridging veins that connect the brain and the dural sinuses i.e. cortical bridging veins.
Memo: Most common cause of extradural hemorrhage is Rupture of middle meningeal artery.

370. Answer is D (Left chronic subdural hematoma): *Schwartz 7th/335*

The presence of progressive hemiparesis and aphasias together with signs of raised ICT (papilloedema) in an elderly patient, developing weeks after sustaining a mild head injury is characteristic of chronic subdural hematoma

Chronic Subdural Hematoma

Gradual accumulation of blood in subdural space and classically presenting 3 weeks after the initial bleed. (Chronic)

Pathogenesis

Rupture of bridging veins
Repeated cycles of recurrent bleeding into subdural space and resorption of the resultant hematoma.

Etiology

Head Trauma (Usually trivial and unnoticed in upto 25% of cases)
- Motor vehicle Accident
- Repeated falls in elderly from syncope, ataxia, weakness or seizures

Patients with bleeding problems
- Anticoagulation
- Thrombocytopenia
- Liver failure
- Alcoholism

Dural lesions
- Sarcoma's AV mat formations and metastatic cancer

Low CSF volume
- CSF Shunts, renal dialysis, excess diuretics

Risk Factors
- *Elderly age*
- *Coagulopathy*
- *Alcoholism*
- *Epilepsy*
- *Metastatic Carcinoma*

Birth trauma and child abuse are risk factors in infants

Clinical Features

Gradual onset of signs and symptoms over several weeks (characteristically>3 weeks for chronic subdural hematomas)

Headache>90%
Impaired consciousness -55%
Hemiparesis – 45%
Papilloedema-25%
CN III involvement -11%

Headache	Deterioration of mental status with confusion lethargy and memory disturbance	Progressive hemiparesis and Aphasias (speech disturbance)	Popilloedema
Constant and relatively mild & usually lateralized to the side of lesion			Others Seizures Cranial Nerve III abnormalities Hemianopsia Others

9

Nervous System

371. Answer is D (Left chronic subdural haematoma) : *Read text below*

Progressively increasing right sided focal neurological signs over a period of one month along with papilloedema suggest a diagnosis of an IntraCranial Space Occurring Lesion. (ICSOL). Given the history of head trauma in an elderly female chronic subdural haematoma is the diagnosis of choice.

Chronic subdural haematoma :
Chronic subdural haematoma is the common in conditions of cerebral atrophy notably old age and alcoholism.
Minor trauma leads to a little insignificant bleeding in subdural space that goes unnoticed.
As the blood breaks down over the next few weeks or months, fluids is drawn into subdural space because the breakdown products are hyperosmolol and membrane forms.
This collection gradually enlarges and compress the brain producing focal neurological defecits mimicking tumor.

372. Answer is A (Craniotomy): *Schwartz Pre-Test/Q.635*

Coma with a ***dilated pupil*** after a ***lucid interval*** following a head injury ***must be assumed to represent an epidural hematoma.***
Emergency evacuation of the clot without time-consuming studies is vital to restore cerebral function.
With a patient in less critical condition, a CT scan is the appropriate diagnostic study.

373. Answer is D (Intraabdominal bleed) : *Read text below*

Although extradural haemorrhage is the most common intracranial complication following head injury, the ***patient in question is suffering from severe hypotension of 90/60, & has tachycardia, which cannot be explained by extradural haemorrhage alone***. A patient with head injury, more than often has other significant injuries and a thorough examination of other systems therefore is a prime necessassity.

An intraabdominal source of bleed, like a ruptured spleen for example is a more likely cause for hypotension in this patient.

374. Answer is C (Altered mental status) : *Harrison's 16th/1633; Harrison 17th/1722; Harrison 18th/p 2257*

'Early signs of elevated ICP include drowsiness and a diminished level of consciousness (altered mental status). Coma and unilateral papillary changes are late signs and require immediate intervention.' *-Harrisons*

375. Answer is D (Decorticate rigidity): *Ref: Fuller 2nd/ 199, 200; Harrison 17th/ 1714, 1715; Harrison 18th/p 2247, 2248*

Decorticate rigidity is not seen as a manifestation of uncal herniation. All other features form part of the spectrum.

'Herniation or coning' is said to be occurring when part of the brain is forced through a rigid hole.

Uncal herniation			**Central herniation**		
The uncus and the temporal lobe are forced through the cerebellar tentorium (tentorium that separates the cerebrum from the cerebellum)			The diencephation i.e. the thalamus and related structures that lie between upper brainstem and cerebral hemispheres are forced through the tentorium.		
What happens			**What happens**		
Sequential compression occurs of the - Ipsilateral third nerve - Contralateral brainstem (later) - Whole brainstem (eventually)			Sequential compression occurs of the - Upper midbrain (first) - Pons (later) - Medulla (finally)		
Physical signs			**Physical signs**		
Early	***Later***	***Still later***	***Early***	***Later***	***Still later***
• I/L dilated pupils • Signs of supra xentorial mass lesions	• I/L hemiplegia • Progressive ptosis & third n palsy • Cheyne- stokes respiration	• Tetraparesis • B/e fixed dilated pupils • Erratic respiration • Death	• Errotic respiration • Small reactive pupils. • Increased limb tone • Bilateral extensor plantar	• Cheyne stokes respiration • Decorticate rigidity	• Fixed dilated pupils • Decerebrate posturing

376. Answer is A (Furosemide): *Ref: Harrison 16th/ 1633; Harrison 17th/ 1734; Harrison 18th/p 2271*

Although all of the following agents may well be used to decrease intracranial pressure furosemide is the answer of exclusion, as Harrisons text mentions all agents except, furosemide in the stepwise approach to treatment of elevated Intracranial pressure.

Stepwise approach to treatment of elevated intracranial pressure – *Harrison*

- Drain CSF via ventriculostomy.
- Elevate head of bed.
- Osmotherapy with **mannitol.**
- **Glucocorticoids** (*avoid glucocorticoids in head trauma, ischaemic and hemorrhagic stroke*).
- Sedation (e.g. morphine, propofol or midazolam).
- **Hyperventilation**
- Pressor therapy (phenylephrine, dopamine or norepinephrine to maintain adequate mean arterial pressure).
- Consider *second tier* therapies for refractory elevated ICP.
  a. High dose barbiturate
  b. Aggressive hyperventilation
  c. Hemicraniotomy

377. Answer is C (Tolosa-Hunt Syndrome): *'Imaging of the Globe and Orbit: A Guide to Differential Diagnosis' by Norbert Hosten (Thieme) 1998/128*

Painful ophthalmoplepia with enlargement of ipsilateral cavernous sinus on imaging (CT/MRI) suggests a diagnosis of Tolosa-Hunt syndrome
Orbital pseudotumors, Gradenigo syndrome and cavernous sinus thrombosis may present with ophthalmoplegia, but enlargement of cavernous sinus is not a characteristic feature of these syndromes

Tolosa-Hunt syndrome

- Tolosa-Hunt Syndrome consists of *painful ophthalmoplegia caused by idiopathic inflammation of the cavernous sinus*
- The idiopathic non-specific inflammation often *results in a mass of granulation tissue around the cavernous sinus* or superior orbital fissure leading to constant pain and ***asymmetrical enlargement of the cavernous sinus.***
- The disorder is usually unilateral although bilateral cases have been reported
- The symptoms show excellent response to steroid therapy and pain is usually relieved within 72 hours of initiation of steroid therapy

378. Answer is A (Allodynia) : *Harrison's 17th/154,155*

Perception of a non-painful stimulus (non-noxious stimulus) as 'pain' is termed as 'allodynia'.

Terminology	Sensory Disturbance
Allodynia	*Situation in which a non painful (non-noxious) stimulus once perceived is experienced as painful.(example is elicitation of a painful sensation by application of a vibrating tuning fork)*
Hyperalgesia	*Situation in which a mildly painful (mildly noxious) stimulus once perceived is experienced as severely painful, often excruciating*
Hyperesthesia	*Increased sensitivity or pain in response to touch*
Hyperpathia	*Broad term that encompasses all above phenomenon, namely, Allodynia, Hyperalgesia and Hyperesthesia*

379. Answer is None (May be associated with all of the above)

'Diagnostic Nuclear Medicine' by Sandler,Coleman & Patton (Lippincott-Williams) 4th (2003)/ 838;
'Imaging in treatment planning for Sino-nasal disease' by Maroldi & Nicoli (Springer) 2005/94

Spontaneous (Non Traumatic CSF Leaks)

High Pressure Leaks	Normal Pressure Leaks
• ***Elevated Intracranial Pressure*** - *Hydrocephalus* - *Intracranial Tumors* • *Benign Intracranial Hypertension* ***(Pseudotumor cerebri)***	• ***Empty Sella syndrome*** • *Congenital anomalies* - ***Encephalocele*** - *Meningocele* - *Focal olfactory Atrophy* - *Cribriform Plate Defects* • *Osteomyelitis (skull base)* • *Connective Tissue Disorder* - *Marfan's syndrome* - *Ehler's Danlos syndrome* - *Osteogenesis Imperfecta*

380. Answer is C (Increased intracranial tension is seen in all cases): *Brain Injury Medicine by Zasler, Katz, Zafonte (2006)/136, Neuroimaging by Zimmerman (2000) /721; Harrisons 17th/2597 (Insufficient information); 18th/p 3377*

Raised intracranial tension (cerebral swelling) may be present in cases of Diffuse Axonal injury (DAI) but it is not seen in all cases of DAI. The presence of raised ICT is not needed for a diagnosis of DAI

Diffuse Axonal Injury (DAI)
• *Diffuse axonal injury represents the presence of wide spread axonal damage (white matter) in both hemispheres, secondary to severe head injury* • *DAI results from application of severe acceleration / deceleration or angular rotational to the brain which* **results in injuries to the axons by a shearing force (shear injuries)**
Pathobiological Features
• *Focal (irreversible) disruption of axons (white matter) at multiple places in both hemisphers (occurs at the moment of injury) –* **white matter tears** • *These white matter tears* **may be haemorrhagic or non haemorrhagic** • *When non haemorrhagic they are edematous (Non haemorrhagic lesions are not detected by CT scan but may be recognized on MRI as it picks up edema)* • **The most frequent location of tears is in the lobar white matter at the junction of grey and white matter**
Frequent location of tears
• *Lobar white matter at junction of grey and white matter (commonest location)* - *Frontal / Temporal lobe > Parietal lobe / Occipital lobes* - *Cerebellum* - **Basal ganglia** - *Internal / External capsule* • **Corpus Callosum** *(Second most commonly involved location)* • *Brain stem (third most commonly involved location)*
Clinical presentation
Clinical presentations may however range from symptoms of concussion to coma Loss of consciousness is a common finding[Q] *and* DAI is the commonest cause of post traumatic vegetative state[Q] **Raised intracranial tension may or may not be associated**[Q]
Diagnosis
• Many of these injuries are likely to go undetected by any imaging modality[Q] • *DAI may be recognized on CT scan and MRI (MRI > CT scan)*

CT scan	*MRI*
CT scan can usually detect only those lesions that are large and haemorrhagic *CT scan often fails to recognize DAI lesions because most lesions are small and non haemorrhagic* (CT scan is often normal[Q])	*MRI is more sensitive than CT scan for detecting DAI* *MRI can recognize smaller lesion than CT scan and also non haemorrhagic lesions from associated edema*

A normal CT scan in light of a neurologically devastated patient following head injury is a classic finding in Diffuse Axonal injury[Q]

Prognosis
Diffuse Axonal injury carries an extremely poor prognosis[Q]

Miscellaneous

381. Answer is A (Neocortex): *Guyton; Ganong*

The first center that gets activated to initiate skilled movements is the neocortex.

The pyramidal system, comprised of precentral motor cortex, spinal motor neurons and the corticospinal tracts that connect the two, is responsible for initiating and carrying signals for voluntary muscle contractions that enable skilled movements.

Neocortex

- *The neocortex is considered to be the newest part of the brain phylogenetically*
- *It is comprised of the most superficial areas of the brain*
- *It includes the primary motor cortex, primary sensory cortex and association cortices*
- *The Neocortex is only found in mammals*

Premotor Cortex (Area 6, 8) (Lateral portion)	Primary Motor Cortex (Area 4)	Supplementary Motor Cortex (Medial portion of area 6)
• Nerve signals generated in the premotor cortex produce more complex pattern of movements (skilled) than the discrete patterns generated by primary motor cortex • ***In general movements in response to external stimuli involve the Premotor Area***	• The primary motor cortex controls specific muscle movements and is the first level of descending control for precise motor movements	• SMC located on the medial surface of the hemisphere in the premotor region (areas 6, 8) is *involved in the performance of complex skillful movements* • ***In general movements initiated by subject involves the SMR***

Pyramidal Tract (Corticospinal Tract)
↓
Spinal motor neurons
↓
Skilled voluntary movements

Cerebellum and Basal ganglia provide important feed back in planning & excution of skilled movements

382. Answer is C (Supplementary motor Area): *Noback's Human Nervous system 7th/436*

The most important area involved in planning and organizing complex sequential skilled movements is the Supplementary Motor Area (SMA).

'The SMA is important for planning and organizing complex sequential movements. For example the sequence of finger movement required to play a muscal instrument such as Clarinet or Piano is planned and organized in the SMA'.

- Noback's Human Nervous System 7th/436

383. Answer is D (Explicit memory): *Basic Neurochemistry (Academic Press) 2010/965; Psychology: Concepts and Applications (Congage Learning) 2008 (3rd)/234; Practical Neurology (Lippincott Williams) 2012 /37*

Hippocampal lesions primarily affect Declarative or Explicit memory.

The Hippocampus is essential to forming new memories for facts and general information (sementic memory) and also for life experiences (episodic memory). But the hippocampus does not appear to play a role in precedural memory, the kind of memory we draw upon while riding bike or using a tool

9

Classification of Memory Based on Anatomy of Temporal Lobe system (Hippocampus)

Declarative Memory or Explicit Memory (Episodic/Sementic Memory)

- ***Declarative memory also known as Explicit memory***, is memory of events, places, facts and people and is ***dependent on the temporal lobe system (Hipppcampus)***
- Declarative memory can be further divided into two classes.

Episodic memory	*Sementic memory*
Refers to memory of episodic events that contain 'what' 'where' 'when' information	*Refers to memory or facts that are no longer ascribable to any particular occasion in life*

- Lesions of the temporal lobe such as hippocampus are known to greatly impair patient's ability to learn new facts, concepts, vacobulary and knowledge about the world

Non-Declarative Memory or Implicit Memory (Procedural memory)

- Non-Declarative memory is also known as procedural memory and does not depend on the structural integrity of the temporal lobe system.
- Non-Declarative memory encompasses a variety of perceptual motor learning skills and mental operations
- Currently the brain regions involved in encoding procedural memory are not clear, atleast in humans (striatum may be engaged)

Temporal (Time based) classification of memory

Short term memory	**Long term memories**
Newly formed memories (Over a time course of seconds or hours)	*Memories from events acquired over course of weeks, months or years*
Patients with Hippocampal lesions may acquire new memories for a short term but are not able to transform them into long term memories They tend to have amnesia for recent events, though they may retain memory acquired a very long time ago since such memory has already been consolidated	Long term memories refers to relatively permanent storage of information resulting from transformation and consolidation of sensory inputs

384. Answer is C (Transformation of short-term memory to long-term memory): *Practical Neurology (Lippintott Williams 2012/37)*

The Hippocampus plays an important rale in the consolidation of memory. It is involved in object memory and placement of memory in time and place Hippocampal lesions greatly impair the consolidation / transformation of short-term memory to long-term memory (producing antegrade amnesia)

Hippocampus and memory

- *The Hippocampus is essential to forming new memories for facts and general information (sementic memory) and also for life experiences (episodic memory). But the hippocampus does not appear to play a role in precedural memory, the kind of memory we draw upon while riding bike or using a tool*

Hippocampus is essential for Declarative or Explicit memory. This includes Sementic and Episodic memory. Hippocampus is not essential for Non-Declarative or Implicit memory. This includes Procedural memory.

- *With Hippocampal lesions long term memory that has already been consolidated (transformed and stored) may be retained*
- *With Hippocampal lesions new short-term memory may be acquired*
- *With Hippocampal lesion newly acquired short term memory is not consolidated and transformed into long term memory (antegrade amnesia)*
- *With Hippocampal lesions previous memory that has not been fully consolidated prior to lesion is lost (retrograde amnesia)*

Hippocampal lesion

Antegrade Amnesia	Retrograds Amnesia
Hippocampal lesions do not allow consolidation or transformation of newly acquired short-term memories to long-term memories producing learining defecits. The impairment is centered on declarative knowledge and non-declarative learning is rarely impaired.	Hippocampal lesions may result in loss of memory immediately before sustaining the lesion. The Information from the time closest to the point of injury is most likely to be lost (memory which has not consolidated)

385. Answer is B (Hypothalamus): *Harrison's 18th/220*

Narcolepsy in humans is caused by deficiency of hypocretin (Orexin) a neurotransmitter produced in the Hypothalamus.

'Recently several convergent lines of evidence suggest that the hypothalamic neuropeptide hypocretin (orexin) is involved in the pathogenesis of Narcolepsy'- Harrison's 18th/220

Narcolepsy

Narcolepsy is a common sleep disorder charachterized by excessive daytime sleepiness, cataplexy (episodes of muscle weakness triggered by emotions), hypnagogic hallucinations and sleep paralysis.

Narcolepsy (classic Tetrad)

1. Excessive day Time somnolence
2. Sudden weakness or loss of muscle tone without loss of consciousness often elicited by emotion (cataptexy)
3. Hallucination at sleep onset (Hypnagogic Hallucination) or upon awakening (Hypnopompic Hallucination)
4. Muscle Paralysis upon awakening

Pathology /Pathogenesis

Most important cause of narcolepsy is believed to be deficiency of neuropeptide Hypocretin (orexin) produced in Hypothalamus

Autoimmune

All narcoleptics with cataplexy are positive for HLA DQB1 (0602)

386. Answer is C (Consensual Light Reflex Normal): *References with text*

Argyll Robertson Pupil is associated with an absent direct and consensual light reflex.

Argyll Robertson Pupil (ARP)

- The Argyll Robertson Pupil (ARP) refers to a *small (miotic), irregular pupil, with an absent light reflex (both direct and consensual) and normal accommodation reflex (normal near reflex)*. This phenomenon is often called *Light Near dissociation.*
- The ARP results from a lesion involving fibers that pass from pretectal area of the midbrain to the Edinger – Westphal nucleus. However only the rostrally placed fibers subserving the light reflex are involved while the more caudally located fibers responsible for near vision / accommodation are unaffected.

The ARP was first described in neuro-syphillis, but this may be seen in several conditions affecting the midbrain including Encephalitis, CVA, M.S. etc

- ARP shares several features with Adie's Tonic pupil from which it must be differentiated.

Comparison between Argyll-Robertson pupil and Adie's pupil:

Features	ARP	Adie's
Vision	*Good*	*Good*
Pupil	*Constricted*	*Dilated*
Laterality	*Bilateral; may be unilateral*	*Unilateral; may become bilateral*
Effect of Illumination	*Nil*	*Larger in bright light*
Light reflex (Direct and consensual)	*Absent*	*Absent/poor*
Near reflex (Accomodation)	*Brisk*	*Tonic*
Atropine	*No mydriasis*	*Mydriasis*
Miotic	*Constrict*	*Constrict with very weak solution*
Lesion	*Pretectal*	*Ciliary ganglion*

387. Answer is A (Multiple sclerosis): *Harrisons 15th/ 2411/293; 16th/272; Harrison 17th/ 2613; Harrison 18th/p 3398*

Multiple sclerosis is associated with erectile dysfunction or impotence

Neurological disorders associated with Erectile dysfunction include:

- Spinal cord injury
- Multiple sclerosis
- Peripheral neuropathy

388. Answer is D (Apparent Exophthalmos): *Localization in Clinical Neurology (Lippincott Williams) 2011/208; Anatomic Basis of Neurological Diagnosis (Thieme) 2009/467*

Horner's Syndrome is associated with 'Apparent Enophthalmos' and not 'Apparent Exophthalmos'

Apparent Enophthalmos may be seen in Horner's syndrome

Horner's syndrome may be associated with apparent enophthalmos as a result of a narrow palpebral fissure, an appearance that the affected eye is located deeper (sunken in) compared with the unaffected eye.

Heterochromia of iris may be seen in Horner's syndrome

Heterochromia refers to a difference in the colour of iris between the two eyes.

Horner's syndrome may be associated with 'sympathetic heterochromia'.

Sympathetic heterochromia is characterized by pallor/progressive fading of the iris on the affected side (Hypochromic Heterochromia) and usually accompanies occulosympathetic paralysis that is sustained early in life (before age 2) (Congenital Horner's Syndrome).

Progressive Heterochromia from acquired Horner's syndrome in adults is rare.

Anhidrosis and Miosis are classical features of Horner's Syndrome

Anhidrosis (ipsilateral facial anhidrosis) is one of the classical features of Horner's Syndrome seen in lesions of sympathetic pathway below the bifurcation of the carotid artery.

Miosis and Ptosis *are the other typical features of Horner's Syndrome*

Clinical Finding In Horner's Syndrome

Classical Triad

- ***Miosis***
- ***Ptosis***
- ***Anhidrosis***

Note:

Anhidrosis *is absent in lesions at the level of internal carotid artery or above sudomotor and vasomotor fibers to the face follow the external carotid artery at the bifurcation.*

Other Signs of Horner's Syndrome

- ***Apparent Enophthalmos*** *(d/t narrow palpebral fissure)*
- Anisocoria
- ***Heterochromia of iris***
- Dilation lag (slow dilation of pupil after lights are dimmed)
- Increased accommodative amplitude or accommodative paresis
- Transient ocular Hypotonia and conjunctival Hyperemia

Horner's Syndrome from lesion of sympathetic Pathway below bifurcation of carotic artery	Horner's syndrome from lesion of sympathetic pathway above bifurcation of carotid artery
• Ptosis • Miosis • ***Anhidrosis***	• Ptosis • Miosis ***(Anhidrosis is absent)***

Clinical Findings in Horner's Syndrome (Taken from *Localization in Clinical Neurology (Lippincott Williams) 2011/208;*
• *Ipsilateral mild (usually < 2 mm) ptosis* (due to denervation of the Muller's muscle of the upper eyelid) • *Reverse Ptosis or 'Upside down ptosis'* (due to sympathetic denervation to the lower eyelid retractors) • ***Apparent enophthalmos*** • ***Miosis*** • *Anisocoria* due to ipsilateral miosis • *Dilation lag* (slow dilation of the pupil after lights are dimmed) • *Increased accommodative amplitude or accommodative paresis* (Patients hold the near card closer to read) • *Transient (acute phase) ocular hypotony and conjunctival hyperemia* • ***Heterochromia of the iris*** • *Variable ipsilateral facial **anhidrosis*** • Ipsilateral straight hair in some congenital cases (usually congenital but rarely acquired) • Rarely neurotrophic corneal endothelial failure with pain and stromal edema (rare). • Ipsilateral nasal obstruction with contralateral rhinorrhea with infantile cases (rare).

389. Answer is B (Medial Medullary Syndrome): *'Neurosurgery Case Reviews' by Sabbagh & Nadar (Thieme) 2009/Case 102; Sapira's Art and Science of Bed side Diagnosis 4th/187; 'Neurophthalmology Illustrated' (Thieme) 2009/290*

Horner's syndrome is associated with Lateral Medullary Syndrome or Wallenberg Syndrome and not with Medial Medullary Syndrome.

Most common causes of Horner's Syndrome in Adults Based on Lesion Location

Central (First order)	Preganglionic (Second order)	Postganglionic (Third order)
Hypothalamus Stroke Tumor Brainstem Stroke ***(lateral medullary infarction)*** Demyelination ***(multiple sclerosis)*** Tumor Spinal cord (cervicothoracic) Trauma Syringomyelia Tumor (intramedullary) Demyelination ***(multiple sclerosis)*** Myelitis Arteriovenous malformation	Cervical spine disease Brachial plexus injury Pulmonary apical lesion Apical lung tumor Mediastinal tumors Cervical rib Trauma Iatrogenic jugular or subclavian cannulation, chest tube, thoracic surgery Subclavian artery aneurysm Thyroid tumors	Superior cervical ganglion Trauma Jugular venous ectasia Iatrogenic (surgical neck dissection) Internal carotid artery Dissection Aneurysm Trauma Arteritis Tumor Skull base lesion Nasopharyngeal carcinoma Lymphoma Cavernous sinus lesion Tumors Pituitary tumor Inflammation Thrombosis Carotid aneurysm Cluster headache

390. Answer is D (Mycophenolate): *Harrisons 17th/3402, 3403, 2404*

Mycophenolate is lymphocyte specific oral immunosuppressant that is presently being studied for its role in Multiple Sclerosis. Presently Mycophenolate is not U.S. FDA approved for use in Multiple Sclerosis and hence this drug cannot be recommended for the treatment of M.S. at present.

Interferon β-1a, Interferon β-1b and Glatiramer Acetate are all U.S. FDA approved disease modifying agents for treatment of Multiple Sclerosis.

Therapy (Treatment) of Multiple Sclerosis

Treatment with Disease Modifying Agents that reduce the biological activity of Multiple Sclerosis

Seven such agents are approved by the U.S. FDA

- *Interferon Beta-1a (IFN-β-1a) (Avonex)*
- ***Interferon Beta -1a** (IFN-β-1a) (Rebif)*
- ***Interferon Beta-1b** (IFN-β-1b) (Betaseron)*
- ***Glatiramer Acetate** (Copaxone)*
- *Natalizumab (Tysabri)*
- *Fingolimod (Gilenya)*
- *Mitoxantrone (Novantrone)*

Cladribine (Leustatin) is the eighth agent currently awaiting FDA approval

Treatment of Acute Attacks
(Acute Exacerbations or Initial Demyelinating Episodes)

- Glucocorticoids
- Plasma exchange
  (Plasma exchange may benefit patients with fulminant attacks of demyelination that are unresponsive to glucocorticoids)

Off Label Treatment options for Relapsing /Remitting MS and Secondary Progressive M.S.

- *Azathioprine*
- *Methotrexate*
- *Cyclophosphamide*
- *Intravenous Immunoglobulin*
- *Methylprednisolone*

391. Answer is A (Hydrocephalus): *Harrison's 18th/3377-3398*

Multiple sclerosis is not associated with Hydrocephalus.
Optic Neuritis, Spasticity and Spinal cord involvement may all be seen with multiple sclerosis.

Multiple Sclerosis

- *Multiple Sclerosis is a chronic disease characterized by inflammation, demyelination, gliosis (scarring) and neuronal loss*
- *The course can be relapsing – remitting or progressive*
- *The clinical manifestations of M.S. are diverse and vary depending on the site and severity of demyelinating lesions within the CNS*

Lesions are disseminated in time and space (Typically occur at different times and different CNS locations)

- *The onset of symptoms may be abrupt or insidious*
- *The lesions may be anywhere in the CNS including the **spinal cord***

Sensory Symptoms

- *Paresthesias, Dystheseas Hypestheseas*
- *Sensory impairment and sensory level indicate spinal cord as site of lesion*
- *Pain (anywhere) is seen upto 50%*

Motor Weakness

Usually UMN type and associated with

- *Spasticity*
- *Hyperreflexia*
- *Babiniski sign +ve*

Occasionally tendon reflex may be lost if an MS lesion disrupts the afferent reflex fibres

Visual Symptoms/Signs

- **Optic Neuritis** *is typical (usually unilateral but may be bilateral)*
- **Diplopia** may result from internuclear *ophthalmoplegia (INO) or from palsy of 6th CN (Rarely IIIrd/IVth CN)*
- **Visual Blurring** *may result from Optic Neuritis or Diplopia*

Bladder Bowel Involvement

- *Bladder dysfunction is seen in > 90% of MS patients*
- *May include Detrusor Hyper-reflexia or Detrusor sphincter dyssynergia*
- *Constipation > Fecal urgency or incontinence*

Sexual Disfunction

Ataxia/Dysarthria

Ataxia usually manifests as cerebellar tremors.

Facial weakness

Usually due to lesion in pons.

Vertigo

From brainstem lesion.

Cognitive Dysfunction and Depression

Fatigue

Experienced by >90% of patients.

Ancillary Symptoms

- *Heat sensitivity* (Uhtoff's symptom)
- *Lhermitte's symptom*
- *Paroxysmal symptoms*
- *Trigeminal neuralgia Hemifacial spsm Glossophoryngeal neuralgia*

392. Answer is A (Optic Neuritis): *Harrison's 18th/3397*

Optic Neuritis is the most frequent initial presenting feature of MS amongst the options provided.

The most common earliest presenting features of multiple sclerosis are transient sensory defects followed by visual disturbances due to optic neuritis.

Initial Symptoms of MS

Symptom	Percent of Cases	Symptom	Percent of Cases
Sensory loss	37	*Lhermitte's*	3
Optic neuritis	36	*Pain*	3
Weakness	35	*Dementia*	2
Paresthesias	24	*Visual loss*	2
Diplopia	15	*Facial palsy*	1
Ataxia	11	*Impotence*	1
Vertigo	6	*Myokymia*	1
Paroxysmal attacks	4	*Epilepsy*	1
Bladder	4	*Falling*	1

393. Answer is B (Interferon Beta) : *Harrison 16th / 2467; Harrison 2616; Harrison 18th/p 3403, 3404*

Interferon Beta should be considered in patients with Relapsing / Remitting MS (RRMS) and Secondary Progressive MS (SPMS) with superimposed relapses.
Interferon Beta reduces the attack rate in M.S. patients and also improves disease severity measures and disease burden.

Interferons

- Interferons are cytokines that exhibit antiviral activities, immunomodulating properties and antiproliferative properties.
- DNA recombinant technology has made available highly purified α, β and γ interferons.
- IFNs are not available for oral administration but must be given intramuscularly, subcutaneously or intravenously.

Interferon Alpha (IFNα)	Interferon Beta (IFNβ)	Interferon (IFNγ)
Considered for :	Considered for :	Considered for :
• Hepatitis B, Hepatitis C • Mucocutaneous manifestations of Behcet's syndrome (H / 2014) • Carcinoid syndrome (H / 2226) • Chronic myeloid leukaemia (CML) (H / 640) • Follicular lymphoma (H / 651) • Malignant melanoma (Adjuvant) (H / 502) • Essential thrombocytosis	Multiple Sclerosis 3 Approved Agents • Aronex (IFN β1a) • Rebif (IFN β1a) • Betaseron (IFN β1b)	• Osteopetrosis , (H / 2282) (suggested benefit) • Systemic sclerosis ((H/1987) (modest improvement but recurrence) • Idiopathic pulmonary fibrosis (therapeutic trial) H/ 1556 • Chronic granulomatous disease leprosy, non tuberculosis mycobacteria & visceral leishmaniosis (H/357) • Multiple myeloma (H / 660) • Renal cell carcinoma (H / 542) • Splenomegaly (H / 628)

Also Note :

Interferon is not curative for any tumor but can induce partial responses in (Harrison 16th / 482)

- Follicular lymphoma
- Hairy cell leukaemia
- CML
- Melanoma
- Kaposi's sarcoma

IFN γ has been successfully used in the treatment of Leprosy, Nontuberculous Mycobacteria and Visceral Leishmaniosis. - Harrison 16th / 357

394. Answer is B (Locked in state): *Harrisons 16th /1629; Harrison 17th/1718*

'Normal α- activity on the EEG in a patient of coma alerts the clinician to the locked in syndrome or to hysteria or catatonia.' – Harrison 16th/1629

All conditions other than the 'locked in state' present characteristic EEG patterns.

EEG Characteristic;

Subacute sclerosing panencephalitis (SSPE)	Creutzfoldt Jackob disease (CJD)	Hepatic encephalopathy
Characteristic periodic pattern with bursts every 3 to 8 seconds of high voltage, sharp slow waves followed by periods of attenuated (falt) background	Characteristic stereotype periodic bursts of < 200 ms duration occurring every 1 to 2 sec. Makes the diagnosis of CJD very likely (Repetitive high voltage, triphasic and polyphasic sharp discharges are seen in most advanced cases)	Characteristic Symmetric high voltage triphasic slow wave infrontal region

Locked in state :

- This represents a pseudocoma in which an awake patient has no means of producing speech or volitional movement in order to indicate that he awake
- Patient may signal with vertical eye movement and lid elevation which remain unimpaired.
- It usually results from infarction or haemorrhage of the ventral pons which transects all descending corticospinal and corticobulbar pathways.
- EEG is normal

395. Answer is A (Hepatic encephalopathy) *Harrison 16th / 1868; Harrison 17th/1979; Harrison 18th/p 2601*

'Symmetric, high voltage, triphasic slow wave (2 – 5 / second) pattern on Electroencephalogram (EEG) is characteristic (but non specific) of Hepatic encephalopathy' – Harrison 16th / 1868

The diagnosis of hepatic encephalopathy should be considered when four major factors are present
1. Acute or chronic hepatocellular disease and / or extensive portal systemic collateral shunts. 2. Disturbance of awareness and mentation which may progress from forgetfulness and confusion to stupor and finally coma. 3. Shifting combinations of neurological signs including asterixis, rigidity, hyperreflexia, extensor plantar signs and rarely seizures. ***4. A characteristic but (nonspecific), symmetric, high voltage, triphasic slow wave (2 to 5 /second) pattern on electroencephalogram.***

396. Answer is A (Anoxic Encephalopathy): *Ultimate Review of Neurology board (Demos Medical publishing) 2011/143; Clinical Neurophysiology (Oxford) 2009/170; Practical Guide for Clinical Neurophysiologycal Testing. EEG' (Lippincott) 2012/232*

Burst Supression Pattern on EEG is typically seen in Anoxic Encephalopathy or Hypoxic Ischemic Encephalopathy.

Burst Supression Pattern on EEG

- The burst suppression pattern on EEG is typically charachterized by an isoelectric background interrupted by periodic / pseudoperiodic or non-periodic bursts of abnormal activity.
- The suppression period is of either no or low amplitude cerebral activity while the bursts can be a mixture of a variety of all types of wave forms including sharp, spike, alpha, beta, theta and delta activities.
- Burst suppression implies the deepest level of coma state before brain death and carries a poor prognosis. *'This pattern is commonly seen in patients with an acute and severe degree of cereberal insult most commonly in severe anoxic encephalopathy, acute intoxication with CNS depressant drugs and severe hypothermia'.*
- This is generally an invariant pattern that does not change with the state of sleep-wakefulness or in response to stimuli.

397. Answer is D (Creutzfeldt Jakob disease): *Ultimate Review of Neorology Boards (Demos medical publishing) Chapter Neurophysiology Q1 / 123, 143 (Answer); Practical Neurology by Biller / 416; Critical care study Guide (Springer) 2010/162*

Creutzfeldt Jakob disease is associated with periodic sharp wave complexes of a frequency of about 1/second. CJD is typically not associated with Burst suppression pattern on EEG.

Typical Causes of Burst Supression Pattern on EEG
• *Anoxic Encephalopathy or Hypoxic-Ischemic Encephalopathy* • *Toxic CNS drugs (High doses of barbiturates etc; High levels of sedation)* • *Anesthesia (Deep Anesthesia)* • *Hypothermia*

Early infantile Epileptic Encephalopathy called Ohtahora's syndrome is typically associated with Burst – Supression pattern on EEG.

398. Answer is B (Anomic aphasia): *Harrison 15th / 143; 16th/148; Harrison 17th/165;*

'Anomic aphasia is the single most common language disturbance seen in head trauma, metabolic encephalopathy and Alzheimer's disease' *– Harrison, 17th / 165*

*Anomic aphasia is dysfunction where a person is **unable to name objects**.* His articulation, comprehension and repetition are intact, but naming, word finding and spellings are impaired.

399. Answer is D (Autonomic dysfunction): *Harrisons 16th / 408, 409; API 7th / 241*

Autonomic dysfunction has not been mentioned as a manifestation of vit E deficiency

Vit E Deficiency Manifestations.

Haematological Manifestation Anaemia	Neurological manifestations
• Haemolytic anaemia with acanthocytosis and thrombocytosis	• Spinocerebellar & Postcolumn dysfunction • Peripheral neuropathy - Areflexia - Ataxic gaunt - Loss of vibration & position sense • Ophthalmoplegia • Skeletal myopathy • Pigmented retinopathy

Note:

- Dietary deficiency of vit-E does not exist.
- Vitamin E deficiency is seen in only severe and prolonged malabsorptive diseases or after small intestinal resection.

400. Answer is A (L_1): *Fuller / 137; Chamberlain's 11th / 389*

Knee jerk is associated with spinal segments L_3, L_4 and according to some L_2 also.

Segmental levels of some common reflexes include:

Deep		***Superficial***
Q Ankle jerk : S_1, S_2	Triceps jerk Q : $C_{7,8}$	Plantar reflex Q : S_1, S_2
Q Knee jerk : $L_{3,4}$	Radial jerk Q : C_6	Abdominal reflex Q : T_7 - T_{11}
Q Biceps jerk : $C_{5,6}$	Jaw Jerk Q : Pons	Cremesteric reflex Q : L_1

401. Answer is C (Resting tremor): Repeat

Resting tremor is a feature of a lesion in the basal ganglia such as Parkinson's disease. Cerebellar lesions are associated with intention tremors and not resting tremors.

Features of Cerebellar dysfunction / lesions
• *Dysmetria* • *Dysarthria* • ***Ataxia*** • ***Incoordination*** • *Past pointing* • *Dysdiadokinesia* • ***Intention Tremor*** • ***Hypotonia*** • *Cerebellar Nystagmus*

402. Answer is C (Hypertonia): *Guyton 10th/ 655, 656*

Hypotonia is a feature of cerebellar disease (not Hypertonia).

403. Answer is D (Cereblium): *Dejong's Neurological Examination 7th/621; Guyton 10th/655, 656*

Dysmetria is a typical feature of cerebellar dysfunction / disease.

Dysmetria *refers to errors in judging distance and gauging the distance, speed, power and direction of movement. It refers to inaccuracy of movement in which the desired target is either unde- reached (hypometria) or over-reached (hypermetria). Dysmetia is feature of cerebellar disease / dysfunction and is evident on 'finger chase' or 'toe to finger' tests.*

Features of Cerebellar Disease / Dysfunction
• *Dysmetria (Inaccuracy of movement, disturbance of rate, range & force of movement)*
• *Dysarthria (Ataxic dysarthria results from disruption of timing, force, range and direction of movement needed to maintain normal articulation)*
• *Ataxia (unsteady to stand or sit without support)*
• *Incoordination*
Pastpointing *Intention tremor (Inability to coordinate fine motor activity)* *Dysdiadokinesia (Inability to perform rapid lternating movements)*
• *Hypotonia*
• *Cerebellar Nystagmus*

404. Answer is B (Inability to identify faces): *Harrison 15th/ 145; Harrison 16th/150; Harrison 17th/ 105, 188*

'Prosopagnosia is a recognition deficit in which patient is unable to recognize familiar faces.
Face and object recognition deficits are known as Prosopagnosia and visual object agnosia respectively.

Prosopagnosia	**Visual Object Agnosia**
• Patient is unable to recognise familiar faces. • However patient can easily tell if two faces are identical or not. i.e. this is not a perceptual deficit. • Thus Prosopagnosis patients characteristically have no difficulty with the generic identification of a face as a face or of a car as a car, but they cannot recognise the identity of an individual face or the make of an individual car.	• This is an object Recognition disorder. • However in contrast to prospagnosia those with this disorder cannot recognise a face as a face or a car as a car.

The characteristic lesions in Prosopagnosia and visual object Agnosia consists of a *bilateral infarction in the territory of the posterior cerebral arteries* and involve *lingual and fusiform gyri.*

405. Answer is D (Pain): *Harrison 15th/ 131*

Lesion of the primary somatosensory area does not lead to loss in pain sensation. Involvement of the secondary somatosensory area is associated with alteration in pain sensation.

Primary Somatosensory area is (Area 3, 1, 2)

Lesions in this area produce *contralateral* impairment of: -	
Touch *Pressure* *Proprioception* *Two point discrimination*	*Sterognosis* *Barognosis* *Cutaneographia*

406. Answer is A (Amygdala): *Guyton 10th/ 687*

Kluver Bucy Syndrome is caused due to bilateral ablation of Amygdala

Features of K.B. syndrome (Experimented on animals)
1. *Is not afraid of anything*
2. *Has extreme curiosity about everything*
3. *Forgets rapidly*
4. *Has tendency to place everything in its mouth and sometimes even tries to eat solid object*
5. *Often has a sex drive so strong that it attempts to copulate with immature animals of the wrong sex or even animals of different species.*

407. Answer is D (Multiple sclerosis): *Ref: API 9th/ 790, API 7th/ 835; Harrison 17th/ 2533 (table 366-2); Harrison 18th/p 3318 (Table: 372.2)*

All options other than multiple sclerosis are mentioned as causes of extrapyramidal syndrome.

Classification of extrapyramidal disorders :

Akinetic rigid syndromes	
Idiopathic Parkinson's disease	
Secondary Parkinson's disease	
Drugs	: Phenothiazines, haloperidol, pimozide, metoclopramide, reserpine, lithium.
Toxins	: Manganese 1-methyl 4-phenyl tetrahydropyridine (MPTP), carbondisulphide
Hypoxia	: Carbonmonooxide, cynaide
Viral	: Japanese B Encephalitis, C-J Disease, SSPE
Vascular	: Athrosclerosis
Metabolic	: Wilson's disease, hypoparathyroidism, GM1 gangliosidosis
Head Injury	: Punch drunk syndrome
Brain tumor	
Parkinson's plus syndromes	
Progressive supranuclear palsy Multiple system atrophy : olivopontocerebellar atrophy, Shy-Drager syndrome, striato nigral degeneration. Cortico basal degeneration Diffuse lewy body disease Familial basal ganglia calcification Huntington's disorder (Juvenile variant)	

408. Answer is B (Absent pupillary light reflex and delated pupils): *Harrison 18th/2252; 'Concise Textbook of Forensic Medicine & Toxicity' by Sharma (Elsevier) 2nd/44; 'The Neurology of Consciousness' (Academic Press) 2009/156; 'Oxford American Handbook of Clinical Medicine' by Flynn (Oxford) 2007/20*

Brainstem death is defined by the absence of all brainstem mediated cranial nerve reflexes.

Pupillary Light Reflex is a brainstem mediated cranial nerve reflex that is absent in brainstem death.

The pupils are usually midsized but may be dilated (should not however be small).

Occulo-cephalic (Doll's eye) reflex and Vestibulo-ocular (Caloric) reflex are both brainstem mediated cranial nerve reflexes that should be absent in Brainstem death.

Criteria for Brain Death/Brainstem death

The definition of Brain stem death requires simultaneous demonstration that the patient has irreversibly lost the capacity of consciousness (Coma) and the capacity to breathe (Apnoea) both of which are dependent on intact brainstem.
Clinical assessment of the integrity of Brainstem has two components including assessment of the integrity of brainstem mediated cranial nerve reflexes and the Apnea test.

Deep Unresponsive Coma	Absence of all Brainstem Cranial Reflexes	Complete Aponea in pressure of hypercarbia (Absence of Brainstem Respiratory Reflex)
Patients with brain death show the deepest coma possible with total unresponsiveness to all stimuli. • No spontaneous movement • No response to external stimuli (Verbal/ Deep pain)	All reflexes mediated by cranial nerve must be absent • Absent Pupillary Light reflex (CN II, III) (*Pupils are usually midsized but may be enlarged but they should not be small*) • Absent Corneal Reflex (CN V, VII) • Absent Vestibulocochlear Reflex (CN III, IV, VI, VIII) (No eye movement in response to caloric irrigation of ears) • Absent Oculocephalic Reflex (Absent Doll's eye reflex) Eyes will move with the head (No occular movements on rapid turning of head). • Absent Gag Reflex (CNIX, X) • Absent Tracheal Cough Reflex (CNX) • Absent Central Motor Response to Pain (CN V, VII) (No response to deep somatic stimulation).	• No respiratory effort in response to hypercarbia needs to be demonstrated to show that aponea is due to brainstem (medullary) damage • Absent respiratory movement during disconnection from the ventilator with the PaCO2 > 60 mm Hg is required for the test to be valid

Cranial nerve reflexes in Brain Stem Death testing:

Reflex	Cranial nerves	Notes
Pupillary light reflex	II, III	Use bright light source (not ophthalmoscope) in a dimmed environment. Look for both direct and consensual reaction. Important reflex that interrogates at level of midbrain
Corneal reflex	V, VII	Stroke cornea with gauze, whilst gently holding eyes open; avoid trauma to cornea. The various nuclei of V are found throughout the whole length of the brainstem, whilst that of VII (facial nerve) is in the upper medulla.
Central response to deep somatic stimulation	V, VII	Apply deep pressure stimulation centrally (e.g. supra-orbital ridge) and peripherally (e.g. nail bed). Look for central motor response in the distribution of the facial nerve. Peripheral stimulation may illicit peripheral spinal reflexes.
Cold caloric vestibulo-ocular reflex	III, IV, VI, VIII	Check patency of external auditory canal with auroscope. Flex head to 30° (or apply 30° head up tilt if cervical spine injury is suspected). Slowly irrigate canal with 50mL ice-cold water over 60s. Observe for nystagmus for a further 30s. Contra-indicated in trauma-related otorrhea. The nuclei of III and IV lie withjin the midbrain, whilst those of VI and VIII are in the medulla.
Oculocephalic reflex (Doll's eye reflex)	VIII, III, VI	Rapid lateral movement of the head normally results in eye deviation to the contralateral side, testing brainstem gaze mechanism. In brainstem death eyes remain in a fixed position within the orbit.
Gag reflex	IX, X	Stimulate uvula under direct vision with throat spatula, observing for contraction of soft palate. The nuclei of IX and X lie in the medulla.
Tracheal cough reflex	X	Expose patient to umblicus. Stimulate trachea to level of carina by introduction of sterile suction catheter down endotracheal tube. Observe for cough response

409. Answer is C (PET Scan) : *Harrison 16th / 129; Harrison 17th/ 142;* Harrison 18th/p 177

PET scan has not been mentioned as a test to investigate syncope in Harrisons text. It is the single best answer of exclusion. Electrophysiological tests and 24 hour ***ECG Holter monitoring*** are indicated in patients where history suggests a cardiac disease. ***Upright tilt table testing*** is indicated for suspected neurogenic / vasodepressor syncope in patients with normal history / examination.

Invasive Cardiac Electrophysiologic testing : provides diagnostic and prognostic information regarding Sinus Node function, AV conduction and Supraventricular and Ventricular arrhythmia.

Holter monitor : provides 24 - 48 hours monitoring of ECG rhythm on an outpatient basis and is indicated for detection of conduction abnormalities.

Upright tilt table testing :

- Is a test for vasodepressor / neurogenic syncope in patients with normal history / examination.
- In susceptible patients upright tilt at an angle between 60^0 to 80^0 for 30 to 60 minutes induces a vasovagal episode.
- Indications for Table Tilt test include :
    - Recurrent syncope
    - Single syncope episode that caused injury
    - Single syncope event in high risk setting (pilot, commercial vehicle driver)

Syncope

The choice of diagnostic test should be guided by the history and physical examination

For All patients

- Serum electrolytes
- Glucose
- Haematocrit

ECG (almost all)

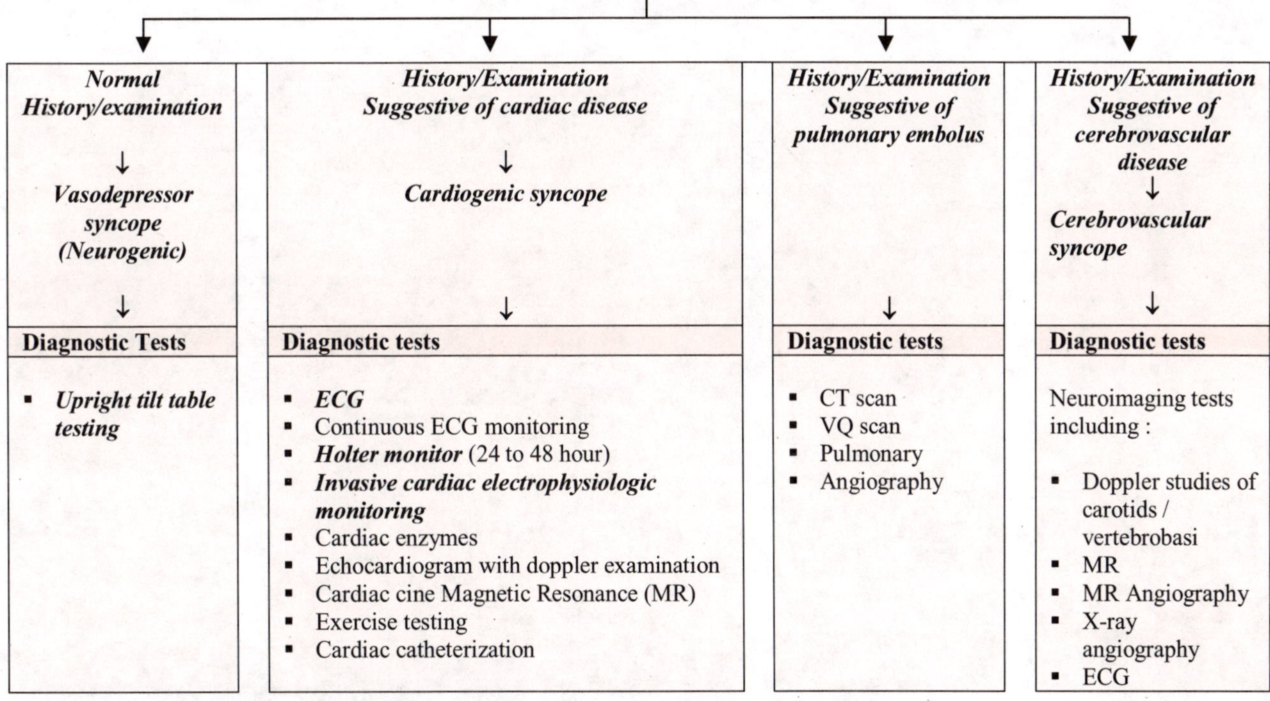

410. Answer is B (Choroid plexus): *Harrison's 17th/95, Neurological Emergencies 2nd/161*

Choroid plexus is a pain insensitive cranial structure.

'The ventricular ependyma, choroids plexus, pial veins and much of brain parenchyma are not pain producing'- Harrison's

Pain Sensitive	Pain Insensitive
Intracranial • *Cranial venous sinuses with afferent veins* • ***Arteries at base of brain and arteries of dura including middle meningeal artery*** • ***Dura around venous sinuses and vessels*** • ***Falx Cerebri*** **Extracranial** • *Skin* • *Scalp Appendages* • *Periostium* • *Muscles* • *Arteries* • *Mucosa* **Nerves** • *Trigeminal (Vth)* • *Facial (VIII)* • *Vagal (X)* • *Glossopharyngeal(IX)* • *Second (II) & Third (IIIrd) C.N.*	**Intracranial** • *Brain parenchyma* • *Ependyma* • ***Choroid plexus*** • *Piamater* • *Arachnoid* • ***Dura over convexity of skull*** • ***(Dura around vascular sinuses and vessels is sensitive to pain)***

NOTES

Miscellaneous

QUESTIONS

Acid Base Disorders and Electrolyte imbalance

1. A 2 year old child is being evaluated for persistent metabolic acidosis. Blood tests show Na+ 140mEq/l. K+ 3mEq/l, Ca2+ 8mg/l, Mg+2 mEq/l. phosphate 3 mEq/l, pH 7.22, bicarbonate 16mEq/l and chloride 112mEq/l. The plasma anion gap is: *(AIIMS Nov 2004)*
   A. 9
   B. 15
   C. 22
   D. 25

2 A normal-anion-gap metabolic acidosis occurs in patients with : *(AIIMS Nov 2003)*
   A. Diarrhoea
   B. Diabetic ketoacidosis
   C. Methyl alcohol poisoning
   D. Acute renal failure

3. Widened anionic gap is ***not*** seen in : *(AI 1996)*
   A. Acute renal failure
   B. Diarrhea
   C. Lactic acidosis
   D. Diabetic ketoacidosis

4. Normal anion gap metabolic is caused by :
   A. Cholera *(AI 2003)*
   B. Starvation
   C. Ethylene glycol poisoning
   D. Lactic acidosis

5. All of the following cause high anion gap metabolic acidosis except: *(AIIMS Nov 2002)*
   A. Lactic acidosis
   B. Salicylate poisoning
   C. Ethylyene glycol poisoning
   D. Ureterosigmoidostomy

6. Increased 'anion gap' is ***not*** seen in : *(AI 1994)*
   A. Salicylate poisoning
   B. Renal tubular acidosis
   C. Lactic acidosis
   D. Ethylene glycol poisoning

7. The following condition is not associated with an increased anion-gap type of metabolic acidosis :
   A. Shock *(AI 2002)*
   B. Ingestion of ante-freeze
   C. Diabetic keto-acidosis
   D. COPD

8. Lactic acidosis is ***not*** seen in *(AI 1996)*
   A. Methanol poisoning
   B. Respiratory failure
   C. Circulatory failure
   D. Tolbutamide

9. A 7 years girl, parents gave history of fever for which she was treated with Paracetamol following which the fever subsided. Later she developed seizures and altered sensorium. The urine examination revealed oxalate crystals on microscopy, Blood anion gap and osmolality were increased. The diagnosis is :
   A. Lactic acidosis *(AIIMS May 2002)*
   B. Ethylene glycol poisoning
   C. Renal tubular acidosis
   D. Paracetamol poisoning

10. A 2 year old boy presents with fever for 3 days which respond to administration of paracetamol. Three days later he developed acute renal failure, marked acidosis and encephalopathy. His urine showed plenty of oxalate crystals. The blood anion gap and osmolal gap were increased. Which of the following is the most likely diagnosis :
   A. Paracetamol poisoning *(AIIMS Nov. 05)*
   B. Diethyl glycol poisoning
   C. Severe malaria
   D. Hanta virus infection

11. Urinary anion gap an indication of excretion of :
   A. Ketoacids *(AI 2002)*
   B. NH4+
   C. H+ ion
   D. Na+ ion

12. Acute metabolic acidosis : *(AI 2002)*
   A. Has biphasic effect on K+ excretion
   B. Does not effect K + excretion
   C. Decreases urinary K+ excretion
   D. Increase urinary K+ excretion

13. A 50kg man with severe metabolic acidosis has thc following parameters : pH 7.05, pCO2 12mm Hg, pO2 108 mm Hg, HCO3 5mEq/L base excess – 30 mEq/L. The approximate quantity of sodium bicarbonate that he should receive in half hour is :
   A. 250 mEq *(AI 2003)*
   B. 350 mEq
   C. 500 mEq
   D. 750 mEq

14. Causes of metabolic alkalosis include all the following ***except*** : *(AI 2003)*
A. Mineralocorticoid deficiency
B. Bartter's syndrome
C. Thiazide diuretic therapy
D. Recurrent vomiting

15. Metabolic alkalosis is seen in all ***except*** : *(AI 1996)*
A. Thaizide diuretic therapy
B. Prolonged vomiting
C. Uretero-sigmoidostomy
D. Cushing's disease

16. A patient with salicylic acid poisoning has the following arterial blood gas analysis report : pH = 7.12 : pCO_2 = 18mmHg; HCO_3 = 12mmol/L. The resulting acid base abnormality can be best labeled as : *(AIIMS Nov 03)*
A. Metabolic acidosis with compensatory respiratory alkalosis
B. Metabolic acidosis with compensatory respiratory alkalosis
C. Respiratory acidosis with metabolic alkalosis
D. Metabolic acidosis

17. In a patient PO_2 is 85 mmHg, PCO_2 – 50mmHg, pH is 7.2 and HCO_3 is 32 meq/l is suffering from :
A. Respiratory acidosis with compensatory metabolic alkalosis *(AIIMS June 2000)*
B. Respiratory acidosis with compensatory metabolic acidosis
C. Metabolic acidosis
D. Metabolic alkalosis

18. Arterial blood gas analysis of a patient reveals pH 7.2, HCO_3 36mmol/L, pCO_2 60mm of Hg. The abnormality is : *(AIIMS June 99)*
A. Respiratory acidosis with compensatory metabolic alkalosis *(AI 1996)*
B. Respiratory acidosis
C. Respiratory alkalosis with compensatory metabolic acidosis
D. Respiratory acidosis with compensatory metabolic acidosis

19. A 40 year old male develops excessive hyperventilation. ABG reveals pH- 7.5, PCO_2 24 mmHg, PO_2 88 mm of Hg. Treatment is :
A. Respiratory alkalosis *(AIIMS June 1999)*
B. Metabolic alkalosis
C. Respiratory acidosis
D. Metabolic acidosis

20. ABG analysis of a patient on ventilator,shows decreased pCO2, normal pO2, pH 7.5; diagnosis is:
A. Respiratory acidosis *(AI 2001)*
B. Metabolic alkalosis
C. Resp alkalosis
D. Metabolic acidosis

21. An ABG analysis shows : pH 7.2, raised pCO_2, decreased HCO_3; diagnosis is : *(AIIMS June 97)*
A. Respiratory acidosis *(AI 2001)*
B. Compensated metabolic acidosis
C. Respiratory and metabolic acidosis
D. Respiratory alkalosis

22. A female patient after injury comes to casualty. Her ABG shows low pH, pCO2 high, bicarbonate normal. The diagnosis is:
A. Respiratory alkalosis *(AIIMS Nov 1999)*
B. Respiratory acidosis
C. Metabolic acidosis
D. Metabolic alkalosis

23. A newly posted junior doctor had difficulty in finding out base deficit/excess for blood in a given patient. An experienced senior resident advised a quick method to determine acid base composition of blood based on pCO_2. Which of the following is the likely method he suggested to predict acid base composition of blood?
A. Red ford nomogram *(AI 2004)*
B. DuBio's nomogram
C. Goldman constant field equation
D. Siggard-Andersen nomogram

Immune Disorders

24. Haptane is : *(AIIMS-98)*
A. Same as epitope
B. Small molecular weight protein
C. Requires carrier for specific antibody production
D. Simple haptens are precipitate

25. All of the following forces are involved in antigen antibody reaction, EXCEPT:
A. Vander Waal's forces *(AIIMS-96, 98)*
B. Electrostatic bond
C. Hydrogen bond
D. Covalent bond

26. TRUE about immunoglobulins is: *(AIIMS-97)*
A. IgE fixes complements
B. IgM fixes complements
C. IgG is found in minimum concentration
D. IgG is elevated in primary immune response

27. The serum concentration of which of the following human IgG subclass is maximum?
A. IgG1. *(AI 2005)*
B. IgG2.
C. IgG3.
D. IgG4

28. Which of the following immunoglobulins can crosses placenta: *(AIIMS-99)*
A. IgA
B. IgM
C. IgG
D. IgD

29. Which of the following statements concerning immunoglobulins is wrong: *(AIIMS-97)*
A. IgM does not cross placenta
B. IgE is increased in parasitic infection
C. IgM increased in primary response
D. Fetal infection is characterized by increase in IgG

30. Which of the following best denotes classical complement pathway activation in immuno inflammatory condition: *(AIIMS-2000)*
A. C_2, C_4 and C_3 decreased
B. C_2 and C_4 normal, C_3 is decreased
C. C_3 normal and C_2, C_4 decreased
D. C_2, C_4, C_3 all are elevated

31. Which is not a macrophage: *(AIIMS-97)*
A. Monocyte
B. Microgila
C. Kupffer cells
D. Lymphocytes

32. Langerhan's cells are: *(AIIMS-98)*
A. Phagocytic cells
B. Antigen presenting cells
C. Seen in auto immune conditions
D. Seen in chronic infection

33. Antigen processing cells are all of the following, EXCEPT: *(AIIMS-02)*
A. Astrocytes
B. Dendritic cells in lymphoid follicles
C. Reticulum cells of lymph nodes
D. Langerhan's cells

34. True statements are all, EXCEPT: *(AIIMS-2000)*
A. Chromosome six harbours the gene for MHC
B. Genes encoding compliments are located adjacent to class I
C. Monocytes have MHC class II antigens on their surfaces
D. Class III MHC does not encode complement

35. Neonatal thymectomy leads to: *(AIIMS-02)*
A. Decreased size of germinal center
B. Decreased size of paracortical areas
C. Increased antibody production
D. Increased bone marrow production of lymphocytes

36. Regarding NK cells, false statement is:
A. It is activated by IL-2 *(AIIMS-01)*
B. Expresses CD3 receptor
C. It is a variant of large lymphocyte
D. There is antibody induced proliferation of NK cells

37. The following feature is common to both cytotoxic T cells and NK cells: *(AIIMS-02)*
A. Synthesize antibody
B. Require antibodies to be present for action
C. Effective against virus infected cells
D. Recognize antigen in association with HLA class II markers

38. The marker for B lymphocyte is: *(AIIMS-2000)*
A. CD19
B. CD68
C. CD34
D. CD4

39. Which of these is false regarding cytokines:
A. Mediators of immune system *(AIIMS-97)*
B. Produced by monocytes
C. Are soluble proteins
D. Does not mediate specific reactions

40. IL-1 produces: *(AIIMS-02)*
A. T lymphocyte activation
B. Delayed wound healing
C. Increased pain perception
D. Decreased PMN release from bone marrow

41. IL-2 is produced by: *(AIIMS-97, 2000)*
A. T cells
B. B cells
C. Monocytes
D. Neutrophils

42. IL-2 is secreted by: *(AIIMS-97)*
A. CD4 and lymphocytes
B. CD8 cells
C. Macrophages
D. Neutrophils

43. Examples of type I hypersensitivity is:
A. Tepromin test *(AIIMS-98)*
B. Tuberculin
C. Casoni's test
D. Arthrus reaction

44. Ram Devi presented with generalized edema, sweating, and flushing tachycardia and fever after bee sting. This is: *(AIIMS-01)*
A. T cell mediated cytotoxicity
B. IgE mediated reaction

C. IgG mediated reaction
D. IgA mediated hypersensitivity reaction

45. Which of the following is an example of type IV hypersensitivity: *(AIIMS-97)*
A. Arthrus reaction
B. Serum sickness
C. Schwartzmann reaction
D. Granulomatous reaction

46. Type of graft, best suited for renal transplantation: *(AIIMS-99)*
A. Allograft
B. Autograft
C. Xenograft
D. Isograft

47. Most common cause of chronic granulomatous disease in children is: *(AIIMS-98)*
A. Myeloperoxidase deficiency
B. Defective phagocytosis
C. Defective H_2O_2 production
D. Job's disease

48. Adenosine deaminase deficiency is seen in the following: *(AIIMS-01)*
A. Common variable immunodeficiency
B. Severe combined immunodeficiency
C. Chronic granulomatous disease
D. Nezelof syndrome

49. Adenosine deaminase (enzyme) deficiency is associated with: *(AI 2005)*
A. Severe combined immunodeficiency (SCID).
B. X-linked agammaglobulinemia.
C. Transient hypogammaglobulinemia of infancy.
D. Chronic granulomatous disease.

50. Recurrent Giardiasis is associated with:
A. Severe combined immunodeficiency
B. Common variable immunodeficiency
C. Digeorge syndrome *(AIIMS-2000)*
D. C8 deficiency

51. Humoral immunodeficiency is suspected in a patient and he is under investigation. Which of the following infections would not be consistent with the diagnosis-
A. Giardiasis *(AIIMS Nov 04)*
B. Pneumocystis carinii pneumonia
C. Recurrent sinusitis
D. Recurrent subcutaneous abscesses

52. Wiskott Aldrich syndrome is associated with all of the following except : *(AIIMS Dec 97)*
A. Thrombocytopenia
B. Recurrent infections
C. Low levels of IgG
D. Deficient cell mediated immunity

53. Ataxaia telengiectasia is associated with all of the following except : *(AI 2004)*
A. Recurrent sinopulmonary infections
B. Lymphatic reticular malignancies
C. Increased fraction of IgA immunoglobulins
D. Insulin resistance

54. Thymoma can be associated with all, EXCEPT:
A. Superior mediastinum syndrome
B. Myasthenia gravis *(AIIMS Dec 95)*
C. Hypergammaglobulinemia
D. Pure red cell aplasia

55. Vertical transmission of antibody can occur in all of the following, EXCEPT :*(AIIMS Sept 96)*
A. Rh incompatibility
B. Isoimmune thrombocytopenia
C. Neonatal toxic erythema
D. Neonatal myasthenia gravis

Genetic Disorders

56. Most common group of diseases following Mendelian inheritance are : *(AI 1999)*
A. Autosomal dominant
B. Autosomal recessive
C. X-linked dominant
D. X- linked recessive

57. Which one of the following is an Autosomal Dominant disorder : *(AI 2002)*
A. Cystic fibrosis
B. Hereditary spherocytosis
C. Sickle cell anemia
D. G-6PD deficiency

58. Which of the following is Autosomal dominant
A. Achondroplasia *(AI 1996)*
B. Hemochromatism
C. Wilson's disease
D. Cystic fibrosis

59. Which of the following is an autosomal dominant disorder? *(AIIMS 96)*
A. Duchenes muscular dystrophy
B. Fragile X syndrome
C. Fanconi's syndrome
D. Hutington's chorea

60. Which of the following is an automsomal dominant metabolic disorder? *(AI 2004)*
A. *Cystic fibrosis*
B. *Phenyl ketonuria*
C. *α-1 antitrypsin deficiency*
D. Familial hyper cholestrolemia

61. Which of the following is Autosomal Dominant:
A. Retinoblastoma (AI 2000)
B. Ataxia telangiectasia
C. Bloom's syndrome
D. Xeroderma pigmentosa

62. Which one of the following is Autosomal recessive
A. Homocystinuria (AI 98)
B. G6PD deficiency
C. Myotonic dystrophy
D. Otospongiosis

63. All of the following are X-linked except:
A. G-6 PD deficiency (AI 1998)
B. Hemophilia –A
C. Von Willebrandt's disease
D. Fragile X syndrome

64. The commonest mode of inheritance of congenital heart disease is (AI 2002)
A. Autosomal dominant
B. Autosomal recessive
C. Sex linked dominant
D. Multifactorial

65. Study the following carefully: (AI 2005)

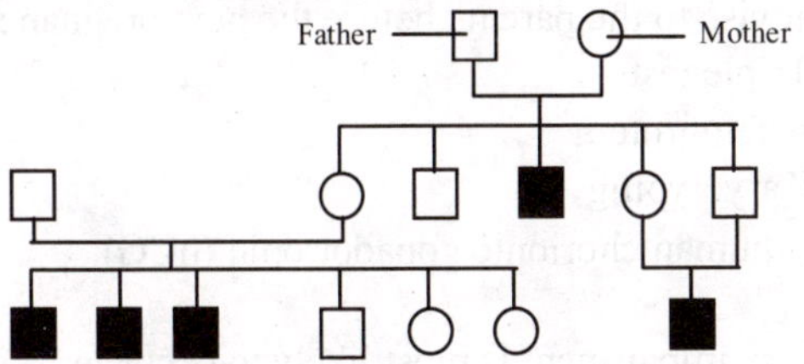

Read the pedigree. Inheritance pattern of the disease in the family is:
A. Autosomal recessive type.
B. Autosomal dominant type.
C. X-Linked dominant type.
D. X linked recessive type.

66. Kinky hair disease is a disorder where an affected child has peculiar white stubby hair, does not grow, brain degenration is seen and dies by age of two years. Mrs A is hesitant about having children because her two sisters had sons who had died from kinky hair disease. Her mother's brother also died of the same condition. Which of the following is the possible mode of inheritance in her family? (AI 2004)
A. X-linked recessive
B. X-linked dominant
C. Autosomal recessive
D. Autosomal dominant

67. An X-linked recessive disease is characterized by the following inheritance : (AI 1997)
A. Vertical transmission
B. 50% female carriers if male is affected and female is normal
C. 50% male affected if female is carrier and male is normal
D. 50% male carriers if female is affected and male is normal.

68. The chances of having an unaffected baby, when both parents have achondroplasia, are: (AI 2005)
A. 0%.
B. 25%
C. 50%
D. 100%

69. An albino girl gets married to a normal boy, What are the chances of their having an affected child and what are the chances of their children being carriers?
A. None affected, all carriers (AI 2003)
B. All normal
C. 50% carriers
D. 50% affected, 50% carriers

70. Father has a blood group B ; Mother has AB ; Children are not likely to have the following blood group: (AI 2001)
A. O
B. A
C. B
D. AB

71. The mother has sickle cell disease; Father is normal; Chances of children having sickle cell disease and sickle cell trait respectively are:
A. 0 and 100% (AI 2001)
B. 25 and 25%
C. 50 and 50%
D. 10 and 50%

72. A couple, with a family history of beta thalassemia major in a distant relative, has come for counseling. The husband has HbA2 of 4.8% and the wife has HbA2 of 2.3%. The risk of having a child with beta thalassemia major is:
A. 50% (AI 2003)
B. 25%
C. 5%
D. 0%

73. Kamlesh, a 2 years old girl, has Down's syndrome. Her karyotype is 21/21 translocation. What is the risk of recurrence in subsequent pregnancies if the father is a balanced translocation carrier : (AI 2002)
A. 100%

B. 50%
C. 25%
D. 0%

74. Most common trisomy among following is :
A. 18 *(AI 1998)*
B. 21
C. 13
D. 5

75. A married middle aged female gives history or repeated abortions for the past 5 years. The given below is conceptions pre-natal karyogram.

1 2 3 4 5
6 7 8 9 10 11 12
13 14 15 16 17 18
19 20 21 22 y x

This karyogram suggests the following :
A. Klinefelter's syndrome *(AI 2003)*
B. Turner's syndrome
C. Down's syndrome
D. Patau's syndrome

76. All the following are features of Down's syndrome *except* *(AI 1994)*
A. Brushfield's spots in iris
B. Simian crease
C. Mental retardation
D. Hypertonicity

77. All of the following may occur in Down's syndrome except : *(AI 06)*
A. Hypothyroidism
B. Undescended testis
C. Ventricular septal defect
D. Brushfield's spots

78. Which of the following is the investigation of choice in a pregnant lady at 18 weeks of pregnancy with past history of delivering a baby with Down's syndrome.
A. Triple screen test *(AI 2004)*
B. Amniocentesis
C. Chorionic villous biopsy
D. Ultrasonography

79. Diagnosis of Down syndrome at 11 weeks is best assessed by: *(AI 1998)*
A. Ultrasonography
B. Aminocentesis
C. Chorionic villous biopsy
D. Doppler Ultrasound

80. A 35 year old female with a previous history of birth of a child with Down's syndrome, presents with 18 weeks Amenorrhoea. The Investigation of choice rule out Down's syndrome in the present pregnancy is:
A. Triple test *(AI 2000)*
B. Amniocentesis
C. Cordocentesis
D. Chorionic villous biopsy

81. Triple test for diagnosis of down's syndrome includes all of the following except : *(AI 1999)*
A. β- HCG
B. α- Fetoprotein
C. Serum HPL level
D. Serum oestriol level

82. Increased nuchal fold thickness is a feature of :
A. Paul-Bunnel syndrome *(AI 1999)*
B. De-pan syndrome
C. Down's syndrome
D. Cri-duchat syndrome

83. Mr. and Mrs. Annadurai have a 2 month old baby suffering with Down's syndrome. Karyotype of Mrs Annadurai shows translocation variety of Down syndrome. Which of the following investigations will you advise to the parents before the next pregnancy ?
A. Triple test *(AI 2004)*
B. α-fetoprotein
C. Karyotyping
D. β-human chorionic gonadotropin (hCG)

84. Memory impairment is most likely to occur in :
A. Downs Syndrome *(AIIMS Nov. 1999)*
B. Alkaptonuria
C. Attention deficit disorder
D. Conduct disorder

85. A chromosomal anomaly associated with Alzheimer's dementia is: *(AI 2001)*
A. Trisomy 18
B. Patau syndrome
C. Trisomy 21
D. Turners syndrome

86. A child present with antimongoloid slant, pulmonary stenosis, short stature and undescended testis. Most likely diagnosis is :
A. Klinefelter's syndrome *(AI 1997)*
B. Noonan's syndrome
C. Turner's syndrome
D. Down syndrome

87. Webbing of neck, increased carrying angle, low posterior hair line and short fourth metacarpal are characteristics of: *(AI 2004)*
A. Klinefelter syndrome
B. Turner syndrome
C. Cri du chat syndrome
D. Noonan syndrome

88. In Turner's syndrome which of the following is NOT seen : *(AIIMS June 2000)*
A. Short stature
B. Widely spaced nipple
C. Webbed neck
D. Mental retardation

89. The following statements regarding Turner syndrome are true except. *(AIIMS May 2003)*
A. Occurrence of Turner syndrome is influenced by maternal age.
B. Most patients have primary amenorrhoea.
C. Most patients have short stature.
D. Edema of hands and feet is an important feature during infancy.

90. A patient with XO chromosomes and short stature is likely to have *(AIIMS June 2000)*
A. Klinefelter's syndrome
B. Turner's syndrome
C. Down's syndrome
D. *Condy syndrome*

91. A nineteen year old female with short stature, wide spread nipples and primary amenorrhoea most likely has a karyotype of : *(AI 2003)*
A. 47, XX+18
B. 46, XXY
C. 47, XXY
D. 45 X

92. Coarctation of the aorta is common in which syndrome *(AI 1995)*
A. Down's
B. Turner's
C. Klinefelter's
D. Noonan's

93. All of the following may occur in Noonan's syndrome except: *(AI 2003)*
A. Hypertrophic cardiomyopathy
B. Cryptoorchidism
C. Infertility in females
D. Autosomal dominant transmission

94. Males who are sexually under developed with rudimentary testes and prostate glands, sparse pubic and facial hair, long arms and legs and large hands & feet are likely to have the chromosome complement of : *(AI 2004)*
A. 45, XYY
B. 46, XY
C. 46, XXY
D. 46, X

95. True in Klinefelter syndrome is
A. Short stature *(AI 1998)*
B. Pituitary adenoma
C. Subnormal intelligence
D. Breast adenoma

96. A patient of 47XXY karyotype with features of hypogonadism; likely diagnosis is :
A. Turners syndrome *(AI 2001)*
B. Kilenfelters syndrome
C. Edwards syndrome
D. Down syndrome

97. In Klippel-Feil syndrome, the patient has all of the following clinical features ***except***:
A. Low hair line. *(AI 2005)*
B. Bilateral Neck webbing.
C. Bilateral shortness of sterno mastoid muscles.
D. Gross limitations of neck movements.

98. Fragile X-syndrome is characterised by all of the following features except :
A. Long face *(AI 1999)*
B. Large ear
C. Large-nose
D. Large-testis

99. Rokitansky Kuster hauser syndrome is associated with: *(AI 2001)*
A. Ovarian agenesis
B. Absent fallopian tube
C. Vaginal atresia
D. Bicornuate uterus

100. Characteristic features of Rokitanski-Kuster Hauser syndrome are all of the following except:
A. Absent uterus *(AI 1999)*
B. Absent vagina
C. Anovulation
D. 46-XX

101. A 16 yr old female presents with Primary Amenorhea. Examination shows a Short Blind Vagina, with absent Uterus. The Next Investigation of choice is :
A. Karyotyping *(AI 2000)*
B. IVP
C. Gonadotrophin levles
D. Serum Prolactin

10 Miscellaneous

102. Pseudohermaphroditism in a female child is most commonly due to: *(AI 1994)*
A. 21-hydroxylase deficiency
B. 17-hydroxylase deficiency
C. 11-hydroxylase deficiency
D. 3-hydroxylase deficiency

103. The most common cause of ambiguous genitalia in a newborn is - *(AI 2002)*
A. 21 hydroxylase deficiency
B. 11 β -hydroxylase deficiency
C. 17 α -hydroxyalse deficiency
D. 3 β–hydroxysteroid deficiency

104. All of the following can be used for establishing antenatal diagnosis except : *(AI 1997)*
A. Fetal blood
B. Maternal blood
C. Amniotic fluid
D. Decidua

105. Screening by using maternal serum alpha fetoproteins helps to detect all of the following except:
A. Neural tube defects *(AI 2004)*
B. Duodenal Artesia
C. Talipes equinovarus
D. Omphalocele

106. Abnormal α-fetoprotein is seen in
A. Trisomy 18 *(AI 1996)*
B. Twin pregnancy
C. Neural tube defect
D. All of the above

107. Ataxia telangiectasia is chracterised by all of the following except : *(AI 2004)*
A. Chronic sinopulmonary disease
B. Decreased level of α-fetoprotein
C. Chromosomal breakage
D. IgA deficiency

108. Which of the following tests on maternal serum is most useful in distinguishing between open neural tube defects and ventral wall defects in a fetus?
A. Carcinoembryogenic antigen *(AI 2004)*
B. Sphingomyelin
C. Alpha-feto protein
D. Pseudocholinesterase

109. Which of following is the feature of Y chromosome?
A. Acrocentric *(AI 2004)*
B. Telocentric
C. Submetacentric
D. Metacentric

110. Which of the following procedures as routine technique for karyotyping using light microscopy:
A. C-banding *(AI 2003)*
B. G-banding
C. Q-banding
D. Brd V-staining

111. RNA fragments are sequenced by: *(AI 1999)*
A. Eastern-blot
B. Western blot
C. Northern blot
D. Southern-blot

112. Differential expression of same gene depending on parent of origin is referred to as: *(AI 2005)*
A. Genomic imprinting.
B. Mosaicism.
C. Anticipation.
D. Nonpenetrance.

113. Which is the most common cytogenetic abnormality in adult myelodysplastic syndrome (MDS)?
A. Trisomy 8 *(AI 2004)*
B. 20q –
C. 5 q-
D. Monosmy 7

114. Hereditary retinoblastomas develop the following chromosomal deletion: *(AI 2003)*
A. 13 q 14
B. 13 p 14
C. 14 p 13
D. 14 q 13

115. The HLA important in IDDM is *(AI 1994)*
A. HLA-A_3
B. HLA-B_{27}
C. HLA-DR_3/DR_4
D. HLA-W_1

116. Which type diabetes is HLA associated
A. Type I diabetes *(AI 2002)*
B. Tyep II diabetes
C. Malnutrition related type disease
D. Pregnancy related type diabetes

117. All the following diseases are associated with HLA B-27 & Uveitis, except : *(AI 2000)*
A. Behcet's syndrome
B. Psoriasis
C. Ankylosing Spondylitis
D. Reiter's syndrome

118. Gluten sensitive enteropathy is most strongly associated with; *(AI 2003)*
   A. HLA-DQ2
   B. HLA-DR4
   C. HLA-DQ3
   D. Blood group 'B'

Miscellaneous Themes

119. Hyperthermia is seen in : *(AIIMS Feb 1997)*
   A. Malignant neuroleptic syndrome
   B. Cannabis poisoning
   C. Opium intoxication
   D. Aspirin toxicity

120. All the following are features of Anorexia Nervosa ***except*** : *(AI 1994)*
   A. Predominantly seen in females
   B. There is loss of weight at the time of presentation
   C. Amenorrhea is rare
   D. Avoidance of high calorie foods

121. Tumor marker relevant with ovarian carcinoma is: *(AIIMS 96)*
   A. CA-125
   B. CA-19.9
   C. CD-30
   D. CD-25

122. Which one of the following is not used as a tumor marker in testicular tumors? *(AI 2005)*
   A. AFP.
   B. LDH.
   C. HCG.
   D. CEA.

123. A 60 year old male presented to the emergency with breathlessness, facial swelling and dilated veins on the chest wall. The most common cause is: *(AI 2003)*
   A. Thymoma
   B. Lung cancer
   C. Hodgkin's lymphoma
   D. Superior vena caval obstruction

124. A man presents with mass at duodenojejunal flexurs invading renal papillae. Histopathology reports it as lymphoma; true statement is: *(AI 2001)*
   A. II E stage
   B. III E Stage
   C. IV E stage
   D. Staging cannot be done until bone marrow examination is performed

ANSWERS, REFERENCES, EXPLANATIONS AND RELEVANT HIGH YIELD FACTS

1. **Answer is B (15) :** *Love & Bailey 24th/45, Harrison 15th/283; 16th/264, 265;17th/289, 290;* Harrison 18th/p 365 *Kumar & Clarke's 5th/692*

Substitution of values for Na^+, K^+, HCO_3^- and Cl^- in the deduction formula gives us an anion gap value of 15

Plasma electrolyte values in patient			Deduction from formula
Na+	:	140meq/l	Anion Gap : $\{[Na^+]+[K^+]\} - \{[HCO_3^-]+[Cl^-]\}$
K+	:	3 meq/l	= {140 + 3} – {16 + 112}
HCO3-	:	16meq/l	= 15
Cl-	:	112 meq/l	anion Gap = 15meq/l

Anion Gap = $\{[Na^+]+[K^+]\} - \{[HCO_3^-] + [Cl^-]\}$

Anion gap

Anion gap represents the unmeasured anions in plasma and serves the first step to identify whether the acidosis is due to retention of H^+ Cl^- or to another acid.

The normal cations present in plasma are Na^+, K^+, Ca^{++}, Mg^{++}[Q]

The normal anions present in plasma are Cl^-, HCO3-, negative charges on albumin, phosphate, sulphate lactate, other organic acids[Q]

The sums of positive and negative charges are equal[Q]

Measurement of plasma Na^+, K^+, Cl^- and HCO_3^- are usually easily available.[Q]

Anion Gap = $\{[Na^+]+[K^+]\} - \{[HCO_3^-] + [Cl^-]\}$

Because there are more unmeasured anions than cations, the normal anion gap is 10-12 mmol/l.[Q]

2. **Answer is B (Diarrhea):** *Davidson's 17th/605; Harrison 17th/292* Harrison 18th/p 368

Diarrhea is associated with normal anion gap metabolic acidosis

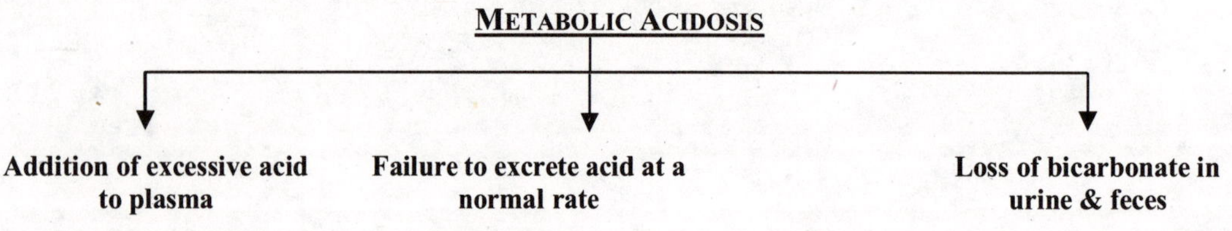

Condition	Anion Gap
Ketoacidosis[Q]	↑ed
Lactic acidosis[Q]	↑ed
Methanol Poisoning[Q]	↑ed
Ethylene glycol Poisoning[Q]	↑ed
Salicylate Poisoning[Q]	↑ed

Condition	Anion Gap
Acute Renal failure[Q]	↑ed ↑ed
Chronic Renal failure[Q]	Normal
Distal renal tubular acidosis	

In Urine	
Condition	**Anion Gap**
Proximal[Q] *Renal Tubular Acidosis*	*Normal*[Q]
Carbonic anhydrase Inhibitors	*Normal*[Q]

In Feces	
Condition	**Anion Gap**
Diarrhea[Q] *Fistula*[Q] *Uretero-sigmoidostomy*[Q]	***Normal***[Q]

Remember:

Four principal causes of high anion gap acidosis – *Harrison*
1. *Lactic Acidosis*[Q]
2. *Ketoacidosis*[Q]
3. *Toxin ingestion*[Q]
4. *Acute and Chronic renal failure*[Q]

3. **Answer is A (Diarrhea) :** *Harrison 15th/286; 16th/265; 17th/290, 292; Kumar &Clarke 5th/693; Refer previous question*

Diarrhea is a cause of normal anion gap metabolic acidosis produced as a result of increased gastrointestinal bicarbonate loss.

4. **Answer is A (Cholera) :** *Kumar & Clark 5th/693;* Harrison 18th/p 368 *Harrison 17th/292*

Cholera is a cause of normal anion gap metabolic acidosis produced as a result of loss of bicarbonate in the faeces.

Metabolic acidosis with normal anion gap :

Normal anion gap in the presence of acidosis suggests that either, $H^+CO_3^-$ is retained or that Na^+ HCO_3^- is being lost.

Increased Gastrointestinal bicarbonate loss	**Decreased renal hydrogen ion excretion**
Diarrhoea Ileostomy Ureterosigmoidostomy	Distal (type 1) renal tubular acidosis Type 4 renal tubular acidosis (aldosterone deficiency)
Increased renal bicarbonate loss	**Increased HCl production**
Acetazolamide Proximal (type 2) renal tubular acidosis Hyperparathyroidism Tubular damage, e.g. drugs, heavy metals, paraproteins	Ammonium chloride ingestion Increased catabolism of lysine, arginine

Causes of normal anion gap metabolic acidosis :
1. Diarrhea (Cholera), Fistula, Ureterosigmoidostomy
2. Renal Tubular Acidosis
3. Ingestion of Ammonium Chloride
4. Mineralocorticoid deficiency

5. **Answer is D (Ureterosigmoidostomy) :** *Refer previous questions*
Ureterosigmoidoscopy is associated with metabolic acidosis but with a normal anion gap.

6. **Answer is B (Renal tubular acidosis) :** *Repeat, Refer previous question*

Both proximal and distal renal tubular acidosis are characterized by a normal anion gap.[Q]

7. **Answer is D (COPD)** *: Harrison 14th/279; Harrison's 15th/285; Harrison 17th/292* Harrison 18th/p 369 *Davidson 17th/605; API 6th/232, 682]*

In COPD Blood pH is usually maintained within normal range in spite of increased $PaCO_2$ because of renal compensation which leads to retention of bicarbonates *- API/6th/232*

8. **Answer is D (Tolbutamide) :** *Harrison's 15th / 286 ; Harrison 17th/290;* Harrison 18th/p 366 *KDT 4th / 279*

Oral hypoglycemics of the biguanide group (Metformin & Phenformin) are known to cause Lactic acidosis. It is not a complication of sulfonylureas such as Tolbutamide, Chlorpropamide etc.

Lactic acidosis

- Lactic acid is produced from pyruvate when oxidative metabolism is reduced and glycolysis is increased.
- Lactic acidosis occurs when the rate of production of lactic acid from pyruvate in muscle, skin brain and erythrocytes exceeds the rate of removal by liver and kidney.

CAUSES OF LACTIC ACIDOSIS	
Defective Oxygenation (Type A – Lactic acidosis)	**Aerobic disorders (Type B-Lactic acidosis)**
• ***Circulatory Insufficiency***[Q] - Shock - Circulatory failure • Anemia • Mitochondrial enzyme defects • Inhibitors – Carbon-monoxide, Cyanide • ***Respiratory failure***[Q] *(Davidson's)*	• Malignancies • Diabetes mellitus • Renal or Hepatic failures • Severe infections - Cholera - Malaria • Seizures • AIDS • Toxins - Biguanides (Oral Hypoglycemics) - ***Methanol***[Q] - Ethanol - INH / AZT / Fructose

The ingestion of methanol (wood alcohol) causes metabolic acidosis and its metabolites formaldehyde and formic acid cause severe optic nerve and central nervous system damage. Lactic acid[Q]*, Aceto-acids and other unidentified organic acids contribute to the acidosis - Harrison 15th/287*

9. Answer is B (Ethylene glycol): *API 7th/1277; Harrison 17th/291* Harrison 18th/p 367

Increased anion gap in the backdrop of Oxalate crystals in urine and seizures suggests a diagnosis of ethylene glycol poisoning.

Ethyleneglycol poisoning :

Results from the ingestion of ethylene glycol used as antifreeze, de lacir car coolant and industrial solvents .

Toxity results from accumulation of four major metbolites :

Glycoaldehyde	Central nervous system manifestation (Seizures)
Glycolate and Formic acid	Cause acidosis (High anion gap metabolic acidosis)
Oxalate	Cause calcium oxalate crystal formation and its deposition in tissues

Four clinical stages of toxity are deliniated :

Stage I	Central nervous system effects and metabolic acidosis depressed reflexes, kussmaul's respiration, nystagmus coma with focal seizures
Stage II	Multisystem complications due to deposition of calcium oxalate crystals renal failure
Stage III	Oliguric renal failure
Stage IV	Delayed neurological sequelle hyperreflexia, ataxia, cranial nerve abnormalities

10. Answer is B (Diethyl glycol poisoning): *Harrison 17th/291; API 7th/1277* Harrison 18th/p 367

Increased anion gap type metabolic acidosis in the backdrop of oxalate crystals in urine, together with central nervous system manifestations and renal failure all suggest and the diagnosis of glycol (Diethyl glycol) poisoning.

11. Answer is B (NH_4^+ ion): *Harrison 15th/1603; Harrison 17th/291, 292* Harrison 18th/p 367, 368

Urinary anion gap ($Na^+ + K^+ - Cl^-$) can be used to estimate renal ammonium production & distinguish RTA from G.I. bicarbonate loss. - *Harrison*

12. Answer is C (Decreases urinary K+ excretion) : *Ganong 19th/690*

When H^+ concentration is increased as in acidosis, H^+ ions are secreted (preferentially over K^+ ions) in exchange of Na^+. ***Thus in acidosis K^+ secretion into tubules (excretion) is inhibited.***

- **K^+ excretion is decreased when :**
  - *amount of Na^+ reaching the distal tubule is small*
  - *H^+ secretion is increased[Q] as in acidosis [Q]*
- **Filtered** K^+ is actively *reabsorbed in proximal tubules[Q]* from the tubular fluid.
  Reabsrobed *K^+ is then secreted into the tubular fluid in distal tubular cells [Q]*
- **The rate of K^+ secretion** is proportionate to the amount of Na^+ reaching the distal tubule, where
  - Na^+ reaching the distal tubule is reabsorbed and this intracellular migration favours K^+ secretion.
  - **Na^+ is however also reabsorbed in associated of H^+ secretion.**

Thus H^+ and K^+ compete for exchange with Na^+ in distal tubular cells.

When H^+ concentration is increased as in acidosis, H^+ ions are the ones to be secreted (preferentially over K^+ ions) in exchange of Na^+. ***Thus in acidosis K^+ secretion into tubules (excretion) is inhibited.***

13. Answer is A (250 mEq.) : *CMDT 2003/914; Nelson 16th/221*

Amount of sodium bicarbonate given in metabolic acidosis is $= \frac{1}{2} \times \text{body weight (kg)} \times \text{Desired } HCO_3 - \text{measured } HCO_3$
Half of this quantity should be administered with in first ½ hr.

Desired HCO_3^- is 25 meq. (Normal =22-25 meq/L) Measured HCO_3^- is 5 meq.	Total amount required is $= \frac{1}{2} \times 50(25 - 5) = 500$ meq
Half of this quantity should be administered with in first ½ hr. and hence answer is 250 meq.	

14. Answer is A (Mineralocorticoid deficiency) : Harrison 18th/p 370 *Harrison 17th/293*

***Mineralo corticoid deficiency is a cause for normal anion gap metabolic acidosis** - Harrison 15th/286*

There is a long list for causes of metabolic alkalosis which includes all other options mentioned in the question.

Recurrent vomiting	Thiazides	Bartter's Syndrome
Gastro intestinal loss of H + from repeated vomitings results in retention of HCO_3^- and hence metabolic alkalosis	Thiazides are diuretics which acutely diminish the ECF volume without altering the total body bicarbonate The serum Bicarbonate concentration therefore increases and hence metabolic alkalosis	Bartter's syndrome is characterized by pathologically by impaired[Q] Cl^- reabsoption in thick ascending loop of Henle and clinically by triad of - Metabolic alkalosis [Q] - Hypokalemia [Q] - Normal or low BP [Q]

15. Answer is C (Uretero-sigmoidostomy): *Harrison 15th/288; Harrison 17th/293* Harrison 18th/p 370

Ureterosigmoidostomy is a cause for normal anion gap type metabolic acidosis produced due to loss of bicarbonate in feces. *All other options mentioned in the question are causes of metabolic alkalosis.*

16. Answer is A (Metabolic acidosis with compensatory respiratory alkalosis): *Oxford handbook of Medicine 5th/684*

With pH < 7.35 (7.12) acidosis is confirmed. Abbnormal CO_2 with change in opposite to expected. (acidosis should have increased CO_2) indicates that the change in compensatory (compensatory respiratory alkalosis), Decreased bicarbonates with change in keeping with change in pH suggests that the problem is metabolic. Thus the whole picture represents metabolic acidosis with compensatory respiratory alkalosis.

Explanation :

Acid base disorders needlessly, confuse many people, but if a few simple rules are applied then interpretation and diagnosis are easy.

pH < 7.35 is acidosis ; pH > 7.45 is alkalosis
1° change in HCO_3^- is termed as metabolic (Normal HCO3- = 22 – 30 meq/l)
if change in HCO_3^- is in keeping with the pH (i.e. if there is acidosis and HCO_3^- decreased) the problem is a Metabolic one. If change in HCO_3^- is opposite with the pH (if there is acidosis and HCO_3^- is increased or normal) the problem is compensatory metabolic.
1° change is CO_2 is termed as respiratory (Normal pCO2 = 35 – 45 mmHg)
If change in CO_2 is in keeping with the pH (if in acidosis CO_2 is raised) the problem is termed respiratory If change in CO_2 is opposite with the pH (if there is acidosis and CO_2 is decreased or normal) problem is termed as compensatory respiratory.

STEP 1 : What is the pH.

Normal pH	pH of patient	Inference	Acidosis
7.35 – 7.45	7.12	pH is decreased	Acidosis

STEP II : Is it a metabolic or respiratory change

Parameter	Inference	Is change towards acidosis or alkalosis	Is change in keeping with change in pH	Final Inference
pCO_2 = 18mm Hg (Respiratory component)	pCO_2 is decreased	Alkalosis	No	Respiratory component is compensatory
pCO_3- = 12 mmol/e (Metabolic component)	HCO_3^- is decreased	Acidosis	Yes	Metabolic component is primary

STEP III : Final deduction

Because metabolic component is primary and respiratory component is compensatory the acid base disorder is Metabolic acidosis with compensatory Respiratory alkalosis.

17. Answer is A (Respiratory acidosis with compensatory metabolic alkalosis) : *Harrison 17th/1590, 288, 289;* Harrison 18th/p 364, 365 *Read text below*

Because primary respiratory component is causing acidosis and metabolic component is compensatory by producing alkaosis, the acid base disorder is Respiratory acidosis with compensatory metabolic alkalosis.

STEP 1 : What is the pH.

Normal pH	pH of patient	Inference	Is it acidosis or alkalosis
7.35 – 7.45	7.2	Decreased pH	Acidosis

STEP II : What component is primary and what is compensatory

Parameter	Inference	Is change towards acidosis or alkalosis	Is change in keeping with change in pH	Final Inference
pCO_2 = 50mm Hg (Respiratory component)	increased	acidosis	Yes (pH=7.2 = Acidosis)	Primary component is respiratory (acidosis)
HCO_3^- = 32 mmHg (metabolic component)	increased	Alkalosis	No (pH=7.2 = Acidosis)	Metabolic component is compensatory (alkalotic)

STEP III : Final deduction

Because the primary component is respiratory and the metabolic component is compensatory the acid base disorder is respiratory acidosis with compensatory metabolic alkalosis.

18. Answer B (Respiratory acidosis) : *Refer previous question*

19. Answer A (Respiratory alkalosis) : *Refer previous questions*

There is alkalosis (pH = 7.5) and CO2 is low (alkalosis). Change in CO2 is inkeeping with change in pH and thus the primary cause is respiratory. The acid base disturbance is thus primary respiratory alkalosis.

20. Answer is C (Respiratory akalosis) : *Refer previous questions*

There is alkalosis (pH = 7.5) and CO2 is low (alkalosis). Change in CO2 is inkeeping with change in pH and thus the primary cause is respiratory. The acid base disturbance is thus primary respiratory alkalosis.

21. Answer is C (Respiratory and metabolic acidosis) *See text below; Refer previous questions*

The acid base disorder is therefore both respiratory and metabolic acidosis.

- There is ***acidosis*** (pH < 7.35).
- Raised PCO_2 (acidosis) indicates that change in CO_2 is in keeping with change in pH. The ***respiratory component is therefore primary***.
- Decreased HCO_3 (acidosis) indicates that ***change in*** HCO_3 ***is also primary*** .

The acid base disorder is therefore both respiratory and metabolic acidosis.

22. Answer is B (Respiratory acidosis) : *Read text below; Refer previous questions*

The acid base disorder is respiratory acidosis.

- There is acidosis (pH : low)
- Raised pCO2 (acidosis) indicates that the change in CO2 is therefore primary
- Normal bicarbonate indicates that there is no alteration in the metabolic component
- The acid base disorder therefore is Respiratory acidosis.

23. Ans D (Siggard-Anderson nomogram) : *Ganong 19th/e P-703 fig 39.8*

Siggard-Anderson nomogram: plots the acid-base characteristics of arterial blood and is helpful in clinical situations.

PCO_2 is plotted on the vertical axis and pH on the horizontal axis.

- **Vertical line through pH 7.40:**
  - Any point to left of this vertical line denotes acidosis.
  - Any point to right denotes alkalosis.
- **Horizontal line through p CO_2 of 40 mmHg:** Position of point above or below this horizontal line defines the effective degree of hypoventilation or hyperventilation.

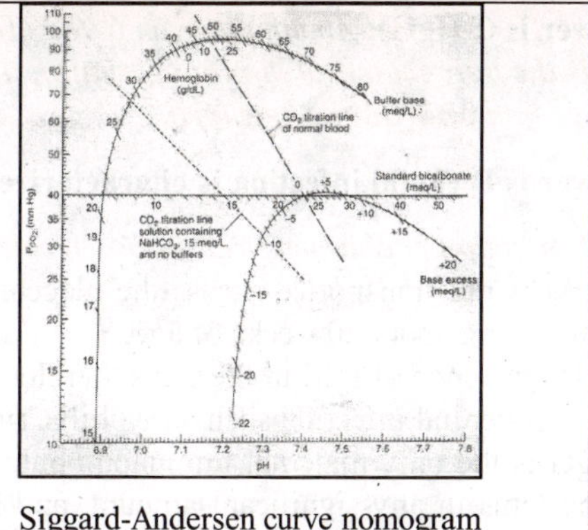

Siggard-Andersen curve nomogram

24. Answer is C (Requires carrier for specific antibody production): *Ananthnarayan 6th/75; Greenwood 14th/131*

Hepatitis become immunogenic only when attached to a large molecule or 'carrier' *- Ananthnarayan*

Antigens can be divided into two groups functionally:

Immunogens	**Haptens**
Substances which are able to generate an immune response by themselves.	Molecules that are able to react with preformed antibodies but unable to stimulate their production directly. Haptens only become immunogenic when attached to large molecule or 'carrier'– *Ananthnarayan 6th/e P-75.*

25. Answer is D (Covalent bond) : *Ananthnarayan 6th/87*

*The combination between antigen and antibody is effected during the primary stage of an Ag-Ab reaction. This reaction is essentially reversible and effected by the weaker intermolecular forces such as: Vander Waal's, Hydrogen bonds, Ionic bonds and **not by the firmer covalent bonds**.*

26. Answer is B (IgM fixes complements): *Ananthnarayan 6th/82*

IgM and IgG fix complement via the classical pathway

Frequently asked questions on immunoglobulins:	
• Immunoglobulin to fix complements via classical pathway	IgG & IgM (IgM > IgG)Q
• Immunoglobulin to fix complements via alternate pathway	IgAQ & IgDQ
• Immunoglobulin with maximum serum conc.	IgGQ
• Immunoglobulin with minimum serum conc.	IgEQ
• Immunoglobulin that in heat labile	IgEQ
• Immunoglobulin in primary immune response	IgMQ
• Immunoglobulin in secondary immune response	IgGQ
• Immunoglobulin with maximum molecular weight	IgMQ
• Immunoglobulin present in milk	IgAQ & IgGQ
• Immunoglobulin with maximum sedimentation coefficient	IgMQ
• Immunoglobulin with shortest ½ life	IgEQ
• Immunoglobulin in seromucinous glands	IgG & IgAQ
• Immunoglobulin resp. for hypersensitive pneumonitis	IgGQ
• Immunoglobulin mediating the prausnitz Kustner reaction	IgEQ
• Homocytotropism is seen in which Ig	IgEQ

27. Answer is A (IgG 1) : *Harrison 17th/2036*

IgG comprises ~ 75 to 85% of total serum immunoglobulin

The four IgG subclasses are numbered in order of their level in serum, IgG_1 being found in greatest amounts and IgG_4 the least *– Harrsison*

28. Answer is C (IgG): *Ananthnarayan 6th/82 (Table 13.1); See previous question*

IgG is the only maternal immunoglobulin, that is normally transported across the placenta and provides natural passive immunity in the newborn.

29. Answer is D (Fetal infection is characterized by increase in IgG) : *Ananthnarayan 6th/182, 184; Read below*

Fetal infection is characterized by an elevated IgM and not by IgG

- IgM is not transported across the placenta Q. It is also the earliest immunoglobulin to be synthesized by the fetus beginning about 20 weeks of age. Q
- The presence of IgM in the fetus therefore indicates intrauterine infection and its detection is useful in the diagnosis of congenital infection such as syphilis, rubella, HIV and toxoplasmosis – *Ananthnarayan 6th/184*
- IgG is the only maternal immunoglobulin that is normally transported across the placenta. It is not synthesized by the fetus in any significant amount, and its presence indicates passive immunity from the mother and not internal infection of the fetus – *Ananthnarayan 6th/182.* Q
- IgM is increased in primary response, and IgG provides for the secondary response. Q – *Park 16th*
- IgE is increased in response to parasitic infection. Q

30. Answer is A (C_2, C_4 and C_3 decreased): *Jawetz 22nd/126*

Classical complement pathway involves reduction of all complement components C_1 to C_9 *while the alternate pathway causes depletion causes depletion of all complements except C_1, C_2 & C_4.*

Complements
(Heat labile proteins found in serum[Q]/ produced by the liver[Q])

Classical pathway	Alternate pathway
• Activated by antigen antibody reaction • Antigen antibody binding activates complement C_1 and initiates the cascade	• Does not require antigen antibody reaction • Activated by • IgG complexes • Complex carbohydrates • Endotoxins • Properidin • Serum factors B & D • Magnesium ions • Activation occurs directly at C_3 level and does not involve early complement factors C_1, C_4 & C_2)

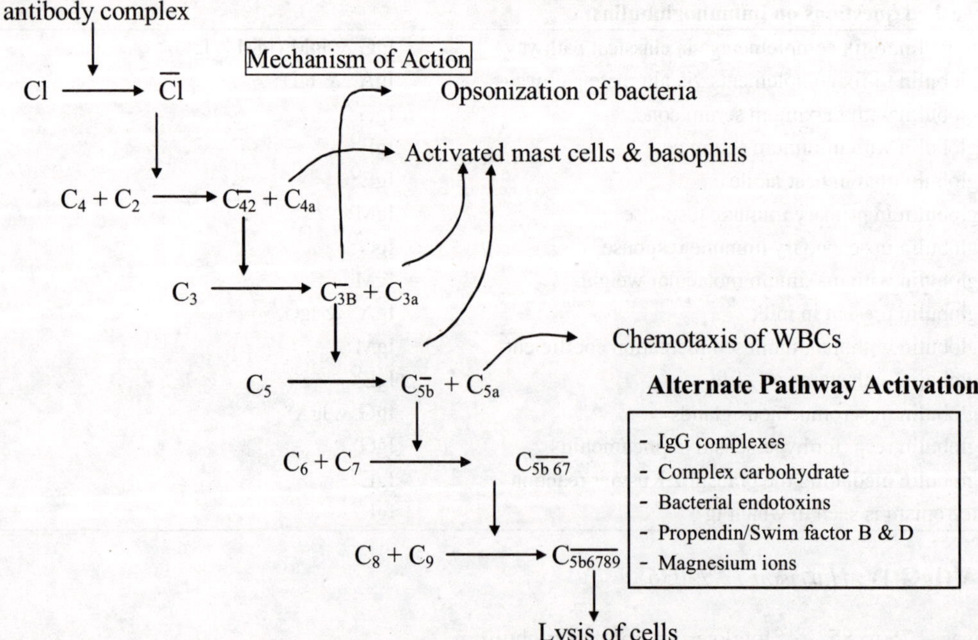

The final outcome of both the pathways is formation of membrane attack complex [C_5b C_6 C_7 C_8 C_9], which causes lysis of cells.

31. Answer is D (Lymphocytes): *Ananthnarayan 6th/186*

Lymphocytes are not classified as macrophages

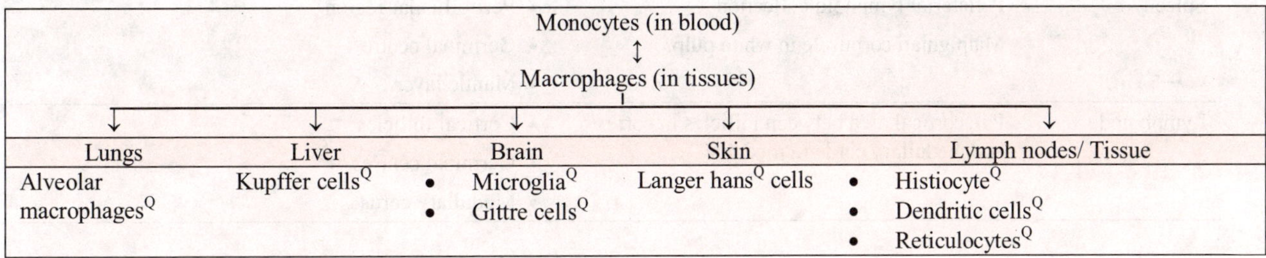

32. Answer is B (Antigen presenting cells) : *Chandrasoma Taylor 3rd/876*

Langerhan's cells are characteristic Antigen presenting cells

- Langerhan's cells are clear dendritic[Q] cells situated among the cells of stratum spinosum (slun).[Q]
- They are believed to be antigen processing cells.[Q]
- They are S100 positive[Q] on immunohistochemical studies.
- On electron microscopy: they lack melanosomes[Q] contain characteristic organelle, the Birbeck's granule.[Q]

33. Answer is A (Astrocytes) : *Robbins 6th/e P-191; Chandrasoma Taylor 3rd/52, 877*

Astrocytes do not function as antigen processing cells.

Foreign antigens must be recognized by the immune system before an immune response can develop. An optimal immune response to most antigens occurs only after introduction of the antigen with certain cells. A macrophage acting in this role is termed as *an antigen processing cell.*

Antigen processing cells include:
1. Macrophages: APC of blood.
2. Modified macrophages:
• Dendritic reticulum cells in follicles of lymph nodes.
• Interdigitating reticulum cells in paracortical zone of lymph nodes.
3. Langerhan's cells: APC of skin.

34. Answer is D (Class III MHC does not encode complement): *Robbins 6th/193*

Class III MHC encode complements of the component system.

Genes coding for histocompatibility antigens are clustered on a small segment of chromosome 6. This cluster constitutes the Human MHC or Human Leucocytes Antigen (HLA) complex.

Class I antigens:
• are expressed on all nucleated cells and platelets.[Q]
• encode cell surface glycoproteins.[Q]
• they are encoded by three closely related loci HLA-A, HLA-B, HLA-C.[Q]
• CD8 + T cells widely express Class I HLA antigens.[Q]
Class II antigens:
• are expressed on macrophages, B cells and T cells.[Q]
• encode cell surface glycoproteins.[Q]
• they have a single loci HLA-D (with three surface loci DR, DQ, DP).[Q]
Class III antigens:
• these encode complements of the complement system.[Q]

Note: That class III molecules loci, are present in between the loci for class I and class II molecules, on the *HLA complex. Thus they lie adjacent to both class I as well as class II molecules.*[Q]

35. Answer is B (Decreased size of paracortical areas): *Ananthnarayan 6th/110, 111*

7Paracortical area of Lymphnodes is thymus dependent and characterized by collection of T-lymphocytes.

The thymus dependent regions as the name suggests are found grossly depleted in neonatal thymectomy.

Tissue	Thymus dependent (Collection of T-Lymphocytes)	Thymus independent Bursa Dependent (Collection of B-Lymphocytes)
Spleen	Periaterial lymphoid collection Malpighian corpuscle in white pulp.	• Perifollicular region • Germinal centre • Mantle layer
Lymph node	Paracortical area between follicles in cortex and medullary cords in medulla	• Cortical follicles • Germinal centres • Medullary cords

36. Answer is D (There is antibody induced proliferation of NK cells) : *Harrison 14th/1754 and See below*

Antibodies do not induce proliferation of NK cells. NK cells express CD3, CD16 & CD56 and also but less commonly CD2 & CD8.

Null cells (NK cells + K cells): Null cells are a heterogeneous group of lymphocytes (non T and non B) called so because :

- They do not form E rosettes[Q] (test to identify T lymphocytes is negative).
- They lack surface immunoglobulins[Q] (test to identify B lymphocytes is negative).
- They account for 5-10% of circulatory lymphocytes.[Q]

NK cells: are also called large granular lymphocytes[Q] as they are morphologically larger & contain azurophillic granules[Q] (which are absent in both T or B cells).

- They are first line defence against:
  - Neoplastic cells[Q]
  - Virus laden cells[Q]
- NK cells are unique in the sense, that, they cause direct cell lysis[Q] which is:
  - Not mediated by an immune response.[Q]
  - Does not involve antigen antibody interaction.[Q]
- They are therefore capable of getting rid of non sensitized organisms[Q] i.e. those that have never been exposed before.
- NK cells are activated to 'lymphocytes activated killer cells' (LAK) in presence of IL 2[Q] but not by antibody.
- NK cells are identified by detection of CD57[Q].

Killer cells: participate in cell destruction with aid of antibody e.g. antibody dependent cell mediated cytotoxicity.

- Mechanism: antibody binds to antigenic determinant on the target cell.
- K cells then attach to target cells by means their Fc receptors and cell lysis results. Even here cell lysis proceeds without phagocytosis. [Q]
- They are CD16 positive. [Q]

Remember that many authors do not believe in the distinction of Null cells into Killer cells and NK cells and attribute both these functions to NK cells (Null cells).

37. Answer is B (Effective against virus infected cells) : *Muir 13th/196 and AIIMS 2001*

Common to both cytotoxic T cells and NK cells is affectivity against virus infected cells.

Natural Killer cells:

- Are first line of defense against virus laden cells and neoplastic cells.
- Cytotoxicity is not MHC restricted.

Cytotoxic T cells:

- They are antigen specific T cells whose function is to produce antigen specific lysis of target cells by direct cell-to-cell contact.
- Are usually CD + class I MHC restricted T cells.
- Are important in defense against viral infections of tissues.

Thus the feature common to both cytotoxic T cells and NK cells is affectivity against virus infected cells.

38. Answer is A (CD19) : *Robbins 6th/654*

CD 19 is a marker for B lymphocytes.

Primarily B cell associated antigens include[Q]	CD10 and CD19 to CD23 i.e. CD10, CD19, CD20, CD21, CD22, CD23
Primarily T cell associated antigens include[Q]	CD1 to CD8 with the exception of CD6 i.e. CD1, CD2, CD3, CD4, CD5, CD6, CD7, CD8.
Primarily monocyte macrophage associated antigens	CD13 to CD15 and CD33 i.e. CD13, CD14, CD15, CD33.
Primarily NK cell associated antigens include[Q]	CD16 and CD56.

(Do remember the antigens associated with NK cells: CD16 and CD56 being the primary ones, and also CD2 which is found expressed in a subset.[Q])

39. Answer is D (Does not mediate specific reactions) : *Robbins 6th/191-193*

"Cytokines mediate their effects by binding to specific high affinity receptors". Such specific binding would obviously mediate specific reactions. Thus cytokines actually do mediate specific reactions.

Cytokines

- Cytokines are short acting, soluble mediators of the immune system which are involved in induction and regulation of the immune response.
- Cytokines are produced by several different cell types:
  - Lymphokines (lymphocyte derived).
  - Monokines (monocyte derived).
- They are short acting.
- They are required for:
  - Regulation of growth.
  - Activation of immune system.
  - Mediation of inflammatory response.

40. Answer is A (T lymphocyte activation) : *Schwartz Q12*

IL-1 in response to injury increases T lymphocyte activation.

It is secreted by phagocytes. It also increases PMN release from bone marrow and its actions include :

- Promotes wound healing.
- Diminishes pain perception.
- Increases body temperature.

41. Answer is A (T cells) : *Ananthnarayan 6th/136 and Jawetz 22nd/129*

IL-2 is produced by T helper cells (CD4 cells). Its actions include:

- Promotes growth and differentiation of T and B cells: interestingly, receptors for IL-2 are present on T cells themselves, and so the secreted IL-2 acts on these very receptors and promotes growth & differentiation of T cells.
- Promotes cytotoxicity of T cells and NK cells.
- Promotes secretion of other lymphokines.

Note: IL-3 is produced by T cells for hematopoiesis.

42. Answer is A (CD4 and lymphocytes) : *Ananthnarayan 6th/134; Jawetz 22nd/129 and See previous question*

IL-2 is produced by T helper (CD4) lymphocytes

43. Answer is C (Casoni's test) : *Ananthnarayan 6th/150; Chandrasoma Taylor 2nd/103 and See below*

Casoni's test is an immediate H.S. type skin test (type I) that detects, positive reaction (wheal) in response to intradermal injection of fresh sterile Hydatid fluid – *Chatterjee 12th/127*

Type I Hypersensitivity (IgE)[Q]	**Type II Hypersensitivity (IgG & IgM)**[Q] **Cytotoxic, complement mediated lysis**[Q]
Includes: • Local: Eczema, Hay fever, Asthma (Atopy).[Q] • Systemic: Anaphylaxis. *Examples based on type I.H.S*[Q]: • Theoblad Smith phenomenon:[Q] This is anaphylaxis in guinea pigs. • PK reaction (Prusnitz Kunster):[Q] Demonstrate that IgE is homocytotropic i.e. species specific. • Casoni's test: Immediate type (IgE) H.S	*Includes:* • Complement mediated lysis.[Q] • Antibody dependent cell mediated toxicity (formerly classified as type I).[Q] • Changes in cellular function (former type V).[Q] - Increased function: Grave's disease.[Q] - Decreased function: M. Gravis.[Q] • Phagocytosis.[Q] *Examples includes:* • Those with Ag on RBC. - Blood transfusion reaction.[Q] - Hemolytic anemia e.g. with I.M. and mycoplasma.[Q] • Those with Ag on Neutrophils: Agranulocytosis.[Q] • Those with Ag on platelets: e.g. ITP.[Q] • Those with Ag on basement membrane: Goodpasture's[Q]
Type III Immune complex (IgM & IgG)	**Type IV Delayed hypersensitivity (cellular immunity)**
Includes: • Local: Arthus reaction.[Q] • Systemic: Serum sickness.[Q] *Examples:* • Shick's test.[Q] • Post streptococcal G.N.[Q] • Detected by RAJI Assay.[Q]	*Includes:* • Tuberculin test.[Q] • Lepromin test.[Q] • Contact dermatitis.[Q] • Jones-Mote reaction (cutaneous basophilic hypersensitivity).[Q] • Graft rejection (chronic).[Q]

44. Answer is B (IgE mediated reaction)

Symptoms of generalized edema, sweating, flushing tachycardia and fever following bee sting point towards on anaphylactic type of reaction. This is a type I hypersensitivity reaction mediated by IgE.

45. Answer is D (Granulomatous reaction): *Ananthnarayan 6th/151*

Granulomatous inflammation/Granuloma formation is typical of reaction to poorly digestible agents elicited by tuberculosis, leprosy, fungal infection etc. It is type IV hypersensitivity[Q] *– Robbins*

- **Arthrus reaction and serum sickness** are forms of type III hypersensitivity.[Q]
- Schwartzmann reaction is not an immune reaction at all. It is rather an alteration in factors affecting intravascular coagulation.

46. Answer is D (Isograft) : *Ananthnarayan 6th/164*

"Although the best graft is an Autograft, a renal graft can obviously not be an Autograft…silly." So the best renal graft is an Isograft from an individual twin.

- *Isograft*: Is a graft from a different individual genetically identical with recipient e.g. identical twin.
- *Autograft*: Is to self.
- *Allograft*: Graft from different species.
- *Xenograft*: Graft from different species.

47. Answer is C (Defective H_2O_2 production) : *Ananthnarayan 6th/147; Harrison 14th/356*

Chronic granulomatous disease is a 'disorder' of microbial killing' characterized by decreased ability of neutrophils to produce H_2O_2.[Q]

• Chronic granulomatous disease is a 'disorder' of microbial killing' characterized by decreased ability of neutrophils to produce H_2O_2.[Q] Patients, here become susceptible to disease caused by organisms that produce 'catalase', which destroys the small amount of H_2O_2 present in these cells and leads to failure of bacterial killing. • The disease is called so, because granulomas, are formed in various tissues, as a second line defence against organisms, that normally would be removed by the acute inflammatory response.
Manifestations:
• Recurrent infections with which catalase +ve Pyogenic bacteria e.g. staph/coliforms.[Q] - catalase negative bacteria e.g. streptococcus, Pneumococcus are often handled normally.[Q] • Normal humoral immune response[Q] but • Defective killing process: Leucocytes are unable to kill bacteria after phagocytosis the major reason being decreased production of H_2O_2.[Q]
Screening method:
• NBT test: Nitroblue retrazolium dye is not reduced by neutrophils in vitro.[Q]

48. Answer is B (Severe combined immunodeficiency): *Ananthnarayan 6th/146; Robbins 6th/235; and Chandrasoma Taylor 2nd/98*

The most common cause of autosomal recessive severe combined immunodeficiency disease (SCID) is the deficiency of the enzyme adenosine deaminase (ADA).

Severe combined immunodeficiency:

- Defect lies in lymphoid stem cells, resulting in both:
  - Failure of T cells.[Q]
  - Failure of B cells.[Q]
- Most common form of inheritance is autosomal recessive.[Q]
- Deficiency of ADA leads to accumulation of deoxyadenosine & its derivatives, which are particularly toxic to immature lymphocytes, especially those of T lineage, and this may account for the marked decrease in T lymphocyte numbers in severe cases.
- Status of adenosine deaminase (ADA) in amniotic cells is helpful in prenatal diagnosis.[Q]

Nezal of syndrome: Review :

- It is a form of combined immunodeficiency.[Q]
- Cellular immunodeficiency with abnormal immunoglobulins.
- Term Nezalof syndrome is applied to disorders with consistent features in the form of:
  - Marked deficiency of T cell immunity.
  - Varying degree of deficient B cell immunity.

49. Answer is A (Severe Combined Immunodeficiency (SCID): *Harrison 16th/1942*

'Patient with severe combined Immunodeficiency Disease (SCID) are deficient in an enzyme involved in purine metabolism, adenosine deaminase (ADA), due to mutation in ADA gene' *- Harrison*

50. Answer is B (Common variable immunodeficiency): *Harrison 15th/1849, 2059*

Common variable deficiency is associated with recurrent chronic intestinal giardiasis.

- Common variable immunodeficiency is characterized by deficient production of antibodies.
- They have normal no. of B lymphocytes but these B lymphocytes fail to mature into plasma cells.
- This results in hypogammaglobulinemia, with reduction in all classes of immunoglobulins but sometimes only IgG is reduced.

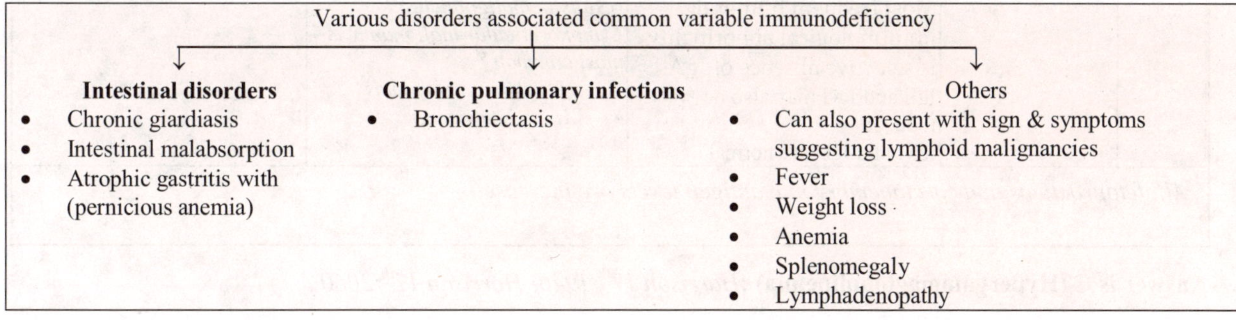

51. Answer is B (Pneumocystis carinii pneumonia) : *Harrison 16th/1940, 1941; 17th/2055; Ananthnarayan 7th/154*

Pneumocystis carinii infections are associated with deficient cell mediated immunity and not with humoral immunodeficiency.

Humoral immunodeficiencies i.e. predominantly antibody deficiencies are associated with recurrent serious infections with pyogenic bacteria and giardiasis. Recurrent sinusitis and recurrent subcutaneous abscess result from infection with pyogenic bacteria and hence are consistent with diagnosis of humoral immunodeficiency.

52. Answer is C (Low levels of IgG) : *Ananthnarayan 7th/156; Harrison 16th/1946; 17th/2056 (t)*

'Immunoglobulin defect in Wiskott-Aldrich syndrome include low serum concentration of IgM. IgA & IgG are normal and IgE is frequently increased' – Harrison

'Serum IgM levels is low but IgG and IgA levels are normal or elevated' - Ananthnarayanan

<u>Wiskott Aldrich Syndrome : Review</u> :

<table>
<tr><td colspan="2">Nature of Disorder & Inheritance</td></tr>
<tr><td colspan="2">Combined immunodeficiency disorder with X-linked inheritance</td></tr>
<tr><td colspan="2">Immunological defects</td></tr>
<tr><td>Humoral immunological defects include
- Low levels of IgM
- Normal (or elevated) IgG & IgA
- Increased IgE</td><td>Cellular immunity undergoes progressive deterioration with depletion of T cells</td></tr>
<tr><td colspan="2">Clinical triad</td></tr>
<tr><td colspan="2">• Eczema
• Thrombocytopenia
• Repeated infections</td></tr>
</table>

53. Answer is C (Increased fraction of IgA immunoglobulins) : *Harrison 16th/1943; 17th/2057, 2058; Various other texts*

***Although B lymphocytic development is normal most patients are deficient in serum IgE and IgA** - Harrison*

Ataxia – Telengiectasia : Review

Autosomal Recessive genetic disorder

↓

Mutation of AT gene (Ataxia telengiectasia gene)
Located on chromosome 11 (11q 22-33)

↓

Defect in DNA Repair
Increased number of chromosomal breaks

↓

Manifestations

↓

Ataxia	**Oculocutaneous Telengiectasias**	**Immunodeficiency**	**Malignancies**	**Endocrinal**
		Immunodeficiency clinically manifests as *chronic recurrent & sinopulmonary infections leading to bronchiectasis* [Q] Most frequent humoral immunological abnormality is selective absence of IgA[Q] IgE and IgG may also be reduced IgM and IgD are normal	Defect in DNA repair mechanisms renders cells *highly susceptible to radiation induced chromosomal damage and results in malignancies*[Q] *Lymphoreticular malignancy is most common* [Q] - *Hodgkins Lymphomas* - *Acute Leukaemia*	*Insulin Resistance*[Q] *Insulin dependent diabetes mellitus*[Q] *Premature aging*

Alfofetoproetiens and carcinoembryonic antigen levels are increased

54. Answer is C (Hypergammaglobulinemia) :*Harrison 17th/1946; Harrison 17th/2060*

Thymoma is associated with Hypogammaglobulinemia and not Hypergammaglobulinemia

<u>Thymomas</u> : are tumors of thymic epithelial cells found in adults and may be benign or malignant

Presentation in Thymomas

Presentation due to mass effect	**Presentation due to associated paraneoplastic syndrome**
Arise in Anterosuperior mediastinum and may present with manifestation of superior mediastinal syndrome	• Myaesthenia gravis[Q] • Acquired Hypogammaglobulinemia[Q] • Pure red cell aplasia [Q] • Graves disease • Perenicious anemia • Dermatomyositis / polymyositis • Cushing's syndrome

55. Answer is C (Neonatal toxic erythema) : *Read text below*

Neonatal toxic erythema is characterized by benign self limiting evanescent eruptions and are seen in about 50% of full term infants. Preterm infants are less affected and the cause of erythema toxicum is not known.
Rh incompatibility isoimmune thrombocytopenia and neonatal myasthenia gravis are all produced due to passive transfer of antibodies from mother to fetus.

56. Ans A (Autosomal dominant) : *Harrison 14th/377, 15th/390, 16th/373; 17th/398*

The most common human monogenetic Mendelian mode of inheritance is autosomal dominant.
Mendelian disorders:
Monogenetic human disorders obey the principles of genetic transmission set forth by Gregor Mendel.
One dominant allele and one recessive allele can display three Mendelian modes of inheritance

Autosomal dominant	:	65%
Autosomal recessive	:	25%
X Linked	:	5%

57. Answer is B (Hereditary Spherocytosis) : *Harrison's 15th/391; 14th/380 (not elaborated in Harrison 16th/17th*

Hereditary spherocytosis is inherited as an autosomal dominant disorder.

Autosomal dominant disorders:	Autosomal recessive disorders:	X-Linked disorders:
- Familial Hypercholesterolemia - Hereditary nonpolyposis colon cancer - Polyposis of the colon - BRCA 1 and BRCA 2 breast cancer - **Marfan's syndrome** [Q] - **Hereditary spherocytosis** [Q] - **Adult polycystic kidney disease** [Q] - **Huntington's chorea** [Q] - **Acute intermittent porphyria** [Q] - **Osteogenesis imperfecta tarda** [Q] - **von Willebrand's disease** [Q] - **Myotonic dystrophy** [Q] - **Neurofibromatosis** [Q] - **Tuberous sclerosis** [Q] - **Otospongiosis** [Q]/**otosclerosis** - **Achondroplasia** [Q]	- Deafness - **Albinism** [Q] - **Wilson's disease** [Q] - **Hemochromatosis** [Q] - **Sickle cell anemia** [Q] - **β thalassemia** [Q] - **Cystic fibrosis** [Q] - **Hereditary emphysema (α_1 antitrypsin deficiency)** - **Homocystinuria** [Q] - **Freidrich's ataxia** [Q] - **Phenylketonuria** [Q] - Fanconi's Syndrome – *[H 14th/e P-2201]* - Gaucher's Disease – *[H 14th/e P-2174]*	- **Hemophilia A** [Q] **(recessive)** - **G6PD deficiency** [Q] **(recessive)** - **Ducchene/Becker muscular dystrophy** [Q] **(recessive)** - Fabry's disease - Ocular albinism - Testicular feminization syndrome - Chronic granulomatous disease - **Hypophosphatemic rickets** [Q] **(dominant)** - **Fragile-X syndrome** [Q] **(recessive)** - **Color-blindness** [Q]

58. Answer is A (Achondroplasia) : *Refer previous question*

Achondroplasia is inherited as an autosomal dominant disorder.

All other disorders mentioned as options follow an autosomal recessive inheritance pattern.

59. Answer is D (Huntington's chorea): *Refer previous question*

Huntington's chorea is inherited as autosomal dominant

Disorder	Inheritance
Fragile X syndrome	X Linked
Fanconi's syndrome	Autosomal recessive
Duchene's dystrophy	X Linked

60. Answer is D (Familial hypercholesterolemia): *Harrison's 15th/2251: Repeat*

'Familial combined Hyperlipidemia' is transmitted as an autosomal dominant disorder

Disorder	Inheritance
Cystic fibrosis	Autosomal recessive
Phenyl ketonuria	Autosomal Recessive
α-1antitrypsin deficiency	Autosomal Recessive

61. Answer A (Retinoblastoma) : *Parson's disease of eye 19th/397; Harrison 15th/386; 16th/385*

Retinoblastoma presents dominant inheritance with variable penetrance

62. Answer is A (Homocystinuria) : *Refer previous question*

Homocystinuria is inherited as an autosomal recessive disorder.

Disorder	Inheritance
G-6 PD deficiency	X-Linked
Myotonic dystrophy	Autosomal dominant
Otospongiosis	Autosomal dominant

63. Answer is C (Von Willebrand disease) : *Refer previous questions*

Von Willebrand disease is inherited as autosomal dominant disorder. It is not X-linked.

64. Ans D (Multifactorial) : *Robbins 6th/592; 5th/57*

Congenital heart disease is the most common type of heart disease among children.[Q]
Multifactorial Genetic and Environmental factors account for the majority of cases. *–Robbins*

65. Answer is D (X-linked recessive type) : *Harrison 16th/374; Harrison 17th/399* Harrison 18th/p 500, 501

Presentation of disease only amongst males identifies the disorder as sex (X) linked. Because carrier mothers are not manifesting the disease, yet their sons do, the disorder can only be recessive. The disorder is thus X-linked recessive.

X-linked disorders:

Males (Father) XY	**Females (mother) XX**
Father have only one X-chromosomes - A daughter always inherits father's X-chromosomes - A son never inherits father's X-chromosomes	Mother (females) have two chromosomes - A daughter always inherits one X chromosome - A son always inherits one X chromosome
↓	↓
• Father to son transmission never occurs in an X-linked disorder • Males always express the phenotype because they have only one X chromosome and the are hemizygos for the allele	• Daughters of an affected male are obligate carriers of the mutant allele. • Females may be homozygos or heterozygous and expose the phenotype dependance on whether the allele is X linked dominant or recessive.

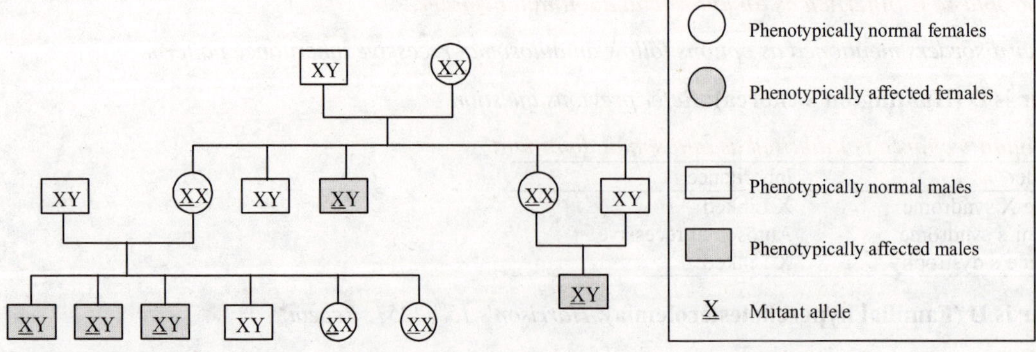

66. Answer is A (X-linked Recessive) : See text below

The transmission of disease follows on X-Linked recessive pattern

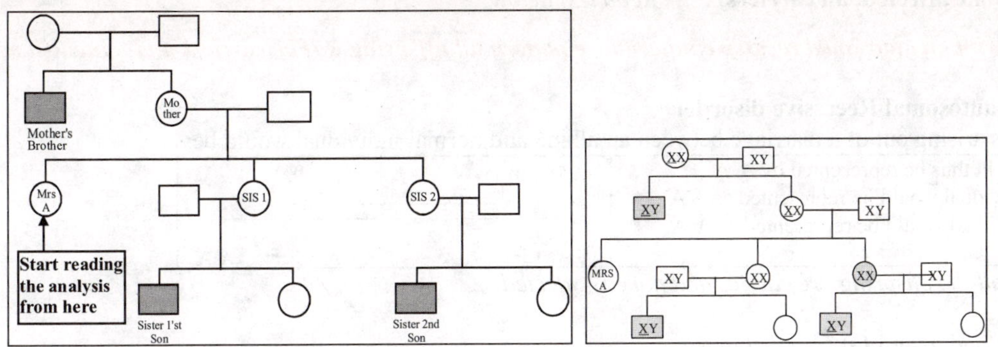

- The pedigree analysis reveals the following:
  - Males only are affected by disease
  - Females are acting as carriers (sister 1 & sister 2)
- The disease is thus likely to be transmitted through the 'X' chromosome in the mother
- *It is a recessive condition and the mother is a carrier, because if it were a dominant condition, the mother would also manifest the disease. So would sister 1 and sister 2 who carry the affection at least on a single X chromosome as is evident by the affection of male children of both sisters.*
  Males having a single X chromosome (XY) manifest a recessive condition as a disease

Also note: females with only one chromosome eg Turner's syndrome can manifest X-linked recessive disorders in the same way as males do.

67. Answer is C (50% male affected if female is carrier) : *Read text below*

50% of males will be affected in transmission of an X-linked recessive disease between a carrier E(female) & a normal Γ (male)

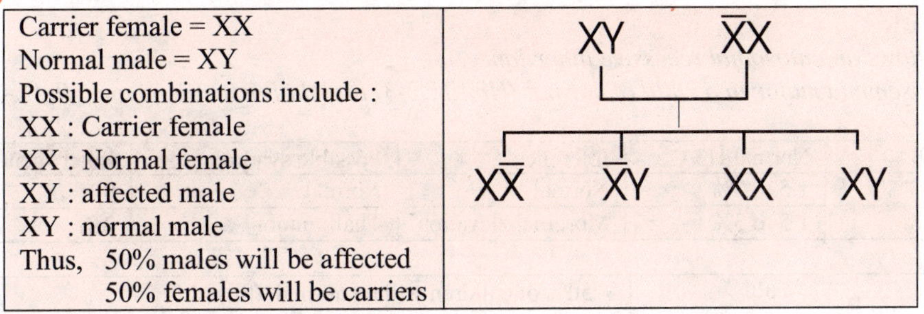

Carrier female = XX Normal male = XY Possible combinations include : XX : Carrier female XX : Normal female XY : affected male XY : normal male Thus, 50% males will be affected 50% females will be carriers	XY X̄X → XX̄, X̄Y, XX, XY

68. Answer is B (25%) : *Harrison's 16th/2235, 2414, 399*

In accordance with an autosomal dominant inheritance pattern the chances of having an anaffected baby are 25%.

Achondroplasia is an **autosomal dominant** condition.

- Let 'a' represent the normal allele and A represent the achondroplasic allele.
  Given that both parents have achondroplasia, the most favourable inheritance would be :

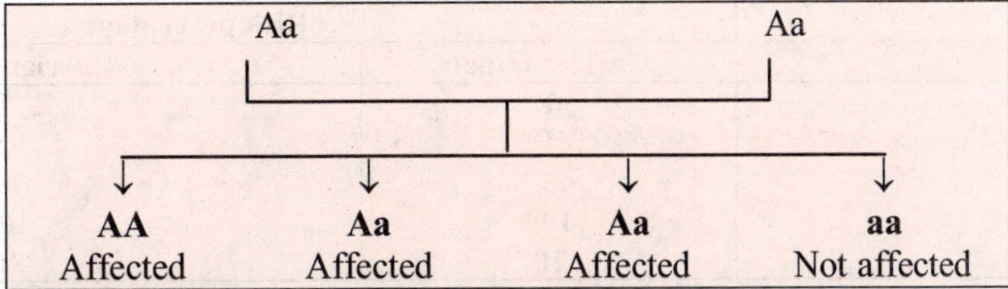

- 3 out of 4 children would be affected or 75% of children will be affected
- 1 out of 4 i.e. 25% children will be unaffected.

Note: *We have chosen only a heterozygous state in both parents as the question is asking about the most favourable outcome possible. If both parents are homozygous 0% children will be unaffected.*

69. Answer is A (None affected, all carriers) : *Read text below*

In accordance with an autosomal recessive inheritance pattern all offspring will be carriers and none will be affected.

Albinism is an autosomal Recessive disorder.

The possibilities arising out of a marriage between an albino and normal individual would be:

- An albino would thus be represented by A^+A^+
- A normal individual would be represented as A^-A^-
- A carrier individual would be represented as A^+A^-

A^+A^+ × A^-A^- → A^+A^-, A^+A^-, A^+A^-, A^+A^-

As we can see, all the offspring are carries and none is affected.

70. Answer is A (Blood group O) : *See below*

There is just no way that children might have blood group O. The answer is obvious so please excuse me on in explanation to this one.

71. Answer is A (O and 100) : *Too obvious for reference*

If the mother has sickle cell disease 'SS' and father is normal 'AA' all the offsprings will be 'SA'

Thus % of sickle cell disease (SS) will be zero and that of sickle cell trait (SA) will be 100%.

- Sickle cell disease is the homozygous state of HbS (SS) where S stands for gene coding HbS
- Sickle cell trait is the heterozygous state of HbS (SA) where A stands for Absent gene.
- Normal individual has no gene for HbS (AA)

If the mother has sickle cell disease 'SS' and father is normal 'AA' all the offsprings will be 'SA'

Thus % of sickle cell disease (SS) will be zero and that of sickle cell trait (SA) will be 100%.

72. Answer is D (0%) : *Harrison's 15th/673; Harrison 17th/399;* Harrison 18th/p 500,501 *Nelson 16th/1486,15-673; Robbins 6th/617*

Thallassemia follows an autosomal recessive inheritance.

The risk of thallasemmia major in a child of normal (HbA2 : 2-3) and thallassemia minor (HbA_2 = 4.8%) parents is zero%.

Parents	HbA2	Normal HbA2	Inference	Possible syndrome	Likely genotype
Wife	2-3%	1.5 to 3%	Normal	Normal	ββ
Husband	4.8%	1.5 to 3%	Morginal elevation	Thall. minor	$\beta^+\beta$

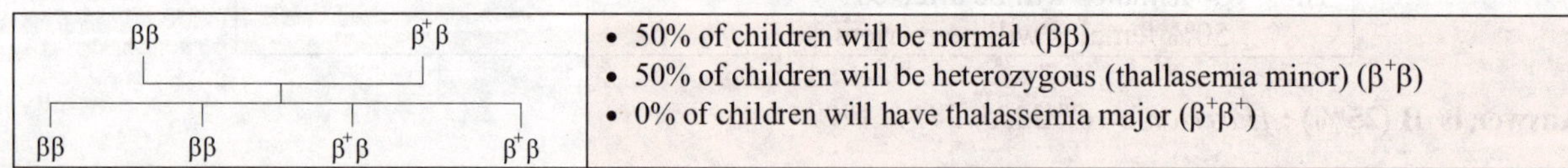

- 50% of children will be normal (ββ)
- 50% of children will be heterozygous (thallasemia minor) ($\beta^+\beta$)
- 0% of children will have thalassemia major ($\beta^+\beta^+$)

73. Answer is A (100%) : *Davidson 17th / 24*

Risk of abnormal offspring for a carrier of balanced translocation of 21:21 is 100% - Davidson

Risk of abnormal offspring for carriers of a balanced translocation:

	Risk percentage	
Translocation	**Carrier father**	**Carrier mother**
Centric fusion 13:14	**1**	1
Centric fusion 14:21	**1**	15
Centric fusion 21:22	**5**	10
Centric fusion 21:21	**100**	100
Reciprocal (any)	**10**	10

74. Answer is B (Trisomy 21) : *Nelson 15th/314; Ghai 6th/591-592*

***The most common abnormalities of chromosome number are 'trisomies'** – Nelson*

***The most frequent and best known trisomy in humans is trisomy 21 or Down's syndrome.** – Nelson*

- *This is the commonest chromosomal disorder occurring with a frequency of 1:800 to 1:1000 new borns.*
- ***Down syndrome occurs more often in offspring of mothers conceiving at older age.***

75. Answer is C (Down's syndrome) :*Robbins 6th/171 Fig. - 27 Pretest Obs & Gynecology/Q31/9th ed*

Trisomy 21 is synonymous with down's syndrome and is the most common of the chromosomal disorders*-Robbins6th/170*

The picture in question is a typical karyogram:

One X & and one Y chromosome are seen (Lower Right)	Indicate a Male phenotype
A third chromosome is seen at the 21st pair	Indicates trisomy 21

Remember :

Trisomy	Syndrome
Trisomy 21	Down syndrome^Q
Trisomy 18	Edward syndrome^Q
Trisomy 13	Patau syndrome^Q

76. Answer is D (Hypertonicity) : *Ghai 5th / 478*

Down's syndrome is typically characterized by Hypotonia (not hypertonia) *– Ghai 5th / 478*

DOWN'S SYNDROME :

It is the most common of chromosomal disorders and a major cause of mental retardation'

- **Phenotypic Features**

Facies :	- **Skull appears small, brachycephalic, with flat occiput** - **Flat facial profile** - ***Oblique palpebral fissure*** ^Q ***and epicanthic folds*** ^Q - *Brushfield's spots* ^Q *are whitish speckling on iris seen in light skinned people* ^Q - **Nose is small and flat** - ***Ears are small and dysplastic*** ^Q
Neck :	- ***Abundant skin is present at the back of neck*** ^Q ***(Neck folds)***
Limbs :	- **Hands are broad and short** - **Clynodactyly : Hypoplasia of middle phalynx with a single flexion crease of 5th finger.** - *Simian crease* ^Q - **Wider gap between 1st and 2nd toe.**

- **Congenital heart diseases**
  - ***Most common cause of death***
  - **ASD, VSD**
- ***Increased risk of developing Leukemia*** ^Q
- ***Increased tendency to senile dementia and Alzheimer's disease*** ^Q **in patients older than 40 year.**
- *Mental retardation* ^Q *: Down's syndrome is a leading cause of mental retardation*
- *Hypotonia* ^Q *: There is a significant hypotonia*

77. Answer is B (Undescended testis): *Ghai 6th/592, http://www.kcdsg.org/AboutDownSyndrome.php*

Health concerns observed in people with Down syndrome :

1. Sixty to 80 per cent of children with Down syndrome have ***hearing deficits.***
2. Forty to 45 per cent of children with Down syndrome have ***congenital heart disease. ASD and VSD are the most common forms of congenital heart diseases seen.***
3. Intestinal abnormalities also occur at a higher frequency in children with Down syndrome. Esophageal atresia, duodenal atresia and anal abnormalities are not uncommon in infants with Down syndrome.
4. Children with Down syndrome often have more eye problems than other children who do not have this chromosome disorder.
   Eye problems such as strabismus, refractive errors and other eye conditions are frequently observed in children with Down syndrome.
   Brushfield's spots are whitish speckling on iris seen in light skinned people.
5. Thyroid dysfunctions are more common in children with Down syndrome than in normal children. Between 15 and 20 per cent of children with Down syndrome have ***hypothyroidism.*** It is important to identify individuals with Down syndrome who have thyroid disorders since hypothyroidism may compromise normal central nervous system functioning.
6. Skeletal problems have also been noted at a higher frequency in children with Down syndrome, including : patellar subluxation (incomplete or partial dislocation), hip dislocation, and atlantoaxial instability. Approximately 15 per cent of people with Down syndrome have atlantoaxial instability.
7. Other important medical aspects in Down syndrome, including immunologic concerns, leukemia, Alzheimer disease, seizure disorders, sleep apnea and skin disorders.

Undescended testis has not been described as an association with Down's syndrome.

78. Answer is B (Amniocentesis): *Harrisons 14th / 408; Ghai 5th / 479 ; Williams 21st / 984*

The ideal investigation in a mother with a pregnancy at risk (previous child with Down's) at 18 weeks gestation is amniocentesis.

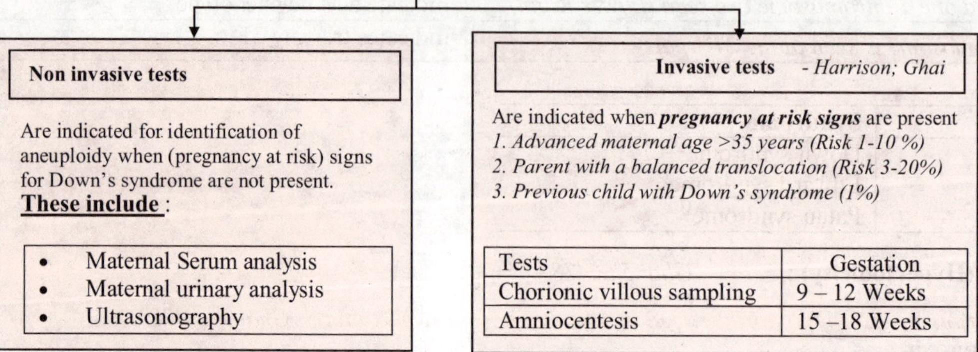

Thus the ideal investigation in a mother with a pregnancy at risk (previous child with Down's) at 18 weeks gestation is undoubtedly amniocentesis.

Non-invasive tests - *Review*

Maternal Serum analysis	Maternal Urinary analysis	Ultrasonography
1. MSAFP (15-18 weeks) : • Maternal serum alphafetoprotein analysis • MSAFP is decreased in Down's **2. Triple test /Expanded MSAFP Multiple marker Screening test (15-18 weeks)** • *MSAFP ↓* • *Unconjugated oestriol ↓* • *HcG ↑*	• **Easy and simple** • Maternal total urinary estriol • Various forms of degraded HcG: - intact & nicked HcG - α & β subunits - β core fragment	• 6-40 weeks • assessment of nuchol fold thickness etc can aid diagnosis

79. Answer is C (Chronic villous biopsy) :

The best investigation for down's syndrome is amniocentesis, but it is not recommended at 11 weeks of gestation. At 11 weeks the best investigation is a chronic villous sampling.

Method	Stage of Gestation	Role in detection of Down's Syndrome
• *Ultrasonography*	*6-40 weeks*	Detects morphological abnormalities of foetus: Skeleton dysplasia, but *not particularly suited for detection of Down's syndrome.*
• **Chorionic villous**	**9-12 weeks**	detects cytogenetic, biochemical and molecular **sampling** fetal disorders. **appropriate for down's syndrome.**
• Amniocentesis	*15-18 weeks*	detects cytogenic, biochemical and molecular: fetal disorders + neural tube defects: *appropriate for down's syndrome.*
• Tripple test	*16-18 weeks*	*helps in detection of down's syndrome (but not diagnostic, only suggestive)*[Q]

Doppler untrasound has no role in diagnosis of down's syndrome.

80. The Answer is B (Amniocentesis) : *Dutta 4, 5th / 530, 112.*

At 18 weeks of pregnancy the best confirmatory test available is amniocentesis

'Triple test only gives a risk ratio. For confirmation of diagnosis, amniocentesis has to be done' - *Dutta*

81. Answer is C (Serum HPL levels) : *Dutta 4th / 530, 112*

Serum HPL is not included as a parameter within the 'triple test' for downs syndrome

Triple test is a combined biochemical test which includes :
- *MSAFP*[Q]
- *HCG*[Q], &
- *Unconjugated Oestriol*[Q]

Triple Test :

• It is used in the detection of Downs syndrome. Q • In an affected pregnancy : - level of MSAFP is decreased Q - level of oestriol is decreased Q - levels of hCG is High (increased) Q • This test only gives a risk ratio and result is considered positive if risk ratio is 1 : 2 *For confirmation Amniocentesis has to be done.* Q • It is performed between *16 to 18 weeks.* Q

82. Answer is C (Down's Syndrome) : *Ghai 5th /479*

Ultrasonography in a case of Down's syndrome Q may reveal increased nuchal fold thickness. Q

(Note that this is also a feature of ***Turner's Syndrome****.)* Q

83. Answer is C (Karyotyping) : *Williams 21st / 944; Ghai 5th / 478, 479*

The question specifically asks for an investigation before the next pregnancy. Out of the options provided only karyotyping is of value prior to pregnancy, the remaining three being of significance during the antenatal period for detection of fetal affection with Down's syndrome.

Down's syndrome a trisomy 21 may arise from

a. **Non-disjunction of chromosome 21:**	b. **Translocation (or mosaicism) :**
• Most common mode accounting for 95% cases • Risk of recurrence is one percent. • ***Parental chromosome study is not necessary*** but ***invasive prenatal diagnosis is indicated by either chorionic villous sampling or amniocentesis.***	• Accounts for remaining cases. • Risk of recurrence is high. • ***Parental chromosome study is indicated***

Karyotyping of Mrs. Annadurai has already been done and a translocation variety of Downs detected. Risk of recurrence however does not depend on mother's karyotype alone, but it also depends on the father's karyotype. Fathers karyotyping is therefore the test of choice prior to next pregnancy to determine the recurrent risk of having another child with Down's syndrome.

84. Answer is A (Down's Syndrome) : *Chandrasoma, 3rd/934*

"Patients with Downs syndrome (Trisomy 21) frequently develop lesions of Alzheimers disease in the third or fourth decade of life." Memory impairment forms an important characteristic of Alzheimer's disease and Down's syndrome thus may be considered as a predictor of memory impairment in later life

85. Answer is C (Trisomy 21) : *Harrison 14th/2350, 15th/2393; 16th/2399; 17th/2542* Harrison 18th/p 3307

Several genetic factors are known to play important roles in pathogenesis of at least some cases of Alzheimers disease. Trisomy 21 is one of them.

Adults with trisomy 21 (Down's) consistently develop the Neuropathologic hallmark's of Alzheimer's disease if they survive beyond age 40.

86. Answer is B (Noonan's Syndrome) : *Harrison 14th / 2121, 2137, 15th/2174, 1332; 17th/375 (t)*

Presence of pulmonary stenosis and 'male' child with features of Turner's syndrome leads us to a diagnosis of Noonan's syndrome.

Noonan's syndrome *is an autosomal dominant syndrome with features mostly identical to Turner's syndrome but in a person with a normal karyotype.*

Turner's syndrome	Noonan's syndrome
• Defect in X chromosome • Karyotype in XO • Phenotypical females only • Cardiac defect is most commonly coarctation of aorta and bicuspid aortic valve • Short fourth metacarpal • No mental retardation	• Autosomal dominant disorder • Karyotype is normal (46XX) • Phenotypically males or females (both) • Cardiac defect is most commonly pulmonary valvular stenosis, hypertrophic cardiomyopathy or ASD. - • Mental retardation present.

10

Miscellaneous

87. Answer is B (Turner's Syndrome) : *Nelson 17th /1925; Harrisons 14th /2122; 17th/2341; 18th/304; Ghai 5th /480*

Noonan syndrome presents with most features similar to Turner's Syndrome. Webbing of neck, increased carrying angle, low hair line are present in both Noonan's and Turner's Syndrome but short fourth metacarpal is characteristic of Turner's Syndrome only.

Term Noonan syndrome has been applied to males and females who present with phenotypic features of Turner's Syndrome but have a normal Karyotype (46X, Y or 46 XX)

Turner's Syndrome	Noonan's Syndrome
• ***Defect in X chromosome***	• ***Autosomal dominant disorder***
• ***Karyotype is XO***	• ***Karyotype is normal (46 X, X or 46 X, Y)***
• ***Phenotypic females only ♀ (female sex only)***	• ***Phenotypic Males or females (seen in both sexes)***
Manifestations	**Manifestations**
• Short stature	• Short stature
• Webbed neck	• Webbed neck
• Low posterior hair line	• Low posterior hair line
• Characteristic facies - Hypertelorism - Epicanthus - Slanted palpebral fissures - Ptosis - Micrognathia - Ear abnormalities	• Characteristic facies - Hypertelrism - Epicanthus - Slanted palpebral fissures - Ptosis - Micrognathia - Ear abnormalities
• Cubitus valgus	• Cubitus valgus
• ***Borad chest with widely spaced nipples***	• Pectus carinatum / Pectus excavatum
• Cardiac defect : - Most commonly coarctation of aorta and bicuspid aortic valve	• Cardiac defect : - Most common cardiac defect is pulmonary valvular stenosis, Hypertrophic cardiomyopathy, ASD
• Sensorineural hearing loss	• Sensorineural hearing loss
• ***Short fourth metacarpal***	-
• *No mental retardation*	• Mental retardation present

88. Answer is D (Mental retardation): *Harrison 18th/p 3048, 3049; Harrison 17th/2341;O.P. Ghai 5th/ 456; (6th/493, 593-594); Refer previous question*

Mental retardation is seen in Down & Klinefelter's syndrome but not in Turner's syndrome.
All other features mentioned as options may be seen in Turner's syndrome.

89. Answer is A (Occurrence of Turner's syndrome is influenced by maternal age) : *Harrison 15th/2174 & 2175, 2341, 669; 16th/2215-2216*

Maternal age constitutes an important influence on the incidence of Down's syndrome. Occurance of Turner's syndrome is not affected by maternal age.

- Turner's syndrome is the most common cause of primary amenorrhea. At puberty sexual maturation fails to occur and primary amenorrhea is common.
- Short stature is characteristic of Turner's syndrome.
- Lymphoedema of the dorsum of hands and feet is also a characteristic finding in patients with Turner's syndrome.

90. Answer is B (Turner's syndrome) : *Refer previous question*

Turner's syndrome is associated with an 'XO' genotype and results from complete or partial loss of one X chromosome.

91. Answer is D (45X): *Robbins 6th/174*

Short stature, widespread nipples and primary amenorrhea characterize Turner's syndrome which is genotypically 45(XO).

92. Answer is B (Turner's syndrome) : *Nelson 16th / 1747*

Congenital Syndromes	Cardiac anomaly
Turner's syndrome	***Coarctation of Aorta*** Q *Pulmonic stenosis* Q *Aortic stenosis* Q
Down's syndrome	*ASD* Q - endocardial cushion type
Noonan's syndrome *(Nelson 6th / 1747)*	*Pulmonary stenosis* Q ASD Hypertrophic cardiomyopathy

93. Answer is C (Infertility in females) : *Nelson 16th/1756; Harrison 15th/2042*

Females usually show normal sexual maturation but it is delayed 2 years on an average.

Males frequently have cryptorchidism and small testes. They may be hypogonadal or normal. Puberty is delayed 2 yr on average

Term 'Noonan Syndrome' *has been applied to males and females who have some phenotypic features that resamble females with turner's syndrome (45 X, O), but themselves have apparently normal sex chromosomes (46XX or 45 XY).*

- These boys and girls have *normal Karyotope*Q
- Inheritance is ***autosomal dominant***Q (gene on chromosome 12q)

Clinical features Q:

- Short stature, webbed neck, pectus carinatum / excavatum
- Hypertelorism, epicanthus, dominant slanted palpebral fissures, ptosis, micrognathia and ear abnormalities.
- Clinodactyly, hernias, vertebral anomalies are less common
- Mental retardation occurs in 25% of patients
- High frequency sensorineural hearing loss is common
- Cardiac Defects : Pulmonary stenosis, ***Hypertrophic Cardiomyopathy***, ASD
- Hepatosplenomegaly and hematological diseases including Leukemia occur

94. Answer is C (46, XXY) : *Harrison's 15th/2173*

The patient in question depicts a hypogonadic male that occurs when there are two or more X chromosomes, (47XXY) and one Y chromosome, and represents the clinical picture of klinefelter's syndrome.

None of the options appear technically correct as an extra X chromosome in the male should increase the total number of chromosomes to 47 and hence 47 XXY should be the most appropriate answer. Within the available options however an extra X-chromosome is the most essential aspect and hence the best answer here is 46 XXY.

Klinefelter's Syndrome: 47 XXY or 46 X,Y / 47 XXY Mosaicism

Q Small firm testes: Hyalinization of seminiferous tubules and azoospermia
Q Gynaecomastia
Q Lack of secondary male characters such as deep voice, beard, male distribution of pubic hair
Q Distinct body habitus: Elongated body: Abnormally long legsQ
Q The mean IQ is some what lower than normal but mental retardation is uncommon
Q Hypogonadism and infertilityQ:
Q Klinefelter's syndrome is produced by non disjunction during meiotic divisions

95. Answer is C (Subnormal intelligence) : *Ghai 5th/479*

'Patients with Klinefelter's syndrome are mentally subnormal. Diagnosis should be considered in all boys with mental retardation' - Ghai

- *Patients are tall and underweight* Q *(not short in stature)*
- *Pubertal development is delayed*Q *- testes are small*Q *occasionally Cryptoarchidism*Q *is associated Secondary sexual characters are delayed or absent*Q*. Growth of pubic hair and facial hair is delayed*Q. No association with breast adenomas or pituitary adenomas has been mentioned.

96. Answer is B (Klinefelter's Syndrome): *Harrison 14th/2120, 15th/2174; 17th/2340, 2341*

Klinefelter's syndrome most commonly presents with 47 (XXY) karyosome and hypogonadism is a common form of presentation and supports the diagnosis.

97. Answer is B (Bilateral Shortness of Sternomastoid): *Nelson 17th/2289*

Bilateral shortness of Sternomastoid' has not been mentioned as a feature of Klippel-Feil Syndrome

Kippel-Feil Syndrome
Refers to an array of clinical disorders associated with congenital fusion of one or more cervical vertebra
Characteristic triad
• Short 'web' neck • Low hair line • Restriction of neck motion
Associations
• Abnormalities of musculoskeletal system - Webbing of neck (prominence of trapezius muscles gives appearance of webbing of neck and may be apparent from mastoid to acromian) - Sprengel shoulder (congenital elevation of scapula) - Torticollis - Scoliosis • Abnormalities of genitourinary tract • Deafness and ocular abnormalities • Abnormalities of cardiovascular system

98. Answer is C (Large Nose): *Nelson 15th/ 318, 16th/331*

Large nose is not a manifestation of Fragile-X syndrome

Fragile X Syndrome
Fragile X sndrome is associated with a fragile site on chromosome X (Xq 29.3) (Fragile sites are regions of chromosomes that show a tendency to separation breakage or attenuation under particular growth conditions.
Inheritance
Inheritance does not follow the usual Mendelian single gene patterns It is due to Allelic expansion[Q].
Clinical Manifestations : *The main clinical manifestations* are :
1. Mental Retardation [Q] : In fact *it is the commonest cause of mental retardation in males.* 2. Macro-orchidism. [Q] 3. Characteristic facial appearance with : - Long face [Q] - Large prominent ears [Q] - Prominant Jaw [Q]

99. Answer is C (Vaginal atresia) : *Harrison 14th/2126, 15th/2182*

Congenital ***hypoplasia or absence of vagina*** in combination with an ***abnormal or absent uterus*** is called ***Meyer Rokitansky Kuster Houser Syndrome.***

This is the second most common cause of Primary amenorrhea after gonadal dysgenesis.[Q]

100. Answer is C (Anovulation) : *Shaws 11th/ 83 ; Shaws 12th/ 216*

Ovaries are normal and there is no reason for anovulation.

Meyer-Rokitansky-Kuster-Hauser Syndrome	Absent vagina in a non functional uterus in a normal female (who is XX)

Absent uterus with vaginal aplasia may thus be a feature of this syndrome.

101. Answer is A (Karyotyping) : *Read text below; Harrison 15th//2179*

A female phenotype along with amenorrhea, absent uterus and short blind vagina may result from either :

- Female (XX) with mullerian agenesis or
- Male pseudo-hermophrodite (XY)

Karyotyping is the investigation of choice, to make such a distinction

102. Answer is A (21-hydroxylase deficiency) : *Harrison 15th / 2178; Harrison 17th/2345* Harrison 18th/p 3053, 3054

Classic 21-hydroxylase deficiency is the most common cause of Ambiguous genitalia in a new born. Virilization is usually apparent at birth in females ***ie. Pseudohermaphroditism of a female child***

103. Answer is A (21 hydroxylase deficiency) : *Harrison 14th / 2124; Harrison 17th/2345* Harrison 18th/p 3053, 3054

Congenital adrenal hyperplasia due to classic 21-Hydroxylase deficiency is the most common cause of ambiguous genitalia in the newborn*. Virilization is apparent at birth in the female and within the first 2-3 years of life in the male.*

104. Answer is D (Decidua) : *Dutta 5th/ 112, 114*

Decidua has not been mentioned to play any role in antenatal diagnosis

Maternal Blood	Amniotic fluid	Fetal Blood
Can be used as in estimation of AFP (MSAFP) : MSAFP level is elevated in a number of conditions. - wrong gestational age Q - open neural tube defects Q - multiple pregnancy Q - Intra uterine fetal death Q - Renal anomalies Q	Forms on important tool for antenatal diagnosis. Following tests may be performed on amniotic fluid : - estimation of Alpha feto-protein (AFP). - culture and chromosomal study of desquamated fetal cells in the amniotic fluid.	May be used for - fetal anemia - Bleeding disorders - Rheusus disease - Non-Immune Hydrops Fetalis

105. Answer is C (Telipes equinovarus) : *Williams 21st / 982 ; Repeat*

Serum alpha fetoproteins have no role in prenatal detection of Telipes equinovaries

Alpha fetoprotein' (AFP) is a glycoprotein synthesized by the fetal yolk sac early in gestation, and by gastrointestinal tract and liver late in gestation.
It circulates in fetal serum and passes into fetal urine and amniotic fluid.
AFP passes into the maternal circulation by diffusion across the placental circulation.
The serum levels of AFP show variation from normal levels in a number of conditions and can thus be used to screen for these conditions.

Condition associated with abnormal maternal serum Alpha fetoprotein concentration :

Elevated Levels		Low Levels
1. Neural tube defects *2. Pilonidal cysts* *3. Esophageal or intestinal obstruction* *4. Liver necrosis* *5. Cystic hygroma* *6. Sacrococcygeal teratoma* *7. Abdominal wall deffects* *- omphalocele* *- gastroschisis* *8. Urinary obstruction* *9. Renal anomalies* *- polycystic* *- absent kidneys*	*10. Congenital nephrosis* *11. Osteogenesis imperfecta* *12. Congenital skin defects* *13. Cloacal exstrophy* *14. Chorioangioma of placenta* *15. Low birth weight* *16. Oligohydramnios* *17. Multifetal gestation* *18. Decreased maternal weight* *19. Underestimated gestational age* *20. Maternal hepatoma or teratoma*	*1. Chromosomal trisomies* *2. Gestational trophoblastic diseases* *3. Fetal death* *4. Increased maternal weight* *5. Overestimated gestational age.*

Confusion : *'Dutta has mentioned IUFD as a cause of increased AFP while 'Williams' mentions fetal death as a cause of decreased AFP.'*

106. Answer is D (All of the above) : *Williams 21st/982; Dutta 4th/112*

All conditions mentioned in options are associated with abnormal Alpha fetoprotein levels.
Open Neural tube defects and multiple gestations (twin pregnancy) are associated with elevated alpha protein levels while chromosomal trisomies (trisomy 18) show decreased alphaprotein levels.

107. Answer is B (Decreased levels of α fetoproteins) : *Nelson 17th/ 699, 2020; Harrisons 15th*

"Persistance of very high levels of oncofetal proteins, including alpha fetoproteins and carcinoembryonic antigens is of diagnostic value" *- Harrison*
All other features mentioned as options are characteristics of Ataxia-telengiectasia

108. Answer is D (Pseudocholinesterase) : *Genetic disorders and the fetus 4th / 673*

Acetyl Cholinesterase and pseudocholinesterase (Butryl cholinesterase) are more useful than alpha-fetoproteins in distinguishing between open neural tube defects and ventral wall defects because alpha-fetoproteins are increased in both of the above conditions.

Neural tube defects	Ventral wall defects
High Acetyl cholinesterase Low pseudocholinesterase (↓ butryl cholinesterase)	Low Acetyl cholinesterase High pseudocholinesterase (↑ butryl cholinesterase)

109. Answer is A (Acrocentric) *Molecular genetics by Precid and Strachan /49, 153*

Human 'Y' chromosome is a large submetacentric chromosome with numerous genes

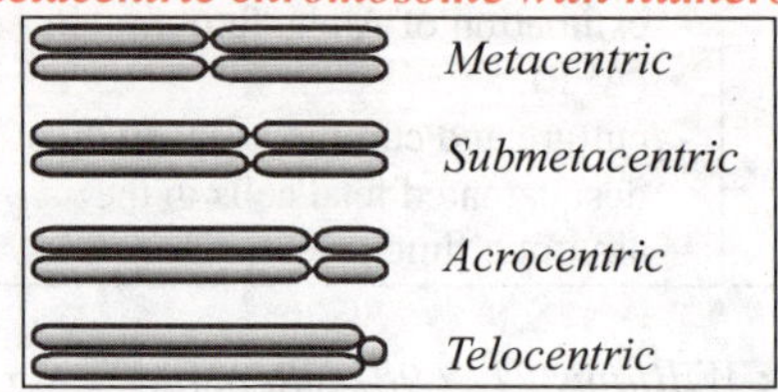

Human X chromosome is large submetacentric chromosome with numerous genes.

110. Answer is B (G-Banding): *Robbins 6th/165, Harshmohan 5th/22*

'The most commonly employed staining method uses a Giemso stain and hence is called G-banding'- *Robbins*

A Karyotype is a standard arrangement of a photographed or image stained chromosomes, where:

- Chromosomes are in *metaphase stage*Q.
  - Mitosis is arrested in dividing cells in metaphase stage by use of colchicineQ
  - In metaphase stage individual chromosomes take the form of two chromatids connected at the centromere
- Chromosomes are *arranged in pairs*Q
- Chromosome pairs are *arranged in decreasing order of length.* Q

STAINING

Staining allows identification of each individual chromosome on the bases of distinctive and reliable pattern of alternating light and dark bands. One of the following banding techniques may be used.

G-Banding (Giemsa banding)	**R – Banding** (Reverse staining Giesma banding)	**Q-Banding** (Quinacrine banding)	**C-Banding** (Constitutive banding)
Most commonly used pattern	Gives pattern opposite to G-Banding	Demonstrates bands along chromosomes	Demonstrates constitutive heterochromatin

111. Answer is C (Northern Blot) :*Harrison 14th/372, 15th/380, 16th/365; 17th/390*

RNA fragments are sequenced by Northern blot tests.

- Blotting techniques combine a fractionation and a detection method to provide a sensitive technique for analysis of DNA, RNA and Protein.

a. *Southern blot:*	For 'DNA' Q
b. *Northern blot:*	For 'RNA' Q
c. *Western blot (Immunoblotting):*	For 'Protein' Q

- *Procedure as Eastern blot is not mentioned anywhere.*

112. Answer is A (Genomic imprinting) : *Harrison 16th/375*

The phenomenon referred to as genomic impriting leads to preferential expression of an allele depending on its parental origin - *Harrison*

113. Answer is D (Monosomy-7) : *Wintrobe's 10th/2329*

'Myelodysplastic syndromes' are a group of clonal haematopoetic stem cell diseases characterized by dysplasia and ineffective hematopoesis in one or more of the major myeloid stem lines.

The cytogenetic abnormalities in Adult myelodysplastic syndromes are

Trisomy 8	**10-15%**
20 q⁻	**3-5%**
5 q	**20%**
Monosomy 7	**10-50%**

Thus monosomy 7 and 5q are the two commonest cytogenetic abnormalities. Although 5q may be commoner than monosomy 7 in some settings, overall monosomy 7 appears more common.

114. Answer is A (13q 14) : *Harrison's 15th/403, Kanski 4th/307*

Retinoblastomas are associated with deletion of part of long arm of chromosome B (Bq 14.11)

Deletion of a small number of tightly clustered genes result in a number of genetic disorders termed as microdeletion syndromes.

Some of the important ones that have been asked include

Syndrome	Deletions	
Wilm's tumor – Aniridia complex[Q] (WAGR syndrome)	11p 13[Q]	Deletion of part of short arm of chromosome 11
Retinoblastoma[Q]	13q 14.11[Q]	Deletion of part of long arm of chromosome 13
Prader - Willi syndrome[Q]	15q 11-13[Q]	Deletion of pa rt of long arm of Angelman syndrome[Q] chromosome 15
Prader - Willi syndrome[Q]	15q 11-13[Q]	Deletion of pa rt of long arm of Angelman syndrome[Q] hromosome 15
DiGeorge's syndrome[Q] Velo-cardiofacial syndrome	22q 11[Q]	Deletion of part of long arm of chromosome 22

Note :

- *Deletions involving the long arm of chromosome 22 (22q 11) ar the most common microdeletions identified to data.*
- *Velo-cardiofacial syndrome*, is the most commonly associated syndrome*

115. Answer is C (HLA DR_3/DR_4) : *Harrison 14th /2065; Harrison 15th/1837; 17th/2279* Harrison 18th/p 2973

95% of IDDM (Type I Diabetes Mellitus) patients express either HLA DR_3 or HLA DR_4 or the heterozygous DR_3 /DR_4 configuration.

No HLA association is seen with Type II Diabetes mellitus or NIDDM.

116. Answer is A (Type I Diabetes) : *Harrison's 15th/2113; 16th/2156; 14th/2065; 17th/2279* Harrison 18th/p 2973

95% of Type I or IDDM patients express either HLA DR3 or HLA DR4 or the heterozygous HLA DR3/DR4 configuration.

No HLA association is seen with Type II Diabetes Mellitus or NIDDM (Robbin's)

117. Answer is A (Behcet's syndrome) : *Harrison 14th/1781, 15th/1956, 16th/2014; 17th/2132* Harrison 18th/p 2801

Behcet's syndrome is associated with HLA B5 and HLA B51

Conditions associated with HLA B27 include: [Q]
1. Ankylosing spondylitis [Q] 2. Reiter's syndrome [Q] 3. Reactive arthritis [Q] 4. Psoriatic arthritis [Q] 5. Juvenile rheumatoid arthritis [Q] 6. Acute anterior uveitis. [Q]

Remember :

Conditions	Associated HLA
• Rheumatoid arthritis	HLA DR 4
• Sjogren's syndrome	HLA DR 3
• SLE	HLA DR 3, DR 2
• Gluten-sensitive enteropathy (Celiac disease)	HLA DR 3
• Type I DM	HLA DR 4
	HLA DR 3
	HLA DR 2
• Hyperthyroidism (Grave's)	HLA B 8, DR 3
• Myasthenia gravis	HLA B8, DR 3
• Multiple sclerosis	HLA DR 2
• Narcolepsy	HLA DR 2
• Goodpasture's syndrome (anti GBM)	HLA DR 2

118. Answer is A (HLA-DQ2): *Harrison's 15th/1674,1836; 17th/118*

"About 95% of patients with coeliac sprue express HLA-DQ2 allele" - *Harrisons*

Gluten sensitive Enteropathy (coeliac disease)

HLA-DQ genes are the primary bases for disease association
HLA - DQ gene present on both DR3[Q] & DR7 haplotypes appear to account for HLA genetic contribution to disease susceptibility

119. Answer is A (Malignant neuroleptic syndrome) : *Harrison 16th/105*

'Malignant Neuroleptic Syndrome is an important cause of Hyperthermia Syndromes' - *Harrisons*

Causes of Hyperthermia

Heat Stroke
Exertional : Exercise in higher-than-normal heat and/or humidity Nonexertional : Anticholinergics, including antihistamines; antiparkinsonian drugs; diuretics; phenothiazines
Drug Induced Hyperthermia
Amphetamines, cocaine, phencyclidine (PCP), methylendioxymethamphetamine (MDMA; "ectasy"), lysergic acid diethylamide (LSD), salicylates, lithium, anticholinergics, sympathomimetics
Neuroleptic Malignant Syndrome
Phenothiazines, butyrophenones, including haloperidol and bromoperidol; fluoxetine; loxapine; tricyclic dibenzodiazepines; metoclopramide; domperidone; thiothixene; molindone; withdrawal of dopaminergic agents
Serotonin Syndrome
Selective serotonin reuptake inhibitors (SSRIs), monoamine oxidase inhibitors (MAOIs), trycyclic antidepressants
Malignant Hyperthermia
Inhalational anesthetics, succinylcholine
Endocraniopathy
Thyrotoxocosis, pheochromocytoma
Central Nervous System Damage
Cerebral hemorrhage, status epilepticus, hypothalamic injury

120. Answer is C (Amenorrhea is rare): *Read text below*

Amenorrhea is associated in almost hundred percent of cases of Anorexia Nervosa.

	Anorexia Nervosa	Bulimia Nervosa
Features [Q]	• *Refusal to maintain body weight above a minimal normal* [Q]	• Irresistible craving for food with episodes of over eating in less time **(Binge eating** [Q]**)**
Method of weight control	• ***Very less eating*** [Q]	• Attempts to counteract the effects of over-eating by - self-induced vomitings - purgative abuse - periods of starvation - appetite suppressants
Ritualized exercise [Q]	• ***Common*** [Q]	• Rare
Amenorrhea [Q]	• ***100%*** [Q]	• 50%
Decreased Vitals [Q] ↓ BP, ↓ Pulse	• ***Common*** [Q]	• Uncommon
Hypothermia [Q]	• ***Common*** [Q]	• Rare
Skin changes [Q] (hirsutism)	• ***Common*** [Q]	• Rare
Medical Complications	• ***Hypokalemia*** [Q] • ***Cardiac arrhythmias*** [Q]	• ***Hypokalemia*** [Q] • ***Cardiac arrhythmias*** [Q]

121. Answer is A (CA 125) : *Harrison 16th/439; 17th/605;* Harrison 18th/p 812 *Manual of Clinical Surgery by Kirk*

CA 125 is the most commonly used tumor marker for ovarian cancer *– Kirk*

CA-125 is found in derivatives of Coelomic epithelium, including pleura pericardium and peritoneum but is not detected in normal ovarian tissue.

Tumor Markers	*Cancer*	*Non-Neoplastic Conditions*
Hormones		
Human chorionic gonadotropin	- Gestational trophoblastic disease, gondal germ cell tumor	Pregnancy
Calcitonin	- Medullary cancer of the thyroid	
Catecholamines	- Pheochromocytoma	
Oncofetal Antigens		
Alphafetoprotein	- Hepatocellular carcinoma, gonadal germ cell tumor	Cirrhosis, hepatitis
Carcinoembryonic antigen	- Adenocarcinomas of the colon, pancreas, lung, breast, ovary	Pancreatitis, prostatic hypertophy Hepatitis, hemolytic anemia, many others
Enzymes		
Prostatic acid phosphatase	- Prostate cancer	Prostatitis, prostatic hypertrophy
Neuron-specif enolase	- Small cell cancer of the lung, neuroblastoma	
Lactate dehydogenase	- Lymphoma, Ewing's sarcoma	Hepatitis, hemolytic anemia, many others
Tumor Associated Proteins		
Prostatic-specific antigen	- Prostate cancer	Prostatitis, prostatic hypertrophy
Monoclonal immunoglobulin	- Myeloma	Infection, MGUS
CA-125	- Ovarian cancer, some lymphomas	Menstuation, peritonitis, pregnancy
CA 19-9	- Colon, pancreatic, breast cancer	Pancreatitis, ulcerative colitis
CD 30	- Hodgkin's disease, anaplastic large cell lymphoma	-
CD 25	- Hairy cell leukemia, adult T cell leukemia/lymphoma	-

122. Answer is D (Carcinoembryonic antigen (CEA)) : *Harrison 16th/551; 561*

CEA is an oncofetal antigen and may be used as a tumor marker in adenocarcinoma of colon, pancreas, lung, breast & ovary. It is however not used as marker for Germ cell tumors.

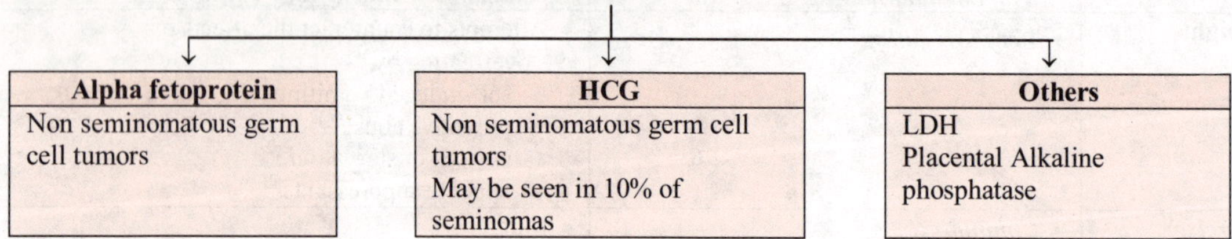

123. Answer is D (Superior Vena cava obsrtuction) : *Harrison 16th/575 (15th/642); 17th/1730* Harrison 18th/p 2266

The patient in question is presenting with classical signs and symptoms of superior mediastinal syndrome or Superior vena caval syndrome.

<u>Clinical manifestations of obstruction of SVC :</u>

Symptoms	Signs
• ***Swelling around neck & face*** especially around the eyes • ***Dyspnea*** • Cough • Others:Hoarseness / Headache / Tongue swelling / Nasal congestion / Epistaxis Haemoptysis / Dysphagia / Pain / Dizziness / Syncope	• Dilated neck veins • ***Increased number of collateral veins over anterior chest wall*** • Cyanosis • Edema of face, arms & chest • Proptosis, glossal and Laryngeal edema and obtundation in severe cases

- *Symptoms are aggravated by bending forwards and lying down.*
- ***Lung cancer is the commonest cause of superior vana caval syndrome or SVC obstruction. As the options provided include superior vena caval obstruction as a distinct entity, it is the option of choice.***

124. Ans C (IV E stage) : *Meningot 10th/1181*

Involvement of another organ (kidney) by Gi lymhon\ma of duodenojejunal flexure classifies it as a stage IV lymphoma.

Gastrointestinal lymphomas are staged using a **modified Ann Arbor Classification:**
IE: Tumor confined to small intestine **IIE:** Spread to regional lymphnodes **IIIE:** Spread to non resectable nodes beyond regional nodes **IVE:** Spread to other organs

NOTES